FIND IT FAST – DISEASES

T5-CCX-588

FIND IT FAST – SUDDEN EMERGENCIES

A Lifetime of Help in Your Home For Less than One Doctor Visit

The Natural Remedies Encyclopedia

VANCE FERRELL • HAROLD M. CHERNE, M.D.

THE SIMPLE, INEXPENSIVE REMEDIES OF NATURE WERE GIVEN BY GOD FOR OUR HEALING

OBEDIENCE TO HIS LAWS BRINGS BLESSINGS

SEVENTH EDITION
NEWLY REVISED - SEVERAL NEW CHAPTERS

OVER 11,000 INEXPENSIVE HOME REMEDIES
COVERS OVER 730 DISEASES AND DISORDERS !
NOW WITH OVER 570 FULL-COLOR PICTURES

Better Health is Worth the Effort to Obtain It
Obedience to the Laws of Nature is a Great Way to Live

OVER 120,000 COPIES IN PRINT

Heritage Edition

Harvestime Books

HB-795

NATURAL REMEDIES ENCYCLOPEDIA

Home Remedies for over 730 diseases

by Vance Ferrell,

Harold M. Cherne, M.D.

Published by Harvestime Books

Box 300, Altamont, TN 37301

Printed and bound in the United States of America

Fourth Edition cover painting: Elfred Lee

"For health-care reform to succeed at reducing costs . . disease prevention must be the ultimate focus of the primary health-care system, rather than disease treatment."
National Institutes of Health
1994 Report

IN THIS ENCYCLOPEDIA —

1 - <u>A lifetime of help</u> in your home - for less than one doctor visit.
2 - Simply explained.
3 - Full of <u>what to do and how to do it</u>.
4 - Topically arranged.
5 - <u>Easy to locate</u> everything. Plus thousands of cross references.
6 - Uses <u>simple, lowest-cost</u>, drugless herbs, water therapy, nutrition.
7 - <u>Step-by-step</u> how to get well !

"The solution to the health problems of the world today is to be found in natural remedies, not in poisoning the system with chemicals. Although they may appear to bring temporary relief, they add a debt of debilitating poison which will later result in serious problems."
John Harvey Kellogg, M.D.

The Natural Remedies Encyclopedia

OVER 150,000 COPIES IN PRINT in all editions!

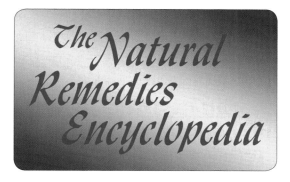

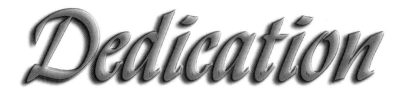

This book is DEDICATED:

First, to the suffering ones who need help, yet so often
do not know where to find it.

As you study and, perhaps, use some of the simple remedies in this volume, go frequently to the Great Physician in prayer and plead for wisdom, strength, and help. He alone can give you what is best for your case. These words are for you:

"Whatever your anxieties and trials, spread out your case before the Lord. Your spirit will be braced for endurance. The way will be opened for you to disentangle yourself from embarrassment and difficulty. The weaker and more helpless you know yourself to be, the stronger will you become in His strength. The heavier your burdens, the more blessed the rest in casting them upon the Burden Bearer."—Desire of Ages, 329.

"Keep your wants, your joys, your sorrows, your cares, and your fears before God. You cannot burden Him; you cannot weary Him. He who numbers the hairs of your head is not indifferent to the wants of His children. 'The Lord is very pitiful, and of tender mercy.' James 5:11. His heart of love is touched by our sorrows and even by our utterances of them. Take to Him everything that perplexes the mind. Nothing is too great for Him to bear, for He holds up worlds. He rules over all the affairs of the universe. Nothing that in any way concerns our peace is too small for Him to notice. There is no chapter in our experience too dark for Him to read; there is no perplexity too difficult for Him to unravel. No calamity can befall the least of His children, no anxiety harass the soul, no joy cheer, no sincere prayer escape the lips, of which our heavenly Father is unobservant, or in which He takes no immediate interest. 'He healeth the broken in heart, and bindeth up their wounds.' Psalm 147:3. The relations between God and each soul are as distinct and full as though there were not another soul upon the earth to share His watchcare, not another soul for whom He gave His beloved Son."
—Steps to Christ, 100.

Second, to the God and Father of us all. The kind Shepherd will lead—all the sheep willing to follow Him—to the heavenly pastures.

We thank Thee for forgiveness as we confess our sins to Thee.
We thank Thee for enabling strength, by the grace of Jesus Christ
Thy Son, to obey Thy Ten Commandment Law.

THE MOST PRACTICAL AND COMPREHENSIVE BOOK OF ITS KIND

Complete information on **VITAMINS, MINERALS, AND OTHER NUTRIENTS**, including regular and therapeutic dosages. [99-128]

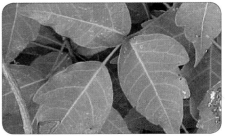 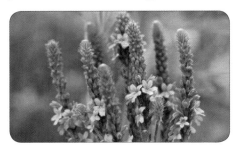 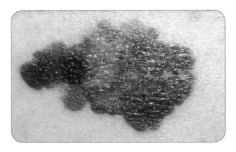

Full coverage of 126 HERBS - Plus two or three color pictures for each herb. Total of 303 color pictures. What each is used for, dosages, and more. [129-189]

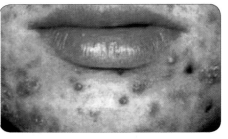 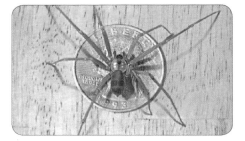 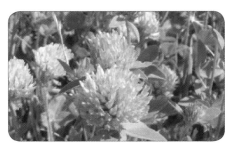

Very large HYDROTHERAPY chapter - How to apply 83 water therapies, effects of hot and cold, the list of the most important ones for your herb shelf. How to gather, store, and prepare them. Plus 195 color photos, showing step-by-step what to do! [208-273]

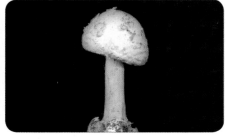 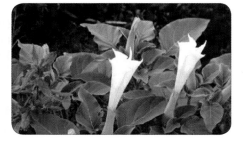 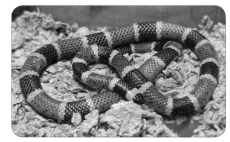

A LIFETIME OF HELP IN YOUR HOME FOR LESS THAN ONE VISIT TO THE DOCTOR

[First line] Poison Ivy (Page 200) Vervain (184) Melanoma (798) [Second line] Acne (356) Brown Recluse (886) Red Cover (177) [Third line] Death Angel (200) Jimsonweed (201) Coral Snake (885)

EVERYTHING IS SIMPLY WRITTEN AND SIMPLY EXPLAINED

<u>Over 11,000 SIMPLE, INEXPENSIVE HOME REMEDIES</u> for over 730 diseases and disorders. Much larger than any other natural remedies book available anywhere. Large nutrient, herb, and water therapy coverage. [278-672]

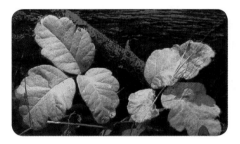 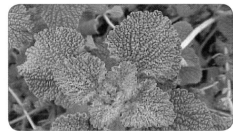 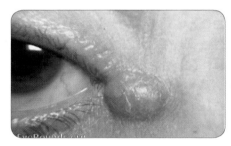

<u>Complete **WOMEN'S SECTIONS**</u>: Special difficulties. Pregnancy and breast-feeding. Infancy and childhood problems and infections. Basic women's herbs. Herbs for pregnancy. How to deliver a baby. [672-779]

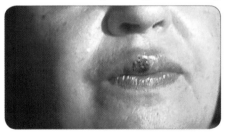 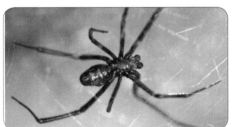 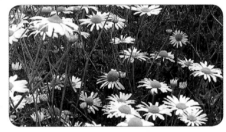

<u>Detailed explanation of **HUMAN PHYSIOLOGY**</u>, plus 16 color pages of <u>50</u> anatomy charts. [1011-1040]

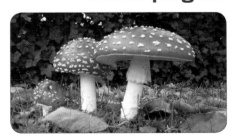 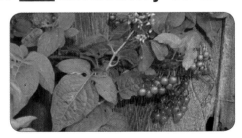 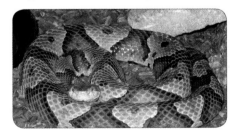

Identifying and explaining <u>over **200 HARMFUL SUBSTANCES**</u> in and around your home, which you should be aware of. [891-972]

<u>Detailed **FIRST AID HANDBOOK**</u>, explaining (with pictures) exactly what to do for choking, drowning, and many other sudden emergencies. [990-1009]

[First line] Poison Oak (Page 200) Horehound (163) Sebaceous Cyst (362) [Second line] Syphilis (809) Black Widow (886) Chamomile (151) [Third line] Fly Amanita (200) Nightshade (200) Copperhead (885)

SAMPLES FROM LETTERS AND PHONE CALLS I HAVE RECEIVED—

"We purchased your Encyclopedia two years ago, and found it such a help. Then in March my beloved husband of 42 years had a sudden heart attack. We quickly turned to page 513—and it saved his life! Now I want another copy to send to my daughter who has two children . . The information in the book got us both on a better diet and way of life. We feel so much better now. That book is a life-changer. I wouldn't part with our copy for a thousand dollars."

—Northern Ohio

"Our Methodist pastor sold me the Encyclopedia about three years ago. It was so beautiful I put it on the coffee table in the living room so it would be easier to use. No other book in the house has that kind of information.

"When our neighbors started looking in it, they found it helped them also. Before long, they were stopping by, one after another, to read in it and write down what they needed to do.

"I tell you, people have been healed by using those low-cost remedies! There's not much money around here, and people appreciate this. —And the book has not one drug or doctor bill in it. Anywhere!

"Since I am home all the time, folk come regularly now, two or three a week. They have found they can care for themselves at home, and that helps a lot. So many are out of work now. I am thankful my husband still has a job." *—Central Georgia*

FIRST - God wants us to be in good health.
"Beloved, I wish above all things that thou mayest prosper and be in health, even as thy soul prospereth." —3 John 2

SECOND - The original diet that God gave to man was plain, simple food. None of it was processed or had chemical additives.
"And God said, Behold, I have given you every herb bearing seed, which is upon the face of all the earth, and every tree, in the which is the fruit of a tree yielding seed; to you it shall be for meat." —Genesis 1:29

THIRD - When we obey God's moral and health laws, we will have better health.
"And ye shall serve the Lord your God, and he shall bless thy bread, and thy water; and I will take sickness away from the midst of thee." —Ex. 23:25
"Bless the Lord, O my soul, and forget not all his benefits: Who forgiveth all thine iniquities; who healeth all thy diseases" —Psalm 103:2-3
"What? know ye not that your body is the temple of the Holy Ghost which is in you, which ye have of God, and ye are not your own? For ye are bought with a price: therefore glorify God in your body, and in your spirit, which are God's." —1 Corinthians 6:19-20

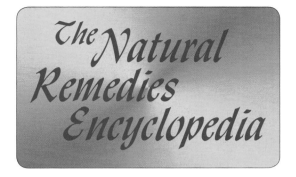

The Natural Remedies Encyclopedia

IMPORTANT
Read This First

This book has the largest collection of drugless, natural, home remedies available anywhere. It provides you with information on more than twice as many diseases (over 730) and far more natural remedies (over 11,000) than any other book. It is urgently needed in your home and will help you for many years to come.

But there is another matter of concern that I must share with you just now.

OUR NATION IS IN DEEP TROUBLE—We deeply love our country. But while a flood of sickness and disease is gradually overwhelming the lives of our people and the economy of our nation,—**there is a far greater crisis confronting us. One which none of our remedies can cure.** Please! Pause a moment and let me tell you of its nature.

A sickness has come upon our nation. It has invaded every aspect of our lives. Few seem to have an answer. Fewer still correctly identify its cause.

You will not hear it in your doctor's office or from the pulpit. Both the secular and religious media are silent about it. Yet it threatens to overwhelm us. **—Our forefathers called it sin. They said it was caused by disobedience to the law of God.**

Since the 1960s, there has been a runaway explosion of every variety of evil, secret and brazenly open. Theft, assault, pillage, murder, gambling, pornography. More and more crazed people are destroying lives or killing themselves. Tiny children are being slain and some want laws enacted to put older people to death. In selfish greed, a few people amass great fortunes and millions suffer in dire need.

While politicians quarrel with one another, terror stalks the streets and illegal drugs are sold on every corner. Strife and bloodshed is filling the land. People trust more in guns and political parties than they trust in God.

None of us live very long. The end of our probation comes with death; this is our final opportunity to make peace with God. —Yet millions have abandoned Him. Lured on by the search for a few hours of excitement, they flock to racetracks, stadiums, pleasure parties, porn sites, bars and nightclubs.

But above the din of traffic jams, personal problems, and international warfare,—God speaks.

It is urgent, my friend! We must return to obedience to God's Ten Commandment law. It is the basis of all human morality! There is no other solution to the mounting problems confronting us.

I agree that nearly everyone will offer some reason for rejecting the idea of obeying God. But unless we do so, we will perish—as individuals, as families, and as a nation. It is our lack of moral principles—moral standards—that is crumbling the very fabric of our society.

Atheists tell us we don't need to keep God's moral law—because society has rejected moral standards. **They ignore the fact that the foundations of society are crumbling away—from the flood of immorality that is pouring in upon us.**

Some pastors tell us that Christ got rid of the Ten Commandments while He was here on earth, so we no longer need try to keep them. But they ignore the fact that, all through the Bible, God requires obedience to His laws. It is the basis of all peaceful society.

Others tell us that, while we are required to obey all the laws of the State, we no longer have to submit to the laws of the God who made us. But the rejection of God's Ten Commandment law lies at the heart of the crisis facing civilization today.

We live in a dangerous hour of Earth's history. Our only solution is to individually come to Christ; surrender our lives to Him; and let Him empower us by His forgiving, enabling grace, to fulfill His will for our lives.

We must let the good work begin in our own hearts and lives, and then extend outward. Friend, it is not too late to begin!

There is a chapter in the back of this book which will help you rededicate your own life to Jesus, your only Saviour, and day by day, draw closer to Him. He is the best Friend you will ever have.

A better Way of Life - p. 1080 - All about how to come to Jesus and remain close by His side. How to live a richer, happier life in Christ. How to prepare for the future.

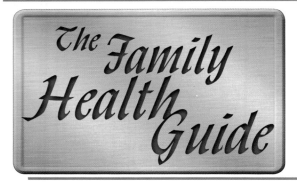

- A Lifetime Investment in Better Living -

Why This Book Was Written

"Our artificial civilization is encouraging evils destructive of sound principles. Custom and fashion are at war with nature. The practices they enjoin, and the indulgences they foster, are steadily lessening both physical and mental strength, and bringing upon the race an intolerable burden. Intemperance and crime, disease and wretchedness, are everywhere.

"Many transgress the laws of health through ignorance, and they need instruction. But the greater number know better than they do. They need to be impressed with the importance of making their knowledge a guide of life. The physician has many opportunities both of imparting a knowledge of health principles and of showing the importance of putting them in practice. By right instruction he can do much to correct evils that are working untold harm.

"A practice that is laying the foundation of a vast amount of disease and of even more serious evils is the free use of poisonous drugs. When attacked by disease, many will not take the trouble to search out the cause of their illness. Their chief anxiety is to rid themselves of pain and inconvenience. So they resort to patent nostrums, of whose real properties they know little, or they apply to a physician for some remedy to counteract the result of their misdoing, but with no thought of making a change in their unhealthful habits. If immediate benefit is not realized, another medicine is tried, and then another. Thus the evil continues.

"People need to be taught that drugs do not cure disease. It is true that they sometimes afford present relief, and the patient appears to recover as the result of their use; this is because nature has sufficient vital force to expel the poison and to correct the conditions that caused the disease. Health is recovered in spite of the drug. But in most cases the drug only changes the form and location of the disease. Often the effect of the poison seems to be overcome for a time, but the results remain in the system and work great harm at some later period.

"By the use of poisonous drugs, many bring upon themselves lifelong illness, and many lives are lost that might be saved by the use of natural methods of healing. The poisons contained in many so-called remedies create habits and appetites that mean ruin to both soul and body. Many of the popular nostrums called patent medicines, and even some of the drugs dispensed by physicians, act a part in laying the foundation of the liquor habit, the opium habit, the morphine habit, that are so terrible a curse to society.

"The only hope of better things is in the education of the people in right principles. Let physicians teach the people that restorative power is not in drugs, but in nature. Disease is an effort of nature to free the system from conditions that result from a violation of the laws of health. In case of sickness, the cause should be ascertained. Unhealthful conditions should be changed, wrong habits corrected. Then nature is to be assisted in her effort to expel impurities and to re-establish right conditions in the system.

"Pure air, sunlight, abstemiousness, rest, exercise, proper diet, the use of water, trust in divine power— these are the true remedies. Every person should have a knowledge of nature's remedial agencies and how to apply them. It is essential both to understand the principles involved in the treatment of the sick and to have a practical training that will enable one rightly to use this knowledge.

"The use of natural remedies requires an amount of care and effort that many are not willing to give. Nature's process of healing and upbuilding is gradual, and to the impatient it seems slow. The surrender of hurtful indulgences requires sacrifice. But in the end it will be found that nature, untrammeled, does her work wisely and well. Those who persevere in obedience to her laws will reap the reward in health of body and health of mind.

"Too little attention is generally given to the preservation of health. It is far better to prevent disease than to know how to treat it when contracted. It is the duty of every person, for his own sake, and for the sake of humanity, to inform himself in regard to the laws of life and conscientiously to obey them. All need to become acquainted with that most wonderful of all organisms, the human body. They should understand the functions of the various organs and the dependence of one upon another for the healthy action of all. They should study the influence of the mind upon the body, and of the body upon the mind, and the laws by which they are governed.

"We cannot be too often reminded that health does not depend on chance. It is a result of obedience to law. . It is not mimic battles in which we are engaged. We are waging a warfare upon which hang eternal results. We have unseen enemies to meet. Evil angels are striving for the dominion of every human being. Whatever injures the health, not only lessens physical vigor, but tends to weaken the mental and moral powers. Indulgence in any unhealthful practice makes it more difficult for one to discriminate between right and wrong, and hence more difficult to resist evil. It increases the danger of failure and defeat."

—Ministry of Healing, 125-128

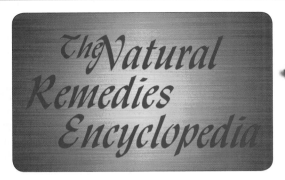

How to Use This Book

LARGEST COVERAGE OF DISEASES—You have in your hands **thousands of easy-to-use solutions to over 730 diseases and physical problems**, far more than any comparable health book on the market. For the cost of what you would pay for one or two prescriptions at the drugstore, **it is now yours—helping your family for a lifetime.**

ARRANGED THE BEST WAY—Instead of being in alphabetical order like most books, the 25 Disease Sections *(276-700)* are arranged topically, just like major medical books written for physicians—because that is the way doctors who treat diseases all the time want them arranged. **Similar diseases and disorders are grouped together on nearby pages. In this way, you can easily compare symptoms, causes, treatments, and prevention.** You will find sections on breast-feeding difficulties, infant problems, skin rashes, and dozens more. In most books, *"Urinary Problems"* is right after *"Ulcer,"* just before *"Urticaria"* (a skin rash). A confusing way to arrange things. But **in this *Encyclopedia*, all the urinary diseases are next to the kidney and bladder disorders.** This outstanding feature is a great help when you are searching for the information you urgently need—*when you need it.*

TWO WAYS TO FIND WHAT YOU WANT—**If you have trouble in the chest, turn to the complete Disease Table of Contents in front of the book. There you will find all the chest problems listed together** under *"Respiratory."* **If you want to find a specific disease (*"Bronchitis,"* for example), you will find it fast in the complete Disease Index at the back of the book.** Black edge tabs quickly help you locate the Table of Contents, the Index, and the section you are looking for. In addition, we have added **thousands of cross-references** to **pages** all through the book. The *Find It Fast* pages in the front of the book also help you get quick results.

EASY TO READ, EASY TO USE—**This outstanding book is simply written, nothing complicated, and in a very readable print size.** Many natural remedies are given for each disease. Simple home remedies never go out of date. They are **always**
low-cost or free. They are not toxic and appeal to common sense.** Here you will find the best natural remedies of earlier generations combined with the latest nutritional facts. **These are simple home remedies you can immediately use to help your family.** This durable *Encyclopedia* comes to you in a washable, casebound edition. It will help your family for a lifetime. And it will bring you assurance every time you see it on the shelf, ready when you need it.

HERBS AND WATER TREATMENTS—This *Encyclopedia* includes two complete chapters on herbal remedies *(129-205)* and hydrotherapy treatments *(206-275)*: **The 126 most important herbs and how to use them** to treat dozens of diseases. **How to use over 100 water treatments in caring for the sick.** This information is of highest value. You will not find this much on these two subjects, as given in those two chapters, in any other full-size natural remedies book dealing with hundreds of diseases. **The skillful use of herbs and water therapy is invaluable** in the recovery from sickness.

HOW TO IMPROVE YOUR HEALTH—But there is more: You not only want to know how to deal with sickness, **you want to know how to rebuild health and maintain it in the future.** The first four chapters in this *Encyclopedia (27-128)* are filled with invaluable information: **Basic health principles *(27-41)*, The Eight Laws of Health** *(42-92)*, **Dietetic Principles** *(93-98)*, **Vitamins, Minerals** *(99-128)*, **and much more.**

SEVEN SPECIAL SECTIONS FOR WOMEN—*Nearly 100 pages of special help:* Diseases of reproductive organs *(677-700)*, Pregnancy and Breast-feeding *(701-754)*, Infant and Childhood Problems *(722-753)*, Women's Herbs *(754-758)*, Pregnancy Herbs *(760-764)*, How to Deliver a Baby *(765-773)*, and Nine Months *(774-779)*.

PLUS MUCH MORE—Terrorist and New Diseases *(811-818)*, Disasters and Emergency Care *(973-989)*, How to Quit Smoking and Drinking *(819-823)*, Hard Drug Warning Signals *(824-827)*, Herb and Seed Sources *(1075-1076)*, Healthful Cookbooks *(1076-1078)*.

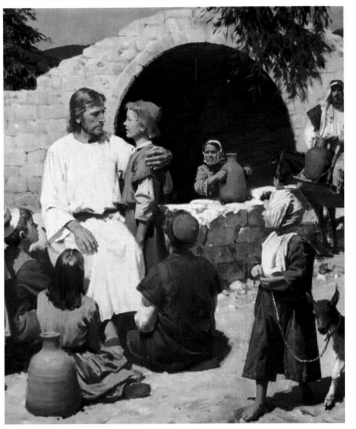

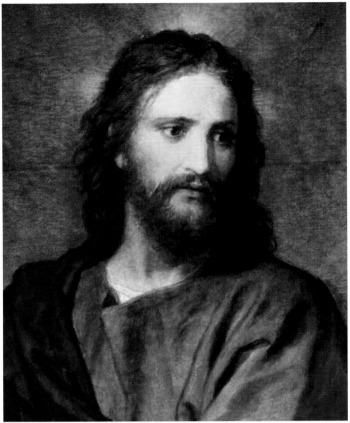

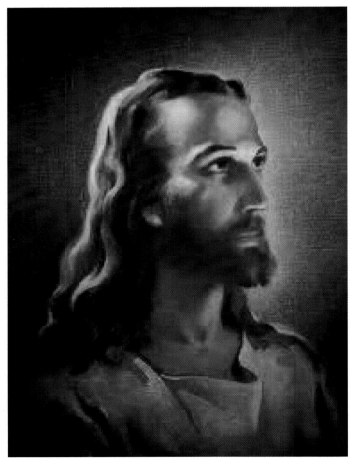

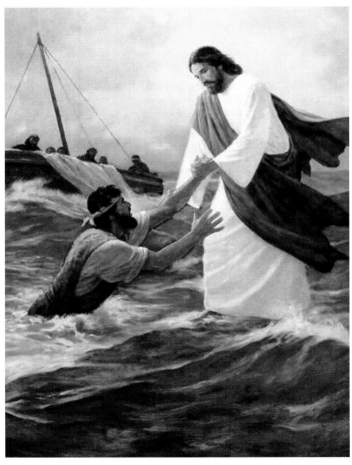

The Natural Remedies Encyclopedia

- A Lifetime Investment in Better Living -

Quick Locator Guide

FIND IT QUICK ! —
THE LARGE TABLE OF CONTENTS IN FRONT
AND THE FULL-SIZE INDEX IN THE BACK

First, there are HUNDREDS OF REMEDIES and how to use them - which are carefully explained in the first part of this Encyclopedia.

—A complete topical listing of remedies is on pp. 4-9.

Second, there are the HUNDREDS OF DISEASES and the simple home remedies needed for them - which are carefully detailed in the second part of this Encyclopedia.

—A complete topical listing of diseases begins on p. 10.

Third, there is the WOMEN'S SECTION, with hundreds of WOMEN'S , CHILDREN'S and PREGNANCY HELPS described in the third part of this Encyclopedia.

—A complete table of contents begins on p. 10-26.

Fourth, there is a special section on BITES, POISONS, ACCIDENTS, FIRST AID, and other helps.

—Bites and poisons begins on p. 22 / FIRST AID on p. 25.

Fifth, there are TWO COMPLETE INDEXES to help you find what you are looking for.

—The DISEASE INDEX begins on p. 1211.

—The GENERAL INDEX begins on p. 1222.

GOD NEEDS US - AND WE NEED HIM—All around us are the sick and the suffering. They need the help we are able to give them. God wants us to learn how to minister to their needs!

In order to do this, we need to draw closer to God, study and obey His Word, the Bible—and also study this book. Continually referring to The Family Health Guide, each one of us can become qualified to become efficient helpers to many others.

And it is urgent that this be done; for terrible crises are ahead of us. More occur every week! We are nearing the end, and Christ is soon to return for His own. We want to be among those who will be ready for His coming. There is information in this book which can help you draw closer to God. This is something that each of us needs.

You will meet with many perplexities as you seek to help others and live more like Jesus; but as you pray earnestly for guidance, God will show you what to do.   -vf

The Natural Remedies Encyclopedia

- A Valued Friend in Time of Need -

Master Table of Contents

Part One - Table of Contents -
to Hundreds of Remedies - and How to Use Them

BASIC PRINCIPLES OF HEALING
Step-by-step through the healing process in the sickroom.

THE EIGHT LAWS OF HEALTH
Fundamental Rules for Better Living:

DIETETIC PRINCIPLES FOR HEALING AND HEALTH
121 Principles of Good Health:

VITAMINS, MINERALS, AND OTHER NUTRIENTS
A Wealth of Nutritional Facts:

HEALING HERBS AND HOW TO USE THEM (303 Color Pictures)
Extremely Thorough and Helpful:

IDENTIFICATION GUIDE: POISON-OUS PLANTS (51 Color Pictures)

Here are 51 color pictures of the 21 most poisonous plants in the field and woods of North America, so you will avoid them, instead of picking them, thinking they might be useful when you are collecting healing herbs in the field and woods:

THE WATER THERAPY MANUAL
(195 Color Pictures)
(Contents: 206-207 / Alphabetical Contents: inside back cover / Special Water Therapy Disease Index: 273-275)
A Complete Book on Hydrotherapy:

The Natural Remedies Encyclopedia

- A Valued Friend in Time of Need -
Complete Disease Table of Contents

If you know the name of the disease you are looking for, quickly find it by turning to the DISEASE INDEX - pages 1211 onward

= Items marked # provide information, but do not discuss diseases.
— Also see = This indicates related topics which are listed elsewhere.

HERE ARE THE 13 BASIC CATAGORIES IN THE DISEASE CHAPTERS:

(A complete table of contents is at the beginning of each chapter / A special Index to all the diseases will be found on pp. 1211-onward)

WHERE TO FIND IMPORTANT THINGS IN THE ENCYCLOPEDIA
DISEASES - List: 10-26 / Indexes: 1211- / HERBS - Contents: 129- / Preparing: 132 / Using: 141-189 (dose:
often 1 tsp. mixed herbs in 1 cup boiled water) / VITAMINS-MINERALS - Index: 100- / Dosages: 124 / HYDRO-
THERAPY - Therapy index: 206- / Disease index: 263- / CARE OF SICK - 28-39 / EMERGENCIES - 973-, 990-

IDENTIFICATION GUIDE: SKIN DISEASES (86 Color Pictures)

Here you will find 86 color pictures of various stages of 38 diseases which produce markings on the skin during the course of the infection:

- SECTION 3 -
EXTREMITIES

- SECTION 4 -
HEAD AND THROAT

WHERE TO FIND IMPORTANT THINGS IN THE ENCYCLOPEDIA
DISEASES - List: 10-26 / Indexes: 1211- / HERBS - Contents: 129- / Preparing: 132 / Using: 141-189 (dose:
often 1 tsp. mixed herbs in 1 cup boiled water) / VITAMINS-MINERALS - Index: 100- / Dosages: 124 / HYDRO-
THERAPY - Therapy index: 206- / Disease index: 263- / CARE OF SICK - 28-39 / EMERGENCIES - 973-, 990-

WHERE TO FIND IMPORTANT THINGS IN THE ENCYCLOPEDIA
DISEASES - List: 10-26 / Indexes: 1211- / HERBS - Contents: 129- / Preparing: 132 / Using: 141-189 (dose:
often 1 tsp. mixed herbs in 1 cup boiled water) / VITAMINS-MINERALS - Index: 100- / Dosages: 124 / HYDRO-
THERAPY - Therapy Index: 206- / Disease index: 263- / CARE OF SICK - 28-39 / EMERGENCIES - 973-, 990-

WHERE TO FIND IMPORTANT THINGS IN THIS FRONT TABLE OF CONTENTS
REMEDIES CHAPTERS - 4-9 / DISEASE CHAPTERS - 10-17 / WOMEN'S CHAPTERS - 18-20 / TOXIC PROBLEMS CHAPTERS - 21-24 / EMERGENCIES CHAPTERS - 24-25 / ADDITIONAL HELPS - 25-26

WHERE TO FIND IMPORTANT THINGS IN THE ENCYCLOPEDIA
DISEASES - List: 10-26 / Indexes: 1211- / HERBS - Contents: 129- / Preparing: 132 / Using: 141-189 (dose:
often 1 tsp. mixed herbs in 1 cup boiled water) / VITAMINS-MINERALS - Index: 100- / Dosages: 124 / HYDRO-
THERAPY - Therapy index: 206- / Disease index: 263- / CARE OF SICK - 28-39 / EMERGENCIES - 973-, 990-

---

WHERE TO FIND IMPORTANT THINGS IN THE ENCYCLOPEDIA

DISEASES - List: 10-26 / Indexes: 1211- / HERBS - Contents: 129- / Preparing: 132 / Using: 141-189 (dose: often 1 tsp. mixed herbs in 1 cup boiled water) / VITAMINS-MINERALS - Index: 100- / Dosages: 124 / HYDRO-THERAPY - Therapy index: 206- / Disease index: 263- / CARE OF SICK - 28-39 / EMERGENCIES - 973-, 990-

WHERE TO FIND IMPORTANT THINGS IN THE ENCYCLOPEDIA
DISEASES - List: 10-26 / Indexes: 1211- / HERBS - Contents: 129- / Preparing: 132 / Using: 141-189 (dose: often 1 tsp. mixed herbs in 1 cup boiled water) / VITAMINS-MINERALS - Index: 100- / Dosages: 124 / HYDRO-THERAPY - Therapy index: 206- / Disease index: 263- / CARE OF SICK - 28-39 / EMERGENCIES - 973-, 990-

WHERE TO FIND IMPORTANT THINGS IN THIS FRONT TABLE OF CONTENTS

WHERE TO FIND IMPORTANT THINGS IN THE ENCYCLOPEDIA

DISEASES - List: 10-26 / Indexes: 1211- / HERBS - Contents: 129- / Preparing: 132 / Using: 141-189 (dose:
often 1 tsp. mixed herbs in 1 cup boiled water) / VITAMINS-MINERALS - Index: 100- / Dosages: 124 / HYDRO-
THERAPY - Therapy index: 206- / Disease index: 263- / CARE OF SICK - 28-39 / EMERGENCIES - 973-, 990-

— EMERGENCIES —

FIRST AID
IS ON THE NEXT PAGE !!

WHERE TO FIND IMPORTANT THINGS IN THE ENCYCLOPEDIA
DISEASES - List: 10-26 / Indexes: 1211- / HERBS - Contents: 129- / Preparing: 132 / Using: 141-189 (dose:
often 1 tsp. mixed herbs in 1 cup boiled water) / VITAMINS-MINERALS - Index: 100- / Dosages: 124 / HYDRO-
THERAPY - Therapy index: 206- / Disease index: 263- / CARE OF SICK - 28-39 / EMERGENCIES - 973-, 990-

A BETTER WAY OF LIFE

An excellent collection of helpful topics which will deepen your walk with God: You will find it to be very helpful and encouraging. Begins on page 1080.

"For God so loved the world, that He gave His only begotten Son, that whosoever believeth in Him should not perish, but have everlasting life."

— John 3:16

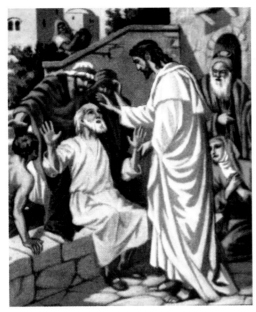

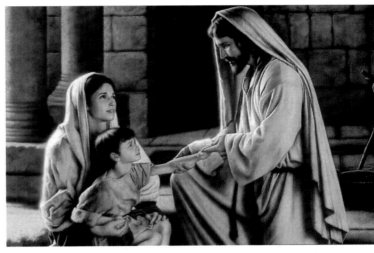

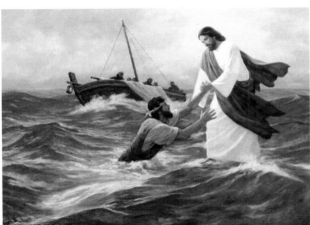

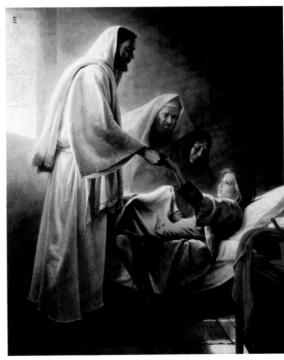

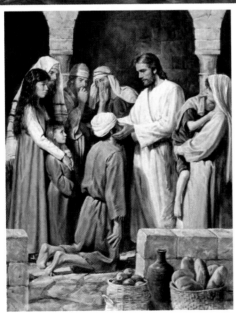

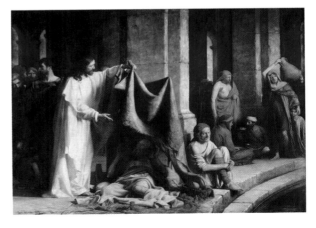

CHRIST OUR WONDERFUL HEALER AND RESTORER

28 **BASIC PRINCIPLES** **BASIC HEALING METHODS** NATURAL REMEDIES ENCYCLOPEDIA
OVER 11,000 REMEDIES - OVER 730 DISEASES

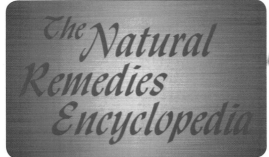

The Natural Remedies Encyclopedia

Basic Principles of Healing

1 - BASIC HEALING PRINCIPLES

The basic principle upon which modern medicine is based is twofold: poisoning and cutting. While in training, every physician and nurse is taught that every drug is poisonous. Two primary types of poisons are used: chemical poisoning and radiation poisoning. The other method is cutting. If something is wrong with an organ, cut it out instead of letting it heal.

In great contrast are the natural healing principles which work with the body's own efforts to restore health. Here we find rest, generally brief liquid fasts, light meals, enemas, water applications, fresh air, sunshine, avoidance of harmful substances, and trust in divine power.

Here is a clarifying passage which is outstanding in its simplicity and breadth of understanding; it was written by a pioneer in natural remedies, Ellen White. Paragraph headings have been added to focus on the points made:

The solution is to teach the people: "The only hope of better things is in the education of the people in right principles. Let the physicians teach the people that restorative power is not in drugs, but in nature."

The true nature of "disease." It is a cleansing process: "Disease is an effort of nature to free the system from conditions that result from a violation of the laws of health."

What we should do when a person is sick: "In case of sickness, the cause should be ascertained. Unhealthful conditions should be changed, wrong habits corrected. Then nature is to be assisted in her effort to expel impurities and to reestablish right conditions in the system."

Here are the eight natural remedies: "Pure air, sunlight, abstemiousness, rest, exercise, proper diet, the use of water, trust in divine power,—these are the true remedies."

Everyone should be taught how to use these remedies: "Every person should have a knowledge of nature's remedial agencies and how to apply them. It is essential both to understand the principles involved in the treatment of the sick and to have a practical training that will enable one rightly to use this knowledge."

The use of natural remedies requires thought and work, but is well-worth it: "The use of natural remedies requires an amount of care and effort that many are not willing to give. Nature's process of healing and upbuilding is gradual, and to the impatient it seems slow . . But in the end it will be found that nature, untrammeled, does her work wisely and well. Those who persevere in obedience to her laws will reap the reward in health of body and health of mind."

Prevention is better than treatment: "Too little attention is generally given to the preservation of health. It is far better to prevent disease than to know how to treat it when contracted."

There are important laws of life which govern every part of our bodies, our diet, and our behavior: "It is the duty of every person, for his own sake, and for the sake of humanity, to inform himself in regard to the laws of life, and conscientiously to obey them."

We need to learn about these laws and how they govern the parts (anatomy) and function (physiology) of our bodies: "All need to become acquainted with that most wonderful of all organisms, the human body. They should understand the functions of the various organs and the dependence of one upon another for the healthy action of all. They should study the influence of the mind upon the body, and of the body upon the mind, and the laws by which they are governed."

Health is not the result of chance, but of obedience to law: "We cannot be too often reminded that health does not depend on chance. It is a result of obedience to law."

Athletes understand this principle better than many others: "This is recognized by the contestants in athletic games and trials of strength. These men make the most

NATURAL REMEDIES ENCYCLOPEDIA
OVER 11,000 REMEDIES - OVER 730 DISEASES   **BASIC HEALING METHODS   BASIC PRINCIPLES**   **29**

PRIN

careful preparation. They submit to thorough training and strict discipline. Every physical habit is carefully regulated. They know that neglect, excess, or carelessness, which weakens or cripples any organ or function of the body, would ensure defeat."

Failure to understand and practice these principles, and obey these laws of nature—can have effects which reach far into the future: "How much more important is such carefulness to ensure success in the conflict of life. It is not mimic battles in which we are engaged. We are waging a warfare upon which hang eternal results. We have unseen enemies to meet. Evil angels are striving for the dominion of every human being."

When we weaken our health, we weaken our mental and moral powers: "Whatever injures the health, not only lessens physical vigor, but tends to weaken the mental and moral powers. Indulgence in any unhealthful practice makes it more difficult for one to discriminate between right and wrong, and hence more difficult to resist evil. It increases the danger of failure and defeat."

Everyone can be a winner, if he will determine to control himself and practice right principles: " 'They which run in a race run all, but one receiveth the prize' *(1 Corinthians 9:24).* In the warfare in which we are engaged, all may win who will discipline themselves by obedience to right principles. The practice of these principles in the details of life is too often looked upon as unimportant—a matter too trivial to demand attention. But in view of the issues at stake, nothing with which we have to do is small. Every act casts its weight into the scale that determines life's victory or defeat. The Scripture bids us, 'So run, that ye may obtain.' "

If we would have success, we must obey the law of God: "The foundation of all enduring reform is the law of God. We are to present in clear, distinct lines the need of obeying this law. Its principles must be kept before the people. They [the moral law of Ten Commandments and the physical laws of nature] are as everlasting and inexorable as God Himself. One of the most deplorable effects of the original apostasy was the loss of man's power of self-control. Only as this power is regained, can there be real progress."

The mind must control the body, or the mind will lose control of itself: "The body is the only medium through which the mind and the soul are developed for the upbuilding of character. Hence it is that the adversary of souls directs his temptations to the enfeebling and degrading of the physical powers. His success here means the surrender to evil of the whole being. The tendencies of our physical nature, unless under the dominion of a higher power, will surely work ruin and death."

The power of the will must be exercised, to bring both body and mind under the control of God: "The body is to be brought into subjection. The higher powers of the being are to rule. The passions are to be controlled by the will, which is itself to be under the control of God. The kingly power of reason, sanctified by divine grace, is to bear sway in our lives."

We must urge upon men and women the vital importance of self-mastery in controlling the appetites and passions, and keeping the body in good health: "The requirements of God must be brought home to the conscience. Men and women must be awakened to the duty of self-mastery, the need of purity, freedom from every depraving appetite and defiling habit. They need to be impressed with the fact that all their powers of mind and body are the gift of God, and are to be preserved in the best possible condition for His service."

Only in the enabling strength of Christ can this be done: "Apart from divine power, no genuine reform can be effected. Human barriers against natural and cultivated tendencies are but as the sand-bank against the torrent. Not until the life of Christ becomes a vitalizing power in our lives can we resist the temptations that assail us from within and without."

Each of us can have strength to bring our appetites and passions under control: "Christ came to this world and lived the law of God, that man might have perfect mastery over the natural inclinations which corrupt the soul. The Physician of soul and body, He gives victory over warring lusts. He has provided every facility, that man may possess completeness of character."

A surrendered life makes obedience a delight, not a drudgery: "When one surrenders to Christ, the mind is brought under the control of the law; but it is the royal law which proclaims liberty to every captive. By becoming one with Christ, man is made free. Subjection to the will of Christ means restoration to perfect manhood."

Obedience to God is freedom to be happy: "Obedience to God is liberty from the thraldom of sin, deliverance from human passion and impulse. Man may stand conqueror of himself, conqueror of his own inclinations, conqueror of principalities and powers, and of 'the rulers of the darkness of this world,' and of 'spiritual wickedness in high places.' "

The above quotations were taken from *Ministry of Healing,* pages 127 to 131, by Ellen White. The book was first published in 1905; yet the health and healing principles in it are needed as much today as then. (Single copies of *Ministry of Healing* may be obtained from the publisher of this present book, for $5.00 a copy, postpaid in the U.S.)

2 - BASIC METHODS OF HEALING

Introduction: You will find, scattered throughout this present volume, the J.H. Kellogg, M.D., formulas for natural healing. Each one is identified as such in the indexes, so you can easily locate them. They deal primarily with water treatments. In addition, John Kellogg also used a variety of other natural remedies.

Another major figure in the natural healing movement was John H. Tilden, M.D. (1866-1940). He was a pioneer in natural remedies; and, along with Trall, Jackson, White, and Kellogg, he made immense strides in providing us today with a systematic regimen for natural healing.

Dr. Tilden had a medical practice in Denver, Colorado, where he operated a 200-bed natural healing hospital; and, on the premises, he conducted the Tilden Health School. For over 25 years, he published a monthly magazine which did not close down until a year before his death at the age of 74, in 1940.

From his writings, and from those of others who have

PRIN

30 **BASIC PRINCIPLES** **BASIC HEALING METHODS** NATURAL REMEDIES ENCYCLOPEDIA
OVER 11,000 REMEDIES - OVER 730 DISEASES

used his methods, the following information has been gathered.

These principles, which are little understood by many in our time, should be taught to every grade school student. A special required two-semester class should be taught in every high school in the land!

The principles you will learn here, if followed, can help you and your loved ones for the rest of your lives. That is how important they are!

Here is a brief summary overview of the Tilden method of natural healing:

Importance of proper care and diet: Flowers, fruits, and vegetables which are grown in good soil will always be superior to those grown on depleted soils. Every experienced farmer knows that proper nourishment of livestock and crops is vital to good production. People who raise show dogs are very careful to give them balanced nutriments, supplemented by significant amounts of vitamins and minerals.

Yet basic scientific knowledge of human nutrition is almost completely ignored in the everyday feeding of children, as well as the diet of teenagers and adults.

Good health can be built, and disease prevented, by eating right and taking proper care of the body. The mind will be vigorous and achieve its greatest development when the body is well.

The body's self-healing mechanism: It is a remarkable fact that, with the help of God, the body can heal itself. It is normal for a person to be well, eat the right food in the proper amount, and have the energy to work hard. The body has built-in ways to process the food into the needed energy.

But when that individual becomes ill, the body also has built-in ways to produce healing. (We say "built-in"; yet this is not entirely correct. It is only the power of God which can make us well and keep us well. Indeed, it is God who not only made us but also the good natural food we so much need!)

The human system is subject to wear and tear; but, when disease strikes, the regular functions are temporarily set aside and the body goes to work to regenerate itself. Instead of using energy for food digestion and muscular activity, it switches over to cleansing, repair, and rebuilding.

When a person becomes sick, his organs have become weary and overloaded with toxins. The word, "Dis-ease," is what the word says: The body is no longer at ease. Disease is actually an effort of nature to cleanse the body of the toxins; let the body rest awhile, and rebuild the organs. Disease is meant to be a friend, not an enemy.

It is at this time that we must help the body cleanse the system of impurities and restore itself to health.

When the sick person rests in bed, while receiving only a *minimum* of the most nourishing and most digestible food, his body turns its attention to carrying on the healing process. Results can be amazing. What the sick need is pure air, wholesome food, gentle help by attendants, rest, and pure water.

The medical route: But, before explaining how that is done, let me answer a question you may have at this point: How is the method used by the medical association

different? Rather than cleanse the system of impurities, it tends to do just the opposite: Chemicals, known to be poisonous, are placed into the body. Yet the body seems to get well! What has happened here?

The body has, as it were, shut down or reduced all extra functions so the healing can take place. You feel weak, you cannot handle much food, you want to lie in bed and rest your mind and body. The healing function is in progress and it needs help in order to succeed.

But, instead, a poisonous drug is introduced into the body. Immediately, the body is aroused. "Hey, I must stop the natural healing process—and fight that poison!"

Everything is now changed. The sickness may apparently end or you may get sicker some other way. Perhaps surgery will be the next step.

But true healing did not take place. Additional poisons are now in the body, which will only weaken it for years to come. They can be very tenacious and are frequently lodged in the body, to bring you grief at a later time.

Let us now return to the natural method of bringing about the healing process. If the condition is serious, we do well to begin with a liquid fast, followed by a juice diet, and then by light meals. We will discuss all of these in this chapter. If the situation is not too serious, we may begin with a light juice diet. Let us first consider that.

The Juice Diet: Wholesome food for the person who is impaired in health consists of fresh, raw fruit juices and fresh, raw vegetable juices. This is a juice diet.

Three or four times a day, a glass of fresh, raw juice is given. It may be fruit juice or it may be vegetable juice. Sometimes it may be a fruit-vegetable juice.

The best fruits are citrus or pineapple. The best vegetables are carrots, beets, and/or celery. These are "salad vegetables." The best fruit-vegetable combination juice is carrot and apple.

When a person is distressed (physically, mentally, or emotionally), this juice diet will bring him back to normal far better than the taking of drugs.

The ordinary staples (such as nuts, bread, cereals, etc.) are set aside for a period of a few days to a few weeks, depending on the nature and severity of the condition.

Sometimes, a longer cleansing program is needed and a *rotation diet* is maintained for a time: This may involve several days of liquid fasting, followed by 1-3 days of light meals.

It is obvious that all this must be done carefully. Pray for guidance and proceed carefully.

Such a program enables the body to cleanse itself of retained wastes instead of allowing those wastes to remain and cause the organs to deteriorate. When drugs are introduced, this only accelerates the deterioration process! Too much unnecessary food clogs the system; eating junk food, smoking cigarettes, and drinking liquor and colas only add to the eventual misery. Taking pills and drugs in order to reduce the stomach trouble, headaches, sleeplessness, and minor ailments which result—does not help the situation. Disaster is sure to result.

Before excessive medication and drastic surgery are considered, it is generally better that a rest and juice diet cure be tried for several weeks.

A person who is ill needs blood cleansing and tissue

CHART 1050: Temperatures at different ages; Respiration, Pulse, Temperature ratios

cleansing. This is done by means of rest and fresh, raw fruit and vegetable juices. Sick people frequently have little or no appetite. This is normal! Work with nature instead of against it.

At such times, we should not use force-feeding by intravenous methods. Such desperate measures do the sick more harm than good. It is true that, at times, the physician must make use of intravenous nourishment—but this is primarily in cases of coma, insulin-shock, or accidental loss of blood. (A similar mistake is made when post-operative cases are fed the same foods that, in a measure, made them sick in the first place. Faulty food is a basic cause of the chronic diseases. Faulty food affects the digestive structures by irritation, inflammation, ulceration, and neoplastic changes, as well as the entire biochemistry of the body.)

We should, instead, let those who are sick rest and get well. Here is how this is done:

Every home should own a food liquefier and juice extractor. A food blender is good when you are in health; but an electric juicer (juicing machine) is needed both in times of health and illness. A glass of freshly made raw carrot, beet, or celery juice will help the well remain well and the sick get well. This is not fruit and vegetable pulp, but juice.

In some hospitals, fruit juices are given in addition to the regular menus of the day. This cannot work. An individual who suffers from an inflammatory disease process (such as hypertension, bronchial asthma, arthritis, nephritis, or endocarditis) can be helped in a really curative manner only when systematically treated by means of raw fruit and raw vegetable juices. They provide an ideal combination of staple food to meet the needs of the sick, so they can regain their health.

Lemon-water fasting: We have looked at the fruit and vegetable juice diet. But there is also the fast. A *"healing crisis"* often occurs at some point in an illness. (More on the healing crisis elsewhere in this book; look it up in the index at the back.) If the person is experiencing an infection, a healing crisis generally occurs near the beginning of the sickness while there is a fever, etc. In most cases, a fast should be given during this fever and/or during the healing crisis.

This fast generally consists of water with lemon juice or grapefruit juice, unsweetened, taken by the sick person as often as it can be enjoyed without forcing.

This is a water-lemon fast. It is not a strict water-only fast, which is not as beneficial. Remember that a water-only fast is generally not the best.

In some cases, it is well to have the fast continue for one to three or more days. This is especially needed during the healing crisis (which is usually about three days duration, but sometimes as long as seven days).

At other times it is best to alternate between fasting and a juice diet, rotating between a day or two on a water and lemon juice fast, a day or two on juices, then back to the water and lemon juice fast.

Sometimes it is best to give only juices for several days. But, at times, it is best to alternate between a juice diet for a day or two, followed by light meals for a day or two.

As a general rule, it is best not to give light meals until after the primary symptoms (fever, etc.) are past, the crisis is over, and the person is ready to start recuperation.

Fasting provides physiological rest for the organism. It provides the body with its best chance for throwing off the retained impurities plaguing the body cells. Organs and structures throughout the system are able to regain, as much as is possible, their former strength. No chemical, cutting, or radiation can provide that healing; only the body's own resources can do it. —And the body will try to do it, if permitted! Work with the body, not against it.

Nature is a wonderful healer and physician. Soon after an individual is put on a fast, the system begins to oxidize (burn up) materials from the tissues of the body. These are used for basic life functions (basal metabolism) while the healing continues.

Obviously, fasting must be used thoughtfully and skillfully. It is not a stereotyped method, to be applied equally to all. One individual may be able to fast with complete comfort while another may become very distressed on one fast—and perhaps not on another. A person who is mildly ill will actually feel better on the fast. But one who is quite sick, or has some organs in poor shape, may feel worse during a first attempt at fasting.

A person who is normally very thin may not be able to fast as long as a person who has average or excess weight. If it is a chronic condition, requiring longer fasts, he may need a three-day fast, alternated with three days on light fruit meals or light meals (both are described below).

Fasting alternated with light fruit meals: A variation which works quite well is to alternate a fast with light fruit meals. The light feeding consists of fresh, raw fruits—mostly oranges, grapefruit, pineapple, and their juices—while the fasting consists of water and lemon juice only. The fast on lemon juice and water gives the whole organism the most effective opportunity to cleanse itself of its accumulated and retained wastes.

But this fasting cannot go on too many days, without the possibility of organic or functional damage. Fasting (living on water and lemon juice) is low-level starvation. So one must be careful and not overdo it.

Do not overdo it! Think, pray, and ask God to help you know what to do next. When in doubt, you may need to move from a fast to a juice diet for a meal or two. Perhaps a light meal is needed before returning to the fast. Thoughtful consideration is needed.

During the fasting process, the body consumes some of its stored chemicals (including calcium, iron, phosphorus, and various other tissue components). The one who is fasting is very weak, even while lying comfortably in a warm bed. He may get severe palpitations of the heart when he tries to sit up or walk to the bathroom. While on a fast, he needs an experienced helper, nurse, or physician. He needs to be observed very carefully. The fast must only be carried to the point where he can take it with psychological comfort.

When in doubt, put him back on additional nourishment. This may be a light fruit meal; it may be best to put him on the juice diet of fresh, raw fruit and vegetable juices. Or he may need a light meal (described below).

If he is in the midst of a healing crisis (which

frequently does not require more than 1-3 days before the fever breaks), it is best to keep him on the water-lemon juice fast, with possible rotation back and forth to fruit and vegetable juice. Remember, if he can remain on the water-lemon fast during the crisis, he will recover more quickly. Yet you must watch him and do what is best in the situation.

But if the crisis is extended longer than three days, you may need to give him a meal of juice or food, on a rotational cycle.

Extra warmth: While the person is fasting, he needs extra warmth. The extremities (the feet and hands) generally get cold during the fasting period. It is therefore necessary to apply one or two electric pads, or an electric blanket, day and night in order to keep him comfortably warm.

Although important, this is often not done, even in the hospitals.

The avenues of elimination: At this juncture, we should consider another aspect of physiology. The body is constantly producing wastes. It tries to throw them off through the *"organs of elimination,"* which are primarily these: the bowels, the kidneys, the lungs, the skin, and spitting.

If too much waste is produced (because of overeating, wrong eating, overwork, and a lack of rest, exercise, and fresh air), then the body becomes overburdened, and sickness and organic breakdown occur.

During natural healing, the system goes into high gear in its efforts to eliminate these poisons. It must be aided in its efforts.

We must *"open all the organs of elimination"*; that is, we must help the body throw off toxins through the four avenues by which it can do it:

The bowels - Daily enemas or colonics must be given.

The kidneys - The sick person must be given an abundance of fluids to drink. (This also helps the other avenues of elimination function better.)

The lungs - There must always be a current of fresh air in the bedroom of the sick person.

The skin - Daily baths must be given.

To the above four, we can add a fifth. This is spitting. Both the blood and lymphatic system carry waste away from the cells to the organs of elimination. The lymphatic system empties part of its load through the right thoracic duct and into the back of the mouth, so the phlegm can be spit out. Try to do this rather than swallowing it. At a time when your body is trying so hard to cleanse itself, do not endlessly recycle phlegm!

And we can add a sixth: cell and tissue cleansing. Like the other five, drinking plenty of water and juices helps here also.

Water is the best way to cleanse the system of impurities. Apply it internally, by drinking water, diluted fruit juices, and raw fruit and vegetable juices. Apply it externally in baths and water treatments.

Drinking fluids to cleanse: In order to cleanse the blood and lymph of impurities, one has to drink fluids. This consists of water-lemon fasts or fresh fruit or vegetable juices; never a water fast alone. Keep in mind that water

alone does not cleanse as well when it is not accompanied by juice. The vitamins and minerals in the juices aid directly in the cleansing and rebuilding process.

Enemas and colonics to cleanse: During a fasting period, two daily enemas (or colonics) should be given. (Instructions on how to make a colonic apparatus are given in the back of the author's book, *The Water Therapy Manual*.) Each enema or colonic consists of plain water that is mixed with the juice of a lemon. Up to 3 pints should be given to the person as a matter of routine—while he is fasting.

At any other time in the healing process that he is not having proper bowel movements, he should also be given enemas or colonics. This is important. But never put soap suds in the water! You may wash the skin with soap, but do not put it in the body. Remember the basic rule: Never place poisons in the body.

Medical knowledge has it that a person does not need a bowel movement when he is not eating. Yet this is not true. During the healing process, toxic substances are being drawn from the tissues. They need to be eliminated from the body; and this cannot be fully done by the kidneys, lungs, and bathing.

(In the disease sections of this book, various herbal enemas will be mentioned. They can be used in place of the water-lemon juice enema formula. An enema, with added catnip tea, works well for children.)

Wastes accumulated in the colon must be washed out once, twice, or even three times a day. During a fast, enemas or colonics must be used for this purpose. If this is not done, wastes are absorbed into the bloodstream and carried throughout the body.

Baths to cleanse: If the person is in the healing crisis, give him a sponge bath once or twice a day while he is in bed. If he is able to do so, give him a couple showers or a tub bath each day. However, tub baths are often too taxing and may cause fainting or weakening of the one who is quite ill.

As a rule, water placed on the skin enables the skin to throw off more poisons than it would otherwise do. Yet water on the skin also has other uses:

• If a person is in a fever, you will need to cool his body with sponging or other methods.

• If he has an inflammatory condition, you will want to apply one or more water treatments.

Light exercises: When a sick person is in bed, he is obtaining the extra rest he so much needs. But a little movement is also required from time to time, to help his lymphatic elimination. The lymph only moves by muscular activity.

Encourage him to move lightly every so often. This may be simply a matter of shifting and flexing the arms and legs. If the person is on a lengthy program of overcoming a chronic disorder, he needs to be taught to regularly extend, flex, and rotate each muscle every so often. This includes the arms, hands, legs, feet, abdomen, shoulders, and neck. Although this may seem complicated, it is not. It is just a matter of some simple body movements. He may do this while in bed or sitting on its edge.

Summary to this point: Let us summarize the typical

regimen.

• *Water-lemon fast*—First comes the fast of water and lemon juice, with no sweetening. Continue this until the fever crisis (typically 1-3 days) is past. Give him *as much* water-lemon as he wants, *as often* as he wants it.

• *Rotational fast: juice*—If there is a need for a longer fast, you may find it best to alternate it with a juice diet of fresh fruit and vegetable juices; perhaps a glass of fresh juice once a day.

• *Rotational fast: light meal*—If the fast is unusually long, as in the case of very chronic diseases, you may alternate it with light meals; perhaps fasting for 3 days, followed by light meals for 3 days.

Always give 1-2 enemas or colonics every day when fasting.

• *Juice diet*—Then comes the juice diet. If the illness is not severe, you may omit the fast and only place him on the juice diet.

Three or four times a day, a glass of fresh, raw juice is given. It may be fruit juice or it may be vegetable juice. Or it may be a fruit-vegetable juice.

• *Light meals*—Next comes some solid food. Let us consider that now.

Light meals: Sometimes a light meal is given alternately with a juice diet (a day of one, followed by a day of the other, etc.).

But, when the crisis from a fever or other inflammatory illness is past, a light diet should be started. The person is now recuperating. Healing is still going on, but he definitely "is on the mend." Or perhaps he is recovering from severe arthritis, will continue receiving care for an extended period, and needs to eat light meals alternated with a juice diet.

Such foods should include some solid fruits that are raw rather than cooked, raw vegetables in the form of a salad, and steamed vegetables once a day. A protein food once a day may be included.

The kind of protein food will depend on the type of ailment, the age of the person, his weight, and other factors. For example, one who has hardening of the arteries should necessarily be fed a lighter protein diet than one who is suffering from a milder problem.

No meat should be given to the person who is cleansing or recovering! No junk food! No processed, white-flour food! No fried, greasy food! No caffeine, tobacco, alcohol, or hard drugs! And, if at all possible, no medicinal drugs! And, after he is well again, he does well not to return to such things.

It is true that eggs have blood-building properties *(cf. Counsels on Diet and Foods, 204, 365, by E.G. White)*. Yet eggs, if used at all, must be used judiciously. People with a tendency to malignancy or actual malignancies must not be given any eggs. Those with skin diseases cannot handle eggs. Eggs have a sulphur-containing protein, so they cannot be given to anyone with a degenerative disease.

Meat contains a variety of substances which weaken and infect the body.

Milk has its own dangers, including contamination. Every public health officer knows that meat and milk are two of the most dangerous foods.

Yet for those who feel they need milk, it is more easily handled by those convalescing from chronic diseases than by those who are very ill. However, the very chronic types of inflammatory diseases (such as arthritis, bronchitis, and sinusitis) react unfavorably to milk and milk products.

Starchy foods and sweet foods are handled much better by the chronically sick than are protein foods. The invalid needs first to have been prepared for a mixed (building-up) diet by having undergone an initial fast, followed by a juice diet. Then he will be able to properly digest starches and sugars to gradually gain body weight and energy.

What are the most easily digested starches? Two are baked potatoes and steamed brown rice. But they must be prepared without salt, butter, oil, or grease. The third is toasted bread, ideally zwieback. Zwieback ("twice-toasted" in German) is made by taking whole-grain bread and, after it has been baked, toasting the slices in the oven until it is firm throughout. (A toaster does not do this as well.) This helps dextrinize the starch and render it more digestible. The heat converts the starch into intermediate dextrines.

The light diet includes a mixture of starchy foods and raw fruits, along with the raw vegetable juices, raw fruit juices, some palatable salads, and those raw vegetables which can be palatably chewed and enjoyed. A certain amount of fat (in the form of unhydrogenated vegetable oil) can be added to the starchy foods to make them more palatable; but this must be added to the food on the plate as it is served, not to the cooking.

Thousands could be helped who would follow this healing procedure of water-lemon fasting, raw fruit and vegetable juice fasting, and the above light meals for a time.

Someone may ask, exactly how many days on this and on that? Each case may be different. Yet if you will pray for help, think, watch, and be ready to make a changeover to a different diet when the need arises, you can have success.

Pointers to keep in mind: Fasting removes cellular wastes from the skin and mucous membranes. A sufferer from the irritation and inflammation of hay fever or asthma can get great relief by a properly managed fast of 7-10 days, followed by a correct diet. (But it may require a month for the wheezing to stop and 4-6 months on this careful program for the problem to be overcome.) A deep-seated disorder, such as arthritis or inflammation of the joints, may require a longer period of fasting for relief.

Individuals with poor kidney elimination may be troubled by mild or severe symptoms of uremic poisoning during a stringent fast, because urinary wastes thrown off by the tissues are more poisonous than bowel wastes. They may irritate the kidneys or bladder. Adding colonic irrigation to the water-lemon juice intake helps to eliminate those toxins more rapidly.

It is remarkable what can be done in the hands of a person who is skilled in caring for people. Using these methods (and obtaining the full cooperation of the patient), here are some of the things which repeatedly have been accomplished:

• Placed on a natural healing program, a drug user can generally stop his medicines; and tobacco / alcohol users can be released from their addictions. After several days of fasting, the tobacco user loses his taste for the tobacco and the coffee drinker loses the craving for caffeine. The alcoholic can lose the craving more quickly and thoroughly by means of fasting than in any other way.

• Skin ailments of prolonged duration, such as psoriasis and other forms of eczema, have responded very well to fasting methods.

• Bronchial asthma in individuals who had been sick for over a decade were cured by a few fasting periods, alternated with a properly chosen diet.

• The chronic disease complex, called arthritis (even when many joints are immobilized and deformed), responds well to the fasting method.

• The younger the person, the quicker the healing occurs.

• There are some conditions which, through long years of abuse, are entrenched. They may require many months of care, sometimes a year. Yet any other approach would require many years of treatment with drugs, as the condition keeps getting worse.

• In some cases, diabetes mellitus requires some insulin during the fast, especially for juvenile diabetics. Short fasting periods are safer and more effective for such people. But, in most other cases, medicinal drugs are not needed on a fast.

• If a child has a cold, he should be placed on a short fast; he should not be given food "to feed the cold to death."

• Children would never have dangerous complications, such as mastoid infections or middle-ear diseases, if they were quickly placed on a short fast to stop the infection at its inception.

• Raw vegetable salads can be given, in extracted juice form, to a stomach-ulcer case. This works quite well.

• In the late stages, the fight to control cancer is difficult. The one with cancer has much to gain by body-cleansing treatments which include fasting. Early stages of the disease are marked by fatigue, weakness, and skin eruptions such as eczema and warts.

• In the late stages of cancer, the body actually shrinks. It loses weight, despite the Jell-O, puddings, meat, gravy, and canned fruit given to the patient in the hospitals. The cancer sufferer may lose 100-150 pounds. This occurs because the body cannot regenerate itself on ordinary food.

• If those individuals were, every day, fed 3-4 glasses of raw vegetable juice and also freshly made fruit juice, their bodies would not suffer from starvation and cachexia.

The extent of the malnutrition is so serious that, in very late stages, spontaneous fractures of various bones occur. This could have been prevented by feeding several glasses of raw vegetable juice every day.

The post-recovery diet: What should I eat after I am well again? Read the two chapters, *Dietetic Principles for Health* and *Healing* and *Vitamins, Minerals, and other Nutrients.* If you are really serious about keeping well—and not slipping back into a diseased state—then your future can be much brighter.

Fasting, as a method of *preventing* disease, should not be ignored. It is as important for people in good health as it is for those who have succumbed to, or been overwhelmed by, disease.

Once or twice a year, an adequately managed fast of 3-10 days can do wonders for the man or woman who has reached the age of 35 or 40. Because your body is not as filled with morbid wastes, you will feel more comfortable while on the fast than will a person who is sick.

Fasting once or twice a year is a powerful tool to help the body cleanse itself of accumulated wastes. Fatigue, constipation, premature aging, and sclerotic changes of the arteries, nerves, and heart could be prevented by occasional fasting periods, followed by correct dietary programs. Everyone over 35 should do this.

But if you are very thin, it is best to have not more than 3 fasts a year, with only 3 days on each fast. Some individuals do best by skipping only a single meal and going to bed during that time.

If properly done, tumors, in their early degenerative condition, may be reabsorbed by bodily reconstructive changes; chronic ear, nose, and throat conditions can be cleared up.

Remember to always take enemas during a fast.

3 - SIX TILDEN FORMULAS

We are here dealing with a subject which is not commonplace to many people. All that some know is drugging, tubes, and surgery. So it would be well to amplify on the above Tilden principles by giving several examples of how he used them in giving his treatments. (Cross references to these examples will be placed in the main disease sections of this book.)

COMMON COLD

For more on the common cold, see p. 289.
Put the person, whether an adult or a young child, to bed right away. Do not feed a cold. Give an enema. A purgative or laxative may take as long as 10 hours before the cleansing effects occur; but an enema will do it in just 10 minutes. During that 10 hours, much toxic absorption from the bowels into the bloodstream can take place.

Follow the enema with a heat application of one or two heating pads or an electric blanket, to warm up the body parts which are chilled. Cold feet and hands are often found in people with a "head cold." They need to be warmed up quickly. This removes excessive amounts of blood from the congested head and chest areas. Turn the heat down only to the degree that the limbs become warmed.

Give him some fruit juice with water (from half a grapefruit in half a glass of cold water or juice of half a lemon in half a glass of cold or hot water, unsweetened). Do not give food, milk, coffee, regular tea, etc. The body cannot properly digest even good food, much less junk food, while fighting an infectious inflammation. One to 3 days on lemon juice and/or grapefruit juice and water is quite safe.

Give only fruit juice and water until the nose has ceased to discharge watery or thick material. Keep him in bed and quiet.

If a headache is present, place a cold moist towel or ice bag on the forehead or on top of the head. When the headache is caused by congestion and nerve strain, it will clear up quickly without any medicines if the person is allowed to rest quietly in bed, even if he cannot sleep.

Convalescing from a cold requires one week, possibly two, to properly build up strength to resist a future cold.

Why so long? Because the whole body is being cleaned out. *This is, in reality, a wonderful process.* Let it work itself out properly; and your life will be more pleasant, freer from later crippling disease, and you will live longer. If you try to stop the process too early, especially by taking drugs, then the problem has been stifled, not eliminated—and years later more serious diseases will result.

Diet during this recovery period will depend on the person's weight and appetite. It is always safe to give a raw fruit diet for several days: lemonade that is sweetened with honey and raw fruits for breakfast, dinner, and supper.

After 3 days on a fruit diet, the noon and evening meal may include steamed vegetables and a small raw salad with some almonds or pecans or a baked potato. Chew it well.

By this time, the bowels should be moving normally and enemas are no longer needed. The cold will have been eliminated without the use of drugs.

ASTHMA

For more on asthma, see p. 852.

Using the Tilden method, the wheezing may be relieved within 4 weeks; but the complete problem will not be eliminated for 2-6 months or more. Asthma tends to be entrenched; and it takes time before it is eliminated.

Breakfast: Juices of two fruits and some solid fruit, for which there is an appetite. The fruit juices are diluted with hot or cold water. A small amount of honey may be added to diluted lemon or orange juice. Asthmatics can eat fresh or stewed fruits, but only in small portions. Cooked fruit must not be sweetened with sugar. Half of the above breakfast is eaten first thing in the morning and the other half in mid-morning.

Lunch: A raw salad is given about noon, as much as he has an appetite for. This salad may be 1/6th of an average head of lettuce, a grated raw carrot, 1/4th of a pear or avocado, some raw celery, and a little orange juice to season it all. No oil or cream dressing. In addition, 2 steamed vegetables (1 green and 1 yellow) may be given instead of bread. No crackers, milk, or cake.

Rest and sleep after this meal, for 2 hours until he is well.

3 or 4 p.m.: Fruit and fruit juice, same as at breakfast.
Supper: An early supper, same as lunch.
No food before bedtime.
No social life, except for a radio by the bed for the first 6 months.

PERNICIOUS ANEMIA

For more on pernicious anemia, see p. 539.

Here is a sample case; remember that the care and diet can vary according to the individual. This person had a good digestive system, did not have a healing crisis, and needed to solve an ongoing problem. So a fuller diet was given to him.

He was given a fresh glass of grapefruit juice first thing in the morning. An hour later, breakfast of raw fruits in season. It consisted of 2-3 kinds of fruit; and he was told to eat only one kind every hour. In addition to the fruit, he was also given a glass of freshly made raw vegetable juice (consisting of celery leaves and stalks, beet tops, carrots, lettuce, and parsley), some almonds (to be chewed slowly

and well), and 2 slices of whole-wheat bread with a little vegetable oil on the bread. He was told to eat the nuts and fruit at one time and the bread and some sweeter fruit an hour or two hours after the nuts. Thus his breakfast was divided into 2-3 periods. In his case, he needed to build his blood.

Noon meal: One glass of raw vegetable juice (same as for breakfast), raw salad materials to chew, 2 slightly steamed vegetables (green, average-portion), lentils, and a few almonds (to be chewed well).

Mid-afternoon: Glass of freshly made orange juice and glass of raw vegetable juice.

Evening meal: Some almonds (chewed slowly and well), raw green salad (lettuce, cucumber, celery), 2 servings of steamed vegetables (1 yellow and 1 green), and raw fruit for dessert.

No drugs of any kind, liver, or liver extract were given. The patient was given showers or sponge baths instead of tub baths, which are more debilitating. He was given enemas when the bowels did not move naturally.

After the first 3 weeks of treatment, instead of the nuts at noon, the patient was given a baked potato twice a week with the noon meal, alternating with brown rice or buckwheat once or twice a week.

Because eggs are needed to build up the blood, his breakfast was modified to include 2 eggs every morning. But the evening meal remained the same.

After 5 weeks, he was strong enough to take his own tub bath and walk around outside.

DIABETES

For more on diabetes, see p. 656.

Here are some helpful hints for treating this condition: Raw, fresh vegetables are the safest foods for the diabetic. Salads that are freshly made of raw cabbage, lettuce, celery, radishes, tomatoes, and seasoned only with lemon juice. Do not give him cooked vegetables, meats, bread, etc. He should eat raw salads for breakfast, dinner, and supper.

Raw fruits which are low in sugar can also be used. This would include grapefruits, apples that are not too sweet, peaches, and pears. The sub-acid and acid fruits help burn up excess sugar from the blood and tissues. The raw salads provide alkaline mineral ash, which tends to soak up cellular wastes and help prevent diabetic gangrene and other complications.

Feeding him a breakfast of sour fruits (such as slightly diluted lemon juice, grapefruit, and raw apple) helps reduce sugar in the blood and urine to an impressive degree. Before insulin was discovered, Dr. Da Costa used lemon juice as a medicine, to oxidize excess blood sugar in the body of the diabetic. This is still very useful. The diabetic relishes pure lemon juice. And it quenches thirst very well, because it burns up excess blood sugar without causing insulin shock.

Fasting is very helpful in treating diabetes. It is given alternately with raw salad and raw fruit feeding. During the fast, only give slightly diluted lemon juice. The juice of 4 lemons is placed in a glass, then filled with water. The diabetic takes this as often he can, without forcing. (Remember not to "chew" lemon juice; swallow it, so as not to injure the teeth.)

Two enemas are given each day (2-3 pints water, plus juice of a lemon).

When he is ready for food other than raw fruits or vegetables, give him slightly cooked leafy green vegetables, without seasoning.

Be very careful about giving him any fats; because he cannot metabolize fat as a normal person can. In him, fats break down in the blood into more severe poisons than excess sugar. Many diabetics are overweight. But if the one you are working with is thin, you must still give him some oil, but only a small amount. Give him a little avocado.

For proteins, give him a few nuts.

Starchy foods must be used in great moderation by diabetics, especially the young. But young people who participate in energy-consuming activities must have some starch.

Insulin may be needed, especially for juvenile diabetics. But, on this diet, they will require only small amounts of insulin. (The less insulin taken, the less likelihood of complications or blindness in later years.) It is much easier to regulate older diabetics without having to give them insulin.

TONSILLITIS

For more on tonsillitis, see p. 740.

Inflamed and infected tonsils can be treated by putting the patient to bed and keeping him there. He should be on a diet of oranges, grapefruit, fresh raw pineapples, and two raw vegetable salads per day. (Anyone, child or adult, can live on such a diet while resting in bed quietly for a month to six weeks.) Within a relatively short time, the tonsillitis problem will be gone. Such a treatment is superior to surgery for diseased tonsils. The bowels must be evacuated twice a day, using enemas if necessary.

ALCOHOLISM

For more on alcoholism, see p. 881.

The food intake during the first three days consists of freshly made orange juice, grapefruit juice, and lemonade (the latter sweetened with a little honey). These are given to the person at 2-hour intervals. At his bedside is always one or two glasses of fruit juice with an ice cube or two in it. Cold drinks are not only soothing, but also a good substitute to satisfy the craving for liquor.

The bowels are cleansed once or twice a day with an enema or colonic.

After 3 days on this program, a building program is begun. By this time, there will be a good appetite for a full breakfast: a slice of toast, a small dish of cereal with almond nut milk on it. Fresh fruit is kept by the bedside, to be eaten whenever desired.

For lunch, a steamed vegetable, baked potato or rice, and a glass of raw vegetable juice.

In the evening, a raw salad, sprinkled with ground nuts (or a small handful is given to be chewed well), steamed vegetables, and a glass of fresh fruit juice.

In concluding this brief overview of one of the giants of the nineteenth and early twentieth centuries' natural healing, it is intriguing to note that Trall, Jackson, Kellogg, or Tilden never used vitamin / mineral supplements. Their nutritional importance was only beginning to be discovered during Kellogg's and Tilden's last years. Nor did those men work much with herbs. Nearly all their remarkable healing work was done with fasting, simple diet, rest, and water therapy.

Therefore, with the additional nutritional information available today (and much of it is included in this book), we should all the more easily be able to resist and overcome disease.

But the counterpoint fact is that, today, we have far more poisons in the air, water, soil, plants, processed foods and animal kingdom than they had back then. In addition, far too many of us pay for high-priced poisons which we regularly take for our many ailments, brought on by the other poisons in our environment and food.

There is no doubt that we need all the help we can get. So, when we become ill, let us not swallow or inject an additional load of toxic substances.

4 - THE HEALING CRISIS

Physicians and laymen have known about the healing crisis for thousands of years. During the healing process, the body tries to throw off toxins and poisons. What is known as the "healing crisis" frequently occurs in illnesses. The body seems overwhelmed with all the toxins and wastes it is trying to throw off. The organs of elimination (bowels, kidneys, lungs, skin, nasal passages, throat, bronchi, and urinary organs) become congested, crowded, and irritated.

During this crisis, that which appears to be disease symptoms appear. These may be open sores, perspiration, diarrhea, boils, colds, kidney and bladder infections, fevers, etc. But this is not a new or intensified disease—it is just part of the healing process. The body knows it must eliminate the wastes before it can begin rebuilding; so it works valiantly to do this.

Physicians sometimes try to stop the process by introducing poisons (drugs) into the system. Immediately, the body stops throwing off wastes—stops the crisis—and turns its attention to the terrible new invader. The body may appear to be resting quietly now, with the symptoms reduced or gone; but, in actuality, it has been prostrated by the drugging.

Let us now return to a healing crisis and its symptoms. They are part of the cure, and should not be feared. Just work with the body, to help eliminate those toxic wastes. Open the channels of elimination by means of drinking water and fruit juices, fasting, enemas, colonics, showers, baths, and water treatments.

Sometimes the pain becomes severe during the crisis. Drugs taken in earlier years are being pulled out of the tissues in an effort to discard them. The damage of many years is being righted.

The body arouses itself in self-defense and brings forth acute elimination of toxins in the form of a fever, cold, inflammations, itching, boils, ulcers, hemorrhages, excessive menstrual discharge, etc. Reactions vary, in accordance with how the person has been living and the condition of the body.

But sometimes this sudden turn in an illness is not a healing crisis, but a change for the worse in a disease. It is important to be able to tell the difference. Consider this:

• Watch the person carefully, as you earnestly work to

help him eliminate toxins (water, juices, enemas, sweating, baths, etc.). If not watched properly and helped, the crisis can be extended and his energies weakened.

• If it is a healing crisis, you will generally see a positive change—a change for the better—after three days. The most severe symptoms begin to decrease. Fevers break. The person becomes more relaxed and begins to feel better.

• But if, after three days, the symptoms do not change for the better, then a new course of treatment must be started. However, if the person has low energy and vitality, the crisis may take three to seven days.

• If the individual has a strong constitution and the organs of elimination are working well and are being helped, he may recover without having undergone a healing crisis.

Are there ways to tell when a healing crisis is about to begin? Certain symptoms will intensify, such as sluggishness, fevers, dark urine, coated tongue, weakness, irritability, headaches, and ringing in the ears.

When you see these signs, immediately set to work to help the person's system cleanse more fully. Herbs, massage, water therapy treatments, and enemas can help him through this time.

If no poisons were introduced into the system (in an effort to block the healing crisis) the person will generally keep improving. Right living, right eating, and rest can bring healing.

Additional healing crises may occur before the patient is fully recovered. Each one will generally be milder, only one to three days in length, and be followed by a new level of feeling better.

The intensity of the crisis will depend on how ill the person was. The nature of the crisis will be keyed to where the illness is centered in his body and how easily he can throw off the poisons.

If the wastes can be eliminated through normal pathways, a fever will develop and burn it out; if it does not, it can store it as boils and acne. If the mucous is thick, there will be nasal drip, colds, flu, etc. Constipation may precede diarrhea; lung congestion may come before a respiratory crisis.

Sometimes we feel pain in our kidneys, bladder, or bowels and imagine it is a disease. But, in fact, often the body has selected the strongest organ of elimination to throw off unwanted and excess wastes.

When the crisis is over, the body needs help rebuilding itself. But, throughout the sickness and recovery, never go to extremes in diet. Carry on with a gradual transition back to regular living. Trying to make the system too pure too fast can overly weaken the patient. Work carefully and keep praying for guidance; and, if the patient fully cooperates, all will go well.

5 - THE KELLOGG FORMULAS

In 1866 the Battle Creek Sanitarium opened its doors; and, in 1875, it was placed under the directorship of John Harvey Kellogg, M.D. He was one of the foremost natural healing experts of the late nineteenth and early twentieth centuries.

Ninety-five of his multiple treatments for disease are included in the disease sections of this book, and are identified as "Kellogg Formulas."

6 - ADDITIONAL HEALING PRINCIPLES

We have included the statements of a number of different natural healing pioneers in this volume. Here are insightful comments from the writings of Ellen G. White, who had a profound understanding of the origin and transmission of pathological problems.

"The transgression of physical law is the transgression of God's law. Our Creator is Jesus Christ. He is the author of our being. He has created the human structure. He is the author of the physical laws, as He is the author of the moral law. And the human being who is careless and reckless of the habits and practices that concern his physical life and health, sins against God."—*Counsels on Diet and Foods, 43 (cf. Ministry of Healing, 131).*

"God's law is written by His own finger upon every nerve, every muscle, every faculty which has been entrusted to man."—*Spalding and Magan's Manuscript Testimonies of Ellen White, 40.*

"Health, strength, and happiness depend upon immutable laws; but these laws cannot be obeyed where there is no anxiety to become acquainted with them."—*Healthful Living, 18.*

"The Lord has made it a part of His plan that man's reaping shall be according to his sowing."—*Healthful Living, 25 (Letter, May 19, 1897).*

"To make plain natural law, and urge the obedience of it, is the work that accompanies the third angel's message to prepare a people for the coming of the Lord."—*3 Testimonies, 161 (Counsel on Diet and Foods, 69).*

"There are many ways of practicing the healing art, but there is only one way that Heaven approves. God's remedies are the simple agencies of nature that will not tax or debilitate the system through their powerful properties. Pure air and water, cleanliness, a proper diet, purity of life, and a firm trust in God are remedies for the want of which thousands are dying; yet these remedies are going out of date because their skillful use requires work that the people do not appreciate."—*5 Testimonies, 443.*

"It is the duty of every human being, for his own sake and for the sake of humanity, to inform himself or herself in regard to the laws of organic life, and conscientiously to obey them . . It is the duty of every person to become intelligent in regard to disease and its causes."—*Healthful Living, 19 (Letter, December 4, 1896).*

"God has formed laws to govern every part of our constitutions, and these laws which He has placed in our being are divine, and for every transgression there is a fixed penalty, which sooner or later must be realized."—*Healthful Living, 20.*

"Our first duty, one which we owe to God, to ourselves, and to our fellow men, is to obey the laws of God, which include the laws of health."—*3 Testimonies, 164.*

"The laws governing the physical nature are as truly divine in their origin and character as the law of the Ten Commandments. Man is fearfully and wonderfully made;

38 **BASIC PRINCIPLES** **ADDITIONAL PRINCIPLES** NATURAL REMEDIES ENCYCLOPEDIA
OVER 11,000 REMEDIES - OVER 730 DISEASES

P
R
I
N

for Jehovah has inscribed His law by His own mighty hand on every part of the physical structure."—*16 Manuscript Releases, 60 (Letter, August 5, 1896).*

" 'Have I not a right to do as I please with my own body?' —No, you have no moral right, because you are violating the laws of life and health which God has given you. You are the Lord's property,—His by creation and His by redemption. Every human being is under obligation to preserve the living machinery that is so fearfully and wonderfully made."— *Healthful Living, 10 (Letter, May 19, 1897).*

"Our very bodies are not our own, to treat as we please, to cripple by habits that lead to decay, making it impossible to render to God perfect service. Our lives and all our faculties belong to Him. He is caring for us every moment; He keeps the living machinery in action. If we were left to run it for one moment, we should die. We are absolutely dependent upon God."—*Medical Ministry, 275-276 (Letter, October 12, 1896).*

"The health should be as sacredly guarded as the character."—*Medical Ministry, 77.*

"Proportionally as nature's laws are transgressed, mind and soul become enfeebled . . Physical suffering of every type is seen . . Suffering must follow this course of action. The vital force of the system cannot bear up under the tax placed upon it, and it finally breaks down."—*Healthful Living, 24 (Letter, August 30, 1896).*

"Sickness is caused by violating the laws of health; it is the result of violating nature's laws."—*3 Testimonies, 164.*

"Health is a great treasure. It is the richest possession that mortals can have. Wealth, honor, or learning is dearly purchased, if it be at the loss of the vigor of health. None of these attainments can secure happiness if health is wanting."—*Fundamentals of Christian Education, 35.*

"That time is well spent which is directed to the establishment and preservation of sound physical and mental health . . It is easy to lose health, but it is difficult to regain it."—*Review, September 23, 1884.*

"Perfect health depends on perfect circulation."—*2 Testimonies, 531.*

"Many have inquired of me, 'What course shall I take to best preserve my health?' My answer is, Cease to transgress the laws of your being; cease to gratify a depraved appetite; eat simple food; dress healthfully, which will require modest simplicity; work healthfully, and you will not be sick."— *Counsels on Health, 37.*

"An aimless life is a living death. The mind should dwell upon themes relating to our eternal interests. This will be conducive to health of body and mind."—*Counsels on Health, 51.*

"God has pledged Himself to keep this living machinery in healthful action, if the human agent will obey His laws and cooperate with God."—*Counsels on Diet and Foods, 17.*

"Let it ever be kept before the mind that the great object of hygienic reform is to secure the highest possible development of mind and soul and body."—*Counsels on Health, 386.*

"Nature will restore their vigor and strength in their sleeping hours, if her laws are not violated."—*Healthful Living, 46.*

"Close confinement indoors makes women pale and feeble, and results in premature death."—*Healthful Living, 61.*

"Indulging in eating too frequently, and in too large quantities, overtaxes the digestive organs, and produces a feverish state of the system. The blood becomes impure, and then diseases of various kinds occur."—*Counsels on Diet and Foods, 189.*

"The effects produced by living in close, ill-ventilated rooms are these . . The mind becomes depressed and gloomy, while the whole system is enervated; and fevers and other acute diseases are liable to be generated . . The system is peculiarly sensitive to the influence of cold. A slight exposure produces serious diseases."—*1 Testimonies, 702-703.*

"What influence does overeating have upon the stomach? It becomes debilitated, the digestive organs are weakened, and disease, with all its train of evils, is brought on as a result."—*2 Testimonies, 364.*

"The free use of sugar in any form tends to clog the system, and is not unfrequently a cause of disease."— *Counsels on Health, 154.*

"The liability to take disease is increased tenfold by meat eating."—*2 Testimonies, 64.*

"Rich and complicated mixtures of food are health destroying. Highly seasoned meats and rich pastry are wearing out the digestive organs."—*Healthful Living, 63.*

"Drugging should be forever abandoned; for while it does not cure any malady, it enfeebles the system, making it more susceptible to disease."—*5 Testimonies, 311.*

"A neglect of cleanliness will induce disease."— *Adventist Home, 22.*

"If you would have your homes sweet and inviting, make them bright with air and sunshine."—*2 Testimonies, 527.*

"Dwellings, if possible, should be built upon high and dry ground. If a house is built where water settles around it, remaining for a time, and then drying away, a poisonous miasma arises, and fever and ague, sore throat, lung diseases, and fevers will be the result."—*Counsels on Health, 58-59.*

"It is important also that the clothing be kept clean. The garments worn absorb the waste matter that passes off through the pores; if they are not frequently changed and washed, the impurities will be reabsorbed."—*Ministry of Healing, 276.*

"When we do all we can on our part to have health, then may we expect that blessed results will follow, and we can ask God in faith to bless our efforts for the preservation of health."—*Medical Ministry, 13.*

The book, Ministry of Healing, is a remarkable analysis of human health and divine healing. It is available from the publishers of this book for $5.00 ppd. Overseas: Send U.S. money order and add $3.00 p&h. In Tennessee, add 9.25% tax.

7 - THE USE OF DRUGS

What is the difference between a medicinal drug and an herb? Herbs contain a variety of chemical compounds placed there by God. Over the centuries, many have been found to be extremely useful for physical problems. Medicinal drugs are different. In order to patent them (for exclusive sales and profits), medicinal drugs cannot have the exact formulas found in herbs. Instead, they contain various man-made combinations of chemicals. Because of this, to one extent or another, they are always poisonous. Their "contraindications" paragraphs verify the fact. The liver, kidneys, and other organs frequently suffer from them.

The following analysis of the nature and effects of medicinal drug medication is taken from the writings of Ellen G. White, an influential author and worker in the field of health and natural healing. She was also the founder of a major medical college.

"Drugs never cure disease; they only change its form and location . . When drugs are introduced into the system, for a time they seem to have a beneficial effect. A change may take place, but the disease is not cured. It will manifest itself in some other form . . The disease which the drug was given to cure may disappear, but only to reappear in a new form, such as skin diseases, ulcers, painful diseased joints, and sometimes in a more dangerous and deadly form . . Nature keeps struggling, and the patient suffers with different ailments, until there is a sudden breaking down in her efforts, and death follows."—*2 Selected Messages, 451-452 (Healthful Living, 243).*

"Although the patient may recover, yet the powerful effort nature was required to make to induce action to overcome the poison, injured the constitution and shortened the life of the patient. There are many who do not die under the influence of drugs, but there are very many who are left useless wrecks, hopeless, gloomy, and miserable sufferers, a burden to themselves and to society."—*2 Selected Messages, 442.*

"Every additional drug given to the patient . . will complicate the case, and make the patient's recovery more hopeless . . An evil, simple in the beginning, which nature aroused herself to overcome, and which she would have done had she been left to herself has been made ten-fold worse by introducing drug poisons into the system, which is a destructive disease of itself, forcing into extraordinary action the remaining life forces to war against and overcome the drug intruder."—*2 Selected Messages, 448.*

"There are more who die from the use of drugs than all who would have died of disease had nature been left to do her own work."—*2 Selected Messages, 452.*

"The endless variety of medicines in the market, the numerous advertisements of new drugs and mixtures, all of which claim to do wonderful cures, kill hundreds where they benefit one . . Yet people keep dosing, and continue

to grow weaker until they die . . God's servants should not administer medicines which they know will leave behind injurious effects upon the system, even if they do relieve present suffering. Every poisonous preparation in the vegetable and mineral kingdoms, taken into the system, will leave its wretched influence, affecting the liver and lungs, and deranging the system generally."—*Healthful Living, 245.*

"Educate away from drugs, use them less and less, and depend more upon hygienic agencies; then nature will respond to God's remedies—pure air, pure water, proper exercise, and a clear conscience."—*Counsels on Health, 261.*

"A great amount of good can be done by enlightening all to whom we have access, as to the best means, not only of curing the sick, but of preventing disease and suffering. The physician who endeavors to enlighten his patients as to the nature and causes of their maladies, and to teach them how to avoid disease, may have uphill work; but if he is a conscientious reformer, he will talk plainly of the ruinous effects of self-indulgence in eating, drinking, and dressing, of the overtaxation of the vital forces that has brought his patients where they are. He will not increase the evil by administering drugs till exhausted nature gives up the struggle, but will teach the patients how to form correct habits and to aid nature in her work of restoration by a wise use of her own remedies."—*Counsels on Diet and Foods, 449.*

"In treating the sick, the physician will seek God for wisdom; then, instead of placing his dependence upon drugs and expecting that medicine will bring health to his patients, he will use nature's restoratives, and employ natural means whereby the sick may be aided to recover."—*Healthful Living, 247-248.*

"Let the instruction be given in simple words [such as hot water, charcoal, or catnip tea]. We have no need to use the many expressions used by worldly physicians which are so difficult to understand that they must be interpreted by the physicians . . Nature's simple remedies will aid in recovery without leaving the deadly aftereffects so often felt by those who use poisonous drugs."—*Loma Linda Messages, 335.*

"Were I sick, I would just as soon call in a lawyer as a physician from among general practitioners. I would not touch their nostrums, to which they give Latin names. I am determined to know, in straight English, the name of everything that I introduce into my system."—*2 Selected Messages, 290; 20 Manuscript Releases, 1.*

"Indulging in eating too frequently, and in too large quantities, overtaxes the digestive organs and produces a feverish state of the system. The blood becomes impure, and then diseases of various kinds occur. A physician is sent for, who prescribes some drug which gives present relief, but which does not cure the disease. It may change the form of the disease, but the real evil is increased ten-fold. Nature was doing her best to rid the system of an accumulation of impurities, and could she have been left to herself, aided by the common blessings of heaven, such as pure air and pure water, a speedy and safe cure could have been effected."—*Medical Ministry, 281.*

"Use nature's remedies,—water, sunshine, and fresh

P R I N

40   BASIC PRINCIPLES   NUTRITIONAL EXPERTS SPEAK   NATURAL REMEDIES ENCYCLOPEDIA
OVER 11,000 REMEDIES - OVER 730 DISEASES

air. Do not use drugs. Drugs never heal; they only change the features of the disease."—*The Paulson Collection of Ellen G. White's Writings, 17.*

"Experimenting in drugs is a very expensive business . . Nothing should be put into the human system that will leave a baleful influence behind."—*Medical Ministry, 228.*

"Nature's simple remedies will aid in recovery without leaving the deadly aftereffects so often felt by those who use poisonous drugs. They destroy the power of the patient to help himself. This power the patients are to be taught to exercise by learning to eat simple, healthful foods, by refusing to overload the stomach with a variety of foods at one meal. All these things should come into the education of the sick. Talks should be given showing how to preserve health, how to shun sickness, how to rest when rest is needed."—*2 Selected Messages, 281 (Letter 82, 1908).*

"Christ's remedies cleanse the system. But Satan has tempted man to introduce into the system that which weakens the human machinery, clogging and destroying the fine, beautiful arrangements of God. The drugs administered to the sick do not restore, but destroy. Drugs never cure. Instead, they place in the system seeds which bear a very bitter harvest."—*2 Selected Messages, 289.*

8 - NUTRITIONAL EXPERTS SPEAK

"Ninety percent of all conditions other than acute infections, contagious diseases, and traumatisms, are traceable to diet."—*Sir William Osler, M.D., quoted in Foods, Nutrition, and Clinical Dietetics, 13.*

"The food question is infinitely the most important problem of the present day . . and if properly dealt with must result in the disappearance of the vast bulk of the disease, misery and death."—*Sir Arthuthnot Lane, M.D., quoted in The Motive, June 1925.*

"At least nine-tenths of all chronic maladies with which doctors are called upon to deal might be successfully treated without the use of drugs by a physician well acquainted with the varied resources afforded by the science of nutrition."—*John H. Kellogg, M.D., in Good Health, June 1940, 69.*

Major General Sir Robert McCarrison, M.D., D.Sc., F.R.C.P., while serving as Director of Nutritional Research, Pasteur Institute, Coonoor, India, fed pigeons, guinea pigs and monkeys the usual "deficiency diets" eaten by so many today in "civilized nations," and induced in them every known disease of the digestive tract and every other body organ. In a major address in which he discussed his findings, he listed over 30 leading diseases, and said this: "All these states of ill-health had a common cause; faulty nutrition with or without infection . . Of all the medicines created out of the earth, food is the chief."—*McCarrison, quoted in Madras Mail, March 16, 1935. Also see the British medical journal, Lancet, May 23, 1931.*

Man is the only creature given to the practice of self-destroying habits.

"The span of human life has not been lengthened, and there is no prospect that it soon will be. The average duration of life is all that has been altered, and that has been accomplished chiefly by giving more babies a fairer start in life's journey than they used to have. Because more of them get by the early and very difficult hurdles, more of them survive to later ages. But the likelihood that any individual aged seventy today can safely say he will be alive at ninety appears to be not quite as good as they were fifty years ago."—*Raymond Pearl, M.D., "The Search for Longevity," Scientific Monthly, May 1938.*

Why is the truth about the superiority of good nutrition rarely discussed today?

There is more money to be made by selling people junk food, which has little or no nutritional value. It is cheaper to manufacture; and it stores well because no bugs want it.

People have become accustomed to eating fast foods, which they do not have to refrigerate or prepare.

As long as it has a combination of one or more of the following, most people will buy and consume it, even though it contains essentially no food value: sugar, salt, cheap protein, carbohydrates, and grease (trans fat).

If it tastes good today, why worry about the long-term effects of junk food later on?

Why is the truth about the superiority of natural remedies rarely mentioned today?

There is more money to be made by selling people chemicals (medicinal drugs), surgical operations, and radiation treatments. Good nutrition and natural remedies cannot be patented and sold for a nice profit. If widely used, good diets and home remedies would heavily reduce the income of pharmacies, physicians, hospitals, pharmaceutical firms, hospital equipment, and supply firms. It would also eliminate the immense grants of money given to universities, to produce research findings favorable to those products.

People have become accustomed to wanting fast recovery from a pill. They want to get back to work quickly and continue to ignore the proper care their bodies urgently need.

Many people prefer remedies which do not require a change of diet or living habits, a putting away of bad habits or taking time to learn about (and use) natural remedies.

Rely on God for help to obey His law, and do what it takes to live right, and you will be richly repaid later on. It is worth any inconvenience to have good health.

More Encouragement

"Jesus saw in every soul one to whom must be given the call to His kingdom. He reached the hearts of the people by going among them as one who desired their good. He sought them in the public streets, in private houses, on the boats, in the synagogue, by the shores of the lake, and at the marriage feast. He met them at their daily vocations, and manifested an interest in their secular affairs. He carried His instruction into the household, bringing families in their own homes under the influence of His divine presence. His strong personal sympathy helped to win hearts. He often repaired to the mountains for solitary prayer, but this was a preparation for His labor among men in active life. From these seasons He came forth to relieve the sick, to instruct the ignorant, and to break the chains from the captives of Satan . .

"As disciples of Christ we shall not mingle with the world from a mere love of pleasure, to unite with them in folly. Such associations can result only in harm. We should never give sanction to sin by our words or our deeds, our silence or our presence. Wherever we go, we are to carry Jesus with us, and to reveal to others the preciousness of our Saviour. But those who try to preserve their religion by hiding it within stone walls lose precious opportunities of doing good. Through the social relations, Christianity comes in contact with the world. Everyone who has received the divine illumination is to brighten the pathway of those who know not the Light of life.

"We should all become witnesses for Jesus . . Let the world see that we are not selfishly absorbed in our own interests, but that we desire others to share our blessings and privileges. Let them see that our religion does not make us unsympathetic or exacting. Let all who profess to have found Christ, minister as He did for the benefit of men.

"We should never give to the world the false impression that Christians are a gloomy, unhappy people. If our eyes are fixed on Jesus, we shall see a compassionate Redeemer, and shall catch light from His countenance. Wherever His Spirit reigns, there peace abides. And there will be joy also, for there is a calm, holy trust in God."
—Desire of Ages, 151-153

THE EIGHT LAWS OF HEALTH
ENABLING US TO OBTAIN IT AND KEEP IT

THE FIRST LAW
CLEAN AIR TO PURIFY OUR BLOOD-STREAM AND CELLS

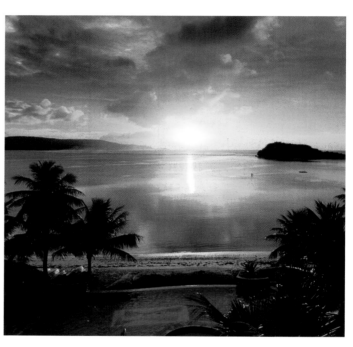

THE SECOND LAW
SUNLIGHT TO PURIFY OUR BODIES AND SURROUNDINGS

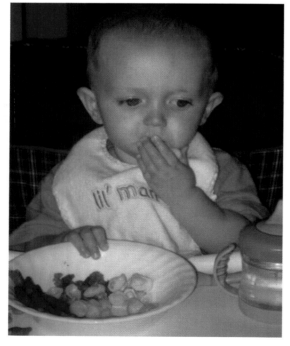

THE THIRD LAW
TEMPERATE LIVING IN ALL OF OUR ACTIVITIES

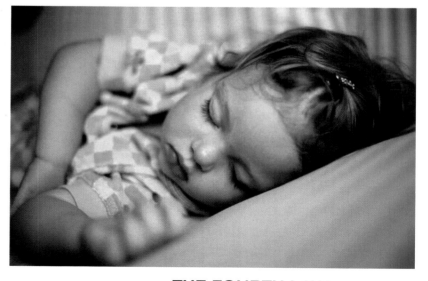

THE FOURTH LAW
ADEQUATE REST TO RESTORE OUR BODIES

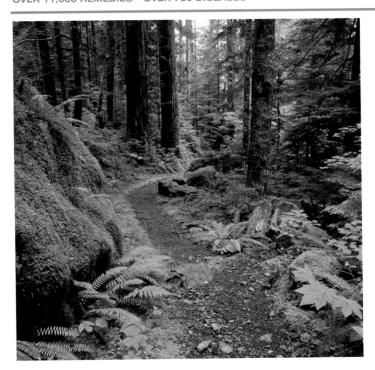

THE FIFTH LAW
EXERCISE, ESPECIALLY OUTDOORS,
TO REBUILD AND STRENGTHEN US

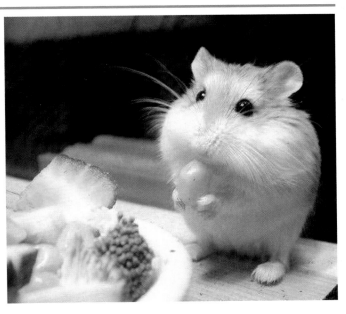

THE SIXTH LAW
THE FOOD GIVEN US BY GOD,
TO MAINTAIN GOOD HEALTH

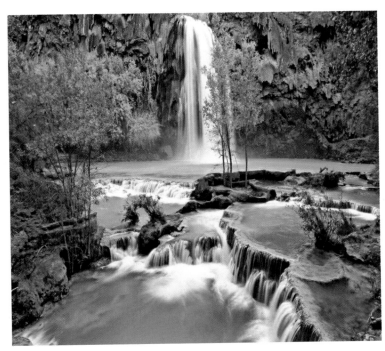

THE SEVENTH LAW
PURE WATER, TO CLEANSE OUR SKIN
AND EVERY CELL IN OUR BODIES

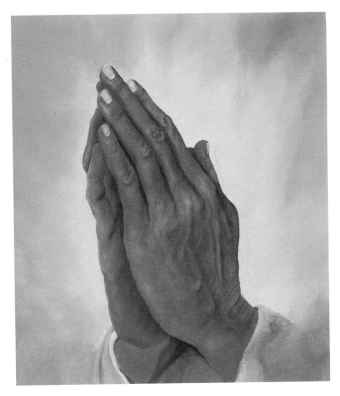

THE EIGHTH LAW
SURRENDERED TRUST AND
OBEDIENCE TO THE GOD OF HEAVEN

The Natural Remedies Encyclopedia

The Eight Laws of Healing

S - Sunlight
t - Temperance
a - Air
r - Rest
t - Trust in God
N - Nutrition
e - Exercise
w - Water

"Pure air, sunlight, abstemiousness, rest, exercise, proper diet, the use of water, trust in divine power,— these are the true remedies."

—*Ministry of Healing, p. 127*

God our Creator has provided, in the simple things of nature, many strengthening and remedial agencies. As we look to Him in faith and use the agencies He has provided for our health, we will have far less suffering and problems.

In this chapter, you will find an overview of these restorative agencies.

The Natural Remedies Encyclopedia

The First Law of Health
The Air You Breathe

The year was 1875; the place, Paris, France. For more than two years, three scientists had worked toward this day; and now they were ready. Carefully, they climbed into the gondola of the balloon, "Zenith," while thousands around them watched.

Determined to set a new altitude record, they wanted to go higher than man had ever risen above the earth. And they did just that,—but at what a cost.

Slowly the large balloon rose into the air, with its human cargo of three men in a basket-shaped gondola swinging just beneath it. All seemed well; they were well on their way toward the goal: to climb higher than any man had ever gone.

Then at 24,430 feet it happened. Tissandier, one of the three, later described it: "Croce is gasping for breath, Sivel is dazed, but can still cut three sandbags loose in order to reach 26,240 feet."

At that point, Tissandier himself was overcome and slumped to the floor, losing consciousness. Some time afterward, as the balloon—freed from the sandbags continued its ascent—he awoke. They had attained a height of 8,600 meters (approximately 28,000 feet)—but two of the scientists lay dead in the gondola of the balloon. Yes, they had conquered the heights, but before it was done the heights had conquered them. There was not enough air, with its precious life-giving oxygen, to sustain life at that great altitude.

Without air, man dies. Air is the most vital element for man and animals. One may live for weeks without food, or for days without water, but deprived of air he will perish within minutes.

Millions of people suffer from a wide variety of ailments that are partly caused by an insufficient supply of oxygen. The problem is that most people do not breathe correctly, and this continually weakens their health, their happiness, and their hold on life itself. One of the finest statements written on the importance of air are these words penned by an outstanding health educator:

"In order to have good blood, we must breathe well. Full, deep inspirations of pure air, which fill the lungs with oxygen, purify the blood. They impart to it a bright color and send it—a life-giving current—to every part of the body.

"A good respiration soothes the nerves; it stimulates the appetite and renders digestion more perfect; and it induces sound, refreshing sleep . . [If] an insufficient supply of oxygen is received, the blood moves sluggishly. The waste, poisonous matter, which should be thrown off in the exhalations from the lungs, is retained, and the blood becomes impure. Not only the lungs, but the stomach, liver, and brain are affected. The skin becomes sallow, digestion is retarded; the heart is depressed; the brain clouded; the thoughts are confused; gloom settles upon the spirits; the whole system becomes depressed and inactive, and peculiarly susceptible to disease."—*Ministry of Healing, pp. 272-273.*

Every cell of your body must receive a constant supply of oxygen—or they will weaken and die. But that air must be fresh in order to help you the most. When you breathe stale or polluted air, the supply of oxygen is insufficient to keep the cells strong and healthy. Apart from oxygen from the air you breathe, they die within a few minutes.

"Air is the free blessing of Heaven, calculated to electrify the whole system. Without it the system will be filled with disease, and become dormant, languid, feeble."—*1 Testimonies, p. 701.*

The life-giving air around us is a most precious blessing from Heaven. On the last day of Creation Week, God created man. Having formed him from the dust of the ground, Adam lay before his Maker inert and lifeless—until he was vitalized by the breath of life. And moment by moment, you and I must have fresh air also.

"Fresh air will prove far more beneficial to sick persons than medicine, and is far more essential to them than their food . . Thousands have died for want of pure water and pure air, who might have lived."—*Counsels on Health, p. 55.*

It is of the highest consequence to your life, health, and happiness, that you keep fresh air in every room in your home, and especially in your sleeping rooms. If you are not able to have your windows open in very cold weather, then leave a door open into another room where a window is open. By day and by night, always keep a current of air flowing through the house. You do not want to sit or sleep in a draft, but some air circulating throughout your home—a lot in the summer, less in the winter—is a necessity to good health.

"The effects produced by living in close, ill-ventilated rooms are these: The system becomes weak and unhealthy, the circulation is depressed, the blood moves sluggishly through the system because it is not purified and vitalized by the pure, invigorating air of heaven. The mind becomes depressed and gloomy, while the whole system is enervated; and fevers and other acute diseases are liable to be generated.

"Your careful exclusion of external air, and fear of free ventilation leaves you to breathe a corrupt, unwholesome air which is exhaled from the lungs of those staying in these rooms, and which is poisonous, unfit for the support of life. The body becomes relaxed; the skin becomes sallow; digestion is retarded, and the system is peculiarly sensitive to the influence of cold. A slight exposure produces serious diseases. Great care should be exercised not to sit in a draft or in a cold room when weary, or when in a perspiration. You should so accustom yourself to the air that you will not be under the necessity of having the mercury higher than sixty-five degrees."—*1 Testimonies, pp. 702-703.*

Fresh air should be inhaled as freely indoors as out-doors in warmer weather. In colder weather, your home will need to be heated. But beware of too much heat, for the burning of the fuel itself takes precious oxygen from the air. If necessary, dress more warmly, so that, as much as possible, you can breathe purer air at all times. Students of body health tell us that it requires an abundance of oxygen in the body and surrounding it in order to keep the physical organism in top condition. Why is this so? It is the oxygen in the air that purifies the blood, contributes to the production of body heat and energy, and conveys electrical energy with which to vitalize every organ and tissue.

H.E. Kirschner, M.D., said this:

"I am also in full agreement with Dr. Philip Welsh, who declares: 'Any form of treatment—any program of health which does not give full and due consideration to the first essential of life—pure air—will absolutely fail to get the best results—yes, this one question of supplying the body with pure air is important enough to determine the difference between health and sickness—between life and death!'

"Contrast this, if you will, with the popular notion that air—especially night air—is harmful to the sick. Many of my colleagues in the medical profession have excluded air from the sick room. This is a great mistake, for air is the food God has provided for the lungs—and your lungs, when deprived of fresh air, will be like a hungry person deprived of food. Therefore, air should not be regarded as an enemy, but as a precious blessing."— *H.E. Kirschner, M.D., Nature's Seven Doctors, p. 18.*

Do you have difficulty in going to sleep at night? Try this simple remedy for sleeplessness; it is a good one: Make sure that there is a current of air coming into the room (best from a window). The room should be comfortable and not chilling, but with some fresh air circulating through it. Now relax, pray as you lie there and give your life anew into the hands of God. Then slowly take several deep breaths, holding each one a moment before exhaling it. Let your mind slow down. Your thoughts are upon God, the peace of being with Him, and the need for deep, full breathing. Very soon you will be sound asleep.

"Those who have not had a free circulation of air in their rooms through the night, generally awake feeling exhausted, feverish, and know not the cause. It was air, vital air, that the whole system required, but which it could not obtain. Upon rising in the morning, most persons would be benefited by taking a sponge-bath, or, if more agreeable, a hand-bath, with merely a wash-bowl of water. This will remove impurities from the skin. Then the clothing should be removed piece by piece from the bed, and exposed to the air. The windows should be opened, and the blinds fastened back, and the air left to circulate freely for several hours, if not all day, through the sleeping apartments. In this manner the bed and clothing will become thoroughly aired, and the impurities will be removed from the room."—*Spiritual Gifts, Vol. 4a, p. 143.*

Actually, this is also a good way to start the morning. When you first awake, take several deep breaths, and then as you arise take several more. Before breakfast, go out-of-doors and look on the things of nature and breathe deeply as you silently thank God for another day of life to work for Him. From time to time, throughout the day, repeat this deep breathing practice. At times, take in very deep breaths of air, in order to expand your lungs. (A method, that this writer uses with excellent results, is to exhale strongly and then allow the fresh new air to enter the lungs in whatever amount and rate the body wishes to take it in; then exhale again, and let more in.)

"Air, air, the precious boon [gift] of Heaven, which all may have, will bless you with its invigorating influence, if you will not refuse it entrance. Welcome it, cultivate a love for it, and it will prove a precious soother of the nerves.

"Air must be in constant circulation to be kept pure. The influence of pure, fresh air is to cause the blood to circulate healthfully through the system. It refreshes the body, and tends to render it strong and healthy, while at the same time its influence is decidedly felt upon the mind, imparting a degree of composure and serenity. It excites the appetite, and renders the digestion of food more perfect, and induces sound and sweet sleep."—*1 Testimonies, p. 702.*

Develop a habit of deep breathing. Shallow breathing is a habit easily developed but harmful in its effects on the entire body. Many people only breathe "at the top of their lungs." Take full, deep inspirations of air. Do not just fill the top of your chest.

Here are some additional suggestions that will help you:

Just after eating, and also before retiring, go outside and take eighteen or twenty deep breaths, using the muscles of the abdomen. Inhale and exhale slowly. Some folk extend the arms above their heads while they do this. Take a walk out-of-doors just before you retire for the night. Breathe that fresh night air, relax your mind, talk to your heavenly Father, and thank Him for His continual care and blessings. Give yourself anew to Him. Then, with contentment of heart, go to sleep, forgetting all your present perplexities. Know and believe that He will work them all out at the right time.

Get outdoors as much as possible. Develop hobbies and avocations that are out in the open air. Especially beware of hobbies and recreation that require being bent over with the chest cramped and the eyes and brain overtaxed.

"A walk, even in the winter, would be more beneficial to health than all the medicine the doctors may prescribe . . There will be increased vitality, which is so necessary to health. The lungs will have needful action, for it is impossible to go out in the bracing air of a winter's morning without inflating the lungs."—*2 Testimonies, p. 529.*

"And while the importance of deep breathing is shown, the practice should be insisted upon. Let exercises be given which will promote this."—*Education, p. 199.*

Colder weather may require additional clothing, but continue to obtain the much needed pure, fresh air.

"In the cool of the evening it may be necessary to guard from chilliness by extra clothing, but they should give their lungs air."—*2 Testimonies, p. 527.*

Keep proper ventilation in mind wherever you may be, whether it be in your home, in the office or shop, at church, etc. Avoid stuffy people who like to sit in stuffy rooms all day talking or watching television. If you are not able to directly help them by word or action, then leave them to their misery and go where there is air.

And beware of tobacco "side stream." Scientific researchers now know that the cigarette smoke in a room can greatly injure adults, and especially children. Only stay with cigarette smokers long enough to help them; then go where you can have a purer atmosphere to breathe.

Do not rent or purchase a home that is in any kind of low concavity. Watch out for homes in hollowed-out places, for they tend to be damp. Research studies by the National Institute of Health in Washington County, Virginia, in the late 1950s and early 1960s, revealed the fact that houses built in such low, miasmic areas frequently had a history of cancer in those who lived in them. This included homes in low places by creeks. Many do not realize the fact that there are continually flowing rivers of air. These currents, flowing into and along narrow valley bottoms, creeks, and rivers, are much more damp than the air found in more elevated places. But living in such damp places induces sickness and disease. If you reside in such a location, you would do well to move somewhere else.

"If we would have our homes the abiding place of health and happiness, we must place them above the miasma and fog of the lowlands."—*Ministry of Healing, p. 275.*

You also do well not to permit too much shrubbery or shading too close to your house. This can keep the purifying air from circulating through the home.

"So far as possible, all buildings intended for human habitation should be placed on high, well-drained ground. This will insure a dry site, and prevent the danger of disease from dampness and miasma. This matter is often too lightly regarded. Continuous ill health, serious diseases, and many deaths result from the dampness . . of low-lying, ill-drained situations.

"In the building of houses it is especially important to secure thorough ventilation and plenty of sunlight. Let there be a current of air and an abundance of light in every room in the house. Sleeping rooms should be so arranged as to have a free circulation of air day and night. No room is fit to be occupied as a sleeping room

unless it can be thrown open daily to the air and sunshine. In most countries bedrooms need to be supplied with conveniences for heating, that they may be thoroughly warmed and dried in cold or wet weather."—*Ministry of Healing, pp. 274-275.*

So we can see that it is very important that we keep our houses properly ventilated. It is the fresh, purifying air inside a home that makes it a healthful place in which to live.

When the day is sunny and warm, take the bedding out, hang it on the clothesline, and air it out. The purifying air and sunlight will do much to sterilize it. Take it back into the house before the dampness of the late afternoon sets in. You will notice that it all smells perfectly fresh.

It is of the utmost importance that every room in the house be open to the sunlight and a current of air throughout the day.

"Some houses are furnished expensively, more to gratify pride, and to receive visitors, than for the comfort, convenience and health of the family. The best rooms are kept dark. The light and air are shut out, lest the light of heaven may injure the rich furniture, fade the carpets, or tarnish the picture frames. When visitors are permitted to be seated in these precious rooms, they are in danger of taking cold, because of the cellar-like atmosphere pervading them. Parlor chambers and bedrooms are kept closed in the same manner and for the same reasons. And whoever occupies these beds which have not been freely exposed to the light and air, do so at the expense of health, and often even of life itself."—*2 Selected Messages, p. 462.*

On pages 16-17 of his book, *"Nature's Seven Doctors,"* Dr. H.E. Kirschner explains that the most successful cure for tuberculosis of the lungs requires an unusually large amount of fresh air for the patients, day and night. "Sleeping porches were provided for all patients and . . they were allowed indoors only for meals and other duties . . This required warm sleeping garments and usually a stocking cap." He explains that a similar program was successfully followed for typhoid.

Of course, such a strenuous cold-air regime would not work for many physical ailments, such as pneumonia. In every sickness, provide the patient with fresh air, but in most cases it should be fresh, warm air.

The healing of wounds takes place more quickly in the presence of fresh air and sunlight. (But there are times when dirt may get into a wound if it is not covered, as when a workman has a cut on his finger.)

"It is a well-known fact that wounds exposed to sunshine and fresh air heal more rapidly than when bandaged. In fact, no wound will heal without air. In order, then, for wounds to heal quickly, it is most important that they be exposed to a constant supply of pure, fresh air."—*Kirschner, p. 23.*

Do all you can to avoid poisonous gases in or near your home. This would include the use of unvented gas heaters, leaks from sewer gases, tobacco fumes, and agricultural sprays, such as defoliants, insecticides, mosquito spraying programs, and similar poisonous fumes and vapors.

Specially treated woods are now being used in new house construction. They are supposed to resist insect attack for decades. But poisonous gases were applied to them; and it has been established that fumes from that wood escape into the house and surrounding air for several years after installation.

Another source of danger is the use of new plastic hard-form insulation panels into walls during house construction or remodeling. Although true that these panels provide better R-factor insulation at a lower price, the fact remains that if the house ever catches on fire,—poisonous fumes from those panels will fill the home!

We live in a chemical age, and the air, water, vegetation, earth, and animal kingdom are being slowly poisoned to death.

In my files I have a clipping that I cut out of a newspaper in July, 1958:

BREATHING HELPS STOP THAT PAIN

It's not the pain-killing properties of aspirin which make it so beneficial for arthritic patients.

"Instead, it's the huffing and puffing produced by large doses of aspirin which really control the aches, pain and stiffness.

"This was suggested here yesterday by Drs. Frederick Kahn, Daniel Simmons, and Howard Weinberger of UCLA and the Los Angeles VA hospitals.

"Physicians have long known, they said, that normal doses of aspirin won't help arthritis patients. It takes dosages of about 15 tablets a day to control arthritic pains.

"But at these doses, they said, aspirin produces what is called "hyper-ventilation"—the patient constantly breathes deeply and rapidly, often while he's at rest. In turn, this hyper-ventilation lowers the amount of carbon dioxide in the blood.

"To check their suspicions, the Los Angeles doctors put victims of arthritis in an iron lung and made them over-breathe without any aspirin.

"The relief of pain and other symptoms, they found, was just as effective as that achieved with aspirin."— *Newsclip, July, 1958.*

The above is valuable information that you and I can use every day of our lives. Deep breathing reduces pain and relaxes the entire system. (But our suggestion is that you not use an aspirin-type product to help you do that breathing: There is a poisonous chemical in "headache pills" which causes the stomach to bleed internally each time it is taken, whether in tablet or powder form.)

It is now known that fallen leaves emit carbon monoxide fumes.

"Shade trees and shrubbery too close and dense around a house are unhealthful; for they prevent a free circulation of air, and shut out the rays of the sun. In consequence of this, dampness gathers in the house. Especially in wet seasons the sleeping rooms become damp, and those who occupy them are troubled with rheumatism, neuralgia, and lung complaints which generally end in consumption. Numerous shade trees cast off many leaves, which, if not immediately removed, decay, and poison the atmosphere. A yard beautified with trees and shrubbery, at a proper distance from the house has a happy, cheerful influence upon the family, and, if well taken care of, will prove no injury to health. Dwellings, if possible, should be built upon high and dry

ground. If a house is built where water settles around it, remaining for a time, then drying away, a poisonous miasma arises, and fever and ague, sore throat, lung diseases, and fevers will be the result."—*Counsels on Health, 1951, pp. 58-59.*

The smog that envelopes homes and offices in and near the large cities is now known to be quite harmful in its effects. During morning and evening rush hours, when so much traffic is on the streets, smog will even be found in smaller cities and towns. A major source of the smog is automobile exhaust fumes, which contain two deadly chemicals: vaporized lead and sulfuric acid. Lead fumes, inhaled into the body, cause the destruction of red blood cells. Sulfuric acid is such a powerful toxic agent that it is the primary reason that stone cathedrals and buildings are crumbling throughout Europe.

What is the solution? Move to the country, and not too close to a large city.

A lack of fresh air is a significant factor in causing people to become ill. Yet how few realize this fact.

"Many labor under the mistaken idea that if they have taken cold, they must carefully exclude the outside air, and increase the temperature of their room until it is excessively hot. The system may be deranged, the pores closed by waste matter, and the internal organs suffering more or less inflammation, because the blood has been chilled back from the surface and thrown upon them. At this time, of all others, the lungs should not be deprived of pure, fresh air. If pure air is ever necessary, it is when any part of the system, as the lungs or stomach, is diseased."—*2 Testimonies, p. 530.*

"Many families suffer with sore throat, lung diseases, and liver complaints, brought upon them by their own course of action. Their sleeping-rooms are small, unfit to sleep in for one night, but they occupy the small apartments for weeks, and months, and years . . They breathe the same air over and over, until it becomes impregnated with the poisonous impurities and waste matter thrown off from their bodies through the lungs and the pores of the skin . . Those who thus abuse their health must suffer with disease."—*Healthful Living, p. 173.*

"The health of the entire system depends upon the healthy action of the respiratory organs."—*2 Selected Messages, p. 473.*

"In order to have good blood, we must breathe well."—*Healthful Living, p. 171.*

Since a lack of fresh air can cause sickness, how very important it is that fresh air be supplied to the ill so that they can become well.

"Fresh air will prove far more beneficial to sick persons than medicine, and is far more essential to them than their food."—*Counsels on Health, p. 55.*

"The sick room, if possible, should have a draft of air through it day and night. The draft should not come directly upon the invalid. While burning fevers are raging, there is but little danger of taking cold . . The sick must have pure, invigorating air. If no other way can be devised, the sick, if possible, should be removed to another room, and another bed, while the sick room, the bed and bedding are being purified by ventilation."—*Counsels on Health, pp. 56-57.*

"Every breath of vital air in the sick-room is of the greatest value, although many of the sick are very ignorant on this point. They feel much depressed, and do not know what the matter is. A draught of pure air through their room would have a happy, invigorating influence upon them."—*Healthful Living, p. 72.*

Those who are aged, infirm, or invalid also have a very definite need of fresh, pure air to breathe.

"Those who have the aged to provide for should remember that these especially need warm, comfortable rooms. Vigor declines as years advance, leaving less vitality with which to resist unhealthful influences; hence the greater necessity for the aged to have plenty of sunlight, and fresh, pure air."—*Ministry of Healing, p. 275.*

"The sick need to be brought into close touch with nature. An outdoor life amid natural surroundings would work wonders for many a helpless and almost hopeless invalid."—*Ministry of Healing, p. 262.*

"How grateful to the invalids weary of city life, the glare of many lights, and the noise of the streets, are the quiet and freedom of the country! How eagerly do they turn to the scenes of nature! How glad would they be to sit in the open air, rejoice in the sunshine, and breathe the fragrance of tree and flower! There are life-giving properties in the balsam of the pine, in the fragrance of the cedar and the fir, and other trees also have properties that are health-restoring."—*Ministry of Healing, p. 264.*

"For invalids who have feeble lungs, nothing can be worse than an overheated atmosphere."—*2 Testimonies, p. 527.*

"The heated, oppressed atmosphere, deprived of vitality, benumbs the sensitive brain. The lungs contract, the liver is inactive."—*1 Testimonies, p. 702.*

It is frequently necessary, especially in cold weather, to warm the air in the home or office. But we must be careful to do this in moderation, since oxygen from the room is generally consumed in providing the heat (with a few exceptions, such as steam heat sent through pipes from a more distant heat ignition source).

"Stove heat destroys the vitality of the air and weakens the lungs."—*Place of Herbs, p. 21.*

How important it is that we ourselves—and our children also—study and work in rooms with adequate ventilation to the fresh outside air.

"Many young children have passed five hours each day in schoolrooms not properly ventilated, nor sufficiently large for the healthful accommodation of the scholars. The air of such rooms soon becomes poison to the lungs that inhale it."—*3 Testimonies, p. 135.*

"The lungs, in order to be healthy, must have pure air."—*Healthful Living, p. 171.*

"The strength of the system is, in a great degree, dependent upon the amount of pure, fresh air breathed. If the lungs are restricted, the quantity of oxygen received into them is also limited, the blood becomes vitiated, and disease follows."—*Healthful Living, p. 176.*

Buildings should be constructed in such a manner that there is always enough fresh air and sunlight entering them.

"In the construction of buildings, whether for public purposes or as dwellings, care should be taken to provide good ventilation and plenty of sunlight. Churches and schoolrooms are often faulty in this respect. Neglect of proper ventilation is responsible for much of the drowsiness and dullness that destroy the effect of many a sermon and make the teacher's work toilsome and ineffective."—*Ministry of Healing, p. 274.*

Yes, fresh air is important to our health—for it is one of the simple remedies of nature, given by God to His people.

"There are many ways of practicing the healing art; but there is only one way that Heaven approves. God's remedies are the simple agencies of nature, that will not tax or debilitate the system through their powerful properties. Pure air and water, cleanliness, a proper diet, purity of life, and a firm trust in God, are remedies for the want of which thousands are dying; yet these remedies are going out of date because their skillful use requires work that the people do not appreciate. Fresh air, exercise, pure water, and clean, sweet premises, are within the reach of all with but little expense; but drugs are expensive, both in the outlay of means, and the effect produced upon the system."—*Counsels on Health, 1951, p. 323.*

SPIRITUAL LESSONS

God asks us to come to Him that we might breathe the air of heaven. The plan of redemption was designed to give us forgiveness of sin, as well as empowerment to resist temptation and obey the commandments of God. It was given to redeem us so we might live with God and the holy angels forever.

Jesus said that He came "not to call the righteous, but sinners to repentance" (Luke 5:32). Only he who acknowledges himself to be a sinner before God can receive pardon and acceptance. The inquiry bursts from the heart: "Men and brethren, what shall we do? . . What must I do to be saved?" (Acts 2:37; 16:30). "The sorrow of the world worketh death," but "godly sorrow worketh repentance to salvation" (2 Corinthians 7:10).

The cry of the soul is, "I will declare mine iniquity; I will be sorry for my sin" (Psalm 38:18). In heartfelt anguish for what he has done against God, he comes to Christ.

"When a man or woman shall commit any sin that men commit, to do a trespass against the Lord, and that person be guilty; then they shall confess their sin which they have done" (Numbers 5:6-7).

How thankful we can be that Jesus forgives the humble repentant sinner. "For Thou, Lord, art good, and ready to forgive; and plenteous in mercy unto all them that call upon Thee" (Psalm 86:5). "If we confess our sins, He is faithful and just to forgive us our sins, and to cleanse us from all unrighteousness" (1 John 1:9).

Thank God that "as the heaven is high above the earth, so great is His mercy toward them that fear Him" (Psalm 103:11). "Let the wicked forsake his way, and the unrighteous man his thoughts: and let him return unto the Lord, and He will have mercy upon him; and to our God, for He will abundantly pardon" (Isaiah 55:7).

Oh, my friend, as we return to the Lord, He is so very happy to receive and accept us! "When he [the prodigal son, returning from years of sin] was yet a great way off, his father saw him, and had compassion, and ran, and fell on his neck, and kissed him" (Luke 15:20) "Who is a God like unto Thee, that pardoneth iniquity, and passeth by the transgression of the remnant of His heritage? He retaineth not His anger for ever, because He delighten in mercy" (Micah 7:18). "Likewise, I say unto you, there is joy in the presence of the angels of God over one sinner that repenteth" (Luke 15:10).

Accepting Christ as his Saviour, the soul experiences the new birth. "Therefore if any man is in Christ, he is a new creature: old things are passed away; behold, all things are become new" (2 Corinthians 5:17).

"Thou hast in love to my soul delivered it from the pit of corruption: for Thou hast cast all my sins behind Thy back" (Isaiah 38:17). "Thou wilt cast all their sins into the depths of the sea" (Micah 7:19).

There is a great blessing for those willing to seek the Lord and forsake their sins. "Blessed is he whose transgression is forgiven, whose sin is covered. Blessed is the man unto whom the Lord imputeth not iniquity, and in whose spirit there is no guile" (Psalm 32:1-2).

This experience is for you and me today! The call of Jesus is clear, and the message is cheering. There is hope for the lowliest. Coming to Christ, we give Him our sins and dedicate our lives to His service. All that He asks of us in His Word, we are now willing to do.

Is this an experience that you want right now? I know it is. Open the doors of your heart and let the fresh air of God's salvation into your heart. It is refreshing and wonderful. It means eternal life.

"Blessed are they that do His commandments, that they may have right to the tree of life, and may enter in through the gates into the city."—Revelation 22:14.

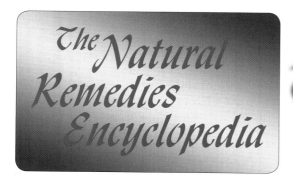

The Natural Remedies Encyclopedia

The Second Law of Health
The Sunlight on Your Body

A miracle factory is at work just beneath your skin. And when the ultraviolet rays of the sun touch the skin, the factory sets to work.

It is a most marvelous system; and, without it, you could not remain alive an hour.

There are millions of red corpuscles constantly flowing through very small blood vessels throughout every part of the 3,000 square inches of your skin. And there are also tiny oil glands just beneath the skin which biochemists call sterols. As sunshine strikes them, substances within them, called ergosterols, are irradiated and transformed into vitamin D. Carried to all parts of your body, it enables you to have strong bones, teeth, and nails.

But we are getting ahead of our story—the fascinating story of what one of God's special gifts, sunlight, can do for you.

Every living thing in our world is dependent upon the sun. Without sunshine, nothing could live. Sunlight is composed of energy wavelengths of various types. We will here focus our attention on the visible rays, along with the infrared and ultraviolet rays. In this brief report—you will learn part of this miracle of what sunlight can do for you,—and how it can bring you better health and even a happier outlook on life.

In 1877, two researchers, Downes and Blunt, discovered that sunlight can destroy harmful bacteria. Today, it is used to treat bacterial infections. Sunlight on the body dramatically lowers high blood pressure, decreases blood cholesterol, lowers excessively high blood sugars, and increases white blood cells.

Adequate sunlight on your body will lower your respiratory rate and will cause your breathing to be slower, deeper, and even easier. Your resting heart rate will decrease, and after exercise it will return to normal much more quickly. Sunlight increases the capacity of the blood to carry more oxygen and take it to your body tissues. Even a single exposure to the ultraviolet light in sunlight will greatly increase the oxygen content of your blood. And this effect will continue for several days. Bronchial asthma patients who could hardly breathe, were able to inhale freely after a sunbath.

It is of interest that many of these beneficial effects of sunlight are heightened if a person combines sunbathing with a regular program of physical exercise. For example, fatigue and exhaustion tend to be lessened and the capacity for work is increased. It is now known that part of this is due to an increase in glycogen content of the blood and muscles following sunlight and exercise.

The strength of the heart is steadied and deepened. The pulse rate is lowered because the heart muscle is pumping more blood at each beat. This enables your heart to rest more between beats. And yet the blood output is increased by an average of 39% for several days after a sunbath. Many people worry about their blood pressure; yet regularly taking sunlight on the body lowers it. Sunbaths alone will lower blood pressure by an average of 8%.

Combined with exercise, it is lowered 15%.

And there are those that worry about their blood sugar because they are diabetic. It has been discovered that exposure to sunshine has an insulin-like effect on the body—it lowers the blood sugar. And it does it in exactly the right proportion. Those who have no diabetic problem experience almost no change in blood sugar while diabetics have a striking lowering of it. It is now known that this lowering is caused by the fact that sunlight on the body causes glycogen (stored sugar) to be increased throughout the body, enabling the blood sugar to be lowered. Higher storage levels of glycogen result in more body energy for longer stretches of physical activity, with more endurance and less fatigue. (Warning: A diabetic taking sunbaths should try reducing his insulin intake, lest he inject too much.)

And then there is stress. We all encounter tensions and problems throughout the day. Sunlight can help you more easily glide through the day. A deepened sense of well-being results and better sleep comes at night. You feel better and live better. Because you are more relaxed, the crises of life are met with less difficulty. Sunlight on the body both calms the nerves and increases adrenalin. This relaxation is not merely mental; it is physical also. Both gastric and duodenal ulcer patients have been found to improve under the beneficial effects of sunshine.

The wealth of new scientific insights on the restorative power of sunlight continues to unfold. Sunlight lowers blood cholesterol; an excess of blood cholesterol is one of the problems leading to heart and artery disease. The basic fact underlying this truth goes back to the year 1904, when it was discovered that sunlight changes the cholesterol just under the skin into vitamin D. Because there is so much cholesterol just under the skin, when it is changed by sunlight into vitamin D, cholesterol from the blood is sent to take its place, thus lowering the cholesterol in the blood. Researchers now know that when cholesterol is removed from the blood—cholesterol stored within the plaques deposited on the artery walls takes its place. The result is a beneficial reduction of the dangerous deposits that accompany hardening of the arteries and lead to strokes. Two hours after a sunbath, an average of 13% reduction in human blood cholesterol occurs.

Research carried out in 1970 in Russia disclosed that sunbaths help people with hardening of the arteries of the brain. Their improved mental performance and memory indicates that those harmful blood vessel deposits were lessened by the exposure to sunlight.

Incidentally, one insight that came out of this and other Russian research was the fact that patients were helped more by frequent short exposures to sunlight than by infrequent longer sunbaths. Proof of this was shown in the electrocardiograms: almost twice as good in those receiving shorter, more frequent sunshine on their bodies.

Dramatic evidence of the importance of sunlight on the body is to be found in the fact that dark-skinned races suffer more from certain diseases than light-skinned races. Of all the races, the Negro race is the most susceptible to rickets. The solution is vitamin D, but in order to manufacture it in the body, blacks must have their bodies in the sunlight more than the light-skinned races.

Because blacks require more sunlight on their bodies for good health than whites, blacks tend to have more jaundice, higher blood pressure, tuberculosis, and diabetes.

In our book, "The Water Therapy Manual" (Part Two of "Better Living for Your Home"), we include a section on sunbathing as a healing principle in the treatment of tuberculosis. Tuberculosis of the skin, bone, and lung are all helped by sunbathing.

Streptococcal infections have been found to be reduced when sunlight regularly reaches the skin. In 1929, Dr. Ude introduced sunbathing into America for the treatment of erysipelas (a streptococcal infection of the skin). In 1938, penicillin was discovered and many researchers turned their eyes from sunlight to the wonder drugs. But the many dangerous side effects of these medicinal drugs are less likely to be found in taking a sunbath.

Fungus infections of the feet and toes are especially helped by sunlight. So many different bacteria and viruses exist that it is neither wise nor safe to attempt vaccination against them all. But sunlight on the body is part of the best solution to many of these problems.

Infectious diseases include many physical problems ranging from the common cold to flu,—and even the dangerous spinal meningitis.

How very important it is that we make sure that we frequently obtain the vital sunlight that our bodies so much need in order to maintain good health.

Some people believe that all of the problems of mankind are due to germs, and others think that germs are no problem at all—as long as one lives properly and eats healthfully. We well agree that right living is the most important of all, but germs in the water and air around us are not always harmless.

In 1935, Daryl Hart noted the frequency with which infections developed in people who had just had operations. He wondered whether air-borne germs might have contaminated them while the operation was in progress. He placed petri dishes in an operating room for an hour during an operation, and found 78 colonies of staphylococcus on one place alone. Was there a way that those germs in the air could have been killed? Dr. Hart placed ultraviolet lights overhead—and discovered that all the germs—including very dangerous ones—were killed within ten minutes, if they were within eight feet of those lamps. And this happened even when the lights were so low in intensity that it required eighty minutes for blond skin to be reddened. A similar experiment was done in a naval training center, in which very low-intensity ultraviolet lights were installed in the barracks. The result was a 25% reduction in respiratory infections among the recruits using those sleeping quarters.

(Please, do not set up sunlamps in your bedroom! They are far too high in intensity, and your eyes will be damaged. Instead, draw back the curtains—and let the sunlight in. For it has been scientifically established that sunlight reduces the danger of open air transmission of disease. Sunlamps must be used with greatest care and for only a few seconds at a time.)

Water purification is now being taken to the sunlight. Chlorination kills many water-borne diseases, but the chlorine has certain carcinogenic (cancer-causing) effects. Researchers are now turning to irradiation with ultraviolet light.

52 **THE EIGHT LAWS** THE SUNLIGHT ON YOUR BODY NATURAL REMEDIES ENCYCLOPEDIA
OVER 11,000 REMEDIES - OVER 730 DISEASES

L
A
W
S

The four most dangerous water-borne bacterial infections are cholera, typhoid, bacillary dysentery, and hepatitis. It has been demonstrated that sunlight can kill such bacteria to some depth, if the flow of water is slow enough so that the ultraviolet radiations can effectively reach them.

What about germs on the skin? Exposure to sunlight increases the skin's resistance to disease. It does this by directly killing the bacteria on the skin. The shorter ultraviolet wave lengths are the most bactericidal, and do not particularly penetrate beneath the skin. But the longer wavelengths also kill germs, though to a lesser extent, and they penetrate more deeply.

Sunlight not only directly kills bacteria on the skin,—but it changes natural body oils on the skin into bactericidal agents! Even the vapors rising from these irradiated natural skin oils are able to kill bacteria.

Psoriasis and acne are two common skin diseases. Both are being treated with sunlight. Sunlight keeps psoriasis under control, and the purifying power of these rays helps to sterilize acne, and bring to it more rapid healing.

Sunlight also strengthens the body's immune system. This is partly due to the fact that sunlight striking the body increases the number of white blood cells in the body. These are the fighter cells that resist infection by gobbling it up wherever found in the body. There is one particular white blood cell that is the most powerful germ killer of them all: the lymphocyte. Science has now come to the startling conclusion that sunlight increases the number of lymphocytes—more than any other kind of white blood cell.

Antibody production, so important to a successful resistance to infection, is also greatly increased after sunbathing. This is due to the fact that it is primarily the lymphocytes that produce the antibodies, such as the very important gamma globulins. In laboratory animals, this antibody increase can last for two or three weeks.

Neutrophils, fairly common white blood cells, are very important. They spend their life within your body eating up bacteria, fungus, and other harmful invaders. After being exposed to the sun, the neutrophils are, in some unknown way, stimulated to chew up harmful bacteria even more rapidly. Research experiments have disclosed that this increase in gobbling action is doubled after a sunbath.

Did you ever notice that people are more likely during the winter months to contract colds, during spells of lessened sunlight?

An interesting study related to this fact is that of the early polar explorers. After spending months in those icy areas with so little sunlight, they would always develop upper respiratory infections upon returning home. The lack of sunlight for eight months had weakened their immune systems, and their antibodies and white blood cells were markedly decreased.

And, of course, sunlight also affects your bones.

In children without adequate sunlight, the vitamin D needed to calcify the bones is not present in proper amounts for the body to lay down calcium in the bones—and they bend more easily. In adults, when there is not enough vitamin D in the body, the calcium leaves the bones and they become softer.

In one research study, over 800 children were studied; and it was noted that they had more dental cavities during the winter and spring months than during the summer months. The lessened sunlight in the winter would be a factor here. However, it should also be noted that those children probably also had less fresh greens, vegetables, and fruit during the winter months. This would also affect their vitamin C and calcium intake—both important to good bones and teeth.

Newborn and young children in areas of the world with less sunlight have a tendency to develop jaundice. It was a nurse in England that first discovered that sunlight could eliminate the problem. Two blood samples taken of the same infant, one shortly after the other—brought the whole matter to the attention of medical science. The sunlight bath given by the nurse, Mrs. Ward, to that infant dramatically changed its condition.

Further study into this revealed that sunlight through glass could partially but not as effectively help the infants with jaundice.

Jaundice in adults can be caused by a number of different factors; sunlight seems to help in every case.

But of all light available, there is none as healthful to the human body as full-spectrum sunlight taken out-of-doors.

It was centuries ago that the beneficial value of sunlight in the treatment of arthritis was first observed. Many examples of this could be cited, but the moral of the story is this: If you have arthritis, take sunbaths.

Gout is also helped by sunlight. It is thought that the ultraviolet rays increase uric acid excretion.

Sunlight helps heal wounds. Under its influence, they heal better and more rapidly. Part of the reason for this is the greater blood supply to the wounded body area when sunlight has fallen on it. Another reason is the purifying effects of the sun's rays. But there are other factors involved of which we are not yet certain.

Sunlight, which can help heal wounds, can also aid in the treatment of sores and surface ulcers. Older folk can develop such problems due to an inadequate blood circulation. But sunlight increases the circulation.

An unusual new development in sunlight research involves that of poisonous chemicals. Sunbathing helps destroy many of them, such as lead, mercury, cobalt, manganese, cadmium, fluoride, benzene, pesticides, and even aids in the elimination of quartz and coal dust.

For example, lead was removed twice as fast from the bodies of animals receiving adequate doses of sunlight. The principle here is that the ultraviolet light in sunlight apparently increases the number of enzymes that eliminate toxic chemicals by metabolizing them. Russians give sunlight therapy daily to miners to help remove coal, quartz, and other rock dusts from their lungs.

Yet, oddly enough, while toxic levels of heavy metal and rock particles are removed by sunlight—the amount of valuable trace minerals in the blood are increased.

One unusual fact that turned up in the course of sunlight research was the insight that experimental animals receiving sunlight treatments undergo some weight loss. It is thought that this is related to increased thyroid production, which sunlight is known to do. Basal body metabolism is thus increased and more calories are burned up.

Sunlight striking the skin also increases muscle tone; and this in turn would use up more calories. Sunlight even helps childbirth. Dr. Robert Bradley, an obstetrician of many years experience, has discovered that women who obtained extra sun over all their body in the months before delivery were less likely to tear at childbirth. He found their skin to be more flexible and less brittle at the time of delivery.

The University of Illinois did research on students, and found that the ones who received regular sunbaths showed greater interest in their classes, attended more regularly, and were more alert. F.A. Kummerow found that sunlight treatments favorably affect the mind and help balance the stimulating and depressing nerve impulses. Try sunbathing yourself—and notice how you will gain a feeling of general well-being and a more cheerful outlook on life.

For the healthiest home, let the light in. Push the curtains back so the sunshine can pour in. Yes, it may fade the rug, but the benefits are far greater than the losses. Sunlight purifies the air in the room. Normal air exchange will carry that air to the north rooms of the house and help purify them. Did you know that patients in hospitals tend to recover more quickly when they are in southern exposure rooms, and less quickly when they are in rooms located on the north side? Let the sunlight into your home, as much as possible, and open the doors between the different rooms, so that its quiet, healing influence may permeate your home.

Rooms can be partially purified by skylight (sunlight reflected from the sky) coming in through the windows. See our book, *"Prophet of the End,* pages 69-70, for more information on this.

HOW TO OBTAIN
THE NEEDED SUNLIGHT

Not too much and often as possible is the best formula. Dr. Zane Kime, whose book, *Sunlight,* is a classic in the field, wrote this:

"If too much sunlight is received, it can have a drying effect, and one may occasionally have flaking, dry skin. Exposure to the sun should be progressive, beginning with only a few minutes a day . . If the tissues of the skin are saturated with the necessary vitamins, the sun will not age the skin, but enhance its beauty."—*Sunlight, p. 89.*

If you would like an abundance of scientific background information on the therapeutic value of sunshine, obtain a copy of Dr. Kime's book, *Sunlight.*

On page 267 of that book, you will find a listing of many of the human diseases that sunlight can help alleviate.

Here is another important quotation from Dr. Kime's book:

"Nutrition and sunlight are intimately related. By striking the skin, sunlight can produce certain hormones and nutrients like vitamin D. Unless one has a proper diet, sunlight has an ill effect on the skin. This must be emphasized: Sunbathing is dangerous for those who are on the standard high-fat American diet or do not get an abundance of vegetables, whole grains, and fresh fruits. Those on the standard high-fat diet should stay out of the sun and protect themselves from it; but, at the same time, they will suffer the consequences of both the high-fat diet and the deficiency of sunlight."—*Zane Kime, Sunlight, p. 117.*

The problem here is skin cancer. (1) If you are not eating a healthful diet, and (2) if you are getting too much sunlight on your skin,—your chances of developing skin cancer are greater.

Fortunately, of all the malignancies that plague mankind, skin cancer is the easiest to detect and the easiest to remove. In relation to its frequency of occurrence, there are fewer deaths from skin cancer than from any other type of carcinoma.

But, in view of the advantages—and dangers—of sunbathing,—what is the best way to obtain it? How long should we sunbathe, and how often? Here are some suggestions:

Some people are more sensitive to sunlight than others. They burn more quickly. Such individuals should take less sunlight to start with and never obtain very much at a time. Others can take more. Dark-skinned people will need to spend more time in the sun in order to obtain enough. The higher in the sky the sun is, the stronger its rays. In the winter months, you will want to sunbathe near noontime, since the sun is lower in the winter skies. In the summer, there is a wider range of hours to select from. Keep in mind that the higher the sun is in the sky, the more ultraviolet rays it sends to your body. And those are the rays that purify; they are also the rays that can bring sunburn. Also keep in mind your latitude. The farther north you live, the lower in the sky the sun will be at noon. People sunburn more quickly at the beach than at home. This is due to the fact that light rays reflect back from the water. (Snow reflects 85% of the ultraviolet; dry sand 17%, water 3-5%, and grass 2.5%.) Wet skin burns more rapidly than dry skin.

Many of the drugs, cosmetics and soaps that people use tend to sensitize the skin so that burning can occur more easily. Another problem is the suntan lotions. These frequently tend to block out the sun's rays, and this you do not want.

Sunbathe under the sun—without any glass or plastic between. Be in the sun regularly; best at about the same time of the day you were last in it. Carefully time yourself. This writer uses a stopwatch and begins at two minutes to a side, and finds that he does best not to later go beyond eight minutes per side. Have it settled in your mind that you want a balanced and regular program of sunbathing, not just a suntan. As we said earlier: You want frequent sunlight on your body, but not too much at a time. This is an ideal that you may not always be able to achieve. But such a program, combined with a good diet, will give you the healing sunlight you need, with little likelihood of skin cancer.

On the first day, start with no more than two minutes to a side, and later lengthen it. Do it every day, every other day, or as often as you are able. Beware: Sunlight is relaxing; do not fall asleep during a sunbath.

If you are able to do so, build an inexpensive solarium where you can take sunbaths in privacy. In this way, each sunbath will bring the healing, purifying, strengthening rays to a larger part of your body than would otherwise be possible.

Carotene and vitamin A in the diet, along with fresh fruits and vegetables, while carefully avoiding free fats (grease, oil, etc.)—will help protect you from the negative effects of sunlight.

Should you use artificial sunlamps? Only if there is absolutely no way you can get out into the sunlight itself.

Never buy or use a sunlamp that produces ultraviolet rays with frequencies below 290 nm. (Only a few firms manufacture sunlamps with safe radiation frequencies—above 290 nm.)

If you use sunlamps, always wear protective glasses to shield your eyes, and work quickly, rotating before the bulb. Sunlamps are dangerous—be careful!

It is possible to purchase ultraviolet window panes—that will let in the ultraviolet from the sun. Apparently, this new development is useful. Overcast skies only filter out about 20% of the ultraviolet rays, so such windows could enable you to take a sunbath in a blizzard.

Sunlight is one of the great blessings given by God to you. Let it help you and your loved ones every day, and thank Him daily for such a wonderful gift.

ADDITIONAL PRINCIPLES

"Shade-trees and shrubbery too close and dense around a house are unhealthy; for they prevent a free circulation of air, and prevent the rays of the sun from shining through sufficiently. In consequence of this a dampness gathers in the house. Especially in wet seasons the sleeping-rooms become damp, and those who sleep in the beds are troubled with rheumatism, neuralgia, and lung complaints, which generally end in consumption. Numerous shade trees cast off many leaves, which, if not immediately removed, decay, and poison the atmosphere. A yard, beautiful with scattering trees and some shrubbery at a proper distance from the house, has a happy, cheerful influence upon the family, and if well taken care of, will prove no injury to health."—*How to Live,* p. 64.

"Rooms that are not exposed to light and air become damp. Beds and bedding gather dampness, and the atmosphere in these rooms is poisonous, because it has not been purified by light and air. Various diseases have been brought on by sleeping in these fashionable, health-destroying apartments . . Sleeping rooms, especially, should be well ventilated, and the atmosphere made healthful by light and air. Blinds should be left open several hours each day, the curtains put aside, and the room thoroughly aired. Nothing should remain, even for a short time, which would destroy the purity of the atmosphere."—*How to Live,* pp. 62-63.

"Life in the open air is good for body and mind. It is God's medicine for the restoration of health. Pure air, good water, sunshine, the beautiful surroundings of nature—these are His means for restoring the sick to health in natural ways. To the sick it is worth more than silver or gold to lie in the sunshine or in the shade of the trees."—*7 Testimonies,* p. 85.

"The guest-chamber should have equal care with the rooms intended for constant use. Like the other bedrooms, it should have air and sunshine, and should be provided with some means of heating to dry out the dampness that always accumulates in a room not in constant use. Whoever sleeps in a sunless room, or occupies a bed that has not been thoroughly dried and aired, does so a the risk of health, and often life."—*Ministry of Healing,* p. 275.

"If those who are well need the blessing of light and air, and need to observe habits of cleanliness in order to remain well, the sick are in still greater need of them in proportion to their debilitated condition."—*How to Live,* p. 60.

"If you would have your homes sweet and inviting, make them bright with air and sunshine. Remove your heavy curtains, open the windows, throw back the blinds, and enjoy the rich sunlight, even if it be at the expense of the colors of your carpets."—*2 Testimonies,* p. 527.

"If the windows were freed from blinds and heavy curtains, and the air and sun permitted to enter freely the darkened rooms, there would be seen a change for the better in the mental and physical health of the children. The pure air would have an invigorating influence upon them, and the sun that carries healing in its beams would soothe and cheer, and make them happy, joyous, and healthy."—*Healthful Living,* p. 229.

"Exercise, and a free use of the air and sunlight . . would give life and strength to many an emaciated invalid."—*Our High Calling,* p. 223.

SPIRITUAL LESSONS

God wants His people to be like the sunshine. They are to be the light of the world. They are to rejoice in His salvation, and share the glorious news of deliverance with everyone they meet.

It is daily consecration which begins this experience. Jesus is calling upon us to make this daily, renewed dedication to Him. "I beseech you therefore, brethren, by the mercies of God, that ye present your bodies a living sacrifice, holy, acceptable unto God, which is your reasonable service" (Romans 12:1).

Each new dedication, lived out in the daily life, makes us more like our Master—the One whom we are trying to be like. "Let this mind be in you, which was also in Christ Jesus" (Philippians 2:5), for He "made Himself of no reputation, and took upon Him the form of a servant" (Philippians 2:7).

The closer we come to Jesus, the more we can understand His character of love, gentleness, and helpfulness. "Take My yoke upon you, and learn of Me; for I am meek and lowly in heart: and ye shall find rest unto your souls" (Matthew 11:29).

It is unselfish ministry to others that makes the difference between the Christian and the worldling. "And whosoever will be chief among you, let him be your servant: even as the Son of man came not to be ministered unto, but to minister, and to give His life a ransom for many." (Matthew 20:27-28). Jesus said, "I am among you as he that serveth" (Luke 22:27).

Sunshine in the life of the Christian means to love God and live to help and bless others. It also means to praise God with all the heart and soul. "By Him therefore let us offer the sacrifice of praise to God continually, that is, the first fruit of our lips giving thanks to His name" (Hebrews 13:15).

Sunshine never stops, but the clouds sometimes keep us from seeing it. Let our praise to the Lord be continual also. "I will bless the Lord at all times: His praise shall continually be in my mouth" (Psalm 34:1). "Every day will I bless Thee; and I will praise Thy name for ever and ever" (Psalm 145:2).

"In every thing give thanks; for this is the will of God in Christ Jesus concerning you" (1 Thessalonians 5:18). "Giving thanks always for all things unto God and the Father in the name of our Lord Jesus Christ" (Ephesians 5:20).

What a wonderful way to live! Always dwelling in the sunshine of God's countenance; always spreading the sunshine to those around you. "Be careful for nothing; but in every thing by prayer and supplication with thanksgiving let your requests be made known unto God" (Philippians 4:6).

When the sunshine of praise is not present, we lapse into doubt, discontent, and darkness. "Because that, when they knew God, they glorified Him not as God, neither were thankful; but became vain in their imaginations, and their foolish heart was darkened" (Romans 1:21).

Whether on the street, about our business, or at church—let us praise the Lord. "My praise shall be of Thee in the great congregation: I will pay my vows before them that fear Him" (Psalm 22:25).

We praise God by telling others how good He has been to us, and the blessings and protection He has brought us. "Come and hear, all ye that fear God, and I will declare what He hath done for my soul" (Psalm 66:16). "My soul shall make her boast in the Lord; the humble shall hear thereof, and be glad" (Psalm 34:2).

In every place and by every means, praise the Lord. "Praise ye the Lord. Praise God in His sanctuary: praise Him in the firmament of His power. Praise Him for His mighty acts: praise Him according to His excellent greatness . . Let everything that hath breath praise the Lord. Praise ye the Lord" (Psalm 150:1, 2, 6). Spread the sunshine.

From age to age, throughout times past and eternity to come, God's people praise Him with song and rejoicing. "Where wast thou when I laid the foundations of the earth? . . when the morning stars sang together, and all the sons of God shouted for joy?" (Job 38:4,7). "Then sang Moses and the children of Israel this song unto the Lord . . The Lord is my strength and song, and He is become my salvation . . and I will exalt Him" (Exodus 15:1-2). "Serve the Lord with gladness" (Psalm 100:2).

"Unto Him that is able to keep you from falling, and to present you faultless before the presence of His glory with exceeding joy."—*Jude 24.*

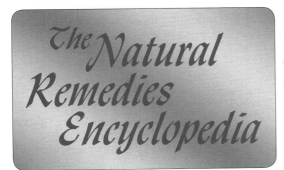

The Natural Remedies Encyclopedia

The Third Law of Health

The Power of Abstemiousness

To be "abstemious" is to be moderate or sparing in the use of certain things, including an excess of even good food. Temperance has a similar meaning: It means to have moderation or self-restraint.

Temperance can also mean to totally avoid certain substances or activities, and so does abstinence.

We are here speaking of self-control. In order to succeed physically, mentally, and morally in life, we must have temperance in regard to things good and abstinence in regard to things harmful.

"In order to preserve health, temperance in all things is necessary,—temperance in labor, temperance in eating and drinking."—*How to Live, p. 57.*

"True temperance teaches us to abstain entirely from that which is injurious, and to use judiciously only healthful and nutritious articles of food."—*Health Reformer, April 1, 1877.*

The evangelist, Paul, counsels us to be "temperate in all things" (1 Corinthians 9:25). This means that we should shun that which is harmful, avoid unneeded extremes, and be moderate in the enjoyment of those things which are lawful. Health of body, mind, and soul is impossible without careful, temperate living.

Even when eating the most careful diet, you can get too much of a good thing. Too much, even of the best food, is harmful. Too much sunshine can result in severe sunburn; too much exercise can cause excessive exhaustion. The Apostle Paul said, "Let your moderation be known unto all men" (Philippians 4:5). Seneca said, "Man does not die; he kills himself!" Much of the tragic shortening of men's lives—that we so often see around us—is unnecessary. Men and women violate the laws of health; and the law of abstemiousness is one of the most important of these laws.

The well-known American writer, William Cullen Bryant, lived to a very old age. When asked the reason for his excellent health at such an advanced age, he replied, "It is all summed up in one word: moderation." If we would be temperate in all things, self-control must be exercised in our conversation, in our daily diet, in our work habits, in our recreation, in our travels, in our time for sleep, and in our study. Throughout life, we must ever be on guard lest we fall into intemperance. The strains and injuries of earlier years add up and reveal themselves in the later years. Live carefully, and if you are not doing so,—then immediately turn about and determine that, by the help of God, you will live a better life. Fortunately, whenever we begin living more healthfully, our future happiness immediately begins improving.

The will power to make the needed changes can be found only in Christ, humble submission to Him, and careful obedience to His Inspired Word. It is the will of our heavenly Father that we not only learn and obey His Moral Law, the Ten Commandments, but that we also learn and obey the physical laws that govern our being.

A little later in this chapter will be found a number of very helpful quotations that will explain the importance of studying and living by the laws of health. Moderation is something that but few value as they should. Yet it is the cord that binds together many other health principles.

The Bible says, "Every man that striveth for the mastery is temperate in all things" (1 Corinthians 9:25). As we have mentioned earlier, true temperance includes moderation in things good as well as abstinence in things harmful.

Here are some of the harmful things that should be avoided: Do not use tobacco in any form, for it is a slow but powerful poison. Totally avoid alcoholic drinks. Stay away from poisonous substances and toxic drugs. This includes not only liquids and solids, but also vapors and fumes. Beware of addicting substances and never indulge in them. Included under this category would be not only alcoholic beverages, but also caffeine products (such as coffee, tea, and cola drinks). Caffeine products injure your organs; and, in addition, cola drinks gradually melt your teeth.

The heavily sugared foods (such as candy, ice cream, cake, and chewing gum) are better left alone.

The Bible says not to eat the blood or the fat. Yet it is practically impossible to prepare meat dishes with any taste—after all the blood, fat, and uric acid (urine in the tissues) has been first soaked and boiled out of the raw meat.

Do not use greasy foods. This includes butter, margarine, and animal fat. Any oil that is solid or semi-solid at room temperature should never be put into the body. Beware of trans-fats. These are the partially hydrogenated oils that have been put into margarine and many other foods. An example of this is the peanut butter sold in regular grocery stores. You will notice that it contains no free-flowing ("runny") oil. All of the oil has been solidified by hydrogenation into a grease form.

Chemically, such grease has the same effect in the body that animal fat has. (In addition, some manufacturers remove the expensive peanut oil from the crushed peanuts, and then add to the peanut pulp a cheap oil that has been hydrogenated into grease. This cheap oil additive is sometimes an animal fat, although marked on the label as "vegetable oil.") Meat in the diet has a tendency to rot in the system. This is due to the fact that our digestive tracts are much longer than those of dogs, tigers, and other flesh-eating animals.

Do not cook or eat food in aluminum. Aluminum salts are poisonous to the body. Avoid foods that have been taken apart (such as white flour, white rice, white sugar, white bread, etc.). Instead, eat the whole foods: whole-grain bread and cereal, brown rice, honey, etc.

Baking powder and soda should not be used in food preparation; for they damage the delicate lining of the stomach. Vinegar is a powerful acid and should never be in any food that you eat.

The use of spices and condiments disturbs the stomach, creates a thirst that is difficult to satisfy with food, can lead to addictive habits, and has been known to cause disease. For example, white and black pepper can lead to intestinal cancer.

Avoid automobile and tobacco fumes. Car exhaust contains lead; and cigarette smoke has many dangerous chemicals, in addition to nicotine. Stay away from spray painters. Metal lacquer (such as is used by auto body refinishers) is especially harmful to the lungs.

Chlorinated water leads to atherosclerosis. And fluoridated water injures your bones, teeth, and nerves.

Do not eat or drink things that are too hot or too cold. Both upset the stomach and weaken the digestive system.

Food preservatives and insecticide residues are both dangerous in food. It is best to wash fresh fruit and vegetables before eating them, in order to eliminate as much of the insecticide as possible. Try to avoid using processed foods that list preservatives on the label.

Both chocolate and cocoa contain harmful substances.

That which is harmful should be avoided; and many of those things which are good should be used in moderation: Maintain a balance of rest and exercise; not too much work or too little. Regularity in scheduling and the daily routines of life will greatly aid in keeping you in the best health. Try to have a set time for rising, morning worship, prayer, drinking your water, mealtime, quitting time in the afternoon, family worship, evening walk time, bedtime, etc. Maintaining simple routines simplifies life, relaxes the mind, and helps us work more efficiently.

Personal cleanliness is actually another type of moderation.

Cleanliness of body, clothing, bedding, and house are important to good health. Open the windows and let in the purifying sunlight and fresh air. Water is the best cleansing agent known to mankind. It is a gift of God. Keep your environment clean and your life will be a happier one.

Closely related to cleanliness is neatness and tidiness. Keeping things neat and in order is both encouraging to the spirits and helpful to mental efficiency.

Tight compressions about the waist (such as belts, corset, etc.) can induce later pelvic organ disease. Suspend the clothing from the shoulders. Wear clothing that will avoid chilling of the arms and legs.

Refuse to live a life of anxious concern. Worry wears out the life forces. If you cannot solve it in five minutes, give it to God in prayer—and then forget it. Later the solutions will come to mind. That simple habit has been a help to this writer.

Have certain times to work and certain times not to; do the same with your mind. Turn it off at times and just relax. Above all things, keep cheerful, and keep close to God and His Written Word. Permit nothing to keep you continually depressed or anxious. People that are cheerful and relaxed always are healthier and have longer, happier lives than they otherwise would—without exception.

A cheerful, relaxed, unworried attitude; trust in God; prayerful and obedient study of His Scriptures; moderation in living habits; the use of the eight natural remedies; the avoidance of addictive and poisonous substances; trying to be a blessing and a help to those around you (regardless of whether they seem to appreciate your efforts);—this is the seven-fold formula for a happy, satisfying, worthwhile, and long life.

ADDITIONAL PRINCIPLES

"God is the owner of the whole man. Soul, body, and spirit are His. God gave His only begotten Son for the body as well as the soul, and our entire life belongs to God, to be consecrated to His service, that through the exercise of every faculty He has given, we may glorify Him."—*Healthful Living, p. 9.*

"The living organism is God's property. It belongs to Him by creation and by redemption; and by a misuse of any of our powers we rob God of the honor due Him."—*Counsels on Diet and Foods, p. 16.*

"The wonderful mechanism of the human body does not receive half the care that is often given to a mere lifeless machine."—*Gospel Workers, p. 175.*

"The health should be as sacredly guarded as the character."—*Counsels to Parents, Teachers and Students, p. 84.*

"Our very bodies are not our own, to treat as we please, to cripple by habits that lead to decay, making it impossible to render to God perfect service. Our lives and all our faculties belong to Him. He is caring for us every moment; He keeps the living machinery in action; if we were left to run it for one moment, we should die. We are absolutely dependent upon God."—*Medical Ministry, p. 13.*

"It is our duty to study the laws that govern our being, and conform to them. Ignorance in these things is sin."—*Healthful Living, p. 13.*

"From the first dawn of reason, the human mind should become intelligent in regard to the physical structure. We may behold and admire the work of God in the natural world, but the human habitation is the most wonderful."—*Counsels to Parents, Teachers, and Students, p. 125.*

"Ignorance of physiology and neglect to observe the laws of health have brought many to the grave who might have lived to labor and study intelligently."—*Special Testimonies on Education, p. 98.*

"To become acquainted with the wonderful human organism,—the bones, muscles, stomach, liver, bowels, heart, and pores of the skin,—and to understand the dependence of one organ upon another for the healthful action of all, is a study in which most mothers take no interest."—*3 Testimonies, p. 136.*

"Study that marvelous organism, the human system, and the laws by which it is governed."—*Christian Temperance, p. 120.*

"If people would reason from cause to effect, and would follow the light which shines upon them, they would pursue a course which would insure health, and the mortality would be far less . . All who possess common capabilities should understand the wants of their own system."—*How to Live, p. 51.*

"He who hungers and thirsts after God will seek for an understanding of the laws which the God of wisdom has impressed upon creation. These laws are a transcript of His character. They must control all who enter the heavenly and better country."—*Unpublished Testimonies, August 30, 1896.*

"God's law is written by His own finger upon every nerve, every muscle, every faculty which has been entrusted to man."—*Unpublished Testimonies, August 30, 1896.*

"The transgression of physical law is transgression of God's law.

"Our Creator is Jesus Christ. He is the author of our being. He is the author of the physical law as He is the author of the Moral Law. And the human being who is careless and reckless of the habits and practices that concern his physical life and health, sins against God. God is not reverenced, respected or recognized.

"This is shown by the injury done to the body in violation of physical law."—*Unpublished Testimonies, May 19, 1897.*

"God loves His creatures with a love that is both tender and strong. He has established the laws of nature; but His laws are not arbitrary exactions. Every 'Thou shalt not,' whether in physical or Moral Law, contains or implies a promise. If it is obeyed, blessings will attend your steps; if it is disobeyed, the result is danger and unhappiness."—*5 Testimonies, p. 545.*

"Health, strength, and happiness depend upon immutable laws; but these laws cannot be obeyed where there is no anxiety to become acquainted with them."—*Health Reformer, September 1, 1881, p.11.*

"God is greatly dishonored by the way in which man treats his organism, and He will not work a miracle to counteract perverse violations of the laws of life and health."—*Unpublished Testimonies, August 30, 1896.*

"The Lord has made it a part of His plan that man's reaping shall be according to his sowing."—*Unpublished Testimonies, May 19, 1897.*

"God calls for reformers to stand in defense of the laws He has established to govern the human system, and to maintain an elevated standard in the training of the mind and culture of the heart."—*Testimonies to Ministers and Workers, p. 195.*

"It is the duty of every human being, for his own sake and for the sake of humanity, to inform himself or herself in regard to the laws of organic life, and conscientiously to obey them . . It is the duty of every person to become intelligent in regard to disease and its causes. You must study your Bible, in order to understand the value that the Lord places on the men whom Christ has purchased at such an infinite price. Then we should become acquainted with the laws of life, that every action of the human agent may be in perfect harmony with the laws of God. When there is so great peril in ignorance, is it not best to be wise in regard to the human habitation fitted up by our Creator, and over which He desires that we shall be faithful stewards?"—*Unpublished Testimonies, December 4, 1896.*

"The transgression of the physical law is transgression of God's law. Our Creator is Jesus Christ."—*Un-*

published Testimonies, May 19, 1897.

"Every law governing the human machinery is to be considered just as truly divine in origin, in character, and in importance as the Word of God. Every careless action, any abuse put upon the wonderful mechanism, by disregarding His specified laws of the human habitation, is a violation of God's law. This law embraces the treatment of the entire being."—*Unpublished Testimonies, January 11, 1897.*

"God has formed laws to govern every part of our constitutions, and these laws which He has placed in our being are divine, and for every transgression there is a fixed penalty, which sooner or later must be realized."—*Healthful Living, p. 20.*

"Our first duty, one which we owe to God, to ourselves, and to our fellow men, is to obey the laws of God, which include the laws of health."—*3 Testimonies, p. 164.*

"The laws governing the physical nature are as truly divine in their origin and character as the law of the Ten Commandments.

"Man is fearfully and wonderfully made; for Jehovah has inscribed His law by His own mighty hand on every part of the human body."—*Unpublished Testimonies, August 5, 1896.*

"It is just as much sin to violate the laws of our being as to break one of the Ten Commandments, for we cannot do either without breaking God's law."—*2 Testimonies, p. 70.*

"A violation of these laws is a violation of the immutable law of God, and the penalty will surely follow."—*Review and Herald, October 16, 1883.*

"All our enjoyment or suffering may be traced to obedience or transgression of natural law."—*3 Testimonies, p. 161.*

"God, the Creator of our bodies, has arranged every fiber and nerve and sinew and muscle, and has pledged Himself to keep the machinery in order if the human agent will co-operate with Him and refuse to work contrary to the laws which govern the human system."—*Unpublished Testimonies, August 30, 1896.*

"Every misuse of any part of our organism is a violation of the law which God designs shall govern us in these matters; and by violating this law, human beings corrupt themselves. Sickness, disease of every kind, ruined constitutions, premature decay, untimely deaths,—these are the result of a violation of nature's laws."—*Unpublished Testimonies, August 30, 1896.*

"Sickness is caused by violating the laws of health; it is the result of violating nature's laws."—*3 Testimonies, p. 164.*

"Everything that conflicts with natural law creates a diseased condition of the soul."—*Review and Herald, January 25, 1881.*

"The moral powers are weakened because men and women will not live in obedience to the laws of health, and make this great subject a personal duty."—*3 Testimonies, p. 140.*

"Satan knows that he cannot overcome man unless he can control his will. He can do this by deceiving men so they will cooperate with him in transgressing the laws of nature, which is transgression of the law of God."—*Temperance, p. 16.*

"If we unnecessarily injure our constitutions, we dishonor God, for we transgress the laws of our being."—*Healthful Living, p. 27.*

"If appetite, which should be strictly guarded and controlled, is indulged to the injury of the body, the penalty of transgression will surely result."—*Unpublished Testimonies, August 30, 1896.*

"Intemperance of any kind is a violation of the laws of our being."—*Review and Herald, September 8, 1874.*

"Eating merely to please the appetite is a transgression of nature's laws."—*Unpublished Testimonies, August 30, 1896.*

"Health is a great treasure. It is the richest possession that mortals can have. Wealth, honor, or learning is dearly purchased, if is be at the loss of the vigor of health. None of these attainments can secure happiness if health is wanting."—*Christian Education, p. 16.*

"The health should be as sacredly guarded as the character."—*Christian Temperance, p. 83.*

"Our physical, mental, and moral powers are not our own, but lent us of God to be used in His service."—*Healthful Living, p. 29.*

"The importance of the health of the body is to be taught as a Bible requirement."—*Unpublished Testimonies, August 30, 1896.*

"All who profess to be followers of Jesus should feel that a duty rests upon them to preserve their bodies in the best condition of health, that their minds may be clear to comprehend heavenly things."—*2 Testimonies, pp. 522-523.*

"That time is well spent which is directed to the establishment and preservation of sound physical and mental health . . It is easy to lose health, but it is difficult to regain it."—*Review and Herald, September 23, 1884.*

"God has not changed, neither does He propose to change our physical organism, in order that we may violate a single law without feeling the effects of its violation . . By indulging their inclinations and appetites, men violate the laws of life and health; and if they obey conscience, they must be controlled by principle in their eating and dressing, rather than be led by inclination, fashion, and appetite."—*Counsels on Diet and Foods, p. 161.*

"Neglecting to exercise the entire body, or a portion of it, will bring on morbid conditions. Inaction of any of the organs of the body will be followed by a decrease in size and strength of the muscles, and will cause the blood to flow sluggishly through the blood vessels."—*3 Testimonies, p. 176.*

"Perfect health depends upon perfect circulation."—*2 Testimonies, p. 531.*

"The health of the entire system depends upon the healthy action of the respiratory organs."—*How to Live, p. 57.*

"If we would have health, we must live for it."—*Health Reformer, December 1, 1870.*

"We can ill afford to dwarf or cripple a single function of mind or body by overwork, or by abuse of any part of the living machinery."—*Review and Herald, September 23, 1884.*

"A sound body is required for a sound intellect."—*Christian Education, p. 17.*

"A careful conformity to the laws God has implanted in our being will insure health, and there will not be a breaking down of the constitution."—*Health Reformer, August 1, 1866.*

"Blindness mingles with the want of moral courage to deny your appetite, to lift the cross, which means to take up the very duties that cut across the natural appetites and passions."—*Unpublished Testimonies, November 5, 1896.*

"Nature's path is the road He [God] marks out, and it is broad enough for any Christian."—*3 Testimonies, p. 63.*

"Overeating prevents the free flow of thought and words, and that intensity of feeling which is so necessary in order to impress the truth upon the heart of the hearer."—*3 Testimonies, p. 310.*

"Excessive eating of even the best of food will produce a morbid condition of the moral feelings . . Wrong habits of eating and drinking lead to errors in thought and action. Indulgence of appetite strengthens the animal propensities, giving them the ascendancy over the mental and spiritual powers . . Everything that conflicts with natural law creates a diseased condition of the soul."—*Review and Herald, January 25, 1881.*

"The foundation of all enduring reform is the law of God. We are to present in clear, distinct lines the need of obeying this law.

"Its principles must be kept before the people. They are as everlasting and inexorable as God Himself.

"One of the most deplorable effects of the original apostasy was the loss of man's power of self-control. Only as this power is regained, can there be real progress."—*Ministry of Healing, p. 129.*

"The less feverish the diet, the more easily can the passions be controlled."—*2 Testimonies, p. 352.*

"A failure to care for the living machinery is an insult to the Creator. There are divinely appointed rules which if observed, will keep human beings from disease and premature death."—*Counsels on Diet and Foods, p. 16.*

"Dearly beloved, I beseech you as strangers and pilgrims, abstain from fleshly lusts, which war against the soul."—*1 Peter 2:11.*

"Parents often make a mistake by giving their children too much food. Children treated in this way will grow up dyspeptics.

"Moderation in the use of even good food is essential."—*Child Guidance, p. 391.*

"Irregularity in eating and drinking, and improper dressing, deprave the mind and corrupt the heart, and bring noble attributes to the soul in slavery to the animal passions."—*Health Reformer, October 1, 1871.*

"A diseased body causes a disordered brain, and hinders the work of sanctifying grace upon the mind and heart."—*Health Reformer, September 1, 1871.*

"If man will cherish the light that God in mercy gives him upon health reform, he may be sanctified through the truth, and fitted for immortality."—*3 Testimonies, p. 162.*

"Every organ of the body is made to be servant of the mind."—*3 Testimonies, p. 136.*

"The brain is the capital of the body, the seat of all the nervous forces and of mental action. The nerves proceeding from the brain control the body. By the brain nerves, mental impressions are conveyed to all the nerves of the body as by telegraph wires; and they control the vital action of every part of the system. All the organs of motion are governed by the communications they receive from the brain."—*3 Testimonies, p. 69.*

"The brain nerves which communicate with the entire system are the only medium through which Heaven can communicate to man and affect his inmost life. Whatever disturbs the circulation of the electric currents in the nervous system, lessens the strength of the vital powers, and the result is a deadening of the sensibilities of the mind."—*2 Testimonies, p. 347.*

"A calm, clear brain and steady nerves are dependent upon a well-balanced circulation of the blood."—*Healthful Living, p. 194.*

"Immediately after eating there is a strong draught upon the nervous energy . . Therefore, when the mind or body is taxed heavily after eating, the process of digestion is hindered. The vitality of the system, which is needed to carry on the work in one direction, is called away and set to work in another."—*2 Testimonies, p. 413.*

"Every wrong habit which injures the health of the body, reacts in effect upon the mind."—*Health Reformer, February 1, 1871.*

"The brain is the citadel of the whole man, and wrong habits of eating, dressing, or sleeping affect the brain, and prevent the attaining of that which the student desires,—a good mental discipline. Any part of the body that is not treated with consideration will telegraph its injury to the brain."—*Christian Education, p. 125.*

"It is impossible for the brain to do its best work when the digestive powers are abused. Many eat hurriedly of various kinds of food, which set up a war in the stomach, and thus confuse the brain . . At mealtime cast off care and taxing thought. Do not be hurried, but eat slowly and with cheerfulness, your heart filled with gratitude to God for all His blessings. And do not engage in brain labor immediately after a meal. Exercise moderately, and give a little time for the stomach to begin its work."—*Gospel Workers, pp. 241-242.*

"The tempted ones need to understand the true force of the will.

"This is the governing power in the nature of man,— the power of decision, of choice. Everything depends on the right action of the will. Desires for goodness and purity are right, so far as they go; but if we stop here, they avail nothing. Many will go down to ruin while hoping and desiring to overcome their evil propensities. They do not yield the will to God. They do not *choose* to serve Him.

"God has given us the power of choice; it is ours to exercise. We can not change our hearts, we can not control our thoughts, our impulses, our affections. We can not make ourselves pure, fit for God's service. But we can *choose* to serve and do according to His good pleasure. Thus our whole nature will be brought under the control of Christ . . A pure and noble life of victory over appetite and lust is possible to every one who will unite his weak, wavering human will to the omnipotent, unwavering will of God."—*Ministry of Healing, p. 176.*

SPIRITUAL LESSONS

Abstemiousness, or temperance, is simply self-control. Only through the continual aid of our Lord and Saviour Jesus Christ can we be empowered, by His grace, to control ourselves, resist temptation, and obey God's will.

The will of God is revealed throughout the Inspired Writings of Scripture, and especially in the Ten Commandments which summarize many basic principles of godliness.

If you would be like Jesus, then, by His enabling grace, obey the Ten Commandments which He gave on Mount Sinai over 3,400 years ago.

Obedience to God is the basis of all true temperance, the foundation of successful, happy living in this life, and the assurance of life on through eternity with God.

"The law of the Lord is perfect, converting the soul: the testimony of the Lord is sure, making wise the simple. The statutes of the Lord are right, rejoicing the heart: the commandment of the Lord is pure, enlightening the eyes" (Psalm 19:7-8).

It is in the law that we learn God's pattern for our conduct and His will for our lives. "And knowest His will . . being instructed out of the law" (Romans 2:18). "Fear God, and keep His commandments: for this is the whole duty of man. For God shall bring every work into judgment, with every secret thing, whether it be good, or whether it be evil" (Ecclesiastes 12:13-14).

Intemperance in life is sin, and sin is the breaking of God's law. "Whosoever committeth sin transgresseth also the law: for sin is the transgression of the law" (1 John 3:4). "For by the law is the knowledge of sin" (Romans 3:20).

Obedience to God is the passport to heaven. Jesus said, "If thou wilt enter into life, keep the commandments" (Matthew 19:17). "Blessed are the undefiled in the way, who walk in the law of the Lord" (Psalm 119:1). "Moreover by them is Thy servant warned: and in keeping of them there is great reward" (Psalm 19:11).

The rewards of obedience are abundant: "Great peace have they which love Thy law: and nothing shall offend them" (Psalm 119:165). "O that thou hadst hearkened to My commandments! Then had thy peace been as a river, and thy righteousness as the waves of the sea" (Isaiah 48:18). "The fear of the Lord is the beginning of wisdom: a good understanding have all they that do His commandments" (Psalm 111:10). "If ye be willing and obedient, ye shall eat the good of the land" (Isaiah 1:19).

Yet it is only through the enabling strength of Christ's grace that we can keep God's law. Apart from Christ, we are helpless to resist sin.

"I am not ashamed of the gospel of Christ: for it is the power of God unto salvation to every one that believeth" (Romans 1:16). Jesus came to earth and died so we might be delivered from falling into sin. "Thou shalt call His name Jesus: for He shall save His people from their sins" (Matthew 1:21). "We preach . . Christ the power of God, and the wisdom of God" (1 Corinthians 1:23-24). "Behold the Lamb of God, which taketh away the sin of the world" (John 1:29).

By believing in Christ as our Saviour, and acting in accordance with our faith, we are enabled to obey all that God asks of us. "Do we then make void the law through faith? God forbid: yea, we establish the law" (Romans 3:31).

This is the basis of the new covenant: God enables us to obey His commandments as we accept and cling to Jesus, His Son. Christ is our Mediator in Heaven, and He strengthens us to resist temptation and obey God's law (Hebrews 8:6, 10).

Law and grace are closely associated in the plan of redemption. To understand grace, we need to understand the law.

In the beginning, God created man and placed him under law. Man was not just to be a wild man, a law unto himself. He was to obey God. The Moral Law of the Ten Commandments were later written down (Exodus 20). Other laws were also given at that time.

There were civil laws which regulated many matters of the nation of Israel. They applied to the governing of the nation.

Then there were the ceremonial, or sanctuary, laws. These governed the religious services of the nation, and were written in a book which was placed beside the Ark of the Covenant. These ceremonial laws were abolished at the cross, for at that time Christ, the great antitypical Lamb of God died for mankind. No longer need lambs be brought to the earthly sanctuary to be sacrificed. In Christ at Calvary, shadow met substance and type met antitype—and the ceremonial laws were abolished.

"Blotting out the handwriting of ordinances that was against us, which was contrary to us, and took it out of the way, nailing it to His cross" (Colossians 2:14). "Which are a shadow of things to come; but the body is of Christ" (Colossians 2:17).

Then, third, there was the Ten Commandments. It is the Moral Law of God, given by Him to all humanity. It is the universal law of mankind. No one is to commit adultery, or the other sins listed in this holy code.

This was the only law written by the finger of God. It was the only law placed inside the Ark of the Covenant. "He wrote on the tables, according to the first writing, the Ten Commandments, which the Lord spake unto you in the mount out of the midst of the fire in the day of the assembly" (Deuteronomy 10:4). "And I turned myself and came down from the mount, and put the tables in the ark which I had made" (Deuteronomy 10:5).

The moral Ten Commandment law is eternal. It is God's own covenant, and it is as everlasting as God Himself. "The law of the Lord is perfect, converting the soul" (Psalm 19:7). "Wherefore the law is holy, and the commandment holy, and just, and good" (Romans 7:12). "Thy law is the truth" (Psalm 119:142). "Concerning Thy testimonies, I have known of old that Thou hast founded them forever" (Psalm 119:152).

What does the law do for the sinner?

First, it gives a knowledge of sin. "By the law is the knowledge of sin" (Romans 3:20).

Second, it brings guilt and condemnation. "Now we know that what things soever the law saith, it saith to them who are under the law: that every mouth may be stopped, and all the world may become guilty before God" (Romans 3:19).

Third, it acts as a spiritual mirror. "If any be a hearer of the Word, and not a doer, he is like unto a man beholding his natural face in a glass: for he beholdeth himself, and goeth his way, and straightway forgetteth what manner of man he was. But whoso looketh into the perfect law of liberty, and continueth therein, he being not a forgetful hearer, but a doer of the work, this man shall be blessed in his deed" (James 1:23-25).

Without the law the sinner is like a man afflicted with a deadly disease, who does not know he has it. Paul said, "I had not known sin, but by the law" (Romans 7:7).

What is the law unable to do for the sinner?

The law of God cannot forgive or justify him; only Jesus can. He died to redeem us. "By the deeds of the law there shall no flesh be justified in His sight" (Romans 3:20).

The law of God cannot keep from sin or sanctify us. "Is the law then against the promises of God? God forbid: for if there had been a law given which could have given life, verily righteousness should have been by the law" (Galatians 3:21).

The law of God cannot cleanse or keep the heart clean. Only Jesus can cast out the evil, and enable man to obey Him.

What does the grace of Christ do for the sinner?

When the law of God and the Spirit of God have made the sinner conscious of his sin, he will feel his need of Jesus Christ. Going to the Saviour, he can receive help. If we come to Him and confess and put away our sin, He forgives us. "If we confess our sins, He is faithful and just to forgive us our sins, and to cleanse us from all unrighteousness" (1 John 1:9).

Through grace, we can receive forgiveness and justification. "Be it known unto you therefore, men and brethren, that through this Man is preached unto you the forgiveness of sins: and by Him all that believe are justified from all things, from which ye could not be justified by the law of Moses" (Acts 13:38-39).

Through grace, we can be saved from sin, or sanctified. "Thou shalt call His name Jesus: for He shall save His people from their sins" (Matthew 1:21). "But of Him are ye in Christ Jesus, who of God is made unto us wisdom, and righteousness, and sanctification, and redemption" (1 Corinthians 1:30).

Grace inspires faith, and encourages us to come to Christ and remain with Him. "By grace are ye saved through faith; and that not of yourselves: it is the gift of God: not of works, lest any man should boast. For we are His workmanship, created in Christ Jesus unto good works, which God hath before ordained that we should walk in them" (Ephesians 2:8-10).

Grace brings us God's power. "I am not ashamed of the gospel of Christ: for it is the power of God unto salvation to every one that believeth; to the Jew first, and also to the Greek" (Romans 1:16).

What is the relationship of a sinner, who is being saved by grace, to the law of God?

The law becomes the standard of his life "This is the love of God, that we keep His commandments" (1 John 5:3).

He permits Christ to fulfill in him the righteousness of the law (Romans 8:3). Christ writes the law on the heart. "This is the covenant that I will make . . I will put My laws into their mind, and write them in their hearts: and I will be to them a God, and they shall be to Me a people" (Hebrews 8:10).

What is the relationship of grace, faith, love and the law?

Grace is unmerited favor, but grace does not sanction continued transgression. "What then? shall we sin, because we are not under the law, but under grace? God forbid" (Romans 6:15).

Faith does not make void, but establishes, the law. "Do we then make void the law through faith? God forbid: yea, we establish the law" (Romans 3:31).

Faith brings overcoming power. "Whatsoever is born of God overcometh the world: and this is the victory that overcometh the world, even our faith" (1 John 5:4).

Love is the fulfilling of the law. "Love worketh no ill to his neighbour: therefore love is the fulfilling of the law" (Romans 13:10).

True love keeps the commandments. "This is the love of God, that we keep His commandments: and His commandments are not grievous" (1 John 5:3).

"The you of the Lord is your strength."—*Philippians 4:19.*

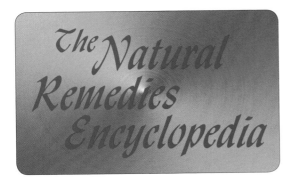

The Fourth Law of Health
The Rest Your Body Needs

"Come ye apart . . and rest" are the words of Jesus. Are you weary and worn with the routine of everyday life? Rest is what you need: physical rest, mental rest. Come rest awhile. It is one of God's special healing remedies; and it is just for you, just now.

Let us, for a few minutes, learn some of the blessings that rest can bring, blessings that you may very much need.

Strangely enough, you can read almost any book on remedies and you will find hardly any mention of rest. Most of the directions are about swallow this or inject that. Yet

62 **THE EIGHT LAWS** THE REST YOUR BODY NEEDS NATURAL REMEDIES ENCYCLOPEDIA OVER 11,000 REMEDIES - OVER 730 DISEASES

L
A
W
S

rest is one of the most basic healers known to mankind. When you become sick, what is the first thing that you do? You lie down. Can you imagine a hospital in which all the patients only go to bed at night? No, they are lying flat in bed most of the day as well as all the night because the restorative power of rest is a key to the success of all other remedial agencies.

But, just now, you are not ill. Do you need rest when you are well? To a startling degree, it is the lack of adequate rest while you are well that causes you to become sick.

Here are some simple principles about rest:

One does not always have to sleep in order to rest. Just a change of pace—doing something different—can bring rest to your mind and body. Different muscles are used, different things are considered, and you begin to relax. The everyday work is set aside and you take time to think more of God and His blessings seen and felt every day of your life.

You can train yourself to relax. Even if you cannot lie down, you can stand by an open window or walk out-of-doors and take several deep breaths. As you do this, think thankful thoughts to God, in heaven, for His blessings. Ask for His help and guidance for the duties just ahead. Believe that He has heard your silent petition and thank Him in advance for giving the help you need.

As you do this, a sense of rest and calm trust will fill your heart; a genuine, quiet relaxation of spirit will come over you.

The "go, go attitude," so common to Western civilization, leads many to nervous breakdowns. They simply did not take time to rest. It was an objectionable word in their thinking. But such an imbalanced pattern of living crowds out thoughts of God and eternal life. And discouragement and despair begins to crowd in.

By the time that George Sheehan, M.D., was 45, he felt ready to collapse. Work, work, work had brought him to the top of the professional ladder, but all he had achieved was a crowded work schedule and little else.

Then one night he recalled to mind something he read in a book: "We never shall have any more time. We have, and we have always had, all the time there is."

George Sheehan vowed then and there that he would immediately change his life style. He began to take time for the healthful exercise and much needed rest he had cheated his body out of for years. And then the better years began for him. They can begin for you just now also.

One reason so many people have nervous breakdowns is that they try to surpass and have the supremacy. So they go at high speed, without adequate rest, until the body machinery breaks under the load. Instead, put Jesus first, others second, and yourself last. Refocus your life. Take time to rest. Just go outside and sit in a chair and do nothing. If the very thought of that sounds ominous to you,—then you are the very one who needs to restudy your attitude toward adequate rest.

Peace of mind does not come by being always in a hurry. And hurry is often concerned with gathering up tomorrow's problems and trying to tackle them all today. All God has given you is one day at a time; how will you use it?

What we want is a better way to live—a new kind of day. Begin the first of your new days by praying to God when you first arise in the morning. Thank Him for His help, dedicate this special day to Him. Ask for His help and thank Him for giving it. Then open His Word—the Bible—and read in it. Where should you read? It is all worthwhile, but, if you wish, start with the book of Ephesians. Read it slowly and thoughtfully, not hurriedly, like a regular book. (On later days, when Ephesians is completed, begin in 1 John, and then the Gospel of John. Try reading in the Psalms—Psalms 37 and 23 for example,—and then go to Genesis, the first chapter. When you finish that, read on through to Revelation 22.)

After time alone with God and His Word, mingling prayer with your reading, arise and begin doing your daily duties, continually sending up little silent prayers of thanks and requests for help. Go out of your way to be a help to others. Too often in the past they have had to go out of their way to adjust to you, but now things are different. It is your concern to help them. Be not concerned if they do not seem to immediately appreciate or even want your help. Keep at it, quietly, thankfully, living to be a blessing to others around you. Even though others may misinterpret your efforts, you can know that you are doing what is right in God's sight. And that awareness will bring a peace and sweet joy into your life that you may not have experienced in years.

If you have children, take time to have morning and evening worship with them. Gather them to you, sing a song of Jesus, kneel down and pray with them, then read a portion from God's Word, and close with prayer, dedicating them that day anew to the care of their heavenly Father.

Yes, true rest of heart and life means taking time for God and living for Him. And such a rest as this will bring tranquillity of mind and lengthening of your days.

Rest with God includes time with Him each day, and it also means time with Him on the Sabbath day. He wisely knew our needs better than we, and back in the beginning (Genesis 2:1-3) He gave us the seventh-day Sabbath as a weekly day for physical, mental, and spiritual rest. So important was it, that He wrote it into the Moral Law of Ten Commandments. It is the Fourth Commandment (Exodus 20:8-11), and is of equal importance with all the rest. In fact, by carefully observing the seventh-day Sabbath, we shall be enabled by His grace to keep all the other commandments as well. There is always a blessing in obeying God. And that which He wants us to obey is written in Scripture.

Here are more principles for obtaining the rest that your body so much needs:

No muscle works continually. After some work there is some rest. Even your heart—the hardest-working muscle in your body—rests after each beat. Your lungs rest at the end of each breath. Your stomach should rest for thirty to sixty minutes after each meal. By this we mean that immediately after a meal you should not do hard physical or mental work. (But rest after a meal does not mean lying down. Be up and active after every meal.)

Your heart works for a lifetime—with only one tenth of a second rest stops. Whatever you do to deprive it of that rest will cause serious trouble later.

Rest should be preceded by exercise, or it may not

NATURAL REMEDIES ENCYCLOPEDIA THE REST YOUR BODY NEEDS THE EIGHT LAWS **63**
OVER 11,000 REMEDIES - OVER 730 DISEASES

L
A
W
S

accomplish its objective. It is the exercise that makes the rest necessary.

And keep in mind that one's best sleep is with the stomach empty, and that sleep out-of-doors in summertime is more restful than sleeping indoors.

It is said that one hour of sleep before midnight is worth two after midnight. They say that some people go to bed with the chickens. Several years ago this writer was told of someone's friend who did it all his adult life. He decided that the chickens knew the best time to retire, and so he went to bed when they did—at sunset—and arose the next morning when they did—long before dawn. That may not fit into your work schedule the best, but let me tell you of another pattern that is very helpful.

Try lying down for a brief rest before lunch every day. Fifteen minutes rest in the middle of the day is equal to 45 minutes or more at night. Oh, but you say, you are not able to fit that into your work schedule. Then do this for sure: When you eventually retire from the 8 to 5 work schedule at the shop or factory,—then give your last years an hour of rest in the middle of the day, just before lunch. And keep active throughout the remainder of the day doing those things which are important. You may thus lengthen your lifespan.

A number of years ago this writer read a report by one of the actuarial experts, at the Social Security Administration, in Washington, D.C. Did you know that the average American dies just three years after he begins receiving social security? This fact is indeed significant. In commenting on it, geriatric authorities believe that it is partly due to the fact that, when retirement is suddenly thrust upon them, many people find that they have lost their purpose in life. The best preparation for retirement is to begin working for God by helping others now. You will then have something very worthwhile to live for when the retirement years come. Rest and work, work and rest is what is needed. But do not slack on the *rest;* you need enough of each in order to fully enjoy both.

The old adage that "a change is good as a vacation" is often true. Overwork, worry, lack of exercise, overeating, and a distressed mind are among the chief causes of fatigue. Living for a purpose—and that purpose being to honor God and help others—helps you rest better at night and makes you feel more restful all through the day.

Adequate rest is necessary in order to protect the alkalinity of the blood. This is due to the fact that waste matter is especially eliminated during those periods when you are resting or sleeping.

The ever active, ever growing child requires more sleep than does the adult. Yet we also need it—more than we often think we do.

"Oh," but you may say, "I don't know how to relax and rest day or night!" Go down by a babbling brook, and lie down and listen to the sounds of nature all about you. Gaze upward through the trees and view the glorious panorama of sunlight striking leaves and limbs, with the blue, cloud-flecked sky beyond. Then shut your eyes and listen to the soft chirps of God's little creatures around you. All are telling you softly that God loves you and will do wonderful things in your life as you yield yourself to Him. By now, as you lie therein—God's great out-of-doors—

you will find that you are becoming wonderfully relaxed.

Amid the hurry and rush of life, our weary bodies and minds need rest. Even metals can become tired. They lose their vitality from repeated shocks and strains, and become exhausted and break under the load. If you feel as if you are nearing the point of breaking under the load, reread this chapter again—and the chapters in this series on the Eight Laws of Health—and put them into practice. There are answers that will work—for you—just now.

Dr. Frederick Rossiter wrote, "Recreation is a vitalized form of rest." Sleep is important and few are getting enough. But rest is not merely sleep. A change of activity is also needed from time to time. Go outdoors for an hour or two and experience this change. Set aside the vexing perplexities of the everyday world, and relax out in nature. Reading a good book—especially God's book—is also restful. The mind is drawn to better things—higher purposes—and the mind and body are rested. Once again you can return to your daily duties refreshed in heart and soul.

But amusement that consists only of foolishness lacks that deep refreshment that you so much need. You must guard your hours for recreation—making sure that you take time for them. And you must guard what you do during those hours. All true recreation is re-creative; it genuinely refreshes, draws us closer to God, and strengthens us for the better performance of our daily duties.

And we all need sleep, good sound sleep every night. But many have a difficult time obtaining it. So they take such medicines a Sominex, Mytol, Sleep-Ease, Compos, Nite Rest, Sure-Sleep, or something similar. But sleep studies reveal that many nonprescription—and almost all prescription sleep medications—drastically alter sleeping cycles, suppressing the very important REM sleep. And this applies to all the "sleeping pills," containing barbiturates or benzodiazepines, as they do. In order to more fully understand why suppression of REM sleep is harmful, we must delve into the physiology of sleep itself.

In the early presleep phase, body temperature falls and alpha brain waves are prominent. Then comes Stage 1 of sleep as the pulse slows and your muscles relax. About 5 to 10 minutes later, Stage 2 begins. The brain waves become larger and the eyes roll from side to side. Another 20 minutes or so and Stage 3 is entered. Brain waves now become slow and fairly large. Muscles are relaxed and breathing is slow and even. Stage 4 begins next, is called delta sleep, and generally lasts about 20 minutes. Then the sleeper enters REM sleep. REM stands for "rapid eye movement." This is a lighter sleep, and it is quite easy to know when a person is in it, for his eyes move very rapidly as if he were watching something. He is,—this is the dream part of his sleep. The heartbeat becomes irregular and brain waves are similar in the waking state. After about 10 minutes, the sleeper returns to Stages 2, 3, and then delta sleep, in a cycle lasting about 90 minutes. Then REM starts again. There is more delta sleep earlier in the night, and more REM sleep toward morning.

Experimenters have discovered that people who do not get their REM sleep awaken irritable and tired. They become depressed, aggressive, angry, restless and/or apathetic. If kept from their REM sleep, as soon as they are asleep again they will try to get longer sessions of REM sleep.

But a condition know as "REM withdrawal sleep" occurs when people take sleeping tablets or most other types of put-you-to-sleep pills. The lack of REM sleep, brought on by taking these sleep medications, makes folk feel bad enough that they are convinced more than ever that they need go-to-sleep tablets in order to survive. So they take more and the problem gets worse.

You need your sleep. Try getting it in the natural way and you will be well rewarded. As we said earlier, work and rest during the day. When evening comes, after your evening worship and just before bedtime, go outside and walk in the fresh air, breathing it in deeply. You may not think that you have time to do this, but you have time to lie in bed trying hard to fall asleep. Just before retiring, take that walk out-of-doors in the quiet of the evening, drinking in the fresh air. Then go inside and immediately take a relaxing shower and go to bed. As you lie there if you find that you want to think about something, think about these two things: First, think about God, how good He is to you all the time, and how thankful you are for His watchcare. Second, think about being relaxed and breathing well. Mouth breathing just then will help clear out your mind so that it can drift off to sleep more quickly.

During the sleeping hours, the body is repaired and invigorated for another day of work. So be regular in obtaining your sleep. Try to go to bed at the same time each night and get up at the same time each morning. The most vigorous, enthusiastic people I know are generally individuals who are quite consistent in getting their full sleep. They are usually the ones who retire on a definite schedule every night.

Oxygen intake is an important part of the rejuvenating effect of sleep. Your body is working less, and the air you breathe is used to restore and rebuild body tissue. Therefore, be sure there is a current of fresh air entering the room—preferably outdoor air—while you sleep. If you do not have that fresh air at night, you will tend to awake tired and exhausted.

Keep in mind the words of the wise man: "The sleep of a laboring man is sweet" (Ecclesiastes 5:12). Only those who use their muscles during the day in physical work can enjoy sweet sleep at night.

Go to bed early and arise early. Staying up late and then sleeping in the next morning is a poor way to live.

Calcium in the diet helps you relax. It relaxes your nerves and is even restful to your heart. If you have a history of poor tooth structure, that is an indication that taking a little calcium each day will make life more restful for you, and will help you sleep better at night. Two facts are well known: Older people need more calcium . . and have more sleeplessness at night.

Pantothenic acid (calcium pantothenate), a vitamin of the B complex, will also help you get to sleep at night. Along with this, take some niacin (best taken in its niacinamide form to avoid face flushing) in your meals to aid in sound sleep at night.

Certain nontoxic natural herb teas have been used for years to help folk to go to sleep at night. Two of the best are hops and chamomile. Others include catnip, lady's slipper, yarrow, and mullein. To our knowledge, herbs are not mixed for this purpose. Select one and use it. The first

two listed above are, by far, the best of them.

Living on micro-sleep is a poor way to go through life. After only a few hours of sleep loss, the body begins experiencing momentary lapses into sleep, each one of which lasts only a split second. As in real sleep, eyelids droop and heartbeat slows. Each micro-sleep is a period of blankness, or it may be filled with wisps of dreams. As the sleep loss increases, the micro-sleeps increase to two or three seconds at a time. If you are driving when it happens, you may die.

Nervous tension, the use of caffeine products, and too much salt in the diet,—all are items found to cause sleeplessness at night. Anything that increases cerebral (brain) activity causes sleeplessness. Neutral temperature baths for 8 minutes or more are excellent for relaxing and calming the mind, and preparing one for sleep. As you leave the tub, blot your skin dry without undue friction, move slowly, climb into bed, think little, breathe relaxed, thank God for peace of heart, go to sleep.

Dr. Samuel W. Gutwirth, in his book, *How to Sleep Well,* describes a method to help insomniacs learn how to go to sleep. In a quiet room, lie on your back, outstretched. Then tense each group of body muscles for several minutes (the arms, legs, trunk, facial muscles, eye muscles), then relax them. Try to relax them even more. The point here is twofold: to learn what it feels like to relax, and then to do it when you want to—so you can go to sleep at night. If there are any diehard insomniacs out there, you might want to try Dr. Gutwirth's approach. He says that, to start with, you need to do it for 45 minutes at a time.

If you cannot sleep, take a warm bath. It is relaxing and will help induce sleep. Never retire soon after eating. Going to bed within an hour or so after supper is hard on the heart and other vital organs, and exhausts the brain. There appears to be a positive correlation between going to sleep at night after a big meal—and the frequency of heart attacks.

For most adults, eight hours of sleep at night is sufficient. Some appear to do well on less. Older people need less sleep, but at the same time they may have a harder time getting it. If you tend to be sleepless at night, get some active exercise in the day, and take that outdoor walk before retiring. If you still feel tired from lack of sleep, the midday nap will do much to solve your problem. Sleep for an hour or two before lunch. It will not hurt you and can only help you.

Sleep should come naturally and not be induced by drugs. If you are napping during the day, do not fear some sleeplessness at night, for just by laying there you are having a good rest. As you lie there, think cheerful thoughts about God and heaven. From time to time send up little prayers for yourself and your loved ones. Keep positive, for it is sad, gloomy thoughts that kill, not sleeplessness.

During the day, rest your eyes by shutting them occasionally or by gazing outdoors upon the things of nature. Rest your ears by avoiding the loud noises of civilization. Noise exhausts the mind and nervous system, and even damages the heart. Rest your mind by not talking so much. Too much talk wears people out: those who do it *and* those who have to listen to it. Rest your mind by not constantly dwelling upon a particular problem and trying endlessly to solve it. If you cannot solve it in five minutes, forget it—is a dictum that has helped this writer. Solutions will come to mind later. Rest your body by not being such a workaholic. Work and rest is what is needed; not work, work, work. Rest your lungs by going out-of-doors every so often through the day and drinking in the fresh air deeply. If you live in a city, move out into the country where there is fresh air. If you smoke, stop; if you do not smoke, refuse to work in rooms where people smoke.

Rest your soul by reading God's Word daily, praying to Him, trusting in Him. Refuse to worry but give all into His hands. Peace of heart, peace with God; this is what you want. Few people have it, but it is as near as your silent prayer to your Creator as you go about your duties throughout the day.

ADDITIONAL PRINCIPLES

"Some make themselves sick by overwork. For these rest, freedom from care, and a spare diet, are essential to restoration of health. To those who are brain weary and nervous because of continual labor and close confinement, a visit to the country, where they can live a simple, carefree life, coming in close contact with the things of nature, will be most helpful. Roaming through the fields and the woods, picking the flowers, listening to the songs of the birds, will do far more than any other agency toward their recovery."—*Ministry of Healing, pp. 236-237.*

"All who are under the training of God need the quiet hour for communion with their own hearts, with nature, and with God . . When every other voice is hushed, and in quietness we wait before Him, the silence of the soul makes more distinct the voice of God. He bids us, 'Be still and know that I am God.' . . Amidst the hurrying throng, and the strain of life's intense activities, he who is thus refreshed, will be surrounded with an atmosphere of light and peace."—*Ministry of Healing, p. 58.*

"Nature will restore their vigor and strength in their sleeping hours, if her laws are not violated."—*Solemn Appeal to Mothers. p. 16*

"The influence of pure, fresh air is to cause the blood to circulate healthfully through the system. It refreshes the body, and tends to render it strong and healthy, while at the same time its influence is decidedly felt upon the mind, imparting a degree of composure and serenity. It excites the appetite, and renders the digestion of food more perfect, and induces sound, sweet sleep."—*1 Testimonies, p. 702.*

"The stomach, when we lie down to rest, should have its work all done, that it may enjoy rest, as well as other portions of the body. The work of digestion should not be carried on through any period of the sleeping hours."—*How to Live, p. 162.*

"Rooms that are not freely ventilated daily, and bedding that has not been thoroughly dried and aired, are not fit for use. We feel confident that disease and great suffering are brought on by sleeping in rooms with closed and curtained windows, not admitting pure air and the rays of the sun . . The room may not have had an airing for months, nor the advantages of a fire for weeks, if at all. It is dangerous to health and life to sleep in these rooms until the outside air shall have circulated through them

for several hours and the bedding shall have been dried by the fire. Unless this precaution is taken, the rooms and bedding will be damp. Every room in the house should be thoroughly ventilated every day, and in damp weather should be warmed by fires . . Every room in your dwelling should be daily thrown open to the healthful rays of the sun, and the purifying air should be invited in. This will be a preventive of disease . . If all would appreciate the sunshine, and expose every article of clothing to its drying, purifying rays, mildew and mold would be prevented."—*Healthful Living, pp. 142-143*

"One great error of the mother in the treatment of her infant is, she deprives it very much of fresh air, that which it ought to have to make it strong. It is a practice of many mothers to cover their infant's head while sleeping, and this, too, in a warm room, which is seldom ventilated as it should be. This alone is sufficient to greatly enfeeble the action of the heart and lungs, thereby affecting the whole system. While care may be needful to protect the infant from a draught of air or from any sudden and too great change, especial care should be taken to have the child breathe a pure, invigorating atmosphere."—*How to Live, p. 66.*

"Much harm has resulted to the sick from the universal custom of having watchers at night. In critical cases this may be necessary; but it is often the case that more harm is done the sick by this practice than good . . Even one watcher will make more or less stir, which disturbs the sick. But where there are two watchers, they often converse together, sometimes aloud, but more frequently in whispered tones, which is far more trying and exciting to the nerves of the sick than talking aloud. Attendants upon the sick should, if possible, leave them to quiet and rest through the night, while they occupy a room adjoining . . The sick as a general thing are taxed with too many visitors and callers, who chat with them, and weary them."—*How to Live, pp. 58-59.*

"Keep the patient free from excitement, and every influence calculated to depress. Her attendants should be cheerful and hopeful. She should have a simple diet, and should be allowed plenty of pure, soft water to drink. Bathe frequently in pure, soft water, followed by gently rubbing. Let the light and air be freely admitted into the room. She must have quiet and undisturbed rest."—*How to Live, pp. 54-55.*

"Many agitated people on the brink of a psychotic break suffer from severe insomnia."—*Archives of Neurology and Psychiatry.*

"I believe it can safely be said that all human beings need a minimum of six hours' sleep to be mentally healthy. Most people need more. Those who think they can get along on less are fooling themselves."—*Dr. George S. Stevenson, National Association for Mental Health.*

"If we do not get enough sleep, we cannot be fully awake during the day."—*Dr. Nathaniel Kleitman.*

SPIRITUAL LESSONS

Our kind, heavenly Father has not only given us a physical law of rest which we need for optimum health; He also knew we needed time to come apart and rest with Him,—time to worship Him and refresh ourselves in the things of God.

66 **THE EIGHT LAWS** THE REST YOUR BODY NEEDS NATURAL REMEDIES ENCYCLOPEDIA
OVER 11,000 REMEDIES - OVER 730 DISEASES

L
A
W
S

As soon as God created man, He gave him the seventh-day Sabbath. The Sabbath was designed to stop our ceaseless turmoil of the week, and draw apart to be with our Creator and with our families.

The Bible explains that the Sabbath was also given to remind us that God is our Creator.

"Wherefore the children of Israel shall keep the Sabbath, to observe the Sabbath throughout their generations, for a perpetual covenant. It is a sign between Me and the children of Israel for ever: for in six days the Lord made heaven and earth, and on the Seventh day He rested, and was refreshed" (Exodus 31:16-17).

It is crucial that we remember and honor our Creator, because it is the fact of God's creatorship that makes Him our God. Because of this we are to worship Him.

"Thou art worthy, O Lord, to receive glory and honour and power: for Thou hast created all things, and for Thy pleasure they are and were created" (Revelation 4:11).

God created all things from nothing (Hebrews 11:3), and hung the earth upon nothing (Job 26:7), upholds all things (Hebrews 1:3), and sustains life (Acts 17:28); He is our owner, ruler, and only God.

The Bible Sabbath—the seventh-day Sabbath—was made before man sinned. It was made on the seventh day of Creation Week.

"On the seventh day God ended His work which He had made; and He rested on the Seventh day from all His work which He had made. And God blessed the Seventh day, and sanctified it: because that in it He had rested from all His work which God created and made" (Genesis 2:2-3).

It is the only day of the week on which God rested, and the only day He blessed. In order to change that day to some other, He would have to abolish this world and create a new one! The Seventh day Sabbath is the day, fixed by the God of heaven, on which we are to worship Him.

When God wrote the Ten Commandments, He gave us the Fourth Commandment in its heart:

"Remember the Sabbath day to keep it holy . . The seventh day is the Sabbath of the Lord thy God . . In six days the Lord made heaven and earth . . and rested the Seventh day: wherefore the Lord blessed the Sabbath day, and hallowed it" (Exodus 20:8-11).

God does not change, and neither does His Sabbath change. "I am the Lord, I change not" (Malachi 3:6). "Thou blessest, O Lord, and it shall be blessed forever" (1 Chronicles 17:27). "God is not a man, that He should lie; neither the son of man, that He should repent . . He hath blessed; and I cannot reverse it" (Numbers 23:19-20).

The Sabbath was made for all men, not just the Jews. It was given to mankind 2,000 years before Abraham, the first Hebrew (Genesis 2:1-3). Jesus said, "The Sabbath was made for man, and not man for the Sabbath" (Mark 2:27). This does not mean for Jews only. Woman was created for man (1 Corinthians 11:9), but that does not mean women were only made for the Jews. The Sabbath is universal.

Abraham knew and obeyed God's laws. "Abraham obeyed My voice, and kept My charge, My commandments, My statutes, and My laws" (Genesis 26:5).

God brought forth Israel from Egypt, that they might obey Him and keep His laws. "He brought forth His people with joy, and His chosen with gladness . . that they might observe His statutes, and keep His laws" (Psalm 105:43-45).

Many blessings were promised to those who kept the Bible Sabbath. "If thou turn away thy foot from the Sabbath, from doing thy pleasure on My holy day; and call the Sabbath a delight, the holy of the Lord, honourable; and shalt honour Him, not doing thine own ways, nor finding thine own pleasure, nor speaking thine own words: then shalt thou delight thyself in the Lord; and I will cause thee to ride upon the high places of the earth, and feed thee with the heritage of Jacob thy father: for the mouth of the Lord hath spoken it" (Isaiah 58:13-14).

The seventh-day Sabbath was also the Sabbath of Jesus. Since Jesus was the Creator, He made the world and the Sabbath too (John 1:1-3, 14). "He came to Nazareth, where He had been brought up: and as His Custom was, He went into the synagogue on the Sabbath day, and stood up for to read" (Luke 4:16).

Jesus kept all His Father's commandments. He did not come to destroy them, but to show how they should be kept. "If ye keep My commandments, ye shall abide in My love; even as I have kept My Father's commandments, and abide in His love" (John 15:10).

He rested in the tomb on the Sabbath (Luke 23:52-54). His followers sacredly kept it also, for He had not taught them to keep any other day of the week.

"The women also, which came with Him from Galilee, followed after, and beheld the sepulchre, and how His body was laid. And they returned, and prepared spices and ointments; and rested the Sabbath day according to the commandment" (Luke 23:55-56).

His followers honored the Sabbath forty years after His death. He had commanded them to do so. "Pray ye that your flight be not in the winter, neither on the Sabbath day" (Matthew 24:20).

In Matthew 24, Jesus told His disciples what would occur at the destruction of the Temple and Jerusalem, and at the end of the world (Matthew 24:1-2). In verse 20, quoted above, Jesus told them to be sure and keep the Sabbath when those terrible events (the destruction of Jerusalem in A.D. 70, and the end of the world) should occur.

"Sin is the transgression of the law" (1 John 3:4), and Jesus never sinned (1 Peter 2:22). He always kept the Ten Commandments.

In Paul's time, the apostles kept the Bible Sabbath also. "When they departed from Perga, they came to Antioch in Pisidia, and went into the synagogue on the Sabbath day, and sat down." "And when the Jews were gone out of the synagogue, the Gentiles besought that these words might be preached to them the next Sabbath." "And the next Sabbath day came almost the whole city together to hear the Word of God" (Acts 13:14, 42, 44).

Paul, a servant of God, would have no more right than you or I to dishonor God and His sign of creatorship. He was a loyal observer of the Bible Sabbath. "This I confess unto thee, that after the way which they call heresy, so worship I the God of my fathers, believing all things which are written in the law and in the prophets" (Acts 24:14; also Acts 25:8).

The Sabbath will also be kept by the saved in the new earth.

NATURAL REMEDIES ENCYCLOPEDIA
OVER 11,000 REMEDIES - OVER 730 DISEASES   THE REST YOUR BODY NEEDS **THE EIGHT LAWS**   **67**

L
A
W
S

"As the new heavens and the new earth, which I will make, shall remain before Me, saith the Lord, so shall your seed and your name remain. And it shall come to pass, that from one new moon to another, and from one Sabbath to another, shall all flesh come to worship before Me, saith the Lord" (Isaiah 66:22-23).

"Blessed are they that do His commandments, that they may have right to the tree of life, and may enter in through the gates into the city" (Revelation 22:14).

How is the Sabbath related to the work of redemption?

First, redemption involves a work of creation. Since it takes creative power to redeem, God used the Sabbath as a sign of sanctification, or redemption. When He creates the new earth the Sabbath will continue on as the sign of God's peace and power. Throughout all eternity it will carry the double significance of a sign of power to create and to redeem (2 Corinthians 5:17; Psalm 51:10).

Second, the Sabbath is a sign of this sanctifying power.

"Verily My Sabbaths ye shall keep: for it is a sign between Me and you throughout your generations; that ye may know that I am the Lord that doth sanctify you" (Exodus 31:13).

"Moreover also I gave them My Sabbaths, to be a sign between Me and them, that they might know that I am the Lord that sanctify them . . And hallow My Sabbaths; and they shall be a sign between Me and you, that ye may know that I am the Lord your God" (Ezekiel 20:12, 20).

The Bible Sabbath is the special symbol of loyalty to God. It is God's flag. We dare not dishonor it. We are not to disregard it, lower it, or trample it beneath our feet. His Sabbath is a sign of loyalty to Him as Lord and Saviour.

What about the first day of the week (Sunday) in the Bible? It is only found eight times in the Bible. Here they are: The first day of Creation week (Genesis 1:3-5). No mention of sacredness here. It is mentioned six times as the day the resurrection occurred (Matthew 28:1; Mark 16:1-2, 9; Luke 24:1; John 20:1, 9), but no word or hint that it was now sacred. The disciples were in the upper room, but not to keep Sunday holy but "for fear of the Jews" (Mark 16:14: Luke 24:33-37). They were hiding from their enemies. The seventh occurrence of the first day is in Acts 20:7—Sunday is only mentioned once in the book of Acts! Paul spoke to the people, then resumed his traveling, and a couple days later held another meeting. The eighth time is the only mention of the first day by Paul: 1 Corinthians 16:1-2, where he asks the believers, while they are figuring up their weekly income from the previous week (which they would not do on the Sabbath, since it was holy time), to set aside some money at home for the poor in Jerusalem. Paul intended to later get the money from them.

So there is no Sunday sacredness in the Bible.

In the centuries since the Bible ended, the seventh day Sabbath has continued to be kept by faithful ones here and there. As for the weekly cycle, it has not changed over the centuries. There is historical, scientific, linguistic, and astronomical proof of that. Look in any encyclopedia. The number of days in the year have been altered, but the number of days in the week has not changed—going back through time immemorial. Everyone keeps the seven-day weekly cycle and it has never changed. The existence of the Jewish people is profound proof of this. All other Near-Eastern groups have disappeared, but the Jews have continued as a distinct people on down to the present time. And they have always kept the seventh-day Sabbath. Ask any Jew what day is the Sabbath, and he will tell you: It is the Seventh day of the week, Saturday.

Sunday is the first day of the week. Saturday is the Seventh day of the week. There is no authority for Sunday sacredness in Sacred Scripture. "To the law and to the testimony: if they speak not according to this Word, there is no light in them" (Isaiah 8:20).

Someone tried to change the Sabbath to Sunday. If the change is valid, who authorized it? Nowhere in the Bible do we find the change. God does not change (Malachi 3:6; James 1:17). The Ten Commandments are His own covenant (Deuteronomy 4:13). He will not break the covenant or alter His words (Psalm 89:34). He keeps His covenant for a thousand generations (Deuteronomy 7:9). His acts stand forever (Ecclesiastes 3:14).

We know that Jesus did not change the law and the Sabbath. Christ is the active agent in God's plans, by whom God created all things (Ephesians 3:9; 1 Corinthians 8:6) Christ, as Creator, made the Sabbath in the beginning, so He could not have come to earth to destroy it (John 1:1-3, 14; Genesis 2:1-3). We know, from Scripture, that it was Christ who led the Israelites in the wilderness, and who therefore gave them the law on Mount Sinai (Nehemiah 9:12-13 with 1 Corinthians 10:4).

While here on earth, Christ kept His Father's commandments (John 15:10). Jesus did no sin (1 Peter 2:22), and "sin is the transgression of the law" (1 John 3:4). Indeed, Christ came to fulfill (keep) the law, not to destroy it.

"Think not that I am come to destroy the law, or the prophets: I am not come to destroy, but to fulfil. For verily I say unto you, Till heaven and earth pass, one jot or one tittle shall in no wise pass from the law, till all be fulfilled. Whosoever therefore shall break one of these least commandments, and shall teach men so, he shall be called the least in the kingdom of heaven: but whosoever shall do and teach them, the same shall be called great in the kingdom of heaven" (Matthew 5:17-19).

The Greek word for "fulfill" means "to give a perfect example of." Christ came to magnify the law (Isaiah 42:21; Matthew 5:21-22, 27-28). He Himself kept the Sabbath (Luke 4:16). He openly ignored the Jewish Sabbath laws not found in the Bible (Luke 6:1-11). He indicated that the Sabbath was to be sacredly observed forty years after Calvary. "But pray ye that your flight be not in the winter, neither on the Sabbath day" (Matthew 24:20).

Did Paul change God's law or Sabbath? He would have no authority to do that; only the God of heaven could do that. And Paul specifically said that he did not attempt to do so. "Do we then make void the law through faith? God forbid: yea, we establish the law." (Romans 3:31).

However, keeping of the yearly sabbaths (the ceremonial sabbaths), was eliminated at Calvary (Colossians 2:16). This includes the Passover, Pentecost, etc.

Do men claim that there is Bible proof for the change? Roman Catholics say there is absolutely no Bible proof.

Cardinal Gibbons declared:

"You may read the Bible from Genesis to Revelation,

and you will not find a single line authorizing the sanctification of Sunday. The Scriptures enforce the religious observance of Saturday."—*Faith of Our Fathers, p. 89.*

Protestants agree:

"There was and is a commandment to keep holy the Sabbath day, but that Sabbath day was not Sunday. It will be said, however, and with some show of triumph, that the Sabbath was transferred from the Seventh to the first day of the week . . Where can the record of such a transaction be found? Not in the New Testament, absolutely not."—*Dr. Edward T. Hiscox, author of the Baptist Manual, in a paper read to a New York Ministers' Conference, November 13, 1893.*

Historians tell us the change did not come until long after the Bible was finished.

"Unquestionably the first law, either ecclesiastical or civil, by which the sabbatical observance of that day is known to have been ordained, is the edict of Constantine, A.D. 321."—*Chamber's Encyclopedia, article, "Sabbath."*

The Roman Catholic Church made the change over three centuries after Calvary.

"Q. Why do we observe Sunday instead of Saturday? A. We observe Sunday instead of Saturday because the Catholic Church, in the council of Laodicea [A.D. 336], transferred the solemnity from Saturday to Sunday."— *Peter Geiermann, Convert's Catechism of Catholic Doctrine, p. 50 [R.C.].*

For a better way of life, we want to enter more fully into God's rest for our souls. That rest is found, not only in physical rest, but also in the Sabbath rest. And our kind heavenly Father has promised that, if we keep His Sabbath holy, we will receive the blessing He placed in the keeping of that day!

Surely, that is not something we want to miss! We can always know that what God wants to give us—is always the best for us!

Thank the Lord for His wonderful blessings to us! He loves us more than we will ever know!

—*For more information on the Sabbath, go to page 1080.*

"My God shall supply all your need according to His riches in glory by Christ Jesus."—*Philippians 4:19.*

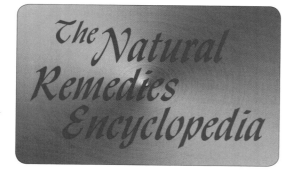

The Fifth Law of Health
The Exercise Your Obtain

God's plan for your life includes active exercise. Just now, for a few minutes, see what it can do for you.

Do you want to live longer? Here is how Dr. Roy J. Shepard, an expert on exercise and aging at the University of Toronto, explains it:

"You'd have to go a long way to find something as good as exercise as a fountain of youth. And you don't have to run marathons to reap the benefits. Little more than rapid walking for 30 minutes at a time three or four times a week can provide ten years of rejuvenation."

One of the early studies on the relationship of exercise to aging was done by Dr. Herbert de Vries. In one study of his, more than 200 men and women, ages 56 to 87 in a California retirement community, participated in a fitness program that included walking, a walk-jog routine, calisthenics, and stretching. After just six weeks, their blood pressure dropped, body fat decreased, maximum oxygen transport increased, and neuromuscular signs of nervous tension diminished. Analyzing the results, de Vries concluded:

"Men and women of 60 to 70 became as fit and energetic as those 20 to 30 years younger." And he added, "The ones who improved most were those who had been the least active and the most out-of-shape."

Later in this chapter we will give more information on how to use exercise to help lengthen your life.

Here is a brief summary of some of the things that regular exercise can begin doing for you right now:

(1) Exercise will improve the tone of your muscles and blood vessels, changing them from weak and flabby tissue to strong and firm tissue, often reducing blood pressure in the process. (2) It will increase the efficiency of your heart in several ways. Gradually it will grow stronger and pump more blood with each stroke, thus reducing the number of strokes needed to supply your body with life-giving blood. (3) It will improve your digestion by quickening the circulation and helping to lift the blood back to the heart from the digestive organs and thus normalizing your bowel action. (4) It will increase the efficiency of your lungs, conditioning them to process more air with less effort. (5) It will increase your maximum oxygen consumption by increasing the amount available and the efficiency of its delivery to body cells. (6) It will improve the overall condition of

NATURAL REMEDIES ENCYCLOPEDIA
OVER 11,000 REMEDIES · OVER 730 DISEASES   THE EXERCISE YOU OBTAIN   **THE EIGHT LAWS**   **69**

L
A
W
S

your body, especially your most vital parts: the lungs, heart, blood vessels, and endocrine system. This will impart added protection against sickness. (7) It can change your whole outlook on life, enabling you to relax, work more efficiently, and handle stress better. When not overdone, it imparts a cheerful quality to the mind. (8) It will enable you to sleep better at night and think better during the day. Exercise strengthens the will. You will be able to get more work done with less fatigue. (9) It will slow down your aging process—by slowing down the natural physical deterioration that old age normally brings. It will give you a new zest for life at a time when you most need it. And there is evidence that it can reduce the likelihood of cancer.

Now, let us look more closely at some of these facts:

Exercise, consistently done with proper moderation as the years advance, can help prevent heart attacks as well as many other ailments.

The blood vessels are carefully lined with smooth muscle fibers and if these special muscles do not receive adequate exercise, they gradually atrophy. The only way you can exercise a blood vessel is to put demand on the blood stream to provide more oxygen. When you exercise, your muscular tissues use up oxygen more rapidly. Your heart has to beat faster to pump along a new supply of oxygen-carrying blood to meet this demand. As your heart increases its pumping action it pushes more blood through the system. The blood vessels expand and contract in order to meet this demand. And this exercises them. Without that exercise, they become flabby and begin to degenerate.

Aside from the physiological benefit that exercise has on the heart, arteries and veins, it also improves muscle tone—which will stand one in good stead in emergencies. Then there is the improvement in digestion that takes place. And, have you had to deal with nervous tension? One of the best ways to counteract tension is the physical fatigue from healthful exercise. And that benefit cannot be stressed too much.

The involuntary muscles of the body—for example those in the stomach and intestinal canal—are strengthened by the exercise of their fibers equally as much as are the voluntary or external muscles. At the same time, the muscular structures of the body, such as the heart and uterus are improved.

Difficult and painful menstruation is often relieved by a general program of physical exercise and a careful diet composed of natural foods.

Physical exercise helps children grow. The proper development of their bones, muscles, and other body organs are keyed to physical activity. For some strange reason, children seem to sense their need of physical exercise more than do their elders.

The nervous system is improved functionally by body movements of any kind.

Exercise provides a powerful increase of oxygen to the body. Ordinarily, a man inhales about 500 cubic inches of air every minute. By walking about four miles per hour, he draws in about 2,500 cubic inches per minute,—or five times more than that absorbed when sitting down.

Physicians are now prescribing exercise as part of the recovery program for speeding up the recovery of surgical and maternity patients; preventing phlebitis, clots,

embolisms, kidney stones, and loss of calcium from the bones of bed patients. They require it for the restoration of physical and mental health in elderly invalids. It is given to help rehabilitate those who have has poliomyelitis, strokes, arthritis, accidental injury, and other neurologic and orthopedic disorders.

Researchers have learned that regular exercise tends to reduce blood pressure slightly, increase the pumping efficiency of the heart, and improve oxygen utilization by all the tissues in the body.

Dr. Richard W. Eckstein of Western Reserve University, conducted a significant series of tests. The coronary arteries of several dogs were surgically narrowed to simulate the atherosclerosis of the coronary artery. Half the dogs were then exercised and half were not. Five to eight weeks later, the exercised group showed decidedly more improvement in "collateral circulation." What had happened was that there was an increase in tiny blood vessels to bypass the narrowed artery. Many heart specialists believe that regular, moderate exercise will do the same for many people with coronary artery disease.

A lack of physical activity leads to abnormal or accelerated clotting of the blood in coronary, cerebral, and other arteries, as well as in the veins. In view of this, it is now felt that regular on-going activity all year long may be important in preventing or reducing strokes and coronary heart attacks. But it is thought that spurts of activity at intervals in an otherwise sedentary life will not accomplish this objective. Such physical exercise may even be harmful over a period of time. Yes, exercise is needed at every age of life, but in the later years we must obtain it in a more careful manner.

Other studies have shown that moderate or vigorous exercise can reduce blood cholesterol levels. And this is an important factor, for in atherosclerotic patients this level is often higher than it should be.

One comparative study was made of elderly men, who in college had been physical athletes. For the most part, they died from heart disease about as quickly as the rest of us. This was due to the fact that after leaving college they did not continue to exercise vigorously. Another research study, conducted by Drs. Paul White and William Pomeroy, analyzed the later living habits of 355 men who had been Harvard football players between 1901 and 1930. Their later exercise program—or lack of it—was compared with their health, longevity, and deaths. Across the board, those men who led sedentary lives did not live longer.

Dr. J.N. Morris, of the British Research Council, found that London bus drivers were more likely to die suddenly from coronary thrombosis than their fellow workers, the conductors, who walked about collecting tickets from the passengers. He also discovered that government clerks more frequently suffered from fatal coronary artery infarction than do the government postmen who were out on the streets delivering mail.

Do you want to live a long time? Exercise—regularly—moderately—but exercise. And do it for the rest of your life.

"Eventually we all decline," says Everett L. Smith, director of the Biogerontology Laboratory at the University of Wisconsin. "But the quality of life is so much higher for the elderly who are physically active than for people who sit waiting for the Grim Reaper."

Aging brings problems. And everyone past twenty is aging, without an exception. Each year after reaching maturity, the heart's ability to pump blood drops about one percent. That is a lot. By the time you are 60, the blood flow is 30 to 40 percent slower than when you were a young adult. With age, the amount of air that you can exhale after a deep breath lessens and your chest wall gradually stiffens. Nerve messages travel through your body at a slower speed: about 10-15% less by the time you have reached the age of 70.

But studies reveal that most of these age-associated declines can be delayed by exercise. For example, exercise lowers the resting heart rate and increases the amount of blood pumped with each beat. Exercise puts stress on the bones and causes them to have more calcium in them, thus making them stronger and less susceptible to fractures.

If you are young, anticipate the aging process and get ahead of it. If you are older, then get to work—begin a moderate exercise program to help keep you in shape for years to come.

Even though you may be older, exercise will improve your heart and respiratory function, increase your muscle strength, give you denser bones, quicker reaction time, and reduced susceptibility to depression and a number of diseases.

But, if you are over 50, exercise carefully. Avoid jumping and pounding activities. Yes, exercise, but do it carefully and properly. A little frequently, with a gradual buildup in your exercise program. And if you get stopped by sickness, start back slowly. The best objective is light exercise, such as walking for 30 minutes, three to five times weekly. Take it slow, gradually move up. Know your limit. Exercise regularly. Warm up first with stretching or slow walking. Cool down afterward by never stopping suddenly when it is done.

One of the great faults of our current civilization is that our young adults at about the age of 25 become "too busy" to exercise. Yet, for the next two decades of their lives, they probably need it even more than when they were children.

Walking is one of the simplest and best exercises. Go outdoors into the open air and walk. Leave all your cares behind you and briskly set off with your arms swinging. Take deep breaths of air as you go. Some people use a pedometer to count the distance walked. Other people, including this writer, employ what to them is a simpler method: clock it. Go for a brisk walk and come back 30 minutes or 60 minutes later.

Jogging is the great way to exercise—or is it? It is fine if you are young and do not stick with it too many years. This is what the experts are now conceding. Even Dr. Kenneth Cooper, the Dallas physician who helped launch the fitness boom in 1968 with his best-selling book, "Aerobics," has shifted gears after suffering from bone fractures and heel problems from years of jogging. "I've changed my mind," he says, "I'm running less and performing better." And that is where the problem lies: the bones and the joints. They were not made to take the punishment of running, day after day, month after month.

People are waking up to the fact that low-impact exercise is more beneficial in the long run than are the high-impact workouts. Instead of weight lifting, basketball, jogging, tennis; more people are turning to walking, hiking, and cycling.

A study published in the spring of 1986, in the "New England Journal of Medicine," described an analysis of nearly 17,000 Harvard alumni who entered the school between 1916 and 1950. It was found that those who engaged in such moderate exercise as walking and climbing stairs lived up to two years longer than their sedentary peers. Most significant of all was the fact that those who engaged in the "high-impact" vigorous exercises, such as jogging, did not gain any significant health advantage or longevity over those whose exercise program was also consistent each day, although less strenuous and exhausting.

The director of the study, Dr. Ralph Paffenbarger, of the Stanford University Medical School, discovered that the major health benefits came with only 2,000 calories burned off by exercise a week—which is only the equivalent of 2 1/2 to 3 hours of brisk walking every week, in addition to normal activity. Jogging may be great for some, but it is well to recognize, in advance, the foot and knee damage that may be developed later because of it.

But do not think that exercise is only for your off hours. Charles F. Kettering, the automotive genius, worked at full speed until his death at 82. Without any formal exercise program, he instead exercised all day long as he worked. There are ways to do this if you will carefully think them through. But it all adds up to more walking and less sitting.

But, please, do not try to get all your exercise at work. You need time to relax, breathe freely out-of-doors, put all your cares and worries behind you and just amble along. Time to look at the birds and listen to them; time to think of all the ways God has helped you; time to thank Him for it. Exercise, when not at work, is re-creative.

Gene Tunney advised his students:

"Take regular exercise—not violent weekends of golf or sporadic bursts of squash, but a daily drill that becomes as much a part of your life as brushing your teeth."

Dr. Arthur H. Steinhause, dean and professor of physiology at George Williams College, developed an exercise program that would also build some muscle in the process. And we can all use some of that.

"In a German laboratory where I worked, it was discovered that a muscle can grow at only a certain rate—and a very small amount of the right exercise will start it growing at that rate. If you contract any one of your muscles to about two-thirds of its maximum power and hold that for six seconds once a day, the muscle will grow just as fast as it can.

"Every day there are bound to be intervals when you have six seconds to relax. They can make a tremendous difference. Pull in your stomach. Pull up your chin. Do these exercises on company time. Do them while going from one place to another. Weave them into the day's routine."

Actually, exercising can be fun. And you need it,—both at your place of business and in your off hours.

Here are eight basic exercises which would fit in with Dr. Steinhaus' recommendations:

(1) Stretch—while sitting, lying, or standing. (2) Straighten your spine—while standing with your back against the wall. (3) Expand your chest. (4) Suck in your stomach—while sitting or bending over. (5) Flex your arms—by pushing, pulling, and reaching. (6) Bend your legs—by squatting, climbing, and walking. (7) Limber your toes and feet. (8) Firm your muscles—by bouncing, pinching, and kneading them.

A SAMPLE EXERCISE PROGRAM

Now, for a few moments, let us consider an ongoing exercise program, designed just for you. There are dozens of ways to do it; here is one:

If necessary, find a friend with whom to do this exercise program. You can help each other stick to it. But, with a friend or without one, the next step is to find your target heart rate (THR).

Your THR will help you exercise at just the right pace for you, so you won't overdo. Your THR is the most effective training pulse rate for maximum cardiovascular function and control of excess fat consumption for a person of your age and current level of fitness.

First, take your pulse. The easiest place to feel it is on the side of your neck. (Or you can take it on the thumbside of your wrist, palm up.) Use your first two fingers (not your thumb). Press lightly and count the number of beats per minute.

Now that you know how to take it, you will want to find your Resting Heart Rate (RHR). To be most accurate, take your pulse for a full minute when you first awake in the morning, while still lying down, on two consecutive mornings. The average of them is your Resting Heart Rate.

You then want to find your Target Heart Rate. Here is how to learn what it is:

Subtract your AGE from 220 to find your Predicted Maximum Heart Rate. This is the fastest that your heart should ever beat at your age. (Example: 220 minus 50 years of age equals 170.)

From your Predicted Maximum Heart Rate, subtract your Resting Heart Rate (the Pulse rate you found while lying in bed upon awakening). (Example: 170 minus 71 equals 99.)

At this point, you will want to select your Target Zone. This is your current level of fitness, and is a percent of your Maximum Heart Rate. If you are a beginning exerciser, this percentage will be 60%. If you are already doing it regularly, it can be 70%. Competitive athletes will use 80%. Now, multiply the above total by this percentage (Example: 99 times .60 equals 59.4, which we will round off to 59.)

Add to this your Resting Heart Rate, and you have your Target Heart Rate. (Example: 59 plus 71 equals 130.)

It only took a few moments to figure, and now you have your Target Heart Rate. In order to quickly determine it later, just now divide your THR by 6. This will give you your 10-second Target Heart Rate. Henceforth, you will only need to take your pulse for ten seconds in order to see how you vary from your THR. (Example: 130 divided by 6 equals 21.6, which rounds to 22.)

Of course, this formula is only a guide. You will want to watch your own body for signs of overexertion (such as pounding in your chest, a dizzy or faint feeling,

or profuse sweating). Breathlessness is another important sign to be alert to.

As time passes on this program, you may find that your Resting Heart Rate will lower somewhat.

During your exercise program of fast walking, etc., you will want to take your pulse as soon as you begin sweating lightly and breathing harder. If you are below your Target Heart Rate, then stride, stroke, pedal, or push a little harder. If you are above your THR, then slow down a bit and take it easy.

Then there is your Recovery Rate. This is how long it takes for your pulse to return to normal. To find this, take your pulse once a minute after you stop your main exercise program each day. It is good for your heart that you cool down slowly, and you are checking on your Recovery Rate at the same time. (Example: Ideally, your pulse should have dropped below 100 beats per minute within 3-5 minutes.)

Before you begin your exercise workout, warm up with a few stretching exercises for 5 minutes. Then begin your active program to keep FIT. F—Frequency: Exercise 3-5 times a week. Four times is ideal, with a day off between workouts to avoid "overuse injury." I—Intensity: Work up to your Target Heart Rate, but do not pass it. T—Time: Do it for at least 20 minutes.

What kind of exercise should this be? Select one that is steady, rhythmic, and continuous. It should place an increased oxygen demand on your heart, lungs, and muscles. And it should use the large-muscle groups of your body (legs, arms, and back). Then comes the cooling down period. This should be for at least 5 minutes. By cooling down slowly, you safely lower your pulse from your Target Heart Rate to normalcy. This both protects your heart and helps prevent injuries from stiff muscles, and is the ideal time for stretching exercises, since warm muscles stretch best and feel better later.

One inventive athletic researcher came up with this way to check yourself while exercising: If you can't talk comfortably while exercising, you're working too hard. If you can sing, then you're not working hard enough.

(Of course, before starting any kind of exercise program, you do best to have a medical evaluation first, if you have a heart condition or family history of heart disease, hypertension, diabetes, other medical problem, or it you are overweight, over 35, or use tobacco.)

Some people do "cross-training." They alternate between, say, walking, one day, and then swimming; then, next time, they work out. Each activity is done twice a week to maintain good physical stamina. But if all you have opportunity to keep up is a brisk walk, then do that. There is no better exercise.

You might want to keep an Exercise Log, jotting down each time what you did, how long you did it, and the date.

If your exercise is walking, be sure and do it in a good pair of shoes that are comfortable, good fitting, with soles that are cushioned and flexible.

Here are some sample stretching exercises to limber you up during your 5-minute warm-up period: (1) Roll your shoulders several times in each direction. Imagine each shoulder is a wheel. First, turn the wheels forward, as though they were car tires taking you down the road;

then put the gears into reverse and rotate them backwards several times. (2) Reach your right arm up straight and then stretch your right side up and over toward your left side, as you tilt your body away from that raised arm, all the while keeping your shoulder straight up from your trunk. Then do the other arm, keeping your hips steady throughout. (3) With your head, hips, and feet in a straight line,—pull one knee up to your chest. Then do the other knee. (4) Keeping your knee pointing straight downward to the ground,—reach back and pull your foot up to your buttocks with your opposite hand. Use the other hand to steady yourself, with a slight lean against a wall or tree. (5) With one foot about 12 inches behind the other, bend your front knee, and keeping both knees aimed forward,—press your back heel unto the ground and stretch your calf muscle.

Each of the above exercises was done while standing, and each stretched certain muscles.

With your warm-up stretching completed, for a minute or two, slowly begin walking. Now you can speed up for your regular 20-minute work out, checking your THR as you go.

After your workout is over, slow down for a minute or two, and then stop and begin your cooling-down stretching exercises. These can be the five described just above.

Exercise is one of the most helpful of the Eight Laws of Health, but it works closely with all of the others, especially rest and proper diet. How thankful we can be to God for these many blessings.

ADDITIONAL PRINCIPLES

"By active exercise in the open air every day, the liver, kidneys, and lungs also will be strengthened to perform their work."—*Counsels on Health, p. 54.*

"Without physical exercise no one can have a sound constitution and vigorous health; and the discipline of well-regulated labor is no less essential to the securing of a strong, active mind and a noble character."—*Counsels to Teachers, p. 307.*

"Exercise aids the dyspeptic by giving the digestive organs a healthy tone. To engage in severe study or violent physical exercise immediately after eating, hinders the work of digestion; but a short walk after a meal, with the head erect and the shoulders back, is a great benefit."—*Ministry of Healing, p. 240.*

"Such exercise would in many cases be better for the health than medicine. Physicians often advise their patients to take an ocean voyage, to go to some mineral spring or to visit different places for change of climate, when in most cases if they would eat temperately, and take cheerful, healthful exercise, they would recover health, and would save time and money."—*Ministry of Healing, p. 240.*

"Exercise in a gymnasium, however well conducted, cannot supply the place of recreation in the open air."—*Education, p. 210.*

"What does a person do who has been sitting at his desk for many hours and is tired? Does he lie down? No! He takes a walk. What do children do when they come home from school and are tired? Do they go to sleep? No! They run to the playground. If the body is completely exhausted by strenuous labor, a long hike, a wash-day, or a moving-day, one recuperates best by lying down and permitting the organism to rest. However, if only a certain part of the body is tired—for instance, the brain by long calculations, the hands from many hours of typing, the eyes by too much reading or sewing, or the legs when one has had to stand very long—the tired limb or organ recuperates best if other rested parts of the body are active.

"If one lies down, all the activities of the body are curtailed; in a manner of speaking, the vital furnace of the body is banked. The heart beats slowly, the blood vessels contract, respiration becomes shallow, and the exhausted brain sleeps, so that all the organs are at rest. On the other hand, if one enters into some new activity, if after a long lecture one goes out into the fresh air, thus exposing oneself to new impressions and stimuli, to the cool air and the fragrance of flower beds, respiration is increased, the blood circulates faster, and the glands are more active, thus facilitating the elimination of waste products from the exhausted organ. If you are totally exhausted, go to sleep! If only part of your body is tired, go for a walk or take a swim, engage in athletics, or occupy yourself with your garden. There is no better form of rest for an exhausted organ than the activity of neighboring organs."—*Fritz Kahn, "Man in Structure and Function," Vol. 1, p. 136.*

SPIRITUAL LESSONS

We not only want to maintain a daily physical exercise program, we also need to stretch our spiritual muscles each day as well. Not only are we to accept Jesus as our Saviour, we are to work with Him to help minister to the needs of others.

Just as God gave, we need also to give. "God so loved the world, that He gave His only begotten son, that whosoever believeth in Him should not perish, but have everlasting life" (John 3:16).

Jesus told His followers: "Freely ye have received, freely give" (Matthew 10:8). He also said, "It is more blessed to give than to receive" (Acts 20:35).

Because we have been comforted, in Christ's strength we are able to comfort others. "[God] who comforteth us in all our tribulation, that we may be able to comfort them which are in any trouble, by the comfort wherewith we ourselves are comforted of God" (2 Corinthians 1:4).

There are many in the world who need our help. God calls for helpers, and we must answer the call. "I heard the voice of the Lord, saying, Whom shall I send, and who will go for us? Then said I, Here am I; send me" (Isaiah 6:8).

We are to do the work which Jesus did. "The Spirit of the Lord God is upon Me; because the Lord hath anointed Me to preach good tidings unto the meek; He hath sent Me to bind up the brokenhearted, to proclaim liberty to the captives, and the opening of the prison to them that are bound" (Isaiah 61:1; *cf.* Luke 4:18).

We live our faith, we share our faith, and we come to Jesus to renew and deepen our faith. As we pray and work, work and pray, our experience deepens, and others are helped.

"Who then is a faithful and wise servant, whom his lord hath made ruler over his household, to give them meat in due season? Blessed is that servant, whom his lord when he cometh shall find so doing. Verily I say unto you, That he shall make him ruler over all his goods" (Matthew

24:45-47).

Every follower of Jesus is assigned the task of helping those around them, and sharing with them the wonderful gospel message of the forgiving and empowering grace of Christ, and the hope of eternal life through Him.

"And He said unto them, Go ye into all the world, and preach the gospel to every creature" (Mark 16:15). "I am not ashamed of the gospel of Christ: for it is the power of God unto salvation to every one that believeth" (Romans 1:16). "And this gospel of the kingdom shall be preached in all the world for a witness unto all nations; and then shall the end come" (Matthew 24:14).

God purposes to use you and me to help many souls who are living in darkness. "I the Lord have called thee in righteousness, and will hold thine hand, and will keep thee, and give thee for a covenant of the people, for a light of the Gentiles; to open the blind eyes, to bring out the prisoners from the prison, and them that sit in darkness out of the prison house" (Isaiah 42:6-7).

We can help the poor and the needy. "I was a father to the poor, and the cause which I knew not I searched out" (Job 29:16). "Pure religion and undefiled before God and the Father is this, To visit the fatherless and widows in their affliction, and to keep himself unspotted from the world" (James 1:27). "He shall deliver the needy when he crieth; the poor also, and him that hath no helper" (Psalm 72:12). "Whoso stoppeth his ears at the cry of the poor, he also shall cry himself, but shall not be heard" (Proverbs 21:13).

We can also minister to the sick, and help them understand the importance of obedience to God's commandments so they might remain in better health. "Pray for one another, that ye may be healed" (James 5:16). "Thou shalt therefore keep the commandments . . and the Lord will take away from thee all sickness" (Deuteronomy 7:11, 15). "[God] who forgiveth all thine iniquities; who healeth all thy diseases" (Psalm 103:3).

As we minister to the needs of others, and bring them the good news of salvation, through the forgiving/enabling grace of Christ, we have the promise that we are working with the angels of God. Even though our efforts may not be appreciated by those on earth, yet the God of heaven accepts us. Thank the Lord!

"For what is our hope, or joy, or crown of rejoicing? Are not even ye in the presence of our Lord Jesus Christ at His coming? For ye are our glory and joy" (1 Thessalonians 2:19-20).

"As the heaven is high above the earth, so great is His mercy toward them that fear Him."—Psalm 103:11.

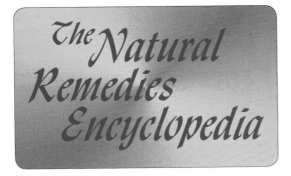

The Natural Remedies Encyclopedia

The Sixth Law of Health
The Food You Eat

The human body was created by the God of heaven on the sixth day of Creation Week. It is marvelously made.

Because of this, we have a special responsibility, as His children, to carefully obey His health laws. He has provided bountifully from the things of nature for our care; and it is our responsibility to use these blessings to keep ourselves in good health, so that we may better minister to the needs of those around us.

We can live as did Daniel, in full obedience to all of God's laws. A basic aspect of this is the diet we choose. Our physical health is maintained by that which we eat; for that which you put into your body affects all of your organs and tissues. A wrong diet, or an indulged appetite of a good one, greatly hinders mental and physical efficiency. An improper diet not only injures our bodies, but keeps our minds from functioning as well as they should. For example, an intemperate man cannot be a patient men.

Eating the right amount of the right food, and only at regular hours, is what is needed. The food should be of a simple, healthful quality, and eaten slowly in an atmosphere of cheerful thankfulness to God for His many blessings. In order to understand these matters aright, we need individually to reason from cause to effect, study the Word of God, and act from principle. We dare not let the fads and fashions of the world become our criteria.

All of our enjoyment or suffering may be traced to obedience or transgression of natural law. To make these laws plain, and to urge their obedience in the strength of God—is the special work for our time in history. Men of God in Bible times carefully obeyed the moral and health laws; and we should obey them today. A significant aspect of this is the fact that the body is the only medium through which the mind and the soul are developed for the upbuilding of character. How important it is, then, that we do all in our power to yield ourselves in obedience to God's pattern for our lives. This is the greatest work we can do. And we can be thankful that He will, by His enabling grace, strengthen us to fulfill His will.

The original diet, given by Heaven to our human family, consisted of grains, fruits, nuts, and vegetables. These foods, prepared in as simple and natural a way as possible, are the most healthful and nourishing. They impart a strength, a power of endurance, and a vigor of intellect, that are not afforded by a more complex and stimulating diet.

This diet that God gave to our first parents did not include meat. It is contrary to His plan to have the life of any of His creatures taken in order to supply us with food. He desires to bring us back to this original plan. He does not want us to subsist upon the flesh of dead animals.

And this diet should be a simple one. It is very easy to take simple food—and make a complicated dish out of it that is hard to digest. Our diet should be simple: composed of simple food, simply prepared. By this is meant simple, healthful food, both raw or properly cooked, free from spices, grease, flesh meats, and complicated mixtures. Raw food is good, but warm food is needed by the system also. Eating only cold food draws vitality from the body to heat it up in the stomach prior to its digestion. Also helpful is the eating of fewer kinds of food at a meal, and eating it with thanksgiving. A cheerful heart will help your food digest better. Simply prepared meals will be more nourishing for your family and guests. Fashionable eating with its many dishes, mixtures, and hurtful foods is an invitation to gluttony. And this, of course, you do not want.

The diet also needs to be adequate. Do not consider it a matter of indifference as to what you eat. Your diet should not be impoverished, but nourishing, for only in this way can your body make good blood. Perfect health is keyed to perfect circulation, and this cannot be done without good blood.

Fruits, grains, vegetables, and nuts, prepared in a simple way—free from meat or spice or grease of every kind,—constitute the most healthful diet. It requires careful thought to prepare nourishing food. This effort requires faith in God, earnestness of purpose, and a willingness to help one another. We are mortal and must supply ourselves with food that will give proper sustenance to the body.

Investigate your habits of diet and study from cause to effect. You do not want a rich, greasy, complicated worldly diet, but neither do you want a skimpy, impoverished one. There are healthful foods that you need. Do not avoid them.

However, in some cases, you will find certain articles of diet that do not agree with you. For example, beans bother some people. In such instances, change the diet; use less of some foods; try other things. And be alert to food combinations; some are healthful and some are not. Individually study this matter for yourself and come to your own decisions as to what you shall eat. There is no doubt but that there is generally an ample variety of foods from which to select.

In making this choice, keep in mind the climate. Certain foods may be suitable for one country and not for another, or for one season of the year and not for another. Then, too, there is the matter of your occupation. If you are engaged in hard, physical labor, you can eat somewhat

more amply than can a more sedentary person.

The warmer the climate, the less severe our physical work should be, and the less food is correspondingly needed. In connection with this, too much sugar in the diet, in hot weather or in a hot climate, can cause trouble.

Yet no precise line of diet is marked out for those living in various seasons, climates, and countries. As you depend on Him for help, God will guide you from day to day.

In those lands in which an abundance of fresh fruits, grains, and nuts are available, flesh food is not necessary. And in countries in which there is an extra abundance of fruit throughout most of the year, we should make use of it.

God will guide His children to develop simple, healthful recipes that will help many others. Develop your talents and learn how to develop more healthful meals.

In order to better understand these things, we need to better understand the process of normal digestion within our bodies. Overeating injures the stomach and weakens all the digestive organs. Disease is thus brought on. Too much vital power is being expended in trying to digest so much food. The immediate effect may be headache, indigestion, pain, or temporary stoppage of digestion. Eat sparingly of the best food. Allow nothing to pass your lips that in any way might weaken your health and life. Constantly study from cause effect, as you go from meal to meal, day to day.

That which we need more of is spiritual food—study in God's Word,—for that will give us overcoming power in controlling our selection and intake of physical food.

Overeating has a worse effect on the body than overworking. The excess food only clogs the system, burdens the life, and, if continued, leads to disease. Too much food, even of the right quality, is harmful. Eat moderately, of the right food, and only at regular periods.

Do not study, or do heavy work or violent exercise immediately after a meal. As soon as it is concluded, both the blood and brain power are needed in aiding in its digestion. When the meal is completed, go outside and take a short walk, with your head erect and your shoulders back. This light exercise will greatly help your digestion. Your mind is thus diverted from yourself to the things of nature about you. And that is another benefit of the after-meal walk.

There are far too many people who worry about their food. Eat it cheerfully, with a sense of thankfulness to God. Do the best you can, and then go about your work believing that He will bring the best. If you are in constant fear that your food will hurt you, it most assuredly will. Forget it—and all your other problems too. Think of something cheerful and trust that all will work out for the best.

Pure, fresh air, breathed in through lungs unhindered by tight clothing or belts or lacing, will greatly help your digestion. This is no unimportant detail. It is better to suspend your clothing from the shoulders, instead of using belts. Avoid cramping or compressing your lungs or your abdomen.

Do not spend most of your time thinking about yourself. Act from principle, and then live to bless others.

There are a number of foods which it is best to eliminate or minimize in our diets. A meal of only cold food should not be partaken. Warm it first. Hot drinks and hot food debilitate the stomach; very cold foods require too much vital force in order to be warmed up in the stomach prior to digestion. Cold water drunk with the meal diminishes the flow of saliva. The colder the food or water, the greater the injury to the stomach. Ice water or ice lemonade stops digestion until it is warmed up. Food that is washed down with liquids results in poor digestion. When liquids are taken with meals, the stomach must absorb the liquid before it can begin to digest the food. Overworking the stomach in many little ways can add up to more serious problems at a later time.

When you sit down to a meal, take time to eat. Chew your food slowly, and do not crowd in a great variety of food at one meal. The benefit derived from food depends less on the quantity eaten than on how thoroughly it was masticated, and digested. The amount of time the food is in the mouth and how well it is chewed are both very important to thorough digestion. In order to do this effectively, it is necessary to eat your food slowly.

Do not have too great a variety at a meal; three or four dishes are plenty. It is more important that we eat that which will agree with us than that we taste of every dish set before us.

It is well not to eat fruit and vegetables at the same meal. Vary the meals from day to day. All mixed and complicated foods are injurious to the health.

And, above all, do not overeat. It is one of the quickest avenues to disease and death. Especially should sedentary workers be careful in regard to this point.

It is best that five hours elapse between meals. Two meals a day are better than three, especially for those who obtain relatively little exercise. Late suppers, just before bedtime, are particularly harmful. If eaten at all, the third meal should be light and several hours before bedtime.

Eat your meals at regular times and between meals eat nothing.

Fruit is a wonderful blessing from God. Whenever it is available, you will want to make use of it. Fresh fruit, freshly picked, is especially good. It would be well to do less cooking and eat more fruit raw. But also preserve them in sealed jars for winter usage. Fruits of different kinds—but not too many kinds—at a meal are very fine. But even fruit should not be eaten after a full meal of other foods.

Never eat fruit if it has any decay on it. Decayed vegetables and fruit ferment in the stomach and poison the blood. As with grains, nuts, and vegetables, prepare the fruit for the table in as simple a manner as possible.

Brain workers do well, from time to time, on a fruit diet for a day or two.

The dried fruits are very helpful in the diet. Apples are one of the best standby storage fruits that you can find.

The grains are another blessing from our Creator. When you eat grains and vegetables, you are obtaining your food first-hand; but when you eat meat, you are getting it second-hand. The needs of the system can be better supplied, and muscular strength maintained without the use of animal flesh. The grains, along with peas, beans, and lentils, are foods that store well. Do not use grease on your grains or in preparing them. This principle applies to the preparation of fruits and vegetables also.

Grains used for porridge or cooked cereal should have several hours' cooking. But even then, they are still less wholesome than dry foods which require careful chewing. For this reason, to eat largely of cereals does not ensure health to the digestive organs, for they are too much like liquid. Instead, eat fruit, vegetables, and bread.

Bread should be thoroughly baked, and should be light and dry. Do not use baking powder or soda when preparing it. The strong alkalinity of soda injures the stomach. Use water in making bread, instead of milk. Milk bread does not keep sweet as long, and ferments in the stomach. The loaves should be small, with no taint of sourness. Never eat fresh raised bread (yeast bread) before it is a day old. And two- or three-day-old bread is more healthful still. (This is because there is no baker's yeast remaining in it by then.) But unleavened bread—without yeast—can be eaten fresh out of the oven.

Zwieback is bread that has been baked a second time. ("Zwieback" means "twice baked.") This transforms the bread into one of the most easily masticated and digestible foods you can find. Simply cut ordinary raised bread into slices and then lay it in a warm oven to dry until the last trace of moisture disappears. Then let it be browned slightly all the way through. If kept dry, zwieback can be kept much longer than regular bread, and it can be reheated before using, to freshen it up. Since it is so easily digested, zwieback does well, along with fruit, for the evening meal.

Beware of partially baked bread. If it is soft, doughy, or sticky inside, do not eat it. Hot, raised biscuits should not be eaten. Sour bread is not healthful either. Do not put sour milk into your bread mix.

Whole wheat bread is far better than white bread. Sweet breads and sweet cookies cause problems in the stomach.

Thank God for the good vegetables that we can serve to our families. They afford us solid nourishment. When picked fresh from the garden, they are the best. Hearty, hard-working men need plenty of vegetables. Such a simple diet is by far the best for us.

God wants to bring His people back to simple fruits, vegetables, and grains. These have the nutritive properties that our bodies need. This is the food needed, not meat or grease.

There are those who are not able to digest certain vegetables as well as others.

Avoid fried foods, or any food that has been prepared with grease or butter (or margarine). These clog the system and lead to serious trouble later on.

Raw and cooked greens are among the most nourishing foods obtainable. Other good foods include such items as tomatoes, corn, or peas. But never use decayed vegetables.

It would be well to obtain a piece of land so you can grow fruits and vegetables.

Sugar is a real problem. People use far too much of it in preparing their food, and yet it causes fermentation in the stomach. Milk and sugar combined is one of the worst combinations you can find, yet the two are mixed into breads, puddings, pastries, and other things.

Sugar clogs the system. Some people try to make sugar supply the place of good food, properly cooked. But the result is sickness and disease. Sugar, overused in the diet, is worse than meat eating. Avoid eating the sweet foods that are prepared. Candies and confections are best kept out of the diet.

A little sweetening, such as honey, mixed in with the preserved fruits is helpful. It is not wrong to use a little milk or a little sweetening. But only a little sugar is all that is needed. Some put a lot of it on their mush, or use milk and sugar mixtures. But this is not healthful. Milk, eggs, and sugar mixed together in recipes are not good either.

Pies, cakes, pastries, and puddings may taste good, but this does not make them good for you. Many of these desserts are detrimental to health. Rich dinners, highly flavored sauces, sweet delicacies, sweet cakes, sweet puddings, and custards would be better omitted from the diet entirely. Often spices are added, which only makes the mixture worse. The jellies, jams, and all the rest are an active cause of indigestion.

Instead, use fruit. Fruit, fresh or stored in jars, can provide your family with the nourishment that the other treats, mentioned above, lack. But plain, simple pies, with a small amount of sweetening is helpful—as long as you stay with only one piece.

Other worthwhile desserts would include plain cake with raisins, rice pudding with raisins, prunes, and figs.

Always be careful in regard to the sweet things. They are not really needed, and they can be harmful to your system.

Spices and condiments, so frequently used in our world today, are ruinous to the digestion. The less exciting the food, the better. Mustard, pepper, spices, pickles, and similar articles only irritate the stomach and fever the blood. Condiments have a similar effect on the stomach as does drinking alcohol. And both begin a subtle craving for something more stimulating to eat or drink.

In reality, the use of spicy food develops a craving that leads many onward to become alcoholics. Yet many place these luxurious foods before their children,—spiced foods, rich gravies, cakes, and pastries. This highly seasoned food irritates the stomach and causes a craving for still stronger stimulants.

Those who have indulged in such foods find it difficult to sit down to a meal of simple, wholesome food. But if they will stick with it, their enjoyment of simple food will return.

Soda, or baking powder, should never be placed in your breads when you are preparing them. Soda inflames the stomach and often poisons the entire system. But good bread can be made without them.

Do not use much salt in your diet. Some people advocate a no-salt regime, but this is not good. A little salt is needed in the diet, but only a little.

Pickles and vinegar should not be eaten. (Soda and baking powder are very high alkaline products that remain excessively alkaline in the system; pickles and vinegar are the opposite; they are excessively acid and likewise derange the delicate gastrointestinal track.) It would be well if pickles, vinegar, mustard, mince pies, and such things were entirely omitted from the diet.

Folk often put vinegar and oil on their salads. (Mayonnaise is a vinegar, oil, and raw egg combination.) Yet the vinegar causes a fermentation in the stomach, and the food does not digest but instead decays or putrefies. As a consequence of such a diet, the blood is not nourished, but instead becomes filled with impurities. Eventually liver and kidney problems develop.

The effect of butter in the body is quite different than that of cream. (Chemically, cream is composed of oil droplets surrounded by water, and thus is relatively more digestible. When churned, cream becomes butter, which is water droplets locked into an ocean of hardened oil. This grease-like substance causes very serious problems in the digestive system, and later in the blood vessels. Never eat anything that is grease-like.) It is best to dispense with butter and not use it at all.

It has been said that a little milk or cream in the diet is helpful, but you need to know that it is well to work away from their use. Soon there will be no safety in using eggs, milk, or cream. This is due to the increase in animal diseases. God will give His people ability to prepare food without these substances.

If eggs are used at all, they should be from hens that you know to be well-cared for and suitably fed. It is best that children have few, if any eggs. Milk should come from livestock that you know to be healthy, be boiled first, and only used in moderate amounts.

Some individuals, in abstaining from milk and eggs, have failed to supply the system with proper nourishment, and as a consequence have become weak and unable to work. Still others cannot afford the better food, such as nuts and fruit. And there are those who do not know how to properly supply the place of milk and eggs with other foods. They need instruction.

The time has not yet come to prescribe the strictest diet for others to follow. But let the diet be progressive. Let the people be taught how to prepare food without the use of milk. Tell them that soon there will be no safety in using eggs, milk, cream, or butter, because disease in animals is increasing. Do know that the time will come when it will not be safe for anyone to use milk and eggs. (Many believe that that time has already come.)

Animals from which milk is obtained are not always healthy. They may be diseased so that a cow, apparently well in the morning, dies before night. Then she was diseased in the morning, and her milk was diseased, but you did not know it.

Cheese should never be introduced into the stomach. It is wholly unfit for food.

Lard and grease clog the system. The body cannot handle them. Keep grease out of your food. It defiles any preparation of food you may make. It renders the food difficult of digestion (and produces a clogging of the arteries, leading to heart attacks later on). For example, fried potatoes are not healthful, for grease or butter is used in preparing them. Instead of this, serve baked or boiled potatoes with cream and a sprinkling of salt.

Eat only food that is free from grease. Such a diet will prove a blessing to you, and will avoid later suffering and grief.

Olives may be so prepared that they may be eaten with good results at each meal. They can take the place of butter. Olives and nuts, along with the other protein vegetables, can supply the place of butter and flesh meats.

Nuts and nut foods are coming largely into use to take the place of flesh foods. Care must be taken not to use too large a proportion of nuts. Time should be spent learning how to prepare the nut foods, but do not eat too heavily of them.

Some kinds of nuts are not as wholesome as others. Do not reduce the diet to a few articles composed largely of nut foods. They should not be used too freely. Combined in large proportions with other articles in recipes, they make the food so rich that it cannot be properly assimilated. One-tenth to one-sixth part of nuts to other foods is sufficient in recipes, varied according to the combination.

Almonds are preferable to peanuts, but peanuts, in limited quantities, may be used with grains to make nourishing food.

Water is the best liquid possible to cleanse the tissues of the body, but take it between meals rather than with your meals. Especially do not use hot drinks or cold drinks at mealtime. Warm or hot water taken a half hour or so before the meal is helpful.

Tea, coffee, tobacco, alcohol, and the narcotics are not good for your body and should never be used. Such things may at first appear to stimulate and excite the nerves, but trembling nerves and lack of self-control will later result. Tired nerves need rest and quiet, not artificial stimulation. Intemperance begins at our tables, in the use of unhealthful food. Then stimulants are resorted to, and the nerves, artificially excited, borrow from the future. Later comes sickness and nervous prostration. The only safety is to leave them totally alone.

Be careful of apple cider. It is often made of wormy or half-rotten apples. And it may have some alcoholic content.

Fresh and properly prepared fruit juices are wholesome and a blessing from God.

How very thankful we can be that the God of heaven has provided us with wonderfully designed bodies, and so many blessings in nature to keep us in good health. He is our Creator and how we love Him. Let us carefully use each of the Eight Laws of Health—pure air, sunlight, abstemiousness, rest, exercise, proper diet, the use of water, and trust in divine power,—to keep ourselves in the best health in our daily service to Him.

A brief summary of some of the basics in this invaluable instruction would include several of these points:

The meal should be simple, appetizing, but not complicated, or hot, cold, or too liquid. Eat unhurriedly and at regular hours, chewing well, and without overeating. The diet itself is best to consist of fruit, vegetables (especially greens), grains, and some nuts. Be cautious about the many highly processed, sweet, and spiced foods. Exercise afterward and eat nothing between meals. Throughout the day, be cheerful, positive, and live to help and bless others. Let gratitude to God fill your thoughts, and praise Him who cares for you.

ADDITIONAL PRINCIPLES

"God gave our first parents the food He designed that the race should eat . . The fruit of the trees in the garden was the food man's wants required [Genesis 1:29: and afterward, field crops also, Genesis 3:17-18]. God gave man no permission to eat animal food until after the Flood. Everything had been destroyed upon which man could subsist, and therefore the Lord in their necessity gave Noah permission to eat of the clean animals which he had taken with him into the ark [Genesis 9:3] . .

"After the Flood the people ate largely of animal food. God saw that the ways of man were corrupt, and that he was disposed to exalt himself proudly against his Creator and to follow the inclinations of his own heart. And He permitted that long-lived race to eat animal food to shorten their sinful lives. Soon after the Flood the race began to rapidly decrease in size, and in length of years. [Compare Genesis 5:3-32 with 11:10-26]."—*Counsels on Diet and Foods, p. 373.*

"In choosing man's food in Eden, the Lord showed what was the best diet; in the choice made for Israel, He taught the same lesson [Psalm 105:37]. He brought the Israelites out of Egypt, and undertook their training, that they might be a people for His own possession. Through them He desired to bless and teach the world. He provided them with the food best adapted for this purpose, not flesh, but manna, 'the bread of heaven' [Exodus 16; Psalm 78:24]. It was only because of their discontent and their murmurings for the fleshpots of Egypt that animal food was granted them, and this only for a short time. Its use brought disease and death to thousands [Numbers 11:4-12, 31-33; Psalm 78:17-37]. Yet the restriction to a nonflesh diet was never heartily accepted. It continued to be the cause of discontent and murmuring, open or secret, and it was not made permanent."—*Counsels on Diet and Foods, p. 374.*

"Had they been willing to deny appetite in obedience to His restrictions, feebleness and disease would have been unknown among them [Exodus 23:25; Psalm 107:4-9]. Their descendants would have possessed physical and mental strength. They would have had clear perceptions of truth and duty, keen discrimination, and sound judgment. But they were unwilling to submit to God's requirements, and they failed to reach the standard He had set for them, and to receive the blessings that might have been theirs. They murmured at God's restrictions, and lusted after the fleshpots of Egypt. [Psalm 106:13-15]. God let them have flesh, but it proved a curse to them [1 Corinthians 10:5-6]."—*Counsels on Diet and foods, p. 378.*

SPIRITUAL LESSONS

We have our physical food which we need to partake of daily. It should be of good quality. But, in addition, we need spiritual food each day.

"And He humbled thee, and suffered thee to hunger, and fed thee with manna, which thou knewest not, neither did thy fathers know; that He might make thee know that man doth not live by bread only, but by every word that proceedeth out of the mouth of the Lord doth man live" (Deuteronomy 8:3).

As the children of Israel journeyed through the wilderness, God provided manna from heaven for their daily food. It was filling and nutritious. But, as the above verse reveals, the giving of the manna was to serve as an object lesson. God's people were always to receive spiritual food from Him every day of their lives.

"But He [Jesus] answered and said, It is written, Man shall not live by bread alone, by every word that proceedeth out of the mouth of God" (Matthew 4:4).

We are to obtain that spiritual food from the Inspired Scriptures. God alone can supply the necessities of the soul. We are to partake of the Word of God. Jesus is the living

Word, and His words are found in the Bible.

"In the beginning was the Word, and the Word was with God and the Word was God . . And the Word was made flesh, and dwelt among us" (John 1:1, 14). "In Him was life; and the life was the light of men" (John 1:4).

"And Jesus said unto them, I am the bread of life: he that cometh to Me shall never hunger; and he that believeth on Me shall never thirst" (John 6:35).

Jesus is the spiritual manna from heaven.

"As the living Father hath sent Me, and I live by the Father: so he that eateth Me, even he shall live by Me. This is that bread which came down from heaven; not as your fathers did eat manna, and are dead: he that eateth of this bread shall live forever" (John 6:57-58). "It is the spirit that quickeneth; the flesh profiteth nothing: the words that I speak unto you, they are spirit, and they are life" (John 6:63).

As we prayerfully study the Bible, we partake of this life in Christ. "And have tasted the good Word of God, and the powers of the world to come" (Hebrews 6:5). "Give us this day our daily bread" (Matthew 6:11). "Thy words were found, and I did eat them; and Thy Word was unto me the joy and rejoicing of mine heart: for I am called by Thy name, O Lord God of hosts" (Jeremiah 15:16).

We have been bought with a price, and are no longer our own (1 Corinthians 6:19-20). We belong to God and are to eat the food He gives us.

Doing so will bring us the deepest happiness in this life, and bring us salvation unto the world to come.

Receive the manna daily. Study God's Word with prayer every day, and live it in your daily life. If you will be humble and submissive, God will use this to change you and, in turn, use you to help others.

"The righteous eateth to the satisfying of his soul."—Proverbs 13:25.

"He will love thee, and bless thee, and multiply thee."—Deuteronomy 7:13.

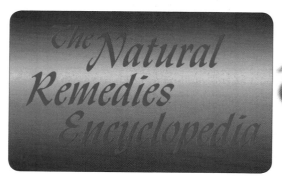

The Seventh Law of Health
The Water that Cleanses

Livestock and wild animals know what to do when physical sickness strikes. They have been observed eating certain plants. Seeking out a stream or lake, they will bathe in the water, or lie in it, to treat their injuries.

A dog that was bitten on the head by a rattlesnake first killed the snake; then he went to a nearby creek, where he lay in the water, off and on, for a week. He recovered completely.

Water is one of the most valuable helpers you have in the daily task of keeping yourself in health or in recovering health when it is lost.

How very important it is that you drink enough water each day! Your kidneys alone filter about 50 gallons of fluid a day. In a 24-hour period, more than 8 quarts of digestive juices flow into the digestive tract. Much of this water is recycled over and over again by your kidneys. But about 2 to 4 quarts of water a day are lost through the urine, lungs, or perspiration. For this reason, if you do not keep drinking water, your kidneys cannot perform their function well, and kidney disease results.

It has been found that water intake can increase physical endurance and ability to work by as much as 80%. When you do not drink enough water, your blood thickens and flows with greater difficulty. This can cause trouble not only in your body tissues and organs, but also to your heart that must pump that sludged blood.

So many people eat far too much salt, sugar, and protein, yet each of these substances requires additional water to process.

In late 1986, the World Health Organization officially stated that the incidence of illness around the globe would fall by 80% if people in the developing nations had access to pure drinking water.

Lack of water not only affects health; it affects work production as well. Athletes, in particular, find that a slight decrease in fluid will greatly affect performance.

It is generally recommended that we drink 8 glasses of water a day. But it is best if you not drink it with your meals, but between them. The very best times for water drinking is first thing upon arising in the morning, and then 30 minutes or so before each meal. One or two warm glasses of water about a half hour before breakfast will help cleanse the stomach and sharpen the appetite. Small amounts drunk from time to time throughout the remainder of the day are also helpful.

Some people drink hot water or cold water drinks with their meal, but this hinders the digestion of the food even more than drinking lukewarm water at mealtime.

The drinking water should be pure, but this is becoming

more difficult to obtain. This is unfortunate. One solution is to purchase a reliable water distiller for your home. This will clean the water. Distilled water will not hurt you; it will only help you, if you are eating a good diet so that you are obtaining your proper amounts of calcium and other minerals from your food. In contrast, regular water often contains an excess of inorganic sodium, chlorine, sulfur, fluorine, iron, chromium, lead, and other undesirable minerals—and in far greater amounts than the body could possibly use. We can be thankful that small, inexpensive home distillers are now easily available.

Joseph M. Price, M.D., has done careful research into the relationship of chlorinated water to atherosclerosis in the arteries. He found so much evidence that he wrote a book about it, entitled, *Coronaries/Cholesterol/Chlorine.* For example, after seven months every chicken fed chlorinated water had developed atherosclerosis, while no chickens fed pure water had it. Here is another interesting fact: American soldiers killed in the Korean War averaged 75% with evidence of coronary atherosclerosis, yet had an average age of only 22! In order to avoid disease, the water given the soldiers in Korea had been very heavily chlorinated.

Cadmium in water increases high blood pressure. Dr. Henry Schroeder has established that people who die of high blood pressure complications tend to have an unusually high level of cadmium in their kidneys. And this most frequently occurs in certain cities with higher cadmium content in the drinking water.

Lead, copper, and sulfur can also be dangerous. Zinc in the water helps to protect the body against cadmium and copper. Patients with either hypertension or atherosclerotic heart disease or an old myocardial infarction generally have higher copper and lower zinc levels in the serum and toenail samples, according to the World Health Organization.

If you have the choice, when drinking water from pipes, it is better to drink hard water than soft water. The hard water, which mainly has calcium and magnesium in it, will lower your chances of acquiring cardiovascular and kidney diseases. The "Journal of the American Medical Association" for October 7, 1974, reported on Monroe County, Florida, where, by changing its source, the hardness of the drinking water was dramatically increased from 0.5 ppm to 200 ppm. "The death rates from cardiovascular disease dropped from a range of 500 to 700 to a range of 200 to 300 only four years after the increase in water hardness."

Oddly enough, you can purchase water-softening equipment and supplies,—but no one sells anything to artificially harden it. Hard water results primarily from the presence of calcium and magnesium salts in the water, while softness is due to the absence of these salts. These two minerals help protect the water from absorbing dangerous minerals from the ground—or from pipes.

The average person will, by the age of 75, have drunk 20,000 gallons of water. Stop and think about it for a moment—and you will agree with the statement of scientists that this is the "water planet." Not only is six tenths of its surface covered by water, but water is the essential factor that makes all life possible. No plant, animal, or living organism can survive long without it.

"When we come to the individual need for water, it is readily realized that water is certainly our most precious mineral. It is the most essential of all minerals for our bodies. An animal can lose all its fat, about half its protein,—but if it loses as much as one-tenth of its water, it will die."—*Jonathan Forman, M.D., in "Water and Man."*

Your body is 80% water. The countless millions of cells inside of you are constantly being bathed in water. And this is not merely a soaking process, but a rewashing activity done by your blood stream. Water in the blood brings nutrition and oxygen to your tissues, and carries off wastes. If injury occurs, coagulants come out of the fluid and stop the bleeding, while white blood cells emerge from the blood stream and begin attacking poisonous substances. Delicate chemical balances are maintained by the flowing blood, as hormones, digestive substances, and many other vital substances are transported through the body fluids to their appointed place.

It is no wonder that this most precious commodity should be needed by mankind—not only inside but outside as well.

Frequent bathing is a very important health practice. It should be done at least once a week, but a daily bath or shower is even better. Warm baths relax; hot baths prepare for cold ones and strengthen and invigorate; all baths help cleanse the skin. There are millions of tiny pores—little mouths—that open out onto your skin. Bathing cleans them and removes the impurities that they bring to the surface.

But, in all your consideration of the values of water, do keep in mind that a better use of water must be accompanied by corresponding improvements in the diet also.

"Rest, freedom from care, light, pure air, pure water, and spare diet, are all that they need to make them well."—*2 Selected Messages, p. 458.*

ADDITIONAL PRINCIPLES

"In health and in sickness, pure water is one of heaven's choicest blessings. Its proper use promotes health. It is the beverage which God provided to quench the thirst of animals and man. Drunk freely, it helps to supply the necessities of the system, and assists nature to resist disease. The external application of water is one of the easiest and most satisfactory ways of regulating the circulation of the blood. A cold or cool bath is an excellent tonic. Warm baths open the pores, and thus aid in the elimination of impurities. Both warm and neutral baths soothe the nerves and equalize the circulation.

"But many have never learned by experience the beneficial effects of the proper use of water, and they are afraid of it. Water treatments are not appreciated as they should be, and to apply them skillfully requires work that many are unwilling to perform. But none should feel excused for ignorance or indifference on this subject. There are many ways in which water can be applied to relieve pain and check disease. All should become intelligent in its use in simple home treatments. Mothers, especially, should know how to care for their families in both health and sickness."—*Ministry of Healing, p. 237.*

80 **THE EIGHT LAWS** **THE WATER THAT CLEANSES** NATURAL REMEDIES ENCYCLOPEDIA
OVER 11,000 REMEDIES - OVER 730 DISEASES

L
A
W
S

"Taken with meals, water diminishes the flow of the salivary glands; and the colder the water, the greater the injury to the stomach. Ice water or iced lemonade, drunk with meals, will arrest digestion until the system has imparted sufficient warmth to the stomach to enable it to take up its work again."—*Review, July 29, 1884.*

"Food should not be washed down; no drink is needed with meals. Eat slowly, and allow the saliva to mingle with the food. The more liquid there is taken into the stomach with the meals, the more difficult it is for the food to digest; for the liquid must be first absorbed . . Hot drinks are debilitating; and besides, those who indulge in their use become slaves to the habit . . Do not eat largely of salt; give up bottled pickles; keep fiery spiced food out of your stomach; eat fruit with your meals, and the irritation which calls for so much drink will cease to exist. But if anything is needed to quench thirst, pure water, drunk some little time before or after a meal, is all that nature requires . . Water is the best liquid possible to cleanse the tissues."—*Review, July 29, 1884.*

"I am advising the people wherever I go to give up liquid food as much as possible."—*Unpublished Testimonies, October 29, 1894.*

"Twice a week . . take a general bath, as cool as will be agreeable, a little cooler every time, until the skin is toned up."—*1 Testimonies, p. 702.*

"Bathe frequently in pure soft water, followed by gentle rubbing."—*Healthful Living, p. 192.*

"Upon rising in the morning, most persons would be benefited by taking a sponge bath, or, if more agreeable, a hand bath, with merely a wash bowl of water; this will remove impurities from the skin."—*Healthful Living, p. 192.*

"Frequent bathing is very beneficial, especially at night just before retiring, or upon rising in the morning."—*Healthful Living, p. 192.*

"Bathing frees the skin from the accumulation of impurities which are constantly collecting, and keeps the skin moist and supple, thereby increasing and equalizing the circulation."—*Healthful Living, p. 789.*

"See that the children have a daily bath, followed by friction till their bodies are aglow."—*Counsels on Health, p. 103.*

"Persons in health should on no account neglect bathing. They should by all means bathe as often as twice a week. Those who are not in health have impurities in the blood, and the skin is not in a healthy condition. The multitude of pores, or little mouths, through which the body breathes, become clogged and filled with waste matter. The skin needs to be carefully and thoroughly cleansed, that the pores may do their work in freeing the body from impurities; therefore, feeble persons who are diseased surely need the advantages and blessings of bathing as often as twice a week, and frequently even more than this is positively necessary. Whether a person is sick or well, respiration is more free and easy if bathing is practiced. By it, the muscles become more flexible, the mind and body are alike invigorated, the intellect is made brighter, and every faculty becomes livelier. The bath is a soother of the nerves. It promotes general perspiration, quickens the circulation, overcomes obstructions in the system, and acts beneficially on the kidneys and urinary organs. Bathing helps the bowels, stomach, and liver, giving energy and new life to each. It also promotes digestion, and instead of the system being weakened it is strengthened. Instead of increasing the liability to cold, a bath, properly taken, fortifies against cold because the circulation is improved, and the uterine organs, which are more or less congested, are relieved; for the blood is brought to the surface, and a more easy and regular flow of the blood through all the blood vessels is obtained."—*3 Testimonies, pp. 70-71.*

"Most persons would receive benefit from a cool or tepid bath every day, morning or evening. Instead of increasing the liability to take cold, a bath, properly taken, fortifies against cold, because it improves the circulation."—*Ministry of Healing, p. 276.*

"If the garments worn are not frequently cleansed from impurities, the pores of the skin absorb again the waste matter thrown off."—*Healthful Living, p. 206.*

"The impurities of the body, if not allowed to escape are taken back into the blood, and forced upon the internal organs. Nature, to relieve herself of poisonous impurities, makes an effort to free the system, which effort produces fevers, and what is termed disease. But even then, if those who are afflicted would assist nature in her efforts, by the use of pure, soft water, much suffering would be prevented. But many, instead of doing this, and seeking to remove the poisonous matter from the system, take a more deadly poison into the system, to remove a poison already there."—*2 Selected Messages, p. 460.*

"Why need anyone be ignorant of God's remedies— hot water fomentations and cold and hot compresses. It is important to become familiar with the benefit of dieting in the case of sickness."—*2 Selected Messages, p. 290.*

"Water can be used in many ways to relieve suffering. Drafts of clear, hot water taken before eating (half a quart, more or less), will never do any harm, but will rather be productive of good. A cup of tea made from catnip herb will quiet the nerves. Hop tea will induce sleep. Hop poultices over the stomach will relieve pain. If the eyes are weak, if there is pain in the eyes, or inflammation, soft flannel cloths wet in hot water and salt, will bring relief quickly. When the head is congested, if the feet and limbs are put in a bath with a little mustard, relief will be obtained. There are many more simple remedies which will do much to restore healthful action to the body. All these simple preparations the Lord expects us to use for ourselves."—*2 Selected Messages, p. 297.*

"Keep the patient free from excitement, and every influence calculated to depress. Her attendants should be cheerful and hopeful. She should have a simple diet, and should be allowed plenty of pure soft water to drink. Bathe frequently in pure soft water followed by gentle rubbing. Let the light, and air, be freely admitted into her room. She must have quiet, and undisturbed rest."—*2 Selected Messages, p. 446.*

SPIRITUAL LESSONS

Not only our bodies need washing, our souls need it as well. We are to be washed by the Word, as we daily study in the Bible. It brings cleansing and strength. "He sent His Word and healed them, and delivered them from their destructions" (Psalm 107:20). "Let the Word of Christ dwell in you richly in all wisdom" (Colossians 3:16).

"Whereby are given unto us exceeding great and precious promises: that by these ye might be partakers of the divine nature, having escaped the corruption that is in the world through lust" (2 Peter 1:4).

There is cleansing power in studying Scripture. By doing it daily, we receive an ongoing washing through the Word. "Wherewithal shall a young man cleanse his way? by taking heed thereto according to Thy Word" (Psalm 119:9). "Now are ye clean through the word which I have spoken unto you" (John 15:3).

This occurs as we pray for help, learn anew His Word,—and bring it into our souls by living it out in our lives each day. "Thy Word have I hid in mine heart, that I might not sin against Thee" (Psalm 119:11). "By the words of Thy lips, I have kept me from the paths of the destroyer" (Psalm 17:4).

While Jesus was here on earth, He also gave us another example—if we would follow in His steps:

"Then cometh Jesus from Galilee to Jordan unto John, to be baptized of him" (Matthew 3:13). He was baptized by John the Baptist, not because He had sinned, but as an example to us. The Father was pleased with what He had done (Matthew 3:17).

Then Jesus later commanded His disciples to baptize converts from all nations. "Go ye therefore, and teach all nations, baptizing them in the name of the Father, and of the Son, and of the Holy Ghost" (Matthew 28:19).

This is a command of Jesus which we are to follow, after learning God's special truths in Scripture and dedicating our lives to Him.

"Verily, verily, I say unto thee, Except a man be born of water and of the Spirit, he cannot enter into the kingdom of God" (John 3:5).

John was baptized at Aenon, "because there was much water there" (John 3:23). Jesus, our example, "went up straightway out of the water" (Matthew 3:16). It is obvious that this was baptism by immersion, not merely sprinkling. Had John used sprinkling, one pail of water would have sufficed for a great host of people. Philip and the eunuch also went into, and came out of, the water (Acts 8:36-39). Philip had immersed the man in a pool of water by the side of the road.

The very word, "baptize" comes from the Greek word, *"baptizo,"* which means "dip under," "immerse," or "plunge under." The meaning is definitely not "sprinkle" or "pour."

It is clear, from the Bible, that baptism represents a complete death to the old way of life, a burial with Christ, and a rising with Him out of death into a new life. The "old man of sin" is dead and, rising, we become a "new creature" in Christ. This is the meaning of baptism—which obviously must be by immersion. Read this carefully:

"Know ye not, that so many of us as were baptized into Jesus Christ were baptized into His death? Therefore we are buried with Him by baptism into death: that like as Christ was raised up from the dead by the glory of the Father, even so we also should walk in newness of life.

"For if we have been planted together in the likeness of His death, we shall be also in the likeness of His resurrection: knowing this, that our old man is crucified with Him, that the body of sin might be destroyed, that henceforth we should not serve sin" (Romans 6:3-6).

"By which also ye are saved, if ye keep in memory what I preached unto you . . how that Christ died for our sins according to the Scriptures; and that He was buried, and that He rose again the third day according to the Scriptures" (1 Corinthians 15:2-4).

"Buried with Him in baptism, wherein also ye are risen with Him through the faith of the operation of God, who hath raised Him from the dead" (Colossians 2:12).

Before baptism, the candidate must be carefully taught (Matthew 28:19-20); he must believe (Mark 16:16); he must repent of his sins (Acts 2:38); he must be willing to die to sin (Romans 6:3, 11-13); He must be ready to live for God (Romans 6:11, 13).

In addition to baptism, there is another water service that we are to perform: the ordinance of foot washing, in connection with the Lord's Supper. God's plan is for us to keep, in memory, Christ's death and resurrection, and our baptism into it.

Some think that Sunday must be kept holy in commemoration of Christ's resurrection. But, according to Scripture (1 Corinthians 15:2-4, quoted above), the ordinance which commemorates Christ's resurrection is Baptism. In addition to baptism, the Lord's Supper commemorates Christ's death.

"The Lord Jesus the same night in which He was betrayed took bread: and when He had given thanks, He brake it, and said, Take, eat: this is My body, which is broken for you: this do in remembrance of Me" (1 Corinthians 11:23-24).

"For as often as ye eat this bread, and drink this cup, ye do shew the Lord's death till He come" (1 Corinthians 11:26).

"If we walk in the light, as He is in the light, we have fellowship one with another, and the blood of Jesus

"When the poor and needy seek water, and there is none, and their tongue faileth for thirst, I the Lord will hear them, I the God of Israel will not forsake them."—Isaiah 41:17.

"Keeping mercy for thousands, forgiving iniquity and transgression and sin."—Exodus 34:7.

"In God will I praise His Word . . in God have I put my trust: I will not be afraid what man can do unto me."—Psalm 56:10-11.

"The Lord God is a sun and shield: the Lord will give grace and glory: no good thing will He withhold from them that walk uprightly."—Psalm 84:11.

The Natural Remedies Encyclopedia

The Eighth Law of Health
Your Trust in God

Individually, you and I need the ministry of God's healing power in our own lives. Oh, how great is our need! Yet, thankfully, it is available.

God has a special healing ministry for you. For it is available to you as you come to Jesus and become His trustful follower, obedient to His Written Word.

Here are the answers that you are looking for, summarized from a special book, *The Ministry of Healing.* **At the close of this book, we will tell you how you may obtain a complete copy of that outstanding book for your very own.**

Our story starts with Jesus. He came to this world at His first advent, to reveal to us the love of God and not only to show us His care for us, but also how we, in His strength, should care for one another.

His work is to give us forgiveness of sin, overcoming power, health, peace, and perfection of character.

Varied were the circumstances and needs of those who besought His aid; and none who came to Him went away unhelped. This help—this healing—is for us today. Wherever there are hearts ready to receive His words—the words of Scripture,—He will bring them the comfort of His own presence, the assurance of their heavenly Father's love.

In all things He brought His wishes into strict alignment with the purpose for His life. He glorified His life by making everything in it subordinate to the will of His Father. His life was one of constant self-sacrifice. He spent His days ministering to the needy and teaching those who desired to learn how to become part of His kingdom. Always patient and cheerful, much of His time was given to minister to the sick and infirm. Yet He made each work of healing an opportunity to implant divine principles of truth in mind and soul. For it was His plan to help men and women physically, so that He could then minister to them spiritually.

At every opportunity He presented the Word—the holy Scriptures—to the people. Never was there such an evangelist as Christ. He was the Majesty of heaven, but He humbled Himself to take our nature, that He might meet men where they were.

He spoke to each one in such kindly, sympathetic, simple words that those words could not fail to be understood. He presented the truth in such a way that it was ever afterward intertwined with their most hallowed memories. His instruction was so direct, His illustrations so appropriate, His words so sympathetic and encouraging,—that His hearers could sense the completeness of His identification with their interests and happiness. What a busy life He led, as He went from home to home ministering to the needy and downcast. Gracious, tenderhearted, pitiful, He went about lifting up the bowed-down and comforting the sorrowful. Wherever He went, He brought blessing and better living.

Jesus sought to reach the poor; He sought also to reach the rich, for they needed His help just as badly. Just now He is seeking to reach you and me and help us in our special needs.

Christ came to this world to show that, by receiving power from on high, one can live an unsullied life. With unwearying patience and sympathetic helpfulness, He met men in their necessities. It mattered not to Him what might be their rank or status in life, for He was not a policy man. That which appealed to His heart was a soul thirsting for the water of life.

"He passed by no human being as worthless, but sought to apply the healing remedy to every soul. In whatever company He found Himself, He presented a lesson appropriate to the time and the circumstances. Every neglect or insult shown by men to their fellow men, only made Him more conscious of their need of His divine-human sympathy.

"He sought to inspire with hope the roughest and most unpromising, setting before them the assurance that they might become blameless and harmless, attaining such a character as would make them manifest as the children of God.

"Often He met those who had drifted under Satan's control, and who had no power to break from his snare. To such a one, discouraged, sick, tempted, fallen, Jesus would speak words of tenderest pity, words that were needed and could be understood. Others He met were fighting a hand-to-hand battle with the adversary of souls. These He encouraged to persevere, assuring them that they would win; for angels of God were on their side, and would give them the victory."—*The Ministry of Healing, pp. 25-26.*

His sympathy, social kindliness, and concern for their best good,—made men and women long to become worthy of His confidence. Upon their thirsty hearts His words fell with blessed, life-giving power. New impulses were awakened and, though they might be outcasts of society, there opened before them the possibility of a new life.

The same Jesus is calling you to His side to-day. Whatever your past may have been, regardless of your weakness,—He wants to forgive your past, transform your weakness by His grace, through obedience to His Written Word, the Holy Scriptures.

Christ neglects no one. Wherever there are hearts open to receive the truth, Christ is ready to instruct them. He reveals to them the Father, and the service acceptable to Him.

Christ was hid in God, and God was revealed in the character of His Son. The evidence of His divinity was seen in His ministry to the needs of suffering humanity. Not by pomp and the overthrowing of kingdoms was Christ to establish His kingdom, but by speaking to the hearts of men by a life of mercy and self-sacrifice. His healing ministry is for you today, that His life might be yours. His objective is that your soul shall be imbued with the principles of heaven; so that then, as you come in contact with others, you will be enabled to impart of Heaven's light to them. Your consistent faithfulness to God and His Word will be a special means of revealing that light.

"Human effort will be efficient in the work of God just according to the consecrated devotion of the worker,—by revealing the power of the grace of Christ to transform the life. We are to be distinguished from the world because God has placed His seal upon us, because He manifests in us His own character of love. Our Redeemer covers us with His righteousness."—*The Ministry of Healing, p. 37.*

If you are a mother, the Master desires to help you in your work to raise your children for God. Come to Him, and tell Him of your needs, and He will impart strength and blessing, just as He did to the mothers who, so long ago, brought their little ones to Him for a blessing. Come to Him for help that you may be empowered to better take up your daily duties again. Instruct your children in the Word of God, and in after years the memory of the words of Scripture will keep many from straying from the pathway to heaven.

But do not let your un-Christlikeness hinder the little ones from coming to Jesus. Plead with God, alone in prayer, for grace and help in time of need, that you may provide them the example of right living that they desire to see in you.

"We should neglect nothing that would serve to benefit a human being. Let everything be gathered up that will relieve the necessities of earth's hungry ones . . By every word of God we are to live. Nothing that God has spoken is to be lost. Not one word that concerns our eternal salvation are we to neglect . . The miracle of the loaves teaches dependence upon God. When Christ fed the five thousand, the food was not nigh at hand . . The providence of God had placed Jesus where He was, and He depended on His heavenly Father for means to relieve the necessity. When we are brought into strait places, we are to depend on God. In every emergency we are to seek help from Him who has infinite resources at His command."—*The Ministry of Healing, pp. 48-49.*

The Saviour's life on earth was a life of communion with nature and with God. In this communion He revealed for us the secret of a life of power. In study of the Inspired Word, earnest prayer, and careful obedience, the soul is ennobled and enabled to fulfill its mission in life.

All day Christ ministered to the people, but in the evening or at dawn He spent hours in prayer to His heavenly Father. Returning from the time spent in prayer, a look of peace, freshness, and power seemed to pervade His whole being. From hours spent alone with God, He came forth morning by morning, to bring the light of heaven to men. And as He opened to men the treasures of truth, they were vitalized by divine power and inspired by hope and courage. Out of the depths of His pure, compassionate heart, the good Shepherd had only love and pity for these restless, thirsting souls.

Take time as Jesus did to be alone with God, that you also may be strengthened in your own battles with temptation, enabled to live a godly life, and minister to the needs of those around you.

"All who are under the training of God need the quiet hour for communion with their own hearts, with nature, and with God. In them is to be revealed a life that is not in harmony with the world, its customs, or its practices; and they need to have a personal experience in obtaining a knowledge of the will of God.

"We must individually hear Him speaking to the heart. When every other voice is hushed, and in quietness we wait before Him, the silence of the soul makes more distinct the voice of God. He bids us, 'Be still, and know that I am God' *(Psalm 46:10).*

"This is the effectual preparation for all labor for God. Amidst the hurrying throng, and the strain of life's intense activities, he who is thus refreshed, will be surrounded with an atmosphere of light and peace. He will receive a new endowment of both physical and mental strength. His life will breathe out a fragrance, and will reveal a divine power that will reach men's hearts."—*The Ministry of Healing, p. 58.*

"If I may but touch His garment, I shall be whole" (Matthew 9:21), said the woman, and by her persistent faith she was healed. Christ realized her great need, and He was helping her to exercise faith. As He passed, she reached forward and succeeded in barely touching the border of His garment. That moment she knew she was healed. It is through contact with Christ that we are strengthened and helped. To believe in Christ merely as the Saviour of the world can never bring healing to the soul. The faith that is unto salvation is not a mere assenting to the truth of the gospel. True faith means that we receive Christ as our personal Saviour from sin.

"Many hold faith as an opinion. Saving faith is a transaction, by which those who receive Christ join themselves in covenant relation with God. A living faith means an increase of vigor, a confiding trust, by which, through the grace of Christ, the soul becomes a conquering power."—*The Ministry of Healing, p. 62.*

There is help for those with evil habits that grip them. That help is to be found in Christ. He can break the chains, transform the mind, and remake us into the image of God. Turn the eye not to the dark cave of despair,—but upward to Christ. Fix the eye upon Jesus, and the glory of His unchanging power will do for you that which you could never do for yourself. The centurion came to Christ for help, not fearing to ask Him for help. Not to his own goodness did he trust, but to the Saviour's mercy. His only argument was his great need. So it is with us. In the same way we may come to Him.

"Remember that Christ came into the world to save sinners. We have nothing to recommend us to God; the plea that we may urge now and ever is our utterly helpless condition which makes His redeeming power a necessity. Renouncing all self-dependence, we may look to the cross of Calvary and say: *'In my hand no price I bring; simply to Thy cross I cling.'*

" 'If thou canst believe, all things are possible to him that believeth' (Mark 9:23). It is faith that connects us with heaven, and brings us strength for coping with the powers of darkness. In Christ, God has provided means for subduing every evil trait, and resisting every temptation, however strong."—*The Ministry of Healing, pp. 65-66.*

But so many feel that they must first make themselves "right" before they can come to Christ. Yet only Jesus can forgive our past and give us strength to overcome in the future. Coming to Him we receive this help; staying with Him continues this help. Look not to self, but to Christ. In your helplessness, cast yourself upon Him. He will receive you and never, except by your own choice, let you go. As you come, believe that He accepts you—simply because He has promised. You can never perish while you do this, never!

When we pray for earthly blessings, the answer to our prayer may be delayed, or God may give us something other than we ask; but not so when we ask for deliverance from sin. Thank God that that is so. It is His will to cleanse us from sin, to make us His children, and to enable us to live a holy life.

Looking upon the distressed and heart-burdened, those whose hopes have been blighted, Jesus calls them to Himself. He sees their wasted years of seeking to quiet the longings of the soul by the trinkets and tinsel of worldliness and sin,—and He invites them to come unto Him for the peace of heart that they so much want, genuine peace of heart that they can find nowhere else.

He is speaking to you just now: "Take My yoke upon you, and learn of Me; for I am meek and lowly in heart: and ye shall find rest unto your souls" (Matthew 11:29). All are weary and heavy laden with the cares of life. Come, He bids you; come. Only Christ can remove the burdens. And the heaviest load that we bear is the burden of sin.

He knows all the weaknesses of humanity, all of our wants, all of our temptations.

"He is watching over you, trembling child of God. Are you tempted? He will deliver. Are you weak? He will strengthen. Are you ignorant? He will enlighten. Are you wounded? He will heal. The Lord 'telleth the number of the stars;' and yet 'He healeth the broken in heart, and bindeth up their wounds' " *(Psalm 147: 3, 4).*

"Whatever your anxieties and trials, spread out your case before the Lord. Your spirit will be braced for endurance. The way will be open for you to disentangle yourself from embarrassment and difficulty. The weaker and more helpless you know yourself to be, the stronger will you become in His strength. The heavier your burdens, the more blessed the rest in casting them upon your Burden bearer.

"Circumstances may separate friends; the restless waters of the wide sea may roll between us and them. But no circumstances, no distance, can separate us from the Saviour. Wherever we may be, He is at our right hand, to support, maintain, uphold, and cheer. Greater than the love of a mother for her child is Christ's love for His redeemed. It is our privilege to rest in His love, to say, 'I will trust Him; for He gave His life for me.' "—*The Ministry of Healing, pp. 71-72.*

As with those that He healed while on earth, Christ watches the first glimmer of faith grow stronger as we are aroused to seek Him. It is Jesus who is convicting your heart, and drawing you to Himself right now. If it were not for the inexpressible love of God and the drawing of His Holy Spirit, none of us would come to Him. Our problems, our sicknesses, are often the result of our own habits. Yet He does not turn us away. He bids us come that He may solve our problems in His own unique way. The solutions may not come in exactly the manner we expected. Sometimes instead of removing the problem, He gives us strength to live with it. In Him we have victory and peace, whatever the circumstances of life around us.

Do not wait to feel that you are made whole. Believe the Saviour's word. Put your will on the side of Christ. Will to serve Him, and in acting upon His word you will receive strength to obey His Moral Ten Commandment Law. Whatever may be the evil practice, the master passion which may bind both soul and body, Christ is able to deliver.

"When temptations assail you, when care and perplexity surround you, when, depressed and discouraged, you are ready to yield to despair, look to Jesus, and the darkness that encompasses you will be dispelled by the bright shining of His presence.

"When sin struggles for the mastery in your soul, and burdens the conscience, look to the Saviour. His grace is sufficient to subdue sin.

"Let your grateful heart, trembling with uncertainty, turn to Him. Lay hold on the hope set before you. Christ waits to adopt you into His family. His strength will help your weakness; He will lead you step by step. Place your hand in His, and let Him guide you.

"Never feel that Christ is far away. He is always near. His loving presence surrounds you. Seek Him as One who desires to be found of you. He desires you not only to touch His garments, but to walk with Him in constant communion."—*The Ministry of Healing, p. 85.*

The soul that turns to Him for refuge, Christ lifts above the accusing and strife of tongues. No man or evil angel can impeach that soul. Christ will unite you to His own divine-human nature, and by faith you will stand beside your Saviour in heavenly places, in the light proceeding from the throne of God.

As a result of the sacrifice of Christ on Calvary, we are henceforth to look on Satan as a conquered foe. Clinging to Christ we are safe, moment by moment.

And now, having found the ark of safety yourself, live now to show others the pathway to it.

"The two restored demoniacs were the first missionaries whom Christ sent to teach the gospel in the region of

Decapolis. For a short time only, these men had listened to His words. Not one sermon from His lips had ever fallen upon their ears. They could not instruct the people as the disciples who had been daily with Christ were able to do.

"But they could tell what they knew; what they themselves had seen, and heard, and felt of the Saviour's power. This is what everyone can do whose heart has been touched by the grace of God. This is the witness for which our Lord calls, and for want of which the world is perishing."—*The Ministry of Healing, p. 99.*

Christ sends the very ones who have been freed from Satan's prison camp—to tell the prisoners who remain behind of the good news. Our confession of what Christ has done for us is Heaven's chosen plan for revealing Him to the world. And everyone has his own unique way of telling that message. Begin sharing it now, for others are waiting to hear it. And as you do so, your own experience will deepen.

"Every true disciple is born into the kingdom of God as a missionary. No sooner does he come to know the Saviour than he desires to make others acquainted with Him. The saving and sanctifying truth can not be shut up in his heart. He who drinks of the water of life becomes a fountain of life. The receiver becomes a giver . . In doing this work a greater blessing is received than if we work merely to benefit ourselves. It is in working to spread the good news of salvation that we are brought near to the Saviour."—*The Ministry of Healing, pp. 102-103.*

In sympathy and compassion we are to minister to those in need of help, seeking with unselfish earnestness to lighten the woes of suffering humanity. We are not to think ourselves detached from the perishing world around us. They are part of the web of humanity; a web that we ourselves are part of.

Millions of human beings, in sickness and ignorance and sin, have never so much as heard of Christ's love for them. Were our condition and theirs to be reversed, what would we desire them to do for us? As far as lies in our power, we must help them. Whatever our talents or abilities, we are, by those abilities, in debt to all less fortunate than ourselves. Our strength must be used to help them in their weakness.

"Jesus did not consider heaven a place to be desired while we were lost. He left the heavenly courts for a life of reproach and insult, and a death of shame. He who was rich in heaven's priceless treasure became poor, that through His poverty we might be rich. We are to follow in the path that He trod."—*The Ministry of Healing, p. 105.*

The strongest evidence of man's fall from a higher state is the fact that it costs so much to return. The pathway of this return can be trod only by hard fighting, inch by inch, hour by hour. One hasty, unguarded act can bring us deep trouble. We dare not act from impulse. Beset with temptations without number, we must resist in the strength of Christ. Live by principle and obedience to the Word of God.

"The life of the apostle Paul was a constant conflict with self. He said, 'I die daily' . . His will and his desires every day conflicted with duty and the will of God. Instead of following inclination, he did God's will, however crucifying to his nature."—*The Ministry of Healing, pp. 452-453.*

It is only by unceasing endeavor that we can maintain the victory over the temptations of Satan. But God will give the strength for this as you cry to Him for help, determining that you will not leave His side.

Only by overcoming as Christ overcame shall we win the crown of life. But we must realize our great need of His help in order to receive it. It is only as we see our utter helplessness and renounce all self-trust, that we can lay hold on divine power.

"It is not only at the beginning of the Christian life that this renunciation of self is to be made. At every advance step heavenward it is to be renewed. All our good works are dependent on a power outside of ourselves; therefore there needs to be a continual reaching out of the heart after God, a constant, earnest confession of sin and humbling of the soul before Him. Perils surround us; and we are safe only as we feel our weakness and cling with the grasp of faith to our mighty Deliverer."—*The Ministry of Healing, pp. 455-456.*

It is faith in Christ and the study of the Inspired Word of God that can bring us this power. The entire Bible is a revelation of what God is like. Within its pages we find the needed strength, and the key with which to unlock it is earnest, humble, dependent, obedient trust in God. It is obedience that makes the difference.

"The truths of the Bible, received, will uplift mind and soul. If the Word of God were appreciated as it should be, both young and old would possess an inward rectitude, a strength of principle, that would enable them to resist temptation."—*The Ministry of Healing, p. 459.*

Apart from the Sacred Scriptures, man's greatest philosophies are only conjectures. It is not men's writings, but the Bible that you need. Let the life, ministry, and death of Christ become your study. And teach Bible principles to your children as well.

"The knowledge of God as revealed in His Word is the knowledge to be given to our children. From the earliest dawn of reason they should be made familiar with the name and life of Jesus. Their first lessons should teach them that God is their Father. Their first training should be that of loving obedience. Reverently and tenderly let the Word of God be read and repeated to them, in portions suited to their comprehension and adapted to awaken their interest. And, above all, let them learn of His love revealed in Christ, and its great lesson: 'If God so loved us, we ought also to love one another' (1 John 4:11)."—*The Ministry of Healing, p. 460.*

Such a humble, prayerful study of the Word of God can bring the character-changing power of the Holy Spirit into your life. You come to know God by an experimental knowledge, and prove, for yourself, the reality of His Word and the truth of His Scriptures. You are tasting and seeing that the Lord is good. You are setting your seal to the fact that God is true (Psalm 34:8; John 3:33). This may be your experience:

"He can bear witness to that which he himself has seen and heard and felt of the power of Christ. He can testify:

" 'I needed help, and I found it in Jesus. Every want was supplied, the hunger of my soul was satisfied; the

Bible is to me the revelation of Christ. I believe in Jesus because He is to me a divine Saviour. I believe the Bible because I have found it to be the voice of God to my soul.' "—*The Ministry of Healing, p. 461.*

It is our privilege to reach higher and still higher for clearer revelations of the character of God. In His light we shall see light, until mind and heart and soul are transformed into the image of His holiness. As we walk in the path of humble obedience, fulfilling His purpose, we will learn more and more of the deep things of His Word.

Take the Bible as your guide, and stand firm for principle,—and you may attain the highest level of usefulness as a servant of the living God. And this is what you want for your life now? As you dwell upon His goodness, His mercy, and His love, clearer and still clearer will be your perceptions of truth. The soul dwelling in the pure atmosphere of holy thought is transformed by such continuous contact with God, through the study of His word. Self is lost sight of, and we become more and more like the One whom we have come so much to love.

"The relation that exists between the mind and the body is very intimate. When one is affected, the other sympathizes. The condition of the mind affects the health to a far greater degree than many realize. Many of the diseases from which men suffer are the result of mental depression. Grief, anxiety, discontent, remorse, guilt, distrust, all tend to break down the life forces and to invite decay and death.

"Disease is sometimes produced, and is often greatly aggravated, by the imagination . . Many imagine that every slight exposure will cause illness, and the evil effect is produced because it is expected."—*The Ministry of Healing, p. 241.*

"Courage, hope, faith, sympathy, love, promote health and prolong life. A contented mind, a cheerful spirit, is health to the body and strength to the soul. 'A merry [rejoicing] heart doeth good like a medicine.' "—*The Ministry of Healing, p. 241.*

"There is, however, a form of mind-cure that is one of the most effective agencies for evil. Through this so-called science, one mind is brought under the control of another, so that the individuality of the weaker is merged in that of the stronger mind. One person acts out the will of another. Thus it is claimed that the tenor of the thought may be changed, that health-giving impulses may be imparted."—*The Ministry of Healing, p. 242.*

"Instead of teaching the sick to depend upon human beings for the cure of soul and body . . direct them to the One who can save to the uttermost all who come unto Him. He who made man's mind knows what the mind needs. God alone is the One who can heal."—*The Ministry of Healing, p. 243.*

"Sympathy and tact will often prove a greater benefit to the sick than will the most skillful treatment given in a cold, indifferent way."—*The Ministry of Healing, p. 244.*

"The power of the will is not valued as it should be. Let the will be kept awake and rightly directed, and it will impart energy to the whole being, and will be a wonderful aid in the maintenance of health. It is a power also in dealing with disease. Exercised in the right direction, it

would control the imagination, and be a potent means of resisting and overcoming disease of both mind and body."—*The Ministry of Healing, p. 246.*

"Nothing tends more to promote health of body and of soul than does a spirit of gratitude and praise. It is a positive duty to resist melancholy, discontented thoughts and feelings,—as much a duty as it is to pray."—*The Ministry of Healing, p. 251.*

"Abiding peace, true rest of spirit, has but one Source. It was of this that Christ spoke when He said, 'Come unto Me, all ye that labor and are heavy laden, and I will give you rest' (Matthew 11:28). 'Peace I leave with you, My peace I give unto you: not as the world giveth, give I unto you' (John 14:27). This peace is not something that He gives apart from Himself. It is in Christ, and we can receive it only by receiving Him . . When the sunlight of God's love illuminates the darkened chambers of the soul, restless weariness and dissatisfaction will cease, and satisfying joys will give vigor to the mind, and health and energy to the body."—*The Ministry of Healing, p. 247.*

SPIRITUAL LESSONS

There are crises in every life. These draw us closer to God as we plead with Him for strength, help, and guidance.

At such times, how very important it is that we learn the deep meaning of faith, prayer, and trust in God.

Here is a brief Bible study to conclude this section. The highest standard of living, something we all want for our lives, is always found in God's holy Word:

1 - HOW DOES THE BIBLE HELP OUR FAITH?

There is yet something important we must mention to help you. Faith, to be strong, must be fed. The Word of God is the food of faith. The Bible is heaven's pantry, on the shelves of which are stored, in unlimited quantity and almost infinite variety, the foods that nourish Christian faith and experience, and abundant delicacies to delight the soul of the Christian (see Jeremiah 15:16). "Sweeter also than honey and the honeycomb" (Psalm 19:10).

But it is so easy to keep on trying to live while neglecting to feed upon this heavenly food. Often the cares and pleasures of this life consume our time and energies to the neglect of God's Word. Sometimes, even in the work of God, it is possible to grow nervous and anxious, to work in haste, if not in fury, to do God's service, while at the same time neglecting to nourish the soul and the spirit with daily, regular feeding on God's Word. The importance of daily Bible reading may be seen by the following:

1. Faith comes by hearing the Word of God.

"So then faith cometh by hearing, and hearing by the Word of God."—*Romans 10:17.*

2. The Christian feeds upon and lives by the Word of God.

"He answered and said, It is written, Man shall not live by bread alone, but by every word that proceedeth out of the mouth of God."—*Matthew 4:4.*

3. His Word is a heavenly light.

"Thy word is a lamp unto my feet, and a light unto

my path."—*Psalm 119:105.*

4. It is powerful to resist evil.

"The word of God is quick, and powerful, and sharper than any twoedged sword."—*Hebrews 4:12.*

5. His Word is the sword of the Spirit.

"Take the helmet of salvation, and the sword of the Spirit, which is the Word of God."—*Ephesians 6:17.*

In the wilderness of temptation, Jesus wielded the "sword of the Spirit" with swift and telling strokes—"It is written . . It is written." "It is written" (Matthew 4:4, 7, 10). "Then the devil leaveth Him, and, behold, angels came and ministered unto Him" (Matthew 4:11). Oh friend, know this Book. Know it well. Use it in temptation to conquer the world and sin. Use it when overwhelmed with sorrow and fear and worry. Use it when doubt and unbelief assail you. Every promise has power. Every command has wisdom. Every warning has deep meaning. Become known as a Bible-believing, Bible-practicing Christian.

2 - WHY IS PRAYER SO ESSENTIAL TO VICTORY?

"Ask, and it shall be given you," said Jesus. "Every one that asketh receiveth" (Matthew 7:7-8). So it is clear that God has made prayer the means for receiving spiritual blessings that we would not otherwise receive unless we asked. We may well remember three things.

3 - PROMISES TO THE OVERCOMER

1. What are we told to overcome?

"Be not overcome of evil, but overcome evil with good."—*Romans 12:21.*

2. What only can overcome the world?

"For whatsoever is born of God overcometh the world."—*1 John 5:4.*

3. What gives us the victory in our conflict with the world?

"And this is the victory that overcometh the world, even our faith."—*1 John 5:4.*

4. What promises are made, by Christ, to the overcomer?

(a) "To him that overcometh will I give to eat of the tree of life, which is in the midst of the paradise of God."—*Revelation 2:7.*

(b) "He that overcometh shall not be hurt of the second death."—*Revelation 2:11.*

(c) "To him that overcometh will I give to eat of the hidden manna, and will give him a white stone, and in the stone a new name written, which no man knoweth saving he that receiveth it."—*Revelation 2:17.*

(d) "He that overcometh and keepeth My works unto the end, to him will I give power over nations: and he shall rule them with a rod of iron; as the vessels of a potter shall they be broken to shivers: even as I received of My Father. And I will give him the morning star."—*Revelation 2:26-28.*

(e) "He that overcometh, the same shall be clothed in white raiment; and I will not blot out his name out of the book of life, but I will confess his name before My Father, and before His angels."—*Revelation 3:5.*

(f) "Him that overcometh will I make a pillar in the temple of My God . . and I will write upon him My new name."—*Revelation 3:12.*

(g) "To him that overcometh will I grant to sit with Me in My throne, even as I also overcame, and am set down with My Father in His throne."—*Revelation 3:21.*

5. In what one promise are all these promises summed up?

"He that overcometh shall inherit all things; and I will be his God, and he shall be My son."—*Revelation 21:7.*

In heaven there will be no parting, no pain to bear;
 No care-worn brow, no sigh, no silvery hair:
No death to snatch our loved ones from our side,
No angry waves, no sea, no treacherous tide.

In heaven there'll be no thirst, no cry for bread;
No soul who knows not where to lay his head;
 No one to feel the winter's chilling blast,
 For there the piercing storms will all be past.

In heaven there'll be no toil without repay;
No building for a brief, ephemeral day;
For all the joys that prophets old have told
'Twill take the endless ages to unfold.

In heaven there'll be no weary pilgrim band;
No seekers for a better, fairer land;
For all who reach that blissful, happy shore,
Will never cry nor sigh, nor wish for more.

4 - IDENTIFYING GOD'S REMNANT (Revelation 14:6-12)

1. God's remnant church in the last days will preach a worldwide judgment-hour message (Revelation 14:6-7).

Heaven's great investigative judgment began in 1844; and at that time God had a people ready to preach that message. Their burden was to reach the whole world; and that work is going forward with lightning speed. This message is being proclaimed in more than seven hundred languages and dialects, and is being printed in more than two hundred languages.

2. It will deliver the message of mystic Babylon's fall (Revelation 14:8).

3. It will give the warning against the beast's image and mark (Revelation 14:9-10).

This unwavering warning has been given from the rise of this movement. Religionists offer first one, then another, explanation of the mark of the beast. But God's remnant people bear the same consistent message through the years.

Fortunately, a people rose up and began the preaching of these three angels' messages. When the time came, in 1844, the people of prophecy arose, bearing the messages of warning.

4. It urges the worship of the Creator above the beast or image (Revelation 14:7).

God foreknew the peculiar times to which His people

would come. Not only would the Sabbath sign of the Creator have been set aside centuries before, but in these closing days the theory of evolution was to become widespread, denying Creation as a series of specific acts of God in six days' time. The observance of the seventh-day Sabbath is therefore, in a special sense, the sign of those who believe in, serve, and worship, the Creator.

5. It keeps the commandments of God (Revelation 14:12).

The only way the keeping of God's commandments could help to identify God's people would be for the world and religion, in general, to be living *contrary* to His commandments. Any particular commandment on which there would be a decided difference would tend to mark them as commandment-keeping people. So, in answer to prophecy, such a people arose in 1844 and 1845 keeping all God's Ten Commandments, including the Sabbath commandment (designating the seventh day).

6. It keeps and exalts the faith of Jesus. (Revelation 14:12).

God knew that modernism would sweep through Christendom. When men deny Creation, they naturally deny the fall of man; and so the law of God is also set aside. If man was not created and had no fall, he would need no atoning blood of Jesus. God's message today is calling men to recognize Creation, the law of God, the Sabbath, and the cross of Christ. God's remnant people proclaim these great doctrines, and cling by faith to Christ the Creator, Christ the Lawgiver, and Christ the Redeemer of Calvary.

7. It believes and holds to the gift of the Spirit of Prophecy.

"The dragon was wroth with the woman, and went to make war with the remnant of her seed, which keep the commandments of God, and have the testimony of Jesus."—*Revelation 12:17.*

"The testimony of Jesus is the Spirit of prophecy."—*Revelation 19:10.*

This church is a church of fulfilling prophecy and believing in God's special direction of His church through a latter-day manifestation of the gift of prophecy and the writings of the Spirit of Prophecy. This is a special feature of this movement.

8. It will endure reproach, scorn, and persecution (Revelation 12:11).

He who keeps God's commandments will meet ridicule at times, and Satan will make war with him; but a new book of Acts is being written as angels record the faithfulness of God's people as they endure whatever comes to them anywhere in the world. A great test awaits them, but also a great reward.

9. It heeds God's voice to come out of Babylon.

"I saw another angel come down from heaven, having great power; and the earth was lightened with His glory. And he cried mightily with a strong voice, saying Babylon the great is fallen, is fallen, and is become the habitation of devils . . And I heard another Voice from heaven, saying, Come out of her, My people, that ye be not partakers of her sins and that ye receive not of her plagues."—*Revelation 18:1, 2, 4.*

Out of confusion, false doctrines, and worldliness,

God is calling His people. Thousands of them are coming from every part of the world. They come because God is calling them, and His "sheep hear His voice." They separate from the ways of the world (1 John 2:15-17), lay aside its pride and vanity (1 Timothy 2:9-10, 1 Peter 3:3-4), give up its evil ways (2 Corinthians 7:1), and turn to Jesus for salvation. Then, by His grace, they "keep the commandments of God, and the faith of Jesus" (Revelation 14:12). The true church, therefore, as you can see, must come out and be separate.

He keeps "the commandments of God," (2) "the faith of Jesus," and (3) "has the testimony of Jesus Christ." He observes the Bible Sabbath, the seventh-day Sabbath.

This is God's true church, according to the prophecies of the Bible; but the majority of His true followers are still in the churches of Babylon, are living according to all the truth they have. Will you yourself not answer the call, "Come out of her My people," make your own decision, and by your example help to gather others into the fold of Christ?

Oh, my friend, every day we need a daily victory in Christ! Here is more information on how to experience it:

5 - DAILY VICTORY IN CHRIST

Jesus said, "I am the way, the truth, and the life: no man cometh unto the Father, but by Me." (John 14:6). And the apostle John wrote, "He that hath the Son hath life." (1 John 5:12). Paul wrote, "For to me to live is Christ." (Philippians 1:21). "Nevertheless I live; yet not I, but Christ liveth in me" (Galatians 2:20). "I can do all things through Christ which strengtheneth me" (Philippians 4:13).

The active exercise of living faith in Christ is the one great essential to obtaining and maintaining an experience in the Lord that will bring increasing satisfaction in this life and ultimate deliverance from this world when Christ comes. "Without faith it is impossible to please Him" (Hebrews 11:6). "This is the victory that overcometh the world, even our faith." (1 John 5:4). "God hath dealt to every man the measure of faith" (Romans 12:3). Faith is a gift of God to every man—rich and poor, high and low, free and bond, wise and simple. It is man's duty to nourish and exercise this faith. Though it be as small as a grain of mustard seed, it can grow and be used to move mountains of evil and build temples of righteousness.

However, it is not merely faith, but primarily the *object* of true faith that counts most. Faith in God, in Christ, in the promises of the Holy Scriptures, and in all God's plans and agencies for the accomplishment of His purposes is what we need. It is what *we must* have if we are to be victorious. Let us now see how faith makes us righteous and holy in God's sight.

6 - HOW MAY A SINNER BECOME RIGHTEOUS?

"Being justified [forgiven and made righteous] by faith, we have peace with God through our Lord Jesus Christ."—*Romans 5:1.*

"Be it known unto you therefore, men and brethren, that through this man is preached unto you the forgiveness of sins: and by Him all that believe are justified from all things, from which ye could not be justified by the law of Moses."—*Acts 13:38-39.*

If you will read the story of the Pharisee and the publican in Luke 18:9-14, you will note that the publican sought forgiveness of sin. "God be merciful to me a sinner," he cried. Jesus adds this comment, "I tell you, this man went down to his house justified." In other words, the "forgiveness" that the publican sought, Jesus called "justification." This includes also the merciful gift of righteousness, which God counts to the credit of the repentant sinner for the simple reason that he has no acceptable righteousness of his own! The great store of righteousness upon which God draws, when imputing (counting) this undeserved credit, is the righteous life of our Lord Jesus Christ.

A man may have been unjust, but by faith he may be counted as just. When an unjust man is thus accounted as a just man, he is "justified." He is forgiven all past sins. God gives him credit as a righteous person (through Christ). Then he has peace. He is counted as though he had never sinned at all.

This justification comes by faith in the blood of a righteous Christ.

"Being justified freely by His grace through the redemption that is in Christ Jesus: whom God hath set forth to be a propitiation through faith in His blood, to declare His righteousness for the remission of sins that are past, through the forbearance of God."—*Romans 3:24-25.*

"If we confess our sins, He is faithful and just to forgive us our sins, and to cleanse us from all unrighteousness."—*1 John 1:9.*

The cleansing from unrighteousness is through the blood of Christ. The sinner is condemned to eternal death for the violation of God's eternal law. The substitute death of another sinner would not atone. No angel of glory could die to save man. Since the divine law is as sacred as God Himself, only one equal with God could make atonement for its transgression.

So Jesus came, lived a sinless life and "died for our sins according to the Scriptures" (1 Corinthians 15:3); and it is He "whom God hath set forth to be a propitiation [satisfaction] through faith in His blood, to declare His righteousness for the remission of sins that are past, through the forbearance of God." (Romans 3:25). Thus do we exercise faith in the blood of a righteous Christ whose righteous life answers for our unrighteous and unjust past. "To declare, I say, at this time, His righteousness: that He [God] might be just, and the justifier of him which believeth in Jesus" (Romans 3:26).

"Him that cometh to Me I will in no wise cast out."—*John 6:37.*

Any man, who will, may come to Christ. Whosoever will, may come. And no sincere seeker will be turned away.

"Come unto Me, all ye that labour and are heavy laden, and I will give you rest."—*Matthew 11:28.*

At conversion, Christ satisfies the claims of the sacred, unchangeable law by counting His righteousness to the sinner's credit. The gracious gift of forgiveness God offers free. It is ours to exercise faith to the point of taking the gift. "Lay hold on eternal life" (1 Timothy 6:12). This is a definite spiritual action and transaction. We give God our sins and He gives us forgiveness. It is by faith that the just shall live (Romans 1:17).

"Do we then make void the law through faith?" This is a very good question. Paul answers, "God forbid: yea, we establish the law." (Romans 3:31). We are forgiven that we might from henceforth be obedient children, walking in all the commandments of the Lord blameless. This life of victory begins by faith in Christ's righteousness. It continues by faith in Christ's righteousness. It ends by faith in Christ's righteousness. It is Christ—Christ—Christ—first, last, and always. He alone is the Saviour—in the beginning, through life, and at death. And faith in Him is the connecting link.

7 - WHAT NEW RELATIONSHIP DOES THE CHRISTIAN ENJOY?

Without reservation the follower of Christ will say to Christ, as Thomas did, "My Lord and my God." (John 20:28). Jesus has a perfect right thus to be honored. He said, "Ye call me Master and Lord: and ye say well; for so I am." (John 13:13). As our Lord and Master, Jesus bids us follow Him.

"He saith unto them, Follow Me . . And they straightway . . followed Him."—*Matthew 4:19-20.*

"Whosoever he be of you that forsaketh not all that he hath, he cannot be My disciple."—*Luke 14:33.*

Too many hear the good news of escape from hell and of a way to heaven, and "with joy" receive it. They want to escape trial and suffering; they have visions of beautiful mansions on high that they will occupy by and by. But they are not concerned with relating themselves to Christ as followers and disciples. They are not prepared to acknowledge Jesus as "my Lord and my God." Jesus gave up heaven, came down here, and risked eternal loss that we might gain heaven. He who would accept this sacrifice intelligently and wholeheartedly will give up this world in order to follow the Saviour (see Philippians 2:5). This means sacrifice. But think—think of the promise:

"Every one that hath forsaken houses, or brethren, or sisters, or father, or mother, or wife, or children, or lands, for My name's sake, shall receive an hundredfold, and shall inherit everlasting life."— *Matthew 19:29.*

For all that we give up, God will return a hundredfold. He takes away, but only to give more and better in return.

"Whosoever heareth these sayings of Mine, and doeth them, I will liken him unto a wise man, which built his house upon a rock: and the rain descended, and the floods came, and the winds blew, and beat upon that house; and it fell not: for it was founded upon a rock."—*Matthew 7:24-25.*

If we hear and obey, we shall be built upon the solid rock, Christ Jesus, not otherwise. Between these two extremes lie all the shades and colors of professed Christianity.

8 - WHAT IS THE SECRET OF SPIRITUAL POWER?

After the transaction has been made in which faith claims forgiveness for past sins, and after the soul by faith makes a complete surrender of all to Christ as Lord and Saviour, to do God's will and obey all His commandments, the next step is to have faith in Christ as a living

Saviour with power to deliver you; yes, and to keep you from the power of sin. To learn this is to discover the secret of spiritual power. It is not enough to believe in the death of Christ. It is not enough to surrender to Christ. We must believe that Christ is a risen, all-powerful Saviour, who can and will bring victory over sin into the life through His indwelling Spirit. All of this is made possible through His resurrection victory. Paul said, "That I may know Him, and the power of His resurrection." (Philippians 3:10). Here are three promises of power made by the risen Saviour.

1. "Jesus came and spake unto them, saying, All power is given unto Me in heaven and in earth . . And, lo, I am with you alway, even unto the end of the world."—*Matthew 28:18, 20.*

2. "Behold, I send the promise of My Father upon you: but tarry ye in the city of Jerusalem, until ye be endued with power from on high."—*Luke 24:49.*

3. "Ye shall receive power, after that the Holy Ghost is come upon you."—*Acts 1:8.*

4. "He is able also to save them to the uttermost that come unto God by Him, seeing He ever liveth to make intercession for them."—*Hebrews 7:25.*

5. "Let us lay aside every weight, and the sin which doth so easily beset us, and let us run with patience the race that is set before us, looking unto Jesus the author and finisher of our faith."—*Hebrews 12:1-2.*

This power, as in the case of all other blessings, comes through active faith. "This is the victory that overcometh the world, even our faith" (1 John 5:4). "A living faith means a confiding trust, by which the soul becomes a conquering power." And by all means, hold on! "Being confident of this very thing, that He which hath begun a good work in you will perform it until the day of Jesus Christ" (Philippians 1:6). In this way, dear friend, we enter upon the life of victory. In this way, we receive spiritual power for an abiding life of conquest in the Saviour!

1. "Let him ask in faith."—*James 1:6.*

2. "Whatsoever we ask, we receive of Him, because we keep His commandments."—*1 John 3:22.*

3. "He that turneth away his ear from hearing the law, even his prayer shall be abomination."—*Proverbs 28:9.*

The promise is made that "they that wait upon the Lord shall renew their strength" (Isaiah 40:31). "He ever liveth to make intercession for them" (Hebrews 7:25). So ask, friend, and receive. Pray morning, noon, and night as David and Daniel did, and learn the sweetness of communion with God in the Secret place of power. Oh, yes, and don't forget to always pray in Jesus' name.

9 - WHY IS EVERY CHRISTIAN CALLED TO BE A WITNESS?

Christian service is necessary for soul prosperity. "Take my yoke upon you," said Jesus (Matthew 11:29). All life is action. We cannot be ever receiving and never giving. By faith we receive forgiveness and appropriate power. We feed on the Word of God and pray for this and that, but we must surrender, not only to do the will of God as between ourselves and Him, but to do His will toward others.

Every soul is born into God's kingdom as a missionary. Every Christian should be a soul winner. Moody said

that if a man will read the Word of God fifteen minutes a day, pray sincerely fifteen minutes a day, and spend fifteen minutes a day talking definitely to help some soul to Christ, or heavenward, he will enjoy a good experience. Not only the ministers but the laymen should work to make others Christians. Think about the following texts:

1. "Go ye into all the world, and preach the gospel."—*Mark 16:15.*

God needs you to help spread abroad the story of the saving gospel and the speedy return of Jesus. If you love Him, the saving truth cannot be sealed up in your heart. It will overflow in blessing to others.

2. "Pure religion and undefiled before God and the Father is this, To visit the fatherless and widows in their affliction, and to keep himself unspotted from the world."—*James 1:27.*

Only "faith which worketh by love" (Galatians 5:6) will purify the soul and keep the channel of blessing open. The true Christian will have a special care for the widows, the fatherless, and the poor (Matthew 25:34-40).

3. "Well done, thou good and faithful servant."—*Matthew 25:21.*

These words of commendation are spoken to servants—faithful servants—who have worked for Christ. These soul-winning Christians are the ones whom He will take to heaven with Him when He comes again. They have exercised the faculties of the soul and become strong even as the muscles of the body become strong by exertion.

10 - ETERNAL LIFE

1. What precious promise has God made to His children?

"And this is the promise that He hath promised us, even eternal life."—*1 John 2:25.*

2. How may we obtain eternal life?

"For God so loved the world, that He gave His only begotten Son, that whosoever believeth in Him should not perish, but have everlasting life."—*John 3:16.*

3. Who has everlasting life?

"He that believeth on the Son hath everlasting life."—*John 3:36.*

4. Where is this everlasting, or eternal, life?

"And this is the record, that God hath given to us eternal life, and this life is in His Son."—*1 John 5:11.*

5. What therefore follows?

"He that hath the Son hath life; and he that hath not the Son of God hath not life."—*1 John 5:12.*

6. What does Christ give His followers?

"I give unto them eternal life; and they shall never perish."—*John 10:28.*

7. Why, after the Fall, was man shut away from the tree of life?

"Lest he put forth his hand, and take also of the tree of life, and eat, and live forever."—*Genesis 3:22.*

8. What has Christ promised the overcomer?

"To him that overcometh will I give to eat of the tree of life, which is in the midst of the paradise of God."—*Revelation 2:7.*

9. To what is the life of the redeemed compared?

"For as the days of a tree are the days of My people,

and Mine elect shall long enjoy the work of their hands."—*Isaiah 65:22.*

10. When will immortality be conferred upon the saints?

"We shall not all sleep, but we shall all be changed, in a moment, in the twinkling of an eye, at the last trump: for the trumpet shall sound, and the dead shall be raised incorruptible, and we shall all be changed. For this corruptible must put on incorruption, and this mortal must put on immortality."—*1 Corinthians 15:51-53.*

11 - THE HOME OF THE SAVED

1. For what purpose was man created?

"For thus saith the Lord that created the heavens; God Himself that formed the earth and made it; He hath established it. He created it not in vain, He formed it to be inhabited."—*Isaiah 45:18.*

2. To whom has God given the earth?

"The heavens, even the heavens, are the Lord's: but the earth hath He given to the children of men."—*Psalm 115:16.*

3. How did man lose his dominion?

Through sin (*Romans 12; 6:23).*

4. When man lost his dominion, to whom did he yield it?

"For of whom a man is overcome, of the same is he brought in bondage."—*2 Peter 2:19.*

5. In tempting Christ, what ownership did Satan claim?

"And the devil, taking Him up into an high mountain, shewed unto Him all the kingdoms of the world in a moment of time. And the devil said unto Him, All this power will I give Thee, and the glory of them: for that is delivered unto me; and to whomsoever I will I give it."—*Luke 4:5-6.*

6. Through whom is this first dominion to be restored?

"And Thou, O tower of the flock, the strong hold of the daughter of Zion, unto thee shall it come, even the first dominion; the kingdom shall come to the daughter of Jerusalem."—*Micah 4:8.*

7. Why did Christ say the meek are blessed?

"Blessed are the meek: for they shall inherit the earth."—*Matthew 5:5.*

8. Whom does David say have the most now?

"For I was envious at the foolish, when I saw the prosperity of the wicked . . Their eyes stand out with fatness: they have more than heart could wish."—*Psalm 73:3, 7.*

9. Where are the righteous to be recompensed?

"Behold, the righteous shall be recompensed in the earth: much more the wicked and the sinner."—*Proverbs 11:31.*

10. What will be the difference between the portion of the righteous and the wicked?

"Wait on the Lord, and keep His way, and He shalt exalt thee to inherit the land: when the wicked are cut off, thou shalt see it."—*Psalm 37:34.*

11. What promise was made to Abraham concerning the land?

"And the Lord said unto Abram, after that Lot was separated from him, Lift up now thine eyes, and look from the place where thou art northward, and southward, and eastward, and westward: for all the land which thou seest, to thee will I give it, and to thy seed for ever."—*Genesis 13: 14-15.*

12. How much did this promise comprehend?

"For the promise, that he should be the heir of the world, was not to Abraham, or to his seed, through the law, but through the righteousness of faith."—*Romans 4:13.*

13. How much of the land of Canaan did Abraham own in his lifetime?

"And He gave him none inheritance in it, no, not so much as to set his foot on: yet He promised that He would give it to him for a possession, and to his seed after him, when as yet he had no child."—*Acts 7:5.*

14. How much of the promised possession did Abraham expect during his lifetime?

"By faith Abraham, when he was called to go out into a place which he should after receive for an inheritance, obeyed; and he went out, not knowing whither he went. By faith he sojourned in the land of promise: . . for he looked for a city which hath foundations, whose builder and maker is God."—*Hebrews 11:8-10.*

15. Who is the seed to whom this promise was made?

"Now to Abraham and his seed were the promises made. He saith not, And to seeds, as of many; but as of one, And to thy seed, which is Christ."—*Galatians 3:16.*

16. Who are heirs of the promise?

"And if ye be Christ's then are ye Abraham's seed, and heirs according to the promise."—*Galatians 3:29.*

17. Why did not these ancient worthies receive the promise?

"And these all, having obtained a good report through faith, received not the promise: God having provided some better thing for us, that they without us should not be made perfect."—*Hebrews 11:39-40.*

18. What is to become of our earth in the day of the Lord?

"But the day of the Lord will come as a thief in the night; in the which the heavens shall pass away with a great noise, and the elements shall melt with fervent heat, the earth also and the works that are therein shall be burned up."—*2 Peter 3:10.*

19. What will follow this great conflagration?

"Nevertheless we, according to His promise, look for new heavens and a new earth, wherein dwelleth righteousness."—*2 Peter 3:13.*

20. To what Old Testament promise did Peter evidently refer?

"For, behold, I create new heavens and a new earth: for the former shall not be remembered, nor come into mind."—*Isaiah 65:17.*

21. What was shown the Apostle John in vision?

"And I saw a new heaven and a new earth: for the first heaven and the first earth were passed away; and there was no more sea."—*Revelation 21:1.*

22. What will the saints do in the new earth?

"And they shall build houses, and inhabit them; and they shall plant vineyards, and eat the fruit of them. They shall not build, and another inhabit; they shall not plant, and another eat: for as the days of a tree are the days of My people, and Mine elect shall long enjoy the work of their hands. They shall not labour in vain, nor bring forth for trouble; for they are the seed of the blessed of the Lord, and their offspring with them."—*Isaiah 65:21-23.*

23. How readily will their wants be supplied?

"And it shall come to pass, that before they call, I will answer; and while they are yet speaking, I will hear."—*Isaiah 65:24.*

24. What peaceful condition will reign throughout the earth then?

"The wolf and the lamb shall feed together, and the lion shall eat straw like the bullock: and dust shall be the serpent's meat. They shall not hurt nor destroy in all My holy mountain, saith the Lord."—*Isaiah 65:25.*

25. What seasons of worship will be observed in the new earth?

"For as the new heavens and the new earth, which I will make, shall remain before Me, saith the Lord, so shall your seed and your name remain. And it shall come to pass, that from one new moon to another, and from one Sabbath to another, shall all flesh come to worship before Me, saith the Lord."—*Isaiah 66:22-23.*

26. What will the ransomed of the Lord then do?

"And the ransomed of the Lord shall return, and come to Zion with songs and everlasting joy upon their heads: they shall obtain joy and gladness, and sorrow and sighing shall flee away."—*Isaiah 35:10.*

27. How extensive will be the reign of Christ?

"And the kingdom and dominion, and the greatness of the kingdom under the whole heaven, shall be given to the people of the saints of the most High, whose kingdom is an everlasting kingdom, and all dominions shall serve and obey Him."—*Daniel 7:27.*

12 - THE CONFLICT ENDED

1. What statement is made about the completion of the creation process?

"Thus the heavens and the earth were finished, and all the host of them. And on the Seventh day God ended His work which He had made."—*Genesis 2:1-2.*

2. When expiring on the cross, what did Christ say?

"When Jesus therefore had received the vinegar, He said, It is finished: and He bowed His head, and gave up the ghost."—*John 19:30.*

3. At the pouring out of the Seventh plague, what announcement will be made?

"And the seventh angel poured out his vial into the air; and there came a great voice out of the temple in heaven, from the throne, saying, "It is done."—*Revelation 16:17.*

4. And when the new heavens and the new earth have appeared, and the holy city, New Jerusalem, has descended from God and become the metropolis of the new creation, what announcement will then be made?

"And He that sat upon the throne said, Behold, I made all things new. And He said unto me, Write: Write: for these words are true and faithful. And He said unto me, It is done. I am Alpha and Omega, the beginning and the end."—*Revelation 21:5-6.*

5. In the new earth, what will be no more?

"And God shall wipe away all tears from their eyes; and there shall be no more death, neither sorrow, nor crying, neither shall their be any more pain: for the former things are passed away."—*Revelation 21:4.*

"And their shall be no more curse."—*Revelation 22:3.*

6. What will then be the condition of all the earth?

"The wolf also shall dwell with the lamb, and the leopard shall lie down with the kid; and the calf and the young lion and the fatling together; and a little child shall lead them. And the cow and the bear shall feed; their young ones shall lie down together: and the lion shall eat straw like the ox. And the sucking child shall play on the hole of the asp, and the weaned child shall put his hand on the cockatrice' den. They shall not hurt not destroy in all My holy mountain: for the earth shall be full of the knowledge of the Lord, as the waters cover the sea."—*Isaiah 11:6-9.*

7. How does the prophet again speak of this time?

"The whole earth is at rest, and is quiet: they break forth into singing."—*Isaiah 14:7.*

8. What will finally be the privilege of God's children?

"And they shall see His face."—*Revelation 22:4.*

9. How perfect will be their knowledge of God?

"For now we see through a glass, darkly; but then face to face: now I know in part; but then shall I know even as also I am known."—*1 Corinthians 13:12.*

10. How long will they possess the future kingdom?

"But the saints of the most High shall take the kingdom, and possess the kingdom for ever."—*Daniel 7:18.*

God's plan for each of us is far greater than we can imagine. The pathway to heaven is found in the Holy Scriptures. Only there will we find the truths which can save the soul, bring the power of Christ into the life, and enable each of us to triumph over all the power of Satan. May our kind Father bless and keep you in the days ahead.

"Ye shall walk in all the ways which the Lord your God hath commanded you, that ye may live, and that it may be well with you, and that ye may prolong your days in the land which ye shall possess."—Deuteronomy 5:33.

"Eye hath not seen, nor ear heard, neither have entered into the heart of man, the things which God hath prepared for them that love Him."—1 Corinthians 2:9.

"God shall wipe away all tears from their eyes; and there shall be no more death, neither sorrow, nor crying, neither shall there be any more pain: for the former things are past away."—Revelation 21:4.

"God is not ashamed to be called their God: for He hath prepared for them a city."—Hebrews 11:16.

FRUITS, VEGETABLES, NUTS, AND GRAINS PROVIDE THE BEST DIET

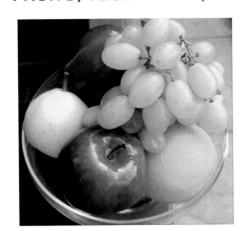

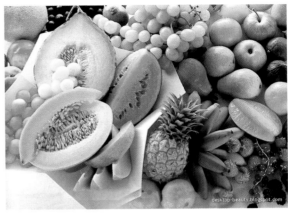

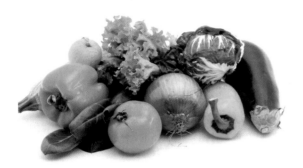

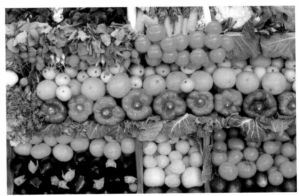

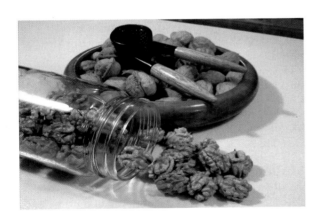

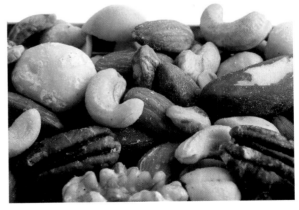

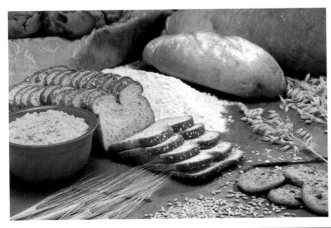

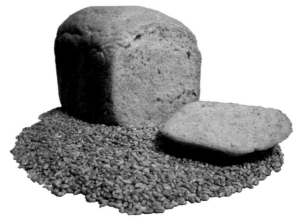

94 **DIETETIC PRINCIPLES** **PRINCIPLES OF DIET** NATURAL REMEDIES ENCYCLOPEDIA
OVER 11,000 REMEDIES - OVER 730 DISEASES

DIET

The Natural Remedies Encyclopedia

Dietetic Principles for Health

Also see Harmful Substances (889-891)

What are the basic principles of right living, to ensure the best health you can have with the limitations imposed by the body you have?

Here are 121 principles of healthful living:

1 - BASIC PRINCIPLES OF HEALTH

1 - Regularity in meals. Do not eat them early or late, but maintain a regular schedule. Your stomach is used to eating at certain times each day.

2 - Moderation. Only eat as much as you need. Never overeat. Only eat to satisfy hunger, and then stop.

3 - Take small bites. Only put a small amount in your mouth at a time. You will chew and salivate it better, and tend to eat less at that meal.

4 - Relax and eat slowly. If you are too rushed to eat, then do not eat. Do not be hurried, anxious, worried, fatigued, or angry.

5 - Chew your food well. You will derive far more energy out of less food, if you do this.

6 - Do not eat too many things at a meal. Three or four items (plus a little salt, oil, etc.) are all you need.

7 - Avoid complicated mixtures. Say no to the gravies, vegetable loaves, gluten foods, and all the rest. Keep your meal simple.

8 - Avoid peculiar additives, such as vinegar, monosodium glutamate, etc., which only upset your stomach and slow digestion.

9 - Vary your diet from meal to meal. If you ate oat-

meal this morning, try rye or wheat tomorrow.

10 - The food should be palatable. But if it is good food, this should not be hard to do.

11 - Never eat anything prepared in aluminum. Never drink water or juice out of an aluminum container. Alzheimer's is worth avoiding.

12 - Aside from fresh, raw juices or the green drink, drink all your liquids (water) between meals, not with your meals.

13 - As a rule, eat your fruits at one meal and vegetables at another. Acid fruits (such as citrus) can be eaten with either.

14 - Greens have more compacted vitamins and minerals than other types of food. They only lack vitamin D, which the body can get from sunlight. But they do not have adequate amounts of trace minerals.

15 - Nova Scotia dulse and Norwegian kelp (two types of seaweed) are the only rich source of trace minerals.

16 - Blackstrap molasses is the only very rich source of iron. It is also a very rich sources of choline and inositol, the two B vitamins used in the largest quantities.

17 - The best pattern is to rest before the meal and walk around after it, not vice versa.

2 - FRUITS

1 - The more natural, the better. Raw fruits and vegetables are better than cooked ones, although some find that a little cooking is necessary. Store-bought canned goods

are even less nutritious.

2 - Wash the fruit before eating it.

3 - Do not eat melons, cantaloupes, and watermelons with other foods; eat them alone.

4 - Always soak dried fruit (prunes, apricots, etc.) before eating them.

5 - Never eat sulphured fruit. It may be golden in color, but the sulphur is not good inside of you.

3 - VEGETABLES

1 - The best is fresh, raw vegetable juice, made from carrots, with some beets, and possibly some celery. This is made in a vegetable juicing machine. It is one of the most valuable appliances you can purchase. Use it every day. The juice is best drunk fresh, within a couple minutes of making it. But, when you know you will be away from home that day, make it in the morning and drink it later as part of a sack lunch.

2 - Also good is the "green drink." This is pineapple juice with some greens whizzed in and is made in a food blender.

3 - Some people's digestive systems cannot tolerate a diet of totally raw vegetables. Each must do that which works best for him.

4 - Eat largely of raw vegetables, with possibly some steamed. A good way to cook vegetables is to keep records on the amount of water used and the time it takes to cook the vegetables, so all the water is gone. For example, broccoli can be lightly cooked for 15 minutes or softer in 30. Find how much water is required to do this; and only have a very small amount of water left in the pan at the end of that time.

5 - Never pour off the vegetable water! Make it part of the meal. For this reason, prepare the food so that very little of the water remains (not over an eighth of a cup) when the cooking is finished. Then drink that water during the meal. Other than the cooking water and a glass of fresh juice, drink no other liquids with the meal.

6 - Beets, potatoes, and squash are excellent foods. Cut out the growing eyes of the white potatoes, but otherwise do not peel them! The outer half inch of the white potato is rich in potassium and is the best part.

7 - All the greens are outstanding, but avoid too much spinach; it is higher in oxalic acid. Enjoy broccoli, brussel sprouts, celery, kale, collards, beet greens, turnip greens, mustard greens, and some lettuce. The deeper the greenness, the more vitamins and minerals it has. (By the way, never eat rhubarb; it is terribly high in oxalic acid.)

8 - Fiber is very important in the diet, for the bowels and the arteries. It can protect you from intestinal problems and heart disease. Oat bran is the best, but whole grains and other vegetable and fruit roughage is very helpful.

4 - GRAINS   (also p. 897)

1 - Only eat whole grains. This includes whole-grain cereals and breads. Never eat processed grains, such as white-flour products.

2 - If you can eat wheat (many cannot), make zwieback of your bread. Place the slices in the oven and toast

them until firm, but not rock-hard. This dextrinizes the starch and renders it more digestible.

3 - Avoid toasted wheat germ; for the oils in it will be rancid. Raw wheat germ should be stored in the refrigerator at the health-food store and in your own refrigerator, when you arrive home. It should smell very fresh.

4 - Oats are one of the best grains. Rye, millet, and buckwheat are also. If you are out on the road and want to have a grain with you which is easily obtained, can be eaten as it is, and is very nourishing, eat Cheerios. Make sure it was recently purchased. Many people are allergic to wheat and products made with wheat.

5 - You are better off having a varied grain diet rather than just rice. Yet rice is a very good food. Make sure it is unpolished (brown rice).

6 - Chew each bite of grain products very well before swallowing. Digestion of starches begins in the mouth.

5 - NUTS AND SEEDS

1 - The nuts and seeds you eat should be fresh. Rancid oil and decaying protein are not good for you.

2 - Nuts, seeds, nut butters, seed butters, and peanut butter are very rich in protein and should only be eaten sparingly. Chew these foods very well. This breaks the food down so the amino acids will be better processed by the stomach acid.

3 - Most commercial peanut butter has the peanut oil removed and cheap oils in its place. These oils are generally hydrogenated; thus they are even more dangerous. Never use peanut butter which does not have floating oil on the top and does not smell fresh.

6 - FATS

According to your body's needs, use little or no added oil. But you do need vitamin F (the essential unsaturated fatty acids). The *best* sources are flaxseed oil (Barleans brand) and wheat germ oil (Viobin Brand); second-best are sunflower seed oil, soy oil, and corn oil. Never use cottonseed oil.

7 - SWEETENING   (also 898-899)

1 - For your sweetening, only use fresh fruit, dried fruit, a little honey, dried cane sugar, organic brown rice syrup, maple syrup, or blackstrap molasses.

2 - Blackstrap is the richest natural source of iron, and one of the richest in calcium and several important B vitamins.

8 - OTHER NUTRIENTS

1 - Salt. Some say that all the salt you need is in the food; but that may or may not be true. You may need to add a little salt; but do not add very much. The best way is to put no salt in the cooking; then add a slight amount of salt to the food at the table. Pour a little into the palm of your hand and sprinkle it where you want it. In this way you will get the exact small amount you need, and no more.

2 - The type of salt to use: Regular store-bought, free-flowing salt has aluminum in it. If you cannot do better,

buy iodized salt at the store (never non-iodized). Better yet, buy a nonfree-flowing salt. It will cake somewhat (salt attracts moisture). Even better, use dulse or kelp!

3 - Nova Scotia dulse comes from western Canada. By checking around, you can locate a food source. This is an outstanding source of trace minerals—including iodine, as well as of common salt (sodium chloride). Eat only enough to satisfy your salt intake needs,—and you will have supplied all your iodine and trace mineral requirements as well. Norwegian kelp is an alternate. California kelp is not as good.

4 - Certain kitchen herbs are helpful; and, when used in small amounts, they can be used to flavor foods. This would include sage, dill, garlic powder, dried parsley, thyme, fennel seed, celery seed, oregano, marjoram, summer savory, basil, rosemary, and ginger.

5 - Cayenne is a very useful medicinal herb; but, if used more than a very little at mealtime, this can lead to pleurisy.

9 - VITAMINS AND MINERALS

Here is a brief introduction to principles concerning the use of vitamins and minerals. More technical information and dosages will be found in the chapter, *"Vitamins Minerals, and Other Nutrients."*

1 - Always take a full vitamin / mineral supplement with every main meal. Buy them from a source you are sure is supplying you with new stock, that has not been on a room temperature shelf for a month or two. Keep the bottle in the refrigerator until it is used.

2 - *Vitamin A:* Unless you are ill and need it right away, use a beta carotene source, not vitamin A. Because it is an oil-soluble vitamin, over a period of time, you can get too much vitamin A.

3 - *Vitamin B complex:* The complete B complex contains a dozen or so different, related, vitamins. Make sure you are getting them all in your supplement(s). These are water soluble, so you can never get too much of them.

4 - *Vitamin C:* Ascorbic acid by itself is not as useful as many believe. Take a "total C" formula, which also contains bioflavonoids (vitamin P). You will pay a little more, but it is worth it. It is also water soluble, so you cannot take too much. (If you oversaturate on C, the excess will be excreted through the bowels as a brief diarrhea. This will tell you that, just then, you have taken a little more than your body needs. This is what it means to take vitamin C "to bowel tolerance.")

5 - *Vitamin D:* Do not take animal or fish liver oil; it can damage your heart muscle. Instead, go out in the sunlight every so often and you will get enough vitamin D. Vitamin D is oil soluble and is the most dangerous vitamin. It is vital that you have some of this for your bones, but you do not want too much.

6 - *Vitamin E:* Make sure your vitamin E supplement says "tocopherols," not "tocopheryls" which is synthetic and worthless. Do not rely on a multivitamin supplement for vitamin E. Take vitamin E capsules, either 200 or 400 IU per capsule. Although it is oil soluble, the possibility of overdosing is rare in the extreme.

7 - *Vitamin F:* This is the essential fatty acids which is best obtained from the flaxseed oil or wheat germ oil, mentioned earlier.

8 - The most important minerals are calcium, potassium, magnesium, iodine, zinc, selenium, and manganese. Avoid phosphorus supplements. Your body always gets all the phosphorus it needs in the food you eat; too much locks with calcium and causes your bones to become weak.

9 - Most people need a calcium supplement. Take half a spoonful of powdered calcium twice or three times a day. Do not use a calcium supplement which has phosphorus in it.

10 - Be careful about iron supplements. They are generally not good for you. Especially avoid them during pregnancy! Use blackstrap instead.

11 - What about the capsules? They are made from animals from the slaughterhouse, generally pigs. If it is a split capsule, open and pour it into a spoon. If it is a sealed capsule, crack it in your mouth and spit out the capsule.
—*For MUCH MORE information! See pp. 99-127.*

10 - SUMMARY

In summary, some of the best foods for you to eat are these:

1 - Fresh, raw fruits. You may also wish to make some fresh, raw fruit juice.

2 - Fresh, raw vegetables and possibly some moderately cooked vegetables prepared in a small amount of water, all of which will be used in the meal.

3 - Fresh, raw vegetable juices made from carrots, beets, and possibly some celery. This drink is outstanding! Green drink (pineapple juice and greens) made in a blender is also good.

4 - Beets, potatoes, and squash are excellent foods. Do not peel white potatoes.

5 - Whole grain cereals or bread toasted in the oven into zwieback. Chew starches extra well.

6 - Add some supplemental fiber to your diet. You will be thankful later that you did. Fiber will help your digestive tract, colon, liver, heart, and blood vessels.

7 - A few fresh nuts and seeds, chewed extra well. Brewer's yeast is another good protein source; so are beans. White potatoes are low in protein, but they are very well assimilated.

8 - A good vitamin / mineral supplement, vitamin E capsules, calcium, plus other nutrients as needed. Each person will have special needs.

9 - Eat some kelp or dulse each day for iodine and other trace minerals. You do well to use it instead of salt.

10 - Drink pure water, and only between meals.

11 - Should you use milk and / or eggs? Each one will have to decide that for himself. Both are known to frequently be contaminated with disease germs. Yet some need the blood-building properties in these products. It is well-known that more people are allergic to cow's milk or wheat than anything else. It is best if you can work away from using them.

12 - Do not eat very much.

13 - Be relaxed and thankful, chew your food well; and, aside from the fresh juices or green drink, drink all your liquids (water) between meals.

11 - THINGS TO AVOID (889-972)

"Avoid" means do not use at all.

1 - Avoid sugar and sugar foods. This is food which has added corn syrup, glucose, or other sugar additives in it. Many canned and processed foods are sugar foods. Do not eat candy.

2 - Do not use white sugar, granulated sugar, or brown sugar.

3 - Avoid spices and condiments which cause stomach upset and worse. This would include black pepper, white pepper, cinnamon, and mustard.

4 - Avoid grease. Grease remains firm at room temperature; this includes Crisco, butter, margarine, and all meat fat.

5 - Avoid hydrogenated oils. An atom of hydrogen has been added to them; so, like grease, they can only be used to coat your arteries and produce fat cells.

6 - Do not use fried foods. Anything fried in oil should be avoided. Your life is too important.

7 - Avoid rich gravies, pastries, ice cream, and all the other delicacies.

8 - Avoid white-flour products: cookies, biscuits, sour bread, bagels, doughnuts, soda crackers, etc. Avoid the glue foods. Along with cheese, these are the sticky, white-flour stuff which is hard on your intestinal tract

9 - Avoid processed foods. This includes a wide variety of "food" which you will find in the store.

10 - Do not eat cheese. In order to normalize your intestinal flora, you may need a little plain yogurt for a time.

11 - Do not eat baker's yeast. This is fresh bread yeast. (Brewer's yeast and torula yeast is all right.)

12 - Avoid junk food and nonfood. This includes soft drinks, cola drinks, potato chips, corn chips, and all the rest. Do not drink non-caffeinated soft drinks.

13 - Do not eat vinegar or foods made with it (pickles and mayonnaise).

14 - Never eat meat or fish! They are heavily contaminated with bacteria, parasites, dangerous fat, and uric acid (urine). As soon as they are slain, the flesh begins rotting.

15 - Avoid the food additives. You will find them listed on the labels of most all processed foods at the store. They lead to arthritic, cardiac, and cancer problems.

16 - Many people are allergic to cow's milk; you may be one of them. Every public health officer knows that meat and milk are the two most contaminated and diseased foods in the country. Eggs rank close behind them. It is best to avoid them also.

17 - Do not use caffeine products. This includes chocolate, coffee, China tea (also called black tea), and caffeinated drinks (such as Coca Cola and Pepsi Cola).

18 - Do not use nicotine products. Tobacco is responsible for an astonishing number of deaths in our world today. Avoid side smoke; do not be in rooms where people are smoking. Chewing snuff causes cancer of the mouth and throat.

19 - Do not drink spiritous liquors: beer, wine, whiskey, or vodka.

20 - Do not use hard (street) drugs.

21 - Avoid medicinal drugs, to whatever extent that you can. Careful living and eating will generally help you avoid having to take them.

22 - Find the foods and other substances you are allergic to, and avoid them. The most common allergenic foods are cow's milk and wheat products.

12 - CAUSES OF INDIGESTION

In his book, *Abundant Health*, Julius Gilbert White lists several special causes of indigestion *(pp. 91-99):*

- Eating too fast. Food needs to be mixed with saliva.
- Overeating. This applies even to good food.
- Meals too close together. For most people, 4 or 5 hours between meals is needed.
- Eating between meals. This weakens the stomach.
- Eating a large evening meal or late at night. Digestion should be nearly finished before retiring.
- Eating when tired, and especially when exhausted.
- Loss of sleep. Nervousness. Mental Depression.
- Eating unripe fruit, spoiled fruit, or condiments.
- Eating bread which was not well baked. If the inside can be squeezed into a dough, do not eat it.
- Eating yeast bread which is not 24 hours old.
- Eating vinegar, fried foods, or complex mixtures.
- Eating vegetables and most fruits at the same meal.
- Eating milk and sugar together, as in ice cream. This is because sugar ferments quickly, yet is enfolded in the milk which digests slowly.
- Eating too much liquid food.
- Eating sugar, tea, coffee, cocoa, liquor, etc.
- Drinking with meals. This dilutes the stomach juices.
- Chewing gum, drinking soft drinks, eating demineralized food or food cooked in aluminum utensils.

13 - ACID-ALKALINE FORMING FOODS

About 80% of your diet should consist of good alkaline-forming foods. The remaining 20% should be good acid foods. Litmus paper, used to test pH, is also called nitrazine paper. It can be purchased at most local pharmacies.

GOOD ACID-FORMING FOODS—Asparagus, beans, brussels sprouts, buckwheat, chickpeas, cornstarch, cranberries, flour, legumes, lentils, oatmeal, olives, plums, and prunes.

GOOD LOW-LEVEL ACID-FORMING FOODS—Canned fruit, dried coconut, dried fruit (most non-sulphured), grains (most), lamb's quarters (type of wild greens), nuts and seeds (most), parsley.

GOOD ALKALINE-FORMING FOODS—Avocados, citrus fruits (become alkaline in body), corn, dates, fresh coconut, fresh fruits (most), fresh vegetables (most, especially onions, potatoes, rutabagas), honey, horseradish, maple syrup, molasses, mushrooms, raisins, soy products, sprouts, watercress.

GOOD LOW-LEVEL ALKALINE FORMING FOODS—Almonds, blackstrap molasses, brazil nuts, chestnuts, lima beans, millet.

BAD ACID-FORMING FOODS—Alcohol, catsup, cocoa, coffee, fish, meat, organ meats, pasta, black pepper, poultry, shellfish, soft drinks, sugar (all foods with added sugar), black tea, vinegar, aspirin, tobacco, drugs (nearly all of them).

BAD LOW LEVEL ACID-FORMING FOODS—Butter, glazed fruit, cheeses, dried sulphured fruit (most).

98 **DIETETIC PRINCIPLES** **OTHER PRINCIPLES** NATURAL REMEDIES ENCYCLOPEDIA
OVER 11,000 REMEDIES - OVER 730 DISEASES

D
I
E
T

14 - OTHER HEALTH PRINCIPLES

1 - Obtain fresh air during the day and while sleeping at night. A slight current of air should pass through your sleeping room at night. When you have the opportunity to go outside, breathe deeply of the fresh air. Practice good posture. Negative ions are important for good health; and they are primarily outside the house.

2 - Sunlight is important. Get a little every day. There is a higher rate of breast cancer in localities where there is less sunlight.

3 - Exercise is important; and, as everybody says, walking outside is the best way to get it. If you are going to do vigorous exercise, warm up first. Do some vigorous walking every day.

4 - Rest is of vital consequence. As you grow older, try to rest a little before preparing the meal. Then, when the meal is over, go outside and walk around a little.

5 - Do not do heavy reading or study just before bedtime, or your brain will be congested and it will be harder to go to sleep. Instead, go outside and walk around in the cool night air, breathing deeply. You will more easily drop right off to sleep.

6 - Maintain a cheerful, sunny, thankful, contented attitude. This is a powerful health-building recipe.

7 - Trust in God; He is the only One who can help you through the problems and trials of life.

8 - You need periods of rest and relaxation every so often. Purposive living, when the objective is to help others, is powerful for good—and excellent for your health. But do not overwork.

9 - Cleanliness is important. Keep your yard clean, your house clean, your clothes clean, and your body clean. Wash the outside with water (take a shower every day); and wash the inside by drinking enough liquids. At certain times, take an enema or colonic when needed, especially when you are sick. Showers are generally better than tub baths; they are quicker and more sanitary.

10 - Do not wear belts, corsets, garters. The clothes should be supported from the shoulders, not at the waist. Men should wear suspenders as part of the way to avoid later prostate problems.

11 - The right exercise of the will is crucial. You are well, you become well, you resist disease, you choose not the wrong, and choose to do the right—through the power of the will, strengthened by firm reliance on God and obedience to His Written Word.

12 - As much as possible, live on a scheduled routine. In this way, you will get your meals, water, rest, exercise, and fresh air. You will have time to eat, to think, and make right decisions. Maintaining regular hours is a great benefit to health. Avoid staying up late at night! Use your will and go to bed when you are supposed to.

13 - Avoid chilling or overheating. Avoid drafts. The danger is in chilling or overheating the blood; either can cause trouble. Dress properly; keep the limbs covered. They should be as warm as the trunk.

14 - Fast occasionally. Skip a meal and just drink fruit or vegetable juice instead. If you are in good health, you can carry on your work on a lighter load till the next meal. If you are frail, go to bed and rest. This will do you wonders in rebuilding and strengthening your body, so you will avoid later development of chronic and degenerative diseases.

15 - Keep your blood circulation equalized. Do not chill the extremities. Do not overeat or eat wrong foods. Maintain moderate exercise. Do what it takes to live right, and you will be richly rewarded.

16 - Avoid anger, fear, worry, and enervation. An excellent way to ruin yourself is by indulging in excess sex or forbidden sex. Happiness comes through self-control, not indulgence.

17 - Never overdo your immune system. It protects you, only as you do not make it work too hard in the process.

18 - Do not overwork one body part more than the others. Many occupational injuries occur because this rule is violated. Take time to rest, when you are not busily working. Look a little closer at athletes, boxers, and karate experts. They are usually physically damaged in their joints by the time they are 50. This is not necessary. Live well by living moderately. Too much food, too much work, and too much relaxation can each be a problem. Learn to balance it all.

19 - Have a careful attitude. Avoid falls, blows, hazards, and dangerous activities. More quadriplegia occurs from diving into shallow water than any other single cause. Get extra rest when you work near sick people.

20 - Learn the distant early warning signs. What are the first indications that you are headed toward sickness? Find out what they are—for yourself, your loved ones, and your children. When you see trouble coming, get extra rest; retire earlier. Skip a meal or two, go to bed, and fast on water and lemon juice.

21 - When able to do so, avoid jet lag and traveling in foreign countries. They have different intestinal bacteria, and you can surely get sick over there.

22 - Avoid loud sounds, such as chain saws and other loud machinery. Wear ear protectors.

23 - Avoid dust, smoke, and chemical vapors.

24 - Move out to the country, if you want the best of health! Away from the noise, the fumes, the rush and turmoil. Out to where there is quietness, peace, fresh air, negative ions, and better sunlight.

25 - Do not live in the lowlands, by a creek. Do not live where it is always damp around the house. Settle in an upper area where it tends to be drier.

26 - Do not have trees close to your house. Do not have your windows covered up with curtains; let the sunlight come through. It purifies every room it enters. Skylight is purifying also, but lesser so.

27 - If possible, avoid pets in, or around, the house. If you want a dog or cat in your house, give it a weekly bath. You can contract diseases from dogs, cats, pigeons, birds, and other animals.

28 - Vegetable, fruit, berry, and flower gardening is an outstanding way to maintain your health—in several ways. But avoid using chemical fertilizers, insecticides, and other garden chemicals.

29 - Learn how to give water therapy (hydrotherapy) treatments. Learn how to prepare and use simple herbs. Keep a few on hand. As we try to help others, our own health improves.

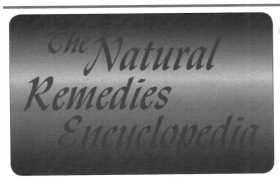

Vitamins, Minerals and Other Nutrients

DOSAGES, SOURCES, FUNCTIONS, USES, DEFICIENCY SYMPTOMS, CAUTIONS

— CONCLUDED ON THE NEXT PAGE

ABOUT DOSAGES: The dosages listed in this chapter are for adults and children weighing 100 pounds and over. Appropriate dosages for children vary according to age and weight. A child weighing between 70 and 100 pounds should be given ¾ the adult dose; a child between 7 and 70 pounds (and *over* the age of six) should be given half the adult dose. A child under the age of six years should be given nutritional formulas designed specifically for young children. Follow the dosage directions on the product label.

RDA (Recommended Daily Allowances) are specified by the government, but are far too small to provide good health, much less physical healing from disordered conditions. **ODA** (optimum daily amount) is the best for regular living, and **TDA** (therapeutic daily allowances) is what is needed when a particular vitamin is needed to help bring healing. All measures are given as amounts needed for one day. But that total daily amount is generally apportioned out into smaller doses, given at 2 or 3 meals.

Dosages are for **adults**. **For a child** between **12-17**, reduce the dose to three-quarters the recommended amount. For a child between **6-12**, use one-half the recommended dose. For a child **under 6**, use one-quarter the amount.

1 - VITAMINS

IMPORTANCE OF VITAMINS—Without vitamins, you would quickly die. They are crucial to all life functions. Vitamins are called *co-enzymes,* because they work with enzymes (chemical catalysts) and enable them to trigger all body processes. *For more on vitamins, see p. 96.*

B-COMPLEX VITAMINS

VITAMIN B COMPLEX—The dozen or so B vitamins are all important, and should be taken together since they work together. They are as follows: B_1 *(Thiamin),* B_2 *(Riboflavin),* B_3 *(Niacin, Niacinamide),* B_5 *(Pantothenic acid),* B_6 *(Pyridoxine),* *(Cobalamin),* B_{13} *(Orotic acid),* B_{15} *(Pangamic acid),* B_{17} *(Nitrilosides, amygdalin [Laetrile]), Biotin, Choline, Folic acid, PABA (Para-aminobensoic acid), Inositol.* For best results with any of them, take all the B vitamins at the same time. This is best done in a multi-vitamin tablet. The B vitamins are excel-

lent for the entire nervous system.

Cautions: Prolonged use of large doses of any one of the isolated B-complex vitamins may result in high urinary losses of other B vitamins, resulting in deficiencies of them.

Functions: Nerves, eyes, skin, hair, liver, mouth, muscle tone.

Needed for assimilation: Vitamins C and E, calcium.

VITAMIN B_1 (THIAMINE)—

Dosage: RDA 1.4 mg / ODA 50 mg / TDA 200-500 mg. *Recommended:* 50-100 mg daily. In the elderly with age-related mental impairment (including Alzheimer's): 3-8 grams daily.

Sources: *Richest sources:* brewer's yeast, torula yeast, wheat germ, sunflower seeds, rice polishings, pine nuts, peanuts with skins. *Other good sources:* wheat germ, wheat bran, rice polishings, most whole-grain cereals (especially wheat, oats, and rice). All nuts, seeds, nut butters. All beans, especially soy. Milk and milk products. Some vegetables, including beets, potatoes, and leafy vegetables.

Functions: Protects and helps heart, muscle, brain, growth, nervous system, peristalsis, red blood count, circulation. Works with other B vitamins in energy metabolism.

Principle uses: Prevents thiamin deficiency, especially in diabetes, Crohn's disease, multiple sclerosis, and other neurological diseases, including epilepsy. Also used to prevent and treat impaired mental function in the elderly, including Alzheimer's.

Deficiency symptoms: Muscular weakness, slow heart beat, defective hydrochloric acid production, chronic constipation, weight loss, mental depression, diabetes, beriberi, neuritis, edema. Eating lots of sugar, alcohol, or refined foods can lead to deficiency. Severe deficiency results in psychosis (up to 30% of those entering psychiatric wards are deficient in thiamin).

Needed for assimilation: Vitamin B, manganese.

Cautions: Destroyed when the diet includes alcohol, tannins in coffee and black tea, sulfites, or uncooked freshwater fish and shellfish. Magnesium is needed for the conversion of thiamine to its active form.

Safety: Thiamine is not associated with any toxicity.

VITAMIN B_2 (RIBOFLAVIN)—

Dosage: RDA 1.6 mg / ODA 50 mg / TDA 200-500 mg. *Recommended:* 5-10 mg daily. Body cannot absorb more than 20 mg in a single dose.

Sources: *Richest sources:* torula yeast, brewer's yeast, almonds wheat germ. *Other good sources:* whole grains, almonds, sunflower seeds, soybeans, cooked leafy vegetables, milk.

Functions: Aids carbohydrate metabolism; works with vitamin A and other B vitamins. Needed for growth, good eyes, nails, skin, and hair. Helps prevent certain cataracts. Important during pregnancy.

Deficiency symptoms: Eye problems: itching, burning, sensitivity to light, bloodshot. Mouth: sore, cracking of the lips and corners of the mouth, burning and itching of the mouth, lips, inflamed tongue. Oily or dull hair, oily skin, premature wrinkles on face and arms, split nails. Visual disturbances such as sensitivity to light and loss of visual acuity, cataract formation. Other disorders of the mucous membranes. Severe anemia, seborrheic dermatitis. Certain esophageal cancers.

Needed for assimilation: Vitamin B complex, vitamin C.

Uses: Crucial in the production of energy. Primarily used in treating migraine headaches, sickle-cell anemia, and cataracts (but for cataracts, do not use more than 10 mg daily).

Cautions: Destroyed by light, but not by cooking.

Toxicity: No toxicity or side effects, except that cataract patients should not take more than 10 mg daily.

Interaction: Riboflavin works closely with thiamin.

VITAMIN B₃ (NIACIN, NIACINAMIDE, NICO-TINIC ACID)—

Dosage: Niacinamide has many of the same effects as niacin; but, for most purposes, is better because it does not cause the flushing of face which niacin will induce for several minutes. Best use niacinamide to avoid face flush). RDA 18 mg / ODA 100 mg / TDA 2,000-6,000 mg (time release). Megadoses are up to 25,000 mg for schizophrenia, high cholesterol, and arteriosclerosis (but prolonged massive doses might induce stomach ulcers, jaundice, liver damage, colitis, and male impotence). *Recommended:* Take it with meals. Of patients given 1.5 grams daily of niacin for 26 weeks, 23% had lowered LDL (bad) cholesterol, and 33% had increased HDL (good) cholesterol. (However, some patients could not tolerate the face flushing.) Hundreds of patients with rheumatoid arthritis and osteoarthritis were given 900-4,000 mg of niacinamide in divided doses daily and experienced good results.

Sources: *Richest sources:* torula yeast, brewer's yeast, rice bran, rice polishings, wheat bran, peanuts. *Other good sources:* wheat germ, brown rice, sunflower seed, whole-wheat products, green vegetables.

Functions: Maintains and strengthens gastro-intestinal tract, circulation, nervous system, skin. Needed for protein and carbohydrate metabolism. Increases blood flow to skin, and extremities. Good for cold feet and hands. Important in energy production, and metabolism of fat, cholesterol, and carbohydrates. It helps the body produce many hormones. Used in over 50 different chemical reactions in the body. Helps regulate blood sugar, antioxidant mechanisms. Helps lower high cholesterol, and reduce early-onset arthritis and diabetes. It is excellent when used in treating early diabetes (but should not

be used for advanced cases).

Deficiency symptoms: *Mild deficiency:* canker sores, irritability, nervousness, diarrhea, insomnia, chronic headaches, digestive problems, and anemia. *Severe:* pellagra, neurasthenia, mental dullness, and disorientation. (The primary symptoms of pellagra are dermatitis, dementia, and diarrhea.)

Needed for assimilation: Vitamin B complex, vitamin C.

Interactions: The body converts tryptophan into niacin. Because niacin works closely with the other B vitamins, they all need to be taken at the same time.

Warning: Do not use sustained-release niacin; it can damage the liver. (In one test, 52% taking it experienced liver damage). Instead, gradually increase dosage of regular pure crystalline niacin over 4-6 weeks (from 100 mg 3 times daily, to 1.5-3 grams daily in divided doses). Inositol hexaniacinate is the safest form of niacin currently taken. Niacin should not be used in advanced diabetes or for those with pre-existing liver disease.

VITAMIN B₅ (PANTOTHENIC ACID, CALCIUM PANTOTHENATE)—

Dosage: RDA 4 mg / ODA 50 mg / TDA 50-200 mg. Researchers have given 1,000 mg daily for 6 months without side effects. Helps in the assimilation of many foods. *Recommended:* 250 mg daily. For rheumatoid arthritis, 2 grams daily. For lowering cholesterol and triglycerides, 300 mg daily.

Sources: *Richest sources:* Brewer's yeast, torula yeast. *Other sources:* wheat bran, wheat germ, whole-grain products, molasses, milk, green vegetables, beans, peas, peanuts, crude molasses, yogurt, and egg yolks. Deficiency is rare since pantothenic acid is found in so many different foods.

Functions: Stimulates metabolism and all life processes, promotes growth. Prevents graying, skin changes. Good for sunburn and skin burns. May protect against skin cancer. Helpful in eczema and lupus. Helps absorption of folic acid. Increases cortisone and other adrenal hormone output. It is an anti-stress factor, and helps the body resist the effects of stress, infection, and premature aging of skin and organs. It helps one recover more rapidly and protects against radiation effects.

Uses: Used to treat adrenal function, rheumatoid arthritis, lower blood cholesterol and triglyceride levels.

Deficiency symptoms: Anemia, eczema, extreme fatigue, infertility, reproductive problems, muscular weakness, stomach distress, constipation, chronic fatigue, tendency to infections, graying and loss of hair, retarded growth, painful and burning feet, insomnia, adrenal exhaustion, low blood sugar, muscle cramps, low blood pressure, skin disorders. Deficiency is one of the causes of asthma. Severe deficiency shown by "burning foot syndrome," and possibly numbness and shooting pains in the feet.

Interactions: Vitamin B complex, vitamins A,C, and E are needed for the assimilation of pantothenic acid. It is used in the manufacture of coenzyme A, and also for ACP. Without this, fats and carbohydrates cannot be used for energy production. It is needed in the production of adrenal hormones and red blood cells.

Cautions: It is possible that continuous ingestion of high doses can cause heart, kidney, and liver problems. Works with folic acid. Also see cautions under *B Complex,* above.

VITAMINS AND MINERALS CONTAIN NUTRIENTS
FOUND IN FRUITS, GRAINS, NUTS, AND VEGETABLES

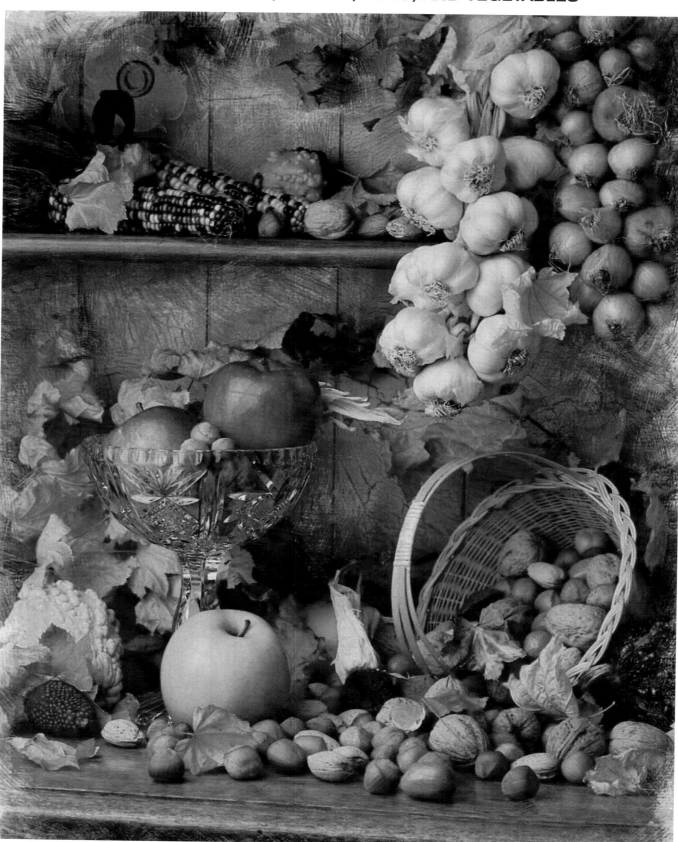

VITAMIN B₆ (PYRIDOXINE)—

Dosage: RDA 2.2 mg / ODA 50 mg / TDA 200-500 mg, combined with other B vitamins. *Recommended:* Therapeutic dosage is 50-100 mg daily, even for long-term use. If use more than 50 mg daily, divide it into 50 mg doses (because the body can only absorb 50 mg at a time). In some instances, 25-50 mg. daily reduces or eliminates epileptic seizures, but must be strictly monitored. It should not be given with anti-seizure drugs. Pregnant women given 30 mg daily experienced significantly less nausea and vomiting. (Ginger root powder did about as well.) In another study, 72% of 106 young women taking 50 mg daily for one week prior and during their period experienced a reduced premenstrual acne flare-up. Over a dozen other studies also produced lowered PMS symptoms.

Sources: *Best sources:* Torula yeast, brewer's yeast, sunflower seeds, wheat germ, soybeans, walnuts, lentils. *Other good sources:* bananas, brown rice, oats, whole wheat, peanuts, avocados, eggs.

Functions: Pyridoxine is used in more body functions than almost any other vitamin. Needed for proper functioning of over 60 different enzymes. Extremely important in the formation of body proteins and structural compounds, red blood cells, chemical transmitters in the nervous system, and prostaglandins. Important in maintaining hormonal balance and proper immune function. Vital in cell multiplication; hence in avoiding miscarriage. Parkinson's has responded to B_6 injections (in combination with magnesium). Vitamin B_6 is required for the absorption of B_{12}, and hydrochloric acid production. Crucial for brain chemistry because involved in production of all amino acid neurotransmitters. Vital to over 100 health conditions, including: asthma, autism, cardiovascular disease, carpal tunnel syndrome, Chinese restaurant syndrome, diabetes, depression, epilepsy, immune enhancement, kidney stones, nausea and vomiting during pregnancy, osteoporosis, premenstrual syndrome.

Deficiency symptoms: Skin disorders, sore mouth and lips, anemia, edema, metal depression, halitosis, eczema, nervousness, kidney stones, insomnia, tooth decay, colon inflammation, migraines, premature senility.

Needed for assimilation: Vitamin B complex, vitamin C, potassium.

Toxicity: This is one of the few B vitamins associated with some toxicity. Doses greater than 2,000 mg daily can produce tingling sensations in the feet, loss of muscle coordination, and degeneration of nerve tissue. Therefore limit dosage to 50 mg. daily.

Interactions: Riboflavin and magnesium are necessary for the body to utilize pyridoxine. Riboflavin interacts with magnesium and zinc, and helps their utilization. Food colorings, certain drugs, oral contraceptives, alcohol, and excess protein intake destroy riboflavin.

VITAMIN B₁₂ (COBALAMIN)—

Dosage: RDA 3 mcg / ODA 200 mcg / TDA 1,000 mcg. It is difficult to assimilate therapeutic doses by mouth, so doctors generally give it by injection. A sublingual tablet, available in a health food store, can be placed under the tongue. *Recommended:* 2 mcg daily. For pernicious anemia, take 300-1,000 mcg daily. Research shows that B_{12} taken orally (1,000-2,000 mcg daily) is just as effective as injections for pernicious anemia. (Ideal dosage: 2,000 mcg daily for 1 month, followed by daily intake of 1,000 mcg thereafter (Methylcobalamin is preferred over cyanocobalamin). Daily intake of 2,000 mcg greatly improved 18 of 20 patients with asthma. Multiple sclerosis patients given 60 mg (not mcg) daily experienced significant improvement.

Sources: B_{12} is present in vegetables in only small amounts. It is in fortified brewer's yeast, milk, eggs. It can also be taken in a vitamin supplement. You need so little of it, that it generally can be obtained from food sources.

Functions: It is needed for production of red blood cells. Prevents anemia and promotes growth in children. B_{12} is especially used in the treatment of impaired mental ability in the elderly, asthma, depression, diabetic neuropathy, low sperm counts, multiple sclerosis, and tinnitus. (In order to absorb the small amounts of B_{12} found in food, the stomach secretes "intrinsic factor," a special digestive secretion that increases its absorption in the small intestine.).

Deficiency symptoms: Chronic fatigue, numbness or stiffness, sore mouth, difficulty in concentrating. If there is enough B_6 and cobalt, the body will make its own B_{12}. Pernicious anemia is largely caused by B_{12} deficiency. Although the classic symptom of B_{12} deficiency is pernicious anemia, a lack of B_{12} actually affects the brain and nervous system first. This can result in numbness, pins-and-needles sensations, or a burning feeling; or in the elderly a mimic-Alzheimer's effect. B_{12} deficiency is a major cause of depression in older people.

Cautions: Be cautious about taking B_{12} if you have folate (folic acid) deficiency, iron deficiency, any kind of infection, Leber's disease, polycythemia vera or uremia. Otherwise, you are not likely to have problems with B_{12}. If there is enough cobalt in the body, the bowel can make its own B_{12}. Unlike other water soluble vitamins, B_{12} is stored in the liver, kidney, and other body tissues. No one has ever reported toxicity from B_{12}. There are two forms of B_{12}. In clinical trials, methylcobalamin (the more active form) produces better results than cyanocobalamin.

Interactions: B_{12} and folic acid work closely together, and should be taken together. A lack of B_{12} causes melatonin to be undersupplied, resulting in inadequate sleep at night.

VITAMIN B₁₃ (OROTIC ACID)—

Dosage: Dosage not known.

Sources: Whey portion of milk.

Functions: Needed for synthesis by the body of nucleic acid. Used in treating multiple sclerosis. Helps cells regenerate.

Deficiency symptoms: Apparently liver disorders, cell degeneration, and premature aging occur. Also overall degeneration, such as multiple sclerosis.

VITAMIN B₁₅ (PANGAMIC ACID, CALCIUM PANGAMATE—

Dosage: Regular dose not known. Therapeutic dose is 100 mg daily: take 50 mg in the morning before breakfast, and 50 mg at night. Used extensively in Russia and certain other countries, but not in America.

Sources: Whole grains, whole-brown rice, seeds and nuts.

Functions: Helps regulate fat metabolism, stimulates glandular and the nervous system. Increases tolerance to insufficient oxygen supply. Used in treating angina, heart disease, blood cholesterol, premature aging, and impaired circulation. Given to people who have experienced carbon monoxide poisoning. Given to drunks to detoxify them.

VITAMIN B$_{17}$ (NITRILOSIDES, AMYGDALIN; known as Laetrile when given as a medical dose for cancer)—

Dosage: No set amount, since it is not yet officially listed as a vitamin. Nutritional deficiency of this factor may be unlikely if whole seeds, grains, nuts, and beans are eaten. Therapeutic doses are given for the treatment of cancer.

Sources: Most whole seeds of fruits and many grains and vegetables. Especially rich in apricot, peach and plum pits; also apple seeds, raspberries, cranberries, blackberries and blueberries. Mung beans, lima beans, garbanzos; millet, buckwheat and flaxseed. Deficiency of this factor may be unlikely if whole seeds, grains, nuts, and beans are eaten.

Functions: Laetrile was discovered and developed by Drs. Ernst Krebs Sr. and Jr., of San Francisco, California, and is used in various countries in the treatment of cancer. Its other nutritive functions have not yet been fully examined.

Cautions: If you eat a bucketful of apricot pits each day, you could experience arsenic cyanide poisoning.

BIOTIN—

Dosage: RDA 200 mcg / ODA 300 mcg / TDA 500-3,000 mcg. *Recommended:* 30-300 mcg daily. For cradle cap, give 3,000 mcg daily to nursing mothers. (If not being breast-fed, give 100-300 mcg daily to the infant.) For stronger nails and healthy hair, 1,000-3,000 mcg daily (in one study, 91% experienced improvement).

Sources: *Richest source:* brewer's yeast. *Other good sources:* soy flower, soybeans, unpolished rice, rice bran, rice, germ, rice polishings, peanut butter, walnuts, pecans, oatmeal, other nuts and whole grains.

Functions: Needed for protein and fat metabolism, and hair growth. Prevents hair loss. Has antiseptic qualities and has been used in the treatment of malaria. Increases the strength of nails.

Deficiency symptoms: Dry, scaly skin. Dandruff, hair loss, and skin disorders, such as eczema, seborrhea. Nausea, anorexia. Pallor, loss of appetite, confusion, extreme fatigue, drowsiness, hallucinations. Lung infections, heart abnormalities, anemia. (The underlying cause of cradle cap in infants is biotin deficiency.)

Needed for assimilation: Vitamin B complex, folic acid, pantothenic acid, vitamin B$_{12}$, vitamin C.

Caution: Biotin is extremely safe, and no one has reported side effects from overdose. Raw egg white contains avidin, a protein which binds biotin and prevents its absorption.

Interactions: Biotin works closely with other B vitamins, and with coenzyme Q$_{10}$ and carnitine. But its absorption is damaged by alcohol, and antibiotics.

CHOLINE—

Dosage: RDA 150 mg / ODA 600 mg / TDA 500-1,000 mg. Choline works closely with inositol in carrying on certain physical functions. Not toxic under 6,000 mg. *Recommended:* Take a lecithin product which has 90% phosphatidylcholine, 3 times daily with meals. For the treatment of liver disorders: 350-500 mg daily. To lower cholesterol: 500-900 mg daily. To treat Alzheimer's disease and bipolar depression: 5,000-10,000 mg.

daily. Choline, in the form of phosphatidylcholine, is usually used to treat these diseases, since it is more useable in the body.

Sources: *Richest sources:* Both choline and inositol are found abundantly in lecithin, which is the richest source for both. However, egg yolks are equally rich. Blackstrap molasses is a rich source of both choline and inositol. *Other sources:* Choline is found in grains, legumes, and egg yolks primarily as lecithin, and as free choline in vegetables (especially cauliflower and lettuce). If a choline supplement is taken, it should be rich in phosphatidylcholine.

Functions: Lecithin helps the body digest, absorb, and carry fat and fat-soluble vitamins in the bloodstream. It helps less fat and cholesterol to be deposited in the arteries and liver. Without it, the arteries become clogged, leading to hypertension and cardiac problems. Lecithin is not only essential for fat metabolism, but it is needed for the synthesis of nucleic acids (DNA and RNA). Needed for the myelin sheaths of the nerves. Helps liver and gallbladder function. Needed for production of phospholipids. Essential for manufacture of certain neurotransmitters, and for proper metabolism of fats. Without it, fats become trapped in the liver, where they block metabolism. Choline is extremely important in brain and memory function, and is helpful in treating Alzheimer's.

Uses: Choline prevents gallstone formation, high blood pressure, atherosclerosis, kidney damage, nephritis, glaucoma, and myasthenia gravis. It is also used in the treatment of bipolar depression (manic depression). In Germany, choline is used to treat a wide variety of serious liver problems; and phosphatidylcholine is used to significantly lower total serum cholesterol and triglyceride levels, and increase HDL cholesterol levels. (HDL is the good kind of fatty acid.)

Deficiency symptoms: Cirrhosis and fatty liver degeneration, atherosclerosis, high blood pressure, hardening of the arteries, kidney damage.

Cautions: Prolonged massive doses of choline (isolated and separated from inositol) may cause depletion of B$_6$. Choline should always be taken with other B vitamins, *especially inositol.* (Lecithin is rich in both choline and inoslitol.) Not toxic under 6,000 mg. Choline helps conserve carnitine and folic acid, and works closely with inositol in carrying on physical functions.

INOSITOL—

Dosage: RDA 75 mg / ODA 100 mg / TDA 500-2,000 mg. Frequently said to be the same dosage as for choline. *Recommended:* 100-500 mg daily for general liver support. 1,000-2,000 mg daily to treat diabetes. 12 grams daily for depression or panic disorder.

Sources: Both choline and inositol are found abundantly in lecithin, which is the richest source for both. See *Choline, Functions,* above. One tablespoon of brewer's yeast provides 40 mg each of choline and inositol. Blackstrap molasses is a rich source. Good plant sources include citrus fruits, whole grains, nuts, seeds, and legumes. Wheat germ, bulgar wheat, brown rice. When phytic acid in plant sources is eaten, intestinal bacteria changes some of it into inositol. (Phytic acid, itself, helps protect the body against cancer.)

Functions: See *Choline,* above, for data on what lecithin does in the body. Inositol prevents hair thinning and baldness, increases hair growth. It is needed for the integrity of the heart muscle. Reduces blood cholesterol. Used in treatment of schizophrenia and obesity, liver disorders, depression, and diabetes. Both choline and inositol are primary components of cell membranes. Like choline, inositol has a "lipotropic" effect; that is, it promotes export of fat from the liver—which must take place or the liver stagnates and cirrhosis, etc., develops. It is used in treating a wide range of liver disorders. Very useful in treating depression.

Deficiency symptoms: Eczema, eye abnormalities, high blood cholesterol, hair loss, constipation.

Needed for assimilation: Vitamins B complex and C.

Side effects: There are no side effects to inositol.

FOLIC ACID—

Dosage: RDA 400 mcg / ODA 1,000 mcg / TDA 20 mg. Use this amount only with a prescription for osteoporosis). (0.4 mg is the normal amount. Therapeutic amounts to correct anemia are 5 mg or more. Unfortunately, potencies higher than 0.1 mg (100 mcg) in one tablet are available only by prescription. Physicians usually prescribe 5-10 mg daily. But it has proven safe in larger amounts, if given with B complex or brewer's yeast, and B_{12}.) *Recommended:* 400 mg daily for general use and prevention of atherosclerosis and osteoporosis. 10 mg daily for treatment of cervical dysplasia and depression. In the U.S., 1-2 babies per 1,000 have neural tube defects; yet 400 mcg given daily in early pregnancy would reduce this by 58%-80%. When 1-2.5 mg daily is given, elevated homocysteine levels are significantly reduced. Yet high levels are significant cause of heart attack or stroke. 10 mg daily normalizes pap smears, reducing cervical dysplasia. High doses (15-50 mg daily) reduce psychotic depression. (Note: FDA restricts folic acid in supplements to 400 mcg., so significantly larger therapeutic doses require a prescription.)

Sources: *Richest source:* Brewer's yeast. *Other good sources:* blackeye peas, rice germ, soy flour, wheat germ, wheat bran, various beans, Deep green leafy vegetables, white potatoes, nuts, peanuts. There are high concentrations of it in green, leafy vegetables.

Functions: Folic acid works with B_{12} in forming red blood cells. Needed for RNA and DNA production, cell growth and division, protein metabolism, healing processes, skin and hair health. Helps prevent graying hair, and builds antibodies to fight infection. Needed in dropsy, diarrhea, menstrual problems, and stomach ulcers. Also atherosclerosis, anemia, radiation burns, circulation problems, and sprue (a tropical anemia and diarrhea).

Deficiency symptoms: Impaired circulation, hair loss, serious skin disorders, grayish-brown skin pigmentation, megaloblastic anemia of pregnancy and mental depression. Reproductive problems such as difficult labor, spontaneous abortion, high infant-death rate. Without folic acid, cells do not divide properly. It is critical for the development of the nervous system of the fetus. Deficiency during pregnancy is linked to several birth defects, including neural tube defects like spina bifida. Because meat is such a poor source, meat eaters are especially likely to develop deficiency symptoms. A lack of folic acid increases homocysteine in the body, which leads to atherosclerosis and osteoporosis. Inadequate folic acid is also involved in the following health problems: acne, AIDS, anemia, atherosclerosis, cancer, candida, canker sores, cataract, celiac

disease, cervical dysplasia, constipation, Crohn's disease, diarrhea, epilepsy, fatigue, gout, hepatitis, infertility, Parkinson's disease, periodontal disease, restless leg syndrome, seborrheic dermatitis, senility, ulcerative colitis. But the principal use of folic acid is in the prevention or treatment of neural tube defects, atherosclerosis, osteoporosis, and cervical dysplasia.

Cautions: Some authorities believe folic acid should not be taken during leukemia and cancer. Folic acid works closely with vitamin B_{12}, and should always be taken with that vitamin. This is because folic acid can mask a B_{12} deficiency, resulting in nerve damage. Folic acid is destroyed by light, heat, drugs, estrogens, barbiturates, and alcohol. High dosage folic acid should not be given to epileptics because it occasionally increases seizure activity.

PABA (PARA-AMINOBENZOIC ACID)—

Dosage: ODA 50 mg. Potencies of PABA higher than 30 mg per tablet are only available by prescription. Yet much higher doses are used, up to several hundred mg.

Sources: Brewer's yeast, whole-grain products, wheat germ, molasses, milk, yogurt, deep greens, and eggs.

Functions: Needed for body growth, metabolism, and all physical functions. Used in combination with pantothenic acid, choline, and folic acid to treat graying of hair and skin changes. When added to salve, it is said to protect against sunburn and skin cancer. (It does this by absorbing ultraviolet-B (UVB) radiation.) Can also be put on burns. Useful in treating various skin disorders, including lupus and eczema. It helps protect against ozone, other air pollutants, and secondhand tobacco smoke. It reduces arthritic inflammation, and increases joint flexibility. It keeps the skin healthy and delays wrinkles.

Deficiency symptoms: Anemia, gray hair, infertility, extreme fatigue, reproductive problems, and patchy areas of white skin (vitiligo).

Needed for assimilation: Vitamin B complex, folic acid, vitamin C.

Cautions: Some authorities suggest that continuous ingestion of PABA can injure the heart, liver, and kidneys. Sulfa drugs block its absorption.

OIL SOLUBLE VITAMINS

VITAMIN A—

Dosage and cautions! RDA 5,000 IU / ODA 5,000 IU / TDA 20,000-300,000 IU. Best to take it only in the form of beta carotene; which is the vegetable-source precursor of vitamin A. The therapeutic dose of Vitamin A (not carotene) would be 25,000 units a day *for only a few days!* It is dangerous to take too much vitamin A (which is oil soluble and stores well). In contrast, carotene is safe. The liver will only convert as much of vitamin A as is needed. During an acute viral infection, a single oral vitamin A dose of 50,000 IU for 1-2 days *(at the most!)* is safe, even in infants. Overdosage of vitamin A is dangerous. *Other dosage cautions!* Do not normally take more than 5,000 IU a day! Do not take large amounts of it for a long period of time! Regular use of 50,000 IU can cause weakness, hair loss, headaches, enlarged liver and spleen, anemia, stiffness, and joint pain. Beware of fish liver oils! They are extremely rich in vitamin A and D, and can damage the heart muscle! Women who might be pregnant must not use vitamin A supplements;

instead, use beta-carotene. Accidental ingestion of a single large dose of vitamin A (100,000-300,000 IU) reduced acute toxicity in children; but, if no more is taken, complete recovery will result. Toxicity occurs in adults who take more than 50,000 IU per day for several years. Women of childbearing age must be careful when taking vitamin A. Daily doses of 10,000 IU (found in some supplements) during the first three months of pregnancy are possibly linked to birth defects.

Toxicity symptoms: Dry and fissured skin, brittle nails, alopecia, gingivitis, chapped lips, anorexia, irritability, fatigue, and nausea. Intracranial pressure with vomiting, headache, joint pain, stupor, papilledema, Prolonged toxicity results in bone fragility and thickening of long bones. *There are never any toxicity symptoms from eating carotenes.*

Sources: Vitamin A (retinol) is a pure yellow, fat-soluble crystal. (Its other name, retinol, comes from the fact that it is found in the retina of the eye.) Vitamin A is found in meat, milk, and eggs.

The safer, and very nutritious carotenes (also called carotenoids) are *pro-vitamin A.* They are found in abundance in fruits and vegetables, and are converted by the liver into vitamin A. It is always safe to take carotene in larger amounts, because the liver only converts the amount needed by the body into vitamin A. *Richest sources:* Dark green leafy vegetables. *Other sources:* Green and orange fruits and vegetables, especially carrots, lighter green vegetables, yams, tomatoes, mangos, Hubbard squash, cantaloupe, apricots. Lesser amounts are in legumes, grains, and seeds.

Beta-carotenes: These are the most active form of carotenes and are most abundant in green plants, carrots, sweet potatoes, squash, apricots, green peppers. (Although it is red, cayenne does not contain pro-vitamin A carotene.) The best supplement form of carotenes is nonhydrogenated palm oil (absorbed 4-10 times better than any other type). In addition, palm oil has minimal fat content.

Carotenes are the most widespread group of naturally occurring pigments in nature, and are intensely colored (red and yellow) fat-soluble compounds. Along with chlorophyl, they are used by plants in photosynthesis to make carbohydrates (sugars, starches, and cellulose). Of the more than 600 carotenes, only 30-50 have vitamin A activity. Beta-carotene has the most pro-vitamin A activity; but several other carotenes have greater antioxidant effects. One of the richest sources of carotenes is freshly made carrot juice.

Functions: Vitamin A (and carotenes) keep mucous membranes healthy; thus it protects against infections, even in infants. Extremely important in fighting infections. It prevents night blindness, eye diseases, weak eyesight. It is important for skin, hair, gastro-intestinal juices and digestion. It prevents premature aging and senility, and increases lifespan. Helps blood capillaries work better and protects against cardiovascular disease. Important in treating skin disorders, dry eyes, cancer, light sensitivity of eyes, and vaginal candidiasis. Affects growth and development, necessary for reproduction, and helps the immune system. Protects against death among children with measles in developing countries. Carotenes provide far more antioxidant effect than vitamin A.

Deficiency symptoms: Prolonged deficiency can produce frequent colds, retarded growth, lack of appetite and vigor, eye infections, poor vision, night blindness, frequent infections,

bad teeth and gums, scaly and dry skin, weakened sense of smell and hearing.

Absorption factors: Conversion of carotenes into vitamin A depends on protein status, thyroid hormones, zinc, and vitamin C, D, E, and choline. Both vitamin A and carotene absorption require essential fatty acids and zinc. When an adequate intake of carotenes is achieved after a meal, no further absorption occurs. Vitamins C, D, E, and choline in the diet, and bile action by the liver is needed for absorption of vitamin A and carotenes. The presence of some fatty acids in the meal (vegetable oil, etc.) increases vitamin A and carotene absorption. Liver disease reduces their utilization by the body.

VITAMIN D (ERGOSTEROL, CALCIFEROL, VIOSTEROL)—

Dosage and cautions! RDA 400 IU / ODA 275 IU / TDA 1,000 IU. *Recommended dosage and cautions!* 200-400 USP units. Therapeutic dose is up to 4,000-5,000 units a day for adults, and half that for children, if taken for not longer than one month. It is dangerous to take too much vitamin D! *This is the most dangerous of the vitamins, if too much is taken (vitamin A is second, but far less of a problem).* Vitamin D can be toxic in excessive doses over a period of time, especially by infants. The best way to get vitamin D is by exposing your body to the sunlight. Doses of 1,800 units a day can cause stunted growth in infants and young children. High intake can lead to a coma. Never take over 600 IU a day; half that for children; even less for infants. However, elderly people, not exposed to any sunlight or living in northern latitudes, should take a daily supplement of 400-600 IU.

Toxicity symptoms: Excessive amounts of vitamin D can produce increased blood concentration of calcium (a serious situation), deposits of calcium on internal organs, or kidney stones. Some researchers believe that long-term use of "vitamin D fortified foods" ("vitamin D milk," etc.) increases the risk of atherosclerosis and heart disease (by decreasing magnesium absorption).

Non-dietetic source: Sunlight on the skin will provide all the vitamin D you need. Muslim women, fully clothed in black cloth, get adequate amounts of D just by exposing their bare feet to the sun for a few minutes each few days.

Sources: Vitamin D and Vitamin B_{12} are the only vitamins never found in fruits and vegetables. Leafy greens have all the vitamins except those two. (However, if there is enough cobalt in the body, the bowel can make its own B_{12}.) Vitamin D food sources include milk and egg yolks. Beware of fish liver oils! They can damage the heart muscle. (Recent research indicates that there is some vitamin D in dark green leafy vegetables.) *Also see Calcium, p. 110.*

Functions: Vitamin D is needed for the absorption of calcium, phosphorous and other minerals out of the digestive tract. Needed by the thyroid gland. Parathyroids use vitamin D in regulating calcium levels in the blood. Needed for proper formation of bones and teeth, especially during childhood. Has many anticancer properties, especially against breast and colon cancer. (Both types of cancer are higher in areas where people are exposed to the least sunlight.)

Deficiency symptoms: Pyorrhea, tooth decay, rickets (in children) and osteomalacia (adults), osteoporosis, retarded growth, muscular weakness, and old-age bone problems. Deficiency symptoms primarily occur in elderly people who do not get any sunlight, especially in nursing homes. The result is lack of bone strength and density, and joint pain.

Absorption factors: Vitamins A, C, calcium, choline, essential fatty acids, and phosphorus are needed for vitamin D absorption. Mineral oil, phenobarbital, Dilantin, and certain other drugs interfere with vitamin D absorption and/or utilization.

VITAMIN E (TOCOPHEROLS: Alpha, Beta, Gamma, Mixed)—

Dosage: RDA 15 IU / ODA 400 IU / TDA 1,200 IU. Usually measured in international units (IU), but sometimes in milligrams (mg). One mg is equal to 1.5 IU. *Recommended:* Normal dosage is 400-800 IU daily. Menopausal patients should take 800 IU daily, until hot flashes subside, and then lower to 400 IU daily. Diabetic patients given 1,350 IU daily experienced lowered insulin need, and their glucose tolerance and insulin activity improved. Of 87,000 nurses, those who took 100 IU of vitamin E for two years had a 41% lower risk of heart disease. Dosages of 400-800 IU provide better oxidative protection for those in high-stress situations.

Natural vs. synthetic forms: Be sure you are getting natural vitamin E, not synthetics. Synthetics are worthless; do not purchase or use them. Read the label: Natural E is written "tocopherols" or "d-tocopherol." Natural alpha-tocopherol (the most active form of E) is "alpha-tocopherol" (or "d-alpha-tocopherol"). The synthetic is "tocopheryl" [with a "y"] or "dl-alpha-tocopherol" [with "dl"]). Mixed tocopherols contain alpha, beta, and delta tocopherol. Alpha tocopherol (d-alpha-tocopherol) has the highest level of activity, and is preferred by many specialists. But mixed tocopherols are also good. Another commercial form is "water-soluble vitamin E." Although much more expensive, it is no more absorbable or useful in the body than the natural oil-soluble type.

Sources: *Best sources:* Fresh, cold-pressed wheat germ oil and flaxseed oil. (Because flaxseed oil is also so rich in omega-3 and omega-6 fatty acids, which prevent cancer, it is the best oil to take. Buy cold-pressed, keep it in the refrigerator, and do not cook it. See section later in this chapter on *Flaxseed Oil) Other sources:* Other unrefined, cold-pressed, crude vegetable oils also have vitamin E. Soy oil and sunflower oil are good; corn oil somewhat lesser so. All whole raw or sprouted seeds, nuts, and grains contain vitamin E. It is also in green, leafy vegetables and eggs.

Functions: The principal use of vitamin E is as an antioxidant in protecting against heart disease, cancer, and strokes. It oxygenates the cells and tissues, reduces the need for oxygen. Prevents unsaturated fatty acids and oil-soluble vitamins from being destroyed in the body. Dilates blood vessels and thus improves circulation. Prevents scar tissue formation in burns. Protects and helps capillaries, lungs, reproductive organs. Used in treating heart disease, varicose veins, burns, angina pectoris, emphysema, hypoglycemia, leg ulcers, reproductive problems, infertility (male and female). Lessens likelihood of miscarriages. Vitamin E enters the fatty portion of cell membranes; there it stabilizes and protects them from compounds (such as lead, mercury, and other heavy metals). Also toxic compounds (such as benzene, carbon tetrachloride, cleaning solvents, drugs, radiation, and the body's free-radical metabolites). Because of its strong antioxidant effects, a high-E diet (or taking of worthwhile vitamin E supplements) exerts a protective effect in many common health conditions. It protects the thymus gland and circulating white blood cells from damage. It is important in immune function, especially during stress and chronic viral illnesses (such as AIDS and chronic viral hepatitis). It reduces LDL cholesterol and increase HDL cholesterol. When taken in high doses, it offers significant protection against cancer. (In one study, patients with low vitamin E levels had a 50% greater risk of cancer.) Vitamin E helps relieve many post-menstrual symptoms, including fibrocystic breast disease. It is effective in relieving hot flashes and menopausal vaginal complaints. The list of diseases it protects against would fill this entire page!

Deficiency symptoms: Nerve damage, muscle weakness, poor coordination, involuntary movement of the eyes, and breaking of red blood cells (leading to hemolytic anemia). In premature infants, vitamin E deficiency is characterized by hemolytic anemia and a severe eye disorder (retrolental fibroplasia). Pulmonary embolism, strokes, heart disease, coronary degeneration, testicle degeneration, miscarriages, sterility, muscular disorders, red-blood cell fragility. Fat malabsorption syndromes, such as celiac disease, cystic fibrosis, and post-gastrectomy syndrome. Premature infants. Hereditary disorders of red blood cells, such as sickle-cell anemia and thalassemia.

Needed for assimilation: Vitamins A, C, D, and E.

Cautions: Iron supplements destroy vitamin E. Rancid oil does also. Do not eat any rancid grains or other foods—and that includes even slightly old wheat germ oil. Many of those interested in better health never eat wheat germ, since it is so difficult to obtain fresh and then keep it from going rancid before being eaten. You can consider toasted wheat germ to be rancid. One study suggested that those with high blood pressure, heart conditions, or rheumatic heart disease do best not taking over 400-600 IU of vitamin E daily. But all other reports indicated vitamin E was safe in any quantity. The healing, strengthening power of vitamin E is not perceived until one takes at least 200-600 mg daily.

VITAMIN F (ESSENTIAL FATTY ACIDS (EFA): linoleic, linolenic, and [less important] archadonic acids)—

Dosage: National Research Council says the diet should include "essential unsaturated fatty acids to extent of at least 1 percent of the total calories." *Recommended:* Therapeutic dose would include at least 1 teaspoon to 1 tablespoon of raw, fresh, cold-pressed wheat germ oil or flaxseed oil at each meal.

What it is: Vitamin F (also called polyunsaturates) is a fat-soluble vitamin and consists of the essential unsaturated fatty acids ("essential" because they cannot be made by the body, yet are vital to normal functions). The body daily needs 10%-20% of its total calorie intake in essential fatty acids (EFA). The most essential of them is linoleic acid. The two primary types of EFA are omega-3 and omega-6. Omega-3 includes alpha-linolenic and eicosapentaenoic acid. They are found in fish (unfortunately, most of which are now caught in polluted waters; the best sources are flaxseed oil and walnut oil. Omega-6 includes linoleic and gamma-linolenic acids. Sources are raw nuts, seeds, legumes, and unsaturated vegetable oils (grape seed oil, primrose oil, evening primrose oil, sesame oil, soybean oil, borage oil). Considering its lower cost and high levels of both omega-3 and -6, the best single source of EFA is raw, fresh, cold-pressed flaxseed oil. Other high-level sources are generally more expensive.

Functions: Essential fatty acids reduce cholesterol and

triglyceride levels. Reduce risk of blood clot formation. Lower blood cholesterol in atherosclerosis, thus preventing heart disease. Needed by the glands, especially adrenals, for proper functioning. Needed for healthy skin and mucous membranes. Needed for metabolism and growth. Enables calcium and phosphorous to be absorbed by the cells. Protects from radiation. Help prevent arthritis. Beneficial for candidiasis, cardiovascular disease, eczema, and psoriasis. Found in high concentrations in the brain, and aid in the transmission of nerve impulses. Needed by every living cell for rebuilding and producing new cells. Used by the body in the production of prostaglandins, which are hormone-like substances which regulate various body processes.

Deficiency symptoms: Skin disorders include acne, rashes, eczema, dry skin. There is kidney, prostate, menstrual, and other reproductive disorders. It also impairs ability to learn and recall information.

Cautions: Very important! The source of supply must be fresh, raw, and cold-pressed. It cannot be labeled "hydrogenated oil." Other, inferior sources (inferior because of the commercial processing they undergo) include soy oil, sunflower seed oil, and corn oil. Never use cottonseed oil; it can damage the optic nerve. Do not use safflower oil. Do not use hardened (solid) vegetable oil (margarine or butter) or animal fat. They only clog the system and help you die younger. In order for the EFA to be used by the body, the oil must be consumed in pure liquid or supplement form and must not be subjected to heat, either in processing or cooking. Heat immediately destroys essential fatty acids, changing them to dangerous free radicals.

VITAMIN K (MENADIONE)—

Dosage: RDA 70 mcg / ODA 140 mcg / TDA 140 mcg. **Dosage:** The best source is eating dark leafy vegetables, either cooked or raw. Possibly take 150-500 mcg of vitamin K_1.

Sources: Green plants, soybean oil, and egg yolks. See sources for vitamin E for more information. Vitamin K is also made by normal bacteria in a healthy colon.

Functions: This is the anti-hemorrhage vitamin. It has essential blood-clotting factors (VII, IX, and X), and it is used in production of prothrombin. It is also needed for normal liver and nerve function. Necessary for building healthy bones, and helps prevent osteoporosis. It converts an important bone protein (osteocalcin) to an active form, so calcium can be retained in the bones. Vitamin K and fat-soluble chlorophyll are used in preventing and treating osteoporosis, excessive menstrual bleeding, and hemorrhagic disease of newborns. (Fat-soluble chlorophyll stimulates hemoglobin and blood-cell production, and relieves excessive menstrual flow.)

Deficiency symptoms: Deficiencies are rare. People normally do not have K deficiencies; yet some individuals do. Hemorrhages (internal or external bleeding) anywhere in the body, due to prolonged blood-clotting time. This would include nosebleeds, bleeding ulcers, etc. Leads to premature aging.

Sources: Dark green leafy vegetables are by far the best. This is because the largest amounts of it are found in chlorophyll, which is fat-soluble. *Richest sources:* kale, turnip greens. *Good sources:* broccoli and other dark green vegetables. *Other sources:* lettuce, cabbage, asparagus.

Cautions: The vitamin has no known side effects or toxicity. Colon bacteria can also produce vitamin K; but their action is stopped by anticoagulant drugs, long-term antibiotics, aspirin,

and Dilantin. Some newborns lack this bacteria, and need an intramuscular injection to provide them. The mother should take vitamin K during pregnancy. Do not use liquid chlorophyll as a vitamin K remedy. Because it is not natural (not in its original oil form), it is only useful in treating skin ulcers. In contrast, fresh vegetable juice (kale, etc.) contains much useable chlorophyll for various healing purposes, as well as providing vitamin K.

C-COMPLEX VITAMINS

VITAMIN C (ASCORBIC ACID)—

"Taking it to bowel tolerance": Whether in sickness or health, you can always know when you are getting too much vitamin C: If your body is saturated with it, the extra will be excreted in the bowel; *i.e.,* you will have a temporary diarrhea. So you can never take too much. Of course, you need far greater amounts when you have any kind of infection. So, when you are ill, take vitamin C *"to bowel tolerance"* (a phrase frequently used in this *Encyclopedia*); that is, until it produces a mild diarrhea effect. Keep in mind that, when you are sick, it will only be a few hours and you may need another large dose of vitamin C. The white blood cells use vitamin C to fight and destroy germs in the system; so do not be skimpy on C when you are ill.

Dosage: RDA 60 mg / ODA 1,000-3,000 mg / TDA 10,000 mg. It is best to always take vitamin C with bioflavonoids, if the amount of bioflavonoids is equal to or greater than the C; they help its absorption. The officially recommended amount is 30-70 mg, but far higher amounts are even better. Therapeutically, vitamin C is given in doses of 1,000 to 10,000 mg a day. In acute poisoning, give 1,000-2,000 mg (preferably by injection) every 1-1/2 or 2 hours. Vitamin C is nontoxic, even in massive doses. *Recommended: When you are well,* take at least 500 mg daily. Nobel Prize winner Linus Pauling, an expert on vitamin C, said to take 2-9 grams daily, to maintain good health. Pregnant women should take at least 500 mg daily. *When you are sick,* it has been proven that, when ill, taking a large dose of vitamin C at one time (say, 2,000-5,000 mg) is far better than taking smaller portions of that total amount over many hours. Several hours after taking a large amount, take another large dose. Many chronic conditions require ongoing high C dosage (such as diabetes, cataracts, glaucoma, cancer, Parkinson's disease, plus many others). Keep in mind that supplements generally do not contain other substances (flavonoids and carotenes) which work to enhance the effects of vitamin C. So it is best that you eat lots of fresh fruits and vegetables.

Sources: The very richest sources are acerola, guavas, red sweet peppers, kale leaves, parsley, collard leaves, turnip greens, green sweet peppers, broccoli, Brussels sprouts, and mustard greens. Good sources are all fresh fruits and vegetables (especially green, leafy vegetables). Early explorers learned that, to avoid scurvy, they needed to eat oranges, lemons, limes, berries, or (as the French explorer Cartier did in 1856) spruce tree needles.

Functions: Adele Davis said that vitamin C would cure every disease. That may be an over-statement; yet she was a deep student of nutrition as it relates to disease. Vitamin C is involved in all vital functions of the body. Needed for production of collagen ("cell cement"), the main protein substance of the body, vitamin C literally holds your body together. This is because it is the basis of connective tissue, cartilage, tendons, etc.

CHART 1064: Vitamin C Content of foods (108-109)

Vitamin C is also important in the manufacture of certain nerve transmitting substances and hormones, carnitine synthesis, and the absorption and utilization of other nutritional factors. It is an extremely important antioxidant. It strengthens various immune functions by enhancing white blood-cell function and activity and increasing interferon levels, antibody responses, and secretion of thyroid hormones. It also resists chemical stress factors, such as water and air pollutants. It is needed by adrenal and thyroid glands; and it protects against all types of stress, physical and mental. It is a natural antibiotic. Wonderful in dealing with fevers and infections. Used for gastro-intestinal problems and treating rattlesnake bites. Counteracts poisonous effects of drugs. Extremely helpful in treating asthma, other allergies, atherosclerosis, high cholesterol, high blood pressure, cataracts, Parkinsons' disease, skin ulcers, wound healing, and pregnancy-related conditions. It overcomes cadmium poisoning. Cancer patients should be urged to take lots of vitamin C. A book could be written on what vitamin C is able to do in your body to help you. It is vital in the treatment of a lengthy list of physical disorders and diseases.

Types of supplements: Vitamin C from the health-food store comes in several forms: powders, crystals, capsules, tablets, and timed-release tablets. *Ascorbic acid* is the most widely used and least expensive. It is usually made from corn. *Buffered vitamin C* has sodium, magnesium, calcium or potassium in it, in order to reduce the immediate acidity of the vitamin C in the mouth and stomach. Sodium ascorbate may not be good for you, since it is best to not eat much sodium. Then there is *"corn-free" vitamin C*, made from the sago palm. This also works well, and is for those who do not have problems eating corn products. *Ester-C* is a new, more expensive product which, it claimed, is absorbed more easily. However, tests reveal that this claim is not correct. Taking supplements containing *vitamin C and bioflavonoids* would be helpful; except that most do not contain enough bioflavonoids to increase absorption of the vitamin. The level of bioflavonoids needs to be equal to or greater than the C content. For most people, plain *ascorbic acid* is the best; by far it is the least expensive and with research-proven effectiveness.

Deficiency symptoms: Soft gums (pyorrhea), tooth decay, skin hemorrhages, anemia, slow healing of sores and wounds, capillary weakness, premature aging, deterioration in collagen, thyroid insufficiency. Also reduced resistance to infections, toxic effects of drugs, and environmental poisons. The classic symptoms of scurvy are bleeding gums, poor wound healing, and extensive bruising; plus susceptibility to infections, hysteria, and depression.

Interactions: Bioflavonoids, calcium, magnesium are needed for vitamin C assimilation. Vitamin C works closely with other nutritional antioxidants, especially vitamin E, selenium, and beta-carotene. When a combination of antioxidants is given, the patient can more easily deal with cancer. Vitamin C increases the absorption of iron, decreases the absorption of copper, and interferes with the blood test for vitamin B_{12}.

Cautions: You cannot get too much vitamin C; the unneeded amount will cause slight diarrhea and be expelled. Exposure to air destroys vitamin C; so it is important to eat fresh foods as quickly as possible. Fresh, sliced cucumbers lose 49% of their C content within 3 hours. A sliced, uncovered cantaloupe in the refrigerator loses 35% within 24 hours.

There is the possibility of "rebound scurvy," which are physical problems caused by suddenly stopping high (500 mg or more) daily dosages. This can especially be a concern to pregnant women; so they should terminate its use slowly. Research does not support the theory that high C intake causes calcium oxalate kidney stones. Pollutants (such as cigarette smoke) increase the need for vitamin C intake.

BIOFLAVONOIDS (Vitamin P)—

The bioflavonoids are part of the vitamin C complex. (They are rarely called vitamin P today.) The bioflavonoids are citrin, eriodictyon, flavones, hesperetin, hesperidin, quercetin, and rutin. All are essential. Because the body cannot produce them, they must be included in the diet. Excessive amounts are excreted in urine and perspiration.

Dosage: RDA not established / ODA 500 mg / TDA Therapeutic dosage is 50-200 mg or more. *Hesperidin:* ODA 100 mg. *Rutin:* ODA 25 mg. TDA 50-200 mg or more. Two weeks of 3,000 mg given to a woman, with severe rheumatoid arthritis, eliminated the pain in 2 weeks. Her blood pressure dropped from 190 to 176; and, in 6 weeks, she had more action in joints and much more endurance. In 36 patients with bleeding duodenal ulcers, 3-9 capsules daily (along with orange juice) totally eliminated the ulcers within 22 days, with no recurrence in a year.

Sources: *Richest sources:* Buckwheat, grapes, apricots, black currants, strawberries, cherries, prunes, blackberries, grapefruit, plums, rose hips, pulp of citrus fruits (especially the white beneath the peel). *Other sources:* Also in other fresh fruits and vegetables. Because they are largely destroyed by cooking, it is important that you eat some raw fruits. There is 10 times the amount of bioflavonoids in fruit pulp than is in the juice.

Functions: Vital in preventing capillary fragility and hemorrhaging by strengthening capillary walls. (The capillaries are the smallest blood vessels.) Protect vitamin C from destruction in the body by oxidation. Work with vitamin C as a synergist, thereby strengthening its properties. Used for hemorrhoids, varicose veins, hypertension, respiratory infections, bleeding gums, hemorrhaging, eczema, psoriasis, radiation sickness, cirrhosis of the liver, coronary thrombosis, arteriosclerosis, and retinal hemorrhages. Often used to treat athletic injuries because they relieve pain, bumps, and bruises. They reduce pain in the legs or across the back, and reduce bleeding and low serum calcium. Promotes circulation, lowers cholesterol levels, stimulates bile production, and prevents and treats cataracts. Useful in treating stomach ulcers and dizziness caused by labyrinthitis, a disease of the inner ear. (Both are caused by capillary weakness.) When taken with vitamin C, they reduce oral herpes, improve muscular dystrophy, improve the disorder of the eye affecting diabetics, and may help prevent habitual miscarriages.

Quercetin (when taken with bromelain and vitamin C, in tablet form) is very useful in treating asthma symptoms. *Rutin,* which comes from buckwheat leaves, is especially helpful in the prevention of recurrent bleeding arising from weakened blood vessels. It is sometimes used in the treatment of hemorrhoids and helps prevent the walls of blood vessels from becoming fragile.

Deficiency symptoms: Purplish or blue spots on the skin, caused by capillary fragility. Reduced vitamin C activity. A deficiency of vitamin C or bioflavonoids may contribute to rheumatism and rheumatic fever.

Interactions: Bioflavonoids are essential for vitamin C absorption; so the two should be taken together. In natural foods, they occur together. In supplements, the C is generally not balanced by enough of the bioflavonoids, which should be equal to or greater than the amount of C. Bioflavonoids are totally nontoxic.

OTHER VITAMINS

VITAMIN T ("Sesame seed factor")—
Dosage: Not established.
Sources: This is an oil-soluble vitamin, found in sesame seeds, raw sesame butter (tahini), some vegetable oils, egg yolks.
Functions: Needed for platelet integrity in the blood. It reestablishes blood coagulation and is useful in correcting nutritional anemia. Promotes the formation of blood platelets (the round disks in the blood) and combats hemophilia, a hereditary blood disease that is characterized by slowed rate of clotting.
Deficiency symptoms: Anemia.

VITAMIN U ("Anti-ulcer factor")—
Dosage: Not established.
Sources: Raw cabbage juice is the best source. Other sources include raw cabbage, and homemade sauerkraut.
Functions: This is the anti-ulcer vitamin. It is a specific for peptic ulcers, especially duodenal ulcers.
Deficiency symptoms: Stomach or duodenal ulcers.

2 - MAJOR MINERALS

At least 18 minerals are essential in human nutrition. They are divided into major minerals and minor minerals. Our bodies daily need more than 100 mg of major minerals and less than 100 mg of minor minerals. The major minerals are calcium, phosphorus, potassium, sodium, chloride, magnesium, and sulfur. The minor (or trace) minerals are boron, chromium, copper, iodine, iron, manganese, molybdenum, selenium, silicon, vanadium, and zinc. Make sure you are obtaining a balanced mineral intake.

CALCIUM (Ca)—
Dosage: *Calcium (Ca):* RDA 2 / ODA 2,000 mg / TDA 2,000-5,000 mg. *Recommended:* 1,000 mg daily. During pregnancy and lactation, 1,200 mg daily. Especially during pregnancy or lactation, take 1,000-1,400 mg. Calcium supplements are generally well-tolerated at dosages less than 2,000 mg; but higher dosages may increase the risk for kidney stones and soft-tissue calcification (although neither problem has conclusively been shown to be caused by taking calcium supplements).
Sources: *Best sources:* Milk, most raw vegetables, especially the green, leafy ones. Sesame seeds are an excellent source, since they have such a good calcium-phosphorus ratio. Brewer's yeast. *Other sources* include oats, almonds, navy beans, walnuts, millet, sunflower seeds. A good calcium source will contain lots of calcium and relatively little phosphorous.
Calcium supplements: *Calcium citrate* is easily absorbed, can be used if you have low stomach acid levels, and is generally the best form to take. But many products contain lower amounts of elemental calcium. It should contain 21% calcium by weight. *Calcium carbonate* contains 40% calcium, but is not easily absorbed. (Refined forms are produced in a laboratory;

unrefined forms are derived from limestone or oyster shells.) *Calcium gluc*onate contains 9% calcium, but sometimes causes diarrhea and nausea. *Calcium lactate* contains 13%, along with lactic acid from milk. It is more acid than some of the other supplements. *Calcium phosphorus* contains 30% calcium; but the phosphorus in it tends to lock with the calcium and carry it on out of the system. Do not take calcium phosphorus tablets or powder. Other forms are *dolomite*, which is calcium and magnesium from dolomitic rock, and *bone meal,* from ground-up animal bones (an inferior product because they also contain phosphorus). Most unrefined calcium products have unacceptably high levels of lead. *Calcium citrate* is probably best for lowest lead level, and is absorbed the best. *Calcium lactate* and *calcium gluconate powder* are useable sources. In the opinion of some, the gluconate formula tastes better than the one with lactate. *Also see Vitamin D, p. 106.*
Functions: Needed to build and repair bones and teeth. Essential for heart and muscle action. Protects against radioactive strontium 90 intake. Needed for enzyme and blood clotting. Very important during pregnancy and lactation. Speeds all healing processes. Helps maintain proper balance between sodium, potassium, and magnesium. Needed for treatment of osteoporosis, reducing high blood pressure. Calms heart action, and tends to reduce pain.
Deficiency symptoms: Retarded growth, tooth decay, rickets, osteomalacia, osteoporosis, irritability, nervousness, heart palpitations, muscle cramps, and insomnia.
Needed for assimilation: Vitamins A, C, D, and E. boron, essential fatty acids, magnesium, manganese, phosphorus, lysine.
Interactions: Calcium interacts with many nutrients, especially vitamin D, Vitamin K, and magnesium. High dosages of magnesium, zinc, phosphates, protein, sodium, and sugar reduce calcium absorption. Caffeine, alcohol, phosphates, sodium, protein, and sugar increase calcium excretion. (The weightlessness of space travel also does.) Antacids containing aluminum increase bone breakdown and excretion of calcium.
Cautions: Too much phosphorus in a meal will lock with calcium and render it ineffective. Too much oil at a meal will lock with calcium, turn it into a kind of soap, and both will go out through the bowels. Much more information on calcium will be found elsewhere in this *Encyclopedia* in the article, titled *"Strengthening the Bones (chapter 10 p. 606)."*

PHOSPHORUS (P)—
Dosage: RDA 800 mg / ODA 0.00 / TDA 0.00. Adults 800 mg. Children and women during pregnancy or lactation: 1,000-1,400 mg.—but everyone gets enough. *Recommended:* This is the one mineral you want to avoid. First, it is practically impossible to have a phosphorus deficiency. Although phosphorus is vitally needed, you always get enough. Second, too much of it at a given meal locks with calcium, rendering it ineffective. Too much phosphorus also causes other difficulties. Avoid supplemental phosphorus whenever possible. *(See Calcium, above.)*
Sources: whole grains, corn, seeds, nuts, legumes, dried fruits, dairy products, egg yolks, meat, fish.
Functions: Phosphorus works with calcium, but only when in proper balance. They work together to build bones and teeth. It is also needed in maintaining an acid-alkali balance

in the blood. It is needed for nerve function and carbohydrate metabolism.

Deficiency symptoms: For practical purposes, hardly ever seen. Symptoms would include poor mineralization of bones, retarded growth, inadequate nerve and brain function, overall weakness.

Needed for assimilation: Vitamin B_6, calcium, iron, manganese, sodium.

MAGNESIUM (Mg)—

Dosage: RDA 350 mg / ODA 1,000 mg / TDA 1,000 mg.
Recommended: Ideal supplement intake should be 6 mg per 2.2 lbs. body weight (154-lb. person should daily obtain 420 mg). For specific problems, described below, take 12 mg per 2.2 lbs. body weight.

Sources: *Richest sources:* kelp, dulse, wheat bran, wheat germ, almonds, cashews, blackstrap molasses, brewer's yeast, buckwheat, Brazil nuts, filberts, peanuts, millet, wheat grain, pecans, English walnuts, rye. *Other sources:* soybeans, other nuts, raw and cooked green leafy vegetables, whole grains, figs, apples, lemons, peaches, apricots, brown rice, collard leaves, other greens. Magnesium chloride is the best form of supplementary magnesium; but other forms can be used.

Functions: Second only to potassium in its concentration within cells. Magnesium is crucial to many functions, including energy production, protein formation, and cellular replication. It participates in more than 300 enzyme reactions in the body. Operates as a catalyst in many functions involving energy (including production of the very crucial ATP); also in utilization of vitamins B and E, calcium, fats, and other minerals. Essential for the heart, muscle tone, bones. It regulates acid-alkaline balances, aids in lecithin production. Like calcium, magnesium is a natural tranquilizer. Because it is required for the activation of the sodium and potassium pump that removes sodium from cells and puts potassium into them, without magnesium, potassium leaves the cells and sodium enters them (which is the basis of a cancer cell). Magnesium also regulates calcium metabolism.

Causes of deficiency: Magnesium deficiency is extremely common in the U.S., especially in the elderly and premenstrual women. Other major causes of deficiency include high calcium intake, surgery, alcohol, diuretics, liver disease, kidney disease, and oral contraceptive use.

Deficiency symptoms: Without adequate magnesium, both calcium and magnesium leave the body. Fatigue, mental confusion, irritability, weakness, muscle cramps, loss of appetite, tendency to stress, nerve problems. Kidney stones, high blood pressure, kidney damage, heart disease, heart attack, insomnia, PMS, menstrual cramps, nervous irritability, confusion and depression, epileptic seizures, premature wrinkles, cancer, and damaged protein metabolism.

Magnesium therapy: helps cardiovascular and heart problems, high blood pressure, acute myocardial infarction, asthma, diabetes, fatigue, glaucoma, hearing loss, kidney stones, migraine, osteoporosis, pregnancy toxemia, premature delivery, premenstrual problems, dysmenorrhea,

Needed for assimilation: Vitamins B_6, C, D, calcium, potassium, phosphorus.

Interactions: Because magnesium, potassium, calcium and other minerals interact extensively, dosages of other minerals reduce the intake of magnesium, and vice versa. High calcium in-

take, fortified with vitamin D, decreases magnesium absorption.

Cautions: Digitalis, insulin (taken by diabetics), antibiotics, diuretics, and hyperthyroidism all tend to cause the body to lose magnesium.

Warning: Although magnesium is usually tolerated well, those with kidney disease or severe heart disease should not take magnesium (or potassium) except by physician's orders. Supplements of magnesium sulfate (Epsom salts), hydroxide, or chloride occasionally causes loose bowel movements.

POTASSIUM (K)—

Dosage: RDA 1,875 mg / ODA 2,500 mg / TDA 5,500 mg.
Recommended: The estimated dietary intake is 1.9-5.6 grams. But this amount will easily be surpassed if you eat largely of fruits and vegetables.

Three electrolytes: Potassium, sodium, and chloride are electrolytes (minerals which, when dissolved in water, conduct electricity). The three are very closely related. They always operate in pairs: a positively charged molecule (sodium or potassium), with a negatively charged one (chloride [chlorine]). Although all are important, potassium is the key—it is the most important of the three.

Sources: It is in all vegetables, especially green leafy ones. Thick white potato peelings are rich in it. Bananas are also excellent.

Functions: There is more potassium in body cells than any other mineral; and you have a great need for *large amounts* of it. Potassium helps maintain proper acid-alkaline balance in the blood and tissues, and prevents over-acidity. It is essential for muscle contraction, promotes hormone secretion, helps kidneys detoxify the blood. Its vital functions include acting as an electrolyte, converting blood sugar into glycogen, and storing blood sugar in the muscles and liver. For example, muscle energy comes from burning glycogen; but, without enough potassium, there is not enough glycogen—and extreme fatigue and muscle weakness results.

Deficiency symptoms: Lack of potassium causes sodium (salt) to accumulate in the body. The result is edema, high blood pressure, and heart failure. The heart muscle can be damaged. Constipation, extreme fatigue, muscular weakness, low blood sugar, and nervous disorders.

Interactions: Potassium works closely with magnesium in many body functions.

Warning: Potassium and sodium must be kept in proper balance at all times, or serious problems develop. Too much sodium in the diet disrupts the potassium / sodium balance in the body. A low-potassium, high-sodium diet helps produce cancer, cardiovascular disease (heart disease, high blood pressure, strokes, etc.). But a diet high in potassium and low in sodium—protects against those diseases! You can easily take too much sodium; but you cannot take too much potassium! *See Sodium, below, for more information.* Restricting salt (sodium chloride) intake does not lower blood pressure, until potassium intake is greatly improved. High-dosage potassium salts (in pill form) can cause nausea, vomiting, diarrhea, and ulcers. There is lots of potassium in fruits and vegetables, and almost none in processed foods. There is relatively little sodium in fruits and vegetables, and far too much (often extremely too much) in processed foods. There are no ill effects from a diet rich in excess potassium, with one exception: If you have kidney

NUTR

disease, you will need to restrict your potassium intake.

SODIUM (Na)—

Dosage: RDA 1,100 mg / ODA 200-600 mg / TDA 300-3,000 mg. Sodium is a mineral to avoid. You need a little, but not very much. If you want to get it from the salt shaker, sprinkle a tiny (tiny) bit on only one or two foods at the table, having put none in the cooking. *Recommended:* Obtain sodium from natural food alone, plus, at the most, only an extremely slight amount of table salt. The best way to do this is to pour a tiny amount into your hand, so you know you only have a very small amount; then pour it onto your food. (If you pour salt directly on your food, you cannot see how much is going on it.)

The salt problem: Sodium is a mineral you should be very cautious about. You need a little, but only a very little. In America, only 5% of the sodium comes from natural food. Prepared foods add 45%, cooking adds 45% more, and condiments add another 5%. All the sodium the body generally needs is found in the natural (unsalted) food which is eaten. *Also see Potassium, above.* A word about table salt: Most of it has added aluminum, to keep the salt free-flowing. You do not want to eat aluminum (Alzheimer's is not easy to live with)! So-called "sea salt" is just regular salt; it has no other minerals in it. If the salt you buy is free-flowing, you do not want to use it (because of the added aluminum)! But, if you insist on buying regular salt, select iodized salt. Because Americans add too much salt to their meals, they have a potassium-to-sodium ratio of 1:2. (They are eating twice as much sodium as potassium.) What is needed is a 5:1 ratio (5 times as much potassium as sodium) to maintain good health. If you eat a natural diet of fruits and vegetables, you will take in 100:1—100 times as much potassium as sodium. If you will look on any food chart, you will find that all the natural foods have a high potassium to sodium ratio, whereas all the junk food will have a high sodium to potassium ratio. Do not be afraid of potassium; you cannot get too much! DO be afraid of sodium.

Sources: Although it is found in a variety of foods, including romaine lettuce, celery, asparagus, and watermelon, most people like to get it out of the salt shaker. The best source of added salt to your diet is Nova Scotia dulse or Norwegian kelp. Both are full of vitally needed trace minerals.

Functions: Sodium works closely with potassium and chlorine in a number of important functions *(see Potassium, above)*. They maintain proper electrolyte balance; for they change into electrically charged ions which carry nerve impulses. They also control and maintain osmotic pressure into, and out of, the cells. This enables the blood to carry nutrients throughout the body. They also keep the amount of body fluid at the proper level. Sodium is an important constituent of stomach acid.

Deficiency symptoms: It is rare for a person to have a sodium deficiency. But it may be caused by excessive sweating, chronic diarrhea, or overuse of diuretics. Muscular weakness, heat exhaustion, mental apathy, nausea, or respiratory failure can result.

Excess symptoms: Too much sodium in the diet is far more common, and is shown in water retention, high blood pressure, stomach ulcers or cancer, hardening of the arteries, and heart disease.

Needed for assimilation: Vitamin D, calcium, potassium, sulfur.

CHLORINE (Cl)—

Dosage: RDA 1,700 mg / ODA 2,500 mg / TDA 500-2,500 mg. You usually obtain enough in food. There is no recommended daily allowance for chlorine because the average person gets about 3-9 grams daily in the table salt he sprinkles on his food and the salt that is added to most processed foods.

Sources: Kelp, dulse, rye flour, ripe olives, tomatoes, cabbage, endive, kale, celery, turnips, cucumbers, asparagus, oats, pineapple, avocado.

Functions: Chlorine mainly occurs in compound form with sodium or potassium, and is widely distributed throughout the body in the form of chloride. It is needed, along with sodium, for production of hydrochloric acid (stomach acid). Without HCl, minerals cannot be properly absorbed and proteins cannot be digested. Chlorine is also involved in fluid and electrolyte balance, and liver function. It helps regulate the balance of acid and alkali in the blood and maintains pressure that causes fluids to pass in and out of cell membranes until the concentration of dissolved particles is equalized on both sides. It stimulates the liver to function as a filter for wastes and helps clean toxic waste products out of the system. It helps keep joints and tendons in youthful shape and aids in distributing hormones. Chlorine is used to treat diarrhea and vomiting.

Deficiency symptoms: Body fluid levels do not function properly, and digestion is poor. Hair and tooth loss can occur. Poor muscular contraction and impaired digestion can occur.

Caution: Chlorine is commonly added to drinking water (chlorinated water); but it is a highly reactive chemical and may join with inorganic minerals and other chemicals, to form harmful substances. Chlorine in drinking water destroys vitamin E, as well as many of the intestinal flora that help digest food.

IRON (Fe)—

Dosage: RDA 10 mg for men; 18 mg for women / ODA 45 mg / TDA 50-100 mg. Do not take iron supplements unless you have to. Blackstrap molasses is the richest food source of iron and is a good food. Of course, take it in moderation because it is so sweet. Do not take iron *supplements* (tablets) unless you have to; they often contain an iron compound which damages the body.

Sources: Black molasses is the richest source. Eat a half teaspoonful twice a day. Other sources include apricots, prunes, raisins, brewer's yeast, beets, dulse, kelp, peaches, whole grain cereals, leafy greens, seeds, nuts, beans, egg yolks, raisins.

Herbal sources: Alfalfa, burdock root, chamomile, chickweed, dandelion, dong quai, fennel seed, lemongrass, fenugreek, mullein, peppermint, plaintain, raspberry leaf, rose hips, uva ursi.

Functions: Needed for hemoglobin formation in the blood. Hemoglobin enables the red blood cells to fill with oxygen and carry it to the cells. It is also needed for myoglobin, the type of hemoglobin in muscle tissue, and the production of many enzymes. It is needed for growth, energy production, and immune protection.

Deficiency causes: Although primarily due to insufficient intake in the diet, it can result from intestinal bleeding, ulcers, poor digestion, a diet high in phosphorus (eating lots of meat), continued use of antacids, or excessive use of coffee or black tea. Heavy and prolonged periods during menstruation, or short menstrual cycles. Rarely a deficiency of pyridoxine (vitamin B_6) or vitamin B_{12}. Heavy perspiration and strenuous exercise depletes body reserves of iron. Taking supplemental calcium with a meal can reduce absorption of iron. Take calcium supplements at bedtime instead. Excessive amounts of zinc and vitamin E can also interfere with iron absorption. Rheumatoid arthritis and cancer can hinder iron utilization in the body.

Deficiency symptoms: Simple iron deficiency (anemia), reduced resistance to disease, headaches, skin that is too pale, brittle hair, digestive disturbances, difficulty in swallowing, fatigue, dizziness, fragile bones, hair loss, inflamed mouth tissues, slowed mental reactions, nervousness, or nails that have lengthwise ridges or are spoon-shaped. People with candidiasis or chronic herpes are likely to be low on iron.

Cautions: Iron is not absorbed unless there is sufficient hydrochloric acid in the stomach. Eating acid fruits helps iron absorption at that meal. Vitamin C also aids absorption while coffee and tea interferes with it. Iron cannot be absorbed without a slight amount of copper. (But an excess of copper destroys vitamin C.). Iron is stored in the body; and excessive amounts of it is another, but less frequent, problem. Too much iron in the tissues results in too many free radicals (increasing the need for vitamin E) and, ultimately, to bronzed skin coloring. (Do not confuse that with the normal—and harmless—slight yellowing of the skin which may occur when carrot juice is drunk.) Do not take iron supplements during an infection; doing so can increase bacterial growth.

Warning: Do not take iron supplements unless absolutely necessary, and definitely not during pregnancy. Avoid multivitamin mineral supplements which contain iron. Never take ferrous sulfate! Instead, choose organic forms of iron (ferrous gluconate or ferrous fumarate). The safer way is to take a daily spoonful of blackstrap molasses.

SULFUR (S)—

Dosage: RDA Not stated / ODA 500 mg / TDA 1,000 mg. *Recommended:* You generally obtain enough in food. Normal intake amount is 500 mg; and therapeutic dosage is 1,000 mg.

Sources: *Best sources:* garlic, cabbage, dried beans, Brussels sprouts, eggs, kale, onions, wheat germ, and the horsetail herb. *Other sources:* It is widely found in vegetables and beans. MSM (methylsufonylmethane) is said to be a good source of sulfur.

Functions: This acid-forming mineral, found in all body tissues, is needed for the formation of four amino acids: cysteine, methionine, glutathione, and taurine. It is needed for healthy hair, skin and nails; and utilization of oxygen by the body. It disinfects the blood, protects cell protoplasm, helps the body resist bacteria, stimulates bile secretion, and protects against harmful effects of pollution and radiation. It is used in the manufacture of collagen, a special protein which strengthens skin.

Deficiency symptoms: Dull hair and brittle nails.

Needed for assimilation: Vitamin B$_1$, pantothenic acid, potassium, biotin.

Cautions: Sulfur is destroyed or damaged by moisture and heat. Do not swallow powdered sulfur! Although thought by some to be a "spring remedy," it may give you a series of boils, extending over a period of many months, as the body tries to discharge this poison from the body.

3 - TRACE MINERALS

Trace minerals are needed by the body in extremely small amounts; yet they are extremely vital to physical function. The richest source is consistently found in sea plants (seaweeds).

IODINE (I)—

Dosage: 150 mcg (which is 0.15 mg). It is crucial that you obtain enough of this mineral. Dulse and kelp (two types of seaweed) are the best sources. Too much iodine can actually inhibit synthesis by the thyroid gland; therefore keep dietary or supplementary levels of iodine (also called iodide) intake below 500 mcg daily. This is a vitally needed element which far too many people do not obtain enough of. The body uses more of this than any other trace mineral.

Sources: *Richest sources:* Nova Scotia dulse and Norwegian kelp (types of seaweed). California kelp is not a good nutritional source. Although Lugol's solution is another source, and is only obtainable by prescription, it is easy to take too much. *Other sources:* garlic, leafy greens, pineapples, pears, artichokes, citrus fruits, egg yolks. Do not use fish liver oils as a source; for they damage the heart muscle!

Bottled iodine can be painted on the bottom of the foot (or elsewhere on the body), and will be partially absorbed. But, of course, you might overdose. It is believed that, if the reddish color of the iodine on the painted area disappears within 24 hours, the body needs the iodine.

One research study found that when cows were given 200 times the "normal" dosage of iodine, they were in better health.

Functions: Thyroxine, the hormone produced by the thyroid gland, is almost pure iodine. Thyroxine (T3 is the most active form) regulates very much of the total functions of the body, including metabolism, energy production, body weight, heat, etc. Plentiful iodine in the diet can block absorption of radioactive iodine from fallout. Iodine modulates the effect of estrogen on breast tissue.

Two forms: Iodine is the elemental form of iodide; and, in the body, it is most efficient in helping estrogen in breast tissue. Iodide is iodine compounded to sodium or potassium (potassium iodide is better than sodium iodide). In either form, it is absorbed well by the thyroid. However, organic sources of iodine (kelp, dulse, iodine caseinate, etc.) are absorbed by the body about as well as inorganic iodides (potassium iodide and sodium iodide). Iodide caseinate is especially effective in treating fibrocystic breast disease.

Deficiency symptoms: Goiter, thyroid gland enlargement or malfunction. Cretinism, anemia, slowed pulse, fatigue, low blood pressure. Frequently a tendency to obesity. In extreme cases, thyroid cancer, high blood cholesterol, and heart disease can result.

Iodine-deficiency disorders: Goiter, cretinism, growth retardation, intellectual disability, neonatal hypothyroidism, increased early and late pregnancy miscarriage, increased infant mortality.

Needed for assimilation: Iron, manganese, phosphorus.

Foods which block iodine absorption: These foods are known as *goitrogens* (goiter producers) and include cabbage, turnips, mustard, soybeans, cassava root, peanuts, pine nuts, and millet. Cooking often inactivates goitrogens.

Cautions: If you are going to sprinkle regular salt on your food, use iodized salt. However, you would maintain better health if you used as little added salt as possible. So-called "sea salt" is just regular sodium chloride, which was produced by ocean water evaporation; it contains no trace minerals, nor iodine. Excessive iodine (or iodide) intake will reduce thyroid absorption, and may cause acne-like skin eruptions. When given at physiological dosages (150-600 mcg), iodine (or iodide) does not interact negatively with any nutrient or drug.

SELENIUM (Se)—
Dosage: RDA not established / ODA 70 mcg / TDA 55 mcg.
Recommended: Supplement the diet with 50-200 mcg selenium and 200-400 IU vitamin E. Intake levels above 1,000 mcg daily can produce toxicity; so it is best not to take more than 400 IU daily. For children: Take 1.5 mcg per pound of body weight. Do not take more than 40 mcg daily during pregnancy.
Sources: *Richest sources:* Nova Scotia dulse and Norwegian kelp. *Other good sources:* wheat germ, Brazil nuts. *Other sources:* brewer's yeast (not primary grown yeast), garlic, organically grown foods, cereals, most vegetables.
Functions: A powerful antioxidant. Works closely with vitamin E and has similar functions. Helps E accomplish more, so not as much is needed. Keeps hemoglobin from being damaged by oxidation. Slows the aging process by inhibiting action of free radicals. Helps regenerate liver, especially after cirrhosis. Essential for activity of glutathione peroxidase, an important enzyme. Protects body from mercury, aluminum, lead, and cadmium poisoning. Involved in thyroid hormone production. A principal function is to reduce the oxidation of lipids (fatty acids).
Primary uses: Prevention of cancer, increases immune function, protects against cardiovascular disease. Treats inflammatory conditions (such as rheumatoid arthritis, eczema, and psoriasis). Treats cataracts. Helps ensure proper fetal growth and development (selenium requirements increase during pregnancy; selenium levels are always low in low birth weight babies). Prevents SIDS (sudden infant death syndrome). Improves male fertility. Helps reduce high blood pressure.
Deficiency symptoms: Muscle degeneration, liver damage, premature aging, heart disturbances, muscle weakness. Severe deficiency, over a period of time, can induce cancer of the digestive and intestinal tracts. Keshan disease is a severe heart disorder in China in areas where selenium levels in the soil are low. The most common risk of selenium deficiency is an increased risk for cancer, heart disease, and low immune function.
Excessive intake symptoms: Brittle nails, garlicky breath, hair loss, irritability, liver and kidney impairment, pallor, metallic taste in mouth, skin eruptions, tooth loss, yellowish skin.
Supplement forms: Inorganic salts (sodium selenite, etc.) are not absorbed as well and are less active than organic forms (selenomethionine and selenium-rich yeast).
Interactions: All other antioxidants work well with selenium in strengthening the system.
Cautions: Selenium absorption and utilization is reduced by heavy metals (mercury, cadmium, lead, etc.), high doses of vitamin C (affects sodium selenite more than organic forms of selenium), high intakes of other trace minerals (especially zinc), and various drugs (especially chemotherapy).

ZINC (Zn)—
Dosage: RDA 15 mg / ODA 30 mg / TDA 50 mg.
Recommended: 15-20 mg daily, in addition to average food intake of 10 mg daily. Therapeutic dosage is 30-60 mg daily for men and 30-45 mg daily for women.
Sources: Richest sources: Nova Scotia dulse and Norwegian kelp (types of seaweed) are the best sources. Pumpkin seeds, ginger root, pecans, split peas, Brazil nuts. Other good sources: whole wheat, rye, oats, peanuts, lima beans, almonds, walnuts, buckwheat, other vegetables. Zinc in grains and seeds tends to be locked by

phytin, but is unlocked by the fermentation process (when making bread) and by sprouting seeds.
Functions: Needed for RNA and DNA formation, and synthesis of proteins. A component in over 200 enzymes, zinc is in every body cell. It functions in more enzyme reactions than any other mineral. Also crucial to many hormones, it is primarily stored in the muscles, and is highly concentrated in red and white blood cells. It is extremely important during fetal development and results in premature births, low birth weight, growth retardation, pre-eclampsia. Zinc is in insulin, so is involved in carbohydrate and energy metabolism. Needed for normal development of reproductive organs and the function of prostate. Speeds up healing of burns and wounds. Needed for vitamin A metabolism. Very helpful in treating acne, macular degeneration, Alzheimer's disease, and Wilson's disease.
Deficiency symptoms: skin changes, diarrhea, mental disturbances, recurrent infections. The elderly are most likely to have marginal zinc deficiencies. Other problems caused by lack of zinc include sleep and behavior disturbances, psychiatric illness, growth retardation, loss of sense of smell or taste, night blindness, abnormal menstruation, alcohol abuse, rheumatoid arthritis, delayed wound healing, mouth ulcers, a white coating on the tongue, marked halitosis. Causes birth defects, retarded growth, reproductive problems, lowered resistance to infections, slow healing of wounds and skin diseases, white spots on finger and toe nails, poor sense of smell and taste. Lethargy, apathy, dandruff, hair loss, atherosclerosis, epilepsy, and osteoporosis.
Supplements: All forms of zinc supplements are absorbed well.
Causes of deficiency: Alcoholism, old age, anorexia nervosa, protein deficiency, acute infections, burns, chronic blood loss, pregnancy and lactation, oral contraceptives, growth spurts and puberty, diarrhea, liver disease.
Needed for assimilation: Vitamin B$_6$, calcium, phosphorus, copper.
Cautions: Toxic effects of zinc occur with prolonged intake of more than 150 mg daily. This is rare; since vomiting usually occurs and flushes out excess amounts. Zinc is probably the least toxic mineral, and does not negatively react with any drug. If taken on an empty stomach, zinc (especially zinc sulfate) supplementation can result in stomach upset and nausea. High dosages of other minerals (especially calcium and iron) can reduce zinc absorption. For best absorption, zinc supplements are best taken apart from high-fiber foods.

COPPER (Cu)—
Dosage: RDA 2 mg / ODA 3-4 mg / TDA 4-6 mg. *Recommended:* Normal need is 1.5-3 mg, and therapeutic dosages are 4-6 mg. But needs are generally supplied by a good diet. Supplemental copper intake is keyed to supplemental zinc intake. The best zinc to copper ratio is 10:1 (If 30 mg zinc is taken daily, you should also take 3 mg. copper.)
Sources: Foods rich in iron are also rich in copper. *(See Iron, just above.)* Nuts (highest in Brazil nuts, almonds, hazelnuts, walnuts, and pecans) and legumes are the richest source. Grains are next best. Copper is widely distributed in foods.
Functions: Copper works closely with iron in accomplishing the same functions *(see Iron, above).* Needed for RNA production, protein metabolism, healing processes, and hair color. Involved in brain, nerve, bone, and connective tissue development. Several enzyme systems require copper. The highest concentration (amount per gram of tissue) is in the brain and liver. The estimated 70-80

mg of copper in the body are distributed throughout all the organs and cells.

Deficiency symptoms: Anemia, weakened respiration, digestion, heart function, and graying of hair. Because copper is needed for iron absorption, insufficient copper also results in iron deficiency.

Needed for assimilation: Folic acid, iron, zinc, cobalt. Copper absorption is decreased by chronic antacid intake, chronic diarrhea, high dosage of supplemental zinc or vitamin C.

Caution: Additional copper is needed during pregnancy, lactation, and the teenage years. Chelation therapy, burns, and nephrosis tend to cause copper to be lost from the body. The danger is generally too much inorganic copper in the diet, due to water from copper water pipes and copper sulfate (added to frozen foods to make them greener, especially peas). Copper is an emetic. As little as 10 mg usually produces nausea; and 60 mg will cause vomiting. Keep copper supplements away from children; 3.5 grams can kill a person. It is estimated that daily consumption of 10-35 mg is continually safe. However, such a high dosage would adversely affect zinc absorption and utilization.

MANGANESE (Mn)—

Dosage: RDA 2.5 mg / ODA 5 mg / TDA 2-50 mg.

Recommended dosage: Most people require 2-5 mg daily. Therapeutic dosages for epilepsy are 15-30 mg daily; and, for diabetes, it is 5-15 mg daily. For strains and sprains, 50-200 mg daily for first 2 weeks, followed by 15-30 mg daily.

Sources: Richest sources: Nova Scotia dulse and Norwegian kelp (types of seaweed). Also good: pecans, Brazil nuts, almonds, barley, avocados. Other sources: other grains, green leafy vegetables, beets, oranges, blueberries, grapefruit, apricots, peas, fresh wheat germ, raw egg yolk.

Functions: Enters into the work of several enzymes which affect metabolism of carbohydrates, proteins, and fats. Aids coordinative action between brain, nerves, and muscles. Involved in reproduction and mammary gland function. Works with choline in fat digestion and utilization. Aids in the formation of mother's milk.

Deficiency symptoms: Digestive disturbances, retarded growth, defects in carbohydrate and fat metabolism, male and female sterility, abnormal bone development, poor equilibrium, myasthenia gravis, and asthma. If manganese deficiency occurs during pregnancy, the offspring exhibit lack of balance, movement incoordination, retraction of the head, hearing problems, heart disorders, high cholesterol, memory loss, muscle contractions, pancreatic damage, rapid pulse, tremors, breast ailments. Deficiencies tend to be rare.

Primary uses: Manganese is primarily used to treat sprains, strains, inflammation, diabetes, and epilepsy.

Absorption: Manganese sulfate or chloride are not as well-absorbed as manganese picolinate, magnesium gluconate, or other chelates.

Needed for assimilation: vitamin B complex, vitamin E, calcium, iron.

Interactions: Needed for utilization of vitamin B_1 (thiamine) and vitamin E. It helps all the B vitamins function better. Essential for people with iron-deficiency anemias.

Cautions: Extremely low toxicity. However, environmental pollution or mining of manganese can lead to "manganese madness" (hyperirritability, hallucinations, and violent acts).

SILICON (Si)—

Dosage: RDA is not established; but 20-40 mg daily is considered safe and probably adequate. Until more is learned, dosages should not exceed 50 mg daily.

Richest sources: Nova Scotia dulse and Norwegian kelp (types of seaweed). *Other very good sources:* oatmeal, brown rice, root vegetables. Oat straw tea and horsetail herb are considered very good sources. *Other sources:* young green plants, such as alfalfa and horsetail. Steel-cut oats, grapes, apples, strawberries, onions, beets, almonds, sunflower seeds, and peanuts.

Functions: Needed for hair, nails, teeth, skin, tendons, and bones. Helps during healing and protects against a variety of diseases, including skin disorders and tuberculosis. Needed for proper development of collagen, the major protein component essential for proper bone and connective tissue integrity. The highest concentrations of silicon is found in the skin and hair. For some unknown reason, the silicon content of the aorta, thymus, and skin declines with age while the amount in other tissues do not.

Deficiency symptoms: Wrinkles, thinning or loss of hair, soft or brittle nails, inferior bone development, osteoporosis, insomnia.

Needed for assimilation: Iron, phosphorus.

Cautions: Silicon is a primary constituent in sand and very hard rocks. Only take it as it naturally occurs in food. Eat nothing which, according to the label, has added silicon in it.

Warning: Avoid exposure to silicon in the air (such as miners inhaled in mines). Silicosis is not a pleasant disease. Increased levels of silicon and aluminum have been found in the neurofibrillary tangle and senile plaque in the brains of Alzheimer's disease patients.

FLUORINE (F)—

Dosage: *Fluorine (F):* RDA 1.5 mg / ODA 1.5 mg / TDA 20 mg (Use this amount only with a prescription for osteoporosis.) Needed only in very small amounts.

Sources: Nova Scotia dulse and Norwegian kelp (types of seaweed) are the best sources. Steel-cut oats, garlic, carrots, sunflower seeds, green vegetables, beet tops, almonds, naturally hard water.

Functions: Needed for bone and tooth formation. An internal antiseptic, it protects against infections.

Deficiency symptoms: Not known.

Cautions: An excess of fluoride (sodium fluoride) is added to drinking water in many cities; but it is a poison. It mottles teeth and does not help them. Only the minute traces of fluorine found in food are safe to ingest. Use some type of filtration device to remove chlorine and fluoride from your drinking water, or buy a water distiller.

CHROMIUM (Cr)—

Dosage: RDA 50 mcg / ODA 200 mcg / TDA 300-1,000 mcg. Apparently, we need at least 200 mcg daily in our diet. Experts recommend 400-600 mg daily, for impaired glucose tolerance patients, and as a help to weight loss.

Sources: *Richest sources:* Nova Scotia dulse and Norwegian kelp. Normally present in natural waters, especially hard (highly mineralized) water, brewer's yeast. *Other good sources:* whole-grain bread, raw sugar and cane juice.

Functions: Part of many enzymes, hormones, and insulin. Needed for sugar utilization, cholesterol metabolism, and synthesis of protein in the heart muscle. Contains what is known as the *glucose tolerance factor.* Chromium's key benefit is helping insulin work properly.

Primary uses: Treatment of impaired glucose tolerance (hypoglycemia and diabetes), elevated blood cholesterol and triglyceride levels, acne, and aiding weight loss.

Deficiency symptoms: High or low blood sugar, diabetes, hypoglycemia, hardening of the arteries, heart disease. The primary sign of chromium deficiency is glucose intolerance characterized by elevated blood sugar and insulin levels.

Cautions: White sugar in the diet induces chromium deficiency. (When sugar is made white, the chromium is removed; so when that white sugar is eaten, it unites with chromium in the body in an attempt to again make itself a normal sugar molecule, thus depleting the body of chromium. In the same way, white sugar removes other minerals from the body.)

MOLYBDENUM (Mo)—
Dosage: RDA 15 mcg / ODA 500 mcg / TDA 1,000 mcg. **Recommended:** 200-500 mcg daily. Higher doses are given for Wilson's disease.

Sources: Richest sources: Nova Scotia dulse and Norwegian kelp (types of seaweed). Very good sources: whole cereals, especially millet, brown rice, and buckwheat, brewer's yeast, legumes (lentils and split peas best), and naturally hard water.

Functions: Part of certain enzymes, especially oxidizing enzymes. Protects somewhat against copper poisoning. Needed for carbohydrate metabolism. It is now known that molybdenum deficiency occurs in cases of cancer.

Primary uses: The treatment of Wilson's disease, protection against dental cavities, and prevention of cancer.

Deficiency symptoms: Sulfite toxicity such as increased heart rate, headache, nausea, vomiting, shortness of breath.

Deficiency causes: A primary cause is total parenteral nutrition (food supplied fully by intravenous feedings in a hospital).

Interactions: Molybdenum interacts with copper and fluoride, and with no other substances.

Cautions: Relatively nontoxic. Toxicity only occurs when more than 100 mg per kg body weight is taken. Daily intake of 10-15 mg sometimes produces symptoms of gout, due to increased uric acid production. Fortunately, molybdenum is most completely absorbed in the intestines, is conserved at low intakes, and rapidly excreted in the urine when too much is taken in.

COBALT (Co)—
Dosage: Not established.

Sources: Nova Scotia dulse and Norwegian kelp (types of seaweed) are the best sources. All green, leafy vegetables.

Functions: Part of the vitamin B_1, (2 molecules). It is therefore necessary for synthesis of this anti-pernicious anemia vitamin. If there is enough cobalt in the system, the body can make its own B_{12}. Working with B_{12}, cobalt is needed to make healthy hemoglobin molecules.

Deficiency symptoms: Pernicious anemia.

LITHIUM (Li)—Measured in milligrams (mg) and micrograms (mcg)
Dosage: Not established. Available in tablets on a prescription basis. Highly toxic in overdoses.

Sources: Nova Scotia dulse and Norwegian kelp (types of seaweed) are the best sources.

Functions: Needed for the metabolism of sodium, and its transport to the nerves and muscles. Important in the proper functioning of the autonomic (involuntary) nervous system. It alters and normalizes the rhythmic cycling of the brain and helps to even out the mood.

Side effects: (when taken as a drug) diarrhea, edema, kidney dysfunction, nausea, tremors, stomach cramps, thirst, thyroid enlargement, weight gain, acne, and psoriasis.

Deficiency symptoms: Mental and nervous disorders, especially paranoid schizophrenia, bipolar disorder (manic depression).

GERMANIUM (Ge)—
Dosage: A dosage of 100-300 mg per day has been used to improve many illnesses, including rheumatoid arthritis, food allergies, candidiasis, elevated cholesterol, chronic viral infections, cancer, and AIDS. A Japanese scientist found that this amount improved many illnesses, including rheumatoid arthritis, food allergies, candidiasis, elevated cholesterol, chronic viral infections, cancer, and AIDS.

Sources: Best sources: Nova Scotia dulse and Norwegian kelp (types of seaweed). Other sources: garlic, onions, shiitake mushrooms, and the following herbs: aloe vera, comfrey, ginseng, and suma. (Now you know part of the reason why those herbs, and garlic, are so beneficial.)

Functions: Improves cellular oxygenation. Keeps immune system functioning properly, helps fight pain and rid body of toxins and poisons. Acts as a carrier of oxygen to the cells.

Deficiency symptoms: Not known.

Cautions: In rare instances, individuals taking excessive amounts have been known to develop kidney problems.

BORON (B)—
Dosage: TDA 2-3 mg. Do not exceed this amount per day.

Sources: *Richest sources:* Nova Scotia dulse and Norwegian kelp. *Other sources:* apples, carrots, grapes, leafy vegetables, nuts, pears, and grains.

Functions: Needed for healthy bones and calcium, phosphorous, and magnesium metabolism. Enhances brain function and promotes alertness. Helps prevent postmenopausal osteoporosis. Aids in the building of muscles. Elderly people do well to take a boron supplement, because of their greater problem with calcium absorption.

Deficiency symptoms: Boron deficiency accentuates vitamin D deficiency. Poor teeth and bones, osteoporosis.

VANADIUM (V)—
Dosage: RDA is not established / 500 mcg / TDA 2-5 mg. *Recommended:* A daily intake of 50-100 mcg is considered safe and adequate to meet nutritional needs. You may already be getting that much in your food. (The problem is that most of that which is eaten is not absorbed.) The amounts promoted by bodybuilding and diabetic advertisers (15-100 mg) are probably unsafe. Of 12 volunteers fed 13.5 mg daily for 2 weeks, followed by 22.5 mg daily for 5 months, 5 developed cramps and diarrhea at the high dosage. But non-insulin-dependent diabetic patients given 100 mg daily experienced no side effects.

Sources: *Richest sources:* Nova Scotia dulse and Norwegian kelp. *Other sources:* dill, parsley, olives, radishes, snap beans, vegetable oils, mushrooms, and whole grains.

Functions: Needed in formation of bones, teeth, and cell structure. Involved in growth and reproduction, inhibits cholesterol synthesis.

Deficiency symptoms: Vanadium is not easily absorbed. Cardiovascular and kidney disease, increased infant mortality, impaired reproductive ability.

Primary uses: Diabetics and bodybuilders take vanadium (usually vanadyl sulfate) because it either improves insulin action or mimics that action. It can also improve oral glucose tolerance.

Interactions: The only known interaction is with lithium.

Cautions: The use of tobacco decreases vanadium absorption. Take chromium supplements at different times than vanadium; they seem to interfere with one another's absorption. Toxic effects of vanadium include elevated blood pressure, reduction of coenzyme A and coenzyme Q_{10} levels, and interference with cellular energy production.

NATURAL REMEDIES ENCYCLOPEDIA
OVER 11,000 REMEDIES - OVER 730 DISEASES   **SPECIAL SUPPLEMENTS**   **NUTRIENTS**   **117**

N
U
T
R

4 - SPECIAL SUPPLEMENTS

Listed below are nutritive elements which have been discovered more recently. Some may be vitamins, not yet recognized as such. Or they may be enzymes. At any rate, they seem to be helping people. As a rule, they are only obtainable in supplemental capsules and tablets.

Sometimes (as in the case of flaxseed) they are only very rich sources of a very important nutrient.

BETA-SITOSTEROL—Measured in milligrams (mg).
Supplementary dosage: 500 mg. (Taking oat bran would probably accomplish the same task more inexpensively.)
Source: Health-food store.
Functions: Inhibits the absorption of cholesterol into the bloodstream.

BOSWELLIA—Measured in milligrams (mg).
Supplementary dosage: 400 mg.
Source: Health-food store.
Functions: Boswellia is an Asian herb which repairs damaged blood vessels, and inhibits swelling and discomfort in joints.

BROMELAIN—Measured in milligrams (mg).
Supplementary dosage: 500 mg. (Eating fresh, raw pineapple may be less expensive.)
Source: Health-food store.
Functions: Aids stomach digestion of proteins and reduces swelling and discomfort in painful joints.

CHROMIUM PICOLINATE—Measured in milligrams (mg).
Supplementary dosage: 200 mcg. (Chromium may be obtainable in multivitamin-mineral supplements at a lower overall cost.)
Sources: Health-food store. Trace minerals are abundant in certain seaweeds.
Functions: The trace mineral, chromium, is required for the body to make insulin. It also contains hydroxylcitric acid, which helps keep body weight down.

COENZYME B_{12}—Measured in micrograms (mcg).
Supplementary dosage: 250 mcg. (It would be cheaper to just make sure you have enough stomach acid, or take lemon with the B_{12}. If there is enough B_6 and cobalt, the body will make its own B_{12}!)
Source: Health-food store.
Functions: B_{12}, an important vitamin, is made into coenzyme B_{12}; but B_{12} is not always absorbed, due to inadequate hydrochloric acid. Coenzyme B_{12} is absorbed more easily than B_{12}.

COENZYME Q_{10} (CoQ$_{10}$)—Measured in milligrams (mg).
Supplementary dosage: 15-30 mg / TDA 90 mg.
Source: Health-food store.
Functions: Needed by heart for proper operation. Helps convert fat into energy. CoQ$_{10}$ is in the mitochondria of all body cells. CoQ$_{10}$ carries into the cells the protons and electrons used to produce ATP, the primary source of cell energy. This is a constant process because only a small supply of ATP is stored at any one time.
Deficiency symptoms: Shortness of breath, chest pain, low energy, heart trouble. An 80-year-old has half the CoQ$_{10}$ levels of a 20-year-old.

CRANBERRY JUICE EXTRACT—Measured in milligrams (mg).
Supplementary dosage: 500 mg. (Cranberry juice would be less expensive.)
Sources: Health-food store. Cranberries.
Functions: Cranberry juice protects the urinary tract from harmful bacterial which can be there.

DEGLYCERINATED LICORICE (DGL)—Measured in milligrams (mg).
Supplementary dosage: 500 mg.
Source: Health-food store. This is licorice, with the glycyrrhizin removed. Glycyrrhiza can affect blood pressure.
Functions: Licorice promotes healing of the stomach.

GERMANIUM SESQUIOXIDE—Measured in milligrams (mg).
Supplementary dosage: 50-250 mg.
Sources: Health-food store. Trace minerals are abundant in certain seaweeds.
Functions: Germanium helps the whole immune system. It stimulates immune cells, including T cells.

GINGER—Measured in milligrams (mg).
Supplementary dosage: 250 mg. This can be purchased less expensively in herbal (whole) form.
Source: Health-food store.
Functions: Helps the body produce enzymes which help the stomach digest proteins.

GINKGO BILOBA—Measured in milligrams (mg).
Supplementary dosage: 40-60 mg. 50 pounds) of the ginkgo biloba herb is used to make 1 pound of the extract used in supplements.
Sources: Health-food store. Ginkgo can also be purchased from herb companies.
Functions: Strengthens and supports blood vessels and helps keep them flexible and resilient.

GLUCOSAMINE SULFATE (or Glucosamine hydrochloride)—Measured in milligrams (mg).
Supplementary dosage: 500 mg.
Source: Health-food store.
Functions: Needed to build cartilage, ligaments, tendons and joint fluid. It also helps lubricate areas around a joint. Used by the body to reduce joint tenderness and regain mobility in damaged joints.

GRAPE SEED EXTRACT—Measured in milligrams (mg).
Supplementary dosage: 5 mg.
Sources: Health-food store. Or chew or grind up grape seeds and swallow them.
Functions: This is probably the most powerful antioxidant known at this time. Antioxidants fight free radicals, and thus lengthen your life.

Other good antioxidants include: Vitamin E, beta-carotene (provitamin A), milk thistle, coenzyme Q_{10}.

HAWTHORN—Measured in milligrams (mg).
Supplementary dosage: Not established
Source: Health-food store.
Functions: Has high concentrations of flavonoids, which promote metabolic processes of the heart.

HYPERICUM (St. John's Wort)—Measured in milligrams (mg).
Supplementary dosage: 450 mg. This is the herb, St. John's wort, which can be purchased less expensively in herbal form.
Source: Health-food store.
Functions: Helps prevent breakdown of neurotransmitters, so the brain works better.

N
U
T
R

IRON CHELATE—Measured in milligrams (mg).
Supplementary dosage: 18 mg.
Source: Health-food store.
Functions: Provides a more easily absorbed iron source, which causes fewer side effects.

L-ARGININE—Measured in milligrams (mg).
Supplementary dosage: 500 mg / TDA 1000 daily.. (Taking oat bran would probably accomplish the same cholesterol task more inexpensively.)
Source: Health-food store.
Functions: L-arginine is a precursor to nitric oxide, which inhibits cholesterol build-up in the arteries. Also aids normal blood pressure.

L-CARNITINE—Measured in milligrams (mg).
Supplementary dosage: 125-250 mg.
Sources: Health-food store. Eggs and green, leafy vegetables (but less).
Functions: L-carnitine is needed for proper metabolism of fatty acids. Helps transport fatty acids into muscle cells.

L-TYROSINE—Measured in milligrams (mg).
Supplementary dosage: 500 mg. This is an essential amino acid and is probably obtainable more inexpensively from brewer's yeast or other higher protein sources.
Source: Health-food store.
Functions: Overcomes fatigue, needed for brain chemicals associated with alertness.

MAGNESIUM CHELATE—Measured in milligrams (mg).
Supplementary dosage: 200 mg.
Source: Health-food store.
Functions: Helps maintain a strong heartbeat. Works closely with calcium and potassium in protecting the heart.

MELATONIN—Measured in milligrams (mg).
Supplementary dosage: 1-5 mg.
Source: Health-food store.
Functions: Melatonin is a hormone, produced by the pineal gland, which is associated with natural body rhythms and sleep / wake patterns.
Cautions: Do not use if you have an autoimmune disease or a depressive disorder.

MILK THISTLE—Measured in milligrams (mg).
Supplementary dosage: 100 mg.
Source: Health-food store. Less expensive when obtained as an herb.
Functions: Milk thistle contains silymarin, which protects the liver against pollutants. It helps inhibit the amount of toxins which can penetrate cell walls of the liver. It also helps the liver produce and maintains healthy cells while promoting better antioxidant levels in the liver. It is also an antioxidant.

QUERCETIN—Measured in milligrams (mg).
Sources: Health-food store. Quercetin is one of the bioflavonoids (vitamin P). The bioflavonoids can be obtained in food and are important for physical health.
Functions: Quercetin helps the body block the allergic response of coughing, breathing difficulties, clogged sinuses, and related reactions.

PYCNOGENOL—Measured in milligrams (mg).
Supplementary dosage: ODA 50 mg / TD 100 mg.
Source: Health-food store.

Functions: This is another powerful antioxidant substance; and it is extracted from an evergreen tree in Northwest U.S.

SOY ISOFLAVONES—Measured in milligrams (mg).
Supplementary dosage: 500 mg. (Eating soybeans would be less expensive, although perhaps not as potent.)
Source: Health-food store.
Functions: These are phytochemicals which mimic the activity of estrogen in the body, without the negative effects of taking estrogen.

WILD YAM—Measured in milligrams (mg).
Supplementary dosage: 200 mg. (The herb would be less expensive.)
Source: Health-food store.
Functions: Wild yam contains a natural precursor to progesterone. It can be taken in capsules or in salve which can be rubbed on the abdomen. It works very well for a number of female problems. Another herb, dong quai, works well with it.

5 - SPECIAL FOODS

VEGETABLE OILS: In contrast, we will first consider animal fats. A triglyceride is a saturated fat because the carbon molecules in the fatty acids are "saturated" with all the hydrogen molecules they can carry. These animal fats (butter, lard, tallow) are semi-solid to solid at room temperature. They should never be eaten!

In contrast, unsaturated fats are typically liquid at room temperature and are therefore often referred to as oils. Most vegetable oils primarily consist of unsaturated fats. But many of them are rendered dangerous during processing. This is done by "hydrogenating" them. During the manufacture of margarine and shortening, a hydrogen molecule is added to the vegetable oil's fatty acid molecules, to make it more saturated. The result is "hydrogenation," which changes them from *"cis fatty- acids"* to *"trans-fatty acids."* They have become *"trans-fat."* (Butter is essentially the same as margarine, and just as problematic for the body.)

Here is part of what these trans-fats can do to you: heart disease, harmful cholesterol levels, abnormal sperm production, increased likelihood of cancer, diabetes, obesity, prostate disease, decreased testosterone in men, low quality and volume of breast milk, low birth weight infants, and immune suppression.

Thus, neither animal fats nor hydrogenated oils should be used. They cause cardiovascular disease, clogged arteries, and strokes.

Next, let us consider non-hydrogenated oils. There are two types of vegetable oils: Cooking oils and medicinal oils. The best *cooking oil* is olive oil. It is composed chiefly of oleic acid, a monounsaturated oil that is more resistant to the damaging effects of heat and light than are the *highly polyunsaturated oils* (like corn, soy oil, and safflower oil). When polyunsaturated oils are exposed to heat or light, their chemical structure is changed to toxic derivatives which are known as lipid peroxides.

In contrast, *medicinal oils* contain gamma-linolenic acid (evening primrose oil, borage oil, and black current oil), or alpha-linolenic acid (flaxseed oil). These oils do not hold up well when exposed to heat; *but they are the very best oils you can take into your body!* Of them, flaxseed is the least expensive and also the richest in Omega-3 while still containing a balanced amount of the very much needed Omega-6. This *Encyclopedia*

20 Important Phyochemicals and their food sources (1072)

highly recommends flaxseed oil.

FLAXSEED OIL: Researchers have found raw, cold-pressed flaxseed oil to be the best nutritional oil you can place in your body. Suggested dosage is 1,000 mg daily. It is the richest plant source of Omega-3 fatty acids. The essential fatty acids help produce hormone-like substances needed for proper functioning of muscular, nervous, cardiovascular, and immune systems. Omega-6 comes from mostly good vegetable oils and eggs; Omega-3 is best found in flaxseed oil.

You can take a few capsules with each meal, along with other oils in your diet. But a better way is to use flaxseed oil alone. Here is how to do this: Purchase a quart of *Barlean's Flaxseed Oil;* and immediately pour some into a small pint jar. Put it into the refrigerator and put the larger container in the freezer. During your meal, pour a little oil into a tablespoon; and either pour it on your plate of food or put it directly into your mouth with some other food. Occasionally refill the small jar (after cleaning it) from the larger one, shaking it first in order to stir up the lignins. You are eating the best oil in the world; and it can only help you. Eat 2-4 tablespoons of it daily and no other fatty acid in any form. Barlean's also contains natural, brown lignins (the dark stuff at the bottom), which are excellent for lowering cholesterol and preventing gallstones.

CHLORELLA AND SPIRULINA: *Chlorella* is a tiny, single-celled water-grown algae filled with chlorophyll, plus protein (58%), carbohydrates, all of the B vitamins, vitamins C and E, and rare trace minerals. It is nearly a complete food and contains more B_{12} than liver. Chlorella is one of the few edible species of water-grown algae. Very high in RNA and DNA, it protects against ultraviolet radiation, and cleanses the bloodstream. It is an excellent source of protein. Take 1 teaspoon or 4 tablets, 1-2 times daily. This outstanding "green food" algae is grown in purified freshwater which contains all essential vitamins (except D), plus alpha-linolenic acid.

Spirulina is another waterborne microalgae. It produces 20 times as much protein as soybeans, grown on an equal amount of land. Spirulina contains as astounding array of nutrition: gamma-linolenic acid, vitamin B_{12}, iron, 60%-70% protein, RNA and DNA, chlorophyll, and phycocyanin (a blue-green pigment which protects against cancer). It increases mineral absorption, protects the immune system, reduces cholesterol, curbs the appetite, and stabilizes blood sugar.

GARLIC: This amazing food has helped people for thousands of years, and (especially raw or in supplement form) should be eaten daily. Garlic aids digestion, lowers blood pressure, thins the blood by keeping platelets from clumping (reducing risk of blood clots and helping prevent heart attacks). It is a natural antibiotic (probably the best among all foods) and stimulates the immune system. It lowers serum cholesterol levels and helps in the recovery from bacterial disease.

It can be used to treat fungal infections (athlete's foot, candidiasis, yeast vaginitis), which can be so hard to eliminate. It reduces arthritis, circulation problems, and certain viruses (such as fever blisters, a type of influenza, the common cold, genital herpes, and smallpox). During World War I, it was used to treat wounds and infections, to prevent gangrene.

To make garlic oil, wash your hands well, peel whole garlic cloves, rinse them, and place them in a quart of olive oil. This will prevent mold from forming. Keep the oil refrigerated; it will last a month. Add it to salad dressings and put in on your food. The active ingredient, *allicin,* is destroyed by heat.

KELP AND DULSE: Nova Scotia dulse and Norwegian kelp are the best natural sources of trace minerals you can find. Both are types of seaweed which can be eaten raw, in leaf form, or ground into powder. Sprinkling a little on your food (about a teaspoonful twice a day) will provide both salt and vital trace minerals. It is also a good source of protein. Excess minerals will be excreted in the skin or urine. California kelp is not as good a product for nutritional purposes; however, it is useful as a fertilizer, to enrich the soil.

LECITHIN: Lecithin primarily consists of choline, plus linoleic acid and inositol. Most lecithin is derived from soybeans. It is a type of lipid needed by every cell in the body; it is especially important in the brain and entire nervous system, where it coats nerve fibers.

Most commercial lecithin contains only 10%-20% phosphatidylcholine; but some newer preparations contain up to 98%. These are the best ones to use when large doses are needed to treat disease.

Lecithin helps prevent cardiovascular disease and arteriosclerosis; improves brain function, and promotes energy. It aids absorption of thiamine by the liver and vitamin A by the intestines, and repairs liver damage caused by alcoholism. An extremely important function is its ability to enable fats (including cholesterol) to be dispersed in water, so they can be removed from the body. Sprinkle 2 tablespoons of lecithin on cereals or soups, or add it to juices or breads. The best kind of lecithin to use is granulated rather than liquid. If you want to spend more money, buy capsules.

BREWER'S AND TORULA YEAST: This is a remarkably rich source of many vitamins and minerals, plus easily absorbed protein. Both contain all the B vitamins (except B_{12}), 16 amino acids, and 14 minerals.

Brewer's yeast is grown on hops; and *torula yeast* is grown on blackstrap molasses or wood pulp. Never use live yeast (called baker's yeast). Because the yeast cells are still alive, they absorb B vitamins in your body. Nutritional yeast is useful in treating eczema, gout, heart disorders, nervousness, and fatigue. It helps control sugar metabolism. It is best to avoid all types of yeast if you have a problem with candidiasis. Because it has large amounts of phosphorus, additional calcium should be taken; however, yeast should be avoided in cases of osteoporosis.

BLACKSTRAP MOLASSES: This is another wonderful substance which you will want to add to your diet. There are several steps in the processing of sugar (either from sugar beets or from sugar cane). The final result is pure white sugar crystals which, because they are totally devoid of vitamins and minerals, are dangerous to eat (because they absorb minerals out of your body). But earlier production stages include molasses, which has some vitamins and minerals, and blackstrap molasses, which is even richer. Add a spoonful to your meal, and you will be the healthier for having done so. Blackstrap molasses is an excellent source of choline, inositol, and calcium. It is an outstanding supplement.

FIBER: Fiber is cellulose. It is needed in the body to help lower blood cholesterol, stabilize blood sugar levels, remove toxic metals from the body. It prevents constipation, colon cancer, obesity, hemorrhoids, and a variety of other problems. Processed foods lack fiber, while whole natural foods have it.

If you are not getting enough fiber gradually add some (such as bran) until your bowel movements are the right consistency. Excessive amounts of fiber may decrease the absorption of iron, calcium, and zinc. Take supplemental fiber separately from other medications or supplements, since it can lessen their effectiveness. Make sure there are high-fiber foods in your diet, such as whole-grain cereals and breads, brown rice, bran, dried prunes, nuts, seeds (especially flaxseed), beans, and fresh raw fruit and vegetables.

GREEN PAPAYA: This is a very good source of vitamins, minerals. It especially contains the papain enzyme which helps digest proteins, carbohydrates, and fats. Papain, in your stomach, has very powerful digestive activity and will help you digest your meals. You can either eat the fresh fruit or take a powdered supplement.

OLIVE LEAF EXTRACT: This remarkable herbal supplement is effective against nearly all the viruses and bacteria. It helps protect against infection by influenza, herpes, and other viruses. It is used to deal with sore throat, rashes, skin diseases, sinusitis, pneumonia, and chronic infections. It is good for bacterial infections, and even stubborn fungal infections.

6 - ANTIOXIDANTS

Although essential to life, oxygen is very active and combines with many compounds in our body. Some of them can cause damage. During cellular respiration (which produces needed energy), some oxygen molecules are converted into free radicals which are oxidizing agents. Because they are unstable, these radicals try to combine with other compounds which can be damaging to the body. You need to obtain antioxidants and avoid free radicals.

Some of the free radicals you want to avoid: saturated fat in your diet, cigarette smoke (active and passive), heavy metals (mercury, cadmium, lead, etc.), hydrogen peroxide, ozone and nitrous oxide (primarily from car exhaust), excessive exposure to the sun, cosmic rays, medical X-rays, and a number of other chemicals and compounds in food, water, and air.

Antioxidant nutrients: Antioxidants destroy free radicals. Vitamins, enzymes, and certain minerals act as antioxidants in your body. Here are some of these antioxidant nutrients which it would be well to include in your diet: vitamins C, E, A, the carotenoids (alpha-carotene, beta-carotene, lycopene, lutein, and zeaxanthin), flavonoids, vitamin B_3 in the form of niacin, vitamin B_2, vitamin B_6, coenzyme Q_{10}, cysteine, silymarin, and pycnogenol.

Herbs which act as antioxidants: These also help eliminate free radicals in your body: garlic, bilberry, burdock, turmeric (which contains curcumin), grape seed extract, pine bark extract, and ginkgo biloba.

Substances made within the body which fight free radicals: glutathione and melatonin. There are also several others.

Two important minerals which act as antioxidants in the body: selenium (working with vitamin E) and zinc.

7 - ENZYMES

Enzymes are catalysts, which are substances that precipitate and hasten hundreds of thousands of biochemical reactions in the body. Without enzymes, these reactions would take place too slowly to sustain life. Enzymes are not destroyed or exhausted during these reactions. Each enzyme has a specific function which no other enzyme can fulfill. The substance an enzyme acts upon is called a *substrate*.

There are two types of enzymes, digestive and metabolic. *Digestive enzymes* are produced in the stomach and small intestines. The three main types are *amylase, protease, and lipase.* These break down carbohydrate, protein, and fat.

Metabolic enzymes catalyze various chemical reactions within the cells, such as energy production, construction of new parts, and detoxification. They work within the blood, organs, and tissues. Each body part has its own set of enzymes. The whole thing is mind-boggling; yet, without each of those millions of enzymes, you could not exist. People who desire a proof that God exists and made our bodies need only consider the enzymes. There is no way that they could have been made by the random changes of so-called evolution. There are literally hundreds of thousands of different enzymes; yet each one is important and vital to life. Each enzyme is made of a different, complicated protein formula. Yet research scientists have discovered that so-called "evolution" (random action over a period of many years) could not produce even one protein molecule in billions and billions of years, much less all the different types of protein in your body.

While the body manufactures many enzymes, it also gets others from food. *—And those are the ones which you can safely eat in order to improve digestion:* Avocados, papayas, pineapples, bananas, and mangoes are all high in enzymes. Pineapples (bromelain) and unripe papaya (papain) are excellent sources. Both bromelain and papain are *proteolytic enzymes* which break down proteins.

Many fat-containing foods contain lipase, an enzyme which helps break down fat in your intestines.

Superoxide dismutase is an important enzyme which is found in broccoli, brussels sprouts, cabbage, and most dark green leaves.

Enzymes require the help of *coenzymes* to do their work. Among the most important are the B vitamins, vitamins C and E, and zinc.

Most commercial enzyme products are made from animal enzymes, such as *pancreatin* and *pepsin*. The problem here is that you will be eating raw meat which may contain mad cow disease or other animal diseases.

Fortunately a number of excellent, and very safe, enzymes are available from plant sources; these include *lipase, amylase, protease, cellulase, glucoamylase, invertase, lactase,* as well as other enzymes. Bromelain and papain are also excellent, plant-based digestive enzymes.

8 - NUTRIENT THIEVES

Here is a partial list of substances which rob your body of important nutrients. Nearly all of them are purchased at your local drugstore. After the dash are listed robbed vitamins and minerals. If you take any of the following deleterious substances, you would do well to take extra amounts of the stolen nutrients.

Allopurinol (zyloprim) – iron
Antibiotics – B complex, vitamin K, friendly colon bacteria

Antacids – B complex, vitamins A, C, calcium, phosphorus

Antihistamines – Vitamin C

Aspirin – B complex, vitamins A, C, folic acid, calcium, potassium, iron

Barbiturates – Vitamin C

Beta-blockers (Corgard, Inderal, Lopressor, etc.) – Pantothenic acid, choline, chromium

Caffeine – Vitamin B_1, biotin, inositol, potassium, zinc

Carbamazepine (Atretol, Tegretol) – Sodium

Chlorthiazide (Aldoclor, Diuril, etc.) – Potassium, magnesium

Cimetidine (Tagamet) – Iron

Clonidine (Catapres, Combipres) – B complex, vitamins, calcium

Corticosteroids – Vitamins A, B_6, C, and D, calcium, potassium, zinc

Digitalis (Crystodigin, Digoxin, etc.) – Vitamins B_1, B_6, zinc

Diuretics – Vitamins B_2, C, calcium, potassium, magnesium, iodine, zinc

Estrogen preparations – Vitamin B_6, folic acid.

Ethanol (alcohol) – Vitamins C, D, E, K, B complex, magnesium

Flouride – Vitamin C

Glutethimide (Doriden) – Vitamin B_6, folic acid

Guanethidine (Esimil, Ismelin) – Vitamins B_2, B_6, potassium, magnesium

Hydralazine (Apresazide) – Vitamin B_6

Indomethacin (INH, etc.) – Niacin, vitamin B_6

Laxatives (not including herbal) – Vitamins A, K, potassium

Lidocaine (Xylocaine) – Calcium, potassium

Nitrate / nitrite coronary vasodilators – Vitamins C, E, niacine, pangamic acid, selenium

Oral contraceptives – B complex, vitamins C, D, and E.

Penicillin – Vitamin B_6, niacin, niacinamide

Phenobarbitol – Vitamins B_6, B_{12}, D, K, folic acid

Phenylbutazone (Cotylbutazone) – Folic acid, iodine

Phenytoin (Dilantin) – Vitamins B_{12}, C, D, K, folic acid, calcium

Prednisone (Deltasone, etc.) – Vitamins B_6, C, potassium, zinc

Quinidine – Vitamin K, pantothenic acid, potassium, choline

Reserpine – Vitamins B_2, B_6, potassium, phenylalanine.

Spironolactone (Aldactone, etc.) – Folic acid, calcium.

Sulfa drugs – Para-aminobenzoic acid, friendly bowel bacteria

Synthetic neurotransmitters – Vitamins B_2, B_6, potassium, magnesium

Thiazide diuretics – Vitamin B_2, potassium, magnesium, zinc

Tobacco – Vitamins A, C, E

Triamterene (Dyrenium) – Folic acid, calcium

Trimethoprim (Bactrim, Septra, etc.) – Folic acid

9 - THESE THREE CAN KILL YOU

According to statistics, most deaths in the United States do not occur in the home: 80% of all deaths occur in the hospital; 70% who die each year are over age 65 and 5% are under age 15.

A 1985 health report disclosed that 50% of all deaths and illnesses are either unnecessary or premature. **After studying the most prevalent deaths in the U.S., the Carter Center at Emory University concluded that a healthy lifestyle is twice as effective as medical technology at increasing life expectancy**.

The number one cause of premature death is *cigarette smoking*: 360,000 deaths each year are directly attributable to smoking. Most occur as heart attacks, strokes, diabetes, cancer, and chronic lung disease. Tobacco is the most deadly carcinogen known, with an estimated 6,000 chemicals (most are poisonous) in cigarette smoke.

Alcohol ranks second in causing death, causing 75,000 per year in the U.S. Of that number, about 20,000 are due to illness. 24,000 are due to motor vehicle accidents. And 32,000 are due to falls, fires, drownings, homocides, and suicides.

It is estimated that 80% of middle-aged men have excessively *high cholesterol* levels, primarily from eating meat. The chance of dying from heart disease rises as the amount of blood cholesterol increases: It is 29% if a person has 182-202 mg. cholesterol. From 203-220 mg., the risk is 73%. From 221-244 mg., the odds skyrocket to 121%. As of 1986, the average cholesterol level among middle-aged U.S. men and women is about 215 mg. Heart attacks rarely occur if the cholesterol level is less than 150 mg.

10 - NUTRIENT COMBINATIONS

The following nutrients work best when taken together:

Vitamins A and C—They work together as water and fat soluble antioxidants. C helps regenerate E, and lipoic acid also helps regenerate E (helps it have stronger effects on any given amount taken).

Vitamins C, E, and CoQ_{10}—Both C and CoQ_{10} help regenerate the antioxidant qualities of E.

Vitamins A and E—A and E inhibit cell growth in human brain cancer cells.

Vitamin A and Zinc—Zinc increases the ability of A to restore night vision in night-blind pregnant women with low initial serum zinc concentrations.

Vitamin C and Soy isoflavones—Work together in increasing levels. Inhibits LDL oxidation.

Vitamins A and D_3—Both together cause leukemia cells to change into stable, noncancerous cells.

L-Carnitine and CoQ_{10}—Increase utilization of fatty acids.

Niacine and Chromium—Combining these causes significant decrease in glucose in normal, healthy people.

Vitamin E and Selenium—E increases the antitumor action of high-dose selenium.

Vitamins C and E—Work together to increase the detoxifying ability of the liver.

Folic acid and Betaine—Folic acid, taken by itself or with B complex, lowers homocysteine to healthy levels. But adding betaine (or trimethylglycine; TMG) enhances this, and is essential for some people. But always take B_{12} along with folic acid, or anemia and serious neurological damage could occur.

Folic acid and Vitamin B12—These work together to reduce homocysteine levels. (Excess homocysteine leads to cardiovascular disease.) But always take folic acid with vitamin B_{12}.

L-cysteine, N-acetylcysteine, and/or Glutathione and Vitamin C—These three amino acid supplements do not function well without vitamin C.

Calcium and magnesium—Although they function somewhat differently, they work together to contract and relax muscles. Because people are often magnesium deficient, it is important that magnesium be taken when extra calcium is eaten.

Evening primrose oil (EPO) and Zinc, vitamin C, and Chromium—In order for EPO to change to anti-inflammatory prostaglandins, vitamin C, zinc, and chromium must be taken in adequate amounts.

Unsaturated oil and vitamin E—Unsaturated oils (flaxseed, primrose, borage, etc.) should be taken with oil-based antioxidants (usually vitamin E as mixed tocopherols). Otherwise the oils are oxidized in the system before they can be utilized.

Bioflavonoids together and Vitamin C, plus Lutein and Lycopene—The various bioflavonoids include the antocyanins, flavins, flavonols, flavones, quercetin, rutin, carotenoids, lutein, and reserveratrol. They tend to work best together, along with vitamin C, which replenishes them in the system. These bioflavonoid mixtures are also more effective when lutein or lycopene is present.

11 - NUTRIENT WARNINGS

These special warnings, mentioned elsewhere in this Encyclopedia, are also given here:

Vitamin A—This is the most dangerous of the vitamins! Levels of 10,000 to 25,000 IU per day may cause headache, fatigue, mouth fissures, increased pressure on the brain, and congenital deformities (if taken during pregnancy). Never take during pregnancy. Cancer patients are sometimes given 100,000-200,000 IU daily. Such high doses could eventually produce toxic problems. Another danger is increased bone fracture risk when higher dosages of vitamin A are taken. One study showed bone mineral density was reduced by 10% in those taking more than 5000 IU of vitamin A from both dietary sources and supplements. Never exceed 5000 IU daily. Symptoms of high dosage of vitamin A includes: headache, dizziness, blurred vision, joint pain, dry lips, scaly and/or dry hair, and excessive hair loss. If any of these symptoms occur, discontinue vitamin A until the symptoms disappear, and then resume the therapy at a lower dosage. Those with thyroid cancer must not take any vitamin A. Pregnant women should not take more than the RDA (recommended daily allowance) of vitamin A, because it is cancer-causing to the fetus.

Arginine—This can neutralize insulin and elevate blood sugar in some Type II diabetics.

Beta carotene—This is pro-vitamin A, which produces yellowing of the skin, which is harmless. But people with liver damage should avoid niacin, vitamin A, and beta-carotene. AIDS patients with hepatitis should not take beta-carotene.

Calcium—Do not take over 2 grams daily. Prolonged ingestion of excess calcium, along with excess vitamin D, may cause hypercalcemia (excess calcium in them) of bone and soft tissue (such as joints and kidneys), and may also cause a mineral imbalance.

Copper—Prolonged ingestion may be toxic, especially with Wilson's disease (a rare disorder which can produce an excess of copper in the liver, red blood cells, and brain.

Curcumin—High doses on an empty stomach can cause stomach ulcers. Do not use if you have an obstruction in your bile tract, because curcumin could reduce the flow of bile.

Evening primrose oil—Those with temporal lobe epilepsy or bipolar disease should use with caution.

Folic acid (Folate, folacin)—Always take B_{12} with folic acid. Those with psychoses should avoid doses above 15 mg/day. An excess intake of folic acid, without taking B_{12}, can mask a B_{12} deficiency, so it is not recognized.

L-glutamine—Because this amino acid promotes cell growth, some say it should not be given to cancer patients. But research studies have found that it provides beneficial effects to cancer patients.

Genistein—This is found in soy extract, and can interfere with the ability of radiation to kill cancer cells. Otherwise, it has no negative effects.

Ginkgo—When massive bleeding from wounds occurs, flavonoids, such as ginkgo, should be avoided; since they could accelerate hemorrhaging.

Iodine—Prolonged ingestion of excess iodine may cause "iodine goiter," an enlargement of the thyroid gland. May also induce acne-like skin lesions or aggravate preexisting acne conditions.

Iron—Be cautious about multi-vitamin supplements which contain "iron." It might be iron sulfate instead of iron gluconate. Only take extra iron if you are known to be deficient. Excessive iron intake can adversely affect the liver, pancreas, heart, and nucleus. And it can increase susceptibility to infection. Poorly utilized iron may cause constipation and/or stomach upset. Iron supplements, if taken at all, should only be taken with food and supplemental vitamin C.

Lysine—If a person has high levels of arginine in the diet, this amino acid may not be as effective.

Magnesium—Extremely high doses (30,000 mg or more) may be toxic in certain individuals with kidney problems. Doses of 400 mg or more may produce diarrhea.

Manganese—Large doses (or occupational exposure) can produce serious neurological toxicity.

Melatonin—Use cautiously, or not at all, in autoimmune diseases, such as rheumatoid arthritis. Avoid in cases of leukemia, Hodgkin's disease, or lymphoma.

Potassium—Extremely high doses (25,000 mg daily) of Potassium chloride may be toxic in kidney failure.

Phosphorus—An extremely large amount, relative to calcium intake, may cause a deficiency in calcium and a mineral imbalance.

Sodium—Prolonged ingestion of excess sodium has been linked to high blood pressure and increased incidence of migraine headaches. Extremely high intake can result in swelling of tissues (edema).

St. John's wort—This herb should be used only in small amounts, if at all. It can produce a wide variety of negative side effects, some of them serious.

Selenium—Doses of 200 mcg. daily are safe. Some take 400 mcg daily. Toxic levels start at more than 1000 mcg a day, causing hair loss, muscle soreness, nausea, fatigue, and brittle nails.

L-Tryptophan—Sometimes causes nausea, excitability, and tremor. Use with caution with other antidepressant drugs or herbs.

Vitamin B1 (Thiamine)—Injections may cause allergic reactions, such as flushing, shortness of breath, and rapid heartbeat.

Vitamin B2 (Riboflavin)—Moderate to high doses may cause nonharmful bright yellow coloration of urine.

Vitamin B3 (Niacin)—Liver toxicity can occur if over 500 mg per day is taken, especially if it is sustained release. Those with severely damaged liver should avoid niacin, vitamin A, and beta-carotene. (The facial flush after even small doses of niacin are harmless; niacinamide does not produce the flush.)

Vitamin B_5 (Pantothenic acid)—extremely high doses (10,000 mg or more) will produce diarrhea.

Vitamin B6 (Pyrodoxine)—High doses (more than 300-500 mg daily) may cause a reversible neuropathy with symptoms of tingling and numbness in the extremities. Never take high doses without also taking the other B complex vitamins. Prescription oral contraceptives may cause deficiency of vitamin B_6.

Vitamin B12 (cyanocobalamin)—No reports of overdosing problems.

Vitamin C (ascorbic acid)—Large doses may cause temporary diarrhea. When that occurs, you know that you have reached the upper limit of your immediate need of vitamin C. Doses over 6 grams a day may increase urinary output of oxalic acid; yet there is no proof that large doses cause renal stones. The buffered ascorbate form of vitamin C is not as acid, so will not disturb the stomach when taken in large doses.

Vitamin D3—Large doses (1400-2000 IU daily) may cause hypercalcemia (an excess of calcium in the blood), a decrease in kidney function, and calcification in the kidney nephrons. Do not take during kidney disease.

Vitamin E—Because it inhibits blood clotting, do not take if excessive bleeding is occurring.

Vitamin K—Unlike the other fat-soluble vitamins, vitamin K is not stored in significant quantity in the liver. Synthetic vitamin K (menadione) is toxic in excess dosages.

Valerian—Only use small amounts of this herb, and infrequently, to help fall asleep. It produces a drug-like, hypnotic effect. If taken regularly, increasing amounts are needed for the same effect. Chronic use could permanently damage the liver and central nervous system.

Zinc—Large doses (over 75 mg daily) displace copper, leading to copper deficiency. Continual doses of more than 100-125 mg daily may reduce immune function.

12 - SOME NUTRIENT DOSAGES

These are the normal daily doses; therapeutic doses may be much higher, as discussed earlier in this chapter.

Be careful not to confuse milligrams (mg) with micrograms (mcg). A microgram is 1/1,000 of a milligram, or 1/1,000,000 of a gram.

VITAMINS

Vitamin A (retinol) — 5,000-10,000 IU

or Carotenoid complex, containing beta-carotene (vegetable form of Vitamin A) — 5,000-25.000 IU

Vitamin B₁ (thiamine) — 50-100 mg

Vitamin B2 (riboflavin) — 15-50 mg

Vitamin B3 (niacin) — 15-50 mg

or Niacinamide form of B3 — 50-100 mg

Pantothenic acid (vitamin B₅) — 50-100 mg

Vitamin B6 (pyridoxine) — 50-100 mg

Vitamin B12 — 200-400 mcg

Biotin — 400-800 mcg

Vitamin D3 (cholecalciferol) — 400 IU

Vitamin E (d-alpha-tocopherol) — 200 IU

Vitamin K (use natural sources such as alfalfa, green leafy vegetables) — 100-500 mcg

Essential fatty acids (EFAs) — (primrose oil, flaxseed oil, salmon oil. and fish oil are good sources) — 1-2 tablespoons daily

MINERALS

Boron (picolinate or citrate) — 3-6 mg

Calcium (citrate. ascorbate, or malate) — 1,500-2,000 mg

Chromium (GTF, picolinate, or polynicotinate) — 150-400 mcg

Copper — 2-3 mg

Iodine (kelp is a good source) — 100-225 mcg

Iron (ferrous gluconate, fumarate, citrate, or amino acid chelate; avoid inorganic forms such as ferrous sulfate, which can oxidize vitamin E) — 18-30 mg

You should take iron supplements only if you have been diagnosed with a deficiency of this mineral. Always take iron supplements separately, rather than in a multivitamin and mineral formula.

Magnesium — 750-1,000 mg

Manganese — 3-10 mg

Molybdenum (ascorbate, aspartate, or picolinate) — 30-100 mcg

Potassium (citrate) — 99-500 mg

Selenium — 100-200 mcg

Vanadium (vanadyl sulfate) — 200 mcg-1 mg

Zinc — 30-50 mg

AMINO ACIDS

You should not take individual amino acids on a regular basis unless you are using them for the treatment of a specific disorder.

Acetyl-L-Carnitine — 100-500 mg

Acetyl-L-Cysteine — 100-500 mg

L-Carnitine — 500 mg

L-Cysteine — 50-100 mg

L-Lysine — 50-100 mg

L-Methionine — 50-100 mg

L-Tyrosine — 500 mg

Taurine — 100-500 mg

Zeaxanthin — 90 mcg

13 - THERAPEUTIC DOSAGES

THERAPEUTIC DOSAGES—

Vitamin B₁ (Thiamin): 200-500 mg.

Vitamin B₂ (Riboflavin): 200-500 mg.

Vitamin B₃ (Niacin or Niacinamide; best use Niacinamide to avoid face flush): 2,000-6,000 mg.

Pantothenic acid (Vitamin B₅): 50-200 mg.

Vitamin B₆ (Pyridoxine): 200-500 mg,

Vitamin B₁₂: 1,000 mcg.

Biotin: 500-3,000 mcg

Choline: 500-1,000 mg.

Inositol: 500-2,000 mg.

Folic acid: 5 mg.

PABA (Para-aminobenzoic acid): 100 mg.

OIL SOLUBLE VITAMINS

Vitamin A (given in form of beta carotene): Take only in the form of beta carotene; which is the vegetable-source precursor of vitamin A. The therapeutic dose of Vitamin A [not carotene] would be 25,000 units a day *for only a few days!*

Vitamin D: 1,000 IU.

Vitamin E: 400-600 IU.

Vitamin F: 2 Tbsp. flaxseed oil.

Vitamin K: 140 mcg.

C COMPLEX VITAMINS

Vitamin C: 1,000-3,000 mg. Take vitamin C "to bowel tolerance;" that is, till it produces a slight diarrhea following the dosage. As long as it does not produce diarrhea, your body needs it and is using all the vitamin C you fill up on.

Bioflavonoids: 50-200 mg.

Hesperidin: ODA 100 mg.

Rutin: ODA 25 mg.

MAJOR MINERALS

Calcium (Ca): 2,000-5,000 mg.

Iron (Fe): 50-100 mg. Do not take iron supplements unless you have to. Blackstrap molasses is the richest food source of iron.

Magnesium (Mg): 1,000 mg.

Potassium (K): 5,500 mg.

TRACE MINERALS

Iodine (I): 150 mcg. Dulse and kelp (two types of seaweed) are the best sources.

Manganese (Mn): 2-50 mg.

Selenium (Se): 500-3,000 mcg.

Zinc (Zn): 150-600 mg.

OTHER SUPPLEMENTS

CoQ10 (Coenzyme Q10): 90 mg

14 - WORTHWHILE FOODS

All **beans** (especially soy) cooked without animal fat or salt (salt- and fat-free).

Herbal teas, fresh vegetable and fruit juices, cereal, grain beverages (often sold as coffee substitutes), **mineral or distilled water**.

All fresh, frozen, stewed. or dried **fruits without sweeteners** (except, for some people, oranges, which are acidic and highly allergenic), **unsulfured fruits, home-canned fruits.**

All **whole grains and products containing whole grains**: cereals. breads, muffins, whole-grain crackers, cream of wheat or rye cereal, buckwheat, millet, oats, brown rice. (Some should limit yeast breads to 3 servings per week.)

All fresh raw **nuts** (peanuts in moderation only).

Cold-pressed oils: corn, safflower, sesame, olive, flaxseed, soybean, sunflower. (The best is **wheat germ oil**, and **flaxseed oil**.)

Garlic, onions. All regular **herbs, dried vegetables, Nova Scotia dulse, Norwegian kelp**.

All slightly cooked **sprouts** (except **alfalfa**. which should be raw and washed thoroughly), **wheatgrass**, all **raw seeds**.

Barley malt or **rice syrup**, small amounts of **raw honey. pure maple syrup, stevia, unsulfured blackstrap molasses**.

Vegetables - all raw, fresh, frozen (no additives), or home-canned without salt (undercook vegetables slightly).

15 - FOODS TO AVOID

Canned pork and beans, canned beans with salt or preservatives, other types of meat.

Alcoholic drinks, coffee, cocoa, pasteurized and/or sweetened juices and fruit drinks, sodas, tea (except herbal tea).

All soft cheeses, all pasteurized or artificially colored cheese products, ice cream.

Fried or pickled.

All fried fish, all shellfish, salted fish, anchovies, herring, fish canned in oil.

Canned, bottled, or frozen fruits with sweeteners added; oranges.

All white flour products, white rice, pasta, crackers, cold cereals, instant types of oatmeal and other hot cereals.

Beef; all forms of pork; hot dogs; luncheon meats; smoked, pickled, and processed meats; corned beef; duck; goose; spare ribs; gravies; organ meats.

All salted or roasted nuts; peanuts (if suffering from any disorder).

All saturated fats, hydrogenated margarine, refined processed oils, shortenings,hardened oils.

Black or white pepper, salt, hot red peppers, all types of vinegar and fermented foods.

Canned soups made with salt, preservatives, MSG, or fat stock; all creamed soups.

All seeds cooked in oil or salt.

White, brown, or raw cane sugar, corn syrups, chocolate, sugar candy, fructose (except that in fresh whole fruit), all syrups (except pure maple syrup), all sugar substitutes, jams and jellies made with sugar.

All canned or frozen with additives or excess salt.

16 - HARMFUL SUBSTANCES WHICH DESTROY NUTRIENTS IN THE BODY

Different substances deplete the body of different nutrients. Here is a list of the supplements you may need if you choose to take medicinal drugs (prescription or over-the-counter). Alcohol and caffeine are also included in this list. In the list below, the first is the harmful substance. This is followed by the nutrient your body needs which that substance tends to destroy.

Allopurinol (Zyloprim) — Iron.

Antacids — B-complex vitamins; calcium; phosphate; vitamins A and D.

Antibiotics, general (See also isoniazid, penicillin, sulfa drugs, and trimethoprim) — B-complex vitamins; vitamin K; "friendly" bacteria

Antihistamines — Vitamin C.

Aspirin — B-complex vitamins; calcium; folic acid; iron; potassium; vitamins A and C.

Barbiturates — Vitamin C.

Beta-blockers (Corgard, Inderal, Lopressor, and others) — Choline; chromium; pantothenic acid (vitamin B_5).

Caffeine — Biotin; inositol; potassium; vitamin B1 (thiamine); zinc.

Carbamazepine (Atretol, Tegretol) — Dilutes blood sodium.

Chlorthiazide (Aldoclor, Diuril, and others) — Magnesium; potassium.

Cimetidine (Tagamet) — Iron.

Clonidine (Catapres, Combipres) — B-complex vitamins; calcium.

Corticosteroids, general (See also prednisone) — Calcium; potassium; vitamins A, B6, C, and D; zinc.

Digitalis preparations (Crystodigin, Digoxin, and others) — Vitamins B_1 (thiamine) and B6 (pyridoxine); zinc.

Diuretics, general (See also chlorthiazide, spironolactone, thiazide diuretics.and triamterene) — Calcium; iodine: magnesium; potassium; vitamins B2 (riboflavin) and C; zinc.

Estrogen preparations — Folic acid; vitamin B6 (pyridoxine).

Ethanol (alcohol) — B-complex vitamins; magnesium; vitamins C, D, E, and K.

Fluoride — Vitamin C.

Glutethimide (Doriden) — Folic acid; vitamin B6 (pyridoxine).

Guanethidine (Esimil, Ismelin) — Magnesium; potassium; vitamins B2 (riboflavin) and B6 (pyridoxine).

Hydralazine (Apresazide, Apresoline, and others) — Vitamin B6 (pyridoxine).

Indomethacin (INH and others) — Vitamins B3 (niacin) and B6 (pyridoxine).

Laxatives (excluding herbs) — Potassium; vitamins A and K.

Lidocaine (Xylocaine) — Calcium; potassium.

Nitrate/nitrite coronary vasodilators — Niacin; pangamic acid; selenium; vitamins C and E.

Oral contraceptives — B-complex vitamins; vitamins C, D, and **E.**

Penicillin preparations — Vitamin B3 (niacin); niacinamide; vitamin B6 (pyridoxine).

Phenobarbital preparations — Folic acid; vitamin B6 (pyridoxine); vitamin B12; vitamins D and K.

Phenylbutazone (Cotylbutazone) — Folic acid; iodine.

Phenytoin (Dilantin) — Calcium; folic acid; vitamins B12, C, D, and K.

Prednisone (Deltasone and others) — Potassium; vitamins B6 (pyridoxine) and C; zinc.

Quinidine preparations — Choline; pantothenic acid (vitamin B_5); potassium; vitamin K.

Reserpine preparations — Phenylalanine; potassium; vitamins B2 (riboflavin) and B6 (pyridoxine).

Spironolactone (Aldactone and others) — Calcium; folic acid.

Sulfa drugs — Para-aminobenzoic acid (PABA); "friendly" bacteria.

Synthetic neurotransmitters — Magnesium; potassium; vitamins B2 (riboflavin) and B6 (pyridoxine).

Thiazide diuretics — Magnesium; potassium; vitamin B2 (riboflavin); zinc.

Tobacco — Vitamins A, C, and E.

Triamterene (Dyrenium) — Calcium; folic acid.

Trimethoprim (Bactrim, Septra, and others) — Folic acid.

17 - YOUR HEART ATTACK RISK

Take this heart health evaluation to determine your risk for cardiovascular disease. In each category circle the one number which reflects your lifestyle:

Cigarette Smoking

Never smoked or inhaled secondhand smoke	0
Quit smoking 3 or more years	1
Don't smoke, but exposed to secondhand smoke	2
Stopped smoking within the past 3 years	3
Smoke regularly	4
Smoke regularly and exposed to secondhand smoke	5

Total Blood Cholesterol

Lower than 160	1
160-199	2
Don't know	3
200-239	4
240 or higher	5

HDL "Good" Cholesterol

60 or higher	1
56-60	2
Don't know	3
35-55	4
Lower than 35	5

Systolic Blood Pressure

Lower than 120	1
120-139	2
Don't know	3
140-159	4
160 or higher	5

Excess Body Weight

Within 10 pounds of desirable weight	1
11-20 pounds above desirable weight	2
21-30 pounds above desirable weight	3
31-50 pounds above desirable weight	4
More than 50 pounds above desirable weight	5

Physical Activity

Job requires very hard physical labor at least 4 hours per day OR exercise 4 or more times per week for 20 or more minutes	1
Exercise 3 times per week for 20 minutes	2
Job requires walking, lifting, carrying, or other moderately hard work for several hours per day OR spend much leisure time doing moderate activities (gardening, walking, housework, etc.) OR exercise 1-2 times per week	3
Occasionally exercise	4
Never exercise	5

Heredity

No known history of heart disease among relatives	1
One relative with heart disease after age 60	2
Two relatives with heart disease after age 60	3
One relative with heart disease before age 60	4
One relatives with heart disease before age 60	5

Age

10-20 years	1
21-30 years	2
31-40 years	3
41-50 years	4
51 or more years	5

Eating Habits

Vegetarian or rarely eats meat and dairy products	1
Eats meat and low-fat milk fewer than 6 times per week	2
Eats most lean meat and low-fat milk 6-12 times per week	3
Eats meat, cheese, eggs, and whole milk 12-24 times per week	4
Eats meat, cheese, eggs, and whole milk over 24 times per week	5

For your Total Score:

Add the numbers you circled to get your total score, which is an estimate. Neither a high nor low score indicates that you will or will not have a heart problem. *If your Total Score was*

9-21 - your heart attack risk is **low**

22-33 - your heart attack risk is **moderate**

34-45 - your heart attack risk is **high**

18 - HOW LONG WILL YOU LIVE?

This life-expectancy quiz is typical of questionnaires used by insurance companies. Of course, it cannot be 100% accurate. But, though exceptions exist (and barring sudden accidents), it is likely that your predicted life span may be somewhere in that range.

You will start with the number **74**. So write down that number at the top of a sheet of paper. If you are a male, **subtract 2**. If a female, **add 4**. If you live in an urban area of over 2 million people, **subtract 2**. If you live in a rural area with a population under 10,000, **add 2**. If any grandparent lived to be 85, **add 2**. If all four grandparents lived to be 80, **add 6**. If either parent died of a stroke or heart attack before the age of 50, **subtract 4**. If any immediate relative (parent, brother, sister) under 50 has—or had—cancer or a heart condition, or has had diabetes since childhood, **subtract 3**. If you earn over $50,000 a year, **subtract 2**. If you finished college, **add 1**. If you have a graduate or professional degree, **add 2 more**. If you live with a spouse or friend, **add 5**. If not, **subtract 1** for every 10 years alone, since age 25. If you work behind a desk, **subtract 3**. If your work is physically demanding, **add 3**. If you exercise 3-5 times a week for at least 30 minutes, **add 4**. If you exercise twice a week, **add 2**. If you sleep more than 10 hours per night, **subtract 4**. If you are generally relaxed and

easygoing, **add 3**. If you are generally happy most of the time, **add 1**. If you are generally unhappy most of the time, **subtract 2**. If you smoke a pack of cigarettes a day, **subtract 7**. If you smoke 2 packs or more a day, **subtract 8**. If you smoke half-a-pack a day, **subtract 3**. If you drink more than 1½ oz. of liquor a day, **subtract 1**. If you are overweight by 10-30 pounds, **subtract 2**. If overweight by 30-50 pounds, **subtract 4**. If overweight by 50 pounds or more, **subtract 8**. If you are between 30-40, **add 2**. If you are between 40-50, **add 3**. If you are between 50-70, **add 4**. If you are over 70, **add 5**.

Your Total Score will be the estimated number of years you may live. But there is more: *You are likely to live even longer if your* blood pressure is less than 130 / 75 and your cholesterol is less than 200. Your resting pulse rate is less than 60 beats per minute, with no breathing problems, asthma, or history of chronic illness. You presently live with a pet and still work after age 62. You are a light eater, do not skip breakfasts, and have social contacts besides your spouse.

Your Life is likely to be shorter if your blood pressure is greater than 140 / 90 and your cholesterol greater than 200. It take a long time to recover after exercise. You are anemic and suffer illnesses more than the average person your age. Also you are easily winded, with a resting pulse rate greater than 80 beats per minute. You are a heavy eater, skip breakfasts, and have no social contacts besides your spouse.

CHART 1069: Life Expectancy Tables - by Race, Gender, Age

What to do if you have a heart attack (513) / How to tell if he is about to have a stroke (529)

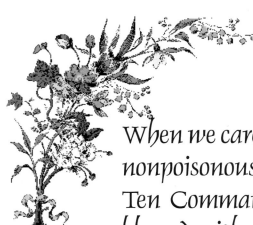

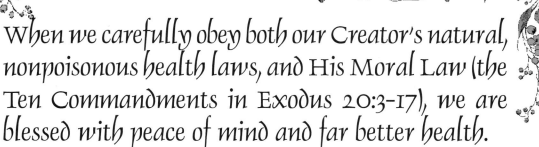

When we carefully obey both our Creator's natural, nonpoisonous health laws, and His Moral Law (the Ten Commandments in Exodus 20:3-17), we are blessed with peace of mind and far better health.

Many of God's simple laws of health and healing are described throughout this Encyclopedia. Each of those ten moral principles governing our lives is explained at the back of this book, starting on 1080.

God loves you deeply, and wants you to be His humble, obedient child; walking by His side and, like Him, living to help and bless others.

May this book be to you a source of help and encouragement as you travel the pathway of life. Study the Bible every day and pray your way through each part of the day, and you will be protected and guided all the way to the end.

—The authors and publishers of this book

The Natural Remedies Encyclopedia

Healing Herbs and How to Use Them

This chapter provides you with a complete, working guide to the use of herbs and their healing power. Here is all the basic information you need: name, part of plant, body parts affected, preparation, amount given, purposes, and warnings.

In addition to listing a large number of herbs (126), there are 303 color pictures. This is the only herb book which has two or three color pictures to help you identify each herb. For quick reference, this complete herb index is also on the inside back cover.

The next chapter explains how an additional 115 herbs are used overseas by scientists and approved by governments as healing agents. They recognize the value of herbs in the recovery of the sick.

130   **HERBS**   **THE 126 MOST IMPORTANT HERBS**   NATURAL REMEDIES ENCYCLOPEDIA
OVER 11,000 REMEDIES - OVER 730 DISEASES

HERBS

What is the difference between a medicinal drug and an herb? Herbs contain a variety of chemical compounds placed there by God. Over the centuries, many have been found to be very extremely useful for physical problems. Medicinal drugs are different. In order to patent them (for exclusive sales and profits), medicinal drugs cannot have the exact formulas found in herbs. Instead, they contain various man made combinations of chemicals. Because of this, to one extent or another, they are always poisonous. Their "contraindications" paragraphs verify the fact. The liver, kidneys, and other organs frequently suffer from them.

2 - PURCHASING HERBS

Try to locate the best sources (a list of herbal sources is at the back of this *Encyclopedia*). Do you want the flowers, leaves, seeds, berries, barks, resins, or roots? What form do you want the herb in: whole form (all of the leaves together, not cut up, etc.), pieces, or powdered?

3 - GATHERING HERBS

Collect herbs in clear, dry weather and in the morning, after the dew has disappeared.

Leaves—Gather the leaves as soon as fully matured, just before the flowers appear, just before they fade, or at the maturing of the fruit. (Biennials do not perfect their leaves until the second year.)

Stems—Cut herbaceous stems after the foliage appears, but before the blossoms develop. Cut ligneous (woody) stems in the autumn, after the foliage falls.

Stalks—Collect stalks in the autumn.

Twigs—Collect twigs in the autumn.

Bulbs—Gather bulbs after the new bulb is developed, just before the leaves decay.

Rhizomes and roots—Gather the roots of *annual plants* just before they flower. Gather the roots of *biennial plants* soon after the leaves have fallen in the autumn of the first year. Gather the roots of *perennials* in the autumn, after the leaves and flowers have fallen, or in the spring, before vegetation begins.

Barks—Gather barks in the spring, before flowering season begins, or in the fall, after the foliage has fallen. Separate and discard all decaying matter. Only use the inner bark of the slippery elm.

Flowers—Gather flowers when they are about to open from the bud. But if it is the buds that you want, gather the buds when they are nicely formed.

Berries, Fruits, and Seeds—Gather them when they are fully mature and ripe.

Aromatic Plants—Peppermint, Spearmint, pennyroyal, etc., are best gathered after the flowers are formed and nearly ready to open. Gather them in dry weather.

4 - DRYING HERBS

How to Dry—Dry the various herb materials in a clean room which has no dust, away from sunlight and where it is not too hot or cold. Do not dry them too fast; for too much heat spoils the herbs.

Guard them from mold—In order to protect them from becoming moldy, turn them occasionally; so no mold will form. Or hang the herbs, so they dry equally throughout.

Leaves—Dry aromatic leaves in the shade. Then place in the sun a short time to prevent fungus. Unscented leaves may be dried in the sunlight; but it is best to dry them in an airy, dry place.

Flowers—The strength of the flower can be judged by the intensity of its color; so dry flowers carefully, but rapidly, in order to preserve the color. Give special care to flowers which have volatile oils. Spread the flowers loosely on white paper (although some can be tied in loose bunches and hung with a string from a rafter, etc., in a airy room). Dry the flowers only in the shade; but place them in the sun a brief time, to prevent fungus growth.

Plants and tops—If the plants are not too juicy, they may be strung in bunches across the top of an airy, dry room.

Bulbs—Peel off the outer membranes. Then cut the bulbs into transverse (straight across) slices, each about ½ inch in length. Stir them every so often while they dry and move several times, to prevent mold from forming.

Barks, twigs, and woods—Dry in the sunlight or in thin layers in the open air. Do not dry wild cherry bark in the sun.

Fleshy roots and rhizomes—As you did with the bulbs, cut them in transverse slices, about ½ inch in length. Stir and move several times during the drying process.

Fibrous roots—Dry these in the sunlight or artificially at temperatures between 65° and 80° F.

5 - STORAGE OF HERBS

Once the herbs are dry, and as long as they remain in a dry place, they should be good for quite some time. It is generally best to store the herbs in paper sacks in a cool, dry area. The fruits and berries, of course, will be jarred or dried. They are all a blessing from God in heaven.

It is important that you store your herbs properly for longest shelf life. An alternative to storing them in brown paper sacks is to place them in a tight container, not made of plastic (which contains formaldehyde). The container can be a waxed carton if it is given a wax seal; but glass bottles are best (unless you are able to seal a steel can). Never store anything in aluminum!

The stored herbs should be labeled, dated, and well-organized in the herbal medicine chest or cabinet. If the particular herb will not be used within a year, then fill the jar to the top, to crowd out oxygen, and then seal it with wax.

Herbal oils must be stored in brown bottles, sealed tightly, and kept out of the sun and extreme heat. Powdered forms of herbs will keep up to a year or more and retain

132 **HERBS** **THE 126 MOST IMPORTANT HERBS** NATURAL REMEDIES ENCYCLOPEDIA
OVER 11,000 REMEDIES - OVER 730 DISEASES

H
E
R
B
S

fairly full potency, when stored in a fairly cool place. Powdered herbs generally do not need refrigeration. At room temperature, they will keep 6 months. When hermetically sealed with wax, they will keep 2 or 3 years. Herbal powders containing oils (such as cayenne) cannot be stored even a short time in paper, but must be wax sealed in a tight container. Tinctures are best kept in tightly capped 3-oz. colored glass bottles.

Flowers may be stored in bunches in a dry, airy room or placed in labeled brown paper bags. Fold bags to prevent insect attacks.

6 - THE PREPARATION OF HERBS

1 - Infusion (steeping): One pint boiling water is poured over 1 oz. dried herb. Cover it with a tight fitting lid, so steam will not escape. Let it stand (steep) 20 minutes. Strain off the clear liquid. Immediately use or keep in the refrigerator a short time till used. Average dose: 1 Tbsp. of the herb per teacup. Take 3 times a day. An infusion is used when the volatile oils in herbs are needed, as in peppermint and spearmint, or when the herb is composed of flowers or leaves.

A "sun tea" is made in this way: Put the 1 oz. of dried herb and a pint of water into a large glass jar. Place this in the sun for 2-4 hours; and the heat from the sun will extract the herb into the liquid.

2 - Decoction (boiling): (1) Place 1 oz. dried herb (or 2 oz. fresh herb) in 1½ pints of cold water. Boil for 20-30 minutes (or longer if roots are very hard). Strain off the clear liquid. (2) Here is an alternative method (which requires more time): Take 1 oz. dry herb or 2 oz. fresh herb (pulverize for best results), soak for 3-12 hours in 1½ pints of cool water. Then simmer in warm water for 30 minutes. Strain liquid into a clean container. Allow to settle and cool slightly. Drink liquid while still warm. *Average dose:* 1 Tbsp. to 1 ounce water. Take 3 times a day. In order to extract the deeper healing qualities of stems, roots, and barks, the herbs must be simmered for 15-25 minutes. Many times it is left uncovered during the simmering, to evaporate some of the water.

Infusions and decoctions require a brief period of time for their preparation; and both must be used before they sour or growth of the undesirable materials starts (usually within 24-72 hours).

3 - Tincture: 1-2 oz. dried herbs are steeped in 1 pint cold grain alcohol (brandy or vodka) for 3-4 weeks. During that time, vigorously shake it 3 times a day. Then strain and store for use. *Average dose:* One tablespoon clear liquid, taken 3 times a day. *Advantage:* The herb or herbal compound (several herbs mixed together) are ready for instant use whenever needed, with no aging problems. But it contains alcohol.

4 - Fluid extracts: This is a tincture which may be as concentrated as a regular tincture, but may be as much as 5 times more concentrated.

5 - Concentrated herbs: These are relatively new products on the market. Some herbs need to be taken in larger doses to be effective. For those who take many capsules of an herb daily, using concentrated herbs is a great help. The concentration is often 4-6 times that of the original herb. Concentrated herbs are taken one step further than herbal extracts; they are freeze-dried to remove the moisture content. The result is a solvent-free product—*with no added alcohol!* This powder has all the nutrients in a form that will digest quickly in the bloodstream. They work quickly for the relief of pain.

6 - Capsules (dry powder): Dry herbs are powdered, then placed in a 2-piece gelatin capsule. A #0 ("one ought") capsule contains about 400-450 mg. But this varies with the density of the herb and whether the herb is a root or leaf. A #00 ("double ought") capsule has about 500-600 mg. The lesser-used #000 ("triple ought") contains about 650-850 mg. The capsule may be opened and emptied into hot water for tea; this can be made into a paste for poultices, tinctures, decoctions, infusions or just swallowed. If there is a problem swallowing the capsules, they can be moistened by dipping them in water or a little vegetable oil. Capsules should be stored in a cool, dry place, so they will not lose moisture and become brittle. Also excess heat and moisture will soften the capsules and they will stick together. *Advantages:* A capsule is ready for use; and strong acrid herbs, like valerian root or wormwood, are more pleasant to take. Capsules can also be inserted in the rectum easier than tablets, to treat hemorrhoids and other rectal diseases. *Disadvantages:* If swallowed, you are taking powder, not the steeped or boiled liquid; and the powder in the capsules gradually ages. A major disadvantage is that many capsules are made from boiled tissues derived from slaughtered livestock; so only use capsules made from vegetable gelatin.

7 - Tablets: Dried herb (plus an excipient [binder or carrier]) is pressed into a tablet shape. The tablet can be used in the same way as a capsule. *Advantages:* Tablets do not tend to stick together and will resist a warmer climate better than capsules. You can make the tablets yourself and know exactly what is in each one. *Disadvantages:* Do not let your supply of herbal powder become too old; for it will be difficult to be dissolved in the stomach.

There are two ways to prepare your own tablets: (1) Purchase an inexpensive tablet machine. It will press them into shape. Mix the herb with 1/10 binder (slippery elm, etc.), before making tablets. (2) Another way is to grind the herb fine and add to it a small amount (1/10 of the total) of slippery elm, an herbal syrup, or other mucilaginous herb. Add small amounts of water while mixing, keeping the preparation firm. Then roll them into small pills, about the size of a pea. Dry (1) by spreading them out onto a pie dish and left to dry at room temperature or (2) by placing them in an oven: Preheat the oven to 250°, then turn it off and place the pie dish in the oven for 15-30 minutes. Check them every 5 minutes. When dry, bottle them and keep in a cool, dry place, such as a refrigerator. When giving them to children, they can be dipped in honey, molasses, or peanut butter to cover the taste.

8 - Electuary: This is an herbal preparation which is mixed with honey, maple syrup, peanut butter, or slippery elm, to form a paste and then rolled into balls. These are then given to children to swallow with juice. Any powdered herb can be mixed with honey and given immediately without any advance preparation. Measure the exact amount of herb and then add the sweetening to it.

7 - IMPORTANT FACTS ABOUT HERBS

1 - Storage: Herbs are best stored in glass jars. Do not expose them to the sunlight for long periods of time.

2 - Weight factor: Larger persons require larger amounts than smaller or underweight individuals. Women generally require smaller doses than men, due to their lower average weight. Children and elderly people need smaller doses.

3 - Climate: The medicinal effect of herbs is intensified in hot climates, therefore give less at such times.

4 - People vary in their reactions: Some people are more intolerant to herbs than others are. It is best to initially give a smaller dose and see the reaction. It is always safe to start with the smaller child's dose, then build up to a larger dose if that seems best. Increase slowly, remaining on each level for 2-3 days, to observe for unusual reactions.

5 - Amounts for children: Here is the formula: Divide 150 (the assumed average adult weight) by the child's weight. Example: A child weighs 50 pounds. This is 1/3 of the average adult weight (of 150 pounds). Therefore give him only a third of the regular dose.

6 - During pregnancy: Women respond to herbs differently when they are pregnant. At such times, it is best to give smaller herbal doses and observe response. Sometimes mild and nutritive herbs are best. Some herbs should not be given during pregnancy (including diuretics, purgatives, and emmenagogues; all of these are active in the pelvic area and should be avoided.)

7 - Nervous people: Give them smaller doses than robust individuals.

8 - People with high blood pressure: These people should avoid herbs that stimulate the heart or constrict the blood capillaries and arteries (licorice root, ephedra, and lily of the valley are examples). But cayenne and garlic can be used in normal amounts.

9 - When herbs are combined: Herbs are frequently combined; but, if not done properly, one herb may overpower or neutralize the effects of others.

10 - Laxative herbs: Give slow-acting laxatives in the morning, so as not to disturb sleep. They may take 1-3 days to work; whereas fast-acting ones usually take 4-8 hours. Do not increase the amount until a 3-day period is over, using the same amount every day. Then, if the desired result is not obtained, you may increase the amount. The desired objective is generally 2 bowel movements a day.

11 - Sedatives and antispasmodic herbs: Give them on an empty stomach or just before bedtime.

12 - Astringents and minerals: Astringent herbs should not be taken at the same time as nutritional supplements containing iron. The tannins in astringent herbs will leach calcium, iron, and other important minerals out of the intestines. Therefore, only give astringent herbs for a short period of time.

13 - Blood-purifying herbs: Take these herbs on an empty stomach.

14 - Strong, bitter herbs: To avoid nausea, be sure and give enough water with them.

15 - Powerful herbs: Be careful in giving herbs which have powerful effects. These include lobelia, juniper berries, black cohosh, poke root, aconite, and shavegrass (horsetail).

16 - Bitter pills: They have a tonic effect on the stomach, digestion, and related organs.

17 - Herbal temperatures: A hot infusion or decoction is used to help induce sweating. Cool teas are used for tonic effect, and warm teas produce a feeling of relaxation. (Vervain is the best for inducing sweating.)

18 - Tablets vs. capsules: Tablets are easier to work with than capsules in hot climates; the latter tend to stick together. Vegetarians either open and empty capsules or use tablets, since capsules are made from slaughterhouse products.

19 - Herbs at mealtime: To avoid taking too much liquid, capsules or tablets are preferable to teas at mealtime.

20 - Varying the intensity of the amount given: Here are several principles to keep in mind:

• For a slow, gradual, general effect, give the herbs in small quantities of syrup or milk between meals. This will retard absorption.

• To aid the appetite, increase digestive secretions or, for a local effect on stomach or intestines, give herbs before meals. Give the herbs in acacia gum or olive oil for a localized effect on stomach or intestines.

• To reduce the irritation of certain herbs, give them in syrup or soy milk.

• To increase absorption of the herbs and produce a more rapid effect, give them 1-2 hours after the meal.

• To reduce the bitter taste of herbs, without reducing the bitterness, take the dose in a large quantity of fluid, syrup, or honey. The bitter taste is often necessary for the proper effect to take place, but the bitterness can be disguised to the taste buds.

• Fluids which do not taste good can be taken more easily by drinking them cold, followed by a drink of plain water.

21 - Weekly rest day: In order for herbs to work best, they should not be taken one day each week. Then, after 2-3 weeks of treatment, no herbs should be taken for 3 days in a row. During this rest period, observe the patient. (1) If his energy remains low during that time or if the symptoms worsen, at the end of the rest period put him back on the herb dosage. (2) If he improves during the rest period, then extend the rest period a day or so and then continue the treatment with smaller doses than were used before. (3) If he seems to completely recover during the rest period, then the treatment can be changed to a more tonic, nutritive approach. (4) New symptoms or problems may reveal themselves at this time. If so, an herb formula or new therapy should be instituted to meet it. (5) If he seems to get stronger during each rest period, begin reducing therapy and extending the rest periods.

22 - Types of teas: When bitter teas are taken, they have a tonic effect on digestion and related organs. A cool infusion or decoction is used for tonic effects. Hot teas are used during sweating therapy. Warm teas will create a feeling of relaxation.

23 - Types of herbs: Flowers and leaves, being more delicate, are usually made into infusions. A decoction is used when trying to extract healing properties from most roots, barks, twigs, and seeds.

24 - Determining the dosage: First study the suggested dosages for each herb. Next consider whether the disease is chronic or acute; whether the patient is a child or an adult; and whether he is strong, weak, or pregnant. Perhaps lactation or menstruation is present. Consider the age, temperament, sex, and size of the individual. It is always safer to start with a smaller dose; and, if that works well, increase it slowly to the normal dosage. If a child will take the herb, give him only part of that which an adult would receive: Assuming 150 pounds for an average adult, if the child is 50 pounds, then 150 divided by 50 = 1/3 of the adult dose.

25 - Herbs for children: Only give mild herbs to children and adults who are experiencing an acute ailment, not harsh laxatives and strong cleansing herbs. Mild herbs can be given in large amounts, usually 1 cup of tea per dose. Here are the mild herbs: peppermint, chamomile, catnip, comfrey leaf, nettles, chickweed, spearmint, and alfalfa. The strength and energy level of the individual tells a lot.

8 - TYPES OF HERBAL APPLICATIONS

1 - Fomentation: These are cotton towels soaked in an herbal tea infusion or decoction which is as hot as can be tolerated. Placed on a body part. This stimulates blood and lymph circulation; warms joints and other body parts; reduces internal inflammations; and relieves colic and pain. By alternating hot and cold fomentations, healing blood moves more rapidly into and out of the affected area. This is especially helpful for sluggish circulation, constipation, urine retention, etc. After soaking it in the herbal tea, fold and wring the hot towel slightly and place it on the affected area. Over that place a layer of plastic. To keep the heat in, place a dry towel or heating pad on top. Every so often, resaturate the hot, soaked towel.

2 - Poultice: This is a small pile of powdered or pulverized herbs, moistened with water (and/or tinctures, infusions, decoctions, salves, oils) and applied to the surface of the skin. Fresh herb can be applied without moistening. If there will be body movement, wrap a cloth around the poultice to hold it in place, perhaps taping it slightly. Poultices are used to reduce inflammation, and withdraw pus and embedded particles. Ginger and cayenne increase circulation; echinacea and garlic reduce infectious sores. Valerian and kava kava reduce pain. Lobelia tincture added to a poultice will reduce pain very well. Clay poultices, with or without herbs, made into a thick, doughy consistency, are good at drawing out poisons. Clay can be purchased at health-food stores. Mixed with mashed cabbage leaves, the clay poultice is good for boils and tumors. Mixed with powdered cayenne or ginger, painful arthritic joints can be treated.

3 - Salves: Salves are used to treat boils and dry or itchy skin. Astringent herbs (white oak bark, bayberry) tone the skin. Demulcent herbs (comfrey) soften and keep the surface moist and healthy looking. Salves are a thick consistency of herbal oil, herbs, and a little oil (never mineral oil) to cover the mixture, baked in a covered pot at 125°-200° for 2-4 hours. Melt beeswax (about 1½ oz. to 1 pint oil) and stir it into the oil. Preserve the salve by adding ½ tsp. vitamin E per cup of solution to 1 oz. of salve.

4 - Oils: Oils are usually made from mints and aromatic herbs, and are applied to increase circulation and warmth to the area, and treat skin diseases and painful joints. They are also used when giving massages, for dry skin; these are to be rubbed on the surface of the skin before a poultice, hot pack or fomentation is applied.

Add 1 oz. olive oil to 2 oz. macerated herb. Mix carefully and bake in the oven at 115°-200° until the herbs become crisp (about 2-4 hours). When that happens, the oils have left the herbs and entered the olive oil. Strain out the herbal oil. Add to it the oil from one 400 I.U. vitamin E capsule to every cup of herbal oil (as a preservative). Put the oil in a dark bottle. Olive oil usually has a long shelf life before it goes rancid.

Certain oils will be absorbed by the skin faster than others. When you want the oil to remain on the skin for a long period to help heal external sores, etc., use olive or peanut oil, or avocado. (Wheat germ, sesame, and sunflower oil absorb much faster.). Essential herbal oils can also be purchased in a health-food store and are more highly concentrated.

5 - Douches: These are used to treat vaginal infections and excessive secretions. They are prepared by making a strong infusion or decoction using herbs such as goldenseal, myrrh, slippery elm, plantain, and (if there are excessive secretions or bleeding) white oak bark. One Tbsp. of apple cider vinegar should be added to 1 quart tea, to help maintain an acid pH. While the tea is warm, carefully insert the douche. Retain for 3-5 minutes. Use once daily for 5-7 days, and only during the infection. Thereafter, only used once a month. Pregnant women should not use douches.

6 - Bolus: This is a suppository inserted into the rectum or vagina, to draw out toxins and treat swellings, infections, cysts, tumors, inflammations, and hemorrhoids. For vaginal infections, boluses are only used when douches are not successful. The herbs used in boluses are astringents (white oak bark, bayberry, witch hazel), demulcents (slippery elm, comfrey root), and antibiotic herbs (garlic, goldenseal, chaparral, myrrh). To make a bolus, add 10% powdered slippery elm (by volume or weight) to your selection of herbs. Mix the herbs well, either by stirring or blending. Slowly pour water into the mixture until it becomes a thick, doughy consistency. Then roll into strips about ½-inch thick and ¾-inch long. If necessary, put the mixture into the refrigerator to cool awhile before rolling the suppositories. When formed, let them dry by being exposed to the sun or in an oven under low heat. Do not burn them. Then put them in a jar and keep in the refrigerator. Before inserting the bolus, let it set at room temperature 15-20 minutes, to warm up. To make insertion easier, dip in olive oil or warm water and quickly insert. Insert before long rest periods in bed.

9 - TWENTY-TWO USEFUL POULTICES

For much more on poultices, go to pp. 243-245.

1 - Cabbage poultice: Pulverize the leaves and lay it on the skin. This will draw out poisons and pus. When it feels hot, replace it with a fresh one. Another way to prepare the cabbage: Wash a leaf, lay it flat on a breadboard, roll it with a rolling pin to break ridges and veins, then attach to the sore.

2 - Garlic poultice: Crush fresh garlic and add warm water and flour. It relieves pain, pus, and infection.

3 - Potato poultice: Place grated raw potato on bruises, sprains, or boils.

4 - Carrot poultice: Take the pulp (remaining after juicing carrots or finely grating carrots) and place it on bruises, sores, chapped skin, and nipples.

5 - Comfrey poultice: Mash the leaves, then moisten them with comfrey tea. It is good for open sores, wounds, or swellings.

6 - Fig poultice: Heat figs for 3 minutes, cut open, and apply to infected sores. It will bring them to a head.

7 - Flaxseed: Boil in water to extract the healing oil in the outer skin of the flaxseed. Stir briskly with a wooden spoon. Stir in a little olive oil (just enough to dissolve hardened lumps). Place in cloth bag, dip in hot water and apply hot to the painful area.

8 - Ginger: Simmer ginger root in water or add powdered ginger to boiling water. Soak a folded cloth in water and apply to relieve pain or to bring blood to the surface of a congested area.

9 - Hops: Steep it for 10 minutes and apply. It soothes inflammations and boils, and reduces the pain of toothache.

10 - Oatmeal poultice: Cool cooked oatmeal; then place it in a soft, cotton cloth. Put it over inflammations and insect bites, and cover with a dry cloth. Apply a heating pad.

11 - Onion: Pack roasted onion on bruised, inflamed, and injured areas. In emergencies, use raw onions. Like carrots and turnips, onions have exceptional drawing power.

12 - Plantain: Apply a leaf of this invaluable weed, either crushed or mashed on a swollen or running sore. Wrap around a finger for whitlow (felon). Attach with tape or bandage. Discard if it gets hot and apply fresh plaintain.

13 - Potato, Flaxseed: Put a piece of raw, grated potato, mixed with flaxseed on a sprain, bruise, boil.

14 - Rice: Soak whole rice in a small amount of water. Either cook it briefly or discard the water and crush the raw rice into a paste. Apply to the wound.

15 - Sage: Apply the cool tea, or hot-leaf mash, to rough abrasions and injuries.

16 - Salt: Heat 1-2 pounds of coarse salt. Put it in a pillow case and apply to the injured or painful area.

17 - Slippery elm: Squeeze out the cake, chop it up, add a teaspoon of ginger, then flour till it thickens. This will draw out inflammation and fever.

18 - Tofu poultice: Squeeze out the soy cake, add a tablespoon or so of wheat flour, and apply to the inflam-mation. Alternate this poultice with a hot ginger poultice to help reduce pain.

19 - Witch hazel: The herb poultice is outstanding for reducing surface swellings on the body or eyes. Distilled witch hazel, obtainable from a drugstore, can be applied to bruises, sunburns, and cuts. Apply it with absorbent cotton to small areas, including the eyes. Use a saturated cloth for larger applications.

20 - Yarrow: Steep the leaves in water and apply. It is good for reducing swellings and eases earaches. It will soothe bruises and abrasions. It can be applied in a tea for nursing mothers with sore nipples or as a wash for rashes, eczema, and poison ivy.

21 - Charcoal: This is an outstanding remedy. Apply dampened charcoal in a poultice to a surface infection. For deeper infections, wrap the charcoal in a pack and apply it overnight; then change again in the morning. This is good for deeper infections, not only for the surface ones.

22 - Clay poultice: Get clay from a place where it is found and sterilize it in the oven. Or buy it at the health-food store (either regular clay or bentonite clay). Mix the clay with just enough water or herb tea to make a consistency that is thick, like bread dough. Apply to bruises and infections. Mix clay with crushed cabbage leaves and place the mixture on boils or tumors. Mix clay with cayenne or ginger and apply to sore arthritic joints.

10 - TWENTY ESSENTIAL OILS

Essential oils are always applied externally; they are never, never swallowed! Taking them internally may be fatal. They are applied to the skin and used as an aroma, to help certain physical conditions.

Purchase small bottles, since the oxygen in the bottle gradually deteriorates the oil. Make sure the label says "pure essential oil." Some oils cannot be extracted (such as peach oil or apple blossom oil); products so advertised are not genuine.

Directions for use: Dilute a small amount of the essential oil in either water or another oil (a carrier oil). Either apply or inhale it. The best carrier oils include olive oil, almond oil, apricot oil, grapeseed oil, or jojoba oil.

Facial oil: Add 6 drops essential oil to 1 oz. jojoba oil.

Massage oil: Add 25 drops essential oil to 2 oz. olive oil, almond oil, or apricot oil.

Baths: Add 8 drops essential oil to 1 cup water and put in bath.

Hair rinse: Add 10 drops essential oil to 16 oz. water.

Hair conditioner: Add 1 drop essential oil to 4-6 oz. unscented conditioner.

Antiseptic cleaning: Add 25 drops essential oil to 2 gallons water.

Cedarwood - Antiseptic, astringent, and sedative. Good for bronchial problems.

Chamomile - Pain reliever, reduce spasms, good for headaches when applied in a compress to the head.

Clary sage - Anti-inflammatory, antidepressant. Helps induce sleep. Do not use during pregnancy.

Cypress - Antiseptic, astringent, antispasmodic. Constricts blood vessels, reduces coughing.

Eucalyptus - Antiseptic, antiviral, decongestant (rubbed on chest), expectorant. Reduces fevers and aches.

Frankincense - Anti-inflammatory, antiseptic, sedative. Useful for bronchitis.

Geranium - Antidiabetic, antidepressant, antiseptic. This mildly sedating oil is useful for nervous tension, PMS.

Grapefruit - Reduces appetite, water retention. Detoxifies the skin and helps weight reduction.

Hyssop - Detoxifies, cleanses, an antiseptic. Clears the lungs of congestion and aids breathing.

Juniper - Detoxifier, diuretic, an antiseptic. Helps arthritic conditions and cellulitis. Do not use during pregnancy.

Lavender - Calms and normalizes, fights bacterial and fungal infections. Good for acne, burns, eczema.

Lemon - Excellent germ killer. Good for varicose veins and reducing swellings.

Peppermint - Useful for headaches, fatigue, congestion, fever, muscle soreness, sinus problems.

Rose - Tonic astringent, antiseptic, antidepressant. Good for nervousness and insomnia.

Rosemary - Among the best of the oils; good for pain, infection, spasms, dandruff, cellulite, headaches.

Rosewood - Good for anxiety, depression, headaches, nausea, tension, and PMS. It is antiseptic and calming.

Sandalwood - Antiseptic, expectorant, antidepressant. Also good for bronchitis, nervousness, and as a skin moisturizer.

Tea Tree - Antiviral, anti-infective, fungicide, antiseptic. Athlete's foot, dandruff, bronchitis, ringworm.

Thyme - Antiseptic, expectorant, antispasmodic. Herpes, skin infections, calming effect.

Yarrow - Improves digestion, reduces blood pressure, fights infection and spasms.

11 - HERBAL PROPERTIES

Medicinal herbs produce certain effects on the body. A list of all these possible effects is called "herbal properties." One herb will produce certain effects while another may produce some of the same ones, plus certain others. Listed below are the major categories of herbal properties. The *"examples"* are some of the best herbs containing those properties.

To this list has been added a *"goes with"* section. This is because herbs with certain properties work best with herbs containing certain other properties. The *"goes with"* sections, below, will tell what these are. Experienced herbalists select one or two herbs which have one target property (example: *antipyretic,* or fever reducing). To this will be added one or two other complementary herbs which accomplish a related objective. As you learn to combine herbs, you become a skilled herbalist!

Basic herbal formula: Here is a general outline for preparing an herbal formula for acute ailments:

(1) Use a large proportion (about 70%-80% by weight) of 1 to 3 herbs that possess the primary property required to treat the ailment (*expectorant* for coughs, *antibiotic* and *blood purifying* properties for infections, *warming* properties for colds, etc.).

(2) Add a small amount of a *stimulant* herb (cayenne works well), to promote the action of the primary herbal medicine.

(3) Add a small amount of an *antispasmodic* herb, to reduce tensions in the body.

(4) Add a small amount of a *carminative* or *demulcent* herb, to provide gentle action and protection to the system.

1 - Alteratives (Blood purifiers): These are herbs which purify the blood. They promote the cleaning action of the spleen, liver, kidneys, and bowels and should be used over a long period of time in order to gradually detoxify the bloodstream; this in turn will improve digestion, assimilation, and glandular secretions. Bad habits must also be corrected. Impure blood causes infections, arthritis, skin disease, cancer, etc. **Examples:** Alfalfa, red clover, garlic, barberry, black cohosh, cayenne, chaparral, comfrey, echinacea, eyebright, goldenseal, gotu kola, plantain, sassafras, uva ursi, wood betony, yellow dock. **Goes with:** Add a *stimulant* herb, such as cayenne, to speed the action of the alterative. Ginger will also do this, plus increase action in the genito-urinary area. Add an *aromatic,* to cover the taste of the *alterative.* Peppermint is both an *aromatic* and an *alterative.*

2 - Anodynes: Herbs which relieve pain by reducing the excitability of the nerves and nerve centers. They can be used as fomentations on the surface or internally as teas, tinctures, or powders. *Anodynes* are closely allied to the *antispasmodics.* **Examples:** Skullcap, chamomile, valerian, echinacea, ginger, hops, lobelia, vervain. **Goes with:** *Antispasmodic* and *nervine* herbs go well with *anodynes*; often using cayenne (a *stimulant* herb) as an accentuator.

3 - Anthelmintics: Herbs which kill or expel intestinal worms and parasites. *Vermicides* destroy worms without always causing their expulsion from the bowels; and vermicides should be followed by, or combined with, laxative or cathartic herbs. **Examples:** Garlic, black walnut. *Vermifuges* expel worms from the bowels. *Examples:* Cascara sagrada, gentian, wormwood. **Goes with:** *Laxatives* are almost always used with anthelmintics. *Nervines* are often added to relax a certain area made tense by worms.

4 - Antacids: Herbs which correct acid conditions in the stomach, blood, and bowels. **Examples:** Comfrey leaves or root, flaxseed, raspberry, slippery elm, wood betony. **Goes with:** *Stimulant* herbs, such as ginger and cayenne, to accentuate. *Demulcent* herbs soothe and relieve pain in specific areas.

5 - Antibiotics: Herbs which not only inhibit the growth of (and destroy) viruses and bacteria, but help promote the body's own immunity. **Examples:** Chaparral, echinacea, garlic, goldenseal, myrrh, pau d'arco.

6 - Anticatarrhals: Herbs which eliminate mucous conditions. **Examples:** Angelica, bayberry, bistort, cayenne, comfrey, elecampane, garlic, ginger, wild cherry, yerba santa. It is best to increase elimination by also including laxative herbs or diuretic teas.

7 - Antiemetics: Herbs which relieve sickness of the stomach and prevent vomiting. **Examples:** Ginger, cloves, goldenseal, lobelia (very small doses), peppermint, red clover, spearmint. **Goes with:** We want to not only relieve the vomiting, but also settle the nerves. Antispasmodics will ease the area and nervines will settle the nerves (for sometimes vomiting is continued from a nervous condition alone). The source of the nausea is key here. A demulcent will soothe the stomach area and hepatic herbs (such as barberry) will ease the liver. A cleansing laxative enema is always used to clean out the bowel, greatly reducing the chance of nausea.

8 - Antipyretics (refrigerants): Herbs which cool the system and reduce fevers. **Examples:** Alfalfa, chickweed, lemons, licorice, limes, oranges, skullcap, valerian. **Goes with:** Stimulant herbs (cayenne, ginger) are used to increase circulation as rapidly as possible and carry off the poisons. Diuretic and diaphoretic herbs (raspberry leaf, peppermint) combine well. Tonic herbs rebuild the entire body.

9 - Antiseptics: Herbs which prevent the growth of bacteria. **Examples:** Garlic, echinacea, goldenseal, myrrh, barberry, bistort, black walnut, saw palmetto, white oak bark. **Goes with:** Stimulant herbs (cayenne, ginger) speed the healing.

10 - Antispasmodics: Herbs used for cramps, muscular spasms, and convulsions. **Examples:** Black cohosh, blue cohosh, cayenne, fennel, garlic, lobelia, peppermint, raspberry, sage, skullcap, valerian, vervain, wild yam. These herbs are helpful during tetany, extreme irritability, feebleness, hysteria, intestinal and leg cramps, menstrual cramps, intestinal worms which cause spasms, infantile convulsions, etc. **Goes with:** A stimulant herb (cayenne, ginger) accentuates and speeds this along.

11 - Aperients: Herbs which produce a mild laxative effect, softening the stool without purging. **Examples:** Figs, flaxseed, fruit, licorice root, olive oil, prunes, raisins. **Goes with:** Use a mild stimulant and a nervine to assist.

12 - Aromatics: Herbs which have a fragrant odor and an agreeable taste. Their essential oils stimulate the gastro-intestinal mucous membrane. Their spicy taste aids digestion and expels wind from the stomach and bowels. They are used to mask the taste of bitter herbs. Do not use them if the stomach is inflamed. **Examples:** Anise seed, barberry, cloves, coriander seed, fennel, ginger, juniper berries, peppermint, rosemary, sage, sassafras, spearmint, wood betony. Also see *Carminatives,* below. **Goes with:** These work well with almost every other class of herbs, not altering their medicinal values, but helping the other herbs taste better.

13 - Astringents: Herbs which increase the tone and firmness of the tissues, and reduce mucous discharge from the nose, intestines, vagina, and draining sores. **Examples:** White oak bark, witch hazel, bayberry, cayenne, eyebright, fenugreek, gravel root, mullein, plantain, raspberry, sage, slippery elm, squaw vine, uva ursi, vervain, wild cherry bark, yarrow, yellow dock, yerba santa. **Goes with:** When taken internally, add an aromatic to improve the taste.

14 - Cardiacs: Herbs that increase the power of the heart. **Examples:** Black cohosh, hawthorn berries, moth-erwort. **Goes with:** Add cleansing herbs which tone the heart, including cayenne. Also add wheat germ oil. Add nutritional and alterative herbs, to help heal the heart. At times a nervine will help reduce pain, but an antispasmodic will work more quickly to cut the pain.

15 - Carminatives: Herbs containing volatile oils which stimulate expulsion of gas from the gastro-intestinal tract. They also increase the tone of its muscular wall, thus stimulating peristalsis. Aromatic herbs are also carminatives. **Examples:** Anise, caraway, coriander, cumin, dill, fennel, sassafras, spearmint, thyme, peppermint, angelica, catnip, cayenne, chamomile, garlic, ginger, juniper berries, myrrh, parsley, sarsaparilla, valerian. **Goes with:** You can speed the action with a stimulant (cayenne, etc.), and antispasmodics help with the pain.

16 - Cathartics: Herbs which produce a rapid evacuation of the contents of the entire intestinal tract and bowel. **Examples:** Cascara sagrada, aloe vera, senna. **Goes with:** Use ginger as a guiding factor to carry into the abdominal area. In addition, stimulant herbs (a little cayenne) accelerate the action, nervines condition the peristaltic muscles, and antispasmodics alleviate any pain. Carminatives (wild yam, celery seed, etc.) will cut the gas. Always add a demulcent or emollient to soothe the area, because cathartics may be sharp in action.

17 - Cholagogues: Herbs which promote the flow of bile. **Examples:** Barberry, beets, bistort, boneset, cascara sagrada, cayenne, elecampane, gentian, goldenseal, hops, hyssop, olive oil, Oregon grape root, vervain, wild yam, wormwood, yellow dock.

18 - Demulcents: Herbs which soften and relieve irritation of the mucous membranes (which are the walls of all inner cavities of the body). **Examples:** Agar-agar, Irish moss, flaxseed, psyllium seed, slippery elm, aloe vera, burdock root, chickweed, coltsfoot, comfrey root (not leaf), corn silk, fenugreek, kelp, licorice root, marshmallow, mullein. (These herbs are also routinely combined with other herb powders, to bind them in making herb tablets.) **Goes with:** Demulcents are compatible with all other herbs.

19 - Deobstruents: Herbs which remove obstructions. **Examples:** Barberry (liver, gallbladder), Culver's root (bowel), goldenseal (glands), gravel root (kidneys), hydrangea root (kidneys), plantain (blood, kidneys). (For treating the intestines, see *Aperients* and *Laxatives.*) **Goes with:** Combine with nervine or antispasmodic herbs and often a demulcent in order to give ease, because some damage is often done to the bowel by the obstruction. Marshmallow or comfrey will help rebuild, or restore, the area.

20 - Diaphoretics (Sudorifics): Herbs which increase perspiration. They affect the entire circulatory system and fall into three subtypes: *Stimulating diaphoretics:* **Examples:** Angelica, blessed thistle, boneset, buchu, garlic, ginger, peppermint, spearmint, yarrow. *Neutral diaphoretics:* **Examples:** Horehound, safflower, sarsaparilla, sassafras. *Relaxing diaphoretics:* **Examples:** *Blue vervain,* catnip, chamomile, lemon balm, motherwort, pleurisy root, thyme, vervain, white willow, wild yam. **Goes with:** Stimulant herbs (ginger, mustard, cayenne) must always be added, to accentuate the sweating and water treatment. Always use moist heat in the cold sheet and whatever therapeutic process you use, also plenty of liquids or teas. Nervines relax the tissues, open the pores, and assist the action. Diaphoretics blend with most herbs.

21 - Discutients: Herbs which dissolve and remove tumors and abnormal growths. These are used in poultices, fomentations (see section on *Hydrotherapy*), and taken internally as teas. **Examples:** Red clover, chaparral, garlic, black walnut, burdock root, devil's claw, poke root (only used externally). **Goes with:** Stimulant herbs (cayenne) and demulcents.

22 - Diuretics: Herbs which increase the flow of urine. Of course, one should drink additional water when taking diuretics. They are generally combined with *demulcents,* to soothe any irritation from acids or gravel. Diuretics are important in helping to care for water retention, bladder ache, kidney stones, scalding urine, obesity, prostatitis, backache, gonorrhea, skin eruptions, and lymphatic swelling. **Examples:** Corn silk, gravel root, pleurisy root, black cohosh, blue cohosh, burdock root, chaparral, cleavers, dandelion, false unicorn, fennel, gotu kola, Hawthorn berries, juniper berries, cranberry, mullein, plantain, squaw vine, white oak bark, white willow. **Goes with:** Ginger will help direct the herb action into the kidney/urethral area. Use stimulant herbs (cayenne) in order to speed up the action; and use nervine tonics, to relax the tube ends and open up the valves for an easier flow of fluids and to tone up the area.

23 - Emetics: Herbs which induce vomiting. They are generally given as teas or tinctures. **Examples:** Lobelia (tincture or ½ cupful tea), bayberry, chaparral, false unicorn (large doses), mandrake (large doses). **Goes with:** Emetics are generally used alone, but a light stimulant (peppermint tea) can be added, to allay pain due to muscular wrenching.

24 - Emmenagogues: Herbs which promote menstrual flow. **Examples:** Squaw vine, motherwort, angelica, black cohosh, blessed thistle, blue cohosh, chamomile, gentian, goldenseal, myrrh, pennyroyal, prickly ash, rue. **Goes with:** These combine well with stimulant herbs, nervines, demulcents and emollients. Emmenagogues depend on the stimulant ginger as a carrier. Sometimes gas is generated, for which a carminative is used.

25 - Emollients: Herbs which soften and soothe, when applied externally in salves, poultices, and fomentations. They may also be taken internally for their *demulcent* quality. **Examples:** Flaxseed, slippery elm, wheat germ oil, Irish moss, chickweed, coltsfoot, comfrey root (not leaf), fenugreek, marshmallow, plantain. **Goes with:** These combine well with almost all herbs or herb combinations.

26 - Expectorants: Herbs which help excrete mucus from the throat and lungs. They are generally combined with demulcents, which are soothing. **Examples:** Garlic, chaparral, comfrey, elecampane, fennel, fenugreek, horehound, lobelia, lungwort, mullein, myrrh, nettles, plantain, pleurisy root, thyme, vervain, wild cherry, yerba santa. **Goes with:** These combine with demulcents, emollients, stimulant herbs, antispasmodics, and nutritives.

27 - Febrifuges: Herbs which reduce fevers. **Ex-** amples: Boneset, catnip, dandelion, hyssop, peppermint, shepherd's purse, white willow, yarrow. **Goes with:** These are compatible with stimulant herbs, antispasmodics, and with most diaphoretics.

28 - Galactagogues: Herbs which help secretion of milk from a nursing mother. **Examples:** Anise seed, blessed thistle, cumin, dandelion, fennel, fenugreek, raspberry, vervain. **Goes with:** Galactagogues work best alone. There are a number of herbs which a nursing mother should not take. *(See the chapter on Herbs for Pregnancy, pp. 722-726)*

29 - Hemostatics: Herbs which stop internal bleeding or hemorrhaging. **Examples:** Bayberry, beet root, blackberry, mullein, nettles, white oak bark, witch hazel, yarrow. Also see *Astringents.* **Goes with:** These combine well with stimulant herbs and antispasmodics, but do not combine with any herb that will expand the pore structure (such as diaphoretics).

30 - Hepatics: Herbs which strengthen, tone, and stimulate the secretive functions of the liver. **Examples:** Aloe vera, barberry, bayberry, buckthorn, carrot, dandelion, wild yam, wood betony, yellow dock. **Goes with:** These work well with stimulant herbs (cayenne, ginger), with antispasmodics, and with carminatives. Often aromatics are added, to cover some of the bitterness.

31 - Laxatives: Cascara sagrada, flaxseed, psyllium seed, agar agar, boneset, buckthorn bark, cleavers, goldenseal, motherwort, Oregon grape root, senna, yellow dock. **Goes with:** Combine with emollients, demulcents, stimulant herbs, nervines, antispasmodics, carminatives; and, often, aromatics are added.

32 - Lithotriptics (Resolvents): Herbs which dissolve and discharge urinary and gallbladder stones and gravel. **Examples:** Gravel root, corn silk, barberry, buchu, cascara sagrada, chaparral, dandelion, juniper berries, marshmallow, Oregon grape root, Uva ursi. **Goes with:** Add demulcents and emollients when cutting stone adhesions loose or breaking them up from a stony mass, because passing them though the urethral or gall ducts is very painful. Olive and natural oils are excellent to ease the passing, but *never* use mineral oil. Nervines relax tension in the tract itself, wherein the tubes expand and the stones are more easily discharged.

33 - Lymphatics: Herbs which stimulate and cleanse the lymphatic system. **Examples:** Garlic, black walnut, chaparral, dandelion, echinacea, Oregon grape root, yellow dock. **Goes with:** Alteratives and stimulants are helpful.

34 - Mucilages: Herbs which soothe inflamed parts. **Examples:** Agar agar, flaxseed, slippery elm, marshmallow root, okra, chickweed, comfrey root, lungwort, mullein. Also see *Demulcents.* **Goes with:** These combine with nutritional herbs, demulcents, and most herbs, as mucilages act as carriers.

35 - Nervines: Herbs which act as a tonic to the nerves. They relieve pain and regulate the nervous system. **Examples:** Hops, lobelia (small amounts), skullcap, cramp bark, gravel root, lady's slipper, mistletoe, motherwort, mugwort, passionflower, peach bark, pleurisy root, vervain, wood betony. **Goes with:** Combine with antispasmodics and stimulant herbs.

36 - Nutritives: Herbs which provide a substantial amount of nutrients and aid in building and toning the body. **Examples:** Alfalfa, spirulina, parsley, comfrey leaves, comfrey root, red clover, rose hips, slippery elm, yellow dock. **Goes with:** All herbs are partially nutritive. With specifically nutritive herbs, add demulcents and emollients, to soothe the digestive area, and sometimes a stimulant herb (cayenne), to seed the absorption.

37 - Opthalmics: Herbs which help heal the eyes. **Examples:** Eyebright (first and foremost), chickweed, fennel, mullein, rue. **Goes with:** These often require nervines because the pain in the eyes is so severe. Also helpful are antispasmodics (an accentuator, such as cayenne) and, in many cases, a demulcent.

38 - Oxytocics (Parturients): Herbs which assist labor and promote easy childbirth. **Examples:** Angelica, black cohosh, blue cohosh, juniper berries, raspberry, squaw vine. **Goes with:** Nervines combine well here, plus antispasmodics; stimulant herbs; and nearly always such an herb as raspberry leaf, to relax the pelvic area.

39 - Parasiticides: Herbs which kill and remove parasites from the skin. **Examples:** Black walnut, cassia, wormwood, cloves, chaparral, echinacea, false unicorn, garlic, gentian, rue, thyme, wood betony. **Goes with:** Add demulcents and emollients, to soothe the digestive area.

40 - Purgatives: Herbs which have a very strong enema effect. **Examples:** Buckthorn bark, castor oil, mandrake root, senna. Combine these with *carminatives,* to lessen griping. **Goes with:** Antispasmodics, emollients, and demulcents are best added. Nervines mix well and carminatives will cut the flatulence.

41 - Rubefacients: Herbs which are applied locally, to stimulate and increase the blood flow to the surface. **Examples:** Cayenne, mustard seed, peppermint oil, rosemary oil, thyme oil, prickly ash, rue. **Goes with:** Stimulant herbs, such as cayenne or ginger.

42 - Sedatives: Herbs which calm the functional activity of an organ or body part. They influence the circulation, reducing nervous expenditure. **Examples:** Catnip, all mints, hops, skullcap, black haw, hawthorn berries, hyssop, kava kava, lemon balm, passionflower, peach bark, red clover, rue, saw palmetto, sorrel, valerian, wild cherry bark, witch hazel, wood betony.

43 - Sialagogues: Herbs which promote an increased flow of saliva. **Examples:** Cayenne, ginger, licorice, prickly ash, echinacea. **Goes with:** Ginger and a few other stimulants work well here; for they excite the salivary glands.

44 - Stimulants: Herbs which assist the functional activity of the body, thereby increasing energy. **Examples:** Cayenne, garlic, ginseng, ginger, red clover, angelica, bayberry, boneset, elder flowers, elecampane, false unicorn, fennel, fo-ti, gravel root, juniper berries, mandrake, myrrh, pennyroyal, prickly ash, raspberry, rosemary, rue, sassafras, shepherd's purse, wild cherry bark, yarrow, yerba santa. **Goes with:** These combine well with most herbs.

45 - Stomachics: Herbs which strengthen the functions of the stomach. Although usually bitter, they promote and improve digestion and appetite. In Britain they are known as "bitters." **Examples:** Agrimony, barberry, blessed thistle, elecampane, juniper berries, mugwort, peach bark, rue, wormwood. **Goes with:** Demulcents and emollients are often needed for soothing. Nutrients; mucilages; and, in most cases, stimulants are also added. If there is severe pain, nervines and antispasmodics can be mixed with them.

46 - Styptics: Herbs (usually astringent) which stop bleeding, hemorrhaging, and draining of wounds. They may be used externally or internally. **Examples:** White oak bark, witch hazel, bistort, shavegrass, plantain leaves, yarrow. **Goes with:** Stimulant herbs will help seed the action.

47 - Tonics: Herbs which increase energy and strengthen the body. They increase muscular strength and tone the nervous system while improving digestion and assimilation, resulting in a general sense of well-being. *Gallbladder tonics:* **Examples:** Goldenseal, Oregon grape root, parsley, wild yam. *Heart tonics:* **Examples:** Bugleweed, hawthorn berries motherwort, ginseng. *Intestinal tonics:* **Examples:** Barberry, blackberry leaves, cascara sagrada, goldenseal. *Kidney tonics:* **Examples:** Buchu, burdock root, cleavers, fo-ti, kava kava, parsley, pipsissewa, saw palmetto, uva ursi. *Liver tonics:* **Examples:** Barberry, buckthorn bark, cascara sagrada, dandelion, eyebright, fo-ti, goldenseal, mandrake. *Lung tonics:* **Examples:** Bethroot, comfrey, elecampane, fenugreek, garlic, lungwort, pleurisy root, wild cherry. *Nerve tonics:* **Examples:** Chamomile, hops, lady's slipper, valerian. *Stomach tonics:* Agrimony, blessed thistle, elecampane, gentian, goldenseal, mugwort, raspberry, wild cherry bark, wormwood. **Goes with:** Use demulcents and emollients, to soothe; and often combine mucilage herbs with stimulant herbs, antispasmodics, and carminatives in order to cut gas. Tonic herbs combine well with most herbs, and usually require aromatics to make them more pleasant.

48 - Vulneraries: Herbs which promote the healing of cuts, wounds, and burns by protecting against infection and stimulating cellular growth. **Examples:** Aloe vera, tee tree oil, garlic, black walnut, comfrey (leaves or root), fenugreek, lungwort, mullein, plantain, slippery elm, yarrow. **Goes with:** Stimulant herbs, such as cayenne, and can be used alone as vulneraries. When there is pain, add antispasmodics and nervines with it. For fresh wounds, oils and mucilage herbs keep the vulneraries fresh for faster healing. A favorite here is slippery elm.

12 - BASIC EFFECTS OF HERBS

Different medicinal herbs have different types of effects and tend to exert their activities on different body systems and organs. The following table classifies some of the best known herbs according to their actions and areas of prime activity

Antibacterial/antiviral — Aloe, anise, annatto, astragalus, black walnut, boneset, boswellia, burdock. catnip, cat's claw, cayenne, cedar, chanca piedra. chaparral. chickweed. echinacea, elder, eucalyptus. garlic. goldenseal, jaborandi, jatoba. kudzu, lady's mantle, lemongrass, licorice, macela, meadowsweet, myrrh. olive leaf, pau d'arco, pleurisy root. puncture vine, red clover.

rose, rosemary. sangre de grado, slippery elm. suma. tea tree, turmeric, uva ursi. valerian. white oak, wild oregano.

Anticancer/antitumor — Astragalus. birch, burdock, cat's claw, chaparral, chuchuhuasi, cranberry. dandelion. fennel. garlic. green tea, licorice, macela. milk thistle, parsley. pau d'arco. rosemary, suma. turmeric.

Antifungal — Acerola. alfalfa, aloe, black walnut. boswellia, burdock, cedar. cinnamon. jatoba. puncture vine, rosemary, sangre de grado, tea tree, wild oregano.

Anti-inflammatory — Alfalfa, aloe, annatto, ashwagandha, bilberry, birch, blessed thistle, boldo. boneset, boswellia, buchu, butcher's broom. calendula. catnip, cat's claw, chamomile. chanca piedra. chuchuhuasi. devil's claw, echinacea, elder, fenugreek. feverfew. flax. ginger. goldenseal. jaborandi, jatoba, juniper, lady's mantle. licorice, macela, meadowsweet, mullein, mustard, pleurisy root, puncture vine, pygeum, rosemary, sangre de grado, suma. turmeric, white willow. wild oregano, wild yam. wintergreen. witch hazel, yellow dock.

Antioxidant — Acerola, annatto. bilberry. burdock, cat's claw, celery, chaparral, elder. ginger. ginkgo, green tea. jatoba, milk thistle, olive leaf, rosemary, sangre de grado, turmeric, wild oregano, yerba mate.

Cleanser/detoxifier — Alfalfa. black walnut, blessed thistle, cascara sagrada. cat's claw. cedar. dandelion, elder. garlic, ginger. goldenseal, guarana, licorice, muira puama. Oregon grape, pau d'arco. rosemary. yellow dock, yerba mate.

Bones/joints — Alfalfa. black cohosh, boswellia, cat's claw, cayenne. celery. chuchuhuasi. dandelion, devil's claw, feverfew, flax, garlic. ginger, horsetail, jatoba, muira puama, nettle, olive leaf. pau d'arco, peppermint. primrose, red raspberry. St. John's wort. sarsaparilla. skullcap. suma, wild oregano, wild yam, wintergreen. yucca.

Brain/nervous system — Ashwagandha, astragalus, bayberry. bilberry, blessed thistle. blue cohosh, catnip. celery, chamomile. chaste tree, devil's claw, dong quai, eyebright, fennel. fenugreek. feverfew, ginger, ginseng. goldenseal. gotu kola, guarana. hops. jaborandi. kava kava, kudzu, lavender. lemongrass, licorice. marshmallow, motherwort, muira puama. oat straw, passionflower. peppermint, plantain, rosemary, sage. St. John's wort, sarsaparilla, skullcap. squawvine. stone root, suma, thyme, valerian, vervain, white willow, wild cherry, wild oregano, wintergreen, wood betony, wormwood, yerba mate.

Circulatory/cardiovascular systems — Aloe, barberry, bayberry, bilberry. black cohosh, black walnut, blessed thistle, borage, boswellia. butcher's broom, cayenne, celery, chickweed, cinnamon, devil's claw, elder. garlic, gentian. ginger. ginkgo, ginseng. gotu kola, green tea, hawthorn, hops, horse chestnut, horsetail, hyssop. jaborandi, kudzu, licorice, motherwort. muira puama. olive leaf. parsley, passionflower, pau d'arco. peppermint. primrose. rosemary. skullcap, suma, uva ursi. valerian. white oak. wintergreen, wood betony.

Gastrointestinal/digestive systems — Acerola. alfalfa. aloe, anise. annatto. bilberry. black walnut. blessed thistle, boldo, boswellia, buchu, burdock, cascara sagrada, catnip. cayenne. chamomile, chanca piedra. chuchuhuasi. cinnamon, clove, dandelion, devil's claw, fennel. fenu-

greek. flax, garlic, gentian. ginger, ginseng. goldenseal, gotu kola, green tea, guarana, horsetail, horehound. jaborandi, juniper. kava kava. kudzu, lady's mantle, lemongrass, licorice, macela, marshmallow, meadowsweet, muira puama, mustard. olive leaf, Oregon grape. papaya. parsley, pau d'arco, peppermint, plantain. puncture vine, red clover, red raspberry, rosemary, sage, slippery elm, stone root, suma. thyme, turmeric, uva ursi, valerian, vervain, white oak, wild cherry. wild oregano, wood betony. wormwood, yellow dock, yerba mate.

Hair/nails/teeth — Borage, burdock clove, hops, horsetail, Irish moss. lemongrass, muira puama, nettle. red raspberry, sage, tea tree. vervain, white willow. wintergreen.

Immune system — Ashwagandha. astragalus. bayberry. burdock. cat's claw. cedar, chuchuhuasi, devil's claw. echinacea, eyebright, elder, garlic, ginseng. goldenseal, green tea. horehound, licorice, maca, macela, milk thistle. myrrh, pau d'arco, puncture vine. red clover, suma, white willow, wild oregano, yerba mate.

Muscles — Blue cohosh. celery, chanca piedra, chuchuhuasi. eucalyptus. feverfew. ginger, hawthorn. horse chestnut, horsetail, kava kava. lady's mantle, licorice. macela, meadowsweet, puncture vine, skullcap, uva ursi, valerian, wild oregano. wild yam. wintergreen, wood betony.

Reproductive system — Menopause: Chaste tree. dandelion. devil's claw, kava kava, licorice, motherwort, puncture vine, sage. suma, wild yam. Menstruation: Black cohosh, blue cohosh. calendula. chamomile, chaste tree. chuchuhuasi, corn silk, crampbark. dong quai, false unicorn root, feverfew, licorice, maca. macela, motherwort, muira puama. primrose, red raspberry, rosemary. sarsaparilla. squawvine. valerian, white willow, wild oregano, wild yam. Prostate: Buchu, goldenseal, gravel root, horsetail, hydrangea. juniper. licorice. milk thistle, parsley, pumpkin. pygeum, saw palmetto, uva ursi. Sexual function/hormones: Alfalfa. ashwagandha. chaste tree, chuchuhuasi, damiana, dong quai. false unicorn root, gotu kola. muira puama. puncture vine. sarsaparilla. saw palmetto.

Respiratory tract — Anise, astragalus, boneset, boswellia. catnip, cayenne, chanca piedra, chuchuhuasi, chickweed. elder, eucalyptus; fennel, fenugreek. feverfew, garlic, ginkgo, ginseng, goldenseal. green tea, horehound, horsetail, Irish moss, jaborandi, jatoba. juniper. licorice. macela, muira puama, mullein. mustard, myrrh. nettle. parsley, plantain, pleurisy root, red clover, stone root, thyme, white oak, wild cherry, wild oregano. yellow dock.

Skin — Acerola, alfalfa, aloe, annatto, barberry, borage, boswellia, calendula, chaparral, chickweed, chuchuhuasi, comfrey, cranberry. elder. flax. green tea, horsetail. Irish moss, lavender, lemongrass, marshmallow, milk thistle, myrrh, oat straw, olive leaf, Oregon grape, primrose, red clover. red raspberry, sangre de grado, sarsaparilla. tea tree, white oak, wild oregano, witch hazel, wormwood, yellow dock.

Urinary tract — Annatto, bilberry. birch, buchu. butcher's broom, cayenne. cedar. celery. chanca piedra, corn silk, cranberry. dandelion. devil's claw, fennel.

ginkgo, goldenseal, gotu kola. gravel root. guarana, hydrangea. jatoba, juniper. kava kava. marshmallow, milk thistle. mullein. nettle. parsley, plantain, puncture vine, pumpkin, rose, red clover, saw palmetto, slippery elm, stone root, uva ursi, wild oregano, wild yam.

12 - THE 50 HERBS WHICH YOU WILL USE THE MOST

One of the biggest problems which people have when they want to use herbs—is where to start! There are so many of them. Which are the most important for my small cupboard space? Here is a list of the herbs you will use the most. You will find every one explained in detail in the next section on the 126 most important herbs.

The five most valuable herbs:
Cayenne, charcoal, garlic, goldenseal, peppermint.
The next five most valuable herbs:
Echinacea, cascara sagrada, catnip, corn silk, hops.
The next five most valuable herbs:
Comfrey, flaxseed, ginger, slippery elm, witch hazel.
The next five most valuable herbs:
Lobelia, myrrh, skullcap, vervain, red clover.
The next ten most valuable herbs:
Chamomile, chickweed, dong quai, eyebright, licorice root, red raspberry, squaw vine, valerian, wild cherry bark, wild yam.
The next twenty most valuable herbs:
Barberry, black cohosh, burdock root, chaparral, cramp bark, cloves, dandelion, fenugreek, mullein, oats, parsley, plantain, pleurisy root, psyllium, sage, sassafras, white oak bark, wormwood, yarrow, yellow dock.

13 - THE 126 MOST IMPORTANT HERBS - PLUS 303 COLOR PICTURES

Here you will find basic information you need to know about the most important medicinal herbs, plus charcoal:

• *Which herbs are the most valuable* • The common name of each plant • *Its scientific name* • The portions of the herb which are used for therapeutic purposes • *The special properties of each herb* • The parts of the body which are affected by the herb • *The several ways to prepare the herb for use* • The amount to take and frequency • *The purposes for which the herb is primarily used* • Additional information about the herb • *Warnings and cautions about the use of the herb.*

This wide-ranging collection of data (especially the medicinal uses), on more than a hundred of the most important herbs, exceeds that which you can find in most other books on herbs. Yet, in the Natural Remedies

Encyclopedia, it is only part of an even larger collection of home remedy information.

AGRIMONY

(Agrimonia eupatoria) Part used: Herb. *Properties:* Hepatic, stomachic, astringent, diuretic, tonic. *What it affects:* Stomach, liver and intestines.

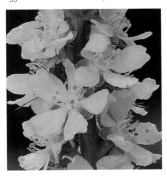 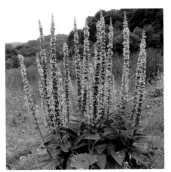

Agrimony Flowers   Agrimony Plant

Preparation and amount: *Decoction:* 1 oz. to 1¼ pints of water. Simmer down to 1 pint. Take 3-5 Tbsp. 3-4 times daily. *Tincture:* Take 30-60 drops 3-4 times daily. *Fluid extract:* Take ¼-1 tsp. 3-4 times daily. *Powder:* Take 5-10 #0 capsules (30-60 grains) 3 times daily.

Purposes: *Internally,* American Indians used agrimony as a tonic to strengthen the whole system. It is specifically used for all digestive disorders and for strengthening the stomach, intestines, liver, gallbladder, and kidneys. A strong decoction of root and leaves is used to treat pimples, skin blotches, and ulcers. An infusion of the leaves can treat jaundice and other liver problems. It is used for inflammatory diseases. When combined with a demulcent (mullein or slippery elm), a douche made from the leaves can be effectively used for excess vaginal secretions.

Externally, a fomentation containing agrimony is applied to athlete's foot, sores, wounds, insect bites, and skin eruptions. It can also be taken internally for bites and stings. A tincture applied to the skin will draw out thorns and splinters.

Note: Gentian root *(Gentiana)* works like agrimony as a bitter tonic, to stimulate the digestive organs. For this purpose, both herbs are prepared as a tea, using one ounce to a pint of water. Agrimony is quite bitter and contains about 5% tannins, which adds to its astringency.

Overseas: The European species *(Small-Flowered Agrimony, Agrimonia eupatoria)* is used to **stop bleeding** and used for **wounds, diarrhea, inflammation of gallbladder, urinary incontinence, jaundice, and gout**. Gargled for **mouth ulcers, throat inflammation**. In France, it is **drunk as much for its flavor** as for its medicinal values. Throughout Europe, the tea is used for **diarrhea, blood disorders, fevers, gout, hepatitis, pimples, sore throats, and even worms**. In Germany, it and a related species *(A. pilosa)* is approved for use in the treatment of **mild diarrhea** and **inflammation of the throat and mouth**; used externally for **mild skin inflammations**. In studies with mice, the European species *(A. pilosa)* have shown

antitumor activity. In Germany it is approved by the government for use in the treatment of **mild diarrhea and inflammations of the throat and mouth**; used externally for **mild skin inflammations**.

Warning: It should not be used when there is a dryness of the body secretions.

ALFALFA

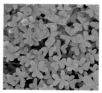 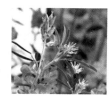 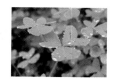

Alfalfa   Alfalfa   Alfalfa

(Medicago sativa) Part used: Tops. *Properties:* Alterative, nutritive, antipyretic. *What it affects:* Stomach and blood.

Preparation and amount: *Infusion:* Steep 5-15 min. Take 6 oz. 3 times daily. *Tincture:* Take 5-15 drops 3 times daily. *Fluid extract:* Take ½ to 1 tsp. 3 times daily. *Powder:* Take 5-10 #0 capsules (30-60 grains) 3 times daily.

Purposes: *Internally,* alfalfa must be used in fresh, raw form in order to provide essential nutrients—which alfalfa is full of. Every vitamin and major mineral is in alfalfa, with the exception of vitamin D. Alfalfa aids in the assimilation of protein, fats, and carbohydrates and is an excellent blood purifier. It can be added to soups and salads. Eight alfalfa tablets, taken at mealtime (preferably chewed before swallowing) provide a fiber bulk which greatly aids in maintaining bowel regularity.

Alfalfa sprouts are a great favorite with many people; but rinse them thoroughly before serving, to remove mold and bacteria. Because it has similar properties, alfalfa has been substituted for red clover blossoms. It is good for lowering fevers. Alfalfa detoxifies the body and alkalinizes it, lowers cholesterol, balances both blood sugar and hormones, and promotes pituitary function. It acts as a diuretic, attacks fungi, reduces inflammations and helps reduce various types of bleeding.

Alfalfa is good for ulcers, disorders of the skin, digestive system, bones, and joints. In addition to reducing cholesterol and balancing hormones and blood sugar, it is good for arthritis and other disorders of the bones and joints. Taken every day, it improves the appetite, relieves urinary and bowel problems, eliminates retained water, and even helps cure peptic ulcers.

It was named *al-falfa,* "father of plants," by the Arabs. They were among the first to recognize its marvelous properties. Alfalfa is commonly added to other herbs for its nutritive qualities. It may be added as 10%-20% of the formula.

ALOE VERA

(Aloe vera, var. officinalis) Part used: Gel from the leaves. *Properties:* Demulcent, emollient, laxative, vulnerary, emmenagogue. *What it affects:* Skin, colon, and stomach.

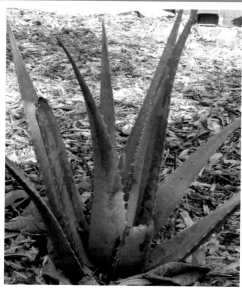

Aloe Vera

Preparation and amount: *Gel:* Take 2 oz. each time, up to 1 pint daily. *Tincture:* Take 10-40 drops 3 times daily. *Fluid extract:* Take ½-1 tsp. 3 times daily.

Purposes: The gel from the leaves of this desert plant is invaluable. It is best used freshly picked from a plant. Keep several plants growing; you cannot have enough! Because of its nauseating taste, when used as a purgative it is generally taken in powder or pill form. It also tends to gripe and cause a constipative reaction, so that it should be combined with a *carminative* herb (such as peppermint) for best results.

Externally, the fresh leaves of the aloe can be split, to expose the gelatinous juice and then rubbed onto the skin. The gel inside the leaves has the capacity to heal even the most severe burns (including sunburns) and irritated skin rashes. It can be used for insect bites and stings, poison oak and ivy, "detergent hands," acne and itchy skin. It is used for abscesses, infection in wounds, skin irritations, and ulcers. It is said to help heal wounds by preventing or drawing out infection. As a first-aid remedy for burns and surface irritations, break off a leaf and squeeze the gel onto the affected area. When applied to the skin for severe burns and skin rashes, it can be left on for two days without changing the application. A tea made from the dried juice makes a good wash for wounds and for the eyes.

Internally, the aloe is good for chronic constipation, gastritis, hyperacidity, and stomach ulcers. It is a laxative and regulator of the bowels. Because, when used alone, it might cause griping (bowel cramping), it is best combined with ginger root. Combine 4 parts aloe powder and 1 part ginger root powder and fill "00" gelatin capsules. Take 2 capsules, 3 times a day. Taken internally, it increases blood-vessel generation in the lower extremities of those with poor circulation. In the 1950s, it was discovered to be invaluable in reducing radioactivity. It is also helpful for eliminating AIDS.

Another way to treat gastro-intestinal ulcers is to take the bitter aloe gel in small quantities at regular intervals (totaling a pint a day for ulcers), along with a tea of ginger and licorice root, to help prevent any adverse reactions to the bitter taste.

Aloe plants are readily obtained and grow well in the home. You only need to water them once a week. Place them in a south window. There are several other aloe plants, but aloe vera is the best for medicinal purposes.

Warning: Do not use it during pregnancy, nor in large doses when there are hemorrhoids. Some people are allergic to aloe. First apply a small amount behind the ear or under the arm. If stinging or rash occurs, do not use it.

ANGELICA

(Angelica archangelica) Parts used: Root and leaf. *Properties:* Carminative, diaphoretic, emmenagogue, stimulant, alterative, expectorant, tonic. *What it affects:* Circulation, heart, stomach, intestines, and lungs.

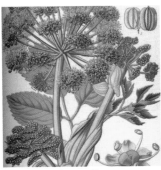
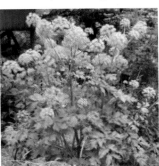

Angelica   Angelica

Preparation and amount: *Infusion (leaf):* Steep herb 15 min. Drink 1-2 oz. 3 times daily. *Decoction (root):* Simmer 10-15 min. Drink 1-2 oz. 3 times daily. *Tincture:* Take 5-15 drops 3 times daily. *Fluid extract:* Take ½-1 tsp. 3 times daily. *Powder:* Take 3-5 #0 (15-30 grains) 3 times daily.

Purposes: *Internally,* angelica tea improves circulation and warms the body. It is one of the best herbs to use for coldness in the winter. Its regular use will create a distaste for alcoholic drinks.

Angelica tea stimulates **appetite**, relieves **flatulence, heartburn,** and **muscle spasms** (including spasms of the stomach and bowels), and stimulates **kidney action**. It is useful for all sorts of **stomach** and **intestinal** difficulties, including **ulcers, vomiting,** and **stomach cramps**. It can also be used for **intermittent fever, nervous headache, colic,** and **general weakness**. It is a good herb to add to treatments for **lung diseases, coughs, colds, fevers, pleurisy,** and **all lung diseases**.

Externally, angelica tea is useful in the treatment of **rheumatism**, with a pint of boiled water poured over an oz. of the bruised root. The usual dose is 2-3 Tbsp. 3 times daily.

Note: Gather the rootstock and roots in the second year.

Warning: Used in large doses, angelica has a negative effect on blood pressure, heart action, and respiration. It is a strong emmenagogue and should not be taken by pregnant women. Diabetics should avoid using angelica, as it tends to increase the sugar in the blood. Be cautious when harvesting the plant in the wild, because it can be confused with European water hemlock, which is a deadly poison. There is a second herb, called "angelica" *(Angelica sylvestris);* but it is a different herb, with different properties, and used far less by herbalists.

ASTRAGALUS

(Huang Chi)—Part used: Root. *Properties:* Stimulant, diuretic, tonic. *What it affects:* Spleen, kidneys, lungs, and blood.

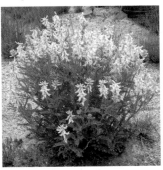
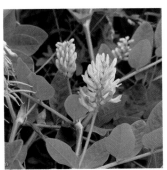

Astragalus   Astragalus

Preparation and amount: Take 4 to 18 grams, several times a day.

Purposes: *Internally,* astragalus helps neutralize **fevers** and improves **digestion**. It is one of the most valuable tonics, especially used for those under 35 years of age. It is a specific for all **wasting and exhausting diseases** because it strengthens the body's resistance. It aids **adrenal gland function** and **digestion**. It increases **metabolism**, produces **spontaneous sweating**, promotes **healing**, and provides energy to combat **fatigue** and **prolonged stress**. It helps protect the **immune system** and increases **stamina**. It is good for **colds, flu,** and **immune-deficiency-related problems**, including AIDS, **cancer,** and **tumors**. Those with **chronic lung weakness** are helped by it.

Warning: Do not use it if a fever is present.

BARBERRY

(Berberis vulgaris) Parts used: Root bark. *Properties:* Antiseptic, hepatic, stomachic, alterative, aromatic, tonic. *What it affects:* Liver, spleen, digestive tract, blood.

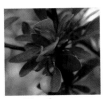
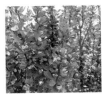
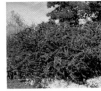

Barberry   Barberry   Barberry

Preparation and amount: *Infusion:* ½ oz. to 1 pint water. Steep 10 min. Take 1-4 cups daily before meals. *Decoction (root bark):* Simmer 10 min. Take 1 Tbsp. as needed. *Tincture:* Take ½-1 tsp. as needed. *Fluid extract:* Take ½-1 tsp. as needed. *Powder:* Take 2-5 #0 capsules (15-30 grains) 3 times daily.

Purposes: *Internally:* The bark of barberry root contains an alkaloid which promotes the secretion of bile.

HERBS

This makes it outstanding for various **liver** complaints. Barberry is primarily used for all sluggish liver conditions; and, because of its bitterness, it is best taken in small quantities. An infusion is very helpful for swollen **spleen** and chronic **stomach** problems when taken in tablespoon amounts several times a day, especially before meals. Barberry **dilates the blood vessels**, thereby lowering **blood pressure**. It decreases the **heart rate**, reduces **bronchial** constriction, and slows breathing. It destroys **bacteria on the skin** and stimulates **intestinal movements**. A teaspoon of the root will **purge the bowels**. Combined with cayenne, goldenseal, and lobelia, it is a specific for **jaundice** and **hepatitis**.

Externally, a decoction of either berries or the bark makes a good **mouthwash** or **gargle** for **mouth and throat irritations**. The fresh juice of the fruit will strengthen the **gums** and relieve **pyorrhea**, when brushed on or applied directly to the gums.

Warning: It should not be taken during pregnancy.

BAYBERRY

(Myrica cerifera) Part used: Root. *Properties:* Astringent, emetic, stimulant. *What it affects:* Circulation, stomach, and intestines.

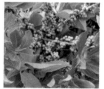 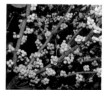 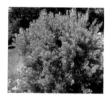

Bayberry   Bayberry   Bayberry

Preparation and amount: *Decoction (root):* Simmer 10-15 min. Take 1 Tbsp. as needed. *Tincture:* Take 15-30 drops as needed. *Fluid extract:* Take ½-1 tsp. as needed. *Powder:* Take 4-10 #0 capsules (25-60 grains) per day.

Purposes: *Internally,* bayberry is useful wherever an **astringent** is required. White oak bark may be substituted, but it does not have the stimulating qualities of the bayberry bark. Bayberry is a stimulating astringent that **raises the vitality of the system**. This valuable herb can be made into a tea using one teaspoon to a cup of hot water. Taken as a warm infusion, bayberry will **induce perspiration, improve circulation, and tone all the tissues** it contacts. In large doses, it acts as an **emetic**. It may be used as a **gargle** for **sore throat**. A fomentation made from this tea can be applied externally at night to relieve, cure, and prevent **varicose veins**. Small amounts are used to aid **digestion** and treat **chronic gastritis, enteritis, diarrhea, leukorrhea,** and **dysentery**. It will reduce **fevers**; and it is good for **circulatory disorders** and **ulcers**. It is also good for the **eyes** and the **immune system**.

Bayberry can be used with all **mucous membrane conditions** and can be substituted for myrrh. It is used to treat **prolapsed uterus**; excessive **menstrual bleeding**; and may be used in a douche, to treat **vaginal discharge**. It will stop **hemorrhage of the bowels, lungs, and uterus**. The powder may be taken in gelatin capsules, two at a time as needed. Direct application of the powder to the gums is good for managing **pyorrhea**.

Externally, bayberry is good for **canker sores, sore throat, varicose veins,** and **leukorrhea**.

Warning: Bayberry should not be used in large quantities or for prolonged periods. It may temporarily irritate sensitive stomachs. Do not confuse bayberry bark with barberry bark; they are very different herbs.

BISTORT

(Polygonum bistorta) Part used: Root. *Properties:* Astringent, styptic, antiseptic. *What it affects:* Bowels, lungs, and stomach.

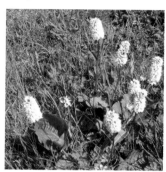 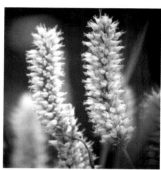

Bistort   Bistort

Preparation and amount: *Decoction:* Simmer 5-15 min. Take 1 Tbsp. several times daily. *Tincture:* Take 5-15 drops several times daily. *Fluid extract:* Take ½-1 tsp. several times daily. *Powder:* Take 1-5 #0 capsules (5-30 grains) several times daily.

Purposes: *Internally,* bistort is a powerful astringent. A teaspoon of the powdered root in a cup of boiling water, steeped for 10 minutes and drinking freely several times a day, is a successful treatment for **diarrhea, dysentery, and hemorrhages** from the lungs and stomach, even **bloody diarrhea**. It can be used as a wash for **internal sores and hemorrhage**. A douche can be used for **leukorrhea**.

Externally, bistort is good for **sprains, tonsillitis, wounds,** and **hemorrhoids**. The decoction can be used as a mouthwash for **gum problems** and for **inflammations of the mouth** (stomatitis). It can be used as a **gargle** for **throat infections**. When directly applied to a wound, the powder will stop the **bleeding**.

BLACKBERRY

(Rubus villosus) Parts used: Leaves, root, bark. *Properties:* Astringent, hemostatic, styptic, diuretic, tonic. *What it affects:* Stomach and intestines.

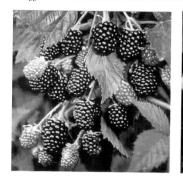 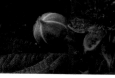

Blackberry   Blackberry

Preparation and amount: *Decoction (root, bark):* Simmer 5-15 min. Take 4 oz. 3-4 times daily. *Tincture:* Take ½-1 tsp. 3-4 times daily. *Fluid extract:* Take ½-1 tsp. 3-4 times daily. *Powder:* Take 2-5 #0 capsules (15-30 grains) 3-4 times daily.

Purposes: *Internally,* blackberry leaves and roots are a long-standing remedy for **watery diarrhea,** especially in children. Prolonged use of the tea is beneficial for **enteritis, chronic appendicitis,** and **leukorrhea.** It has **expectorant** properties as well. The leaves made into an infusion are helpful for milder cases of **diarrhea** and for **sore throats.** Both root and leaves are good for poor **digestion,** when caused by deficient **glandular secretions of the stomach and intestines.** Made into a syrup, it is useful for children with **weak stomachs,** no **appetite,** and **skin pallor.**

BLACK COHOSH

(Cimicufuga racemosa) Part used: Rhizome. *Properties:* Antispasmodic, emmenagogue, alterative, diuretic. *What it affects:* Uterus, nerves, lungs, and heart.

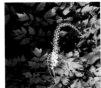
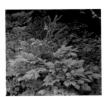

Black Cohosh   Black Cohosh   Black Cohosh

Preparation and amount: *Infusion:* Take 1 tsp. every 30 min., up to 3 Tbsp. every 3 hours, according to need. *Decoction (root):* Simmer 5-15 min. Take 1-2 oz. 3-4 times daily. *Tincture:* Take ½-1 tsp. 3 times daily. *Fluid extract:* Take 5-30 drops 3 times daily. *Syrup:* Take ½-1 Tbsp. 3-4 times daily. *Powder:* Take 1-5 #0 capsules (5-30 grains) 3 times daily.

Purposes: *Internally,* black cohosh is a helpful antispasmodic for all **nervous conditions, fits, convulsions, spasmodic afflictions, cramps,** and **pains.** American Indians used it for all **pelvic conditions, uterine troubles,** to relieve the **pains of childbirth** and the **menstrual cycle,** including **back pain.** It will help to bring about **menstrual flow** that has been retarded by exposure to cold. It lowers **blood pressure** and **cholesterol** levels. It induces **labor** and aids in **childbirth.** Many herbalists recommend taking it 2 weeks before childbirth. It is good for **morning sickness and pain.**

Black cohosh **reduces mucous** production. It is a potent remedy for **hysteria** and **spasmodic problems** such as **whooping cough, consumption,** and **chorea** (St. Vitus' Dance). Both the infusion and decoction have been used for **rheumatism** and **chronic bronchitis,** as well as **neuralgia** and **bronchial spasms.** It has a **sedative effect on the nervous system,** but it also acts as a **cardiac stimulant.** Small doses are helpful for **diarrhea** in children. It has been used for **dropsy, spinal meningitis,** and as an **emetic.** It even helps in case of poisonous **snakebites.** It can be used for **eruptive diseases,** such as **measles**; and, by **equalizing the circulation,** it is an excellent remedy for **high blood pressure.** Combined in a tincture or in capsules with equal parts of elecampane and wild cherry

bark and taken with a tea of yerba santa, it is an excellent remedy for **whooping cough, respiratory spasms, asthma,** and **bronchitis.**

Note: Black cohosh is often combined with blue cohosh, since they complement one another.

Warning: Large doses can cause nausea and dizziness. Some herbalists say not to use either blue cohosh or black cohosh in teas, because some of the active principles are not soluble in water.

BLACK HAW

(Viburnum prunifolium) Part used: Bark of the root. *Properties:* Antispasmodic, emmenagogue, sedative, tonic. *What it affects:* Uterus, nerves, stomach, and intestines.

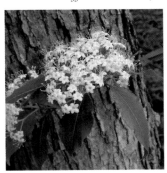
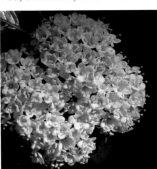

Black Haw   Black Haw

Preparation and amount: *Infusion:* Steep 30 min. Take 3 oz. 3-4 times daily. *Decoction:* Take 1 oz. herb to 1 quart water. Simmer 30 min. Take 1 Tbsp. 3-4 times daily or as needed. *Tincture:* Take ½-1 tsp. 3-4 times daily. *Fluid extract:* Take ½-2 tsp. 3-4 times daily. *Powder:* Take 5-10 #0 capsules (30-60 grains) 3-4 times daily.

Purposes: *Internally,* black haw is another very helpful herb for **female problems.** It acts as a tonic and sedative to **female reproductive organs.** It eases **cramps and contractions in the pelvic organs.** It is excellent for **painful menstruation,** whether due to nerve debility or congested tissue. It is extremely helpful for **scanty menstrual flow** accompanied by a severe bearing-down feeling with intermittent pain. It is valuable in **chronic uterine inflammation, congested uterus,** and **leukorrhea.** Lastly, unlike some other "female herbs," black haw **can be used during pregnancy,** and gives a **tonic effect.**

BLACK WALNUT

(Juglans nigra) Parts used: Leaves and bark. *Properties:* Antiseptic, astringent, vermicide, alterative. *What it affects:* Blood, intestines, and nerves.

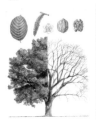
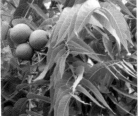
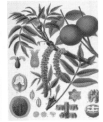

Black Walnut   Black Walnut   Black Walnut

Preparation and amount: *Infusion (leaves):* Take 6 oz. 1-4 times daily. *Decoction (inner bark):* Simmer 10-15 min. Take 1 Tbsp. 3-4 times daily. *Tincture:* Take 10-20 drops 3 times daily. *Fluid extract:* Take 1-2 tsp. 3-4 times daily. *Syrup:* Take 1 Tbsp. 1-2 times daily. *Powder:* Take 5-10 #0 capsules (30-60 grains) 3 times daily.

Purposes: Black walnut is rich in organic iodine and tannins which provide **antiseptic** qualities. *Internally,* It helps heal **mouth and throat sores**, aids **digestion** and acts as a **laxative**. It cleanses the body of some types of **parasites**. As an infusion, it is good for all **toxic blood conditions**. It may help **lower blood pressure and cholesterol** levels. Use the infusion as an injection for **vaginitis, bleeding, piles, intestinal worms, dysentery, prolapsed intestines,** and **prolapsed uterus**.

Externally, black walnut is good for **bruising, fungal infection, herpes, poison ivy, warts, ringworm,** and **scabies**. The tincture can be used to paint **sores and pimples**. Apply tincture or powdered leaves to **bleeding** surfaces or **moist skin diseases**.

WARNING: Fruit husks and leaves can cause contact dermatitis.

BLESSED THISTLE

(Cerbenia benedicta) Part used: Tops. *Properties:* Emmenagogue, galactagogue, stomachic, tonic, alterative. *What it affects:* Stomach, heart, blood, mammary glands, and uterus.

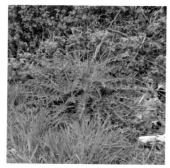
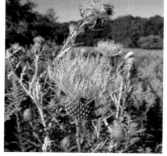

Blessed Thistle   Blessed Thistle

Preparation and amount: *Infusion:* Steep 5-15 min. Take 3 oz. as needed. *Tincture:* Take 5-20 drops as needed. *Fluid Extract:* Take ½-1 tsp. as needed. *Powder:* Take 5-10 #0 capsules (30-60 grains) as needed.

Purposes: *Internally,* blessed thistle is an excellent **stimulant tonic for the stomach,** by **increasing stomach secretions**. It is a tonic for the **heart**, for it strengthens it. It aids **circulation** and helps resolve all **liver** problems. It is useful for all **lung and kidney** problems also. It stimulates the **appetite**, acts as a **brain** food, and stimulates **memory**. It lessens **inflammation** and cleanses the blood. As a **blood purifier**, combine it with yellow dock and burdock root. It is good for **female disorders** and increases **milk flow** in nursing mothers. The warm tea, mixed with equal parts of raspberry leaves and marshmallow root, increases **mother's milk**.

Warning: If taken in excess, blessed thistle will act as an emetic. Do not use it during the first two trimesters of pregnancy. It should not be taken alone or in large amounts during the remainder of pregnancy.

Overseas: The whole plant is used as a weak tea (2 teaspoons to 1 cup of water) of dried flowering plant traditionally used in Europe to **stimulate sweating, appetite, milk production; diuretic**. Folk reputation as remedy for **boils, indigestion, colds, deafness, gout, headaches, migraines, suppressed menses, chilblains, jaundice, and ringworm**. Experimentally, it **increases gastric and bile secretions; antibacterial, anti-inflammatory**. Approved by the government in Germany for treatment of **loss of appetite and dyspeptic discomfort**. Seeds have served as emergency **oil seeds**.

BLUE COHOSH

(Caulophyllum thalictroides) Part used: Rhizome. *Properties:* Antispasmodic, emmenagogue, oxytocic, diuretic. *What it affects:* Uterus, nerves, joints, and urinary tract.

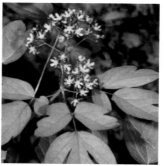
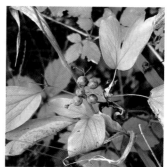

Blue Cohosh   Blue Cohosh

Preparation and amount: *Infusion:* Take 3 oz. 3-4 times daily. *Decoction:* Simmer 5-15 min. Take 1-2 oz. 3-4 times daily. *Tincture:* Take ½-1 tsp. 3-4 times daily. *Fluid extract:* Take 10-30 drops (1/6 to ½ tsp.) 3-4 times daily. *Powder:* Take 1-5 #0 capsules (5-30 grains) 3-4 times daily.

Purposes: *Internally,* blue cohosh is used to regulate **menstrual flow**, especially for suppressed menstruation. The Indians used it to **induce labor**, for **children's colic**, and for **cramps**. Indian women made sure they took it during the **last month of pregnancy**, to aid in a **speedy and painless delivery**.

Blue cohosh eases **muscle spasms** and stimulates **uterine contractions** for childbirth. It is useful for **nervous disorders** and **memory problems**. It is used as an antispasmodic in **cough medicines** and to treat **lung problems** and all **female spasms**.

Note: Blue cohosh is often combined with black cohosh because the herbs have complementary properties beneficial for the **nerves** and a strong **antispasmodic** effect on the entire system. It is also combined with other herbs, to promote their effects in treating **bronchitis, nervous disorders, urinary tract ailments,** and **rheumatism**.

Warning: Blue cohosh should always be given only in combination with other herbs indicated for the condition being treated. Blue cohosh can be very irritating to mucous surfaces and can cause dermatitis on contact. Children have been poisoned by the berries. It is best not to use either blue cohosh or black cohosh in teas, because some of the active principles are not soluble in water. Because of its emmenagogue properties, it is not to be used by pregnant women, except during the last month of pregnancy.

BONESET

(Eupatorium perfoliatum) Part used: Tops. *Properties:* Diaphoretic, stimulant, antipyretic, laxative. *What it affects:* Stomach, liver, intestines, and circulation.

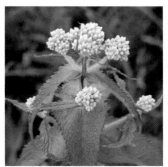
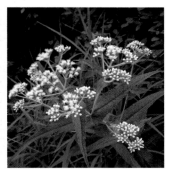

Boneset   Boneset

Preparation and amount: *Infusion:* Steep 5-15 min. Take 3 oz. 3 times daily. *Tincture:* Take 10-40 drops 3 times daily. *Fluid extract:* Take ½-1 tsp. 3 times daily. *Powder:* Take 4-10 #0 capsules (20-60 grains) 3 times daily

Purposes: *Internally,* boneset is a specific for treating **severe fevers**, especially **intermittent fevers**. Taken as a warm infusion (drink 4-5 cups while in bed, to encourage **sweating**), it is widely used for **flu, catarrh, and bronchitis**. It helps relieve **fever-induced aches and pains**. It is a decongestant, **loosening phlegm, reducing fever, increasing perspiration,** and **calming the body**. An American Indian in Colonial times became famous for curing **typhoid** with boneset. For decades thereafter, the plant was named after him: Joe Pye weed.

The tea is made using an ounce of herb to a pint of water, steeped 10 minutes. One-half cup is taken 3 times daily. When taken cold, it is a tonic stimulant and a mild laxative. Taken warm, it is diaphoretic and emetic; it can be used to break up a common cold, an intermittent fever, and the flu. The hot tea is both emetic and cathartic; and is used for sweating therapy, using 4-5 half-cup doses while in bed.

Warning: Long-term use can result in toxicity.

BUCHU

(Barosma betulina) Part used: Leaves. *Properties:* Antiseptic, diuretic, diaphoretic. *What it affects:* Kidneys and bladder.

Preparation and amount: *Infusion:* Steep 5-15 min. Take 3 oz. 3-4 times daily (do not boil leaves). *Tincture:* Take ½ tsp. 3 times daily. *Fluid extract:* Take ½-1 tsp. 3 times daily. *Powder:* Take 2-3 #0 capsules (10-15 grains) 3 times daily.

Purposes: *Internally,* buchu leaves are one of the best **diuretics** known. The herb is used for all **acute and chronic bladder and kidney disorders**, including **inflammation of the urethra, nephritis, cystitis,** and **catarrh of the bladder**. It is a specific for **bladder infection** and good for **urine retention**. It lessens **inflammation of the colon, gums, mucous membranes, prostate, sinuses, and vagina**. It is good for **diabetes** in the first stages, **digestive disorders, fluid retention,** and **prostate disorders**.

As with most diuretics, buchu works better if it is given as a cool infusion. Buchu is commonly combined with uva ursi for the treatment of **water retention** and **urinary tract infections**. Make an infusion, using one ounce of buchu leaves to a pint of water.

When given warm, buchu is used to treat **enlargement of the prostate gland, burning urine, and irritation of the membrane of the urethra**. It can be used in **fever** remedies. It is also used for **venereal disease**.

Some herbalists recommend it as an after-dinner beverage, to **replace coffee**: Buchu leaves (2 parts), uva ursi (2 parts), orange peel (1 part), peppermint (1 part), chamomile (1 part), comfrey leaves (1 part). Use ¼ oz. of the herb mixture in a pint of boiled water and steep 10 minutes. This will strengthen the **kidneys**.

Note: Do not boil buchu leaves or uva ursi, because their active principles are volatile oils.

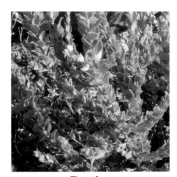
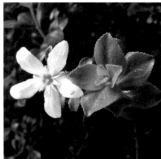

Buchu   Buchu

BUCKTHORN

(Rhamnus frangula) Part used: Bark. *Properties:* Hepatic, laxative, galactagogue, emollient. *What it affects:* Liver, gallbladder, intestines, and blood.

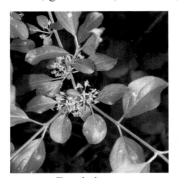
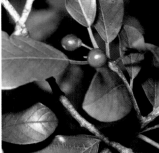

Buckthorn   Buckthorn

Preparation and amount: *Decoction:* 1 oz. bark to 1 quart water, boiled down to 1 pint. Take as needed. *Tinc-*

H
E
R
B
S

ture: Take 5-60 drops 3 times daily. *Fluid extract:* Take ½-2 tsp. 3 times daily. *Powder:* Take 4-10 #0 capsules (20-60 grains) 3 times daily.

Purposes: *Internally,* buckthorn is a **purgative** and works without irritating the system. It can be used for all conditions caused or associated with **constipation**, including **liver and gallbladder problems**. It produces no constipative backlash during purgation as some other remedies do; neither does it become less effective with repeated use. The decoction will produce **sweating**, when taken hot. Internally, it will keep the **bowels** regulated. It is helpful for **colic, obesity, dropsy, hemorrhoids, rheumatism, gout, and** all **skin diseases**.

Externally, use buckthorn as a fomentation for **dry or itchy skin problems**, and **skin diseases**. It is also used for **warts**.

Note: Do not confuse this buckthorn *(Rhamnus frangula)* with its relative, cascara sagrada *(Rhamnus purshiana),* called "California buckthorn," which is a different herb.

Warning: Fresh bark and unripe fruit can cause symptoms of poisoning. Storage for a year or heating to 212° F. will render the bark safe to use. Do not use during pregnancy.

BUGLEWEED

(Lycopus virginicus) Part used: Whole herb. *Properties:* Astringent, sedative, tonic. What it affects: Heart, lungs, and circulation.

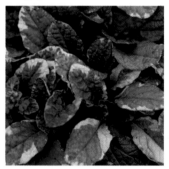 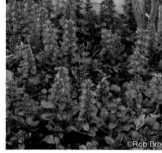

Bugleweed   Bugleweed

Preparation and amount: *Infusion:* Steep 5-15 min. Take 6 oz. frequently. *Tincture:* Take ½-1 tsp. frequently. *Fluid extract:* Take ¼-1 tsp. frequently. *Powder:* Take 5-10 #0 capsules (30-60 grains) frequently.

Purposes: *Internally,* bugleweed is especially good for **hemorrhages from the lungs and bowels**. It is excellent for **heart diseases** marked by **irregular heartbeat** (whether functional or organic). Because it acts like digitalis in quieting the pulse, it is useful for **pericarditis** and **endocarditis**. Bugleweed is also good for **chronic inflammation of the lungs**, all **chest congestive diseases**, and **coughs**. In addition, it is used for conditions in which the blood flow needs to be reduced, such as reducing **hemorrhoids**, stopping **intestinal bleeding, nosebleeds, excessive menstruation,** or **blood in the urine**. When treating these conditions, it is best to add demulcent herbs (slippery elm) to the mixture.

BURDOCK

(Arctium lappa) Parts used: Root (especially), seeds, and leaves. *Properties: Root:* Alterative, diaphoretic, diuretic, demulcent. *Seeds:* Alterative, diuretic. *Leaves:* Tonic.

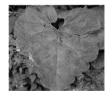 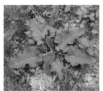 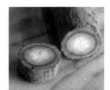

Burdock Root   Burdock Root   Burdock Root

Preparation and amount: *Infusion (leaves):* Take 1 cup 3-4 times daily. *Decoction (root or seeds):* 1 oz. root to 1½ pints water, boiled down to 1 pint. Take 3 oz. 3-4 times daily. *Tincture:* Take 30-60 drops 3-4 times daily. *Fluid extract:* Take ½-1 tsp. 3-4 times daily. *Powder (root or seed):* Take 10-20 #0 capsules (60-120 grains) daily. *Powder (leaves):* Take 5-10 #0 capsules (30-60 grains) 3 times daily.

Purposes: *Internally,* burdock is used to promote **kidney** function and works through the kidneys to help clear the blood of harmful acids. It is one of the best **blood purifiers for chronic infection, rheumatism, arthritis, skin diseases, and sciatica**.

Burdock is used for **skin** disorders, such as **carbuncles** and **boils**, and relieves **gout** and **menopausal problems**. It aids elimination of excess fluid, **uric acid**, and toxins; and it has **antibacterial and antifungal** properties. It acts as an **antioxidant** and may help protect against **cancer**, by helping control **cell mutation**.

The diaphoretic property of burdock is due to a volatile oil which, taken internally, is eliminated from the sweat glands, thus removing toxic waste. **Sweating** has a **cooling effect** on the body. So it is used to reduce **fevers** and **heat conditions such as boils, sties, carbuncles, canker sores, and infections**. For this purpose, use ½ cup of the decoction 3 times daily. An infusion of the leaves is used as a **stomach tonic** and for **indigestion**.

Burdock contains 27%-45% *inulin*, the source of most of its curative ability. Inulin is a form of starch. Burdock also has an abundance of iron, which makes it of special value for the blood. It is also a **blood purifier**. That is why it is so helpful in treating **arthritis, rheumatism, sciatica, and lumbago**. When the seeds are made into a tincture or extract, they are good for **skin and kidney diseases**. It is excellent for all skin diseases, taken alone or with other blood purifiers, such as sarsaparilla. Take it internally for **acne, boils, chicken pox, eczema, psoriasis**. Make a decoction of the root, using 1 oz. to 1½ pints of water, and simmer until the volume is reduced to 1 pint. Take ½ cup 3 times daily. For **sweating**, simmer in covered pan for 10 minutes; then drink 1 cup of the tea before taking a hot bath.

Externally, take it for **boils, eczema, itching, poison ivy,** and **poison oak**.

Warning: May interfere with iron absorption, when taken internally.

NATURAL REMEDIES ENCYCLOPEDIA
OVER 11,000 REMEDIES - OVER 730 DISEASES
THE 126 MOST IMPORTANT HERBS **HERBS** **149**

H
E
R
B
S

CALENDULA

(Calendula officinalis) Part used: Flower. *Properties:* Astringent, vulnerary, antispasmodic, diaphoretic. *What it affects:* Blood and skin.

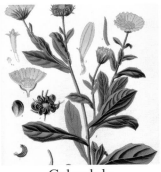
Calendula

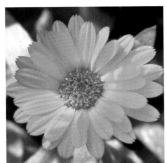
Calendula

Preparation and amount: *Infusion:* Steep 5-15 min. Take 1 Tbsp. each hour or 1 cup daily. *Fluid extract:* Take ½-1 tsp. 3 times daily. *Powder:* Take 3-10 #0 capsules (15-60 grains) 3 times daily.

Purposes: *Internally,* calendula can be used as a non-irritating **fomentation or salve for sores, burns, bleeding hemorrhoids, and wounds**. It reduces **inflammation** and is soothing to the **skin**. It is used internally as a warm infusion—to treat **fevers, ulcers, cramps,** and **eruptive skin diseases**. It has been successfully used as a **nasal wash** for **sinus problems**.

An infusion of the flowers (either the rays or the whole head) can be used for such **gastro-intestinal problems** as **ulcers, stomach cramps, colitis, and diarrhea**. As a warm infusion, it is useful internally for **fever, boils, abscesses,** and to prevent **recurrent vomiting**. The fresh juice of the herb or flowers can substitute for the infusion.

Calendula tincture helps **gastritis** and **menstrual difficulties, vaginal infections, ulcers,** and **cramps**. An infusion can be used in treating **smallpox** and **measles**.

The tea, made with 1 oz. of herb per pint of water, may be taken hourly for acute ailments. It is commonly used in making salves and is a very good first-aid remedy.

Internally, Calendula can be used with oil in a salve or poultice in order to **stop bleeding**, soothe pain and irritation, and promote mending and **healing of wounds**. A very good salve for wounds can be made from the dried flowers or leaves, from the juice pressed out of the fresh flowers, or from the tincture. The salve or diluted tincture is also good for **bruises, sprains, pulled muscles, sores, and boils**. To get rid of **warts**, rub on the fresh juice. The oil is put in ears and left overnight for **earaches**. A strong tea can be used as a sitz bath for **bleeding hemorrhoids**. A fomentation is good for varicose veins. It is also good for **bee stings** and **skin ulcers**. You can wash wounds with it.

CASCARA SAGRADA

(California Buckthorn)—*(Rhamnus purshiana) Part used:* Bark. *Properties:* Hepatic, laxative, antispasmodic. *What it affects:* Colon, stomach, liver, gallbladder, and pancreas.

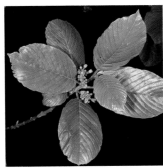
Cascara Sagrada

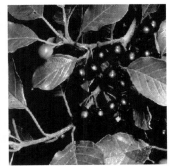
Cascara Sagrada

Preparation and amount: *Decoction (bark):* Simmer 5-15 min. Take 1 tsp. 3-4 times daily before meals or 1 cup during the day, cold. *Tincture:* Take 5-20 drops, morning and evening. *Fluid extract:* Take ½-1 tsp. at night before retiring. *Syrup:* Take ½-2 tsp. 2-3 times daily. *Powder:* Take 6-12 #0 capsules (10-100 grains) daily.

Purposes: *Internally,* cascara is one of the safest laxatives for **chronic constipation**. If used too much, it is habit forming. It is one of the best, commonest, and safest plant **laxatives**. It encourages peristalsis by irritating the bowels. The bitter principles in cascara stimulate the secretions of the entire digestive system—including the liver, gallbladder, stomach, and pancreas.

Cascara is excellent for i**ntestinal gas, liver, and gallbladder problems,** especially **enlarged liver**. It is also used for **gastric and intestinal disorders, indigestion, and jaundice.**

In order to use it for its gentle, laxative effect, cascara is best taken not as a tea, but as tincture or in capsules. This is because it is so bitter.

Note: The bark must be at least a year old before being used. Do not confuse cascara segrada *(Rhamnus purshiana),* sometimes called "buckthorn," with buckthorn *(Rhamnus frangula).* They are both good, but different herbs.

CATNIP

(Nepata cataria) Part used: Tops. *Properties:* Carminative, diaphoretic, sedative, nervine. *What it affects:* Nerves and intestines.

Catnip

Catnip

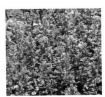
Catnip

Preparation and amount: *Infusion:* Steep 5-15 min. Take 1 oz. to 1 cup as needed (do not boil herb). *Tincture:* Take ½-1 tsp. as needed. *Fluid extract:* Take ¼-1 tsp. as needed. *Powder:* Take 5-10 #0 capsules (30-60 grains) 3 times daily.

Purposes: *Internally,* it is wonderful for **children and infants when gas, stomach cramps, or nervousness** occur. This is the children's herb, but it is also helpful to grown-ups. It is famous for its **gentle sedative effect** on the nervous system, reducing **nervous tension**.

Catnip is used for **mumps, painful swellings, chronic bronchitis, and diarrhea**. Use catnip as an enema, to **expel worms**. Drink the tea for headaches caused by indigestion. It is frequently used **in enemas, to relax** and gently restore the tone of the bowels. It is an excellent herb for children, especially when mixed in a tea with chamomile, spearmint, and lemon balm. It is also good for **insomnia**.

Catnip is also used for **colds, bronchitis, dizziness, fevers, gas, diarrhea, headaches, hysteria, insomnia, morning sickness, mumps, smallpox,** and **urine retention**. It quickly reduces **fevers** when a catnip tea enema is taken. It stimulates the **appetite**.

Externally, use catnip as a fomentation for mumps and painful swellings.

CAYENNE

(Capsicum anuum) Part used: Fruit. *Properties:* Carminative, stimulant, antispasmodic, astringent. *What it affects:* Heart, circulation, stomach, and kidneys.

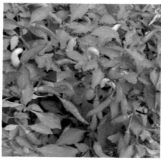 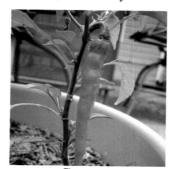

Cayenne   Cayenne

Preparation and amount: *Infusion:* 1 tsp. to 1 cup boiling water, taken in ½ fluid oz. doses. Pour water over cayenne. *Tincture:* Take 5-15 drops 3 times daily. *Fluid extract:* Take 10-15 drops 3 times daily. *Oil:* For **toothache**, clean the cavity and place cotton, saturated with the oil, into the cavity; use sparingly, as it is very potent. *Powder (internal):* Take 1-2 #0 capsules (1-10 grains) 3 times daily. *Powder (external):* For **external bleeding**, powder may be placed directly on the wound.

Purposes: Dr. Christopher, a well-known herbalist of the mid-twentieth century, said that if he only had two herbs, he would select charcoal and cayenne. Cayenne is powerful in its ability to **attract blood to a body part.** Since it is the blood which brings healing, this is an important quality.

Internally, When added to herbal formulas, cayenne **stimulates the action of other herbs**. It stops **heart attacks**; and is used for **flus, colds, indigestion, and lack of vitality**. It is good for treating the **spleen, pancreas, kidneys**; and it is effective as a fomentation for **rheumatism, inflammation, pleurisy, sores, and wounds.**

Cayenne is useful for **arteriosclerosis, arthritis, asthma, bleeding, high or low blood pressure, bronchitis, chills, colds, convulsions, coughs, indigestion, infections, jaundice, ulcers,** and **varicose veins**.

Externally, cayenne is used for **frostbite, painful joints, swellings,** and **varicose veins**. It can be rubbed on **toothaches** and **swellings**. Sprinkled on **bleeding cuts**, it

will immediately stop the bleeding.

Warning: Very excessive use can damage the kidneys and lead to pleurisy or gastro-enteritis. Prolonged application to the skin can cause dermatitis and raise blisters. When cooked, it becomes an irritant. It is best to use cayenne primarily as a medicine, and only very small amounts as a food additive. Apply it with a glove.

WILD CELERY

(Apium graveolens) Parts used: Root, seeds. *Properties:* Carminative, diuretic, nervine, stimulant, tonic. *What it affects:* Kidneys, bladder, and nerves.

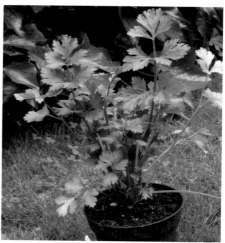

Wild Celery

Preparation and amount: *Decoction (root, seeds):* Simmer 5-15 min. Take 1 oz. 3 times daily. *Fluid extract:* Take 10-30 drops as needed. *Essential oil:* Take 1-2 drops 3 times daily. *Powder:* Take 4-10 #0 capsules 3 times daily.

Purposes: *Internally,* wild celery is good for **arthritis, gout,** and **kidney** problems. It acts as a diuretic, antioxidant, and sedative. It reduces **blood pressure**, relieves **muscle spasms**, and **improves appetite**. A decoction of celery seed is useful for **incontinence** of urine, **dropsy, rheumatism, neuralgia**, and to aid in ridding the body of **excess acid**. It can be used for **gout**, tendencies toward **overweight, flatulence, chronic pulmonary catarrh, and deficiency diseases**. The root can be eaten raw or made into broth, to treat the same problems. The whole plant can be used to treat **kidney** ailments and **rheumatism**. It also promotes the onset of **menstruation**. When eaten as a salad vegetable or made into a tea, it will help clear up skin problems.

Warning: During pregnancy, the seeds of wild celery should not be used, nor large amounts of the herb. It is a strong diuretic and should not be used when acute kidney problems exist (but moderate use is all right when kidney problems are not chronic).

CHAMOMILE

(Camomile)—*(Matricaria chamomilla) Part used:* Flowers. *Properties:* Emmenagogue, nervine, sedative, carminative, diaphoretic, tonic. *What it affects:* Nerves, stomach, kidneys, spleen, and liver.

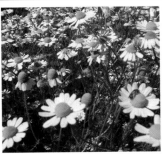

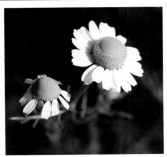

Chamomile   Chamomile

Preparation and amount: *Infusion:* Steep 10-30 min. (do not boil flowers). Take 6 oz. 2-3 times daily. *Tincture:* Take 30-60 drops 3 times daily. *Fluid extract:* Take ½-1 tsp. 3 times daily. *Powder:* Take 5-10 #0 capsules (30-60 grains) 3 times daily.

Purposes: *Internally,* chamomile is good for **insomnia** and **nervousness**. It **increases appetite** and helps those with **weak stomachs**. It reduces **inflammation**, and aids digestion and sleep. Six ounces of the infusion or 1-2 teaspoons of the tincture at a time is good for **menstrual cramps, kidney, spleen, or bladder problems**. It acts as a **diuretic** and **nerve** tonic, and is a useful remedy for **stress, anxiety, and indigestion**.

Chamomile can be safely used **for children with colds, indigestion, and nervous disorders**. It helps relieve **cramping** associated with the **menstrual cycle** and will bring on the period. It can also be used as a relaxing **antispasmodic, anodyne bath additive**. It is good for **dizziness, gas, hysteria, jaundice, kidney problems, measles,** and **swellings**. It is also good for **lumbago, rheumatic problems,** and **rashes**.

Externally, chamomile can be used as a **mouthwash** for **minor mouth and gum infections**. The tea is a good wash for **sore eyes and open sores**. Use it as a wash or compress for **skin** problems and **inflammations**, including inflammations of the **mucous tissues**. Keeping a mouthful in the mouth for a time will temporarily relieve **toothache**. Use it for a sitz (sitting) bath, to help **hemorrhoids**, or as a foot- or hand-bath for **sweaty feet or hands**. For **hemorrhoids and wounds**, the flowers are also made into a salve. To help **asthma** in children or to relieve the symptoms of a **cold**, try a vapor bath of the tea. A fomentation can be used for **cramps, gas, and swellings**.

Note: This is German chamomile *(Matricaria chamomilla)*. Do not confuse it with Roman chamomile *(Anthemis nobilis),* which is also a good but lesser-used herb; it is quite different in its properties and applications, yet sometimes it is also called chamomile.

Overseas: In Germany, its name means "capable of anything." Dried flowers make a famous **beverage tea**, used for **colic, diarrhea, insomnia, indigestion, gout, sciatica, headaches, colds, fevers, flu, cramps, and arthritis**. Its essential oil is antifungal, antibacterial, anodyne, antispasmodic, anti-inflammatory, and anti-allergenic. This oil contains two dozen different anti-inflammatory compounds which work together to **reduce fevers, inflammation**, etc. Heavily used to treat **inflammation or spasms of the gastrointestinal tract**

and **inflammation of the respiratory tract**. *Externally,* used for inflammatory cojnditions of the **mouth, gums, and bacterial-induced skin diseases**.

Warning: Chamomile should not be used daily for a lengthy period, for this could lead to constipation, or ragweed allergy. Those allergic to ragweed should use it with caution (same family). It should not be used with sedatives or alcohol.

CHAPARRAL

(Larrea divaricata) Part used: Leaves. *Properties:* Alterative, antibiotic, antiseptic, parasiticide. *What it affects:* Stomach, intestines, and blood.

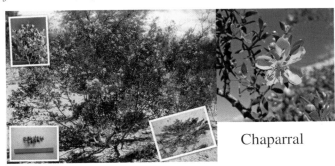

Chaparral

Preparation and amount: *Infusion:* Steep 5-15 min. Take 6 oz. 3 times daily. *Tincture:* Take 10-20 drops 3 times daily. *Powder:* Take 2-10 #0 capsules (10-60 grains) 3 times daily.

Purposes: *Internally,* chaparral is one of the best herbal antibiotics. It is useful against **bacteria, viruses, and parasites**, both internally and externally. It fights **free radicals** and **chelates heavy metals**. It has **anti-HIV** activity. It protects against harmful effects of **radiation**. It may be taken internally for **colds and flus, inflammations of the respiratory and intestinal tracts, diarrhea,** and **urinary tract infections**.

Chaparral protects against the formation of **tumors, cancer cells**, and **over-exposure to sunlight**. It contains a substance called NDGA (nordihydroguararaetic acid), which is a powerful antioxidant, useful in preserving fats and oils, and a powerful anti-tumor agent. American Indians used it to treat **cancer**. It **relieves pain** and is good for **skin disorders**. It is excellent as an addition to an herbal formula in the treatment of **kidney and bladder infections**.

Externally, chaparral is applied to **wounds** as an antiseptic. As a fomentation, it is applied to the skin for **skin diseases, psoriasis, herpes, scabies, eczema, arthritic pains, skin parasites**; it is to the scalp as a **hair tonic** and for **dandruff**. It makes a good hair rinse. A liniment made from chaparral or a bath made by soaking the leaves in the water is used for **rheumatism**.

Note: Chaparral is very bitter and is usually mixed with other herbs or taken in tincture form. Pau d'arco *(Tabebuia heptaphylla),* also called lapacho or taheebo, has similar antibiotic and anti-cancer properties, but is less harsh than chaparral.

H
E
R
B
S

CHARCOAL

(Carbon) **Preparation and amount:** *Powder:* Take ½-1½ tsp. in ½-1 cup water—swallowed, spread onto a poultice, or taken as a slurry (see below for details). *Tablets:* 4-8 chewed in mouth and then swallowed.

Although not an herb, yet charcoal is invaluable in a number of ways. It is pure carbon and **will adsorb (not absorb, but bind with) 29 of the 30 most dangerous poisons, thus neutralizing them.**

Purposes: Usually obtained from a hard wood, charcoal is produced by slow combustion in a relative absence of oxygen. If you do not have any available, in an emergency, you can burn a piece of hard wood and scrape or chip the charcoal from the charred wood. After moistening it with water, force it through a food grinder. Commercial sources are usually made from coconut shells. (Burnt toast or charcoal briquettes *are not* charcoal!) Treatment with superheated steam can produce "activated" charcoal, which is capable of much greater adsorptive effect. This is because more surfaces of the charcoal have been exposed. The surface area of charcoal is astounding, for it has millions of micropores with surface areas ranging from 400 to over 1,800 square meters per gram! There are 50 million charcoal particles in one pound.

Internally, charcoal cannot adsorb all poisons, but it can bind with, and thus neutralize many of them. Here are but a few of the many things it adsorbs: *Many industrial toxins, including:* **DDT, dieldrin, strychnine, malathion, and parathion.** *Many medicinal drugs, including:* **aspirin, barbiturates, cocaine, opium, nicotine, morphine, penicillin, and sulfas.** *Many inorganic chemicals, including:* **mercury, phosphorus, chlorine, iron, lead, and silver.**

In any type of **acute poisoning**, the best thing to do is to induce vomiting, followed with a large dose of activated charcoal, diluted in water, to render most substances harmless. Usually 30-60 grams (about ½ cup) is needed, suspended in water and taken as soon as possible after the injection of any toxin.

Charcoal can also be taken to stop **intestinal gas** (about a spoonful in half a glass of water, followed by another glass of water). It is also very good for **diarrhea.**

In cases of **colitis** or unusual chronic **inflammations of the bowel**, a charcoal slurry solution can be made by stirring powdered activated charcoal into water. Then use only the cloudy solution which results after the liquid has set for a couple hours. This "slurry enema" will reduce inflammation locally, giving considerable relief.

Externally, you can use it as a poultice on **wounds, skin infections,** and above inflamed body areas.

CHICKWEED

(Stellaria media) Part used: Tops. *Properties:* Antipyretic, demulcent; alterative. *What it affects:* Blood, liver, lungs, kidneys, and bladder.

Preparation and amount: *Infusion:* Steep 5-15 min. Take 6 oz. 3-4 times daily, between meals. *Decoction:* 1 oz. to 1½ pints boiling water, simmered down to 1 pint. Take 3 oz. 3-4 times for every 2-3 hours when needed. *Tincture:* Take ½ tsp. as needed. *Fluid extract:* Take ½-1

tsp. as needed. *Powder:* Take 5-10 #0 capsules (30-60 grains) 3 times daily.

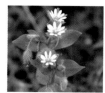 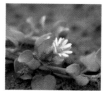 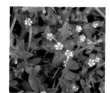

Chickweed   Chickweed   Chickweed

Purposes: *Internally,* this common weed is invaluable for treating **blood toxicity, fevers, inflammations,** and **other "hot" diseases.** Chickweed relieves **nasal congestion.** Useful for **bronchitis, pleurisy, circulatory problems, bowel inflammation, colds, coughs, skin diseases, and hoarseness.** This mild herb is as safe to take as any garden vegetable, and is full of vitamins and minerals. People often eat it as a salad green. Therefore it can be used in high dosages. Because it lowers blood lipids, it is particularly useful in **reducing excess fat** having both mild **diuretic and laxative** properties. Drink the tea, to build the blood.

Externally, chickweed can be applied as a poultice to **warts, boils, and abscesses.** Made into an oil and ointment, it is used for a wide variety of **sores** and other **skin diseases.** Add the tea to a bath, to soothe **rashes and skin irritations.** Make it into a salve for **dry, itchy skin.** It can also be used for **mouth sores.**

Europeans use as a cooling demulcent and expectorant to relieve coughs; also externally for skin diseases and reduce itching.

CLEAVERS

(Galium aparine) Part used: Tops. *Properties:* Alterative, astringent, diuretic, antipyretic, laxative. *What it affects:* Kidneys, bladder, blood, and skin.

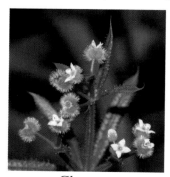 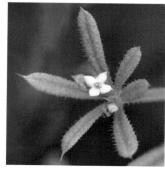

Cleavers   Cleavers

Preparation and amount: *Infusion:* Let 3 oz. to 2 pints cold water stand 3-4 hours. Take 3 oz. (cold) 3-4 times daily or 1½ oz. to 1 pint of warm water. Steep 2 hours. Take 1 cup 3-4 times daily. *Tincture:* Take ½-1 tsp. 3-4 times daily. *Fluid extract:* Take ½-1 tsp. 3-4 times daily. *Powder:* Take 5-10 #0 capsules (30-60 grains) 3-4 times daily.

Purposes: *Internally,* cleavers is excellent for breaking up fevers. Highly recommended for **kidney** problems, including **suppressed urine, inflammations of the kidneys and bladder, obstructions of the urinary tract (stones and gravel), and scalding urine during gonorrhea**. It is a powerful diuretic and will rid the body of excess fluid. It will **clean the blood** and strengthen the **liver**. Combine it with equal parts uva ursi, buchu, and one-quarter part marshmallow root for **urinary** problems. Because it is a powerful diuretic, it is useful in **reducing weight** and **treating edema**. It is also good, taken internally, for **skin diseases and eruptions**. Its cooling properties make it a good treatment for **fevers**.

Externally, cleavers is used in a salve for **scalds, burns, and external tumors**.

CLOVES

(Caryophyllus aromaticus) Part used: Fruit. *Properties:* Antiseptic, aromatic, carminative, stimulant, anodyne, antiemetic. *What it affects:* Mouth, stomach, intestines, circulation, and lungs.

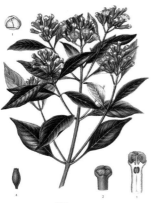
Cloves

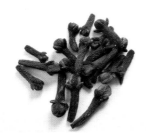
dried Cloves

Preparation and amount: *Infusion:* Steep 5-15 min. Take 1-2 Tbsp. 3 times daily. *Fluid extract:* Take 8-30 drops 3 times daily. *Oil:* Take 1-2 drops 3 times daily. *Powder:* Take 1-5 #0 capsules (2-10 grains) 3 times daily.

Purposes: *Internally,* a few drops of the oil in warm water will stop nausea and vomiting. Cloves have **antiseptic and antiparasitic** properties, and also aid **digestion**. It **stimulates and warms** the system, helping those with cold extremities. If you have a bitter herb formula, add cloves to cover the taste and **improve digestion and circulation**. It promotes **sweating** in colds, flus, and fevers and can be used to treat **whooping cough**. As a carminative, it is good for **expelling gas and stopping intestinal spasms**.

Externally, apply clove oil directly to a **toothache**, to stop the pain.

Warning: Clove oil is very strong and can cause irritation if used in its pure form. Dilute the oil in olive oil or distilled water. Do not take the undiluted oil internally.

COLTSFOOT

(Tussilago farfara) Part used: Leaf. *Properties:* Demulcent, emollient, expectorant. *What it affects:* Lungs, stomach, intestines.

Preparation and amount: *Infusion:* Steep 30 min.

Take 6 oz. frequently. *Tincture:* Take ½-1 tsp. as needed. *Fluid extract:* Take ½-1 tsp. as needed. *Powder:* Take 10-20 #0 capsules (60-120 grains) as needed.

Purposes: *Internally,* coltsfoot is a long-used remedy for **respiratory** problems. Use it for **coughs, colds, hoarseness, bronchitis, bronchial asthma, pleurisy, and throat catarrh**. It can also be used for **diarrhea**. Its name, *tussilago,* means "cough dispeller," and it is one of the best cough remedies available. For relief of **asthma, bronchitis and difficulty in breathing**, it can be taken as a tea, especially in combination with horehound and marshmallow. As a **cough syrup** combination, combine coltsfoot with horehound, ginger, and licorice root. Add it to all spasmodic lung problem remedies. It is **soothing to the stomach and intestines** when there is inflammation and bleeding.

Externally, it speeds the **healing of wounds** and many skin conditions. It is helpful for **bedsores, bites, stings, bruises, inflamed bunions, burns, dermatitis, and dry skin**. The crushed leaves, or a decoction, can be applied externally for **insect bites, inflammations, general swellings, burns, erysipelas, leg ulcers, and phlebitis**. It is good for **bleeding hemorrhoids, leg ulcers, nosebleeds, psoriasis, scabies, sunburn, and skin rashes**.

Overseas: Mucous membranes and that leaves have anti-spasm activity. Leaf is approved in Germany for treatment of **cough and hoarseness, inflammation of the respiratory tract, and mild inflammation of the mouth or throat**.

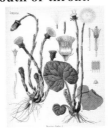
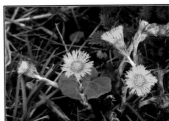
Coltsfoot   Coltsfoot

WARNING: Contains traces of liver-affecting pyrrolizidine alkaloids; potentially toxic in large doses. In Germany use is limited to 4 to 6 weeks per year, except under advice of a physician.

COMFREY

(Symphytum officinale) Parts used: Leaves and root. *Properties:* Demulcent, expectorate, mucilage, vulnerary; alterative, astringent, nutritive. *What it affects:* Bones and muscles, general effects on whole body.

Comfrey

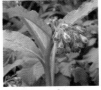
Comfrey

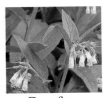
Comfrey

Preparation and amount: *Infusion (leaves):* Steep 30 min. Take 6 oz. 3 times daily. *Decoction (root):* Simmer

30 minutes. Take 3 oz. frequently. *Tincture:* Take ½-1 tsp. 3 times daily. *Fluid extract:* Take ½-2 tsp. 3 times daily. *Powder:* Take 5-10 #0 capsules (30-60 grains) 3 times daily.

Purposes: Comfrey is an all-around good remedy. It has a healing, soothing effect on every organ it contacts. It may be used both *internally* and *externally* for the healing of **fractures, wounds, sores, and ulcers**. It aids cell proliferation, helping to **heal wounds** rapidly.

Internally, comfrey is excellent for **dysentery**; one of the best for **internal bleeding**; excellent for **coughs; catarrh; ulcerated bowels, stomach, and lungs**. It helps the **pancreas** in regulating blood sugar levels. It helps relieve irritations associated with the **gallbladder, kidneys, small intestines, and stomach.** It helps promote the secretion of pepsin and is a general aid to the **digestion**. Comfrey has the highest content of mucilage of any of the herbs. Its demulcent properties, especially of the root, have been used to treat **lung troubles and coughs**. It is used for **anemia, arthritis, asthma, internal bleeding, as a blood purifier, bronchitis, calcium deficiency, colitis, coughs, diarrhea, dysentery, emphysema, and gallbladder inflammation**.

Externally, comfrey is used for **boils, bruises, burns, psoriasis, and sprains. It is good for bedsores, bites and stings, leg ulcers, nosebleeds, psoriasis, scabies, skin rashes, and sunburn**. For **bleeding**, use a strong decoction of the root, using ½-1 oz. of the root every two hours until the bleeding has stopped. Bruise the fresh leaves and apply as a poultice to **wounds, burns, open sores, gangrene, and moist ulcers**. The tea can also be put on them.

Keep some comfrey growing in your garden. Once established, it will keep coming up year after year. It is extremely prolific and versatile. A small piece of the root will reproduce itself in any shady, moist area in a very short time.

Ovrseas: In Germany, external application of the leaf is approved for the treatment of **bruises and sprains**; root poultice approved for **bruising, pulled muscles and ligaments, and sprains**.

CORN SILK

(Zea mays) Part used: Leaves. *Properties:* Diuretic, lithotriptic, demulcent. *What it affects:* Kidneys, bladder, and prostate.

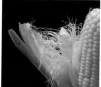

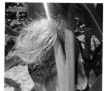
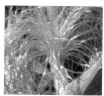

Corn Silk   Corn Silk   Corn Silk

Preparation and amount: *Infusion:* Steep 5-15 min. Take 3 oz. as needed. *Tincture:* Take 5-20 drops 3 times daily. *Fluid extract:* Take ¼-½ tsp. 3 times daily. *Powder:* Take 1-5 #0 capsules (5-30 grains) 3 times daily.

Purposes: Corn silk is the best single herb for increasing **urine flow**, thus helping to eliminate **kidney and bladder** problems.

Internally, corn silk tea is used for **bed-wetting, chronic cystitis, inflammation of kidneys and bladder, kidney stones, prostatitis, excess uric acid, and urine retention**.

It is a good remedy for all **inflammatory conditions of the urethra, bladder, prostate, and kidney**; it can **remove gravel from the kidneys, bladder, and prostate**. It helps the aged, when their urine is scanty and has heavy sediment. Use it with other kidney herbs, **when the urinary tract needs to be opened up or when there is mucus in the urine**. It lessens the frequency of bed-wetting, when taken several hours before bedtime. It is good for **dropsy and edema**, when a weak heart is the cause. It is used for **carpal tunnel syndrome** and **prostate disorders**.

CRAMP BARK

(Viburnum opulus) Part used: Bark. *Properties:* Antispasmodic, astringent, nervine. *What it affects:* Nerves, heart, and reproductive organs.

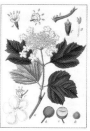

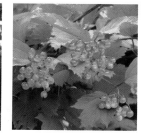

Crampbark   Crampbark   Crampbark

Preparation and amount: *Infusion:* Steep 30 min. Take 3 oz. 3-4 times daily. *Decoction:* 1 oz. herb to 1 qt. water. Simmer 30 min. Take 1 Tbsp. 3-4 times daily or as needed. *Tincture:* ½-1 tsp. 3-4 times daily. *Fluid extract:* Take ½-2 tsp. 3-4 times daily. *Powder:* Take 5-10 #0 capsules (30-60 grains) 3-4 times daily.

Purposes: Cramp bark is especially helpful for the relief of **menstrual cramps**. It can be combined with equal parts of ginger, angelica root, three parts chamomile and taken as a warm tea for all cramps and **convulsions**. It is also useful for any **spasms of involuntary muscles, hysteria**, and **painful or excessive uterine bleeding**. It helps alleviate **acute heart palpitation** and **rheumatism**. For **asthma**, make a decoction of ½ oz. of the bark to a pint of water; take 1 Tbsp. frequently as needed.

Note: Cramp bark has properties very similar to black haw; one can generally substitute for the other.

In Europe, bark tea has been used to relieve **all types of spasms**, including menstrual cramps; astringent, uterine sedative. Science confirms antispasmodic activity. In China, leaves and fruit arc used as an **emetic, laxative, and antiscorbutic** (anti-scurvy).

Warning: It is useful for heart palpitations, cramps during pregnancy, and to prevent miscarriage. Avoid using it in the third trimester of pregnancy. Berries are considered potentially poisonous; they contain chlorogenic acid, *betasitosterol*, and ursolic acid, at least when they are unripe.

DANDELION

(Taraxacum officinale) Parts used: Leaf and root. *Properties:* Cholagogue, diuretic, hepatic, lithotriptic, stomachic, alterative, astringent, galactagogue. *What it affects:* Liver, kidneys, gallbladder, stomach, pancreas,

H
E
R
B
S

intestines, and blood.

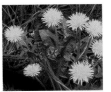 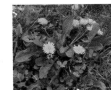 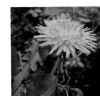

Dandelion   Dandelion   Dandelion

Preparation and amount: *Infusion:* Steep 30 min. Take 3-4 cups daily, hot or cold. *Decoction:* Simmer root 30 min. Take 6 oz. frequently or 3-4 times daily, hot or cold. *Tincture:* Take 30-60 drops (½-1 tsp.) frequently. *Powder (leaves):* Take 10-20 #0 capsules (60-120 grains) frequently. *Powder (root):* Take 5-10 #0 capsules 30-60 grains frequently.

Purposes: *Internally,* dandelion is especially important in promoting the formation of **bile** and **removing excess water** from the body in edematous conditions resulting from liver problems. The root decidedly affects all forms of secretion and excretion from the body. By removing poisons from the system, it acts as a tonic and stimulant as well. It **cleanses the blood and liver.** It is especially good as a blood cleanser for **diabetes, dropsy,** and **eczema.** Because of its high mineral content, it is used to treat **anemia.** It reduces serum **cholesterol** and **uric acid** levels. Lukewarm dandelion tea is useful for **dyspepsia with constipation, fever, and insomnia.**

Dandelion improves the functioning of the **pancreas, kidneys, spleen, and stomach.** An infusion of the fresh root is good for **gallstones, jaundice, and other liver problems.** For **stomachaches,** drink ½ cup of the infusion every ½ hour until relief is obtained. The root is a specific for **hypoglycemia.** Take a cup of the tea 2-3 times a day and maintain a balanced diet. With a good diet, the root tea can eliminate adult-onset **diabetes.** The root tea will also help lower **blood pressure,** thus aiding the action of the heart.

Dandelion relieves **menopausal symptoms** and is useful for **boils** (taken internally), **breast tumors, cirrhosis of the liver, constipation, liver and spleen enlargement, fluid retention, hepatitis, jaundice, bronchitis, low blood sugar, and rheumatism.** It may help prevent **age spots** on the skin. Serious cases of **hepatitis** have been cured with the use of **dandelion** root tea within a week or two when the diet is controlled properly and limited to easily digested foods.

The fresh juice is particularly effective, but a tea can also be prepared. Dandelion leaves are healthful as **salad greens,** especially in springtime. The roasted root is a **coffee substitute.**

Overseas: The leaf approved in Germany for treatment of **loss of appetite and dyspepsia** with a feeling of fullness and flatulence. The root is approved for treatment of **bile flow disturbances, as a diuretic, to stimulate appetite,** and to treat **dyspepsia.** One of Europe's mostly popular **cough remedies;** dried leaves smoked for **coughs and asthma.** Smoke is believed to impede impulse of fibers of parasympathetic nerves and to act as an antihistamine. Research indicates that leaf mucilage **soothes inflamed tissues.**

DEVIL'S CLAW

(Harpagophytum procumbens) Part used. Root. *Properties:* Alterative, discutient, lithotriptic, stimulant. *What it affects:* Liver, stomach, joints, and kidneys.

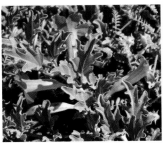 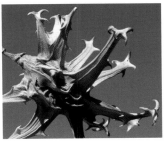

Devil's Claw

Preparation and amount: *Infusion:* Steep 30 min. 1-2 cups daily. *Decoction:* Simmer 15 min. Take 6 oz. 3 times daily. *Tincture:* Take ½-1 tsp. 3 times daily. *Powder:* Take 2-3 #0 capsules (15-30 grains) 3 times daily.

Purposes: *Internally,* devil's claw is primarily used for **rheumatism, gout, lumbago, and arthritis.** It is a **blood cleanser** which removes **deposits in the joints** and aids in elimination of **uric acid** from the body. It reduces **inflammation** and **relieves pain.** Acting as a **diuretic, sedative, and digestive stimulant,** it is good for **allergies, liver, gallbladder, kidneys, arteriosclerosis, and menopausal symptoms.**

Warning: Do not use during pregnancy.

DONG QUAI

(Tang Kwei, Dong Kwei, Dang Quai)—(Angelica sinensis) Part used: Root. *Properties:* Diuretic, antispasmodic, anodyne, uterine alterative. *What it affects:* Uterus, blood, and muscles.

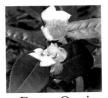 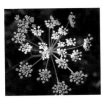

Dong Quai   Dong Quai   Dong Quai

Preparation and amount: Take 4-7 grams, several times a day.

Purposes: *Internally,* dong quai is useful for **almost every female gynecological problem.** It is especially useful for **menstrual cramps, irregularity, delayed flow and weakness during the menstrual period.** It also helps relieve the symptoms of **menopause.** It is useful in treating **hot flashes, premenstrual syndrome, and vaginal dryness.** It **strengthens the reproductive system** and **helps the body use hormones.**

Dong quai is useful for treating **insomnia, hypertension, and cramps.** It **nourishes the blood, helps treat anemia, and is a valuable blood purifier.** It acts as a **mild sedative, laxative, diuretic; and it relieves spasms and pain.** It is **warming to the circulation** and is used to **moisten the intestines** and thus treat **constipation.**

Warning: It should not be used during pregnancy or with excessive menstrual flow.

ECHINACEA

(Echinacea angustifolia) Part used: Root. *Properties:* Alterative, antiseptic, lymphatic, parasiticide, sialagogue. *What it affects:* Blood, lymph, and kidneys.

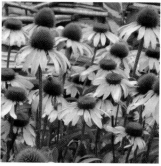
Echinacea

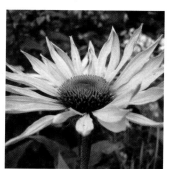
Echinacea

Preparation and amount: *Decoction:* Simmer 5-15 min. Take 1 Tbsp. 3-6 times daily. *Tincture:* Take 30-60 drops 3-6 times daily. *Fluid extract:* Take ½-1 tsp. 3-6 times daily. *Powder:* Take 2-5 #0 capsules (15-30 grains) 3-6 times daily.

Purposes: Echinacea is **the most effective blood and lymphatic cleanser of all the herbs**; and it is tolerated by the system in fairly large amounts. The plant is apparently nontoxic; although, in some people, it may cause mild dizziness and nausea for a time. But combining it with a small amount of licorice root, or making the tea with 2-3 dates, will reduce those symptoms.

Use echinacea *internally* and *externally* for **acne, bad breath, boils, gangrene, infections, skin diseases, tonsillitis**. It is said to be effective against all **venomous bites from insects, snakes, other animals, and reactions to poison oak and ivy**. It is used for **open wounds** and **painful surface swellings**.

Internally, echinacea is used for **bladder infections, blood poisoning, blood purifier, fevers, inflammation of mammary glands, intestinal antiseptic, leukopenia** (reduction in blood leukocytes), **lymphatic congestion, uremic poisoning, venereal disease, and all chronic and acute bacterial and viral infections**. It has been used for years for **syphilis, gonorrhea**, and in douches for **all vaginal infections**. Combine it with myrrh, to rid the body of **pus, abscess formations, and for typhoid fever**. The rootstock helps dispel **flatulence**. Echinacea aids **digestion** and is a **digestive tonic**.

Echinacea is **an excellent antibiotic, and ranks with goldenseal and red clover**. For acute ailments, it must be taken every hour or two, as a tincture (one tsp.) or a powder in two #00 capsules.

Externally, echinacea is used for **acne**.

Note: Do not use the rootstock once it has lost its odor.

Warning: It should be used with caution by those who are pregnant, or allergic to ragweed or plants in the sunflower family. Because it stimulates the immune system, it should *not* be taken for lengthy periods by those with autoimmune disorders. Only take 1 week at a time.

ELDER

(Black Elder)—*(Sambucus nigra) Parts used:* Flowers, bark, berries, and root. *Properties:* Diaphoretic, alterative, laxative, stimulant. *What it affects:* Blood, circulation, lungs, bowels, and skin.

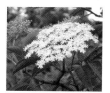
Elder

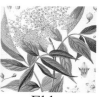
Elder

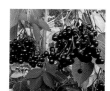
Elder

Preparation and amount: Infusion (flowers): Steep 15 min. Take 6 oz. 3 times daily. *Decoction (bark, berries, root):* Simmer 15 min. Take 1 cup at a time. *Tincture (flowers):* Take 15-30 drops 3 times daily. *Fluid extract (flowers):* Take ½-1 tsp. 3 times daily. *Powder (bark):* Take 5-10 #0 capsules (30-60 grains) 3 times daily. *Powder (leaves):* 10 #0 capsules (60 grains) 3 times daily.

Purposes: *Internally,* both the bark of young branches and the root (the inner bark which is used) are purgative and diuretic in proper dosage. In large doses they are **emetic**, strongly purgative, and can cause inflammation in the gastro-intestinal tract.

Elder flowers taken warm **induce sweating**. They are used in the **first stages of colds and flus**. Combine equal parts of the flowers with peppermint, to make a tea (1 oz. per pint of water) and drink as hot as possible. Take the tea in bed or just before taking a hot bath; and then sweat out the cold or flu during sleep.

For cases of **neuralgia, sciatica, or lumbago**, follow a juice cure regimen, taking about 2 Tbsp. warm or cold juice 2 times a day until results are obtained.

Externally, elder flowers are also used in salves for the treatment of **burns, rashes, and minor and serious skin ailments**, as well as **hemorrhoids, sprains, and wounds**.

Note: The "elder" described here is black elder *(Sambucus nigra)*. Do not confuse it with three other "elders," used less frequently by herbalists as "elder"; which are elder *(Sambucus canadensis)*, elder *(Sambucus racemosa)*, and elder *(Sambucus ebulus)*—all of which are different herbs, less often used, and each containing different properties.

Warning: Because it is used by many herbalists, black elder is described here. But, because it can be difficult and toxic, the author advises that you use other herbs internally instead of black elder. Here are additional significant warnings about this plant: Only use black elder bark and root which has been grown in Europe. The bark and root in North America contain larger amounts of both hydrocyanic acid and sambuline, a nauseating alkaloid also found in fresh paint. The stems of the plant should always be avoided, since they contain cyanide and can be very toxic. North American black elder flowers appear safe, but other parts may cause a toxic reaction. Do not use any part of the elder herb during pregnancy. All parts of the fresh plant can cause poisoning. Fresh juice will cause vomiting and diarrhea. Children have been poisoned by chewing or sucking on the bark. Cooked berries are safe and are commonly used in pies and jam.

ELECAMPANE

(Inula heminum) Part used: Root. *Properties:* Cholagogue, diuretic, expectorate, stomachic, astringent, stimulant. *What it affects:* Lungs, stomach, and spleen.

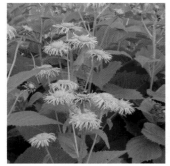
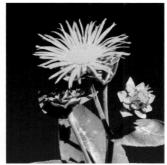

Elecampane   Elecampane

Preparation and amount: *Infusion:* Steep 15-30 min. Take 1-2 cups daily, hot or cold. *Decoction:* Simmer 15-30 min. Take 1 Tbsp., as needed or 1-2 cups daily. *Tincture:* Take 30-60 drops (½-1 tsp.) 1-2 times daily. *Fluid extract:* Take ½-1 tsp. 1-2 times daily. *Powder:* Take 3-10 #0 capsules (20-60 grains) 1-2 times daily.

Purposes: *Internally,* Elecampane tea is frequently used to quiet **coughing**, to stimulate **digestion**, and to tone the **stomach**. It is useful for all **respiratory** problems, including **bronchitis, urinary and respiratory** tract inflammation. For **chronic lung ailments**, combine with wild cherry bark, white pine bark, comfrey root, and licorice. The oil is excellent for treating **respiratory and intestinal catarrh, chronic diarrhea, chronic bronchitis, and whooping cough**.

Elecampane promotes **expectoration** and is good for **whooping cough, weak digestion, and poor assimilation**. The decoction taken in 1 Tbsp. dosages will counteract stomach poisons and increase digestive power.

The Chinese use it to counteract ingested poisons. A decoction is made using 1 ounce of the root, simmered in a pint of water for 1 hour, then taken in doses of 2 tsp. as needed. The powdered root is taken in capsules (1 capsule) or ½ tsp. of the tincture for each dose, 3 times daily. The decoction or tincture also expels worms. When combined with echinacea, it is excellent for tuberculosis.

Externally, elecampane can be used as a wash or fomentation for skin problems, such as scabies, itches, and skin diseases.

EYEBRIGHT

(Euphrasia officinalis) Part used: All that is above ground. *Properties:* Alterative, astringent, tonic. *What it affects:* Eyes, liver, and blood.

Preparation and amount: *Infusion:* Steep 5-15 min. Take 6 oz. frequently. *Tincture:* Take 30-60 drops frequently. *Fluid extract:* Take 1 tsp. frequently. *Powder:* Take 10 #0 capsules (60 grains) frequently.

Purposes: *Internally,* eyebright is the best single herb

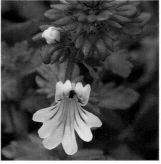
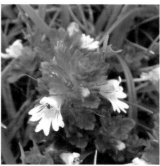

Eyebright   Eyebright

for the eyes. Drink the tea liberally and on a daily basis, to treat **all eye problems**. It aids in stimulating the **liver** to clear the blood and relieve those conditions that affect the **clarity of vision**. It relieves discomfort from eyestrain or minor eye irritation. It is good for itchy and or watery eyes. It has a cooling and detoxifying property that makes it especially useful in combating inflammation. It is also useful with inflammations of the nose and throat.

Eyebright is also used for **allergies, diabetes, cataracts, hay fever, impure blood, indigestion, nose and throat congestion, and upper respiratory problems**.

Externally, eyebright is used as an **eyewash**, especially combined with goldenseal, rue, or fennel for **conjunctivitis, eye weakness, ophthalmia, burning and sore eyes, and other eye diseases**. The infusion is made using 1 oz. herb to a pint of boiled water, steeped 20 minutes. A beverage tea can be made, using ½ oz. herb steeped in a pint of water.

FALSE UNICORN

(Chamailirium luteum [Helonias]) Part used: Root. *Properties:* Emmenagogue, tonic, diuretic, emetic, parasiticide, stimulant. *What it affects:* Uterus and kidneys.

Preparation and amount: *Decoction:* Simmer 5-15 min. Take 6 oz. 3 times daily. *Tincture:* Take 15-30 drops 3 times daily. *Fluid extract:* Take ½-1 tsp. 3 times daily. *Powder:* Take 2-5 #0 capsules (15-30 grains) 3 times daily.

Purposes: *Internally,* the primary use of this herb is in the treatment of **female sterility and impotence**. Taking it is said to increase the likelihood of getting pregnant.

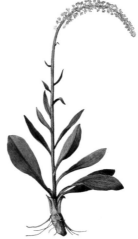

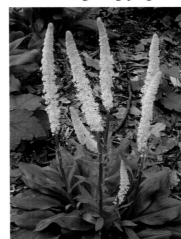

False Unicorn   False Unicorn

It **balances sexual hormones, helps treat infertility, and prevent miscarriage**. For these purposes, it may be taken daily for several months. One or 2 #00 capsules of the powdered root are taken 3 times daily for a number of months, either alone or in combination with other herbs.

The root is also used in the treatment of **painful or irregular menstruation, or the lack of it**. It is also good for **leukorrhea and menorrhagia**. Small amounts may be taken during the early part of pregnancy, to relieve **morning sickness**.

False unicorn is used for glandular tonic, prolapsed uterus, uterine and ovarian problems, and uterine displacement.

This herb is also used for **prostrate disorders, spermatorrhea, diabetes, digestive tonic, intestinal weakness, and urinary tract tonic.**

False unicorn root is usually combined with other herbs, such as cramp bark or black haw; but it can be taken alone. During threatening situations, 15 drops of the tincture or ½ tsp. of the fluid extract can be taken every hour.

Note: Do not confuse false unicorn root with true unicorn root *(Aletris farinosa),* also known as star grass; this has similar properties, but is primarily used as a diuretic.

FENNEL

(Foeniculum vulgare) Part used: Seed. *Properties:* Antispasmodic, aromatic, carminative, diuretic, expectorant, galactagogue, stimulant. *What it affects:* Stomach, nerves, intestines, and eyes.

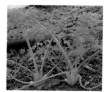 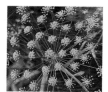 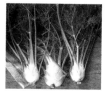

Fennel   Fennel   Fennel

Preparation and amount: *Infusion:* Steep 5-15 min. Take 6 oz. 3 times daily. *Fluid extract:* Take 5-60 drops 3 times daily. *Oil:* Take 1-5 drops 3 times daily. *Powder:* Take the average dose of 3 #0 capsules (15 grains).

Purposes: *Internally,* although the seeds are mainly used, both the seeds and root of fennel are excellent **stomach and intestinal remedies**. It promotes the function of the **kidneys, liver, and spleen**, and helps **clear the lungs**. It helps to arouse the appetite, and relieve colic and abdominal cramps. It relieves **abdominal and colon disorders**. It expels **mucous accumulations**. It is especially used to reduce **gastro-intestinal tract spasms** and **expel flatulence**. For this purpose, take fennel oil with honey or as a saturated solution in water. Add it also to gargle for **coughing** and **hoarseness**. It is used to treat **acid stomach, colic, and cramps**. In larger doses, it removes **obstructions of the liver, spleen, and gallbladder**. Fennel will **increase the flow of urine, menstrual blood, and mother's milk**.

Externally, fennel can be used as an **eyewash**.

Overseas: Seeds are eaten in Middle East to **increase milk secretion, and promote menstruation**. Powdered

seeds are poulticed in China for **snakebites**. Seed oil **relieves spasms of smooth muscles, kills bacteria, removes hookworms**. Seeds approved in Germany for treatment of **gastrointestinal fullness and spasms, catarrh of the upper respiratory tract**. Experimentally, seed oil relieves **spasms of smooth muscles, kills bacteria, removes hookworms**. Fennel seed is our best source of *anethole,* used commercially as "licorice" (actually anise) flavor. Seed extracts stimulate gastrointestinal motility.

FENUGREEK

(Trigonella foenum graecum) Part used: Seed. *Properties:* Demulcent, emollient, expectorant, aphrodisiac, astringent, galactagogue, tonic. *What it affects:* Lungs, stomach, intestines, and reproductive organs.

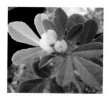 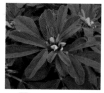 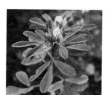

Fenugreek   Fenugreek   Fenugreek

Preparation and amount: *Infusion:* Steep 5-15 min. Take 1 cup during the day, hot or cold. *Decoction:* Simmer 5-15 min. Take 6 oz. 3 times daily. *Tincture:* 30-60 drops 3 times daily. *Fluid extract:* Take ½-1 tsp. 3 times daily. *Powder:* Take 2-10 #0 capsules (10-60 grains) 3 times daily.

Purposes: *Internally,* Fenugreek is one of the oldest medicinal plants, dating back to Hippocrates and the ancient Egyptians. It is useful for all **mucous conditions of the lungs**. Large amounts of the decoction are given to strengthen those suffering from **tuberculosis** or **recovering from an illness**. It is also good for **fevers, bronchitis, stomach, ulcers, diabetes, gout, asthma, emphysema, hay fever, heartburn, hoarseness, migraines, neuralgia, sciatica, and gas**. By reducing mucus, it helps **asthma and sinus problems**. Promotes **lactation** in nursing mothers. Helps **lower cholesterol and blood sugar levels**. Good for the **eyes**.

Externally, fenugreek is used for **boils, carbuncles, abscesses, sore throat, dry skin conditions**. The tea is excellent for **sore throats** (drink and gargle). Make a poultice of pulverized seeds and place over **wounds, fistulas, tumors, sores, areas of gouty pains, swollen glands, and skin irritations**.

Note: The taste can be improved by mixing it with peppermint oil, lemon extract, or honey.

FLAXSEED

(Linum usitatissimum) Part used: Seed. *Properties:* Demulcent, emollient, laxative, mucilage, nutritional. *What it affects:* Lungs, throat, intestines, and stomach.

Preparation and amount: *Infusion:* Steep 5-15 min. Take 1 cup daily. *Decoction:* Take 2 oz. 3 times daily. *Tincture:* Take 15-40 drops 3 times daily or as needed. *Fluid extract:* Take 15-30 drops 3 times daily or as needed. *Powder:* Take 10-20 #0 capsules (60-120 grains) once daily.

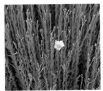
Flaxseed

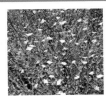
Flaxseed

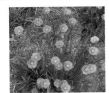
Flaxseed

Purposes: Flaxseed is even more mucilaginous than slippery elm and useful for a variety of problems. It is **better than olive oil**, for the purposes for which it is used.

Internally, flaxseed is used for **asthma, bronchitis, catarrh, constipation, coughs, diarrhea, enteritis, flatulence, hemorrhoids, stomach ulcers, pleurisy, and lung, and chest problems**. It is also good for all **intestinal inflammations**.

Eating the seeds intact is good for **constipation**. Take 1-2 Tbsp. whole seeds and swallow with lots of water if necessary. Then eat stewed prunes. The seeds swell up in the intestines, encouraging elimination by increasing the volume of fecal matter.

To eliminate **gallstones**, take 1½-2 Tbsp. flaxseed oil and lie down on your left side for half an hour. The gallstones will pass into the intestines and be eliminated from there.

Externally, flaxseed is excellent in poultices for sores, **boils, inflammations, and tumors**. Combine it with slippery elm for **boils, oozing sores, and burns**.

Caution: It is best to avoid flaxseed if you have diverticulitis.

FO-TI (Ho Shou Wu)

(Polygonum multiflorum) Part used: Root. *Properties:* Stimulant, tonic, astringent, diuretic. *What it affects:* Liver, stomach, kidneys, and reproductive organs.

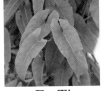
Fo-Ti

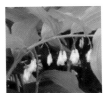
Fo-Ti

Fo-Ti

Preparation and amount: *Decoction:* Simmer 5-15 min. Take 2 oz. 2-4 times daily. *Tincture:* Take 15-30 drops 3 times daily. *Fluid extract:* Take 5-20 drops 3 times daily. *Powder:* Take 2-3 #0 capsules (10-15 grains) 3 times daily.

Purposes: *Internally,* fo-ti focuses on helping the **endocrine glands** by strengthening them. It acts as a tonic and nutritive herb. It is also a **digestive tonic.** Take it either as a decoction or as a powder.

GARLIC

(Allium sativum) Part used: Bulb. *Properties:* Alterative, antibiotic, antispasmodic, diaphoretic, expectorant, stimulant. *What it affects:* Lungs, circulation, nerves, and sinuses.

Preparation and amount: *Tincture:* Take 30-60 drops (½-1 tsp.) 3-4 times daily. *Juice:* Take 10-30 drops 3-4 times daily. *Oil:* Take 2-3 drops or 1 tsp. *Syrup:* Take

1 Tbsp. 3-4 times daily. *Powder:* Take 5-10 #0 capsules (30-60 grains) 3-4 times daily.

Garlic

Garlic

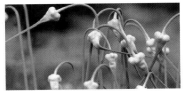
Garlic

Purposes: Garlic is **one of the most powerful antiseptic substances ever discovered**. It is also one of the most readily available, easily used medicinal substances.

In the 1950s, Soviet scientists found it to be equal to penicillin, yet without the harmful effects of that powerful drug.

Internally, garlic **detoxifies** the entire body and **protects against infection** by **enhancing immune function**. It is good for **virtually every infection and disease**. Its beneficial effect on **blood circulation** and **heart action** can bring relief for many common body complaints. It is used for **all lung and respiratory ailments, colds, tuberculosis, fevers, and blood diseases**; and it can be used as a tea or added to syrups for coughs.

It is used for **arteriosclerosis, cancer, contagious disease, coughs, cramps, diverticulitis, emphysema, gas, heart problems, high blood pressure, indigestion, liver congestion, rheumatism, sinus congestion, and ulcers**. It aids in the treatment of **arthritis, asthma, circulatory problems, cold and flu, digestive problems, heart disorders, insomnia, liver diseases, sinusitis, ulcers, and yeast infections**.

Garlic regularizes the action of the **liver** and **gallbladder**. It stimulates the **digestive** organs and thereby relieves various problems associated with poor digestion. It helps stabilize **blood sugar levels**. As an **expectorant**, it is useful for **chronic stomach and intestinal catarrh**, as well as **chronic bronchitis**. A cold tea can be taken as an enema for **worms and pinworms**. A warm enema tea is good for **bowel infections**. Use the fresh extract oil or eat the raw cloves.

Garlic is helpful in **all intestinal infections,** including **dysentery, typhoid, cholera, and paratyphoid fever**. It **lowers blood lipid** levels. It works to **eliminate putrefactive intestinal bacteria**. Because garlic **lowers blood pressure**, it helps to counteract **arteriosclerosis**.

Externally, garlic is used for **ringworm, skin parasites, tumors, and warts**.

Overseas: In China, used for **digestive difficulties, diarrhea, dysentery, colds, whooping cough, pinworms, old ulcers, swellings, and snake bites**. Also to **lower blood pressure and serum cholesterol**. Also **hypertension, heart ailments, and arteriosclerosis**.

Warning: People who take anticoagulant (blood-thinning) drugs should not take garlic, since it also thins the blood somewhat.

GENTIAN

(Gentiana lutea) Part used: Root. *Properties:* Cholagogue, stomachic, tonic, anthelmintic. *What it affects:*

Stomach, liver, blood, spleen, and circulation.

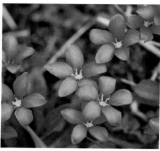 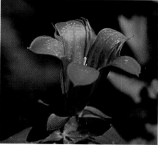

Gentian   Gentian

Preparation and amount: *Decoction:* Simmer 5-15 min. Take ¼-1 tsp. 3 times daily to ½-1 cup daily. *Tincture:* Take ½-2 tsp. 3 times daily. *Fluid extract:* Take ¼-½ tsp. 3 times daily. *Powder:* Take 2-4 #0 capsules (10-30 grains) 3 times daily.

Purposes: *Internally,* gentian primarily works on the **liver** and **stomach**. Because it is a bitter tonic herb, it **quickens intestinal action** and tends to **overcome slow digestion**. It improves the **appetite**, increases **digestion**, and improves **circulation**. It is good for **pancreatitis, female problems, slow urination, colds, and gout**.

Note: Because of its bitterness, combine gentian with aromatic herbs, such as ginger, peppermint, sassafras, spearmint, or wood betony.

GINGER

(Zingiberis officinalis) Part used: Rhizome. *Properties:* Aromatic, carminative, diaphoretic, stimulant, diuretic. *What it affects:* Stomach, intestines, joints, muscles, and circulation.

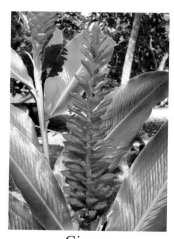 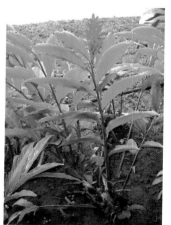

Ginger   Ginger

Preparation and amount: *Infusion:* Steep 5-15 min. Take 1 fluid oz. at a time. *Decoction:* Simmer 5-15 min. Take 2 oz. 3 times daily. *Tincture:* Take 15-60 drops 3 times daily. *Fluid extract:* Take 5-20 drops 3 times daily. *Syrup:* Take ½-1 tsp. 3 times daily. *Powder:* Take 2-4 #0 capsules (10-20 grains) 3 times daily. Take every 2 hours for nausea and vomiting.

Purposes: *Internally,* ginger promotes **cleansing of the system through perspiration**. Taken hot, the tea is good for **suppressed menstruation and scanty urine**. It **brings heat** into the system and **stimulates digestion**. Taken in frequent doses, it will **raise body temperature**. **It is** *without a peer* among herbs dealing with sea sickness, air sickness, and every other kind of motion sickness. It is helpful in reducing **flatulent colic**; and, when taken with laxative herbs, it makes their effect milder. It fights **inflammation, cleanses the colon, reduces spasms and cramps, and stimulates circulation**. Take it at the onset of a **cold**, to ease the effects of the usual symptoms. It is used for **contagious diseases, coughs, cramps, indigestion, gas, headache, colon spasms, morning sickness, nausea, sinus congestion, and stomach spasms**. It is a *strong antioxidant* and **germ killer for sores and wounds**. To s**timulate the flow of saliva** and **soothe a sore throat**, chew the rootstock as is. It protects the liver and stomach, and is useful for **bowel disorders, arthritis, fever, hot flashes, indigestion, muscle pain, and vomiting**.

Externally, ginger is used as a fomentation in cases of **mumps**.

GINSENG

(Panax ginseng) Part used: Root. *Properties:* Alterative, stimulant, stomachic, tonic. *What it affects:* Heart and circulation, general effects on the whole body.

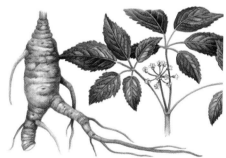 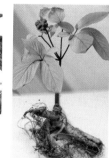

Ginseng   Ginseng

Preparation and amount: *Decoction:* Simmer 15-60 min. Use about ¼ oz. of herb to 1 pint water. Take 4 oz. 3 times daily. *Tincture:* 20-60 drops 3 times daily. *Fluid extract:* ½-2 tsp. 3 times daily. *Powder:* 2-5 #0 capsules (15-30 grains) 3 times daily.

Purposes: *Internally,* ginseng is especially used for **feverish and inflammatory illnesses,** for **hemorrhage,** and for **blood diseases**. Women take it for **everything from normalizing menstruation to easing childbirth**. It strengthens the **adrenal and reproductive glands**. It **promotes lung functioning, enhances immune function, and stimulates the appetite**. It helps **digestive disturbances**. It is mildly stimulating to the **central nervous system** and the **endocrines**. It is useful for **bronchitis, diabetes, infertility, lack of energy, and stress**. It protects against the effects of **radiation exposure** and helps in **withdrawal from cocaine**. Because it is a demulcent, the tea taken hot is effective for **colds, chest troubles and coughs**. It helps to normalize **blood pressure, tone the heart, increase circulation and reduce cholesterol**. It **reduces blood sugar**, which is helpful for **diabetics**. Its nutritional qualities help alleviate **anemia**.

Note: Only use thoroughly dried roots. The value of ginseng is overblown, but it is still a useful herb. Do not take it at night, for it will keep you awake.

Chinese ginseng *(Panax ginseng)* is thought to be far better than the North American variety. But, in reality, American ginseng *(Panax quinquefolius)* is essentially the same as the Chinese version! So much so, that the bulk of the U.S. crop (most of which is grown under cultivation in Wisconsin) is shipped to Europe and Asia, to supplement the supply from the Orient (which is primarily grown in Korea).

GOLDENSEAL

(Hydrastis canadensis) Part used: Rhizome. Properties: Alterative, antibiotic, antiseptic, emmenagogue, stomachic, tonic, laxative. *What it affects:* Stomach, intestines, spleen, liver, eyes, all mucous membranes.

 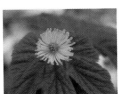 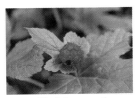

Goldenseal   Goldenseal   Goldenseal

Preparation and amount: *Infusion* (powered root): Steep powder until cold. Take 1-2 tsp. 3-4 times daily. *Decoction:* Simmer 15-30 min. Take 1-2 tsp. 3-4 times daily. *Tincture:* Take 20-90 drops (1/3 to 1½ tsp.) 3 times daily. *Powder:* Take 2-5 #0 capsules (10-30 grains) 3 times daily or 2-3 #00 capsules (5 is average dose) per day.

Purposes: Goldenseal is a powerful **antiseptic** (germ killer). **Like echinacea, it is good for nearly every disease. Taken with any herb, it increases the tonic effects on the specific organs being treated.** Add it when giving eyebright for the **eyes,** squaw vine for the **female genito-urinary system,** gotu kola for the **brain,** and **cascara segrada** for the lower bowel. Add it to salves for the **skin,** douches for **vaginal infections,** and reducing **hemorrhoids.** It especially acts on **mucous membranes** and can be used for all **catarrhal conditions,** including those in the intestines. Used at the first sign of possible symptoms, it can **stop a cold, flu, or sore throat.**

Internally, goldenseal is good for **alcoholism, allergies, asthma, bad breath, bladder diseases, bronchitis, canker sores, chicken pox, colds, diabetes, eczema, hay fever, stomach ailments, heart weakness, hemorrhoids, herpes, indigestion, infections, inflammations, leukorrhea, liver problems, lymph congestion, measles, mammary and ovarian tumors, ulcers.** It is a douche for **vaginal infections.** Used with cascara sagrada, it is a **bowel tonic.** As a retention enema, it will reduce swollen **hemorrhoids.** It is good for **allergies, ulcers,** and disorders affecting the **bladder, prostate, stomach, or vagina.** Small doses will relieve **nausea** (morning sickness) during **pregnancy,** but see the warning below. Combine it with myrrh when treating **ulcers of the stomach.** For **hemorrhoids and prostate problems,** combine 2 parts goldenseal and 1 part wild alum. It **increases the effectiveness of insulin** and strengthens the **immune** system. It reduces

blood pressure, stimulates the **central nervous system,** regulates the **menses,** and decreases **uterine bleeding.**

Externally, goldenseal is used for **burns, canker sores, eye inflammations, herpes sores, leukorrhea, mouth sores, ringworm, skin inflammation, tonsillitis, and wounds.** Use it with a toothbrush or as an antiseptic **mouthwash** for **bleeding gums or gum infections.** Use it as a gargle for **tonsillitis** and other **throat problems.** Goldenseal can be used on **open sores, inflammations, eczema, ringworm, or itchy skin conditions.** It is a specific for all kinds of **mucous membrane** problems. Snuffed up the nose, the powder is good for **nasal congestion or catarrh.** For **ringworm,** wash it with the tea, then sprinkle powdered root on it. For a soothing **eyewash,** mix it with boric acid (1 tsp. powdered root and 1 tsp. boric acid to 1 pint boiling-hot water); stir; let cool; and pour off the liquid. Add 1 tsp. of the liquid to ½ cup of water for the eyewash.

Warning: Goldenseal is a powerful alkaloid and should not be overused. Two or three #00 capsules per day are safe and adequate for most conditions. Normally, **do not use it more than a week at a time, then switch to echinacea** or another antibiotic herb (myrrh, chaparral, pau d'arco). Excessive use diminishes vitamin B absorption, by killing certain intestinal bacteria. Over a prolonged period, use no more than 2-3 #00 capsules a day. Do not use large amounts during hypoglycemia. Those with high blood pressure or insomnia should not use it. Eating the fresh plant produces ulcerations and inflammation of mucous tissue.

Because large doses of goldenseal contract the uterus, women who have a tendency to miscarry should avoid the use of it unless, for **morning sickness,** it is used in this formula: Less than ¼ tsp. goldenseal, plus ¼ tsp. cloves; the powders taken in gelatin capsules are not to exceed 2 capsules per day and taken with spearmint tea.

GOTU KOLA

(Centella Asiatica) Part used: Tops. *Properties:* Nervine, tonic, alterative, antipyretic, diuretic. *What it affects:* Brain, nerves, kidneys, bladder, heart, and circulation.

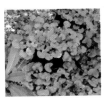 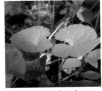 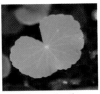

Gotu kola   Gotu kola   Gotu kola

Preparation and amount: *Infusion:* Steep 5-15 min. Take 3 oz. 3 times daily. *Tincture:* Take 15-30 drops 3 times daily. *Fluid extract:* Take ½-1 tsp. 3 times daily. *Powder:* 5-10 #0 capsules (30-60 grains) 3 times daily.

Purposes: Gotu kola is a very common medicinal plant throughout India and the tropical countries. *Internally,* it is one of the best herbs for the **nerves and brain,** including **epilepsy, schizophrenia, and loss of memory.** It decreases **fatigue and depression,** and stimulates the **central nervous system.** To treat **nervous disorders,** gotu kola oil is applied externally over the entire body, including the scalp. This oil (called Brahmi oil) is an herbal extract in sesame oil. To make it, add enough sesame oil to cover the herb; cover and let stand 14 days; then squeeze out the oil.

Gotu kola has remarkable rejuvenating properties similar to those of fo-ti and ginseng. It **neutralizes blood acids and cools the blood**, thus making it of great value in **all fevers and inflammations**. It is both a **blood purifier and diuretic**. It is good for **heart and liver** function. It helps **eliminate excess fluids**. It promotes the healing of **wounds** and is good for **varicose veins**. It is used to treat **rheumatism, blood diseases, connective tissue disorders, poor appetite, kidney stones, and sleep problems**.

GRAVEL ROOT

(Queen of the Meadow)—(Eupatorium purpureum) Part used: Root. *Properties:* Diuretic, lithotriptic, astringent, nervine, stimulant. *What it affects:* Kidneys, bladder, nerves, and joints.

  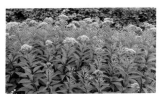

Gravel Root Gravel Root   Gravel Root

Preparation and amount: *Infusion (herb):* Steep 5-15 min. Take 1-2 cups daily. *Decoction (root):* Simmer 6-15 min. Take 1-2 oz. as needed up to 2 cups daily. *Tincture:* Take 30-60 drops (½-1 tsp.) 3 times daily. *Fluid extract:* Take ½-1 tsp. 3 times daily. *Powder:* 5 #0 capsules (30 grains) 3 times daily.

Purposes: *Internally,* gravel root is one of the best remedies for **gravel and stones in the kidneys and bladder**. It is also used to treat the **uric acid deposits in joints**, which make them so painful. It also works to reduce **water retention** and deal with **prostate** disorders. A strong decoction is used: 1 oz. of the root boiled in a pint of water for one hour. Take a quarter cup at a time, as needed. When using a tincture, take 1 tsp. at a time.

In addition, gravel root is a **nerve tonic** and used for many **female problems**, alone or in combination. This includes **dysmenorrhea, endometritis, leukorrhea, chronic uterine disease, labor pains, and threatened abortions**. Gravel root is also used for **cystitis, edema, gout, rheumatism, weak pelvic organs, gonorrhea, cystitis, bright's disease, bloody urine, and backache**.

HAWTHORN (Hawthorne)

(Crataegus oxycantha) Part used: Fruit. *Properties:* Tonic, antispasmodic, astringent, diuretic, sedative. *What it affects:* Heart, circulation, nerves, and kidneys.

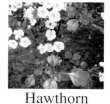 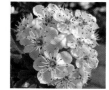 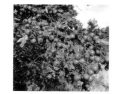

Hawthorn   Hawthorn   Hawthorn

Preparation and amount: *Infusion:* Steep 5-15 min. Take 1 cup 2-3 times daily. *Decoction:* Simmer 5-15 min. Take 6 oz. 3 times daily. *Tincture:* Take 15-30 drops (½-1 tsp.) 3 times daily. *Fluid extract:* Take 10-15 drops 3 times daily. *Powder:* Take 10 #0 capsules (60 grains) 3 times daily.

Purposes: This is the herb for the heart! *Internally,* hawthorn **normalizes blood pressure** by regulating heart action. It dilates the coronary blood vessels. Those are the ones that nourish the heart itself. Taking the herb over a period of time will generally **lower blood pressure**. (Keep in mind that a key factor in lowering blood pressure is drinking enough water every day!) But it normalizes blood pressure, helping to **elevate low blood pressure**. It helps **rapid or arrhythmic heartbeat, inflammation of the heart muscle** (myocarditis), **arteriosclerosis, and nervous heart problems**. It is good for **heart muscles** weakened by age. Taking it regularly strengthens the heart muscle. It helps prevent **hardening of the arteries**; it is excellent for **feeble heart action, valvular insufficiency, and irregular pulse**.

Hawthorn tea is also good for **nervous conditions**, particularly **insomnia**. A decoction of the berries is good for **sore throats** and **acid conditions of the blood**. American Indians used it to treat **rheumatism**. In China, it is used to aid **digestion**.

HOPS

(Humulus lupulus) Part used: Strobiles. *Properties:* Nervine, stomachic, anodyne, antibiotic, carminative, cholagogue, tonic. *What it affects:* Nerves, stomach, blood, liver, and gallbladder.

 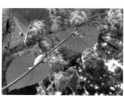 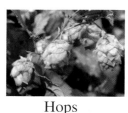

Hops   Hops   Hops

Preparation and amount: *Infusion:* Steep 5-15 min. Take 6 oz. 3 times daily, hot or cold. *Tincture:* Take 15-30 drops (½-1 tsp.) 3 times daily. *Fluid extract:* Take 10-15 drops 3 times daily. *Powder:* Take 5-10 #0 capsules (30-60 grains) 3 times daily.

Purposes: Hops is an excellent nervine and will produce sleep when **insomnia** is present. *Internally,* it has a very calming effect on the entire system. It is used for **nervous diarrhea, insomnia, restlessness, headaches, shock, weak nerves, hyperactivity, nervousness, pain, stress, nervous stomach, and relieves anxiety**.

But it also has other uses. Hops is used for **coughs, fever, indigestion, jaundice, morning sickness, stomach tonic, throat, bronchial tubes, chest ailments, toothache, and ulcers**. It will **stimulate the appetite, dispel flatulence, and relieve intestinal cramps**. It is useful for **cardiovascular disorders, sexually transmitted diseases, toothaches, and ulcers**. Cold tea before meals will increase **digestion**. The dry herb that is placed inside a pillow will induce sleep.

Externally, it is used for **boils, bruises, earaches, inflammations, rheumatic pains, skin ailments, and ulcers**.

Note: Hops lose their effectiveness as internal medication rapidly when stored.

Overseas: Approved in Germany to treat discomfort from **restlessness or anxiety and sleep disturbances**. Considered **calming** and **helpful in promoting sleep**. Tea of fruits (strobiles) traditionally used as **sedative, antispasmodic, diuretic**; for **insomnia, cramps, coughs, fevers; externally, for bruises, boils, inflammation, rheumatism**. Experimentally anti-microbial, relieves **spasms of smooth muscles**, acts as **sedative**. Hops contains several sedative and pain-relieving components. Used to **relieve mood disturbances, nervous tension, anxiety, and unrest**. Japanese hops *(Hunnihis japonicas)*, is a weedy annual with 5-9 leaf lobes. Leaves much rougher than common hops. Used for the same purposes.

HOREHOUND

(Marrubium vulgare) Part used: Tops. *Properties:* Diaphoretic, expectorant, tonic. *What it affects:* Lungs, chest, and stomach.

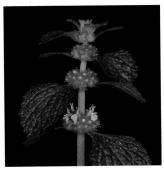
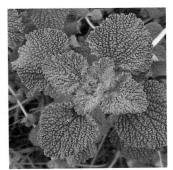

Horehound   Horehound

Preparation and amount: *Infusion:* Steep 20 min. Take 6 oz. at a time, frequently. *Tincture:* Take 20-60 drops 3 times daily. *Fluid extract:* Take ½-1 tsp. 3 times daily. *Syrup:* Take ½-1 tsp. 3 times daily. *Powder:* Take 5-10 #0 capsules (30-60 grains) 3 times daily.

Purposes: *Internally,* horehound is especially useful as a remedy for **coughing and bronchial problems**. As an **expectorant for bronchial catarrh**, it can be taken as a tea or syrup. It is used for acute and chronic **bronchitis**, as well as **coughs and hoarseness**. It is useful in **chronic sore throats and pulmonary problems**. Use it in syrup form for children.

Horehound is also used for **typhoid fever**. It is said to restore the normal balance of secretions by various organs and glands. It is used for **heart conditions, to calm heart action**. It is also used for **asthma, dyspepsia, hay fever, bloating, fevers, and jaundice**. It **boosts the immune system**. Taken warm, it is **diuretic**; taken cold, it makes a good **stomach** tonic.

Externally, the tea or the crushed leaves of horehound can be applied for temporary or persistent **skin problems**.

Overseas: In Europe, the malodorous, bitter leaves are used in **cough syrups**. Also as a bitter stomach to **stimulate digestion** and an expectorant to break **up-**phlegm, relieve coughs, soothe sore throats, and relieve bronchitis** and **other upper-resoiratory ailments**. Also used for **stomach and gallbladderdisorders, jaundice, hepatitis; fesh leaves poulticed on cuts, wounds. It also increases bile flow**. In Germany, it si approved for **coughs and colds** and as a **digestive aid and appetitie stimulant**.

HORSERADISH

(Cochleria armoracia) Part used: Root. *Properties:* Diaphoretic, diuretic, expectorant, stomachic. *What it affects:* Sinuses, stomach, gallbladder, and urinary tract.

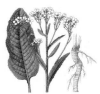
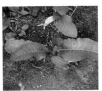
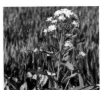

Horseradish   Horseradish   Horseradish

Preparation and amount: *Decoction:* Simmer 5-15 minutes. Take 6 oz. 1-2 times daily, cold; or take warm, 2-3 Tbsp., 3 times daily.

Purposes: *Internally,* promotes **stomach secretions**. A syrup of horseradish is excellent for **sinus** congestion and promotes **digestion**. Good for **dropsy, urine retention, and helps the pancreas**. Used for **colds, coughs, asthma, arthritis, dropsy, hoarseness, sciatica, worms**.

Externally, it is used for **liver and spleen swellings**.

Overseas: In Germany, root is used for treatment of inflammation of the respiratory tract, and urinary tract infections.

Warning: Left in contact with the skin, it will cause blistering. Avoid contact with the eyes.

HORSETAIL

(Shavegrass, Scouring Rush)—(Equisetum arvense) Part used: Tops. *Properties:* Astringent, diuretic, lithotriptic, emmenagogue, galactagogue, nutritive, vulnerary. *What it affects:* Kidneys, blood, heart, and lungs.

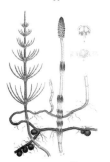
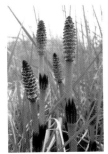
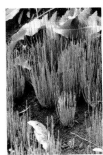

Horsetail   Horsetail   Horsetail

Preparation and amount: *Infusion:* Steep 45 min. Take a mouthful 4 times daily or 1-2 cups daily. *Decoction:* Simmer 5-15 min. Take 2 oz. 3-4 times daily. *Tincture:* Take 5-30 drops 3-4 times daily. *Fluid extract:* Take 5 drops 3-4 times daily. *Powder:* Take 5-10 #0 capsules (30-60 grains) 3-4 times daily.

Purposes: *Internally,* shavegrass is a reliable diuretic and used for all **urinary** disorders. Take a decoction of

1 cup 2-3 times a day or 2 Tbsp. every hour. The early settlers used shavegrass as a **diuretic** in kidney problems and dropsy. It is specific, not only for urine retention, but for **internal bleeding**. It **stops bleeding** by helping to coagulate the blood.

Shavegrass can be used for **skin** and **eye** conditions, and is good for **glandular swellings** and discharges of **pus**. It clears **fevers, releases nervous tension**, and calms an **overactive liver**. It strengthens the **heart and lungs** and removes **gravel** from the bladder and kidneys. **Fractured bones** heal more quickly when shavegrass is taken. The Chinese use it as a **healing eyewash**. It can also be used for **bed-wetting, gallbladder diseases, skin diseases, edema, and spitting of blood**. Use it for **muscle cramps and spasms**. It is used for **bone diseases**, including **osteoporosis and rickets**.

Early settlers used shavegrass to scour their pots and pans, hence its other name. Because it is ridged with silica, it is an outstanding scouring pad. Fine cabinetmakers use it for polishing wood finishes.

Externally, a fomentation can be placed on **bleeding wounds, ulcers, and burns**.

Note: Early spring shavegrass is the best to use.

Warning: Excessive use of shavegrass will irritate the kidneys and intestines; so only take it infrequently and in small doses for a short time. After 2-3 weeks, do not use it for a week. Then the treatment can be repeated. Continued use interferes with the absorption of thiamine (vitamin B_1).

HYSSOP

(Hyssopus officinalis) Part used: Leaves. *Properties:* Diaphoretic, expectorant, cholagogue, stimulant, vulnerary. *What it affects:* Lungs, sinuses, and circulation.

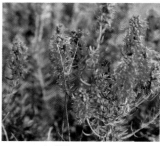

Hyssop

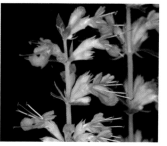

Hyssop

Preparation and amount: *Infusion:* Steep 5-15 min. 1-2 cups daily or frequently. *Tincture:* Take ½-1 tsp. frequently. *Fluid extract:* Take 1-2 tsp. frequently. *Powder:* Take 10 #0 capsules frequently.

Purposes: *Internally,* hyssop is used in the treatment of **lung** ailments, especially **chronic catarrh**. It is a valuable **expectorant**, promoting expulsion of mucus from the respiratory tract and thus relieving congestion. It is used for **coughs and colds**, due to congestion.

Hyssop is used the same as sage, with which it is sometimes combined, to make a gargle for a sore throat. It is used for **colds, coughs, asthma, sluggish circulation, and weak digestion**. It regulates **blood pressure, dispels gas**, and helps with **breast and lung problems, nose and throat infections, mucous congestion in the**

intestines, asthma, scrofula, dropsy, and jaundice. A warm infusion, mixed with equal parts of horehound, is good for **asthma** and **heavy mucous** conditions. The infusion of hyssop alone is helpful for **gas** and to promote **sweating**, when trying to **break fevers**. A decoction will help relieve **inflammations**. It is used for **epilepsy, gout, and weight problems**.

Externally, hyssop is used for the healing of **wounds**. Poultices from fresh green hyssop help heal **cuts**. A fomentation made from the leaves will relieve **muscular rheumatism and bruises**. A decoction can be used as a wash for **burns, bruises, skin irritations**, and as a gargle for **sore throat or chronic catarrh**.

Overseas: Gargled for **sore throats**. Also tea thought to **relieve gas, stomachaches, loosen phlegm**; used with Horehound for **bronchitis, coughs, and asthma**. The herb has been used externally to treat **rheumatism, muscle aches, wounds, and sprains**. Experimentally, extracts are useful against **herpes simplex; anti- inflammatory**. Contains at least 8 **antiviral** compounds. In 1990 researchers found that a Hyssop extract inhibited replication of **human immunodeficiency virus (HIV)**.

Warning: Do not use extensively for extended periods.

IRISH MOSS

(Chondius crispus) Part used: Whole plant. *Properties:* Demulcent, emollient, nutritive. *What it affects:* Lungs, kidneys, and skin.

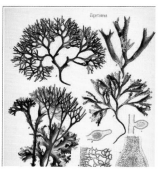

Irish Moss

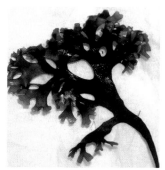

Irish Moss

Preparation and amount: *Infusion:* Steep 5-15 min. Take 2 oz. 2-3 times daily, up to 2 cups daily. *Tincture:* Take 30-60 drops (½-1 tsp.) 2-3 times daily. *Fluid extract:* Take ½-1 tsp. 2-3 times daily. *Powder:* Take 4-6 #0 capsules (20-40 grains) 2-3 times daily.

Purposes: Irish moss is a seaweed that grows among submerged rocks off the coast of France and Ireland. A significant factor in its healing qualities is its high nutritional mineral content.

Internally, it is a remedy for **tuberculosis, coughs, bronchitis, and intestinal problems**. Because it is very high in mucilage, it is an excellent demulcent for **soothing inflamed tissues** and is used in all **lung and kidney** complaints. When making a decoction, you may wish to sweeten it with licorice root, honey, or an aromatic herb. Irish moss is also used for **anemia, thyroid difficulties, goiter, and throat and stomach ulcers**.

Externally, use Irish moss in hair rinses for **dry hair**.

It is also used for **dry and burning skin diseases**, and **surface inflammations**. It can be used externally, to **soften skin** and **prevent premature wrinkling**.

Note: Irish moss and other seaweeds (especially Nova Scotia dulse and Norwegian kelp) are rich sources of minerals and the best sources of trace minerals. Include a little every day in your diet.

JUNIPER BERRIES

(Juniperus communis) Part used: Fruit. *Properties:* Antispasmodic, diuretic, anodyne, aromatic, astringent, carminative, lithotriptic, stimulant. *What it affects:* Kidneys and stomach.

 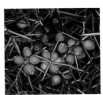 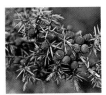

Juniper   Juniper   Juniper

Preparation and amount: *Infusion:* Steep 5-15 min. Take 3 oz. 1-3 times daily. *Decoction:* Simmer 5-15 min. Take 1-2 cups daily. *Tincture:* Take 5-20 drops 3 times daily. *Fluid extract:* Take ½-1 tsp. 3 times daily. *Oil:* Take 1-3 drops 2 times daily. *Powder:* Take up to 10 #0 capsules (up to 60 grains) daily.

Purposes: *Internally,* juniper berries act as a stimulating diuretic and are beneficial in the treatment of **urine retention, catarrh of the bladder, gravel, and pains in the lower back**. It is also good for **bladder discharges** and **uric acid buildup**. Take 1-3 drops of the oil, plus honey, 2 times a day. It is usually taken internally by eating the berries or making a tea from them. The berries eliminate **excess water**. The tea is a good douche for **vaginal infections**. It is helpful in the treatment of **asthma, fluid retention, and prostate disorders**. It is also used for **diabetes, cystitis, bladder diseases, allergies, arthritis, bed-wetting, hay fever, lumbago, and nephritis**.

Juniper berries are used for **gastro-intestinal infections and cramps, leukorrhea, gonorrhea, gouty and rheumatic pains**. It is an excellent **digestive** tonic. It helps in cases of reduced production of **stomach acid** (hydrochloric acid) and in regulating **blood sugar** levels.

As a spice, the berries are used to enhance flavor, **stimulate appetite**, and counteract **flatulence**. The berries can be made into a jam or syrup as an appetizer. A few dried berries can be chewed and taste good.

Externally, juniper oil, derived from the berries, penetrates the skin easily and is good for **bone and joint problems**. Inhaled in a vapor bath, it is useful for **bronchitis and infection in the lungs**. The berries can be boiled and then **sprayed in a room where sick people have been, to disinfect it**. It is said that those who are nursing patients with serious diseases should chew a few berries, to protect themselves from pathogenic substances which might be inhaled.J

Overseas: Juniper berries are one of the most widely used herbal **diuretics**. Approved in Germany in teas for **stomach complaints and to simulate appetite**. Science

confirms **anti-inflammatory and spasm-reducing** activity, which may contribute to diuretic activity. Fruits eaten raw or in tea are a folk remedy used. as a **diuretic and urinary antiseptic for cystitis, carminative for flatulence, antiseptic for intestinal infections**; Also for **colic, coughs, stomachaches, colds, and bronchitis**. Externally, used for **sores, aches, rheumatism, arthritis, snakebites, and cancer**. Volatile oil is responsible for **diuretic and intestinal antiseptic** activity. Diuretic activity results from irritation of renal tissue.

WARNING: Potentially toxic. Large or frequent doses cause kidney failure, convulsions, and digestive irritation. In Germany, use limited to four weeks. Avoid during pregnancy. Oil may cause blistering.

Large doses of juniper berries can be irritating to the kidneys and urinary passages. It may interfere with the absorption of iron and certain other minerals. It should not be used during pregnancy, nor by persons with kidney disease. It should not be used for a lengthy period of time by those with urinary tract or inflammatory diseases. The pure oil, placed on the skin in large quantities, can cause inflammation and blisters.

KELP

(Fucus vesiculosus) Part used: Whole plant. *Properties:* Demulcent, nutritive, alterative, diuretic. *What it affects:* Thyroid, nerves, brain, kidneys, and bladder.

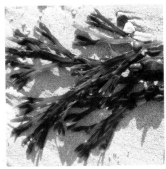 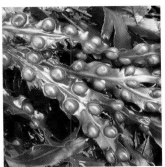

Kelp   Kelp

Preparation and amount: *Infusion:* Steep 5-15 min. Take 1-2 cups daily. *Tincture:* Take 5-10 drops 1-2 times daily. *Fluid extract:* Take 10 drops 1-2 times daily. *Powder:* Sprinkle on food. Take 1 tsp. 1-2 times daily. *Powder:* Take 3-5 #0 capsules (10-30 grains) 1-2 times daily.

Purposes: California kelp, Norwegian kelp, Nova Scotia dulse, and European Irish moss are all primarily useful for the trace minerals they contain. (California kelp is not as nutritionally good as the others.)

Internally, this seaweed provides an abundance of natural **iodine** which is missing from much of the soil on the continents. In addition to their nutritive value, when eaten, the seaweed **absorbs waste** from the body fluids, **binds with poisons**, and carries them off. A factor, called sodium alginate, in kelp binds with **radioactive strontium-90** in the intestines and carries it out of the body. This is an extremely important discovery.

Warning: It is said that, because of their high iodine content, very large quantities of seaweed could produce goiter-like symptoms. But, in reality, the excess trace minerals tend, rather quickly, to be eliminated in the sweat and through the kidneys.

LADY'S SLIPPER

(Cypredium pubescens) Part used: Root (fresh). *Properties:* Antispasmodic, nervine, sedative. *What it affects:* Nerves.

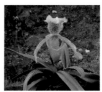 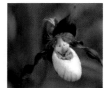 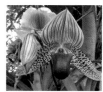

Lady's Slipper   Lady's Slipper   Lady's Slipper

Preparation and amount: *Infusion:* Steep 60 min. Take 1 Tbsp. every hour. *Decoction:* Simmer 60 min. Take 1 Tbsp. in 6 oz. water 3-4 times daily. *Tincture:* Take 5-30 drops 3 times daily. *Fluid extract:* Take ¼ tsp. 3 times daily. *Powder:* Take 2-10 #0 capsules (5-60 grains) 3 times daily.

Purposes: *Internally,* lady's slipper is **an excellent nervine** and acts as a tonic to an exhausted nervous system. It is said to be the best nervine relied upon for **chorea, epilepsy, hysteria, headache, insomnia, and general nervousness**. It is good for **nervous indigestion**. It has no narcotic (addictive) properties. Combined with ginger and a small amount of lobelia, it can be used for **nervousness associated with fevers**. Combined with chamomile or dandelion, it is a useful treatment for **stomach or liver problems**, including **hepatitis**. Combined with skullcap, it is used for **headaches and hysteria**. It is also good for **cholera, epilepsy, and nervous exhaustion**.

LEMON BALM

(Melissa officinalis) Part used: Tops. *Properties:* Diaphoretic, sedative, antitryptic, antispasmodic. *What it affects:* Nerves and circulation.

 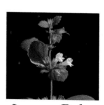 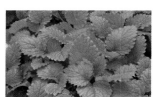

Lemon Balm Lemon Balm   Lemon Balm

Preparation and amount: *Infusion:* Steep 5-15 min. Take 6 oz. as needed frequently. *Tincture:* Take 30-60 drops (½-1 tsp.) as needed. *Fluid extract:* Take ½-2 tsp. as needed. *Powder:* Take 10 #0 Capsules (60 grains) as needed.

Purposes: *Internally,* lemon balm is a specific **for children and infants when indications of colds, flus, or fever** appear. Sweeten the tea with honey and give it hot to feverish children while they are covered with warm blankets. Or first put them into a hot bath with copious amounts of the tea; and then bundle them under blankets, to sweat it out.

Lemon balm is frequently used to cure **melancholy**

and **depression-induced sicknesses**. It is also good for **hysteria, cholera, insomnia, epilepsy, headache, nervous indigestion, and hepatitis**.

LICORICE ROOT

(Glycyrrhiza glabra) Part used: Root. *Properties:* Demulcent, expectorant, laxative, alterative. *What it affects:* Lungs, stomach, intestines, spleen, and liver.

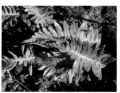 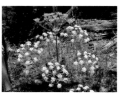

Licorice   Licorice   Licorice

Preparation and amount: *Decoction:* Simmer 5-15 min. Take 1 Tbsp. as needed. *Tincture:* Take 30-60 drops (½-1 tsp.) 2-3 times daily. *Fluid extract:* ½-1 tsp. 2-3 times daily. *Syrup:* Take 1 tsp. to 1 Tbsp. as needed. *Powder:* Take up to 10 #0 capsules (60 grains) daily.

Purposes: *Internally,* licorice is primarily used for **bronchial problems, coughs, hoarseness, mucous congestion, and similar problems**. It can also be taken for **stomach** problems, such as **peptic ulcers and bladder and kidney ailments**.

Added to bitter tonics, licorice root makes them more palatable and helps balance the herbal formula. It is excellent for all kinds of **stomach and intestinal ulcers**. It fights **inflammation and viral, bacterial, and parasitic infection**. It is a specific for **colds, flu, and lung congestion**, and is frequently added to cough syrups. It **cleanses the colon, reduces muscle spasms, increases the fluidity of mucus in the lungs and bronchial tubes**. It is a **mild laxative** and is effective for children and the elderly. It **helps to inhibit the formation of plaque and prevents bacteria from sticking to tooth enamel**. For **hoarseness and throat problems**, combine it with sage, ginger, horehound, and coltsfoot.

Licorice root is useful for **asthma, allergies, chronic fatigue, emphysema, depression, enlarged prostate, fever, herpesvirus, hypoglycemia, and glandular infection**. For **children's throat and lung problems**, combine licorice root powder with other herbs. Use it for **inflammatory bowel disorders, premenstual syndrome, and menopausal symptoms**. A strong decoction makes a good laxative for children and may also help **reduce fever**. Add it to other herbal medicines (and even drug medications), to make them more palatable. Use it for **upper respiratory tract infections**. It protects against **atherosclerosis**.

Licorice stimulates the production of interferon and may **help inhibit replication of HIV**. There is also evidence that it may **prevent hepatitis C from causing liver cancer and cirrhosis**.

Licorice extract has been shown to have **activities similar to those of cortisone** and, to a lesser extent, **estrogen**. It induces the adrenal cortex to produce larger amounts of cortisone and aldosterone. Glycyrrhizin, a chemical in licorice, has a chemical structure similar to human steroid hormones. Three other herbs (ginseng, wild yam, and sarsaparilla), all of which combine well with licorice, also have hormone-like substances in them. In Europe, licorice is used to help those with ulcers to recover.

Note: Licorice candy is useless because of its white sugar content and because it primarily consists of anise, not licorice.

Overseas: European forms of this (Wild Licorice, *Glcyrrhiza lepidota*) are used in Germany for **gastric and duodenal ulcers** and **congestion of upper respiratory tract**. Chinese research finds it **better than codeine**. Used for **gastric and duodenal ulcers, bronchial asthma, coughs**. One of the extensively used herbs in Chinese herbal prescriptions. Use it to **detoxify potentially poisonous drugs**. But in Germany not used for more than 4-6 weeks at a time, because longer use can increase blood pressure.

Warning: Licorice should not be used by persons with diabetes, glaucoma, heart disease, high blood pressure, or those who have had strokes. It should not be taken by those with severe menstrual problems or who are pregnant. It should not be used over seven days; for it can cause high blood pressure, even in those who have low or normal pressure. In addition, extended use can result in water retention or low potassium levels.

LOBELIA

(Lobelia inflata) Parts used: Plant and seeds. *Properties:* Antispasmodic, emetic, nervine, expectorant. *What it affects:* Nerves, lungs, stomach, muscles, and circulation.

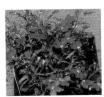 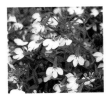 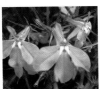

Lobelia   Lobelia   Lobelia

Preparation and amount: *Infusion:* Steep 5-15 min. Take 1 Tbsp. as needed. *Tincture:* Take 10-30 drops as needed. *Fluid extract:* Take 5-30 drops as needed. *Powder:* Take 1-2 #0 capsules (1-10 grains) as needed.

Purposes: Lobelia is both a relaxant and stimulant, and is a powerful helper.

Internally, in *very small doses* (5-10 drops of the tincture or one gelatin capsule), it is extremely relaxing for all **spasms**, both internally and externally; and it is used for **lung congestion** and as an **antispasmodic** in herbal formulas. In *slightly larger doses* (15 drops), it acts as a sedative. In *large doses* (40 drops of the tincture, or 2 gelatin capsules or more), it is a powerful **emetic**, and can be used to vomit up something which you want to get out of the stomach fast! For most conditions (unless you want to induce vomiting), you will only use *small doses*.

In small doses: Lobelia is very good for **asthma** and **whooping cough**. It is outstanding for **relieving spasms** associated with lung and respiratory conditions. As an **expectorant**, it is useful in all respiratory treatments, especially the spasmodic type, in expelling **phlegm**. Add it to all cough medicines. Combine it with lady's slipper for **convulsions**. Lobelia is also used for **headache, heart**

palpitation, indigestion, allergies, arthritis, asthma, chicken pox, contagious diseases, fevers (all kinds), jaundice, pleurisy, pneumonia, St. Vitus dance, teething, toothache**. It **relaxes the heart** and **lowers rapid pulse**. Combined with skullcap and lady's slipper, it is good for **lock jaw**.

In large doses: It is invaluable for **clearing the stomach** of its contents, food poisoning, etc.

Small doses: Externally, lobelia is a **wash for infected or itchy skin diseases**. It is put in baths, fomentations, poultices, and liniments for **muscle spasms**. A few drops of the tincture placed in the ear will relieve **earaches**. It is used in poultices for **bruises, sprains, felons, ringworm, erysipelas, poison ivy, snake and insect bites, poison ivy, and tumors**. Add it to liniments for **sore muscles, pains, and rheumatism**.

Overseas: Lobeline, a chemical cousin of nicotine, one of 14 alkaloids in the lobelia plant, until recently was used in the U.S. in commercial "quit smoking" lozenges, patches, and chewing gums—said **to appease physical need for nicotine without addictive effects**. Still used in other countries. Also produces **dilation of the bronchioles and increased respiration**.

Warning: Do not give very large doses of lobelia! Although it is poisonous in large amounts, it will be vomited so fast as to unlikely cause any permanent harm.

LUNGWORT

(Pulmonaria officinalis) Part used: Leaves. *Properties:* Demulcent, emollient, expectorant, mucilage, astringent, tonic, vulnerary. *What it affects:* Lungs, bronchials, intestines, and liver.

 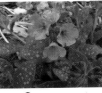 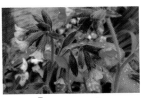

Lungwort   Lungwort   Lungwort

Preparation and amount: *Infusion:* Steep 5-15 min. Take 6 oz. at a time. *Tincture:* Take 15-30 drops 3 times daily. *Fluid extract:* Take ½-1 tsp. 3 times daily. *Powder:* Take 10 #0 capsules (60 grains) 3 times daily.

Purposes: *Internally,* lungwort tea is used primarily for the respiratory system, especially when there is **bleeding of the lungs**. It is reliable for **coughs, asthma, colds, and bronchial and catarrhal problems**. It will help **heal tissues** and **counteract inflammation**. It is also used for **diarrhea, hemorrhoids, and hoarseness**. It is also **mildly diuretic**.

Externally, lungwort tea is used for all kinds **wounds and swellings**. It is a good wash for **infected sores**.

MANDRAKE

(American)—*(Podophyllum peltatum) Part used:* Root. *Properties:* Cholagogue, hepatic, laxative, alterative, emetic, stimulant. *What it affects:* Liver, gallbladder, intestines, and skin.

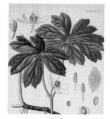
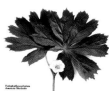
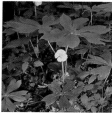

Mandrake   Mandrake   Mandrake

Preparation and amount: *Decoction:* Simmer 5-15 min. Take 1 Tbsp. (cold) 2 times daily. *Tincture:* Take 1-10 drops 2 times daily. *Fluid extract:* Take ¼-½ tsp. 2 times daily. *Powder:* Take 1-3 #0 Capsules 2 times daily.

Purposes: *Internally,* mandrake is a powerful **glandular stimulant** and should be taken in small amounts. It is used for **lymphatic problems, all skin diseases, liver diseases, and obstructions of the liver and gallbladder** (gallstones and jaundice), as well as **digestive problems**. It is best taken in small doses in combination with ginger, licorice, or Oregon grape root. American Indians used it as a **cathartic**. It is said to eliminate poisoning from **mercury** ingestion.

Externally, the concentrated tincture (by gently cooking it down) is directly applied to **warts**, to rapidly remove them. But it must only be put on the wart and not on the surrounding skin. Indians used the crushed rootstock on warts, but doing so could produce dermatitis. A diluted solution is applied to **skin diseases**.

Note: European mandrake *(Mandragora officinarum)* is a different herb, with different properties.

Warning: Only take mandrake in small doses. Large doses, even applied externally, produces nausea, vomiting, and inflammation of the intestines and the stomach lining. An overdose could be fatal. Taking it during pregnancy could cause birth defects. Placing it undiluted on the skin may cause dermatitis.

MARSHMALLOW

(Althea officinalis) Parts used: Root, flowers, and leaves. *Properties:* Demulcent, diuretic, emollient, lithotriptic, alterative, nutritive, vulnerary. *What it affects:* Intestines, kidneys, and bladder.

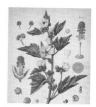

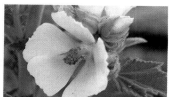

Marshmallow   Marshmallow   Marshmallow

Preparation and amount: *Infusion (flowers and leaves):* Steep 5-15 min. Take 1 cup at a time, frequently. *Decoction (root):* Simmer 5-15 min. Take 6 oz. 3 times daily. *Tincture:* Take 30-60 drops (½-1 tsp.) 3 times daily. *Fluid extract:* Take 1-2 tsp. 3 times daily. *Powder:* Take 5-10 #0 capsules (30-60 grains) 3 times daily.

Purposes: Marshmallow **soothes and heals skin, mucous membranes, and other tissues**, externally and internally. *Internally,* it is the best source of easily digested mucilage. It helps the body **lubricate joints, to protect them against dryness and irritation**. Because digestive fluids contain mucilage, marshmallow also acts as a **counter-irritant to the digestive tract** and aids in **diarrhea, dysentery, and ulcers**. It is also used for **lung problems** and as a douche in **vaginal infections**. It is good for **bladder infection**.

Use marshmallow with other laxative herbs for **chronic constipation** that is associated with dryness or lack of roughage. In combination with other diuretic herbs, such as parsley root, use it as tea for **kidney stone** attack and to help **expel gravel**. It is also used for **headache, sinusitis, sore throat, asthma, allergies**. Marshmallow is often used as 10% of the formula in various herbal mixtures.

Externally, as a poultice, marshmallow can be applied with a pinch of cayenne on a daily basis in order to treat **open wounds, burns, gangrene, septic wounds, bruises, and blood poisoning**. The tea is good to bathe **sore eyes**.

Ovrseas: Marshmallow roots and leaves traditionally used in tea for **sore throat** and **expectorant in bronchitis**. Externally poulticed for **bruises, sprains, aching muscles, and inflammations**. Root (up to 30 percent) and leaves (up to 16 percent) are high in mucilagin, responsible for demulcent or **soothing effect to irritated mucous membranes and skin**. Has **immuno-stimulating activity**. The German health authorities allow use of the leaf and root preparations to relieve local irritation (such as **digestive-tract inflammatory conditions**) and to soothe mucous membrane irritation, such as a **sore throat accompanied by dry cough**.

MOTHERWORT

(Leonurus cardiaca) Part used: Tops. *Properties:* Emmenagogue, nervine, tonic, antispasmodic, diaphoretic, laxative. *What it affects:* Nerves, heart, and uterus.

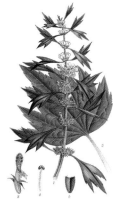
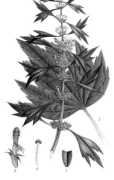

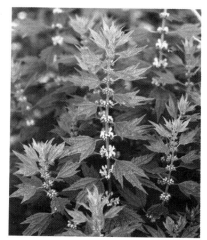

Motherwort   Motherwort

Preparation and amount: *Infusion:* Steep 5-15 min. Take 6 oz. 3-4 times daily. *Tincture:* Take 30-60 drops (½-1 tsp.) 3-4 times daily. *Fluid extract:* Take ½-1 tsp. 3-4 times daily. *Powder:* Take 5-10 #0 capsules (30-60 grains) 3-4 times daily.

Purposes: *Internally,* motherwort is most commonly

used for **nervous heart problems** and for **stomach gas and cramps**. For this purpose, a good combination is equal parts of motherwort, cramp bark, and calendula. It relieves **childbirth pain** and is excellent for **suppressed menstruation** and **other female problems**, including amenorrhea. It is a good tonic for the heart and may be combined with hawthorn berries for an effective **heart tonic** and **antispasmodic**. This can be used to prevent **heart attack** and treat **palpitations, pericarditis, and neuralgia**. It is good for **all nervous conditions, sleeplessness, convulsions, neuritis, neuralgia, and hysteria**. It is used for **shortness of breath, goiter, and congestion of respiratory passages**. It is also used for **menopausal symptoms and vaginitis**. It is used for headache, thyroid, insomnia, verti**go, fevers, rheumatism, and suppressed urine**. In general, it has similar properties to valerian, and can be used like it.

Overseas: Extracts approved in Germany for **nervous heart conditions** and in the supportive treatment of **hyperthyroidism**. Experimentally, *leonurine*, a leaf constituent, is a **uterine tonic**. Chinese species, well documented with laboratory and clinical reports, have been used similarly.

Warning: Contact with the plant may cause dermatitis in some individuals.

MUGWORT

(Artemisia vulgaris) Part used: Tops. *Properties:* Emmenagogue, nervine, stomachic, diaphoretic, diuretic. *What it affects:* Nerves, circulation, stomach, and uterus.

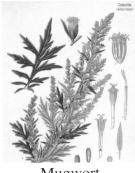
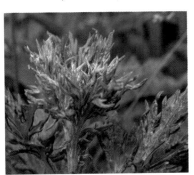

Mugwort   Mugwort

Preparation and amount: *Infusion:* Steep 20 min. Take 1 tsp. as needed. *Tincture:* Take 30-60 (½-1 tsp.) as needed. *Fluid extract:* Take 1 tsp. as needed. *Powder:* Take up to 10 #0 capsules (up to 60 grains) as needed.

Purposes: *Internally,* mugwort is excellent for **nervousness, insomnia, and controllable shaking**. It is also good for **female problems**, such as **suppressed menstruation and menstrual cramps**. It is especially good when combined with cramp bark, marigold, and black haw for these problems. It will **bring on the menstrual period**; and it is used with cramp bark to treat **menstrual cramps** and **other female problems**. The tea is useful in treating stomach disorders. For this purpose, it is diluted 3 times, to overcome the strong taste. For pains in the stomach and bowels, drink the tea in small frequent doses and apply a fomentation of the infusion over the painful area. It is good in kidney herb combinations for **stones or gravel**.

American Indians used it for **colds and flus, bronchitis and fevers**. Drink it hot for a **sweating therapy**. It is also used for **asthma, difficulty in breathing, bronchitis, hay fever, earache, epilepsy, and swollen glands**.

Externally, mugwort may be applied as a poultice to **boils, carbuncles, and abscesses**.

Overseas: Experiments reveal that it **lowers blood sugar**. Components have **antibacterial and antifungal** activity.

MULLEIN

(Great Mullein)—*(Verbascum thapsus) Part used:* Leaf. *Properties:* Demulcent, expectorant, antispasmodic, astringent, diuretic, vulnerary. *What it affects:* Lungs, glands, and lymph.

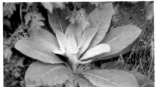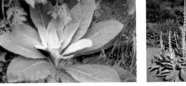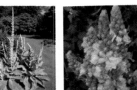

Mullein   Mullein   Mullein

Preparation and amount: *Infusion:* Steep 5-15 min. Take 3 oz. frequently. *Tincture:* Take 30-60 drops (½-1 tsp.) frequently. *Fluid extract:* Take ½-1 tsp. frequently. *Oil:* Take 2-3 drops 2-3 times daily. *Powder:* Take up to 10 #0 capsules (60 grains) frequently.

Purposes: *Internally,* mullein tea is a good remedy for **coughs, bronchitis, bronchial catarrh, and whooping cough**. It is commonly used as a **nervine and antispasmodic**. It can be used for **gastro-intestinal catarrh** and **cramps in the digestive tract**. It is useful for **hemorrhoids, diarrhea, hemorrhages of the lungs, and shortness of breath**. For **lungs and coughs**, use a tea made of mullein, yerba santa, wild cherry bark, licorice, and comfrey root. It is used in **kidney formulas**, to soothe inflammations. The leaves are also used to treat **lymphatic congestion**. It is also used for **hay fever, swollen glands, diarrhea, asthma, sinus congestion, and tumors**.

Externally, mullein oil is one of the best remedies for **ear infection**. Put 2-3 drops of the warm oil in the ear overnight or 2-3 times daily. It is also used for the lymphatic congestion that results in **earaches**, as well as **toothaches**. For external use on **inflammations or painful skin conditions**, use the tea or a fomentation of the leaves boiled or steeped in vinegar and water. It is also used for **diaper rashes** and **inflamed eyes**.

Four different herbs are called "mullein." The primary medicinal one is described here. The others are black mullein *(Verbascum nigrum)* and two European species: common mullein *(Verbascum phlomoides)* and orange mullein *(Verbascum phlomoides)*. The last two have medicinal properties similar to great mullein.

Overseas: Common Mullein *(Verbascum thapsus)* is originally from Europe, Flowers are there preferred over leaves; both are used in European **cough remedies**. Leaves high in mucilage, **soothing to inflamed mucous membranes**. In Germany, approved by the government as an **expectorant in inflammations of the upper respira-**

tory tract. Folk in India used the stalk for **cramps, fevers, and migraine**. Leaves high in mucilage, soothing to **inflamed mucous membranes**; experimentally, strongly **anti-inflammatory**. Science confirms **mild expectorant and antiviral activity against herpes simplex and influenza viruses**; used against both. Contains *verbascoside*, which has **antiseptic, antitumor, antibacterial, and immunosuppressant activity**. They also used the stalk for **cramps, fevers, and migraine**. The seed is used as a narcotic fish poison.

MYRRH

(Commiphora mayrrha) Part used: Gum. *Properties:* Antiseptic, emmenagogue, carminative, expectorant, stimulant. *What it affects:* Stomach and lungs.

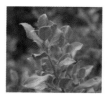 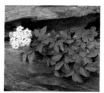 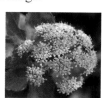

Myrrh   Myrrh   Myrrh

Preparation and amount: *Infusion:* Steep 5-15 min. Take 3 oz. 3-4 times daily. *Tincture:* 30-60 drops (½-1 tsp.) 3-4 times daily. *Powder:* Take 2-6 #0 capsules (10-40 grains) 3-4 times daily.

Purposes: Myrrh is a strong antiseptic and works well with goldenseal. Mix them in equal parts.

Internally, **myrrh is a powerful antiseptic, and ranks with goldenseal and echinacea**. It is often combined in equal parts with goldenseal as a specific for **intestinal ulcers, intestinal catarrh, bad breath, and other mucous membrane problems**. It is an antiseptic, disinfectant, expectorant, and deodorizer. Myrrh destroys **putrefaction in the intestines** and **prevents blood absorption of toxins**. The tincture added to water is an excellent mouth wash for **spongy gums, pyorrhea, and all throat diseases**. It destroys **putrefication in the intestines**. It stimulates the **immune system and gastric secretions**; and it is good for **sinusitis, sore throat, herpes simplex, and ulcers**. It **treats chronic diarrhea, lung disease, and general body weaknesses**.

Use myrrh for **hemorrhoids, bedsores, asthma, boils, cankers, chronic catarrh, colitis, coughs, digestive tonic, bleeding gums, herpes, indigestion, infections, leukorrhea, mouth sores, skin disease, thrush, and ulcers**. Small doses will help **remove toxins from the stomach and intestines**.

Externally, myrrh is used for **cankers, cuts, bleeding gums, leukorrhea, abscesses, boils, mouth sores, skin disease, thrush, and wounds**. It is a good wash for **wounds and skin diseases**. The powder will **dry up most skin problems**. It is excellent for most problems involving **pus**, externally or internally. It helps fight **harmful bacteria in the mouth**. Insert the tincture of myrrh in the sinuses for **all sinus infections and inflammations.** If the sinuses are too sensitive, dilute it with water.

Note: Other gums and resinous materials from conifers, such as pine and fir, have similar properties.

Warning: Myrrh and other gums should not be used in large amounts over a long period of time, for they contain potent volatile oils that are toxic in large amounts.

NETTLES

(Urtica urens) Part used: Tops. *Properties:* Alterative, nutritive, antiseptic, expectorant, hemostatic. *What it affects:* Lungs, kidneys, bladder, and blood.

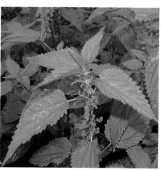 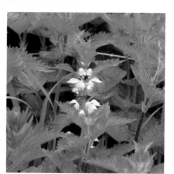

Nettles   Nettles

Preparation and amount: *Infusion:* Steep 5-15 min. Take 3 oz. frequently. *Tincture:* Take 5-15 drops frequently. *Fluid extract:* Take ½-1 tsp. frequently. *Powder:* Take 3-10 #0 capsules (20-60 grains) frequently. *Juice:* 1 tsp. as needed.

Purposes: *Internally,* nettles is considered a specific for **asthma** when taken over a prolonged period, providing an **expectorant and antispasmodic**. The tea will **expel phlegm from the lungs**. Combine it with equal parts of comfrey, mullein, and a pinch of lobelia. Make a tea from this formula; and, using an ounce of herbs steeped in a pint of boiled water, take 4 times a day. The seeds are used in **cough** medicines. The leaves can be pounded and used as a poultice for **rheumatic pains**. The tea made from the root will help cure **dropsy**.

Nettles is good for **benign prostatic hyperplasia, anemia, hay fever, and other allergic disorders**. The tea is good for **kidney problems, diarrhea, dysentery, arthritis, inflammatory conditions, hemorrhoids, goiter, mucous conditions of the lungs, and gravel in the kidneys**. To stop **intestinal bleeding**, extract the fresh juice and take 1 tsp. every hour. Use it as a tea for **anemia** in children. The fresh leaves may be used in **salads**.

Externally, a poultice of nettles and slippery elm will **stop bleeding** when applied to the skin. Use fresh leaves. It stimulates **hair follicle growth**, and reduces a buildup of **scalp oils**. Use it as a hair rinse, to restore **natural color**.

Note: An antidote to poisoning from nettle sting is fresh bruised yellow dock that is rubbed over the affected area.

OAT STRAW

(Avena sataiva) Parts used: Stem and fruit. *Properties:* Nervine, tonic, antispasmodic, stimulant. *What it affects:* Nerves, uterus, stomach, and lungs.

Preparation and amount: *Infusion:* Steep 5-15 min. Take 6 oz. 3 times daily. *Tincture:* Take 30-60 drops 3 times daily. *Fluid extract:* Take 1 tsp. 3 times daily. *Powder:* Take up to 10 #0 capsules (60 grains) 3 times daily.

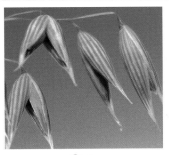

Oats

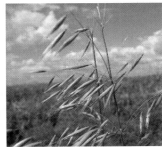

Oats

Purposes: *Internally,* oat straw tea is recommended for **chest and kidney** problems. It acts as an **antidepressant** and a **restorative nerve tonic**. It **increases perspiration**. For **bed-wetting,** give this tea to children. It is also good for **insomnia, colic, depression, stress, epilepsy, heart palpitation, occipital headaches, weak muscles from nerve exhaustion, nervous diseases, and stomach problems**.

Externally, oat straw tea is used in Europe for **various baths** which, when taken regularly, is helpful for a number of ailments. *Full bath* (adding a gallon of the tea to the bath): good for **rheumatic problems, paralysis, lumbago, liver ailments, gout, kidney and gravel problems**. *Sitz bath:* **bladder and abdominal problems, intestinal colic, and bed-wetting**. *Local wash:* **skin diseases, frostbite, flaky skin, wounds, chilblains, and eye problems**.

Fresh oats (not oat straw): An extract made from fresh oat berries, picked when the milky substance is in the grain, is good for the **brain** and functions of the body. It is a specific for **weak nerves** and can be used as a nerve tonic. It will overcome **most diseases caused by nervous disorders and physical exhaustion,** including **ovarian and uterine disorders**.

OLIVE

(Olea europaea) Parts used: Leaves, bark, fruit. *Properties: Oil:* Cholagogue, demulcent, emollient, laxative. *Leaves:* Antiseptic, astringent, febrifuge, tranquilizer. *What it affects:* Digestive tract, other internal organs, blood.

Olive

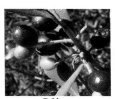

Olive

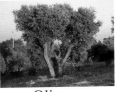

Olive

Preparation and amount: *Infusion:* Steep 1-2 tsp. of leaves in 1 cup of water for 10 min. Take 2 tsp. *Decoction:* Boil 2 handfuls of leaves or bark in 1 quart water until 1 cup of liquid remains. *Oil:* As a laxative, take 1-2 fluid oz.; as a cholagogue, take 1-2 tsp. at a time.

Purposes: The olive has been used for food and medicine from earliest times. *Internally,* a decoction of the leaves or inner bark of the tree is effective against **fever**. An infusion of the leaves has a **calming effect** on nervous people.

Olive oil, taken internally, **increases the secretion of bile** and acts as a **laxative** by encouraging muscular contraction in the bowels. It is soothing to the **mucous membranes** and is said to dissolve **cholesterol**.

The leaf of the olive helps the system resist **colds and flus**. It fights **bacteria, viruses, fungi, and parasites**; and it is good for **most infectious diseases**. It appears to **lower blood pressure**. It is also used for **diarrheal diseases, inflammatory arthritis, psoriasis, and chronic fatigue syndrome**.

Externally, olive oil is useful for **insect bites, sprains, burns, bruises, and intense itching** (pruritus). Combined with rosemary, it is helpful in treating **dandruff**.

Note: Olive oil is frequently used as a base for liniments and ointments. Only use cold-pressed olive oil.

ONION

(Allium cepa) Part used: Bulb. *Properties:* Anthelmintic, antiseptic, antispasmodic, carminative, diuretic, expectorant, stomachic, tonic. *What it affects:* Digestive tract, other internal organs, blood.

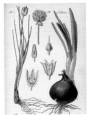

Onion

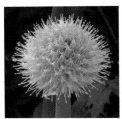

Onion

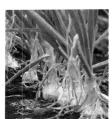

Onion

Preparation and amount: *Juice:* Take 1 tsp. 3-4 times a day. *Cold extract:* Soak a chopped onion in 1 cup of water for 24 hours and strain. Take ½ cup daily. *Decoction:* Boil a medium-size, chopped onion in a little more than a cup of water until 1 cup of liquid remains. Take 1 Tbsp. several times a day for several days.

Purposes: *Internally,* onion juice is most often used as a **diuretic** or **expectorant**. But it has been used, for ages, for **worms** and **spasms**. It **expels gas**, is a **general tonic**, and **tones the stomach**. As an **antiseptic**, it helps to **eliminate putrefaction and fermentation processes in the gastro-intestinal tract**. It helps **strengthen the heart and lower blood pressure**. Mixed with honey, onion juice is good for **hoarseness and coughs**.

Externally, onion juice can be placed on **suppurating wounds**.

Warning: A California research study of volunteers found that onion oil, used heavily over a period of time, will cause very serious iron anemia.

OREGON GRAPE ROOT

(Berberis aquifolium) Part used: Root. *Properties:* Alterative, antiseptic, cholagogue, laxative, tonic. *What it affects:* Liver, stomach, intestines, blood, and skin.

Preparation and amount: *Infusion:* Simmer 10 min. Take 3 oz. 3 times daily. *Decoction:* Steep 10 min. Take 3 oz. 3 times daily (before meals, made fresh each day). *Tincture:* Take 30-60 drops (½-1 tsp.) 3 times daily. *Fluid* *extract:* Take ½-1 tsp. 3 times daily. *Powder:* Take 2-5 capsules (15-30 grains) several times a day.

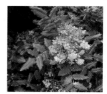 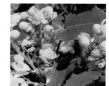 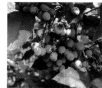

Oregon Grape   Oregon Grape   Oregon Grape

Purposes: *Internally,* Oregon grape root stimulates the **secretion of bile**. In this way, it aids in digestion and is a good blood purifier. It **cleanses the liver**. By stimulating the liver and gallbladder, it helps to overcome **constipation**.

Although almost identical to barberry in its action, Oregon grape root affects the **liver** more strongly and stimulates the **thyroid**. It is a **tonic for all the glands** and helps the **assimilation of nutrients**. Its antiseptic qualities favorably affect the **kidneys**.

Oregon grape root is useful in the treatment of all **skin diseases** which are due to toxins in the blood. This includes **psoriasis, eczema, herpes, and acne**. It is also used in treating **bronchial congestion, hepatitis, and rheumatoid arthritis**. Its mild antiseptic effects makes it useful in douches for **vaginitis**. It acts as a **laxative**.

Note: Oregon grape root acts on the body in a manner quite similar to goldenseal and barberry. It is good for chronic skin problems, including acne, eczema, herpes, and psoriasis.

PARSLEY

(Petroselinum sativum) Parts used: Root, leaves, seeds. *Properties:* Nutritive, diuretic; carminative, expectorant, nervine, tonic. *What it affects:* Kidneys, bladder, stomach, liver, and gallbladder.

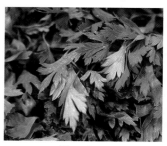 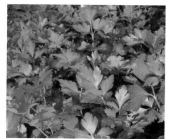

Parsley   Parsley

Preparation and amount: *Infusion (leaves):* Steep 5-15 min. Take 6 oz. 2-3 times daily. *Decoction (root and seeds):* Simmer 5-15 min. Take 6 oz. 2-3 times daily. *Tincture:* Take 30-60 drops (½-1 tsp.) 2-3 times daily. *Fluid extract:* Take ½-1 tsp. 2-3 times daily. *Fresh juice:* Take 2 oz. 2 times daily. *Powder:* Take 2-5 #0 capsules (10-30 grains) several times daily.

Purposes: *Internally,* parsley tea (especially that made from the seeds, leaves, and also the fresh juice) is used for **dropsy, asthma, coughs, and suppressed or difficult menstruation**. The root is good for **jaundice**. It is excellent for **difficult urination, stones, and obstruc-**

tions of the liver and spleen**. It helps the function of the **thyroid**. The leaves have repeatedly been used for **bladder infections**, especially when taken with equal parts of echinacea and marshmallow root. However, parsley is a warming herb; so it is best avoided during acute infections and inflammations, especially in the kidneys. It **expels worms, relieves gas, and freshens breath**.

A few slices of parsley root, cooked in soup, will strengthen weak or sensitive persons. The fresh juice of the leaves (2 oz. daily in apple juice) is an excellent **blood tonic** and remedy for **simple anemia**. It is good for **bedwetting, fluid retention, high blood pressure, indigestion, obesity, and prostate disorders**. The root can be prepared as a decoction, in combination with dandelion, chicory, and burdock, making a total of 1 oz. of roots per pint of water simmered for about 1 hour.

Parsley contains a substance that **prevents the spread of cancer cells**. In addition, the high chlorophyll content of the leaves makes this herb very useful in treating **cancer**. The seeds contain *apiol*, which is considered a safe and efficient emmenagogue, used for **amenorrhea** and **dysmenorrhea**. Combine it with buchu, cramp bark, and black haw for **female problems**. It is good to drink the fresh juice daily.

Externally, parsley juice has been used successfully in treating conjunctivitis and inflammation of the eyelids (blepharitis).

PASSIONFLOWER

(Passifloria incarnata) Parts used: Plant and flower. *Properties:* Antispasmodic, sedative, diaphoretic. *What it affects:* Nerves and circulation.

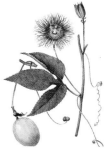 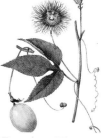

Passion Flower   Passion Flower

Preparation and amount: *Infusion:* Steep 5-15 min. Take 1 cup during the day. *Tincture:* Take 15-60 drops in water as needed. *Fluid extract:* Take 10-20 drops as needed. *Powder:* Take 1-2 #0 capsules (3 -10 grains) as needed.

Purposes: *Internally,* Passionflower is most commonly used for **nervous conditions**—such as **restlessness, insomnia, nervous headaches, and hysteria**. It is normally used with other herbs as part of a prolonged treatment. It is helpful for **anxiety, neuritis, anxiety, and stress-related disorders**. It is used for **nervousness** in children, such as **muscle twitching and irritability**. In the elderly, it is good for **nerve debility and sciatica**. It has a **gentle sedative effect** and helps **reduce blood pressure**.

Passionflower is also used for **hiccups, spasms, coughs, eye tension, convulsions, and back tension**. It is used for **headaches, fevers, and reduced pulse during high fevers**. It stimulates **perspiration**.

Note: Some herbalists recommend that you only use professionally prepared herbal medications.

Overseas: The whole plant is approved in Germany for **nervous restlessness, nervous tension**; considered especially useful in **sleep disturbances or anxiety arising from restlessness. Fruits edible, delicious**.

Warning: Passionflower should not be taken during pregnancy, since it may cause uterine stimulation.

PAU D'ARCO

(Lapacho or Taheebo) (Tabebuia heptaphylla)—Pau d'arco is a South American herb which, *internally,* fights **bacterial and viral infections; cleanses the blood**; and is useful for **AIDS, cancer, tumors, ulcers, candidiasis, smoker's cough, allergies, cardiovascular problems, inflammatory bowel disease, rheumatism, and all types of infections**. Only the inner bark is used. It has similar **antibiotic and anti-cancer properties** to chaparral, but is less harsh.

 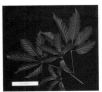 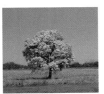

Pau D'Arco   Pau D'Arco   Pau D'Arco

PENNYROYAL

(American Pennyroyal)—*(Hedeoma pulegioides) Part used:* Tops. *Properties:* Diaphoretic, emmenagogue, carminative, stimulant. *What it affects:* Circulation, uterus, and lungs.

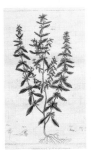 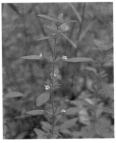 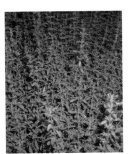

Pennyroyal   Pennyroyal   Pennyroyal

Preparation and amount: *Infusion:* Steep 5-15 min. Take 6 oz. frequently. *Tincture:* Take 30-60 drops (½-1 tsp.) frequently. *Fluid extract:* Take 1-2 drops frequently. *Powder:* Take 3-10 #0 capsules (20-60 grains) frequently.

Purposes: *Internally,* pennyroyal is especially used for **all fevers and lung infections**. It drives out the heat and inflammation through the pores of the skin and helps the circulation. The warm infusion used freely will promote **perspiration**. It is good for **nervous headaches, intestinal pains, cramps, hysteria, nervousness, and colds**. It is also used for **convulsions, lung congestion, and colic**.

A warm infusion promotes **menstruation**. Use hot footbaths of the tea, to **bring on the menstrual flow**. It is thus useful in regulating menstrual flow and for **relieving cramps**. But it should not be used by those who have a tendency toward excessive menstruation.

Externally, because it is a very strong smelling mint, pennyroyal is used to **repel insects** such as mosquitoes, flies, and fleas. It is also used for **itching and skin diseases**.

Note: The American species *(Hedeoma pulegioides)* and the European species *(Mentha pulegium)* have similar properties. So either one can be used.

Warning: It is urgent that penneyroyal not be taken during pregnancy!

PEPPERMINT

(Mentha piperita) Part used: Leaves. *Properties:* Aromatic, carminative, diaphoretic, stimulant, antispasmodic. *What it affects:* Stomach, intestines, muscles, and circulation.

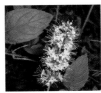 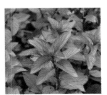

Peppermint   Peppermint   Peppermint

Preparation and amount: *Infusion:* Steep 5-15 min. Take 6 oz. 3 times daily. *Tincture:* Take 30-60 drops 3 times daily. *Fluid extract:* Take ½-2 tsp. 3 times daily. *Oil:* Take 5-10 drops 3 times daily. *Powder:* Take up to 10 #0 capsules (up to 60 grains) 3 times daily.

Purposes: Peppermint is an old household remedy and useful for a variety of conditions.

Internally, peppermint **slightly anesthetizes mucous membranes and the gastro-intestinal tract**. The tea or oil is useful for **insomnia, migraine, measles, menstrual cramps, migraines, morning sickness, muscle spasms, chills, headache, nausea, nervous disorders, colic, fevers, dizziness, gas, vomiting, diarrhea, dysentery, heart trouble, poor appetite, rheumatism, spasms, and hysteria**. It increases **stomach acidity, aiding digestion, and is useful for irritable bowel syndrome**. It will **stop vomiting due to nervous causes**.

Externally, peppermint leaves make a **cooling and slightly anodyne application**. They can also be made into a salve or a bath additive for **itching skin conditions**. Peppermint is used for **toothache** and to provide **local anesthetic to pains and inflamed joints**. For example, to **open up the sinuses**, put 5-10 drops into 2 quarts hot water and breathe it in through the mouth and nostrils. Cover the head with a cloth as you do this.

Note: Peppermint tea makes a good **substitute for coffee or tea**. The other mints are spearmint and catnip; both of these are included in this herb list.

Overseas: Peppermint capsules are used in Europe for **irritable bowel syndrome**. Peppermint leaf is approved by the government in Germany for use in **muscle spasms of the gastrointestinal tract**, as well as **spasms of the**

H E R B S

gallbladder and bile ducts. The essential oil is used externally to treat **neuralgia and myalgia**. Menthol is an approved ingredient in cough drops. The oil **stops spasms of smooth muscles**. Animal experiments show that *azulene*, a minor component of distilled Peppermint oil residues, is **anti-inflammatory** and has **anti-ulcer** activity.

WARNING: Oil is toxic if taken internally; causes dermatitis. Menthol, the major chemical component of Peppermint oil, may cause allergic reactions. Infants should never be exposed to menthol-containing products, as they can cause the lungs to collapse. Use should be avoided in cases of gallbladder or bile duct obstruction.

PIPSISSEWA

(Prince's Pine)—(Chimaphila umbellata) Part used: Tops. *Properties:* Alterative, diuretic, astringent, tonic. *What it affects:* Urinary tract, liver, skin, and circulation.

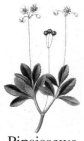
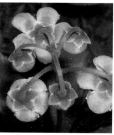
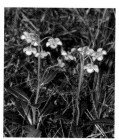

Pipsissewa   Pipsissewa   Pipsissewa

Preparation and amount: *Infusion:* Steep 5-15 min. Take 3 oz. as needed. *Tincture:* Take 15-60 drops as needed. *Fluid extract:* Take ½-1 tsp. as needed. *Powder:* Take 5-10 #0 capsules (30-90 grains) as needed.

Purposes: *Internally,* pipsissewa is a good remedy for **kidney and bladder** problems. It is especially good at producing diuretic action without irritant side-effects. Combined with dandelion, goldenseal, and yellow dock, it is good for all blood troubles and **diseases of the urinary organs**. It excellent for **burning urine, urethral and prostate irritation, catarrh of the bladder, and relaxed bladder**. Prolonged use of the leaf tea is said to **dissolve bladder stones**. For most **liver, kidney, joint, and skin problems**, a combination of this herb with Oregon grape root, taken frequently throughout the day, will prove very helpful.

It is also used for **rheumatic problems, scrofula, dropsy, albuminuria, hematuria, chronic kidney problems, and gonorrhea**. One cup of tea, 3 times daily (or 20 drops of tincture, 3 times a day), is the usual dosage. Karok Indian women in their late eighties would drink a quart or two a day for **stiffness and genito-urinary problems**.

Externally, a tea or poultice made from pipsissewa can be applied to **blisters, ulcerous sores, tumors, and swellings**.

PLANTAIN

Common Plantain (Plantago major) and *Lance-leaf Plantain (plantago lanceolata). Parts used:* Leaves and seeds. *Properties:* Diuretic, emollient, alterative, antiseptic, astringent, deobstruent, expectorant, vulnerary.

What it affects: Kidneys, veins, intestines, and externally on the skin.

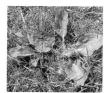
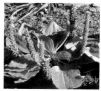
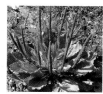

Plantain   Plantain   Plantain

Preparation and amount: *Infusion (leaf):* Steep 5-15 min. 3 oz. 3-4 times daily. *Decoction (seed):* Simmer 1 oz. seeds in 1½ pints of water; reduce to 1 pint; sweeten with honey. Take 1 Tbsp. 3-4 times daily. *Tincture:* Take 2-60 drops 3-4 times daily. *Fluid extract:* Take ½-1 tsp. 3-4 times daily. *Powder:* Take up to 10 #0 capsules (up to 60 grains) 3-4 times daily.

Purposes: There are several plantains, but they all have the same properties. The two primary ones are common plantain *(plantago major),* which has an almost circular leaf, and the lesser-used lance-leaf plantain *(plantago lanceolata),* which has very narrow leaves. The wider the leaf, the greater the diuretic effect.

Internally, plantain has **soothing, cooling properties** which make it effective in a wide range of maladies, including **infections, inflammations, diarrhea, ulcers, bronchitis, and excessive menstrual discharge**. Make an infusion using an ounce of the herb in a pint of water. It acts as a **diuretic** and is soothing to the **lungs and urinary tract**. It is excellent for **acute neuralgia**; for this, take 2-5 drops of tincture every 20 minutes. It is a good remedy for **cough irritations, hoarseness, gastritis, and enteritis**. It is helpful for all **respiratory problems**, especially those involving **mucous congestion**. It is useful for **indigestion and heartburn**.

It is useful in the treatment of **water retention and kidney and bladder infections**. It will **neutralize stomach acids** and normalize all **stomach secretions**. It may slow the growth of tuberculosis bacteria.

The seeds are similar to psyllium seeds. And, if taken in amounts of 1 tsp. of powdered juice 3 times a day, it will provide an excellent bulk **laxative**. Soaked overnight in water, this will produce a gel. Then bring it to a boil, turn off the fire, and let it steep for 10 minutes. Press the gel through a strainer and use for ulcers, intestinal pains, and spitting up of blood. Inject a cup of the tea several times a day into the colon for **hemorrhoids**. Use it as a douche for **vaginal difficulties**. The fresh juice, pressed from the whole plant, is good for **chronic catarrhal problems, gastro-intestinal difficulties, and worms**.

Externally, plantain has a healing, antibiotic, and styptic (**blood stanching**) effect when applied to **sores and wounds**. It is commonly known to **neutralize the toxins of insect and snakebites**. Put freshly ground leaves (or chewed slightly) onto the bites of **snakes, insects, and bees**. A decoction of the dried leaves promotes **coagulation of blood**. Place a salve of it on **boils, carbuncles, and eczema**. The fresh juice extract is good for **itchy skin**. At the same time, swallow a tablespoon of the fresh juice. Plantain is an excellent remedy for **skin infections, cuts,** scratches, and chronic skin problems. It is used in a variety of salves and ointments, alone or in combination with other herbs (such as chickweed, comfrey, mugwort, and angelica). Apply the fresh leaves to **wounds, sores, insect bites, ringworm, and even hemorrhoids**. Chewing the rootstock will give temporary relief from **toothache**.

Overseas: The Asian form, *P asiatica* is used clinically in China to **reduce blood pressure** (50% success rate). Common Plantain *(Plantago major)* is a prominent folk **cancer remedy** in Latin America. Used widely for this purpose throughout the world. Is both **antimicrobial** and **stimulates healing process**.

PLEURISY ROOT

(Asclepias tuberosa) Part used: Root. *Properties:* Diaphoretic, expectorant, antispasmodic, carminative, diuretic, nervine, tonic. *What it affects:* Lungs, kidneys, and nerves.

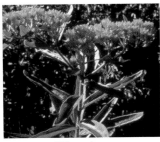
Pleurisy

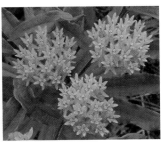
Pleurisy

Preparation and amount: *Infusion:* Steep 30 min. Take 1-2 cups daily; children should take 1-5 drops in hot water every 1-2 hours. *Decoction:* Simmer 5-15 min. Take 2-3 oz. as needed. *Tincture:* Take 30-60 drops every 3 hours. *Fluid extract:* Take ½-1 tsp. 3-4 times daily. *Powder:* Take 3-5 # 0 capsules (20-30 grains) 3-4 times daily.

Purposes: *Internally,* pleurisy root was widely used as an **expectorant** in the nineteenth century. It is ideal for **pleurisy and pneumonia**. In severe cases, combine equal parts of it with an infusion of skullcap, given in small amounts (2 oz.) every half hour while the patient is warmly tucked in bed. It is an excellent sweating agent to **break up colds, flus, pleurisy, and bronchial problems**. Sometimes it is given with cayenne at the beginning of a cold. American Indians chewed the dried root or made a tea, by boiling the root, as a remedy for **chest problems or dysentery**. It **reduces the inflammation of the pleural membranes of the lungs, stimulates the lymphatic system, and encourages the flow of normal lung fluids**. It is also good for **children's stomach and bowel disorders**. For bowel problems, use 1 tablespoon to a quart of boiling water; steep for 30 minutes and use warm as an enema for this.

Warning: Animals have been poisoned by eating the leaves and stems. The fresh root may also produce toxic effects.

PRICKLY ASH

(Xanthoxylum americanum) Part used: Bark. *Properties:* Stimulant, alterative, antispasmodic/astringent, emmenagogue, rubefacient. *What it affects:* Blood, circulation, and stomach.

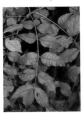
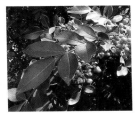
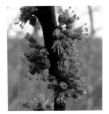
Prickly Ash   Prickly Ash   Prickly Ash

Preparation and amount: *Decoction:* Simmer 5-15 min. Take 1-2 oz. 3-4 times daily. *Tincture:* Take 5-20 drops 3-4 times daily. *Fluid extract:* Take ½-1 tsp. 3-4 times daily. *Powder:* Take 2-5 #0 capsules (10-30 grains) 3-4 times daily.

Purposes: *Internally,* prickly ash is a stimulant that **greatly increases blood circulation** throughout the body. For this reason, it is used for **impaired circulation, cold extremities and joints, wounds that are slow to heal, lethargy, rheumatism, and arthritis**. It will **promote warmth during chills**. Add a carminative herb (such as peppermint or catnip) to prickly ash, to increase the effect. Because it is so warming to the stomach, it is used for **weak digestion**, as well as **colic and cramps**. If an excess amount of unwanted sweating occurs, reduce the amount by a fourth, until the amount taken is producing the desired effect. This herb will produce **sweating** when all else fails.

Externally, prickly ash bark was a **toothache** remedy for both the Indians and early settlers. Indians also boiled the inner bark to make a wash for **itching skin**. Herbalists today use boiled fresh bark (inner and outer) for the same purpose. It is applied as a poultice, to help **dry up and heal wounds**.

Note: As a stimulant, prickly ash bark is very similar to bayberry bark.

PSYLLIUM

(Plantago psyllium) Part used: Seeds. *Properties:* Demulcent, laxative. *What it affects:* Intestines.

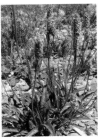
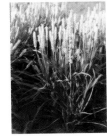
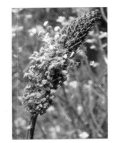
Psyllium   Psyllium   Psyllium

Preparation and amount: *Infusion:* Steep 5-15 min. Take 2-4 tsp. after each meal; children take 1 tsp. after each meal. *Powder:* Take 1 tsp. in warm water or juice, 3 times daily. *Powder:* Take 6-8 #0 capsules (50-60 grains) 3 times daily.

Purposes: *Internally,* psyllium seed is a faithful standby. Either the powder or the soaked seed will assist

H
E
R
B
S

easy bowel movements during colitis, inflamed ulcers, and hemorrhoids by increasing water content in the colon. Take a teaspoon of the powder in warm water or juice 3 times a day, to **clean the intestines and remove putrefactive toxins**. Make the dose one-half teaspoon for children.

Externally, psyllium seed powder is very often **added to poultices as a binder** (to hold it all together). For this purpose, add a small amount while pouring water over the ingredients and stir until it becomes thick, similar to dough. Psyllium will **draw pus from boils, sores and carbuncles**.

Note: Psyllium seed powder can also be added to unleavened bread as a binder.

PUMPKIN SEEDS

(Curcubita pepo) Part used: Seeds. *Properties:* Anthelmintic. *What it affects:* Intestines.

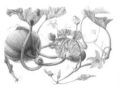
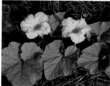
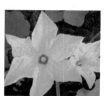

Pumpkin   Pumpkin   Pumpkin

Preparation and amount: Crush 7-14 oz. of seeds for children and up to 25 oz. for adults; stir into fruit juice, to make a mash to be eaten. Two or three hours later, take castor oil to drive out the worms.

Purposes: *Internally,* pumpkin seed is the classic means of **eliminating parasites—worms—from intestines and large bowel**. These are the seeds from the pumpkins harvested in your garden in the fall. As you know, each pumpkin is full of them. Take large amounts of pumpkin seeds as a safe anthelmintic (worm expeller). It is safe for both children and adults. The seed is also used to treat **prostate disorders and irritable bladder**.

Externally, pumpkin seed oil is used for **healing wounds, especially burns**, as well as for **chapped skin**.

Note: Take care with tapeworms, that the entire worm is expelled.

QUASSIA

(Picraena excelsa) Part used: Wood. *Properties:* Anthelmintic, febrifuge, stomachic, bitter tonic. *What it affects:* Gastro-intestinal system.

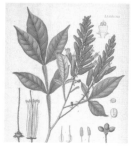
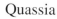
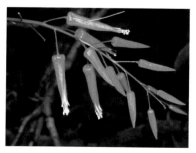

Quassia   Quassia

Preparation and amount: *Infusion:* steep 1 tsp. quassia wood in 1 cup water. Take 1 cup a day. *Tincture:* One dose is 2-5 drops.

Purposes: *Internally,* the primary value of quassia is to **kill round worms**. Taken as an enema, it kills **pinworms**. An infusion of quassia wood is used to treat **fever, rheumatism, and dyspepsia**. A bitter tonic for the stomach can be obtained by letting water stand overnight in a cup made of quassia wood or glass cup with many wood chips. The result is a weak infusion which, in a drink, will help **strengthen the stomach**. The tea is also said to **destroy an appetite for alcohol**.

Externally, an infusion can be used as a scalp rinse, to counteract **dandruff**.

RED RASPBERRY

(Rubus strigosus) Part used: Leaf. *Properties:* Antispasmodic, astringent, alterative, stimulant, tonic. *What it affects:* Stomach, liver, blood, genito-urinary system, and muscles.

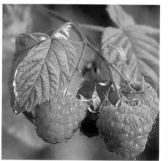
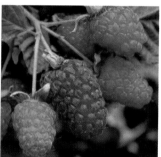

Raspberry   Raspberry

Preparation and amount: *Infusion:* Steep 5-15 min. Take 6 oz. frequently. *Tincture:* 30 drops (½-1 tsp.) frequently. *Fluid extract:* Take 1-2 tsp. frequently. *Powder:* Take 5-10 #0 capsules (30-60 grains) frequently.

Purposes: *Rubus idaeus* is the regular red raspberry you like to grow in your garden. *Internally,* the leaf tea is good for **diarrhea** and one can also drink it as a beverage. Because it is perfectly safe, it is one of the best herbal teas for **pregnancy**: to relieve **nausea, prevent hemorrhage, reduce pain, and ease childbirth**. It is also used freely to **reduce menstrual cramps**. Combined with other herbs, such as uva ursi and squaw vine, it is used for the treatment of **vaginal discharge, hot flashes, and other female problems**. Combine it with peppermint, to treat **uterine hemorrhage or morning sickness**. It is a stimulating, astringent tonic to the **mucous membranes**. As a douche or enema for **dysentery, combine it with myrrh or goldenseal** in equal parts. It will stop **uterine hemorrhages**. It is also used for **measles**.

Raspberry relieves **urinary irritation**, and **soothes the kidneys and entire urinary tract**. For relief of kidney infection, chronic dysentery, and hemorrhage, mix 1 part raspberry, slightly over 1 part goldenseal, and 2½ parts witch hazel.

Raspberry is also a reliable treatment for **acute stomach problems, fevers, colds, and flus**. The fresh juice, mixed with a little honey, makes an excellent **refrigerant beverage, to be taken in the heat of a fever in order to**

reduce it. Steep an ounce of the herb in a pint of boiled water for 20 minutes. It promotes **healthy nails, bones, teeth, and skin**.

Externally, because of its astringent qualities, raspberry is used as a **gargle, mouthwash, or an external wash for sores, wounds, burns, canker sores, and skin rashes**. It is also used as an **eyewash**. The above formula, using goldenseal and witch hazel, is also a helpful gargle for **throat diseases**.

Note: Wild red raspberry *(Rubus strigosus)* has somewhat similar properties, but is not used very much; since the garden variety is so easy to obtain.

RED CLOVER

(Trifolium pratense) Part used: Flowering tops. *Properties:* Alterative, nutritive, sedative, stimulant. *What it affects:* Nerves, lungs, blood, liver, and lymph.

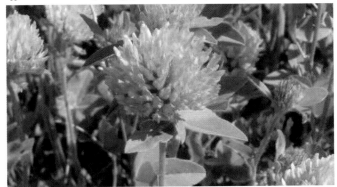

Red Clover

Preparation and amount: *Infusion:* Steep 30 min. Take 1-2 oz. frequently or 4-6 cups daily. *Tincture:* 5-30 drops frequently. *Fluid extract:* Take 1 tsp. frequently. *Powder;* Take 5-10 #0 capsules (30-60 grains) frequently.

Purposes: *Internally,* red clover is **considered among the very best anti-cancer herbs**. It is a powerful **blood purifier**, either used alone or in combination with yellow dock, dandelion root, sassafras, or other blood purifiers. It **fights infection, suppresses appetite, relaxes the system, stops spasms, and induces expectoration**. It is **soothing to the nerves** and is good for **whooping cough, psoriasis, rheumatism, and stomach problems**. It is used for **coughs, bronchitis, inflamed lungs, kidney problems, liver disease, weakened immune system, bacterial infections, HIV, and AIDS**.

Externally, it can be applied as a poultice or fomentation on **cancerous growths**.

RUE

(Ruta graveolens) Parts used: Herb, leaves. *Properties:* Antispasmodic, emmenagogue, rubefacient, stimulant. *What it affects:* Nerves, tendons, circulation, and uterus.

Preparation and amount: *Infusion:* Steep 5-15 min. Take 2 oz. 3 times daily between meals. *Tincture:* Take 5-20 drops 3 times daily. *Fluid extract:* Take ½-1 tsp. 3 times daily. *Oil:* Take 1-5 drops 3 times daily. *Powder:* Take 2-5 #0 capsules (10-30 grains) 3 times daily.

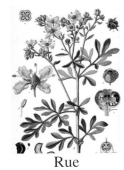 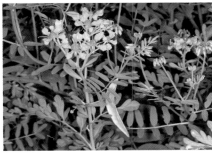

Rue   Rue

Purposes: *Internally,* rue is a valuable antispasmodic herb useful in treating **hypertension, nervous complaints, neuralgia, trauma, and bowel cramps**. As a warm infusion, it is an excellent help for **stomach problems, gas pains, colic, spasms, dizziness, nervousness, and congestion in the female organs**. It relieves **gouty and rheumatic pains** and treats **nervous heart problems**, such as **palpitations** in women going through menopause. It **improves appetite and digestion**. It is a good herb to add to **cough** medicines, especially when **poor digestion and gas** are also present. It is widely prescribed as a first-aid medicine for **strained tendons and muscles**. The Chinese use a tincture of rue for sedation and rheumatism. It is used by them to **decrease swelling, increase local circulation, and improve metabolism**.

Externally, an infusion will help eliminate **worms**. A poultice placed on the forehead will relieve certain types of **headaches**. Used as a poultice, the fresh, bruised herb is an irritant which helps **sciatica**. It is used as a rubefacient, to **promote local circulation**. (A rubefacient increases the flow of blood to the surface and increases redness of the skin.) It is best to first rub a vegetable oil on the body part where the poultice will be placed.

Warning: Do not take too much rue at a time; small, frequent doses are best. If adverse symptoms develop from overuse, a small amount of goldenseal root will act as an antidote. Because it is an emmenagogic, it should not be used during pregnancy.

SAGE

(Salvia officinalis) Part used: Leaves: *Properties:* Antispasmodic, astringent, anthelmintic, aromatic, vulnerary. *What it affects:* Bowels, sinuses, bladder, mucous membranes, and nerves.

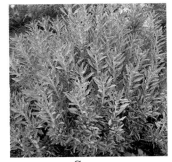 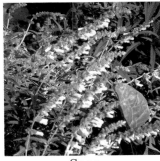

Sage   Sage

Preparation and amount: *Infusion (leaves):* Steep

178 **HERBS** **THE 126 MOST IMPORTANT HERBS** NATURAL REMEDIES ENCYCLOPEDIA
OVER 11,000 REMEDIES - OVER 730 DISEASES

H
E
R
B
S

5-15 min. Take 1 Tbsp. as needed or 1-2 cups daily, hot or cold. *Tincture:* Take 20-60 drops 3-4 times daily. *Fluid extract:* Take ¼-1 tsp. 3-4 times daily. *Powder:* Take 2-5 #0 capsules (10-30 grains) 3-4 times daily.

Purposes: *Internally,* sage's best-known effect is its ability to **reduce perspiration**, which will begin about 2 hours after it is taken. The effect may last several days. This makes it useful in treating **night sweats** which often occur in tuberculosis. A nursing mother, whose child has been weaned, can take sage tea for a few days, to help **stop the flow of milk**. It also **reduces salivation and decreases secretions of the lungs, sinuses, throat and mucous membranes**. It also helps **eliminate mucous congestion** in the respirator passages and the stomach.

Sage tea is good for **stomach troubles, diarrhea, gas, dysentery, colds, and flus**. It is good for **hot flashes and other symptoms of estrogen deficiency**, whether in menopause or following hysterectomy. It will **expel worms** in children and adults. It is used for **nervous conditions, trembling, depression, and vertigo**. It is used for **inflamed throat and tonsils, laryngitis, and tonsillitis**.

Sage tea can be combined with equal parts of peppermint, rosemary, and wood betony for a very helpful **headache** remedy. It is used for **leukorrhea, dysmenorrhea, and amenorrhea**. As an astringent, it is used for **diarrhea, gastritis, and enteritis**.

Externally, sage tea is an excellent gargle when combined with freshly squeezed lemon juice and honey for all **mouth diseases**. It is a good wash for **wounds** that are slow to heal. It is a useful hair rinse to eliminate **dandruff**, stimulate **hair growth**, and promote **shine in the hair**. As a gargle, the tea is good for **laryngitis, tonsillitis, and sore throat**. Crushed, fresh sage leaves can be used as first aid for **insect bites**.

Warning: Extended or excessive use of sage can cause symptoms of poisoning.

SARSAPARILLA

(Smilax ornata) Part used: Root. *Properties:* Alterative, carminative, tonic, diaphoretic. *What it affects:*

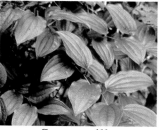
Sarsaparilla

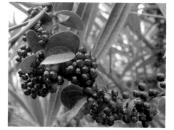
Sarsaparilla

Blood, skin, circulation, and intestines.

Preparation and amount: *Decoction:* Simmer 15-30 min. Take 3 oz. 3 times daily. *Tincture:* Take 5-15 drops 3 times daily. *Fluid extract:* Take 2-4 tsp. 3 times daily. *Powder:* Take 5-10 #0 capsules (30-60 grains) 3 times daily.

Purposes: *Internally,* sarsaparilla tea **increases the flow of urine**; and, taken hot, it **induces sweating to help break fevers**. It is good for **skin problems, flatulence, catarrhal problems, and scrofu**la. It is used for **disor-ders of the nervous system**. Steep 1 tsp. rootstock in 1 cup water; take 1-2 cups a day. It is used for **arthritis, rheumatism, and gout**.

Sarsaparilla tea is a **blood cleanser**, and is often taken as a "spring tonic." It **promotes the excretion of fluids, increases energy, protects against radiation exposure**, and **regulates hormones**.

It contains a hormone-like substance which makes it useful in **glandular formulas**. It is useful for **frigidity, hives, infertility, impotence, and psoriasis**.

Externally, sarsaparilla tea is a good eyewash. Use it as a wash or poultice on **ringworm**. **Pustules and sores** may be washed with a tea made from the root. Use it for **ringworm and skin eruptions**.

SASSAFRAS

(Sassafras officinale) Parts used: Root, bark. *Properties:* Alterative, aromatic, carminative, diaphoretic, diuretic, stimulant. *What it affects:* Blood, skin, circulation, and intestines.

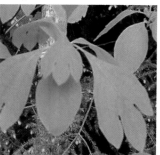
Sassafras

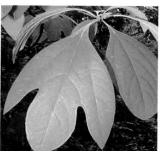
Sassafras

Preparation and amount: *Decoction:* Simmer 5-15 min. Take 3 oz. 3-4 times daily. *Tincture:* Take 15-30 drops 3-4 times daily. *Fluid extract:* Take ¼ to 1 tsp. 3-4 times daily. *Powder:* Take 5-10 #0 capsules (30-60 grains) 3-4 times daily.

Purposes: *Internally,* sassafras is one of the oldest and most respected herbal remedies in America. It is a **spring tonic and blood purifier**. After a heavy winter, it thins the blood, **stimulates and cleans the liver** of toxins, and **promotes perspiration and urination**. When used to purify the blood, it is usually combined with other alterative herbs. Therefore, it is recommended for **rheumatism, gout, arthritis, and skin problems**. Indians used it as an infusion, to **reduce fevers**.

The bark of the root contains a volatile oil that has anodyne and antiseptic properties. The bark has been used as a **pain reliever** and also to treat **venereal disease**. It is given during **painful menstruation**, and will **relieve suffering in childbirth and the afterpains**.

For **chronic blood disorders**, sassafras is often combined with other alteratives—such as sarsaparilla, licorice, burdock, and echinacea.

Internally and externally, use sassafras to treat **skin problems and ulcers** of various kinds, including **acne**. Apply the oil externally as a disinfectant and for **rheumatic pains**.

Warning: Sassafras oil can be used externally, but must never be used internally.

SAW PALMETTO

(Serenoa serrulata) Part used: Fruit. *Properties:* Diuretic, tonic, antiseptic, sedative. *What it affects:* Lungs, throat, reproductive organs, and kidneys.

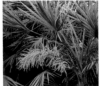 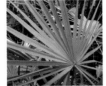 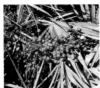

Saw Palmetto   Saw Palmetto   Saw Palmetto

Preparation and amount: *Infusion:* Steep 5-15 min. Take 6 oz. 2-3 times daily. *Tincture:* Take 15-16 drops 2-3 times daily. *Fluid extract:* Take 10 drops 2-3 times daily. *Powder:* Take 2-4 #0 capsules (10-20 grains) 2-3 times daily.

Purposes: *Internally,* saw palmetto berries are especially useful for **colds, asthma, and bronchitis**. They are good in **all throat conditions, whooping cough, and head and nose congestion. Catarrhal problems and mucous congestion** respond to a tea made from the dried berries. It is a **diuretic and urinary antiseptic**. The tea is a general tonic, to **build strength during convalescence from illness**. It is used to treat **diseases of the male and female reproductive organs**. It is especially helpful in promoting a **quicker recovery from glandular diseases**. It inhibits production of dihydrotestosterone, a form of testosterone that contributes to **enlargement of the prostate**. Steep 1 tsp. dried berries in 1 cup water. Take 1-2 cups a day.

SENNA

(Cassia acutifolia) Parts used: Leaves, pods. *Properties:* Laxative, vermifuge, diuretic. *What it affects:* Intestines.

 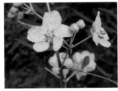 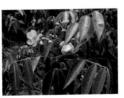

Senna   Senna   Senna

Preparation and amount: *Infusion:* Steep 30 min. Take 2 oz. 3 times daily. *Tincture:* Take 30-40 drops 2-3 times daily. *Fluid extract:* Take ½ tsp. 2-3 times daily. *Powder:* Take 2-10 #0 capsules (10-60 grains) 2-3 times daily.

Purposes: *Internally,* senna is one of the most reliable **laxatives** and increases the intestinal peristaltic movements.

It should be combined with a carminative herb (such as ginger, anise, fennel, or coriander), to avoid griping (bowel cramps). Use 6-12 pods for adults and 3-6 pods for children. (The pods are preferred, since they are milder than the leaves.) Make an infusion of an ounce of senna to 1 pint water. To this add 10% of an aromatic herb. Steep for 20 minutes and drink it cold. (There is less cramping if one drinks it cold.) Do not make more than will be immediately used (about ½-1 cup at a time.) Senna is also combined with other anthelmintics, to get rid of **intestinal worms**.

Externally, senna is useful as a mouthwash for **halitosis** and a **bad taste in your mouth**.

Note: There are four primary senna herbs: Alexandrian senna *(Cassia acutifolia),* from northern Africa, and the lesser-used American senna *(Cassia marilandica).* Both have the same properties, work in the same manner, and have the same cautions. There are also two other senna herbs: tinnevelly senna *(Cassia angustifolia)* which is weaker in its properties, and not sold very often, and purging cassia *(Cassia fistula)* which is grown in India. It is stronger and the herb generally included in most commercial cassia pods and many packaged preparations.

Warning: Senna should not be used if there is inflammation anywhere in the intestinal tract, if there are prolapsed intestines, rectum, or piles. It should not be used during pregnancy. It is addictive if used too long.

SHEPHERD'S PURSE

(Capsella bursa-pastoris) Part used: Tops. *Properties:* Astringent, diuretic, stimulant. *What it affects:* Kidneys, bladder, and blood.

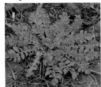 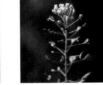 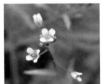

Shepherd's   Shepherd's   Shepherd's
Purse   Purse   Purse

Preparation and amount: *Infusion:* Steep 30 min. Take 6 oz. 1-2 times daily. *Tincture:* 20-60 drops 1-2 times daily. *Fluid extract:* ¼-½ tsp. 1-2 times daily. *Powder:* 2-10 #0 capsules (15-60 grains) 1-2 times daily.

Purposes: Shepherd's purse is an outstanding blood coagulant which can be used to **stop internal or external bleeding**. *Internally,* it is an excellent astringent which will **stop bleeding of the lungs, colon, kidneys, and bladder**. The tops should be used fresh for this purpose, but an infusion of dried herb can also be used. It is also good for **excessive menstrual bleeding** and **bed-wetting**. Because it acts to constrict the blood vessels, it **raises blood pressure**. But it will also **regulate blood pressure and heart action**, whether the pressure is too high or too low.

It is good for **intermittent fevers, hemorrhoids,** and especially good for **stopping diarrhea**. It promotes **uterine contracts during childbirth and can improve intestinal and bowel action**. Steep 1 tsp. fresh or 2 tsp. dried herb in ½ cup water. Take 1 cup a day, unsweetened, a mouthful at a time.

Externally, put the juice **in an ear to stop pain**. Doing this will also **stop strange noises** in the ear. It is also used in washes and poultices for **wounds** on the body **and especially on the head**. It will also stop **surface bleeding**.

Note: Do not store shepherd's purse longer than a year.

H
E
R
B
S

SKULLCAP

(Scutellaria lateriflora) Part used: Tops. *Properties:* Antispasmodic, nervine, antipyretic. *What it affects:* Nerves and stomach.

  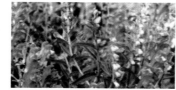

Skullcap   Skullcap   Skullcap

Preparation and amount: *Infusion:* Steep 15-30 min. Take 3 oz. 4-5 times daily. *Tincture:* Take 10-40 drops 3-4 times daily. *Fluid extract:* Take ¼ tsp. 3-4 times daily. *Powder:* Take 3-5 capsules (15-30 grains) 2-3 or more times daily.

Purposes: Skullcap is one of most needed herbs for your collection, and is **very good for almost any nervous problem**. It is a very safe and reliable nerve sedative. It is food for the nerves, supporting and strengthening them as it gives i**mmediate relief of all chronic and acute diseases stemming from nervous affections and debility.** Whatever the nerve problem, mild or chronic, skullcap can provide help. Combine it with other tonic, nervine, and antispasmodic herbs (such as hops, wood betony, lady's slipper, and passionflower). It may be used freely and is essentially nontoxic. Use an ounce of the herb steeped in a pint of boiled water, for 10 minutes.

Internally, skullcap is good for **drug and alcoholic withdrawal symptoms, insomnia, epilepsy, neuralgia, convulsions, coughs, indigestion, insanity, muscle cramps, pain, stress, anxiety, fatigue, headache, nervous headache, hyperactivity, hysteria, restlessness, spasms, or excitability.** It is used to **wean people from barbiturates, excessive use of valium, and other addictions.** In combination with American ginseng (¼ oz.) and skullcap (½ oz.), taken in small frequent doses, it is a good treatment for **alcoholism.** First make a decoction of ginseng root, then an infusion of skullcap, then combine the two.

American Indians used skullcap to promote **menstruation.** It will **reduce pains of ovarian or uterine origin.** It **strengthens the heart muscle.** It is said to be effective against **rabies.**

Note: Skullcap should be used as fresh as possible, otherwise its activity rather quickly dissipates.

SLIPPERY ELM

(Ulmus fulva) Part used: Inner (not outer) bark. *Properties:* Demulcent, emollient, nutritive, astringent. *What it affects:* Generally effects the whole body.

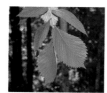 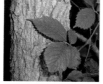 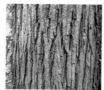

Slippery Elm   Slippery Elm   Slippery Elm

Preparation and amount: *Infusion (powder):* Slowly pour 1 pint of boiling water over 1 oz. powdered bark, stirring constantly. Simmer 5-15 min. Take 6 oz. 3-4 times daily. *Decoction (whole bark):* Simmer 5-15 min. Take 3 oz. 3-4 times daily. *Tincture:* Take 15-30 drops 3-4 times daily. *Fluid extract:* Take ½-1 tsp. 3-4 times daily. *Gruel:* Mix 1 tsp. powder with sufficient cold water to make a thin and very smooth paste. Stirring steadily, pour 1 pint of boiling water onto the paste. Flavor with honey and lemon rind. Take ½-1 pint (warm) 1-3 times daily. *Syrup:* 1 Tbsp. as needed. *Powder:* Take 5-10 #0 capsules (30-60 grains) 3-4 times daily.

Purposes: It is the inner *white* bark of the slippery elm tree that should be kept on hand. (The outer *dark* bark is also sold, but is useless.)

Internally, slippery elm is used for **bladder inflammation, bronchitis, colitis, constipation, ovarian cramps, coughs, cystitis, diarrhea, diverticulitis, dysentery, eczema, flu, gas, hemorrhage, hemorrhoids, hoarseness, lung congestion, stomach problems, tonsillitis, ulcers, ulcerative colitis, gastritis, leukorrhea, rheumatoid and gouty afflictions.** It is beneficial for **Crohn's disease.** It is an excellent cleanser and can be used in a douche or enema.

Slippery elm makes a **nourishing gruel for children,** for the **elderly with weak stomachs,** for **those with ulcers,** and **those who are recovering from diseases.** It can be made into a gruel by gradually adding a small amount of water and mixing until the proper consistency is obtained. This can be sweetened with a little honey. It is **an excellent food whenever there is difficulty holding and digesting food.**

Externally, slippery elm is used for **burns, gangrenous wounds, hemorrhoids, tumors, open sores, and wounds.** It is also used to treat **painful rheumatic and gouty areas.**

Note: Slippery elm is an excellent binder. A small amount can be added to other herbs with a little water, and then rolled into small pills. By adding a little maple syrup, it can be used to make lozenges for **coughs and sore throats.** It can also be used to make suppositories, boluses, and to hold unleavened bread together. If used as a douche or enema, it must be diluted with water, so it will not plug the apparatus (since it is a mucilaginous herb).

SPEARMINT

(Mentha viridis) Part used: Leaves. *Properties:* Aromatic, carminative, diaphoretic, stimulate, antispasmodic, diuretic. *What it affects:* Stomach, intestines, muscles, and circulation.

 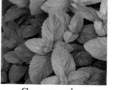 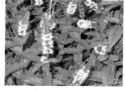

Spearmint   Spearmint   Spearmint

Preparation and amount: *Infusion:* Steep 5-15 min. Take 6 oz. 3-4 times daily. *Tincture:* Take ½-1 tsp.

3-4 times daily. *Fluid extract:* Take ¼-½ tsp. 3-4 times daily. *Powder:* Take 5-10 #0 capsules (30-60 grains) 3-4 times daily.

Purposes: *Internally,* the *Mentha spicata* species of spearmint shares many of the properties of peppermint. It is often given for common women's problems and for **suppressed or painful urination**. An infusion combined with horehound is sometimes given to children for **fever**.

The *Menta viridus* species is also nontoxic, and similar to peppermint in its uses. This herb is mainly used during **colds, flus, cramps, indigestion, gas, and slight spasms**. Combined with horehound, it is used to **break fevers in children**. It is good to **stop vomiting and excellent when used as an enema for restlessness**. Combined with pleurisy root and skullcap, it is a good remedy for **pneumonia and pleurisy**.

Note: Do not boil the herb, for the volatile oil will be steamed off. Use it in bitter herb combinations, to add flavor.

The other mints are peppermint *(Mentha piperita)* and catnip *(Nepeta cataria);* both of these are dealt with elsewhere in this herb list.

Overseas: Spearmint and Spearmint oil are used as carminatives (to **relieve gas**), and primarily to **disguise the flavor of other medicines**. Spearmint has been traditionally valued as a **stomachic, antiseptic, and antispasmodic**. The leaf tea has been used for **stomachaches, diarrhea, nausea, colds, headaches, cramps, fevers**, and is a folk **cancer remedy**.

WARNING: Oil is toxic if taken internally; causes dermatitis.

SPIKENARD

(American)—*(Aralia racemosa)* Parts used: Rootstock and roots. *Properties:* Diaphoretic, expectorant, stimulant.

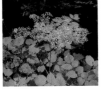 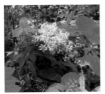

Spikenard   Spikenard   Spikenard

Preparation and amount: *Infusion:* steep 1-2 tsp. powdered rootstock and roots in 1 cup water. Take 1-2 cups daily.

Purposes: *Internally,* the powdered root of spikenard is for **rheumatism, asthma, and coughs**. Taking the tea for some time before labor will **make childbirth easier**. American Indians used the plant for **backache**.

Externally, Indians would pound the root into a pulp and use it for poultices. It is used for **skin problems, wounds, swellings, bruises, and inflammations**. A fomentation is placed **over the chest, to reduce internal pains**.

Note: Spikenard is a close relative of sarsaparilla. There is also a second herb called "spikenard" *(Aralia nudicaulis)*, or wild sarsaparilla. Its properties are much like those of sarsaparilla, discussed elsewhere in this herb list.

SQUAW VINE (Partridge Berry)

(Mitchella repens) Part used: Whole plant. *Properties:* Emmenagogue, astringent, diuretic. *What it affects:* Uterus, bladder, colon.

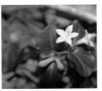

Squaw Vine   Squaw Vine   Squaw Vine

Preparation and amount: *Infusion:* Steep 5-15 min. Take 3 oz. 3-4 times daily. *Tincture:* Take 15-60 drops 3-4 times daily. *Fluid extract:* Take ½-1 tsp. 3-4 times daily. *Powder:* Take 5-10 #0 capsules (30-60 grains) 3-4 times daily.

Purposes: *Internally,* American Indians used squaw vine **throughout pregnancy and especially during the last few weeks, to make childbirth faster and easier**. It was also used to **improve lactation**. It is used for the same purposes today. It is a **uterine tonic** and also relieves **congestion of the ovaries**. It is also good for **painful or absent menstruation**. As a fomentation for **sore nipples**, crush the berries, mix them with myrrh, boil, and then let steep for 3 days and strain. During pregnancy, combine it with raspberry leaf. Mix it with cramp bark, raspberry leaves, and a small portion of lobelia in order to **prevent miscarriages**. The same formula is good for **vaginal discharges**.

Squaw vine (especially combined with witch hazel) is also used for **leukorrhea**. Also use this combination for **dysentery and bleeding piles**.

As a diuretic, it can be used for **gravel and urinary problems**. It is also used for **insomnia**. For general use, make a decoction, using an ounce of herb in a pint of water. Take ½ cup 3 times a day.

Externally, squaw vine tea makes a good wash for **sore eyes and skin problems**.

Note: Squaw vine is similar in properties and effects of pipsissewa.

ST. JOHN'S WORT

(Hypericum perforatum) Part used: Tops. *Properties:* Astringent, alterative, diuretic, nervine, sedative. *What it affects:* Stomach, bladder, blood, liver, and nerves.

 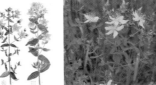 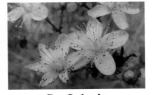

St. John's Wort   St. John's Wort   St. John's Wort

Preparation and amount: *Infusion:* Steep the leaves 5-15 min. Take 1 oz. when needed, up to 1 cup daily. *Tincture:* 10-20 drops as needed. *Fluid extract:* Take ½-1 tsp. as needed. *Powder:* Take 5-10 #0 capsules (30-60 grains) as needed.

Purposes: *Internally,* St. John's wort **purifies the blood** and is used for **diarrhea, dysentery, jaundice, boils, suppressed urine**, as well as **uterine and afterbirth pains**. It is good for **bed-wetting, hysteria, coughs, irregular menstruation, uterine disorders, muscle pains and bruises, tenderness and pain in the spine**. It is a good expectorant for **bronchial and lung problems**. The herb should be taken close to meals.

Externally, Steep the flowers in olive oil for 2 weeks and then apply. The extracted oil of St. John's wort can be applied to **bruises, wounds, and other skin problems**, especially those that are sensitive. Also apply the oil to **hard tumors, ulcers, burns, and swollen breasts**.

Warning: St. John's wort makes the skin more light-sensitive. Those who have light skin should avoid exposure of the area (where the herb has been applied) to strong sunlight and other sources of ultraviolet light, including tanning beds. If used to support treatment of depression, its effectiveness should be checked by a nutritionally oriented doctor after 4-6 weeks. It should not be used at the same time as prescription anti-depressants, or during pregnancy or lactation.

STONEROOT

(Collinsonia canadensis) Part used: Root. *Properties:* Astringent, diuretic, hepatic. *What it affects:* Veins, liver, and colon.

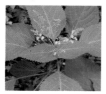 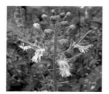 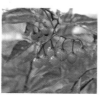

Stoneroot   Stoneroot   Stoneroot

Preparation and amount: *Decoction:* Simmer 5-15 min. Take 1 Tbsp. 3 times daily or up to 1 cup during the day. *Tincture:* Take 30-60 drops 3 times daily. *Fluid extract:* Take ¼ to 1 tsp. 3 times daily. *Powder:* Take 2 #0 capsules (5 grains) 3 times daily.

Purposes: *Internally,* stoneroot is **primarily used in the treatment of hemorrhoids**. Its astringency restores the tone of flaccid veins and is thus useful for both **hemorrhoids and varicose veins**. An infusion makes a good diuretic for **urinary problems, constipation, and excessive water retention**. It is often included with other herbs as part of a **urinary formula**. Use it with bladder root in the **removal of bladder stones**. It is very good taken for **pain after surgical operations of the rectum for piles, ulcers, or fistula. It breaks up mucus and is helpful for headache, cramps, indigestion, and bronchitis**. Its continued use **strengthens the heart** through improvements in the circulation. It is **especially good for the heart when it has been tired from sickness or fever**.

Externally, in addition to taking stoneroot internally for **varicose veins**, apply it externally to them. Mix a salve with equal parts goldenseal and a small amount of tea tree oil. The fresh leaves of stoneroot can be used as a poultice or fomentation, to **help heal bruises and wounds**. Small amounts are good for a **hoarse voice**.

Note: The fresh rootstock of stoneroot is better than the dried herb.

Warning: If used in large doses, it may cause nausea.

TANSY

(Tanacetum vulgare) Parts used: Herb, seed, root. *Properties:* Anthelmintic, emmenagogue, stimulant, tonic. *What it affects:* Intestines.

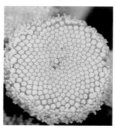 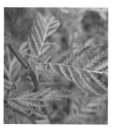 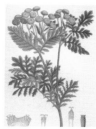

Tansy   Tansy   Tansy

Preparation and amount: *Infusion (herb):* Steep 30 min. Take 1 tsp. 3-4 times daily. *Decoction (seed, root):* Simmer 5-15 min. Take 3 oz. 3 times daily. *Tincture:* ½-1 tsp. 2-3 times daily. *Fluid extract:* Take ½-2 tsp. 2-3 times daily. *Syrup (root):* Take 1 tsp. 2-3 times daily. *Powder:* Take 5-10 #0 capsules (30-60 grains) 2-3 times daily.

Purposes: *Internally,* tansy is **primarily used for expelling worms in children and adults**. Take an infusion teaspoonful morning, noon, and evening. Pour 1 cup of the infusion over ½ cup raisins. Let the raisins swell with the liquid. Then take 3 tsp. doses of the liquid daily.

Tansy is used to **promote suppressed menstruation, hysteria, kidney weaknesses, nervousness, and fever**.

Externally, an infusion of leaves and flowers is a good wash for **skin problems and blemishes**, as well as for **bruises and sprains**. A hot fomentation is used for **arthritic and rheumatic pains**.

Warning: Tansy is a mild irritant when used in small doses. It can be poisonous, even when applied externally. An overdose of tansy oil or tea can be fatal. It would probably be best to avoid using tansy.

TEA TREE

(Tee Tree) (Leptospermum scoparium)—Part used: Essential oil. Properties: Disinfectant.

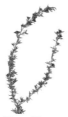 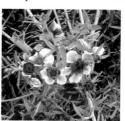 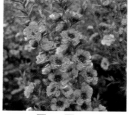

Tea Tree   Tea Tree   Tea Tree

Preparation and amount: Pure or diluted oil, used in poultices, fomentations, and douches.

Purposes: *Externally,* tea tree oil is a powerful **disinfectant of wounds**. It is the "skin herb," and **heals all skin conditions, including cuts and scrapes, acne, boils, fungal infections, athlete's foot**. It is used for **hair and scalp problems, herpes, scabies, warts, and insect**

and spider bites. Add it to water and use as a douche for **vaginitis** and a **gargle for colds, sore throat, and mouth sores**. But do not swallow it.

Warning: Only use tea tree oil externally. It can be toxic if swallowed. If irritation occurs, discontinue its use, or dilute it with distilled water, vegetable oil, primrose oil, or vitamin E oil. If irritation continues after its dilution, discontinue its use.

THYME, GARDEN

(Thymus vulgaris) Part used: Tops. *Properties:* Antiseptic, carminative, diuretic, antispasmodic, expectorant, parasiticide. *What it affects:* Intestines, lungs, throat, stomach, and skin.

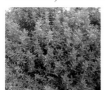 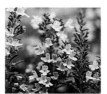 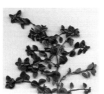
Thyme   Thyme   Thyme

Preparation and amount: *Infusion:* Steep 30 min. Take 1 oz. frequently, up to 2 cups a day. *Tincture:* Take 30-60 drops (½-1 tsp.) 2-3 times daily. *Fluid extract:* Take 1 tsp. 2-3 times daily. *Powder:* Take 5-10 #0 capsules (30-60 grains) 2-3 times daily.

Purposes: *Internally,* thyme is **especially used in throat and bronchial problems, including laryngitis, bronchitis, croup, and whooping cough**. It **eliminates gas and reduces fever, headache, and mucus**. A warm infusion **promotes perspiration and relieves flatulence**. It is used for **all stomach and intestinal problems, including diarrhea, chronic gastritis, lack of appetite, and colic**. It is also used for **asthma, and fever**. An infusion of the leaves will relieve **headache**. For **coughs and spasms**, use the fresh plant. It has strong antiseptic properties and **lowers cholesterol** levels.

Externally, thyme is used for **itching of the scalp and flaking caused by candidiasis**. A salve of thyme, goldenseal, and myrrh is good for **herpes and other skin problems**. Use it as a useful antiseptic wash for all **wounds**. The tincture or oil, diluted with vegetable oil (1 part thyme to 10 parts oil) is a helpful antiseptic for **scabies, athlete's foot, ringworm, crabs, and lice**. For **itchy skin**, add 15 drops of tansy oil to a hot bath and soak 45 minutes.

THYME, MOTHER OF

(Thymus serpyllum) Parts used: Leaf and flower. *Properties:* Antispasmodic, carminative, expectorant, rubefacient, tonic.

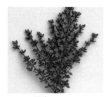 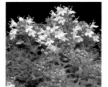 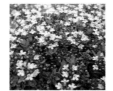
Thyme   Thyme   Thyme

Preparation and amount: *Infusion:* Steep 1-2 tsp. herb in 1 cup water. Take 1-1½ cups daily. *Bath additive:* Add 3-4 oz. flowers for a strong decoction of the herb to the bath water. *Alcohol cure:* Add a handful of the herb to 1 qt. boiling-hot water. Steep in a covered pot for 30 minutes. Give (or take) 1 Tbsp. every 15 minutes.

Purposes: *Internally,* mother of thyme is useful for **respiratory problems** and **helps clear mucous congestion from the lungs and respiratory passages**.

As a bath additive, it **stimulates the flow of blood toward the surface, thus alleviating nervous exhaustion**. An infusion of leaves relieves the **headache of a hangover**.

A **tonic for the stomach and nerves**, it is used for **gastro-intestinal problems—such as enteritis, stomach cramps, and mild gastritis**. It is also good for **anemia, insomnia, and painful menstruation**.

Mother of thyme is useful in **breaking the alcohol habit by inducing vomiting, diarrhea, sweating, thirst, and hunger, along with a revulsion for alcohol**. This may have to be repeated several times (generally at longer and longer intervals), until the person is weaned from the habit.

Externally, mother of thyme is used for **bruises, tumors, stab wounds, arthritis, and rheumatism**.

Note: Except when used for gastro-intestinal problems, it can be sweetened with honey.

UVA URSI

(Arctostaphylos uva ursi) Part used: Leaves. *Properties:* Astringent, diuretic, alterative, tonic. *What it affects:* Kidneys and urinary tract.

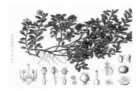 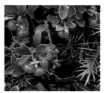
Uva Ursi   Uva Ursi   Uva Ursi

Preparation and amount: *Infusion:* Steep 30 min. Take 3 oz. as needed, up to 3 cups a day. *Tincture:* Take 10-20 drops 3 or more times daily. *Fluid extract:* Take ½-1 tsp. 3 times daily.

Purposes: *Internally,* uva ursi is a **specific for kidney and bladder infections**. When combined with marshmallow root, it will **eliminate stones** from those organs. It is useful as a **postoperative medicine, to reduce hemorrhaging**. Put a cup of leaves in a stocking and add to a hot tub of water as a good bath for immediately after childbirth. Also use this bath **after inflammations, hemorrhoids, and skin infections**. It is used as a douche for **vaginal infections** and **other pelvic problems**.

It also **helps restore the womb to normal size**. Because of its astringent qualities, uva ursi leaves are good as a tonic for **chronic diarrhea, piles, and diabetes, dysentery, and profuse menstruation**. Use it for **gonorrhea**.

Note: Uva ursi is often used with buchu leaves; but do not boil buchu leaves or uva ursi, because their active principles are in their volatile oils.

VALERIAN

(Valeriana officinalis) Part used: Root. *Properties:* Antispasmodic, nervine, carminative, stimulant. *What it affects:* Nerves.

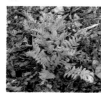
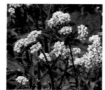
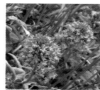

Valerian   Valerian   Valerian

Preparation and amount: *Decoction:* Simmer 5-15 min. Take 3 oz. 3 times daily. *Tincture:* Take ½-1 tsp. 3 times daily. *Fluid extract:* Take ½ tsp. 3 times daily. *Oil:* 5 drops 3 times daily. *Powder:* Take 2-3 #0 capsules (10-15 grains) 3 times daily.

Purposes: *Internally,* valerian is a **very calming and sedating** herb **for all emotional disturbances and pain**. However, it stimulates a few people (because the essential oils were not changed into valerianic acid, the calming principle). In everyone, it will be stimulating for a little while until the oils are changed.

Valerian is **especially useful when under emotional stress and pain**. It is good for **nervous conditions, migraine, and insomnia**. It is also helpful for **fatigue, low fevers, colds, colic, hysteria, neurasthenia, gravel in the bladder, as an enema for pinworms, and stomach cramps that cause vomiting.** The tea will **lessen menstrual cramps, intestinal cramps, stomach cramps, bronchial spasms, and muscle pains**. It is also used for **afterbirth pains, gas, hangover, measles, palsy, paralysis, high blood pressure, irritable bowel syndrome, and ulcers.** It **reduces mucus from colds**.

Valerian is widely used in many nervine herbal formulas. A well-known bedtime tea for **insomnia** is ½ tsp. valerian root and ½ tsp. hops, steeped in a cup of hot water.

Externally, valerian can be used as a **wash for pimples and sores**; and, at the same time, take it internally.

Note: Valerian should not be boiled, for this will dissipate the essential oils. Hops has very similar properties and may be substituted.

Overseas: Valerian is a leading over-the-counter **tranquilizer** and **sleep aid** in Europe. Ten controlled clinical studies have been published on Valerian preparations; a recent study found it worked best as a sleep aid over a period of a month rather than on a single-dose basis. Approved in Germany for use as a **sedative**, in sleep-inducing preparations for **nervous restlessness**, and to **aid in falling asleep.** Cats arc said to be attracted to the scent of the root as they are to Catnip. In eighteenth-century apothecaries, the quality of Valerian root was determined by the way in which cats reacted to it.

Warning: Large doses or extended use of valerian may produce symptoms of poisoning. Take the tea twice daily for no more than 2 weeks at a time. Large doses can bring on depression. Do not combine it with alcohol.

VERVAIN, BLUE

(Blue Vervain)—*(Verbena officinalis) Part used:* Tops. *Properties:* Antipyretic, antispasmodic, diaphoretic, astringent, expectorant, galactagogue, vulnerary. *What it affects:* Circulation, lungs, and intestines.

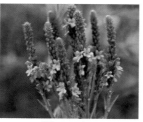
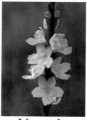
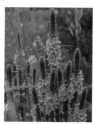

Vervain   Vervain   Vervain

Preparation and amount: *Infusion:* Steep 5-15 min. Take 3 oz. frequently. *Tincture:* Take 10-20 drops frequently. *Fluid extract:* Take ½-1 tsp. frequently. *Powder:* Take 3 #0 capsules (15 grains) frequently.

Purposes: *Internally,* vervain is **excellent for inducing sweating** and, in this way, **reducing fevers**; but **large amounts will act as an emetic**. Take the hot tea every few hours, to induce **good sweating**. Combine it with boneset for **fevers**, and take ½-1 hot cup every hour. By strengthening the nervous system, it is a **natural tranquilizer** and is used for **nervous problems and insomnia**. The warm tea, taken often, is recommended for **fevers and colds**, and especially good for getting rid of all types of **congestion in the throat and chest**, including **pneumonia**. It is used for most lung ailments. It **promotes liver and gallbladder health**, as well as **menstruation**. It increases mother's milk. The tea will settle a nervous stomach.

It is used for **convulsions, coughs, fevers, headaches, measles, nerve weakness, pain in the bowels, and pleurisy**. It is helpful for **rheumatism, neuralgia, sciatica, and swellings of the spleen**. It is often effective in **eliminating intestinal worms**. It is a popular remedy for griping (**intestinal cramps**).

Vervain is good for **pneumonia, asthma, and other chest diseases**. Put the tea on **sores**, to aid in healing. Use it for **coughs and upper respiratory inflammations**. It is good for **mild depression**. Use it as a poultice (mixed with wheat flour or bran) on **swellings of the spleen**. Vervain is bitter and can be made more palatable if combined with lemon grass or peppermint and honey. Start with 1 tsp., when treating children, and increase as needed. For adults, give 1 Tbsp. to 1 cup.

Externally, vervain tea can be applied to **sores and wounds, to increase healing**. Put it on **toothaches**.

Warning: Large amounts act as an emetic. Taken in large doses, the herb is poisonous. It should not be used during pregnancy, as it stimulates uterine contractions.

WHITE OAK BARK

(Quercus alba) Part used: bark. *Properties:* Astringent, antiseptic, diuretic. *What it affects:* Skin, gastrointestinal tract, and kidneys.

Preparation and amount: *Decoction:* Simmer 5-10 min. Take 3 oz. as needed. *Tincture:* Take 15-30 drops as needed. *Fluid extract:* Take ½-1 tsp. as needed. *Powder:* Take 3-10 #0 capsules (15-60 grains) as needed.

Purposes: *Internally,* white oak bark is **the most commonly used astringent and is extremely good for**

this purpose. It is used for **ulcers, spleen problems, and diarrhea**. The tea is taken for **bleeding of the stomach, lungs, and rectum**. It will **stop the spitting up of blood**. It will remove **gallstones and kidney stones, and increase the flow of urine**. Use it for **diarrhea**. Simmer an ounce of the bark in a pint of water for an hour. The decoction is good as an injection for **vaginal infections or hemorrhoids**. It is also used for **bladder weakness, herpes, leukorrhea, nose bleeds, and prolapsed uterus**.

Externally, white oak bark is applied to **poison oak, bee stings, insect and snakebites**. Use it to **bathe sores, scabs, burns, and wounds**. Use it **on the gums, to tighten them and prevent the loss of teeth**. Apply a fomentation of it, overnight, to **swollen glands, canker sores, tumors, goiter, mumps, fever blisters, and lymphatic swellings**. Use it for **herpes, leukorrhea, mouth ulcers, pyorrhea, ringworm, skin diseases, thrush, and tonsillitis**. Tie a fomentation over **broken capillaries and weak blood vessels**. It is excellent for **varicose veins**. For this purpose, use the tea internally as well as externally.

Overseas: In Germany, a related species, English Oak, *Quercus robur,* is approved for external use for the treatment of **inflammatory skin diseases**.

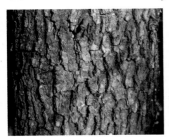 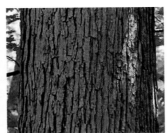

White Oak   White Oak

Warning: Do not use during pregnancy. It may interfere with the absorption of iron and other minerals, when taken internally. It should not be used by people who are allergic to aspirin. Tannic acid is potentially toxic.

WHITE PINE

(Pinus strobus) Parts used: Inner bark, young shoots, sap. *Properties:* Expectorant, antiseptic.

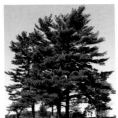 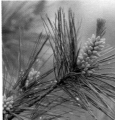 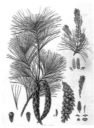

White Pine   White Pine   White Pine

Preparation and amount: *Infusion:* Steep 1 tsp. of the inner bark or young shoots in 1 cup water. Take a mouthful at a time, as needed. *Tincture:* 2-10 drops in water is a dose. *Mixture:* Steep 1 tsp. white pine bark and 1 Tbsp. each of wild cherry bark, sassafras bark, and American spikenard root in 1 pint boiling-hot water for 30 minutes. Take 1 tsp. every hour.

Purposes: *Internally,* the inner bark is valued as a remedy for **coughs and congestion due to colds**. It is used as a tea (or as an ingredient) in cough syrup. The resinous sap and young leaves are used as **cold remedies**.

Externally, make a poultice of the inner bark or the sap of the white pine as a dressing for **wounds and sores**. The sap of the white pine is legendary for its ability to **heal surface cuts and wounds**.

WHITE WILLOW

(Salix alba) Part used: Bark. *Properties:* Anodyne, antispasmodic, tonic, astringent, diaphoretic, diuretic, febrifuge. *What it affects:* Stomach, kidneys, intestines, and head.

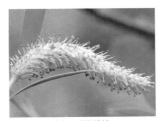 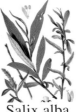 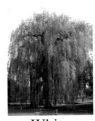

White Willow   Salix alba   White Willow

Preparation and amount: *Infusion:* Steep 5-15 min. Take 1 cup during the day. *Decoction (bark):* Simmer 5-15 min. Take 1 cup during the day. *Tincture:* Take 15-60 drops as needed. *Fluid extract:* Take ¼-1 tsp. as needed. *Powder:* Take 6-10 #0 capsules (30-50 grains) as needed.

Purposes: *Internally,* white willow **alleviates pain and reduces fevers**. Because it contains *salicin,* it is a natural alternative to aspirin. It is the "pain herb," and good for **headache, allergies, nerve pain, pains in the joints, backache, inflammation, and menstrual pain**. It is used for **fevers, neuralgia, gout, rheumatism, and arthritic pains**. It is especially useful for **kidney, urethra, bladder irritabilities**, and acts as an analgesic to those tissues.

Externally, apply it to **injuries and toothache**. Use the tea as a good **eyewash**. Sniff it up your nose, to stop **nose bleeds**. Willow bark is a strong antiseptic and a good fomentation and poultice for **infected wounds, ulcerations, eczema, and all other skin diseases**. Gargle with it for **throat and tonsil infections**. Use it for other **surface bleeding**.

Warning: Not recommended for use during pregnancy. Should not be used by those allergic to aspirin.

WILD CHERRY BARK

(Prunus serotina) Part used: Dried inner bark. *Properties:* Sedative, stomachic, astringent, stimulant tonic. *What it affects:* Lungs, stomach, and nerves.

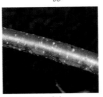 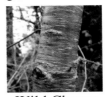 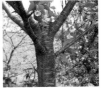

Wild Cherry   Wild Cherry   Wild Cherry

Preparation and amount: *Infusion:* Steep 5-15 min. Take 6 oz. 3-4 times daily between meals. *Decoction:*

Simmer 5-15 min. Take 2 oz. 3 times daily. *Tincture:* Take 30-60 drops 3 times daily. *Fluid extract:* Take ½-1 tsp. 3 times daily. *Syrup:* Take ½-2 tsp. 3 times daily. *Powder:* Take 5 #0 capsules 3 times daily.

Purposes: *Internally,* wild cherry bark is frequently used in the treatment of **chronic coughs**, especially those with a lot of mucus. It acts as **an expectorant, a mild sedative, and is a tonic to the respiratory and digestive tracts**. It is a good remedy for **heart palpitations**, when caused by a stomach disorder. It soothes **nerve irritations of both the stomach and lungs**, and **loosens mucus in the throat and chest**. It **improves digestion** by stimulating the gastric glands. It is good for **coughs, colds, asthma, bronchitis, diarrhea, dyspepsia, tuberculosis, whooping cough, and a nervous stomach**.

Warning: Wild cherry bark should not be used during pregnancy. The leaves, bark, and fruit contain hydrocyanic acid, which can be poisonous.

WILD YAM

(Dioscorea villosa) Part used: Root. *Properties:* Cholagogue, antispasmodic, diaphoretic. *What it affects:* Muscles, joints, uterus, liver, and gallbladder.

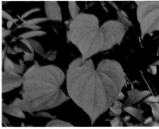 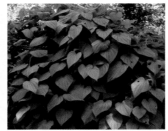
Wild Yam Wild Yam

Preparation and amount: *Decoction:* Simmer 5-15 min. Take 2-3 oz. in water 3-4 times daily, up to 2 cups per day. *Tincture:* Take 10-40 drops 3-4 times daily. *Fluid extract:* Take 1 tsp. 3-4 times daily. *Powder:* Take 5-10 #0 capsules (30-60 grains) 3-4 times daily.

Purposes: *Internally,* wild yam **relaxes muscle spasms** and is a valuable antispasmodic used for **colic, bowel spasms, abdominal cramps, and menstrual cramps**. It **contains steroid-like substances** which are used in many birth control pills. It is included in many gland-balancing formulas. It **promotes perspiration and reduces inflammation**; and it is good for **gallbladder disorders, hypoglycema, kidney stones, irritable bowel syndrome, neuralgia, and rheumatism**. It is used for a variety of **female problems**, including **premenstrual syndrome and menopause-related symptoms**.

Combined with other blood cleaners, wild yam will aid in **removing wastes** from the system, and relieving **stiff and sore joints**. It strengthens the function of the **gallbladder and liver**. To **prevent miscarriage**, combine it with ½ teaspoon of dried ginger and 1 tsp. of raspberry. Steep in 1 pint of water for 20 minutes, strain, and take a mouthful every half hour when threatened by miscarriage. Use 2 oz. with added honey, to counteract nausea. For **arthritic and other pains**, take the following tinctures in a cup of warm water 3 times a day: 20-30 drops of wild yam, 20 drops of burdock root, 15 drops of motherwort,

and 15 drops of black cohosh.

Warning: Wild yam is used in many commercial hormonal products; but the wild yam in them is often extracted from plants treated with fertilizers and pesticides, which could end up in the products. While some herbalists suggest using wild yam to avoid miscarriage (see above), others say not to use it during pregnancy.

Overseas: Contains *diosgenin*, used to manufacture progesterone and other steroid drugs. Research and production of this both in Germany and the U.S. Of all plant genera, there is perhaps none with greater impact on modern life but whose dramatic story is as little known as Wild Yam *(Dioscorea villosa)*. Most of the **steroid hormones** used in modern medicine, especially those in contraceptives, were developed from elaborately processed chemical components derived from yams. Drugs made with yam-derived components *(diosgenins)* relieve **asthma, arthritis, eczema**; they also **regulate metabolism and control fertility**. Synthetic products manufactured from *diosgenins* include **human sex hormones** (contraceptive pills), drugs to treat **menopause, dysmenorrhea, premenstrual syndrome, testicular deficiency, impotency, prostate hypertrophy, and psycho-sexual problems**, as well as **high blood pressure, arterial spasms, migraines**, and other ailments. Widely prescribed **cortisones and hydrocortisones** were indirect products of the genus *Dioscorea*. They are used for **Addison's disease, some allergies, bursitis, contact dermatitis, psoriasis, rheumatoid arthritis, sciatica, brown recluse spider bites, insect stings, and other diseases and ailmeats**. Wild yam has appeared in the American market in recent years as a "source" of estrogen or progesterone, prompting some to call this marketing effort the "wild yam scam," since the root does not contain human sex hormones.

WARNING: Fresh plant may induce vomiting and other undesirable side effects.

WINTERGREEN

(Gaultheria procumbens) Part used: Leaves. *Properties:* Analgesic, astringent, carminative, diuretic, stimulant.

 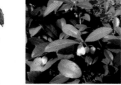 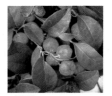
Wintergreen Wintergreen Wintergreen

Preparation and amount: *Infusion:* Steep 1 tsp. of leaves in 1 cup water. Take 1 cup daily, a mouthful at a time.

Purposes: The medicinal qualities of wintergreen are in the oil of wintergreen which can be obtained by steam distillation. That active principle consists primarily of *methyl salicylate* (90%), a close relative of aspirin.

Internally, wintergreen leaves have long been used for **headache, toothache, muscle pain, rheumatic pain, other aches, and inflammations**. It **stimulates the circulation and is good for arthritis**. The leaves are also used for **urinary problems and flatulence**.

Externally, wintergreen leaf tea can be used as a gargle for **sore mouth and throat,** as a poultice for **skin diseases,** and a douche for **leukorrhea.** Place a cloth soaked with the oil over painful joints.

Note: Collect the leaves in the fall.

Warning: The pure oil can cause irritation, so it must be used cautiously.

WITCH HAZEL

(Hamamelis virginiana) Parts used: Bark, leaves. *Properties:* Astringent, hemostatic, tonic, sedative. *What it affects:* Skin, stomach, and intestines.

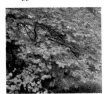 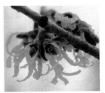

Witch Hazel   Witch Hazel   Witch Hazel

Preparation and amount: *Infusion (leaves):* Steep 10-15 min. Take 6 oz. as needed. *Decoction (bark):* Simmer 10-15 min. Take 3 oz. as needed, up to 2 cups daily. *Tincture (bark):* Take 15-60 drops as needed. *Fluid extract (bark):* Take ½ tsp. as needed. *Powder (bark):* Take 5-10 #0 capsules (30-60 grains) as needed.

Purposes: Witch hazel is **an excellent astringent herb and one of the best remedies for stopping excessive menstruation, hemorrhages from the lungs, stomach, uterus, and bowels.** It is also very good for **stopping bleeding from the lungs, uterus, and other internal organs.** It is because the inner bark has sedative and hemostatic properties, that it is so good for stopping bleeding.

Internally, witch hazel is used for **diarrhea, diphtheria, hemorrhoids, leukorrhea, prolapsed bowel, varicose veins, and uterine problems.** It is used as a vaginal douche.

Externally, witch hazel is primarily used for **insect bites, varicose veins, minor burns, and to stop bleeding of wounds.** It is also used for **bruises, poison ivy, sore breasts, sore muscles, and tonsillitis.** A poultice made from the inner bark is used for **hemorrhoids, varicose veins, and eye inflammation.**

Witch hazel can be used as an injection for **bleeding piles, vaginal discharges, and infections.** As a fomentation or poultice, it is good for **bedsores, oozing skin diseases, and sore and inflamed eyes.** It is good for **almost any internal or external inflamed condition.** Mixed with a small amount of peppermint oil, it is useful as a **mouthwash,** for a **sore throat, or inflamed gums.**

Overseas: Twig tea **rubbed on athletes' legs to keep muscles limber. Relieve lameness.** Tea drunk for **bloody dysentery, cholera, cough, and asthma.** Astringent bark tea taken internally for **lung ailments;** used externally for **bruises and sore muscles.** Widely used today (in distilled extracts, ointments, eyewashes) as an astringent for **piles, toning skin, suppressing profuse menstrual flow, eye ailments.** Used commercially in preparations to treat **hemorrhoids, irritations, minor pain, and itching.** Tannins *(hamamelitannin* and *proanthocyanidins)*

in the leaves and bark are thought to be responsible for astringent and hemostatic properties, antioxidant activity. In the U.S., approved as a nonprescription drug for use in external **analgesic and skin protectant** products, and as an external anorectal, primarily used for symptomatic relief of **hemorrhoids, irritation, minor pain, and itching.** Products are available in every pharmacy. Approved in Germany for treatment of **burns, dermatitis, piles, local inflammation of mucous membranes, minor skin injuries, varicose veins and venous conditions,** among others. Bottled Witch-hazel water, widely available, is a steam distillate that does not contain the astringent tannins of the shrub. More than five *Hamamelis* species also occur in Japan and China, and are there used for similar purposes as the above.

WOOD BETONY

(Betonica officinalis) Part used: Tops. *Properties:* Nervine, alterative, aromatic, hepatic, parasiticide. *What it affects:* Nerves and liver.

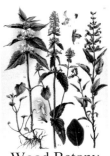 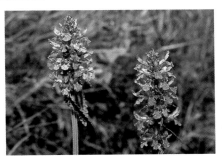

Wood Betony   Wood Betony

Preparation and amount: *Infusion:* Steep 5-15 min. Take 3 oz. 3-4 times daily. *Tincture:* Take 30-60 drops (½-1 tsp.) 3-4 times daily. *Fluid extract:* Take ½-1 tsp. 3 times daily. *Powder:* Take 5-10 #0 capsules (30-60 grains) 3-4 times daily.

Purposes: *Internally,* wood betony is excellent for **headaches, hysteria, and other nervous afflictions.** It is most frequently used in combination with other nervines, to **calm the nerves.** It benefits the function of the liver. It is also useful in treating **diarrhea, convulsions, and nerve twitching in the face, as well as palsy, insanity, neuralgia, and cramps.** Prepare powder herbs of equal parts of wood betony, marjoram, plus a pinch of eyebright, and sniff it up the nose. It is said that this will **stop the most stubborn headaches.** It **stimulates the heart and relaxes muscles.** It **improves appetite and digestion.** Combine it with other blood purifying herbs, in the treatment of **rheumatism and gout.** Combine it with other nervines in the treatment of **nerve diseases and to calm the nerves, when stress is present from sickness and disease.** An infusion, taken 3-4 times a day in 3 oz. doses, will kill **worms** and **open up obstructions of the liver and gallbladder.** It is good for **colds, hyperactivity, nerve pain, anxiety attacks, and cardiovascular disorders.**

Externally, a poultice of the fresh green herb will **draw out splinters, help heal open wounds, and relieve back pains and stitches in the side.**

Note: Because it has a similar flavor, but lacks the

H
E
R
B
S

caffeine and harmful acids, wood betony can be used as a **substitute for commercial black tea**. Use ½ oz. and steep in a pint of boiled water for 10 minutes.

Warning: Avoid the use of wood betony during pregnancy.

WORMWOOD

(Artemisia absinthium) Parts used: Tops, leaves. *Properties:* Antihelmintic, antiseptic, aromatic, diaphoretic, tonic. *What it affects:* Liver, gallbladder, stomach, intestines, uterus, and joints.

 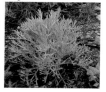

Wormwood   Wormwood   Wormwood

Preparation and amount: *Infusion:* Steep 5-15 min. Take 3 oz. as needed, up to 2 cups daily. *Tincture:* Take 10-30 drops 3-4 times daily. *Fluid extract:* Take 15-60 drops 3-4 times daily. *Powder:* Take 2-4 #0 capsules (5-20 grains) 3-4 times daily.

Purposes: *Internally,* because it is an intensely bitter herb, the special work of wormwood is that of a **stomach medicine**. It is useful for **indigestion, gastric pain, increasing stomach acidity, and improving appetite**, as well as related problems of **heartburn and flatulence**. It **stimulates the uterus** and will **help bring on suppressed menstruation**. It is helpful for **liver insufficiency** by **stimulating liver and gallbladder secretions**. It induces sweating and lowers fevers. It can reduce migraine headaches and will relieve pain during childbirth.

Wormwood tea has been used for years for **gastritis, stomach ulcers, dysentery, tuberculosis, liver and spleen conditions, and kidney and bladder problems**. It **expels roundworms and pinworms**; and it is often used with black walnut, to remove **parasites**. If there is **bleeding from the bowel**, inject the tea and hold it for 5 minutes several times daily as needed.

Externally, it is good for **healing wounds, blemishes, skin ulcers, and insect bites**.

Warning: Wormwood definitely must not be used during pregnancy. With long-term use, it can be habit forming.

YARROW (Milfoil)

(Achillea millefolium) Parts used: Flowers and leaves. *Properties:* Astringent, diaphoretic, hemostatic, stimulant. *What it affects:* Circulation.

Preparation and amount: *Infusion:* Steep 5-15 min. Take 6 oz. 3-4 times daily. *Tincture:* Take 5-20 drops 3-4 times daily. *Fluid extract:* Take ½-1 tsp. 3-4 times daily. *Oil:* Take 5-20 drops 3-4 times daily. *Powder:* Take 5-9 #0 capsules (30-60 grains) 3-4 times daily.

Purposes: *Internally,* yarrow is extremely good for the **early stages of flus and colds**. It is also given as a strong infusion for **children with the measles and other eruptive diseases**. It is also excellent for s**tomach upset, stopping hemorrhages and bleeding from the lungs,**

and shrinking hemorrhoids. Take it as a warm infusion (an oz. of the herb steeped in a pint of boiled water for 20 minutes) for **cramps and to help stop menstrual bleeding**. For **piles, hemorrhage, or vaginal secretions**, use as a douche or enema. If there is **swelling or bleeding of the bowel**, inject 2 oz. into the colon after each bowel movement. If there is much **pain**, inject a warm tea (112°-115° F.), to soothe and reduce that pain. Make a bolus or salve for **bleeding piles**. It is used for **anemia and liver disease**. It is also used for **blood in the urine, epididymitis, leukorrhea, menorrhagia, amenorrhea, measles, and uremic poisoning**.

Externally, it can be **applied directly to wounds, to stop bleeeding**.

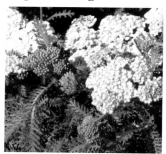 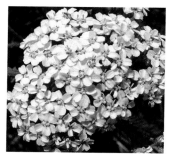

Yarrow   Yarrow

YELLOW DOCK

(Rumex crispus) Part used: Root. *Properties:* Alterative, astringent, cholagogue, laxative, nutritive. *What it affects:* Blood, skin, spleen, liver, and gallbladder.

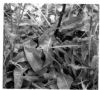 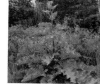 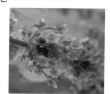

Yellow Dock   Yellow Dock   Yellow Dock

Preparation and amount: *Decoction:* Simmer 5-15 min. Take 1 Tbsp. in 6 oz. water 3 times daily. *Tincture:* Take 5-30 drops 3 times daily. *Fluid extract:* Take ½-1 tsp. 3 times daily. *Syrup:* Take 1 tsp. 3-4 times daily. *Powder:* Take 5-10 #0 capsules (30-60 grains) 3 times daily.

Purposes: *Internally,* yellow dock acts as a **blood purifier and cleanser**, as well as a general tonic. It is an astringent blood purifier used in treating **diseases of the blood**. It tones up the entire system. Because it **stimulates the flow of bile**, it **acts as a laxative**. It improves **colon and liver functions**; and it is good for **tumors, liver, gallbladder problems, and ulcers**.

Use it in formulas for **jaundice and hepatitis**. Because of its high iron content, it is used in the treatment of **anemia**. It is good for inflammation of the **nasal passages and respiratory tract**. It is good for the **spleen**. Combine it in teas and salves with echinacea, burdock root, and sarsaparilla.

It is also used for **cancer, acne, boils, jaundice, leukorrhea, psoriasis, and piles**.

Externally, yellow dock is used for **skin diseases such as eczema, psoriasis, skin itch, ulcers, rashes,** and hives. Combined with sarsaparilla, it makes a tea for **chronic skin disorders**. It makes a good salve for **itchy skin diseases and swellings of glands**. Apply it to **bleeding piles and wounds**. It is good for **running of the ears, scurvy, ulcerated eyelids**. In addition, drink 3 cups of the tea daily. Indians applied crushed yellow dock leaves to boils and pulverized roots to cuts.

Warning: Do not put yellow dock in salads, soups, etc. Its high oxalic acid content can cause poisoning.

YERBA SANTA

(Eriodictyon californisum) Part used: Leaves. *Properties:* Expectorant, astringent, stimulant. *What it affects:* Lungs and stomach.

Preparation and amount: *Infusion:* Steep 30 min. Take 2-3 oz. 3 times daily. *Tincture:* Take 10-30 drops, 3-4 times daily. *Fluid extract:* Take ½-1 tsp. 3-4 times daily. *Powder:* Take 2-10 #0 capsules (15-60 grains) 3-4 times daily.

Purposes: *Internally,* yerba santa is used for all types of **bronchial congestion**. It is used in all types of **chronic skin disorders**. It is a good treatment for **diarrhea and dysentery**, as well as colds and flus. It is an excellent remedy for acute and chronic chest conditions, including asthma. Combine it with equal parts of nettles, mullein, comfrey root, and a small amount of licorice in a tea.

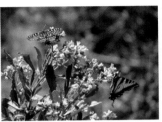
Yerba Santa

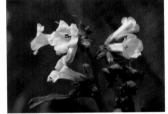
Yerba Santa

WHAT THE BIBLE SAYS ABOUT HERBS

"And God said, Let the earth bring forth grass, the herb yielding seed, and the fruit tree yielding fruit after his kind, whose seed is in itself, upon the earth: and it was so. And the earth brought forth grass, and herb yielding seed after his kind, and the tree yielding fruit, whose seed was in itself, after his kind: and God saw that it was good. And the evening and the morning were the third day"
—Genesis 1:11-13

"And God said, Behold, I have given you every herb bearing seed, which is upon the face of all the earth, and every tree, in the which is the fruit of a tree yielding seed; to you it shall be for meat. And to every beast of the earth, and to every fowl of the air, and to every thing that creepeth upon the earth, wherein there is life, I have given every green herb for meat: and it was so. And God saw every thing that He had made, and, behold, it was very good. And the evening and the morning were the sixth day."
—Genesis 1:29-31

"The fruit thereof shall be for meat, and the leaf thereof for medicine."
—Ezekiel 47:12

"The hay appeareth, and the tender grass sheweth itself, and herbs of the mountains are gathered."
—Proverbs 27:25

"Who cut up mallows by the bushes, and juniper roots for their meat."
—Job 30:4

Applying a poultice: "And Isaiah said, Take a lump of figs. And they took and laid it on the boil, and he recovered."
—2 Kings 20:7 (also in Isaiah 38:21)

"At our gates are all manner of pleasant fruits, new and old."
—Song of Solomon, 7:13

"Ye shall know them by their fruits. Do men gather grapes of thorns, or figs of thistles? Even so every good tree bringeth forth good fruit; but a corrupt tree bringeth forth evil fruit."
—Matthew 7:16-17

"In the midst of the street of it, and on either side of the river, was there the tree of life, which bare twelve manner of fruits, and yielded her fruit every month: and the leaves of the tree were for the healing of the nations."
—Revelation 22:2

The Natural Remedies Encyclopedia

Herbs Overseas

THROUGHOUT THE WORLD, HERBS ARE USED, AND EVEN APPROVED BY GOVERNMENTS AS MEDICINE

A complete table of contents to this chapter will be found on page 11.

How are American herbs, and similar varieties, used by scientists and common folk in Europe, Asia, and elsewhere in the world?

For example, medicinal plants have become extremely popular among doctors and patients in Germany in recent years. Around 75 percent of customers in German pharmacies reach for a natural product when they buy nonprescription medications. In 2006, so-called phytopharmaceuticals accounted for around 2 billion euros ($2.9 billion) worth of revenue, or about a third of the total revenue in nonprescription medications. There is a high demand for these medicinal plants and their leaves, flowers, roots, and seeds.

In total, 45,000 tons of medicinal plants are consumed in Germany each year, making it the market leader in Europe. According to statistics from the *Federal Agency for Nature Conservation* (BfN), around 1,500 types of plants are traded, in Germany, in larger or smaller amounts.

Here are 115 examples of widely used, and frequently government approved, legal herbs sold and heavily used in other countries:

Water Plantain—*Alisma subcordatum* and *Alisma plantago-aquatica*—Used in China for dysuria, edema, disention, diarrhea, and other ailments. Used to lower blood pressure, reduce blood glucose levels, and inhibit storage of fat in the liver.

Garlic—*Allium sativum*—In China, used for digestive difficulties, diarrhea, dysentery, colds, whooping cough, pinworms, old ulcers, swellings, and snakebites. Also to lower blood pressure and serum cholesterol, hypertension, heart ailments, and arteriosclerosis.

Shepherd's Purse—*Capsella bursa-pastoris*—In Germany, fruit is used for excessive or irregular menstrual bleeding and to stop nosebleeds; also used externally to stop bleeding from injuries.

Watercress—*Rorippa nasturtium-aquaticum*—In Germany, watercress is used for inflammation of the respiratory tract. (But do not harvest leaves from polluted waterways.)

Horseradish—*Armoracia rustican*—In Germany, the root is used for treatment of inflammation of the respiratory tract and urinary tract infections.

Buckwheat—*Fagopyrum esculenium*—Used in Europe to treat venous and capillary problems because it increases tone of veins and is taken to prevent hardening of the arteries. Also used to reduce water retention (edema), improve blood flow through the femoral (leg) vein, and enhance capillary resistance.

Horehound—*Morrubium vulgare*—In Germany, used for coughs, colds, and as a digestive aid, and appetite stimulant.

Seneca Snakeroot—*Polygala senega*—Roots of this North American plant are widely used in Japan and Germany to relieve pain, rheumatism, and as an expectorant for inflammation of the upper respiratory tract.

Roundheaded Bush Clover—*Lespediza capitata* — Used in Europe to lower blood cholesterol levels.

Wild Licorice—*Glcyrrhiza lepidota*—European forms of this are used in Germany for gastric and duodenal ulcers, and congestion of the upper respiratory tract. Chinese research finds it better than codeine. Used for gastric and duodenal ulcers, bronchial asthma, and coughs. One of the extensively used herbs in Chinese herbal prescriptions. Use it to detoxify potentially poisonous drugs. But, in Germany, it is not used for more than 4-6 weeks at a time because longer use can increase blood pressure.

Eclipta—*Eclipta prostrata*—Used in China to control internal and external bleeding, dysentery, premature gray hair, bleeding gums, loosening of teeth. In India, leaves are used as a tonic, to treat liver and spleen disease. Plant juice is used for toothaches; this is applied externally with oil, to relieve headaches. Also used to treat abscesses and snakebites. It neutralizes the venom of the South American rattlesnake (Crotalus Durissus terrificus).

Ox-Eye Daisy—*Chrysanthemum vulgare*—In Europe, it is used as a tonic for its antispasmodic effects against whooping cough, to regulate the menses, induce vomiting, and as a diuretic and astringent.

Wild Chamomile—*Chamomilla recutita*—In Germany, its name means "capable of anything." Dried flowers make a famous beverage tea that is used for colic, diarrhea, insomnia, indigestion, gout, sciatica, headaches, colds, fevers, flu, cramps, and arthritis. Its essential oil is antifungal, antibacterial, anodyne, antispasmodic, anti-inflammatory, and antiallergenic. This oil contains two dozen different anti-inflammatory compounds which work together to reduce fevers, inflammation, etc. Heavily used to treat inflammation or spasms of the gastrointestinal tract and inflammation of the respiratory tract. Used externally for inflammatory conditions of the mouth, gums, and bacterial induced skin diseases.

Feverfew—*Tanacetum parthenium*—Five British studies showed that it can prevent 70% of migraines; and it is approved in Canada and England for this. Another indicated that it can profoundly reduce pain intensity.

Prickly Pear Cactus—*Opuntia humifusa*—Mexican physicians use it to help noninsulin-dependent diabetics. An Israeli research group found the dried flowers useful in reducing the urgency to urinate in cases of benign prostatic hyperplasia.

Common Evening Primrose—*Oenatera biennis*—Approved in Britain for treatment of atopic eczema, premenstrual syndrome, and prostatitis.

Indian Strawberry—*Duchesnea indica*—In Asia, the whole-plant poultice or wash (astringent) is used for abscesses, boils, burns, insect stings, eczema, ringworm, rheumatism, traumatic injuries. Whole-plant tea is used for laryngitis, coughs, and lung ailments. The flower tea was traditionally used to stimulate blood circulation.

Small flowered Agrimony—The European species (*Agrimonia eupatoria*) is used to stop bleeding and for wounds, diarrhea, inflammation of the gallbladder, urinary incontinence, jaundice, and gout. Gargled for mouth ulcers and throat inflammation. In France, the drink is used as much for its flavor as for its medicinal values. Throughout Europe, the tea is used for diarrhea, blood disorders, fevers, gout, hepatitis, pimples, sore throat, and even worms. In Germany, small flowered agrimony and a related species (*A. pilosa*) is approved for use in the treatment of mild diarrhea and inflammation of the throat and mouth; it is also externally used for mild skin inflammations.

Fennel—*Foeniculum vulgare*—Seeds are eaten in the Middle East to increase milk secretion and promote menstruation. Powdered seeds are poulticed in China for snakebites. Seed oil relieves spasms of smooth muscles, kills bacteria, removes hookworms. They are also approved in Germany for treatment of gastrointestinal fullness and spasms, as well as catarrh of the upper respiratory tract.

Common Mullein—*Verbascum thapsus*—Originally from Europe, where flowers and leaves are used in cough remedies. Leaves are high in mucilage, soothing to the inflamed mucous membranes, and used for herpes simplex and influenza viruses. In Germany, common mullein is approved as an expectorant in inflammations of the upper respiratory tract. Folk in India used the stalk for cramps, fever, and migraine headaches.

Sicklepod—*Senna obtusifolia*—Chinese seeds are used for internal and external boils and eye diseases. Fruit tea is used for headaches, hepatitis, herpes, and arthritis.

Chickweed—*Stellaria media*—Europeans use this as a cooling demulcent and expectorant, to relieve coughs; also it is used externally for skin diseases and to reduce itching.

Tall Cinquefoil—*Potentilla arguila*—In Germany, the herb is used to treat mild cases of excessive menstual bleeding, diarrhea, and mild inflammations of the throat and mouth.

Lemon Balm—*Melissa officinalis*—Used as an ointment in Europe, to treat cold sores and genital herpes. In Germany, lemon balm is approved for sleeplessness caused by nervous conditions and digestive tract spasms.

Horehound—*Marrubium vulgare*—In Europe, the malodorous, bitter leaves are used in cough syrups, to stimulate digestion and as an expectorant to break up phlegm, relieve coughs, soothe sore throats, and relieve bronchitis and other upper respiratory ailments. Also used for stomach and gallbladder disorders, jaundice, hepatitis; fresh leaves are poulticed on cuts and wounds. It also increases bile flow. In Germany, it is approved for coughs and colds and as a digestive aid and appetitie stimulant.

Narrow Leaved Plantain—*Plantago lanceolata*—The Asian form, *P asiatica,* is used clinically in China to reduce blood pressure (50% success rate).

Common Plantain—*Plantago major*—Prominent folk cancer remedy in Latin America. Used widely for this purpose throughout the world. Is both antimicrobial and stimulates the healing process.

Asparagus—*Asparagus officinalis*—Asians use the shoots as a diuretic in dropsy and gout. Papanese use green asparagus; it aids protein conversion into amino acids. Chinese use it to lower blood pressure. Approved in Germany as a diuretic for irrigation therapy in the treatment of urinary tract infections and to prevent kidney stones.

Indian Strawberry—*Duchesnea indica*—In Asia, whole-plant poultice or wash (astringent) is used for abscesses, boils, burns, insect stings, eczema, ringworm, rheumatism, and traumatic injuries. Whole-plant tea is used for laryngitis, coughs, and lung ailments. Flower tea is used to stimulate blood circulation.

Velvet Leaf—*Helianthemum canadense*—The Chinese use 1 oz. of dried leaves in tea for dysentery and fevers, also as a poultice for ulcers. Dried root is used in tea for dysentery and urinary incontinence. Seed powder is a diuretic and eaten for dysentery and stamachaches.

Small flowered Agrimony—*Agrimonia eupatoria* (European alien)—In France, the drink is used as much for its flavor as for its medicinal virtues. Tea of the European species is believed to be helpful in diarrhea, blood disorders, fevers, gout, hepatitis, pimples, sore throats, and even worms. In studies with mice, the European species, *A. pilosa,* has shown antitumor activity. In Germany, it is approved for use in the treatment of mild diarrhea and inflammations of the throat and mouth; it is also used externally for mild skin inflammations.

Dill—*Anethum grareolens* (leaves, seeds)—In Europe, dill leaves are typically used for flavoring; they are considered digestive, carminative, and a folk medicine for conditions of the gastrointestinal and urinary tract. Dill also reduces spasms.

Fennel—*Foeniculum vulgare* (seeds)—Seeds eaten in the Middle East are used to increase milk secretion, promote menstruation, and increase libido. Powdered seeds are poulticed in China for snakebites. Experimentally, seed oil relieves spasms of smooth muscles, kills bacteria, and removes hookworms. Fennel seed is our best source of anethole and is used commercially as "licorice" (actually anise) flavor. Seeds are approved in Germany for treatment of gastrointestinal fullness, spasms, and catarrh of the upper respiratory tract. Seed extracts stimulate gastrointestinal motility.

Common St. John's Wort—*Typericum perforatum* (leaves, flowers)—St. John's Wort has emerged as the

H
E
R
B
S

best-known herbal treatment for mild to moderate forms of depression. Reportedly outselling the conventional antidepressant Prozac by as much as 20 to 1 in Germany, it is approved in that country for treatment of depression. More than 20 controlled clinical trials have confirmed its safety and effectiveness.

Common Mullein—*Verbascurn thapsus* (leaves, flowering tops)—In Europe, flowers are preferred over leaves; both are used in European cough remedies. Leaves are high in mucilage, soothing to inflamed mucous membranes, and strongly anti-inflammatory. Science confirms the mild expectorant and antiviral activity against herpes simplex and influenza viruses. Contains verbascoside, which has antiseptic, antitumor, antibacterial, and immunosuppressant activity. In Germany, the flowers are approved as an expectorant in inflammations of the upper respiratory tract. Folk in India used the stalk for cramps, fevers, and migraine. The seed is a narcotic fish poison. They also used the stalk for cramps, fevers, and migraine.

Blessed Thistle—*Cnicus benedictus*—(whole plant)—This weak tea (2 teaspoons to 1 cup of water) of the dried flowering plant was traditionally used in Europe to stimulate sweating, appetite, and milk production; it is a diuretic. It has a folk reputation as a remedy for boils, indigestion, colds, deafness, gout, headaches, migraines, suppressed menses, chilblains, jaundice, and ringworm. Experimentally, it increases gastric and bile secretions; and it is antibacterial and anti-inflammatory. Approved in Germany for treatment of loss of appetite and dyspeptic discomfort. Seeds have served as emergency oil seeds.

Golden Ragwort, Squaw Weed—*Senecio allretts* (leaves, roots)—Approved in Germany for treatment of loss of appetite and dyspeptic discomfort. Seeds have served as emergency oil seeds. The root and leaf tea was traditionally used by herbalists to treat delayed and irregular menses, leukorrhea, childbirth complications, lung ailments, dysentery, and difficult urination. Its traditional use in treating a variety of female diseases led to its common name, squaw weed.

Gumweed, Rosinweed—*Grindelia squarrosa* (leaves, flowers)—Approved in Germany for treatment of catarrhs of the upper respiratory tract.

Elecampane—*Intact helenium* (roots, leaves, flowers)—Used in China for certain cancers.

Canada Goldenrod—*Solidago canadensis* (roots, flowers)—Like the European *Solidago virgaurea L*, the leaves of Canada goldenrod are approved in Germany for use as a diuretic in treatment of inflammatory diseases of the lower urinary tract. Also used in irrigation therapy, to prevent and treat urinary and kidney gravel.

Dandelion—*Taraxacum officinale* (roots, leaves)—Leaves are approved in Germany for treatment of loss of appetite and dyspepsia with a feeling of fullness and flatulence. The root is approved for treatment of bile flow disturbances, as a diuretic, to stimulate appetite, and to treat dyspepsia. The dandelion is one of Europe's most popular cough remedies; the dried leaves are smoked for coughs and asthma. Smoke is believed to impede impulse of fibers of parasympathetic nerves and to act as an antihistamine.

Coltsfoot—*Tussilago farfitra* (leaves, flowers)—

Mucous membranes and leaves have spasmolytic activity. The leaves are approved in Germany for treatment of cough, hoarseness, inflammation of the respiratory tract, and mild inflammation of the mouth or throat. WARNING: Contains traces of liver-affecting pyrrolizidine alkaloids; and it is potentially toxic in large doses. In Germany, the use is limited to 4 to 6 weeks per year, except under advice of a physician.

Daylily—*Hemerocallis fulva* (roots, young shoots)—The roots and young shoots of this naturalized lily, from eastern Asia, are an ancient medicinal of Traditional Chinese Medicine and used for more than 2,000 years for mastitis, breast cancer, and a variety of other ailments. In China, the root tea is used as a diuretic in turbid urine and edema; it is used to treat poor or difficult urination, jaundice, nosebleeds, leukorrhea, uterine bleeding; and poultice for mastitis. This is a folk cancer remedy for breast cancer. Experimentally, Chinese studies indicate that root extracts are antibacterial, useful for blood flukes (parasites), and a diuretic. The edible flower buds are used for its diuretic and astringent properties in jaundice and to "relieve oppression and heat in the chest"; also poulticed for piles.

Cypress Vine   *Ipomoea quamoclit* (herb)—A South American folk medicine for its pain-relieving and purgative effects. Externally applied to carbuncles, snakebites, sores, and piles. In India, the leaves are eaten as a potherb. In Australia, it has been used as a purgative and snakebite remedy.

Valarian—*Valeriana officinalis* (root)—Valerian is a leading over-the-counter tranquilizer and sleep aid in Europe. Ten controlled clinical studies have been published on valerian preparations; a recent study found it worked best as a sleep aid over a period of a month rather than on a single-dose basis. Approved in Germany for use as a sedative in sleep-inducing preparations for nervous restlessness and to aid in falling asleep. Cats arc said to be attracted to the scent of the root as they are to catnip. In eighteenth-century apothecaries, the quality of valerian root was determined by the way in which cats reacted to it.

Water or Purple Avens—*Geum rivale* (leaves, root)—In China and Japan, a tea of the whole plant of *Geum japonicum* (a related species) is used as a diuretic and as an astringent to treat coughs and the spitting up of blood. The root and leaves of G. japonicum are used as a poultice or wash for skin diseases and boils. Possesses proven antiviral activity.

Fireweed—*Epilobium angustifolium* (leaves, root)—Leaves are used in Russia as "kaporie" tea (10 percent tannin). Leaf extract is antibacterial and shown to reduce inflammation.

Corn Cockle—*Agrostemma githago* (seeds)—Europeans use it for cancers, warts, hard swellings in uterus.

Soapwort—*Saponaria officinalis* (root)—The root is approved in Germany to treat catarrhs of the upper respiratory tract.

Marshmallow—*Althaea officinalis* (leaves, root)—German health authorities allow use of the leaves and root preparations to relieve local irritation (such as digestive-tract inflammatory conditions) and to soothe mucous membrane irritation, such as a sore throat accompanied by a dry cough. Marshmallow roots and leaves were traditionally used in tea for sore throat and as an expectorant in bronchitis.

They are externally poulticed for bruises, sprains, aching muscles, and inflammations. 30 percent of the root and 16 percent of the leaves are high in mucilagin; and they are responsible for the demulcent or soothing effect to irritated mucous membranes and skin. Marshmallow has immuno-stimulating activity.

High Mallow—*Malva sylvestris* (leaves, flowers, root)—The leaves of Common Mallow *(Callirhoe involucrata)* and *High Mallow (Malva sylvestris)* are approved in Germany for treatment of irritations of the mouth and throat associated with an irritating, dry cough. In China, the leaves and flowers have been used as an expectorant, a gargle for sore throats, and a mouthwash. Diuretic properties are also attributed to the plant; and it is said to be good for the stomach and spleen. Other Malva species are similarly used.

Lady's Thumb, Heart's Ease—*Polygonum persicaria* (leaves)—In Europe, leaf tea is used for inflammation, stomachaches, and sore throats.

Salad Burnet—*Sanguisorba officinalis* (leaves, root)—In Europe, leaf tea is used for fevers and as a styptic. Root tea is astringent and allays menstrual bleeding. In China, the root tea is used to stop bleeding and "cool" the blood. It is taken for piles, uterine bleeding, and dysentery; also it is externally used for sores, swelling, and burns. Experimentally, the plant is antibacterial (in China); it stops bleeding and vomiting. Powdered root is clinically used for second- and third-degree burns.

Motherwort—*Leonurus cardiaca* (leaves)—Extracts are approved in Germany for nervous heart conditions and in the supportive treatment of hyperthyroidism. Experimentally, leonurine, a leaf constituent, is a uterine tonic. Chinese species, well-documented with laboratory and clinical reports, have been used similarly.

Great Burdock—*Arctium lappa* (leaves, root, seeds)—This widespread Eurasian weed is used in traditional medicine in China, Japan, Europe, and N. America. Root tea (2 ounces of dried root in a quart of water) was traditionally used as a "blood purifier." This is a diuretic and stimulates bile secretion, digestion, and sweating; also used for gout, liver and kidney ailments, rheumatism, and gonorrhea. Root is 50 percent inulin. It is was traditionally used for diabetes. Bitter compounds in roots, particularly artipicrin, are antibacterial; this also explains its use as a digestive stimulant. In China, a tea of leafy branches is used for vertigo and rheumatism; and a tea mixed with brown sugar is used for measles. This is externally used as a wash for hives, eczema, and other skin eruptions. Juice of the fresh plant has been shown to protect against chromosome aberrations. Both flowers and leaves have antibacterial activity. Seeds are diuretic and thought to be an antiseptic. They are used for abscesses, sore throats, insect bites, snakebites, flu, and constipation; also once used to treat scarlet fever, smallpox, and scrofula. Crushed seeds are poulticed on bruises. Leaves are poulticed on burns, ulcers, and sores. Japanese studies suggest that roots contain compounds that may curb mutations.

Asiatic Dayflower—*Commelina communis* (leaves)—In China, leaf tea is gargled for sore throats and used for its cooling, detoxifying, and diuretic properties in flu, acute tonsillitis, urinary infections, dysentery, and acute intestinal enteritis. Other *commelina* species are similarly used.

Passionflower, May-Pop—*Passiflora incarnata* (whole plant)—Approved in Germany for nervous restlessness and tension; it is considered especially useful in sleep disturbances or anxiety arising from restlessness. Edible fruits are delicious.

Kudzu—*Pueraria montana* (root, flowers, seeds, stems, root starch)—A Chinese plant, now in the U.S. In China, root tea is used for headaches, diarrhea, dysentery, acute intestinal obstruction, gastroenteritis, deafness, to promote measles eruptions, and induce sweating. Experimentally, plant extracts lower blood sugar and blood pressure. Flower tea is used for stomach acidity; it "awakens the spleen" and "expels drunkenness." Seeds are used for dysentery. Root, flowers, and seeds are used in China to treat drunkenness or sober an intoxicated person. The stem is poulticed for sores, swellings, mastitis; and tea is gargled for sore throats. Root starch (used to stimulate production of body fluids) is eaten as food. Roots are richer in estrogenic isoflavones, daidzein, and genistein than soybeans are. Genistein may prevent development of tumors by preventing the formation of new blood vessels that nourish the tumors. Daidzein and daidzin have been shown to inhibit the desire for alcohol and to reduce blood pressure and venous obstruction. An extract of the root was found to have 100 times the antioxidant activity of vitamin E.

Purple or Spike Loosestrife—*Lythrum salicaria* (whole flowering plant)—Tea is made from the whole flowering plant (fresh or dried) and used as a European folk remedy (demulcent, astringent) for diarrhea and dysentery; it is a gargle for sore throats, a douche for leukorrhea, and a cleansing wash for wounds. Experimentally, it stops bleeding and is antibacterial and anti-inflammatory. This contains tannins and other components, with bactericidal activity in the gastrointestinal tract.

Common Speedwell—*Veronica officinalis* (leaves, root)—In Europe, astringent root or leaf tea was traditionally used to promote urination, sweating, menstruation, and as a "blood purifier." It was also used for skin and kidney ailments, coughs, asthma, lung diseases, gout, rheumatism, and jaundice. Also considered to be an expectorant, diuretic, and a tonic. Extracts of this are found to prevent and speed healing of ulcers in experiments on animals.

Johnny-Jump-Up, Heart's Ease—*Viola tricolor* (leaves)—In Europe, this leaf tea is a folk medicine for fevers, a mild laxative, and a gargle for sore throats; it is considered a diuretic, an expectorant, and a mild sedative. It is a "blood purifier" and used for asthma, heart palpitations, and skin eruptions (such as eczema). Rat experiments confirm possible use for skin eruptions. It is approved for external use in Germany in treatment of mild seborrhea and related skin disorders.

Sharp Lobed Hepatica, Liverleaf—*Hepatica nobilis* (leaves)—American Indians used liverleaf tea for liver ailments, poor digestion, and as a laxative; they used it externally as a wash for swollen breasts. In folk tradition, tea was used for fevers, liver ailments, and coughs. It is thought to be mildly astringent, demulcent, and a diuretic.

Flax—*Linum usitatissimum* (seeds)—Seeds are used in European phytomedicine as a mild, lubricating laxative in constipation, for irritable bowel syndrome, diverticulitis, and for relief of gastritis and enteritis. Flaxseed is also used to correct problems caused from abuse of stimulant laxatives. Flax oil is a folk remedy used for pleurisy and pneumonia; it is high in omega-3 fatty acids.

Comfrey—Symphytum officinale (leaves, root)—In Germany, external application of the leaf is approved for the treatment of bruises and sprains; root poultice is approved for bruising, pulled muscles and ligaments, and sprains.

Lobelia—Lobelia inflata (whole plant)—Used in other countries. *Lobeline*, a chemical cousin of nicotine, is one of 14 alkaloids in the plant; until recently it was used in the U.S. in commercial "quit smoking" lozenges, patches, and chewing gums. It is said to appease a physical need for nicotine without addictive effects. It also produces dilation of the bronchioles and increased respiration.

Perilla—Perilla frutescens (leaves, seed)—One Chinese clinical study found application of the fresh leaves (rubbing on infection) for ten to fifteen minutes a day made warts disappear in two to six days. A favorite culinary herb of some Asian cultures. Seed oil is a rich source of alpha-linolenic acid, an omega-3 essential fatty acid. WARNING: Avoid during pregnancy. A component in the leaves was found to induce severe lung lesions in mice, rats, and sheep.

Peppermint—Mentha piperita (leaf, oil)—Peppermint capsules are used in Europe for irritable bowel syndrome. Peppermint leaf is approved in Germany for use in muscle spasms of the gastrointestinal tract, as well as spasms of the gallbladder and bile ducts. The essential oil is used externally to treat neuralgia and myalgia. Menthol is an approved ingredient in cough drops. The oil stops spasms of smooth muscles. Animal experiments show that azulene, a minor component of distilled peppermint oil residue, is anti-inflammatory and has antiulcer activity. WARNING: Peppermint oil is toxic if taken internally; it causes dermatitis. Menthol, the major chemical component of peppermint oil, may cause allergic reactions. Infants should never be exposed to menthol-containing products because they can cause the lungs to collapse. Use should be avoided in cases of gallbladder or bile duct obstruction.

Hyssop—Hyssopus officinalis (leaves)—Experimentally, extracts are useful for herpes simplex and is anti-inflammatory. This contains at least 8 antiviral compounds. In 1990, researchers found that a hyssop extract inhibited replication of the human immunodeficiency virus. Used with horehound for bronchitis, coughs, and asthma. The herb has been used externally to treat rheumatism, muscle aches, wounds, and sprains.

Heal-All, Self-Heal—Prunella vulgaris (whole plant)—In Europe and Asia, leaf tea was traditionally used as a gargle for sore throats and mouth sores, fevers, and diarrhea; it was used externally for ulcers, wounds, bruises, and sores. In China, a tea made from the flowering plant is considered cooling. The plant was also used in China to treat heat in the liver and aid in circulation; it is used for conjunctivitis, boils, and scrofula; and it is a diuretic for kidney ailments. Research suggests the plant possesses antibiotic, hypotensive, and antimutagenic qualities. This contains the antitumor and diuretic compound, ursolic acid.

New England Aster—Aster novaeangliae (root, leaves)—Root and leaves are approved in Germany for

treatment of loss of appetite and dyspepsia. Root extracts are antibacterial. In experiments, animals given chicory root extract exhibit a slower and weaker heart rate (pulse).

Milk Thistle—Ilybum mariannin (seeds, whole plant)—*Silymarin* is a seed extract that dramatically improves liver regeneration in hepatitis, cirrhosis, mushroom poisoning, and other liver diseases. In the form of an intravenous preparation, silvbin (a flavonoid component of the seed) is clinically useful in treating severe Amanita mushroom poisoning in Germany. While clinically used in Europe, its use in the U.S. is not well-known. Oral commercial preparations of the seed extracts are manufactured in Europe, now widely available in the U.S., and also approved in Germany and other countries for the supportive treatment of chronic inflammatory liver disorders (such as hepatitis, cirrhosis, and fatty infiltration caused by alcohol or other toxins). In addition to treating liver disease, it also has a preventive effect, helping to prevent liver damage from exposure to toxic chemicals. Young leaves (with spines removed) are eaten as a vegetable. Tea was tradionally made from the whole plant; now it is used to improve appetite, allay indigestion, and restore liver function. The tea is used for cirrhosis, jaundice, hepatitis, and liver poisoning from chemicals, drug abuse, and alcohol abuse.

Echinacea, Coneflower—Echinacea angustifolia (**echinacea pallida**, and **echinacea purpurea** have similar effects) (plant)—More than 300 pharmaceutical preparations are made from echinacea plants in Germany (including extracts, salves, and tinctures). Echinacea is used for wounds, herpes sores, canker sores, and throat infections; it is preventive for influenza and colds. This is a folk remedy for brown recluse spider bites. Science confirms many traditional uses, plus cortisone-like activity and insecticidal, bactericidal, and immuno-stimulant activities. It is considered a nonspecific immune system stimulant.

Purple Coneflower—Echinacea purpurea (whole plant)—Purple Coneflower is widely used in Europe, but not native there. Most commercial German echinacea preparations utilize extracts of above-ground parts and/or roots of E. purpurea. Extracts enhance particle ingestion capacity of white blood cells and other specialized immune system cells, increasing their ability to attack foreign particles (such as cold or flu viruses). German studies show significant immune-system stimulating activity with orally administered extracts of *E. purpurea, E. angustifolia,* and *E. pallida* in mice and laboratory experiments. Several clinical studies have revealed that *E. purpurea* reduces severity and duration of cold and flu symptoms. However, recent clinical studies found that ethanolic extracts of *E.angustifolia* and *E. purpurea* did not prevent colds and flu. Different preparations (water versus alcoholic extracts) may have different active components. *Cichoric acid, polysaccharides, alkylamides*, and other compounds have attributed immuno-stimulating activity. Tops (not roots) are approved in Germany as an immuno-stimulant for colds and flu, and are used externally for hard-to-heal wounds and sores. In topical preparations, *echinacoside* has antioxidant activity, reducing degradation of skin when exposed to sunlight.

Dragon or Green Arum—Arisaema dracontium

H
E
R
B
S

(plant)—The Chinese use related *Arisaerna* species for epilepsy and hemiplegia (paralysis), and externally as a local anesthetic or in ointment for swellings and small tumors.

Wild Yam—Dioscorea villosa (roots)—Research and production is in Germany and the U.S. Of all plant genera, there is perhaps none with greater impact on modern life and whose dramatic story is as little known as *Dioscorea*. Most of the steroid hormones used in modern medicine, especially those in contraceptives, were developed from elaborately processed chemical components derived from yams. Drugs made with yam derived components *(diosgenins)* relieve asthma, arthritis, and eczema; they also regulate metabolism and control fertility. Synthetic products manufactured from *diosgenins* include human sex hormones (contraceptive pills) and drugs to treat menopause, dysmenorrhea, premenstrual syndrome, testicular deficiency, impotency, prostate hypertrophy, psychosexual problems, high blood pressure, arterial spasms, migraines, and other ailments. Widely prescribed cortisones and hydrocortisones are indirect products of the genus, *Dioscorea*. They are used for Addison's disease, some allergies, bursitis, contact dermatitis, psoriasis, rheumatoid arthritis, sciatica, brown recluse spider bites, insect stings, and other diseases and ailments. Wild yam has appeared in the American market in recent years as a "source" of estrogen or progesterone, prompting some to call this marketing effort the "wild yam scam" because the root does not contain human sex hormones. WARNING: The fresh plant may induce vomiting and other undesirable side effects.

Hops—Humulus lupulus (leaf, fruit)—Hops is approved in Germany to treat discomfort from restlessness or anxiety and sleep disturbances. It is considered calming and helpful in promoting sleep. Tea of fruits (strobiles) were traditionally used as sedative, antispasmodic, and a diuretic for insomnia, cramps, coughs, fevers; it was used externally for bruises, boils, inflammation, and rheumatism. Experimentally, it is antimicrobial, relieves spasms of smooth muscles, and acts as sedative (disputed). Hops contains several sedative and pain-relieving components and is used to relieve mood disturbances, nervous tension, anxiety, and unrest. Japanese hops, *Hunnihis japonicas*, is a weedy annual with 5-9 leaf lobes. Leaves are much rougher than common hops.

Horseweed, Canada Fleabane—Conyza canadensis (whole plant)—Africans use it for eczema and ringworm. This essential oil was traditionally used for bronchial ailments and cystitis. It is pain-relieving, antioxidant, spasm-relieving, and antibacterial. Plant tea is used as a folk diuretic; astringent for diarrhea; "gravel" (kidney stones); diabetes; painful urination; and hemorrhages of stomach, bowels, bladder, and kidneys; it is also used for nosebleeds, fevers, bronchitis, tumors, piles, and coughs.

Stinging Nettle—Urtica dioica (whole plant)—Leaf tea was traditionally used in Europe as a "blood purifier," "blood builder," diuretic, and an astringent for anemia, gout, glandular diseases, rheumatism, poor circulation, enlarged spleen, mucous discharges of lungs, internal bleeding, diarrhea, and dysentery. Its effect involves the action of white blood cells, aiding coagulation and formation of hemoglobin in red blood corpuscles. Iron-rich leaves have been cooked as a potherb. Studies suggest CNS-depressant, antibacterial, and mitogenic activity; it inhibits effects of adrenaline. This plant should be studied further for possible uses against kidney and urinary system ailments. Recently, Germans have been using the root in treatments for prostate cancer. Russians are using the leaves in alcohol for cholecystitis (inflammation of the gallbladder) and hepatitis. Some people keep potted stinging nettle in the kitchen window, alongside an aloe plant, in the belief that an occasional sting alleviates arthritis. Leaves are approved in Germany for supportive treatment of rheumatism and kidney infections. Root preparations are approved for symptomatic relief of urinary difficulties associated with early stages of benign prostatic hyperplasia which affects a majority of men over 50 years of age. WARNING: Fresh plants sting. Dried plant (used in tea) does not sting.

Cocklebur—Xanthium strumarium (leaves, root)—Chinese use leaf tea for kidney disease, rheumatism, tuberculosis, diarrhea, and as a blood tonic. Historically the root was used for scrofulous tumors (*strumae;* hence the species name). This plant and the related species *(Xanthium spinosum)* were formerly used for rabies, fevers, malaria; they were considered diuretic, fever-reducing, and a sedative. WARNING: Most cocklebur species are toxic to grazing animals and are usually avoided by them. Seeds contain toxins, but the seed oil has served as lamp fuel.

Sheep Sorrel—Rumex acetosella (leaves, root)—Leaf tea of this common European alien (originally in Europe and now in America) is used for fevers, inflammation, scurvy. Fresh leaves are considered cooling and a diuretic. Leaves are poulticed (after roasting) for tumors and wens (sebaceous cysts); this is a folk cancer remedy. Root tea is used for diarrhea and excessive menstrual bleeding. It has become popular in recent years as a component of the reputedly anticancer Essiac formula and Ojibwa Indian teas. Sheep sorrel is rich in cancer-preventive vitamins; it also includes four antimutagenic and four antioxidant compounds, perhaps laying the foundation for reported anticancer (cancer preventing) folk uses. WARNING: May cause poisoning when used in large doses, due to high oxalic acid and tannin content.

Spiny Amaranth—Amaranthus spinosus (leaves)—First used in South America. This weed is found throughout the tropics and is spreading into N. America. Leaves are astringent. They were adopted by American Indian groups for the treatment of profuse menstruation. Many Amaranth species are valued for astringency; most often they are used to stop internal and external bleeding.

Annual Wormwood—Artemisia annua (leaves, seeds)—Used by U.S. Army and Chinese as a powerful treatment of malaria. Leaf tea (gather before flowering) was originally used by American Indians for colds, flu, malarial fevers, dysentery, diarrhea. Externally was poulticed on abscesses and boils. Since then, it has been discovered that this herb is effective against malaria. For quinine and/or *chlorquinine*-resistant malaria (of interest to U.S. Army), clinical use of derivative compounds in China (tested with 8,000 patients) shows near 100 percent efficacy. Seeds are used for night sweats, indigestion, and flatulence. The compound is responsible for the antimalarial activity and also demonstrates marked herbicidal activity. It contains six or more antiviral compounds; some are proven synergetic. WARNING: May cause allergic reactions or dermatitis.

**H
E
R
B
S**

Common Juniper—*Juniperus communis* (fruits)—Juniper berries are one of the most widely used herbal diuretics. They are approved in Germany in teas for stomach complaints and to simulate appetite. Science confirms anti-inflammatory and spasm-reducing activity, which may contribute to diuretic activity. Fruits eaten raw or in a drink of tea are a folk remedy used as a diuretic and urinary antiseptic for cystitis, carminative for flatulence, and antiseptic for intestinal infections; these fruits were once used for colic, coughs, stomachaches, colds, and bronchitis. It is used externally for sores, aches, rheumatism, arthritis, snakebites, and cancer. Volatile oil is responsible for diuretic and intestinal antiseptic activity. Diuretic activity results from irritation of renal tissue. WARNING: Potentially toxic. Large or frequent doses cause kidney failure, convulsions, and digestive irritation. In Germany, use is limited to four weeks. Avoid during pregnancy. Oil may cause blistering.

Saw Palmetto—*Serenoa repens* (fruits)—Both in Germany and the U.S., pharmacological and clinical studies show that the fruits are useful in the treatment of prostate disorders. In the 1990s, saw palmetto berry extracts have emerged as the most important natural treatment for benign prostatic hyperplasia, a nonmalignant enlargement of the prostate that affects a majority of men over 50 years of age. Evaluated in several thousand men in more then two dozen controlled clinical trials, alone or in comparison with a conventional drug, saw palmetto preparations have been found equally effective as the conventional use in relieving symptoms of benign prostatic hyperplasia while producing fewer side effects. Saw palmetto fruit preparations are approved in Germany, France, Italy, and other countries for treatment of symptoms related to benign prostatic hyperplasia. Fruit extracts, tablets, and tincture were traditionally used to treat prostate enlargement and inflammation. It was also used for colds, coughs, irritated mucous membranes, tickling feeling in throat, asthma, chronic bronchitis, head colds, and migraine. A suppository of the powdered fruits in cocoa butter was used as a uterine and vaginal tonic. It is considered as a expectorant, a sedative, and as a diuretic.

Yucca, Soapweed—*Yucca glauca* (root)—In European experiments with mice, water extracts have shown antitumor activity against melanoma. One human clinical study suggests that saponin extracts of the root were effective in the treatment of arthritis.

Rose—*Rosa rugosa* (fruit, rose hips)—This is the largest rose in the U.S. This Asian introduction has larger fruits (rose hips) than any of our native roses. The Chinese use flower tea to "regulate vital energy" and promote blood circulation for stomachaches, liver pains, mastitis, dysentery, leukorrthea, and rheumatic pains. This rose is also thought to "soothe a restless fetus." Fruits (rose hips) make a pleasant, somewhat tart, tea. High in vitamin C, the fruits have been used to treat scurvy (a disease caused by deficiency of vitamin C).

Black Raspberry—*Rufus occidentalis* (root, leaves, fruit)—This astringent root tea was traditionally used for diarrhea, dysentery, stomach pain, gonorrhea, back pain, a "female tonic," and a blood tonic for boils. Leaf tea is a wash for sores, ulcers, and boils. This tea is approved in Germany for treatment of diarrhea and mild inflammation of the mouth and throat. It is astringent because of the tannins in both leaf and root. RELATED SPECIES: The same parts of most blackberry plants (other Rubus species) have been similarly used.

Common Barberry—*Berberis vulgaris* (berries, root bark)—Barberry is used in Chinese medicine for treating lowered white blood cell counts following chemotherapy or radiation therapy in cancer patients. Berry tea is used to promote appetite; it is a diuretic, an expectorant, a laxative. It also relieves itching. Root-bark tea promotes sweating; it is astringent, an antiseptic, and a "blood purifier." It is used for jaundice, hepatitis (stimulates bile production), fevers, hemorrhage, and diarrhea. Leaf tea is for coughs. Root-bark tincture is used for arthritis, rheumatism, and sciatica. This common barbarry contains *berberine*, which has a wide spectrum of biological activity that includes antibacterial activity; and it is useful for infection. It also contains *berbamine*, which increases white blood cell and platelet counts. WARNING: Large doses are harmful.

Hawthorn—Hawthorn *Crataegus* species. This is a highly variable plant group (fruits, flowers)—Fruits and flowers are famous in herbal medicine (American Indian, Chinese, European) as a heart tonic. Research studies confirm its use in hypertension with a weak heart, angina pectoris, and arteriosclerosis. Dilates coronary vessels, reducing blood pressure; it acts as a direct and mild heart tonic. Prolonged use is necessary for efficacy. Tea or tincture is used. Hawthorn products are very popular in Europe and China. Hawthorn leaf and flower (though not the fruits) are approved in Germany for treating early stages of congestive heart failure that is characterized by diminished cardiac function, a sensation of pressure or anxiety in the heart area, age-related heart disorders that do not require digitalis, and mild arrhythmias. Use is confirmed by at least 14 controlled clinical studies. WARNING: Eye scratches from thorns can cause blindness. Contains heart-affecting compounds that may affect blood pressure and heart rate.

Devil's-walking-stick, Angelica Tree—*Aralia spinosa* (root, berries)—Diabetic Koreans in the Washington, D.C., area take the plant to lower their insulin requirements. Tincture of berries is used for toothaches and rheumatic pain. The root is poulticed for boils, skin eruptions, and swelling. Fresh bark is strongly emetic and purgative; it is thought to cause salivation. WARNING: Handling roots may cause dermatitis. Large amount of berries are poisonous.

Southern Prickly Ash—*Zanthoxylum clava-herculis* (bark, berries)—Used in European herbal medicine for treating rheumatic conditions, Raynaud's disease, and as a circulatory stimulant in intermittent claudication. An alkylamide, *neoherculin*, produces a localized numbing effect. Most research on the genus relates to Asian or African species. A folk cancer remedy, it contains the alkaloid, *chelerythrine*, with antibacterial and anti-inflammatory activity. Affects muscle contractility by blocking or stimulating neuromuscular transmissions, rather than through a direct effect on smooth muscle tissue.

Northern prickly ash—*Z. americanurn* (fruit)—An Israeli research group has conducted clinical studies on the use of a fruit extract of European Elder *(Sambucus nigra)* with positive results for colds and flu. Flowers are approved in Germany for use in treating colds because they reduce fever while increasing bronchial secretions. In West Virginia, concentrated fruit syrup is made as a wintertime remedy for colds and flu. WARNING: Bark, root, leaves, and unripe berries are toxic and said to cause cyanide poisoning and severe diarrhea. Fruits are edible when cooked. Flowers are not thought to be toxic and are eaten in pancakes and fritters.

American Indians used inner-bark tea as a diuretic, strong laxative, and emetic; it was poulticed on cuts, sore or swollen limbs, newborn's navel, boils to relieve pain and swelling, and for headaches. Leaves are poulticed on bruises and on cuts, to stop bleeding. Bark tea was formerly used as a wash for eczema, old ulcers, and skin eruptions. A tea with peppermint in water is a folk remedy for colds; it induces sweating and nausea. Considered a mild stimulant, carminative, and diaphoretic.

Chaste Tree—*Vitex agnus-castus* (fruit)—Fruit preparations are approved in Germany for menstrual disorders, pressure and swelling in the breasts, and premenstrual syndrome. WARNING: May cause rare dermatitis. Avoid during pregnancy or hormone replacement therapy. Seeds (fruits) were used for more than 2,500 years for menstrual difficulties. In medieval Europe, seeds were thought to allay sexual desire; hence the name, chaste tree. In the late nineteenth century, American physicians used tincture to increase milk secretion and treat menstrual irregularities. Today it is widely prescribed by European gynecologists for treatment of the premenstrual syndrome, heavy or too frequent periods, acyclic bleeding, infertility, suppressed menses, and to stimulate milk flow.

French Mulberry—Callicarpa americana (leaves, root, berries)—The Chinese use the leaves of a related *Callicarpa* species as a vulnary to stop bleeding of wounds. It is also used to treat flu in children and menstrual disorders. Root and berry tea is used for colic.

Crampbark—*Viburnum Opulus* (bark, leaves, fruit)—In Europe, bark tea has been used to relieve all types of spasms, including menstrual cramps; it is an astringent and uterine sedative. Science confirms its antispasmodic activity. In China, leaves and fruit arc used as an emetic, laxative, and antiscorbutic. WARNING: Berries are considered potentially poisonous; they contain the chlorogenic acid, *betasitosterol*, and ursolic acid, at least when they are unripe.

Blackhaw—Viburnum prunifolium (bark)—Root- or stem-bark tea was originally used by the American Indians; then it was adopted by Europeans for painful menses, and to prevent miscarriage and relieve spasms after childbirth. It is considered a uterine tonic, sedative, antispasmodic, and nervine. Also used for asthma. Research has confirmed that it has uterine-sedative, pain-relieving (like willows, it contains salicin), anti-inflammatory, and spasm-reducing properties. Most of the dozen or so species in our range are similarly used. WARNING: Berries may produce nausea and other discomforting symptoms.

Spicebush—*Lindera benzoin* (leaves, bark, berries, twigs)—American Indians used berry tea for coughs, cramps, delayed menses, croup, and measles; bark tea was used as a "blood purifier" and for sweating, colds, rheumatism, and anemia. Settlers used berries as an allspice substitute. Medicinally, the berries were used as a carminative for flatulence and colic. The oil from the fruits was applied to bruises and muscles or joints (for chronic rheumatism). Twig tea was popular for colds, fevers, worms, gas, and colic. The bark tea was once used to expel worms, for typhoid fevers, and as a diaphoretic for other forms of fevers. An extract of the stem bark has been found to strongly inhibit yeast *(Candida albicans)* much better than any of the other 53 various herb species studied.

Witch Hazel—*Lanianielis virginiana* (bark, leaves)—Leaf tea was originally used for colds and sore throats. But, in modern times, many other uses were found for it. Twig tea was rubbed on athletes' legs, to keep muscles limber and relieve lameness; tea drink was for bloody dysentery, cholera, cough, and asthma. Astringent bark tea was taken internally for lung ailments and used externally for bruises and sore muscles. It is widely used today (in distilled extracts, ointments, and eyewashes) as an astringent for piles, toning skin, suppressing profuse menstrual flow, and eye ailments. It is used commercially in preparations to treat hemorrhoids, irritations, minor pain, and itching. Tannins *(hamamelitannin* and *proanthocyanidins)* in the leaves and bark are thought to be responsible for astringent and hemostatic properties, and antioxidant activity. In the U.S., it is approved as a nonprescription drug for use in external, analgesic, and skin protectant products; also it is an external anorectal that is primarily used for symptomatic relief of hemorrhoids, irritation, minor pain, and itching. Products are available in every pharmacy.

Witch Hazel is approved in Germany for treatment of burns, dermatitis, piles, local inflammation of mucous membranes, minor skin injuries, varicose veins, venous conditions, and more. Bottled witch hazel water, widely available, is a steam distillate that does not contain the astringent tannins of the shrub. RELATED SPECIES: Vernal Witch Hazel H. vernalis, with a range centered in the Ozarks, blooms from December to March. Leaves and bark are indiscriminately harvested as witch hazel, without distinguishing species. More than five *Hamamelis* species also occur in Japan and China.

Southern Magnolia—*Magnolia grandiflora* (bark, leaves, seeds)—Seeds are used in Mexican traditions for antispasmodic activity. Also used for high blood pressure, heart problems, abdominal discomfort, muscle spasms, infertility, and epilepsy. Contains magnolol and honokiol, with antispasmodic activity. Scientific research confirms sedative activity of seeds. American Indians used a wash of the bark to treat prickly heat itching and a wash for sores. Crushed bark was used in steam baths to treat water retention. In nineteenth-century America, bark was used to treat malaria and rheumatism. Fruits were used as a digestive tonic for dyspepsia and general debility. WARNING: Leaves have caused severe contact dermatitis.

Horse Chestnut—Aesulus hippocastanum (seeds)—Horse chestnut seed extracts are widely prescribed in European herbal medicine for edema with venous insufficiency, for varicose veins, and to improve vascular tone; It helps to strengthen weak veins and arteries, in reducing leg edema, nighttime calf muscle spasms, thrombosis, and hemorrhoids. Its uses are backed by clinical studies. Contains *aescin*; this reduces capillary wall permeability, lessening diameter and number of capillary wall openings, regulating the flow of fluids to surrounding tissue, and increasing blood circulation. Also used in gastritis and gastroenteritis. Topically, *aescin*-containing gels or creams are widely used to allay swelling and pain in bruising, sprains, and contusions. Injectable forms of aescin are used in European trauma centers, to help stabilize brain-trauma patients. WARNING: Outer husks are poisonous; all parts can be toxic. Fatalities are reported. Seeds (nuts) contain 30-60 percent starch, but can be used as a foodstuff only after the toxins have been removed.

Paulownia, Princess Tree—Paulownia tomentosa (leaves, inner bark, flowers)—A Chinese native introduced this as an ornamental that has made itself quite at home, especially in the American South. The wood is highly valued by the Japanese and is exported at a high price. In China, a wash of the leaves and capsules was used in daily applications, to promote the growth of hair and prevent graying. Leaf tea was used as a footbath for swollen feet. Inner-bark tincture (after being soaked in alcohol) was given for fevers and delirium. Leaves or ground bark were fried in vinegar and poulticed on bruises. Flowers were mixed with other herbs, to treat liver ailments. In Japan, the leaf juice is used to treat warts. WARNING: Contains potentially toxic compounds.

Sugar Maple—Acer saccharum (inner bark, sap)—American Indians used the inner bark in tea for coughs and diarrhea; also as a diuretic, a expectorant, and a "blood purifier." Maple syrup is said to be a liver tonic and kidney cleanser, and used in cough syrups. During the maple sap-gathering process in spring, New Englanders once drank the sap collected in buckets as a spring tonic. Now it is being used in Europe also.

Flowering Dogwood—Cornus florida (inner bark, berries, twigs)—Astringent root-bark tea or tincture was widely used in the South, especially during the Civil War, for malarial fevers (substitute for quinine); also for chronic diarrhea. Root bark was also poulticed onto external ulcers. Twigs were used as "chewing sticks"—forerunners of modern toothbrushes. An 1830 herbal reported that the American Indians and captive Africans in Virginia were remarkable for the whiteness of their teeth, and attributed it to the use of dogwood chewing sticks. Once chewed for a few minutes, the tough fibers at the ends of twigs split into a fine soft "brush." Contains verbenalin, which has reported pain-reducing, anti-inflammatory, cough suppressant, uterotonic, and laxative qualities. WARNING: As with hard toothbrushes, dogwood chewing sticks can cause receding gums.

Tree of Heaven—Ailanthus altissima (bark, root) —This Chinese native was introduced in the late nineteenth century as an ornamental. It quickly established itself. In cities like New York and Boston, it grows in harsh conditions where no other plants seem able to survive. Considered a weed tree in many American cities. USES: Two ounces of bark infused in 1 quart of water, given in teaspoonfuls for diarrhea, dysentery; leukorrhea, and tapeworm. Used in Chinese healing for these purposes.

National Cancer Institute researchers have reported several antimalarial compounds; five of these are more potent than the standard antimalarial drug, *chloroquine.* WARNING: Large doses are potentially poisonous. Gardeners who cut the tree may suffer from rashes.

Silk Tree, Mimosa—Albizia julibrissin (bark, flowers)—In Chinese medicine, bark *(he-ituan-pi)* and the flowers *(he-huan-litua)* are used. Bark is used in tea (mostly in combination with other herbs) for depression, restlessness, and insomnia caused by anxiety. The poultice is externally used for traumatic injuries. Flowers are used as a sedative for insomnia.

Ginkgo—Ginkgo biloba (seeds, leaves)—Seeds (after removal of toxic flesh with obnoxious odor) are cooked and used in Traditional Chinese Medicine for treatment of lung ailments. Leaves were rarely used historically for cough, asthma, or diarrhea. They were used externally as a wash for skin sores and to remove freckles. Today, complex, highly processed, concentrated Ginkgo leaf extracts (calibrated to 24 percent flavonoids; 6 percent *ginkgolides*, with toxic components removed) are the best-selling herbal preparations in Europe. The subject of hundreds of scientific studies, Ginkgo leaf extracts increase circulation and improve oxygen metabolism to the extremities and the brain; it is an antioxidant. Clinically shown to improve short-term memory, attention span, and mood in the early stages of Alzheimer's. This extract is approved in Germany for memory deficits, poor concentration, peripheral arterial occlusive disease (improving pain-free walking distance), and for vertigo and ringing in the ears (tinnitus) caused by vascular disturbances. WARNING: Leaf extracts may cause relatively rare gastrointestinal upset, headaches, or skin allergies. Fleshy seed coat causes severe contact dermatitis (like poison ivy). Fruits and seeds are handled with rubber gloves.

Sassafras—Sassafras albidum (leaves, twigs, pith, root, bark)—In the early days of European settlement in New England, sassafras was a major export to Europe and is still used there today. In fact, the Plymouth colonies were partly founded on speculation of Sassafras exports. Root-bark tea, which the American Indians told them about, was a famous spring blood tonic and "blood purifier"; it was also a folk remedy for stomachaches, gout, arthritis, high blood pressure, rheumatism, kidney ailments, colds, fevers, and skin eruptions. The mucilaginous twig pith has been used as a wash or poultice for eye ailments and also taken internally (in tea) for chest, bowel, kidney, and liver ailments. Mucilaginous leaves were once used to treat stomachaches and was widely used as a base for soup stocks. WARNING: *Safrole* (found in oil of Sassafras) reportedly is carcinogenic; it is banned by the FDA. However, the *safrole* in a 12-ounce can of old-fashioned root beer is not as carcinogenic as the alcohol (ethanol)

H
E
R
B
S

in a can of beer.

Redbud—*Cercis canadensis* (bark, flowers)—Use of bark is approved in Germany for fever, rheumatic complaints, and headaches. In short, it is used similarly to aspirin; also as an antipyretic, antiphlogistic, and an analgesic. The bark of this willow, and the very bitter and astringent bark of other willows, has traditionally been used for diarrhea, fevers, pain, arthritis, and rheumatism; the poultice or wash is used for corns, cuts, cancers, ulcers, and poison ivy rashes. *Salicylic acid*, derived from *salicin* (found in bark), is a precursor to the most widely used semisynthetic drug, *acetylsalicylic acid* (aspirin), which reduces pain, inflammation, and fever. In the intestines, compounds in the bark are transformed to *saligenin*, which is oxidized in the liver and blood to produce *salicylic acid*. Pain is reduced by inhibition of prostaglandin synthesis in sensory nerves. RELATED SPECIES: While many herbalists list white willow as the most common *Salix* species used, many *Salix* species are involved in the commercial supply of willow bark. In fact, other species contain ten times as much active constituents as white willow. Crack willow *(S. fragilis)*, basket willow, and purple osier *(S. purpurea)* are native to Europe, cultivated, and escaped to the wild in the U.S. Both are higher in *salicin* than white willow and are used as official sources of willow bark in Europe.

Weeping Willow—*Salix babylonica* (bark, leaves)—Traditionally was used in Europe for its tonic, antiseptic, fever-reducing, and astringent qualities. Bark was used for at least 2,000 years in China for rheumatoid arthritis, jaundice, and fevers. Leaves were used in China to reduce heat (fevers), treat skin eruptions, regulate urination, and as a blood purifier. They were used in the treatment of mastitis, toothache, scalds, and other conditions. Like most willows, leaves contain *salicin* and tannins.

White Mulberry—*Morus alba* (leaves, inner bark)—In China, leaf tea is used for headaches, hyperemia (congestion of blood), thirst, coughs, and as a "liver cleanser." Experimentally, leaf extracts are antibacterial. Young-twig tea is used for arthralgia and edema. Fruits are eaten for blood deficiency, to improve vision and circulation, and for diabetes. Inner-bark tea is used for lung ailments, asthma, coughs, and edema.

American Basswood, Linden—*Tilia americana* (flowers, bark)—American Indians used inner-bark tea for lung ailments, heartburn, and weak stomach; bark poultice was used to draw out boils. Leaves, flower and bud tea, or tincture was traditionally used for nervous headaches, restlessness, painful digestion. WARNING: Frequent consumption of flower tea may cause heart damage. RELATED SPECIES: Small-leaved European Linden *T cordata* and large-leaved European Linden *T platyphyllos,* cultivated and sometimes naturalized in N. America, are used in European herbal medicine.

In Germany, the flowers are approved for treatment of colds and cold-related coughs. They are primarily used as a diaphoretic. Preparations of the leaves and wood were also traditionally used for fevers and cellulitis; they were not approved because claimed applications are not scientifically evaluated. Despite lack of scientific proof, the leaves are widely used in herbal products for colds and coughs.

Japanese Honeysuckle—*Lonicera japonica* (bark, flowers, leaves)—In China, it is called the "gold and silver flower." Leaves and flowers are a beverage tea in Japan. Flowers were traditionally used in East Asia in tea for bacterial dysentery, enteritis, laryngitis, colds, fevers, and flu; it is externally used as a wash for rheumatism, sores, tumors (especially breast cancer), infected boils, scabies, swelling. Stem tea is weaker. Experimentally, flower extracts lower cholesterol; they are antiviral, antibacterial, and tuberculostatic. Widely used in prescriptions and patent medicines in Chinese medicine to treat colds and flu. Pills are made from floral concentrates. Used for bronchitis, colds, and flu. When echinacea or garlic have failed against flu, some professional herbalists have used this plant as a last resort. Flowers contain at least a dozen antiviral compounds. With the rapid evolution of viruses, the synergistic combinations of phytochemicals (such as those found in the Japanese Honeysuckle) are less liable to lead to resistant viral strains than solitary chemical compounds.

Field Horsetail—*Equisetum arvense* (whole plant)—Approved in Germany for treatment of post-traumatic edema, irrigation therapy for bacterial and inflammatory diseases of the lower urinary tract, and kidney and bladder gravel; used externally for wounds and burns. Folk in India consider the field horsetail as a diuretic and hemostatic. Root is given to teething babies. American Indians used plant tea for ailments, such as kidney and bladder constipation. This is a folk remedy for bloody urine, gout, gonorrhea, and stomach disorders. Poultice is used for wounds. Field horsetale has a high silica content. Also once used in tea for tubercular lung lesions. Shown to be valuable for inflammation. WARNING: Toxic to livestock, questionable for humans, and may disturb thiamine metabolism.

Common or Running Club Moss—*Lycopodium clavatum* (leaves, spores)—Chinese species in the club moss family is being researched as a potential treatment for Alzheimer's disease. American Indians used plant tea for postpartum pains, fever, and weakness. In folk medicine, spores were used for diarrhea, dysentery, and rheumatism; Its use is as a diuretic and gastric sedative, aphrodisiac, and styptic; it is also used externally in powders for a baby's chafing, tangled or matted hair with vermin, herpes, eczema, dermatitis in folds of skin, and erysipelas. Spores, called vegetable sulphur, were formerly used to coat pills and suppositories. WARNING: This club moss (*L. clavatum*) contains a toxic alkaloid.

Venus Maidenhair Fern—*Adiantum capillus-veneris (whole fern)—In traditional Chinese medicine, a handful of dried leaves are steeped to make a tea drink as an expectorant, astringent, and tonic for coughs, throat afflictions, and bronchitis. Used as a hair wash for dandruff and to promote hair growth. The leaves are similarly used for bronchial diseases and as an expectorant. This fern has also been used as a worm expellent, an emetic, and an agent to reduce fevers. Externally, it has been poulticed on snakebites and used as a treatment for impetigo.*

The Natural Remedies Encyclopedia

Poisonous Plants In Field and Woods

Here are 51 color pictures of the 21 most poisonous plants in the field and woods of North America: This Identification Guide is invaluable, for it will enable you to identify those plants which are extremely poisonous—so you will not pick them, thinking they might be useful, when you are collecting healing herbs in the field and woods: Poison Ivy (2 pics) 200 / Poison Sumac (2) 200 / Death Angel (3) 200 / Fly Amanita (2) 200 / Orange Amanita (3) 200-201 / Buttercups (2) 201 / Death Camas (3) 201 / Horse Nettle (2) 201 / Iris (1) 201 / Jack in the Pulpit (2) 201 / Jimsonweed (2) 201 / Lady Slipper (3) 201-202 / Mayapple (Mandrake) (1) 202 / Mistletoe (1) 202 / Moonseed (1) 202 / Nettles (5) 202 / Wild Parsnip (1) 202, 203 / Nightshade (2) 202 / Poison Hemlock (2) 203 / Skunk Cabbage (2) 203 / Pokeweed (1) 203 / Spurges (2) 203 / Water Hemlock (3) 203 *—5 more plants; 20 more pictures: 204-205*

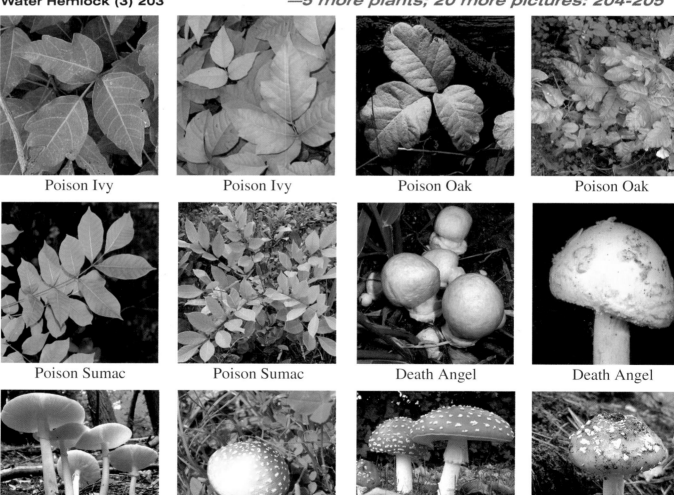

Poison Ivy	Poison Ivy	Poison Oak	Poison Oak
Poison Sumac	Poison Sumac	Death Angel	Death Angel
Death Angel	Fly Amanita	Fly Amanita	Orange Amanita

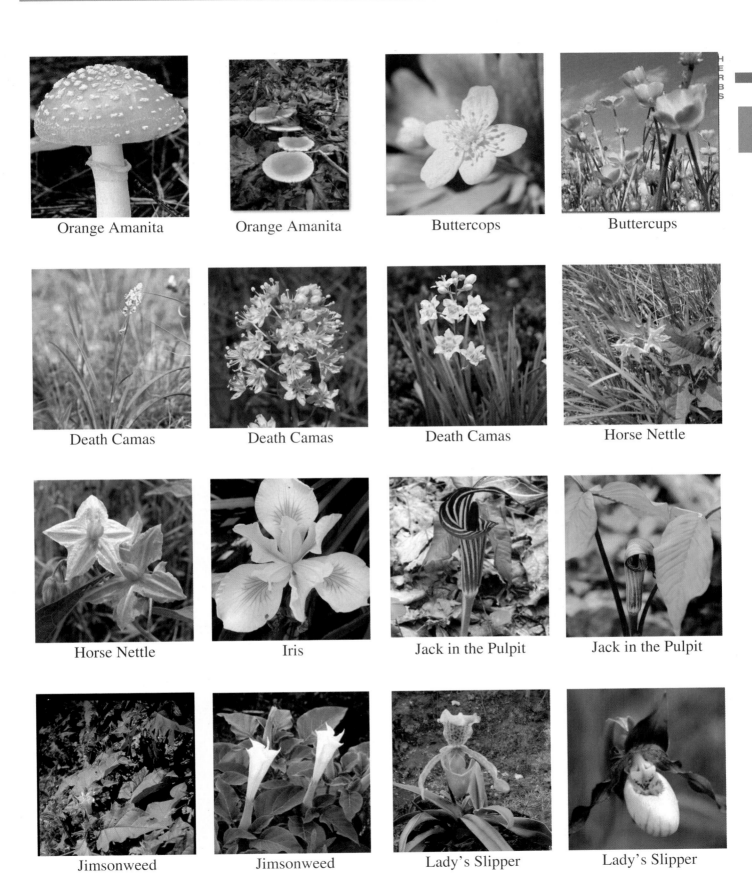

Orange Amanita

Orange Amanita

Buttercops

Buttercups

Death Camas

Death Camas

Death Camas

Horse Nettle

Horse Nettle

Iris

Jack in the Pulpit

Jack in the Pulpit

Jimsonweed

Jimsonweed

Lady's Slipper

Lady's Slipper

HERBS

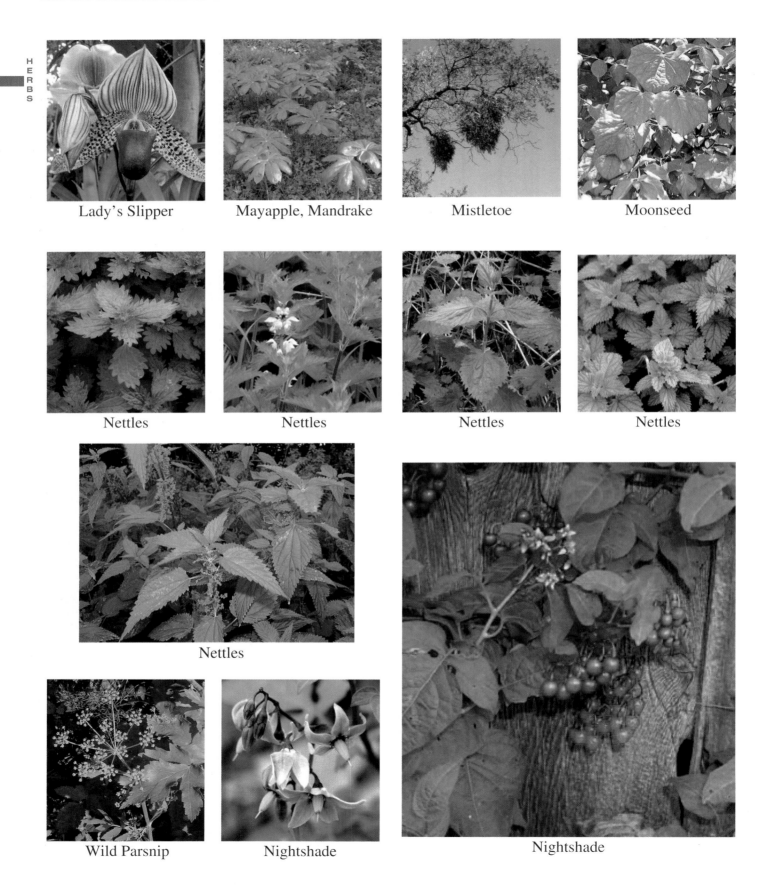

Lady's Slipper

Mayapple, Mandrake

Mistletoe

Moonseed

Nettles

Nettles

Nettles

Nettles

Nettles

Wild Parsnip

Nightshade

Nightshade

HERBS

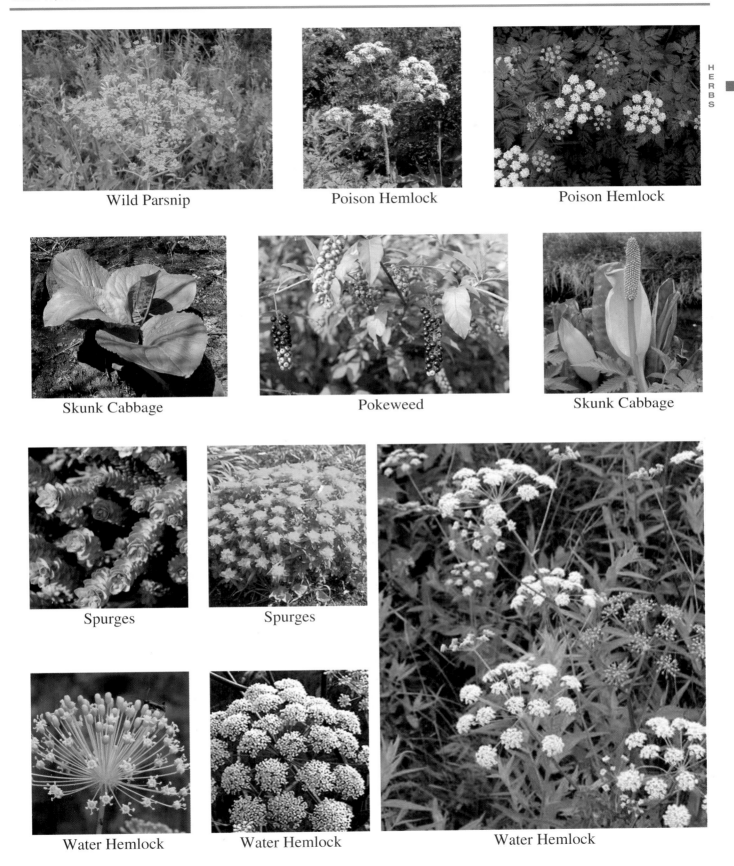

Wild Parsnip

Poison Hemlock

Poison Hemlock

Skunk Cabbage

Pokeweed

Skunk Cabbage

Spurges

Spurges

Water Hemlock

Water Hemlock

Water Hemlock

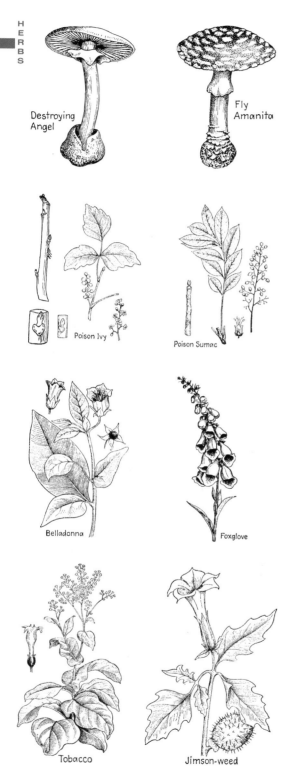

Destroying Angel

Fly Amanita

Poison Ivy

Poison Sumac

Belladonna

Foxglove

Tobacco

Jimson-weed

THE AMANITA AND DESTROYING ANGEL—The two mushrooms sketched on the left are the most deadly of mushrooms. They are found in open woods or clearings in summer or fall. Some mushrooms are edible (yet contain little nourishment because they are fungi) and some are mildly or strongly poisonous. But the Amanita is the worst killer of all. Here are the identifying marks of a full-grown Amanita: (1) A bulb-like root (a cup-like vulva) in the ground. (However, you may break the mushroom off just above the bulb and not notice this identifier.) (2) A small ring on the stem just below the cap. (3) There may be small flecks, or spots on top of the cap. Amanitas have white spores and free gills which are not attached to the stem. The Fly Amanita may be yellow to orange (or even greenish) while the Death Angel (also called the Destroying Angel) is usually white. But, for the Amanitas, color is not a guide. The Amanita first sends up a small round globe which splits on the sides as the stem inside it keeps growing. This causes the cap to break off from the ring and the base. There are bad effects felt 3-4 hours after eating the Fly Amanita and 10 to 40 hours after eating the Death Angel (the most deadly of the Amanitas). Call a physician immediately!

POISON IVY AND OAK—The sketch on the left shows what the leaves of both look like. Poison Ivy, in the Eastern States, is a crawling, climbing vine. Poison Oak, in the West, is a woody shrub. The roots of Poison Ivy are shallow but widely spread. Both prefer part shade, part sunlight. The leaves of both (along with Poison Sumac, below) have an oily contact poison which you can get by touching the leaves, (later) your shoes, or the smoke from the burning plant. Treatment of poison: Wash immediately, several times with non-oily soap and water (or wash with 5% ferric chloride in 50% alcohol). To the itching area, apply baking powder, Epsom salts (1-2 tsp. to cup of water). Also good: wet nutritional calcium powder in water or oil and apply, to stop the itching.

POISON SUMAC—Tree or shrub, height to 25 feet, trunk to 6 inches. Limited to swampy lands throughout Eastern States. Many other sumacs are safe. Treat as above.

BELLADONNA—Height to 6 feet. It is extremely poisonous; yet, unfortunately, it is grown for use as a medicinal drug! Contains two deadly poisons (hyoscyamine and hyoscine) which are used in medicines. For the effects caused by these poisons, see Jimson Weed, below.

FOXGLOVE—Height to 5 feet. Although often raised as an ornamental flower, it is extremely poisonous. The leaves contain three poisons used in medical drugs: digitoxin, digitonin, and digitalin.

TOBACCO—Height to 8 feet or more. One of the most deadly of poisonous plants. A tiny amount, injected, will instantly kill an adult. The only reason cigarettes are not immediately fatal is because the nicotine is absorbed more slowly. Tobacco contains over 3,000 poisons. Beginning in 1612 in Virginia, it has been cultivated as a narcotic. But its use gradually ruins various organs and leads to a startling variety of diseases and eventual death.

JIMSON WEED—Height to 5 feet. Grows wild in Eastern States. All parts of the plant are poisonous to cattle, horses, sheep, and humans. Even contact with the leaves may produce a severe dermatitis (skin rash). Unfortunately, it is also cultivated as a medicinal drug. Contains the same two poisons found in Belladonna: the akaloid hyscyamine is in the leaves, fruit, and roots, and seeds; and hyoscine is in the roots. The poison causes headache, vertigo, thirst, nausea, loss of sight and of coordination, mania, convulsions, and death.

HERBS

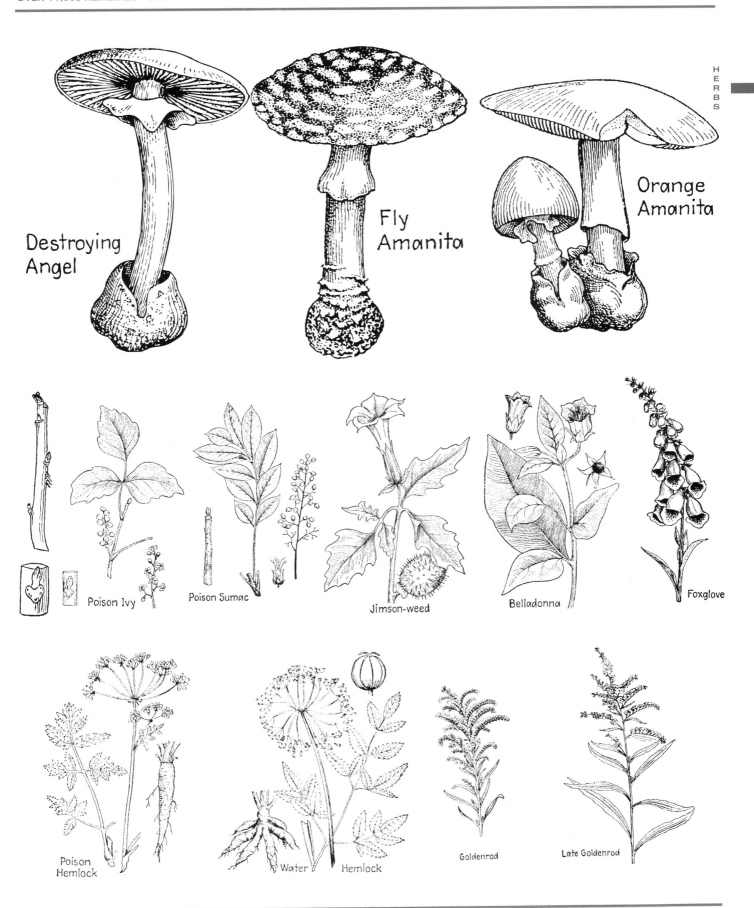

Destroying Angel

Fly Amanita

Orange Amanita

Poison Ivy

Poison Sumac

Jimson-weed

Belladonna

Foxglove

Poison Hemlock

Water Hemlock

Goldenrod

Late Goldenrod

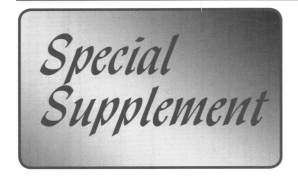

Basic Hydrotherapy

This chapter, in the *The Natural Remedies Encyclopedia,* is a reprint of a full-length book, *The Water Therapy Manual* (now out of print) by the present author.

In order to simplify the step-by-step presentation even more, this chapter now has 195 color pictures.

God has placed in the simple things of nature—clean water, nonpoisonous herbs, rest, nourishing food, sunlight, fresh air, moderate exercise, and trust in Him—the elements needed to bring health to our human bodies. Let us thank Him for these simple methods and use them carefully and wisely. Let us dedicate our lives anew to Him each day and obey His laws of health; for He has given us these blessings because He loves us.

— *The Publisher*

TABLE OF CONTENTS

INTRODUCTION: IMPORTANT

The material in this *Encyclopedia Supplement on Basic Hydrotherapy* is from the 294 page *Water Therapy Manual*, written by the author of this *Encyclopedia*.

It is important that you understand that this material was written by a reporter, not by a trained physician. It provides source material for those who enjoy reading historical monographs in the medical field. It has also been prepared for use in your own home, under the direction of a qualified physician (or his nurse or physical therapist) in one of the following ways: (1) as emergency therapy during an acute attack; (2) as more prolonged therapy in a chronic condition, whether temporary or permanent; (3) as convalescent therapy following a period of sickness; and (4) as tonic applications to rebuild strength and vitality, both in those who are convalescing and those who are well.

This chapter will provide you with information as to the manner in which certain qualified physicians, nurses, and physiotherapists use water applications. And it will also provide you with warnings, cautions, and contraindications that these experts in this field have expressed in regard to various hydrotherapy applications and complicating conditions and situations.

Everything in this chapter, with the exception of several Biblical and historical quotations, is based on the writings of twentieth-century medical personnel who are qualified in the field of *physiotherapy* (the modern name for *hydrotherapy*, or *water therapy*,— the giving of *water treatments*).

This entire chapter is the result of a careful study of over 2,700 pages of hydrotherapy material; most it now out-of-print.

This chapter is based on the writings of the fol-

H
Y
D
R
O

lowing thirteen authorities: George Knapp Abbott, M.D.; Clarence W. Dail, M.D.; Kathryn Jensen-Nelson, R.N., M.A.; John Harvey Kellogg, M.D.; Ethel M. Manwell, B.S., RN., A.R.P.T.; J. Wayne McFarland, M.D.; Gertrude Muench, R.N., R.P.T.; Fred B. Moor, M.D.; Mary C. Noble, B.S., R.N.; Stella C. Peterson, R.N., B.S.N.E.; Charles S. Thomas, Ph.D.; Agatha M. Thrash, M.D.; Calvin L. Thrash, M.D. Most, and probably all of the above medical authorities, were (at the time of their writing) either teachers in medical schools or directors of physical therapy departments in leading hospitals or sanitariums. John Kellogg's 1,193-page *Rational Hydrotherapy,* which has been out-of-print for over half a century, was an especially rich source.

You have a right to care for sickness within your home; but you should realize that it is current medical opinion that anything you do to regain or improve your health should be done under the direction of a qualified physician.

As stated above, this chapter is here provided to be used in your home, under the direction of the physician of your choice. If difficulties of any kind develop, immediately contact him. Treatments carried on without his aid or counsel are treatments carried on at your own risk.   —*Vance Ferrell*

HOW TO USE THIS SECTION

This section on hydrotherapy is remarkably complete in providing you with **HOW to do the water treatments**. In order to find what you are looking for, you can use its table of contents *(pp. 206-207)* and Disease Index *(pp. 273-275).* This section also tells **WHAT conditions to use the therapies on.** But you will find a great abundance of additional information in the Kellogg formulas, scattered throughout this *Encyclopedia.* They tell what diseases to use hydrotherapy on. To locate it, use the large *Encyclopedia* Disease Index at the back of the book to locate them. Water therapy is a most wonderful blessing.

— PART ONE —

THE LIVING STREAM

Within the Sacred Scriptures is to be found one of the most basic laws of the human body:

"For the life of the flesh is in the blood."—*Leviticus 17:11.*

What is it that makes you alive? According to the Bible, it is the blood flowing through your body. Your brain and nerves, glands, and internal organs, are all very important. But there is no "Life" intrinsically in any of them. They are only alive because living blood is flowing through them every moment—bathing and nourishing their every fiber, tissue, and cell.

The life is not in your heart; for it is only a fluid pump. Neither is it in your body secretions, limbs,

lymphatic tissue, eyes, or nerve cells. The only life in your body—which imparts life to all your body by a continual drenching process—is in your blood.

"Flesh with the life thereof, which is the blood thereof, shall ye not eat."—*Genesis 9:4.* "Be sure that ye eat not the blood: for the blood is the life; and thou mayest not eat the life with the flesh."—*Deuteronomy 12:23.*

How does healing come to afflicted parts of your body? Your internal organs, especially your liver, are very important. So also is your brain. But it is the blood that brings the healing to your body. Not only does it contain life, it is also the only means of bringing vital nutrition from your digested food to all of your body parts. And it also brings that spark of life, precious oxygen, without which you would quickly die.

But more: Blood, as it rapidly moves through your body, not only brings food and oxygen; it also carries away waste products from each cell in your body. Thus, the blood not only imparts life, it also heals and restores. And it does this continually. Your blood pump (the heart) need only skip one beat, and you may not recover; two beats skipped and you are dead. That is how important the flow of blood is within your body. Every day, your heart pumps an amazing quantity of blood throughout your body. But without it you would die. For flowing from your heart—issuing from it—is your very life.

"Keep thy heart with all diligence; for out of it are the issues of life [for, flowing from it, is the life]."—*Proverbs 4:23.* What does water therapy do? It is the most powerful, natural, nonpoisonous means of quickly moving the nourishing, healing blood into and out of afflicted, diseased body parts. Let us now turn our attention to how and why water therapy can do this so well:

First, let us take a brief look at two of the many important things that are in the blood. This miraculous fluid contains several different types of cells. One is the *Red Blood Cell* (RBC). This cell, which is the red color of the blood, is the carrier of nutrition and oxygen to every tissue and fiber of your body. And it also takes away carbon dioxide and other waste products. Thus it both nourishes and cleanses. RBCs are so tiny that 3,000 of them could lie side by side in a distance of but one inch. In an amount of blood smaller than a tiny drop (one cubic millimeter), there are about 4½ to 5 million RBCs. Then there is the *White Blood Cell* (WBC). These colorless micro-dots protect the body against toxins, disease organisms, and various irritants. Our heavenly Father gave us the RBCs to bring nourishment to the entire system; and He gave us the WBCs to attack and destroy disease wherever it may be found throughout the body. When a person is well, there are normally about 7,000 to 9,000 WBCs in every tiny blood drop. But when infection is present, this increases to 15,000 to 25,000.

There are many types of cells and factors in the blood; but we will not mention them here, even though they are also important. All in all, there are about 25 trillion blood cells in your body. Laid end-to-end, they would reach to nearly four times around the earth.

As the healing, life-giving blood enters the injured or infected area, it brings nourishment and oxygen. It also brings phagocytes (another name for the White Blood Cells), which literally gobble up the infection and foreign substances. And the blood also provides the materials with which the body can rebuild the torn, diseased structures in the body.

But there are two limitations to the blood:

(1) There really is not enough of it. Your heart would have to be several times larger than it is, in order to provide you with all the blood you need. This is why you should not swim for thirty minutes after a meal: There is not enough blood to care for initial digestion and muscle activity at the same time. It is the same when there is a problem in part of your body: You need more blood—or a quicker flow of blood—than normal in order to bring healing. In connection with this, keep in mind that, at any given time, at least one quarter of all the blood in your body is in your lungs. And what is it doing there? It is rapidly moving past the 1,200 square yards of lung surface area in order to receive a fresh supply of air. Every second, 2 trillion blood cells pass by the air chambers of the lungs. But, at any one time, one-fourth of your body's five quarts of blood are in the lungs, being refreshed there.

(2) The blood has a tendency to congest, or pool, in a damaged or infected part of your body. The result is a clogging up of too much blood in one place. The blood circulation to that part has slowed and the pooled blood has less ability to nourish and heal.

So, we need to bring larger quantities of blood to the afflicted areas; and we need to move it in and out again more rapidly. We need to loosen up, speed up, and equalize the blood circulation. We do not want it pooling in one area. We want it moving back and forth through the body at a good pace; for this is what keeps the blood healthy, full of fresh oxygen from the lungs and abundant nourishment from the liver and portal vein.

And, interestingly enough, as the blood quickens in healthy activity, the bone marrow begins to make more blood than it normally would!

God has provided that carefully given applications of hot and cold to the body will provide the needed help. But what shall we use to place this hot and cold in contact with the body? The answer, in large measure, is water—the most abundant, natural source of hot and cold to be found on our planet. Water: the substance that can retain heat and cold better than any other common element around us. Water: the substance that can cleanse better than anything else in the world.

Water, like blood, is a very special gift of God to mankind.

You, yourself, are about 65 percent water and this wonderful liquid is a continual necessity to your existence both within your body and outside of it.

Fortunately, water is one of the most common substances on Planet Earth. It covers more than 70 percent of the earth's surface and fills the oceans, rivers, and lakes; also it is in the ground and the air we breathe.

— PART TWO —

PRINCIPLES AND CAUTIONS

In order to make the best use of water therapy, we need to understand a number of principles and cautions. In this present section, we will provide you with an overview of these basic principles and cautions.

Hot and cold water can powerfully help to bring healing to your body. The following statement by medical and nursing authorities in the field, although written in somewhat technical language, will give you an idea of the effective help that water therapy can bring you in your own home. Here are some of the effects of water when applied to your body:

"Following all sorts of cold procedures associated with mechanical stimulation, and after hot baths or douches [the name in hydrotherapy for water sprays], when they are followed by cold applications, there is a decided increase in the number of [blood] cells in the peripheral circulation. This increase often amounts to from 20 to 35 percent in the red corpuscles [RBCs] and from 200 to 300 percent in the white corpuscles [WBCs]; the hemoglobin also shows an increase of 5 percent or more.

"Not only does the activity of the peripheral blood vessels keep the blood cells evenly distributed, but the normal movements of the spleen (*ie.,* its alternate dilation and contraction) are also a factor in distributing the white blood cells evenly throughout the body. Various applications to the abdomen and over the spleen stimulate this organ to increased activity. The splenic douche [water spray], alternate hot and cold applications, and cold friction to the abdomen are especially efficient in this respect.

"Another factor in changes in blood counts is the increase of blood volume (fluid) found to occur with applications of heat, so that heat alone may result in a relative lowering of the hemoglobin and the red cells. Strange as it may seem, both hot and cold baths cause an absolute increase in the white blood cells. But, in induced fever therapy, the white cells in the periphery increase up to 10,000 or 15,000. The more or less permanent increases in these elements after a course

HYDRO

or series of tonic treatments must be attributed to an entirely different mechanism and can scarcely be explained in any other way than by the stimulation of the blood-forming organs.

"The earlier experiments done by the Winternitz school [of water therapy studies] indicated a rather notable increase in the completeness of absorption of nitrogenous food and the hastening of nitrogenous catabolism, as shown by the lessening of nitrogen in the feces on days when tonic cold baths were given, and an increase in the percent of nitrogen in the urine at the same time. On these treatment days the excretion of urea was increased about 20 percent and uric acid about 30 percent. The excretion of ammonia was increased as much as 50 percent, and the alkaline phosphates 25-30 percent. After the bath period the more completely burned nitrogenous extractives of the urine sank as low as 0.5 or 1.0 percent of the total nitrogen excreted; whereas the extractives usually take up from 3 to 4 percent of the total nitrogen. With hot treatment these changes were very slight unless it was much prolonged or frequently repeated.

"In one experiment the middle finger was able before complete fatigue to execute work equal to 5.139 kilogram-meters (a kilogram-meter is equal to 1/75 of a horsepower). After a cold bath at 50° F. for fifteen seconds, the same muscles were able to do work equivalent to 9.126 kg-m before complete fatigue . . Even after the muscles have been fatigued by active work and are able to work but a very short time longer, the giving of cold treatment restores them to their usual capacity for work, or the working ability may even be increased over the normal.

"Hot baths have the opposite effect; *i.e.*, the muscles become more quickly fatigued and are able to do less work. On an average, various cold treatments increase the working ability about 30 percent, and hot treatments decrease muscular capacity to the same extent . .

"All alternate hot and [then] cold applications have the same effect in varying degree, according to the nature of each treatment. General cold treatments, such as the cold-mitten friction, cold-towel rub, wet-sheet rub, cold shallow bath, pail pour, and even the salt glow, are powerful means of restoring the muscles to conditions for renewed activity.

"Sugar from foods is the source of muscle energy. In muscular activity it is changed to lactic acid, the accumulation of which produces fatigue. But increased circulation carrying plenty of oxygen quickly changes the lactic acid back into a source of energy. Tea and coffee, while acting as muscle stimulants, add a fatigue poison, which is not easily or quickly gotten rid of, thus lengthening the recovery time, lessening the work done, and decreasing endurance.

"Mechanical effects alone, such as massage, also raise the working capacity of the muscles, but

to a lesser degree than hydriatic [water therapy] procedures. Cold applications should be properly graduated to suit the needs and reactive ability of each individual case.

"These beneficial effects cannot be produced by any medicinal stimulus reputed to possess the power of increasing working capacity. The effects of strychnine [for example] are irregular and transient. It is a whip only, and in no sense a real tonic, since it does not tend to restore to a normal condition.

"On the other hand, those drugs which are used to give relief from fatigue, such as the coal-tar products, bromides, caffeine, etc., do not promote normal rest, but only deaden the nerve centers so that there is not a true appreciation of the worn-out condition of the body. For this reason, the body when under the influence of tea or coffee (caffeine), goes on working when it should rest, and hence to its own damage. A warm bath, however, gives no such false sense of energy, but is conducive to the perfect relaxation and quiet which normal rest and sleep require in order that the powers of the body may be recuperated."—*G.K. Abbott, M.D., F.B. Moor, M.D., K.L. Jensen-Nelson, R.N., Physical Therapy in Nursing Cure, pp. 52-53, 50-51, 54-55, 55-56.*

We mentioned, earlier, that there were two problems about the blood: (1) *There may not be enough of it for emergency needs* and (2) *it has a tendency to congest, or pool, in infected or damaged areas.* But water therapy can help provide solutions to both of these situations. For water treatments can speed up the circulation of the blood; bring it more powerfully into and out of the afflicted area; and, over a period of time, even increase the total amount of blood in the body. Water therapy brings the blood where it is most needed. But when a congestion of blood has occurred, the skillful use of water applications drains away the congestion and brings a refreshing quantity of fresh newly circulating blood to the area needing it. In addition, there is the *"peripheral heart"* factor. The heart, itself, pumps the blood all over the body. But in the more distant parts, the pumping action of the heart cannot send the blood along very fast. But the blood vessels, themselves, have the ability to dilate (enlarge) and contract (reduce) in size and thus pump the blood along also. Oh, how wondrously our God has made us! This is called the "peripheral circulation." And in reaction to hot or cold water applications, this peripheral circulation really jumps into high gear. This pumping action of the heart, which normally occurs four or five times a minute, powerfully increases under many different water treatments.

Here are a few additional principles that will help you to better understand some of the effects of hot, cold, and neutral (lukewarm) water on the human body:

1 - It is the *heat* and *cold* of the water that produces the results. *Neutral* temperatures are quite relaxing, but they do not produce the powerful effects that hot and cold can give.

2 - Heat is measured in degrees by a thermometer. In this chapter on water therapy, we will only use *Fahrenheit*. Scientists may prefer centigrade, but your home and my home only has Fahrenheit thermometers; so that is what we will use. On this scale, normal body temperature taken by the mouth is 98.6° F. Temperature is important in water therapy, and so we will provide you with some very helpful temperature information later in this supplement.

3 - Water is capable of absorbing and storing a larger amount of heat than nearly any other substance. It has high *"specific heat."* This means that when water is applied to the body (in a cloth, bath, shower, etc.), it will impart more heat (or cold) than any other substance at the same temperature. Because water stores so much heat and gives it off so readily, it will seem to the body to be hotter or colder than other substances. (Example: Step from a room at 75° F. into a bathtub at the same temperature!) One substance has a higher specific heat at body temperature—and that is paraffin *(see page 238)*.

4 - Without going into the technical details, ice is, in its effects, far colder than its temperature of 32° F.; and steam is far hotter than 212° F. This is known as *"latent heat."* This gives water a very wide heat and cold range. (In connection with this, keep in mind that steam can burn!)

5 - Water must be in contact with the body for awhile in order to impart heat or cold. But it only needs contact for a moment in order to give a *"thermic impression"* that can be quite strong. For example, plunge your arm for only a moment into a pail of very cold water. It was only there for a moment, but the effect on the circulating blood in the arm will be powerful. This is "thermic impression," and it is important; for you do not have to cool the body with lengthy cold in order to have it react strongly to that cold.

6 - In the Cold Mitten Friction, the impression of cold from the brief application of water is combined with the mechanical stimulus of *"friction"* (the rubbing of the cloth on the arm). Both acting together produce a much greater effect on the body than either alone. The same is true of sprayed water and pail pours. The water "hits" the skin (there is *"percussion"* on the skin) and deepens the reaction of the body to the cold.

7 - Water is the world's greatest *solvent*. As a result it can cleanse better than anything else. It can remove wastes. But it can also hold nutrients placed within it for the body to absorb. Keep this in mind: Many of the diseases of mankind would not exist if people drank an adequate amount of water.

8 - When the body remains in contact with *cold for a long time*, its real effects are seen. Body functions are slowed or depressed; the respiration and pulse are less rapid; the circulation slows; sense of touch is blunted; muscles move sluggishly and clumsily; digestion is retarded or stopped. These are the effects of long-continued cold; but, in water therapy, we rarely give a "long cold" to the body. (Dangerously high fevers are among the only exception.).

9 - *Moderate heat* stimulates the life processes. It quickens the circulation, pulse rate, respiration, digestion. It makes the muscles more active and the skin sensations more sensitive. Many water treatments consist of moderate heat.

10 - *Brief cold* has dramatic, powerful effects and is one of the primary types of water treatment. These effects are caused by *"reaction."* The body receives only a quick cold application that makes the body react to the "thermic impression." Recognizing cold as a depressing agent, the body reacts in several ways: The heart beats more rapidly and forcibly, the circulation is quickened, the nerves tingle with new life. Breathing becomes at first rapid, then slow and deeper. Muscles are energized and have new power for work.

11 - A *prolonged hot* application to the body will, eventuality, depress all body processes. Therefore, we only apply a very hot application for a fairly short period of time; and we generally *conclude it* with a brief cold application, to strengthen the body and equalize its circulation.

12 - When giving a brief cold application, be sure the one receiving it has a good reaction. *This will be shown by* the reddening of the skin, the increase of body heat, and the tingling of the nerves to new life. An *"incomplete reaction"* will result in duskiness of the skin, goose flesh, chilliness, shivering, cold hands or feet, a feeling of fullness in the head, or faintness. Immediately do something about this! First, warm him up with a hot application and then give another, less severe, brief cold application. Or, give no cold at all. Quickly dry him and put him into a warm bed in a warm room, free from drafts. (Normally, if healthy and having had a good reaction, he will dry, dress, and then exercise.)

13 - A set of two or three cycles of hot and cold may be given. This is called *"repeated reactions."* But after two or three, give no more immediately. Note that in order to maintain or increase the height of reaction, the *second and third* applications of hot and cold must either be more intense than the first,

HYDRO

14 - Sometimes it is best to "suppress the reaction." This is frequently done in local applications of intense cold, such as an ice bag. Sometimes overactivity in an area, because of infection or inflammation, requires a cooling effect. An ice pack, ice bag, or a cold cloth (frequently renewed) may be applied. When this is done the usual changes produced by reaction do not occur, simply because the cold has been continued so long.

15 - If it is desired to suppress or prevent a reaction, following the *removal* of a prolonged application, a brief application of heat may be immediately given after the cold is removed.

16 - Neither *infants* nor *aged persons* bear cold treatment well. Some people chill after almost any kind of cold application. Remember: They are only being helped if they react well to the cold application. If they don't, then they are not being helped! Conditions which do not always react well to cold would include anemia, emaciation, asthenia, extreme thinness, etc. If they cannot be benefited by cold, then apply mild heat alone.

17 - The body should be warm before the cold is applied. Exercise, friction, percussion all help bring a good reaction. Hot given beforehand to warm the body also aids it. (Remember: The body should always be warm before the cold is briefly applied, or there will not be a good reaction. It is very important that the skin and feet be warm.) He should receive the cold in a room with warm air and no drafts, and he should remain in a warm room without drafts until the desired reaction occurs.

18 - Another excellent help is to apply hot to the feet before the cold is given and—if needed—after the cold is given. After the cold is given, it may be necessary to provide him with additional covering (either bedding or clothing) in order to secure the full reaction.

19 - The *colder* the water, the greater the reaction. The reaction will come more quickly if the cold is accompanied by friction (rubbing) or percussion (the splashing, pouring, or spraying sensation of the water on the skin). The *larger* the cold application or the more general the surface treated, the less promptly will the reaction appear. A *"combination treatment"* is the keeping of hot on part of the body at the same time that the cold is given for purposes of reaction. This will help the reaction. (Example: Continue to keep hot applications, such as a hot foot bath and fomentations, in place while a cold mitten friction is given.)

20 - The cold treatment should be given quickly. As soon as it is completed, *quickly* dry him. Friction with the dry hand or the rubbing of a rough towel, following the drying, will help the developing reaction to be a good one. Percussion (light slapping on the skin) has the same effect. He must be dried well and very quickly. If moisture is left on the surface, the resulting evaporation will cool his body, delay the reaction, and make it less complete. Dry him in a warm room near the place where the last application of cold water was given. Have his clothes all ready for him to put on or have a warm bed in a warm room ready for him. This requires planning ahead! *Carelessness after the cold* can undo all the value that could have been gained from it.

21 - By *alternating the hot and cold* applications, the beneficial properties of both hot and

RELIEVING SURFACE CONGESTIONS

The illustrations above show superficial (at or near skin surface) congestions and sample ways they are dealt with. (1) A congested skin area has the congestion reduced by a cold compress over it. (2) A small cutaneous (skin) congestion (such as a boil) is relieved by a fomentation which dilates (enlarges) the surrounding blood vessels.

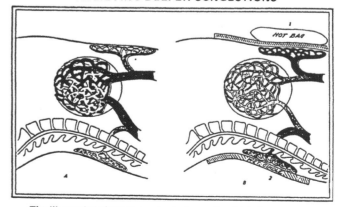

RELIEVING DEEPER CONGESTIONS

The illustration above shows typical ways in which the congestion in a deeper organ is relieved: (1) A hot water bottle (or a fomentation, hot blanket pack, moist abdominal bandage, etc.) is placed above the inflamed organ (or it is placed over a surface area reflexly related to that organ). (2) A wet girdle (a wrap-around moist abdominal bandage), given at the same time, aids in diverting blood from the congested area. (3) A hot foot and leg pack [not shown] will draw the blood away from the congested organ to the legs and feet by derivation.

cold may be obtained without many of the disadvantages of either. Thus, the congestion that tends to come with the application of heat is overcome by the cold application following it. The depressant effect of the cold is counter-balanced by the heat preceding it (and following it, if a series is given). The reaction will stimulate metabolism; this increases circulation, oxidation of toxins, enzyme action, and nerve tone. One example is the contrast bath (hot and cold bath to a limb) as an aid in the healing of fractures. Heat alone may hinder the calcification process, and even induce decalcification. But hot and cold together speeds up the formation of new bone. Another example is alternate hot and cold applications in conquering infections in the extremities. A powerful new surge of blood is brought to the infected hand, arm, foot, or leg, as it is alternately plunged into the hot pail of water and then into the cold. A more speedy recovery is the result.

22 - Water therapy tends to do one or more of six things: (1) Bring blood to an afflicted part. Frequently, this will be an area that is closer to the surface and outside of the trunk. **(2) Pull blood from a deeper internal organ to the skin just above it.** This deeper, congested area is often in the trunk; and the hot application (or a cold-to-heating application) was placed on the skin just above that organ. **(3) Draw blood away from a deeper congested organ** by placing the application on a *reflex area* somewhere else on the body instead of on the skin just above the internal organ. We will discuss this more below. **(4) Pull blood from the internal organ to a distant body part** (usually the legs and/ or feet). This is called *"derivation"* and is frequently done at the same time that an application, just above the internal organ (or to a reflex area connected to it by nerves), is given to also pull blood away from that congested organ. The Hot-Hip-and-Leg Pack is one of the best therapies for *"derivative treatments."*

REFLEXIVE AND DERIVATION EFFECTS COMBINED

Ice Bag over lower abdomen reflexly draws blood from congested uterus; Hot Hip and Leg Pack draws it by derivation.

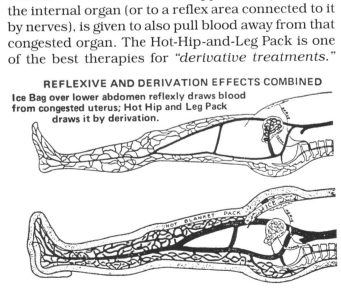

Depletion by Simultaneous Hot and Cold. Upper Figure Shows a Congested Uterus. Lower Figure Shows Depletion of the Uterus secured by the Harmonious Action of an Ice Bag Acting Reflexly, and a Hot Hip and Leg Pack Acting Hydrostatically (Derivation)

(5) A *"proximal compress,"* **consisting of a cold application, may be placed on an extremity.** Here is how this works: Place an ice bag on your upper forearm, and you will lessen the amount of blood supplied to everything below it (the lower arm and the hand). Place an ice compress around the neck, and you will greatly reduce the amount of blood flowing into the head. More information on proximal compresses is given later. **(6) A full application to most of the body, to relieve congestion, equalizes the circulation and brings warmth** from that application (a hot pack—applying heat) or by reaction to it (a heating compress—applying cold for the body to heat).

23 - We will now consider the principle of *"reflex areas."* Internal organs are connected by reflex nerves to various surface portions of the body. In most instances, the area they are connected with is the skin surface directly above that organ. But it has long been known that there are other special reflex areas. These exceptions are primarily the brain, the mucous membrane of the upper respiratory tract, and the organs within the pelvis. But before describing them, here is an example of reflex nerve action: Place the left hand in hot water, and the right hand (as well as the left) will quicken in its blood flow; place either hand in cold water, and the circulation of blood will lessen in both hands.

24 - The special reflex areas normally used are shown on a nearby chart. Here is a brief description of them:

"1. The skin areas of the face, scalp, and back

MAJOR BODY REFLEX AREAS

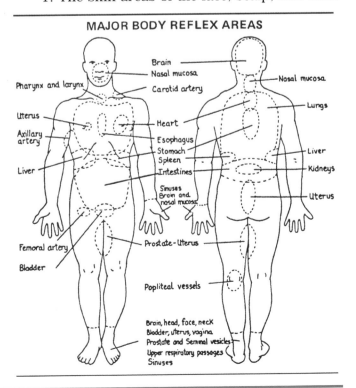

of the neck are reflexly related to the **brain**. 2. The skin of the neck is reflexly related to the **pharynx** and **larynx**. 3. The back of the neck is reflexly related to the mucous membrane of the **nose**. 4. The skin of the chest (front, back, and sides), dorsal region, and shoulders has reflex relations with the **lungs**. 5. The precordia (area above the heart) is in very perfect reflex relation with the **heart** through its accelerator nerves (sympathetic). 6. The hands are reflexly related to the **brain** and the **nasal** mucous membrane. 7. The skin over the lower right chest relates to the **liver**. 8. The skin over the lower left chest relates to the **spleen**. 9. The lower dorsal and lumbar spine relates to the **kidneys** and **intestines**. 10. The skin of the central abdomen, from the naval to the pubes [pubis], is in reflex relation with **kidneys** and **ureters**. 11. The lower lumbar and sacral spine [both on lower back] relate to the **pelvic organs** (uterus, ovaries, bladder, and rectum). 12. The epigastrium [see "stomach" on chart] relates to the **stomach**. 13. The skin of the entire abdomen, especially that of the umbilical [naval] region, is reflexly related to the **intestines**. The fact that the pain of colic, appendicitis, etc., is referred to the region of the umbilicus [naval] is an evidence of a similar nervous connection. 14. The lower abdomen, including the groin and the upper inner surfaces of the thighs, are reflexly related to the **pelvic organs**. 15. The saddle-shaped area covered by a sitz (sitting) bath is in reflex relation with the **prostate** and **seminal vesicles**. 16. The skin of the feet and legs is reflexly related to the **brain**, the **lungs**, and the **pelvic organs**. 17. The breasts are reflexly related to the **pelvic organs**."—*G.K. Abbott, M.D., F.A.C.S., F.B. Moor, M.D., K.L. Jensen-Nelson, R.N., M.A., Physical Therapy in Nursing Care, pp. 60-61.*

In some instances, heat to a reflex area will produce a different response than cold: Cold to the thighs will cause vigorous movement of the stomach, with little or none in the small or large intestines. Cold to the thighs will decidedly increase stomach acidity in most people.

— PART THREE —
SPECIAL CAUTIONS

There are a number of **CAUTIONS** that should be observed in giving hydrotherapy treatments. The next several paragraphs will provide you with far more general cautions than you will find in many modern textbooks on hydrotherapy. (In addition, many cautions relating to specific therapies and diseases will be found later in this chapter.) You MUST KNOW the following paragraphs:

1 - Always keep the feet warm. In case of any kind of heart problem, keep cold over the heart. It is **often necessary to keep cold to the forehead and back of the neck. Too lengthy a water treatment may cause "hydrotherapy headache"** for a while afterward. Dry him quickly and well. He should be kept warm after that for a time. **Here are three things that could cause this headache:** (1) Applications that are too long, an incomplete or an excessive reaction, or insufficient time in bed afterward to obtain the needed reaction. (2) Failure to place a cold compress on the head or neck, when giving a heating treatment. Any time the body temperature goes over 100° F., a cool washcloth should be laid on the forehead, with the face and neck sponged occasionally. Do this for all kinds of elevated temperatures: fevers as well as fevers induced by water treatment.

2 - The lower the temperature, the shorter should be the application: only 1-5 seconds for very cold applications. Neutral and warm applications can be continued for quite some time. **Very hot applications should rarely be more than a minute in length.** When used to reduce fevers, cool applications without percussion or friction can be prolonged to 15-20 minutes. **The neutral bath** can continue for any length of time. It has been used for months on people afflicted with insanity. But in such instances, the temperature was **carefully watched, so that there would be no negative reaction or chilling.** Normally, from 30 minutes to 1-2 hours is the usual time for a neutral bath.

3 - Try to train him to progressively react to the coldest applications. The best and most durable effects come from short cold applications, frequently repeated. **Few people are helped by long cold**; remember that. Exercise before and after a cold treatment is good, but not always feasible.

4 - Here is a list of the people that perhaps should not receive certain water treatments: those who are **anemic**, very **thin**, overly **feeble**, **neurasthenics**, **chronic inebriates** (alcoholics), **hysterical** or **exhausted** by loss of sleep, or other causes: These should only receive short cold treatments. This would also include those with **neuralgia**, **myalgia**, **painful congestions**, or **chronic rheumatism** with **painful joints**. Some, such as those with **painful neuritis**, cannot take any cold. Those that can only take a very brief cold should first receive a hot application. This would also apply to those who are very **sensitive**, **timid**, or **hypochondriac** in temperament. In connection with this, be sure to **always explain what you are going to do next**.

5 - Only give mild cold to those with a weak heart, organic heart disease, Bright's disease and other forms of kidney disease, diabetes, or to children under seven. Avoid cold baths during menstruation, pregnancy, and old age (especially if the aged have **arteriosclerosis** and **similar degenera-**

tion, cardiac weakness, emphysema, or bronchitis). Those with **aneurism of the aorta, advanced arteriosclerosis, or a tendency to apoplexy (stroke)** should also avoid it.

6 - **Very hot applications should be avoided in such conditions as cardiac disease, aneurysm of the aorta, advanced arteriosclerosis, apoplexic tendency, or aortic stenosis.** For such, non-percussion of moderate temperature applications should be used. In giving hot applications, keep in mind that you should **never apply heat at a temperature higher than 102°-104° F. to the feet of an insulin-dependent diabetic.** This is because, not sensing heat as well in their extremities, they can be more easily burned. **Do not apply heat to an abscess in a closed space.** An example of this would be an inflamed **appendix. Heat over it can cause the appendix to swell and burst.** Contrariwise, moist heat over a boil will soften it, bring it to a head better, and help the pus to come up and out.

7 - Regarding ability to give a good **reaction to cold water,** we have already discussed this; however, we will here mention that **very fleshy persons do not at first react so well as lean people, but they bear prolonged application much better,** due to their large heat-making resources. **Lean folk react well, but their powers of reaction are very quickly exhausted; hence they are more likely to suffer from secondary chill,** etc. Thick-skinned people of calm temperament readily tolerate very cold applied with strong pressure in the stream of water; that is, if no other negative symptom is present (such as heart disease, etc.).

8 - On the topic of hot and cold precautions, here is some additional counsel from Dr. John Harvey Kellogg:

"Precautions: 1. **When fatigued** as the result of the loss of sleep or severe muscular exercise, a cold application should be preceded by a hot immersion bath for 3 to 7 minutes. 2. **If but slightly fatigued,** a cold friction may be substituted for the cold bath. 3. **A very cold bath should always be short, and should never be administered when the body surface is cold or chilly.** The hot bath carried to the point of gentle perspiration is an excellent preparation for a cold application. 4. The temperature of the **air of the room in which the cold bath is taken should always be higher [hotter] than that of the bath.** 5. **Avoid frequent hot baths** at all seasons, and especially in winter, as they are depressing, and lessen vital resistance to cold and other disturbing influences. The best time for hot or warm bath in cold weather is just before retiring."—*J.H. Kellogg, M.D., "Rational Hydrotherapy," p. 396.*

9 - Here are still more cautions in regard to *cold applications,* whether for tonic or recovery purposes: **Extremely feeble persons** are the ones most needing tonic treatment, especially those who have the least tolerance for cold water. Therefore, begin with very gentle measures, such as the Cold Wet-hand Rub, Salt Glow, Cold Mitten Friction, Alternate Hot and Cold to the spine, etc. Confine the first applications to small areas, rubbing each, drying it well, then passing on to the next. Do this symmetrically: right arm and hand and then left arm and hand, etc. Feeble people often experience a very unpleasant and discouraging sense of fatigue after tonic applications, especially when the course of treatments first begin. So **use great care to avoid exhausting him with much cold.** This will discourage him and blight his prospects for recovery. (In his writings, Kellogg tells of the time when the famed Bavarian water therapist, Joseph Kneipp, was called to the Vatican to treat an aged pope who had chronic rheumatism. Upon his arrival, he was received with great honors; but the first cold bath given to the aged prelate, entirely unaccustomed to such heroic treatment, caused the pope to quickly send Kneipp back home.) Instead, **begin with mild cold applications while his feet are in a hot foot bath.** The impression of heat on his feet helps him take the cold elsewhere. Also he can be **prepared for the cold by giving him a very hot spray or shower (110°-120° F.) for 1-3 minutes beforehand.** This hot application should be of gradually increasing temperature, then turned off and the cold applied.

10 - [Special attention needed in this paragraph: These external sprays, in hydrotherapy called "douches," are not explained in this Supplement.] Be on guard to avoid the cold douche (cold hand-held spray, not the modern meaning of "douche") with strong pressure to the upper part of the chest. The effect on the respiratory nerve centers can cause temporary coughing and a sense of distress. Also avoid the cold douche over the stomach, loins, and abdomen in cases of hyperpepsia, ulceration of the stomach, hemorrhage from the bowels or any form of uterine hemorrhage, as menorrhagia or metrorrhagia. (Obviously, because it would increase blood circulation, and hence internal bleeding, in the afflicted part.) Again, care must be taken to avoid the abdomen, the chest, and particularly the region of the heart in nervous cases—especially those in which hysteria, heart disease, or asthma is a well-known symptom.

11 - In certain instances, **one water application can nullify the effect of another.** Kellogg was a master in the field of water treatments, so we will let him give us the following cautions:

"Hydriatic [hydrotherapy] Incompatibilities: Wise discretion must be used in the combination of

procedures, lest one measure shall undo the therapeutic work accomplished by another. The combination of hydriatic [water therapy] processes in such a manner as to enable one procedure to intensify or to prolong the effect of another is perhaps the best test of a physician's experience and skill. The following meager suggestions barely touch the surface of the subject:

"1. **Tonic procedures** [quick cold and/or rubbing] must be carefully avoided when a sedative effect is desired, such as cold and neutral baths or other measures. The tonic application may be accidental. The contact with pure cold air after a neutral bath or of the feet with a cold floor may destroy the sedative effect of the bath altogether.

"2. **Sedative** [relaxing, sleep-inducing] measures must be as carefully suppressed when tonic procedures are employed for their specific effects. When a hot bath precedes a cold bath, if too prolonged, or if the cold application is too short, or if the patient is exposed to an overheated atmosphere after the bath, the tonic effect will be lost.

"3. In the use of **antipyretic** [fever reducing] measures, the procedures must be so managed that heat production will not be increased so much as to more than counter-balance the increase in heat elimination; hence . . short cold or cool applications may be injurious [by making him hotter]. Cool sponging often raises the temperature by increasing heat production."—Kellogg, *"Rational Hydrotherapy,"* pp. 978-979,

— PART FOUR —
COMPARATIVE SUMMARY
THE CHIEF EFFECTS OF COLD AND HEAT

To conclude this chapter of basic principles, we will give you several **water therapy classifications** that may help you more clearly obtain a broad view of the general categories they fall into and their relationships to one another.

1 - Scientists have discovered that water therapy can help the human body in so many ways. For example, Crawford was the first to observe that brief cold applications will increase the difference in color between arterial and venous blood. This is the result of increased oxidation. Liebig discovered that cold air, cold water, and exercise, habitually employed, are the most powerful of all means of stimulating tissue activity. And Strasser has shown that general cold applications increase the alkalinity of the blood, the reduction in acid phosphate amounting sometimes to fifty percent. On *page 216* is a special chart. It is Dr. J.H. Kellogg's *"Comparative Summary of the Chief Effects of Cold and Heat."* It is taken from pages 194-195 of his immense book, *Rational Hydrotherapy.*

2 - Charles S. Thomas has, for years, made a care-

ful study of the field of hydrotherapy. As a university professor teaching the subject, he is uniquely qualified to speak. *Here, slightly adapted, is his classification of the water therapies by their effects:*

SHORT COLD and CONTRASTS: The predominate effect is that of a reaction—

General applications that give a tonic effect: Tonic sprays, tonic frictions, hot and cold and revulsive compresses, pail pours, plunges, cold shallow bath.

Local applications that give a stimulating effect: Contrast baths, hot and cold and revulsive compress, local tonic frictions.

Reflex applications that give a tonic effect: Contrast baths, hot and cold and revulsive compresses, local tonic frictions.

PROLONGED COLD: The predominate effect is that of intrinsic action—

General applications that give an antipyretic (fever-reducing) effect: Graduated spray and bath, sponges, ice pack and rub, enemas and colonics, wet-sheet pack, exposure to air, fanning.

Local applications that give a decongestive and depressant effect: Ice pack, ice bag, cold local bath, cold compress, direct ice application.

Reflex applications that give a constriction (lessening of blood) effect: Ice pack, ice bag, cold local bath, cold compress, direct ice application.

MILD HEATING (without perspiration): The predominate effect is that of a reaction—

General applications that give a sedation (sleep-inducing) effect: Continuous flowing bath, wet-sheet pack, local warm bath, fomentations.

Reflex applications that give a relaxing effect: Heating compresses, Kenny packs, mild fomentations, warm bath.

MODERATE HEATING (with only a moderate rise in body temperature): The predominate effect is that of a reaction—

General applications that give a diaphoresis (increase of sweating) effect: Hot bath (partial and general), Hot blanket pack, wet-sheet pack, fomentations.

MARKED HEATING: The predominant effect is that of a reaction with a marked intrinsic action—

General applications that give a peripheral vasodilation (enlargement of blood vessels distant from the heart) effect: Warm full bath, hot local bath. Hot blanket pack, wet-sheet pack, steam bath, fomentations.

General applications that give a stimulation of blood circulation and body metabolism: Hot full bath, steam bath, fever cabinet (for fever therapy), insulating blanket.

Local applications that give a stimulation of circulation and metabolism: Whirlpool (circulating) partial bath, Fomentations, Kenny packs (5 minutes),

COMPARATIVE SUMMARY OF THE CHIEF EFFECTS OF COLD AND HEAT

COLD

General

Primary: depressant
Short: excitant by tonic reaction
Prolonged: depressant

Special

Skin: Action, diminished activity
Reaction: increased activity
Diminished sensibility
Heart: First quickened, then slowed
   Increased force
Vessels: Action, contraction
   Reaction, dilatation
   Increased tone and activity
   Local anemia, collateral hyperemia
   With reaction, local hyperemia, collateral anemia
   Short, reflex dilatation of visceral vessels
Nerves: Benumbs and paralyzes
   Excites by tonic reaction
Muscles: Short, increased excitability and capacity
   Prolonged, lessened excitability, capacity
Lungs: Slows and deepens respiration
   Increased amount of respired air
   Increased CO_2
   Increased respiratory quotient
Stomach: Increased HCL and motor activity
Kidneys: Congests and excites
Animal Heat: Short, increased heat production
   Prolonged, diminished heat production
Blood: Increased blood count
   especially leucocytes
Metabolism: Increased CO_2
   Increased urea, and improved oxidation

Tonic Reaction

1. Vasodilatation
2. Skin red
3. Pulse slowed
4. Arterial tension increased
5. Skin action increased
6. Temperature lowered
7. Feeling of invigoration
8. Muscular capacity increased
9. Amount of respired air increased
10. Heat production increased

HEAT

General

Primary: excitant
Short: depressant by atonic reaction
Prolonged: mixed, excitant, and depressant

Special

Skin: Action, increased activity
Reaction: diminished activity
Diminished sensibility
Heart: First slowed, then quickened
   Decreased force
Vessels: Action, contraction, then dilatation
   Reaction, contraction
   Lowered tone-paralysis. Local hyperemia, collateral anemia
   With reaction, local anemia, collateral hyperemia
   Short, reflex fluxion and derivative effects
Nerves: Excites
   Depresses by atonic reaction
Muscles: Short, lessening fatigue effects
   Prolonged, diminished capacity, excitability
Lungs: Quickens and facilitates respiration
   Diminished amount of respired air
   Decreased CO_2
   Diminished respiratory quotient
Stomach: Decreased HCl and motor activity
Kidneys: renders anemic and lessens activity
Animal Heat: Short, diminished heat production
   Prolonged, increased heat production
Blood: Decrease in number of red cells
   Increase in number of leucocytes
Metabolism: Decreased CO_2
   Increased urea and general protein waste

Atonic Reaction

1. Vasoconstriction
2. Skin pale
3. Pulse rate increased
4. Arterial tension diminished
5. Skin action decreased
6. Temperature lowered
7. Languor
8. Muscular capacity decreased
9. Amount of respired air decreased
10. Heat production decreased

—J.H. Kellogg, M.D., "Rational Hydrotherapy," pp. 188-189

hot-water bottle, paraffin bath, thermal mud baths, heating appliances, hot air applications.

Reflex applications that give a relaxation and counter-irritation effect: same as those listed immediately above.

—The preceding is adapted from Simple Water Treatments for the Home, by Charles Thomas, Ph.D., Loma Linda, California, 1983 Revision, pp. 100, 47-48.

3 - Water, applied to the body, can do seventeen different things. Dr. Abbott called them the *"remedial properties"* of water. Here they are:

"**Remedial Properties of Water** - The terms listed below are commonly used to designate the various physiologic or therapeutic effects of water. The definitions given should be studied thoroughly and memorized.

"**1. TONIC** - A tonic effect is one in which vital activities are increased so as to restore the body to a normal tone or condition. The nutrition, circulation, and other body functions are promoted.

"**2. PURE STIMULANT** - A stimulant arouses the body to unusual activities. It may be compared to a whip, and is used chiefly in emergencies. Like a tonic it increases vital activities, but to a much greater degree. Between a pure stimulant and a tonic there are various graduations which might be designated as mild stimulant, extreme tonic, etc.

"**3. SEDATIVE** - A sedative or calmative agent is one which lessens vital activity and is conducive to relaxation and rest.

"**4. ANTISPASMODIC** - The relaxing of spasm or relieving of convulsions.

"**5. DEPRESSANT** - A depressant effect is one in which heightened or normal body activities are decreased to a marked degree. Such an effect is desirable only in cases in which a function is greatly overactive.

"**6. ANODYNE** - An anodyne effect refers to the relief of pain.

"**7. SPOLIATIVE** - A spoliative treatment is one which increases the oxidation and breaking down (catabolism) of tissue, which tends to reduce weight.

"**8. DIAPHORESIS** - The production of sweating. An agent that produces sweating is said to have a diaphoretic or sudorific effect.

"**9. DIURESIS** - Increasing the excretion of urine.

"**10. ELIMINATIVE** - An eliminative effect consists in promoting and hastening excretion from the kidneys (diuresis), the skin (diaphoresis), and the lungs.

"**11. DEPLETION** - Depletion is the lessening of the amount of blood in a given part. Practically, it is the reduction of congestion.

"**12. DERIVATIVE** - Derivation is the drawing of blood or lymph from one part of the body by increasing the amount in another part. The term "depletion" is also applied to this process, but refers particularly to the result produced. [The blood was pulled away by derivation; the result was depletion, or less blood in the congested part.]

"**13. FLUXION** - Fluxion consists in greatly increasing the rapidity of the blood current in a particular part. It is the production of active or arterial hyperemia.

"**14. ANTIPYRETIC** - The lowering of body temperature in fever.

"**15. REFRIGERANT** - Relieving of thirst and restoring the alkalinity of the blood by such means as free water drinking and the use of fruit juices.

"**16. REVULSIVE** - A term used to designate a treatment consisting of a single prolonged application of heat followed by a single very brief application of cold. This meaning is not strictly adhered to, as the term is also used where three applications of such proportionate duration are made.

"**17. ALTERNATE** - The expression "alternate hot and cold" is used in this text to describe treatments in which the duration of the cold application is from one-fourth to one half that of the heat (in a few cases equal to it), and in which three or more changes from heat to cold are made."—*G.K. Abbott, F.B. Moor, K.L. Jensen-Nelson, Physical Therapy in Nursing Care, pp. 70-72.*

4 - Throughout the treatment, give him the best of care: The room should be warm, free of drafts, and with no bright lights shining in his eyes. Avoid possible water damage by covering bedding, rugs, furniture, etc. Avoid distracting noise (such as overly talkative people, radios, etc.) where the treatment is being given. Plan ahead in the giving of each treatment; this will help everything go smoothly and will eliminate undue delays that might overheat or chill the one you are working with. This includes assembling everything you need ahead of time. Briefly explain beforehand what you are going to do. Stay with him or within easy calling distance throughout the treatment. Quietly tell him at each step what is coming next and the effect desired. While not too talkative, you are continually studying your patient—noting his words, feelings, and actions. Are the applications helping him or not? Why? Make the changes quickly. Be neat and pick up, clean up, as you work. Use both time and materials carefully and economically, and put everything away when finished.

Know when to talk and when to keep quiet. Talking and extra noise wearies the sick. But do keep a cheerful outlook and express cheerful, hopeful comments from time to time. Pray with and for the one you are helping. Bring him to God; there he will find the strength and courage that he needs.

5 - Helping him is what it is all about: He must be warm before you begin. Apply a cold compress to the head or neck when giving a heating application. Do not unnecessarily expose him,—but rather only the part under immediate treatment. He should be comfortable at all times. Protect him from falling, burns, chilling, and uncomfortable positions. He should not be chilled or sweating when the treatment ends, but should be warm and dry. When cold is given, he must have a good reaction or you must do something to restore proper warmth to his body. If necessary, put him in a warm bed in a warm room for 30-60 minutes.

6 - Here are some basic nursing observations that you should keep in mind: Note signs and symptoms without his realizing it; otherwise he will tend to exaggerate every little ache and pain. It is equally important to note the symptoms and signs that are not present. The general appearance of his face, skin, expression, movements, along with what he says will tell you a lot. Keep in mind that symptoms can point to a number of different things; so do not quickly jump to conclusions. (Indicators of a common cold, such as runny nose, sneezing, coughing, hoarseness, difficulty in breathing, and sore throat can be symptoms of other conditions also).

Here are additional things to watch for: **Skin** - Any discoloration, itching, swelling, rash, etc.? **Mouth** - Are the gums pink and firm? How about the **tongue**? **Voice** - Anything unusual about it? **Appetite** - Any loss of appetite? **Weight** - Unusual weight changes? Continued loss or gain? Is **Sleep** easy or difficult to obtain? General **fatigue** indicators - and why? **Fever** - Is the skin moist or dry? Cool or hot, or alternating cool and hot?

Take his temperature (1) when he complains of feeling ill or shows signs of it, (2) once or twice daily during illness, (3) when there is a sudden change in his condition (chills, restlessness, pain, etc.) or (4) when he has a headache, chest or abdominal pain, sore throat, chills, vomiting, diarrhea, or skin rash. A fever in addition to the above signs indicates a significant illness or condition demanding immediate attention.

Pulse and respiration - Is it different than normal for him? **Pain** - Another warning indicator. Pain in the abdomen should be relieved quickly by rest, drinking charcoal in water, and skipping a meal; if not—call a physician. **Nausea and vomiting** - What is the color, general appearance, and amount of material vomited? **Bowel movements** - Note number, frequency, color and consistency. **Urinary problems** - Is there inability to urinate, pain or burning sensation, incontinence, presence of blood? Are they too frequent?

7 - In the next chapter, we shall discuss a large number of practical water therapy applications. But just before concluding this present chapter, **we shall let three experts in the field tell us how useful such simple water treatments can be in the home:**

"Hydrotherapy may be given with very meager facilities. The procedures are not so difficult but that a layman of average intelligence may be taught how to give them with a little practical instruction. **With the following materials available in the home, all the effects of hydrotherapy may be accomplished:**

"**Procedures:** Fomentations, compresses, hot-water bottle, ice bag, heating compress, cold mitten friction, cold hand and towel rubs, sponging, alcohol rub, partial bath, sitz bath, hot half bath, full immersion bath, hot blanket pack, wet-sheet pack, shower (optional), pail pour, enema, vaginal irrigation. **Materials [needed to give the treatments]:** Blankets, old blanket that may be cut up (part wool), hand towels, Turkish towels (towels made of cotton terry cloth), sheets, old sheet that may be cut up, newspapers, hot-

water bottle, ice bag, bathtub, shower (optional), pails, washtub, small basins, enema can and tube with rectal and vaginal tips, ice, hot and cold water."—*Fred B. Moor, M.D., Clarence W. Dail, M.D., J. Wayne McFarland, M.D., Hydrotherapy, 1980, p. 2829. (This book is a partial reprint of their medical college textbook, Physical Therapy, Textbook for Medical Students and Practitioners of Medicine, 1944.)*

— PART FIVE —

21 BASIC OBJECTIVES

Before turning to the individual water therapy applications, we need to understand the 21 objectives of water therapy. This knowledge will better help us use hydrotherapy in our own homes. *The following section is summarized from pp. 327-329, 968-978, and 194-200 of Kellogg's 1,199-page Rational Hydrotherapy:*

WATER THERAPIES WHICH INCREASE BOTH HEAT PRODUCTION AND HEAT ELIMINATION - This listing is arranged in order from the most to the least powerful, and is primarily composed of tonic and fever-reducing applications:

Graduated bath. Cooling wet-sheet pack. Cold friction bath. Prolonged tepid full bath at 88° F. Cold full bath followed by a short hot full bath, pail pour, or sprinkling (shower). Tepid pail pour. Cold pail pour. Cold compress. Graduated compress. Evaporating sheet. Cold to head and neck. Cold to spine. Cold to abdomen. Cold over heart. Cold colonic. Tepid or cold enema. Cold water drinking, a measure that should be combined with all the others named above. Cold air bath.

WATER THERAPIES WHICH INCREASE THE ELIMINATION OF HEAT - These are the best methods to use when a fever is present and the cold bath should be avoided. This one is also arranged in a list from the most to the least powerful:

Hot bath for 2-3 minutes, followed by a cold bath with friction for 1 minute. Hot blanket pack. Hot evaporating sheet. Hot sponge bath. Fomentation to the back. Fomentation to the abdomen, followed by the cold enema. Fomentation to the back, followed by a cold wet-sheet pack. Hot blanket pack, followed by graduated bath. Hot blanket pack, followed by prolonged tepid bath. Hot blanket pack, followed by cold friction. Dry friction (rubbing the skin with a dry cloth). Cold friction.

WATER THERAPIES WHICH ENCOURAGE THE DESTRUCTION OF TOXINS - These are procedures which encourage vital resistance to disease while, at the same time, encouraging the destruction of toxins by stimulating the toxin-destroying cells of the thyroid, liver, spleen, lymphatics, and other tissues. (From this point forward, the listings will not be in order of decreasing strength, unless otherwise stated.)

WATER THERAPIES WHICH ENCOURAGE THE ELIMINATION OF TOXINS - Radiant Heat Bath. Sweating wet-sheet pack. Steam bath. The elimination of producing sweat and washing it away is very important:

"In observations made upon rabbits some seven or eight years ago, the writer demonstrated that the perspiration of the ordinary healthy man contains toxic substances in such quantity that from 100 to 200 c.c. of the liquid collected from the surface of a sweating man is, when injected intravenously, capable of killing a rabbit weighing one kilogram."—*Kellogg, Rational Hydrotherapy, p. 970.*

WATER THERAPIES WHICH GREATLY INCREASE LEUCOCYTIC ACTION - The following applications help increase white blood cell formation. WBCs, as you know, are a primary body fighter against toxins and bacterial infection. General cold bath. Heating compress frequently renewed. Alternate heating compress.

WATER THERAPIES WHICH GREATLY ENCOURAGE ELIMINATION OF BACTERIA BY THE SKIN AND KIDNEYS - Especially: Steam bath. Sweating wet-sheet pack. Prolonged neutral bath. Also good: Sweating baths. Copious water drinking. Each of these should be followed by a cold mitten friction, cold towel rub, or some other cold procedure.

WATER THERAPIES WHICH INCREASE OXIDATION - Cold baths increase the absorption of oxygen, the elimination of carbon dioxide, and the oxidation of fat and carbohydrates. Thus, all cold applications will tend to do this; but here are some of the best: Prolonged cold baths, such as: Dripping sheet rub. Rubbing shallow bath. Cold full bath. Plunge (quick dip into a bathtub of cold water). Cooling wet-sheet pack.

WATER THERAPIES WHICH ARE THE MOST EFFICIENT MEANS OF STIMULATING NITROGEN OXIDATION - Hot applications are what are needed for this, and here are Kellogg's top recommendations:

Hot full bath. Heating wet-sheet pack. Dry pack. Steam bath. Hot air. Sunbath. Radiant Heat Bath. (Kellogg called this the "electric-light bath," a device he invented consisting of a boxful of incandescent bulbs for heating purposes.) We have changed it to "Radiant Heat Bath," with the thought in mind that electric space heaters, or something similar, could be used in your home for this same purpose.) In each case, follow these general hot applications with a very short general cold application.

WATER THERAPIES WHICH EXCITE THE CENTRAL NERVE GANGLIA - The following are especially helpful in adynamic fevers, many neurasthenic conditions, hypopepsia, kidney insufficiency, and various visceral congestions; these are primarily very hot followed by very cold applications. But, of course, much of the time you will have to gradually work up to "very" hot

and "very" cold. Alternate spinal sponging. Alternate spinal compresses. Alternate full bath, followed by various forms of cold. Alternate localized compresses.

WATER THERAPIES WHICH ENCOURAGE METABOLIC PROCESSES - In most forms of chronic disease, there is a grave disturbance of the general nutrition, arising from failure of the tissues to maintain normal metabolism. The most permanent effects toward improving the metabolism, either locally or generally, come from somewhat prolonged hot applications followed by a brief cold application. Here are the most effective:

Apply one or more of the following to the skin area affecting the body part(s) you wish to help: Alternate or heating compress.

WATER THERAPIES WHICH INCREASE BLOOD FORMATION - General cold applications, whether mild or more severe, are the best hydriatic means of promoting the processes of blood formation. The metabolic applications listed, just above, also increase blood formation and glandular activity, but the following ones are especially helpful for anemia. Short general cold baths are the best; the lower the temperature, the better, but the applications must be very short. The cold mitten friction and the cold towel rub applied 2-3 times daily are especially valuable for this purpose.

WATER THERAPIES WHICH INCREASE GENERAL BLOOD MOVEMENT AND LOCAL BLOOD SUPPLY - The ability to move fresh vitalized blood into and out of key areas is very important in providing nutrition and oxygen, carrying away wastes and toxins, and in fighting disease. Here are some suggestions:

Cold applications to the surface of the body excite the heart, increase blood pressure, and increase blood and lymph movement throughout the body. All tonic measures may be used for this purpose. The cold compress over the heart area can be used in many cases, when general cold applications are ruled out. In cases of fever, heart or kidney disease, in neurasthenia with general feebleness, and in chronic tuberculosis and other wasting diseases, the cold mitten friction and the cold towel rub are especially useful in reinforcing the energy of the heart and strengthening the circulation.

General hot applications are not helpful here. They ultimately lower the blood pressure, diminish heart energy, and lessen blood flow. So avoid them. If a hot application must be made, guard against heart failure by applying a cold compress to the heart area while the hot application is being given. This especially applies to steam baths and hot full baths.

WATER THERAPIES WHICH INCREASE HEAT PRODUCTION - It is the impression of cold on the thermic nerves of the skin that best increases heat production. The more intense (and sometimes prolonged) this impression, the greater the desired effect. The most intense effects are produced by prolonging the application until the temperature of the body has been slightly lowered. But if the cold is greatly prolonged, or is repeated at short intervals, the heat-rise effect fails.

WATER THERAPIES WHICH INCREASE THE ELIMINATION OF HEAT - Nearly all types of fever cases need an increase of heat elimination. Elevation of temperature in fever is due less to increased heat production than to decreased heat elimination.

Vigorous rubbing in a cold full or shallow bath. Wet-sheet rub. Wet-sheet pack. Very short hot applications followed by short cold to the surface. Cold friction bath. Cold towel rub. Cold water drinking. Cold enema. Cold applications to the spine. In certain cases, the hot blanket pack, evaporating wet-sheet pack, and similar measures may also be used.

WATER THERAPIES WHICH RELIEVE PAIN AND NERVOUS IRRITABILITY - Hydrotherapy applications can greatly help in this area also.

The general neutral bath is very effective in relieving nervous irritability, inducing sleep, in insomnia, delirium, and even acute fevers. Moist abdominal bandage. Cool head cap. Heating spinal compress, in certain cases. For relieving localized pain and irritability, the hot fomentation and the heating compress are both good. The cold compress and ice compress are both valuable in those instances in which the pain is in superficial (near the surface) parts and the applications can be made directly to the area of pain.

WATER THERAPIES WHICH COMBAT BACTERIAL DEVELOPMENT - This is done by increasing blood movement through the infected parts while, at the same time, increasing white blood cell activity.

Prolonged applications of cold, when it can be applied directly to the parts involved. For deeper areas of infection, it is best to increase blood alkalinity by means of general cold applications and by measures for increasing local leucocytic action, such as the frequently renewed heating compress and the alternate compress.

WATER THERAPIES WHICH CONTROL BLOOD MOVEMENT AND VOLUME - The slowing of blood and lymph encourages morbid processes as waste and toxic materials accumulate in the tissues.

Apply to inflamed or congested parts the measures (mentioned earlier) which encourage leucocytic (white blood cell) activity. Also helpful: Derivative measures (such as hot leg-and-foot pack, hot foot bath, etc.). Cold compress over the affected part. Revulsive measures of all sorts.

WATER THERAPIES WHICH LESSEN HEAT PRODUCTION - Heat production must be discouraged in fever cases; it is best inhibited by short hot applications to the surface and by prolonged or frequently repeated cold applications.

The best heat applications for this purpose would be: short hot full bath. Hot blanket pack. Fomentations to the spine. Hot evaporating sheet. The best cold applications would be: Graduated bath. Prolonged tepid bath. Cooling wet-sheet pack.

WATER THERAPIES WHICH LESSEN HEAT ELIMINATION - It is seldom necessary to discourage the elimination of heat by the body. But fainting is an exception.

These help prevent excessive heat loss: Dry pack. Hot blanket pack. Hot enema. Hot water drinking. Avoid exposing him to cold while changing applications. It is wise to alternate the hot application by a short cold application, such as vigorous cold wet-hand rubbing and cold mitten friction.

WATER THERAPIES WHICH DIMINISH GENERAL METABOLIC ACTIVITY - Above all, maintain absolute rest in bed. Also good is the neutral bath. Diminishing activity of an overexcited gland (such as in hypopepsia [inadequate stomach HCl] or catarrh of the intestines or uterus) may be lessened by various derivative measures (leg and foot baths, etc.) which will draw blood away from the part.

WATER THERAPIES WHICH CONTROL BLEEDING - Hemostatic (stopping of bleeding) effects may be obtained either directly by application to the bleeding area or indirectly through applications to a reflex area.

To obtain direct effects, either very hot (110°-115° F.) or very cold (32°-40° F.) applications must be used. The most valuable hot applications is the hot compress. A jet of hot vapor has also been used successfully. Here are some examples of hot applications: Hot nasal spray and sponging the face with very hot water for nose bleed; hot vaginal douche for menorrhagia; hot uterine irrigation in metrorrhagia and postpartum hemorrhage.

The most convenient cold applications are ice and ice compresses. These should be applied directly to the bleeding area or (as a proximal compress) across the trunk of a main artery supplying the bleeding part. An example of this would be an ice collar (ice cravat) for nosebleed.

Here are some indirect or reflex applications: Cold applications to the upper spine is a most excellent measure for checking nosebleed. Placing the hands in ice water while applying ice to the base of the cranium (lower back of head) and to upper part of the spine. Placing the feet in cold water will also help stop nosebleed. For hemorrhage of the lungs, place cold compresses over the chest and very hot fomentations between the shoulders and over back of the neck and upper spine. Ice applied to the nostrils will also contract the blood vessels in the lungs. For stomach hemorrhage, swallow lumps of ice, and place ice compresses over the reflex area that affects the stomach *(see reflex chart on page 213)*. In apoplexy, the ice cap and ice-cold compresses to the head, face, and neck are very helpful.

H
Y
D
R
O

THE WATER THERAPIES

— PART ONE —
CLOTH AND BLANKET APPLICATIONS

In the preceding section, we learned the great importance of blood and of the careful use of water in aiding the blood to bring both restoration and increased physical capacity. And we learned many basic facts about how to apply neutral, hot, and cold to the human body.

In this present chapter, we shall consider over a hundred different water therapy applications, under fifteen major categories. In preparing this list of the water therapies, as in the rest of this chapter, the author has tried to combine simplicity with thoroughness and clarity with cautions. This entire chapter is the result of a careful study of over 2,700 pages of hydrotherapy material. Extracting the best and making it as simple and usable as possible is the objective of the present writer.

That which in centuries past was called "home remedies" or "water treatments," became known in the early and mid-nineteenth century as "water cure," as Drs. Thatcher Trall and James Jackson helped thousands in their "water-cure institutes." By the beginning of the twentieth century, it gained the title of "hydrotherapy" and "hydriatics"; and, for several decades now, it has been called "physical therapy" or "physiotherapy" by the medical world.

We will here use the humble title of "water therapy." Yet whatever name you care to give it,—it is still a most wonderful blessing of God to mankind.

Here is the first of the two sections that will explain to you over one hundred water therapies:

— SECTION ONE —
LOCAL COLD

WHAT THEY ARE—These are localized applications of cold water, which means that they are applied only to smaller parts of the body.

These cold applications can also be used as a "proximal compress" (pp. 213, 225) to reduce blood flow to a limb.

1 - COLD COMPRESS

WHAT IT IS—A Cold Compress is a local application of cold given by means of a cloth wrung out of cold water. Either hand towels or cotton cloths may be used.

HOW IT CAN HELP YOU—The Cold Compress is very helpful in cases of fever, pain due to edema or trauma (such as sprains). And they are used for congestion in the sinuses and for congestive headaches (for both of these, use a Cold Compress along with a

Hot Foot bath *(p. 256)*. In addition, they are helpful for tachycardia (heartbeat over a 100 per minute).

   HOW TO APPLY IT—*(See picture below.)*

1 - Use Turkish towels to protect the bedding, as well as his clothing, from becoming wet.

2 - Fold the towels (or cloth) to a desired size; then dip into cold water and wring them out—but only enough to prevent dripping. (Better: Take the wet cloths off a block of ice and quickly apply them. In this way the compresses will be far colder.)

3 - Lay them on the afflicted part.

4 - Change the compress for a fresh cold one every 1-5 minutes. A set of two compresses will be needed, so they can be continually alternated. If this is not done, the compress quickly warms up. The thicker the compress, the less often will it have to be changed for a new one.

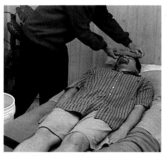 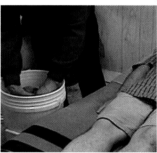

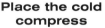

| **Place the cold compress** | **Replace the cold compress frequently** |

5 - Cold compresses can be placed on the head, neck, over the heart or lungs, and to the abdomen, spine, etc. When applied to the head, they need to be pressed down firmly—especially over the forehead and temporal arteries (these arteries are to the right and left of the front forehead, just above and to the front of the ears). The compresses can be placed over the abdomen in typhoid fever.

ADDITIONAL POINTS—Unless the application is quite thick, and always when it is left on too long (over 3-5 minutes), the application changes from a cold compress to a heating compress. And when you are applying a Cold Compress, you do not want it to turn into a Heating Compress! *(For more information on Heating Compresses, see pages 225-229.)*

COLD COMPRESS

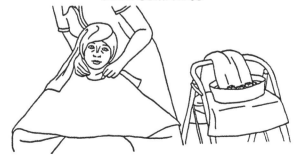

HYDRO

2 - ICE PACK

WHAT IT IS—Although not given that name, this is actually an ice compress; and it will always produce a stronger cold effect than cold cloths wrung out of water.

HOW IT CAN HELP YOU—It can be used over the heart and chest, to slow the heart. It has been used for sprains or torn ligaments, acute joint inflammation, in rheumatic fever, acute infectious arthritis, bursitis, and burns. (In hospitals, it has been used successfully to slow the heart and limit thermic reaction following surgical operations for exophthalmic goiter.)

HOW TO APPLY IT—

1 - Pound ice into snowy bits and pieces or use snow itself.

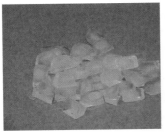
Place ice on towel or flannel

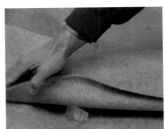
Wrap ice

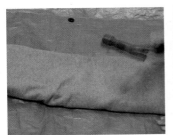
Crush Ice with side of hammer

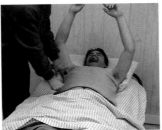
Protect the surface with flannel

ICE PACK and ICE CRAVAT

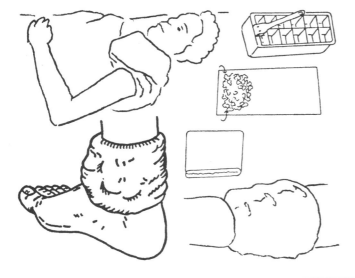

2 - Wrap the body part in flannel (to keep it from freezing).

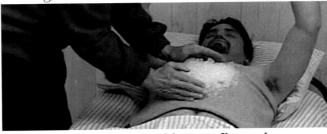
Place crushed ice on flannel

3 - Pack the snow or pounded ice very closely around it, until the pack is about one inch thick.

4 - Wrap a large flannel cloth over it all to keep everything in place. Pin it together.

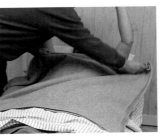
Wrap another flannel over the crushed ice

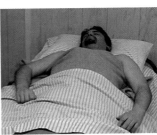
See *Point 5* for the next step

5 - Interrupt the ice pack frequently in order to prevent freezing. Rub the part with snow or apply a hot fomentation over the body part, to bring a local heating reaction.

3 - ICE CRAVAT

WHAT IT IS—The Ice Cravat is basically the same as the Ice Pack, described just above. Instead of being laid around part of the body and then wrapped, the snow or crushed ice is placed inside a towel and then wrapped around the neck or another joint area of the body. The Ice Cravat is thus easier to work with than is the Ice Pack.

When wrapped around the neck, the Ice Cravat becomes an Ice Collar (ice neck pack). But it can also be laid around a shoulder, elbow, knee, or ankle.

The effect is that of a proximal application (*Proximal Compresses are explained on page 225*); the carotid arteries in the neck and the vertebral arteries by the spine that go into the head, along with their small branch arteries, are all contracted. Thus the blood supply to the brain and the head is lessened.

HOW IT CAN HELP YOU—The Ice Cravat is frequently used in fever, congestive headache, acute epidemic meningitis, sunstroke, and whenever prolonged sweating treatments are given, as in eclampsia and uremia. Contraction of the blood vessels slows down the oozing of blood into the injured tissues; thus edema is prevented. It can also help prevent black-and-blue swelling when tissue has been injured (by sprains, contusions, etc.). In addition, it is used for rheumatoid arthritis, acute infectious arthritis, and the acute joint inflammation of rheumatic fever.

HOW TO APPLY IT—*(See picture on page 223.)*

1 - Crush ice and place it in a towel. (Instead of placing snow or crushed ice inside of a dry towel, you can wring the towel from cold water without putting ice or snow inside it. But this will not be as cold and must be changed much more frequently.)

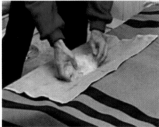
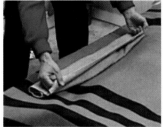

Place crushed ice in towel   **Wrap the ice in the towel**

2 - Fold the towel until it is about 3 inches wide, and long enough to encircle the neck.

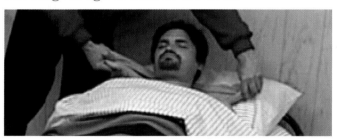

wrap the afflicted area

3 - Put it in place around the neck.

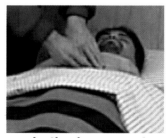
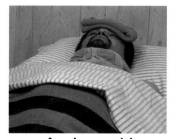

pin the ice cravat   **Apply a cold compress**

4 - If, instead of being applied to the neck, it is to be placed on a different body joint area: Use a piece of flannel that is at least 12 by 12 inches for the shoulders and knees and 8 by 9 inches for the elbows or ankles.

4 - ICE BAG (ICE CAP)

WHAT IT IS—Ice bags and ice caps can be purchased or ordered from your local drugstore. Ice bags come in various shapes and sizes. (One example is the spinal ice bag, which is about 3 inches wide by 7-10 inches long.) The best ones are made of pure natural gum rubber, and all come with screw caps.

HOW IT CAN HELP YOU—The Ice Bag (or Ice Cap) prevents or reduces swelling, relieves pain, checks bleeding, and reduces congestion and inflammation.

A second value lies in their reflex effects: They can relieve congestion and inflammation of deeper internal organs, such as in appendicitis and salpingitis. For this purpose, the application must be placed over the reflex area that affects that deeper organ. *(See pages 213-214 for additional information on reflex effects.)*

A third use is to strengthen and slow the activity of the heart when the pulse is rapid and weak.

HOW TO APPLY IT—*(See pictures on page 225.)*

1 - Fill the ice cap or ice bag about one-half full with finely chopped ice. Press it down to expel the air; and, then, screw the cap on tightly. Dry it and test for leaks.

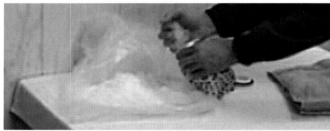

Fill ice bag with crushed ice

2 - Cover it with a flannel or hand towel, and apply it where needed. Never apply an ice bag or ice cap directly to the skin; always place a cloth over the body part first.

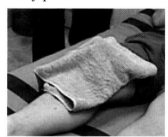
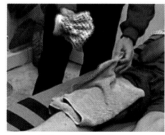

Apply to affected area   **Place ice bag in a towel**

3 - Continually watch to see that there is no danger of injuring the skin through frostbite.

4 - When the ice melts, refill it with more ground ice.

SPECIAL POINTS—Choose a bag that is light in weight; if it is used continually (especially on the abdomen or chest), you may want to suspend it in a cradle, to take off part of the weight. When it is filled, if all the air is not expelled, the ice will melt more rapidly.

HYDRO

5 - PROXIMAL COMPRESS

WHAT IT IS—A Proximal Compress is any type of cold compress, ice bag, etc., that is placed over a large artery in order to reduce blood circulation in the part of the body or limb served by that artery. It is not always convenient to apply a wet cloth to an afflicted part. This is especially true with open wounds, which need to be kept very clean.

HOW TO APPLY IT—

1 - A Cold Compress *(page 222)* is wrung out of water (60°-70° F.) and then placed over the artery supplying the afflicted part. Instead of a Cold Compress, an Ice Bag *(page 224)*, filled with ice or ice water, can be used.

2 - The compress must be frequently changed in order to maintain the cold effect.

WHERE TO APPLY IT—What one needs to know is where to apply the cold Proximal Compress. Here are the most useful places to put it and the corresponding areas in which the temperature and blood supply will be reduced:

1 - To the knee and the calf of the leg (to affect the foot).

2 - To the femoral artery on the inside of the leg, to the whole thigh, or an ice bag to the back side of the knee (to affect the portion of the leg below the knee).

3 - An ice bag to the groin (to affect the whole leg).

4 - A cold compress around the elbow joint (to affect the hand).

5 - To the whole upper arm (to affect the forearm).

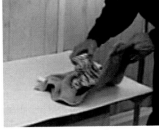 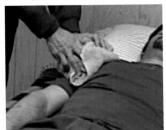

Place ice bag   **Apply to the**
in a towel   **afflicted area**

6 - An ice bag to the arm pit (to affect the whole arm).

7 - An ice bag at the bend of the elbow (to affect the hand).

8 - An ice collar or cold, wet towel, around the neck (to affect the brain). This application helps reduce congestion in the brain, reduce laryngeal inflammation, and aids in meningitis.

ICE BAR

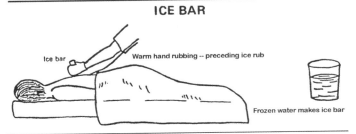

Ice bar   Warm hand rubbing -- preceding ice rub

Frozen water makes ice bar

9 - Over the carotid arteries, which are located on both sides of the neck (to affect the brain).

—SECTION TWO—
COLD-TO-HEATING

WHAT IT IS—These are applications of cold cloths, covered with flannel, to a body area. The body reacts and heats up the pack; and the result is improved circulation and a better flow of healing blood in and out of the afflicted area.

1 - HEATING THROAT COMPRESS AND DRY THROAT COMPRESS

WHAT IT IS—This is a cold compress that is so covered up that warming soon takes place. The effect produced is that of a mild, prolonged application of moist heat.

HOW IT CAN HELP YOU—Gradually, over several hours, a throat compress can reduce inflammation and bring healing to a body part. A cold, wet cloth is placed about the throat, then covered with dry flannel to prevent air circulation, thus increasing body heat in that area. Mothers will often place a heating compress on a child with a sore throat in the evening and take it off the next morning. The compress should be dry by then.

PROBLEMS IT CAN HELP SOLVE—The Throat Compress is a very common household remedy for sore throat, hoarseness, tonsillitis, pharyngitis, laryngitis, quinsy, and eustachian tube inflammation.

WHAT YOU WILL NEED—2 or 3 thicknesses of ordinary cotton cloth about 3 inches wide and long enough to encircle the neck twice. Two thicknesses of flannel not less than 4 inches wide. Safety pins. Possibly a piece of bandage.

HOW TO APPLY IT—*(See picture below.)*

1 - Prepare your materials for the neck compress. If it is to go on one who is too frail to warm it up, then use a Dry Throat Compress, which is prepared in the same manner as the regular Heating Throat Compress, but without being first wrung out of cold water.

2 - In giving a regular Heating Throat Compress, wring the cotton cloth from cold water and place it around the neck. This should be about 2-3 thicknesses about the neck.

THROAT COMPRESS / JOINT COMPRESS

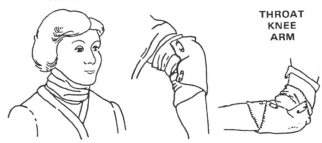

THROAT
KNEE
ARM

H
Y
D
R
O

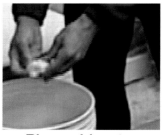

**Ring cold water
from cloth**

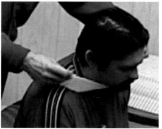

**Wrap cloth
around neck**

3 - Cover it well with the flannel (single or double thick, depending on the weight of the material). Fit the flannel snugly but not too tightly that it will be uncomfortable. Pin it securely.

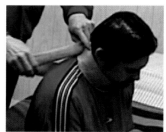

**Wrap flannel
around the cloth**

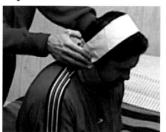

**Wrap a cloth over
the head, to secure
the throat wrap**

4 - In tonsillitis, quinsy, and inflammation of the eustachian tube, the compress should extend upward about the lower part of the ear. You may need to hold up this part of the compress (that is by the lower part of the ear) with a bandage that is fastened to it and goes over the top part of the head and back down to it on the other side.

5 - Remove it the next morning. It should be entirely dry. When first put on, it can be quite wet but should not drip. But the next morning it must be dry.

6 - As soon as you have removed the compress, rub the neck with a cloth wrung out of cold water.

2 - HEATING JOINT COMPRESS AND DRY JOINT COMPRESS

WHAT IT IS—This compress is quite similar to the Heating Throat Compress, described above. The primary difference lies in the fact that this heating compress is applied to one of the joints (foot, ankle, knee, elbow, hand, or wrist) instead of to the neck.

PROBLEMS IT CAN HELP SOLVE—The Heating Joint Compress is most frequently used in cases of rheumatism and rheumatic fever. But there are other painful joint conditions that it may also alleviate.

HOW TO APPLY IT—*(See picture on page 225.)*

1 - You will need similar materials to those listed above under the Heating Throat Compress. If the one it is to be placed upon is too weak or frail to heat up a wet compress, it may be best to make it a Dry Joint Compress (several layers of flannel, with or without dry cotton beneath it).

2 - You may wish to place solution (such as oil of wintergreen, camphorated oil, menthol, mustard water, etc.) on the cotton before it is wrapped around the joint. This helps relieve pain; and, by its counter-irritant action, it enhances the heating effect by increasing the blood circulation at the painful joint.

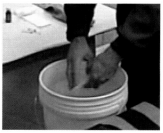

**Wring cloth
in cold water**

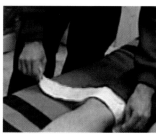

**Apply to the
afflicted joint**

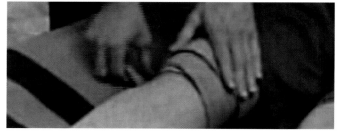

Wrap with flannel and pin together

3 - Two thicknesses of cotton cloth are wrapped around the afflicted joint(s). Sometimes gauze is used, but cotton will enable you to bring the material closer to the skin surface. This is then held in place either with a three-inch roller bandage (obtainable from a drugstore) or with a broad flannel cloth.

3 - MOIST ABDOMINAL BANDAGE, PARTIAL ABDOMINAL BANDAGE, PROTECTED JOINT BANDAGE, AND WET GIRDLE

WHAT IT IS—This is a heating compress applied over the stomach and intestinal area. It is an application of cold, wet sheeting, covered up with dry flannel, which the body then warms up into a very helpful heating pack. This Moist Abdominal "Bandage" is also called a "binder," "girdle," or "pack." When only the front part is moistened, it is called a Partial Abdominal Bandage.

HOW IT CAN HELP YOU—The Moist Abdominal Bandage (or Binder) is one of the most useful of the heating compresses. It is recommended in nearly all forms of atonic indigestion, neurasthenia, anemia of the liver, insomnia, catarrhal jaundice, constipation, and similar conditions. For these purposes, it is generally worn only at night.

With a hot-water bottle *(pages 238)* placed over the stomach, it is also useful in milder cases of nausea and vomiting. If plastic is placed over the flannel to prevent the cotton from drying out, it is called a Protected Binder; and it is used for hyperacidity and also to obtain relaxation in the abdominal organs. A protected binder, by keeping the cotton from drying out, will induce a stronger perspiration than would otherwise occur.

WHAT YOU WILL NEED—One thickness of cotton sheeting, linen, or 3-4 thicknesses of gauze. It should be 8-9 inches wide, no matter what this material is made of, and a little longer than 1½ times around the body. Over this will go an outer flannel covering that is about 12 inches wide, about the same length as the linen or slightly longer. Safety pins, and possibly plastic, will also be needed.

HOW TO APPLY IT—(*See picture below.*)

1 - Prepare the sheeting for a Moist Abdominal Bandage by dipping it into cold water.

2 - (If the one receiving the treatment is too frail to warm up the large wet surface of the cotton wrapping, give him a Partial Abdominal Bandage: Only wet that portion of the cloth that is over the front (over the abdomen). Or, only place a smaller, wet cloth over the abdomen, and let the rest of the encircling covering be flannel alone. These two variations of the Partial Abdominal Bandage are milder forms of the Moist Abdominal Bandage.)

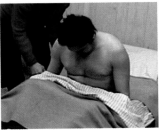

Lay out flannel material

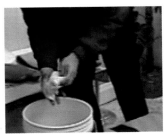

Wring cold water from cotton cloth

3 - The dry flannel is placed across a table; the linen (or gauze), wrung nearly dry from cold water, is placed over it.

4 - The one not feeling well now lies back on the bandage. The lower edge of the cloth and flannel should touch below his hipbones (below the iliac crests).

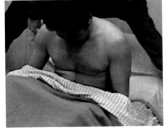

Lay wet cloth on top of flannel material

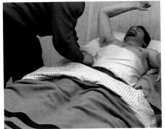

Wrap wet cloth around the body

5 - Pull each end of the wet cloth tightly over his abdomen and tuck them under the opposite side.

6 - Cover quickly and snugly with both ends of

the flannel, and securely fasten the ends with safety pins. Also pin darts at each side, to make the binder fit better. The flannel piece should project 1½-2 inches beyond the wet gauze or linen.

7 - (If plastic is now placed over the flannel to keep it from drying out (for hyperacidity), it now becomes a Protected Bandage; but understand that this is not the usual way of preparing Moist Abdominal Bandages.)

8 - A hot-water bottle is sometimes placed outside the flannel, over the stomach area.

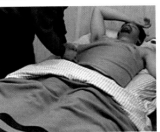

Overlay the flannel material and pin securely

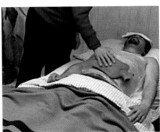

Place hot water bottle and cold compress

9 - When you later remove the binder, wash the area with cold water and dry thoroughly.

THE WET GIRDLE—The Moist Abdominal Bandage is a heating compress over the front of the abdominal area. Kellogg frequently made use of the "Wet Girdle." This is a wraparound Moist Abdominal Bandage. It covers the front, sides, and back of the lower trunk. "The region to which it is applied is bounded by the nipple line above and the hip joints below" (Kellogg). In nearly every instance in which the "Hot Abdominal Pack" is given in the Kellogg Water Remedies section of this chapter, the "Wet Girdle" is the application referred to. (*See picture below.*)

4 - HEATING CHEST PACK

WHAT IT IS—The Heating Chest Pack is similar in some respects to a fomentation over the chest. The difference lies in the fact that, instead of continually applying and changing fomentation cloths, a piece of wet cotton sheeting is wrapped around the chest and then covered. Thus, a slow buildup of heat occurs over a longer period of time.

MOIST ABDOMINAL BANDAGE

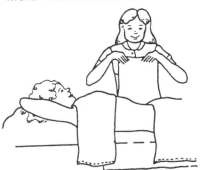

One alternative is the **Partial Chest Pack** *(see pictures on this page)*, in which a wet cloth is placed only over the chest. This is used when the person would be too frail to heat up the full wet pack. Another alternative is the **Dry Chest Pack** *(see picture on next page)*, which has no moist compress within it. It is especially helpful between other treatments; however, those who are thin, aged, and those in the early stages of pneumonia do not react well to cold applications. The **Hot Trunk Pack** *(page 247)* is a chest pack that covers the entire chest, abdomen, and pelvic area.

HOW IT WORKS—These chest packs gradually build up heat in the skin above the chest, and thus aid in relieving various congestions in the chest and lungs.

Of the above packs, the Heating Chest Pack is the most powerful (but not immediately as powerful as Fomentations to the chest: *See pages 234-237*); the Partial Chest Pack has far less strength; the Dry Chest Pack is the mildest.

PROBLEMS IT CAN HELP SOLVE—Here are some of the conditions the Chest Pack is used for: Bronchial and respiratory colds that hang on. Influenza of the respiratory type. Pneumonia. Only use a Dry Chest Pack during the acute stage of pneumonia; only use a Heating or Partial Chest Pack during later convalescence from it. During pneumonia, the skin does not have its normal ability to adjust to changes in outside temperature. Pleurisy: When treating this condition, if he is robust, use the heating pack immediately after an application of heat, such as a Fomentation *(page 234)*; but if he has lessened vitality, only use a Dry Chest Pack, with a hot-water bottle applied outside the pack. These chest packs are also helpful for whooping cough, croup, asthma, and similar conditions.

WHAT YOU WILL NEED—The chest pack can be made in several ways; but, since you will be using it many times on the same person, we will here describe the simplest: the fitted chest pack.

Take flannel material and cut it with scissors into two fitted pieces. One will go over his chest, upper shoulders, and sides; the other will cover his back, lower shoulders, and side. Allow for overlapping under the arms and on the shoulders. This will be pinned together each time it is used.

You will also need a cotton cloth (such as old sheeting material) if a wet cloth (inside a regular Heating or Partial Chest Pack) is to be used. You will not need it if a Dry Chest Pack is being applied.

HOW TO APPLY IT—*(See picture to right.)*

1 - Warm up his chest with fomentations or a heat lamp over his chest.

2 - If a moist cloth is to be applied, wring it thoroughly from tap water and place it on his chest (Partial Pack), or wrap it about his chest and upper back (Heating Pack).

3 - (At this point, you may wish to put warm camphorated oil, or something similar, on the wet sheeting over his chest.)

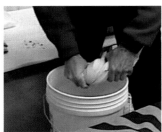
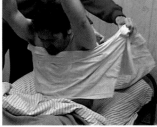

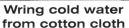
Wring cold water from cotton cloth **Wrap around the trunk of the body**

4 - (If you wish to increase the sweating, place plastic over the moistened cloth.)

5 - Cover quickly with the fitted flannel that you earlier cut out for this purpose. He should be covered well, but not too tightly. Pin securely.

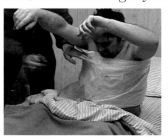
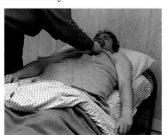

Wrap with plastic sheet **Wrap with flannel material**

CAUTIONS—The wet compress should be wrung out thoroughly and then covered well, to avoid chilling and to aid in a prompt reaction. The pack must be snugly applied at all places, but not so tight as to restrict the movements of the chest in breathing. The pack should be comfortable and should feel warm in a very short time. If not, remove it and apply a milder pack (a Partial or Dry Chest Pack). Use a Dry Chest Pack (not a Heating Chest Pack) during the acute stages of pneumonia. When caring for pleurisy, it is best to only use the Dry Chest Pack. Both the Partial and Dry Chest Pack are described just below:

5 - PARTIAL CHEST PACK

WHAT IT IS—The Partial Chest Pack is identical to the Heating Chest Pack, described just above, with the exception that the wet cloth is only placed over the chest.

HEATING CHEST PACK

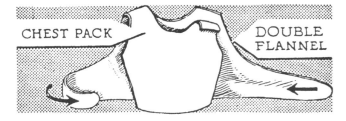

CHEST PACK   DOUBLE FLANNEL

HYDRO

HOW IT CAN HELP YOU—This pack can enable you to give a heating-type chest pack to one who is too frail to warm up the full wet pack (the Heating Chest Pack).

HOW TO APPLY IT—

1 - The cotton covering for the partial pack can be cut to any desired shape, since it will only go over part of the chest.

2 - Wring it out wet and apply it over the chest.

3 - Cover it with the flannel.

Since most of the chest is covered with dry material, this pack is quite similar in effect to the Dry Chest Pack.

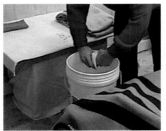

Wring cold water from cotton cloth

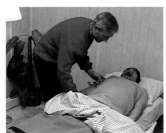

Place wet cloth on chest

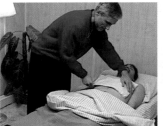

Wrap with flannel material

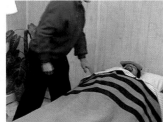

Use cold compress on the forehead

CAUTION—Only use the Dry Chest Pack during the acute stage of pneumonia; only use a Heating or Partial Chest Pack during later convalescence from it.

6 - DRY CHEST PACK

WHAT IT IS—The Dry Chest Pack is also like the Heating Chest Pack, with one primary exception: It does not have any wet cloth between the skin and the blanket.

HOW IT CAN HELP YOU—This pack is especially helpful between other water treatments. It is also well-adapted to the special needs of the thin and the aged who are not able to react and heat up the moist cloth used in the Heating Chest Pack. The dry pack is also the best method for the early stages of pneumonia.

HOW TO APPLY IT—

Only the flannel is used, and should be applied over a thin undergarment that he is wearing.

The dry Pack is necessary for thin, weak people because it is almost impossible to pin the wet pack tightly enough to prevent air from circulating under the edges of the pack and yet be loose enough to be comfortable and not restrict the breathing.

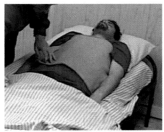

Wrap flannel material around the body

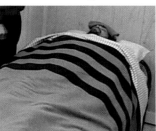

Apply cold compress to the forehead

CAUTION—Only use the Dry Chest Pack during the acute stage of pneumonia; only use a Heating or Partial Chest Pack during later convalescence from it.

— SECTION THREE —
LARGER COLD-TO-HEATING

WET-SHEET PACK

STAGE ONE: COOLING WET-SHEET PACK
STAGE TWO: NEUTRAL WET-SHEET PACK
STAGE THREE: HEATING WET-SHEET PACK
STAGE FOUR: SWEATING WET-SHEET PACK

WHAT IT IS—This is a bed sheet wrung out of cold water and then quickly draped around a person who is covered with a blanket or two. The body, in reaction, quickly begins warming up the sheet; and fairly soon it turns into a moist heating pack.

HOW IT CAN HELP YOU—According to how long it is left on, the Wet-sheet Pack has one or more of four different effects. This is due to the fact that, according to the degree of warming that it undergoes, the Wet-sheet Pack passes through four stages: (1) the Cooling Stage, (2) the Neutral Stage, (3) the Heating Stage, and (4) the Sweating Stage. The stage that you stop at—or prolong—is determined by the effect that you wish to produce. We will conclude this explanation of the Wet-sheet Pack with a careful look at each of these four stages.

HOW TO APPLY IT—*(See picture on next page.)*

1 - Having all the materials ready, explain the treatment to him. An enema *(page 268)* or colonic *(page 269)* is considered to be an important preliminary step. Also, if needed, give him a 10 - minute Hot Foot bath *(page 256)*, with a Cold Compress *(page 222)* to his head; for the entire body should be warm

---

HEATING CHEST PACK / DRY CHEST PACK

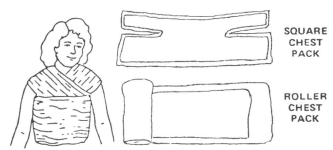

SQUARE CHEST PACK

ROLLER CHEST PACK

H
Y
D
R
O

before beginning the Wet-sheet Pack. If not, precede it with a Hot Full (tub) Bath.

2 - Place a plastic or rubber sheet on the bed. Over it, place a double blanket, folded lengthwise, with the edge of the far side hanging longer than the near edge. The upper end of the blanket should cover the lower half of the pillow.

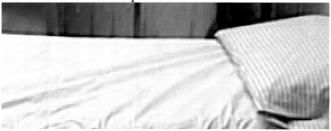
Cover matress with a plastic sheet

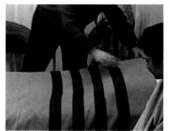
Cover plastic sheet with a blanket

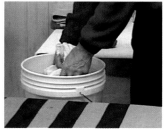
Wring cold water from cotton cloth

3 - Take the wet sheet from the cold water and wring it as dry as possible. Place it on the blanket, with the upper end a little below the top of the blanket.

4 - Now help him lie on his back on the sheet, with his shoulders 3-4 inches below the upper edge of the sheet.

5 - As his arms are held up, you quickly wrap the short side of the sheet around his trunk, and also around his nearest leg.

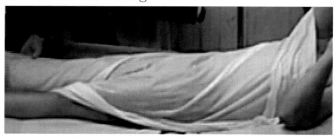
Wrap first leg and the trunk of the body

6 - Draw the sheet smoothly in contact with the skin in all places. Tuck it under on the opposite side.

7 - Lower his arms, and then wrap the other side of the sheet smoothly over his arms, trunk, and his farther leg. Fold the sheet over his shoulders, and across his neck. Tuck it in. Important: Wrap him in the sheet quickly. The wet sheet must come in close contact with the skin at all points.

8 - Wrap the narrower edge of the blanket around his body and tuck it in. Do the same on the opposite

edge, pulling it snugly around him. At this point, pull the remainder of the blanket over and tuck it also under his body and under his feet. Important: Wrap him in the blanket quickly. The dry blanket must prevent circulating air or he may become chilled. Warming up should begin immediately.

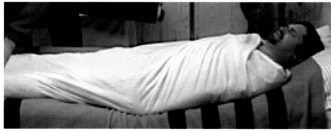
Finish wrapping the body

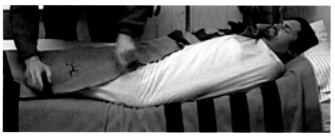
Wrap in blanket

9 - It may be best to now cover him with a second blanket. Additional blankets may be laid over him and tucked in on the sides and about the feet, if needed.

10 - Place a Turkish towel around his neck, to protect him from the blanket and to keep out the air. Put the hot-water bottle to his feet to hasten warming.

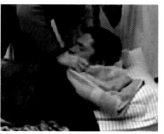
Cover with additional blanket and wrap neck with towel

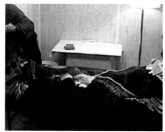
Place hot water bottle under the feet

11 - Sponge his face with a Cold Compress (*page 222*) at the beginning of the pack and also after the first 10 minutes when the reaction begins (when he

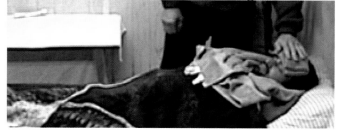
Apply cold compress to the forehead

begins sweating).

12 - His feet must be kept warm at all times. Take his temperature before and after the pack is given.

13 - When the pack is removed, give a Cool Sponge, with brisk drying to the body.

14 - Repeat with another Wet-sheet Pack later that day or give it daily until the fever comes down. Duration of each Wet-sheet Pack is 15-20 minutes. Have him rest afterward. Liquid nourishment is best.

FOUR TYPES OF WET-SHEET PACK—As mentioned at the beginning of this section, there are four stages to the Wet-sheet Pack. The stage you bring him up to and stop at—or prolong—will determine the objectives you are going to achieve:

1 - Cooling Wet-sheet Pack—This is the first stage of the pack before the sheet has been warmed to the temperature of the body. 5-12 minutes is needed to reach this stage. At the end of this time the effect can be intensified by removing the sheet and applying another (wet, cold) sheet or by folding back the blanket and sprinkling cold water on the wet sheet that covers him.

This cooling pack is a powerful way to lower a high temperature, and is especially useful in typhoid fever and other continued fevers.

2 - Neutral Wet-sheet Pack—This begins when the temperature of the pack reaches, or slightly exceeds, skin temperature. After body warming has well begun, this second stage can be prolonged by removing all but one or two dry coverings over the wet sheet. But the body must continue to be evenly warm, with no circulating air reaching it.

This neutral pack is excellent for insomnia, and helps put the sleepless to sleep. It is also used for mania, alcoholic delirium, and restlessness. A neutral bath will accomplish the same purpose as a neutral pack—and probably do it better.

3 - Heating Wet-sheet Pack—This begins when the warming pack has raised the body temperature slightly above its usual degree; and it ends when general perspiration begins. Once achieved, this should, for best results, be continued for about 20 minutes.

This heating pack helps warm the body and lessens localized congestions, wherever they may be in the body.

4 - Sweating Wet-sheet Pack—This last stage begins with the onset of general sweating. The sweating

may be increased or prolonged by additional coverings, hot-water bottles between blanket layers, or by drinking hot water or lemonade. The cold compresses on the head should not be very cold or renewed too frequently.

This sweating pack is excellent for childhood fevers, capillary bronchitis, colds, and also for obesity and obese rheumatism.

Heating and sweating packs are also used for alcoholism, gout, influenza, and the elimination of nicotine from the body (which lessens the physical craving for more tobacco).

One of the most useful treatments for the fevers of early childhood is this: Give him a Full Hot Tub Bath *(page 259)*, followed by a cold Wet-sheet Pack, as described above. The child, so exhausted by the fever on his body and head, will often fall into a quiet sleep after the pack reaches the heating stage.

— SECTION FOUR —
LOCAL HOT AND COLD

1 - ALTERNATE COMPRESS

WHAT IT IS—This is an application of very hot and very cold compresses in alternation (one following the other).

HOW IT CAN HELP YOU—There is probably no other procedure which is capable of so intensely and rapidly exciting the flow of blood in various parts of the body. Thus it helps to eliminate pus formation, avoid bed sores (which are so likely to appear in typhoid fever, tuberculosis, and other wasting diseases). It can also be applied to paralyzed limbs and to parts affected by chilblains as a means of stimulating absorption in dropsy of the abdomen or of the chest. It is also used in chronic pleurisy and pneumonia, in which the parts damaged by the acute inflammatory process have not been fully restored.

Alternate Compresses to the spine are a very effective means of arousing one from morphine-derivative poisoning, alcoholic intoxication, and similar problems.

"The author recalls very vividly a case of opium poisoning to which he was called in consultation some twenty-five years ago, in which a patient's pulse was reduced to less than twenty and respiration to four per minute. Thoroughgoing hot and cold applications to the spine quickly brought the pulse to a nearly normal count. The respiration became twelve per minute within five minutes; and the change in the entire aspect of the case was so marvelous as to seem little short of a miracle to the bystanders who had never before witnessed the powerful stimulating effects of thermic applications properly managed."—*Kellogg.*

HOW TO APPLY IT—

1 - This is a Fomentation application *(page 234)*, with the addition of a Cold Compress *(page 222)* after

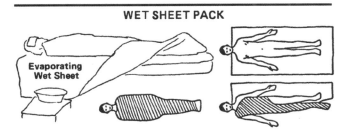

WET SHEET PACK

Evaporating
Wet Sheet

it: When the fomentation cloth is removed, a hand towel, wrung from cold water or ice water, is placed on the body part. The cold application will need to be renewed frequently in order to keep it cold; but it may be left on nearly as long, or as long as the hot

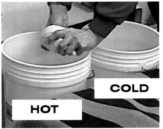

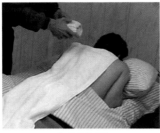

Wring hot water from fomentation cloth

Lay hot fomentation cloth in between towel

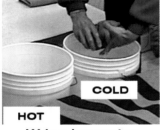

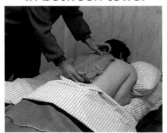

Wring ice water from face towel

Place cold towel directly to the afflicted body part

application (but never longer).

2 - Then it is removed and the surface dried well. Another fomentation is then applied. Three changes from hot to cold are usually given. The procedure must always begin with a hot application and end

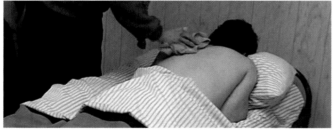

Dry and repeat the first steps again

with a cold one.

2 - REVULSIVE COMPRESS

WHAT IT IS—This hot and cold application differs from the Alternate Compress, described just above, only in the different timing of the heat and cold. In the Alternate Compress, the applications are of equal time; or, at least, the hot application does not exceed the cold. In the Revulsive Compress, the hot application is decidedly longer.

HOW IT CAN HELP YOU—This compress is very helpful in relieving pain in many, many physical problems. (Neuralgia is but one example.)

(It should be understood that pain is sometimes

best relieved by very hot applications, in others by cold ones, and in still others by alternate hot and cold. But in many instances, pain is increased as the affected nerves are excited—especially when inflammation is present. At such times, alternate hot and cold will best help reduce the pain.)

The Revulsive Compress is also a powerful aid in reducing congestion, such as gastric congestion, gastritis, enteralgia, acute sciatica, neuritis, painful affections of the eye, and spinal irritation. It often affords immediate relief from the heavy pain of toothache.

HOW TO APPLY IT—

1 - Follow the directions for giving a Fomentation *(page 234)*. But when each hot application has been lifted off, place a hand towel, wrung from cold water or ice water (according to his ability to react to cold) on the surface. Let it remain there a few seconds; then turn it over to remain a few seconds more.

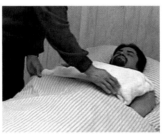

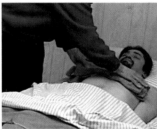

Apply hot fomentation

Apply cold, wet towel for a few moments

2 - The skin is now dried and the next fomentation is applied. Three changes of hot and three of cold are usually given.

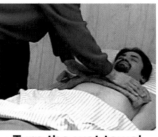

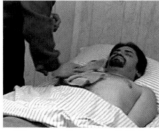

Turn the wet towel over for a few moments

Dry and repeat this process three times

3 - ALTERNATE HOT AND COLD TO THE HEAD

There are two totally different hot and cold applications to the head. We are placing them here together, one right after the other, so that you will make no mistake regarding which one to use. First, we shall describe the Alternate Hot and Cold to the Head:

WHAT IT IS—This is an alternation of hot and cold to the head. It means that first you place hot to the head and then cold; then hot and then cold again, for three complete cycles.

HOW IT CAN HELP YOU—This set of applications

causes fluxion, or an increase of blood, to the afflicted area. Thus it can work to improve the circulation of blood within the head and relieve an anemic headache (a headache caused by a lack of blood in the brain). It is also helpful in remitting passive congestion and cold in the head.

WHAT YOU WILL NEED—Two pieces of Turkish toweling or thick hand towels (about 12 inches square) for wet compresses. Two ice bags, filled with finely chopped ice and then covered with a thin cotton cloth (or cheesecloth). A hot-water bottle, partly filled with hot water and then covered either with a dry fomentation cloth or with a towel. A bowl of ice water and a pail of boiling water.

HOW TO APPLY IT—

1 - Place the hot-water bottle crosswise over the back of the neck, bringing it well up under the back of the head and over the neck.

2 - Wring the toweling compress out, lightly, from ice water and then apply it to the face. It should cover the face, top of the head, and the ears. Press down firmly over the forehead and the temporal arteries (these arteries are just above and in front of the ears).

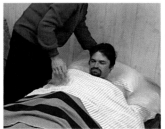

Use plastic sheet to protect the pillow

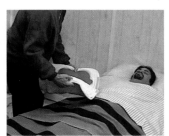

Place hot water bottle inside a fomentation cloth

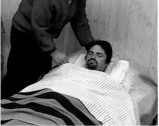

Place the fomentation cloth with the hot water bottle behind the neck

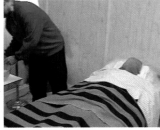

Place face cloth into ice water; then wring water from it; apply to the face - Change once every 60 seconds

3 - Renew this compress every minute.

4 - After three minutes, remove the hot-water bottle and put two cloth-covered ice bags where it had been. And also replace the cold compress over the face by another wrung, quite dry, from hot water. Follow the cautions listed under "cautions," below, in applying hot cloths to the face.) Renew this hot compress every minute.

5 - In another three minutes begin the cycle over again: Replace with the first applications of the hot-water bottle to the back of the neck and the cold compress to the face.

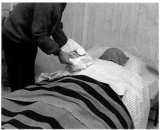

Replace fomentation cloth with an ice bag wrapped in a towel

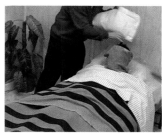

Replace ice bag wrapped in towel with hot water bottle wrapped in fomenation cloth

Reverse this order and repeat every 3 minutes

6 - Continue these alternations for three complete cycles. Then cool all the parts by wiping off with a cold compress and dry thoroughly, especially the hair.

CAUTIONS—The bed should be protected with plastic sheeting. The hot compress should not be pressed to the face. The eyes should be protected from the heat with a thick compress or towel.

4 - SIMULTANEOUS HOT AND COLD TO THE HEAD

WHAT IT IS—Once again, hot and cold is placed to the head; but, instead of alternating back and forth (first hot and then cold) to those places, the hot is kept on certain areas and the cold is kept on others. A primary difference is that the cold application is placed over a reflex area of a deeper part, or over a large artery supplying blood to it. This produces depletion, or a removal of blood from the head. Thus, the effect produced is the exact opposite of that produced by alternate hot and cold to the head.

HOW IT CAN HELP YOU—This treatment is very effective in reducing congestion in the head and relieving congestive headache (headache caused by an excess of blood in the brain).

WHAT YOU WILL NEED—Essentially the same articles are needed for this, the Simultaneous Hot and Cold, as were used for the Alternate Hot and Cold, described just above.

HOW TO APPLY IT—

1 - Place an ice bag to the base of the brain (the back of the neck) and a second ice bag (or better, an ice cap [both are obtainable at your local drugstore]) to the top of the head. A cold, wet towel on the hair will intensify the cold application to the top of the head (do this instead of wetting the hair).

2 - Also place ice bags or ice compresses (ice inside a folded towel) over the carotids. (The carotid arteries are on both sides of the neck, and are the

H
Y
D
R
O

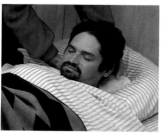

Place an ice bag to the base of the neck

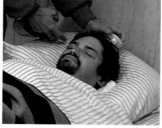

Place ice bag to the top of the head

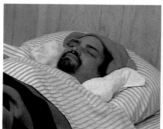

Place ice packs on either side of the neck and a cold, wet cloth over the hair

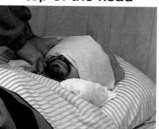

Apply a hot fomentation over the face while making sure the person can breath through the nose

arteries near the surface that bring blood to the brain.)

3 - Then apply a Fomentation *(this page)* to the face, covering the ears and forehead. Cotton sheeting material (or gauze or cheesecloth) should be used under the fomentation when it is applied to the face. The nose should not be covered by the fomentation, for it is better that he be able to breathe cooler air.

4 - Conclude the treatment by first pouring hot, and then cold, water onto the feet. Keep a cold neck and head compress (cold, damp toweling) on him while pouring the water on the feet.

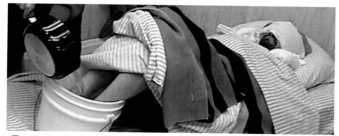

Pour hot water, then cold water, over the feet

5 - ALTERNATE HOT AND COLD TO THE SPINE

WHAT IT IS—This is a Revulsive Compress *(page 176);* except that, instead of the cold compress, a small piece of ice is rubbed over the part. Thus, it is a regular set of Fomentation applications *(this page),* plus the use of ice between each hot application.

HOW IT CAN HELP YOU—This alternate hot and cold application to the spine acts as a strong stimulant and tonic, and is used in a large number of conditions which are helped by such a general treatment.

It improves the circulation, increases muscular tone, and stimulates vasomotor nerve action.

HOW TO APPLY IT—

1 - The Revulsive Compress is described on page 232, and is a variation of the standard Fomentation *(below).* Give Alternate Hot and Cold to the Spine in the same manner as the Revulsive Compress, with the following exception:

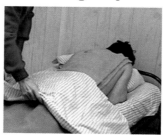

Begin with a hot fomentation

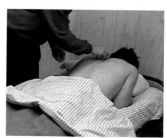

Rub ice up and down the back 3 to 5 times

2 - When each fomentation is removed, instead of briefly placing a cold compress on the part, as is done in the Revulsive Compress, a small piece of ice is quickly rubbed back and forth over the area, making three to five or more to-and-fro movements. The part is then dried and another fomentation is placed there. (In making these applications, it IS important that the next fomentation be ready before the ice is applied.)

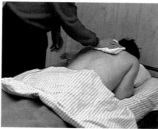

Dry the back

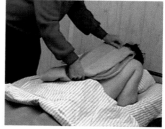

Repeat the previous steps as before

— SECTION FIVE — LOCAL HOT

1 - FOMENTATIONS

WHAT IT IS—A Fomentation is an application of moist heat to part of the body. The moist heat is produced by cloths wrung from hot water and then laid upon the afflicted part. Of all methods of applying heat to the body, there is no more effective or simpler method than the use of cloths wrung out of very hot water.

Heat can be applied as dry heat or moist heat, but moist heat is the more powerful of the two. When given to relieve pain, this heat is best given locally, that is, to only part of the body. A fomentation is one of the simplest and most effective means of applying moist heat to various parts of the body.

HOW IT CAN HELP YOU—A fomentation can re-

H
Y
D
R
O

lieve pain; but, if the heat is more moderate and the application more prolonged before being renewed, it can also relax and enable a person to go to sleep. It also increases the circulation of white blood cells and the flow of blood to the skin, thus relieving internal congestion. It relieves muscle tension and spasms, and pain in muscle joints and internal organs. It promotes sweating, thus increasing the elimination of toxins. And it either stimulates or relaxes, according to the temperature of the application. Fomentations are excellent for chest congestion due to colds, bronchitis, or pleurisy.

WHAT YOU WILL NEED—You will need a kettle of boiling water (or a steamer), at least four fomentation cloths, one or two Turkish towels, a washcloth, and a basin of cold water. Here is how to make your own fomentation cloths: The material can be cut from blankets or purchased especially for this purpose. The size should be 30-36 inches square, so four cloths can be cut from one regular-sized blanket. It is best when it is part wool and never all cotton. In fact, it is ideal when it is 50% wool (to retain heat) and 50% cotton (to retain moisture). Some folk use quilted 36-inch-square cloths made of 50-50 wool and cotton. These are considered best if a steamer is used to heat the cloths; yet, ultimately, they are somewhat less effective than the single folded cloths (cut from blankets) wrung out of boiling water.

(If the cloths are placed in a steamer to heat up instead of being wrung out from a pot of boiling water, there is also more danger of burns; since steam is so much hotter than boiling water. With all this in mind, we will only describe below the boiling water, not the steamer method.)

HOW TO APPLY IT—(See pictures on page 236.)

1 - The room should be warm (75°-80° F.), with no drafts; and the water on the stove should be boiling. Fold one fomentation cloth into about three thicknesses.

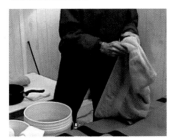

Lay out a towel on
the side of the bed

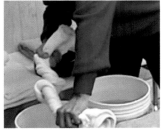

Carefully wring boil-
ing hot water from
another towel

2 - Grasp the ends and partially twist them. Now immerse all, but the ends you are holding, into the boiling water. Lift out and twist tightly, as you hold the dry ends. Stretch or pull the twisted fomentation, to wring it as dry as possible. Then untwist it quickly

(by dropping one end while holding the other end) and wrap it in a dry fomentation cloth. For moderate heat, use only one wrung-out cloth inside the dry one; for stronger moist heat, place two inside the dry fomentation cloth.

3 - With the hot, moist fomentation quickly placed inside it, quickly fold over the dry fomentation cloth onto itself and carry it to the bedside.

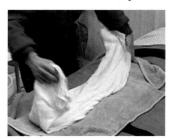

Fold the hot,
wet towel in
the dry towel

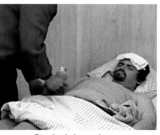

Quickly place
the fomentation
on the chest and
cover with blanket

4 - Unfold and place the inner side of the dry cloth on the area to be treated. (The moist ones are still inside it.) Cover with a towel. A fomentation should be large enough to cover a much larger area than the afflicted part of the body.

(If the treatment is to be given at some distance from the stove, three sets of fomentation cloths may be wrung out and placed in the bottom of a pail lined with large, dry fomentation cloths. They will preserve their heat for 30 minutes or longer. If thought necessary, a hot-water bottle can be placed at the bottom of the pail and a second one at the top, over the three cloth sets.)

5 - If the fomentation is unbearably hot to the one it is placed upon, rub underneath it until it can be tolerated. Always ask if the fomentation is burning him. If it is too hot, place another towel (best a rough or Turkish towel) between him and the fomentation.

6 - The outer, dry, fomentation cloth should lie in close contact with the skin and should be changed every 3-5 minutes, unless a relaxing effect is all that is desired (see next paragraph). In case of pain, very

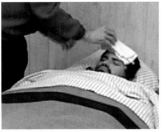

Apply cold compress
to the forehead

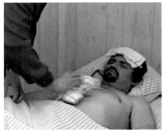

Dry the skin
before changing
the fomentation -
It should be changed
every 3-5 minutes

hot applications should be used; they should be changed as soon as they begin feeling comfortable.

7 - When given for insomnia or only to remove pain, milder heat should be applied for a longer time (6-10 minutes); it is best placed over the spine or, if there is spasticity of the bowel, over the abdomen.

8 - Have another fomentation ready to replace the one being removed. Be sure and quickly wipe the moisture from the skin before applying the next application. Work quickly to expose the area as little as possible.

9 - Usually three successive applications are made. When the last fomentation is removed, cool the area with a washcloth wrung from cold water (or a wet-hand rub, a cold compress, or a rub with a cold and wet towel); then dry thoroughly and cover at once, to prevent chilling.

IMPORTANT POINTS—It is important that the room be warm. Be especially careful when working with thin or aged persons, or with children. Avoid chilling him during or after the treatment. Keep his feet warm. Wipe moisture from the skin before applying each fomentation (it is moisture on the skin that can cause burns). All changes should be made quickly. A cool cloth on the forehead or neck may be necessary. Keep the head cool. In fomentations to the face or other sensitive parts, first apply gauze next to the skin. If perspiration continues after the treatment is ended, give a general cold friction, wet-hand rub, or wet-towel rub. Sensitive surfaces, especially bony prominences (and also scars and metal implants) should

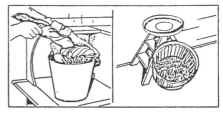

LEFT & BELOW: The fomentation can be heated in boiling water, then wrung out.
RIGHT: An alternate method is to place quilted cloths in a canner. Above is pictured an improvised "steamer"—a can with a lid with a false (second bottom) in it to keep the cloths out of the boiling water (so only steam penetrates them).

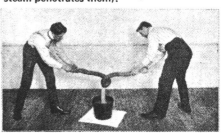

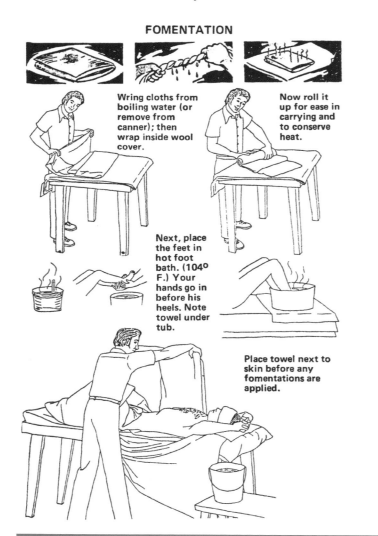

FOMENTATION

Wring cloths from boiling water (or remove from canner); then wrap inside wool cover.

Now roll it up for ease in carrying and to conserve heat.

Next, place the feet in hot foot bath. (104° F.) Your hands go in before his heels. Note towel under tub.

Place towel next to skin before any fomentations are applied.

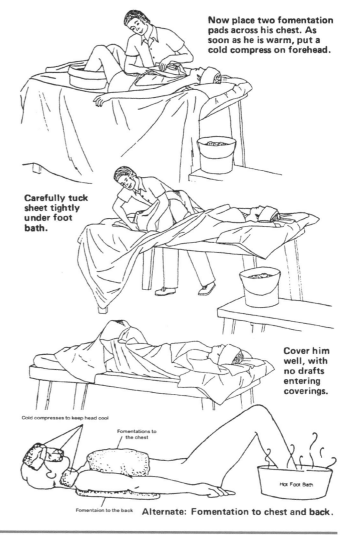

Now place two fomentation pads across his chest. As soon as he is warm, put a cold compress on forehead.

Carefully tuck sheet tightly under foot bath.

Cover him well, with no drafts entering coverings.

Cold compresses to keep head cool
Fomentations to the chest
Fomentation to the back
Hot Foot Bath
Alternate: Fomentation to chest and back.

HYDRO

be protected by extra coverings of flannel or Turkish towel. If he is liable to congestion in the head, always in case of fever or general perspiration, lay cold compresses (cloths wrung out from cold water) on his head and neck. In case of heart disease, usually in fever and with rapid pulse from any cause, place an ice bag over the heart. Where there is extreme pain, have the fomentation as hot as can be tolerated. Omit the cold afterward in extreme pain, as in pleurisy, kidney pain, and dysmenorrhea. In such cases, at the end of the fomentations, the part is dried—without the cold application—and immediately covered with flannel or other dry covering.

STEAMER METHOD—An alternate method is the use of a steamer. This is also a good method and is often easier to do; but one must remember that the cloths have been taken out of a steamer pot and therefore are much hotter than the regular method. Be careful not to burn yourself or the one receiving the Fomentation! Here is how it is done: Sprinkle the fomentation cloths (the cut-up blankets) as you would do to clothes you are about to iron. Then place them in the steamer. (This is the type of steamer, or canner, used to cook jars of fruit or vegetables for canning. It should have a second bottom in it (above the floor of the steamer), with approximately 3-inch diameter holes in it. Below this second bottom is water in the bottom of the steamer.) After sprinkling, roll up the cloths and stack them in the steamer vertically. Cover and let it steam for 20 minutes. Then remove and proceed as normally, except that you need not now wring out excess moisture.

CAUTIONS—Do not give fomentations when the sick person is unconscious, has paralyzed body parts, malignancy, tendency to bleed (hemorrhage), or stomach or bowel ulcers. Do not place fomentations on the legs or feet of a diabetic, or on the legs or feet of one with edema, varicose veins, or advanced vascular disease in these extremities. Never place hot of any kind directly on an open eyeball.

2 - HOT GAUZE COMPRESS

WHAT IT IS—This is an application of heat to a small and delicate part of the body, such as an eye or a fresh wound.

And for both, sterile (perfectly clean) dressings should be used. This small heating compress of gauze has an effect similar to that of a Fomentation. (See pictures on facing page).

HOW IT CAN HELP YOU—These small compresses are most generally used to relieve localized congestion and inflammation, and to stimulate circulation in the afflicted part.

HOW TO APPLY IT—

1 - Dip the gauze into boiling water and then wring it out.

This is done in a manner similar to that of Fo-

mentations (page 234), in which the ends are kept dry and the boiling hot center part is twisted. Care must be taken not to apply too hot a compress. For this purpose, a temperature of 120° F. is best.

2 - Be very careful to place no pressure on the cloth; for you do not want it to touch the eyeball. While one eye is being treated, the other should be protected with a clean, dry dressing or with a shield of some kind.

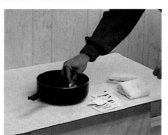

Wring boiling water from gauze cloth

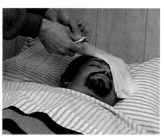

Protect the eye not being treated with a covering cloth

3 - The eye should be dried well before the next hot compress is applied, in order that burning will not occur. Because the compress is usually quite small and uncovered, it cools quickly, and must be changed about once a minute. 10-15 minutes of such compress changes will usually bring the desired results.

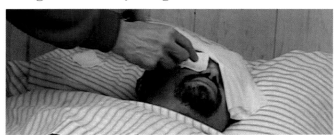

Apply hot, wet guaze to the eye - This should be changed once every 60 seconds for 10 - 15 minutes

4 - The treatment should be concluded by cooling the body part with a cool cloth, then drying thoroughly and covering it to keep it warm.

CAUTION—Memorize this sentence: No hot cloth should ever directly touch an eyeball, with the eye open.

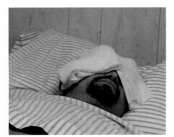

Cover the hot guaze with a dry cloth, to keep heat in

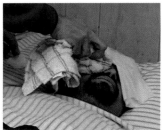

It is important to dry the eye before changing guazes, to avoid burning

3 - HOT-WATER BOTTLE

WHAT IT IS—This is a soft rubber bag filled with hot water that is laid on or beside a body part. Most people are well-acquainted with hot-water bottles; but many do not realize the several precautions that should accompany their use.

HOW IT CAN HELP YOU—The hot-water bottle provides localized heat just where it is needed; and it does it with relatively little effort. A hot-water bottle can be used to relieve pain and congestion, provide relaxation and rest (if prolonged), and reinforce or prolong the effect of Fomentations *(pages 234)*.

WHAT YOU WILL NEED—A hot-water bottle (obtainable at your local drugstore), a flannel cover or a Turkish (rough surface) towel, a pitcher or jar with water (at 115°-125° F.), and a bath thermometer if you need to test its temperature.

HOW TO APPLY IT—*(See picture on this page.)*

1 - Fill the pitcher with water (115°-125° F.); and, from the pitcher, fill the hot-water bottle a third to half full. Place the bottle on its side, tip up its mouth, and press lightly until the water comes up to the top; this expels the air within it. (Expelling the air from the bottle enables it to lie flat, be less bulky and difficult to use, and thus provide the most heat.) Then close it tightly and test for leaks. Cover the bottle with a flannel cover or a Turkish towel. (It is best to sew a cover with a button flap for the bottle instead of wrapping it in a towel. This is because movement can cause it to become separated from the towel and possibly burn him.)

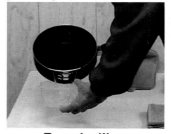
Pour boiling hot water into a pitcher or similar container

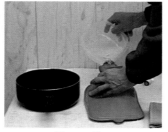
Pour the water into the hot water bottle until it is a third full

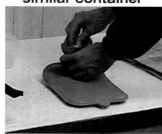
Expel the air

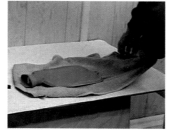
Wrap in a towel

2 - The value of a hot-water bottle is in the temperature of the water within it. Therefore you will need to refill it regularly during the time it is being used.

3 - Later, store the hot-water bottle by hanging it up, bottom up, with the stopper out.

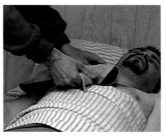
Apply to afflicted area

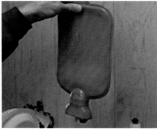
When finished, be sure to empty and hang upside down with the cap removed

ADDITIONAL POINTS—The hot-water bottle can be wrapped in a moist cloth, which is then covered by a dry one. This will give the effect of a mild Fomentation *(page 234)*. And Fomentations, themselves, may be reinforced or prolonged by the use of hot-water bottles placed outside of them.

CAUTIONS—The hot-water bottle should only be partly filled with water, never full. Test the water temperature in some way (thermometer is best), so that you are not placing water that is too hot inside it. Water temperature is especially important if the bottle will be warming a dazed, unconscious, or overly weak person. Be very careful about placing a bottle by a paralyzed or diabetic person, lest he be burned. Always test the bottle for leaks; and always cover it with flannel or toweling. Watch the position of the bottle; for, if he is restless, it may be moved and burn him. Avoid unnecessary weight on him. Never leave the hot-water bottle doubled on itself or in contact with anything oily (oil rots rubber).

4 - HOT PARAFFIN BATH, PACK, DRESSING, AND WRAP

WHAT IT IS—This is a warm bath for an extremity (often an arthritic hand). It is especially helpful because of certain properties of paraffin, described just below.

PARAFFIN AND HEAT—Paraffin is a waxy, white, tasteless, odorless substance that can be a real blessing in your home. One of the important properties of water is its high heat conduction. This means that it can quickly transfer heat to something else. But paraf-

HOT WATER BOTTLE and ICE CAP

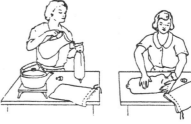
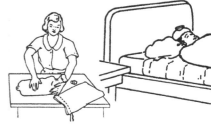

HYDRO

fin has a low heat conduction. This means that it can be used to apply heat for a longer period of time to a local area. Paraffin will hold heat longer than water, because it has a heat capacity of .62 as compared with 1.0 for water. Thus it is about half that of water. But its heat-retaining qualities are greatly increased by the fact that it solidifies only a few degrees above tolerable temperature. Therefore if you place your hand in paraffin just above the melting point, a solid layer, or glove, of paraffin quickly coats the skin, and just as quickly becomes a temperature that is not too hot. All the rest of the paraffin in the bowl will continue to be too hot for your hand; however, the hand will continue to feel nicely warm for quite some time. This is due to the low heat conductivity of the paraffin and the absence of convection currents next to the skin. Also, the actual skin temperature can be hotter than otherwise possible without burning, pain, or any injury because the covering of the paraffin will not permit the coated skin to sweat. Paraffin does not lose heat by evaporation or by convection once it is hardened. Last but not least, it has a "latent heat" of 35 calories, and water has no latent heat so near to body temperature.

HOW IT CAN HELP YOU—The Paraffin Bath is used for painful, arthritic-type joints in the arms or the legs. Most often it is used on the hand. It soothingly relieves pain as it greatly increases the blood circulation to the afflicted body part. Even the smallest blood vessels become dilated as the nourishing, healing blood courses through the painful extremity. In addition, the temperature of the surrounding areas are elevated, thus helping them to resist the disease.

The Paraffin Bath (or Paraffin Pack, Dressing, and Wrap) can help in conditions of arthritis, gout, and sciatica. It is also helpful for stiff joints, tendon repair, sprains, strains, tenosynovitis, old burns, skin grafts, and following fractures. —But do not use it if there are open sores or lesions on the area to be treated. Those with diabetes, or any tendency to lessened skin sensibility, must use it with caution.

WHAT YOU WILL NEED—2-4 pounds of paraffin wax and 4 tablespoons of mineral oil. Double boiler. Bath towel. Piece of oiled silk. Thermometer.

PARAFFIN BATH

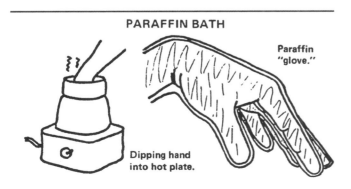

Paraffin "glove."

Dipping hand into hot plate.

Paraffin wax which is used in household preserving can be used. It is best to add some mineral oil to it, so that the solid paraffin is less brittle and melts more easily. The added oil also helps the tissues to be softened, preparatory for later massage. Use 1 pint mineral oil to 5 pounds of paraffin.

HOW TO APPLY IT—(*See picture on this page.*)

[1] THE PARAFFIN BATH

1 - Melt the paraffin in a double boiler or crock pot, and let it cool until a thin film begins to form on top.

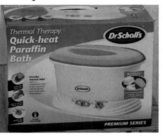
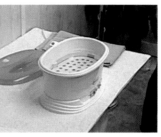

We are using the Dr. Scholl's Paraffin Bath which we found at Walmart

Heat the paraffin just until a small amount of film is left on the surface, to prevent overheating

2 - Examine the skin for open sores, lesions, unhealed scars, and skin infections. Never use the paraffin bath if there are sores, open wounds, etc. Hairy areas on the part to receive the paraffin should previously be clipped, shaved, or oiled. Now wash and dry very carefully the hand (hands, foot, etc.) to be treated. (We will here assume that only one hand is be treated.)

3 - Dip the hand quickly into the paraffin, keeping the fingers separate. If the wrist needs to be coated also (because it also is in pain), the container should be deep enough for this to be done. (Or paint the paraffin with a brush over the parts that cannot be dipped.) If both hands are to be treated, then dip one hand in first, remove and wrap it in plastic while the other hand is being coated. The effect is prolonged by treating the opposite hand also. Instruct him to hold the fingers or toes in a relaxed position without moving - in order to avoid cracks in the paraffin "glove."

4 - Remove the hand until the paraffin hardens; then dip it again. Repeat this (10 times) until a thick glove forms.

5 - When the glove is thick enough, immerse the hand into the paraffin in the pot for 10-15, or up to 30, minutes or longer (or wrap the hand in plastic, towel, and wool fomentation cloth and leave for 15 minutes). Be careful with elderly or weak people. Have a rack in the tank, so their fingers do not touch the bottom. Read all of the directions below in order to learn additional variations.

6 - Leaving the hand in the paraffin bath does

H
Y
D
R
O

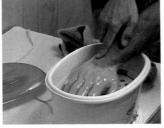

Submerge the hand;
and then raise,
allowing to cool
and harden -
Repeat 10 times
until a glove forms

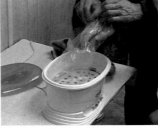

Wrap hand
with plastic bag

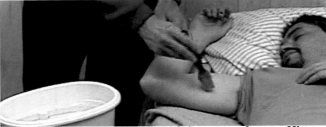

Using a brush, apply 10 layers of paraffin.
Allow to cool between application of layers

[3] HOT PARAFFIN DRESSING

This is similar to the Pack, except that the layers of paraffin are alternated with a gauze bandage. Such dressings are applied to arthritic joints which are acutely inflamed, for they furnish both heat and immobilization. This Dressing may be kept on overnight.

not macerate the skin as might happen if it were left in water for the same amount of time.

7 - When finished, remove the wax by peeling off the "glove," and put the glove back into the pot of paraffin.

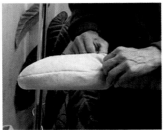

Wrap in mitten,
to maintain
heat longer

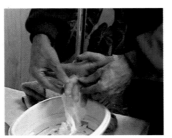

Remove the
paraffin, placing it
back in the bath

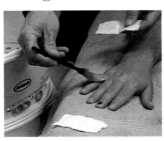

Using a brush, apply
a couple layers
of paraffin directly
to the skin

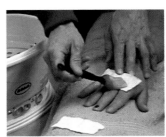

Place a dressing
and begin applying
several layers

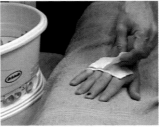

Place a second
bandage and
continue applying
several layers

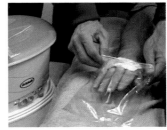

Protect with plastic

[4] HOT PARAFFIN WRAP

This is yet another variation that is especially helpful for sciatica. The paraffin is applied rapidly

8 - Massage and exercise can now be given to the hand; this will help it retain the better blood circulation that it received during the bath. For exercise, squeeze and mold a piece of warm paraffin in the hand.

9 - While the paraffin was on the hand, it absorbed some of the acids in the hand. You can clean this "glove" by placing it in a different pot, if you wish, and then heating it to the boiling point, then removing from the fire. The acids and other wastes quickly boil off. When cold, place the chunk of paraffin back into the regular paraffin pot. When not in use, keep this pot covered at all times.

[2] HOT PARAFFIN PACK

1 - Heat the paraffin in the double boiler (or any double container with water in the lower pot and the paraffin in the upper one). Again, add some oil.

2 - By means of a soft paint brush, about 3 inches wide, the paraffin is applied to the area in successive coats, each of which is allowed to harden enough so that the next one can be put on. Usually about ten coats are sufficient. You have now made a "hot Paraffin Pack" on the afflicted part. It will remain warm for about an hour.

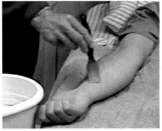

Rapidly apply 10 - 12
coats of paraffin

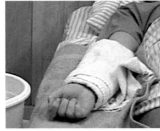

Wrap with plastic
and then a towel

with a brush, 10-12 coats, then covered with oiled silk or wax paper, then a towel or flannel. It may be kept warm with a heat lamp for 10-30 minutes.

5 - KIDNEY STONE PACK

WHAT IT IS—This is a hot application over a painful kidney when sharp pains from a kidney stone are felt.

HOW IT CAN HELP YOU—A Kidney Stone Pack is placed over the painful kidney area at a time of a kidney stone attack (sharp pain from the stone). The pack, renewed as frequently as needed, is kept on for hours until the stone passes or the pain stops.

WHAT YOU WILL NEED—Heating pad. Plastic square or garbage bag. Hot fomentation pack. Towel. Sheet. Blankets. Cold compresses. Radio.

HOW TO APPLY IT—

1 - Spread a half-sheet across the middle of the bed. Over this place a heating pad turned up high, with a plastic square or garbage bag over it. On top of this, place a hot pack *(see Fomentation on page 234)*, with a towel over it. This is a large, very hot fomentation and should be applied quickly while the heat is still almost unbearable. The electric heating pad will keep it hot.

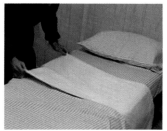

Lay folded sheet on the bed

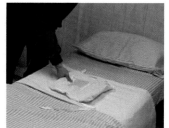

Place heat pad, set it to high, place in center of sheet

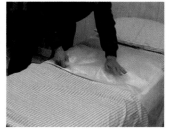

Place plastic sheet over the heat pad and sheet

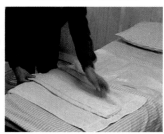

Make a fomentation and lay on the plastic

2 - Position the sufferer on the bed so that his painful kidney is centered over this fomentation. Bring up the sheet on each side and pin it snugly around the body, to help hold the pack in place.

3 - Plug a radio into the same electrical outlet that the heating pad is connected to. Tune the dial to an area of no radio reception, and then turn the volume to high. (If moisture accidentally gets on the electrical

units of the heating pad, the short will cause static on the radio, thus alerting you.)

4 - Keep the head cool with cold compresses.

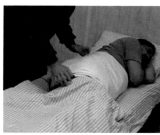

Lay sufferer down; wrap and pin the pack securely

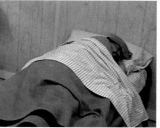

Cover with blankets and use a cold compress to the head

5 - Conclude the application when the stone passes or the pain ceases. Then keep him covered and warm. It is well to let him sleep awhile afterward.

6 - SINUS PACK

WHAT IT IS—This is a combined set of applications applied simultaneously, to reduce sinus pain.

HOW IT CAN HELP YOU—These applications can help relieve the pain of a sinus attack.

WHAT YOU WILL NEED—Fomentation cloths. Two trays of ice cubes. Two small dry towels. Hot foot bath. Hot spinal fomentation.

HOW TO APPLY IT—*(See picture on next page.)*

1 - Put one end of the bed (or treatment table) against the wall. Then place a set of three hot fomentations to the chest (3 minutes hot, with 30 second cold applications between them). There should be no delay between the removal of the hot fomentation and the placement of the cold compress on the chest. Leave it there a full thirty seconds. The third fomentation should remain on the chest throughout the remainder of the treatment.

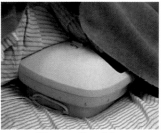

Place feet in hot footbath under the blankets

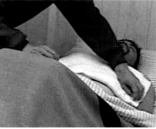

Perform three successive fomentations to the chest, leaving the third in place

2 - Put one tray of ice cubes in a small dry towel; fold it over to a 5" x 10" size. Then make a second ice pack in the same manner.

3 - Place one ice pack under the back of the neck, centered over the lower edge of the skull. Wet the top

HYDRO

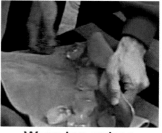

Wrap ice cubes inside two towels

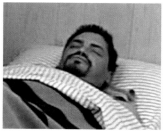

Place one of the ice packs behind the neck

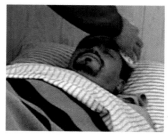

Dampen the forehead

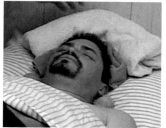

Apply Second ice pack to the head and hold in place with a towel

of the head slightly and then place the second ice pack on the top of the head. Hold the pack in place with a pillow.

4 - Fold a small towel lengthwise; and, holding it in its center edge with one hand, fold the ends down 90° from the central point. *(See picture below.)*

5 - Place it on the face for protection (especially to protect the eyes), leaving the nose exposed through

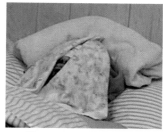

Protect the face with a towel, exposing nose and mouth

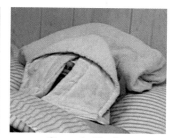

Carefully lay hot femenation over the towel

SINUS PACK

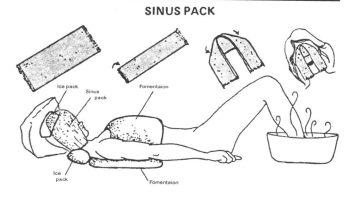

the opening made in the middle *(see picture)*.

6 - Using a single hot fomentation, fold it as the towel was folded, and place it over the towel on the face for exactly three minutes. Then remove both the fomentation and the towel beneath it.

7 - Wring another small towel from ice water and place it on the face over the reddened area. Make this change quickly and leave it on for a full thirty seconds.

8 - End by drying briskly—and then repeat steps 4 through 7 three times. Conclude with a cold mitten friction, beginning with the face. A hot and cold shower can be taken instead of the mitten friction.

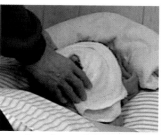

Apply cold, wet towel to the reddened areas for 30 seconds and then dry

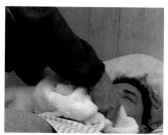

Dry the skin

7 - HEAT LAMP

WHAT IT IS—This is an ordinary incandescent light (or an infrared heat lamp, if you prefer), used as a local hot application. Either way, we will here call it a "heat lamp," but we highly recommend that, in most cases, you use an incandescent and not an infrared lamp (and never an ultraviolet lamp for this purpose). *Do NOT use a sun lamp as a heat lamp!*

HOW IT CAN HELP YOU—Some conditions are best cared for with a heat lamp. An outstanding example is its use in clearing out stuffy, swollen nasal passages. Another example would be earaches. It can also be used for other local heating applications, such as limbs, perineal care, etc.

WHAT YOU WILL NEED—The simplest and least expensive is a shop lamp with a wire screen over it. Screwed into this is a regular incandescent light bulb. Different size wattages may be used for different heating effects; but, normally, a 100-watt bulb will suffice for most purposes. The shop lamp should have a

HEAT LAMP

Wet, folded facial tissue

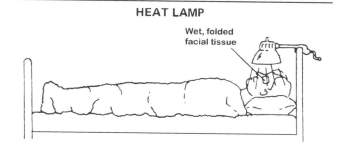

clamp attached to it or should be attached to a clamp. This clamp can then be attached to a bed headboard, chair, or some other bracket above the bed.

An infrared bulb can also be used. But this is more expensive and actually somewhat less useful over an extended period of time, due to its intense heat. (Be very careful to follow the directions on the package.) But in certain situations an infrared lamp can be helpful in the house.

Do NOT use an ultraviolet lamp as a heat lamp! It can cause severe sunburn and permanently damage the eyesight. Ultraviolet rays are powerful; they are intended only for sunbathing purposes in the wintertime. When used (if at all), they should only be turned on for a few moments and at a distance from the body.)

HOW TO APPLY IT—

1 - Firmly set the incandescent heat lamp over the part to be treated. The lamp can be clamped either to the bed headboard or to a temporary arm or bracket.

2 - A folded, wet facial tissue or thin cotton cloth should be laid over the part to be heated with the lamp. If he is laying down in bed, the rest of his body should be covered and kept warm.

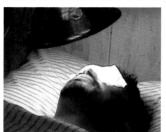 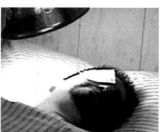

Cover eyes with wet cloth **Rotate the head when applying for earache**

3 - The average timing is 20-30 minutes; but, in certain conditions, such as earache, it might be used for several hours, so that he can obtain rest.

SPECIAL APPLICATIONS—Here are several specialized uses for a heat lamp:

1 - Opening nasal passages - Place a 100-watt (incandescent) shop lamp about 2 inches from the nose. Two small squares of moistened tissue can be placed over the eyes to protect them. The heat wonderfully opens up the stuffed nose and lets it drain. (Be sure that the person is drinking enough water; this alone will open up many stuffed noses!)

2 - Earache - Use a 100-watt regular light bulb. Even children and small babies will lie still as they quickly feel the relief from the pain.

3 - Postpartum perineal care - Following a childbirth, pain from damaged tissue can be relieved during the healing process by occasional use of the lamp. No assistance is needed; it is simple to use. The lamp is also helpful and soothing after a hot sitz bath.

8 - POULTICES
CHARCOAL POULTICE, CLAY AND GLYCERIN POULTICE, CLAY POULTICE, FLAXSEED POULTICE, GARLIC POULTICE, COMFREY AND SMARTWEED POULTICE, HOPS POULTICE, MUSTARD POULTICE, AND CHARCOAL AS A NON-POULTICE

WHAT IT IS—This is a salve of one or several things combined with a little hot water, which is then spread on a damp cloth and placed over an infection which is generally, but not always, on or just below the surface of the skin. *—More poultices on pp. 234.*

HOW IT CAN HELP YOU—Poultices can help in a number of ways in dealing with problems in local, surface portions of the body. Here are some of them: (1) To reduce inflammation. (2) To relieve pain and congestion and act as a counter-irritant. (3) To absorb poison (one of its outstanding advantages!). (4) To adsorb and thus neutralize chemical toxins, insect bites, and stings. (5) To hasten the formation of a head in an abscess or boil. (6) to reduce swelling and tension. (7) To deodorize in the best way: by eliminating the cause of the odor. (8) To help treat wounds. (9) Because of the above help, to act as an effective and safe antiseptic and disinfectant.

WHAT YOU WILL NEED—You will need warm water, a bowl, a spoon, clean muslin sheeting or flannel, wool cloth, piece of plastic, pin or tape, ice or a cold wet cloth. You will also need the ingredients of the salve to be used in this poultice. This may include one or more of the following: charcoal; clay and glycerin; flaxseed; comfrey and smartweed; hops; mustard; garlic.

HOW TO APPLY IT—*(See picture on next page.)*

1 - Assemble everything and prepare the poultice in a warm room.

2 - Several poultice formulas are given below.

3 - Place the salve on a damp cloth; then place that on the area to be treated. Cover with the plastic, and then with the wool cloth over that. Pin or tape it in place. Leave it on overnight.

4 - When removing it, be careful not to spill charcoal, etc., on the floor. Rub the part with ice or with a very cold, wet washcloth. You may wish to renew the poultice with fresh salve and clean cloths.

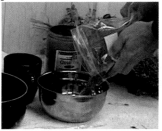 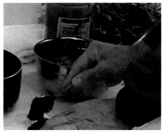

Mix appropriate ingredients **Apply salve (or paste) from your mixture to the cloth**

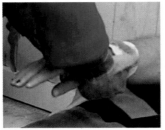

Wrap around the afflicted body part

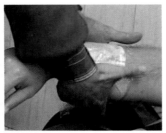

Overlay with plastic wrap

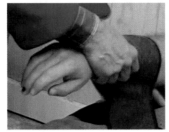

Wrap with wool

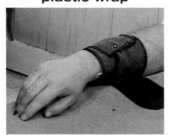

Secure with Safety pin

POULTICE FORMULAS—A number of different mixtures can be prepared for use in poultices. Here are several of the more common ones:

1 - Charcoal Poultice - Charcoal has an amazing absorptive (adsorptive, the experts call it) ability to pull into itself toxins and poisons, thus neutralizing them. This is due to its large chemical surface and the fact that charcoal is pure carbon. The carbon hungrily unites with other substances. Poisons, gases, chemicals, toxins, bee and insect stings and bites—all can be adsorbed by charcoal. Charcoal can also be put in a poultice and placed over the abdomen, in instances of diarrhea and similar intestinal problems (see "Charcoal as a non-poultice," on facing page). Charcoal can adsorb far more than its own weight. A cube that is 2/5 of one inch square can adsorb 33 square yards of poison! Most of the major poisons known to mankind can be adsorbed and thus neutralized by charcoal.

With a spoon in a bowl, mix equal parts of powdered charcoal and ground flaxseed. Add enough hot water to make a paste. Quickly place this salve on a piece of warm, damp cloth before it cools. Spread it to the desired size; and place the cloth on the afflicted area. Follow the remaining directions as described

CHARCOAL POULTICE

CHARCOAL POULTICE

Flax seed   Charcoal   Water   1. Poultice 2. Plastic 3. Wool   arm

above, under "How to Apply It."

2 - Clay and Glycerin Poultice - Dig up some good-quality clay from several inches below the surface. It should be fine and with no pebbles, etc., in it. Heat and sterilize it in the oven at 350° F. Add some water to moisten it again; add several tablespoons glycerin. It is best to use this only once, after which renewing the poultice with a fresh mixture. Clay also absorbs. It is the primary ingredient in mud baths for arthritis.

3 - Clay Poultice - Prepare the clay as described above, but do not mix with glycerin. Cover and keep moist with frequent applications of water (because no glycerin was used as a moisturizer).

4 - Flaxseed Poultice - Obtainable from a health-food store, one tablespoon of flaxseed should be ground up, mixed with a small amount of water, and brought to a boil. This yields enough paste to cover the front of the abdomen. Spread the mixture on a strip of dampened, wrung out, old sheet, or directly on skin. Cover with a larger piece of plastic; hold in place with a 50-60 inch strip of cloth (or an ace bandage, obtainable at the drugstore). Leave it on for 30 minutes or longer (even overnight). Remove it, wash the area with a washcloth, then give a cold mitten friction to it. Shower if necessary. Dry thoroughly.

5 - Garlic Poultice - This is a powerful way to neutralize certain poisons. It can help reduce abscesses, fungus skin infections, eczema, dermatitis, boils, and is used to neutralize the acids in arthritis and similar conditions. Make a pulp of raw garlic and place it on a cloth and then over the affected part. This is not a painless remedy, but the results are usually well-worth the effort.

6 - Comfrey and Smartweed Poultice - Fresh or dried leaves of comfrey and smartweed are whizzed in a blender with a little water and then spread on the area needing attention. Apply as for Flaxseed poultice, above.

7 - Hops Poultice—Using the same methods as for Comfrey and Smartweed Poultice, and Flaxseed Poultice, above, apply the hops poultice. Hops is a plant; the dried, powdered leaves of this are obtainable from your health-food store.

8 - Mustard Plaster—Mix 1 tablespoon dry mustard to 4 tablespoons wheat flour (for a child: 1 to 8; for an infant: 1 to 12). Add enough lukewarm water to make a thin paste that is not runny. Spread it on a cloth that is on a dinner plate. Place one thin cotton cloth over the affected part (use a mustard plaster for arthritic joint pain, backache, and to improve circulation). Put on the poultice; and, over it, place a large piece of plastic and then a towel. A fomentation can be applied over this, to increase the heat. Do not leave the plaster on for more than 20 minutes. Remove it earlier if it is burning or stinging, or the skin has become well-reddened. Wipe the area with a cloth or paper tissue dipped in vegetable oil, to remove all mustard traces! Cover the area with a warm blanket; pin in place and leave on overnight.

CAUTIONS—Certain poultices (especially mustard) can cause blistering. Especially use mustard with caution, and be ready to remove it as soon as needed. A poultice applied after pus develops is sometimes a detriment; for the salve can cause bacterial development. Do not use poultices over active suppuration (pussing). Keep in mind that the heat in the poultice is often as important as the poultice, so keep it warm. In pneumonia, peritonitis, and other deeper inflammations, the poultice should be large enough to cover a surface area as large as the organ being treated. The poultice should be covered with plastic and removed if it becomes cold. A cold poultice or an old poultice do not accomplish much.

CHARCOAL AS A NON-POULTICE—Charcoal can also be used without being placed in a poultice. Here are two of the ways: (1) In case of stomach or small intestinal upset, obtain five (or so) charcoal tablets and a glassful of water. Chew up the first tablet in some of the water and swallow it. Repeat this with the remaining tablets. Include at least 3/4 of a glassful of water—for it is the water that carries the charcoal to the stomach and intestines. (2) In case of diarrhea, drink one tablespoon (or 12 tablets) of charcoal powder to one glass hot water, twice a day. An alternate method is to mix the charcoal in olive oil, and take it 3 times a day. When the stomach or bowels are very tender and irritated, let the charcoal stand in 2 quarts of water and only use the water off the top. This, of course, will not provide as powerful a mixture. See your doctor if the diarrhea is not promptly stopped.

— SECTION SIX —
LOCAL AND LARGER HOT

WHAT IT IS—Hot blankets are wrapped around part of the body in order to impart heat to it. There are several types of Hot Blanket Packs. We will here describe each of the important ones.

"HOT ABDOMINAL PACK"—That which is listed in Kellogg's *Rational Hydrotherapy* as "Hot Abdominal Pack" should read "Wet Girdle." The Wet Girdle (a heating trunk pack) is described on *page 226* of this chapter.

1 - FULL HOT BLANKET PACK

HOW IT CAN HELP YOU—The Hot Blanket Pack is a vigorous sweating measure, and also is very helpful in drawing blood away from congested internal organs. (The congested internal organs are generally the ones beneath where the Hot Blanket Pack is placed.) Any sweating treatment reduces internal congestion, but this application is much more effective when the wet blanket is placed next to the skin. In those

instances in which the congestion is not localized in some particular part, but consists of a general internal congestion, a general sweating treatment is usually sufficient for its relief. And this is especially true in the first stages of many fevers, in colds, gripe, etc.

Thus, the Hot Blanket Pack helps in two ways: (1) induce vigorous sweating, and (2) reduce congestion.

PROBLEMS IT CAN HELP SOLVE—The strong sweating effect of the Hot Blanket Pack is a decided help in uremia, eclampsia, acute Bright's disease, kidney insufficiency and congestion, pneumonia, and sometimes typhoid fever. It is especially helpful for kidney and gallstone pain.

This will help illustrate how hot blanket packs work: When there is congestion and high blood pressure in the kidney, a Hot Blanket Pack laid over it will reduce both of these problems. And with the alleviation of these two conditions, the kidney will soon be able to function again.

WHAT YOU WILL NEED—Two double blankets or one single blanket and one double blanket. Four hot-water bottles half filled with hot water (160° F.). A pail, bowl or wash basin of ice water. Compresses for the head, neck, and heart *(see Cold Compress, page 222)*. Also needed are two Turkish towels, a tumbler, drinking tube, and a pitcher of hot water for drinking.

HOW TO APPLY IT—*(See picture on next page.)*

1 - Give a Hot Foot bath *(page 256)* and have him drink hot water.

2 - Spread a double blanket on a table or bed. Place a Cold Compress *(page 222)* to his head while his feet are still in the Hot Foot bath.

3 - Fold the single blanket (or another double blanket - for holding the heat longer) lengthwise in a convenient width for wringing them (either by hand or through a wringer).

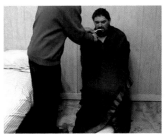
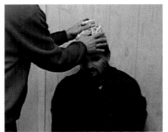

Drink hot water and use hot footbath   **Apply Ice Bag to the head**

4 - Dip the center of the folded blanket in boiling water; and then wring it by twisting. *(See page 235 of "Fomentation" for how to do this.)* Too much water left in the pack will make it feel very hot at first, but it will then cool much more rapidly than if it had been wrung nearly dry. Therefore, wring it as dry as possible. *(For an alternate method, see "Fomentation, Steamer Method" on pages 234-237.)*

5 - Quickly unfold and spread out the moist

blanket over the dry blanket on the table.

6 - Help him to lie on the hot blanket. If he is too weak, you may need to lift him onto it. As quickly as possible (or as rapidly as he can bear it), cover the entire body (except the head) in the hot blanket. The wet blanket should come in contact with the body over its entire surface, so that no air spaces will be left.

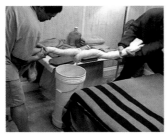
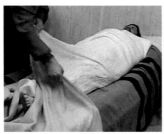

Wring hot water from blanket   **Wrap the body with the hot, wet blanket**

7 - Place a hot-water bottle between the legs with one thickness of dry blanket between it and the moist blanket. Place a second hot-water bottle at the feet. The other two hot-water bottles should be placed along the sides of the trunk. Each one should have the dry flannel between it and the moist flannel. Fomentations *(page 234)* may be used to reinforce the pack instead of hot-water bottles. If used, the fomentations should be changed for fresh ones about every 10 minutes. If there is not enough covering between the hot-water bottles and the skin, there is danger of burns. If he complains, immediately place more covers between the bottles and his body.

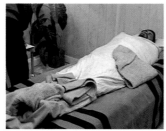
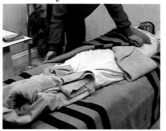

Wrap each of 4 hot water bottles in a towel   **Place a hot water bottle between the legs at the feet and on either side of the trunk of the body**

HOT BLANKET PACK

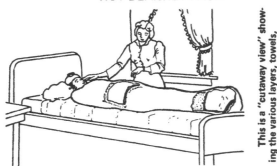

This is a "cutaway view" showing the various layers, towels, fomentations, plastic sheeting and blankets. An ice bag is on his head and a helper is taking the pulse at the temple.

8 - Tuck in the wet blanket well, and then the dry blanket over it. Be sure both are tucked in well about the feet, shoulders, and neck.

9 - Place Cold Compresses *(page 222)* about the head and neck, and use a soft dry towel in order to protect the chin from being touched. Change the compresses to fresh ones before they are warmed very much.

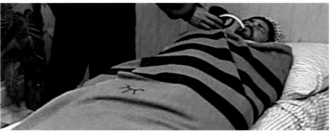

Wrap the body in the dry blanket and give hot water to drink. Wait 20-30 minutes before ending this treatment

10 - (If the pulse becomes too rapid, also place a Cold Compress or an Ice Bag *(page 224)* to the heart.)

11 - General, free perspiration should be induced by the pack. Important: Long-continued heat without perspiration is not good for him. For general sweating purposes, a dry blanket may be placed between him and the wet blanket. But for stronger effects, the wet blanket should be next to the skin.

12 - He should begin perspiring very soon, within 10 minutes. If not, give hot water to drink or a Hot Foot bath, or both. In giving the Hot Foot bath, the blankets should hang down over the legs to keep air from circulating inside.

13 - For sweating effects, continue the pack for 20-30 minutes or until it ceases to have a heating effect. (If only given to tone up the body for tonic effect, the pack should only last 5-10 minutes.)

14 - When finished, remove one part of the blanket at a time and give that body part a Cold Mitten Friction *(pages 249-250)* or a Cold Towel Rub *(pages 250-251)*. Then recover it with a dry blanket or bedding.

15 - Remove the blanket from another body part and repeat the process. Best: Begin with the arms, then chest and abdomen, then legs. Entirely remove the wet blanket and do his back last of all.

CAUTIONS—Be careful that you not burn him with a blanket, initially too hot, next to his skin. Be equally watchful of the hot-water bottles. Give attention to his pulse and apply cold to his heart, if necessary. He must begin perspiring within 10 minutes!

When giving packs to those having paralyzed sensations, are unconscious, or have diabetes or dropsy (edema), it is safer if a thickness of dry blanket intervene between the person and the wet blanket. Hot-water bottles should be more thoroughly covered, and should contain water at a lower temperature.

HYDRO

2 - HOT TRUNK PACK

WHAT IT IS—The Hot Trunk Pack is a Hot Blanket Pack applied only to the trunk of the body, not to the limbs.

HOW IT CAN HELP YOU—Its general effects are similar to those of the Full Hot Blanket Pack, described above. It is especially helpful in digestive disturbances and relieving kidney, bile, and intestinal pain.

HOW TO APPLY IT—

1 - Begin with a Hot Foot bath, both before and during the time that the pack is given.

2 - The hot, wet blanket should cover the body from the arm pits down to the bottom of the pelvis. It should not cover the arms or legs. Under it should be a large dry Fomentation cloth (*see pages 234-237 for details on these cloths*).

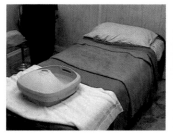

Prepare the bed
with the
hot, wet blanket
and hot footbath

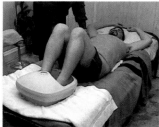

Wrap the body with
the hot, wet blanket
and soak the feet
in the hot footbath

3 - The outside dry blanket should cover the whole body, but this is only to provide the protection of uniform warmth; so it should not be wrapped tightly about the arms and legs.

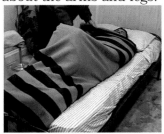

Wrap the body with
the dry blanket -
This can be
done loosely

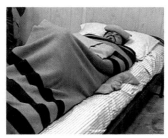

Place a hot water
bottle, wrapped in a
towel, on the stom-
ach and on both
sides of the trunk

4 - Place one hot-water bottle over the abdomen between the folds of the dry blanket. Put two more on either side of the trunk.

5 - The Hot Trunk Pack should last 20-30 minutes, and should normally close with a cold friction treatment. But if the pack is given for the relief of pain, omit the cold friction.

(*For many more details on the giving of Hot Blanket Packs, see Full Hot Blanket Pack, above,* *on page 245.*)

3 - HOT HIP-AND-LEG PACK

WHAT IT IS—This is a Hot Blanket Pack that is applied to a number of problems in the pelvis, legs, and feet. It is also one of the most efficient derivative measures used in water therapy.

HOW IT CAN HELP YOU—Not only is the Hot Hip-and-Leg Pack useful for a number of lower body conditions, but it is extremely helpful in derivation: the application of heat to one area in order to draw blood from a congested area somewhere else. (*For more on "derivation," see pages 213-214.*)

HOW TO APPLY IT—(*See Illustration on facing page.*)

1 - The hot, wet blanket, and the dry blanket over it, should reach from slightly above the top of the hipbone (the crests of the iliac) on down to the full covering of the feet.

2 - One hot-water bottle should be placed at the feet, within the folds of the dry blanket, and another one between the legs.

3 - In order to powerfully increase the derivation effects, place an ice bag over the congested part. The

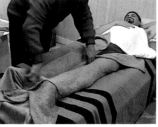

Wrap the legs
and hip with a
hot, wet blanket

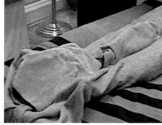

Place a hot water
bottle, wrapped in
a towel, between
the feet and legs

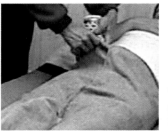

Place ice bag over
the congested part

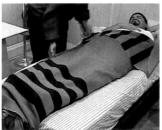

Wrap with
dry blanket

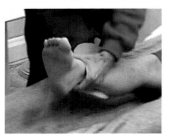

Conclude with a
cold mitten friction

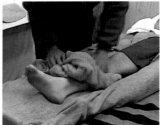

Dry the skin well

pack draws the blood away from this congested part (derivation); and the ice bag drives it away (depletion).

4 - Conclude with a Cold Mitten Friction, applying it to one limb at a time. This will help retain the blood in the legs after the treatment is ended.

(For much more detail on Hot Blanket Packs, see page 245.)

4 - HOT LEG PACK

WHAT IT IS—The Hot Leg Pack includes the feet, legs, and half or more of the thighs.

HOW IT CAN HELP YOU—This pack is given for the same purposes as the Hot Hip-and-Leg Pack, above; yet it is less efficient than the Hot Hip-and-Leg Pack. Why then is it used? It is used when it is undesirable to move the pelvis.

HOW TO APPLY IT—

1 - It is given in the same manner as the Hot Hip-and-Leg Pack, above. You will also want to read about the Full Hot Blanket Pack *(on page 245)* for much more complete details.

2 - Except for the smaller coverage (the hips are not included), the application of the moist blanket, dry blanket, hot-water bottles, and concluding cold friction are all the same.

3 - A large Fomentation *(page 234)* may be used over the front and sides of the pelvis at the same time that the pack is given. In this way, almost as much surface is covered as in the Hot Hip-and-Leg Pack.

5 - HOT PACKS WITH ICE BAGS

WHAT IT IS—This is the most powerful and efficient means of *derivation* known to hydrotherapy. Blood can so concentrate in a state of congestion in a deep organ within the body, that it is difficult to restore a normal flow of blood in and out of that organ. "Derivation" does it by pulling the excess blood away from the congested part.

HOW IT CAN HELP YOU—These packs are especially helpful in reducing internal congestions, reducing or terminating local inflammation of deep parts, and relieving the pain that accompanies the inflammation. For all of these purposes, these packs are used only in the acute stage of the inflammatory process.

PROBLEMS IT CAN HELP SOLVE—The hot pack draws the blood away from the congested area that is choked with an excess of blood. You can call this a "pull effect." The ice bag drives the blood away from the afflicted area by reflexively contracting its deep blood vessels. This is a "push effect." The Cold Mitten Friction (given at the close) causes the extremity, where the packs were placed, to hold the excess blood longer than they otherwise would; this helps the body to maintain the restored organic circulation for a longer period of time.

HOW TO APPLY IT—

1 - This water therapy can be used with any of

the three Hot Blanket Packs, described above *(page 245)*. Simply follow the instructions given under each one while adding the ice bag over the congested area.

2 - Do remember that it is best to use the Hot Packs with Ice Bags only in the acute stage of the infection.

EXAMPLES OF HOW IT CAN BE USED—Here are but a few of the many ways in which Hot Packs with Ice Bags can be employed to reduce inflammation:

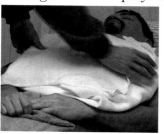

**Begin with
a fomenation**

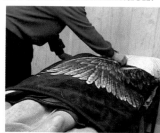

**Cover the upper body
with a blanket**

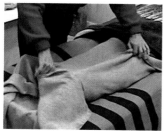

**Wrap the
lower body in
a hot, wet blanket**

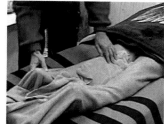

**Place a hot water
bottle, wrapped in
a towel, at the feet
and another
between the legs**

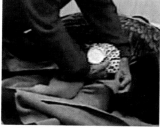

**Place an ice bag,
to create derivation**

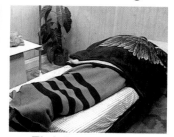

**Finish wrapping
the lower body**

1 - Mastoiditis - Hot Hip-and-leg Pack or a Full Blanket Pack and Ice Cravat *(page 223)* or Ice Bag *(page 170)* over the carotid artery (slightly to the right and above each ear), plus Ice Cap *(page 224)* to the head and Fomentations *(page 234)* to the mastoid (just below the ear).

2 - Alveolar Abscess - Same treatment as for Mastoiditis, except that you give a Fomentation to the jaw.

3 - Kidney Congestion - Hot Trunk Pack or Full Blanket Pack and Ice Bag to lower third of sternum.

4 - Peritonitis - Hot Hip-and-leg Pack, leg Pack only, ice compress *(see Ice Pack, 223)* or Ice Cap *(224)* to abdomen. See a physician!

5 - Appendicitis - Hot Hip-and-leg Pack and Ice Bag to the appendix region. See a physician!

6 - Puerperal Infections and Acute Salpingitis - Full Hot Blanket Pack or Hip-and-leg Pack and ice to pelvis (over pubic area).

— SECTION SEVEN —
TONIC FRICTIONS

WHAT THEY ARE—These are applications of cold water that are given with friction (vigorous rubbing of the body) in order to increase body circulation and heat. From the mildest to the most vigorous, these applications are: (1) the Wet-hand Rub, (2) the Cold Mitten Friction, (3) the Cold-towel Rub, (4) the Wet-sheet Rub, (5) the Dripping-sheet Rub, and (6) the Ice Rub. In addition to this, the Salt Glow is often used on those who have a difficult time reacting well to the Cold Mitten Friction.

One or more of the first four frictions, listed above, are often given in an advancing pattern, aimed at building up the body. When the person is able to react with sufficient heat to one tonic measure, one may wish to begin treatments with the next one that is more severe.

HOW THEY CAN HELP YOU—Each of these water treatments can produce a vigorous stimulation of the whole body, depending upon: (1) which tonic friction is used, (2) the amount of "vigor" put into it as you give it, and (3) the body's general reaction to the vigorous cold rub. With this in mind, these tonic frictions can provide a wholesome and vigorous circulation. They stimulate blood-vessel activity and circulation, heighten muscular tone and activity, increase nerve tone and sensibility. They also stimulate muscular, glandular, and metabolic activities of internal organs. And they increase heat production and oxidation, increase phagocytosis and bactericidal antibody production in infectious fevers, and increase oxidation and elimination of bacterial toxins in infectious fevers.

But, more commonly, they are used to build up general body resistance, improve sluggish circulation, overcome generalized weakness, lack of endurance, low blood pressure, and strengthen one who has frequent colds.

WHAT YOU WILL NEED—The items needed for all of the tonic frictions are simple enough; depending on the treatment given, it will require several of the following:

A wash basin or small tub of water. 1-3 pails. Cold water or ice water for a more vigorous effect. Possibly ice, snow, or salt. 1-3 sheets. 1-2 small washcloths or one or two "friction mitts" made of rough Turkish toweling. (If done frequently, the mitts are well-worth sewing together; for they are so much easier to use than hand-held washcloths.) Plastic sheeting and towels for the bed and bedding, if the friction is given to one who is in bed. A warm, dry towel to dry him

with afterward.

Here are the seven types of tonic frictions:

1 - WET-HAND RUB

WHAT IT IS—This is the mildest of the frictions and is only given to those who are too weak or infirm for a more vigorous tonic friction.

HOW TO APPLY IT—

1 - The Wet-hand Rub should be given in the same order and manner as the Cold Mitten Friction (explained just below), with the following exceptions:

2 - The Body should only be rubbed with a wet hand, dipped several times in cold water. Only one part is exposed for rubbing at a time; it is rubbed, then dried, then briskly rubbed with the dry towel and with the hands.

2 - COLD MITTEN FRICTION

WHAT IT IS—This is the most commonly used tonic friction, and is applied with a washcloth or two friction mitts, rubbed on the skin.

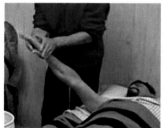 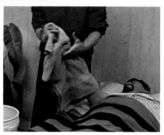

Dip hands in cold water and rub vigorously   **Follow up by drying thoroughly**

WHAT YOU WILL NEED—Pail or wash bowl of ice water at 50°-60° F. A sheet and three Turkish towels. Two friction mitts or two washcloths. Compresses (wet cloths) for the head and neck, if he is ill or infirm. Protective bed coverings, such as plastic sheeting is laid down (or special blankets that will later be dried out).

How to make your own friction mitts: The Cold Mitten Friction is such an invaluable help, to be used so frequently, that you will want to make your own

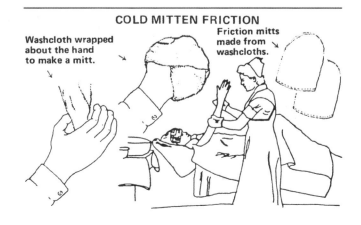

COLD MITTEN FRICTION

Washcloth wrapped about the hand to make a mitt.

Friction mitts made from washcloths.

mitts, since they are so much easier to work with then a hand-held washcloth. Have someone handy with a sewing machine make you some mittens out of rough (Turkish-type) toweling material. Simply cut apart an old pair of mittens and use it for a pattern.

HOW TO APPLY IT—*(See picture on page 249.)*

1 - The room should be warm and without drafts. If he is ill, first bathe his face and neck with cold water, or apply cold cloths to the head and neck. If he has valvular heart disease, place an ice bag over the heart before beginning the tonic friction. (If the person is feeling better, the friction can be given to him as he stands. Many people give it to themselves each morning.)

2 - Wring the washcloths or mitts from cold water, so that they are as dry as possible. Then begin quickly rubbing, drying, re-dipping, wringing, etc. Here is the order to follow:

[1] **Arm and forearm:** Rub vigorously until the skin is pink. This should require only a few seconds. Then dry them thoroughly and cover them well.

[2] **The other arm and forearm:** Dip and wring the cloths and do the other arm and forearm; dry thoroughly and cover with bedcovers.

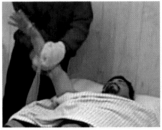 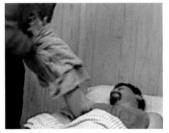

Use cold, wet friction mittens and rub arm vigorously   **Follow up each application by drying thoroughly**

[3] **Chest:** Repeat the dipping, wringing, rubbing, drying, and covering.

[4] **Trunk, thighs, and then legs.**

(When giving the treatment to a person with heart disease, some prefer to begin with the chest instead of the arms.)

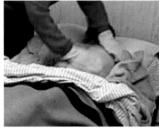 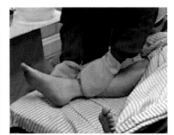

Freshly wring cold water from mittens and rub the chest vigorously   **Freshly wring cold water from them again and rub each leg vigorously**

3 - The entire tonic rub must be given rapidly,

especially during the time that the part is bared and the cloth or mitten is in contact with the skin.

ADDITIONAL POINTS—The severity and tonic effect can be varied by the temperature of the water, frequency of dipping, amount of water left in the cloth after wringing, and the vigor with which the skin is rubbed.

3 - COLD TOWEL RUB

WHAT IT IS—This is the third most vigorous friction; but is not used as often as the Cold Mitten Friction (described above) or the wet-sheet rub (described below), or the Salt Glow *(page 252).*

HOW TO APPLY IT—*(See picture below.)*

Give the Cold Towel Rub in the same manner as the Cold Mitten Friction, described just above, with the exception that a plain hand towel is used instead of the washcloth or mitts.

4 - WET-SHEET RUB

WHAT IT IS—This is a vigorous tonic that, used in a continuing buildup with the other frictions, will help improve one's overall health.

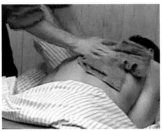 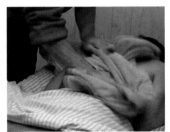

Wring towel in ice water and then rub his back vigorously   **Follow up each application by drying thoroughly**

WHAT YOU WILL NEED—Three sheets. Foot tub of hot water at 105° F. Pail of water at 60°-70° F. Two compress cloths (light hand towels). Pail of ice water. Turkish towel.

HOW TO APPLY IT—*(See picture on next page.)*

1 - The room should be warm, without drafts. The one receiving the Wet-sheet Rub should come to the room with a good circulation and feeling warm.

COLD TOWEL RUB / DRIPPING SHEET RUB

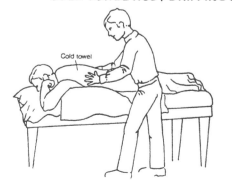 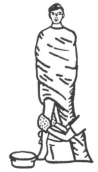

Cold towel

Otherwise the treatment should not be given.

2 - He should stand in the foot tub of hot water, and a cold compress should be put on his head and neck.

3 - Lightly wring a sheet out of the cold water (60°-70° F.) and quickly wrap it about him in the following manner: As he holds up both arms (or someone holds them up for him), the upper left-hand corner of the sheet is placed under his right arm. He then lowers the right arm, thus holding the sheet in place.

4 - Pass the sheet quickly across the front of his body and then under his right arm. He then lowers his right arm, thus holding the sheet in place.

5 - Pass the sheet quickly across the front of his body and under his left arm, which is then lowered to hold it.

6 - The sheet is carried across his back (behind him) and then up and over his right shoulder. From there it goes across his chest, around his neck, and over his left shoulder. The corner is then tucked under the edge of the sheet toward the back.

7 - Then tuck the sheet between his legs, thus bringing the wet sheet in close contact with every part of his body.

8 - Rub vigorously and give percussion (slight slapping) over the sheet. But note: Do not rub him with the sheet, but over the sheet. Work quickly, covering the whole surface as quickly as possible.

9 - The sheet should quickly become warm. When the treatment is finished, follow it by drying him thoroughly with a dry sheet and towels.

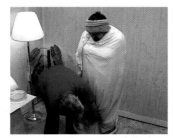

Apply a cold compress and wrap the body in a cold, wet sheet while standing in a bathtub or bucket

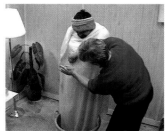

Do not rub with the sheet; but rub over the sheet and also pat your hand against the sheet

SPECIAL POINTS—He must be warm before it begins, and should previously have shown a good ability to react to cold towel rubs, pail pours, or cold percussion sprays. Do not expose him anymore than necessary, but work quickly to avoid chilling him. If he does not obtain a decidedly warm reaction, and soon, the value of the treatment is lost. Two helpers are needed to give the best results in Wet-sheet Rubs.

5 - DRIPPING SHEET RUB

WHAT IT IS—This is a Wet-sheet Rub, with the addition of a second and third pail pour.

WHAT YOU WILL NEED—3 pails of cold water (70°, 65°, and 60° F. respectively) in addition to what you would use for a Wet-sheet Rub (*page 250*),

HOW TO APPLY IT—

1 - Follow the same procedure as with the Wet-sheet Rub, described just above, but with the following exceptions:

2 - Use the water from the 70° F. pail, to wring the sheet from. Give the Wet-sheet Rub treatment (as explained above), but after he and the sheet are warmed by rubbing and percussion. Without removing the sheet, pour the second pail of water (65°) over his shoulders and, again, rub vigorously until he is warm. Then pour the coldest pail (60°) of water over him; and, again, rub till warm.

3 - Conclude with the usual drying.

SPECIAL POINTS—Obviously, this and the next friction are the most severe; so, when given as a tonic measure, they should only be given to those who have shown themselves able to react with sufficient heat in response to milder cold friction treatments. (Do understand that the Dripping Sheet Rub is as strong a tonic as you will normally give. The Ice Rub, below, is generally used, to bring down fevers, not as a tonic treatment.)

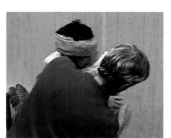

Wrap in a cold, wet sheet and pad; and rub over the sheet

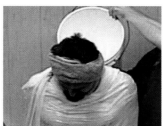

Pour 70 degree water over the person and sheet; and then continue padding and rubbing

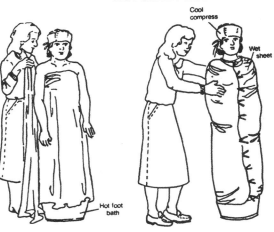

WET SHEET RUB

HYDRO

6 - ICE RUB

WHAT IT IS—This is a rub that uses a piece of ice instead of a wet hand or cold mitten.

HOW IT CAN HELP YOU—The Ice Rub is not used very often for general tonic purposes. Its value lies in its powerful fever-reducing ability. When given to lower a fever, each part should be rubbed for some time and then dried without friction or percussion with the hands. Its prolonged application to the spine is more powerfully antipyretic (fever reducing) than the same length of ice rub elsewhere on the body.

HOW TO APPLY IT—

The Ice Rub is given in about the same manner as the Wet-hand Rub *(page 249)* and Cold Mitten Friction *(pages 249-250)*. But the Ice Rub will require much more careful covering of the bedding with plastic and towels. Tuck Turkish towels about each part, so that the water will be absorbed as it runs off the skin. The cake of ice may be held in the hand, but it is better if wrapped in a thickness or two of gauze.

CAUTIONS—Cold compresses (hand towels wrung out from cold water) should be applied to the head and the neck, and also to the heart, if necessary. In cases of typhoid fever, do not apply the cold treatment to the abdomen.

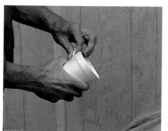

Freeze water in a styrofoam cup, then peel back enough to expose the ice

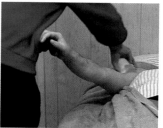

Rub the ice around - keep it moving

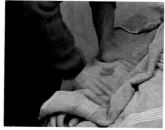

Dry thoroughly

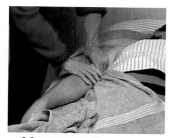

Massage the area

7 - SALT GLOW

WHAT IT IS—This is a tonic friction that has the same general mildness as a Cold Mitten Friction in its effect,—but less body heat reaction is needed to favorably respond to it.

The Cold Mitten Friction is somewhat easier to use and is most often used. But for those who have a difficult time reacting to cold, the Salt Glow is ideal.

HOW IT CAN HELP YOU—Since no great amount of cold water is applied to the body, the Salt Glow does not require as much ability to react to cold. This is what makes it so helpful. It is useful in building up general body resistance, improving sluggish circulation, low blood pressure. And it helps those with generalized weakness, low endurance, and frequent colds.

WHAT YOU WILL NEED—Two pounds of salt (best if it is coarse salt). Foot tub of water at 105° F. Two Turkish Towel Washclothes. Shower cap. One sheet.

HOW TO APPLY IT—*(See picture below.)*

1 - Make sure the room is definitely warm, without drafts.

Moisten the salt with cold water. (Moisten it just enough that it will cling to the skin when applied. If it is too wet, it will not produce the needed friction. This is important; so test it out on your own arm ahead of time, so you will know how moist to make it.)

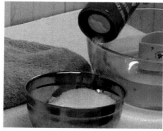

Add sea salt   **Mix with water**

2 - The one receiving the Salt Glow can stand or sit on a stool. Either way, his feet should be in a tub of hot water.

3 - Standing by his side, do each body part separately. Wet the entire skin surface of the shoulder, arm, and hand with hot water from the foot tub. Next apply some of the wet salt, spreading it evenly over the skin. With one hand holding the arm, rub with back-and-forth motions until the skin is in a glow. Use less friction if his skin is sensitive.

4 - Do the next body part, in this order: right arm, left arm, right leg, left leg, front and back of trunk (both done at once), sides of trunk and hips, front and back of hips (he must stand while his hips are done).

5 - Conclude with a shower or a dip in the bathtub to thoroughly wash off the salt. Then dry him with Turkish towels, rubbing briskly.

SALT GLOW

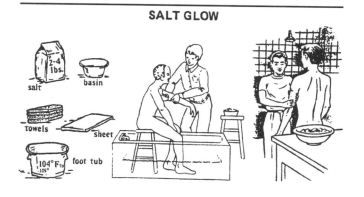

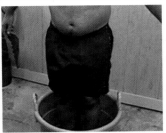
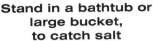

Stand in a bathtub or large bucket, to catch salt

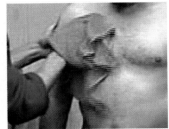

Wring cloth in salt-water solution and rub the skin

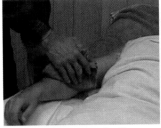

Rub wet cloth thoroughly over both arms

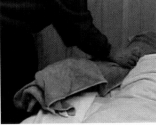

Dry the limbs afterward

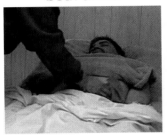

Rub the chest and then the stomach. Then dry them

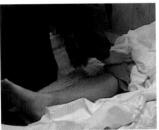

Sponge bathe both legs. Then dry them

— SECTION EIGHT —
SPONGING

FEVER SPONGES

HOT SPONGE
COLD SPONGE
TEPID SPONGE
NEUTRAL SPONGE

WHAT IT IS—Sponging a person when in fever is an old-time remedial help that has been forgotten by many in our modern generation. For this purpose, a wet washcloth is normally used instead of a "sponge."

HOW IT CAN HELP YOU—Sponging greatly helps to reduce fevers; we all know how dangerous they can be if body temperature goes too high. It is important to keep in mind that a person with a fever may (1) have a hot, dry skin (because his body is not giving off heat as rapidly as it is being produced) or (2) he may have cold, clammy skin (because his temperature-regulating mechanism is not working properly, due to the infection). The sponging will be different for hot, dry skin than it will be for cold, clammy skin. And always remember: When in a fever, a person needs water to drink. As in burning buildings, water helps put out the fire.

WHAT YOU WILL NEED—You will need a blanket or extra sheet, a basin of water, two or three Turkish (rough) towels, one or two washcoths (or a soft sea sponge), a hot-water bottle, and a bath thermometer.

HOW TO APPLY IT—(*See picture on this page.*)

1 - Cover him with a cotton blanket instead of the regular bedcovers (so they will not become wet). Protect the bed with towels as each part is sponged.

2 - Sponge one part at a time, in this order: arms, chest, abdomen, legs, feet, and finally the back.

3 - Sponge each part with no rubbing or friction. (The water left on the skin will evaporate, taking heat from the fevered body.)

4 - When you have completed sponging each part, cover it with a dry towel and dry it lightly. The skin may be left slightly moist, unless he shows a tendency to chill. Be sure he is dry before his bedclothes are put on again.

5 - Be certain that there are no drafts in the room during or after the sponging; and watch for a tendency for him to chill.

6 - A hot-water bottle may be placed at his feet afterward if he is likely to chill easily. Take his temperature about 30 minutes later.

FOUR TYPES OF SPONGES—Here are the four basic types of fever sponges:

Hot Sponge - The water should be as hot as he can tolerate. The Hot Sponge relaxes and helps one go to sleep. But it is primarily used to reduce fever in those instances in which chilliness exists. And if he is chilling, also give him a Hot Foot bath (*page 256*) or Fomentations (*page 234*) in order to help him perspire and increase the blood supply to the skin.

When the Hot Sponge is continued for 40-45 minutes, his temperature will not rise as rapidly afterward, as it would have done after a Cold Sponge. When giving any sponge, always do it in the following order: arms, chest, abdomen, legs, thighs, back. Bare one part at a time; then dry thoroughly and cover before doing the next. For the Hot Sponge, the cloth should be dipped several times for each part.

SPONGE

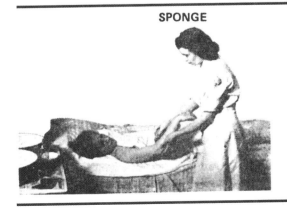

Cold Sponge (70°-80° F.) - This is the sponging temperature most frequently used when the skin is hot and dry and there is no tendency to chilliness. Each part should be gone over several times and/or the entire process can be repeated until the desired effect is obtained. The temperature of the water and the duration of the treatment will determine the results.

A cold compress or washcloth may be placed on the forehead or in the armpit. Friction (rubbing) is used to bring blood to the surface, to increase the rate of circulation, and to hasten the cooling process.

Tepid Sponge (80°-92° F.) and Neutral Sponge (94°-98° F.) - Both of these are given to rest, relax, and help him to go to sleep. The effects are those of the Neutral Bath (see page 259). Sometimes these two sponges are used to reduce fever, but they are not very effective for that purpose. Their primary value lies in bringing relaxation to one who is unable to go to sleep.

As you apply either of these two sponges, dry the skin gently, with as little rubbing as possible. To cool him, the treatment may be prolonged to allow for more evaporation. Then, quietly cover and let him go to sleep.

THE WATER THERAPIES

— PART TWO —
DIRECT WATER APPLICATIONS
— SECTION NINE —
PAIL POURS

WHAT IT IS—This is the pouring of water from a pail over part of the body or all of it. Quick and relatively easy to do, the Pail Pour is often used with other water therapies, often to conclude them.

HOW IT CAN HELP YOU—The Pail Pour (today termed "affusions" by the professionals) can produce an effect unequaled by that of any other water therapy. It is a flow of a considerable amount of water over part or all of the body; no other application has exactly this effect. Also, it is easily used in any home.

1 - GENERAL PAIL POUR

WHAT IT IS—This is a Pail Pour to the entire body.
HOW IT CAN HELP YOU—The General Pail Pour is normally used as a tonic measure, to strengthen the body. For this purpose, over a period of time, these pail pours may be given at gradually lowered water temperatures.

HOW TO APPLY IT—(See picture on this page.)
1 - This may follow or conclude another water therapy, or it may be the entire treatment. If is often used after a Full Bath (page 259), Salt Glow (page

252), etc. See the Tonic Frictions for more information on many of these tonic applications (pages 249-253).

2 - He should be warm beforehand. If given in a bathtub, he may sit or stand. If standing, his feet should be in a tub of hot water. Either way, a Cold Compress (page 222) should be placed on his head.

3 - Prepare three pails of water, each at a different temperature, according to the effect you wish to obtain.

4 - For the first pour, use pails of water at 100°, 90°, and 85,° or 80° F. respectively. This will provide a mild tonic effect. (If he has just come from a warm bath, a lower temperature may be used for each of the three pails or only two pails may be used.)

5 - In succeeding pail pours, lower the temperature of the pails until the third pail is 50°-60° F.

6 - Each time, after the last pail is poured, rub him vigorously, and dry him well with a sheet and towels.

2 - LOCAL PAIL POURS INCLUDING
LOCAL HOT POUR
LOCAL NEUTRAL POUR
LOCAL COLD POUR
LOCAL ALTERNATE HOT AND COLD POUR
SPECIAL APPLICATIONS

WHAT IT IS—These are "water pours" upon only part of the body.

HOW IT CAN HELP YOU—These are simple, brief water applications that are used in a number of situations. Primary among these is (1) a cold pail pour to the hips, after a hot half (shallow) bath, and after a Hot Sitz Bath (page 258). In both instances, this pail pour is given to balance the circulation in the pelvis, which could afterward become chilled. (2) Smaller or larger pours to local body areas for specific physical problems. These special applications are discussed just below.

PAIL POUR

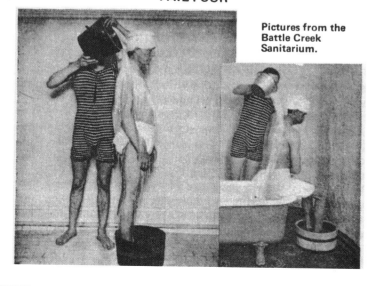

Pictures from the Battle Creek Sanitarium.

HOW TO APPLY IT—*(See pictures below.)* (In giving local pours, the water should fall a distance of at least 3-4 inches, on up to 1-2 feet, before it strikes the body part. The condition of the part and the effect desired will determine this distance.)

Local Hot Pour—Relieves pain, wherever applied. Because the hot is so quickly given, the prompt after-effect is tonic and strengthening.

Local Neutral Pour—This is relaxing; and, especially when applied to the spine, it helps relax nerves and induce sound sleep.

Local Cold Pour—If very brief, it is stimulating and tonic in effect; but, if prolonged, it reduces congestion and inflammation, and encourages white-blood cell activity in overcoming disease. A long, cold pour to the head is strongly fever-reducing.

Local Alternate Hot and Cold Pour—This is a powerful tonic and stimulant. It produces fluxion (an increase of blood) in the part treated and derivation (drawing of blood) from other parts. It also increases white-blood cell activity. Thus, it is very helpful in treating an infected body part, when it is impossible or impractical to immerse the part in water (as with boils or carbuncles about the trunk or thighs).

PAIL POUR - SPECIAL

SPECIAL APPLICATIONS—Here are several special uses for these localized water pours: 1 - Local Pour to the Arm, Hand, Foot, etc.: Hold the body part over a small tub while the water is poured from a pail or large container. 2 - Local Pour to the Spine: Let him sit on the edge of a bathtub or on a stool in the bathtub. Then pour the water over the affected part. 3 - Local Pour to the Head: He should lie down on a bed or table, with his head resting over the end and a tub underneath. You may want to place a hand beneath his head to help support it.

— SECTION TEN —
PARTIAL BATHS

1 - CONTRAST BATHS
CONTRAST BATH TO THE HAND OR ARM, CONTRAST BATH TO THE FEET, CONTRAST BATH TO THE LEGS

SPECIAL APPLICATIONS—

WHAT IT IS—This is the immersion of the hand, arm and hand, foot, or leg and foot into a basin or tub of water. It is both simple and effective.

HOW IT CAN HELP YOU—A Contrast Bath (also known as Alternate Hot and Cold) is an alternating plunge of part of the body into hot water, then into cold, and back again. This results in a powerful alternate contraction, then dilatation of the blood vessels, and a general improvement of body circulation. For the particular body area being treated, it removes waste products and greatly improves rapidity of blood flow. And the quantity of fresh oxygen, nutriments,

and white and red blood cells is also increased.

Contrast Baths to the hands, feet, arms, or legs are very helpful for fractures, arthritis (both rheumatoid and osteoarthritis), congestive headaches, edema, sprains, strains, trauma (after 24 hours), infections, lymphangitis (2-3 times a day), impaired venous circulation, and indolent ulcers.

WHAT YOU WILL NEED—For a contrast bath, you will need two containers, large enough for the water in them to come up over the extremities to be treated. If necessary, thoroughly cleaned buckets can be used. Medical personnel recommend that an antiseptic be placed in the water if there are open wounds. You will also need a bath thermometer and a bath towel. You may also need a pitcher, to add more hot water from time to time, and ice cubes for the cold water bucket. Sometimes a cold compress (hand towel wrung from

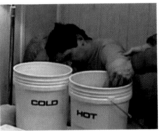

Use hot water between 105-110 degrees and soak 3-4 minutes

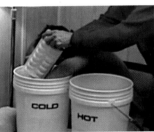

Use ice cold water and soak 30-60 seconds

cold water) or ice bag is also needed.

HOW TO APPLY IT—*(See pictures below.)*

1 - Place the limb in the hot water (105°-110° F.) for 3-4 minutes. Then put it into the cold (cold tap water or ice water) for one-half to one minute.

2 - Begin with the hot water and end with the cold. Change from one temperature to the other 6-8 times (3-4 complete cycles). Time spans are generally 3-4

CONTRAST BATHS

minutes in the hot and, then, one-half to one minute in the cold. Begin hot immersion at lower temperature limits, increasing the temperature as you continue on through the treatment. Add hot water by pouring it over your own hand; add it while the limb is in the cold water. A cold compress (hand towel wrung out of cold water) or ice bag may be needed on the head or back of neck, if a large part of the body is being treated and always if he feels faint. Place an ice bag to the heart if his pulse is over 80 beats per minute. (In serious cases, it is best to check his pulse every 5 minutes during treatment.)

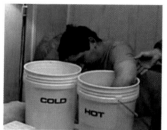 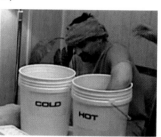

Alternate back and forth 3-4 times. Always end on cold   **Apply cold compress to the forehead**

3 - End by drying the limb thoroughly. Have him rest afterward for a half hour.

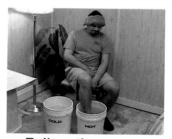 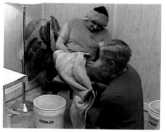

Follow the same procedure for the legs   **Dry the limbs when finished**

ADDITIONAL POINTS—Do not normally use hot water temperatures above 110° F.; in blood vessel disease of the legs and feet, do not go over 105° F. Extremes of hot and cold should not be used in diabetes or in peripheral vascular disease. When working with rheumatoid arthritis, end with the hot instead of the cold.

THREE SPECIAL CONTRAST BATHS—Here are three special Contrast Baths which may prove to be of help to you:

Contrast Bath to the Hand or Arm—Two very deep pails may be used. Use the procedure described above. The hot water should be as hot as can be borne. This bath is very helpful for blood poisoning in an infected arm or hand. It is also of value in controlling nosebleed.

Contrast Bath to the Feet—This bath, consisting of alternate hot and cold to the feet (using two tubs),

is especially helpful in congestive headache, in which case it is well to apply a cold compress to the head (or head and neck) at the same time. It is also used in treating infections of the foot, Charcot's joint at the ankle, tuberculosis of the ankle, bones of the foot, and in gangrene (to hasten the formation of the line of demarcation).

Contrast Bath to the Legs—This is an alternate hot and cold leg bath, and requires two tubs deep enough to immerse the legs to the knees, or deeper. (Galvanized garbage cans, thoroughly cleaned, can be used.) Cold head and neck compresses will be needed, and perhaps an ice bag over the heart. 2-3 minutes in the hot followed by 20-30 seconds in the cold, for 5-30 minutes. (When used for varicose ulcer, the hot should only be one minute in length, or the ulcer will become worse!) This contrast bath is especially useful in treating edema of the legs. After 2-3 treatments, pieces of ice may be added to the cold water. The treatment may be concluded with heavy friction to the feet and legs.

FIVE SPECIAL APPLICATIONS FOR CONTRAST BATHS—Here is information you may be able to use:

1 - Arthritis (osteoarthritis) - Begin with a temperature of 110° F.; then, after four minutes, change to tap water for one minute. Change back and forth 4-6 times, and end with the hot water. The hot water should gradually be raised to 115°-120° F., and the tap water gradually lowered to that of ice water. Give this treatment once or twice a day.

2 - Infections and cellulitis - The contrast of (difference between) the hot and cold should be as great as can be tolerated. Begin with 110° F. and increase temperature to tolerance. One can usually start with ice water. End with ice water. Change 5 to 6 times. Give 2-3 times daily.

3 - Poor circulation caused by blood vessel disease - Begin with a temperature of 105° F. for 3 minutes; change to cold for one-half minute.

4 - Sprained ankle - Use hot water at 110° F. and ice water for the cold application. End with ice water. (Note that an alternation of hot and cold is here used. When cold water alone is used, both the pain and recovery time is lengthened.)

5 - Weak, pronated feet - Use the same treatment as for arthritis.

2 - HOT Foot bath

WHAT IT IS—This is not a contrast bath for the feet, as described in the previous therapy ("Contrast Baths"); it is a continuous bath in hot water.

HOW IT CAN HELP YOU—When the feet are placed in hot water, the excess blood which is congesting other parts of the body is brought to the legs and feet. This helps the entire blood circulation in the body and relieves congestion in the brain, lungs, abdominal, and pelvic organs. The blood is shifted from one

HYDRO

part of the body to another; the entire body is helped.

The Hot footbath also helps to ward off infection and sickness in cold weather, when one is beginning to catch a cold, sore throat, etc. The body has become chilled, and a hot footbath warms the entire body and stimulates the circulation.

Lastly, when an individual is nervously fatigued, the feet are generally cold and the blood circulation is poor and unequal. A hot foot bath will relieve the nervous tension, lessen congestion in the brain, and balance the circulation.

Thus, the Hot Footbath can prevent or shorten colds, relieve headaches, stimulate the circulation when the feet are cold, relieve pelvic cramps, relieve chest and pelvic congestion, stop nosebleed, aid relaxation, and prepare one for a cold water treatment (such as a cold shower, etc.).

WHAT YOU WILL NEED—A foot tub or similar container large enough and deep enough—such as a five-gallon can, large mouthed bucket, or deep dishpan. Thermometer to test the water or test it with your elbow (103°-110° F.). Bath towel. Teakettle or pan for boiling water. Basin of cold water. Pitcher or dipper to add hot water. Two blankets to wrap about him. Cold compress (hand towel wrung out of cold water), if needed for the neck. Floor or bedding protection (rubber sheeting, plastic, or newspaper).

HOW TO APPLY IT—(*See picture on next page.*)

1 - The room should be warm with no drafts. Place the plastic, with towel over it, on the floor under the feet. Fill the foot tub with water (about 104° F.), so that the ankles are fully covered. Test with the thermometer or your elbow.

2 - Instruct him beforehand as to what you are going to do. Place his feet in the tub and cover him with the blanket. (If he is sitting up, wrap him well.) If he is lying down, do not let the calf of his leg touch the foot tub.

3 - Slowly add hot water, to increase the temperature up to 112° or 115° F. Pour the water against the inside of the tub with your hand between the flowing water and his feet, stirring the water as it is added.

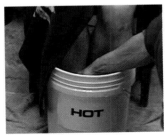 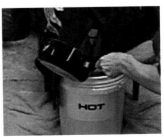

Begin treatment with water at 104 degrees F.   **Slowly add hot water (Increases temperature)**

4 - Continue the bath for 10-30 minutes, depend-

ing on the effect desired. Keep his head cool with a cold compress. A cold head compress is especially important if the foot bath is continued for any length of time, if he is in a sitting position, and always if there is a tendency to faintness.

5 - When the feet are removed from the hot water, pour a dash of cold water over them quickly. This cold water should come in contact with both the dorsal (side) and plantar (bottom) surfaces of the feet. In some cases, the cold water is omitted.

6 - Quickly place the feet on the towel and remove the foot tub. Dry the feet well, especially between the toes. If he is perspiring, dry him thoroughly with a towel.

CAUTION—Do not give a Hot Foot bath to one who has hardening of the arteries of the feet or if there is a loss of skin sensation (no sense of feeling) in the feet.

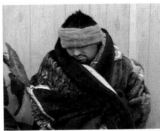 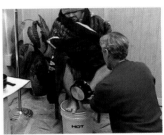

Use a cold compress to the head   **Conclude by pouring cold water on the feet, and then dry thoroughly**

3 - (SHALLOW) COLD Footbath

WHAT IT IS—This is a footbath in a tub of shallow cold water.

HOW IT CAN HELP YOU—The shallow Cold Footbath causes reflex contraction of the blood vessels of the brain, pelvic organs, and liver. It also contracts the muscles of the uterus, bladder, stomach, and intestines.

HOW TO APPLY IT—

1 - This foot bath is given in practically the same way, with the same equipment, as for the Hot Footbath.

2 - The water should only be about 2-4 inches deep; its temperature should be about 45°-60° F.

3 - Everything should be ready beforehand. His feet should be previously warmed. During the bath the feet should be rubbed with the hands or one foot against the other.

4 - The bath should last from 1-5 minutes. When completed, dry the feet well, and make sure that they are warm afterward.

CAUTION—The Cold Footbath should not be given during the menstrual period or in case of acute pulmonary, abdominal, or pelvic inflammation.

4 - SITZ BATHS
COLD SITZ BATH
COLD RUBBING SITZ BATH
PROLONGED COLD SITZ BATH
NEUTRAL SITZ BATH
VERY HOT SITZ BATH
REVULSIVE SITZ BATH
ALTERNATE HOT AND COLD SITZ BATH

WHAT IT IS—"Sitz" comes from the German word, "sitzen," and means to sit. Sitting in water is taking a sitz, or sitting, bath. Priessnitz, the Austrian who used water as a curative remedy, used the Sitz Bath in treating constipation and other abdominal and pelvic conditions.

HOW IT CAN HELP YOU—The Sitz Bath is very helpful for many different pelvic problems. These are more fully described below under "Five Different Sitz Baths."

WHAT YOU WILL NEED—Natural therapy hospitals (they are called "sanitariums") use special sitz tubs (with a second foot-bathtub beside it), but you can use an ordinary washtub. It should be slightly tipped and set up with blocks of wood to make it immovable. A smaller tub or bath pan may be used to give the foot bath (which should always be given with the Sitz Bath). An ordinary bathtub can be used for a Hot Sitz Bath, but the water should be deep enough to reach to the navel. (Technically, this latter is called a Hot Half Bath, not a Sitz Bath; but the effects are pretty much the same.)

HOW TO APPLY IT—*(See picture on this page.)*

The temperature of the water changes the effect of the Sitz Bath. First, we will explain how to give a Sitz Bath; then we will tell you about the five types of Sitz Baths and how they can help in time of need.

1 - Help him into the tub and protect him from contact with it by placing towels behind his back and under his knees. Then cover him with a blanket, arranging it so that it will not become wet. Sufficient water should be used to cover the hips and reach to the abdomen. The temperature of the foot bath *(see pages 256-257 for Foot baths)* should be several degrees hotter than that of the Sitz Bath.

2 - The duration of the Sitz Bath depends on the temperature used and the effect desired. It is most often 3-8 minutes.

3 - Friction (rubbing) can be used with the Cold Sitz Bath if he feels chilly or to intensify the effect. Hot Sitz Baths may be concluded by cooling the water to neutral for a minute or two or by pouring cold water over the hips and thighs. Cold compresses (hand towels wrung out of cold water) to the head and neck must be used with the Hot Sitz.

SIX DIFFERENT SITZ BATHS—Here are the five primary ways in which Sitz Baths are given:

Cold Sitz Bath—55°-75° F. (The foot bath is 105°-110° F.) Time: 1-8 minutes. Enough water should be used to cover the hips and come up on the abdomen. Rub the hips to promote circulation. Friction mitts may be used. If the water is kept circulating (moving) in the tub, the effect will be heightened. If it is only 2-4 minutes in length, the Cold Sitz Bath greatly stimulates pelvic circulation and the muscles of the bowels, bladder, and uterus. These effects are intensified if the water is 55°-65° F. and vigorous friction (rubbing) is given. This makes it the Cold Rubbing Sitz Bath, which is very helpful in constipation, sub-involution, and hastening the absorption of residual thickening after pelvic inflammations.

Prolonged Cold Sitz Bath—If it is 15-40 minutes in length, the Cold Sitz Bath is called the Prolonged Cold Sitz Bath. This sitz bath is 70°-85° F. and the foot bath is 105°-110° F., but it may be started at a higher temperature and slowly lowered to that point. This bath should not at any time cause chilliness, and rubbing is not desirable. If needed to give a sensation of warmth, a fomentation or wrapped hot-water bottle can be placed to the spine. This Prolonged Cold Sitz Bath causes powerful and lasting contraction of the pelvic blood vessels and of the muscular wall of the uterus. It is used in sub-involution.

Neutral Sitz Bath—92°-97° F. (with 102°-106° F. for the foot bath). This bath is 20 minutes to 1-2 hours in length. It relaxes and helps one go to sleep.

Very Hot Sitz—Begin at 100° and rapidly go up to 106°-115° F. (Foot bath: 110°-120° F. As usual, always keep the foot bath two degrees hotter than the Sitz bath it accompanies). The normal length is 3-8 minutes. Keep the head cool. End by cooling the bath to neutral for 1-3 minutes. If sweating has been produced, pour cold water over the shoulders and chest. Very helpful for dysmenorrhea and pelvic pain from various causes. In dysmenorrhea, the bath should not be cooled.

Revulsive Sitz Bath—Begin at 100° and increase rapidly to 106°-115° F. (Foot bath: 110°-120° F.), for 3-8 minutes. Keep the head cool with cold cloths over the forehead or around the back of the neck. Finish with a cold (55°-65° F.) pail pour on the hips. The Revulsive Sitz is a powerful help in heating chronic inflammatory pelvic problems (salpingitis, parametritis, cellulitis, prostatic hypertrophic nocturia, etc.).

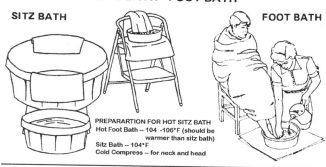

SITZ BATH - FOOT BATH

SITZ BATH   FOOT BATH

PREPARARTION FOR HOT SITZ BATH
Hot Foot Bath -- 104 -106°F (should be warmer than sitz bath)
Sitz Bath - 104°F
Cold Compress -- for neck and head

Alternate Hot and Cold Sitz Bath—For this bath you will need two sitz tubs, side by side. Fill one with hot (106°-115° F.) water and the other with cold (55°-65° F.) water. (Foot baths for both: 105°-115° F.) Apply cold compresses to the head and neck.

— SECTION ELEVEN —
FULL BATHS

WHAT IT IS—Full Tub Baths (also called Full Immersion Baths) are just tub baths, with most of the body immersed in the water. The difference between these and regular tub baths lies in the careful control of the water temperature and a careful observation to see that the desired effects are obtained.

Many different kinds of full immersion baths can be used, but there are only six that you will probably need in your home. Here they are:

1 - HOT TUB BATH (HOT FULL BATH) AND MODERATE HOT BATH

HOW IT CAN HELP YOU—The temperature and duration of the tub bath will determine the effect produced. The temperature of this bath is generally 100°-106° F. The time is usually 2-30 minutes. It may be used as a preparation for a cold treatment. If it is much prolonged (or the temperature is quite high), profuse sweating will be produced.

The Hot Bath can induce perspiration, relieve the pain of muscular rheumatism, reduce the muscular spasm of arthritis and its pain as well. It helps induce mild fever effects, when needed (as in undulant fever). It can also help increase metabolism and peripheral circulation. It can elevate body temperature and relieve pain, fatigue, and congestion of the internal organs.

If it is only a Moderate Hot Bath (100°-102° F.), it will be helpful in relieving opisthotonos (tetanus dorsalis) in tuberculosis meningitis and other diseases associated with spasticity of the muscles.

HOW TO APPLY IT—

1 - Place him in a full hot bath at about 98° F., and then gradually raise it to 100°-106° F. The bath should normally continue for two minutes onward, not over 20 minutes. Give him cold water to drink freely and keep his head cool. You may need to ap-

ply an ice bag to the heart and the back of the neck. Watch him closely.

2 - The bath may be finished by gradually cooling it, by a cold pour (if he is vigorous enough for it), or a shower immediately after he rises from the bath.

CAUTIONS—Do not give this bath where there is heart and valvular diseases, diabetes, vascular disorders, high blood pressure, or malignancies.

2 - NEUTRAL BATH (NEUTRAL FULL BATH) AND CONTINUOUS BATH

HOW IT CAN HELP YOU—The Neutral Bath (94°-97° F.) is given to relax people and help them go to sleep. It does this by equalizing the circulation and thus reducing the amount of blood in the brain and spinal chord. When used for insomnia, give it just before retiring for the night.

It is also excellent for relaxing nervous tension. Try it on yourself when you are full of nervous tension and see how nicely it relaxes you!

The Neutral Tub Bath is also used for anxiety, chronic diarrhea, multiple neuritis, burns (only the area burned need be in the water), nervous exhaustion or irritability, and diseases of the blood and blood vessels (when more extreme hot or cold cannot be used, as in diabetes and arteriosclerosis).

Last but not least, the Neutral Tub Bath has been successfully used by experts in treating insanity. In this condition, there is an excess of blood in the brain (because of the highly tense and excited state of the mind). The Neutral Bath quietly, but inexorably, equalizes the blood circulation throughout the body. Experts have placed a person in a Neutral Tub for days at a time. Proper circulation removes the fevered state of the brain and brings better nourishment to it, thus helping to restore him to a normal condition.

"As this bath is used chiefly in maniacal cases, the patient must be watched constantly. Very excited or violent patients should be wrapped in a sheet or blanket pack, which must be securely pinned about them, before they are placed in the tub. The duration of the bath depends upon the degree of sedative [quieting] effect obtained. It [the neutral bath) may last for hours or days. In the latter case the patient must be removed once or twice in twenty-four hours, the bowels given proper attention, and the skin anointed with oil in order to prevent too great maceration. The continuous-flowing bath is perhaps the most useful treatment in excited cases of insanity. It, together with the wet-sheet pack, has revolutionized the treatment of mania."—*Abbott, et al.*

HOW TO APPLY IT—*(See picture on this page.)*

1 - Place him in a full bathtub with the water temperature at 94°-97° F. The water should, if possible, cover his shoulders. Place a folded towel on the edge of the bathtub under his head for a pillow, and cover his body with a bath towel. Keep his face cool and

NEUTRAL BATH and CONTINUOUS [Neutral] BATH

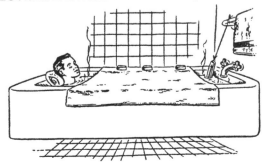

evenly maintain the temperature of the bathwater. Wet his forehead and face in cool water.

2 - The bath is usually 15-30 minutes in length, but it can go on for 34 hours.

3 - End the bath by cooling the water 2°-3° F. at the close. Dry him with no unnecessary rubbing and avoid unnecessary conversation. Dim the lights, if possible, and help him into bed so that he can go to sleep.

ADDITIONAL POINTS—A bath thermometer is needed to keep the temperature constant. He should be warm before beginning, during, and after the bath. If necessary, give a Hot Foot bath *(page 256)* before the Neutral Tub Bath begins. He should be comfortable in the tub. An invalid rubber ring may be placed under his buttocks if he is very thin. A rolled bath towel under his knees is also helpful. And be sure to place the folded towel on the edge of the bathtub under his head.

CAUTIONS—Certain cases of eczema and great weakness of the heart should not receive Neutral Tub Baths.

CONTINUOUS BATH—Here is some additional information on the Neutral Bath, when it is continued for a lengthy period of time: Suspend a hammock or sheet within the bathtub. It should not touch the bottom when a person is in it. Place a rubber pillow beneath the head and heels. Some authorities recommend keeping the feet out of the water.

Once a day, help him out of the tub; give him a cleansing bath with soap and a soft brush or cloth. He should then exercise somewhat, followed by having Vaseline or lanolin rubbed on him. During the time out of the continuous bath, the tub should be cleaned with soap and water. Some suggest placing an antiseptic on it, especially if infection is a problem. After thoroughly (thorough!) rinsing it, run fresh water into the tub so he can again enter it.

The Continuous Bath has been successfully used to aid in very difficult problems, such as extensive burns, pain, paresthesia, spasms, itching, pemphigus, extensive gangrene, profuse or offensive pus from various open abscesses, foul-smelling fistulas, and to bring quiet and rest to agitated mental problems, mania, or alcoholic delirium tremens.

3 - COLD TUB BATH (COLD FULL BATH) AND COLD RUBBING BATH

HOW IT CAN HELP YOU—When given for only a few minutes, the Cold Tub Bath is a stimulant and tonic. But when it is used for a longer time, it becomes antipyretic (fever reducing). And, thirdly, when it is given as a Cold Rubbing Bath, it becomes a most excellent method of treating typhoid fever.

This bath is most frequently used for colds, flu, and fevers.

HOW TO APPLY IT—

1 - The temperature of the water will be 55°-90°

F. And the length of time will be a plunge only, on up to 20 minutes or more (depending on the temperature, the effect desired, and the robustness of the one receiving it).

2 - His face should be bathed in cold water before he enters the bath; and his skin must be warm before it begins.

3 - Throughout this tub bath, it will be necessary to rub him constantly or at frequent intervals.

CAUTION—He must be warm before the bath begins. Test by feeling the warmth of his skin. Afterward, place him in bed and make sure he is warm. The short cold bath is very helpful in cases of diabetes, obesity, skin diseases, infections, scarlet fever, and poor blood circulation. Also chronic diseases, when the body functions are below normal.

But the short cold bath should not be used on those who are cold, have excessive fatigue, poor kidney function, heart or blood vessel disease, or hyperthyroidism (overactive thyroid).

4 - COLD SHALLOW BATH (COLD SHALLOW RUBBING BATH)

HOW IT CAN HELP YOU—The Cold Shallow Bath is one of the most powerful tonics used in water therapy.

HOW TO APPLY IT—

1 - Fill the tub only 4-6 inches deep with water at 65°-75° F.

His feet should be warm before entering the tub, and his head should be kept warm by cold wet towels.

2 - He sits down in the cold water and rubs his arms, legs, and chest vigorously while you rub his hips and back. Cold water dipped, from the tub, is splashed over his shoulders and back; and they are rubbed again. Then he lies down in the tub and rubs his chest and abdomen while you rub his legs. This can be repeated once or twice, as desired.

3 - It should last for 24 minutes; he should leave the tub with a definite glow to his skin. If not, the desired effect has not been obtained. He should be warm afterward, with no tendency to chilliness.

5 - PLUNGE BATH

WHAT IT IS—This is a quick dip into a bathtub of cold water. It can be a shallow or full tub of water. In some respects, the shallow tub is better for most people; for it involves more splashing and less actual coldness on the body. But those built up to it may desire a fuller tub of water.

HOW IT CAN HELP YOU—The effects of the Plunge Bath would be those of any of the other tonic baths and frictions. Actually, this bath is very similar to the Cold Shallow Bath *(above)*. The primary difference is that the Plunge Bath is more of a quick-in and quick-out, and thus a less powerful tonic than the Cold Shallow Bath.

6 - GRADUATED BATH

WHAT IT IS—This is a prolonged bath that begins with warm water which is gradually lowered to a fairly cool temperature.

HOW IT CAN HELP YOU—The Graduated Bath is especially designed to lower fever temperature in a manner that is easier to take than a prolonged cool bath would be. Most often used to lower fevers, such as in typhoid, this bath can also be used for tonic purposes on someone who is well.

HOW TO APPLY IT—

1 - The initial temperature of the tub water should be about 98° F. or higher. His body temperature will determine this. The water temperature should be about 3-5 degrees lower than his mouth temperature. His skin should be warm before the bath is begun.

2 - Help him into the tub, where he can be laid on an air pillow and a hammock (made by tying a sheet across the tub, and then fastening the corners and sides underneath).

3 - Apply cold compresses (cloths wrung out of cold water) to his head. Begin to reduce the bath temperature. Gradually lower it to about 85° F.

4 - When it is below 90° F., or as soon as he feels chilly or shows goose flesh, he should be rubbed constantly to keep the blood in the skin. This will prevent or overcome chilling. A spine bag (a long-narrow hot-water bottle) may be laid along his spine for the same purpose. Both his pulse and temperature should be closely watched throughout the bath. His temperature should be taken every 12-15 minutes.

5 - As soon as he is taken out of the bath, wrap him in a sheet and dry him briskly. If there is any tendency to goose flesh or chilliness, rub him briskly with your hands until the blood returns to the skin. If he is very cyanotic (bluish), put him into a Hot Blanket Pack *(page 245)* for a few minutes, and then, upon removing it, give him a Cold Mitten Friction *(page 249)*.

— SECTION TWELVE — SHOWER BATHS

WHAT IT IS—Special showers are used in natural-healing sanitariums; but the shower in the average home can give similar results.

1 - HOT SHOWER

HOW IT CAN HELP YOU—The Hot Shower is mainly used as a preparation for a Cold Shower *(this page)*.

HOW TO APPLY IT—

1 - Begin the Hot Shower with very warm water (100°-105° F.), and gradually raise the temperature to 110°-115° F. or slightly higher. Time: thirty seconds to two minutes.

2 - A Cold Compress *(page 222)* to the head may be needed during the shower.

3 - If no other treatment is to follow the Hot Shower, then conclude by rapidly cooling the water to 90° or

85° F.

4 - Dry quickly with towels and a sheet. You may wish to finish by fanning the patient cool with a dry sheet.

2 - CONTINUOUS HOT SHOWER

WHAT IT IS—This is a continuous fine stream of hot water for several hours to a body part.

HOW IT CAN HELP YOU—This shower is used for sciatica, brachial neuritis, refractory lumbago, and similar conditions. It is also used with good success on limbs that have painful edema. It does not matter if open ulcers and unhealed wounds are present.

HOW TO APPLY IT—

1 - Make him comfortable on a chair, couch or mat. Over it, a special showerhead produces a fine (not course) stream of water. Special precautions must be taken that the water will not appreciably change in temperature throughout the shower (particularly that it cannot burn him).

2 - The temperature is kept at the upper limit of comfort; and the shower will continue for 24 hours.

3 - Conclude by drying him. Sometimes a dash of cold water from the shower is used before drying.

3 - COLD OR COOL SHOWER

HOW IT CAN HELP YOU—This shower is used for its tonic effect of strengthening the body.

HOW TO APPLY IT—

Give him a Hot Shower *(this page)*. When he is sufficiently warmed, lower the temperature rapidly from hot to as much cold as he can take. This will be about 70°-90° F., for a cool shower, and 55°-70° F. for a cold one.

SPECIAL POINTS—A series of cool or cold showers are often given. When this is done, the first one should only be cool; then, in subsequent showers, gradually lower the final temperature.

4 - NEUTRAL SHOWER

HOW IT CAN HELP YOU—This shower is given at a lukewarm temperature and is chiefly used to calm, relax, and help one go to sleep.

HOW TO APPLY IT—

1 - Begin the shower at 100° F., and very slowly lower it to 97° to 94° F.

2 - The shower should normally last about 3-5 minutes.

3 - Dry him quickly, without any percussion or unnecessary friction. You may then wish to place him in a warm bed, so that he can go to sleep.

5 - GRADUATED SHOWER

WHAT IT IS—This is a shower bath that employs a greater variety of temperature changes.

HOW IT CAN HELP YOU—The objective is to gradually lower the temperature of the body, with as little shock effect as possible.

HOW TO APPLY IT—

1 - Give a prolonged or vigorous sweating bath. Place a Cold Compress *(page 222)* on his head before he leaves.

2 - Begin the Graduated Shower with very warm water (108°-110° F.), and then quickly raise it to a hot shower (115°-118° F.).

3 - Maintain this temperature until he feels warm and is ready for the cold. Then, slowly lower the temperature until it is fairly cool (80°-90° F.)

4 - Conclude the shower in 2-6 minutes; and then quickly dry with sheets and towels.

5 - Do not let him be exposed to cold air or drafts for at least one hour afterward.

6 - REVULSIVE SHOWER

WHAT IT IS—This shower is like the Graduated Shower, described just above, in that the water temperature is first raised and then lowered. It is different, in that the temperature is not slowly, but quickly, lowered to cold.

HOW IT CAN HELP YOU—The purpose is to cool and stimulate the body. Thus, a mild tonic effect is the result. The Revulsive Shower is also used in order to build up the body; so that it can take an alternate hot and cold shower in order to help build resistance.

HOW TO APPLY IT—

1 - Begin the shower at 105°-108° F. Then gradually raise it to 110°-115° F. or slightly higher. Continue at this temperature for two minutes.

2 - When he is fully warm, turn the valve quickly to a cold temperature of about 60°-85° F.

3 - After 5-10 seconds, turn the mixer valve back to the earlier temperature (110°-115° F.) for 1-2 minutes.

4 - Do this cycle three complete times (three complete changes from hot to cold).

5 - Dry quickly with sheets and towels.

SPECIAL POINTS—As a preparation for beginning to take Alternate Hot and Cold Showers, one should become accustomed to Revulsive Showers first. And, gradually, the cold part of the Revulsive Shower should become longer.

7 - ALTERNATE HOT AND COLD SHOWER

WHAT IT IS—Abrupt changes back and forth from hot to cold.

HOW IT CAN HELP YOU—This is a vigorous tonic and physical stimulant. It should not be taken without much preliminary taking of less intense showers.

HOW TO APPLY IT—

1 - Begin with the hot water at a temperature of 106°-110° F.; then quickly raise the temperature to the upper limit of tolerance. Hold it there about one minute.

2 - Turn the valve quickly to full cold. Hold it there for 15-30 seconds.

3 - Reverse again to hot for about one minute; then back to cold for 15-30 seconds again.

4 - Do three complete cycles of hot and cold, finishing with the cold.

5 - Dry well with sheet and towels, and fan dry with a sheet.

— SECTION THIRTEEN — MISCELLANEOUS BATHS

1 - STEAM BATHS INCLUDING RUSSIAN BATH AND SAUNA

WHAT IT IS—This is an application of hot water vapor to the skin. It is not an application of steam; for the temperature of steam is so high that it would immediately cause severe burns.

HOW IT CAN HELP YOU—The so-called "steam" bath produces vigorous sweating. This greatly increases the breakdown of excess fats and carbohydrates—and thus aids in taking off extra weight. Thus, the Steam Bath is very helpful in obesity. But it is also used in chronic rheumatism with obesity, gout, Bright's disease, chronic alcoholism, tobacco addictions, and in arteriosclerosis unless that condition is extreme.

CAUTIONS—Unless one drinks enough water before, during, and afterward, there is a "washed out" effect that can cause a feeling of weakness. It should

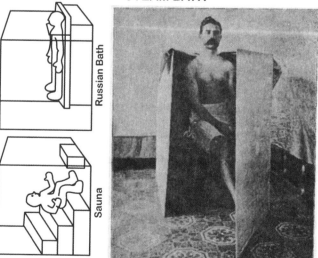

STEAM BATH

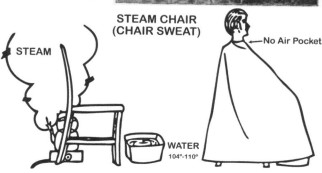

STEAM CHAIR (CHAIR SWEAT)

be noted that a 20-minute steam bath will raise the body temperature about two degrees F. and produce a definite rise in blood pressure.

Do not use the Steam Bath in diabetes, valvular heart disease, extreme arteriosclerosis, and all conditions associated with emaciation.

HOW TO MAKE YOUR OWN—Most homes do not have access to steam-bath rooms, but it is possible to make your own:

1 - A room can be made for this purpose. The walls should be of nonporous material, with wooden benches and a floor drain. A source of heat should be provided outside the room. In addition, a shower or bathtub should be in an adjacent room.

2 - A small, but very functional, steam bath can be made out of secondhand sheet metal. An arc welder and some welding skill can turn it out in a day or two. If you are a handyman, you will have no trouble with it.

3 - Set an old chair on the floor. Have the one needing a steam bath sit on it. Place a heavy blanket around him, that should cover him from the neck on down to the floor. Under the chair, place an electric teakettle. It should be three-quarter's full of hot water and already steaming. Place a cold cloth to the head and put the feet in hot water. End this about 20-30 minutes later with a cold friction *(page 249)* or a cold shower. Be sure that the spout of the teakettle is turned toward the back of chair. Always stay by a person receiving a steam bath.

HOW TO APPLY IT—*(See pictures on this and facing page.)*

1 - Give a preliminary Hot Foot bath *(page 256)* as he drinks several glasses of water.

2 - The steam room should be ready for usage. If the bench is not warm, throw several pails of hot water on it. Warm the room to about 100° F. and cover the bench with a folded cotton sheet.

3 - Assist him to the bench and help him lie on his back, with his head on an air pillow and just outside the opening (as in a steam cabinet or Russian steam Vapor).

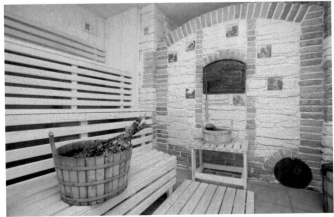

RUSSIAN STEAM BATH

Many homes do not have facilities for steam baths. But some will have homemade steam cabinets, steam rooms, or sheet-metal steam units. Therefore, we will here give directions for steam baths. These directions can be used for a steam cabinet or in a steam room with a small window in it for the head.

4 - The head opening is lowered; and a towel wrung from ice water is placed about the neck or hung across the end of the neck window and tucked about the neck.

5 - A second cold, wet cloth is placed to the head, covering the temporal arteries (which are slightly in front of and above the ears). A third one should be placed above the heart. (Sometimes an ice bag over the heart is necessary).

6 - Turn on the heated vapor, gradually raising the temperature to 115°-120° F. A small amount of vapor must constantly escape in order to maintain this high temperature.

7 - Closely watch him; frequently change the cold, wet cloths on the head and neck. Keep him drinking water before, and frequently during, the steam bath.

8 - The steam bath should continue for 10-30 minutes. A fresh ice-water cloth should be placed on his head just before he rises.

9 - End with a Graduated Shower: Begin with a warm shower (108°-119° F.), quickly raising it to a hot one (115°-118° F.). When he feels warm and is ready for the cold, gradually lower the temperature till it is quite cool (80°-90° F.). This shower should be located close to the steam bath and should take about 2-6 minutes.

DEFINING TERMS—What is a "Russian Bath" and what is a "Sauna," and are they the same? To take a Sauna, one sits on a bench in a room containing hot water vapor ("steam"). His entire body is in that room. For a Russian Bath, he instead lays on a wooden "slab" or bench, with his head protruding from a small opening in the side of the room. In this way, his body receives the benefit of the hot vapor, but his head can remain outside. Obviously, since the Russian Bath keeps the head cooler and the lungs filled with fresher air, it has definite advantages over the Sauna. A Chair Steam Bath (Chair Sweat) combines some of both advantages. The head is vertical and outside the area of vapor; in addition, the entire unit is both inexpensive and portable.

2 - STEAM CHAIR (STEAM SWEAT)

WHAT IT IS—This is a steam bath "in a chair." As such, it is probably the simplest way of giving a "steam bath" to a person. And it has the advantage of keeping his head out of the hot vapor, which a sauna-type steam bath cannot do.

HOW IT CAN HELP YOU—This is a simply erected, very portable, steam bath that can provide the help of a regular steam bath. *(See "Steam Bath, How It Can*

Help You" on pages 262-263 for further information on these benefits.)

WHAT YOU WILL NEED—Hot plate. Kettle or pot filled with hot water. Sheet or blanket. Three towels. Ice bag. Cup of hot water (for drinking). Basin for hot foot bath. If medicated steam bath: Oil of eucalyptus or mint.

HOW TO APPLY IT—*(See picture on page 262.)*

1 - Set the chair in position where you want it (not far from an electric outlet for the hot plate, and arranged so no one will trip over the cord and spill the hot water under the chair). Place the hot plate under the chair and carefully put the kettle or pot on it. The spout should face toward the rear; neither the pot nor hot plate should be able to burn him or set the blanket on fire. The water in the kettle should already be boiling hot. Fold a towel and place it on the seat of the chair. Set a basin or tub of hot water in place for the hot foot bath. (If medication is added to the kettle water: Add about 1 teaspoon of Eucalyptus oil or 2 tablespoons of dried mint leaves to each potful of water.)

2 - Wrap the second towel as a turban around the head of the one to receive the steam bath. Undressed, he should now be seated on the chair and begin the hot foot bath.

3 - Wrap the blanket or sheet (a blanket would be best) around him. Do this by wrapping it about his back and shoulders, covering his body below the neck to the floor.

Fold a towel lengthwise and place it as a snug collar about his neck, thus holding the blanket or sheet in place. When he begins to sweat or his oral temperature goes past 100° F., apply the cold compress (cold, wet cloth) to his head. You will need to keep renewing the cold cloth and adding hot water to the hot foot bath (instructions under "Hot Foot bath" *(page 256)* will explain how to add this water without burning him).

4 - Every 5-10 minutes, he should be encouraged to drink some of the hot water. Offer it to him in a cup or glass with a flexible straw in it.

5 - A very frequent check on temperature and pulse is crucial. Oral (mouth) temperature should be kept under 104° F. Check it every 10 minutes until it is above 103° F.; then check it every 5 minutes until it is again below 103° F. Pulse should be checked at the large artery in his temple or the one at the front side of the neck; this should not go over 140. Air temperature inside the "tent" should be kept between 120°-130° F. until his oral temperature goes up to 102°-104° F.; at which point the tent temperature should be brought down to 105°-110° F.

6 - At the conclusion of the steam bath, carefully remove the basin, kettle, and hot plate. Then dry the feet. If it seems best to prolong the effects, place him

in bed with the tent blanket or sheet still wrapped about him. He should be covered well in order to continue the sweating.

7 - Finally, terminate the treatment with a shower or cold mitten friction. Then place him in bed for 30-60 minutes, so that he will have enough time to react well to the concluding cold tonic. If he sweats during this time, give him an ordinary shower when he leaves the bed. He should receive large amounts of water during and after the treatment.

CAUTION—Only give this chair steam bath to one who is basically healthy, but not feeble or debilitated.

3 - VAPOR INHALATION (STEAM INHALATION)

WHAT IT IS—This is a means of supplying warm, moist air to the congested membranes of the nose and sinuses during a head cold.

HOW IT CAN HELP YOU—After being chilled, the temperature of the respiratory tract is lowered. A cold in the head is the result; soon it may go into bronchitis or chest cold with its harsh, dry cough.

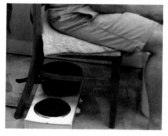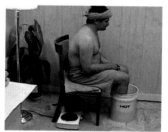
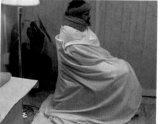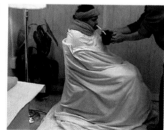

Please carefully read instructions for this treatment before proceeding

Vapor inhalation warms and soothes the respiratory tract, relieves inflammation and congestion in the nasal membranes, relieves "throat tickle" by moistening the air, loosens secretions and stimulates expectoration (spitting); also water drinking will help solve this problem and relieve spasmodic breathing, lessen coughing by relaxing the affected muscles, increase blood flow to this area, and prevent excessive dryness of the mucous membranes.

WHAT YOU WILL NEED—A vaporizer or a kettle with a spout. Boiling water. A chair or bedside stand. Hot plate (if continuous inhalation is desired). An umbrella. A newspaper rolled into a cone-shape. Medication, such as Oil of Eucalyptus (1 teaspoon to a pint of water), Vick's VaporRub, Oil of Wintergreen,

HYDRO

etc. Some use 1-2 tablespoons of fresh or dried mint leaves per pint of water.

HOW TO APPLY IT—*(See picture on this page.)*

1 - Fill the vaporizer or kettle with the boiling water. Add the eucalyptus oil, etc., either to the kettle water or to the newspaper of the cone (to avoid putting the heavy odor of the oil into the kettle). Place it on the stand by the bed or on the floor (according to the arrangement which works best for you).

2 - Arrange an umbrella on the bed, covered partly with a sheet. Place the paper cone over the kettle spout, with its upper, narrower opening, into the umbrella in such a manner that it will not point into the face. Understand that this procedure may work best for you with the kettle on a nightstand without the cone, or on the floor or low chair with it. Or, in a smaller room, the kettle can be placed on the floor without the cone.

3 - Lying on one side of the bed, he can place his head into the "tent" and breathe the vapors.

CAUTIONS—Check the water level in the kettle frequently. Avoid all possibility of burning him. Avoid drafts in the room while the vaporizer is operating. Be especially careful when children are receiving the treatment. Be on guard lest they knock over the kettle and burn themselves. Do not let the hot plate (electric burner) come in contact with the bedding, cone, etc., and start a fire. Individuals with cardiovascular or heart problems may find difficulty in breathing amid the vapors.

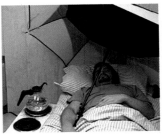
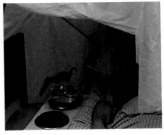
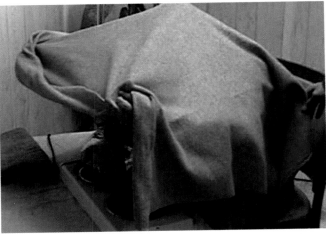

Please carefully read instructions for this treatment before proceeding

4 - RADIANT HEAT BATH (ELECTRIC LIGHT BATH)

WHAT IT IS—This is a heating of the body, not with an immersion bath in water, but an immersion in radiant heat. The heat source can be electric space heaters; but, the original Kellogg arrangement was a box with incandescent bulbs.

NOTE—A steam bath is generally more practical, available, and effective.

HOW IT CAN HELP YOU—Kellogg found that these radiant heat baths could provide an intensity of dry heat not to be obtained in any other way.

The Electric Light Cabinet is a very efficient way to treat acute or chronic conditions requiring fever therapy. (Fever therapy is an artificial raising of body temperature in order to increase white blood cell action and eliminate toxins and bacteria.) A person with an inflammation, or already with a fever, will have a temperature drop of 1°-2° F. within 15 minutes or so after the bath is completed. Thus, the use of this cabinet is very helpful in mild fevers, inflammations, colds, flu, or any condition in which sweating is helpful. It helps in withdrawal from addicting drugs (including tobacco and alcohol), and will lower blood pressure.

WHAT YOU WILL NEED—In order to achieve the full effects of this, you would need to construct a cabinet with these dimensions: 5 x 5 feet square by about 4½ feet high. This will hold 80 bare-filament incandescent light bulbs of about 60-100 watts each. These are arranged in four vertical strips, one on each corner of the cabinet. The four strips are designed on several different switches. In this way a varying amount of heat can be provided, according to how many are switched on. Six switches are recommend-

VAPOR INHALATION

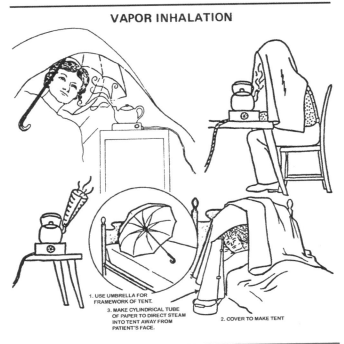

1. USE UMBRELLA FOR FRAMEWORK OF TENT.

2. COVER TO MAKE TENT

3. MAKE CYLINDRICAL TUBE OF PAPER TO DIRECT STEAM INTO TENT AWAY FROM PATIENT'S FACE.

ed. (Avoid circuit overload by placing half the bulbs on one circuit and the other half on a different one.

One vertical side of the box is missing. This is the "door" to the cabinet. After entering and being seated in a chair, a blanket, canvas or heavy sheet is placed over the doorway. At the top, there are two small hinged "doors" with semicircular openings in them. These are now folded down, thus providing a circular opening in the middle, for the head to project through.

HOW TO APPLY IT—*(See picture on next page.)*

1 - After entering the cabinet and seating himself, the front and top is closed and a towel is placed about his neck. Be certain that the bulbs cannot touch him, lest he be burned.

2 - The light switches are turned on and the air in the cabinet will go from about 70° F. to 125°-130° F. within a few minutes. Why so high? Because the body can tolerate a higher dry heat temperature than it can a vapor or water temperature. The body temperature will rise to 101°-102° F. in approximately 20 minutes. This artificial fever effect will help increase white blood cell number and activity, thus hastening the elimination of bacteria and toxins.

3 - Sweating will begin in 5-8 minutes, at which time facial sponging with a cool, wet cloth should begin. Lay a cold, wet cloth over the forehead, eyes, nose, and cheeks.

4 - Always know how he is feeling. Control the heat with the switches. Conclude the bath either when the desired temperature is achieved or after a total of 10-20 minutes.

5 - Follow up with a Cold Mitten Friction, or cool shower.

5 - OATMEAL BATH

WHAT IT IS—This is a full warm tub bath with oatmeal liquid in it.

HOW IT CAN HELP YOU—The oatmeal bath can help reduce the itching and burning from skin rashes of various kinds.

WHAT YOU WILL NEED—Three bath towels. Washcloth. Cloth for head compress. Bath mat. Basin of cool water for the compress. Shower cap to keep the hair dry. 1-2 pounds of quick-cooking oatmeal.

OATMEAL AND OTHER MEDICINAL BATHS

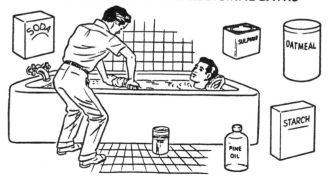

HOW TO DO IT—*(See picture on this page.)*

1 - Put the oatmeal in a thin cloth bag; then place it in the tub, so that the in flowing water will run over the bag into the tub. Fill the tub about two-thirds full with water at 96° F. The water should be the correct temperature, not too warm or too cool. The water should be deep enough for the one taking the bath to be immersed to the neck. When full, squeeze the oatmeal bag into the water. The water should by now be milky and very soft.

2 - Help him into the tub (and out again afterward). This is because the oatmeal water is slippery. Make him comfortable with a folded towel under his neck. The washcloth can be used to bath the parts not immersed.

3 - When finished, help him out of the tub and dry him by patting (do not rub).

CAUTION—Some types of skin conditions are made worse by water.

6 - SODA ALKALINE BATH

WHAT IT IS—This is a full bath to which baking soda has been added.

HOW IT CAN HELP YOU—The partially anesthetic aspect of baking soda, when applied to the skin, provides help in dealing with poison ivy, itching, hives, heat rash, sunburns, eczema, drug reaction rashes, ant and bee stings, and plant sensitivity (nettles, etc.). The alkaline factor helps to counteract acidity in the rashes, stings, poison ivy, etc.

WHAT YOU WILL NEED—Baking soda or commercial grade sodium bicarbonate.

HOW TO APPLY IT—*(See picture on this page.)*

1 - Fill a bathtub with water at 95°-98° F. Add about a cup of baking soda (or an equivalent amount of sodium bicarbonate).

2 - Sitting in the tub, he should dip and pour the alkaline water onto his body, continually covering it. After 30-60 minutes, he stands in the tub and partially "drip drys"; then he pats the skin dry.

7 - STARCH ALKALINE BATH

WHAT IT IS—This is shallow tub bath with a solution of corn starch in it.

HOW IT CAN HELP YOU—This is another type of alkaline bath; it is used for the same purposes as the Soda Bath, described just above. Many may prefer the starch bath; since it is even more of a natural substance on the skin than is baking soda.

WHAT YOU WILL NEED—Dry starch, such as corn starch.

HOW TO APPLY IT—*(See picture on this page.)*

1 - Add about one cup of a dry starch into a shallow tub of water (at 95°-98° F.).

2 - The remainder of the directions are the same as for the Soda Bath, above. Length of time in the bath can be 20-35 minutes or longer.

8 - SUNBATH

WHAT IT IS—This is simply exposing part or all of the body to the sunlight.

HOW IT CAN HELP YOU—Direct sunlight has a wide range of wave energies. The ultraviolet ones are the most important for both healing and maintaining good health. The longer heat waves (infrared) are also helpful for their heating effect.

Ultraviolet rays stimulate various life processes, destroy bacteria, and aid in the manufacture of Vitamin D by the body. Ergosterol is a fat found in the skin that has the capacity for absorbing certain ultraviolet radiations; in the process, it becomes changed into Vitamin D. Without adequate Vitamin D, the human body cannot utilize calcium in the diet to make strong bones.

It has been found that the treatment of pulmonary tuberculosis has been greatly helped by extensive sunbathing. And it has been discovered that sunbathing at higher altitudes (in mountain country) greatly improves the likelihood of healing from this disease. These "higher altitudes" need be only 1,000 feet above sea level, but can be as high as 6,000 feet.

In addition to pulmonary tuberculosis, sunbaths are also of great help in tuberculosis of the bones and joints, and in Pott's disease (tuberculosis of the spine).

Both the red blood cells and blood hemoglobin increase in sunbathing; the increase is proportional to the altitude. In the higher Alps and on Pikes Peak, this amounts to a 30-40 percent increase in both of these very important blood factors. Mountain sunbathing also increases lymphocytes, blood alkalinity, respiratory volume, energy, and a feeling of well-being. It also lowers blood pressure; significantly increases muscular strength; and definitely improves the feelings of hope, courage, and cheerfulness. All these effects will, to a lesser extent, be achieved by sunbaths at lower altitudes or at sea level. Smog in the air at lower altitudes greatly hinders the values of sunbathing.

ELECTRIC LIGHT BATH

On the RIGHT is the Kellogg Electric Light Bath (ELB) for the feet. BOTTOM RIGHT is his ELB for joints. LEFT is a sample of the trunk-and-limb ELB used in homes today.

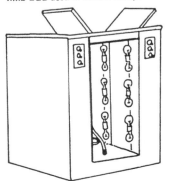
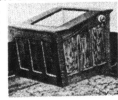
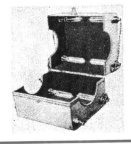

HOW TO APPLY IT—

1 - At a mountain altitude, 7-10 days of rest may be needed to adjust to the physical adaptation needed at higher altitudes. At lower altitudes (3,000 feet or below), this is not necessary.

2 - For normal people, begin with 5 minutes of sunlight a day, and increase 5 minutes each day. In hotter climates, only increase 2-3 minutes a day. For invalids, begin with the feet; give them 5 minutes a day, and gradually increase the exposure and the amount of the body exposed.

3 - Ultimately, never go beyond 3-4 hours a day. Blond people especially lack the "sunscreen" factor in the skin; therefore they must be more careful.

4 - The sunbath should produce a feeling of warmth, but should be given in relatively cool surroundings; for a heat bath is depressing.

9 - SEA BATHING

WHAT IT IS—This is bathing in the ocean.

HOW IT CAN HELP YOU—Sea bathing strengthens and builds the body in several ways: The percussion of the moving, cool water invigorates the body; the ocean water contains trace minerals that are needed by the body. The eating of Nova Scotia Dulse or Norwegian Kelp can help to supply these trace minerals, but sea bathing is also helpful.

(It is interesting to note that, if all the water in your body could somehow be squeezed out, there would be about 11 gallons of seawater. For the mixture would be found to contain the same salts that are dissolved in the ocean, and in almost the same proportions (about 80 percent sodium, 4 percent calcium, 4 percent potassium, etc. The exception is that blood has 2 percent magnesium while seawater has 10 percent.)

WARNING—Sea bathing is becoming more dangerous, due to waste pollution in the waters, from city dumping and runoff from polluted rivers. North Carolina rivers are notorious for its polluted rivers, from swine farm runoff.

10 - SUN, AIR, AND WATER BATH

WHAT IT IS—In northern Mexico, there are natural healing centers which have shallow out-of-door depressions with water in them. Patients sit or lay in them and splash the water over their bodies. The effect of the combined sunlight, fresh air, and water upon the skin provides a pleasant tonic to the body. Try it in your own backyard on a warm summer day. Use a galvanized or plastic tub, or something similar.

11 - WET GRASS WALK

WHAT IT IS—This early-morning tonic is to be found in some natural healing centers. Try it in the privacy of your own backyard: Walk barefoot on the lawn in the early morning while the dew is still on the grass. This is such a nice tonic, that you will thoroughly enjoy it. One of the effects, of course, is a strengthening of the feet. Fortunately, there are lawns all over the nation.

12 - SUMMER SPRAY

WHAT IT IS—Children enjoy it every summer; why not join them? Go out in your backyard on a hot summer day and turn the water hose on each other. The water percussion, cool water on a warm day, the air upon the skin, and the light exercise will all combine to bring a vigorous tonic effect to your body.

— SECTION FOURTEEN —
IRRIGATIONS

WHAT IS AN IRRIGATION?—In hydrotherapy, an "irrigation" is when we put water onto or into the body through a tube. There are irrigations of the ear, nose, eye, throat, etc., but the most common is the rectal irrigation: the enema and the colonic. We will give the most attention to enemas and colonics; but, in the third subsection, we will discuss several other types of irrigations.

WHAT IS AN ENEMA AND A COLONIC—Water is placed in the large bowel (the large intestine) in order to remove impacted wastes and toxic substances. Either an enema bag or a colonic apparatus can be used for this purpose.

WHAT YOU WILL NEED—An enema bag is a hot-water bottle with a rubber tube and plastic tip; this is obtainable at your local drugstore. For more thorough cleansing and removal of toxic substances from the bowel, a colonic is given. Whereas an enema bag can provide cleansing for a minute or two, before renewal, a colonic can do it for twenty minutes or more.

HOW IT CAN HELP YOU—The body primarily eliminates waste through the bowel, bladder, skin, and lungs. When a person is ill, he has far more toxic waste than normal; and the kidneys (cleansed by drinking pure water), the bowel (cleansed by enemas or colonies), the skin (cleansed by bathing), and the lungs (cleansed by fresh air) are very important in the disposing of that waste matter. Of these, the largest amount of wastes will be discharged through the urine (kidneys and bladder) and feces (bowel, or large intestine). An enema or colonic can be of great help in aiding the body in throwing off these excess body wastes.

1 - ENEMAS
INCLUDING: HOT, WARM, TEPID, AND COLD

WHAT YOU WILL NEED—In order to give an enema, you will need the following items: a bedpan and cover (if the one who is ill cannot easily leave the bed), an enema bag with a hard-rubber or plastic enema tip, small rectal tube, lubricant (such as vasoline), toilet paper, and newspapers or plastic sheeting.

HOW TO APPLY IT—(*See picture on this page.*)

1 - Place the enema bag under the faucet and put in water that is lukewarm or slightly cool to the touch. Fill it to the top, press down in order to expel air, and then screw on the cap (which is attached to about 5-6 feet of tubing).

2 - (In the following directions, we will assume that the one receiving the enema is in bed. If he is able to receive the enema in the bathroom, the entire procedure will, understandably, be much simpler.)

3 - Set up the equipment so that it is ready to flow. Fold the bedcovers back and cover him with a cotton blanket. He should be warm throughout the treatment, especially his feet. All clothing that is not removed should be loose. He can lay on his back, on his side, with knees partially or fully raised, or he can sit up during the treatment.

4 - Place a rubber or plastic sheet (or newspapers) on the bed under him. Turn him on his left side, with knees flexed. Allow the solution to flow through the tubing, so that it just begins to come out; then pinch it off. This removes the air from the tubing.

5 - Release the cutoff clamp; and let some of the water flow until the stream is the same temperature as that in the bag. Close the cutoff and place a little lubricant (Vaseline, etc.) on the tip (which you have earlier cleaned). Then let him insert the tip; or, if he is unable to, gently do it for him.

6 - Instruct him to take as much water as possible. To make it easier to do this, stop the flow by pinching the tube two or three times during the taking of the enema. Ask him if it is coming in too fast; if so, lower the enema bag or pinch off the tube more frequently.

7 - Give the solution slowly, and pinch it off for a few seconds when asked. (If he cannot retain the solution, place him on the bedpan while giving it.) When he feels that it is time to terminate the enema, close the tubing clamp, gently remove the tip and wrap it in toilet tissue. Small amounts of water given several times, are better than a large amount all at once.

8 - If possible, he should retain the water a few minutes before expelling it. Place him on the bedpan and stay within call. If he is unable to relax enough to take sufficient fluid, instruct him to breathe deeply

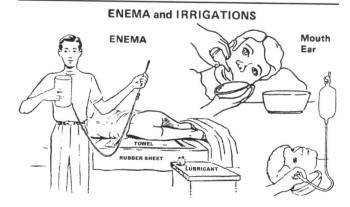

ENEMA and IRRIGATIONS

or to bring his knees upward. Stay with him if he is very ill, so that you can assist him. Note his condition and the results of the enema.

9 - Remove the bed protector, replace the bed covers, and make him comfortable. Then clean all the equipment well and put it away.

WATER TEMPERATURE—What should be the temperature of the water? 104° F. is frequently recommended, but other temperatures can also be used; and, actually, a temperature of 96°-100° F. (just below body temperature) is the ideal, as you will see below.

Hot Enema - (103°-110° F.) The temperature will vary according to his condition and the desired results. The Hot Enema helps relieve irritation, the pain of inflammation in the rectum or prostate, and pain of hemorrhoids. It also aids in expelling gas, and helps to check diarrhea by decreasing rectal tenesmus. It may be used as a preliminary measure in the treatment of dysmenorrhea. It is also used to warm and stimulate the body in shock.

Warm Enema and Tepid Enema - (95°-100° F.) The Warm Enema is the ordinary enema for cleansing purposes. It is at, or slightly below, body temperature. If slightly less, it helps facilitate bowel action during the enema. But if the enema is prolonged, or repeated frequently, it is better to use a still cooler enema or the Tepid Enema (80°-92° F.) in order to avoid the relaxing effects that the warm water has. When the bowel becomes too relaxed, it does not want to move; thus begins what is called the "enema habit."

Cold Enema - (55°-80° F.) 55°-70° F. is considered cold; whereas 70°-80° F. is considered cool. The Cold Enema is a powerful stimulant to bowel movements, and should be more generally used for this purpose instead of the warm enema. It is thus the best for overcoming both the enema habit and the cathartic habit. If retained 10-15 minutes or frequently repeated, it is useful in shrinking hemorrhoids. It may also be used in fever; but, for this purpose, a prolonged colonic would be much more convenient and effective.

2 - COLONICS

WHAT IT IS—A colonic apparatus is an arrangement for taking water into colon, expelling it into a toilet, taking in more and expelling it, for about twenty minutes or so. It is much more practical and helpful than an enema bag.

WHAT YOU WILL NEED—You will need a colonic board, bucket with a hole near the bottom, tubing, and a colonic tip. Years ago, it was difficult to purchase these and so they had to be handmade at home. Doing so is not difficult,—except for making the tip.

But at the present time, they are easy to locate on Google. Just type in "colonic board," and purchase the one you want.

1 - Set up the colonic board, so that its head rests on a chair and its foot rests over a toilet bowl (with the toilet lid raised). Over the board, place a folded blanket wrapped in plastic (or two black-plastic garbage can bags: one covering each end and thus overlapping each other in the middle). Above this blanket, at the head, place a pillow. And, at the foot, lay a bath towel crosswise; and then tuck it underneath on each side.

2 - Set up the colonic bucket near the toilet. (The ideal height for it would be this: bottom of the bucket about 15-20 inches above the tip.) Connect all the plastic and metal tubing together; so that water from the bucket can flow through the tubing to the colonic tip. Snap the tube clamp closed.

3 - Fill the bucket with warm water and open the clamp. As soon as the water begins to come out, snap the clamp closed. Make sure the room is warm; and have a bath towel and a blanket or two ready.

4 - Help the one about to receive the colonic to the board; assist him in lying down on it, with his head on the pillow and his feet flexed and straddling the opening at the foot of the board that is just above the mouth of the toilet.

5 - He should be suitably clothed with both tops and bottoms. You now drape the bath towel crosswise over his lower pelvic and pubic area; and then cover him with the blanket (unless he is warm enough without it). You may need an electric space heater in the bathroom, to provide additional heat.

6 - Lubricate the colonic tip and, if necessary, assist him in inserting it. Then, loosen the clamp and let the water begin flowing. Ask him whether it is too warm or too cool. (It is best if he is able to take it very slightly on the cool side.)

7 - Either remain nearby or give him a bell to ring (have it tested to be certain you can hear it where you are elsewhere in the home). If it is a one-gallon bucket, you will want to check it about every 10 minutes. It is best not to refill it more than twice, at the most. If it is a five-gallon bucket, place about 3½ gallons in it; and you will probably not need to refill it.

8 - When he is finished, clamp off the tubing and remove towel and blanket. Help him arise and to get into the shower or bath.

9 - Clean up everything and put all the equipment away.

3 - OTHER IRRIGATIONS
INCLUDING
IRRIGATION OF THE EAR,
NASAL IRRIGATION,
IRRIGATION OF THE EYE,
THROAT IRRIGATION

WHAT IT IS—Both enemas and colonics are methods of bringing water into the body through a tube. In hydrotherapy, these are classified as "irrigations." There are several other types of irrigations used in water therapy. While not taking the space to explain them in detail, we will here briefly consider several of them:

1 - Irrigation of the Ear - A clean rubber tube is used to gently (gently!) introduce a flow of water onto the outer ear. The water is never applied with any pressure! It flows to the ear and thence out to the side. The temperature may be from 100° to 120° F., depending upon the effect desired. The source of water should be on a level with the top of the head. Never use force, because perforation of the ear often exists; serious injury could result from introduction of water into the middle ear with any degree of force. The head should be inclined to the side as the water is applied.

The canal of the ear should afterward be carefully dried and covered with a napkin or a warm hand for a few minutes. In cold weather, the ear should not be exposed out-of-doors for at least an hour after warm ear irrigation is applied; even after that, a small piece of cotton should be placed in the outer passageway.

"This measure affords great relief in the pain of acute otitis media and earache due to other causes. In chronic suppurative disease of the ear, this measure is indispensable as a means of cleansing and disinfection."—*Kellogg.*

2 - Nasal Irrigation - An ordinary hard-rubber syringe is attached to a rubber tube which has been carefully inserted into one nostril. The water is allowed to gentle flow into one and out the other, as the head is held forward. Kellogg says that he has concluded that it is best NOT to use the Nasal irrigation, because it might cause ear problems (through the eustachian tubes). He suggests using vaporizers or atomizers instead.

3 - Irrigation of the Eye - For this, the eyes are closed; and water is allowed to fall on the lids and also the forehead above the brow. Kellogg considers the hot eye irrigation to be "very valuable in cases of chronic inflammation of the mucous lining of the eyelids." But he does not tell us what temperature to use. Obviously, you would want to proceed with caution in irrigating over the closed eye.

"Hot irrigation of the eye has been proved to be more useful as a means of relieving even acute inflammatory troubles of the eye than cold applications."—*Kellogg.*

4 - Throat Irrigation - This is the same as "gargling."

"The application of very hot water by this means may be recommended in cases of chronic pharyngitis with tickling of the mucous membrane and dryness of the throat, irritation, hacking cough, and rawness, giving rise to frequent clearing of the throat or a tickling cough."—*Kellogg.*

In each of the above irrigations, it is important that it be done with great care, especially as hotter water is used.

— SECTION FIFTEEN —

DOUCHES (HAND-HELD SPRAYS)

WHAT IT IS—This is a spray or jet of water coming out of a flexible hose. Body parts needing a water therapy treatment are sprayed with water by another person who is standing nearby. The person receiving them must be ambulatory (able to walk about). This is NOT the modern meaning of the word: a washing out of an internal orifice.

EQUIPMENT NEEDED—There are three types of professional spray nozzles:

1 - The Jet Douche - A straight (or jet) nozzle lets the water flow out in a hard, solid jet of water. There is no spray to it.

2 - The Spray Douche - This nozzle is round like the sprinkler on a garden watering pot. It produces a circular spray of water that is similar to the showerhead in your bathroom shower.

3 - The Fan Douche - This nozzle also sprays; but, because it has a flattened head, the spray comes out in a fan or linear pattern.

You may be able to substitute a good garden hose changeable nozzle for the first two of the above three nozzles. Other equipment needed for the douches is a stool with an open seat (similar to a toilet seat).

HOW TO APPLY IT -

The Jet Nozzle - When percussion (a definite hitting on the skin) is wanted, the jet nozzle is used. Both cold water and percussion impact on the skin produce a strong thermic reaction in the body. This increases the vigor and permanency of the entire circulatory reaction.

The Spray Nozzle - This nozzle is used whenever percussion is not wanted. It can apply hot and cold to body parts just as well as the jet nozzle; but it does it without percussion.

The Fan Nozzle - This produces the lightest striking effect on the skin. It is best used when the tonic effects of the hot or cold water are not wanted. For example: when applying very cold water to sensitive surfaces, over painful nerves, and painfully inflamed body parts. A spray nozzle, turned on very low, would come the nearest to approximating the fan nozzle.

SPECIAL NOTE—There are (1) five basic douches (Hot, Neutral, Cold, Revulsive, and Alternate Hot and Cold), (2) thirteen local douches (Ascending, Head, Spinal [Dorsal], Lumbar, Shoulder, Thoracic, Epigastric, Hypogastric, Abdominal, Foot, Plantar, Perineal, and Anal), and (3) twelve reflexive.

These hand-held sprays are not included in this chapter in the Natural Remedies Encyclopedia, because they fill many pages and are generally used only by professionals. Most people would never use these (sprays) at home. Therefore this lengthy section is omitted from this *Encyclopedia.* If you wish this data, you would need to order a copy of the author's 204-page book, *The Water Therapy Manual.* They are explained on pp. 152-175 of that book. But the author wishes to assure you that you probably do not need that advanced data.

— SECTION SIXTEEN —
TEMPERATURE TABLES

Temperature is an important subject in water therapy. Here are several useful temperature formulas and tables:

FAHRENHEIT VS. CENTIGRADE—Only the Fahrenheit scale is used in this chapter because that is the thermal measure generally found in most homes. But centigrade has become the thermal standard of science and medicine. As you may know, centigrade is a graduation based on 0° C. at the freezing point of water, with 100° C. at its boiling point (at sea level). Fahrenheit is keyed to 32° F. as the freezing point of water, with 212° F. as its boiling point. (This is based on sea-level temperatures; higher altitudes will yield lower numbers.)

CONVERSION TABLE—Here is how to change one figure for the other:

To change centigrade to Fahrenheit, multiple the centigrade numeral by 9/5 and add 32 (example: 37° C. x 9/5 + 32 = 98.6° F.).

To change Fahrenheit to centigrade, subtract 32 from Fahrenheit numeral and multiply by 5/9 (example: 98.6° F. – 32 x 5/9 = 37° C.).

AVERAGE BATH TEMPERATURES—John Harvey Kellogg, M.D., in his book, *Rational Hydrotherapy*, also provides us with average bath temperatures:

Douche: cold, 50° to 70°, **60°**; hot, 104° to 125°, **115°**; neutral, 92° to 97°, **95°**.

Affusion: cold, 55° to 65°, **60°**; cool, 70° to 80°, **75°**; hot, 104° to 122°, **113°**.

Plunge: cold, 50° to 70°, **60°**.

Immersion: cold, 50° to 70°, **60°**; cool, 70° to 80°, **75°**; hot, 100° to 106°, **102°**; very hot, 104° to 115°; **108°**; neutral, 92° to 97°, **95°**.

Brand bath: **70° F.**

Shallow: cold, 50° to 65°, **60°**; cool, 70° to 80°, **75°**.

Cold wet-sheet pack: **60° F.**

Hot-blanket pack: **130° F.**

Sponge bath: 60° to 75°, **70°**.

Wet-hand rubbing: 45° to 75°, **60°**.

Cold towel rubbing: 40° to 75°, **60°**.

Wet-sheet rubbing: **60°**.

Hot-air bath: 110° to 180°, **160°**.

Local hot-air bath: 200° to 300°, **250°**.

Turkish bath: 140° to 250°, **180°**.

Russian bath: 110° to 140°, **125°**.

Vapor bath: 110° to 140°, **130°**.

Foot bath: cold, 45° to 65°, **55°**; hot, 105° to 120°, **115°**.

Sitz bath: cold, 55° to 65°, **60°**; hot, 105° to 120°, **115°**; neutral, 92° to 97°, **95°**.

Fomentation: 120° to 160°, **140°**.

–Kellog, "Rational Hydrotherapy" page 422.

COMMON NAMES FOR TEMPERATURE—People feel heat and cold differently. What is cool to one is cold to another. Here are some common names for the basic temperature graduations:

Very cold	32° - 55° F.
Cold	55° - 70° F.
Cool	70° - 80° F.
Tepid	80° - 92° F.
Neutral	94° - 97° F.
Warm	92° - 100° F.
Hot	100° - 104° F.
Very hot	104° F. and above

TESTING THE WATER—Here is how Kellogg tells us to quickly estimate water temperature:

"First, test the water to be sure it is not so hot it will burn you. Then test it further: The hand gives unreliable information respecting the temperature of water, but a more accurate judgment may be formed by plunging the whole arm to the elbow into the water, as the arm is usually protected by the clothing, and hence its temperature is more equable. When the temperature of the water is so high as to produce redness of the skin, it may be said to be hot. When there is simply a comfortable sensation of heat, it is warm. A lightly lower temperature is tepid. When the temperature is low enough to produce a goose-flesh appearance, it is cool; and a lower temperature is cold while a temperature which, within a few seconds, produces pain or numbness of the parts immersed is very cold. Water the temperature of which is so high that the hand can be held in but a fraction of a second, perhaps, is very hot."—*Kellogg, Rational Hydrotherapy, p. 49.*

BASIC BODY TEMPERATURES—Body temperature varies with different parts of the body and with the time of day. The temperature under the tongue (oral temperature) is usually 98.6° F. The temperature under the arm (axial temperature), at 2 p.m., may be 99.9° F.; and the temperature may be 96.7° F. at 2 a.m. A thermometer placed in the rectum (rectal temperature) is likely to be 0.5° to 0.75° F. above the oral. Body temperature is usually highest in the early evening and lowest at about 4 a.m. Changes in the range between 97.6° F. and 99° F. are usually not very important. Some people are always a little below or a little above normal. The temperature balance is upset more easily in children than in adults. Mouth temperature should not be taken for 10 minutes or more after a person has had hot or cold food or drink.

Here are several body temperature indications: 93° F.

CHART 1050: Temperatures at different ages; Respiration, Pulse, Temperature ratios is fatal (except in cholera). 94° F. is algid collapse. 96° F. is collapse. 98° F. is subnormal. 98.6° F. is normal. 101° F. is slight fever. 102° F. is moderate fever. 104° F. is severe fever. 105° F. is high fever and dangerous. 106° F. is intense fever. 107° F. is generally fatal, except in intermittent fever.

The God of heaven gave us water, not only to drink and bathe in, but also to help restore us to health when we become ill. How thankful we can be for such a wonderful blessing! Thank Him every day for this, and all the other blessings that He gives you.

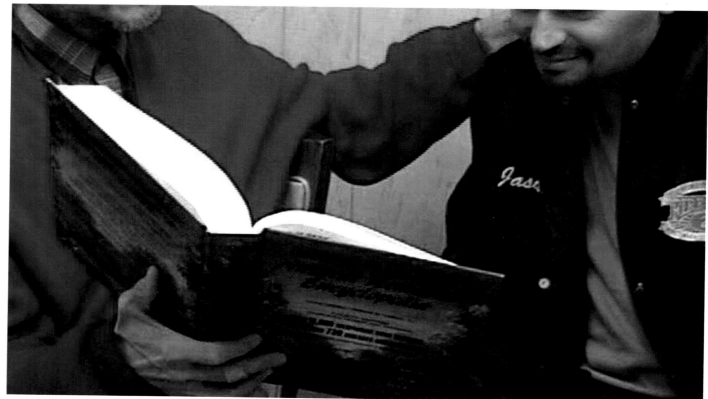

After undergoing countless water therapies (as shown in the color pictures all through this chapter), Jason said he is now totally well! In fact he wants a copy of the book for himself - so he can help still more people get well.

More Encouragement

"In the Saviour's manner of healing there were lessons for His disciples. On one occasion He anointed the eyes of a blind man with clay, and bade him, 'Go, wash in the pool of Siloam . . He went his way therefore, and washed, and came seeing.' John 9:7. The cure could be wrought only by the power of the Great Healer, yet Christ made use of the simple agencies of nature. While He did not give countenance to drug medication, He sanctioned the use of simple and natural remedies.

"To many of the afflicted ones who received healing, Christ said, 'Sin no more, lest a worse thing come unto thee.' John 5:14. Thus He taught that disease is the result of violating God's laws, both natural and spiritual. The great misery in the world would not exist did men but live in harmony with the Creator's plan.

"We should teach others how to preserve and to recover health. For the sick we should use the remedies which God has provided in nature, and we should point them to Him who alone can restore. It is our work to present the sick and suffering to Christ in the arms of our faith." — *Desire of Ages, 824*

Two editions of Desire of Ages, the classic (and best) book on the life of Christ are available from us.

DISEASE INDEX

This index only lists the conditions mentioned in the water therapies section *(pp. 273-275)*. In addition to them, you will want to check the Kellogg prescriptions for specific diseases in the main part of the *Encyclopedia*. They contain many, many suggestions of physical problems which water therapy can be used to relieve. You will find dozens of them scattered all through the 25 disease chapters of this *Encyclopedia*.

When turning to a therapy, read the entire section (example: Different Sponges are used for different fevers). Also check the related ones (example: the various Chest Packs). Some are better than others for certain conditions. You might prefer one to another (example: Oatmeal or Alkaline Bath instead of Soda Alkaline Bath). Also, by reading the entire section, you will find cautions (example: Hot Tub Bath). Be sure to carefully read all the principles and cautions at the front of this hydrotherapy section *(pp. 209-216). If you have a serious condition, see your physician!*

Topics are alphabetized; but, within a topic, the order is often arranged in book order, so you can easily turn pages and decide what you want to do (examples: pelvic, rheumatism). Water therapy is a wonderful blessing of God to mankind.

Alcoholic delirium: Neutral Wet-sheet Pack 229-231

Alcoholic intoxication: Alternate Compress 231

Alcoholism, chronic: Steam Bath 264

Alcoholism: Sweating Wet-sheet Pack 229-231

Alveolar Abscess: Hot Packs with Ice Bags 248

Ankle, sprained: Contrast Bath 255

Appendicitis: Hot Packs with Ice Bags 248

Arthritic joints, painful: Paraffin Bath 239

Arthritis, acute infectious: Ice Cravat 223

Arthritis, acute infectious: Ice Pack 223

Arthritis: Contrast Bath 255

Arthritis, rheumatoid: Ice Cravat 223

Anxiety: Neutral Tub Bath 259

Asthma: Heating Chest Pack 229

Black-and-blue swelling, prevent: Ice Cravat 223

Bed sores: Alternate Compress 231

Bile pain: Hot Trunk Pack 247

Bleeding, checks: Ice Bag 224

Blood poisoning in arm or leg: Contrast Bath 255

Boil, bring to a head: Poultices 243

Bowels, stimulate muscles of: Cold Sitz Bath 258

Brachial neuritis: Hot Shower 261

Bright's disease, acute: Full Hot Blanket Pack 245

Bright's disease: Steam Bath 262

Bronchial colds: Heating Chest Pack 227

Bronchitis, capillary: Sweating Wet-sheet Pack 229

Bronchitis, congestion in: Fomentation 234-237

Bronchitis: Vapor Inhalation 264

Burns: Ice Pack 223

Burns: Neutral Tub Bath 259

Bursitis: Ice Pack 223

Catarrhal jaundice: Abdominal Bandage 226

Cellulitis: Contrast Bath 255

Cellulitis: Revulsive Sitz Bath 258

Charcot's joint at the ankle: Contrast Bath 255

Chemical toxins, neutralize: Poultices 243

Chest cold: Vapor Inhalation 264

Chest congestion: Hot Foot bath 256

Chest congestion due to colds, bronchitis, pleurisy: Fomentation 234-237

Chilblains: Alternate Compress 231

Circulation, improve: Alternative Hot and Cold to Spine 234

Circulation, poor: Contrast Bath 255

Cold in the head: Vapor Inhalation 264

Colds, shorten length of: Hot Foot bath 256

Colds: Sweating Wet-sheet Pack 229-231

Congestion: Ice Bag 224

Congestion of internal organ: Ice Bag 224

Congestion, relieve internal: Fomentation 234-237

Congestion, various types: Revulsive Compress 232

Constipation: Abdominal Bandage 226

Contusions: Ice Cravat 223

Coughing: Vapor Inhalation 264

Croup: Heating Chest Pack 227

Diarrhea, chronic: Neutral Tub Bath 259

Dropsy of abdomen: Alternate Compress 231

Dropsy of chest: Alternate Compress 231

Drug reaction rashes: Soda Alkaline Bath 266

Dysmenorrhea: Very Hot Sitz Bath 258

Eclampsia: Full Hot Blanket Pack 245

Eclampsia: Ice Cravat 223

Eczema: Soda Alkaline Bath 266

Edema: Ice Cravat 223

Edema of legs: Contrast Bath 255

Edema, painful in limbs: Continuous Hot Shower 261

Eustachian tube inflammation: Throat Compress 225

Eye, painful affections of: Revulsive Compress 232

Feet, weak, pronated: Contrast Bath 255

Fever: Cold Compress 222

Fever: Ice Cravat 223

Fever, lower temperature of: Graduated Bath 261

Fever: Sponging 253

Fevers, childhood: Sweating Wet-sheet Pack 229-231

Fever, continued: Cooling Wet-sheet Pack 229-231

Fever, reduce high temperature of: Cooling Wet-sheet Pack 229-231

Gallstone pain: Full Hot Blanket Pack 245

Gangrene: Contrast Bath 255

Gout: Paraffin Bath 239

Gout: Steam Bath 262

Gout: Sweating Wet-sheet Pack 229

Headache, anemic: Alternate Hot

and Cold to Head 232

Headache, congestive: Cold Compress 222

Headache, congestive: Ice Cravat 223

Headache, congestive: Contrast Bath 255

Headache, congestive: Simultaneous Hot and Cold to Head 233

Head, improve circulation within: Alternate Hot and Cold to Head 232

Head, passive congestions in: Alternate Hot and Cold to Head 232

Heat rash: Soda Alkaline Bath 266

Hives: Soda Alkaline Bath 266

Hoarseness: Throat Compress 225

Indigestion, atonic: Abdominal Bandage 226

Infections: Contrast Bath 255

Inflammation: Ice Bag 224

Inflammation: Throat Compress 225

Influenza, respiratory type: Heating Chest Pack 227

Influenza: Sweating Wet-sheet Pack 229

Insanity: Neutral Tub Bath 259 (see Mania)

Insect bites and stings: Poultices 243

Insect bites and stings: Soda Alkaline Bath 266

Insomnia: Abdominal Bandage 226

Insomnia: Neutral Wet-sheet Pack 229-231

Insomnia: Neutral Tub Bath 195-259

Intestinal pain: Hot Trunk Pack 247

Itching: Soda Alkaline Bath 266

Joint conditions, painful: Joint Compress 226

Joint inflammation, acute: Ice Pack 223

Joints, stiff: Paraffin Bath 239

Kidney Congestion: Hot Packs with Ice Bags 248

Kidney insufficiency and congestion: Full Hot Blanket 245

Kidney pain: Hot Trunk Pack 247

Kidney stone attack: Kidney Stone Pack 241

Kidney stone pain: Full Hot Blanket Pack 245

Laryngitis: Throat Compress 225

Ligaments, torn: Ice Pack 223

Liver anemia: Abdominal Bandage 226

Lumbago, refractory: Continuous Hot Shower 261

Mania: Neutral Wet-sheet Pack 229

Mania: Neutral Tub Bath 259

Mastoiditis: Hot Packs with Ice Bags 248

Meningitis: Ice Cravat 223

Morphine-derivative poisoning, arousing from: Alternate Compress 231

Muscle tone, improve: Alternative Hot and Cold to Spine 234

Nasal passages, stuffy and painful: Heat Lamp 242

Nerve action, improve: Alternative Hot and Cold to Spine 234

Nervous exhaustion or irritability: Neutral Tub Bath 259

Neuralgia: Revulsive Compress 232

Neurasthenia: Abdominal Bandage 226

Neuritis, Brachial: Hot Shower 261

Neuritis, multiple: Neutral Tub Bath 259

Neuritis: Revulsive Compress 232

Nicotine elimination: Sweating Wet-sheet Pack 229-231

Nosebleed: Hot Foot bath 256

Obesity: Steam Bath 262

Obesity: Sweating Wet-sheet Pack 229-231

Pain from edema, sprains: Cold Compress 222

Pain, reduce swelling in: Ice Bag 224

Paralyzed limbs: Alternate Compress 231

Parametritis: Revulsive Sitz Bath 258

Pharyngitis: Throat Compress 225

Peritonitis: Hot Packs with Ice Bags 248

Pelvic cramps, relieve: Hot Foot bath 256

Pelvic congestion: Hot Foot bath 256

Pelvic circulation, stimulate: Cold Sitz Bath 258

Pelvic inflammations, hasten absorption of residual thickening

after: Cold Sitz Bath 258

Pelvic pain: Very Hot Sitz Bath 258

Pelvic problems—many different kinds: Sitz Bath 258

Plants, sensitivity to (nettles, etc.): Soda Alkaline Bath 266

Pleurisy, chronic: Alternate Compress 231

Pleurisy, congestion in: Fomentation 234

Pleurisy: Heating Chest Pack 227

Pneumonia, acute (early) stage only: Dry Chest Pack 229

Pneumonia: Alternate Compress 231

Pneumonia: Full Hot Blanket Pack 245

Pneumonia: Heating Chest Pack 227

Poison, absorb: Poultices 243

Poison ivy: Soda Alkaline Bath 266

Nocturia, prostatic hypertropic: Revulsive Sitz Bath 258

Pott's disease (TB of spine): Sunbath 267

Puerperal infections: Hot Packs with Ice Bags 248

Pus formation, avoid: Alternate Compress 231

Quinsy: Throat Compress 225

Respiratory colds: Heating Chest Pack 227

Restlessness: Neutral Wet-sheet Pack 229-231

Rheumatic fever: Ice Pack 223

Rheumatic fever: Joint Compress 226

Rheumatic fever, joint inflammation: Ice Cravat 223

Rheumatoid arthritis: Ice Cravat 223

Rheumatism, chronic: Steam Bath 262

Rheumatism: Joint Compress 226

Rheumatism, obese: Sweating Wet-sheet Pack 229-231

Rheumatism, muscular, relieve pain: Hot Tub Bath 259

Salpingitis, acute: Hot Packs with Ice Bags 248

Salpingitis: Revulsive Sitz Bath 258

Sciatica, acute: Revulsive Compress 232

Sciatica: Continuous Hot Shower 261

HYDRO

The objective of hydrotherapy is to bring the blood to, and remove it from, an affected area. This is because the healing life is in the blood. The life is not in the heart; for that is only a blood pump. It is not in the glands; they only supply regulating hormones. It is not in the bones, organs, or muscles. And it is not in the brain. That only has thinking areas and switching stations. Life ceases in the foot, brain, or heart when the blood no longer reaches it.

The Bible says that out of the heart flows life. That which flows from the heart is the blood; it contains the life.

"Keep thy heart with all diligence, for out of it are the issues of life [issues forth life]."—*Proverbs 4:23.*

Here is another passage which shows that the word, "issue," in the Bible means "to flow forth":

"A fiery stream issued and came forth from before Him."—*Daniel 7:10.*

So the healing power is in the blood. **When your leg or liver becomes afflicted with a disease, you need to move a fresh supply of blood into and out of that body part**, so it can heal more rapidly.

Water therapy is the best way to do this. Nothing else so efficiently and powerfully moves the blood into and out of a weakened, sickly body part.

The Bible says that the life within you is in your blood:

"For the life of the flesh is in the blood."—*Leviticus 17:11.*

Here are other Bible passages discussing the importance of the blood:

"For the life of the flesh is in the blood; and I have given it to you upon the altar to make an atonement for your souls: for it is the blood that maketh an atonement for the souls."—*Leviticus 17:11.*

"Without shedding of blood is no remission [of sin]."—*Hebrews 9:22.*

"The blood of Jesus Christ His Son cleanseth us from all sin."—*1 John 1:7.*

"Whosoever committeth sin transgresseth also the law: for sin is the transgression of the law. And ye know that He was manifested to take away our sins; and in Him is no sin."—*1 John 3:4-5.*

"Unto Him that loved us, and washed us from our sins in His own blood."—*Revelation 1:5.*

"For this is My blood of the new testament, which is shed for many for the remission of sins."—*Matthew 26:28.*

"Whom God hath set forth to be a propitiation through faith in His blood."—*Romans 3:25.*

"In whom we have redemption through His blood."—*Ephesians 1:7, Colossians 1:14.*

"Now the God of peace, that brought again from the dead our Lord Jesus, that Great Shepherd of the sheep, through the Blood of the Everlasting Covenant, make you perfect in every good work to do His will, working in you that which is well-pleasing in His sight, through Jesus Christ; to whom be glory for ever and ever. Amen."—*Hebrews 13:20-21.*

GEN

SPECIAL INFORMATION YOU CAN USE

It is helpful to be able to compare symptoms and physical indicators which are able to differentiate between different diseases, show their progress, or provide other useful information.

There are 39 very helpful Disease Comparison (and other) Charts near the back of this Encyclopedia. In the coming years, you will find many of these charts to be extremely helpful as you minister to the needs of your sick family and friends.

ALL OF THE CHARTS HAVE BEEN CROSS REFERENCED TO THE BOOK

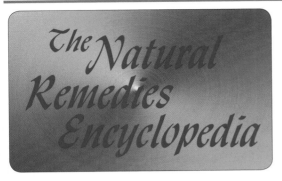

- Disease Section 1 -
Generalized Problems

 # = Information, not a disease

"In all thy ways acknowledge Him, and He shall direct thy paths."
—Proverbs 3:6

FOR MORE NATURAL REMEDIES:
HERBS: Herb Contents (pp. 129-130) will help
    you locate the 126 most important herbs and
    the diseases each one can treat. How to pre-
    pare herbs (132). How to use them (141-189)
HYDROTHERAPY: Therapy Contents (pp. 206-
    207) and its Disease Index (263-265) will
    lead you to over 100 water therapies and
    many more remedies. DIS. INDEX: 1211- /
    GEN. INDEX: 1222-

VITAMINS AND MINERALS: Contents (100-101).
    Using 101-124. Dosages (124). Others (117-
)
CARING FOR THE SICK: Home care for a sick
    person (28-36). The healing crisis (36-39)
WOMEN'S SECTIONS: Female Organs (672)
    Pregnancy (701). Childbirth (765). Infancy,
    Childhood (722). Women's Herbs (754, 760)
EMERGENCIES: (973-). FIRST AID: (990-)

Section 1 - General

G
E
N

GENERAL - 1 - FATIGUE

DEBILITY
(Weak, Debilitated Conditions)

SYMPTOMS—A feeling of exhaustion all, or much, of the time.

CAUSES—This can be caused by **a number of dietetic, physical, or hormonal problems**. Some of which are mentioned below. See *Chronic Fatigue (279-280)* for much more information.

NATURAL REMEDIES

• Some weak individuals only need **rest, fresh air, sunshine, pure water, nutritious meals, and freedom from worry**.

• **Clean the toxins** from the body. You may feel weaker for a few days. But, afterward, you will generally feel much better and stronger.

• **Over-indulgence** in sex debilitates the body. **Worry** wears out the life forces. The use of **coffee, tea, tobacco, alcohol, and processed and junk foods** are also sources of trouble.

• A good program of better nutrition, more rest, less tension, and **taking time to go outdoors and work or walk** 30-60 minutes at a time will do much to build the body.

• A **cold morning shower** invigorates the body.

• You may have **chemical or food sensitivities**. People today are exposed to enormous numbers of chemicals. Try to find what is causing your problem: in your food, your home, your environment.

• **Do not smoke** or be around smokers.

• **Avoid chocolate, soft drinks, caffeine, and highly processed foods**.

• Include **vitamin C** (2,000 mg) **and magnesium** (350 mg) in your diet. Eat lots of **green foods**. Drink **plenty of water** each day.

• Trust in God, obey the Ten Commandments, and live as healthfully as you can.

HERBS

• In some cases the whole digestion must be rebuilt. There can be a speedy recovery with **juice therapy** alone or with **slippery elm gruel.** Other nutritional herbs such as **Irish moss or comfrey** may be used successfully.

• As an aid in rebuilding the body after acute or

chronic illnesses, the following **herbal formula** is quite helpful. It combines nutritional benefits with herbal tonics. Mix together 1 oz. **parsley root**, 1 oz. **alfalfa**, and ½ oz. of each of the following: **dandelion root, comfrey root, yellow dock root, burdock root, nettles leaves, and dulse**. Place in an uncovered pot with a quart of water and simmer for 20 minutes. Let it cool, then strain. Place the liquid back in the pot and simmer uncovered for one hour or until it is reduced to one cup. Stir in one cup of unsulphured blackstrap molasses and refrigerate. Take one Tbsp. 3 times a day.

• Or take the above powdered, mixed, dry herbs (not having gone through the cooking stage). **Place them in #00 capsules** and take 2-4 capsules with each meal.

• Mix the following herbs well: 5 parts **white poplar bark**; 1 part each of **barberry bark, balmony bark** and ½ part: **golden seal, cloves**; ¼ part: **cayenne**. Add **honey**. Put 1 heaping Tbsp. into 1 quart boiling, distilled water. Cover and steep 15 minutes. Strain and sweeten to taste.

HYDROTHERAPY

• **Water treatments** are explained in the chapter on hydrotherapy *(206-275)*. These will increase endurance. Tonic frictions include **Wet-hand Rub, Cold Mitten Friction, Cold Towel Rub, Wet-sheet Rub, Dripping Sheet Rub, Ice Rub, and Salt Glow**.

• In cases of severe exhaustion: **Bed rest** for a time, **proper diet**, plus carefully graduated (increasing) **tonic cold applications** will provide needed help.

—Also see Emotional Fatigue Syndrome (bellow), Chronic Fatigue (279), Epstein-Barr Virus (280), and Neurasthenia (551). Also see Depression (596).

ENCOURAGEMENT—No one understands, as well as Jesus, your problems. He is watching over you. If you are willing to be guided by Him, He will throw around you influences for good that will enable you to accomplish all His will for you. Psalm 27:1.

EMOTIONAL FATIGUE SYNDROME

SYMPTOMS—A variety of symptoms could be involved: continual tension and stress, anxiety, depression, loss of interest, no zest for life, inability to cope with everyday problems, mental and physical fatigue, loss of confidence, fear of failure, panic attacks, a sense of hopelessness, mood swings, muscle spasms, sensitivity to noise, negative attitudes, and constant worrying.

CAUSES—Emotional stress depletes the nervous system, weakens emotional stability, and fatigues the body. Such stress weakens the functions of the body organs (such as the stomach and liver). This in turn results in malnourishment and a release of toxins into the system. Primary causes would include **constipation, autointoxication, nutritional deficiencies, a negative outlook** on people and circumstances, and **negative input** from other people.

NATURAL REMEDIES

• Learn to **relax**, as well as **exercise outdoors**. Do everything with an attitude of thankfulness toward, and trust in, God, believing that He will work everything out for the best.

• Eat **nutritious, high-fiber foods**: fruits, vegetables, sprouts, grains, nuts, seeds, beans, and drink juices.

• **Vitamin A** (5,000 IU), **vitamin D** (1,000 IU), **vitamin C** (2,000 mg), and **vitamin E** (400 IU) are important. Take a multivitamin tablet twice a day. Make sure you are getting enough **calcium** (2,000 mg), **magnesium** (1,000 mg), **and potassium** (1,000 mg).

• **For more natural remedies**, go to *Chronic Fatigue (bellow), Epstein-Barr Virus (280), and Neurasthenia (551).*

ENCOURAGEMENT—Learn all you can about the laws of health and obey them. Nothing is apparently more helpless, yet really more invincible, than the soul that feels its nothingness and relies wholly on Jesus for help. God can help you. Psalm 55:22.

CHRONIC FATIGUE

SYMPTOMS—A continual feeling of exhaustion.

CAUSES—Fatigue is a symptom pointing to other problems; it is not a disease of itself. Chronic fatigue is generally caused by a high-fat and refined carbohydrate diet, along with emotional stress. Any of the following only adds to the exhaustion: drugs, caffeine products, smoking, alcohol, poor eating habits.

Chronic fatigue can forewarn of an undetected problem such as anemia, hypoglycemia, diabetes, allergies, malabsorption of nutrients, candidiasis, poor circulation, hypothyroidism, Epstein-Barr virus (EBV), mononucleosis, or cancer.

It can also be caused by weight loss; obesity; and, if characterized only by a lack of energy, boredom.

Fatigue is usually caused by insufficient oxygen in the body through diet, wearing synthetic clothes, or through improper breathing. It may be caused by being in congested areas, where there is insufficient good air for breathing. The oxygen supply to the body is very important because waste matter accumulates if there is a lack of oxygen to every cell. Overeating also robs the body of the oxygen that should be distributed to various other places. Not only should one use proper herbs and proper foods to rebuild the body, but it is also necessary to take steps to avoid overtiring the body and learn the science of breathing properly.

NATURAL REMEDIES

• Obtain adequate **rest, exercise, and a well-balanced diet**. Eat a well-balanced diet of 50% raw foods and fresh **"live" juices**, especially carrot juice. **Wheatgrass juice** is also recommended for fatigue. Eat a supplement rich in **chlorophyll**: chlorella, Green-Life, Kyo-Green, etc.

• Deficiencies of **vitamin B complex, vitamin C** (2,000 mg), **vitamin D** (1,000 IU), **or iron** (50 mg) may cause fatigue. Also needed: **vitamins A** (1,000 IU), **pantothenic acid** (50 mg), **vitamin B$_{12}$** (1,000 mcg), **folic acid** (5 mg), **iron** (50 mg), **calcium** (2,000 mg), **and magnesium** (1,000 mg). **Acidophilus** is very helpful in improving digestion and the production of certain B vitamins in the bowel.

• **Exercise** everyday outdoors. Try to induce some perspiration.

• Many experts agree that **a vegetarian diet** can greatly reduce chronic fatigue.

• Helpful herbs include **American ginseng, lavender, rosemary, sweet flag, pasqueflower**.

• Brigham tea, carrot juice, cayenne, ginseng, grape juice, lobelia, sarsaparillas.

• Combining several **antiviral herbs** has been successful in many cases. Select several from among **goldenseal, echinacea, licorice, lemon balm, and ginger**. Make a tea using a tsp. or two of 2 or 3 of these, and drink a cup 2 or 3 times a day.

• Improving your **immune system** is important; since with CFS (Chronic Fatigue Syndrome) it is easier for you to become sick. **Astragalus and echinacea** increase immune function and are good for cold and flu symptoms. (But do not use astragalus if you have a fever.)

• In case of **parasites**, use **garlic, gentian root, fresh ginger root, or quassia chips** to help eliminate them.

• In case of **infection**, do this: At the first signs of a sore throat, take a few drops of alcohol-free **goldenseal** extract, hold it in your mouth for a moment, then swallow. Do not use goldenseal for more than a week at a time; during pregnancy; or if you have cardiovascular disease, diabetes, or glaucoma.

• If a **viral infection** occurs, do not take aspirin, for you could develop Reyes' Syndrome *(750)*.

• Many people with CFS are infected with **candida** *(281)*. Take **pau d'arco** in capsule or tea form to counteract this. Adding **acidophilus** to your diet also helps.

• Water therapies are helpful: **ice-cold footbaths, daily morning barefoot grass walks, alternative hot and** cold showers, "salt glow" skin rubs, and a dry-friction rub with a skin brush.

• **Change your way of life.** You will have to make some changes in order to live with this problem. **Reduce stress.** Researchers have found that stress reduces immune function, resulting in many of the changes that occur in chronic fatigue syndrome. Stress can even increase vulnerability for a viral infection or for reactivation of latent viruses, such as herpes. **Get more rest**, especially during flare-ups. This will involve some scheduling changes. **Exercise lightly.** Although too much physical activity can trigger a relapse, too little can weaken skeletal and heart muscles, further aggravating fatigue. **Eat carefully of good food.** Eat a varied whole-food diet that includes ample protein and complex carbohydrates. Avoid junk food. Frequent, small meals will help you maintain energy levels. **Avoid stimulants**. Stay away from caffeine, black tea, and coffee. **Stop smoking.** Avoid secondhand smoke. Both smoking and secondhand smoke increase susceptibility to respiratory tract infections, reduce how much oxygen gets to your cells, and weaken your immune system.

HERBAL RECIPE—In Chinese medicine, a strong tea of the reishi mushroom is used as a remedy for fatigue. Here is the formula: one-third ounce chopped or powdered reishi mushroom and 3 cups of water.

Combine the water and mushroom in a pot with a lid. Bring to a boil. reduce the heat, cover and simmer for 30 minutes. Strain. Drink in divided doses throughout the day; refrigerate for up to three days.

• **For more natural remedies**, go to *Emotional Fatigue (278)* and *Epstein-Barr Virus (bellow). Also see Depression (596).*

ENCOURAGEMENT—The whole family of heaven is interested in the family here below, messengers from the throne of God attend our steps every day. They seek to protect us from our mistakes amid the problems we daily encounter. By faith in Christ, obey God's Ten Commandments and know that He will work everything out for the best. 2 Peter 1:3-4.

EPSTEIN-BARR VIRUS
(Chronic Fatigue Syndrome)

SYMPTOMS—Recurrent upper-respiratory tract infections, exhaustion, extreme fatigue, sore throat, swollen lymph nodes, achy joints and muscles, memory loss, low-grade fevers, headaches, poor concentration, night sweats, irritability, and deep depression. Because the symptoms resemble flu and other viral symptoms, EBV is not always diagnosed correctly. In fact, it is frequently misdiagnosed as hypochondria, depression, or psychosomatic illness.

CAUSES—Chronic fatigue syndrome is caused by the Epstein-Barr virus (EBV). This condition has become widespread in America. The CDC in Atlanta estimates that tens of thousands of people are infected with it. Yet they are unaware of it, since symptoms are frequently not prominent.

This virus is also the cause of infectious mononucleosis. When mononucleosis occurs, the person becomes very ill for two to four weeks or longer if the diet is not corrected. *See Mononucleosis (664).*

EBV is a type of herpes virus, and is related to the viruses that cause genital herpes and shingles.

Keep in mind that chronic fatigue syndrome can also be caused by certain other factors: **candida albicans (yeast infection), anemia, chronic mercury poisoning from dental amalgam tooth fillings, hypoglycemia, insomnia, and hypothyroidism.** *(All of the above problems are dealt with in articles in this book.)*

Once EBV is contracted, it always remains in the body. Fortunately, most people develop antibodies to it. The problem occurs when they become rundown and overworked—and then the dormant EBV strikes. It is more likely to reveal its presence when other diseases are also present, such as **arthritis, lupus, multiple sclerosis, cancer, or AIDS.**

EBV causes the body to overreact, resulting in a burnout of the immune system.

Epstein-Barr virus is very contagious, and can be transmitted by **close contact, kissing, sharing food, coughing, and through sex.**

Blood tests for antibodies against candida albicans and EBV are available for specific diagnosis. Yet the fact remains that EBV symptoms are similar to those of many infections, anemia, parasites, endocrine diseases, and AIDS.

NATURAL REMEDIES

• Antibiotics do not help, since EBV is a virus. Recovery takes time, rest, and good nutrition. Drink **lots of water**, at least 8 glasses a day. **Regularity** in bowel movements is essential. Add **fiber** to the diet. **Cleansing enemas** should be used occasionally.

• It is vital that you get **plenty of rest**. Throughout the day, take relaxation breaks. If possible, try to lay down and rest before meals.

• **Exercise each day** is invigorating. Keep taking a little more. Outdoors exercise is best. Avoid overexertion, but also avoid being too sedentary. You will not recover by remaining in bed!

• Use your energy carefully. **Do not overdo** and then collapse for a time. You may have exhausted adrenal glands.

• Your problem may be partly or wholly caused by the **prescription drugs** you are taking.

DIET

• **Remove** from the diet all junk foods, processed foods, fried foods, stimulants (coffee, tea, soft drinks, sugar), and white-flour products (bread, spaghetti, etc.).

• It is said that 60 percent of those with EBV also have **candida** *(see Candidiasis)*; therefore it is best to eat some form of acidophilus. **Eliminate sugar, alcohol, mushrooms, all fungi, molds, yeast, fermented foods such as sauerkraut, soy sauce, dry roasted nuts, po-**

tato chips, soda pop, bacon, pork, lunch meats, and all types of cheese**.

• Eat some brand of **"greens" tablets. Chlorophyll** is vital to proper diet and healing. Make **green drinks** from whizzed up greens and pineapple juice.

• Take 2,000 mg **vitamin C**, twice a day, and 400 mg **magnesium** daily.

OTHER

• Take **no aspirin**, since it may induce Reye's Syndrome *(750)* in children.

• Helpful herbs include **red clover**, to cleanse the blood; **echinacea**, to help the glands; **garlic**, as an antibiotic; and **saffron**, to help reduce pain.

• Epstein-Barr can be combatted with massive doses of **vitamin C**, immediately **followed by exercise**.

• **For more natural remedies**, go to *Emotional Fatigue (278)* and *Chronic Fatigue (279)*.

• **Similar symptoms:** *Lyme Disease (840), Chronic Fatigue Syndrome (279),* and *Neurasthenia (551)*.

ENCOURAGEMENT—The heart that has once tasted the love of Christ cries out continually for a deeper draught. How thankful we can be for His love and care over us. Hebrews 10:19-20.

CANDIDIASIS
(Yeast Infection, Candida, Thrush, Chronic Fatigue Syndrome)

SYMPTOMS—Symptoms include bad breath, constipation, chronic infections, depression, fatigue, food cravings, gas, headaches, adrenal and thyroid problems, hiatal hernias, indigestion, insomnia, mental confusion, discomforting odors, panic attacks, and menstrual problems. Vaginal infection produces intense itching, accompanied by an odorless, white, cheesy discharge.

CAUSES—This is an infection caused by *candida albicans*, a normally harmless yeast *(saprophyte)* found in your intestines. Some of it is also regularly found in your mouth, throat, and genital tract. But this organism goes wild when its competitors, the normal bacteria of the intestines, are killed by **long-term use of antibiotics**. This enables the candida to greatly increase in number. Yeast infection is caused by a group of yeast-like fungi called candida. The most common of these is *Candida albicans*, but it is not the only one. Yeast live on moist areas of the body, such as the lining of the mouth and the vagina.

In the vagina, the ailment is caused by an alteration of the normal **pH balance** from slightly acid to more alkaline.

Stress causes a reduced production of stomach acid, which lets candida enter the stomach—a place where it normally is never found. As a result, less digested food enters the intestines, much to the liking of the candida which feeds upon it.

Several modern **prescription drugs** cause yeast infection. **Sugary and junk food** adds to the problem.

This yeast-like substance proliferates so massively that it enters the bloodstream and is carried to many parts of the body, weakening the immune system and causing various problems.

In the oral cavity, candida is called *thrush*. White sores may develop on the tongue, gums, and inside the cheeks.

In the vagina, it results in *vaginitis (695)*. Large amounts of a white, cheesy discharge and intense itching occur.

Other effects are *food allergies (858-860), athlete's foot (377), ringworm (335), jock itch (335),* and even *diaper rash (727)*.

Candida is not transmitted sexually, but mothers may pass thrush on to their newborn children. The baby's tongue will appear red and be covered with white spots (generally noticed 8-9 days after delivery) that will appear like milk spots. On the buttocks, thrush may resemble diaper rash. *See Infant Thrush (732)*.

Three out of four adult females have at least one attack of candidia. Because their vaginal environment is more conducive to the growth of yeast, women with **diabetes** can contract candida easier than diabetic men.

You may wish to request a blood test for antibodies against *candida albicans*. A skin test, similar to a TB test, is also available. A positive result confirms that you have candidiasis. But a negative skin test may not be reliable. Candida is difficult to diagnose, since a culture cannot be used. This is because this yeast is a normal constituent of everyone's intestines.

• Although drugstores now boast several competing brands of over-the-counter yeast infection cures, it's important to be sure **what kind of vaginal infection you have**. Why? Some infections can be transmitted sexually, so your partner could inadvertently reinfect you. And some microorganisms can travel up the fallopian tubes, causing painful pelvic inflammatory disease (PID), which can have an impact on fertility and future health.

The most common vaginal infections are:

• **Yeast infections**—This is caused by the yeast organism, *Candida albicans*. Once you've had one of these, you seldom forget the symptoms—white curdish discharge and a miserable itch. If you are experiencing your first yeast infection, however, it's a good idea to consult a doctor for a diagnosis; so you'll know your own symptoms in case of a recurrence.

• **Trichomoniasis**—This is caused by a protozoan.

This infection produces yellowish discharge and a burning itch, occasionally accompanied by frequent, burning urination.

• **Bacterial vaginosis**—This common vaginal infection is often caused by the bacterium, *Gardnerella vaginalis*. This infection can spread to the uterus and fallopian tubes. It's usually accompanied by a thin, gray or greenish discharge.

NATURAL REMEDIES

THINGS TO AVOID

• Try to eliminate **food allergies, hypoglycemia, any infections,** and **indigestion**.

• The **woodpile** by the woodburning stove and fireplace can be a problem; for all wood contains fungi.

• Do not use **insecticides, tobacco,** or **perfumes**.

• Avoid **damp, moldy environments**. Do not use **oral contraceptives** while you have candida.

• Avoid **antibiotics** and **steroids**, because they destroy the competing bacteria and allow candida to overgrow. Avoid **birth control pills** and **cortisone types of drugs**, including Prednisone.

• Do not use the following foods: **Sugary foods, Cheese, alcohol, chocolate, fermented food, gluten grains (wheat, oats, rye, and barley). Meat, pickles, raw mushrooms, vinegar, or any yeast products**.

• Yeast thrives on sugars and carbohydrates. A **vegetarian nondairy diet of protein, unrefined grains, and vegetables** is best. **Onions** and **garlic** are very helpful. Fresh, raw garlic is the best. Avoid meat-based proteins, since these are associated with abnormal bowel flora development. **Avoid yeasted grain foods**.

FOODS

Stay on a **low carbohydrate** diet. Lower it to 80 grams per day. A yeast-infected person may crave such foods. Limit the use of all **yeast foods**; this includes mushrooms, baked goods containing baker's yeast, and foods enriched with vitamins (often made from brewer's yeast). Only use B vitamin supplements from rice bran. **Avoid** mushrooms, **fermented foods** and drinks (sauerkraut, ginger ale, alcohol), **foods with molds** (yogurt, sour cream, buttermilk, all cheeses), **malted products**, and **dried fruit**. Avoid **milk products** (because of lactose in them).

• **These foods inhibit candida** growth: **garlic, broccoli, turnips, kale, collards, cabbage. Safe foods include millet, brown rice, whole grains, beans, and vegetables. Almonds and nuts** are okay, but avoid peanuts.

• **Clean all fresh foods** carefully to remove chemicals, sprays, bacteria, and fungi. Add fiber to the diet; it helps clean the colon.

NUTRIENTS

• **Replant** *Lactobacillus acidophilus*. This is the friendly bacteria in your intestines which the "wonder drugs" you earlier took killed off. Lactobacillus is a primary competitor of candida for food in the intestines. It also helps keep the colon slightly acid. Use a retention enema containing 4 oz. warm water and 10 billion organisms (empty twenty 500,000 organism capsules into the water). Use 3 times weekly, 10 minutes each time. Acidophilus is a preventive and remedy.

• Useful **nutrients** include vitamin **B complex** with extra biotin (100 mg, 3 times a day) and B_{12} lozenges. Place 2,000 mcg lozenges under tongue 3 times a day, between meals. Take **vitamin C** to bowel tolerance (up to 5,000 mg) and **essential fatty acids** such as wheat germ oil (2 Tbsp.), primrose oil, **garlic capsules** (2 capsules, 3 times a day), etc.

• Also helpful: **vitamin A** (25,000 IU, 1-2 times a day, for a week), B_6 (100-250 mg, 1-2 times, daily), **vitamin E** (400-800 IU, daily), **biotin**, and aloe vera juice (2 oz., four times per day).

DIET

• Eat **vegetables** and **gluten-free grains**, such as brown rice and millet. Also some **fiber** (oat bran or flax seed). Eat **plain** (unsweetened) **yogurt**.

HERBS

• Important: *Also see Antifungal Herbs (299) for important information.*

• **Helpful herbs** include **burdock, echinacea, ginger, goldenseal, bee pollen, kelp, lobelia, passionflower, pau d'arco, psyllium, slippery elm, ginkgo, and suma**.

• The immune-stimulating action of **echinacea** is particularly helpful for treating yeast infection. In a German study, 60% of those who took prescription antifungal drugs had yeast recurrences; but only 10% of those who took echinacea had yeast recurrences.

• Also very good is **garlic**, which is an antibacterial, antifungal antibiotic. Take up to a dozen raw, chopped cloves 2-3 times a day in juice. It is not easy to take, but effective. Blend it with carrots and it is much easier to take. **Cranberry juice** is also opposed to candida; so try taking your garlic with that.

• **Goldenseal** contains the antibiotic berberine, which is very effective against yeast. Other helpful antibiotics include **Oregon grape** and **pau d'arco**.

• **Aloe vera** juice increases white blood cell ability to kill yeast germs.

• **Pau d'arco** (other names are lapacho and taheebo) can help destroy the candida. If it does not agree with you, switch to **clove tea**. The ideal is to alternate between the two; for they nicely supplement one another. **Maitake tea** is another good alternative to pau d'arco.

• **Wild oregano oil** is another powerful antiseptic for killing fungi.

• **Olive leaf extract** is a good healer of microbial infections.

MORE HELP

• Place plain **yogurt in the vagina**, or mix one small pan of plain yogurt with an equal amount of water and use it as a douche once or twice daily until the problem is solved. Another way is to open two capsules of acidophilus and add it to a douche. This helps inhibit the growth of the fungus.

• Wear **white cotton underwear**, instead of synthetic fibers which trap the fungus and help it grow in body openings. Change underclothing daily.

• Avoid **household chemicals; cleaners; chlorinated water; mothballs; and damp and moldy places**, such as basements.

• High levels of **mercury** in the body can induce candida. If necessary, have the mercury (**amalgum**) fillings taken out of your teeth.

• **Important: Read** Vaginitis (695), which is very similar. You will there find additional natural remedies against albicans. Also see Chronic Fatigue Syndrome (279), which has similar symptoms.

ENCOURAGEMENT—God's love for His people is infinite. His care for His people is unending.

JET LAG

SYMPTOMS—Fatigue, lethargy, irritability, inability to sleep, trouble concentrating and making decisions, perhaps even diarrhea and a lack of appetite.

CAUSES—Circadian rhythms control your daily cycles of sleep and certain other body functions. **Jetting across several time zones** produces a sudden violation of your body's inner clock. If, from America for example, you fly to Australia or Europe, you will experience jet lag; for you will suddenly be thrust into meals and wakefulness in the middle of "your night" and awake when your body tells you it is time for sleep. North-south trips only produce normal weariness. Traveling westward more than two time zones often results in exhaustion, diminished alertness, disorientation, irritability, loss of appetite, sleepiness during the day, wakefulness at night, and perhaps constipation or diarrhea.

NATURAL REMEDIES

Advance preparation: 1-3 weeks before traveling to a warmer climate, start eating more of **the foods** you will eat at your destination. Start eating **meals closer to the time** you will eat them when you arrive.

TAKING THE TRIP

• Get **extra sleep** beforehand. Drink **plenty of fluids** and be **quiet and relaxed** during the flight. **Fly by day**, arrive at night, and then soak up some **extra rest**. You tend to dehydrate in the plane; so drink enough water: 32 oz. for every 6 hours of flying. But **no coffee or alcohol**; they are both diuretic and flush fluids from the body. Frequently **walk up and down the aisle** in order to avoid the blood clots that can develope in your legs on long trips (especially across the Pacific). Try to break up a long flight by a **one-day layover**. **Do not smoke**. Doing so puts carbon monoxide in your blood; and, at 5,000 feet (the altitude the cabin is pressurized to), you

will have a 10,000 foot oxygen lack. Keep away from others who smoke. **Eat lightly, avoiding heavy proteins, refined starches, and sweet deserts**. If you fly at night: **Eat before you fly** and avoid the meal served. **Put on eyeshades** and stimulate a normal bedtime. It works!

WHEN YOU ARRIVE

• Get out in the **sunshine** the next day; this will help your body adapt. Obtain some **exercise** after arriving. Try to **walk outside in the sunlight,** to help reset your inner clock. If going from west to east, take that walk the next morning in order to help shift your body. Some people try living by their home clock—but most cannot do that. **Do not take a sleeping pill** when you arrive. It will usually cause a hangover or grogginess. Take a 500 mcg **melatonin** tablet.

• Try to **avoid important decisions** during the adjustment days. The general rule is that it will take one day of adjustment for each time zone crossed. So be prepared. If it is a short stay, remain on **home time**.

• When crossing only two or three time zones, it is known that going west is easier on the body than going east. This is because it is easier to get more sleep on arriving, since you experience more hours that particular day.

ENCOURAGEMENT—We should ever seek to realize that the Lord is very near to us. He can help us as no other one can. Trusting Him and obeying His Word, we can have the help we need. Isaiah 12:2.

TONIC EFFECTS, OBTAINING

HYDRO—In the section on hydrotherapy (231-234), **Hot and Cold to the Spine** is a revulsive compress and acts as a strong stimulant and tonic; it is used in a large number of conditions needing such a treatment.

The **Wet-hand Rub, the Cold Mitten Friction, the Cold-towel Rub, the Wet-sheet Rub, the Dripping Sheet Rub, and the Ice Rub** are all used to increase body circulation and heat. The first four are the mildest and best.

The **Revulsive Shower** and **Alternate Hot and Cold Shower** are also beneficial.

The **Sun Bath** and **Sea Bathing** are helpful.

The **Sun, Air, and Water Bath; Wet Grass Walk; and Summer Spray** are equally useful.

Caution should be exercised in giving the above treatments if the patient is frail, diabetic, or has a heart condition. See the Hydrotherapy section of this Encyclopedia for much more information on these and other invaluable water treatments. (206-275).

ENCOURAGEMENT—It is God's plan that we live pure, clean lives and living only to honor Him.

TONIC HERBS

Back in old times, every spring our forebears would clean up the house and take a spring tonic in order to clean and rejuvinate their bodies after the rigors of winter.

Spring tonic: 8 oz. **sarsaparilla root**, 2 oz. **licorice root**, 1 oz. **burdock root**, 3 tsp. **senna leaves**, 1 oz. **cascara or sacred bark**, fluid extract, 5 oz. **glycerine**.

Spring tonic: 1 part **sarsaparilla**, 1 part **sassafras**, ½ part **mezereon bark**, ½ part **guaiac**. Make it into a decoction and simmer for 10 minutes. Dosage would be ½ cup or more, 3-4 times a day.

Spring tonic: 1 part each of the following: **senna, juniper berries, celandine, sarsaparilla, dandelion root, uva ursi, spikenard, burdock root, yellow dock**.

Hops tonic: 1 oz. each of **buchu leaves, hops, dandelion root**, and 1 tsp. **ginger**. Boil the hops and dandelion root slowly for 30 minutes in 1 gallon water. Add 1 lb. honey. Bring to a second boil and skim off impurities. Pour the hot mixture over the buchu and ginger. Cover tightly and steep until cool. Strain, bottle, and keep in a cool place.

General tonic: ½ oz. each of **gentian root, calumba root, licorice root, Peruvian bark**, 1/3 tsp. **cayenne**. Simmer in a covered container for 15 minutes in 1 quart of water. Cool, strain, and give 1 teacup every 3 hours during the day.

Whole body tonic: Here is a tonic which can be used daily as a dietary supplement. It will increase the vitality of the entire body, especially its resistance to disease and ability to rebound from illness or poor health. Mix equal amounts of the following herbal powders: **sarsaparilla root, Siberian ginseng, gotu kola, fo-ti, licorice root, saw palmetto berries, kelp, stillingia, alfalfa**, plus a pinch of **cayenne**. Place in capsules and take 2-12 daily. Use more during periods of convalescence, poor health, or heightened stress.

— Also see *Stomach Tonic (444)*.

ENCOURAGEMENT—In the plan of redemption, God has revealed His love to mankind in a sacrifice so broad and deep and high that it is immeasurable.

LINIMENTS

This is a liniment which can be rubbed onto a person's skin, to help relax and invigorate him. Apply one of the following formulas with a gentle friction of the hand. A liniment is usually thicker than water, but thinner than an ointment, and is usually applied as a liquid at the temperature of the body.

Stimulating liniment: 1 part oil of **cloves**, 1 part **oil of cinnamon**, 1 part **oil of sassafras**. Mix and then massage well into the affected areas.

Relaxing and stimulating liniment: 4 oz. **ladies slipper**, fluid extract; 4 oz. **lobelia**, fluid extract; 1 oz.

oil of sassafras. Mix together well. Massage well into the affected area.

Camphorated oil: Purchase **camphor** (USP grade) from the drug store, and dissolve 1 oz. in 4 fl. oz. **olive oil**. This is good oil for sprains, bruises, pain relief, rheumatic or gouty joint pains. Check for skin sensitivity to camphor before using.

Vinegar liniment for rheumatism: Pour 1 tsp. **oil of wintergreen** into 1 pint **apple cider vinegar**. Soak a folded cloth in the fluid, wring out, and apply. The wintergreen will bring blood to the area, and the vinegar reduces pain. First check for skin sensitivity to the wintergreen oil. It can also be applied to a sore throat in a wrung-out compress, covered with a larger, dry wool cloth or large sock, and pinned so no air penetrates all night long.

ENCOURAGEMENT—If you have given yourself to Christ, you are a member of the family of God, and everything in the Father's house is for you. What a promise this is! May we each one prove faithful to the end. Romans 2:7, 10-11.

"As many as received Him, to them gave He power to become the sons of God, even to them that believe on His name." John 1:12.

GENERAL -   2 - NAUSEA

NAUSEA

SYMPTOMS—A sick feeling in the stomach, similar to motion sickness.

CAUSE—The problem has a number of origins—such as bilious attacks, pregnancy, undigested food, etc. A variety of things can induce nausea, including **nutritional deficiencies, food intoxication, food allergies, pregnancy, and cancer**. Repeated bouts of nausea may be due to food allergies. A common cause of nausea is **worms** (861) **or constipation** (456). See both topics.

NATURAL REMEDIES

• Use the treatments suggested for *Motion Sickness (287)*, especially the **charcoal and ginger root** formula. Powdered ginger root is a definite help in eliminating nausea.

• Do not forget the final solution: Go ahead and **vomit**. That is best if the nausea is caused by something recently eaten. Read *Vomiting (437)*. It will provide very helpful information. It will also tell what to do if you have been nauseated and vomiting for days.

• Eat a small amount of **dry toast or crackers** to clear nausea caused by excess exercise. If you are hypoglycemic, add some **protein**. For post-operative nausea, take two 500-mg capsules of **ginger**.

• Add a **pinch of ginger to other teas**, to help reduce nausea. **Ginger compress** on the head (made from the mild tea) will help relieve headaches due to nausea.

• Drink a mild tea of **goldenseal and honey** on rising to offset the nausea of pregnancy. Put a pinch of goldenseal powder in a cup of just-boiled water, and add a little honey to offset the taste.

• A cup of hot **peppermint tea** will reduce a feeling of nausea. You can add a pinch of basil and/or ginger. Peppermint tea is a powerful antispasmodic. It stops muscle spasms in the digestive tract, including those involved in vomiting. (But large amounts of this tea, during pregnancy, can lead to miscarriage.)

• Here is an excellent herbal formula for nausea: **ginger root, plus a very small amount of licorice root and cayenne**. Dr. Mowrey found it worked for most people. Ginger seems to produce no toxic symptoms, even when taken in large amounts.

• "Carminative" means "stomach soothing"; for these herbs help settle the stomach. Here are the best ones to use: **chamomile, fennel, dill, lemon balm, and any of the mints (peppermint, spearmint, catnip)**. Make a tea of one or more of these.

• With some people, the discomfort can be cleared up quickly by chewing hard, common **cloves**. With others, it takes something a little more potent such as **catnip, peach leaves, peppermint, raspberry leaves, spearmint, or sweet balm**. A few drops of tincture of **lobelia** is very good. A combination of **cinnamon, cloves, spearmint, and Turkey rhubarb** will bring good results when used as prescribed later in the book.

• Sometimes nausea makes it difficult to keep even fluids down. If that's the case, remember to drink liquids in small, frequent sips, not big gulps. Fortunately, the healing chemicals in **many herbs can be absorbed through the skin**. This fact comes in handy when nausea makes it hard to drink teas or tinctures. If your stomach turns at the idea of the recommended teas, make one of them but don't drink it. Instead, let it cool, then soak a clean cloth or hand towel with the tea and apply the cloth to your stomach.

Or make a large pot of **bath tea** by tossing a handful of any of the recommended herbs into a quart of just-boiled water. Allow to steep off heat for 10 to 15 minutes, strain the tea into a warm bath, and soak.

You may, after this, be able to keep down some much-needed fluids.

ENCOURAGEMENT—Angels of God are waiting to show you the path of life. It is outlined in the Bible; and as you seek, through the grace of Christ, to obey His Word, you will find the strength needed to meet your problems. Jeremiah 31:12-13.

Through the study of the sacred Scriptures, your trust will be deepened; and you will have the strength to carry on.

FAINTING
(Syncope)

SYMPTOMS—The person passes out and becomes unconscious.

CAUSES—Fainting points to some other problem, such as **hysteria, epilepsy, insulin shock, heat exhaustion, lack of oxygen, anemia, dehydration, carotid artery obstruction.**

NATURAL REMEDIES

WHAT TO DO IMMEDIATELY

• **Check** the pulse, heart beat, and breathing. Often a dash of **cold water in the face** helps. **Get air to him:** Loosen tight clothing; open windows and doors; and have others stand back, so the person can get more air. **Stimulate the heart:** Use your fist to pound slightly on the back between the shoulders. When able to drink, give him a little cold water.

• If you have it available, place 8 drops of **antispasmodic tincture** on the back of the tongue. If you know in advance that the person has these fainting problems, you may want to prepare the tincture and keep it on hand. Information is at *Antispasmodic Tincture (576)*.

• Sometimes **artificial respiration or oxygen** is needed. As soon as the person is conscious, try to find the cause and deal with it.

• If a person has frequent fainting spells, give him an **herb tea** of mint, skullcap, catnip, rue, mistletoe, rosemary, and small amounts of cayenne.

• For those who have collapsed, here are **water therapy techniques** which will prove helpful. They are described in the *Hydrotherapy* chapter *(206-275)*: **Alternate Hot and Cold Compress over the Spine; Cold Friction; Hot Enema; Alternate Compress over the Heart; Hot Blanket Pack** for 15 minutes, followed by **Cold Mitten Friction**.

• **Heat to neck and short cold application to chest and face. Alternate Compress to spine; percussion of the chest with the hands dipped in cold water** or with the end of a cold towel; vigorous friction, rhythmically moving the tongue back and forth to help wake him up.

ENCOURAGEMENT—We must ever set the Lord before us and trust implicitly in Him. He will guide and care for us to the end. As we obey His Inspired Writings, we shall have the help we need. Joel 3:1.

In His strength, we can do all that He requires of us. How thankful we can be that we have such a wonderful heavenly Father who is always attentive to our cry! Cling to Him and keep reading the sacred Scriptures, and He will open before you a bright path.

HEAT EXHAUSTION

SYMPTOMS—Thirst is generally the first symptom of heat exhaustion, followed by general malaise, weakness, tiredness, a loss of appetite, headache, pallor, dizziness, and a general flu-like feeling that may include nausea and even vomiting. Sometimes the heart races and concentration becomes more difficult.

Heat exhaustion is less severe than heat stroke, and may occur over several days out in the sun. Dehydration may eventually lead to blood volume loss, poor heat regulation, and shock.

CAUSE—Heat exhaustion is generally caused by **water depletion** (dehydration) and, more rarely, by a **lack of salt** in the diet (salt depletion). When we sweat, we lose both water and salt (sodium, as well as potassium).

NATURAL REMEDIES

IMMEDIATELY

• **Get out of the sun immediately**, so body temperature will not continue to rise and the body will not lose more water and salt. If you remain in the sun, even though resting and drinking fluids, your temperature will continue to rise! Do not return to the sun for many hours!

• In the early stages, drink large amounts of **mineral-rich vegetable and fruit juices**, to replace water and electrolyte loss in perspiration. Water, by itself, does not replace electrolytes. **Potassium-rich vegetable broths** are helpful. Make a broth of thick potato peelings.

PREVENTION

• Plan ahead, so you will not come down with heat stroke later. Drink water. **Drink diluted electrolyte drinks**. **Avoid salt tablets**. They do the opposite of what they are supposed to do. The increased salt in the stomach keeps fluids there longer. Use water-based supplements which include magnesium, calcium, and manganese. The dosage is ½ tsp. in 4 oz. water, 3 times a day.

• **Do not use caffeine, alcohol, or tobacco**. The first two accelerate dehydration and the smoking constricts blood vessels.

• Over several days' time, **adapt yourself slowly to the sun**. **Do not overexert** when out in it. Avoid working in the mid day. **Wear a hat**, and keep on a **light-colored shirt**.

• Pour **water over your head and shirt**, especially if the air is not humid. Keep drinking lots of water.

• In hot weather, add ¼ cup dried **lemon balm herb** to 1 quart boiled water. Steep for 30 minutes, strain, and refrigerate until chilled. It is cooling to the body.

J.H. KELLOGG, M.D., PRESCRIPTION *(how to give these water therapies: pp. 206-275 / list of treatments: pp. 206-207 / Hydrotherapy Disease Index: pp. 273-275)*

HEAT EXHAUSTION—Hot Full Bath, 3-8 minutes; **Hot Blanket Pack; Hot Enema**, followed immediately by short **Cold Mitten Friction**, *Afterward:* **Cold Wet Sheet Rub**, wrapping in warm blankets.

—*Read Heat Stroke (286)*, which is different.

ENCOURAGEMENT—Our God delights to do abundantly above all that we ask or think. He will care for you through this crisis. Trust Him. When a soul receives Christ, he receives power to live the life of Christ.

HEAT STROKE
(Sunstroke)

SYMPTOMS—The body temperature goes very high (105° F. or more!). Sweating is reduced. There is a strong headache, accompanied by tingling, numbness, confusion of mind, and delirium. The pulse becomes rapid and breathing is faster. Blood pressure rises.

DANGER—Heat stroke is a *serious emergency*. If not properly cared for, the person can go into convulsions, permanent brain damage, and even death.

NATURAL REMEDIES

• You must **begin the cooling treatments immediately**; do not wait!

• *If near a hospital*, **wrap him in an ice-cold sheet and immediately take him to the hospital. Apply more ice water** as you travel. At least every 5-10 minutes, **take his temperature**. Do not give the cold treatment if it begins to drop below 101° F.

• *If you are not near a hospital*, put him into an **ice-cold bath** and use **fans** to aid cooling. If an ice bath is not available, use a **cold stream or lake** until medical help can be obtained. While he is in the cold bath, **rub the arms, legs, hands, and feet** in order to increase the circulation.

J.H. KELLOGG, M.D., PRESCRIPTIONS FOR HEAT STROKE AND ITS COMPLICATIONS *(how to give these water therapies: pp. 206-275 / list of treatments: pp. 206-207 / Hydrotherapy Disease Index: pp. 273-275)*

SUNSTROKE—Increase the body's heat elimination. From a height, **pour water** (60° F., or less) onto him while two people **rub him** vigorously. Give special attention to the spine. **Ice Compress** to the head and neck. Continue until the temperature falls to 101° F., **Cool Enema, cold water drinking** when possible. **Ice Bag** to the head and neck during the Cold Pail Pour. *As soon as the temperature falls to near the normal point*, give a **sweating Wet Sheet Pack**.

AFTER TREATMENT—Should consist of **daily graduated cold applications** (Tonic Frictions), to slowly build up the body. The **head** should be thoroughly cooled before each application.

—*See Heat Exhaustion (286)*.

ENCOURAGEMENT—Treat God as your honored Friend, giving Him the first place in your affections. He is your Lord and your God. As you do this, you will have the support and help you need to meet each day's trials and afflictions. 2 Timothy 1:7.

MOTION SICKNESS
(Car Sickness, Sea Sickness)

SYMPTOMS—Nausea, excessive salivation, vomiting, cold sweat, queasy feeling, stomach churning. Possible dizziness, sometimes fainting.

CAUSE—The semicircular canals in the inner ears detect your vertical position. When there is **too much jostling back and forth**, movement which you do not have control over (as when riding in cars, planes, or boats), your sensory system may become overloaded. Since **your eyes** also sense vertical balance, what you see does not seem to agree with what your labyrinthine receptors in the inner ear sense. Then mental confusion results. Nausea occurs when the brain does not know what to tell the body to do. This weakens the stomach.

The experts say that nausea at such a time also indicates that **your liver is not doing well**.

NATURAL REMEDIES

• *If at sea*, **lie down and close your eyes**. *If in a car seat*, **rest your head back** on the headrest, so it is somewhat faced upward. This relaxes the semicircular canals.

• **Charcoal tablets** may help settle the stomach. **Ginger capsules** are highly recommended.

• **Raspberry leaf tea** is also recommended for the nausea of motion sickness. It can also be mixed with ginger. **Black horehound** can reduce nausea.

PREVENTION

• Prevention is the best. **Do not eat heavily processed meals, drink liquor, or eat junk food**. Some people do well eating **a few whole-grain crackers** before and during the trip. **Avoid smoke and food odors**. **Stay cool** and **get fresh air**! Cool air is best.

• You may wish to take 5 **charcoal** tablets, one hour before the trip begins. Another method is 2 **ginger** tablets every 3 hours, beginning one hour before the trip. Ginger helps prevent motion sickness, by absorbing acids and thus preventing nausea.

• Some recommend additional **magnesium** (500 mg, one hour before trip) and **vitamin B₆** (100 mg, one hour prior to the trip), to relieve anticipated nausea.

• In order to settle the stomach before a trip, use the nervine herbs: **hops, skullcap, chamomile, and valerian root**.

• **Grab your earlobes and pull down**. This increases circulation to the inner ear and helps prevent motion sickness. Do this often during the trip.

• Lean back and breathe deeply; try to relax and **take a sip of water** from a cup every few minutes. **Avoid rapid changes** in body position or head motion.

• Do not use products that impair circulation: **nicotine, caffeine, and salt**.

Here are more preventive suggestions:

• **Travel at night**. When it is dark, what you see conflicts less with what you sense and the air tends to be fresher.

• If possible, **keep a window open and stay near it**, all the while breathing that fresh air.

• **Sit still and do not look around** very much. Look straight ahead. If you are in the driver's seat, you will sense (and have) better control of the movements taking place. **Do not read** while riding. **Keep your eyes on something stationary far ahead**.

• Take a daily **B-complex supplement** and **vitamin C** (2,000 mg) for 2 weeks before traveling.

ENCOURAGEMENT—He loves you deeply, and wants you as His own precious child.

ALTITUDE SICKNESS

SYMPTOMS—A sickish feeling as you move upward, higher above sea level. The result is headache, fatigue, malaise, fainting, as well as extreme thirst.

Any of the following symptoms are very serious and may indicate altitude induced accumulation of fluid in the brain or lungs. Arrange to descend immediately.

• Lack of coordination or stumbling gait
• Bad headache unrelieved by pain medication
• Severe nausea and vomiting
• Impaired judgment, confusion
• Shortness of breath at rest
• Coughing or gurgling sounds when breathing
• Coughing of white or pink foamy sputum

CAUSE—The higher you go, the **less oxygen** there is. At 8,000 feet, the atmosphere contains half the oxygen of the air at sea level. If you ascend slowly, a few thousand feet a day, your body will probably adjust to the decreased oxygen, with few ill effects. But rapid ascents deprive your body of oxygen, and altitude sickness results. You also tend to become dehydrated.

NATURAL REMEDIES

• **Drink plenty of water** before you start your ascent. Continue drinking as you climb. Drinking enough liquids is extremely important!

• **Ginger** is the best single herb for motion-type sickness. **Peppermint** tea soothes and calms the stomach. Place a drop of the oil on the tongue for quick relief.

• **Clove oil** is rich in eugenol, which tends to thin the blood. Other eugenol herbs include **allspice** and **marjoram**.

• **Garlic** contains 9 compounds that thin the blood. That makes it outstanding in preventing heart attacks—

and altitude sickness. **Tomato, dill, and fennel** also have this property.

• Do not eat heavy, spicy, sugary, dried, or fatty foods. When traveling, take **whole-grain crackers** with you. **Olives** help reduce nausea because they decrease salivation.

ENCOURAGEMENT—In the strength of God, we can keep pressing forward; and He will comfort and help us, even to the end. Jude 21, 24.

GENERAL - 3 - COLDS

CATARRH
(Excess Mucus)

SYMPTOMS—
• Runny nose, headaches, postnasal drip, sore throat, sinusitis, gastritis, glue ear syndrome, and respiratory problems.

CAUSE—Catarrh is the excess mucous which occurs with many different nasal, throat, tracheal, and bronchial infections—for example, croup, whooping cough, or allergies.

Mucus must not be confused with the mucous membrane, the latter being part of the body. Mucus accumulates excessively on top of the membrane. This mucoid filth is caused by improper diet.

NATURAL REMEDIES
FOOD
• **DIET**—Eat a **fruit diet and drink fruit juices** for a few days.

• **NUTRIENTS**—Vitamin A (5,000 IU), **vitamin D** (1,000 IU), **vitamin C** (2,000 mg), and **vitamin E** (400 IU) are important. Make sure you are getting enough **calcium** (2,000 mg), **magnesium** (1,000 mg), **and potassium** (1,000 mg).

• **AVOID**—Excess mucous is normal with some diseases; yet **avoiding certain foods** will lessen the amount of mucous produced. Some foods are high mucous-forming. Overcooking of food is part of the problem. **Avoid pasteurized milk, white flour, sugar foods, cold drinks, and meat** if you want to cut down on mucous. **Eat more fresh fruit, vegetables, whole grains, nuts, and legumes**. If you have cooked food at a meal, **begin with raw food**. This will help the digestive system handle the increased load that cooked food places upon it.

• **Avoid indigestible food**; it forms higher levels of mucous in the body. Any specific **allergen,** food, or substance which you are allergic to may cause catarrh. Orientals are particularly sensitive to **milk products** (up to 85% of them lack the digestive enzyme, lactase, needed to handle milk sugar, which is lactose).

• **Lemon juice and honey** are highly recommended. **Tomato juice** or **onion and garlic** will cut mucus rap-

idly. Many anticatarrhal herbs are available which will do the job. Useful herbs include **bayberry, bistort, bitter root, coltsfoot, cranesbill root, fire weed, goldenseal, gum arabic, hyssop, red raspberry, white pond lily, and yarrow.**

• Other irritants include **fumes, smoke, foreign objects, chemicals, drugs, spicy foods, salt, pepper, alcohol, and poor food combinations.**

DURING THE ILLNESS
• Put **1 tsp. salt in a pint of soft lukewarm water**. Bend over a wash bowl, pour your hand full of it, and **sniff it up your nose**. Keep doing this until it comes out your mouth. Then gently blow the nose, holding one nostril shut and then the other. Repeat this until the nose is entirely clean. **Then gargle** with the salt water. If the nose refuses to unplug, **jump up and down** for a minute, and sniff and blow again.

• **Use steam** (from a humidifier in the room) to break up the mucous, so you can sleep well. **Eucalyptus oil** also helps.

• Be sure and **drink enough water**. As intake decreases, the mucous thickens and cuts off breathing.

• During the illness, you may **drink primarily of fluids**, with **fruit juices** at times. But at those times **when you eat, emphasize a high-fiber diet, using raw food. When grains are eaten, they should be whole grains**, such as brown rice, millet, and buckwheat.

HERBS
• Each day, take at least **one high herb enema** (such bayberry bark tea).

• You may wish to take a **psyllium seed and herbal mixture,** to clean out the digestive tract of mucous. Herbs for this purpose could include **burdock, aloe vera, ginger, alfalfa, cascara sagrada, kelp, and slippery elm.**

• **Black cohosh, calamus, and valerian** are good, cleansing herbs to drink. **Goldenseal** is excellent. Put a teaspoonful of this in a pint of boiling water; steep, cool, and take 2-3 swallows during the day.

• Other helpful herbs include **chickweed, mullein, plantain, sorrel, white oak bark, bayberry bark, comfrey, eucalyptus leaves, white pine needles, and oregano**.

• An herbal formula which helps reduce catarrh: 1 part white **poplar bark** and 2 parts **uva ursi**. Use 1 tsp. to a cup of boiling water. Take ½-1 cupful 3 times daily.

Catarrh is caused by eating devitalized or processed foods; by eating **excess starches and glutinous foods**; by **poor circulation, lack of sunshine, fresh air, exercise**; by eating **wrong food combinations**; by eating **many soft and cooked foods**; by **drinking with meals**; and by **poor elimination**. When foods are not digested, fermentation takes place in the digestive tract, Alcohol and acetic acid are formed, and various forms of catarrh clog the membranes. When this thickened mucoid matter is dispatched to the skin, the skin glands become obstructed, resulting in colds and fevers. The fibrinous and glutinous substances (excess starches and carbohydrates, especially those rendered inorganic in cooking) overload the blood and tissues and cannot be passed off fast enough through the intestinal tract. The eliminative system becomes clogged and the mucus is forced into the various mucous glands or membranes. Although there is only one basic cause, the manifest symptoms are varied according to the form and location. The problem induces such diseases as **arthritis, asthma, biliousness, Bright's disease, bronchitis, cystitis, diphtheria, dysuria, gravel, jaundice, laryngitis, pleurisy, rheumatism, tonsillitis,** etc. If catarrhal matter collects in the bloodstream and congests circulation, it becomes **high blood pressure** and finally **apoplexy.**

• One should keep away from the **mucous forming foods;** and the diet should consist entirely of **leafy, juicy vegetables and fresh fruits.** As catarrh is a general mucoid complaint, one must thoroughly cleanse the stomach, liver and intestines. One must keep the mucous membrane in the nasal passage clean. The "musts" for catarrh are **proper diet, outdoor exercise, and good elimination.** If one doesn't get enough **fresh air and exercise,** the catarrh will develop into **hay fever, asthma, or tuberculosis.** Take **lemon juice and honey** copiously, especially for children. (You may add some glycerine.)

PREVENTION

Take **exercise, plenty of fresh air, and proper diet** in order to prevent catarrh from going into hay fever, asthma, or tuberculosis. **Wash the nose,** to keep the catarrh from going down into the lungs.

ENCOURAGEMENT—It is vital that we exercise faith moment by moment and hour by hour. Only in the strength of Christ can we be enabled to obey His Ten Commandment law, live clean lives, and prepare our hearts for a home in heaven. Isaiah 3:10.

COMMON COLD

NOTE—Most of the following recommendations would also apply to coughs and flu.

SYMPTOMS—Colds are a general inflammation of the mucous membranes of the respiratory passages. Symptoms include nose and throat irritations, watery eyes, fever, headaches, chills, muscle aches, and temporary loss of smell and taste.

A heavy cold may take the form of acute or chronic infection—such as grippe, tonsillitis, sinusitis, bronchial catarrh, chronic cold, or a similar virus-type infection.

Children who frequently have colds or flus may have thyroid malfunctions.

A COLD OR THE FLU?—How can you tell whether it is a heavy cold—or the flu? Here is the difference:

• *Headache* - prominent in flu, but rare in a cold.
• *Fever* - frequent and sudden in flu, but rare in a cold.
• *Fatigue* - extreme in flu and can last 2-3 weeks; there is only mild fatigue with a cold.
• *General aches* - common and often severe in flu; slight in a cold.
• *Runny nose* - occasionally in flu; common with a cold.
• *Cough* - common with flu and can become severe; only mild to moderate in a cold.
• *Sore throat* - sometimes with the flu; common with a cold.
    —Also see Flu (294). Also see p. 289.

CAUSES—In one sense, the cause is a variety of viruses. But in another, the person has allowed himself to **become rundown;** so the virus was able to take hold. Factors which lower the body's resistance to virus infection are **overexposure to cold, fatigue, recent or present infections, lack of rest, allergic reactions, inhalation of irritating dust or gas, overeating, sugar consumption, and wrong eating.**

The common cold is not an infection that leaps out and attacks an innocent passerby. It is not even a disease. A cold is the cure of a pre-diseased condition. And the symptoms are attempts by the body to reestablish normal conditions. The body is carrying out a "spring cleaning." A cold is the result of not living on the best level. Once it arrives, it cleanses toxins from the system and, along with rest, enables the person to get back into better shape. A cold is actually a blessing; for it forces people to rest who, otherwise, would prematurely develop debilitating, chronic, and life-threatening diseases.

The cold virus can change size and shape, making it impossible to produce a suitable vaccine. There are more than 100 different viruses which cause colds. Symptoms last for 7-14 days, regardless of therapy. The incubation period is very short (1-3 days) instead of the 10-21 days for most viruses. The cold seems to suddenly appear.

A cold is always in the upper respiratory tract (nose, mouth, throat, and upper bronchials). If congestion develops in the chest, the cold is worsening into something far more serious!

If you do not know how to take care of yourself, you had better contact a physician, especially if: (1) chills and shortness of breath occur. (2) An accompanying fever goes above 101° F. for more than three days or any fever above 103° F. (3) Yellow or white spots appear in the throat. (4) The lymph nodes under the jaw and in the neck become enlarged. (5) Any hot, extreme pain, such as earache, swollen tonsils, sinus pain, or aching lungs or chest occur. (6) There is excessively large amounts of sputum that is greenish or bloody. (7) There is extreme difficulty when swallowing. (8) Wheezing occurs. (9) There is shortness of breath.

If you have a sore throat, beware of white or yellow

CHART 1056: Is it a Cold (288-293), Flu (294), or Allergy (848-860) ?

GEN

patches on the throat. These can be *Group A beta-hemolytic streptococci*, which can damage the heart muscle. Have a throat swab done when there might be a question about this.

Children with high fevers should see a physician within 24 hours.

When you get a tingling nose and throat, nasal mucous, or scratchy throat—do not wait for the coughing, weakness, and fever to begin!

NATURAL REMEDIES

ACUTE STAGE

• Do not ignore a cold and drag on with your work. As soon it develops—**go to bed, drink fresh lemon juice in water, and settle down to getting well!**

• Treatment should include as much **vitamin C** as you can take, without producing diarrhea (up to 5,000 mg at a time). In acute cases, 1,000 mg of C every other hour. Also take **bioflavonoids** (200-600 mg). Along with vitamin C, small amounts of **garlic** are excellent germ fighters. **Vitamin A** (25,000) units for not more than a few days. **Calcium** lactate or gluconate (6 tablets). **Brewer's yeast. B$_6$** (100 mg). It is a natural antihistamine, as well as providing helpful protein. **Vitamin E** (600 units). **Betaine hydrochloride. Zinc** gluconate lozenges. **Vitamin F** (unsaturated fatty acids) reduces the frequency and duration of colds.

• *In acute stages* **when fever is present, abstain from all solid foods and only drink fresh fruit and vegetable juices, diluted** (50-50) with water, **plus herb teas.** The proper treatment of colds is to **encourage elimination** through all channels so that elimination through one channel does not become excessive (urine, bowel, sweating, showers).

• **Avoid chills; get adequate bed rest**; and take a slight amount of **salt**, to replace that lost in sweat.

• **Gargle** three times a day with saltwater (1 glass of warm water with one-half teaspoon of salt mixed in). Take a hot shower.

• **Avoid aspirin** (especially dangerous for children), since it causes internal bleeding. What you think is of little consequence may be flu or chicken pox—which are caused by a virus. Colds are also. When children who have certain viral infections take aspirin, their risk of developing Reye's Syndrome is greatly increased! This is a rare but fatal brain and liver disease. The same warning applies to cold medications containing aspirin.

• Avoid being depressed; try to **be cheerful.** There is healing in this. Keep looking to Jesus and praying to God. Let a friend read a Bible promise to you every so often; think about it. **Rest, relax,** and do not worry. **Keep warm, but get fresh air** from time to time. Take a lot of **liquids.**

HERBS

• Herb teas can include **rose hip, goldenseal, chamomile, peppermint, slippery elm, ginger, desert tea. Eucalyptus oil** is helpful. Put 5 drops in a hot bath or 6 drops in a cup of boiling water. Put a towel over your head and, without burning yourself, **inhale it**.

• Daily drinking **licorice root tea** soothes an irritated throat and relieves coughing. You might wish to take **hop tea**, to help you get to sleep at night.

Echinacea (coneflower) greatly strengthens the immune system and is a powerful antibiotic. Shortly after drinking the tea, the tongue may become numb and tingly for a time, but this reaction is harmless.

• Pour a cup of boiling water over 2 Tbsp. fresh, shredded **ginger root**; cool and drink it. It contains a dozen antiviral compounds.

• **Goldenseal tea** is excellent. It increases the blood supply to the spleen, a center of your immune system. Goldenseal contains **berberine**, which activates the white blood cells (macrophages) which destroy bacteria, fungi, viruses and tumor cells.

• Often all that is needed is copious amounts of **raspberry leaf tea** and some **bowel cleaning**. A very powerful remedy is the infusion of dried **elderberry flowers** and dried **peppermint leaves,** taken internally as hot as possible. The diaphoretic herbs will open the pores and discharge waste obstructions. When a cold occurs, the whole system is involved. At the first sign of a cold, one should **clean the nose and mouth** of the toxic accumulations (through snuffing and gargling); and after the cold is broken with the **sweating aids (blue vervain tea)**, the patient should be sponged with cold water to close the pores, put to bed, and given **fruits or fruit juices**.

WHEN THE CRISIS SUBSIDES

• When the fever subsides, a low calorie **raw fruit and vegetable diet** can now be eaten. This should include **plenty of raw juices and herb teas**, sweetened with a little honey. Some **raw seeds and nuts** can be eaten, but should be chewed well.

• Drink **potato peeling broth** twice a day. The peelings, rich in potassium, should be one-half inch thick (throw away the centers). Boil it for about 20-30 minutes; strain, cool, and drink. Make it fresh everyday.

WATER THERAPY

There are a variety of water treatments which can be applied. They are described in the hydrotherapy section (206-275).

• Take a **hot mustard footbath**, to increase eliminations and reduce head and sinus congestion.

• Take a **hot Epsom salt bath** while drinking sweating teas. Pour Epsom salt (1-2 pounds) into a hot tub. While soaking, drink 2-3 cups hot pleurisy root tea. Immediately after the bath, get into bed and cover with plenty of blankets, so profuse sweating can begin.

• Take a **hot ginger chest compress**.

• Bromelain is a protein-digesting enzyme in **pineapple**. If you have suffered a serious injury accompanied by bruising. Drink the juice. Bromelain should be taken as soon as possible after the injury and continued for several days afterward. *Caution:* if you have gastric or duodenal ulcers or gastritis, you should not take bromelain.

One study found that it reduced swelling, pain, and tenderness in patients who had suffered blunt trauma.

• Crush **parsley leaves** and apply repeatedly to a bruise. This remedy may help speed the disappearance of black-and-blue marks.

• Slice a raw, cool **white potato** and place it on the bruise. This is also good for black eyes.

• Apply a **trunk pack**. Apply a full cold trunk pack each evening. The objective is to stimulate skin elimination and induce perspiration. Leave it on for at least 3 hours at night.

• Apply a **cold compress to the neck** and leave it on for 1-3 hours or all night. It must—must—dry out before morning, or the value has been lost. If it does not change into a heating compress, it can intensify the sore throat.

• Use a **saltwater nasal douche**, to open the sinuses. Read the article on *Nasal Catarrh (404)*.

• Take a **steam inhalation**, using eucalyptus, pine needles, cloves, and/or thyme. —*Here is how to do it:*

Steam is an old-fashioned remedy for colds, coughs, and congestion. You can increase the steam's effectiveness by adding herbs or their essential oils to the pot. When herbal steams are inhaled, antiseptic, decongestant, airway-relaxing herbal ingredients get right where they're needed.

To prepare: Use 4 cups water, 3 tablespoons eucalyptus leaves, 2 tablespoons thyme leaves, 1 tablespoon rosemary leaves, and 1 tablespoon peppermint leaves.

In a large saucepan (not a teakettle), bring the water to a boil. Remove from heat and add the herbs; allow to steep, covered, for 3 to 5 minutes. (You can substitute 3 to 5 drops of essential oil of any of those same herbs; just make sure you use a total of 3 to 5 drops, not 5 drops of each.)

Remove the pot from the burner. Carefully pour the water into a heat resistant bowl and place it on a sturdy table. Put a towel over your head and hold your face at least 12 inches away from the steam. If the temper-ature feels comfortable, take an experimental breath. If the steam feels good, drape a towel around your head and breathe deeply—through your nose if you have a cold or sinus infection, through your mouth if you have a cough.

After you're finished inhaling the steam, strain out the herbs and pour the solution into the bath. If you used essential oils for your steam, just run a hot bath and add 5 to 10 drops before stepping in.

A basic **cold and flu tea:** This blend combines herbs to soothe the symptoms of the usual cold and flu; it also fight viruses and bacteria.

To make one cup of tea blend: Use 4 cups dried peppermint leaves, 4 cups dried lemon balm leaves, 1¼ cups dried elder flowers, and 4 cups dried yarrow flowers.

Store in an airtight jar away from the heat and light

for up to a year. To make 1 cup of tea: Use 1 cup water. 1-2 teaspoons tea blend, ½ to 1 teaspoon fresh grated ginger (optional), honey (optional), and lemon juice (optional)

Bring water to a boil and remove from heat. Add tea and ginger, if using ginger. (Ginger helps chase away that chilled feeling and adds a sweet/hot taste to the tea). Steep for 5 to 10 minutes. Strain. Add honey and/or lemon, if desired.

• Another **cold-flu tea** can help boost immunity and ease the discomfort of a cold or flu.

To prepare: Use 2¼ teaspoons echinacea leaves, 2¼ teaspoons elder flowers, 2¼ teaspoons yarrow leaves and flowers, 1¼ teaspoons peppermint, and 3 cups water.

Place all the herbs except the peppermint leaves in the water and simmer, covered, for 10 to 15 minutes. Remove from heat and add the peppermint leaves. Steep, covered, for 10 more minutes. Strain herbs and discard. Drink up to 3 cups of tea per day as needed. Store in the refrigerator for up to 3 days.

—*Also see Flu (294).*

PREVENTION—Once contracted, a cold must run its course. So it is better, far better, to prevent it than cure it. The best prevention is to **live right; eat right; get enough outdoor exercise, to strengthen the body; and enough rest**. Do not skimp on sleep at night, especially in the colder months. Do not share food with someone who has a cold. Be sure and **dress warmly** enough when it is cold. **Do not sit in a draft. Do not go outside with a wet head**.

Many people, who are seemingly susceptible to colds, never get them. They have learned to live above the level where they contract such infections. Learn the early warning signs; and, when they come, get extra bed rest!

ENCOURAGEMENT—Christ died so you could be forgiven of your sins and, by His grace, be enabled to obey His revealed will, as given in the Bible and the Ten Commandments (Exodus 20). Isaiah 50:10.

COUGHS

SYMPTOMS—Frequent coughing, productive (producing phlegm) or not.

CAUSES—Coughs often accompany colds and other infections; they are a reflex action to clear the airways of mucous, foreign bodies, an irritant, or some type of blockage. Productive coughs bring up mucous; nonproductive or dry, hacking coughs do not.

A bronchial cough is tight and painful. A sinus infection generally drips mucous down the throat, producing a cough.

Croupy coughs produce a loud raspy sound, bringing

up phlegm with difficulty. Damage to the lung tissues, caused by pneumonia, can result in a chronic cough.

There are two other kinds of cough: Lung cancer or tumors can produce a mild cough which gradually becomes worse and is possibly accompanied by blood. There is also smoker's cough. Lung cancer may follow, unless the tobacco is thrown away.

If there is any suspicion of tuberculosis *(505)*, read that article.

• This is often caused by a stomach disorder that comes from overloading the system with food, wherein fermentation in the stomach causes phlegm. It may also be induced by inflammation in the bronchial tubes, due to a neglected cold. Worms may be the cause. Many coughs are from a nervous condition, where coughing may eventually become habitual. Coughs are highly misunderstood. Usually a sore throat and coughing are caused by the sinuses draining the eustachian tubes, which is like pouring acid down the throat. A cough usually comes from a lowered vitality in the system, from improper diet, loss of sleep, lack of exercise and fresh air, improper breathing, poor elimination, or improper night clothing and bedding.

NATURAL REMEDIES

WHAT YOU CAN DO

• A few drops of **lobelia** herb under the tongue every few minutes will relax the cough muscles and may loosen the mucous. Be sure and **drink enough water** and other liquids, so the mucous does not become thick.

• Applying **eucalyptus oil inhalations** for 10 minutes a day will help.

• An excellent **cough syrup** is made by mixing equal parts **lemon juice and honey, with a little cayenne** into a tea. Take 1 teaspoon when needed.

• **Cayenne neck compress:** Boil a quart of water. Lower the fire as much as possible and add a half teaspoon of cayenne. Wait a few minutes. Then wet a towel in the water; wring it out, and wrap it around the neck. Keep the water hot and change this fomentation every 3-4 minutes, doing this for a half hour while feet are soaked in hot water.

• Helpful herbs include **licorice, fig leaves, mullein, vervain, oregano, bay leaves, hyssop, and thyme**. Take 3 cups a day (1 tsp. granulated herbs per cup of boiling water. Never boil the herbs. Never use aluminum ware).

• Mix thick **flaxseed tea** with 1-2 drops **of eucalyptus oil** and drink it slowly.

• Whenever there is a cold, **keep the nose and mouth clean**. This will tend to keep the cold from going down into the lungs. Add 1 tsp. salt to a pint of soft, warm water. **Sniff it up the nose**; then blow it out gently. Repeat till the nose is entirely clean of mucous. Then **gargle** the throat and rinse the mouth out thoroughly with saltwater.

• Cleanse the colon with **high enemas**. Continue until they reach the upper part, where the transverse colon is.

• If there is any nausea or bad feeling in the stomach, take an **emetic** to vomit it out. Lukewarm water or **water with a little salt** in it will generally help do this. Drink all the water possible and then **run the finger down the throat**. Repeat till the stomach is clean. Then drink a few cups of a **hot herb tea** (such as **sage, hyssop, yarrow, black cohosh, peppermint, or chamomile**). Later in the day, drink some more.

• Acute coughs can often be relieved with a little **honey and onion syrup**. When it is the result of an old acute condition, clear out the morbid condition as rapidly as possible without causing irritation. In old cough conditions, **comfrey with vervain or mullein** are very good. If this is due to a neglected cold, any of the diaphoretic herbs are excellent. To relieve the coughing spasms, use **horehound, comfrey**, or a small amount of **lobelia**. High enemas of herbal laxatives will relieve congestion of the bowels; and, if the cough is severe (**asthma, whooping cough**), load the stomach with liquids and induce vomiting.

• **Keep quiet and stay in bed**. Take only **fruit juices or lemon juice** in hot water. Later drink the broth of thick white **potato peeling soup** (also called potassium broth).

WATER THERAPY

The following suggestions are from the section on *Hydrotherapy (206-275)* in this *Encyclopedia:*

• **Heating Chest pack**, to be changed every 6 hours. If temperature is elevated, change chest pack every 2-4 hours. Copious water drinking.

• **Fomentation to spine**, sipping hot water, **Chest Pack. Cold Compress to the throat, gargling hot water** several times daily, **Steam Inhalation** for 15 minutes every hour, sipping half a glass of hot water when inclined to cough.

• *For irritable cough, without expectoration:* **Sipping very hot water; gargle hot water; Steam Inhalations. Also** avoid mouth breathing; keep air in the room warm (75°-80° F.) and moist with steam; carefully avoid exposure of back of neck, chest, or shoulders to drafts or to chill by evaporation during treatment.

• *For cough with viscid expectoration:* **Copious hot water drinking; fluid diet; Fomentation to chest** every 2 hours, followed by **Heating Chest Pack**.

• *For painful cough:* **Fomentation** to chest every 2 hours and tight bandage about chest, to restrain movement if necessary. **Revulsive Compress** for 15 minutes every 2 hours or often as needed. **Dry cotton Chest Pack** between applications.

• *For ineffective cough:* Increase expulsive power by **rubbing and percussion of the chest** with the hand dipped in ice water or slapping the chest with a cold, wet towel.

ENCOURAGEMENT—Christ knows every temptation that comes to man and the capabilities of each human agent. He can help you overcome and obey His Ten Commandment law. He died to take away your sins and give you strength to live right. Isaiah 43:25.

CHILLS

SYMPTOMS—Sweating, shaking, trembling, and unable to feel warm even when bundled up with blankets.

CAUSES—Chills often occur with flu and other viral infections.

NATURAL REMEDIES
• With clothing covering your head and neck, **do warm-up movements** and exercise.

• If the chilling seems unusual, it is very likely that something serious is developing. Immediately start on a cleansing program. **Go to bed; fast on fruit and vegetable juices or lemon juice. Soak the feet in hot water, get into a tub of hot water, or take a steam bath**.

• Helpful herbs include **blue vervain, cayenne, chamomile, oregano, hyssop, skullcap, peppermint, white willow, and catnip**.

—*Also see Poor Circulation and Chills (536).*

ENCOURAGEMENT—Provision has been made for us to come into close connection with Christ and to better receive the constant protection of the angels of God. Our faith must reach within the veil, where Jesus has entered for us. We can trust Him implicitly for the help we need. Daniel 9:4.

INCREASE HEAT PRODUCTION

HYDRO—Here are hydrotherapy treatments discussed in the Hydrotherapy chapter *(206-275):*

To warm up the body: The **Heating Wet Sheet Pack**, which begins when the warming pack has raised the body temperature slightly above its usual degree and ends when general perspiration begins. Once achieved, for best results this should be continued for about 20 minutes.

To increase heat production: The **Tonic Frictions**, which include the Wet-hand Rub, the Cold Mitten Friction, and other specific ones.

The following list of heat-producing water treatments is arranged from most to the least powerful, and is primarily composed of tonic and fever-reducing applications (see the hydrotherapy chapter for directions): **Graduated bath, Cooling Wet Sheet Pack, Cold Friction Bath**. Prolonged Tepid Full Bath, at 88° F. Cold Full Bath, followed by a short Hot Full Bath. Pail Pour, or Shower. Tepid Pail Pour. Cold Pail Pour. Cold Compress. Graduated Compress. Evaporating Sheet. Cold to head and neck. Cold to spine. Cold to abdomen.

CHART - 1062: Information on the 21 types of infectious diseases

Cold over heart. Cold colonic. Tepid or cold enema. Cold water drinking, a measure that should be combined with all the others named above. And Cold Air Bath.

It is the impression of cold on the thermic nerves of the skin that best increases heat production. The more intense (and sometimes prolonged) this impression, the greater the desired effect. The most intense effects are produced by prolonging the application until the temperature of the body has been slightly lowered. But if the cold is greatly prolonged or is repeated at short intervals, the heat-rise effect fails.

ENCOURAGEMENT—Amid the perplexities that press upon the soul, there is only One who can help us out of all our difficulties and bring us peace of heart. Jeremiah 29:11.

GENERAL - 4 - INFECTIONS
Also: Section on Childhood Infections (724-752)

INFLAMMATION

SYMPTOMS—Swelling, heat, pain, tenderness, induration, reduced range of motion, fever, discharges, edema, and/or allergies.

CAUSES—Inflammation can result from injury, strain, arthritis, bacterial infection, and cancer. A part of the body is reacting to trauma or infection. Any organ or tissue can become inflamed. When internal, it is often associated with bacteria.

Inflammation is a reaction of the body to defend and heal itself after something occurs (a bruise or injury, etc.). Heat, redness, and swelling are generally present. A fever may accompany a severe inflammation. If not cared for promptly, infection could develop.

Other things which trigger inflammation include environmental toxins, drug overuse, infections, free radicals, and injuries.

NATURAL REMEDIES
The treatment is similar to that of other conditions discussed in this section on infections.

• Important nutrients include **vitamin C** (3,000-6,000 mg, daily), **vitamin B complex** daily, **vitamin E** (400-600 IU, daily), **beta-carotenes** (carrot juice and green and yellow vegetables), **flaxseed oil** (2 Tbsp), and **grape seed extract**.

• **Bromelain** (the substance in pineapples), taken on an empty stomach and with a small amount of **magnesium** and **L-cysteine**, has anti-inflammatory activity. **Calcium, kelp,** and **alfalfa** are also important. Primarily eat **raw foods**, and **avoid all junk food**.

GEN

• **Charcoal poultices** or **clay packs** are helpful.

• Drink a **tea of hyssop, chickweed, vervain, mint, and sage**. Read again the section on the common cold *(289)*.

• Place a **compress of fenugreek or chamomile** on the area.

• In case of obstinate inflammation and threatened mortification (gangrene), apply a poultice of powdered or fresh crushed roots of **marshmallow** on the affected area, as hot as possible and renew it before it dries. Add **slippery elm**, to make it even more effective.

• Here are herbs which research studies have shown to be excellent in reducing inflammation: **bilberry, bromelain, echinacea, devil's claw, feverfew, licorice root,** and **onion**. Also outstanding: **goldenseal, pau d'arco, red clover,** and **ginger**.

• **Aloe vera juice, cayenne, echinacea, ginger, goldenseal, pau d'arco,** and **red clover** reduce inflammation.

• This condition must be aided instead of inhibited. If the process is stopped, it can be compared to putting the cork on the poison bottle. When inflammation is accompanied by blood poisoning, use **plantain** to purge the poisons from the body. If inflammation is caused by a rheumatoid or arthritic condition, either **burdock leaves or mullein** in combination with **lobelia** will facilitate cleansing.

—*Also see Common Cold (289).*

ENCOURAGEMENT—Christ is ever seeking to draw souls to Himself; but Satan is seeking to draw them away. We must resist the temptation to separate from our Lord and Saviour. He is the only One who can help us amid all our trials and needs. Psalm 9:9.

FLU
(Influenza, La Grippe)

SYMPTOMS—Prostration, fever, chills, sore throat, headache, aching behind the eyes with sensitivity to light, abdominal pain, hoarseness, cough, enlarged lymph nodes, aching of the back and limbs, and frequent vomiting and diarrhea. The person feels cold and shaky, but is sweating. Serious complications, such as pneumonia, sinus infections, and ear infections, can develop.

The earliest signs are similar to those for the common cold: weakness, headache, and aching in the arms, legs, and back. He may feel feverish, and then chilly. The flu also generally brings on a dry throat, cough, and extreme weariness.

CAUSE—Also known as "the flu," influenza is a highly contagious viral infection of the respiratory tract. It is easily spread by sneezing and coughing. Individual strains continually change, so vaccines are not very successful.

There are three main types of influenza: A, B, and

CHART 1056: Is it a Cold (288-293), Flu (294), or Allergy (848-860) ?

C. Type A is the most common; all are airborne and most frequently spread by droplets (coughing, sneezing, kissing, and sharing drinking glasses and towels). Flu epidemics occur every 1-3 years, generally in the autumn or winter. A major epidemic occurs about every 10 years, because the virus type has changed.

Because it is a viral infection, influenza may appear suddenly after an incubation of only 1 to 3 days (most frequently 48 hours after exposure). So begin treating it as soon as you can. The quicker you start treating a physical problem, the easier and more quickly it can be eliminated. After 2-3 days, the fever usually subsides; and, if cared for properly, the other acute symptoms rapidly diminish. But the cough, weakness, and fatigue may persist for several days or weeks.

Flu is an advanced cold condition. A body catches flu when it is full of waste matter and toxins through lowered vitality and by body exposure to cold and dampness. This is due to mucus in a weak spot in the body--in this case, the respiratory tract. The contributing factors to this weakness are shallow breathing and a lack of oxygen to that particular area.

NATURAL REMEDIES
WHAT YOU CAN DO

• The fastest way to eliminate this body condition is by **proper diet and rest**, and by **flushing the body system with diaphoretic herbs**. Take a ginger bath (using up to a pound of **ginger** to a tub of water), or a **mustard-cayenne bath** with **cold sheeting** afterward under covers in bed. The **antispasmodic herbs** relax the cell structure, loosen and discharge the mucoid matter. **Fruit juices** (especially **hot lemon juice**) should be taken alternately with the **herbal teas**. After the cleansing crisis, the body system should be built up with **tonic herbs** and with **nutritious, non-mucus forming foods**.

• **Take an enema** at the first symptom. *For fever,* take **catnip tea** enemas, plus a ¼ to ½ teaspoon of **lobelia** tincture every 3-4 hours until the fever drops. This is also for children.

• **Give fluids (fruit juices, vegetable soups)** to replace fluid and electrolytes lost through sweating, diarrhea, fever, and vomiting. **Drink at least 10 glasses of water a day**, to keep lung secretions thin. Give **vitamin C**, to bowel tolerance (3,000 mg or more, spaced throughout the day). Also **vitamin A** (25,000 IU for 1 week) **and B complex**. Vitamin A protects the lining of the throat (best to take it in the form of carotenes: carrot juice and green and yellow vegetables). **zinc** (15 mg, three times daily).

• **Do not take antibiotics**, for they have no effect on the flu virus. **Do not smoke, drink liquor, use coffee, or eat junk food**.

• Take **echinacea** and **goldenseal**, because influenza can lead to secondary bacterial pneumonia,

• **Eucalyptus oil vapors** are also good. *See "Com-*

mon Cold" (289) for directions.

• A useful herb is **slippery elm bark** powder (1 tablespoon) mixed with boiling water (1 quart) and honey (half a cup). Put in a jar and give one teaspoon every 3-4 hours for cough and sore throat.

• **Gargle with saltwater**, to help relieve the sore throat (1 teaspoon salt in 1 pint of warm water). **Soak the feet in hot water**, to ease a headache or nasal congestion. **Occasionally breathe deeply** in and out, to refresh and strengthen the lungs and remove wastes.

• **Humidify the air** in the room. **Make sure the air is warm, but also has a current of air** to keep it oxygenated. But it should not be drafty. (A draft on the patient is defined as occurring when the skin becomes cooler than the forehead or the patient is not comfortable.) **Keep warm**. Wear warm, close-fitted bed clothes. Back rubs may be given, to increase comfort.

• Helpful herbs include **cinchona bark, ginger, eucalyptus, slippery elm, sea buckthorn, yarrow, white willow, and wormwood.**

• During the 1918 flu epidemic, about 20 people in one area ate raw **garlic** daily with their meals. None of the 20 contracted the flu.

• Another flu remedy is to place 1 oz. each of **peppermint leaves and elder flowers** in a pan. Pour ½ pint boiling water over these herbs, cover tightly, and keep warm on stove for 15 minutes; strain and cover immediately to keep warm. Take 1 teacupful every 30-45 minutes until there is perspiration; then 2 Tbsp. every 1-2 hours. (For children, give smaller doses and sweeten.) This tea taken hot will break down congestions and equalize circulation. (Or substitute pennyroyal and elder flowers instead of the above two herbs.)

• Pour boiling water over a handful each of **wormwood, sage, alpine speedwell, and licorice root**. Steep for 30 minutes; then take a spoonful every half hour or sip it morning and evening. Recovery time is usually 2 days.

• Boil a 5-inch piece of **fresh ginger** (from the health-food store) in 2 cups water for 5-10 minutes. Drink a cup every 2-3 hours until the flu is gone. It will relieve nasal congestion, improve blood flow, help eliminate chills and aches, and reduce sore throat pain.

• Here is Dr. Holyk's formula: Chop 1-2 cloves **garlic** very fine. Add 3 droppers each of echinacea tincture, **goldenseal** tincture, **cat's claw** tincture, a pinch of **cayenne**, the juice of ½ **lemon**, and 6-8 oz. organic **tomato or vegetable juice**. Put it all into a blender along with 2 ice cubes (to make the drink more palatable). Blend, then sip slowly for a few minutes. Drink it twice a day till the flu is gone.

• Medicinal mushrooms, such as **shiitake** *(Lentinus edodes)* and **reishi** *(Gano-derma lucidum)*, all possess substances called *polysaccharides* that stimulate the immune system. Shiitake also increases the body's production of the antiviral substance, called *interferon*. If you want the healing compounds in these mushrooms to help you fight a cold that you've already gotten, take them in supplement form. *Typical dosage:* 500 milligrams of standardized extract capsules or tablets, twice per day.

• **Reishi's** anti-inflammatory components may help ease the respiratory-tract inflammation that often comes with colds and flu. This mushroom is a long-used and well-respected tonic in Asian medicine. *Typical dosage:* up to five 420-milligram capsules per day; or up to three 1,000 milligram tablets three times per day.

• **Expectorants** help loosen respiratory secretions; so they can be coughed up. Herbal expectorants include **horehound** *(Marrubium vulgare)*, **eucalyptus** *(Eucalyptus globulus)*, and **thyme** *(Thymus vulgaris)*. Thyme is also antimicrobial and relaxes smooth muscles, a property that can help open tight airways. That is why you will often see these herbs in combination for colds with coughs.

• When it is time to make the transition from liquids to food, emphasize **bland, starchy foods**. This would include **dry toast** (so it will be chewed better), **bananas, applesauce, boiled rice, cooked cereal, and baked potatoes**. Eat lightly and carefully.

• If you need to lower the fever, take **catnip tea** enemas and ¼ to ½ tsp. **lobelia** tincture every 3-4 hours until the fever drops. This is also good for children.

• At the first indication of a cough, place 1 dropperful of alcohol-free **echinacea** and **goldenseal** extract in your mouth; and hold it there for 5-10 minutes. Repeat every hour for 3-4 hours. This will keep the virus from multiplying. This extract (4-6 drops) can be given to children every 4 hours for 3 days.

• For a sore throat and cough, mix 1 tablespoon of **slippery elm** bark powder with 1 cup boiling water and ½ cup **honey**. Take 1 tsp. every 3-4 hours, either hot or cold.

• A pinch of **cayenne** added to soups and other foods will help keep mucus flowing, to reduce congestion and headaches.

• **Water therapy:** Take a 5-minute hot shower. Quickly dry. Then place a large towel in cold water, wring it out, and wrap it around your body from your armpits to your groin. Put plastic around that. Crawl into bed under a wool blanket and stay there for 20 minutes or until warmed. Do this 1-2 times daily.

PREVENTION—Be careful; for influenza is sometimes fatal, especially for children and the elderly. Those who are not hardy and are poorly nourished are especially susceptible. If you have a respiratory ailment (asthma, emphysema, pneumonia, etc.), solve it as soon as possible. One thing can lead to another till you are prostrated with sickness. The flu can often lead to ear infections, pneumonia, and sinus infection.

Children who frequently come down with the flu should be checked for hypothyroidism. Check his temperature under the arm with a thermometer.

A case of flu is becoming serious if the voice becomes hoarse, he develops pains in his chest, he has difficulty breathing, or he starts bringing up yellow- or green-colored phlegm. It may be best to see a physician, if this has not already been done. Avoid the flu vaccine!

J.H. KELLOGG, M.D., PRESCRIPTIONS FOR FLU AND ITS COMPLICATIONS *(how to give these water therapies: pp. 207-272 / list of treatments: pp. 206-207 / Hydrotherapy Disease Index: pp. 273-275)*

INCREASE GENERAL VITAL RESISTANCE AND AID ELIMINATION OF POISONS—**Sweating** (Full) **Baths**, followed by **vigorous cold applications** (Cold Pail Pours, Showers, Frictions, etc.); **Hot blanket Pack** or Hot Full Bath; **Hot Leg Bath with Fomentations** to chest or spine, **followed by Cold** Mitten Friction, Cold Towel Rub or Wet Sheet Rub; Sweating Wet Sheet Pack; copious **water** drinking; **large Enema** once or twice daily.

PAIN IN HEAD, BACK, AND LEGS—Very **Hot Leg Pack** till general perspiration begins, **followed by Cold** Mitten Friction or Cold Towel Rub, keeping limbs very warm.

FEVER—**Sweating Wet Sheet Pack** and Neutral Bath, **Cold** Mitten Friction, Cold Towel Rub, copious water drinking, cooling Enema.

HEADACHE—**Hot and Cold Head Compress, Fomentation to face** and especially over eyes (but be sure eyes are closed and covered with dry cloth).

NAUSEA—**Ice Bag** over stomach.

VOMITING—**Hot and Cold Trunk Pack**; withhold liquids.

ENEMA—**Neutral Enema** after each bowel movement. **Cold Abdominal Compress**, changing every 15 minutes.

COLIC—**Hot Enema**, **hot Fomentation** over abdomen.

INFLAMMATION OF EYE OR EAR—Fomentation over affected part, derivative treatment to legs, **Hot Leg Bath**, Hot Footbath, Prolonged Leg Pack.

RHEUMATOID INFLUENZA—Hot Blanket Pack 2-3 hours once or twice daily, followed by **Cold Mitten Friction** carefully given and wrapping in dry flannels. Repeat pack twice a day. **Fomentation** over especially painful parts, several times daily, followed by **Heating Compress** in interval between.

GENERAL METHOD—Combat lung and visceral congestion by maintaining warmth and activity of the whole cutaneous surface; give special attention to the lower extremities, so as to divert blood away from the cranial and pulmonary cavities. Sweating procedures may be employed with vigor and frequently repeated if followed by short Cold Frictions given in such a way as to avoid general chilling of the surface.

If any of the following related problems exist, see under their respective headings: Bronchitis, Bronchopneumonia, Pleurisy, Neuritis, Typhoid Influenza, Thoracic Influenza, Lobar pneumonia, Catarrhal jaundice, Meningitis, Nephritis.

—See Common Cold (289) for how to differentiate between a heavy cold and the flu. Also see Sore Throat (415).

ENCOURAGEMENT—We must have faith that will not be denied, faith that will take hold of the unseen, faith that is steadfast and immovable. Christ can help you, right where you are. Not only can He solve your physical problems, He can guide you all the way to the Holy City above. Lamentations 3:25.

VIRAL INFECTIONS

SYMPTOMS—fever, muscular aches, joint aches, chills, and headaches.

CAUSES—Viruses can be especially serious. Viral infections include the common cold, measles, chicken pox, mumps, influenza, tonsillitis, croup, infectious hepatitis, mononucleosis, spinal meningitis, asthma, and certain bladder infections.

Antibiotics fight bacterial invasion, but are useless against viral infections. There are a few antiviral medications which are useful. In remarkable contrast, the body uses the same variety of powerful defenses—to resist and overcome *both* bacterial and viral crises! So help your body win the battle. The Lord has placed strong defenses against sickness within each of us. We can claim them more fully if we are living according to the laws of health.

NATURAL REMEDIES

• **Vitamin C** (2,000 mg) and **vitamin B$_6$** (200 mg) are especially helpful. Also see the rather complete list of suggestions under Common Cold *(289)*.

• **Vitamin A** (10,000 IU) is a powerful antioxidant and free radical eliminator. **Vitamin B complex** and **selenium** (500-1,000 mcg/day) are other effective agents.

• **Vitamin C** (2,000-10,000 mg daily, in divided doses) works in the white blood cells, to produce a powerful antiviral task force.

• **Zinc** (30 mg daily) is also important in adding to the body's own immune functions.

• Helpful herbs include **goldenseal, garlic, echinacea, red raspberry**.

• Drinking enough **water** is also important.

• Also see *Special Water Therapies which Fight Infectious Diseases (219-221), Special Antibiotic Herbs (297), Four Powerful Antidotes (830).*

PREVENTION—Trouble begins when the invaders are strong and many, and the body is in a weakened condition. Keep yourself in good health. Get **enough rest, exercise in the open air, and maintain a balanced, nourishing diet**.

ENCOURAGEMENT—God can help you, if you will daily seek Him for that help. Unless we continually cherish a close walk with God, we will be tempted to separate from Him and walk alone. Psalm 91:3-6.

STAPH INFECTIONS
(Staphylococcal Infection)

SYMPTOMS—Staph infections produces symptoms ranging from minor to severe to life-threatening. They can include pimples, abscesses, boils, furuncles, carbuncles, osteomyelitis, enterocolitis pneumonia, and bacteremia. They cause a wide range of problems, from skin infections to serious internal disorders.

CAUSES—These infections are produced by the staphylococcus family of bacteria, which is probably the most common bacteria in existence. Under a microscope, they appear as grape-like clusters.

Although present on the skin of most people, inside the body they can produce pustules, sties, etc., on the skin. Affecting the nose, throat, and lungs, they can weaken the body, leading to viral infections such as pneumonia. Infected needles can produce septic shock, infectious arthritis, osteomyelitis, or bacterial endocarditis. Contaminated food can also pass them into the body.

NATURAL REMEDIES
• Eat **whole grains and green vegetables**. **Avoid** sugar in all forms (including honey), oils, dairy products, and meat.
• Take **vitamin C** (1,000-5,000 mg, daily), **vitamin E** (100-400 IU, daily), **beta-carotene** (15-30 mg, daily), and **zinc** (15 mg, daily).
• Herbs which are especially useful in treating staph infections include: **raw garlic, honeysuckle,** and **bear lichen**.
• **Clean all wounds and cuts** with soap and water, flush with **hydrogen peroxide**, rinse with water, apply **tea tree oil** full strength. Repeat every 2 waking hours and before retiring at night. (Do not use iodine or alcohol; for they also kill living cells.) Expose wound to **fresh air and sunlight**. Apply warm **goldenseal** tea compresses to firmly adherent crust. **Change sheets**, pillow slips, towels, and clothing frequently to prevent reinfection.

PREVENTION
• It is important that, through **proper hygiene, diet, rest, exercise, and sunlight**, you maintain a strong immune system. Here are remedies which boost the immune system and help the body fight staph infections:

ENCOURAGEMENT—"Herein is love, not that we loved God, but that He loved us, and sent His Son to be the propitiation for our sins." 1 John 4:10.

SPECIAL ANTIBIOTIC HERBS
(Antimicrobial Herbs)

Read this article carefully and remember how to find it again when you need it.
No antibiotic drugs are useful against virus infections, but all of the following herbs are. Although this article tends to focus on natural antibiotics for viral infections, the following herbs are equally powerful fighters against bacterial infections as well.

NATURAL REMEDIES
• **Echinacea** contains *properdin*, which strengthens the immune system. It is also antibiotic and acts like *interferon*, the body's own antiviral compound. *(Turn to p. 156 for warnings about echinacea.)*
• **Garlic** contains *allicin*, one of the plant kingdom's most potent, broad-spectrum antibiotics (but only if eaten raw). Dice it up raw (or put it in a garlic press) and put it in juice or spread it on surface infections. Or take garlic oil or garlic concentrate tablets. Here is another successful formula: Put a can of tomato (or V-8) juice into a blender, along with 3 cloves of garlic. Drink it at various times throughout the day. Keep the leftover juice in the refrigerator. Cooked garlic lacks the antibiotic factors. Garlic is powerful against bacterial, viral, and fungal infections.
• **Goldenseal** contains *berberine* and *hydrastine*, and is a broad-spectrum herbal antibiotic. *Berberine*, is an immune stimulant. (*Berberine* is also in **barberry root bark** and **Oregon grape root**, two other antibiotics. *Turn to p. 161 for warnings about goldenseal.*)
• **Juniper berries** contain *deoxypodophyllotoxin*, which inhibits a number of different viruses. *(Turn to pp. 165 for warnings about juniper berries.)*
• **Licorice** has eight active antiviral compounds, including *glycyrrhizin*, which keeps viruses from replicating. Licorice has the most bactericidal compounds (up to 33% antibacterial compounds on a dry-weight basis). It also has *saponins*, which increase the availability of other antibiotic compounds. *(Turn to pp. 166-167 for warnings about licorice.)*
• **Ginger** contains 10 antiviral compounds, called *sesquiterpenes*.
• **Lemon balm** is also antiviral.
• **Shiitake** is a tasty Asian mushroom which contains *lentinan*, an antiviral, immune-stimulating and anti-tumor compound.
• **Astragalus** is a Chinese herb which increases the natural killing function of the body's immune system.

(Turn to p. 143 for a warning about astragalus.)

• **Dragon's Blood** is a South American herb which has *dimethylcedrusine* and *taspine*; these have antiviral and wound-healing properties.

• **Eucalyptus** contains *hyperoside, quercitrin* and *tannic acid*, which have virus-killing functions.

• **Olive leaf extract** is a powerful antibiotic, and is excellent for viral infections, the common cold, arthritis, skin diseases, heart trouble, and much more.

• Other herbs rich in bactericidal compounds, in descending order of potency, include **thyme, hops, oregano, and rosemary**.

• Remember that you can always use **licorice** extract, and/or **ginger** (both of which are antibiotic herbs), to help sweeten and flavor your tea with other antibiotic herbs.

ENCOURAGEMENT—We are to keep our minds stayed upon God. In our weakness, He will be our strength; in our ignorance, He will be our wisdom; in our frailty, He will be our enduring might. Exodus 19:5.

SPECIAL HERBAL ANTISEPTICS

Here are several natural antiseptic herbs which you can use to kill germs and hasten healing:

Clove: The oil is a strong germicide. It can be placed on gums, where there are toothaches. Do not swallow the oil.

False unicorn: This valuable herb contains *chamaelirin*, which is a strong antiseptic. It will help eliminate tapeworms from the intestinal tract.

Carrots: Boil and mash carrots; then apply to a sore, to help draw out pus and provide healing.

Lemons: A powerful antiseptic which destroys bacteria. It also helps fade freckles, when applied to the skin.

Thyme: This useful herb contains *thymol*. Put small amounts on wounds. Crush and add to boiling water. Then steep, strain, and apply to sprains and bruises.

Goldenseal: This invaluable herb contains *berberine*, and can be used for gum and mouth infections. It will also help eliminate worms in the bowels.

Black walnut: This is good for internal parasites, infection, tonsillitis, and other internal or external applications.

Cabbage leaves: Containing *rapine*, this is a strong antibiotic. Place warm leaves on an ulcerated sore to draw out the pus.

Myrrh: This herb has excellent antiseptic properties. Is good for dysentery and uterine and vaginal infections. Apply it to the gums for toothaches and paeridontal diseases. It is an outstanding antibacterial and antiviral herb.

Queen of the meadow: This antiseptic herb is used for diseases of the uterus.

Garlic: This powerful herb contains *allicin*. Garlic oil is useful for ear infections. Crushed garlic is useful

for many problems.

SPECIAL WATER THERAPIES WHICH FIGHT INFECTIOUS DISEASES

NATURAL REMEDIES

For specific information on a great variety of water therapy treatments, turn to the chapter on hydrotherapy *(206-275)*.

Water therapies which encourage the elimination of toxins: **Radiant Heat Bath, Sweating wet-sheet pack, Steam bath**. The elimination of sweat production and washing it away is very important.

Water therapies which greatly increase leucocytic activity: The following applications help increase white blood cell formation. WBCs, as you know, are a primary body fighter against toxins and bacterial infection. **General cold bath. Heating compress,** frequently renewed. **Alternate heating compress**.

Water therapies which greatly encourage elimination of bacteria by the skin and kidneys: **Steam bath, Sweating wet-sheet pack, Prolonged neutral bath**. Also good: **Sweating baths.** Copious **water drinking**. Each of these should be followed by a **cold mitten friction, cold towel rub**, or some other cold procedure.

ENCOURAGEMENT—"I will receive you, and will be a Father unto you, and ye shall be My sons and daughters, saith the Lord Almighty." 2 Corinthians 6:17-18. What a promise is made here. What a relationship this is; higher and holier than any earthly tie.

FUNGAL INFECTIONS

SYMPTOMS—Moist, possibly itchy, red patches on the skin, mucous membranes, under the nails, between the toes, or on internal surfaces of the colon, vagina, or throat.

CAUSES—Fungal infections grow most frequently in moist, hot areas on the skin, especially in crevices where the skin touches skin or nails and on the surfaces of the colon, vagina, or throat: Athlete's foot *(377)* occurs between the toes. Candida *(281)* in the throat or colon. Ringworm *(335)*, also known as tinea infection, is a fungal infection of the skin or scalp.

If, while treating the fungal infection, you develop symptoms of a worse infection (such as increased redness and swelling or fever) you may have contracted a bacterial infection—in addition to the fungal infection.

NATURAL REMEDIES

• Avoid applying soap to the area.

NUTRITION

• Eat a nourishing diet of **fruits, vegetables, whole grains, legumes, and nuts**. While treating the infection, a diet primarily of **raw food** is best.

• Avoid **tobacco, alcohol, caffeine**. Do not eat **meat**

or dairy products. Avoid **sugary, fried, and processed foods**. Eat nothing **greasy**.

HERBS

• **Goldenseal** contains *berberine*, which destroys fungi. It can be used against every type of fungus infection. It can be used in a drink or topically applied. Only use goldenseal for a week; then switch, for a time, to another fungicide herb.

• **Pau d'arco** is strongly antifungal. Drink 3 cups daily.

• **Bloodroot** also contain *berberine* and has been shown to be quite effective as a fungicide.

• **Yellowroot, barberry, and Oregon grape** also contain *berberine*.

• **Tea tree** oil is excellent when applied externally, but do not drink it. Apply it several times a day to the affected area, either full strength or diluted with a little distilled water or cold-pressed oil. **Black walnut** extract can also be used.

• A powerful antifungicide is **wild oregano oil**. The most resistent forms of fungus infection can generally be eliminated by it.

• The **pepper tree** (horopito) is a New Zealand shrub which contains *polygodial*; this is useful against both fungi and bacteria. Another antifungal herb is the *Licaria puchuri-major*, a Brazilian plant.

• Research studies have found that raw **garlic** inhibited every type of fungal infection it was applied to.

• **If you're prone to fungal infections, here are several ways to avoid them:** Keep the skin clean and dry. Because fungal infections can spread, don't share combs, brushes, hats, towels, clothes, or shoes with others. To reduce the risk of getting athlete's foot, have a spare pair of socks handy and change into them if your feet become sweaty. Better yet, wear sandals. Disinfect shower stalls and tubs frequently. To prevent groin itch, change into dry clothes after exercising; choose loose clothing that improves air circulation; and wear fabrics that breathe or wick away perspiration.

ENCOURAGEMENT—The Lord, our Redeemer, is heir of God; and those who are co-laborers with Him, in the work of saving souls, are joint heirs with Him. Rom 8:17. To be an overcomer is to be placed in the ranks of those who have the far more exceeding and eternal weight of glory.

SPECIAL ANTIFUNGAL HERBS

Here are some of the best antifungal, antiyeast herbs:

• **Garlic** is excellent, both internally and externally. Clinical trials of people taking 25 milliliters (5-6 tsp.) of garlic extract daily revealed that their blood serum showed significant antifungal activity against several common fungi. Garlic extract is even more powerful when applied externally to fungal infections. Liquefy raw garlic in a blender; put it on a clean cloth and apply it to the area 3 times a day.

• **Licorice** contains 25 fungicidal compounds, more than most other herbs. Add 5-7 tsp. powdered licorice root to a cup of boiling water and simmer about 20 minutes. Strain out the pulp. Apply the liquid on a cloth to the affected area 1-3 times daily. *(Turn to pp. 166-167 for warnings about licorice.)*

• **Tea tree oil** is very good on athlete's foot and candida. Research studies found it better than drugs for eliminating candida. For skin infections, apply 2-3 drops directly to the area 2-3 times a day. If it is irritating to the skin, mix it with some vegetable oil. But do not swallow tea tree oil. It can be fatal. This is one of the strongest of the antifungal herbs. You may first want to try a milder one. *(Turn to p. 182 for a warning about swallowing tea tree oil.)*

• **Chamomile** is another powerful fungicide. It is widely used in Europe, especially against candida. Make a strong tea and apply it directly to the area. *(Turn to pp. 151 for a warning about chamomile.)*

• **Goldenseal, Oregon grape root, barberry, goldthread, and yellow root** all contain *berberine*, a powerful fungicide and antibacterial compound.

• **Pau d'arco** contains three antifungal compounds: *lapachol, beta-lapachone,* and *xyloidine.*

• **Turmeric oil**, even at very low concentrations, inhibits fungi. Purchase commercial oil of turmeric, dilute it (1 part oil to 2 parts water), and apply directly to the area. Do not swallow this oil!

• **Lemongrass.** You can drink 1-4 cups of lemongrass tea daily. It tastes good. Apply the spent tea bags directly to the affected area.

• **Black walnut.** The powdered fresh husk destroys candida and other fungi. Mix 1 oz. of the tincture with a few drops of valerian root, pau d'arco, and 10 drops of tea tree oil. Apply it to the area.

ENCOURAGEMENT—God loves you as He loves His own Son.

HERPES VIRUS INFECTIONS

SYMPTOMS—Infections that can cause painful blisters on, or around, the lips and genitals. Small, painful blisters on the skin and mucous membranes.

CAUSES—Herpes simplex viruses (HSV) are highly contagious and cause a number of different disorders. The infection is transmitted by contact with a blister.

Even though one has been infected with HSV, this does not give immunity. The viruses remain dormant in the nerves and may be reactivated at times of stress or illness. Like many viral infections, outbreaks are more frequent and severe in people with reduced immunity, such as those with AIDS.

There are at least seven types of herpes viruses. The two primary ones are HSV1 and HSV2.

HSV1 (also called herpes, type I) usually causes infections of the lips, mouth, and face (cold sores, *322*). Most people have been infected with HSV1 by the time they are adults. Infections tend to be of minor consequence. But some children, with the skin disorder, eczema *(345)*, may develop eczema herpeticum. After the initial infection, the virus becomes dormant but may periodically reactivate later in life, causing cold sores. Many researchers believe that HSV1 is involved in causing Bell's Palsy *(565)*.

HSV2 (also called herpes, type II) typically causes infections of the genitals (genital herpes, *805-806*).

Both HSV1 and HSV2 can affect the eyes, causing herpes keratoconjunctivitis (see conjunctivitis, *400*). In rare cases, the viruses can cause severe viral inflammation of the brain.

Herpes zoster *(350)* causes chicken pox *(742)*, in children, and shingles *(350)* in adults. The drug companies urgently want to require children to obtain vaccinations against chicken pox. But the fact is that children who get chicken pox quickly recover and are thereafter immune to shingles. But those who never contract chicken pox as children are in danger of getting shingles—a very dangerous disease—when they grow up.

Epstein-Barr virus *(280)* is the virus which also produces infectious mononucleosis *(664)*.

NATURAL REMEDIES

• For natural remedies, go to the specific herpes infection, listed above.

ENCOURAGEMENT—God watches over us with more tenderness than does a mother over an afflicted child. "Your Father knoweth what things ye have need of, before ye ask Him." Matthew 6:8.

IATROGENIC DISEASES

In this, the only section of the Encyclopedia discussing general infections, mention should be made about two new emerging causes of illness:

"Iatrogenic diseases" are defined by an American Medical Association as **"physician-induced diseases."** The July 26, 2000, issue of the *Journal of the American Medical Association* discussed this problem.

This is an unfortunate situation; however, it is best that you are aware of the difficulty. The *Journal* would not have printed the article if they did not want people to know about it. We value our physicians and the care they provide. Yet they are only human and, from time to time, the modern system of rapidly seeing one patient right after another causes difficulties. Here are a few of the research findings in the article:

"As many as 20% to 30% of patients receive contraindicated care" *(ibid.)*. "Contraindicated" is a big word which means care the patients definitely should not have received.

The Institute of Medicine (IOM) has released a report (*"To Err is Human"*), quoted in the JAMA article, which stated that **"millions of Americans [have] learned, for the first time, that an estimated 44,000 to 98,000 among them died each year as a result of medical errors"** *(ibid.)*.

"U.S. estimates of the combined effect of errors and adverse effects that occur because of iatrogenic [physician-caused] damage, not associated with recognizable error, include 12,000 deaths/year from unnecessary surgery. 7,000 deaths/year from medication errors in hospitals. 20,000 deaths/year from other errors in hospitals. 80,000 deaths/year from nosocomial infections in hospitals. 106,000 deaths/year from non-error, adverse effects of medications.

"These total to 225,000 deaths per year from iatrogenic causes. Three caveats [warnings] should be noted. First, most of the data are derived from studies in hospitalized patients. Second, **these estimates are for deaths only and do not include adverse effects that are associated with disability or discomfort.** Third, the estimates of death due to error are lower than those in the IOM report.

"If the higher estimates are used, the deaths due to iatrogenic causes would range from 230,000 to 284,000. In any case, 225,000 deaths per year constitutes the third leading cause of death in the United States, after deaths from heart disease and cancer.

"Even if these figures are overestimated, there is a wide margin between these numbers of deaths and the next [fourth] leading cause of death [cerebrovascular disease]" *(ibid.)*.

A different analysis was mentioned in the JAMA article which estimated negative effects on outpatients (those not in hospitals), without including deaths. It concluded that **a surprising number of patients are so damaged by the drug and other treatments, that they must make an immense number of additional trips to see the doctor or go to the hospital.** Here is this remarkable statement in JAMA:

"One analysis . . [which did not include deaths] concluded that **between 4% and 18% of consecutive patients experience adverse effects in outpatient settings,** with [resulting in] 116 million extra physician visits, 77 million extra prescriptions, 17 million emergency department visits, 8 million hospitalizations, 3 million long-term admissions, 199,000 additional deaths, and $77 billion in extra costs" *(ibid.)*.

ENCOURAGEMENT—God is a friend in perplexity and affliction, a protector in distress, a preserver in the thousand dangers that are unseen to us.

NOSOCOMIAL INFECTIONS

There is a fast-growing hospital crisis in America. And if you live in Canada or overseas, think not that you have escaped the problem. Many of the same factors are affecting foreign hospitals. The following information comes from CDC (Centers for Disease Control) records and a series of articles in the *Chicago Tribune*. Go to chicagotribune.com and especially request the July 22, 2002 issue.

It is vital that you understand that our hospitals urgently need your help! First, we will overview the problem; then we will present several solutions. We want our hospitals to succeed. Yet it is unlikely to occur as long as the public is ignorant of the nature of the problem.

There are 900 fewer U.S. hospitals today, in the new century, than there were in 1980. That fact, plus greatly reduced federal subsidizing of hospital patient expenses since the mid-1980s, has led to unfortunate results.

Federal, state, and other public records reveal that **75,000 of the dangerous infections that patients acquired in hospitals in the year 2000 could have been prevented** if proper patient care and sanitary maintenance had been done. That figure (75,000) represents three-fourths of the 100,000 infections which occurred that year in hospitals. **These are infections which the patient *did not bring* to the hospital—but which he contracted during his stay there.**

Yet most of those infections were often preventable by simple, inexpensive measures. Unfortunately, as a "cost-cutting expedient," they are not done. **A key problem is the hospital cutbacks in the number of staff and subsequent carelessness by overworked physicians, nurses, and cleaning personnel.**

Such a large number of people are becoming infected because they go to hospitals, even for as little as one day, that the CDC has given those infections a special name: They are called ***"nosocomial infections."*** You may have had an acquaintance who mysteriously died while in a hospital. The CDC says that person acquired a "nosocomial infection." That is Latin for "hospital-acquired." The CDC admits it invented the term to shield hospitals from "embarrassment."

Did you know that **the fourth leading cause of death in America (behind heart disease, cancer, and strokes)—is bacteria or viruses given to patients in hospitals—germs which they did not have before they entered those hospitals!** This is astonishing.

At the present time, **more people die because of infections they acquired at U.S. hospitals than those who die from automobile accidents**, fires, or drowning—combined.

Using analytic methods commonly used by epidemiologists, **the *Tribune* found an estimated 103,000 deaths linked to hospital infections in the year 2000 alone.** The Centers for Disease Control and Prevention (CDC), in Atlanta, based its figures on 315 hospitals and an estimated 90,000 deaths caused by infections acquired at U.S. hospitals that same year.

It was found that repeated cost-cutting measures, including nurse layoffs, led to infection-control violations and injury or death to patients.

Since 1995, **over 75% of all hospitals in the United States have been cited for significant cleanliness and sanitation violations.** That totals about 4,350 hospitals, or about three out of every four in the land.

In order to cut costs, U.S. hospitals have reduced cleaning staffs by 25% since 1995 alone.

The CDC and HHS declare that a **clean-hands policy** in our hospitals would, alone, prevent the deaths of up to 20,000 patients each year.

Medical instruments, designed to be slipped into body openings (throat, urethra, vagina, colon, etc.) are frequently contaminated, producing infection.

Doctors wear **germ-laden clothes** from home into the hospital, and even into the operating room. In many hospitals, staff members regularly wear their scrubs home and back to work the next day.

Another serious problem is **adverse drug reactions** (ADR) in hospitalized patients. The situation has become so serious that the *Journal of the American Medical Association* (JAMA) published a report on the problem in its April 15, 1998, issue. This problem generally occurs because **wrong drug (or wrong dosage)** is given to the patient. The article said this:

"In 1994, overall, 2,216,000 hospitalized patients had serious ADRs and 106,000 had fatal ADRs, making these reactions between the fourth and sixth leading cause of death."

According to CDC and *Tribune* findings, in the year 2000 alone, the deaths of 2,610 infants were caused by preventable hospital-acquired infections.

A national study of 799 hospitals, by the Harvard University School of Public Health, found that hospital-acquired infections were directly linked to inadequate nursing staff levels.

What are your chances of acquiring a hospital-induced infection the next time you, or a loved one, goes to the hospital? According to CDC records, you have one chance in 16 of becoming infected with something very serious which could disable or kill you. About 2.1 million patients each year are becoming infected at hospitals. That is 6% of the 35 million admissions annually.

Our hospitals need your help, but there is a solution: Write your U.S. senator and representative and urge that bills be introduced into Congress, mandating better care of patients. We need our hospitals, but they need to be safe!

ENCOURAGEMENT—The gifts of Him who has all power in heaven and earth are in store for the children of God. Gifts so precious that they come to us through the costly sacrifice of the Redeemer's blood; gifts that will satisfy the deepest craving of the heart; gifts lasting as eternity. They are for all who will come to God as little children, submitting to His will for their lives.

CONVALESCENCE

After one has experienced an illness that is more or less severe, there is a period of convalescence, during which the body corrects the losses suffered and normalizes the weakened functions. This period of recovery generally follows any infectious disease. Here are several helpers:

An infusion or decoction of **angelica root** will increase appetite and aid the digestive process. Cooked **oatmeal** flakes will invigorate and balance the nervous system, while nourishing the body. **Spirulina** will invigorate and help revitalize the system. **Ginseng** root powder will provide general invigoration. Raw or toasted **sesame seed** is extremely helpful and nutritive.

ENCOURAGEMENT—Take God's promises as your own, plead them before Him as His own words, and you will receive fullness of joy.

POST-OPERATIVE RECOVERY

Any surgical procedure requires special nutritional attention. Major surgeries, especially abdominal surgery, should be followed by methods designed to reduce inflammation and swelling while promoting proper wound healing. Such measures will not only improve recovery but also help prevent adhesions and excessive scar formation.

To help prevent scarring, apply warm-to-hot **castor oil** over an incision *after* the stitches are removed.

Vitamin E (400 IU), to help reduce scar formation. High-potency **vitamin C** (1,000 mg, 3 times daily), to reduce infection. **Flaxseed oil** (1 Tbsp., daily). **Multivitamin supplement**.

Begin the above regime at least 2 weeks prior to surgery. After surgery, continue it for a month, adding **bromelain** (500 mg, twice daily after meals), to aid in protein digestion.

Barley broth is quite restorative and tasty. Simmer 1 cup barley in 6 cups water. Bring to a boil for 2 minutes, let stand for 15 minutes. Strain out the barley and set aside. Drink the water for strength during convalescence. If hungry, the barley can be eaten and, if desired, blended with a little honey.

ENCOURAGEMENT—The power of God is manifested in the beating of the heart, in the action of the lungs, and in the living currents that circulate through the thousand different channels of the body. We are indebted to Him for every moment of existence and for all the comforts of life. James 1:17.

GENERAL - 5 - FEVER

Related data: Diphtheria (747),
Rocky Mountain Spotted Fever (840),
Typhus (839), Childhood Diseases (724-753)

FEVER

SYMPTOMS—A fever is an elevation of body temperature above normal. A fever is not a disease, but a sign that an infection or disease is present. Fevers are common in a wide variety of diseases, from mild to severe.

Symptoms include headache, flushed face, body aches, nausea, little or no appetite, and sometimes diarrhea or vomiting. Skin may be warm, with some perspiration, or hot and dry. The elevated temperature is an effort by the body to burn out infection, and the perspiration helps eliminate toxins. Therefore a partial fever may be helpful to the body, in fighting the infection. If the fever does not get too high, let it run its course. Many enzymes, antibodies, and white blood cell responses are better during slightly elevated temperatures.

MORE ABOUT FEVERS—Normal temperature is generally considered to be within a range of 97° to 99° F., but it can vary among individuals. If it is 100° F. or above, it is a fever. A fever is defined as body temperature above 98.6° F., measured orally, or 99.8° F. measured from the rectum. One should not have undue concern unless the body temperature rises above 102° F. in adults or 103° F. in children. Then give a tepid bath, and call a doctor immediately. Most fevers never go above 102° F. and most only for a few days.

When body temperature is not more than 5° above normal, it does not completely interfere with body functions. *But levels above 105° F. are dangerous*. At 106° F., convulsions are common; at 108° F., irreversible brain damage frequently results.

Fevers help destroy the bacteria and viruses. But fevers in an infant or small child needs special care, to avoid seizures.

Keep in mind that the fever is not the infection; the infection must be healed as well as the fever.

Putting too many clothes on a child can actually cause a fever.

CAUSE—Fever is not a disease; but it is a condition in the body, wherein the balance of circulation has become disturbed. This is nature's way of trying to burn out the toxic poisons. When the body becomes exposed to excessive chilling or dampness, the capillaries near the surface contract and the pores close by becoming obstructed with body waste matter. This results in a containment of body heat and a sudden rise of body

CHART 1057: Termination of Fever Crisis and Lysis - Fevers 302-309 temperature. In fever, the natural body function is to increase the heat to a point wherein the thick glutinous and fibrinous matters loading and congesting the system are made liquid enough to pass through the fine and delicate excretory membranes and tubules.

NATURAL REMEDIES

DURING THE FEVER

• *If the fever gets too high* (above 102° F. in adults or 103° F. in children), **immediately immerse the body in tepid water**, to lower the temperature. *If it then goes to 103° F.—contact a doctor!*

• Other suggestions would include: **ice packs on the forehead, running cool water over the wrists, cool baths, and drinking certain herb teas**, such as feverfew, cinchona bark, and/or white willow. Others include meadowsweet, sea buckthorn, European holly, and mugwort. A poultice to lower fever can be made from **echinacea** root. **Linden** tea can induce sweating to break a fever. **Black elder** tea is also good.

• **Enemas of catnip tea** are an outstanding way to lower fevers. They bring a high fever down quickly and keep it down. They also relieve constipation and congestion, which tend to keep fevers up. When body temperature goes above 102° F., (103° F. in children over two), give a catnip tea enema. Repeat it ever 4-6 hours, and continue taking them twice a day as long as the fever persists. Do not give catnip tea enemas to children under two.

• **Liquids** are especially beneficial. He should take liquids for 3-5 days.

• **Drink diluted fruit juices,** if fever dominates over chills, **and vegetable or grain soup** if chills dominate over fever. **Hot teas** induce sweating.

• **Vitamin C** (2,000 mg) **and lemon juice** are especially helpful. Other nutrients include **vitamins A (25,000 IU for only a few days), B complex, vitamin B$_1$ (200 mg), vitamin D (4,000 IU, daily for not more than a month), calcium (2,000 mg), magnesium (500 mg), and potassium (2,500 mg).**

• There is a loss of protein during a fever. Caloric needs are higher, and metabolism is increased. **Greater fluid intake** is required. As fluid is lost, sodium and potassium are lost. Drink plenty of distilled **water**, also **fruit and vegetable juices**. It is important that solid food be avoided until the fever reduces.

• Nutrient-rich juices are especially helpful: **beet juice, carrot juice**, etc.

• *For a feverish child,* place a grape or strawberry within a cube of frozen fruit juice, and let him suck on it.

• **Never give aspirin** to children. It can trigger Reye's Syndrome, a potentially fatal neurological illness.

• He needs lots of **oxygen**. Make sure there is a current of air in the room; open the window. Get smokers out of the house.

• **Wet compresses** help to reduce temperature. Keep removing them and applying new ones as he heats up the old ones. Apply them to the forehead, wrists, and calves of the legs. Keep the rest of the body covered.

• **Cool tap water** can be sponged on the skin, to dissipate excess heat. Wring out a sponge and wipe one section at a time, keeping the rest of the body covered. Because of rapid evaporation, you will not need to dry him with a towel.

• Some people shiver when they have a fever. *If he shivers,* immerse him in a tub of warm water. This will also lower temperature. *For babies,* give **room-temperature baths**. Sandwich them between **wet towels**, which are changed every 15 minutes.

• *If very hot,* remove more covers and clothes; *if chilly,* add them.

• **Lemon** juice and lemon drinks are used in the Mediterranean to control fevers. Lemon is cooling. Take hot lemon tea and honey as often as desired.

• If you have a fever, add **peppermint** to fever-fighting herb teas, including one or more of the following: **willow, ginger, elder, and meadowsweet**. All are excellent fever-reducing herbs. Other outstanding fever reducers include **echinacea, garlic, myrrh gum, licorice root, and goldenseal**. Use singly or together.

• **Blue vervain** tea is excellent for inducing a sweat, which helps the patient's temperature lower.

• To reduce a fever, drink **feverfew** tea. To break a high fever, drink hot **ginger** tea.

• **Catnip** tea (a nerve tonic) can be used as an enema to relax the person and reduce fever. **Dandelion** tea has a long history in the treatment of fever.

• Drinking **barley water** helps patients with high fevers. Because it has no irritating properties, it is helpful when the chest lining or intestinal lining is inflamed. Or cook **rice** with lots of water, and drink the water.

• American Indians use **cayenne** to reduce fevers. Add a pinch to any herbal drink. It will bring the blood to the stomach, reducing the fever.

• **Carrot-beet-cucumber juice** is a specific to clean the kidneys and help bring a fever down.

• A unexplained fever of 99-99.8° F. may be due to a food allergy.

• If the fever is from a cold or flu, eliminate the mucoid condition and eliminate the problem. **Raspberry, and other sweetening herbs**, are very beneficial. **Cautiously raise the body heat** with moisture, a stimulant, and diaphoretic herbs; so the restricted blood vessels relax, the obstructed pores open, and the morbid material washes out in the subsequent profuse perspiration.

• As mentioned earlier, one should not have undue concern unless the body temperature rises above 102° F. in adults or 103° F. in children. Then give a tepid bath, and call a doctor immediately. Most fevers never go above 102° F. and most only for a few days.

AFTER THE FEVER

• *When signs of fever are gone*, be sure to **prevent chilling**.

• *After the fever has subsided*, eat easily digested foods: **soybean milk, potassium broth (thick potato peeling soup), zwieback, baked white potato, natural brown rice, and very ripe bananas**.

R.T. Trall, M.D. made this statement: "Fevers, if left to themselves, run a certain course and terminate in a given time by a sudden increase of symptoms, called sinking, or a complete subsidence [elimination] of them, and the commencement of convalescence. This change has been called the *crisis*, and the days on which it occurs, *critical days*. The 3, 5, 7, 9, 11, 14, 17, and 20 have been regarded as critical days."—*Hydropathic Encyclopedia, p. 79.*

RECURRENCE

If feverish flu-like symptoms keep recurring: In children this might indicate diabetes; and, in teenagers and adults, Epstein-Barr virus.

J.H. KELLOGG, M.D., PRESCRIPTIONS FOR VARIOUS TYPES OF FEVERS *(how to give these water therapies: pp. 207-272 / list of treatments: pp. 206-207 / Hydrotherapy Disease Index: pp. 273-275)*

FEVER DISEASES (ACUTE): COMPLICATIONS—This section deals with a number of complications that commonly arise during febrile (fever) disorders.

GASTRITIS—**Fomentation** every 3 hours, followed in intervals between by **Heating Compress** at 60° F., to be changed every 30 minutes.

ENTEROCOLITIS—Large **Hot Enema** (100° F.), followed by **Neutral Enema** (96° F.) after each bowel movement. Fomentation to abdomen every 3 hours. **Heating Compress** at 60° F. during intervals in between, changed every 30 minutes.

PERITONITIS—**Hot Enema,** 3 times daily; **Fomentation** every 3 hours; **Heating Compress** at 60° F. during the intervals between, changing every 30 minutes.

PERICARDITIS AND ENDOCARDITIS—**Fomentation** for 30 minutes every hour, followed by Ice Bag or **Cold Compress**, to be removed for 5 minutes every 15 minutes. **Hot Hip and Leg Pack** if extremities are cold. **Cold Mitten Friction**, to maintain surface circulation.

PHLEBITIS, ARTHRITIS—**Hot Blanket Pack** followed by **Cold Mitten Friction**, carefully avoiding the affected part, or **Hot Pack** to affected limb for 15 minutes every 3 hours. The Hot application should be followed by the **Heating Compress** which is changed after the next hot application and retained during the interval between.

LARYNGITIS—**Steam Inhalation**. **Fomentation** to the throat every 3 hours with **Heating Compress** during the interval in between. Renew this every 15 minutes at first and later once an hour. Derivative applications to legs: **Hot Footbaths**, **Hot Leg Packs**, **Heating Leg Pack**. Repeat 3-4 times daily. **Fomentation** for 15 minutes every 3 hours, with well-protected **Heating Compress** between, changing once an hour. Derivative treatment to lower extremities. **Steam Inhalation** for 15 minutes every hour.

BRONCHO-PNEUMONIA—**Fomentation** to chest every 2 hours, **Heating Compress** at 60° F., during the interval in between, changing every 30 minutes; **Hot Blanket Pack** for 15 minutes, followed by **Heating or Sweating Wet Sheet Pack**. Give 1-3 applications each 24 hours.

PLEURISY—**Fomentation** every 15 minutes until pain is relieved. Repeat every 3 hours. Well-protected **Heating Compress** during the interval between. Tight bandage about chest, if needed to control pain.

NEPHRITIS, ALBUMINURIA—**Hot Blanket Pack** for 30- 60 minutes, 2-3 times in 24 hours. Follow by **Cold Friction**. Protect the surface and maintain vigorous surface circulation. **Large Enema,** 3 times a day; copious water drinking; **Fomentation** to lower back region every 4 hours for 30 minutes, followed by **Heating Compress** during interim between; **Ice Bag** over lower sternum.

EDEMA—The same treatment as for Nephritis and Albuminuria, just above, with the addition of the **Cold Compress over the heart** for 15 minutes every 2 hours.

DELIRIUM—**Ice Cap, Ice Collar, and Heating Wet Sheet Pack** continued 1-2 hours. **Prolonged Tepid or Neutral Bath**.

PARALYSIS—**Ice Cap, ice to spine**; alternate with **Fomentation** for 3 minutes every 15 minutes, repeating 4 times. Repeat every 4 hours.

CONVULSIONS—**Ice Cap; ice to spine; Hot Hip and Leg Pack. Hot Full Bath** 105° F., 5-8 minutes, with **ice to head and neck**.

ABSCESS—**Fomentation** for 15 minutes every 2 hours; **Heating Compress** at 60° F. during the interval between. Renew every 15-30 minutes.

VISCERAL INFLAMMATION—Large hot **Fomentation** over inflamed part for 15 minutes every 2 hours. During the interval between, **Heating Compress** at 60° F., renewed every 15 minutes during the acute stage. Later, **Fomentation** 3 times a day, with continuous **Heating Compress** during intervals between.

THREATENED GANGRENE—**Alternate Compress** every 3 hours, **Heating Compress** or dry heat during the intervals between.

TYPHOID STATE—**Aseptic diet**, copious **water** drinking, daily **Neutral Enema** at 95° F., prolonged **Neutral or Tepid Bath**; and **Graduated Bath**.

—*See Fever Diseases (233-239). Also see diseases listed under "Childhood Problems (Chicken pox, Diphtheria, Measles, Mumps, Scarlet Fever, etc.). They are on pp. 734-763.*

ENCOURAGEMENT—Christ came so that whosoever believeth in Him may be saved. As the flower turns to the sun, so our eyes should turn to Him. We dare not leave Him, lest we fall away. God can help you just now. Proverbs 24:16.

SMALLPOX
(Variola)

SYMPTOMS—It takes 12-14 days for the disease to develop after exposure. Several days of discomfort is followed by a severe chill, intense headache, terrible pain in the back and limbs, vomiting, fever, loss of appetite, and sometimes convulsions.

Then the fever lowers and the eruptions appear. The pain disappears, but the highly contagious disease can still be given to others.

The rash of smallpox initially consists of hard red papules, especially on the forehead, neck, and wrists. They gradually fill with clear serum, becoming vesicles, which become depressed at their centers and then fill with pus (called pustules).

CAUSES—Unsanitary living conditions and poor diet. The disease is highly contagious.

NATURAL REMEDIES
Call a physician.
• Keep the sick person **in bed with the windows darkened**, yet maintaining ventilation and an **even, moderate, temperature** of not over 70° F.
• Put him on a **fast of juices**. During the fever stage, give him plenty of **lemonade** without sweetening.
• Give **high herb enemas** and clean out the bowels. But, during the second to the fourth day, while the skin is producing the eruptions, do not meddle with the stomach and bowels. Give no emetics or strong purgatives during that time.
• *When the skin is hot and dry,* give him **fluids every hour** until there is free perspiration.
• *When the skin is hot and dry,* place equal parts of **pleurisy root and ginger** (or equal parts of **yarrow and valerian**) in a cup of boiling water, steep for 20 minutes, give a cupful every hour or until there is free perspiration.
• *If the fever rises above 103° F.,* reduce it by means of **tepid sponges** and **tepid enemas**. Give a **wet sheet pack**, which the patient warms up. Until the temperature lowers sufficiently, change it as soon as he warms it up.
• *If there is pain in the back and legs,* **hot fomentations** can partially relieve the pain.
• *If there is itching of the skin,* bathe him with **goldenseal root tea, yellow dock root, or burdock root**. Another formula: Mix 1 oz. **goldenseal** and 9 oz. **flaxseed oil**, and apply freely as needed.
• *If the extremities become cold,* warm them with hot water bottles.
• Use the same remedies on the second fever as you did on the first; do this with the same good results, if the first has been properly managed.
• **Open the pustules** by pricking with a sterilized needle, about 4 days after they come to a head. Then bathe them with **hydrogen peroxide**.
• **Bathing the pustules with goldenseal** tea will often keep pitting from occurring. Another formula is to **mix goldenseal with Vasoline** and apply to the pustules, to keep from pitting. Yet another formula is bathing the skin with a tea of **yellow dock root and goldenseal**.
• *During the fever,* **give no food save wheat-meal gruel**; but do not do this unless the appetite calls for it.
• Follow with a light diet of vegetable broth, oatmeal water, and fruit juices.
• *Prevention:* If there is danger of exposure to smallpox, **obtain adequate rest, eat carefully and lightly of good food**, and cleanse your system with **high enemas**.
• *To short the course of the disease:* **Hot baths**, taken before or after contracting smallpox will make the skin active and shorten its duration.

J.H. KELLOGG, M.D., PRESCRIPTIONS FOR SMALLPOX AND ITS COMPLICATIONS *(how to give these water therapies: pp. 207-275 / list of treatments: pp. 206-207 / Hydrotherapy Disease Index: pp. 273-275)*

GENERAL—Spare, aseptic diet; water drinking. See "Scarlet Fever. Build General Resistance."

LUMBAR (LOWER-BACK) PAIN—Fomentation or **Hot Trunk Pack** every 3 hours; **Heating Pack** during interval between, changing every 30-40 minutes.

NAUSEA AND VOMITING—Ice Bag over stomach, **Hot and Cold Trunk Pack**.

CONSTIPATION—Cold Enema daily, colonic at 70° F. daily.

DIARRHEA—Enema at 95° F. after each movement; **Fomentation** to abdomen; **Cold Compress** to be changed every hour.

DELAYED ERUPTION—Hot Blanket Pack or Hot Bath followed by **Sweating Wet Sheet Pack**.

FEVER—Graduated Bath; Prolonged Tepid Bath; Cooling Wet Sheet Pack; Cool Enema, with simultaneous **Fomentation** to back if necessary, to prevent chill; large **Cooling Compress**.

STAGE OF SUPPURATION (PUS FLOW)—Prolonged or Continuous **Neutral Bath**.

SWELLING OF FACE—Hot Compress to face for 5 minutes every hour; **Cold Compress** during intervals at 60° F., renewed every 20 minutes.

PITTING—Cooling Compress, using red cloth, covering face completely; Red curtains on windows.

HEADACHE AND DELIRIUM—Ice Cap, Ice Collar. Hot and **Cold Head Compress**.

CONTRAINDICATIONS—After the eruptions appear, **avoid** the Wet Hand Rub, Cold Mitten Friction, and all Friction Baths.

GENERAL METHOD—Keep the temperature down and maintain activity of the skin by Prolonged Neutral and Tepid Baths. Aid elimination by copious water drinking.

Prevent visceral complications by continuous cold to the head and the frequently changed Abdominal Compress. In confluent cases, general septicemia is prevented by Prolonged Full Baths.

If any of the following related problems exist, see under their respective headings: Broncho-Pneumonia, Endocarditis, Laryngitis, Nephritis, Inflammation of Eye.

ENCOURAGEMENT—It is beyond our power to conceive the blessings that are brought within our reach through Christ; we must unite our human effort with divine grace. As we do this, God enables us to fulfill His will for our lives. Isaiah 44:22.

CHOLERA
(Cholera Morbus)

SYMPTOMS—A few hours or days after contracting the disease, it suddenly begins, often with sudden cramps in the back, legs, or arms. Often there is severe vomiting. So much fluid is lost that he becomes extremely thirsty, and the skin becomes dry. Stools become thin and contain small, white curd-like masses.

Some cases of cholera are very light and have few symptoms other than the diarrhea.

CAUSES—Cholera occurs especially in hot, tropical climates. Filthy living conditions is generally the primary factor. Flies, cockroaches, ants, and mice all carry the disease.

A person cannot get it if he only eats and drinks that which has been boiled. Water and milk must be boiled. Vegetables and fruits must be washed and immersed in boiling water for a few seconds, then peeled.

NATURAL REMEDIES
Call a physician.
• Keep him **quiet in bed**. Provide **fluids** to compensate for the vomiting and fever. **Diluted peppermint or spearmint tea** is helpful. Have him drink a pint, then put your finger down his throat and help him vomit it out. This cleanses the stomach. (Do not do it if he is too weak.) Then give him a cup of **hot peppermint tea** to settle the stomach.
• If vomiting of mucous resumes, repeat the process.
• **Goldenseal** tea is also helpful.
• Give **enemas with white oak bark, bayberry bark, and wild cherry**.
• Give hot **fomentations** over the bowels and the full length of the spine.
• Simmer 2-3 Tbsp. **of cloves** in ½ pint **soymilk** for 5 minutes, Take 1 Tbsp. hot every 15 minutes.
• An infusion of **nettle tea** aids the healing of cholera and dysentery.
• All stools and discharges should be burned or disinfected. No one should touch what is used by the patient. Caregivers should wash their hands frequently.
• A diet of **oatmeal water or slippery elm water** is both nourishing and soothing. Combine with some soy

milk, to provide a balanced protein.
• **Rice water** will check the diarrhea as will **peach leaves, raspberry leaves, and sunflower leaves**. A warm **bayberry and catnip enema** is very soothing. **Antispasmodic tincture** is soothing and relaxing; and the **slippery elm** tea is nutritional and cleansing.
• Other useful herbs include **Uva Ursi, prickly ash, queen of the meadow, raspberry leaves, red clover, rhubarb, saleratus, smartweed, tormentil root, wild alum root, and wild yam**.

J.H. KELLOGG, M.D., PRESCRIPTIONS FOR CHOLERA AND ITS COMPLICATIONS *(how to give these water therapies: pp. 206-275 / list of treatments: pp. 206-207 / Hydrotherapy Disease Index: pp. 273-275)*

IMMEDIATE CONSIDERATION—Secure rest to the stomach and bowels by withholding food. Rest in bed.
VOMITING—Ice Bag over stomach, Ice pills, Ice Compress to the throat, Fomentation to spine, Ice Bag to spine, Hot and Cold Trunk Pack.
DIARRHEA—Hot Enema after each bowel movement; Fomentation over abdomen every 2 hours, duration 20 minutes during intervals between Heating Compress at 60° F., renewed every 30 minutes. If the temperature is above 102° F., Prolonged Neutral Bath or Hot Blanket Pack followed by Cold Mitten Friction or Cold Towel Rub.
COLLAPSE—Hot Blanket Pack for 15 minutes, followed by Cold Mitten Friction.
CARDIAC WEAKNESS—Ice Bag over heart.

ENCOURAGEMENT—If we will but seek God with all our hearts, if we will work with determined zeal to be a blessing each day, the light of heaven will shine upon us, even as it shone upon faithful Enoch. Hebrews 11:5-6.

MALARIA

SYMPTOMS—Chills occur for several hours, followed by drenching sweats every 1-3 days.

CAUSES—There are four types of parasites which are introduced into the bloodstream by the anopheles mosquito. If the disease becomes chronic (recurrent), it results in general debility, anemia, and an enlarged spleen.

Severe cases can be very debilitating. An especially deadly form is called blackwater fever. The skin takes on a yellow tint and the urine becomes progressively darker in color (caused by the excretion of blood in the urine). Few people survive attacks of blackwater fever.

This disease affects more people in the world than any other, and generally occurs only in tropical climates. But it can, and does, occur in the United States as well.

NATURAL REMEDIES
Call a physician.
There are two primary ways to treat malaria:
• One way is by taking **quinine**. This is an extract of the bark of the cinchona tree. Quinine will generally

CHART 1056: Malaria (306) / Mosquito Bite (832)

eliminate the malaria, but a mild to severe hearing loss may result.

• The other way is to give **hot and cold water treatments** to the person. This takes work. The result is equally good, but no hearing loss occurs.

• *During the fever*, give **cold applications** (cool wet sheet packs, sponge him off with cool water, etc.). *During the chills*, give him **hot applications** (hot packs).

• Give **goldenseal** tea.

A cold extract, decoction, powder, or extract of **gentian root** destroys the protozoa causing malaria. A decoction of **black alder** bark decreases the fever. A decoction of **quassia bark** is recommended for this tropical fever.

* **Cinchona bark** tea decreases the fever and is strongly anti-malarial. It eliminates toxins from the blood through sweat and urine. Use a cold extract or an infusion of the bark. Quinine is derived from cinchona, but cinchona is not as harmful as quinine (which is a patented product).

• An equally good substitute for cinchona is **willow bark** (various species). As bitter as quinine, it is also a good pain reliever and fever fighter. **Meadowsweet** also contains *salicin*, the effective chemical in willow.

• Use 2-3 tsp. **elder flowers** daily in tea for feverish chills. To strengthen the effect and add flavor to any fever-fighting herb tea, add **peppermint**.

• **Artemisinin** has been used by the Chinese for centuries to eliminate malaria.

—*See Fevers for additional help (302-309).*

ENCOURAGEMENT—Christ alone can place our feet in the right path. His perfection alone can avail for our imperfection. As we seek, by His enabling grace, to obey His Written Word, He will do for us what we could never do for ourselves. Proverbs 12:20.

TYPHOID FEVER

SYMPTOMS—Onset comes 1-4 weeks after the germs enter the body. First a tired feeling and general weakness, then possibly a headache and nosebleed. The fever rises higher each day until, by the end of the first week, it is 104° F. The evening temperature is distinctly higher than in the morning. Appetite is poor, the tongue is coated, and the teeth and lips have a brownish coat. There is either diarrhea or constipation, and stools are offensive. The abdomen is distended.

CAUSES—Typhoid fever is an acute infectious disease caused by the typhoid bacillus. It is an infectious affliction that is characterized by an enlargement of the spleen and the mesenteric lymph nodes, and catarrhal inflammation of the intestinal mucous membrane. After two or three weeks incubation, there is weakness, headache, vague pains, tendency to diarrhea, nosebleed, and

pronounced stupor. The stools have a peculiar pea-soup color. At times there is constipation; and usually there is slight congestion of the lung, accompanied by a cough. On the seventh to ninth day, peculiar eruptions of small, slightly elevated, rose-colored spots appear on the chest and abdomen. Frequently there is a complication of intestinal hemorrhoids, peritonitis, pneumonia, nephritis, and perforation of the bowel.

Germs are taken into the body through food or drink that has been directly, or indirectly, contaminated by bowel or kidney discharges from a typhoid fever patient.

If the body was kept clean and only pure food and water was consumed, there would by no typhoid.

NATURAL REMEDIES
Call a physician.

• Put him to **bed**; give him air, moderate **warmth**, and **lots of water** to drink.

• Place him on a diet of **fruit juices and vegetable broths**. All patients with typhoid fever must have **raw garlic** to eat.

• Give at least one **hot bath** every day. Have him remain in the tub as long as possible (30 minutes or longer). Put **cold cloths** on the head and throat if he is weak or faint. Finish with a **cold towel rub or spray**.

• Give a daily **high enema**.

• **Red clover** tea and **goldenseal** tea are both good. Add 1 teaspoon of red clover blossoms to a cup of boiling water. Steep and drink 5-12 cups a day.

• Drink hot **echinacea tea** until sweating occurs; then give hourly thereafter until the system is relieved of toxic buildup. Echinacea increases defenses against infections and stimulates processes of detoxification of the liver and kidneys.

• For congestion with nerve irritation and delirium of typhoid, combine **lady slipper** with **cayenne** and give frequently.

• Give **pleurisy root** tea when the skin is dry and hot. Give **wild cherry bark** tea when there is diarrhea.

• **Orange juice** and **oatmeal water** taken at separate intervals are good nourishment. Make a **vegetable broth** from several vegetables (carrot, celery, greens, and a little onion) and give it as a liquid broth.

• With fevers, use **moist heat** to facilitate the cleansing and elimination of the toxic backlog in the system. Induce profuse perspiration by the use of **hot yarrow or raspberry leaf tea** and by **soaking** in a tub of hot water, with up to a pound of **ginger** and a teaspoon each of **mustard and cayenne**. Follow with the **cold sheet treatment**.

• Other useful herbs are **bitterroot, bloodroot, chamomile, cranesbill root, goldenseal, mimosa gum, myrrh, Peruvian bark, pleurisy root, quince seed and fruit, red raspberry leaves, red sage, white oak bark, wild cherry bark, yarrow.**

—*Follow directions under Fevers (302-309).*

GEN

ENCOURAGEMENT—Christ is strong to deliver. Help has been laid on One that is mighty. He encircles man with His long human arm while with His divine arm He lays hold of all the power of heaven. Trust and obey; for there is no other way to be happy in Jesus. Psalm 103:9-12.

YELLOW FEVER

SYMPTOMS—Illness begins about 3-6 days after the mosquito bite. Onset is extremely abrupt (within a few hours), with a rapid rise in temperature from normalcy to 103° F. or more. The face is flushed and swollen; and the eyes are bloodshot. There are severe pains in the head, down the spine, and to the legs. Early in the disease, the pulse is rapid.

CAUSES—An acute, infectious, often fatal, febrile affliction of the tropical and subtropical regions of America, characterized by jaundice, hemorrhages, vomiting, etc. The affliction begins with a chill and pain in the head, sudden onset of fever (103°105° F), vomiting, constipation, scanty and albuminous urine. A period of diminution (remission) occurs; another fever attack; jaundice develops; and the vomit becomes darkened from the presence of blood. The disease is often fatal, occurring in the typhoid state or from uremia. Caused by a virus and transmitted by the bite of the *Aedes aegypti* mosquito or one of several closely related species. It rarely occurs today in North America; but, if you travel in Central and South America, it is more common there. Mosquito netting should be used.

Caused by a thick and sluggish bloodstream. Mucus clogs the body to the point that a fever takes over (without which it cannot clear itself). Yellow fever or other forms of fever do not occur when the body is in a healthy condition. The clogged condition is triggered by an organism carried by a mosquito.

The underlying cause is contagious cleansing-organisms that are introduced through contaminated foods.

NATURAL REMEDIES

• Read the article on *Fevers (302-309)* and apply it to control high fever (above 103° F.). *Reduce fever* with gently given **tepid sponges** over the body.

• Give a **high enema** (preferably a saline enema), and put the patient to bed. He should eat **no food for 3 days**; instead, squeeze juice of 2-3 **lemons** into a quart of water and drink 2 quarts unsweetened every day. Drink a quart of an **herb tea** (*listed under Fevers*).

• *If vomiting is severe,* so water cannot be retained in the stomach, give an **enema** every 2 hours of about a half pint of **tepid water** with a half teaspoon of **baking soda** dissolved in it. Give these enemas slowly.

• Give an **emetic** if there is a lot of phlegm.

• *On the fourth day,* begin giving him **light nutritious food**. Give **fomentations** to the spine; with a **footbath and cold compress** to the head, twice a day.

• Work the fever out through the skin by the use of **diaphoretics, vapor baths, heat baths, cold sheeting;** and **change to a correct diet**.

• To avoid liver damage, do not use tobacco, alcohol, drugs, excess salt, cooked foods, fried foods, processed foods, etc.

J.H. KELLOGG, M.D., PRESCRIPTIONS FOR YELLOW FEVER AND ITS COMPLICATIONS (*how to give these water therapies: pp. 206-275 / list of treatments: pp. 206-207 / Hydrotherapy Disease Index: pp. 273-275*)

MAINTAIN GENERAL VITAL RESISTANCE—**Short hot** applications, followed by **Cold** Mitten Friction or Wet Towel Rub every 3-6 hours. Copious **water** drinking; **Cool Enema** twice a day, more often if vomiting is persistent.

ELIMINATION OF POISONS—Prolonged **Neutral Bath**, **water** drinking, and **Enemas**.

CHILL—**Dry Pack** and hot **water** drinking.

HEADACHE—Ice Cap and **Hot and Cold Head Compress**.

PAIN IN LOINS AND LEGS—Hot Hip, **Leg Pack**, Trunk Pack, and **Fomentation** over lower back.

DELIRIUM—Ice Cap, **Wet Sheet Pack** to heating stage.

CEREBRAL CONGESTION—Ice Cap or Ice Collar; Hot Leg Pack; **Prolonged Neutral Bath**.

GASTRIC IRRITATION—**Fomentation** over stomach every 2 hours. In between: **Heating Compress** at 60° F., renewed every 20 minutes. **Ice Bag** above stomach. **Hot and Cold Compress** over stomach or Hot and Cold Trunk Pack.

VOMITING—**Ice Pills**. If necessary, withhold liquid foods and give food and water by enema. Ice Bag over sternum. Ice to spine. **Fomentation** over stomach.

CONSTIPATION—**Cold Enema** twice daily.

ALBUMINURIA—**Fomentation** to the back every 2 hours for 15 minutes each time. In between: **Heating Compress**, well-protected; **Hot Blanket Pack** for 30 minutes. Followed by short **Cold Friction** and wrapping in dry blankets, repeat every 4 hours. **Ice Bag** over sternum. Continuous **Moist Abdominal Bandage**, changing every 2-3 minutes. Copious **water** drinking and **Enema** twice daily.

COLLAPSE—**Hot Blanket Pack**, Hot Enema, Cold Mitten Friction, **Cold Compress** over heart, **Fomentation** over heart for 30 seconds, Cold Compress for 10 minutes, repeat.

JAUNDICE—Prolonged **Neutral Bath**; large **Hot Enema** twice daily; copious **water** drinking; **Fomentation** over liver every 3-6 hours for 15 minutes each time, with **Heating Compress** in intervals between.

CONVULSIONS—Short **Hot Bath**, followed or accompanied by **Cold Pail Pour** to head and spine. **Alternate Compress** to spine, Heating Wet Sheet Pack.

COMA—**Alternate Compress** to spine or **Sponging** to spine; **Hot Enema**; **Cold Friction**; Ice Cap.

GENERAL METHOD—Combat visceral congestion from the start by maintaining a warm and active skin. Copious water drinking and Enemas will encourage elimination of the poison while the frequently repeated cold rubs (Cold Frictions) stimulate vital resistance.

ENCOURAGEMENT—Christ is our present, all-sufficient Saviour. In Him all fullness dwells. It is our

GEN

privilege to know that Christ will be with us, guiding us even to the end. Trust and obey Him. He will impart to you the grace needed to do it. Psalm 121:1-8. How very thankful we can be that we have such a wonderful God! In Him we trust.

DENGUE
(Breakbone Fever)

SYMPTOMS—Symptoms appear about 4-10 days after the bite of an *Aedes aegypti* mosquito. Onset is abrupt, with the fever rising rapidly and in severe cases sometimes reaching as high as 106° F. The face becomes congested and there is marked soreness in the eyeballs. There are severe pains in the head, lower back, and joints. The pulse is relatively slow and blood pressure is low. After 1-3 days, the temperature rises again; and pains and mental depression reappear. But this second wave of illness is shorter. During this period, an eruption, looking like measles, appears on the body. Convalescence is slow. Death rarely occurs.

CAUSES—This illness primarily occurs in many tropical areas of the world. An estimated 40-80 million people, including many travelers from North America and Europe, become infected each year. Occasionally it occurs in North America.

The virus is carried and transmitted by the *Aedes aegypti* mosquito, which is found in rural and suburban areas and usually bites during daylight hours.

The illness can usually be diagnosed from the symptoms; but there is no specific medicinal treatment, other than rest and drinking plenty of liquids. Recovery usually takes several weeks. An attack of dengue fever gives immunity for about a year. There is no vaccine against the virus.

NATURAL REMEDIES
Call a physician.
• Keep the patient in **bed** and on a **light diet**, drinking plenty of **water**. Keep the bowels open by **enemas**.
• *If the fever goes above 103° F.,* reduce it with **cool enemas** or **tepid sponges**. Very hot **fomentations** over painful areas may bring relief. To relieve headaches, place an **icebag** to the head.
• Giving **cold mitten frictions** or **salt glows** daily after the acute symptoms are past will hasten convalescence.
• Travelers to areas where dengue fever is common, should use **mosquito repellents** and wear **clothing that covers** arms and legs.
• Very helpful information will be found in Fevers (302-309) and Antibiotic Herbs (297).

ENCOURAGEMENT—Every manifestation of creative power is an expression of infinite love. The sovereignty of God involves fullness of blessing to all created beings. 1 John 4:9.

"He giveth power to the faint; and to them that have no might he increaseth strength. Even the youths shall faint and be weary, and the young men shall utterly fall. But they that wait upon the LORD shall renew their strength; they shall mount up with wings as eagles; they shall run, and not be weary; and they shall walk, and not faint."—Isaiah 40:29-31.

GENERAL -
6 - IMMUNE PROBLEMS

WEAKENED AUTOIMMUNE SYSTEM
(Immune Disorders)

SYMPTOMS—It is the immune system which fights infections; this is done by triggering defenses against invading bacteria. The antibodies and antitoxins of this system recognize the foreign bodies and send white blood cells to attack them. When his immune system is weakened, a person is less able to withstand Epstein-Barr virus, candidiasis, food allergies, arthritis, multiple sclerosis, cancer, etc. Infections occur more easily. The person is more susceptible to colds, infections, and viruses.

CAUSES—*There are two types of immune disorders:* One type stems from immune deficiency in which the body's defenses fail to respond properly to a pathogen, allowing the disease to take over. HIV and candida are examples of this. The other type arises from an overreaction of the immune system, when it is hypersensitive to antigens (allergies), or when the body attacks its own tissues (multiple sclerosis).

Autoimmune disorders can result from conditions ranging from rheumatoid arthritis to kidney disease. Unrelenting stress, chronic allergies, and chronic infections can exhaust the immune system. **Medicinal drugs**—such as cortisone, prednisone and chemotherapy—cause immune depression! Beware of them! Other causes of a weakened immune system are **vaccinations** and immunizations against common childhood and epidemic diseases. The thymus gland seems to be the most affected by this weakening. This is especially important, due to its production of T-helper cells.

Prolonged stress, toxic exposure to chemicals, and radiation can weaken the immune system. **Severe infections** can both cause and be a result of it. An example of this would be **allergies** (resulting from immune malfunction) which follow a severe case of rheumatic fever, hepatitis, mononucleosis, or other acute viral or bacterial diseases. Lack of proper rest is yet another cause.

Yet another cause is **nutritional deficiencies**. Some natural healing specialists believe that any infectious disease may be considered an immune deficiency problem.

The taking of **aspirin** has been linked as a cause of Reye's Syndrome, asthma, low birth weight, and birth defects. **Meat** contains hormones, antibiotics, and bacteria which bring on disease. **Alcohol, nicotine, caffeine, chocolate, and a high-sugar diet** weaken the immune system. **Air pollution** is yet another problem (move out of the city!) **Hypothyroidism** can also result in immune deficiency. **Narcotics** (marijuana, cocaine, and the morphine family) are other culprits. **Mercury amalgam tooth fillings** are another incipient cause.

NATURAL REMEDIES

• Eat lots of **fresh fruits and vegetables**. Obtain adequate protein from vegetables, not from meat. Eat broccoli, Brussels sprouts, cabbage, onions, garlic, and similar worthwhile food. Eat **whole grains, nuts, and legumes**. **Skip the junk food**. Maintain a balanced lifestyle, obtaining enough sunlight, exercise, and rest.

• High doses of vitamin A in the form of **carrot juice** (beta-carotene) are especially helpful. That, along with **vitamin C** (2,000 mg), may be the most important vitamins for the immune system. Essential fatty acids (**flaxseed oil**, 2 Tbsp.); **zinc** (15 mg, 3 times a day), **selenium** (300-900 mcg per day), **germanium** (50 mg daily).

• **Vitamin B complex**, especially B$_6$ (300 mg), B$_{12}$ (1,000 mcg.), **folic acid** (2,000 mcg.), **pantothenic acid** (50 mcg.), and **vitamin E** (400-800 IU).

• Immunostimulant herbs include **echinacea root, dandelion, red clover, kelp, garlic, astragalus, and alfalfa**.

ENCOURAGEMENT—When the soul surrenders itself to God, a new power takes possession of the new heart. A change is wrought which man could never accomplish for himself. By faith in His overcoming strength, obey all the Word of God and you will be blessed. Revelation 22:14.

LUPUS
(Systemic Lupus Erythematosus)

SYMPTOMS—Lupus usually begins suddenly with fever, fatigue, arthritis and/or joint pain. Those with it are frequently misdiagnosed as having rheumatoid arthritis. Ninety percent of lupus occurs in women in their 30s. Other symptoms include a characteristic facial "butterfly" rash, severe hair loss, and papular skin lesions. This rash forms over the nose and cheeks in something of a butterfly shape (which tends to intensify because of sunlight).

The skin lesions are small yellowish lumps. They leave scars when they disappear. ("Lupus" means "wolf" in Latin, indicating the rough appearance it gives to the skin.)

Kidney disease (in 50% of those with lupus) and **low white blood cell count** are generally present.

All this, in turn, produces inflammation of the joints and/or blood vessels, affecting many parts of the body.

Sometimes the first appearance of the problem is an arthritic-like condition, with swelling and pain in the joints and fingers. Severe cases can affect the brain and heart.

Sometimes the central nervous system is affected; and deep depression, amnesia, seizures, or psychosis can result.

CAUSES—Lupus is an inflammatory (and autoimmune) disease of the connective tissue. It has been classified as an autoimmune disease, since the body is attacking itself.

Ultraviolet rays in the sun can trigger the first attack. **Stress, childbirth, fatigue, infection, chemicals, and certain drugs** can also bring it on.

NATURAL REMEDIES

Max Gerson, M.D., used a careful, very nourishing diet, including **vegetable and fruit juices and vitamin-mineral supplementation** to eliminate lupus in his patients; but the dietary change had to be total or no progress was made. **All meat, gravy, fats, junk food, fried food, soft drinks, caffeine, alcohol, etc. had to be eliminated** from the Gerson diet. The diet had to be **low in fat and salt** (which helped the weakened kidneys).

• A **vegetable juice fast** would be very helpful.

• Obtain enough **rest and exercise**.

• **Echinacea, yucca, red clover, pau d'arco, and goldenseal** are helpful herbs.

• Follow the arthritis cleansing diet (619).

• The diet should be **70% fresh foods**. Eat **potassium broth** (thick potato peeling soup). Eat no fats other than **flaxseed oil** (because of its high omega-3 content).

• **Goldenseal, burdock root,** and **red clover** placed in gauze on the sores, help fight the inflammation. Do not take goldenseal longer than one week at a time, or during pregnancy.

Drink 3-4 cups of **pau d' arco tea** daily. **Licorice root** tea helps reduce the symptoms. Only use for seven days, and not if you have high blood pressure.

AVOID

• Avoid eating **alfalfa sprouts**, for they contain *canavain* which, in your body, replaces its arginine. *Canavain* can itself produce a lupus-like syndrome. It is only found in the seeds and sprouts of alfalfa, not in the tops. (**Alfalfa tablets** help eliminate the disease.)

• Avoid nightshade plants (**eggplant, tomatoes, tobacco**). Do not eat **sugar** products or **high starch** foods.

• Do not take **birth control pills**; they can intensify the lupus. Do not take **corticosteroid drugs. They weaken the bones and immune system.** Avoid **penicillin, allergenic cosmetics**, and ultraviolet rays (especially **fluorescent lighting** and **strong sunlight**).

• Up to 10% of the lupus cases originate by taking **medicinal drugs** (*New England Journal of Medicine*). **Pollutants, additives, chemicals, and certain foods** can also bring it on. When the cause is drugs, the kidneys or nervous system are generally not affected; the lupus is a milder case, and it tends to stop when the drug is no longer taken.

• Avoid the nightshade vegetables (**tomatoes, white potatoes, eggplant, and peppers**). They contain *solanine*, which will increase the inflammation and pain.

• **Parasites** are associated with lupus. The parasites excrete droppings which interfere with body functions. Until the bloodstream is cleansed and the parasites removed, healing cannot commence.

• **Allergies** can be another causative factor. Search them out and eliminate them. Here are several causes to consider: **beef, cow's milk, wheat, corn, ammonia, hair spray, formaldehyde, perfume, ethanol, pesticides**.

• Avoid **caffeine** and all **stress**.

• Those with **Raynaud's disease** should live carefully; for they are also prone to contracting lupus. Those with lupus are often misdiagnosed as having syphilis. Lupus is not AIDS. HIV destroys the body's immune system, but lupus is a person's immune system destroying the connective system in his own body.

ENCOURAGEMENT—God's faithful ones have ever been able to obtain help from Him. Give Him your heart, and He will fulfill all your needs. In His strength, you can obey all that He commands in the Bible. Matthew 5:2-11.

SJÖGREN'S SYNDROME

SYMPTOMS—A variety of symptoms keyed to a lack of mucous-secreting glands that do not function properly: dry or parched mouth, burning throat, trouble chewing or swallowing, gritty or sandy eyes, eyes which feel like they have a film over them.

Other symptoms include tooth decay, joint pain, digestive problems, dry nose, dry skin, lung problems, vaginal irritations, muscular weakness, kidney problems, burning tongue, and extreme fatigue.

CAUSES—Sjögren's Syndrome (pronounced *SHOW-grens*) is a chronic autoimmune disease which was first identified by a Swedish physician, Henrik Sjögren, in 1933.

As an autoimmune disorder, Sjögren's Syndrome causes the body's immune system to work against itself, destroying mucous-secreting glands, including salivary and tear-producing tissues.

Although not life-threatening, Sjögren's is progressive, debilitating, and can permanently damage the eyes and mouth if symptoms are not treated.

When Sjögren's occurs alone it is considered "primary." When patients also have an additional connective disease, Sjögren's is called "secondary." These other diseases include rheumatoid arthritis, lupus, polymyositis (inflammation of the muscles), scleroderma (thickening and stiffening of the skin), or polyarthritis (inflammation of the arteries).

Anyone at any age can be afflicted with this disease. In the U.S., estimates run from 200,000 to 4 million; 90% are women.

Because each symptom affects different parts of the body, physicians and dentists often treat the symptom which applies to their field as minor and of little consequence.

Tests are available to diagnose the disease. The cause is, so far, unknown. And, to date, there are no known cures. The treatments, some of which are noted below, only help a person live with the condition rather than solving it. Yet, if it can save your eyesight or an internal organ, it is worth it.

NATURAL REMEDIES

You can learn much more about this condition by contacting the National Sjögren's Syndrome Association, P.O. Box 42207, Phoenix, AZ 85023 (Ph: 800-395-NSSA); they will send you free literature. Or contact the Sjögren's Syndrome Foundation, 333 North Broadway, Suite 2000, Jericho, NY 11753 (Ph: 516-933-6365).

• They will tell you that artificial tears (**eye drops**), salves, ointments, and anti-inflammatory drugs are among the treatments prescribed. One individual who regularly uses natural remedies and has this problem told the author this:

• Women with this problem produce **too much estrogen, in relation to the amount of progesterone** they make. So purchase **progesterone cream** and rub in on the abdomen.

• For the eyes, add ¼ teaspoon of **salt** from the health-food store (or its equivalent in **seawater**) to one cup of water; bring it to a boil, then let it set until it is tepid. Put some of this in the eyes every so often. Do not use store-bought salt, because it contains aluminum, which may damage the eyes. Take **emulsified vitamin A** (5,000 IU) and use **torula yeast**. **Black walnut husk tea** may help.

—*Also see Dry Tear Ducts (394).*

ENCOURAGEMENT—It is faith that connects us with heaven and brings us strength for coping with the powers of darkness. In Christ, God has provided means for subduing every evil trait and resisting every temptation, however strong. 1 Peter 3:10-11.

GENERAL - 7 - AGING

AGING

SYMPTOMS—You are experiencing the normal symptoms of aging.

WHAT TO DO ABOUT IT—Some people age more rapidly than others. Causes can include heredity or a debilitating disease. But there can be other reasons.

• **Exercise** is important. Lack of it causes loss of bone and muscle mass. Inevitable physical degeneration results. **Walk out of doors everyday!** Your life depends on it. **Breathe deeply**. **Be positive and cheerful** as you walk. Hold your head up and enjoy it.

• **Go to bed on time**. **If you cannot sleep** in the middle of the night, pray and thank God for your blessings. Go outside and breathe deeply of the good night air; then go back to bed and you will fall sleep.

• A person who is depressed or negative will age faster. Cheer up, go to God, and surrender your life to Him. Obey His Ten Commandment law and trust your life to Him. Be peaceful in Christ. Find in Him your strength and hope.

• It can be more difficult to deal with **stress** as you get older. God can help you with that also.

• **Find someone to help**, write to, and pray for.

NUTRITION

• Hearing loss can accompany aging. **Too much fat** in the diet and **lack of vitamin A** can cause hearing problems. (Best take vitamin A in the form of beta-carotene: carrot juice, green and yellow vegetables.) Some physicians suggest that hearing loss is a sign of later heart disease.

• Older people do not absorb nutrients as well as younger people. This includes vitamins, minerals, and amino acids. Enzymes and co-enzymes are not produced as abundantly as they formerly were. **Food supplements** are needed even more than in earlier years.

• Eat good, **nourishing food**, but **do not overeat**. You are not working hard physically, as you once did. Experimental rats were given much less in food calories and lived 50% longer.

• **Systematic undereating** is one of the key secrets of longevity. **Lose weight** and keep slim. Extra weight rapidly ages you.

• Eat lots of **fresh fruits and vegetables**. Eat **whole grains, nuts, and legumes**. A **high- fiber diet** is important. If you are not hungry, then do not eat very much. Eat one big salad every day. The greener the leaf, the more antioxidants (120) it contains. Broccoli is outstanding.

• Brittleness and fragility of bones result as calcium is more poorly absorbed. Make sure you are obtaining an adequate supply of **calcium** (2,000 mg), **vitamin D** (1,000 IU), **and copper** (4 mg).

• Drink freshly made **carrot juice** everyday.

• If possible, drink only **spring or steam-distilled water**. Keep your body's water table high. It will go a long way toward protecting you against later heart and blood vessel problems.

• There is increased oxidation of cells with the advance of years. Take **vitamin E** (400 IU), to help safeguard against this. **Vitamins A** (taken as **carotene**) **and C** (2,000 mg) are also antioxidants. Drink 2 **antioxidant**

herb teas daily (lemon balm, peppermint, thyme, sage).

• The **B complex** vitamins are needed for good brain function, proper digestion, sound nerves, and physical stamina.

• **Vitamin C** (2,000 mg) in your diet will lessen the likelihood of strokes and blood vessel ruptures. It strengthens the body, and promotes healing of wounds. It fights infection.

• Make sure you are obtaining enough minerals. Take a **vitamin/mineral supplement**—so you will get enough potassium, magnesium, selenium, and zinc.

• Eat a little **Nova Scotia dulse** or **Norway kelp** each day, to get those needed trace minerals.

• Helpful herbs include **ginseng, echinacea, cayenne, pau d'arco, hawthorn, and suma**.

• **Garlic** helps the heart and the immune system.

AVOID

• Processes of aging are accelerated by **poor living, wrong eating and drinking habits, and dangerous activities**. Some people make themselves prematurely old.

• **Stop smoking, drinking, and living in excess**. Throw out the **caffeine** and **processed foods**.

• As much as you can, **stay away from medicinal drugs**, and you will be happier for it.

ENCOURAGEMENT—What a privilege is ours—to be connected with the Majesty of heaven, the One who loved us and gave His life for us. Never forsake Him, and you will be deeply blessed. Exodus 23:25. "The Lord also will be a refuge for the oppressed, a refuge in times of trouble." Psalm 9:9. You can put your whole weight upon Him. He will carry you safely.

—FORMULA FOR ANTI-SPASMODIC TINCTURE

Taken internally, this special herbal formula is extremely useful in treating violent cases of epilepsy, convulsions, lockjaw, delirium tremens, fainting, hysteria, cramps, and unconsciousness. It is very effective for cramps in the bowels, snake bites, pyorrhea, mouth sores, tonsillitis, diphtheria, other throat problems, Gargle with it for these throat problems. In case of croup, give it in full teaspoon doses of warm water, repeating every 10-15 minutes until free vomiting begins.

Applied externally, it is good for any kind of swelling, cramps, rheumatism, lumbago, etc. It is excellent for lockjaw. Put it between the teeth, so it will get on the tongue and the mouth will unlock within a few minutes. If a baby is in convulsions, wet a finger in the tincture and thrust it into the baby's mouth; almost immediately the convulsions will end. For infants, rub the liquid well into the neck, chest, and between the shoulders at the same time. The lobelia causes immediate relaxation. The cayenne warms and stimulates the blood. The skullcap and valerian soothe the nerves and prevent rupture of small blood vessels.

How to prepare anti-spasmodic tincture:
Mix 1 oz., each, of the following powdered herbs:

lobelia seed, skullcap, skunk cabbage, myrrh gum, black cohosh, and ½ oz. cayenne.

Prepare 1 pint boiling water and 1 pint apple cider vinegar. Steep the herbs in the pint of water that is brought to a boil for 30 minutes, strain, add the vinegar, and bottle for later use. *(Go to pp. 132 for herbal preparation.)*

An alternate formula, used in England, is as follows: one-half oz. each of powdered lobelia herb, lobelia seed, skullcap, valerian, skunk cabbage, gum myrrh, and cayenne.

Go to p. 576 for more on anti-spasmodic tincture.

More Encouragement

"From eternal ages it was God's purpose that every created being, from the bright and holy seraph to man, should be a temple for the indwelling of the Creator. Because of sin, humanity ceased to be a temple for God. Darkened and defiled by evil, the heart of man no longer revealed the glory of the Divine One. But by the incarnation of the Son of God, the purpose of Heaven is fulfilled. God dwells in humanity, and through saving grace the heart of man becomes again His temple . .

" 'Know ye not that ye are the temple of God, and that the Spirit of God dwelleth in you? If any man defile the temple of God, him shall God destroy; for the temple of God is holy, which temple ye are.' 1 Corinthians 3:16, 17. No man can of himself cast out the evil throng that have taken possession of the heart. Only Christ can cleanse the soul temple. But He will not force an entrance. He comes not into the heart as to the temple of old; but He says, 'Behold, I stand at the door, and knock: if any man hear My voice, and open the door, I will come in to him.' Revelation 3:20. He will come, not for one day merely; for He says, 'I will dwell in them, and walk in them; . . and they shall be My people.' 'He will subdue our iniquities; and Thou wilt cast all their sins into the depths of the sea.' 2 Corinthians 6:16; Micah 7:19. His presence will cleanse and sanctify the soul, so that it may be a holy temple unto the Lord, and 'an habitation of God through the Spirit.' Ephesians 2:21, 22."
—Desire of Ages, 161-162

"Not by seeking a holy mountain or a sacred temple are men brought into communion with heaven. Religion is not to be confined to external forms and ceremonies. The religion that comes from God is the only religion that will lead to God. . . . Wherever a soul reaches out after God, there the Spirit's working is manifest, and God will reveal Himself to that soul. For such worshipers He is seeking. He waits to receive them, and to make them His sons and daughters."
—Desire of Ages, 189

Two editions of Desire of Ages, the classic (and best) book on the life of Christ are available from us.

The Natural Remedies Encyclopedia

- Disease Section 2 - Skin

Skin: Physiology 1011 / Anatomy Pictures 1035

FOR MORE NATURAL REMEDIES:

HERBS: Herb Contents (pp. 129-130) will help you
   locate the 126 most important herbs and the
   diseases each one can treat. How to prepare
   herbs (132). How to use them (141-189)

HYDROTHERAPY: Therapy Contents (pp. 206-207)
   and its Disease Index (263-265) will lead you to
   over 100 water therapies and many more remedies. DIS. INDEX: 1211- / GEN. INDEX: 1222

VITAMINS AND MINERALS: Contents (100-101).
   Using 101-124. Dosages (124). Others (117-)

CARING FOR THE SICK: Home care for a sick
   person (28-36). The healing crisis (36-39)

WOMEN'S SECTIONS: Female Organs (672)
   Pregnancy (701). Childbirth (765). Infancy,
   Childhood (722). Women's Herbs (754, 760)

EMERGENCIES: (973-). FIRST AID: (990-)

SK
I
N

Section 2 - Skin

For more skin problems, turn to: *Infant Problems (726-734), Childhood Problems (734-739), and Pregnancy problems (706-721).*

SKIN - 1 - WOUNDS, BRUISING

SKIN PROBLEMS

NATURAL REMEDIES

J.H. KELLOGG, M.D., PRESCRIPTIONS FOR SKIN PROBLEMS AND THEIR COMPLICATIONS *(Water therapies: how to give: pp. 206-275 / Disease index: pp. 273-275).*

GENERAL SKIN CARE—The condition of your skin is a window to your lifestyle. Eat, work, rest, exercise properly, and **take care of your liver. Avoid oils, fats, and fried foods.** Take a **cold shower every morning and a warm shower at night. Use less soap** and never use strong soaps.

SKIN DISEASES—Short, **Cold Full Bath** is helpful. But there are those who are not able to tolerate it.

BURNS—The **Evaporating Compress.** The **Cold Irrigating Compress** (cool, wet cloth over the area, to reduce heat or sprinkle water over it, to intensify the cooling effect). If very extensive, the **Prolonged or Continuous Neutral Bath.**

DRY SKIN—**Sweating Wet Sheet Pack, oil rubbed on skin,** Cold Mitten Friction, **Cold Towel Rub,** Wet Sheet Rub, Steam Bath, Hot-air Bath, Electric Light Bath, Sun Bath.

ERUPTIONS—If *dry,* not irritable, give **prolonged Neutral Bath.** If *scaly,* **alkaline bath** (soda bath or oatmeal bath). If *moist* and irritable, **cool evaporating compress** moistened with soda solution (1 ounce to 1 gallon). If skin is *thickened,* as in chronic eczema, **Hot or Alternate Hot and Cold Compress** or Spray Douche for 10-15 minutes, 3 times a day. If *extensively damaged* skin (as in pemphigus, confluent smallpox, bad burns), give the **Continuous Neutral Full Bath** until the skin is healed.

ERYTHEMA—**Cool Evaporating Compress** or Irrigating Compress.

SWEATING FEET—Revulsive Douche to feet, with extremes in temperature as great as possible. Alternate **Hot and Cold Footbath,** Heating Compress to feet during night, with **Cold Mitten Friction** of feet in the morning on arising.

INACTIVE SKIN—**Sweating** water therapy, followed by a **cold bath.**

INCREASE SKIN CIRCULATION AND TONE—Short **sweating** procedures, followed by **short cold** applications—such as Wet-sheet Rub, Shallow Bath, or Cold

CHART - 1045: Skin (314-355)

Douche. Daily Cold morning Bath, Cold Towel Rub, Cold Shower, or Shallow Rubbing Bath.

PRURITUS—**Prolonged Neutral Bath,** copious **water** drinking, large **enema,** daily **aseptic dietary.**

SKIN GRAFTS—Paraffin Bath.

SKIN SCALING—Soda **Alkaline Bath** daily for 15 minutes to 1 hour.

ENCOURAGEMENT—To have fellowship with God the Father and God the Son is to be ennobled and elevated. They can do for you that which you never could do for yourself.

BRUISES
(Contusions)

SYMPTOMS—Although the skin is not broken, the underlying tissue is injured. The result is some pain and swelling, and perhaps black and blue marks.

CAUSE—Contusions occur when the skin is injured, but the skin is not broken. Blood vessels have been ruptured and have released blood into the surrounding tissue, including the skin.

NATURAL REMEDIES

• As soon as possible after an injury, place an **ice pack** on the bruised area and keep it there for 30 minutes. If done right away, this will keep it from swelling. Often the swelling does more damage than the bruise. Later apply a **poultice of greens** (fresh or dry), **oatmeal, wheat bran, comfrey,** or **charcoal.** Pulverize the charcoal, tie it in a cloth, wet it in warm water, and lay it over the bruise for several hours. Repeat until the affected area is better.

• A research study found that placing **bromelain** over bruises received by boxers accelerated healing. Those receiving the bromelain healed much faster. (Pure bromelain can be purchased from a health-food store. Pineapple contains 14% bromelain.)

• Swallow 150-400 mg **bromelain,** 3 times daily on an empty stomach to treat bruises, swelling, and many sports injuries.

• Take **vitamin C** (2,000 mg) and **bioflavinoids** (100 mg). Also **vitamin E** (400 IU), **selenium** (500 mcg), and **zinc** (30 mg).

• Eat a lot of fresh, uncooked foods. This will help you avoid bruise marks. Dark, green leafy vegetables are especially helpful.

• Helpful herbs: **Comfrey** has been used to treat bruises since ancient Greece. **Parsley** leaves usually eliminate black and blue marks within a day or two.

Put a raw potato over a bruise or black eye. **Witch**

SKIN

hazel was used by in the early American Colonies to treat bruises. Saturate a ball of it and place it over the bruise. Both **agrimony** and **yarrow** have been used for centuries to treat bruises.

• Here is a poultice for bruises: 4 parts each of **slippery elm** powder and **wild indigo** powder, 2 parts **myrrh gum**, and 1 part **prickly ash** powder. Wet and mix to paste consistency with good brewer's yeast. Apply over the affected area and cover it.

• **Oil of oregano, dandelion, yellow dock, comfrey root** help with the problem of bruising. Make a tea of one or several to reduce the swelling, pain, and discoloration. Place a cloth that is soaked in the fluid over the bruised area.

• Here is another poultice: wet brown paper. Dip it in **blackstrap molasses** and place it on the bruise.

• More poultices: **Bread blended with water or milk**. A paste of **arrowroot and water** or **cornstarch and castor oil**. Boiled **slippery elm bark**. Grated **raw cabbage**. Chopped boiled **onion**. Raw **potato**.

• **Hydro:** Soak one washcloth in water that is hot, but not enough to burn the skin, and the other washcloth in water with ice cubes. Wring out both, put the hot one on for 3 minutes, then the cold for 30 seconds. Repeat this 4 times, resoaking the washcloths each time.

PREVENTION—

• Strengthen the blood and vessels by eating a **nourishing diet**, rich in **green leafy vegetables and fresh fruit**. **Buckwheat** is helpful. Also **vegetable juices** containing carrot, celery, and beet. Eat **whole grains, nuts, and legumes**.

• Take **vitamin C**, to bowel tolerance (be sure bioflavonoids are included), and **vitamin E** (800-1,200 units). Go out in the sun and absorb some **vitamin D**. People with vitamin C deficiencies bruise more easily than do others; for their blood vessels are weaker. Also important for cell integrity are the bioflavonoids.

• Avoid **aspirin** or **ibuprofen** for pain;, for these drugs can worsen the discoloration, due to their blood-thinning quanities.

—*Also see Easy Bruising (below).*

ENCOURAGEMENT—Jesus is ministering on your behalf in the heavenly Sanctuary. He provides you with enabling grace to obey His Ten Commandment law. Thank God for salvation in Christ! He is all we need now and for eternity. Exodus 15:26.

EASY BRUISING
(Ecchymosis)

SYMPTOMS—Frequent and easily made bruising, when others around you do not seem to have this problem.

CAUSE—Low-fiber diets containing **little fruit and vegetables**. In other words, **junk food** such as coffee, tea, white-flour products, and soft drinks.

• Some people are more prone than others to produce bruise spots. This can be a sign of **kidney and liver disorders**.

• Both **anemia** and **allergies** can cause bruising.

• Other factors that make one more susceptible to bruising are **overweight, menstruation,** and **menopause**.

• Frequent or large bruises can be caused by **leukemia**. Purplish bumps under the skin which do not heal and look like bruises could be a sign of **AIDS**.

• **Aspirin** causes internal bleeding and can increase surface bruise marks. Also beware of **anti-clotting drugs, anti-inflammatory drugs, anti-depressants,** and **asthma medicines. Alcohol** and **hard drugs** weaken the clotting factors.

NATURAL REMEDIES

• Try to make changes listed under "causes," above.

• Eat **citrus fruit** each day, including the **pulp** and **white** under the peeling. This has bioflavinoids.

• Improve your **diet**. Take **alfalfa tablets** and a good **vitamin-mineral supplement** 2-3 times a day.

• Frequent bruising indicates that the body's clotting factors are not strong. Take more **vitamin K** (140 mcg). **Vitamin D** (obtained from the sun) is another natural clotting factor. Take care of yourself—and don't bang yourself against things!

• Helpful herbs include **burdock, aloe vera, cayenne, kelp,** and **white oak bark**.

• **Garlic, alfalfa,** and **rose hips** are useful.

—*Also see Bruises (315).*

ENCOURAGEMENT—This is the victory that overcometh the world, even our faith. This faith can penetrate the darkest cloud and bring rays of light and hope to the desponding soul. It is the absence of this faith and trust which brings perplexity and distressing fears. Psalm 121:1-8.

WOUNDS, CUTS, SCRAPES

PAIN IN DEEP SURFACE WOUND—Wash the deep cut with fairly hot water, to clean wound. Then pour pure **peppermint** extract (same fluid as sold in grocery or health food store) on the wound, to relieve pain. Also put extract on bandage till it soaks through bandage. If pain returns, 3-4 hours later, soak it with more extract without removing bandage.

SYMPTOMS AND CAUSES—Cuts, scrapes, and

torn skin from collisions and falls.

NATURAL REMEDIES

• *If the wound is small:* **Let the blood flow for a short time as you clean it.** This helps cleanse the wound better. *If the wound is larger,* then you need to **stop the bleeding** first and **then cleanse the wound.** Superficial cuts can be cleaned with **soap and water** or **3% hydrogen peroxide**.

The best herb is comfrey (which is also called "knit bone") or you may use **all-heal, chickweed, goldenseal, or mullein** without recourse to the orthodox method of needle and stitches. **Walnut** combinations assist in healing; but **comfrey** is probably the most effective because it possesses a powerful cell proliferative.

• **Goldenseal** root powder helps stop bleeding and promote healing.

• Wounds may be bathed with several herbal washes or poultices (including **aloe vera, comfrey, plantain,** or **tea tree oil**).

• Squeeze together the edges of the wound and place a **butterfly bandage**, or something similar, over it. Apply one for every inch of the cut. A small cut can be closed up and sealed with a **Band-Aid or gauze** wrapped tightly enough to seal it, but not tight enough to hinder circulation.

• *To stop bleeding*—Apply **direct pressure**. If an artery has been cut, the blood will spurt with each heart beat. Small artery cuts should receive direct pressure by your finger, pressed down over a clean cloth on the wound. Larger ones may require a **tourniquet** to control it until you get help. But do not use a tourniquet unless you have to; for they can be dangerous if left too tight and too long. Placing the wound in **ice-cold water** will also tend to stop the bleeding.

• If blood soaks through your bandage, add a new one over the old one. If applying pressure does not solve the problem, **elevate the limb** above the level of the heart, all the while applying pressure with your finger.

• *If inflammation or redness occurs later*— where the cut occurred, make a strong tea of a non-poisonous, green herb (**Goldenseal** powder is the best) and soak the injured area in this hot tea for about an hour everyday until it is all right. Rebandage after each soaking.

• *If a finger, etc., is cut all the way off*—and there is no help available, quickly place it right back in its own blood and hold it in place with a wrapping till you can get help. Healing will often occur. Go to the nearest hospital emergency room.

• Give **vitamin C** orally, to bowel tolerance (1,000-5,000 mg).

• Apply **tea tree oil,** to prevent infection, and reapply every 2-3 hours. To accelerate healing, apply locally one or more of the following: **vitamin E** (600 IU; it will also reduce scarring), fresh **aloe vera juice,** or a **comfrey** poultice.

—Also see Bleeding (541).

—Also see Bleeding (541).

ENCOURAGEMENT—Trusting in God, we can have victory in our lives over the sins which so easily beset us. Through faith, we today can reach the heights of God's purpose for us. Ever trust Him. Isaiah 57:15.

HEMATOMA

SYMPTOMS AND CAUSES—A hematoma is an accumulation of blood in the tissues, outside of the blood vessels. The ones you will deal with are just under the top of the skin. These are caused by injuries and bruises, often by a blow which pinched the skin.

NATURAL REMEDIES

The following herbs, placed on top of the hematoma, will promote reabsorption and reduce local inflammation:

• Apply a tincture of **arnica**. This is a remedy widely used in Europe, by physicians and farmers, for bruises and hematomas. This plant can only be used externally. Do not swallow it.

• **Kidney vetch** is excellent for healing wounds, bruises, and hematomas.

• Compresses of **Solomon's Seal** not only make facial skin more beautiful, but it reabsorbs hematomas.

• A poultice of fresh, mashed leaves of **sanicle** also promotes hematoma reabsorption.

ENCOURAGEMENT—Repentance, faith, and (by the enabling grace of Christ), obedience to God's commands—can open the door to a much happier life on earth and a home with God in heaven.

INTERTRIGO

SYMPTOMS—This is an eruption of the skin, caused by two skin surfaces rubbing together (groin, breasts, underarms, or inner thighs).

CAUSE—Bacteria and yeast can grow in those areas and start an ulceration. Intertrigo primarily affects **overweight** women who perspire heavily or anyone who has urinary **incontinence**. In people with **diabetes**, it is more likely to develop into secondary infections. It most often occurs **in warm climates** and **during the summer**.

TREATMENT—

• Keep the **skin surface clean, dry, and free of friction.** Use only **natural, chemical-free soaps, deodorants**, and other products you place on your skin. These are available from a health-food store.

• To add dryness, **starch** can be applied. But never use **talcum** (baby) **powder**. It is ground talc, a soft rock which can cause cancer. Do not use it on your body, in body openings, or on a baby.

• **Improve the diet** and the general health. Eat **garlic** products and **acidophilus**.

• **Avoid sugar and refined foods**; for they nourish bacteria.

• Avoid **sitting in one position** too long. Wear **loose fitting, all-cotton clothing**. Make sure it is not rubbing on the skin.

• Helpful herbs include **chamomile tea**. This soothes the skin, fights bacteria, and helps healing occur. **Aloe vera gel** is also good. **Tea tree oil** will help the skin heal more quickly.

ENCOURAGEMENT—He who could not see human beings exposed to destruction, without pouring out His soul unto death to save them from eternal ruin, will look with pity and compassion upon every soul who realizes that he cannot save himself.

SWELLING

SYMPTOMS—Swellings occur in various parts of the body.

CAUSE—This can be caused by bruising, sprains, infections, arthritis, or edema.

NATURAL REMEDIES

• Take **bromelain** (which is the proteolytic enzyme in fresh pineapple), either in tablet form or in fresh pineapple juice. Bromelain blocks the production of *kinins*, the compounds produced during inflammation that increase swelling and induce pain. Take 400-500 mg, 3 times a day, on an empty stomach.

• Make a tea out of **chamomile, comfrey, white oak bark, mugwort, dill, or oregano**. Drink it and apply it externally to the swelling.

• A **contrast (hot and cold) bath or shower** may help relieve it. **Cold water** alone may do it. A **raw potato poultice** over the area is helpful.

• Place an ice cravat (**ice bag**) over the area.

• For swelling caused by arthritis, take **ginger** to reduce it. One researcher found that ginger produced better relief of arthritic swelling, pain, and stiffness than nonsteroidal anti-inflammatory drugs.

• **Arnica** (mountain daisy) is widely used by sports physicians to reduce swelling.

• **Corn silk** tea has been used for centuries by the Chinese to reduce swelling.

• Like corn silk, **dandelion** will also remove some of the excess fluids in swellings.

ENCOURAGEMENT—Man is erring and frail. But God is kind and patient, and of tender compassion. He has heaven and earth at His command. He knows just what we need even before we present our necessities and desires before Him. Psalm 84:11.

SCARRING

SYMPTOMS AND CAUSES—A cut or wound has occurred and you want to avoid later scarring or you want to reduce a scar that is already there. Scar tissue can form into keloids which are large, hard growths above the skin surface. They are harmless. Yet they are unsightly, tender, and sometimes itchy. Dark-skinned people are especially at risk for keloids.

NATURAL REMEDIES

TO REDUCE A SCAR

• **Vitamin E** (400 IU) is recommended. Take both internally and externally. Break vitamin E capsules and apply to the scar. In some instances, this will cause even old scars to reduce in size and possibly disappear.

TO AVOID SCARRING

• Put a few drops of undiluted **lavender essential oil** on the skin area immediately. Or mix it with **aloe vera gel**, apply, and cover with a sterile pad.

• To accelerate healing, without the development of scar formation, apply locally one or more of the following: vitamin E, fresh aloe vera juice, or a comfrey poultice. Of these, vitamin E is especially good in avoiding later scarring. Apply vitamin E locally (topically) and include it in the diet. Prick an E capsule and let the oil ooze over the cut or scar.

• **Clean and care for all wounds**, so that they heal properly. Close gaps with a **butterfly bandage**. This will lessen scarring. **Do not pick at scabs**. Let healing progress naturally. **Eat healthfully**. Be gentle on healing wounds, when rubbing the skin, bathing, etc.

ENCOURAGEMENT—Christ is your Advocate, your Helper, and your Friend. He alone is your Saviour from sin. He can enable you, by His grace, to keep His Ten Commandment law and do all that is pleasing in His sight. In His enabling strength, you can conquer all the forces of evil and come off more than victorious. But you must yield yourself fully to God.

ADHESIONS

SYMPTOMS AND CAUSES—Scar tissue from a surgical operation can form an adhesion, where tissue binds to tissue. This can be painful and limit body movement.

NATURAL REMEDIES

TO REDUCE AN ADHESION

• After an operation, when the stitches have been removed and the incision is completely closed, you can **use massage to help prevent adhesions from forming**.

Place the flat of your fingers (not your fingertips, but the pads where your fingerprints are) on either side of the incision. Then, without lifting the fingers, **gently move them around**.

Normal tissue will glide with ease in all directions. But at a point of adhesion, there will be a rapid increase in resistance. The gliding motion will stop.

Do not push beyond that point. But **return to it many times**, a few minutes at a time every day or every other day, and keep gently massaging it. Until the surgical site is well-healed (about 2-3 weeks), never pull on or across the incision itself.

• A Chinese remedy is to **massage Tiger Balm herb tea** in a 1-inch area around, but never on, the incision. Until the incision is completely healed, do this 5 minutes a day with a repeating, circular motion that moves close to the incision and then away from it.
—*Also see Scarring (318).*

ENCOURAGEMENT—Holiness of heart and purity of life were special subjects of Christ's teachings. He wants you to live with Him forever in heaven!

SKIN GRAFTS

SYMPTOMS AND CAUSES—A skin graft has been made, and you want it to heal well with a reduction of pain.

NATURAL REMEDIES
• Turn to *pp. 239-241* and read how to prepare and use a **paraffin bath**. This simple home remedy is ideal for the treatment of skin grafts.

ENCOURAGEMENT—Through the enabling grace of Christ, as God is pure in His sphere, so man can be pure in His. By faith in Christ, you can be more than an overcomer.

SKIN -
2 - SORES, ULCERS, BURNS

BLISTERS

SYMPTOMS—Rounded, fluid-filled spots on the skin. They are small areas of broken cells where leaking fluid has pooled and separated the outer layer of skin from the underlying tissue.

CAUSES—They are most frequently caused by wearing different or loose-fitting shoes and the excessive handling of tools.

NATURAL REMEDIES
• **Clean the area** by soaking it briefly in warm water; you can also apply a small amount of **hydrogen peroxide** solution. Pat dry. Do not drain an intact blister unless it is very large or is interfering with

movement at a joint.

• If you need **to drain the blister**, pierce it with a sterilized needle; allow the fluid to drain and pat dry. Do not remove the protective covering of the skin until it begins to dry and peel on its own; you can then remove it with your fingers or a pair of clean scissors. Apply a small amount of herbal salve or cream to a bandage or soft piece of gauze, and gently cover the blister. Avoid further stress to the area for several days. Repeat the cleaning and application of the herb cream and dressings two or three times per day until the blister is healed.

• Once again, do not prick the blister and let the fluid out, It is best to leave it intact, because a broken blister can more easily become infected. However, if it does break, leave the roof on afterward. This protects the skin while healing occurs.

• Blisters and rashes in babies, which are caused by the high ammonia content in their urine, are greatly helped by the amino acid, **methionine**, in their diet. **Lysine**, another amino acid, has helped heal fever blisters when given 500 mg daily. Also change the baby's diaper more frequently.

• Put **ice** on the blister. Or put a **cool washcloth** on the area to help relieve the pain and itching.

• Apply **peach-pit tea** to the blister.

• **Lavender essential oil**, placed on the blister, will help heal it. This is one of the few essential oils which can be applied to the skin, without first being diluted. Apply it 2-3 times a day until the blister is healed.

• The sap in **dandelion stems** is full of vitamin A. If you have dandelions in your yard, which have not been sprayed with insecticides, pick a few and squeeze the white, milky juice onto the blister and cover it with a bandage. Reapply once a day until healed. (Some are sensitive to the juice. If you are, wash it off immediately and do not put any more on.)

• Here is another excellent formula: This **herbal ointment** is also appropriate for minor cuts, abrasions, burns, and fungal infections.

Use ¼ ounce dried calendula blossoms; ¼ ounce dried comfrey root; 2 cups almond, olive, or other vegetable oil; and ¼ cup finely chopped beeswax. Mix 10 drops lavender essential oil and 10 drops tea tree essential oil.

Combine the herbs and vegetable oil in a Crock-Pot. Turn the Crock-Pot to its lowest setting, cover, and allow to heat gently two to four hours, checking and stirring frequently to prevent burning. When the oil is yellow in color and has an "herby" smell, it is done. Strain through a coffee filter or piece of clean cloth into a large measuring cup. This oil is now an infused herbal oil.

To each cup of infused oil (you'll lose some in the straining process), add ¼ cup of the beeswax. Heat the oil and beeswax together over very low heat until the beeswax is completely melted. Do not allow to boil or burn. Test the consistency by placing one tablespoon

S
K
I
N

of the mixture in the freezer for a minute or two until cool. The balm should be the consistency of an easily spreadable paste. If it seems too thin, add a little more beeswax; if too thick, add a little oil. Remove from the heat. Quickly add the essential oils. Pour into clean glass containers and cover tightly. Cool to room temperature.

ENCOURAGEMENT—Take the hand of Christ and hold it firmly. He will hold you with a grip that will not let go—unless you choose to wander away after the devil's trinkets. Romans 8:17, 35-37.

SORES, ABSCESSES, PUS

SYMPTOMS—A place on the skin that is ruptured, bruised, tender, and painful. This could be an ulcer, boil, wound, etc. Included here are sores that will not heal. Also abscesses which are large, have pus and, because they do not heal, become open skin ulcers. The swollen part becomes inflamed and tender. There may be alternate fever and chills. *Also see Boils (323).*

An abscess can form on the surface of the skin or within the body—in the sinuses, teeth, gums, tonsils, lungs, brain, abdominal wall, intestinal tract, breasts, kidneys, etc.

CAUSES—include **poor hygiene, bad diet, enervation, lack of rest, worry, exhaustion**, as well as **toxic poisoning**. It may also be caused by an **infected wound, an illness, lowered resistance, certain drugs, food allergies, stress, or junk foods**. **Drugs containing sulfur** can produce boils.

Leg ulcers are a special problem. These are open sores which develop on the legs, and are more likely to occur in **those with varicose veins**. Poor circulation causes the skin tissue to break down. The following treatments may, or may not, benefit the patient with such circulatory problems.

Sores can be caused from problems that are internal or external, from abrasion, from running into an object, irritation of shoes on the foot. The hands can become sore from a specific type of tool or some excessive use of a piece of equipment. Internal sores can come from pimples that have been picked, from boils, or from an acid condition of the body. There are many possible causes which can be aggravated by poor diet.

NATURAL REMEDIES
• For sores that will not heal: **vitamin E** (200 IU a day). Apply a dressing of fresh **comfrey** leaves and root or a paste made from raw **garlic** on gauze for 8-10 hours.
• *For a boil (furuncle or carbuncle),* follow the

directions below for an abscess.
• *For a surface abscess:* Keep the infected area **clean with soap and water**. Bring it to a "head" by placing **hot compresses** on it. This will make it soft in the center. (Hot compresses or ice bags will also help relieve the pain. And hot compresses promote healing.) A poultice with 3% **boric acid** can be used or a hot **Epsom salt compress** (dissolve Epsom salt in hot water and apply as a compress all night). **Echinacea** can be used or a **clay** poultice. Some use a **flaxseed** poultice to soften and mature the head. Either it will open itself or, when "ripe," you can open it with a sterile needle. Then flush it clean by a syringe with pure water or one of the above solutions. If bits of pus or dead flesh still remain, apply 3% **hydrogen peroxide**. Then flush out with pure water. The cavity will gradually fill in and heal.

DIET AND NUTRIENTS
• An abscess is a sign that the body is trying to rid itself of impurities. These may be half-starved cells that are deficient in nutrients, such as sulfur or toxins that accumulate because of a lack of normal eliminative processes. Eating junk food clutters the system with foodless-food and deprives it of needed nourishment.
• Take **vitamin C** orally to bowel tolerance (take as much as you can without producing diarrhea, which shows the excess is being excreted). Take **vitamin A** (best taken as beta carotene: carrot juice and green and yellow vegetables), **vitamin B complex, and vitamin E** (400 IU). Get plenty of bed **rest** and drink lots of **fluids**, to help flush the system. Clean the bowels with an **enema** once a week. Stay on a **vegetarian diet— avoiding heavy starches, chocolate, excess sweets, and too many saturated or hydrogenated fats**.
• Go on a **liquid fast** (fruit juice and water is the best) for 24 to 72 hours and stay in bed as much as possible during that time. This will cleanse the system and prepare it for a nourishing diet. This also helps reduce excess weight. Take **alternate hot and cold showers** every morning and evening (or cool baths every evening). Drink distilled water with fresh **lemon juice**, plus 3 cups of **goldenseal** or **echinacea** tea, each day.
• A **nutritious diet** with adequate vitamins and minerals is needed to correct the problems in the body which led to the abscessed condition. Also good: **garlic and kelp**.
• **Garlic and onions** in your diet provide extra sulfur and help to both heal and prevent abscesses.
• Go on a **liquid fast** of fresh juices for 24 to 72 hours.
• Apply **chlorophyll** liquid mixed with water

sevral times a day, to cleanse the affected area.

• If the abscess is external, apply **honey** to it to destroy the bacteria and viruses. This is done by drawing the moisture out of the abscess.

• Most skin sores can be aided by the use of comfrey. Use three parts comfrey with one part lobelia to relieve pain and restore the skin. For ulcers, boils, or wounds, see the index.

POULTICES

• A **slippery elm bark and lobelia poultice** soothes and helps promote healing. Apply **honey** externally to the area. It is believed that honey destroys bacteria by drawing the moisture out of those sores. Applying **chlorophyll** water to the area several times a day will keep it cleansed.

• Wrap a bruised, wet **plantain** leaf around the inflamed area. Keep it wet with plastic covering. Apply large, soaking **witch hazel** compresses to any swelling or inflammation.

• On such open skin ulcers, you can also place herbal poultices—such as **German chamomile, marigold, arnica, cliff rose, snake root, and/or witch hazel.** Also helpful is **red clover tea and carrot and beet juice.** Also good: **Burdock root, cayenne, and yellow dock root. Chamomile** is widely used in Europe to treat leg ulcers. **Tee tree oil** is outstanding, but dilute it. (Never take any herbal oil internally.)

• **Tea tree oil**, applied externally, is a powerful natural antiseptic that kills infectious organisms without harming healthy cells. Mix 1 part tea tree oil with 4 parts water and apply the mixture with a cotton ball 3 times a day. This will destroy bacteria, promote healing, and prevent the infection from spreading.

• Simmer several **peach pits**, wash the infected area with an herb tea, apply a compress of the peach-pit juice.

• **Goldenseal, myrrh, and comfrey** can be made into a paste which will heal almost any sore.

• You can usually **bathe or shower** with an abscess. But first remove bandages, gently wash the wound with a mild, unscented soap.

• The use of poultices, to bring an abscess to a head and clear it out, is the most important method of relief. A poultice of slippery elm, wild sage, and lobelia (equal parts) is good; another poultice that will draw it out very rapidly, and relieve pain at the same time, is mullein (three parts) and lobelia (one part). Others are flaxseed, lobelia, and goldenseal; leek boiled in milk; sour dock, hyssop, green fennel, ground ivy, yarrow; carrot; and potato.

Other useful herbs are bayberry bark, cayenne, cloves, garlic, ginger, hemlock bark, lobelia, mugwort, mullein, sassafras, slippery elm, stinging nettle leaves.

—*Also see Boils (323).*

ENCOURAGEMENT—Christ revealed the love of God to mankind. As Jesus was in human nature, so God means His followers to be. In His strength,

we are to live the life of purity and nobility which the Saviour lived. Romans 8:1, 33-34.

SKIN ULCERS

SYMPTOMS—An interrupted surface or superficial sore having an inflamed base which discharges pus. It is distinguished from abscess, which is a localized collection of pus in any part of the body, and has its origin deep in the tissues.

CAUSES—An ulcer is a large accumulation of dead cells that have decayed and formed pus.

NATURAL REMEDIES

• An ulcer is similar to a tumor. It is an accumulation of foreign material in the body; but, with an ulcer, a drawing agent must be used. Use a poultice of powdered **slippery elm or mullein** (three parts) and **lobelia** (one part), or **wild sage. Cayenne** will speed the process.

• Other helpful herbs include agrimony, bayberry bark, bistort root, burdock root, calamus, cayenne, celandine, chickweed, comfrey root, fenugreek, garlic, golden seal, yarrow.

—*Also see Sores, Abscesses, Pus (320).*

CANKER SORES
(Aphthous Ulcers)

SYMPTOMS—Small oval or round white ulcers that can be very painful. They appear on the tongue, gums, inner or outer lips, or on the insides of the cheeks.

At first it appears as a red, warm spot which ulcerates and has a yellowish border. Next, a yellowish mixture of fluid, bacteria, and white blood cells are seen. There is often burning or tingling at the place for 1-3 days before the canker sore appears.

Canker sores are different in appearance from cold sores, in that canker sores do not form blisters.

CAUSES—The Greek word, *aphthae*, means "to set on fire." **Allergies, stress, vitamin deficiencies, endocrine imbalance, and viral infections** are considered to be possible causes.

You are more likely to have them if your parents had them. They generally do not begin appearing till the age of 20, and occur equally among men and women. Older people have them less frequently. Canker sores generally heal by themselves within a week or two. It is said that as much as 40% of the adult population experiences them. Some people seem to have one after the other. People with **Crohn's Disease** (an illness of the bowels) are more likely to have them. **Vaccines and antibiotics** may cause them.

Gastrointestinal symptoms often accompany cankers. So **food allergies** may frequently be the cause. Most frequent problems: **citrus, apple, spices**

CHART 1054: Comparing different kinds of ulcers - Stomach 442-443 / Skin 321 (especially **cinnamon**), **acidic or salted foods, nuts, English walnuts, caraway, chocolate, coffee, shellfish**.

Other causes include poor dentures, rough tooth fillings, or braces

NATURAL REMEDIES

• As soon as the first tingle is felt, take 500 mg of **vitamin C** with **bioflavonoids** (50 mg), 3 times a day, for 3 days.

• **Goldenseal** powder or a moistened goldenseal tea bag applied over the ulcer is one of best treatments. It may also bring relief of the pain.

• Wash your mouth with plain **hot water**, to draw healing blood and help relieve pain. This is a simple hydrotherapy treatment.

• Squeeze **vitamin E** oil (from a capsule) on the sore several times a day. Apply **baking soda** to the sore.

• **Zinc** (30 mg) helps it heal faster. And **myrrh** or **witch hazel** repairs damage. **Bayberry** and **burdock** are good.

• Gargle with **chlorophyll** or **wheatgrass** juice. Rinse the mouth with **aloe vera** juice 3 times a day.

• In the Midwest, they put a little **earwax** on the sore to help heal it.

• At the first indication of a canker sore, put an activated **charcoal tablet** on the spot and hold it there till the sensation goes away (within 15-20 minutes). The charcoal absorbs the virus, stopping the eruption.

• Put a blob of **blackstrap molasses** on it several times a day. Place a drop of 3% **hydrogen peroxide** on each canker sore or dilute the peroxide (3 parts water and one part peroxide) and swish it in the mouth. Then spit it out and rinse with water.

• **Salads with raw onions** provide sulfur which will help help the canker sore. Eat a good diet of **fruits and vegetables**.

• The following herbs, alone or in a mixture, are all good for canker sores: **Burdock, goldenseal, pau d'arco tea, and red clover** to cleanse the bloodstream and decrease infection. (Do not take goldenseal longer than one week at a time or if pregnant.) **Cayenne, comfrey, garlic, and peppermint** are also extremely helpful.

• Here is a **canker sore gel**: You can use it often throughout the day, until your canker sore heals. Here is the formula: 1 teaspoon echinacea tincture, 1 teaspoon goldenseal tincture, 1 teaspoon calendula tincture, 1 teaspoon grapefruit seed extract 1 tablespoon aloe vera gel. Mix all ingredients in a small jar with a tight seal. To use, place a pea-size amount of the gel on a clean piece of gauze; hold in the mouth against the sore.

PREVENTION—

• Things which tend to cause canker sores include **mouthwashes, citrus fruit, coffee**, or certain other foods—especially **highly seasoned or tart foods**. Do not **smoke** or chew **snuff**!

• **Folic acid (20 mg) and vitamin B$_{12}$** (1,000 mcg.) deficiencies may cause it. **Onions** help reduce their number. Include them in your food preparation. **Lysine, vitamin B$_{12}$, and folic acid** also help.

• **Do not eat meat** for two weeks. Meat increases body acidity. Stop eating it entirely, and you are less likely to have canker sores.

• Avoid **sugar** and **processed foods**. **Citrus fruit** causes them in some people.

• Do not take **iron supplements**. Only obtain it from natural sources.

• Avoid **physical damage** to the area immediately in, and around, the mouth. Avoid **sharp foods**, such as peanut brittle. Use a **soft toothbrush** with no toothpaste.

• **Do not bite** the tongue or cheek. Do this by not talking or turning your head while chewing.

• A **hair analysis** will help you determine your mineral and pH balance. Maintaining a proper balance can help you avoid canker sores.

• If you have repeated attacks of canker sores, something is wrong. With careful checking, you should be able to find it. For example, with some people, it is simply a matter of not overeating on **sweet foods**, even naturally sweet fruit.

• *Beware!* If you have a mouth sore which does not heal, see a dentist. There are certain other diseases which first appear somewhat like canker or cold sores—yet which are much more dangerous.

—Also see Cold Sore (below). You may also wish to turn to Syphilis (804), which often initially appears around the mouth. However, the appearance of the hard chancre of syphilis is much different than that of canker or cold sores.

ENCOURAGEMENT—God is pleased when we keep our faces turned toward the Sun of Righteousness. When we are in trouble and pressed down with anxieties, the Lord is near. He bids us cast all our care upon Him, because He cares for us. "The Lord preserveth the simple. I was brought low, and He helped me." Psalm 116:6.

COLD SORES
(Fever Blisters, Herpes Simplex Type I)

SYMPTOMS—These are thin-walled inflamed pimples which have a tendency to recur in the same area, most frequently at the borders of the mouth, but sometimes on the gums or conjunctiva (the lining of the inner surface of the eyelid). It tends to occur at, or close to, where the skin and mucous membrane meet. First comes a local tenderness with a small bump. Then this bump changes into a blister; and the tenderness may increase. Nearby lymph nodes may become swollen. After about 48 hours, the blisters crust over. Sometimes pus oozes, making eating difficult. Cold sores appear 3-10 days after exposure and may last up to 3 weeks, but generally only 7-10 days.

There are six stages in the development of an average cold sore: (1) No visible cold sore, but a feeling of prickling. (2) Swelling may start and the area may be slightly red. (3) First signs of the blister(s). (4) The most painful stage, generally beginning on the fourth day.

CAUSE—This is an infectious disease caused by herpes simplex *(herpes simplex virus 1, Herpes virus hominis).* It is caused by a life-long virus which you get by kissing or drinking out of someone else's glass, etc. But, for practical purposes, there are other immediate causes as well.

Some people never have cold sores and others frequently have them. **Stress** is a significant cause. Eating too much **sugar** is another. Excess **ultraviolet light** or **acid foods** cause them in some people. For some women, the onset of **menstruation** can be a cause. **Drinking alcoholic beverages** and **poor diet** also bring them on. Local irritation can be an incipient factor. For some, cold sores tend to occur with a fever, infection, or a cold, after exposure to the **sun and wind,** or when the **immune system** is depressed.

If cold sores occur frequently, the problem may be **low-thyroid** function.

Cold sores seem somewhat like canker sores *(above),* but they are different in several ways. They form blisters, but canker sores do not. They can form anywhere on the body, especially on the mouth area or on the genitals. Although we are not certain of the bacterial or viral origins of canker sores, cold sores are caused by herpes simplex virus 1.

NATURAL REMEDIES

• Eat plenty of **raw vegetables**. Strengthen the immune system with a **nutritious diet**.

• Apply **ice** for 15-20 minutes at the first sign of tingling. If possible, repeat it frequently. Apply **vitamin E** between applications. Get enough **vitamin A** (50,000 IU for a few days) and **B complex. Zinc** is also important (zinc gluconate lozenges). Dissolve in mouth every 3 hours for 2 days or take 20-30 mg daily. Daily take 2,000-3,000 mg of the amino acid **lysine** till the cold sore is gone. It is an effective virus blocker.

• **Protect your lips** from sunburn and wind. **Exercise**, plus adequate **rest**, bolsters the immune system, so it can better resist cold sores. Drink lots of **water**.

• Also helpful are **goldenseal, echinacea, red clover, astragalus**, and **pau d'arco**. Along with **black walnut** tincture, they boost your immune system and kill viruses. **Lemon balm** (or **ice**) soothes the pain.

Lemon balm contains *polyphenols* and reduces outbreaks.

Avoid high-arginine foods (**chocolate, peanuts, nuts, seeds, meat, and fish**).

• If it is not bothering you very much, leaving a cold sore alone is a good idea.

• Trust in God and **stop worrying** about so many things. **Eat better**, take time to **walk outside**, and **get enough sleep** at night. Studies have shown a definite link between stress and cold sores.

—*Also see Canker Sores (321).*

PREVENTION—

• **Protect yourself from the sun**. Sun exposure is a known trigger of cold sores. An hour before going outside, apply sunscreen to your face and lips and reapply it frequently. (The exception is products that contain titanium dioxide or zinc oxide; such sunblocks do not need to be applied in advance.) Large-brimmed hats can help but are not a substitute for sun-screen. And if you're taking St. John's wort internally, be doubly careful, as this herb can increase your skin's reactions to sun exposure.

ENCOURAGEMENT—He that keepeth Israel neither slumbers nor sleeps. He is kept in perfect peace whose mind is stayed on God. Isaiah 26:3.

We, too, are to walk with God. When we do this, our faces will be lighted up by the brightness of His presence; and, when we meet one another, we shall speak of His power and say, Praise God. Good is the Lord, and good is the word of the Lord.

BOILS
(Furuncles, Carbuncles)

SYMPTOMS—Itching, mild pain, and local swelling, often on the scalp, buttocks, face, or underarms. Within 24 hours, the boil becomes red and filled with pus. Fever and swelling of the lymph glands nearest the boil may occur. Boils are tender, red, painful, and appear suddenly.

CAUSES—Boils are small pus-filled bumps. The medical name for them is *furuncles*. They are generally caused by a staph infection: hemolytic *Staphylococcus aureus* bacteria.

In contrast, *carbuncles* are many-headed boils which tend to combine and enlarge. They begin as a painful, localized infection, producing pus-filled areas in the deeper layers of the skin. Carbuncles are slower healing than boils. They are both treated alike.

Boils are contagious. Do not let the draining pus (which contains both dead and live bacteria) get on the skin elsewhere! When it spreads to nearby areas, the result is a *carbuncle*. A boil on an eyelid is a *sty (394).*

Untreated boils tend to exude their poisons and disappear within 10-24 days. But, given careful treatment, they are contained and less severe.

S
K
I
N

Keep in mind that if the body is trying to expel a poison (especially sulfur!) through the skin, you may continue to have a string of boils for a time. The body is trying to cleanse itself of something bad. Inorganic sulfur in the body is especially prone to come out in skin boils.

NATURAL REMEDIES
• Go on a **brief cleansing fast**, to rid the system of impurities. The problem may be toxins, but it may be chemical poisoning. One example would be **sulfur**. Whenever it is taken into the body, it tries to leave (but not through the bowels or kidneys)—through the skin.
• While on a liquid fast for a couple days, you may drink 3 cups of an herb tea daily of one or more of the following: **comfrey, red clover blossoms, yellow dock root, chickweed, plantain, and wild cherry bark**.
• Every night apply a poultice of **raw potato** mixed with **flaxseed**. If you apply a poultice during the day, use **whole-wheat flour** and stiffen it with enough **honey**, so it will not run.
• Apply **moist heat** (a clean towel, cloth, or gauze that is wet in warm water) 3-4 times daily to the boil. This will reduce pain and help bring it to a head more quickly. Avoid irritating the area or spreading the pus. **Avoid exercise** which might cause sweating until it heals. Keep it protected, but not with an adhesive bandage. Severe cases may require **bed rest**.
• Squeezing a boil can force infectious bacteria into the bloodstream. Instead use hot compresses to bring a boil to a head quicker. Apply **Hot and Cold Compresses** to draw out the pus. Soak washcloth in hot water, wring it out, place it on boil for 10 minutes. Apply cloth from cold water for 10 minutes. Repeat this 3 times, twice a day.
• Keep the skin clean by **washing** it several times a day. The area around the boil may be sterilized by wiping it carefully with 70% rubbing **alcohol**. Or apply a solution of 1 tsp. **bleach** to 1 quart water.
• Mix **honey with flour** and place directly over the boil. Alternates would be **clay, charcoal, and/or chlorophyll**.
• *More poultices:* Split a **fig** and apply hot. This is especially useful for a boil on the gum. Many Europeans place sliced **radish** on large boils. American Indians applied **slippery elm**. Add cool water to the powder and make a paste. Place wet **cabbage** leaves over it and replace when warm. **Onion** poultices. **Tea tree oil** compresses.
• Apply **vitamin E** oil to the area. Take **garlic** tablets 1-3 times a day.
• Some boils are large and persistent. There is a poison in the body trying to get out. **Bed rest, a short fast**, followed by a **light, nutritious diet** will greatly help.

• Other helpful herb teas include **oat straw, goldenseal, dandelion, and burdock root**.
• **Red clover** is a natural antibiotic and good for bacterial infections, for it cleanses the liver and bloodstream. Drink the tea, and apply directly to the boil.
• **Fenugreek and flaxseed**, simmered together and mashed into a pulp, is then placed as a compress over the boil.
• **Tea tree oil** compresses act as an actiseptic. Add 9-10 drops of the oil to 1 quart of warm water. Soak a clean cloth in the warm liquid and apply directly to the boil. Leave it on for as long as 30 minutes or more. It can be applied 3-4 times a day.
• Take **echinacea and goldenseal** tea 3 times daily until the boil is gone. It kills the bacteria.
• Apply pieces of **onion** wrapped in a piece of cloth—but not directly to the area.
Do not squeeze boils! This causes them to spread. Wash laundry and dishes carefully. Keep the skin clean. Wash the infected area several times a day and swab it with one of the above **herbal antiseptics**. You can also apply **honey** directly to the boil.
• *The most dangerous boil:* One around the nose can lead to internal infection. Beware of red streaks from the boil, or the development of fever or chills. As explained above, apply hot compresses until the boil heads. Then alternate hot and cold to drain it. Contact a physician.
—*Also see Abscesses (320).*

ENCOURAGEMENT—If we were left to ourselves, we would make many tragic mistakes. But we can go to God, our kind Father in heaven, and receive all the help in time of need. Psalm 56:4-5.

BED SORES
(Pressure Sores, Decubitus Ulcers)

SYMPTOMS—These are deep skin ulcers—especially found on buttocks, hips, sacrum, shoulder blades, elbows, and heels.

CAUSES—These ulcers form during periods of prolonged bed rest, as pressure is continually applied to bony parts of the body. The bedridden elderly, the unconscious, and the paraplegic are those most likely to experience this problem.

Also known as pressure sores, these deep ulcers form when pressure is exerted over bony ares of the body for long periods of time, restricting circulation and and leading to the death of cells in the underlying tissue. They are mostly found on the heels, buttocks, hips, sacrum, and shoulder blades.

Such individuals generally have a high pH (too alkaline) and are deficient in vitamins A, B_2 (riboflavin), E, and C, as well as zinc.

NATURAL REMEDIES

TO ELIMINATE THE SORES

• Apply **sugar or honey poultice** to the sore. It will help draw out the poisons. Local applications can also include **zinc oxide ointment, aloe vera, wheat germ oil, or comfrey**. Make a paste out of crushed **comfrey leaves and slippery elm**, and cover the sores. **Wash the sores** 3-4 times a day with a combination tea (**witch hazel and myrrh or goldenseal**). Mix powdered **comfrey leaves and slippery elm** in equal parts, mix with water, make a paste, spread on a cloth, and tie it over the sore. It can be left on overnight. When dry, sprinkle some powdered **goldenseal or echinacea** over the sores to disinfect the area. Cover with **cotton or wool** (not a synthetic fabric).

• **Improve the diet**. This is crucial to solving the problem. Drink enough **liquids**, even when not thirsty, and also at night. **Avoid processed, fried, and junk food. Do not eat meat**. The diet should include enough **fiber**. Oat bran is especially good. The **bowels** should move each day. Lower the pH with acid foods. **Cranberries** are ideal. Never drink vinegar! Eat a simple, well-balanced diet. including plenty of **raw, fresh fruit and green and yellow vegetables**.

• Sprinkle a thick layer of **granulated sugar** over an open bedsore and cover it with an airtight dressing. Place **raw honey** on a gauze pad and over the sore. Either method will probably produce healing within 2 weeks. Sponge with **hydrogen peroxide** or fresh, ripe **cucumber** juice. Dust the sores with **cornstarch**. Apply **aloe vera gel**.

• **Goldenseal, myrrh gum, and pau d'arco** taken in tea or extract form, are beneficial for bedsores. Also useful is **buckwheat tea and lime flower** tea. Do not take goldenseal for more than a week at a time, or during pregnancy.

• Mix equal amounts of **goldenseal** powder or extract and **vitamin E oil** with a small amount of **honey**. Apply this paste to the sores whenever necessary. Alternate this with **raw honey, vitamin E cream, and aloe vera gel**.

PREVENTION

Prevention is much easier than treatment. **Removing the pressure** at the first signs of redness usually aborts the sores. Use **protective padding** on the bed, **massage the skin** to stimulate the circulation. Avoid moist skin. Keep the **skin dry and clean** (especially avoid urine on the skin). **Turn the patient** regularly. **Watch** for signs of redness. Occasional **sunlight** to the skin is beneficial. **Sponge bathe** daily with a mild herbal soap (never with harsh soaps). The **bed** must be kept clean and the **sheet** without wrinkles. **Sheepskin** bed covers help disperse weight more evenly. The use of air or water mattresses can be helpful. **Loose-fitting clothing** allows air to penetrate to the skin (cotton is best). If the patient can **sit up**, have him do it 3-4 times a day. Sometimes prop him up with a pillow. Gentle **massage with petroleum jelly** over the pressured points.

• Give a well-balanced, adequate **diet**. Give plenty of **greens** and **carrot juice**. Give **vitamins A** (one-half **beta-carotene**), **B complex, vitamin C** (1,000 mg), **Bioflavinoids**, and **vitamin E** (400 IU). Also **copper** (4 mg) **and zinc** (20 mg).

• Apply **vitamin E oil** to the skin area.

• The **Alternate Hot and Cold Compress** is very helpful.

ENCOURAGEMENT—Whatever may be the burdens that you bear, cast them upon the Lord. He can solve your problems. He can provide for your deepest needs, as you trust wholly in Him. Isaiah 25:9. God can care for you as no one on earth can.

BURNS
(Scalds)

SYMPTOMS—There are *first degree* burns (redness), *second degree* burns (redness and blisters), and *third degree* burns (the entire skin and some of the underlying muscle is destroyed). For third degree burns, immediately go to a doctor or an emergency room. Even more extreme is a *fourth degree* burn. Instead of oozing flesh, the area is dry and charred.

CAUSES—Tissue damage to the skin as a result of heat, chemical, electrical, or radiational injury. *First degree burn:* usually from sun or water. *Second degree burn:* generally from hot metal objects, flame-contact burns, or severe sunburn. *Third degree burn:* hot-fluid burns, steam from a pressure cooker, electrical burns, or high-flame contact. (Third degree burns are often not painful because the nerves have been destroyed.) Each year, 2 million Americans get burned, 50,000 are hospitalized, and 5,000 die. So be careful.

NATURAL REMEDIES

• **First degree:** Mix equal parts of **white vinegar with water** and cover the burn surface, twice a day. Also apply **aloe vera, tea tree oil,** or **vitamin E oil** locally. **Tannic acid** has been used in clinics for surface burns that have begun to heal. At home, you can effectively use **white oak bark tea**. Apply locally as a tea and wet compress.

• *Second degree:* Apply **vitamin E oil or zinc oxide**. Take **vitamin C** to bowel tolerance. Apply **aloe vera** after healing begins.

• *Third and fourth degrees:* **Immediately take the person to a professional!** Do not try to remove clothing stuck to the burned area. Apply **aloe vera** after healing has begun.

MORE HELP

• **Soak the clothes**, so hot cloth will not increase the burn. **Apply cold until the pain subsides**.

• Immediately apply **cold water or cold, wet cloths** on the area to reduce pain and swelling. Immerse in cold water (not ice or ice water!) immediately until there is no pain. This will prevent blister formation, if first degree, and reduce damage in second degree. **Cover the burn**, to reduce likelihood of infection. Mix and apply **olive oil with baking soda** to the area. **Elevate** the area, to reduce swelling, and keep it **out of the sun**. Do not break the blisters, and **never put salves or butter** on burns. **Watch** for indications of infection, odor, pus, or angry redness. **Cold clay poultices** are useful.

• Second degree, on up, requires a **high protein diet** and **5,000 calories** per day. Increase **fluid intake**. Also important: **vitamins A, B, C, E, and F**. **Calcium** and **magnesium** help structure proteins for healing.

• Applying **vitamin E oil** and spraying on a 1% to 3% solution of **vitamin C** every 2-4 hours is very helpful for pain. This reduces pain and accelerates healing. Take 1,000 mg of **vitamin C** orally, every hour.

• Have the patient **breathe deeply** every so often. He needs the vital oxygen for the healing of the burn.

• **Fresh aloe vera juice** is outstanding on burns, to hasten healing. But this can only be done if you have a growing plant to cut the leaves from.

• **Lavender essential oil** is a wonderful remedy for burns. This includes 2 oz. each of **distilled water**, **witch hazel**, and 25 drops lavender from a glass spray bottle (dark glass best). Store in refrigerator. Give a shake and spray on burn area. Do not use it on broken skin.

• Make a paste of **wheat germ oil and honey** (in blender at low speed). Then add **comfrey** leaves to make a thick paste. Apply to burn. Keep rest in refrigerator.

• Apply fresh **ginger** juice to the burned area, using cotton balls or a compress.

• **Horsetail and slippery elm** help skin tissues to heal.

• Taking **echinacea** stimulates immune responses. Since ancient times, mashed **garlic** has been applied directly to burns. **Plaintain** juice is widely used on burns.

• **Tea tree oil** is effective for minor burns, primarily as an antiseptic and to help soothe the burned area. It is safe for both children and adults. Apply directly to the burned area.

• Burns dehydrate the body quickly. If it is a minor burn, give him drinking **water**. Add a little **cayenne** to the water to help against shock. **Ice water** compresses or applications help relieve pain.

IF SPLATTERED

• *If splattered with hot grease or hot soup*, remove soiled clothing first. Then wash grease off skin. Soak burn in cold water. If clothing sticks to skin, rinse water over clothing and go to a medical facility. Do not pull clothing off the skin! Do not put butter, honey, or vegetable peelings on a burn. If you do, it will seal the heat in. Greasy substances may cause infection. Do not break blisters. Keep bandages loose. With your fingers,

gently move burned area of skin immediately. This will keep skin supple and bring blood to area.

• *To remove hot tar, wax, or melted plastic from the skin,* use ice water to harden the heated substance. But no ice water after that, only cold water. For acid or chemical burns, use baking soda or apple cider vinegar added to warm water. Apply 5 minutes once a day. Keep burn injuries elevated to minimize swelling and aid healing. To avoid bacterial infection, keep burn lightly covered.

• The following hydrotherapy treatments for burns are listed in the *Hydrotherapy* chapter of this *Encyclopedia* (123-259): **Ice Pack**, **Neutral Full Bath**, **Evaporating Compress**, and the **Cool Irrigating Compress**. Extensive burns can be treated with the **Prolonged or Continuous Neutral Bath**. Old burns can be treated with the **Paraffin Bath**. These are excellent helps in time of need.

ENCOURAGEMENT—We can only see a little way before us; but God sees everything. He knows all about our needs; and He cares for us. He sits above the confusion and distractions of the earth. All things are opened to His divine survey. From His great and calm eternity, He orders that which His providence sees best. It is His plan that you grow in grace and in the knowledge of Jesus Christ every day of your life. The more fully we live for Him, the happier are our lives. Titus 3:7.

SUNBURN

SYMPTOMS—*First degree* sunburns cause reddening of the skin and possibly slight fever. *Second degree* sunburns make reddening and water blisters. *Third degree* sunburns produce damage to lower cells and the release of fluid. This results in eruptions and skin breaks, through which bacteria and infection can enter. Symptoms may not begin until one to 24 hours after sun exposure, and usually reach their peak in two or three days.

CAUSES—There has been **excessive exposure to ultraviolet light rays** which first burn the surface skin and, later, the lower cell layers. Ultraviolet rays can penetrate clouds. So be careful even on hazy days. Sunburn is bad for you. It ages your skin and increases your risk of later developing skin cancer. Many drugstore remedies for sunburn numb the pain but do little to support the body's own healing systems. Natural methods are better. Fair-skinned people are more prone to sunburn than darker skinned individuals, but everyone will burn if they get too much sunlight.

PREVENTION—**Do not expose yourself** to the sun for extended periods of time between 10 a.m. and 2 p.m., when the highest concentration of ultraviolet rays are present. Reflections from snow water, metal, sand, or white- and aluminum-painted surfaces can intensify the effect.

• Apply a **sunscreen** about 30 minutes before going out (SPF 15, or higher). Protect your lips, hands, ears, and the back of the neck. Reapply as needed after swimming and sweating. (Be aware of the fact that there are substances in sunscreen which your body should not absorb, but inevitably will.)

• **Get a tan gradually**, beginning with only a few minutes (never over 15). **Wear protective clothing** whenever possible. Keep a **hat** with you, and use it. **Long sleeves** help. If you wear **sunglasses**, get a pair which protects your eyes from both UVA and UVB rays.

NATURAL REMEDIES

SECOND OR THIRD DEGREE SUNBURNS

• *A third degree sunburn is serious. See a doctor.* **Water applications** help. **Keep the muscles flexible**. A strong sunburn can cause underlying muscles to contract somewhat.

• For both *second and third degree* burns, be sure to eat **high-protein foods**. A lot of tissue needs to be repaired because your body is hard at work. Drink a lot of **fluids**.

FIRST OR SECOND DEGREE SUNBURNS

• Put **cold water** on the burn. Lie in a **cool bath**.

• Place dry **oatmeal** in a bag, run cool water through it, and save the water. Throw away the contents of the bag and use the water in compresses. Apply every 2-4 hours.

• Here are more **oatmeal** suggestions; for it is soothing to irritated skin. You can use it in one of four ways:

1 - Cook 3 tablespoons of dry **oatmeal** in ½ cup of water, let cool, wrap in a gauze cloth, and apply to the burn.

2 - Wrap ½ cup of dry **oatmeal** in cheesecloth and let steep in 3 cups water for 15 minutes. Apply the cool liquid to the burn.

3 - Wrap 1 cup of dry **oatmeal** in a cloth or pour into a clean athletic sock. Tie a knot at the top. Put it in a tub of tepid water to soak for 10 minutes, then apply yourself.

4 - Purchase a commercial **oatmeal** product that dissolves in water and add to your bath.

• Massage **aloe vera or tea tree oil** on the area. The inner gel of the aloe vera leaf has also been shown to speed the healing of radiation-induced burns.

• Here is more information on how to use aloe vera: **Aloe vera gel** is very effective for any kind of burn. It is even used in the burn units of some hospitals. It relieves discomfort, speeds healing, and helps moisturize the skin and relieve dryness. Gently apply a thin layer of aloe vera gel to the sunburned area. Reapply it every hour until the pain is gone. Pulp taken directly from inside the fresh plant is best. If you use a commercial aloe product, make sure it has no mineral oil, paraffin

waxes, alcohol, or coloring.

• Here are other suggestions: **Clay** poultices can be used. Moisten a cloth with **witch hazel** and apply often for temporary relief. For small areas, apply with cotton balls. Apply plain **yogurt** to the area. Make a paste of **cornstarch** and water, and apply it. An **ice pack** can help reduce pain. Get lots of sleep.

• Make a large pot of strong **comfrey or gotu kola** tea and let it cool. Soak sterile cotton gauze in the tea to make a compress; and apply it to the affected area. Leave the compress in place for up to 30 minutes.

• A cream with at least 5 percent **tea tree oil** helps to heal sunburn and other skin irritations.

• Mix a cup of **skim milk** with 4 cups water (with ice cubes in it). Every few hours, apply compresses of this solution for 15-20 minutes.

• The cool **cucumber** is often used for scalding burns. Slice it open and apply. Apply **raw eggplant**. In Australia, it is used to treat skin cancer. Apply **plantain**. It contains *allantoin*, which heals injured skin cells.

• More than any other nutrient, experts recommend the placing of vitamin E oil on skin burns.

• Do **not** apply any product which has **alcohol, mineral oil, coloring, or waxes** in it.

• If the legs are burned, **elevate** them above the heart level.

The burned skin area will be delicate for 3-6 months, so be careful.

ENCOURAGEMENT—God helps the feeble and strengthens those who have no strength. The Lord is your shade upon the right hand and upon the left. Trusting in Him, you will be safe. Psalm 46:1.

LEG ULCERS
(and other skin ulcers)

SYMPTOMS—Open sores which develop on areas of the legs. (They may also occur elsewhere on the body.)

CAUSES—Leg ulcers occur when the **blood circulation to the legs is inadequate**. Skin tissue tends to erode and ulcers can form. Individuals with **varicose veins**, **thrombophlebitis**, or other conditions caused by poor circulation, are most likely to develop this problem.

An atherosclerotic plaque or embolism can block an artery, causing an *arterial ulcer* in bony areas of the feet and ankles. When leg veins cease functioning properly, venous stasis occurs, producing a *venous ulcer*. Diabetes can result in insufficient blood supply and a *diabetic ulcer* on the skin.

NATURAL REMEDIES

• Eat a **light, nourishing diet** with adequate **vitamins and minerals**. Much of it should be raw. Leafy, dark **green vegetables** and **garlic** are important.

• **Do not eat meat**, and avoid **alcohol** and **nicotine**!

• Make a gallon of **goldenseal** tea (stronger than

you would drink). And, after straining out the herb, put the leg in it for an hour. When finished, let it dry for 10 minutes. Apply **olive oil** in, and around, the ulcer. Dust a little powdered **goldenseal** on it. If needed to keep out insects, put a light gauze bandage over it while letting the air in. It will heal, but slowly. As much as two months may be required. But do not take goldenseal more than a week at a time—and not if you have glaucoma, diabetes, or cardiovascular problems.

• Keep the ulcer **clean,** so it will not become infected.

—*Also see Abscesses (320) and Boils (323).*

ENCOURAGEMENT—God is pleased when we keep our faces turned toward His Son, Jesus Christ, our only Saviour. When we are in trouble and pressed down with anxieties, the Lord is near. He bids us cast all our care upon Him, for He careth for us. Psalm 55:22.

SKIN - 3 - SKIN SPOTS

MOLES
(and unknown spots)

CAUSE—Most moles are harmless. But those that are flat, or nearly flat, larger than the top of a pencil eraser, or have a mottled color should be checked. If an existing mole turns blue, white, or red and begins to bleed or develops a crust—have it checked. It may be skin cancer.

NATURAL REMEDIES

To remove a suspected skin cancer (before it has continued long enough to go into the system), fasten a thin slice of **garlic** to it in the evening and leave on overnight. Do this for 2-4 nights. The spot will slough off. And, as it heals, new flesh will take its place.

—*For more on this, see Skin Cancer (787).*

ENCOURAGEMENT—Jesus has said that He has set before us an open door; and no man can shut it. The open door is before us. And, through the grace of Christ, beams of merciful light stream forth from the gates ajar. Be faithful, trust and obey, and your future is bright. Proverbs 19:20.

ACNE
(Acne Vulgaris)

SYMPTOMS—Blackheads, whiteheads, pustules, inflamed and infected nodules, sacs, and cysts. They occur where the sebaceous (oil) glands are most nu-merous: face, neck, chest, and back. Permanently expanded pores, as well as scarring, can result.

CAUSES—A sebaceous gland is located in every hair follicle and produces oil which lubricates the skin. **Some of the oil becomes clogged**, bacteria multiply, and inflammation results. This occurs during adolescence (between 12 and 24), when androgens (male hormones) are released in increased amounts in both boys and girls. A few have acne all their lives.

Other causes include **junk foods, oral contraceptives, cosmetics, allergies, stress, and heredity**.

Skin eruptions are often caused by consuming **too much meat, white sugar, denatured flours, eggs and stimulants (including spices), or by the lack of wholesome foods such as fresh vegetables, whole grains, fruits, nuts, and legumes**. Skin ailments will often follow or accompany **diseases of the lung or colon**.

Eggs, peanuts, nuts, colas, and chocolate tend to induce acne. **Milk** is frequently responsible when it is **combined with sugar and eggs** in snacks and ice cream.

The problem is intensified when **sebum, combined with skin pigments, plugs the pores**—and produces blackheads. If scales below the surface fill with sebum, whiteheads are formed.

Canadian Eskimos, prior to 1950, never had acne. When "modern foods" were brought in, acne became common.

Acne is rarely caused by a serious hormonal disorder caused by **tumors in the adrenal glands or ovaries**. Other symptoms of this possibility include **excess facial hair** and **irregular menstrual periods**.

NATURAL REMEDIES
GENERAL

• **Cleanliness** is important. Keep the skin washed and clean. Keep the infected area **free of all oils**. Wash or pat the face with lemon juice 3 times a day. **Shampoo** the hair frequently.

• **Do not squeeze** the spots. Blackheads must be removed (not with picking by the fingers) with a specially designed instrument. Keep hands clean and **avoid touching the face**. Do not touch the affected area unless your hands are thoroughly cleaned. *See Blackheads (330).*

• **Wash the pillowcase** regularly in chemical-free (no added colors or fragrances) detergents,

• Get early morning **sun** on the face daily. Get **fresh air** and **exercise** daily, and plenty of **rest** to eliminate toxins.

• **Avoid irritating the skin**. Avoid clothing which rubs against the affected areas. Do not hold a telephone against your cheek for long periods. Keep your hair from your face, so hair oil and bacteria will not be deposited on the skin.

• **Avoid stress**; for it can cause hormonal changes.

• **Do not put oil on your face**. Avoid the use of greasy creams or cosmetics. **Avoid makeup**. If you feel you must use some, use a natural, water-based product. Wash and dip makeup brushes and sponges in alcohol after each use.

• **Avoid oral or topical steroids**. They will worsen the problem.

• Men should **shave with a blade** and in the direction of hair growth. Shavers can cause scarring.

SPECIAL APPLICATIONS

• Place alternating **hot and cold cloths** on affected area, to bring up cleansing circulation.

• Rub on **lemon juice** at night and wash in the morning.

• Apply **white clay** (from health food-store) and let dry, 3 times daily to bring to a head. Then use once a week.

• Mix 1 part **apple cider** with 10 parts quality water. Apply to the affected areas. This will help balance the skin's pH.

• For acne scars, place **fresh pineapple** on the scars for enzyme therapy; and take 750 mg **bromelain** daily.

• *Here are additional external food poultices to place on the affected areas:* Cook **oatmeal in milk** until thickened, cool, and apply to area. Another method is to **cook carrots** in as little water as possible. Mash, cool, and apply. Or one can apply a whizzed, chopped, ripe **tomato** in a blender with 1 Tbsp. of dry **oatmeal** and 1 tsp. **lemon** juice.

• **Fruit acids** help get rid of excess amounts of the protein, keratin, and those dead skin cells that may otherwise clog pores. They act like commercial salicylic acid formulas without the side effects. Put fruits, such as **grapes** and **strawberries** or **pineapple husks** into a blender. Apply the mixture like a mask; leave on for 10 to 15 minutes, and wash off. Or look for natural face products that contain fruit acids.

• If your acne is severe, take a **steam bath** 2-3 times a week. Take it once a week, to prevent further outbreaks.

• The next two recipes use the antibacterial properties of two berberine-containing herbs.

(1) *To make a wash:* 2 teaspoons chopped dried **Oregon graperoot or goldenseal root** 2 cups water. Simmer all ingredients for 10 to 15 minutes. Strain and cool; use to wash face or soak a clean cloth and use as a compress.

(2) *To make a paste:* 1 teaspoon powdered **Oregon graperoot or goldenseal root.** A few drops of water, plus 5 drops lavender oil. Mix all ingredients. Apply to pimples, let dry. Rinse or gently wash off. NOTE: Oregon graperoot stains fabric

NUTRITION

Proper nutrition is extremely important.

• Drink **6 glasses of pure water** daily.

• Mix 2 oz. each of **beet juice, celery juice and tomato juice**. Take 2-3 times a day. As a general blood purifier, take several times a week.

• **Eliminate all refined and/or concentrated sugars** from the diet.

• Eat a **good, balanced diet.** Exercise regularly and get adequate sleep at night.

• **Eliminate** all **saturated fats** from the diet, along with **junk food, fried food, refined food, dairy foods, carbonated drinks, caffeine, alcohol, and tobacco.** Do not eat foods containing **trans-fatty acids** (milk, milk products, **margarine, shortening**, and other synthetically **hydrogenated vegetable oils**).

• Increase **raw vegetable** intake. The more you eat, the faster the skin will clear and heal. Eat plenty of **non-citrus fruits, raw vegetable juice, cooked vegetables, salads, whole grains, legumes,** and **a few seeds and nuts**. Include some **seaweed** (for iodine) and **pumpkin seed** (for zinc).

• Two servings of **beets or beet juice** weekly, and/or 2 glasses of **carrot juice** daily reportedly improve acne within a few weeks.

• Eat a **high-fiber diet.** This helps the colon eliminate toxins.

• Go on a **short vegetable juice fast** of 1-3 days, along with enemas. It would be well to do this every 2 to 4 weeks, until the skin is perfectly clear.

• Beware of **all oily foods** which have saturated fats. This would include **peanut butter, cheese, milk, and cream**. A small amount of unsaturated vegetable oil would be acceptable.

SPECIAL NUTRIENTS

Certain dietary deficiencies have been linked to acne.

• **Niacinamide** is important in repairing the skin, because it increases the supply of fresh blood to the surface.

• **Vitamin C**, 500-1,000 mg, 3 times daily. Also taking 200-1,000 mg **bioflavonoids** in divided daily doses speed healing and retard spreading.

• **Vitamin E.**, 200-400 IU daily, to protect vitamin A from destruction in the body.

• **Vitamin A** (best taken in the form of carotenes: carrot juice and green and yellow leafy vegetables). Women of childbearing age should not use high-dosage vitamin A.

• Take one **B complex** tablet daily, plus up to 300 mg each of B_6, **niacin**, and **pantothenic acid** in divided doses daily for no longer than a month. B_6, taken in small doses throughout the month, is especially helpful for acne that flares up during menstrual periods.

• **Chromium**, 400-600 mcg daily; plus potassium, 99 mg daily.

• **Zinc**, 30 mg daily for a few months, then 15 mg daily thereafter. In addition to being an effective bacterial suppressor, it aids healing and is essential for gland efficiency. In one study, zinc was found to be an oral antibiotic.

• Too much **iodine** can stimulate the sebaceous glands to produce too much oil.

• **Essential fatty acids** are important. Flaxseed oil is the best.

• If milk and dairy products are reduced, take 800 mg of **calcium** daily to maintain the pH balance for a clear complexion.

• Take 1-2 Tbsp. **brewer's yeast** and 2 **lecithin** capsules daily.

• Take 2 activated **charcoal tablets** after each meal, for 2 weeks, and 2 tablets daily afterward. Clinical tests reveal this to give good results. Do not continue for extended periods because it can block nutrient absorption.

HERBAL FORMULAS - Internal

Here are several which are recommended by leading herbalists:

• Make a tea of 1 part **burdock**, 1 part **dandelion**, 1 part **sassafras**, 1 part **sarsaparilla**, ½ part **licorice**. Simmer 1 oz. of herbs in 1 pint water for 30 minutes. Take 1 cup, 3 times daily.

• Mix the following in equal parts: **elecampane** root, **elder** leaves and flowers, **witch grass** root, **juniper berries**, **ground ivy**. Steep 1 tsp. in ½ cup boiling-hot water. Take ½-1 cup daily, unsweetened in mouthful doses, over an extended period of time.

• Use a good blood purifier, such as 1 part **red clover**, 1 part **kelp**, 2 parts **echinacea**, 1 part **dandelion** root, 1 part **burdock**, 1 part **red clover**, ½ part **licorice**. Fill gelatin capsules with the powder and take 2 capsules every 2 hours until the condition is greatly improved.

• Herbal specifics include **chickweed**, **echinacea**, **burdock**, **dandelion**, **white oak bark**, **yellow dock**, **red clover**, and **valerian**. Take 1-2 capsules of one of these herbs daily for a week or so at a time. Or sip 1-2 cups of the tea. (Also sponge some of the juice over the lesions.)

HERBAL FORMULAS - External

• Apply golden seal and myrrh **solution** to the affected areas.

• **Chaparral** and **comfrey** tea are good **facial rinses**.

• Apply **tea tree oil** on sores 3 times daily. This is known to be very healing to acne.

• Herbs which could be applied to the skin include **dandelion** root, **echinacea**, **alfalfa**, **chaparral**, and **red clover**.

• Apply a poultice of ground **chaparral**, **dandelion** or **yellow dock root**, mixed with hot water and cooled, to the affected areas and allow to remain for several hours. Then rinse off with tepid water.

• **Steam:** Put 1 part **eucalyptus** leaves and 2 parts **elder** flowers in 1 pint of boiled water in a bowl. Cover the head with a cloth and lean over the bowl of aromatic steam.

• Here is another "facial sauna." Cover the head with a towel and lean over a bowl of **steaming tea of red clover, strawberry leaf, and lavender**.

• Steep an 8 oz. cup (with 1 tsp. **yarrow**) for 30 minutes. Then add it to a basin of steaming water and lean over it for 5-10 minutes, with a towel over your head. You should be close enough to feel the steam (about 12 inches) without burning.

ENCOURAGEMENT—At times it will seem that you cannot take another step. Well, wait and know that "I am God," He tells you. "Be strong and of a good courage. Be not afraid, neither be thou dismayed, for the Lord thy God is with thee whithersoever thou goest." Trust Him. Psalm 112:7-8.

BLACKHEADS

SYMPTOMS—Blackheads are small, tallow-like plugs formed in the pores by the accumulation of dirt, oil, and bacteria. They are black at the exposed end, because of oxidation rather than the presence of germs. They generally cause no itching or pain, but are unsightly.

CAUSES—The duct of an oil gland becomes plugged with partly dried oil mixed with, more or less, dust or dirt. Most cases occur between 12 and 30 years of age.

Problems with digestion, constipation, or underactive thyroid and anemia seem to be contributing factors.

Although germs do not cause them, blackheads can easily become infected.

NATURAL REMEDIES

• Squeeze out the visible blackhead very gently, with a **blackhead remover** (available in a drugstore). Never use fingers to do it. Then **wash with mild soap and water**.

• **Sunlight** kills the surface bacteria, thus clearing the condition temporarily. But sunlight can also stimulate the oil glands, possibly making the condition worse later.

• **Do not overeat. Avoid fat, greasy, or fried foods. Avoid ice cream, cream, butter, margarine, chocolate, pastry, sweets, or much starchy food**.

• Eat a **nourishing diet of vegetables**, but **avoid corn**. Only eat a **moderate amount of protein foods** (nuts and legumes). Supplement the diet with **vitamins and minerals**. **Vitamin A** is important.

• **Avoid alcohol, tobacco, coffee, or cocoa**.

• Obtain **adequate rest** at night and keep the bowels open.

• **Exercise** outdoors; but avoid exercise which causes perspiration.

• Put **no creams, oils, or ointments** on the face. **Keep hands away** from the face.

• **Wash the hair** two or three times a week.

ENCOURAGEMENT—We can have access to God, and be accepted by Him, through Christ our Lord. Jesus can strengthen us to obey commands given in the Bible. In Christ, we can overcome our sins. Revelation 2:7.

"Herein is love, not that we loved God, but that He loved us, and sent his Son [to be] the propitiation for our sins." 1 John 4:10.

AGE SPOTS
(Liver Spots, Lentigo, Senile Lentigines)

SYMPTOMS—Age spots (also called liver spots) are the flat brown spots which appear on the skin. They are especially noticeable on the back of the hands.

CAUSES—Liver spots are different than freckles. Freckles are caused by melanin pigments which react to the sunlight in fair-skinned people. Liver spots are the result of a *ceroid* pigment buildup in the skin of older people.

These latter spots are the outward signs of **free radical destruction** within the body. There is pre-oxidation of fats—in the cells instead of in the liver. Free radical damage produces waste materials in cells throughout the body, including the brain and liver. The causes are **poor diet, eating rancid fats, lack of exercise, excess exposure to the sun, autointoxication, and sluggish liver function**.

Exposure to the sun's ultraviolet rays are also involved in this problem. As a result, special cells, called *melanocytes*, produce too much color.

NATURAL REMEDIES
• Eat **high quality food** (especially **green, leafy vegetables**), purify the blood, nourish the glands, and keep the **bowels** open. **Exercise** the body and the mind. Keep the **immune system** in good shape. Take nutritional **supplements**. Drink lots of **water**.

• A powerful helper is the use of **vitamin E** (800-1,200 units per day), which tends to destroy free radicals. Also take **vitamin A** as beta carotene. Take a daily **B complex** supplement, plus additional B_2. Take **grapefruit seed extract** daily.

• Eat quality protein foods and **avoid old seeds and nuts**. The oils in them may be rancid. **Do not use meat or milk**. Obtain all your fats as **unsaturated fatty acids**.

• Drink enough **water**, making sure it is either pure or distilled. Practice deep **breathing**. Learn how to **relax**.

• **Avoid all white flour, white sugar, alcohol, coffee, salt, tobacco, cigarette smoke, hydrogenated oils, fried foods, chemicals, drugs**. **Do not overeat**.

• Center your diet around **broccoli, cabbage, fruits, whole gains, nuts, oats, seeds, and soybeans**. A **high-fiber** diet is important.

• Go on a **brief fast**, to cleanse the liver.

• Avoid too much exposure to the **sun**.

• Do not use commercial **skin creams** or **cleansing creams**. Use **olive oil** and a warm, wet washcloth; then rinse with **lemon juice** and water.

• Apply **lemon oil**. It has bleaching properties that help fade the spots. Take **gotu kola**, to help fade them. Rub on **aloe vera gel**, the milky sap from crushed **dandelion** stems, a slice of **red onion**, fresh **pineapple juice**, **lemon juice**, or **comfrey** root tea.

• Take **burdock, milk thistle, and red clover** to help cleanse the bloodstream.

ENCOURAGEMENT—The gifts of Him, who has all power in heaven and earth, are in store for the children of God. These gifts are precious; for they come to us through the costly sacrifice of the Redeemer's blood. In Christ, we can be overcomers. 1 John 1:7.

SKIN - 4 - CHAPPING, CRACKING, ITCHING

CHAPPED HANDS

SYMPTOMS—Red, dry, cracked hands.

CAUSES—The low humidity in the fall and winter dries and irritates the skin. The skin of older people has less natural oils. This prepares a person for problems. But something can be done about the other causes, listed below.

NATURAL REMEDIES
If you find you have this problem, there are several things you can do, to prevent or lessen it.

• Water removes oils from the skin. A special kind of water is especially devastating: **soapy water**. Dish water not only removes oil from the plates, but also from your hands. That is part of the reason why your hands are chapped and your arms are not! When you must wash your hands, **wash only the palms and not the backs**—which, having thinner skin, tend to dry out more easily.

• **Soak your hands** in warm (not soapy) water for a few moments. As you do this, some of the water is absorbed by the dry skin. Then **pat dry and gently rub a little vegetable oil** on your hands.

• What you place on your skin is absorbed into your body. So **beware of all the creams and lotions** on the market. The makers of those products are not required by the FDA to include food grade ingredients. Yet all those lotions are absorbed into your system for the body to have to deal with.

• Massage a few drops of **glycerin or olive oil**, combined with a few drops of **lemon oil** (both are available at pharmacies), into your hands at bedtime.

• Put oil on your hands at night and then slip **cotton gloves** over the oily hands.

• Hot-air blowers tend to chap the hands. Use a **towel** instead.

• Wear **white cotton gloves** while doing dry work. For harder work, use **leather gloves**. Regarding gloves, **avoid vinyl ones**, if you can. They makes the hands worse! The rubber traps the moisture and keeps the skin from breathing.

• Use a long-handled **brush**, when washing dishes.

• Blend uncooked (or cooked) **oatmeal** into fine particles. Place it on the hands to soften and heal the chapped skin. It can also be added to bathwater.

• Apply the gel from the inside of the leaves of **aloe vera** to heal chapped hands, chapped lips, and minor burns.

• Blend the juice of a fresh **leek** into a vegetable oil and put it on your hands.

—*Also see Chapped Lips (below).*

ENCOURAGEMENT—Through Jesus, we can have access to God and be accepted by Him. Take God's promises as your own. Plead them before Him as His own words, and you will receive fullness of joy. Proverbs 2:3-5.

CHAPPED LIPS

SYMPTOMS—Chapped and cracked lips.

CAUSES—**Low humidity, sunlight, wind, cold temperatures, and lack of oil on the lips**. In addition, there are several other factors you can control:

NATURAL REMEDIES
NUTRITION

• **Vitamin B$_2$, B$_6$,** and **brewer's yeast** both help cracked lips. A lack of **B$_2$** makes lips crinkle, flake, and feel chapped, can cause cracks in the corners of the mouth (cheilosis), and eventually shrink the size of the upper lip. A deficiency of **B$_6$** produces sore lips.

• **Folic acid** (400 mcg) and **pantothenic acid** (100 mg), taken in addition to other B vitamins, often prevent lip ulcers and other sore-lip problems.

• Apply **vitamin E** from a pierced capsule to help heal the lips. Also take 400 IU daily.

• **Calcium** helps hold cells together. And unsaturated fatty acids (**flaxseed oil** is the best) and **magnesium** help your body absorb it. Take 1,000 mg calcium, 500 mg magnesium, and 1 Tbsp. flaxseed oil daily.

• Take a high-potency **vitamin-mineral supplement**.

OTHER HELPS

• **Avoid licking** your lips. It dries them out. Occasionally place a little **vegetable oil** on your lips.

• Your lips are dry because you are not drinking enough **water**. Drink at least 8 glasses a day.

• Toothpaste dries the lips. Instead, use a toothbrush and **baking soda**.

• Chronically sore lips may be due to **allergic reactions to foods, ingredients in chewing gum, cosmetics, mouthwash, or toothpaste**. Experiment, by withholding this or that for a time, and see what is causing your problem.

• Rub your finger alongside of your nose and then on your lips. That puts **natural oils** back in them.

• Finish your meal with a small amount of **lecithin** (which your brain, nerves, and blood vessels need anyway). When you do this, be sure and leave a small amount of it on your lips.

• Do not use "lip balms"; for they generally contain strong antiseptic chemicals. Instead, use **cocoa butter**. It will help rehydrate your lips.

• Rub **beeswax** or unwaxed **cucumber skin** over dry lips to help lubricate them.

• Mix 30 drops **lavender essential oil** (to reduce lip inflammation), 16 drops **sandalwood essential oil** (to moisten your lips), and 2 oz. **cocoa butter** or **flaxseed oil**. Every so often, put some on your lips.

• Place a heat-proof dish in a pan of boiling water. Stir 3 Tbsp. **olive oil** into 1 Tbsp. melted **beeswax** or **paraffin**. Pour this lip salve into small containers with tight lids. Dip into it occasionally and put some on your lips. If the mixture becomes too hardened, reheat it over hot water and stir in a few drops of olive oil.

• When you sip **hot water**, this draws the blood and more water is absorbed into your lips. Take 1-2 sips every 10 minutes throughout the day.

—*Also see Chapped Hands (331).*

ENCOURAGEMENT—We may come into the audience chamber, reach up the hand of faith, and cast our helpless souls upon the One mighty to save. He can help us fulfill His beautiful plan for our lives. Jeremiah 29:1.

DRY SKIN, CHAFING

SYMPTOMS—The skin is overly dry; and there can be a tendency to chafing (more so during winter).

CAUSES—There is both a **water loss** and an **oil loss** in the skin. This may seem to be a matter of little concern. But it can be a sign of a more serious problem: **essential fatty acid deficiency** that can result in cardiovascular disease (stroke, heart attack, etc.). Dry skin can be a sign of an **underactive thyroid.**

If you are daily supplementing with 100,000 units or more of **vitamin A**, dry skin may be the first warning of overdose. It is dangerous to take too much vitamin A!

NATURAL REMEDIES
DIET AND NUTRIENTS

• Eat a nutritious diet of **vegetables, fruit, grains, seeds, legumes, and nuts**. High sulfur foods (**garlic, onions, asparagus**) help keep the skin smooth and youthful.

• **Avoid animal fats, hydrogenated oils, and fried food**. Use no oils that have been heated.

• **Use no sugar, chocolate, junk food, alcohol, or caffeine**.

• The solution to this problem is not superficial creams (which contain vasoline or aluminum), but obtaining enough **unsaturated fatty acids** in the diet. These would be the uncooked vegetable oils, such as **wheat germ oil, flaxseed oil, sesame seed oil, corn oil**, and **soy oil**. The oil should be fairly fresh. Never use rancid oil, for it destroys the vitamin E in that meal. Take additional **vitamin E** supplementation (800-1,200 units a day).

• If you are not taking supplemental **vitamin A**, begin taking a moderate amount (not over 25,000 units a day for a few days). **Carrot juice** (or 15 mg **beta-carotene** daily) will also help.

• Take a **B-complex** supplement, **vitamin C** (1,000 mg 2-3 times daily), and **zinc** (15 mg daily).

• Cut out all **greases** and other **saturated fatty acids**. And, in their place, put a Tbsp. of a good oil (**flaxseed oil** and **wheat germ oil** are the best) on your food after it is cooked.

APPLICATIONS

• "Misting" is helpful. **Spray your face** with a fine mist of water at least 3 times a day. To increase the effect, add some **aloe vera** to the mist water. Or you can add an **essential oil** to the water. But, if you do, you must not spray into your eyes.

• For your shower, rinse off everyday with **lukewarm water**, using as **little soap** as possible. Do not use **hot water**.

• Pour 2 cups of **oatmeal**, ground to a fine powder, into a bathtub of warm water. Tie some oatmeal in a washcloth and use it as a washcloth. Oatmeal is extremely soothing to the body.

• For itchy skin, add **vinegar** to the bathwater and take 2 Tbsp. of **vegetable oil** daily. Helpful herbs include **yarrow, violet**, and **marjoram. Dry-brush massage your skin**, to tone it up.

• Add 2-3 drops lavender essential oil to warm water and apply a **warm compress** to your face. This will hydrate the skin and stimulate the water and oil glands. Only use a washcloth that has all soap and detergent residues thoroughly rinsed out. Lean over the basin, dip the cloth in the water, and hold it to your face and neck for a few moments. Do this 10 times.

• Certain herbs are mucilaginous and help soothe dry skin. Mix an equal amount of **marshmallow root, fennel seed, dried plantain, and violet leaves**. Steep, strain, and sip a quart of the tea daily.

• **Ripe, mashed avocado** alone or mixed with **ripe banana** is an excellent moisturizing mask. It will deep-moisturize desert-dry skin after cleansing. Pat it over the throat and face (except the eye area). Wait 10-15 minutes. Then rinse off.

MISCELLANEOUS

• Drink an adequate amount of **water**. If necessary, gently rub a small amount of **oil** over your body after the bath. **Avoid commercial lotions and saturated fats (greases)**. These are all absorbed by your body. Avoid too much **sunlight**.

• Stop using **coffee and alcohol**. Both are diuretic, forcing water from your body. **Smoking** or **breathing smoke** makes the skin dry, leathery, and wrinkled.

• For the chafing, wear **cotton clothes. Australian wool** (the wool which does not scratch) is also good. **Wash** new inner clothing before you wear it. This softens the fabric. **Do not wear coarse cloth** next to the skin. Do not wear **synthetics**.

• Use **soap** which has cocoa butter, coconut oil, or another vegetable oil. They do not clean as well, but are more soothing to the skin.

• Keep the **house cooler**, and it will not be as dry. Put a **pan of water** on the stove or use a **humidifier**, to put moisture back into the house.

ENCOURAGEMENT—We shall never know, until we reach heaven, what Christ went through to enable us to overcome sin here on earth and live with Him forever. Thank God for His inexpressible, but constantly accessible, Gift. 1 John 1:3.

ITCHING
(Itchy Skin)

SYMPTOMS—The skin is itchy, and you want to scratch it. But this only makes the condition worse.

CAUSES—The itch may (among other things) be caused by an **allergy, shingles, chicken pox, hives, sunburn, diabetes, anemia, or glandular malfunction**.

NATURAL REMEDIES

• Add 2 cups of apple cider **vinegar** to bathwater to relieve itching. Or apply it, full-strength, to the area that is itching—but not near the eyes or genitals. For vaginal itching, douche with diluted vinegar, *see vaginitis (695)*.

• **Soak a towel in ice water** and place it over the itching area. Repeat as needed. Or apply an **ice pack**. For overall itching, slowly enter a **tub of cold water** and remain immersed till you feel better. Or rub an **ice cube** over the area.

• After taking a tub bath, apply a thin amount of **oil on the body**. This will trap water on the skin beneath the oil.

• Wear **cotton clothing** or **Australian wool** instead of **synthetics**. Do not wear tight or poorly fitted clothing.

• Apply freshly squeezed **lemon juice** (but diluted in the genital area).

• Pour uncooked, blended **oatmeal** into bathwater, or apply an **oatmeal compress** to the itching area. This is very soothing and relieves the itch of poison ivy, hives, and other allergic reactions. Do not slip in the tub!

• Soak a cloth in **cool milk** and apply it to the area.

• Apply **anise oil** directly to the area, to destroy lice and similar insects.

• Apply **slippery elm ointment**. Take ½ cup olive oil and 3 Tbsp. slippery elm powder. Heat this for 5 minutes and add 2 Tbsp. cocoa butter. When melted, cook for 10 minutes. Strain through a cheesecloth, pour into a tight-fitting jar, and refrigerate till firm. It will keep for 2 months.

• Dip a finger in **wet salt** and rub the itch. There will first be a sensation of burning, then coolness; and then the itch will disappear.

• Mix **juniper wood oil** and **yellow wax**; and apply to heal eczema and psoriatic skin sores.

• **Avoid violent exercise** which produces sweating. **Do not use soap, hot water, and abrasive cleansing** procedures which injure or remove natural oils. Avoid rapid changes in **temperature** or **emotional upsets**.

ENCOURAGEMENT—In the Plan of Redemption, God has revealed His love in sacrifice, a sacrifice so broad and deep and high that it is immeasurable.

SCABIES
(The Itch)

SYMPTOMS—An itching in a body part which tends to continue, then let up, then continue again. Most frequent areas are finger webs, hands, wrists, elbows, underarms, waist, and feet. Skin above the neck is rarely involved, except in infants. In men, it may also occur in the scrotum and penis. In women, the nipples are most often affected. Peak time is late summer and early autumn. Symptoms begin 2-6 weeks after infestation, with severe itching. Gray or skin-colored ridges appear on the skin. Mites are most active at night in warm beds.

CAUSE—Scabies is an infectious skin disease caused by an almost microscopic **mite**, called *Sarcoptes scabiei*. Although he is a little fellow, you know he is there. This eight-legged mite matures in 10-14 days and lives for about 30 days, all the while laying eggs in tunnels under the skin. They hatch in 4-5 days. Children infested with them usually have about 20. If they fall off the body, they live for 36 hours to 8 days.

Scabies is found on all social levels. Contact, even by a handshake, is all that is needed to acquire it. It can also be transmitted through **clothing** and **bed linen**. It is more common in older adolescents and young people, and in girls rather than boys. People can also get it from **touching dogs, other animals, or their bedding**. It is a special problem in institutions, such as nursing homes, etc. Warmth stimulates mite activity.

Scabies can only be accurately diagnosed by taking skin scrapings and viewing them under a microscope. If one person in a family has them, it is generally well to treat everyone. Children under 15 are often the first to contract them. It is usually best to treat everyone in the family at the same time.

NATURAL REMEDIES

• Mix flowers of **sulfur** with petrolatum (**petroleum jelly**). Sulfur is a poison, so do not swallow it! In addition, it will stain clothing and does not smell good. But it will work to kill the scabies mites. For children, use a 5% sulfur (5% sulfur and 95% petrolatum) mixture; for adults, a 10% mixture. Take a warm, soaking bath before applying the mixture. Apply it for 3-5 nights before retiring. Cover from neck to toes. Have someone else apply it to you, so everything is covered. (Sulfur will stain clothing.)

• During this period, **launder** your clothes frequently in hot water (140° F.). The mite cannot survive temperatures above 120° F. for more than 5 minutes. Dry cleaning or ironing will also kill them.

OTHER HELP

• **Pennyroyal** is also called "fleabane," because it is so effective against fleas. The ancient Romans used it for that purpose. Apply a strong tea of it directly to the affected area.

• Add 2 drops of **tea tree oil** and/or **plaintain leaves** to 2 Tbsp. vegetable oil and apply it to the area. Like pennyroyal, it will kill the mites and reduce itching.

• **Turmeric** has been used for centuries in Asia to kill scabies. Make a paste and spread it on the affected area, at the same time you boil clothes and bedding.

• *To reduce the itching sensation*, soak in a **cool bath, starch bath, or oatmeal bath** (*see directions under Dry Skin, p. 332; Itching Skin, p. 333*). Mix powdered **calcium** with a little oil and apply to the area. The gel of **aloe vera** contains *bradykininase*, which is soothing.

• **Onion skins** contain 3% *quercetin*, which is soothing to itching skin. Boil 6 onions for 15-20 minutes in a quart of water, When the liquid is cool, apply it all over the body. A strong solution of **tansy tea** kills scabies.

• For a bath which both soothes the skin and kills the mites, mix **peppermint, pennyroyal, rosemary, sage, spearmint and thyme** together. Make two quarts of tea, toss it in bathwater, and climb in.

• Eat foods high in **zinc** (such as soybeans, sunflower seeds, whole-grain products, yeast, wheat bran, and blackstrap molasses).

• **Avoid processed, fried, and junk foods.** Use no **sugar, chocolate, soft drinks, alcohol, or tobacco.**

• Apply oil of **St. John's wort** extracted in **evening primrose oil**. To make it, combine approximately a cup of fresh St. John's wort flowering tops in enough evening primrose oil to cover them. Steep for two weeks. Strain out the herbs and apply the oil to scabies lesions up to three times per day.

• After washing the infested area with an herbal skin wash, apply a generous amount of **one of the essential oils** that you have available. In addition to any mite-killing power that the preparation may have, the oil helps to smother the pests.

It's important to dilute essential oils before applying them to the skin. For most oils, mix no more than 1 teaspoon of essential oil with 1 cup of what's called a carrier oil—you can use any neutral vegetable oil such as almond, olive, sesame, or even corn oil.

• Keep fingernails short and discourage scratching.

• **Note:** Do not use Lindane or Kwell. These chemicals can be absorbed through the skin and cause convulsions.

ENCOURAGEMENT—God's love is revealed in all His dealings with His earthly children. He loved us or He would not have paid such an expensive price to redeem us from sin. Thank Him everyday for His wonderful gift of Jesus Christ.

JOCK ITCH

SYMPTOMS—A moist, itchy patch of reddened infection on the surface of the groin.

CAUSES—Fungal infections occur most frequently in moist places on the skin. This is a fungus infection in the area where the top of your legs meet your trunk.

If, while treating the fungal infection, you develop symptoms of a worse infection (such as increased redness and swelling or fever) you may have contracted a bacterial infection—in addition to the fungal infection.

NATURAL REMEDIES

NUTRITION

• Eat a nourishing diet of **fruits, vegetables, whole grains, legumes, and nuts**. While treating the infection, a diet primarily of **raw food** is best.

• Avoid **tobacco, alcohol, caffeine**. Do not eat **meat or dairy products**. Avoid **sugary, fried, and processed foods**. Eat nothing **greasy**.

HERBS

• **Goldenseal** contains *berberine*, which destroys fungi. It can be used against every type of fungus infection. It can be used as a drink or applied topically. Only use goldenseal for a week; then switch for a time to another fungicide herb.

• **Pau d'arco** is strongly antifungal. Drink 3 cups daily.

• **Bloodroot** also contain *berberine* and has been shown to be quite effective as a fungicide.

• **Yellowroot, barberry, and Oregon grape** also contain *berberine*.

• Treat the area with a mixture of **goldenseal and pau d'arco**.

• **Tea tree** oil is excellent when applied externally, but do not drink it. Apply it several times a day to the affected area, either full strength or diluted with a little distilled water or cold-pressed oil. **Black walnut** extract can also be used.

• A powerful antifungicide is **wild oregano oil**. The most resistent forms of fungus infection can generally be eliminated by it.

• The **pepper tree** (horopito) is a New Zealand shrub which contains *polygodial*, which is useful against both fungi and bacteria. Another antifungal herb is the *Licaria puchuri-major*, a Brazilian plant.

OTHER HELPS

• Keep the **skin clean and dry**. Expose the affected area to air as much as possible. Your **clothing** should be kept clean.

—See Candida (281), Athletes Foot (377).

ENCOURAGEMENT—God's gift of Jesus Christ to mankind is beyond all computation. Nothing was withheld that was needed to save mankind, if we will but accept the gift and, by faith in the enabling grace of Christ, obey God's commandments.

RINGWORM

SYMPTOMS—Small, flat, red, slightly elevated ring or oval-shaped sores which may be crusted, dry, scaly, or moist. The centers of the sores heal as the sores spread outward. The result is an infected ring. Itching, burning, or pain may be present. The lesions appear to be circular. The area is often covered with small blisters.

When the scalp is affected, the hair falls out in circular patches. The fingers can also be affected.

CAUSES—Ringworm is a very contagious disease, caused by a parasitic fungus. It can infect children or adults, and is caused by **unsanitary conditions**. **Keep the hands clean!** Pet the dog and then rub your face, and you may regret it.

Ringworm of the beard (face) is more persistent than ringworm of the scalp. Ringworm of the body is the easiest to eliminate.

Dogs, cats, rabbits, children, and contaminated clothing are generally the carriers of the disease.

There are several different types of ringworm, all of which are of fungal origin:

Ringworm of the scalp—This can be on the scalp and on the face. It is the most noticeable kind. It is highly contagious, and often found on schoolchildren. It frequently induces baldness, which may become permanent if hair shafts are destroyed by the fungus. It can be transmitted in unsanitary conditions, from child to child, in hair brushes, barbers' tools, hats, and theater seats.

Ringworm of the trunk—This includes "jockey itch," and is spread by contact with people or their clothing. Dogs and cats can also spread it.

Ringworm of the nails—This consists of a fungus growing under the nails of the hands or feet. It produces thickened, misshapen, brittle, discolored, chalky, pitted, or grooved nails. This type of ringworm is quite difficult to eliminate.

Ringworm of the feet—This is also known as athlete's foot. *See Athlete's Foot (377).*

NATURAL REMEDIES

• **Vitamins A, E, and zinc** are important.
• Put **plantain** and **castor oil,** or **tea tree oil** on the affected area.
• Place **ultraviolet light** on the area: sunlight for at least 6 minutes a day. If you use a sunlamp, never place it closer than 18 inches from the skin, and only for 10-20 seconds at a time.
• Apply **apple cider vinegar** to the area several times a day.
• Equally useful is **castor oil, goldenseal tea, and borax.** Rub the area with **borax** and **castor oil.**
• A 3-day **citrus fast** is very helpful, **cleansing the bowels** daily. Follow this with a **nutritious diet.**
• Eat plenty of **garlic.** Place freshly cut, raw **garlic** 3 times a day on the area. This is a very good remedy. Blend the garlic with a little water and apply as a soak, compress, or poultice. But this remedy is too powerful to apply to raw flesh between the toes. It can burn lower layers of skin. You can also use **black walnut** extract. Wash the area with **garlic juice** or **wormwood.**
• Take 2 **chaparral** or **wormwood** capsules daily.
• Make a strong tea of equal parts **plantain** and **yellow dock,** and bathe the affected area frequently.
• The scalp can be shampooed with **tar soap** and **borax.** Moisten the area every morning and evening with **goldenseal** (1 tsp.) and **myrrh** (½ tsp.) which has been steeped in a pint of boiling water.
• An herb tea can also be taken internally: **goldenseal** or **plantain,** twice a day. **Garlic** is good.
• Make a salve from equal parts of **burdock** root, **chaparral, wormwood, and chickweed.** Apply to the area. Some of it can also be made into a tea to drink in order to fight the fungus internally.
Apply undiluted **lemon juice** every few hours. Adults should drink a solution of 1 tsp. **goldenseal** to a cup of water 2 times a day.
• Keep the skin clean and dry. Ringworm likes damp skin. Take **frequent baths,** but **dry thoroughly** each time. **Rub briskly** with a towel, to remove the outer dead layers of skin that the ringworm initially attacks.
• **Do not scratch.** Keep **fingernails cut short,**

to lessen accidental scratching and spreading of the infection.
• *To remove crusts:* Soak the area in a **saline solution.** An alternate method is to apply **moist cloths** for 10-15 minutes, 3 times a day.
• *To treat nails:* **Pare and scrape** the infected area. Try to remove as much of the loose material beneath the nails as possible. Apply **vinegar** with a Q-tip twice a day. Keep at it, even though it may require months to eliminate. Fungus of the nails is the slowest to conquer.
• *To treat scalp:* **Shampoo** the hair daily, and keep it **short,** but not necessarily shaved. If hair is cut at home, **burn** the hair clippings. **Boil** scissors, combs, etc. after use. **Sterilize** clothing. Kloss suggests washing the hair with **tar soap and borax.** And every morning and evening moisten the area with a solution of 1 tsp. **goldenseal** and ½ tsp. **myrrh,** steeped in a pint of boiled water.
• **Heat and moisture** encourage fungus growth. So it is best for the child to avoid getting **hot and sweaty** during periods of infection. If the **skin is bruised or broken,** the fungi can more easily enter the body.
• Keep in mind that a fungicide parasite (which is what all forms of ringworm are) is best stopped by **sealing off the air.**
—*Also see Athlete's Foot (377), which is a type of ringworm fungus. Also see Antifungal herbs (299).*

ENCOURAGEMENT—Nothing of the world can make you sad, when you have submitted your heart to be molded by the Spirit of Christ. He alone can provide you with the answers you need. Ezekiel 13:22-23.
"But He [Christ] was wounded for our transgressions, He was bruised for our iniquities: the chastisement of our peace was upon Him; and with His stripes we are healed.
"All we like sheep have gone astray; we have turned every one to his own way; and the Lord hath laid on Him the iniquity of us all."—Isaiah 53:5-6.

SKIN - 5 - GROWTHS
Also: Section on Tumors and Cancer (780-796).

WARTS
(Papillomas, Verrucae)

SYMPTOMS AND CAUSES—With the exception of plantar warts (which are flat), warts are always raised bumps. Where there is constant contact, they can cause discomfort and even pain. Venereal (genital) warts are single or clusters of soft cauliflower-like growths. Warts appear more frequently in adolescents who are experiencing hormonal changes, especially between the ages of 12 and 16, and 70% between 10 and 39. There are three primary types of skin warts:

1 - *Contagious warts:* Also called viral warts, these are benign skin warts *(verruca vulgaris), which* are also called *common warts*, and may be found on the hands, arms, face, or body. These hard, irregular, or round warts can be dark or flesh-colored and may range in size from a pinhead to a bean. They most frequently occur on the hands, face, knees, and scalp, where the skin is in friction with clothing, etc. They can also occur on the larynx (voice box) and produce hoarseness. They can be spread by **picking, trimming, or touching them**. On the face, they can be spread by **shaving**.

There are three types of common warts: *flat warts*. These are flat-topped and flesh-colored. They appear on the wrists, backs of the hands, face, and may itch. *Digitate warts* are dark-colored growths with fingerlike projections. *Filiform warts* are long, slender growths appearing on the eyelids, armpits, or neck. They often appear on people who are overweight and middle-aged.

2 - *Plantar warts:* This is another type of *verrucum*, which appears on the sole of the foot. These are actually benign epithelial tumors caused by a virus.

3 - *Venereal warts:* These warts *(condylomatum acuminata)* may be found on the vulva and penis. Venereal warts are caused by the human papilloma virus (HPV), of which there are more than 35 types. These warts are pink, cauliflower-shaped growths on the genitals of men and women. Genital warts on a woman can change into cancer of the cervix or genital area. They should be removed! One study showed they can increase the risk of cervical cancer by 200 percent! The incubation period for genital warts is generally 3 months. It can spread to others even before the person realizes he or she has it. Do not have sexual intercourse until the warts are eliminated.

Physicians use liquid nitrogen, corrosive salicylic acids, and surgery to remove warts.

NATURAL REMEDIES

• As with any infection, warts appear because the body has **lowered vitality and lack of resistance. Eat right, keep proper hours, exercise in the open air, and breathe deep**. Tone up your whole body.

DIET AND NUTRITION

• The usual methods of removing warts (surgery, acids, burning, electrotherapy, or freezing) often results in their reappearance. The underlying causes should be eliminated. Improve the diet. And eat foods high in **vitamins A, B complex, C, and zinc**. Deficiencies in all four are related to an increased incidence of viral infections. Also increase the sufur-containing amino acids in the diet, such as are found in **asparagus, citrus fruits, garlic, and onions**. Eat **raw garlic**.

GETTING RID OF WARTS

Since everyone seems to get better using a different treatment, here are lots of them. It is said that no form of wart treatment is 100% effective.

• Place thin sections of **garlic** on the wart. Try to avoid touching the garlic to normal tissue. Hold it in place with cloth and tape, and leave it there overnight. Do this for 2 or 3 nights. Within a week the wart will fall off.

• Apply **castor oil** to the wart for half an hour, 3 times a day for 3 weeks.

• Cover the wart with **honey** for 15 days.

• Put 1 drop **hydrochloric acid** (historically called muriatic acid or spirits of salt) on the wart once a day, for 8 days.

• Dissolve as much **sodium carbonate** (washing soda) in water as will stay in solution. Swab this onto the warts for 2 minutes, 4 times a day, and let it dry in the air. Very large warts have responded to this.

• Mix **castor oil and baking soda** into a paste and apply to the wart, cover, and keep on all night. Do not pick at it, but let it slough off within 3-6 weeks.

• Apply an **iron** formula, such as **Ironite** or **black walnut** tincture.

• Apply powdered **vitamin C**, as paste, and cover.

• Soak the wart in a concentrated **saltwater** solution: 1½ tsp. of salt to ½ cup water equals a 30% solution. Soak the wart for 20 minutes, 2-3 times a day for a few weeks.

• Soaking the wart for 30-90 minutes twice a week in **hot water** (113°-118° F.) eliminated half the warts in one study.

• Here are several other helpful applications: **green fig juice**; that is, juice from barely ripe figs will destroy warts. **Milkweed sap** applied several times a day. Fresh grated **celandine** juice. Cut a **raw potato**, rub it on, and repeat several times a day for several weeks. **Chickweed** juice. **Sassafras oil**. **Marigold** juice. **Green papaya** juice. **Aloe vera**. **Onion and salt** compress. The juice of **white cabbage**. **Wheat germ oil**. Fresh **pineapple juice**. Mashed **cashew nut**. Spread the juice of a *sour* apple on it. In England, the juice from a **Dandelion** stalk is applied. Houseleek (**Hen and Chickens**) is a succulent rock-garden plant with thick, fleshy leaves containing a large amount of supermalate of calcium which eliminates warts. **Watercress** juice. **Caster bean** oil. The FDA has approved *salicylic acid*, which is abundant in **willow**, for wart removal.

• Plain **salicylic acid**, available over the counter, is an inexpensive home treatment for warts. To use it, first soak the area in water in order to soften the wart. Then apply the salicylic acid. But, because it *is* an acid, apply it to only the wart, not to any irritated or infected skin, mucous membranes, moles, or birthmarks. (Also do not use it on warts with hair, genital warts, or facial warts.) The next morning, you can use a nail file to remove dead skin from the wart. Then repeat the process as often as directed on the label. Soaking the area in water between treatments can further soften a wart. Each morning, you can file away the dead skin with a nail file. Afterward, wash the file with soap and plenty of hot water. (If you have dabetes or a circulatory disorder, it may be best not to use salicylic acid.)

• *For plantar warts* (warts on the bottom of the foot), apply a **plantain** poultice (the leaf itself) to the wart. Another method is to place the inner side of a fresh piece of the inner white part of **banana peel** over the wart and hold it there with tape or rub it on 2-4 times a day for 5-7 days. Change daily after washing the entire area. Once a week the thickened outer horny layer is removed. Maximum time for complete disappearance of a wart is 6 weeks, with no recurrence within 2 years.

• *To prevent warts from forming*, reduce the amount of **protein foods** you eat. Most people eat too much.

ENCOURAGEMENT—Do your duty and trust in God; for He knows what things you need. He watches over you with more tenderness than does a mother over an afflicted child. Mark 9:23.

WENS
(Sebaceous cysts, Steatomas)

SYMPTOMS—These are slow-growing benign cystic cutaneous tumor-like formations. They contain sebaceous material (skin oil and protein) and are often found on the scalp (wen), ears, back, or scrotum. Ranging in size from a pea to a golf ball, a wen is painless and feels soft but firm. Included here are whiteheads. They can become infected with bacteria and form an abscess.

NATURAL REMEDIES

• A "stab" incision is made at the lowest edge of the cyst. The contents are then sucked out and the insides are flushed with **hydrogen peroxide**. If the cyst is large, the wall will have to be removed so it does not refill. Then place a daily changed sterile gauze over, and within, it to keep it draining for a week to 10 days.

• Apply **goldenseal** or **tee tree oil** to eliminate infection. Apply herb tea of **witch hazel** or **white oak bark** to absorb the oil in the cyst.

• *To keep them from growing or returning*, eat lightly, avoiding heavy **protein foods. Avoid fats—especially saturated fats and all fried foods, cheese, chocolate, butter, margarine, and dairy products.** Do not use **alcohol, nicotine, or caffeine** products.

—*Also see Warts (336) and Skin Cancer (787).*

ENCOURAGEMENT—God is a Friend in perplexity and affliction, a protector in distress, and a preserver in a thousand dangers that are unseen to us. Trust Him ever. And, by His grace, obey His Written Word.

Hebrews 6:18-19.

SKIN - 6 - OTHER MINOR SKIN PROBLEMS

OILY SKIN

SYMPTOMS—Excessively oily skin, a shiny appearance, and a tendency to have blackheads and blemishes.

CAUSES—The sebaceous glands, which secrete oil onto the skin, produce more oil than they should—and the oil they produce is the wrong oil. The excess oil clogs pores. Heredity is a factor, but diet and hormones affect it. Oil gland secretions can be increased by stress, hormonal activity changes, hot weather, pregnancy, or taking certain types of birth control pills.

The forehead, nose, chin, and upper back tend to have more sebaceous glands. Hence these areas can be the sites of the most problems. Oily skin is most common among teenagers.

The cause is frequently too much of the wrong type of oil in your diet or, merely, a lack of the right kind.

NATURAL REMEDIES
DIET AND NUTRITION

• Take 1-3 tsp. of **flaxseed oil** every day. It is rich in the right kind of oil needed by your body.

• For healthier skin, eat lots of **fresh fruit, vegetables, whole grains, legumes, nuts, and seeds**.

• Eating 1 tsp. of granulated **lecithin** each day will help emulsify (break apart and eliminate) the saturated fat in your body.

• Eating **red meat and dairy products** puts the wrong oils (saturated fats) into your body. The result is oilier skin, clogged pores, and more blemishes.

• **Keep your skin clean**. Beware of certain **cosmetics**. They aggravate a problem which might not otherwise exist.

OTHER THINGS TO DO

• **Wash twice a day with soap**. It was made to remove oil. **Hot soapy water** is even better. Ivory soap is a more drying soap than many others. To remove leftover cleanser and dirt from oily skin, apply a gentle, astringent herb tea, such as **yarrow, sage, or peppermint**.

• Some people apply **mud masks** to remove oil. White or rose-colored clays are best for sensitive skin.

• **Avoid smoking**. It increases the size of your skin pores and weakens the skin generally.

• If you have areas of oily skin and dry skin, treat

each part separately. —*See Dry Skin (332).*

Fortunately, oily skin tends to age better than dry skin, producing less wrinkles. So, in one way, you can count yourself fortunate.

—*Also see Acne (328).*

ENCOURAGEMENT—God cares for our necessities. His love and grace are continually flowing, to satisfy our needs. In His care, we may safely rest. Luke 12:32.

PRICKLY HEAT

SYMPTOMS—The skin feels hot and prickly.

CAUSES—Dry skin and sweaty skin in hot weather.

NATURAL REMEDIES

• Wash with mild soap, twice a day. After a bath, use ½ teaspoon of cider vinegar in a glass of water. Take vitamin C orally (1,000 mg or more).

ENCOURAGEMENT—Too often we grieve our kind heavenly Father by our unbelief. If we will but trust His guiding hand, all our difficulties will work to our best good. Psalm 95:7-10.

HEAT RASH

SYMPTOMS—An itchy skin rash can occur in the heat of midsummer. These are tiny red or pink, blister-like bumps that are extremely itchy on your chest, back, and even your armpits or the creases of the elbows or groin.

CAUSES—As a result of poor diet, overwork, and lack of proper rest, the skin has become too acid. Sweat becomes stuck in the pores and spreads into surrounding tissue, irritating it.

NATURAL REMEDIES

• Stay **cool and dry, wear light-cotton clothing, and expose the affected area to the air**. Then the heat rash will probably go away by itself in 3-4 days.

• Eat a more **nutritious diet**, obtain adequate **rest**, **avoid meat and junk food**. **Do not smoke or drink liquor**.

• Take a **soda alkaline bath**. This helps counteract acidity in the rash. Fill a bathtub with water at 95°-98° F. Add a cup of baking soda. Sit in the tub and continually pour the water over yourself. About 30-60 minutes later, stand in the tub and partially drip-dry. Then pat yourself dry and get out.

• Put 1-2 cups of fresh **peppermint leaves** in thin cloth, fill the tub with cool water, immerse the mint for 3-5 minutes, and climb in and soak for 5-10 minutes. Do this as often as necessary to relieve the itching.

ENCOURAGEMENT—God loves His children. He longs to see them overcoming the discouragement which Satan would overpower them. Do not give way to unbelief. Remember the love and power that God has shown in times past. How thankful we can be for the gift of God in Jesus Christ His Son! Acts 16:31.

ROSACEA
(Acne Rosacea)

SYMPTOMS—A reddening of the skin—generally on the forehead, nose, cheekbones, and chin. Pustules may appear on the nose and are tender. The skin may thicken. Groups of small blood vessels, close to the surface, become enlarged, resulting in blotchy red areas with small bumps. Red spider veins (telangiectases) and cherry angiomas (red spots caused by tiny tumors in dilated blood vessels) appear. Pimples may accompany the problem. The rosacea may disappear or become permanent. Blackheads or whiteheads are rarely present.

It often begins with a frequent flushing, or reddening, of the face. This is most often seen on the nose and cheeks. A burning, or grittiness, in the eyes may be felt.

CAUSE—Rosacea, which usually begins in the 40s, is a skin disorder which can become chronic. It is important that you try to eliminate the underlying causes which are closely related to a **wrong diet and way of life**.

People who flush easily are more likely to develop this problem. White women between 30-50 have it the most. When men have it, the appearance of the face is worse, often accompanied by a roughened, enlarged nose (rhinophyma). Middle-aged and older people are most likely to have rosacea.

NATURAL REMEDIES

• **Alcohol, stress, excessive heat or cold, sunlight, hot liquids, sugar, or spicy food** may trigger a reaction. Avoid trans-fatty acids (**margarine, shortening, hydrogenated vegetable oils**). It is believed that a **B complex deficiency** is involved, along with a **poor diet**, resulting from too much **junk food. Alcoholics**, who perennially lack in B vitamins and good food, often have reddened faces.

• Each day, take 25 mg of **B₂**, 1,000 mg of **vitamin C**, 400-800 mg of **bioflavonoids**, 400 IU of **vitamin E**, and 15 mg of **zinc**.

• Once or twice a month, go on a **short fast**, to clean out the body. Eat **nourishing food**.

• After washing your face, rinse with cool water in which you earlier boiled **potatoes**. Or use a mixture of ½ cup water and 1 Tbsp. apple cider **vinegar**.

• For 5 minutes each evening, massage **olive oil** outward from nose to ears with circular movements.

• **Avoid strenuous exercise** which produces sweating. Avoid **exposure to heat** from the sun, an open fireplace, oven door, or facial steaming. They can burst dilated capillaries on the face. Avoid **icy chilling, after-shave lotions, skin toners, harsh soaps, or hard**

skin scrubbing. (Pat the skin dry after washing.) Do not drink **hot liquids**. Avoid **friction** on the face, including clothing (turtlenecks, etc.) touching it.

• Avoid **commercial skin creams** and **greasy cosmetics**. Wash your **pillow case** regularly in chemical-free detergents.

ENCOURAGEMENT—Heirs of God and joint heirs with Christ—what a wonderful hope is set before us! May we prove faithful everyday. As we cling to Christ and, by His enabling grace, obey His Ten Commandment law, we will rejoice in His light. Galatians 4:7-8.

ENLARGED PORES

SYMPTOMS—Unsightly larger pores in the face and on the skin, which gives an appearance of premature aging.

CAUSE—Using **nicotine** in any form.

NATURAL REMEDIES

• Stop believing those ads which show beautiful people smoking. The beautiful people in the ads do not smoke. If the ads showed pictures of women who have smoked for ten years, no one would buy their products.

• If you want to start looking better, **quit all tobacco products** and **stop breathing sidestream (second-hand) smoke**. Do not drink **soft drinks or eat sugar, chocolate, potato chips,** and other **junk foods. Begin a good nutritious program with exercise and rest.** Take **vitamin-mineral supplements**, including **vitamins A, C, and the entire B complex**.

ENCOURAGEMENT—All who enter into a covenant with Jesus Christ become, by adoption, the children of God. They are cleansed from sin, as they submit to His rule and obey His Word. Ever trust Him. 2 Chronicles 20:20.

WRINKLES

SYMPTOMS—Wrinkles on the face. The skin tells what is inside. If you have healthful, youthful skin, it is a good sign of a healthy body inside.

CAUSE—The skin loses its elasticity and suppleness. It becomes thinner and dryer. With age, wrinkles are inevitable. But there are ways to avoid getting them earlier than necessary.

NATURAL REMEDIES

• **Stay out of the sun. Avoid tanning booths.** They produce the same wrinkling as the sun. **Wear a hat** when out in the sunlight. **Avoid sunburns.**

• Eat carefully of **good food. Exercise,** drink enough **fluids**, and get adequate **sleep**.

• Wrinkles result from changes in collagen, the "cell cement" protein that is the fibrous portion of your skin. This is about one-third of your body's total protein and 70% of your connective tissue. Without **vitamin C**, you cannot produce collagen. So you begin falling apart.

• **Vitamin A** is important for good skin health. Drink fresh **carrot juice** daily.

• **Cocoa butter** melts at body temperature and re-moisturizes dry skin, especially around the eyes (crows' feet), corners of the mouth, and on the neck (turkey neck). **Coconut oil** helps in a similar way. For centuries, **olive oil** has been used for this purpose.

• Place cool cucumber slices on your face to help eliminate wrinkles. Put mashed purslane on your face and wash it off 15-30 minutes later.

• Purchase an 8-oz. atomizer and, a minimum of 3 times a day, **mist your face** with clean water. Avoid living in a **dry home**. Place a dish of water on your stove.

• **Avoid massaging** your face roughly. It can cause a breakdown of the collagen fibers in your skin.

• **Pressing your face** against a pillow adds more wrinkles. Do not **scrunch up** your face when you talk. That makes new wrinkle patterns.

• **Avoid alcohol and nicotine.** Tobacco dramatically ages the skin! Smoking makes a 25-year-old woman look like a 35-year-old! Smoking also decreases blood supply to the face and skin.

• **Dampen the skin**, and then apply a little **vegetable oil** to lubricate it. That will help put water and oil into your skin cells.

• **Massage your face** as the Orientals do. Doing so exercises the skin and facial muscles, strengthening them.

Now, don't laugh, and I will give you more suggestions:

To soften and nourish your skin, mash half an **avocado** and put it on your face. Leave it there until it dries. And then wipe it off with water. Avocado has essential oils. It is an outstanding facial emollient for those with dry skin.

• To reduce puffiness under your eyes, place cool slices of **cucumber** over them for 10 minutes.

• To get the dead skin cells from your face, mash fresh **grapes** and put them on your face. They contain AHA, the over-the-counter active ingredient in skin lotions.

• To remove dead surface skin cells and improve skin texture, Japanese women gently rub a small handful of dry **short-grain rice** against their faces.

• To cleanse the pores, rub mashed **tomato** over your face.

ENCOURAGEMENT—Only to those who receive Jesus Christ as their Saviour are given the power to become sons and daughters of God. By ourselves, we cannot overcome sin. But, in the strength of Christ, we can be overcomers. 2 Corinthians 13:11.

NIGHT SWEATS
(Excess Sweating, Hyperhidrosis)

SYMPTOMS—Sweating during sleeping hours which seems abnormal. The sweating may begin all at once.

CAUSES—There may be a **lack of air** in the sleeping room. The body may be eliminating **toxins** and needs help. You may have a **thyroid problem**.

NATURAL REMEDIES

• A lack of fresh air in a room can cause you to break out in an abnormal sweat. Make sure **a current of air** flows through your bed chamber when you are sleeping. It does not have to be much, but you need a slight amount of moving fresh air. In some instances, there may be enough air in the room; but, when you breathe out air, it tends to remain in a hollow formed by the bedding. Open a window and **breathe through your mouth**, and you may find that your brain feels more relaxed and ready to go to sleep.

• If you are not living right and eating right, then the sweating can be the result of a toxic overload. **Avoid meat, salt, tobacco, and junk food**.

• Drink 2 oz. **green drink** (whizzed up greens in pineapple or apple juice) everyday. **Do not eat closer than four hours before bedtime**. One day each week, **fast** on distilled water or fruit and vegetable juices.

• Take **Epsom salt baths** (2 cups in the bathtub) at night and **hot / cold showers** in the morning. *After the night sweats are past*, take 10-minute **cool baths** in the morning, to tone the system.

• An alternative is to take a **hot saltwater sponge** before retiring. Use 2 Tbsp. of salt per quart of water. A hot bath followed by a **salt glow** is also good.

• Boil a quart of water, turn off the fire, put 1 tsp. **white oak bark** or **wild alum root** in it, let steep 20 minutes, pour into a cool tub, and get in.

• Steep 1 tsp. **goldenseal** in a pint of boiled water and drink 2 cups upon retiring. This will do much to prevent night sweats.

• Keep the **bowels loose** and the colon clean. Use herbal laxatives and herb enemas if necessary.

• You may be experiencing **hot flashes**, caused by irregular thyroid activity. If so, you will suddenly get hot.

ENCOURAGEMENT—Christ alone has power to cleanse the heart. He alone can make you a child of God. He can transform your life and bring you peace and happiness in the midst of every trial. 2 Corinthians 8:12.

BODY ODOR
(Bromhidrosis)

SYMPTOMS—The secretion of foul-smelling perspiration.

CAUSES AND TREATMENT—The *apocrine* sweat glands produce fluid which has no odor for several hours until bacterial action give it an odor. These glands began working at puberty and are more active in men than women. Most of them are under your arms.

NATURAL REMEDIES

• A lack of soap and water applications cause the sweat to accumulate. **Wash your body** more often, especially in the axial areas (under arms and groin), and change underwear daily. Make sure your clothes are clean. Choose natural fabrics. **Cotton and wool** enable the absorbed sweat to evaporate from the body.

• Foot odors can be caused either by not **changing the socks** often enough or by wearing **rubber or plastic shoes**. They will make your feet smell like an old rubber tire. The problem may be the shoes, not your feet. Many people today wear such shoes, since they are less expensive than leather ones.

• Body odors can also be caused by an excess of **toxins in the body** which it is trying to eliminate. Are you eating **too much food** or **the wrong food**? Are you **staying up late at night, drinking alcohol, or smoking cigarettes**? Apply a **wet sheet pack overnight**. It will help pull the toxins out of a heavy meat eater. By morning, the sheet will be stained by the eliminated poisons. **Fast** one day a week on juice, vegetable juices or water. **Epsom-salt baths** help the body eliminate toxins. Repeat daily for one week. Then reduce to once a week.

• Not eating enough **unsaturated fatty acids** (quality vegetable oils) or not getting enough **zinc** can also produce body odor.

• **Zinc** deficiency may contribute to body odor. If this might be the case for you, check out the following foods, which are rich in zinc, to add your diet: Spinach, whole grains, legumes, rice, nuts.

• Drink lots of **water**. Take **chlorophyll** (1 tsp. 2-3 times daily). It is absorbed from the intestinal tract into the bloodstream and deodorizes the body.

• Take a tip from hunters who wash with **pine soap**, so their odor will not be detected by wildlife. Old-fashioned **glycerin soap** is also good.

• Another cause of body odor is **excessive sexual activity**.

• Pouring tomato juice on a dog to de-skunk him has been done for generations. Some have found that they can pour some **tomato juice** in a tub of water, sit in it for a time, shower off, and get out—and they also smell fine!

• Both **coriander** and **licorice** contain 20 chemicals with antibacterial action. **Ginger** has 17. **Licorice** contains up to 33% bactericidal compounds, on a dry weight basis. Powder one, or all of them, and rub them under your arms.

• Rub **baking soda** under your arms. It instantly neutralizes the acid fluid there which bacteria need.

• Here is a formula using baking soda: You can use this powder under the arms or wherever odor originates: ½ cup **cornstarch**, ½ cup **baking soda**, 1 tablespoon

S
K
I
N

ground sage. 1 tablespoon ground rosemary. Mix ingredients together.

• The herb **goldenseal** can kill bacteria in the intestines, which will reduce body odors.

• Excessive body odor can be caused by **liver disease, diabetes, chronic constipation,** and **certain parasites. Meat eaters** have more odor than vegetarians.

ENCOURAGEMENT—The promise of sonship is made to all who believe on His name. Everyone who comes to Jesus, in faith, will receive pardon and power to obey. Hebrews 13:15-16. Trusting Him is always safe. He will ever guide those who surrender their lives to Him.

SKIN RASH

SYMPTOMS—Reddening of various kinds on the skin, with possible bumps, scaling, and thickening.

CAUSES—In our modern world, skin rashes can have many causes which include **reactions to chemicals, sun, wind, insect bites, alcohol, detergents, and friction**.

Skin rashes in children are often caused by food rashes from **chocolate, peanuts, dairy products, wheat, eggs, or meat**. It has been estimated that 75% of children's skin rashes are caused by sensitivity to eggs, peanuts, or milk.

NATURAL REMEDIES

• Quick relief from many rashes may be obtained by soaking a clean cloth in **cool water**, wringing it out, and applying it to the area for 10 minutes. Repeat as often as needed.

• Better yet, soak the cloth in **comfrey tea** or in **calcium water**. To make calcium water, take a spoonful of calcium gluconate powder (obtainable at a health-food store) and stir it into a cup of water. **Oatmeal water** works just as well.

• A wash of **chamomile tea** helps reduce rashes. A poultice made from **dandelion, yellow dock root, and chaparral** helps alleviate many of them.

ENCOURAGEMENT—When a soul receives Christ, he receives power to live the life of Christ. Just as Christ resisted sin, so you and I can resist temptation to wrongdoing. Psalm 10:13, James 4:9-10.

ERYTHEMA MULTIFORME

SYMPTOMS—Numerous small red spots distributed symmetrically over the body. These may enlarge to form red rings with purplish centers, called target lesions. The lesions may blister in the middle. There

may be itching in the affected area. Other possible symptoms include painful, inflamed lesions within the mouth and nose; fever; headache; sore throat; and, occasionally, diarrhea. Rare: Most of the mucous membranes throughout the body become severely inflamed and ulcerated.

CAUSES—The cause is usually unknown. But the rash can be triggered by infection with a **virus** such as herpes simplex, the virus that produces **cold sores** *(322)*. Other factors include certain **drugs**—such as sulfonamide antibiotics; phenytoin; **cancer**; **radiation** therapy; or **vaccines**, such as the one for polio.

NATURAL REMEDIES

• Did the rash suddenly appear shortly after you took a prescribed drug? If so, that is probably the cause. And you need to **stop taking the drug**. Either switch to a natural remedy or ask your physician to give you a different drug. Although all drugs ultimately injure the body, they do not all produce rashes.

—*See Drug-induced Rashes (349).*

ENCOURAGEMENT—In Christ, God gave us all the treasures of heaven that the moral image of God might be restored in man. Psalm 51:12.

PITYRIASIS ROSEA

SYMPTOMS—It gradually becomes a mild, pink rash. An oval patch, ¾-2½ in. (2-6 cm) in diameter appears, known as a *herald patch*. This patch resembles those that occur in ringworm *(335)*. About 3 to 10 days later, a number of smaller oval, pink, flat spots, 3/8-3/4 inch (1-2 cm) in diameter, appears. This rash begins on the trunk and spreads across the abdomen, along the thighs and upper arms, and up toward the neck. A scaly margin may appear around the edges of the patches after a week. Occasionally, there is mild itching. Rarely are the feet, hands, and scalp affected.

CAUSES—The cause is not known. But **chemicals in the diet, air, or water** may be the cause. It primarily occurs in young adults.

This rash is not serious and usually clears up after about 6-8 weeks without treatment and is unlikely to reappear.

The reason for noting it here is so that you can identify it. The rash could, instead, be psoriasis *(351)* or eczema *(345)*, both of which are serious.

ENCOURAGEMENT—The promise of sonship to God is made to all who believe on the name of Jesus Christ and, by faith in Him, let Him work His will in their lives. How thankful we can be that God has done so much for us all these years! Trusting in Him daily, our future can be even brighter!

DISCOID LUPUS ERYTHEMATOSUS (DLE)

SYMPTOMS—Itchy, red, scaly patches usually develop on the face, scalp, and behind the ears. Over several years, DLE may subside and recur with different degrees of severity. Occasionally, it can also affect other organs of the body. In some instances, the rash disappears, but leaves behind a scarred area in which the skin is thin and discolored. If it occurs on the scalp, the result may be permanent loss of hair and patchy baldness.

CAUSES—DLE is an autoimmune disorder, most commonly occurring in women between the ages of 25 and 45. The problem tends to run in families. Exposure to **sunlight** tends to trigger the onset of the rash or to make it worse.

In about 1 in 10 afflicted with DLE, systemic lupus erythematosus occurs. This condition affects many parts of the body, including the lungs, kidneys, and joints.

NATURAL REMEDIES

• If this problem has occurred to others in your family, it is best that you **avoid too much direct sunlight**.

• Eat a **nourishing diet** and take **vitamin-mineral supplements**. Physical problems are far less likely to overtake those who are have a healthy lifestyle.

ENCOURAGEMENT—When a soul receives Christ, he receives power to live a life such as Christ lived. God can help him live a good, clean life. Hebrews 4:16.

NEEDLE-STICK INJURY

SYMPTOMS—You accidently punctured your skin with a used hypodermic needle.

CAUSES—Although it may cause little pain or bleeding, **a stick by a used needle** ("used" meaning it previously was used on another person) can be dangerous.

Needle-stick injuries need to be investigated, because of the risk that the needle carries organisms such as HIV, the virus that causes AIDS, or the hepatitis B virus. Such sticks can occur among hospital staff or those who visit public places and find a discarded hypodermic needle. But those who take street drugs are the ones who usually are infected from sticks of used needles. They frequently, and purposely, inject themselves with someone else's needle.

NATURAL REMEDIES

• **Never try to put a needle back in the holder** it originally came out of. Instead, carefully **place all the parts in a designated trash container**.

• If a needle stick occurs, you will want to have **tests** run to see if you have contracted HIV or hepatitis B.

ENCOURAGEMENT—God is our Father, and a tender parent. He loves each of us deeply. No one can care for you as well as your Creator, the One who loved you so much that He sent His Son to die to redeem you.

ERUPTIVE AND SKIN RASH DISEASES
(Symptoms of 23 Diseases)

SYMPTOMS—Eruptive diseases are skin diseases which produce spots, medically known as eruptions. Rash diseases produce rashes on the body. Some diseases develop both rashes and eruptions.

Here is a comparative list of many of these diseases:

SEVEN SKIN DISEASES WHICH PRIMARILY AFFECT CHILDREN:

Chicken pox - Small, round, pimples that form blisters and crust over as they heal. Generally appears first on the trunk, followed 1-2 days later by fever and headache. It then spreads to the face and extremities. Extremely itchy. Primarily on children. —*See Chicken pox (742).*

Measles (Rubeola) - After several days of fever, cough, sneezing, runny nose, and possibly conjunctivitis—a raised red rash generally begins on forehead, neck, and ears. This spreads to rest of body as well. As it spreads, fever usually subsides. Sometimes there are tiny red spots with white centers on the insides of the cheeks. —*See Measles (Rubeola) (744).*

Measles (Rubella) - There is fatigue, coughing, headache, mild fever, muscle aches, and stiffness in the neck. A pink rash often develops 1-5 days later, appearing first on face and neck, and spreading to the rest of the body. —*See German Measles (Rubella) (745).*

Scarlet Fever - Vomiting, sore throat, headache, high fever. On the second day reddened raised points show through a white tongue, especially at the tip and sides. Then rash begins on the chest and extends to other parts of body. —*See Scarlet Fever (745).*

Erysipelas - Redness, discoloration, blisters, and swelling usually on face and accompanied by high fever. Skin is deep red or pink and appears glazed. It itches and burns. There is a definite edge or margin to the affected area. Blisters may develop. Swollen area feels firm and hot. Condition tends to spread in all directions from where it started. Face is usually swollen. Eyes are closed. And lips and ears are thickened and feverish. —*See Erysipelas (352).*

Ringworm - Small, itchy round red spots that grow to about ¼-inch in size, with slightly raised, scaly borders. As they expand, they clear in the center and produce a reddish ring. —*See Ringworm (335).*

Impetigo - Redness in cuts or bruises, followed by blister-like swellings. Fluid is straw-colored. If not scratched, lesions break down in 4-6 days and form a honey-colored crust which heals slowly. Skin beneath may lose color, not to be regained for months. Scratching generally results in more skin injury. —*See Impetigo (349).*

    —*Also see Tonsillitis (740), Adenitis (740), Strep Throat (740), Quinsy (740), Adenoids (742), Mumps (743), Diphtheria (747), Whooping Cough (748), Rheumatic Fever (750), and Reye's Syndrome (750).*

SIXTEEN SKIN DISEASES WHICH PRIMARILY AFFECT ADULTS:

Eczema (Dermatitis) - Patches of scaling, flaking, thickening skin which often itches. Skin color in the affected area may change. Appears anywhere on body.— *See Eczema (345).*

Mononucleosis - A red rash with bumps, plus achiness, headache, sore throat, low fever, and persistent fatigue.
    —*See Mononeucleosis (664).*

Lyme Disease - A red, circular lesion that widens as the center heals. Often followed by a rash of small, raised bumps on the trunk. Flu-like symptoms (chills, fever, nausea) may be present. —*See Lyme Disease (813).*

Candidiasis (fungal infection) - Moist, red patches which may be itchy. Usually where skin surfaces rub together. In babies, it will be an inflamed diaper rash. —*See Candidiasis (281).*

Hives - Rash that suddenly appears and looks like tiny goose-bump patches, spots, or red and itchy welts. They cover sizeable areas of the body. —*See Hives (346).*

Athlete's Foot - Scaling, cracking, and inflamed blisters between the toes of the feet. Often severe itching and burning sensation. —*See Athlete's Foot (377).*

Psoriasis - Silvery, scaly patches usually on the scalp under the hair or on the ears, arms, legs, knees, elbows, and back. But it may appear elsewhere on the body. —*See Psoriasis (351).*

Shingles - Groups of tiny, painful blisters which are sensitive to the touch and eventually crust over, scab, then fall off. Usually on abdomen below ribs, but can occur elsewhere. May be accompanied by achiness, chills, and fever. —*See Shingles (350).*

Rosacea - Small, reddening bumps and pimples, usually on the nose and center of face. Although resembling acne, it is a chronic condition. Usually in people over 40 years of age. —*See Rosacea (339).*

Scabies - Persistent, itchy rash with small, red lumps which may become dry and scaly. Fine, wavy dark lines go outward from some bumps. Usually between fingers, forearms, wrists, breasts, or genitals. —*See Scabies (334).*

Seborrhea - Yellowish, greasy, flaky patches of skin that becomes scaly and forms crusts. Usually on scalp, face, and/or chest, but may appear anywhere. —*See Seborrhea (346).*

Leukoderma (Vitiligo) - Loss of skin color, especially in black or dark-skinned people. White patches, surrounded by a dark border (353).

Keratosis (Sharkskin) - The rough goose bump skin on your elbows, back, arms, thighs, and buttocks. It feels somewhat like sandpaper. —*See Keratosis (353).*

Lupus Vulgaris - Great fatigue and depression; rough, red skin patches; chronic nail fungus; low-grade, chronic fever; rheumatoid arthritis symptoms. —*See Lupus (310).*

Food or Drug Allergy - Generally appears as a reddish or pink, flat rash; sometimes with itching and/ or **swelling.** —*See Allergies (848).*

Poison Ivy / Oak / Sumac - An intensely itchy red rash, with oozing blisters. Sometimes, only a few, tiny, itching spots. Can be spread by itching. —*See Poison Ivy (854).*

ENCOURAGEMENT—All who enter into a covenant with Jesus Christ become by adoption the children of God. Angels of God are commissioned to minister to them and guide them.

SKIN - 7 - MAJOR DERMAL PROBLEMS

MAJOR SKIN DISORDERS

NATURAL REMEDIES

J.H. KELLOGG, M.D., PRESCRIPTIONS FOR MAJOR SKIN DISEASES AND THEIR COMPLICATIONS *(how to give these water therapies: pp. 206-275 / list of treatments: pp. 206-207 / Hydrotherapy Disease Index: pp. 273-275)*

    CHILBLAINS—Alternate Footbath; Revulsive Douche to feet; Alternate Douche; Hot Footbath, followed by Footbath under flowing (cold) water; foot pack.

    BURNS—The **evaporating compress**; the cool irrigating compress (cool, wet cloth over it to reduce heat or sprinkle water over it ["irrigate"] to intensify the cooling effect); if very extensive, the prolonged or continuous **Neutral Bath.**

    ERYTHEMA—Cool **evaporating compress** or irrigating compress (explained just above), **neutral compress.**

    PRURITUS—Prolonged Neutral Bath, copious **water** drinking, large **enema**, daily aseptic **dietary.**

    ERUPTIONS—*If dry*, not irritable, give **prolonged Neutral Bath**. If scaly, **alkaline bath** (soda bath or Oatmeal Bath). *If moist and irritable*, **cool evaporating compress** moistened with soda solution (1 ounce to 1 gallon). *If skin is thickened*, as in chronic eczema, **Hot or Alternate Hot and Cold Compress** or Spray Douche for 10-15 minutes, 3 times a day. *If extensively damaged skin* (as in pemphigus, confluent smallpox, bad burns), the **Continuous Neutral Full Bath** until the skin is healed. [*Author's note:* One of

Jethro Kloss' workers personally told me that when Kloss' son was injured in an automobile accident, he gave him a Continuous Bath of water with goldenseal in it for several days.]

JAUNDICE—Copious **water** drinking, large **Enema** twice daily, **sweating hot bath** for 15 minutes—such as Radiant Heat Bath, Steam Bath, Hot Full Bath, Wet Sheet Pack, followed by prolonged Neutral Bath. Give the sweating bath once daily, or even twice, if he is not too weak. For general tonic effects, apply Cold Mitten Friction or **Cold Towel Rub** twice daily. **Alternate Hot and Cold Compress** over the liver twice daily, with **Heating Compress** over the liver or flannel-covered **Hot Abdominal Pack** during intervals between.

DRY SKIN—**Short sweating bath**, such as Radiant Heat Bath, Steam Bath, hot-air bath, Hot Full Bath, Hot Blanket Pack, Dry Pack, sweating Wet Sheet Pack, followed by a **cold bath** suited to his general condition, and this followed by massage with friction.

HYPERHIDROSIS—**Steam Bath**, sweating Radiant Heat Bath, followed by Revulsive Douche (Spray) to spine, and general Cold Douche.

SWEATING FEET—Revulsive Douche to feet, with extremes in temperature as great as possible; **Alternate Hot and Cold Footbath**; Heating Compress to feet during the night, with Cold Mitten Friction to the feet in the morning on rising.

ENCOURAGEMENT—What greater honor could we have than to be called the children of God? What greater rank could we hold, what greater inheritance could we find, than that which comes to those who are heirs of God and joint heirs with Christ? Titus 3:7.

ECZEMA
(Dermatitis, Atopic Dermatitis)

SYMPTOMS—Dermatitis, also called eczema, is a skin problem indicated by reddened skin; thickening and itching when touched; the formation of dry, patchy scales; and flaking.

CAUSES AND TREATMENT—This skin problem can be caused by a number of things. They are listed below under "Things to Avoid."

Oddly enough, hair loss (alopecia) is commonly associated with dermatitis, especially if a there exists a concurrent unsaturated fatty acid deficiency in the diet.

• If the dermatitis is not terminated, it can so weaken the system, so that more serious infections occur. This is because, at the same time that you are having skin problems, your intestines are developing lesions which can greatly weaken your ability to digest and absorb nutrients!

• It is a fact that 13% of those with severe dermatitis later develop cataracts.

NATURAL REMEDIES

THINGS TO AVOID

• Dermatitis is an inflammatory skin condition that generally keeps reoccurring. Dermatitis is actually an allergy which may be caused by contact with **perfumes, cosmetics, rubber, medicated creams, ointments, poison ivy,** or contact with metal alloys (including nickel, silver, and gold**). Some type of **food** could be the problem. If the irritant continues to be in constant contact with the skin, the dermatitis will spread and get worse. Obviously, if you have this problem you want to solve it! Avoid **dust, industrial chemicals, fumes, sprays, paints, cutting oils, varnishes, and solvents**.

• Avoid **cleansers, cosmetics, body oils, and lotions that contain lanolin, benzocaine, or antihistamines**. It causes allergies, plugs up oil glands, and causes dermatitis and acne. Do not wear **rubber gloves** for household chores. Your skin will absorb some of the chemicals in them.

• Do not use **petroleum jelly** and other **greasy ointments**. They prevent sweating and intensify the itching. Avoid **scratching**. It only makes the problem worse.

• The condition can be intensified by **emotional stress, tension, and fatigue**. Avoid **colds and respiratory infections**. They lower body resistance and intensify eczema. Avoid people with **cold sores** because the virus in them can cause serious skin eruptions, if you have dermatitis.

• Here are some of the allergies which the experts have found to especially cause dermatitis: **Cow's milk**. Either stop drinking cow's milk or try switching to goat's milk. **Wheat gluten** (wheat protein). There are other grains you can eat instead. **Nickel**. The experts call this "nickel rash." Women who have their ears pierced and the nickel post placed in them can produce various rashes on the body—especially where any other metal jewelry touches the skin. By the way, any gold jewelry less than 24-karats has some nickel in it.

• Beware of **bubble bath** and similar **soapy tub baths**. Never take a **bath in hot water**. **Pat yourself dry** after bathing. Do not rub.

• **Children's rashes**: A skin rash in children may be caused by eating **eggs, peanuts, milk, wheat, fish, chicken, pork, or beef**. Eggs, peanuts, and milk account for 75 percent of the skin rashes in children.

• Regardless of what may be the cause, omit **wheat, rye, oats, and barley** for six weeks. Then slowly add one back at a time—and see how all this effects the dermatitis.

• If you know how to do so, you may wish to do a *pulse test* after each meal, in an attempt to ascertain which foods increase heartbeat. Those which do are the problematic ones. —*See "Pulse Test" (847).*

• Avoid **dairy products, white flour, fried foods, other processed fats,** and sugar. Avoid **antiperspirants**, for they have metal in them. Use **cotton undergarments**. **Fake fingernails** cause skin rashes. Always use **white bathroom tissue** only. Those with dyes irritate the skin. Be sure and **rinse the soap out of your clothes** which have just been washed. Reduce **sugar and salt** intake.

• **Cow's milk** allergy is the most common cause of dermatitis in infancy. The milk can be taken by the infant or the mother breast-feeding it. Do not eat foods containing **raw eggs**. They contain *avidin*, a protein which binds with biotin and keeps the body from absorbing and using it to heal skin problems.

THINGS TO DO

• Deficiency of any of the **B complex vitamins** can cause dermatitis. Another important item is **unsaturated fatty acids** (1-2 Tbsp. **flaxseed oil** daily is the best). If you are not getting enough, you can begin itching wherever you rub on your skin. Adequate **vitamin A** and enough **protein** are also essential. A deficiency of **selenium** is another definite cause.

• **Antioxidants** help damaged skin heal. The best ones for skin are **beta-carotene** (carrot juice of 12-18 mg daily), **vitamin C** (3,000 mg daily), **vitamin E** (600-800 mg daily), and **zinc** (20-30 mg daily).

• If you want to feel good, soak in an **oatmeal bath**. Add 2 cups of oatmeal to a tub of lukewarm water. Stay in 20 minutes and you will feel fine when you get out! Do not slip in the tub!

• Instead of soap, put **oatmeal in a cloth** and tie the ends. Dip it in water and wash yourself clean.

• Both winter and summer, keep the **relative humidity** above 40%. Eliminate fuzzy and rough clothing. Wear soft, loose cotton clothes. Get rid of feather pillows, furry and fuzzy toys, and long-haired dogs and cats. Get regular exercise.

• Research studies have found the following herbs to be outstanding for treating eczema: **Chamomile, ginkgo biloba, licorice root, and witch hazel**.

• Mix **goldenseal** root powder with **vitamin E oil** and put some on the affected area. This will reduce the itching.

• **Primrose oil** and **vitamin B6** (pyridoxine) have helped infants with dermatitis.

• Some people with eczema have **fatty acid imbalances**. They need more of the **omega-3** fatty acids (the kind found in **flaxseed**) and more of an **omega-6** fatty acid (found in **borage, black currant, and evening primrose seeds**). Some studies—not all—have found that medicinal oils rich in gamma-linolenic acid (omega-3), such as **evening primrose oil**, help reduce eczema. One suggested dose for evening primrose oil is 3,000 mg in capsules per day. **Flaxseed oil** contains alpha-linolenic acid, which the body can convert to omega-3 fatty acid.

• An **oatmeal bath** is another helpful measure, to reduce the itching during the time required to solve the underlying cause. Use 2 cups of colloidal (powdered) oatmeal per tubful. Colloidal oatmeal can be obtained at a pharmacy. Do not slip in the tub!

• Herbs that may help include **comfrey, dandelion, red clover, pau d'arco, plantain, chickweed, burdock root, yarrow, and strawberry leaves**. One can either drink the tea made from any of them or apply it to the affected area.

• Steep a Tbsp. each of **burdock root, yarrow, and yellow dock** root in a pint of boiling water for half an hour. Strain, add a pound of **cocoa fat**, and keep boiling and stirring until it is a salve. Use this for eczema.

• **Sunlight** often helps clear up eczema. To reduce the risk of sunburn, either keep sun exposure short or wear a hypoallergenic sunblock. Go indoors if you start to feel hot and sweaty, which can aggravate itching.

—See Seborrhea (below), Drug Rash (877), and Skin Diseases (314-355).

ENCOURAGEMENT—Christ, having redeemed man from the condemnation of the law, could now enable man to fulfill its requirements. Rejoice that, in Christ, you can stand an overcomer over the temptations which have oppressed you. Psalm 30:5.

SEBORRHEA
(Seborrheic Dermatitis)

SYMPTOMS—Scaly patches of skin most often on the scalp, face, and chest. But these can appear elsewhere. It may or may not be itchy and consist of small bumbs or patches. The affected area may be yellowish and/or greasy, or dry and flaky. Although it can occur at any age, it is most common in infancy (cradle cap) and middle age.

CAUSES—This is a disorder of the oil-secreting (sebaceous) glands of the skin. Causes include **stress and anxiety, nutritional deficiencies (especially vitamin A and biotin), heredity, hot weather, oily skin, acne, rosacea, psoriasis, Parkinson's disease, and AIDS**.

NATURAL REMEDIES

• An **oatmeal bath** is excellent. *See Eczema (above) for how to prepare it.*

• Primarily eat **raw, fresh foods** and **avoid diary products, white flour, chocolate, seafood**, and anything with **sugar** or **raw eggs** in it. **Fast** a day or two each month. Take **vitamins A, C**, and **B-complex**. Eat a **gluten-free** diet.

• Do not use commercial seborrhea **ointments**, irritating **soaps**, or chemical **hair shampoos** (which most are). **Colloidal silver** is useful in reducing seborrhea.

• **Do not squeeze or pick** at your skin.
—See Eczema (345).

ENCOURAGEMENT—By repentance toward God and faith in Jesus Christ, the fallen sons of Adam may become sons of God.

HIVES
(Urticaria)

SYMPTOMS—Strong itching (pruritus) may suddenly occur. Elevated wheals (itchy red skin welts with whitish centers) result, along with swollen eyes. The subsequent scratching makes you appear swollen and scratchy. The intense itchy wheals which may result may disappear in minutes, hours, or several days.

CAUSES—Also known as hives, urticaria is an intensely itchy rash that may affect the whole body or just a small area of skin. Although it usually lasts only a few hours, chronic urticaria can last for sever months.

Both acute and chronic forms can recur.

Sometimes it occurs at the same time as **angio-edema**, which is swelling of body tissues, usually about the face and generally due to an allergic reaction. This can be life-threatening. *See your physician.*

But urticaria can also be an early symptom of **anaphylaxis** *(846)*, which is a severe and potentially fatal allergic reaction to a substance. *See a physician.*

One cause is contact with the **nettle plant**, which pricks a poison into the skin. *(See Nettle Rash, 830).* But more often, the cause is some other allergic substance which may include: **wheat, milk, eggs, chocolate, nuts**, and other food allergens. It may be due to a **drug allergy**. Or it may develop after an **insect bite or sting**.

The first time it occurs in an adult, it is often difficult to identify the cause. It is less common in elderly people and sometimes runs in families.

The acute form of urticaria usually disappears without treatment within a few hours.

The skin is reacting to **allergies, physical irritation, stress, or emotions**. Special dermal cells begin releasing histamine, which causes internal blood vessels to leak fluid into the deepest layers of the skin.

Meat, dairy, and poultry products (especially in frozen or fast foods) are frequent causes of hives. This is due to the chemicals, antibiotics, and hormones given to farm animals.

Some 15%-20% of Americans experience hives at some point in their lives, generally as young adults.

Touching the leaves of the stinging nettle plant can also produce a temporary rash. *See Nettle Rash (830).*

It is important that you try to **identify the cause** of the attack, so you can henceforth avoid it.

• A person need never get hives if the body is in good condition and the bloodstream is clear, free, and clean. Hives can come from the sting of an insect. This irritates the system and causes it to throw off poisons rapidly in the form of large welts. Sometimes hives will be as large as the palm of the hand and swell up with considerable puffiness. In some cases, a person will eat certain combinations of food and come down with hives after exercise. This cuts the poison loose from the body and brings it to the surface. Hives can be so intense that the eyes will close and swell the tissue over the entire body. This is caused by an acid condition.

SUBSTANCES WHICH PRODUCE HIVES IN SOME PEOPLE

Animals, especially animal dander and dog saliva.
Aspirin.
Allopurinol (Zyloprim), a gout medication.
Antimony, a metallic element that is present in various metal alloys.
Antipyrine, an agent used to relieve pain and inflamma-tion.
Barbiturates.
BHA and BHT, preservatives used in many food products.
Chloral hydrate, a sedative used in the treatment of tetany. *Chlorpromazine* (Thorazine), a tranquilizer and antiemetic. *Cologne or perfume.*
Corticotropin (also known as adrenocorticotropic hor-mone, or ACTH, and sold for medicinal purposes under the brand names Acthar and Cortrosyn).
Environmental factors, especially heat, cold, water, and sunlight.
Eucalyptus, a tree whose leaves yield an aromatic oil that is used in cough remedies and other medicines.
Exercise.
Fluorides, which are found in certain dental care prod-ucts and in fluoridated drinking water.
Food allergies, especially allergies to shellfish, eggs, fruits, and various nuts.

Food colorings and preservatives. Gold.
Griseofulvin (Fulvicin, Grisactin, and others), an anti-fungal medication.
Hyperthyroidism.
Infections, especially strep infections, hepatitis, and para-sites.
Insect bites.
Insulin.
Iodines, used in certain antiseptics and dyes. *Liver extract.*
Makeup.
Menthol, an extract of peppermint oil used in perfumes, as a mild anesthetic, and as a mint flavoring in candy and cigarettes.
Meprobamate (Miltown, Equanil, Meprospan), a tranquilizer.
Mercury, a toxic metallic element found in dental fillings, certain antacids, and some first-aid preparations, among other things.
Morphine.
Opium.
Para-aminosalicylic acid, an anti-inflammatory drug. *Penicillin.*
Phenacetin, an ingredient in some pain medications. *Phenobarbital*, a sedative and anticonvulsant. *Pilocarpine*, a glaucoma medication.
Plants.
Poliomyelitis vaccine.

NATURAL REMEDIES

IMMEDIATE HELP

• Any alkaline substance generally helps the itching. Place a **calcium gluconate** paste on the skin or apply **milk, calamine, or milk of magnesia**.

• An **oatmeal** or **bran bath** will help relieve the itching. Place 2 pounds of ether in a muslin bag and sit in a hot bath (104°-106° F.). Do not slip in the tub!

• A paste of **cream of tartar** and **water** can be applied to the area.

• **Cold compresses or cool baths** will immediately help also.

• Rubbing **wheat germ oil** onto the area is a great help. Use **elder leaf tea** or **chickweed,** as a wash, and chickweed or elder ointment to heal the condition. Quick relief can be obtained by drinking **celery seed, comfrey, chickweed, burdock root or seed**, etc. **Burdock seed** is one of the most potent to relieve the skin and lymph areas rapidly. A half-pound to a pound of **ginger** in a tub of hot water will help give relief. The bowels must be cleared; since the worse cases of hives can come from constipation. The mucusless diet is the most important thing for rashes and hives.

LONGER TERM SOLUTIONS

Try to find the cause or causes of this problem and remove them from your diet and environment.

• *Here are some of the things which result in hives in others:* **Stress**, food allergy (**milk, wheat, eggs, peanuts, shellfish, pork, onions, chocolate, some fruits**), **chlorine** in drinking water, adrenal exhaustion and/or liver congestion resulting from an **allergy, hydrochloric acid deficiency, food dyes, preservatives, spices, flavoring, coloring agents, drug allergy, acid conditions, insect stings, chronic infection, penicillin in the milk you drink, aspirin, coffee, alcohol, and tobacco.**

• *Here are more things known to cause hives in some people:* **Aspirin, antimony,** or **bismuth** (in various metal alloys), antipyrine or phenacetin (**pain relievers**), **barbiturates**, BHA and BHT (**preservatives**), phenobarbital or chloral hydrate (**sedatives**), chlorpromazine and meprobamate (**tranquilizers**), **fluoride** (dental products and fluoridated drinking water), **food colorings**, griseofulvin (antifungal), **insulin, liver extract, menthol** (in perfumes, candy, cigarettes), **mercury** (dental fillings), **morphine, penicillin,** pilocarpine (**glaucoma medication**), **preservatives**, procaine (anesthetic, known as **novocaine**), **quinine,** (**quinine** water and malaria medication), **reserpine** (heart medication), **sulfites** (food preservatives, especially in dried fruit), **tartrazine** (food dye and in Alka-Seltzer), **saccharin** (artificial sweetener), **salicylates** (flavoring and preservative), thiamine hydrochloride (**cough medications**), **animal dander, dog saliva, barbiturates, cancer, eucalyptus leaves, hyperthyroidism, insulin, iodines** (in antiseptics and dyes), **cosmetics, tranquilizers,** and **phenacetin** (pain

medication).

• Secondary factors will be **spinal lesions, stoppage of lymph flow, imbalance between deep and surface blood circulation, and adrenal exhaustion**.

• **Insect bites** may induce hives in sensitive children.

• Another factor is **too hurriedly weaning a child** from breast milk. Yet another cause is **sun-induced** hives. They strike 30 minutes after being out in the sun.

Reading over the above lists, it appears that the primary cause is frequently a physical reaction to a substance which the body cannot tolerate being put into it. *We live in a chemical age.* One cannot even drive down the highway without breathing dangerous fumes.

• Do not use **steroids, alcohol, or processed foods**.

• Lymph stasis and poor circulation may result from **poor skin function, lack of exercise, fresh air, and poor elimination**. But ingesting poisonous substances top the list.

TO STOP RECURRENT HIVES

• Aside from trying to find the chemical offenders, **prolonged fasting** is generally considered the best method of terminating recurrent hives. This cleans out the body and enables it to better deal with the chemicals it is daily confronted with. Fasting will help the intestines and other organs to heal. It will eliminate toxins and help the bowels begin working properly again. Trunk packs will help induce sweating. Moderate sunbaths will help also.

• As a rule, each fast should not be over 1-3 days in length. If you are overweight, longer fasts might be considered. If you are thin, never go over 3 days; indeed, one meal or one-day fasts are best for frail individuals. A **carrot, beet, and green vegetable juice fast** is better than a straight water fast.

• Use **enemas** during the fast, and even afterward, until the hives do not return. **Maintain good bowel action** thereafter.

• Also important are **dietary changes**. Be sure to get nutritional supplements, including **vitamins A, B complex, B_6, B_{12}, C, and calcium**. You may need to take **hydrochloric acid** with meals. Massive amounts of **vitamin C** (2,000 mg every 4 hours) stop it in many people. Take 500 mg of **quercetin** twice a day. It has good anti-histamine activity.

• There is one other important, possible cause: a lack of **unsaturated fatty acids**. The best is **flaxseed oil or wheat germ oil**. In addition to including only such oils in your diet, you would do well to rub wheat germ oil on the affected area.

• When the problem exists for weeks or months, it is vital that you **identify the cause**, so you can eliminate the hives.

• Chronic hives can be linked to **candida**.

When severe anaphylactic reactions occur, immediately take the person to the hospital. It is best not to let situations come to such a crisis. Solve the problem before hives produces such an emergency.

OTHER SUGGESTIONS

• Take a **hot shower,** as hot as you can take. It releases anti-histamines which attack the surface hives.

• **Jewelweed** is excellent. It contains *lawsone*, which has anti-hive activity. Make a tea of it and apply it to the affected area.

• The following herbs have good anti-histamine activity: **Chamomile, wild oregano, rue, parsley, basil, echinacea, fennel, yarrow.**

• Simmer ½ pound of **ginger** in a gallon of water for 5 minutes. Pour into a hot bath. After the bath, sponge off with **chamomile** tea. It works well for some people.

• Drink **burdock** seed tea as a diaphoretic to open skin pores from the inside. Also wash the affected areas with a strong decoction of the tea 2-3 times a day. Apply **chickweed** ointment. Take a chickweed bath.

• To draw out toxins from the skin, take a hot bath with 1 pound of **baking soda or Epsom salts** added to the water.

• Other helps include applying **aloe vera gel** to the area and wearing **loose-fitting clothing.** The problem may be linked to **candida.**

• While hot baths draw out the poisons, **cool baths** are soothing. Take a cool shower at the first sign of hives.

—*Also see Nettle Rash (830).*

ENCOURAGEMENT—In the work of redemption, God has revealed His love in sacrifice, a sacrifice so broad and deep and high that it is immeasurable. For God so loved the world, that He gave His only begotten Son—that you and I could have eternal life!

DRUG-INDUCED RASHES

SYMPTOMS—Many different types of skin rashes. Some mimic other disorders, such as lichen planus or erythema multiforme *(342).* But most appear as raised areas of skin spread widely over the body. They may cause intense itching. Sometimes wheezing occurs. Or the person collapses and is taken to the hospital.

CAUSES—**Medicinal drugs** frequently cause rashes to appear on the body. The body wants to quickly get rid of poisonous substances in the drugs. So, in some cases, they are pushed out through the skin. In other instances, they are excreted in the kidneys, sometimes causing kidney damage in the process.

The drugs most often producing the rashes are the **antibiotics,** such as **penicillin.** Drug-induced rashes usually begin within a few days after the drug is first given, but sometimes do not occur until after drug treatments have ended. The rash may not leave until weeks after the drug is discontinued.

NATURAL REMEDIES

• If you develop a rash immediately after taking a drug, your physician is likely to advise that you **stop taking that drug** immediately. It is possible that two or more medicinal drugs are being taken at the same time or a "recreational" drug is also being taken.

• Notify future physicians about your problem with certain drugs. In instances, where a drug caused serious physical problems, you may wish to wear a medical alert drug tag.

—*See Erythema Multiforme (342).*

ENCOURAGEMENT—If God, the divine Artist, gives to the simple flowers that perish in a day their delicate and varied colors, how much greater care will He have for those who are created in His own image?

IMPETIGO
(Impetigo Contagiosa, Echthyma)

SYMPTOMS AND CAUSES—Cuts, abrasions, insect bites, and stings allow entry of the bacteria. An area of redness is seen, followed by blister-like swellings. The fluid is straw-colored. If not scratched, the lesions break down in 4-6 days and form a honey-colored crust which heals slowly. The skin beneath may lose its color and remain pale for months. The scratching generally results in more skin injury and a spread of the infection. It is more frequently found on the face, hands, arms next, and feet and legs third.

Impetigo is a skin disease caused by a streptococcal bacteria. It occurs primarily in children (especially ages 2-8, especially in **undernourished** ones), and in the summer months. Lower economic groups living in **crowded conditions** are the most likely to contract it. Impetigo is not something to ignore. Neglected, it can produce boils, ulcers, or other skin complications. Untreated, it can result in deep infections of the tissue beneath the skin.

NATURAL REMEDIES

• Impetigo is actually an early sign of immune depression, which allows organisms normally on everyone's skin to produce disease. The body's **immune system needs to be strengthened.**

• **Proper nutrition** is needed, along with **sanitary living conditions**.

• In some individuals, a **food allergy** (such as **milk, wheat,** or **soy**) or a **contact dermatitis** (such as **detergents** in the clothes) weakens the immune system—permitting the impetigo to gain a foothold.

• Strict **sanitary hygiene** is necessary to prevent the spread of the infection to other parts of the body—or to other people.

• **Vitamin A** is necessary for good skin health. Give the child a good **multivitamin supplement**. Give **vitamin C,** to bowel tolerance.

• Put a wash of **boric acid** and herbs such as **comfrey, golden seal, or echinacea** on the affected area.

• Place **garlic oil,** squeezed from capsules, on the area.

• **Bathing in soapy water** every 4 hours during the day is helpful. Severe cases may require a slightly **salty or hydrogen peroxide application** (3 parts water to 1 part 3% peroxide). Apply soaks or **warm compresses** to the attached crusts.

• *Removal of the crusts* results in a more rapid cure. Stubborn scabs may require a solution of 1 tsp. **bleach** to 1 quart water to loosen them. A small amount of **dishwashing detergent**, added to the bleach solution, will improve penetration of the solution.

• *After removing the crusts*, apply hot and cold compresses: **Hot compresses** (110°-115° F.) for 3 minutes, alternating with **cold compresses** wrung from ice water for 30 seconds, with 5 changes in each treatment. Do not burn the child. At night, **charcoal poultices** can be attached and left overnight.

• Use **disposable tissues** instead of cloth handkerchiefs. Each person should be given **his own towel and washcloth**. **Wash the hands** frequently. While the infection lasts, keep the **fingernails short and clean**. **Change pillowcases and bed sheet**s daily, and **boil all linens** for 10 minutes. If possible, **isolate the child**.

• Exposure to the **air** and **sunlight** will help, but **do not swim**.

• If impetigo is on the scalp, **cut the hair** so you can treat it.

—*Also see Skin Diseases (314-355).*

ENCOURAGEMENT—God gave His Son to become bone of our bone and flesh of our flesh. The gift of God to man is beyond all computation. Nothing was withheld. God has done, and is doing, everything possible to save us from sin. Psalm 34:19.

SHINGLES
(Herpes Zoster)

SYMPTOMS—Sharp, burning pain along a nerve route somewhere in your body for 3-4 days. There are angry red blisters at that pain site several days later. These are very painful and itchy. Later the bumps blister, turn cloudy, and form scabs. It usually lasts 7-14 days from the time the blisters appear before the scabs drop off. This is no ordinary rash. It is shingles, which is a viral infection of a nerve. It most often occurs on the skin of the abdomen, under the ribs, and above the navel. But it can appear anywhere on the body. It most frequently occurs after the age of 50.

If shingles starts near an eye, beware! The cornea can become infected and blindness may result. You would then do well to consult an eye specialist.

CAUSES—This infection consists of small, round clusters of the same virus which causes chicken pox *(742)* in childhood. But, in adulthood, it causes the far more dangerous condition known as shingles.

What triggers the attack? It is known that **poisonous substances in food, metals, drugs, and other toxic substances** can do it. For example, risk of shingles increases with the use of **anti-cancer drugs**. **Anything that weakens the immune system** can bring on an attack of shingles. Once it occurs, the pain can continue on for months or years. So it is better to prevent an attack.

NATURAL REMEDIES

• Massive doses of **vitamins C** (1,000 mg, 3 times a day, and 200 mg, 5-6 times a day), **rutin**, and **B complex**. In addition, take **vitamin F, calcium, and lecithin**. The amino acid, **lysine**, can help inhibit the spread of the herpes virus. The diet must include **raw fruits and vegetables, brewer's yeast, brown rice, and whole grains**. Be sure and eat enough **protein (legumes and nuts)**.

• Place one or more of the following on them: **tea tree oil with plaintain, calamine**, or other calcium preparation on them. **Calcium** is always soothing to skin rash conditions. Apply **vitamin E oil** from a capsule to the area. Take 500 mg of **lysine** 2 times daily.

• Put **cold water** on a cloth and place it over the area. The cooler it is, the better it feels. Avoid anything that will make your blistered skin hotter.

• Put apple cider **vinegar** on it daily. Take **hot baths** 2-3 times a week. Take a **starch bath** (one cup of cornstarch or colloidal **oatmeal** into a hot tub). Colloidal oatmeal is powdered and can be obtained at the pharmacy. Do not slip in the tub!

• Clean out the **bowels** frequently. **Light fruit and vegetable fasts** will also help clean out and strengthen the body. Wear only **cotton clothing** while the condition exists.

• Dab the infection with **hydrogen peroxide**, to purify it. If pain exists after the blisters are gone, put **ice** on the area.

• Applying **cayenne** blocks pain signals from nerves just under the skin. It works so well, the FDA has approved commercial creams containing it.

• Applied **licorice** eliminates pain and inflammation within 3 days in some people. Drink a weak tea and apply a strong tea directly to the rash.

• If you have access to fresh leaves of lemon balm or flowering tops of St. John's wort, double the quantities of them in this recipe. (Flowering tops are the flowers in bloom, plus about 3 to 5 inches of the stem.): 2 cups **aloe vera gel**, ½ cup lemon balm leaves, ½ cup **St. John's wort** flowering tops, one-eighth cup cut dried **licorice root**, 2 tablespoons **cayenne** or **turmeric**, 8 drops of **bergamot**, **lemon**, **tea tree**, or **lavender** essential oil.

Blend the first five ingredients in a quart-sized jar. Let this mixture sit for 24 hours at room temperature. Strain through a tightly woven cloth into a clean jar. Add the essential oil and cap tightly. Store in the refrigerator.

Apply to a test patch of normal skin. If it burns on contact, add more aloe vera gel. If it doesn't, you can try blending in a bit more cayenne. Apply to the rash three to five times per day as needed.

After applying the gel, be sure to wash your hands with soap to avoid spreading the compounds that burn.

For most people with shingles, cayenne may be too irritating to apply during the blister phase. In addition, some people with pain that lingers after the shingles rash has healed find that cayenne burns too much. If this is true for you, you can still use this gel, but omit the cayenne.

•Olive leaf extract powerfully heals shingles. Produced by Olivus in California, it consists of ground-up, concentrated **olive leaves (Oea europaea).** (*olivus.us*, 888-654-8871) It is available as a tea, as a capsule, or as an extract (OliveLeafMAX), which is the most powerful of all. Twice a day, take 1-2 capsules of **OliveLeafMAX** with 5,000 mg. **vitamin C** powder. Obtain plenty of **water and rest.**

Another firm is *naturallyguaranteed.com/shingles. html.* It offers a product called, **"Heal Shingles",** to be applied topically.

• **Avoid drafts**. Allow **sunlight** on the area for short intervals. **When bathing**, gently wash the blisters and avoid touching or scratching them.

• *Warning:* If the shingles appear on the forehead, tip of the nose, or near the eyes, contact an ophthalmologist. Such cases can lead to blindness.

—*Also see Skin Diseases (314-355).*

ENCOURAGEMENT—As John thought of the love of Christ, he was led to exclaim, "Behold, what manner of love the Father hath bestowed upon us, that we should be called the sons of God." Oh, may we praise Him everyday for the overcoming strength He imparts, so we can resist temptation and fulfill His will. Psalm 34:6, 15, 17.

PSORIASIS

SYMPTOMS—It appears like patches of silvery scales or red areas and is found on the scalp, arms, legs, knees, elbows, ears, and back. There are cycles of flare-ups and remission. It especially occurs in winter months, but sometimes it disappears for months or years. In some, aging makes it better; in others, worse. It is most common between 15 and 25. And it is not infectious. It affects the white race more than any other.

CAUSES—The skin cells seem to run out of control. Instead of skin renewing itself in 28-30 days, the new cells reach the top layer in 3 days. This produces raised areas of skin, called plaques, which are red and often itchy. Cells normally rise and die. But, because so many cells are doing this, they have a raised, silvery, patchy appearance.

Psoriasis may be linked to **faulty fat utilization**. Attacks are related to times of **stress, illness, surgery, cuts, certain viral and bacterial infections, sunburn, poison ivy, or poison oak**. The **drugs such as chloro-**quine, lithium, and beta-blockers also cause it to flare up. Do not use **steroids, alcohol, or processed foods**. There may be a **hereditary factor** involved. Previous **immunizations** seem to be a causative factor for some people. The various medicinal drugs recommended for psoriasis all have potentially dangerous side effects.

There is no certainty that one can totally eliminate psoriasis. Do not spend time worrying over the matter. For the resultant stress may only aggravate it.

NATURAL REMEDIES
• An increased intake of **animal protein** can make it spread outward. Conversely, a reduction tends to shrink it. Consider becoming a vegetarian. **Citrus juices** may also be a problem.

• Since psoriasis is a metabolic disease, a cleansing **juice fast**, 2-3 times for the first week, is a good way to begin working toward its recession. Four weeks later, the fast can be carried out again. But in the meantime, an extremely **nourishing diet** should have been started. All **junk food** should have been discarded. Search out and eliminate **allergy foods**. Beware of **milk and wheat**. It may be well to exclude them for 6 months. Eat a diet of 50% **raw food**, with plenty of **fruits and vegetables**. Eat **whole grains, nuts, and legumes**.

• **Avoid fats (butter, milk, cream, eggs, meat), processed food, white flour, sugar, and citrus fruit. Milk, cheese, eggs, meat, and poultry** contain arachidonic acid, which causes psoriatic lesions to turn red and swell. **Primrose oil** (1 capsule 3 times daily) helps counteract arachidonic acid. Get your food oils from natural foods, such as **flaxseed, sesame seed, and soybeans**. **Flaxseed oil** contains a chemical which tends to reduce psoriasis. Take 3-4 Tbsp. **lecithin** granules each day for 2 months. Then reduce dosage by one-half.

• **Vitamins A, B complex, C, and D** all help the skin and appear to be of help in reducing psoriasis. **Calcium, magnesium, and zinc** are also important.

• Only the scales and skin debris can be removed. Because psoriatic skin is dry, it is well to **put petroleum jelly or vegetable oil on the area**.

• **Lose weight** if you are overweight. Weight loss helps many who have psoriasis.

• Heavy stress can make it worse. Try to retain a **calm, cheerful outlook** on life. Existing psoriasis tends to get worse when you come down with some other **infection**.

• Exposure to **sunlight or ultraviolet light** reduces the scaling and redness. With regular amounts of intense sunlight, 95% of psoriasis sufferers improve. But keep in mind that too much ultraviolet light also produces skin cancer. Sunlight definitely helps many.

• You may wish to consider moving to a **warmer climate**, since the problem becomes much worse in the winter. If you live in a colder climate, maintain higher humidity in the house during the winter.

• **Swimming in the ocean** is good for reducing psoriasis. Bathing in **heated baths** is also helpful, but it also tends to increase the itching. Put **seawater**, several times a day, on the area. Regular **ocean bathing combined with sunlight** heavily reduces psoriasis. (Substitute: 1-4 pounds of **sea salt** (from health-food store) dissolved in bathwater. If you have a second bathtub, you might wish to leave the water in there and bathe in it repeatedly (if you have a way to warm it).

• A **cream containing capsicum** (the active ingredient in cayenne) reduces both scaling and redness. But that causes some burning, stinging, and itching. The chemical relieves pain by acting on sensory nerves. There may be a burning sensation for the first several times it is applied, but this will lessen.

• Apply **vitamin D₃ cream** for good results.

• A combination of **milk thistle seed, dandelion root, oregon grape root, yellow dock and garlic** (combined in a tea) generally eliminates psoriasis within 1-3 months.

• **Angelica** contains *psoralens*, which fight psoriasis. Make a tea and drink it. Food plants containing *psoralens* include **carrots, celery, figs, fennel, and parsnips**.

• Rub mashed **avocado** on psoriasis patches. It is cool and soothing. In Europe, **Chamomile** is used to treat psoriasis, eczema, skin that is dry and flaky. Apply it externally. (But this herb is in the ragweed family, so it might cause a reaction in you.)

• **Licorice** contains *glycyrrhetenic acid*, which works better than *hydrocortisone* in treating psoriasis and eczema. Apply it directly to the affected area. **Sarsaparilla** contains *saponins* which bind to endotoxins and improve psoriasis. Take as a tea and apply to area.

• To relieve itching, toss a few handfuls of **oatmeal** in a warm bath or tie it into cheesecloth, to prevent the sticky oatmeal from clogging the drain.

• Make a strong decoction of 8 oz. each of **garlic juice** and **glycerine**, and 1 pint **burdock seeds**. Mix together, saturate a cotton cloth and place over area, cover with plastic and secure with adhesive tape. Change 2-3 times daily. Also drink 1 tsp. 3-4 times daily till psoriasis is gone.

John Pagano, D.C., has spent 30 years successfully helping people eliminate psoriasis. He says it is caused by leaky gut syndrome, allowing toxic materials to pass through an acid bowel wall. *Here is his formula:*

Drink 6-8 8-oz. glasses of **water** daily. Twice a day, eat **stewed figs, apples, raisins, apricots, pears, peaches, or prunes**. This will help clean the bowels. **Exercise** fairly vigorously outdoors 30-40 minutes a day. Rub **castor oil** on thick skin lesions, and apply a mixture of **olive oil** and **peanut oil** on thinner ones. Stop using all **antiperspirants**, because they block normal elimination through sweat glands.

By this time, an increased amount of toxins will be thrown off, causing increased burning and itching. Take a **lukewarm bath** containing 1 cup **apple cider vinegar** (if your skin is not cracked from scratching), 2/3 cup **rolled oats**, and 1/3 cup **cornstarch**. You might also add 1 pound **baking soda**. Bathe in this 15-20 minutes a day, to wonderfully soothe the nerve endings.

The diet should be 70%-80% **fruits and vegetables**, including many **leafy greens**. The high fiber content will greatly help the bowel. Eat **no meat, shellfish, butter, margarine, or hydrogenated fats** (in most processed foods). Do not eat anything in the nightshade family (**tomatoes, white potatoes, eggplant, peppers, paprika, tobacco**). This includes no **ketchup, pizza**, etc. Also no **processed, pickled, smoked, fried, or junk foods**. No **processed foods with coconut oil or palm oil**. No **excess sweets, candies, pastries, or pies**. Take 4-6 tsp. flaxseed oil daily. The *omega-3* in it helps heal the bowel.

Coat the inner lining of the bowel with **slippery elm**, promoting its healing. Take 1 Tbsp. granular **lecithin** 3 times daily, 5 days a week.

Add ½ tsp. **slippery elm** powder to 1 cup warm water, let stand 15 minutes, stir and drink. Do not eat for the next 30 minutes. Drink this for the first 10 days of the program, then every other day until the psoriasis clears. **American yellow saffron** also help heal the bowel wall, as it flushes toxins from the kidneys and liver. Add boiling water to cup containing ¼ tsp. saffron and let stand 15 minutes. Drink it 5 days a week until psoriasis clears. Stop using it if you have excessive urination or bladder irritation.

—*Also see Skin Diseases (314-355).*

ENCOURAGEMENT—What greater privilege could be ours than to enter the family of God. Trust God and, by the enabling grace of Christ, obey His Ten Commandment law, even though many around you may despise it. Proverbs 29:25.

ERYSIPELAS

SYMPTOMS—Redness, discoloration, blisters, and swelling that most commonly attack the face, and accompanied by high fever and other indications of acute illness. The skin is deep red or pink and appears glazed. It has a combined itching and burning sensation. There is a definite edge or margin to the affected area. Blisters may develop. The swollen area feels firm and hot. The condition tends to spread in all directions from where it first began. Even in cases moderately severe, generally the face is swollen. Eyes are closed. And the lips and ears are thickened and feverish.

CAUSES—Erysipelas is serious. And, in babies, the aged, and women who have recently given birth, it may prove fatal. It is likely to cause abortion in pregnant women. This is obviously a very serious condition.

NATURAL REMEDIES

IMMEDIATELY

You will want to contact a physician. If you have contacted a physician, apply **ice bags or ice-cold compresses** (20 minutes on and 10 minutes off) to the affected area until he arrives. Cold compresses to the head help reduce the headaches.

OTHER HELPS

• Go on a thorough cleansing program, with **fruit and vegetable juice fasting**, followed by a careful **nutritious diet**.

• In addition to the liquid diet, he must drink at least 3 quarts of **water** everyday.

• **Avoid constipation**. When eating, there should be 3 bowel movements a day, or use an **enema**.

• Do not wash with soap and water. Only use a saturated solution of **boric acid**.

• Helpful herbs include **plantain, yellow dock, chickweed, burdock root, chamomile, mullein, and yarrow**. Dissolve herbs in a quart of boiling water. Dip a cloth in cool water and lightly touch the affected areas. Do not wipe the skin. **Chickweed** tea is excellent for this purpose. Add 1 Tbsp. per pint of boiling water.

• Another good wash is equal parts **gum myrrh, echinacea, witch hazel, and goldenseal**. Mix and use 1 Tbsp. to 1 pint boiling water, steep ½ hour, strain, apply with cotton.

• A **raw cranberry poultice**, applied cold, will help remove the burning. Dilute **lemon juice** 50-50 with water and apply gently.

• Cover the area with **grated potatoes**, about a fourth inch thick. When dry, remove, and do it again.
—*Also Skin Diseases (314-355).*

J.H. KELLOGG, M.D., PRESCRIPTIONS FOR ERYSIPELAS AND ITS COMPLICATIONS (*how to give these water therapies: pp. 206-275 / list of treatments: pp. 206-207 / Hydrotherapy Disease Index: pp. 273-275*)

GENERAL—Cold Mitten Friction or Towel Rub every 3 hours.

COMBAT LOCAL INFLAMMATION AND EXTENSION OF THE DISEASE—Cold Compress during the early stage of the disease, renewing before it becomes warm. Later, give it less frequently. **Avoid Ice** Bags or Ice Compresses which involve risk of sloughing. **Fomentations** for 2-5 minutes every 2 hours. Ice Collar when the skin of the head or face is affected.

FEVER—Graduated Bath, Prolonged Neutral Bath, **Cooling Enema**, Cooling **Wet Sheet Pack**.

RECURRING CHILLS—Dry Pack and hot **water** drinking.

VOMITING—Ice Bag over stomach, Hot and Cold **Trunk Pack**.

PERICARDITIS, ENDOCARDITIS—Fomentation over heart for 30 seconds, followed by **Compress** above heart at 60° F.; change every half hour.

GENERAL METHOD—During the early stage of the disease, while the surface is bright red and the inflammation is extending, apply **cooling measures**, changing every few minutes (3-5 minutes), as often as the fomentation is warm. Prevent extreme depression by a **Fomentation** that is not too hot, every hour or two. When the parts become a dull red color or the rapid extension is checked, employ the **Heating Compress**, changing it at intervals of 15-30 minutes, prolonging the interval as the fever and inflammation subside.

If any of the following related problems exist, see under their respective headings: Myocarditis, Arthritis, Acute Nephritis, Delirium.

ENCOURAGEMENT—In the gift of Christ, God gave all heaven, that the moral image of God might be restored in man. His enabling grace, in all its vastness, is offered to us—so that we might live clean, good lives, in obedience to His ten commandment law.. Faithfully trusting in Christ, we will soon be with Him in heaven. Psalm 91:1-2, 4, 10.

KERATOSIS
(Sharkskin)

SYMPTOMS—This is the rough "goose bump" skin you will find on your elbows and also on the backs of your arms, thighs, and buttocks. It feels like a sandpaper surface.

CAUSES—This is a sebaceous and keratinized buildup of hard granular plugs in the openings of hair follicles. Many physicians claim that this is a normal condition, but it is actually a deficiency of **vitamin A and zinc**.

NATURAL REMEDIES

• Take **vitamin A** supplementation. This should be 25,000 units per day. However, keep in mind that vitamin A can be dangerous. Since it is an oil-soluble vitamin, it is stored very well by the body. Never take over 30,000 units a day, and only for a limited period of time.

• Increase **zinc** to 15 mg, three times a day, and essential fatty acids to 5 gm, three times a day.

ENCOURAGEMENT—Give God the most precious offering that it is possible for you to give. Give Him your heart. He offers to make you a member of His family, a child of the heavenly King. What earthly inheritance can equal this! Psalm 42:11.

LEUKODERMA
(Vitiligo)

SYMPTOMS—This is a loss of skin color, especially in black or dark-skinned people. When occurring in Europeans, it is less likely to be noticed. It is most commonly seen as white patches, surrounded by a dark border.

CAUSES—The skin is no longer producing melanin, the dark-coloring pigment. It most frequently occurs to someone who has **thyroid** problems. Premature gray or white hair may also occur. All this points to a deficiency of certain **B complex vitamins**.

When treatment is effective, small spots of pigment will appear in the white patches which gradually fill in. But only a few experience a complete return to the original color. Vitiligo is difficult to eradicate.

NATURAL REMEDIES

• **B complex supplementation**, plus emphasis on two special B vitamins: Para-aminobenzoic acid (**PABA**, 100 mg four times a day. Do not take more than 400 mg per day) and **pantothenic acid**. PABA injections may be needed. Also be sure and take **hydrochloric acid** if it is needed. Other helpful nutrients include **vitamins A, B complex, magnesium, zinc, and copper**.

• One study found that folic acid and vitamin B_{12} were low in those with this condition. High dosages of **folic acid** (1-10 mg daily) and B_{12} (1000 mcg every 2 weeks) produced increased pigmentation (normal skin coloring) within 8 months.

• The amino acid **L-phenylalanine** (50 mg per kg body weight), combined with **ultraviolet** radiation therapy also greatly helped, especially in children. But do not use UV lamps or tanning beds!

• Many with this vitiligo lack sufficient stomach **hydrochloric acid**. If there is a burning sensation, stop taking it. (The normal stomach produces as much HCl as found in 20 10-grain tablets. But no one should take more than 10 grains (650 mg). Do not take HCl if you have heartburn.

• Only two herbs have been found useful for leukoderma: The best is **khella** *(Ammi visnaga)*. The active ingredient in this stimulates repigmentation of the skin. Take 120-160 mg khella per day. But use khella with caution, for it may cause side effects (nausea and insomnia). Another herb that may help is **St. John's wort**. For it also increases the skin's response to sunlight, producing coloring. Do not use this herb during pregnancy or lactation.

• **Avoid cheese, yeast, wine, and pickled herring.**

ENCOURAGEMENT—We need a living faith. We must know that Jesus is indeed ours and that His Spirit is purifying and refining our hearts, and enabling us to keep the Ten Commandments. May we press closer to our God, so He can fulfill His will more fully in our lives. Romans 8:24.

CELLULITIS

SYMPTOMS—This is a bacterial infection of the skin and underlying tissues that causes redness, swelling, pain, and tenderness.

CAUSES—An area of skin and the underlying tissues become infected by bacteria that enter through a small, possibly unnoticed **wound**. The infection causes redness, pain, and swelling and most commonly affects the legs. When it occurs on the scalp, it is a nonlocalized inflammation without suppuration. Symptoms appear gradually over several hours.

Elderly people are especially vulnerable to cellulitis because many of them have **poor circulation**, which leads to edema or leg ulcers. These problems increase the risk of infection. Others at increased risk of cellulitis include **intravenous drug abusers** and those with **diabetes**. Untreated cellulitis may cause septicemia, a serious blood infection. Cellulitis may recur if you have a persistent immune or circulatory problem.

NATURAL REMEDIES

• If your leg is infected, you should **keep it elevated** to reduce swelling.

• Herbs are applied locally to the area, to cleanse skin impurities. To eliminate any excess of liquids and purify the blood, it is taken internally. These include **dandelion**, which improves liver function and prevents internal toxicity. Prepare an infusion of the fresh juice from leaves and roots.

• An infusion of leaves and/or buds from the **white birch** also cleans skin impurities. From a decoction of the rhizome and root of kneeholly, prepare a lotion or compress. This will invigorate the tissues, promote venous circulation, and reduce cellulitis.

ENCOURAGEMENT—Our Lord adapts Himself to our special needs. He is a shade on our right hand. He walks close by our side, ready to supply that which we need. He comes very near to those who are engaged in willing service for Him. He knows every one by name. Oh what assurances we have of the tender love of God! Cling to Him and, by faith in Christ's enabling grace, obey Him.

LUPUS VULGARIS
(local TB of the skin,
Lupus Erythematosis)

SYMPTOMS—Joints and blood vessels are affected, producing arthritis-like symptoms. The kidneys and lymph nodes become inflamed. And in severe cases there is heart, brain, and central nervous system degeneration. The skin and kidneys can be affected.

CAUSES—Lupus is a classic example of an autoimmune-type disease in which the body's immune system attacks connective tissue. It affects women nine times as often as men and becomes life-threatening, when the kidneys become involved. The word "lupus" means "wolf," because of the rough way it causes the skin over the cheeks and nose of some people to appear.

Orthodox medicine does not know what to do for this condition. But natural remedies can help rebuild a stable immune system. Those taking them tend to feel worse for 1-2 months until the toxins are neuturalized.

NATURAL REMEDIES

• Follow a natural remedies arthritis cleansing program.

• Drink 48 oz. **water** daily. The diet should be 60%-75% **fresh foods**. Take **potassium broth** (from thick potato peelings) daily for 1 month, then every other day for another month, then once a week for the third month. Take 1-2 glasses **aloe vera juice** daily. Take 4 tsp. **flaxseed** oil daily. Take a good walk every day for **exercise**. Take **alfalfa tablets** to increase fiber and add minerals. Eat **garlic**. Eat **fresh pineapple** to reduce inflammation. Use **hypoallergenic soaps**.

• Take 500-1,000 mg **vitamin C,** 3 times daily; 400-800 IU; **vitamin E**; and 1-2 Tbsp. **flaxseed oil**.

• Make sure your diet is very **low in fat**. Do not eat **meat** or **fish**. Avoid refined **sugars** and **starches**. Avoid **nightshade plants** (eggplant, tomatoes, peppers, tobacco).

• Avoid **birth control pills, cortico-steroid drugs, penicillin, allergenic cosmetics, UV rays**. Any of them can cause a flare-up of lupus. Avoid **fluorescent lights**. They make lupus symptoms worse. Eliminate **alcohol, caffeine, and sugar**.

• Helpful herbs include **red clover, pau d-arco, and feverfew**. But do not use feverfew during pregnancy. **Licorice** root tea may reduce lupus symptoms. Licorice works better than immunosuppressive drugs, such as steroids. But, if overused, licorice can elevate blood pressure.

ENCOURAGEMENT—The gifts of Him who has all power in heaven and earth are in store for the children of God. Gifts so precious that they come to us through the costly sacrifice of the Redeemer's blood; gifts as lasting as eternity will be received and enjoyed by all who will come to God as little children. Matthew 11:28-30.

ACTINIC KERATOSES

SYMPTOMS—Spots which are dry, red, and scaly. These are most frequently found on the face, neck, or backs of hands.

CAUSES—These are lesions which result from years of **overexposure to the sun**. They may appear to be age spots (above), but are actinic (solar) keratoses. These spots can be precancerous. In fact, they turn malignant roughly 25% of the time. Later they may become hard to the touch and grayish or brown in color.

NATURAL REMEDIES

PREVENTION

Low-fat diets reduce the risk of actinic keratoses. Patients whose diets contain only 21% fat are five times less likely to develop actinic keratoses than those who eat a high-fat diet.

ENCOURAGEMENT—Take God's promises as your own, plead them before Him as His own words, and you will receive fullness of joy.

SCLERODERMA

SYMPTOMS AND CAUSES—Thickening and hardening of the connective tissues in the skin, joints, and internal organs. A rare autoimmune disorder, more common in people of African descent. The skin on fingers and hands may thicken, become swollen, or contract. Also called multiple sclerosis (see 580).

NATURAL REMEDIES

Follow the recommendations given in the chapters on diet, vitamins, and minerals (100-127).

"... Believe in the LORD your God, so shall ye be established; believe his prophets, so shall ye prosper."   —2 Chronicles 20:20

"Finally, brethren, farewell. Be perfect, be of good comfort, be of one mind, live in peace; and the God of love and peace shall be with you."   —2 Corinthians 13:11

"...to do good and to communicate forget not: for with such sacrifices God is well pleased."   —Hebrews 13:16

"...I will look unto the LORD; I will wait for the God of my salvation: my God will hear me." —Micah 7:7

"If ye keep my commandments, ye shall abide in my love; even as I have kept my Father's commandments, and abide in his love."   —John 15:10

"The LORD redeemeth the soul of his servants: and none of them that trust in him shall be desolate."   —Psalm 34:22

"... My grace is sufficient for thee: for my strength is made perfect in weakness. Most gladly therefore will I rather glory in my infirmities, that the power of Christ may rest upon me."   —2 Corinthians 12:9

SKIN

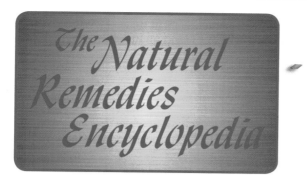

The Natural Remedies Encyclopedia

- Identification Guide -
Skin Diseases

Here you will find 86 color pictures of 45 diseases which produce markings on the skin during the infection:

Acne 356 / Actinic Keratoses 356 / Allergic Prupura 356 / Alergic Reaction 356-357 / Boils 357 / Bruise 357 / Cellulitis 357 / Chicken Pox 357 / Cradle Cap 358 / Dermatitis Herpetifomis 358 / Erythema Annulare Centrifugum (EAC) 358 / Erythema Multiforme 358 / Erythema Nodosum 358 / Hives 359 / Impetigo 359 / Irritant contact Dermatitis 359 / Jaundice or sign of Hepatitis 359 / Hypertrophic Scar 359-360 / Keloid Scar 360 / Lipoma 360 / Lupus Erythmatosus 360 / Measles (Rubeola) 360 / German Measles (Rubela) 358 / Molluscum or Contagiosum 360 / Mumps 361 / Pityriasis Rosea 361 / Poison Ivy Rash 361 / Psoriasis 361 / Ringworm 361-362 / Rocky Mountain Spotted Fever 362 / Scabies 362 / Sebaceous Cyst 362 / Seborrheic Dermatitis 362 / Shingles 363 / Tinea Versicolor 363 / Warts 363 / (Melanoma 363)

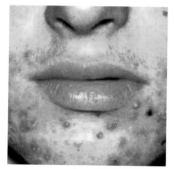
Acne

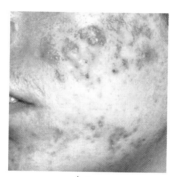
Acne

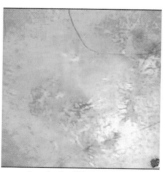
Actinic Keratoses

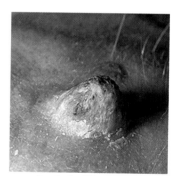
Actinic Keratoses

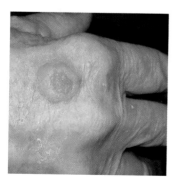
Actinic Keratoses

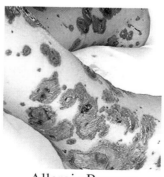
Allergic Prupura

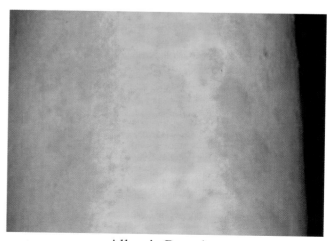
Allergic Reaction

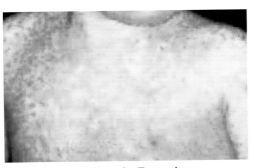

Allergic Reaction

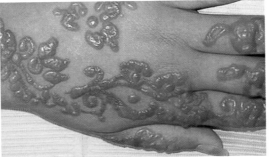

Allergic Reaction

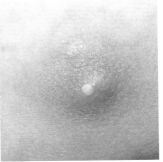

Boil

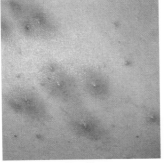

Boils

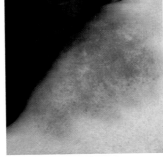

Bruise

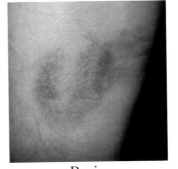

Bruise

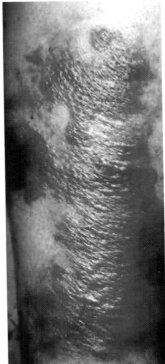

Cellulitis

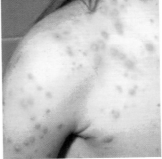

Cellulitis

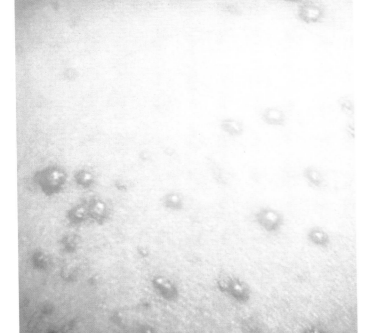

Chicken Pox - First Day

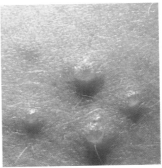

Chicken Pox -
Fourth Day

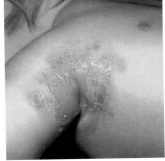

Chicken Pox

S
K
I
N

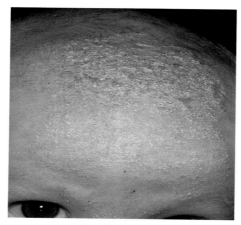

Cradle Cap

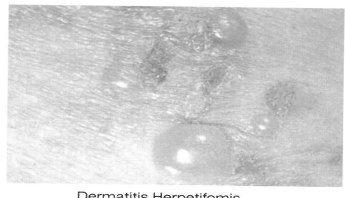

Dermatitis Herpetifomis

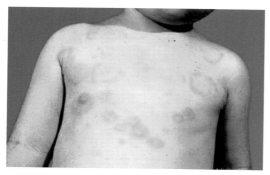

Erythema Annulare Centrifugum (EAC)

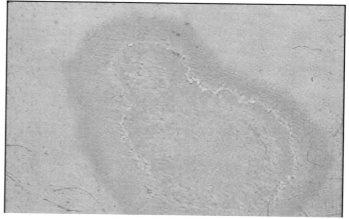

Erythema Annulare Centrifugum (EAC)

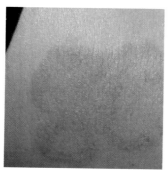

Erythema Annulare
Centrifugum (EAC)

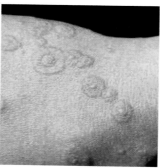

Erythema Multiforme

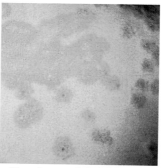

Erythema Multiforme

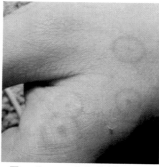

Erythema Multiforme

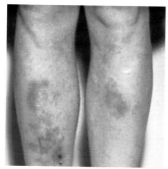

Erythema Nodosum

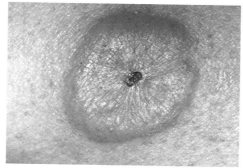

Erythema Nodosum

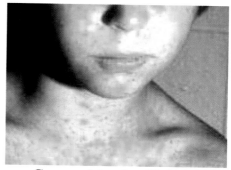

German Measles (Rubela)

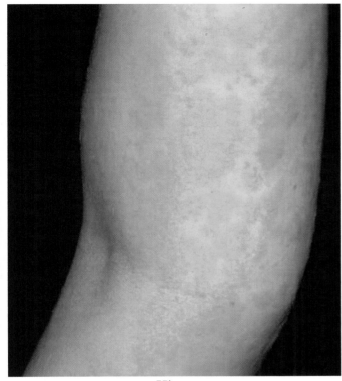

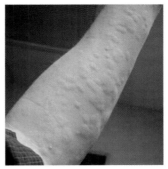

Hives

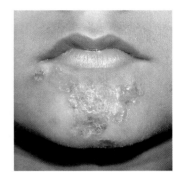

Impetigo

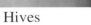

Hives

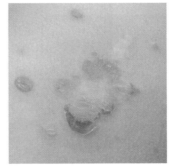

Impetigo

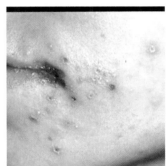

Impetigo

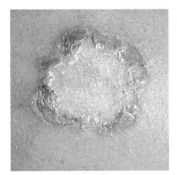

Impetigo

Irritant contact
Dermatitis

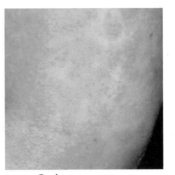

Irritant contact
Dermatitis

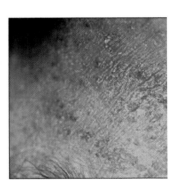

Irritant contact
Dermatitis

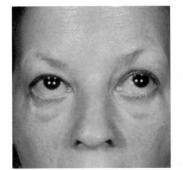

Jaundice

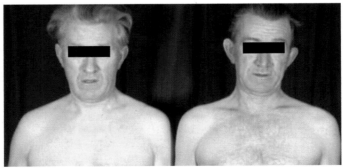

Jaundice (on right); sign of Hepititis

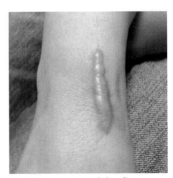

Hypertrophic Scar

SKIN

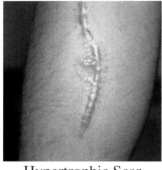

Hypertrophic Scar

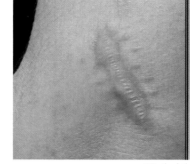

Keloid Scar

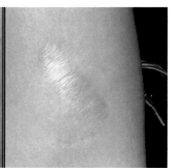

Keloid Scar

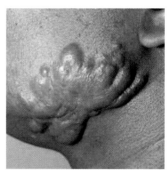

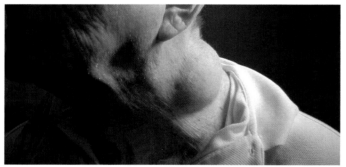

Lipoma

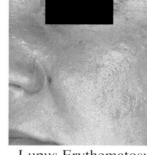

Lupus Erythematosus

Lupus Erythematosus

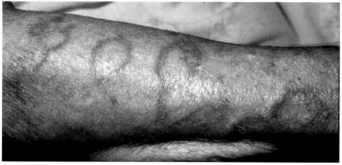

Lupus Erythematosus

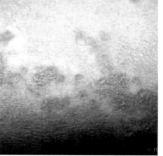

Lupus Erythematosus

Measles (Rubeola)

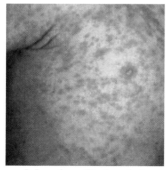

Measles (Rubeola)

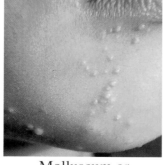

Molluscum or
Contagiosum

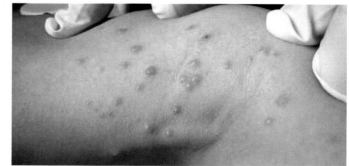

Molluscum or Contagiosum

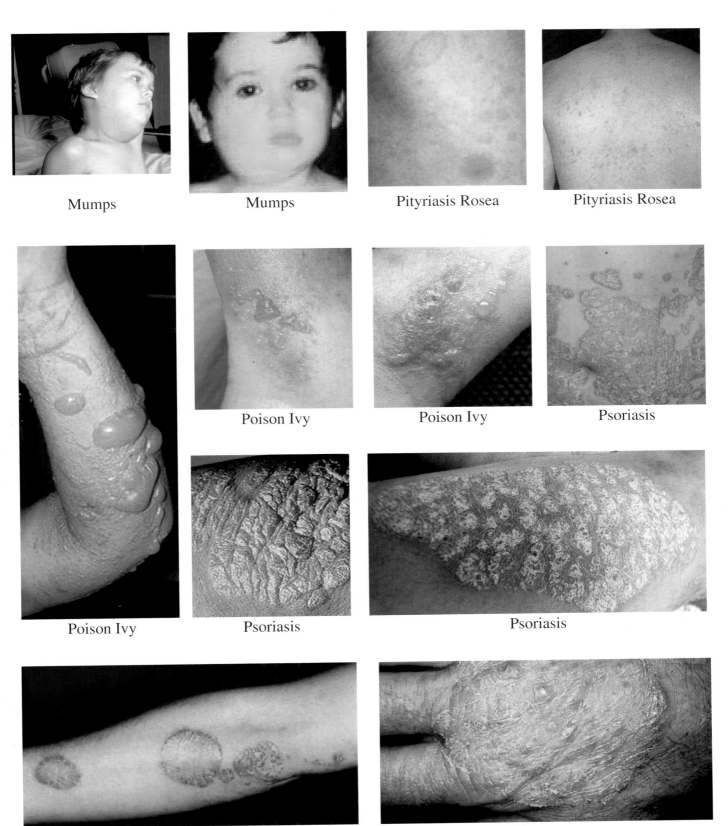

Mumps

Mumps

Pityriasis Rosea

Pityriasis Rosea

Poison Ivy

Poison Ivy

Psoriasis

Poison Ivy

Psoriasis

Psoriasis

Psoriasis

Ringworm

S
K
I
N

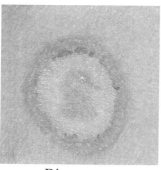

Ringworm

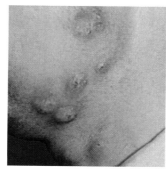

Ringworm

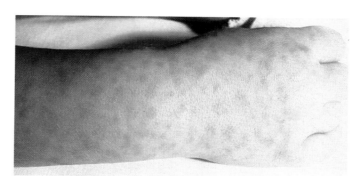

Rocky Mountain Spotted Fever

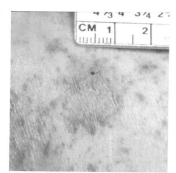

Rocky Mountain
Spotted Fever

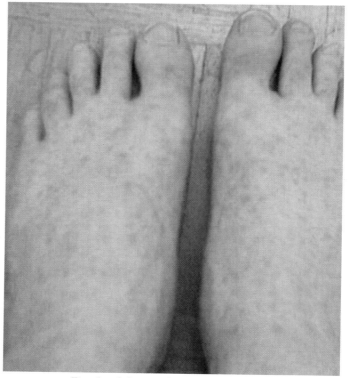

Rocky Mountain Spotted Fever

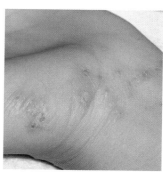

Scabies

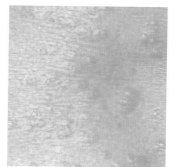

Scabies

Sebaceous Cyst

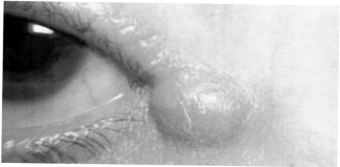

Sebaceous Cyst

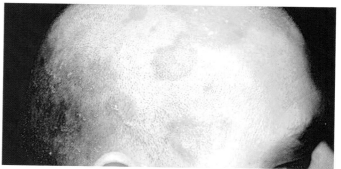

Seborrheic Dermatitis

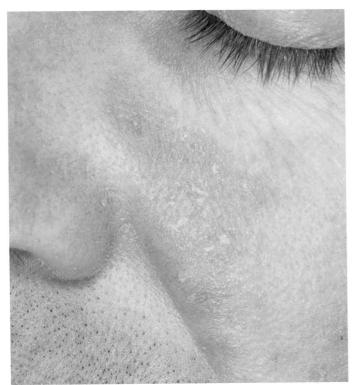

Seborrheic Dermatitis

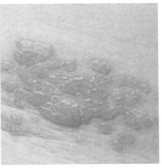

Shingles

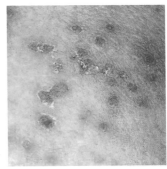

Shingles

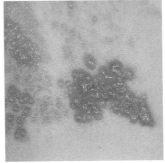

Shingles

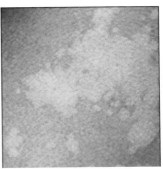

Tinea Versicolor

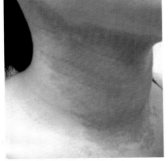

Tinea Versicolor

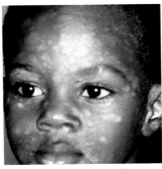

Tinea Versicolor

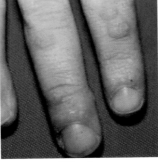

Warts

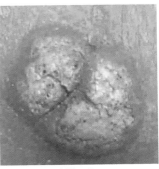

Warts

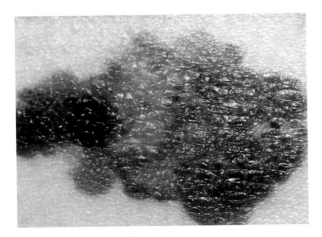

Melanoma

Melanoma (the basic skin cancer) is included here for the purpose of comparrison with the benign diseases shown here. Melanoma is described in the chapter on cancer and color pictures of it will be found in the chapter on skin cancers.

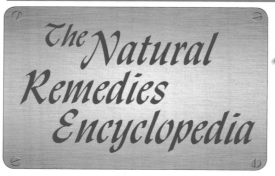

The Natural Remedies Encyclopedia

- Disease Section 3 - Extremities

EXTR

 # = Information, not a disease

Special Senses: Physiology 1023/ Pictures 1036-1037

"I know the thoughts that I think toward you, saith the Lord, thoughts of peace, and not of evil, to give you an expected end."   *—Jeremiah 29:11*

"O Lord, the great and dreadful God, keeping the covenant and mercy to them that love Him, and to them that keep His commandments."   *—Daniel 9:4*

"God hath not given us the spirit of fear; but of power, and of love, and of a sound mind."   *—2 Timothy 1:7*

FOR MORE NATURAL REMEDIES:
HERBS: Herb Contents (pp. 129-130) will help you locate the 126 most important herbs and the diseases each one can treat. How to prepare herbs (132). How to use them (141-189)
HYDROTHERAPY: Therapy Contents (pp. 206-207) and its Disease Index (263-265) will lead you to over 100 water therapies and many more remedies. DIS. INDEX: 1211- / GEN. INDEX: 1221-

VITAMINS AND MINERALS: Contents (100-101). Using 101-124. Dosages (124). Others (117-)
CARING FOR THE SICK: Home care for a sick person (28-36). The healing crisis (36-39)
WOMEN'S SECTIONS: Female Organs (672) Pregnancy (701). Childbirth (765). Infancy, Childhood (722). Women's Herbs (754, 760)
EMERGENCIES: (973-). FIRST AID: (990-)

Section 3 — Extremities

EXTREMITIES - 1 - EXTREMITIES
Also: Claudication (637)

NUMB EXTREMITIES

SYMPTOMS—There is a lack of feeling in the toes, fingers, arms, or legs.

CAUSES—Aside from serious nerve diseases, this temporary condition usually results from pinching off the nerve and blood supply leading to an extremity.

But it could be an initial warning of something serious. If the problem is *not* immediately resolved, check the disorders listed under *Paralysis (576-585)* in *Section 9 (Neuro-Mental)* or contact your physician.

NATURAL REMEDIES
• **Avoid** tight clothing and strained positions.
• Be sure to get an adequate supply of the **B complex vitamins, including B$_6$.**
• A water treatment useful for numb, tingling feet would be a **fomentation to the spine**, along with **hot or alternate sponging of the limbs**.

ENCOURAGEMENT—How lovingly the angels of God guard His earthly children who cry to Him for help. You cannot now understand all the mysteries of Providence. But you can know that all things work together for your best good. Nahum 1:7.

COLD EXTREMITIES

SYMPTOMS—Hands and feet frequently, or always, feeling cold.

NATURAL REMEDIES
• Be sure to **dress warmly** enough. Fashionable clothing often dictates, leaving the arms and legs improperly clad. The blood supply is chilled back from the extremities and pooled in the trunk. This breakdown in proper body circulation can produce diseased conditions in the chest, and in the intestinal and abdominal organs.
• Are your nerves being fed properly? Take a **B complex supplement,** including **niacin and B$_2$.** Also take **ribonucleic acid.**
• You may have a **sluggish thyroid.** *See Hypothyroidism (659).*

• If a sudden coldness comes to your hands and/or feet, and they blanch white, you may have Raynaud's disease *(284).*

ENCOURAGEMENT—The heart in which Jesus makes His abode will be quickened, purified, guided, and ruled by the Holy Spirit. And the soul will be enabled to overcome those sins which he could never put away by himself. Thank God for His enabling grace. 1 Peter 5:6-7.

FROSTBITE (CHILBLAINS)

SYMPTOMS—The first warning is a tingling, followed by a redness. Then comes a paleness and numbness in a body part (generally the fingers, toes, cheeks, nose, or ears). If not immediately cared for, tissue can die and gangrene will set in.

CAUSES—This is partial or total freezing of a portion of the body. *Frostnip* is superficial frostbite and leaves the area firm, white, and cold. It can result in peeling and blistering, 24-72 hours later, and perhaps cold sensitivity in the area.

In contrast, deep *frostbite* produces a cold, hard, white condition which is painless while it remains frozen. On rewarming, it becomes blotchy red, swollen, and can be quite painful.

Dry, non-infected gangrene occurs when the skin becomes so cold so long that the blood flow stops. Tissue becomes numb, oxygen-deprived, and dies. If treated right away, this can be successfully treated. (Wet gangrene is different. It is the result of an infected wound which prevents drainage and deprives the area of blood and oxygen. This requires different treatment. See a physician.)

NATURAL REMEDIES
WHILE OUTSIDE
• To warm the hands, the person should **place them under his armpits**. Have him **roll himself into a ball** to conserve heat. **He should stay out of the wind and not get wet. He should not drink or smoke**. Both block circulation to the extremities. And alcohol gives an artificial feeling of warmth while actually removing it.
• If outside, he should **stay in a car or truck** until help comes. He should **not take off his boots** until it is safe to do so. The foot may be swollen and he might not get it back on. If considerable walking must be done to find a place of safety, leave the feet unthawed until arriving at the destination.

EXTR

• **Do not rub ice** on the area! This only extracts more heat. In the early stages, you can **rub the area with a cloth dipped in cold water or snow**.

• Get the person to a heated room immediately.

INITIAL TREATMENT

• **Cover warmly** in a warm place, so frostbitten areas can warm up gradually.

• Proceed with caution! Rewarming should be done slowly! Rapid rewarming dilates blood vessels near the skin, further lowering blood pressure and sending more cold blood to the body core. As soon as possible, get the person into a slightly **warm tub** (100°-110° F.). The area is numb, so he will not feel the heat.

• **Do not apply more heat** than mentioned above. For the skin is numb and can be burned without anyone realizing it. Unless it is all you have, do not use dry radiant heat (such as a heat lamp or campfire). Frostbitten skin can easily burn; for it does not feel the heat. Living tissue is dying. So **thaw the area quickly. Do not allow it to refreeze**. Move the person to a warmer place. Wrap him in blankets. Give him warm liquids, but no alcohol. **Avoid sedatives, tranquilizers, or pain relievers**. They slow down body processes.

• For frostbite, paint on (but do not rub in) warm **olive oil**. If infective bacterial development has occurred, paint on **honey** to arrest infection.

• Sponge the area with the **water in which potatoes have been boiled**. Give a **hand or footbath**, being very careful how warm the water is. Gently rub the frostbitten skin with a **raw onion, potato slices**, or **raw radishes that are liquefied**. To relieve pain, cover the area with cooked, **mashed potatoes or turnips** which are at room temperature.

• **Gently stroke the kidneys** toward the middle of the back. Use alternating **warm and cool hydrotherapy** to stimulate circulation. **No hot-water bottles, hair dryers, or heating pads**. Only slow warming is needed.

• *If case is severe,* **wrap the area** in gauze. So blisters do not break. **Elevate legs**. Do not rub blisters.

• *If case is very severe,* **immerse areas** in warm water and **massage** very gently under water for 5-10 minutes.

• *After being treated* for frostbite, **aloe vera gel** should be spread on the frostbitten area 4 times a day, to hasten healing and prevent permanent damage. Use the gel from a cut leaf or purchase it. Or apply the inner sides of **cucumber peelings**.

• *For two weeks thereafter,* eat a high **protein diet**, with plenty of **whole grains**.

PREVENTION

• Before heading out into the cold, put **cayenne** pepper in your shoes. In third-world countries this is a much-used remedy for frostbite. Swallowing a little, will speed up the circulation to your extremities. Fill each #00 gelatin capsule with about ¼ Tbsp. powdered cayenne. Carry several with you. And take one a day.

• **Dress warmly in loose-fitting, layered, light-weight wool clothing. Outer garments should be tightly woven and water repellent. Protect your head, ears, face, hands, and feet.** Wear a **thick ski cap (wool is best), gloves (mittens are warmer), and very warm, moisture-absorbing socks and undergarments**. (At least 1/3 of the heat lost from the body is from the head.) If it is cold enough, you may need **goggles** to protect your eyeballs.

• If you get wet, immediately **get out of your wet clothing**, or stand or sit by a strong heat source. Remain indoors when it is extremely cold and windy.

• Taking massive amounts of **vitamin C** (1,500 mg for each 65 pounds body weight) with **bioflavonoids** in divided daily doses, will help the body maintain its normal temperature to prevent frostbite and hyperthermia.

• If you cannot escape from the cold, **wiggle your fingers, cover your face,** and **move or jump about. Do not smoke or drink**.

• **At bedtime,** have enough warm blankets. Have flannel sheets above a sheepskin or wool mattress, warm cap, long underwear, and socks. And, if feasible, use an electric blanket. Extremely warm sleeping bags can be purchased.

• Whether awake or asleep, **room temperatures below 70° F.** can be dangerous, unless you are properly covered.

ENCOURAGEMENT—The sovereignty of God involves fullness of blessing to all created beings. Only in obedience to Him can we be happy.

HYPOTHERMIA

SYMPTOMS—A lowering of the overall body temperature. If the temperature is below 96° F. (35.5° C.), it may be hypothermia. Other symptoms include confusion, disorientation, drowsiness, slurred speech, shallow and very slow breathing, weak pulse, poor muscle coordination, and uncontrollable shivering.

In severe cases, body temperature can drop below 84° F., muscles become rigid, extremities are purple, and loss of consciousness may occur.

CAUSES—This is a lowering of the entire body temperature. But because it so often centers in the extremities, we are including it in this section. The same treatment should be applied as for "Frostbite" *(365)*. The elderly are especially vulnerable.

The temperature is lowered to subnormal levels for some length of time, resulting in near frostbite. Severe numbness and loss of function may occur if the problem is not dealt with. Colds, flu, and infection can result.

NATURAL REMEDIES

• Follow recommendations given for *Frostbite (365)*.

ENCOURAGEMENT—Hide within your heart the precious promises of God's Word, and you will be strengthened in time of need. Cling to Christ and trust Him to care for you to the end. Micah 7:7.

FELON
(Whitlow)

SYMPTOMS—A swelling on an abscess of a thumb or finger (sometimes a toe), which includes throbbing pain and extreme tenderness. It may, at first, seem to be an infection or inflammation of the skin.

CAUSES—The germs causing the infection are usually carried under the skin by a deep pinprick, thorn, sliver, or some other sharp object. The inflammation and pus are deep among the tendons, tendon sheaths, or even next to the bone.

If the felon is not carefully and thoroughly lanced promptly, the tendons could slough or the bone be damaged. This would result in a permanently crippled body part. Moreover, if the pus is not drained, there is danger that the infection may travel to the hand and more extensive crippling occur. Or the infection may infect the blood; and blood poisoning will result. *See Blood Poisoning" (544).*

NATURAL REMEDIES
• Call a physician and **have the felon lanced**. Deep lancing through very painful flesh must be done. So it may be necessary for the patient to be anesthetized.
• An alternate remedy, used by the old timers on the frontier, is as follows: Warm some **kerosene** and immerse the affected part into it for at least 10-15 minutes at a time, 4-5 times a day. This will eliminate the felon.
• To relieve pain, put a piece of **lemon** on it. If on the end of a finger, cut a small hole in the lemon and place it over the finger. If elsewhere, bandage on a thick slice. This may solve the problem if kerosene is not available.
• Jethro Kloss recommends a poultice of equal parts of **slippery elm, lady's slipper,** and **lobelia**.
• Dr. Christopher prescribes boiling the roots of equal parts **blue flag** and **American hellebore** 20 minutes in equal parts of milk and water. Then soak the felon for 20 minutes as hot as can be tolerated. After this, bind on the roots for 1 hour.

ENCOURAGEMENT—Those who take the name of Christian should come to God in earnestness and humility, pleading for help. Jesus has told us to pray without ceasing. And so many need our prayers. James 5:16.

ERYTHROMELALGIA

SYMPTOMS—A skin neurosis, accompanied by burning and throbbing which comes and goes and affects any of the extremities, but especially the feet.

CAUSES—Although this is a nerve problem, it is listed here because it rather consistently affects the extremities.

NATURAL REMEDIES
• Let the patient **rest. Elevate** the affected part. Place a **cold compress** on it. And change this every 20-30 minutes. Apply graduated tonic frictions (such as the **wet hand rub, the cold mitten friction, or the cold towel rub**). See the chapter on *Hydrotherapy* in this *Encyclopedia*, for further information on how to apply these treatments *(206-275)*.

ENCOURAGEMENT—Let your affections center upon God. Think of His goodness and let His Spirit guide you into deeper appreciation of His Ten Commandment law. "If there be first a willing mind, it is accepted according to that a man hath, and not according to that he hath not." 2 Corinthians 8:12.

GANGRENE

SYMPTOMS—The skin darkens, and either remains soft and moist or becomes dry and shrivels. Eventually it sloughs off. As *wet gangrene* progresses, the tissue changes from pink to deep red to gray-green or purple. Symptoms of *dry gangrene* are a dull aching pain, coldness, and eventual numbness in the area.

CAUSES—Tissues affected by gangrene die if not treated in time.

Dry gangrene is caused by a stoppage of blood flow. Lack of blood and oxygen causes the tissues to die. There is no bacterial infection. This most often occurs in the fingers, toes, nose, or ears. If not treated, the gangrenous area will have to be amputated, but the person will not die. Causes include **frostbite, hardening of the arteries, poor circulation, Raynaud's disease, diabetes, injury,** or **blockage within a blood vessel**.

Wet gangrene (also called *gas gangrene*) is caused by a **wound** which becomes infected from lack of oxygen. Bacteria are present. If not treated, the person will go into shock and die within a few days.

NATURAL REMEDIES
Consult a physician. In addition to primary treatment for the gangrene (*see Frostbite, 365*), the following suggestions will help:
• Eat a **nourishing, high-protein diet** to rebuild tissue. Include **kelp,** to strengthen the thyroid. Drink **carrot juice**. Take 25,000 units of **vitamin A** daily for a week. Take **vitamin C** (2,000-5,000 mg daily) until the problem is solved. Drink lots of quality **water** and **green drinks**.
• **Stop eating junk food, all meat, tobacco, alcohol, and nearly all salt**.
• Take an **enema** containing powdered psyllium seed in water daily, to assure good bowel movements.
• If the skin is dry, lightly **rub wheat germ or olive**

oil on it. When pus is oozing, dab warm **hydrogen peroxide** over the area and wipe off carefully.

• Either keep **walking** or **massage** the area (usually the legs) to improve circulation.

• Apply **cool baths** to the extremity or cool whole baths. **Chaparral tea** or **apple cider vinegar** can be added to the water, to help disinfect it (1 Tbsp. per quart). Also very helpful are **alternate hot and cold footbaths** or **fomentation** packs to improve blood flow.

• **Chelation therapy** *(869)* is able to help solve gangrene problems.

If you have hardening of the arteries or diabetes, be especially diligent in treating this condition.

If an injured area becomes red, swollen, painful, or has an odor, contact a physician.

• Gangrene is the advanced condition of blood poisoning. This condition will never happen to a person who has good blood circulation and whose blood has been cleansed. Soak the afflicted area with **marshmallow root tea**, covering the area with tea as hot as the patient can take; and leave it there for long periods of time. Soaking works faster than the poultice or the tea, but drinking the tea along with the soaking will speed the action. **Plantain** used as a poultice is also excellent. Pain in the infected part can be relieved by adding a small amount of **lobelia**. Be sure that the bowels move properly by cleansing them with the lower bowel tonic.

ENCOURAGEMENT—It is difficult to exercise living faith when we are discouraged. Yet this, of all others, is the very time when we should exercise faith. When you have the greatest need, that is the time to seek God the most earnestly. He will hear, He will answer, He will help. Psalm 37:25-26.

RAYNAUD'S DISEASE

SYMPTOMS—The small arteries in the extremities constrict or tighten. The hands and feet are extremely sensitive to the cold and suddenly contract. Lack of oxygenated blood causes the fingers or toes to become whitish or bluish in hue. As a result, the affected area may temporarily shrink in size!

Unless these attacks are reduced, ulcers may form, which further damage the tissue and produce chronic infection under, and near, the fingernails and toenails.

The hands are the areas most often affected. But it can occur in the fingers and possibly toes, nose, tongue, cheeks, ears, or chin. A blood spasm may initially blanch the area. Tingling, and then swelling, may occur and become painful. The appearance may change to a bright red, as the blood vessels again distend and fresh blood is sent back into the area.

The attacks usually do not last long. But, in those instances in which they do, gangrene can develop.

CAUSES—A cold attack is generally brought on by **exposure to cold** or **emotional upset**. But it can also be brought on when the **hands go into the refrigerator** for a moment, a difficult written exam must be taken, or a **verbal conflict** occurs. Spasms of small arteries result.

The underlying cause may be less easy to identify. It might be **high blood pressure, drugs, connective tissue disease, inflammation of the arteries,** or **equipment vibrations** which injure the blood vessels. In some, the problem is a localized oversensitivity to **hormones** that cause blood vessels to constrict.

Some individuals have lived in a **cold, improperly heated environment** for too many months or years, and the problem developed. Try to avoid resting or sleeping in ice cold places. It can also be caused by **not clothing the limbs** properly in cold weather over an extended period of time. Women as well as men should clothe their limbs in the winter.

Food allergies, junk food, or a poor diet which is high in starches and low in greens, vitamins, and minerals may cause it.

Antihypertensives, ergot drugs, channel blockers, or **alpha-and beta-adrenergic blockers** can be the cause.

There are two forms of this condition:

(1) *Raynaud's phenomenon:* This may be due to **various bodily disorders**. It occurs evenly in both men and women, and usually begins after the age of 30. Symptoms in the phenomenon may affect only one side of the body.

(2) *Raynaud's disease:* This is the primary disease, and occurs mainly in women. The disease generally begins in the teens or early twenties. But it can occur at any time in the life. Attacks normally affect both sides of the body equally.

Frequency of the attacks are significant. They may be rare or occur as often as several times a day. Mild occurrences only last a few minutes. Severe ones may continue for hours. Between attacks the hands will at first appear normal. Later they may remain slightly bluish. Gradually the attacks will be more frequent and last longer.

In later years, the hands will be slightly bluish all the time. The fingers become swollen. The skin turns pale, discolored, shiny, taut, and smooth. The nails become clubbed and deformed. In advanced stages, poor blood supply can weaken the fingers and damage the sense of touch. The sense of feel may decrease and delicate movements become more difficult to perform. Infections and gangrene may occur more frequently in the affected area.

Instead of Raynaud's, you might have **Buerger's disease** *(285)*, a nerve disorder which gradually cuts off the nerve supply to the extremities. Buerger's disease is primarily caused by using tobacco products. Buerger's is a steady cutting off of nerve flow. Whereas Raynaud's is an intermittent blood flow.

This may be a symptom of *Scleroderma (355)*, a rare and serious disease that involves hardening of the skin and damage to the internal organs. Or it could be *Claudication (637)*, which involves a narrowing of the arteries in the legs.

NATURAL REMEDIES

DIET

• Drink enough **water**, but **not soft drinks**.

• Eat a **high-fiber diet** which includes some **psyllium seed**, to help clean the colon. Eat slow-cooked **grains** and a **low-protein** diet.

• By increasing your intake of the right **essential fatty acids**, you can combat processes of inflammation that sometimes play a role in disorders, such as Raynaud's. So far, essential fatty acid treatment has shown a mild positive effect in relieving Raynaud's. **Flaxseed oil** is rich in two main types of essential fatty acids and is also inexpensive. *Typical dosage:* 1 to 2 tablespoons of flaxseed oil per day. Animal studies have shown that **evening primrose oil** can reduce blood vessel constriction.

• One study found that a dose of 4,000 milligrams per day of **inositol hexanicotinate** (one form of **niacin** which will not cause flushing) during cold weather reduced Raynaud's attacks. *Typical dosage:* 500 milligrams three times daily for the first two weeks, then 1,000 milligrams three times per day.

• Take **vitamin E** (80-1,200 units per day), **unsaturated fatty acids** (wheat germ oil, etc.), **tryptophan**. Take **calcium** (2,000 mg daily) and **magnesium** (1,000 mg daily). Get enough **iron** in your diet.

• When circulation slows significantly, tissue-damaging substances, called free radicals, are generated. **Antioxidants** can capture and eliminate these free radicals in order to prevent injury. Dietary supplements that might help include **vitamin C** (500 mg once or twice per day) and **vitamin E** (1400 IU per day).

• Deficiency of **magnesium** appears to play a significant role in Raynaud's phenomenon. Even in people without Raynaud's, decreased magnesium levels can induce small arteries to constrict. So make sure you are obtaining the daily value of magnesium: 350 milligrams for men and 280 milligrams for women (320 if pregnant). Good food sources include **kelp, wheat bran, wheat germ, molasses, brewer's yeast, nuts, peanuts, tofu, buckwheat**, and other **whole grains**.

• Sprinkle a small amount of **cayenne** on your food, to increase circulation. Other helpful herbs include **garlic, ginkgo, ginger, biloba extract,** and **pau d'arco**.

• Eat a warm soup which includes **cayenne, garlic, and ginger**. It will really warm you! The warming power of cayenne is legendary. A research study found that garlic improves blood flow in the legs. Chinese herbalists give ginger to treat cold fingers and feet.

• Sprinkle **cayenne** in your shoes, to keep your feet warm.

• **Avoid fatty, fried, and junk foods**. At least 50% of your diet should be **raw food**. Avoid food items which tend to bother you (**allergenic foods**). Avoid caffeine (**caffeine, tea, soft drinks, chocolate**). Caffeine restricts blood flow. Use a **fat-free, sugar-free diet**. Sugar increases blood viscosity as well as triglycerides. Avoid food **seasonings**.

• Do not take any **tobacco** product or use **alcohol**. Nicotine causes constriction of the blood vessels and it produces plaque in them, both of which reduce blood flow. Do not even be in the same room where someone is smoking.

OTHER HELPS

• **Keep hands and feet warm**. This is important. It might be well to select a **warmer climate** in which to live. **Dress warmly** at all times. Always wear **gloves** in cold weather (mittens will keep you even warmer). Wear **shoes**. Do not walk without them when it is cooler, even in the house. Wear extra warm **socks** in the winter. Gloves, mittens, and shoes should be warm before putting them on, since it is difficult for one with this problem to warm them. Wear **shoes** which breathe, so you do not end up with damp, cold feet. If you have a tendency for your socks to become damp, try to change them halfway through the day. It is important that you wear a **warm hat** in cold weather. An uncovered head loses a lot of heat.

• Avoid contact with **cold objects**, even for brief moments. While preparing meals, use **tepid**, not cold, **water**.

• *When an attack occurs*, **immerse the body part** in warm (not hot) water, no warmer than 90° F. Why not warmer water? During an attack, without realizing it, one's skin can more easily burn.

• **Massaging the hands and fingers** every evening helps reduce the severity of the attacks, by stimulating blood circulation in that area.

• **Stressful situations** produce a spasm of the blood vessels. As much as possible, avoid such situations. **Keep calm, cheerful, and relaxed**. **Plan ahead** and avoid scheduling pressures. Trust in God and believe He will care for you. Vigorous outdoor **exercise** will strengthen the entire body and also relax it. Exercise tends to neutralize the attitude and effects of stress.

• Medicinal drugs for Raynaud's do not seem to help. The side effects outweigh the benefits (ergot, beta-blocking drugs, cytotoxic agents, etc.). Do not take **birth control pills**.

• Avoid **machinery which vibrates** the hands. In one study, 50% of pneumatic drill workers had Raynaud's, compared with 5.6% for the average population. Such equipment includes chain saws, metal grinders, stone cutters, lathes, and manual typewriters.

• **Sunbathing** is helpful; for it strengthens both the body and the blood.

• Donald McIntyre, M.D. suggests occasionally **swinging the arms in circles**, 80 twirls per minute, to throw blood into the hands. He says to do it as a pitcher does it: swinging the arm up from the back and then hard downward in front. It has been found that those with back problems can swing their arms entirely in front of the body with the same beneficial effect on the hands (upward from the trunk and downward to the side).

• *Here are several* **practical suggestions** *during cold weather:* Before driving to work in the morning, start your car. Turn on the heater and let it warm up. Arrange for parking close to your employment. Dress warmly, including warm hat and gloves, outdoors. Even indoors, put on extra clothing if you need to. Purchase thermal gloves and socks. Try not to touch cold metal with your bare hands. Cover outside door knobs and keys with rubber caps. Wash produce in lukewarm, not cold, water. Check whether you are taking drugs which interfere with your circulation. Do not drink cold drinks. Drink enough fluids, to maintain a good blood volume and circulation.

—*Also see Buerger's Disease (below).*

ENCOURAGEMENT—Talk with Jesus as though He were right by your side. If there is a place you cannot go with Jesus, then do not go there. If there is anything you cannot watch or listen to with Him, then turn away from it immediately. John 1:12.

BUERGER'S DISEASE
(Thromboangiitis Obliterans)

SYMPTOMS—Continual coldness of the extremity is frequently the first symptom. But numbness, tingling, and aching may also be noticed. When lowered for long periods of time, the feet may turn blue. The problem generally begins in the feet. But it can, and will, occur in the hands and eventually the whole body—if the cause is not stopped.

Asians and Jews develop this problem more frequently than others. And 75 men have it for every one woman who develops it. It most frequently begins at the ages of 20 to 45. There are alternate periods of worsening and inactivity of the disease.

CAUSES—This is an inflammation of the blood vessel walls, accompanied by blood clots and thickening of the blood vessel walls. Eventually they close entirely.

The primary cause is the use of **tobacco** products. Rarely does a non-nicotine user get Buerger's disease.

NATURAL REMEDIES
• Stop using **nicotine** in every form. It is killing you in more ways than one.
• *Use the treatment outlined for Raynaud's disease.* **Walking** is one of the best exercises for increasing blood flow in the legs.
• Lie on the bed and **elevate the legs** for 1-2 minutes or until they blanch. Then sit on the side of the bed and hold them down till they become pink. Do this 5 times each, 3 times a day.

• **Do not sit for long periods of time** without getting up and walking. Sleep on a **firm mattress**. **Never cross the legs** at the knees.

Forty years ago, the present author read a true story written by physician. A man had came to him with a serious physical problem. The doctor diagnosed it as Buerger's. And he warned him that, if he did not stop smoking, he would eventually lose an extremity. Several years later, the physician was walking down the street when he heard a voice, "Would you light me a cigarette, Chum?" Startled, he looked around and then down. There was the same man. He was now on a sliding board, without any arms or feet, and wanted someone to stick a cigarette in his mouth and light it for him.

—*Read Raynaud's Disease (368).*

ENCOURAGEMENT—When we learn to walk by faith and not by feeling, we shall have help from God just when we need it. And His peace will come into our hearts. Proverbs 11:24-25, 27.

DUPUYTREN'S CONTRACTURE

SYMPTOMS—A thickening and shortening of tissues in the palm of the hand, resulting in deformity of the fingers.

CAUSES—In Dupuytren's contracture, the fibrous tissue in the palm of the hand becomes thickened and shortened. As a result, one or more fingers, often the fourth and fifth fingers, are pulled toward the palm in a bent position. Sometimes painful lumps develop in the palm, and the overlying skin becomes puckered.

In about half of the cases, both hands are involved. Very rarely, the disorder affects the feet and toes.

The changes occur very slowly over many months or years. It occurs more frequently in men and those over 50 with Diabetes Mellitus, epilepsy, or who drink alcohol.

NATURAL REMEDIES
• Over 50 years ago, researchers first found that taking **vitamin E** reduced the severity of Dupuytren's Contracture. Several studies reported that 200-2,000 IU of the vitamin per day for several months was definitely helpful. Overall, there are more positive studies than negative ones. However, that earlier research has not been followed up on. The reason is that pharmaceutical firms make no money selling vitamin E. The disease progresses so slowly. Taking large doses of vitamin E should be a definite help. There apparently is no known toxic dose of vitamin E. You probably can take as much as you want each day.

• Exercise your fingers and practice stretching exercises.

ENCOURAGEMENT—God is pleased when we keep

our faces turned toward Christ, the Sun of Righteousness. When we are in trouble and pressed down with anxieties, the Lord is near. And He bids us cast all our care upon Him, because He cares for us.

ELEPHANTIASIS

SYMPTOMS—A thick, livid, reddish, tuberculated, and insensible condition of the skin. This is usually in the lower leg. But the disease can also affect the feet, arms, scrotum, breasts, and vulva. It is accompanied by great debility and several morbid symptoms, including offensive perspiration and fierce, staring eyes.

CAUSES—Elephantiasis is the name given to a firm, somewhat rubbery, slowly developing swelling of various parts of the body. Either one of two species of filarial worms may cause it: Wuchereria bancrofti and Wuchereria malayi. The immature parasites are transmitted by many different species of mosquitoes. The legs are most often affected. Because they become so large, the disease is named after elephants.

The enlargement is due to chronic obstruction of lymph drainage. The deeper layers of skin, together with underlying connective tissues, are enormously thickened and changed into a blubbery mass which oozes lymph freely when punctured or cut.

Travelers to a tropical country, primarily Africa or Southeastern Asia, can contract this disease.

NATURAL REMEDIES
• R.T. Trall, M.D., recommends the following natural remedies for this condition. A diet restricted to **plain vegetables, fruits, and grains**. Absolutely **no meat or fish** of any kind. **Absolute cleanliness, frequent cool or tepid bathing or washing** of the entire surface, along with copious **water** drinking.

ENCOURAGEMENT—God knows just what we need, just what we can bear; and He will give us grace to endure every trial and test.

EXTREMITIES - 2 - NAILS

NAIL PROBLEMS
(Fingernails and Toenails)

SYMPTOMS AND CAUSES—Your fingernails help reveal how well you are absorbing nutrients. A deficient diet can affect your nails. Although fingernails and toenails are primarily composed of protein, other nutrients are also needed. Here are some of the symptoms, followed by the deficient nutrient:
Poor nail growth: zinc.
Dry, brittle nails: protein, vitamin A, calcium, iron.

Fragile and showing horizontal or vertical ridges: B vitamins.
Half moons absent: protein deficiency.
Thin, flat, and even moon-shaped (concave or spoon-shaped) nails: iron deficiency.
Pale nail beds: anemia.
Poor nail growth: zinc deficiency.
Excessively dry, very rounded, and curved nail ends which are darkened: vitamin B12 deficiency.
Splitting nails: lack of hydrochloric acid and amino acid deficiency.
Washboard ridges: Iron, calcium, zinc deficiency.
Hangnails: Protein, folic acid, and vitamin C deficiencies.
White bands on the nails: protein deficiency.
White nails: liver disease, copper excess.
White spots: zinc deficiency, thyroid deficiency, and hydrochloric acid deficiency.
Fungus under nails: lack of lactobacillus in colon.
Bluish nails: chronic lung conditions (not enough oxygen).

NATURAL REMEDIES
• **Supply the indicated deficiencies, listed above**, which apply to you.
• Eat an adequate **protein** diet, which includes **brewer's yeast, calcium, silica**. And, if necessary, add supplementary **hydrochloric acid**.
• **Water** causes the nails to swell. Upon drying, the result can be loose, brittle nails. In addition, avoid immersing the hands in **detergent water**.
• **Never cut the cuticles**. This damages the nail and invites infections. **Do not push them back**.
• *Brittle nails* are common among teenagers, pregnant women, and those with food allergies. The problem is malabsorption or nutritional deficiencies (**unsaturated essential fatty acids, amino acids, calcium, iron**, or **zinc**).
• *Hangnails* are caused by an **essential fatty acid deficiency**. Put **vitamin E oil** or **aloe vera** directly on it, to reduce further breaking and likelihood of infection. They are particularly common among women who have their hands in water a lot or who bite their nails. Keep nails clipped short. Rub **vegetable oil** into the hands occasionally.
• If you tend to pick at your nails, wear clothes with pockets. When you find yourself starting to do it, **put your hands in your pockets**.

ENCOURAGEMENT—If we commit the keeping of our souls to God by living faith, His promises will not fail us. We are limited only through our lack of faith, submission, and obedience. How thankful we can be that we have Christ as our Saviour and God as our Father! 1 John 3:1-2.

INGROWN NAILS

SYMPTOMS—The nail (usually on the big toe) has pushed into the soft tissue alongside it. Soon it results in sharp pain. Infection can result.

CAUSES—Knowing the causes reveals the remedies. Here they are:

NATURAL REMEDIES
• **Wear large enough shoes!** This is the underlying problem for many cases of ingrown nails! If you cannot solve the problem any other way, cut out the front of the shoe so the ingrown nail can heal! Podiatrists know that people who wear shoes which are large enough rarely have foot problems.
• **Never cut your nails too short! Cut toenails straight across**, not rounded. The outside edge of the nail should be parallel to the skin. Do not trim the nail deeper than the tip of the toe.
• **Soak your foot in warm water**, to soften the nail. **Dry** carefully and then **insert a tiny wisp of sterile cotton** under the burrowing edge of the nail. This will slightly lift the nail, so it can grow past the tissue. Apply some **peroxide** as a safeguard against infection. Change the cotton insert daily, until the nail has grown past the problem area.
• **Do not cut a "v"-shaped wedge** out of the center of your toenail! Doing so only worsens the problem. Nails grow from back to front, not from inward to outward or vice versa.
• If you accidentally cut or break a nail too short, **carefully smooth the edges** with an emery board.
• **Never cut nails with scissors**. None are small enough to do the job right. They often leave a sharp edge.

ENCOURAGEMENT—Prayer and faith can do what no power on earth could ever accomplish. In Christ, we can resist temptation and obey the Ten Commandments. 2 Timothy 2:12.

YELLOW NAIL SYNDROME

SYMPTOMS—Thickened nails with yellow or greenish discoloration, often accompanied by stunted growth and swelling of the ankles and sometimes other parts of the body.

CAUSES—This is a nutritional deficiency.

NATURAL REMEDIES
• Take 800 IU of **vitamin E** internally. As often as is practical, apply a little to the nails. After several months of this treatment, you will begin to see results.
Vitamin E is the specific for this problem. There are no herbs or water treatments which can accomplish the task.

ENCOURAGEMENT—God comes to all His children in their affliction. In time of danger He is their refuge. In sorrow, He offers them joy and consolation.

Shall we turn from the Redeemer, the fountain of living water, to hew out for ourselves broken cisterns which can hold no water?

EXTREMITIES - 3 - LEGS
Also: Knee Pain (615)

LEG CRAMPS

SYMPTOMS—Sudden cramping in the leg muscles.

CAUSES—The usual causes are nutritional deficiencies, circulatory problems, strain placed on the legs by excessive weight, and electrolyte imbalances.

NATURAL REMEDIES
IMMEDIATELY
A key immediate factor is inadequate or imbalanced blood circulation.
• When you leg goes into a cramp, get up and move about. Flex your feet, with your toes pointing upward.
• Apply a hot-water bottle or heating pad to the cramping area and apply pressure with your hands.
• If in bed (when the cramping begins) and you know your legs are overheated, put the hurting leg out of the covers and the cramp may immediately stop.

OTHER HELPS
• Begin eating a better diet, primarily consisting of **fresh fruits, vegetables, whole grains, legumes, and nuts**. Do not overeat.
• It is important that you take **calcium** (2,000 mg), **magnesium** (1,000 mg), and **potassium** (5,500 mg) and that you take them in balanced amounts. Without enough calcium, muscles tend to go into spasms.
• Do not stand in one place too long. **Move about**. Shift your weight from one foot to the other. Wiggle your toes. Keep the circulation moving.
Take a **long walk** every day. Relax as you do it and breath well.
• When sleeping or sitting, sometimes **elevate your feet** above your heart.

ENCOURAGEMENT—When danger approaches, shall we seek for help from those as weak as ourselves, or shall we flee to Him who is mighty to save? His arms are open wide, and He utters the gracious invitation, "Come unto me, all ye that labour and are heavy laden, and I will give you rest." How very thankful we can be that we have such a wonderful heavenly Father!

LEG ULCERS

SYMPTOMS—Open sores which develop on deteriorated patches of skin.

CAUSES—Leg ulcers are primarily caused by **poor blood circulation** in the legs. The flow of blood is restricted, and poorly nourished skin tissue can become ulcerated.

The poor circulation restricts the open sore to very slow healing.

Other causes include **varicose veins** *(535)*, and/or **thrombophlebitis** *(533)*.

When veins in the legs stop functioning properly, venous ulcers can result. Blood is not returning to the heart as it should; the skin above the veins becomes inflamed and sores develop. *Venous ulcers* are generally located on the lowest one-third of the leg.

Arterial ulcers are different. An **embolism** or **atheroscleroitic plaque** blocks the proper flow of blood through an artery, causing ulcers on bony areas around the feet and ankles.

Diabetic ulcers are surface ulcers on the skin (usually the feet), caused by **diabetes** *(656)*.

NATURAL REMEDIES
• Improve your diet and way of life. Eat **fresh fruits, vegetables, whole grains, legumes, and nuts**. Do not overeat.
• Avoid **sugary, fatty, starchy, fried, and processed foods**. Do not use **caffeine, alcohol, or tobacco**. If **overweight**, reduce.
• **Garlic** improves blood circulation. **Vitamin C** (1,000 mg) and **vitamin K** (140 mcg) strengthens tissues. Take a full **multivitamin supplement**.

ENCOURAGEMENT—Those who turn to God with heart and soul and mind will find in Him peaceful security. John 14:27.

EXTREMITIES - 4 - FEET
Also: Bone Spur (612)

FOOT PROBLEMS

SYMPTOMS—Feet that hurt all the time. Toes which are curling and become twisted.

NATURAL REMEDIES
• **Shoes that are too small,** shoes that are **too narrow in the toes,** and **high heel shoes** are the source of most foot problems. When you select shoes, purchase **walking shoes, not stylish ones.**

WATER THERAPY
• Here are summaries of some of the information in the chapter on *Hydrotherapy (206-275)*:
Numbness in feet: Give a hot **Fomentation** to the spine, accompanied by **Hot or Alternate Sponging** of the limbs. Repeat this 3 times a day.
Sweating feet: Give **Alternate** very hot and very cold **Footbaths**. During the night, apply a **Heating Chest Pack** to the feet. Give a **Cold Mitten Friction** to the feet in the morning, on arising.
Weak, pronated feet: Put the feet and part of the legs in tubs for **Contrast Baths**. Begin with a temperature of 110° F., and then after four minutes, change to tap water for 1 minute. Change back and forth 4-6 times, and end with the hot water. During the treatment, the temperature of the hot water should be gradually raised to 115°-120° F. The tap water should be gradually lowered to the temperature of ice water. Give the treatment twice a day.
Infections in the feet: Give the same treatment as for pronated feet, above.

ENCOURAGEMENT—It is Jesus that we need. His presence and help must be ours continually. God wants every one of us perfect in Christ. Through His strengthening grace, we can overcome sin and the devil. How thankful we can be for enabling grace! Were it not for the help of God, we could not resist the temptations of the devil. Matthew 19:29.

CORNS AND CALLUSES
(Bunions, Calluses, Warts)

SYMPTOMS AND CAUSES—Pressure and rubbing causes calluses on the bottoms and sides of the feet. They can also form on the hands, and even on the elbows and knees.

Corns form between toes and remain soft from foot perspiration. They occur from the rubbing of adjacent digit bones.

Corns are more painful than calluses.

NATURAL REMEDIES
• Wear proper shoes! **Never wear tight-fitting footwear!**
• **Do not use "corn plasters."** These contain acids intended to eat away at the corns. But they also eat into nearby normal flesh.
• **Do not cut** corns and calluses! This only makes the situation worse. This especially applies to diabetics.
• A corn or callus is hard, dry skin. Regularly moisturizing that skin is the key to healing. As soon as a corn develops, **apply oil** to soften. Or soak your feet in very diluted **chamomile** tea. It will both soothe and soften the hard skin. (The stain the tea makes on the feet will come off easily with soap and water.) Or just soak the feet in comfortably **hot water** for several minutes. Then apply a **hand cream which contains 20% urea**. This will help dissolve the hard skin. Do this daily. Another daily formula is to soak the area in a mixture of **oil of wintergreen, witch hazel, and black walnut** tincture. Use a pumice stone and emery board to trim down the corn or callus.

EXTR

• Open a **fresh fig** and tape the pulp to the corn overnight. Or cut a square of **pineapple peel** and tape the inner side to the corn overnight. Next morning, remove it and soak the foot in hot water. An hour or two later you should be able to remove the corn fairly easily. Or rub it gently with a **pumice stone**.

• Herbalists in many lands apply **calendula** oil or salve. Or massage the corns twice a day with **caster oil**, **vitamin E** oil, or a salve prepared from equal parts **soft soap** and **roasted onions**.

• Another method is to crush 5-6 **aspirin tablets** and mix into a paste, by adding a half tsp. each of **water** and **lemon juice**. Apply this to the hard-skin areas. Put the foot in a **plastic bag**, wrap a warm towel around it, and sit for 10 minutes. Then unwrap the foot and scrub the area with a **pumice stone**. The dead, hardened flesh should come loose and flake off.

• Put a few drops of **citric acid** on the area. The next morning, use an **emery board or pumice stone** and rub off the dead skin.

• A variant method is to soak a piece of cotton in fresh **lemon or pineapple juice**. **Bandage** the cotton over the area. This will dissolve it, but you must be persistent.

• Any **sweet oil** rubbed on the area several times a day, plus the use of the **emery board or pumice stone**, will skim off the dead flesh.

• Other ways to soften the skin: Soak your feet in water from cooked **oatmeal**. Bandage the corns overnight with a paste of **bread crumbs, apple cider vinegar, brewer's yeast, and lemon juice**.

• Apply a non-medicated **corn pad** (a small oval or round pad with a hole in the middle) to the corn. If necessary, stretch the pad so it does not touch the corn in the center. Apply **vitamin E** oil, cover, and tape. Repeat frequently.

IMPROVING YOUR SHOES

• After purchasing larger shoes, put some **lamb's wool between the toes**, separating them.

• You can purchase Stella's Stretch All (or another **leather-stretching solution**) from a shoe store. Apply it to the shoes and then walk in them while wet. Repeat this frequently and the leather shoe will widen out.

• Women should **never wear high-heel shoes**. They ruin the feet, damage the spine, and throw the pelvic organs out of place.

• Women should **not wear pumps**. These are shoes which cause the foot to slide forward, jamming everything into the front. Instead, wear an **oxford-style shoe, with laces**. This properly cradles the foot.

• Always buy **shoes which breathe. Leather** is the best.

• An **undersized shoe** will damage the toes and cause corns, etc. An **oversized shoe** will produce friction and break the skin. But, of the two, oversized shoes are the less harmful.

Some calluses are useful, never painful, and should not be disturbed.

ENCOURAGEMENT—We are seldom placed in the same position twice. There are continually new experiences to be encountered. But, if we will trust in Christ, He will enable us to overcome sin in spite of all that comes our way. James 4:7.

FOOT ACHES

SYMPTOMS—Tired, aching feet.

CAUSES—Inadequate diet and rest, ill-fitting or small shoes, hard ground and floor surfaces, plus being on your feet all day long.

The average person walks 45,000 miles by the age of 35. Each step places a force that is one-third greater than full body weight on each foot. The feet contain 56 bones, plus 107 ligaments, 31 tendons, and 18 muscles. Your feet need good nutrition, plus some other helps.

NATURAL REMEDIES

• Improve the **diet**. Get enough **protein, calcium, and B vitamins**. Stop eating **junk food**. It isn't worth taking the time to chew and swallow. Your diet should be rich in **whole foods, vegetables, and fiber**. Eat **whole grains, nuts, and legumes**.

• **Avoid saturated fats, fried foods, sugars, alcohol, meat, caffeine, chocolate, sodas, salt, and oxalic acid-forming foods**.

• Lose that excess **weight**. It is hard on your feet.

DURING THE DAY

• Always wear **low shoes**, shoes which **fasten firmly**.

• During the day, **lift one foot** and **give it a good shake**. Then lift the other and do likewise. Then relax and **flex your toes** up and down.

• When standing in one place, **keep changing your stance. Try to keep moving** about. If possible, stand on a **carpet or a rubber mat**. Ask the boss if you can buy a rubber mat and lay it on the floor in your work area.

• Take an **ice chest** with you to work. While eating lunch, put your feet in the cold water. Then dry and put on a fresh pair of **dry socks**.

IN THE EVENING

• **Elevate your feet** when you come home at night. Then **soak them** in a basin of warm water, containing 1-2 Tsp. of **Epsom salt**. Rinse with clear, cool water.

• Make a **footbath** with 2 handfuls of **comfrey** root to 1 gallon warm water. Soak your feet 15 minutes.

• Sit on the edge of the bathtub and alternately run (to your comfort) **hot and cold water** over your feet, ending with the cold. (If you have diabetes, be careful about extremes in temperature.)

• Wrap some **ice cubes** in a wet washcloth and rub it over your feet and ankles for a few minutes.

• **Remove your shoes, sit in a chair, and stretch your feet out**. Then, below the ankle, **move each foot in ten circles. Point your toes down and then up**.

• Gently **roll your foot over a golf ball, tennis ball, or rolling pin** for a couple minutes.

• Scatter a few pencils on the floor and **pick them up with your toes**.

• For a terrific **foot massage**, toss a handful of beans in a moccasin-style shoe, and walk gently around the room on them.

• In the evening, sit down and put on a pair of **soft slippers**.

ENCOURAGEMENT—It is a part of God's plan to grant us, in answer to the prayer of faith, that which He would not bestow did we not thus ask. Oh, please, my friend, believe and know that God is your best Friend! Ecclesiastes 8:12.

HEEL PAIN

SYMPTOMS—Your heel hurts.

CAUSES—Underlying causes frequently include **standing, walking, exercising on hard surfaces,** and **excessive walking or athletic activity.** Other causes include these: **Arthritis, gout,** an **infection**. It is rare to be caused by a **benign tumor**.

• **Irritation from the back of a shoe** produces painful bumps on the back of the heel (called pump bumps).

There are several types of heel problems:

• Simple **bruises**. If your heel hurts only when you push down on it or press it with your fingers, it may just be bruised.

• Then there are **heel spurs**. These are bony and sometimes painful growths on the heel. These occur when the plantar fascia is pulled slightly off the heel bone.

• *Plantar fasciitis* is an **inflammation of the band of tissue (fascia)** that runs from the heel bone to the metatarsal bones at the base of the toes. This causes pain on the bottom of the foot near the heel. The pain is worse upon awakening and better later in the day.

• **Stress fractures** are microscopic cracks in the bone. They hurt in the morning and get worse as the day progresses.

NATURAL REMEDIES

You may need to see a medical specialist.

• Recommended herbs include **valerian, turmeric, and boswellia**. Soak the foot in **peppermint** and **skullcap**.

• Try to **reduce the intensity of your daily foot work** and foot load.

• Holding onto a railing for support, **stretch the**

calf muscles by placing both feet on a bottom stair, with half of the feet extended out from the stair. Then carefully rise up on the toes and down about 5 times, gradually building up to 15 or 20. This stretching will help flex the calf muscle. Do this exercise after walking outdoors to warm up the muscles.

ENCOURAGEMENT—He knows just what we need, just what we can bear; and He will give us grace to endure every trial and test that He brings upon us. Our constant prayer should be for a greater nearness to God.

BURNING FEET

SYMPTOMS—Feet which seem to burn at night.

CAUSES—There is a specific factor affecting this. It is a lack of **niacin** (vitamin B3). However, there are also several other possible causes, discussed below.

NATURAL REMEDIES

• **Add niacin or niacinamide to your diet**. Either one will accomplish the task of eliminating the sense of burning feet. But niacin will cause your face to flush red and hot for a couple minutes when you swallow it while niacinamide will not.

• A secondary cause would be **air-excluding shoes** or **perspiration-retaining cotton or wool socks**. Wear leather shoes, not synthetic ones. If possible, change your socks halfway through each day.

• There can also be **allergic reactions** to the dye in new hosiery, the chemicals used in tanning leather, or the rubber compounds in athletic shoes. Did you ever notice that synthetic shoes smell like rubber tires?

• Another possible cause of scorching soles and tingling feet could be **nerve inflammation**, which would be reduced or eliminated by taking a **B complex supplement**—specifically, B_1, B_2, panthothenic acid for burning feet, B_6, and B_{12} to eliminate the pins-and-needles sensation. Drink **brewer's yeast**, stirred into water or juice.

• **Cool or cold foot baths** will invigorate and strengthen the feet.

If the foot only "burns" in one place (especially between your toes), a blister (*319*) or athlete's foot (*377*) may be developing.

Burning feet that do not respond to the above care might be an early warning of the onset of diabetes (*656*).

ENCOURAGEMENT—To have a new heart is to have a new mind, new purposes, and new motives. What is the sign of a new heart? It is a changed life. Through the merits of Christ's righteousness, we can overcome temptation to doubt and sin. We can live clean, godly lives.

SWELLING FEET

SYMPTOMS—Feet that seem swollen and achy.

E
X
T
R

CAUSES—Our feet receive a lot of pounding all day long. Sometimes they need a little special care, plus more rest and an improvement of your overall diet.

NATURAL REMEDIES

• Improve your diet. Stop the **junk food** and eat a **nutritious diet** which includes **vitamin-mineral supplementation**.

• Alternate 5 minutes of comfortably hot **saltwater soaking** with 2 minutes in **cool** water. Repeat the sequence and then rinse with **cold** water. Dry the feet and put on **fresh socks**.

• Occasionally sit with your **feet elevated**.

• While sitting down, **roll your bare feet** over tennis balls or a rolling pin. Using your feet and toes alone, **scrunch up** a terry cloth towel on the floor or try to **pick up** marbles or pencils.

• Here is an herbal tea to reduce swelling feet: Mix equal parts **white oak bark, wormwood, and shave grass**. Steep 1 Tbsp. in ½ cup boiling-hot water. Take in tsp. doses.

ENCOURAGEMENT—Every provision has been made to meet the needs of our spiritual and our moral nature. Light and immortality are brought to light through the Lord Jesus Christ. Jesus has said that He has set before us an open door; and no man can shut it.

FOOT ODOR

SYMPTOMS—Feet that do not smell very nice.

CAUSES—Bacteria on the feet, cheap shoes, or eating meat.

NATURAL REMEDIES

• **Wash your feet** frequently. Keep them clean. Scrub gently with a soft brush, including between the toes. Dry them well when finished.

• Put **talcum powder** in your shoes, to help keep them dry.

• **Change your socks** often, several times a day if necessary. This is one of the best things you can do. You do not want to walk around in wet socks.

• Some find help in wearing **two pairs** of socks at a time. This increases the elimination of sweat.

• **Soak your feet** (15 minutes, twice a week) in ½ cup **vinegar** added to 1 quart of water.

• Soak them in pans or pails of alternate **hot and cold water**. But if you are diabetic or have impaired circulation, it may be best that you not do this.

• Sprinkle some dry, crumbled **sage leaves** into your shoes, to control odor.

• Buy **leather shoes**, for they breathe. This reduces the perspiration. **Avoid rubber or synthetic shoes**. They cause your feet to smell like rubber tires at the end of the day—yet the odor is not from the feet! Even expensive rubber shoes, "endorsed by the athletes," can do this.

• Do not use **antiperspirants**. For they contain aluminum (a cause of Alzheimer's disease). **Spray deodorants** are breathed into the lungs.

• **Avoid spicy, pungent foods**. For their odor will be found in your feet later on.

• **Avoid stress**. It increases sweating, which multiplies bacterial action.

ENCOURAGEMENT—To love as Christ loved means to reveal unselfishness at all times, in all places, by kind words and pleasant looks. The Lord will help every one of us where we need help the most in overcoming and conquering self. Psalm 110:3. How very thankful we can be that we have such a wonderful heavenly Father! He is always kind to His earthly children. We may safely go to Him and entrust our case with Him. If faithful, soon we will be with Him in heaven. Oh happy thought!

COLD FEET

SYMPTOMS—Feet which seem cold too much of the time.

CAUSES—This might be caused by some deeper problem—such as **diabetes** *(656)*, **hypothyroidism** *(659)*, **Raynaud's disease** *(368)*, **Buerger's disease** *(370)*, etc.

NATURAL REMEDIES

• Put your feet in **cold water** for 1 minute, dry them, then **jump rope, run, or walk** for 1-2 minutes. Do this 3-4 times a day.

• If you have a lawn by your house, **walk barefoot** for a few minutes on the cool, wet lawn when you arise. Then quickly dry the feet, put on fresh socks, put on your shoes, and keep active until the feet thoroughly warm. Forget about the neighbors when you do this. You are having more fun than they are. Perhaps they will start doing it too. Better yet, move to the country and exercise.

ENCOURAGEMENT—The pure in heart will see God. It is only God that can, by grace, enable us to choose to be pure. By faith, we walk and talk with our Redeemer, and live His life. Jeremiah 31:18

FLATFEET
(Pes Planus)

SYMPTOMS—The concave arch supporting the bottom of the feet is flattening out, resulting in more exhaustion during the day when you are on your feet.

CAUSES—**Inadequate circulation, impoverished diet, and junk food** may be involved. It can also be caused when frail children **carry heavy weights** in their youth. Once this problem develops it is generally not solved later, especially since it often occurs in childhood when parents are not aware of what is happening until it is too late. So awareness and prevention are especially important.

NATURAL REMEDIES

• Try walking upstairs **barefoot on your toes**, and then back down the same way. Support yourself on a railing as you do this. Do this 10 minutes each day, for a month while eating a **nourishing, moderate diet**. The muscles in your feet may strengthen. By helping your flat feet, your eyesight may also improve.

• If you cannot solve your flatfoot problem (perhaps because it occurred when you were a child and you did not discover it till later), **learn to adapt your step to the condition**. When you take a step, land very slightly on the outer rear portion of the foot. Then, as the foot moves back, keep the weight slightly (very slightly) on the outer part of the foot. In this way, you will make an artificial arch and your foot will not tire as quickly throughout the day.

• Use a low **arch support** and gradually increase its height.

• Try to **do part of your everyday work while sitting down** occasionally. This will help rest the feet.

ENCOURAGEMENT—We may speak with Jesus wherever we may be. There is no time or place where prayer cannot be offered. Prayer rises above the noise of machinery and traffic. We are speaking to God, and He hears us. Psalm 4:3-8.

ATHLETE'S FOOT
(Tinea Pedis)

SYMPTOMS—Blisters and/or cracks on the skin of the foot, especially between the toes. This is accompanied by itching, burning, and (in extreme cases) pustules, and ulcers. As it develops, the blisters and/or cracks soften, turn white, and tend to peel off in flakes. In severe cases, there may be pain. It is worse in warmer weather.

CAUSES—Athlete's foot is caused by one or more parasitic fungi. Fungus infections on the skin are more difficult to eliminate than bacterial ones. Any condition which keeps the **feet both warm and moist** can lead to this problem. By **scratching the sores** on the foot, the disease can be spread on the hands, under the nails, and to other parts of the body.

The fungus causing athlete's foot spreads rapidly when beneficial bacteria are destroyed by **antibiotics, drugs, or radiation**.

The organisms causing it are spread by walking barefoot on the **contaminated floors surrounding pools, showers, and other public places**.

NATURAL REMEDIES

• Eat a **nourishing diet**, including lots of **fruits and vegetables**, and **skip the processed and junk foods**. Obtain **vitamins A, B complex, and C**. Eat **whole grains, nuts, and legumes**.

• **Avoid meat, cola drinks, caffeine, sugary foods, and fried foods.**

• Eat a nourishing diet; and skip the processed and junk foods. Obtain vitamins **A, B complex, and C**.

• **Keep your feet dry**. After bathing, **dry carefully between the toes**. Wear **cotton socks** and **change them daily** (ideally, twice a day).

• **Shoes:** To help keep your feet cool and dry, only wear shoes that will not make your feet sweat. **Leather shoes** are best. **Avoid rubber shoes**, even the expensive ones. Do not use **plastic or waterproof shoes**. They create a warm, moist place for fungi to breed. Never wear heavy **boots** all day.

• Do not wear the same shoes 2 days in a row. This gives a pair of shoes 2 days to thoroughly dry out. Spray Lysol on a cloth and wipe the inside of the shoe.

• **Socks:** To help keep your feet cool and dry, change your socks 3-4 times a day. Boil socks to kill the fungus. After washing them, rinse the socks well, to get out the detergent (which the fungus likes). Put on clean socks before dressing. In this way you avoid infecting the groin area.

• **Sunlight:** Fungi hates sunlight. When in the acute stage, try to **leave your feet uncovered**. Every so often, **put them in the sunlight**. **Walking barefoot outside in the sunlight** is excellent. Place your shoes in the sunlight, angled toward the sun. Ultraviolet light kills fungus.

• **Do not walk barefoot** around the house, so others will not become infected. Also, **never walk barefoot in public places** (public showers, locker rooms, pool decks, motels, hotels). Wear shoes or slippers.

HERBS

Cut raw **garlic** into tiny pieces and, for several days, put some minced pieces in the closed toe of your shoes. Purchase **garlic powder** and twice a day dust your feet with it. Garlic is better than antifungal drugs! Other outstanding antifungal herbs include **ginger, licorice, chamomile, echinacea, goldenseal, astragalus, and oil of turmeric**.

• Apply natural antifungicides, such as **pau d'arco** or **tea tree oil** to your feet. **Drink** 3 cups of pau d'arco tea daily. Also put a strong mixture of it **on your feet**.

• Add 20 drops of **tea tree oil** to a small tub of water. **Soak your feet in it** for 15 minutes, 3 times a day. Dry well afterward and place some undiluted tea tree oil on the feet.

• Apply **plantain and tea tree oil** to the affected area.

• Apply **lemon juice** 1-2 times a day to the area and let it dry. Another method is to apply a strong tea of crushed **juniper berries**. Mash **garlic** with some oil and apply to the area.

• Apply a **baking soda** paste to the area, especially between the toes. Mix 1 Tbsp. of baking soda with a little warm water. Apply, then dry well, and dust feet with **talcum powder**. It is rock dust and not digestible to fungi.

• Twice daily, coat the area with **aloe vera gel, onion juice,** or **vitamin E oil**.

• Once a day, soak your feet in an herb tea **footbath of goldenseal, thyme**, or a half-and-half mixture of **thyme and chamomile tea**.

• Bathe the feet daily in 50-50 **vinegar** and water. Dry well. Then apply a **vegetable oil** to the affected area.

• Soak your foot in a mixture of 2 tsp. of **salt** per pint of warm water, for 5-10 minutes. Dry well and repeat till the problem is solved.

• Apply **goldenseal** powder to the area. At bedtime, cover the area with raw **honey**. Sleep in cotton socks and wash the feet in the morning.

• Crush a green plant juice—such as **chickweed, plantain, Swiss chard,** etc., and apply the juice to the area. Then walk about barefooted in the sun.

Keep in mind that applying overly strong applications to athlete's foot can result in rashes breaking out on hands and elsewhere. If you have unknowingly done this, treat the feet more gently. And, as the foot infection clears, the sympathetic rashes will also.

• In case there is pain, place **cold compresses** on the area. If the problem worsens and pus or a fever develops, see a professional.

—*Also see Antifungal herbs (299) and Ringworm (335), which is a closely related fungal skin disease.*

ENCOURAGEMENT—When we receive Christ as an abiding guest in the soul, the peace of God (which passeth all understanding) keeps our hearts and minds through faith in Christ. How thankful we can be that in Him we can have peace of heart amid trials and turmoil.

More Encouragement

"Like Nicodemus, we must be willing to enter into life in the same way as the chief of sinners. Than Christ, 'there is none other name under heaven given among men, whereby we must be saved.' Acts 4:12. Through faith we receive the grace of God; but faith is not our Saviour. It earns nothing. It is the hand by which we lay hold upon Christ, and appropriate His merits, the remedy for sin. And we cannot even repent without the aid of the Spirit of God. The Scripture says of Christ, 'Him hath God exalted with His right hand to be a Prince and a Saviour, for to give repentance to Israel, and forgiveness of sins.' Acts 5:31. Repentance comes from Christ as truly as does pardon.

"How, then, are we to be saved? 'As Moses lifted up the serpent in the wilderness,' so the Son of man has been lifted up, and everyone who has been deceived and bitten by the serpent may look and live. 'Behold the Lamb of God, which taketh away the sin of the world.' John 1:29. The light shining from the cross reveals the love of God. His love is drawing us to Himself. If we do not resist this drawing, we shall be led to the foot of the cross in repentance for the sins that have crucified the Saviour. Then the Spirit of God through faith produces a new life in the soul. The thoughts and desires are brought into obedience to the will of Christ. The heart, the mind, are created anew in the image of Him who works in us to subdue all things to Himself. Then the law of God is written in the mind and heart, and we can say with Christ, 'I delight to do Thy will, O my God.' Psalm 40:8."

—**Desire of Ages, 175-176**

Two editions of Desire of Ages, the classic (and best) book on the life of Christ are available from us.

More Encouragement

"There are many whose hearts are aching under a load of care because they seek to reach the world's standard. They have chosen its service, accepted its perplexities, adopted its customs. Thus their character is marred, and their life made a weariness. In order to gratify ambition and worldly desires, they wound the conscience, and bring upon themselves an additional burden of remorse. The continual worry is wearing out the life forces. Our Lord desires them to lay aside this yoke of bondage. He invites them to accept His yoke; He says, 'My yoke is easy, and My burden is light.' He bids them seek first the kingdom of God and His righteousness, and His promise is that all things needful to them for this life shall be added.

"Worry is blind, and cannot discern the future; but Jesus sees the end from the beginning. In every difficulty He has His way prepared to bring relief. Our heavenly Father has a thousand ways to provide for us, of which we know nothing. Those who accept the one principle of making the service and honor of God supreme will find perplexities vanish, and a plain path before their feet.

" 'Learn of Me,' says Jesus; 'for I am meek and lowly in heart: and ye shall find rest.' We are to enter the school of Christ, to learn from Him meekness and lowliness. Redemption is that process by which the soul is trained for heaven. This training means a knowledge of Christ. It means emancipation from ideas, habits, and practices that have been gained in the school of the prince of darkness. The soul must be delivered from all that is opposed to loyalty to God.

"In the heart of Christ, where reigned perfect harmony with God, there was perfect peace. He was never elated by applause, nor dejected by censure or disappointment. Amid the greatest opposition and the most cruel treatment, He was still of good courage. But many who profess to be His followers have an anxious, troubled heart, because they are afraid to trust themselves with God. They do not make a complete surrender to Him; for they shrink from the consequences that such a surrender may involve. Unless they do make this surrender, they cannot find peace."

—Desire of Ages, 330

Two editions of Desire of Ages, the classic (and best) book on the life of Christ are available from us.

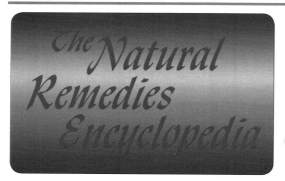

The Natural Remedies Encyclopedia

- Disease Section 4 -
Head and Throat

H E A D

= *Information, not a disease*

Special Senses: Physiology 1023/ Pictures 1036-1037

"Fear thou not; for I am with thee."—*Isaiah 41:10.*

"The name of the Lord is a strong tower: the righteous runneth into it, and is safe."—*Proverbs 18:10.*

Section 4 - Head and Throat

— HEAD AND THROAT —
1 - HEAD

See Headache (556) and
Common Cold (289).

SINUS TROUBLE
(Sinusitis)

SYMPTOMS—One or more of the following symptoms: facial pain and tenderness on the cheekbones, face, and forehead. Also earache, headache, dry cough, bad breath, fever, dazed feeling in the head, loss of smell, and burning and tearing eyes. Sometimes it results in a swollen face, stuffy nose, and a thick mucous discharge. Congestion and pressure in the interior passageways of the skull behind the nose, forehead, and cheeks. It may result in a throbbing pain or a sinus headache.

CAUSES—The nasal sinuses are located in the bones surrounding the eyes and nose. They help your voice sound fuller and richer. They also help store overflow phlegm in time of illness. These five sinus cavities (frontal, maxillary, nasal, ethnoidal, and sphenoidal) humidify and warm the air you inhale.

Sinusitis is an inflammation of the nasal sinuses that generally occurs together with upper respiratory infection. Colds or bacterial and viral infections spread into the sinuses.

Sinus problems which have become chronic may be caused by **injury** of the nasal bones, **smoking, small growths in the nose, or irritant fumes and odors**.

Allergenic sinusitis may result from plant **pollens** (hay fever) and allergies to **milk** or **dairy products**; but this is less likely from **wheat**.

An **overacid condition** in the stomach can cause sinus troubles. **Poor digestion** of starch, sugar, and dairy products can produce a runny nose. When force is used in **blowing the nose**, phlegm is pushed up into the sinuses.

Swimming or **diving** can force phlegm up into the sinuses.

Allergic rhinitis is a common cause of sinusitis. Avoid substances which might be giving you allergies.

Decayed teeth, enlarged and infected adenoids, cigarette smoke, perfume, household cleansers, and dusty air can cause irritation to the sinuses.

It can also be caused by **infection**. If drainage is clear after a week, you probably do not have an infection. But, if mucus is greenish or yellowish, you do. If drainage is clear and there are no accompanying symptoms of a common cold, you probably have an **allergy**. Few people with sinus trouble have actual sinus infection (sinusitis).

Beware of swelling around the eyes! If left untreated, this can lead to bronchitis, asthma, throat infection, or pneumonia.

If you are interested in figuring out which sinuses may be bothering you, here is some helpful data:

Frontal sinuses produce frontal headaches which are most severe between 8 a.m. and 5 p.m.

Maxillary sinuses make pain in the upper teeth and cheek, and sometimes eye pain as well. It generally lasts from 11 a.m. to 6 p.m.

Ethmoid sinuses induce a dull pain behind the eyes, pain in eye movements, tearing, light sensitivity, and occasionally sore throat and nighttime cough.

NATURAL REMEDIES

• **Do not ignore** a cold, flu, sore throat, infected tonsils, other acute disease, or try to suppress it with drugs. **Go to bed, take juices and light meals, rest, and get well**. When suppressed, the phlegm does not flow out, but hardens in the sinuses and trouble begins.

• Take a **short fast** on citrus juices, vegetable juices, and herb teas.

• Drink lots of **water and juices**. This keeps the fluids in your nose loose and flowing instead of hardening.

• As soon as you are able, begin eating **nourishing**

FOR MORE NATURAL REMEDIES:

HERBS: <u>Herb Contents</u> (pp. 129-130) will help you locate the 126 most important herbs and the diseases each one can treat. <u>How to prepare herbs</u> (132). <u>How to use them</u> (141-189)

HYDROTHERAPY: <u>Therapy Contents</u> (pp. 206-207) and its <u>Disease Index</u> (263-265) will lead you to over 100 water therapies and many more remedies. DIS. INDEX: 1211- / GEN. INDEX: 1221-

VITAMINS AND MINERALS: <u>Contents</u> (100-101). <u>Using</u> 101-124. <u>Dosages</u> (124). Others (117)

CARING FOR THE SICK: <u>Home care</u> for a sick person (28-36). The healing crisis (36-39)

WOMEN'S SECTIONS: Female Organs (672) Pregnancy (701). Childbirth (765). Infancy, Childhood (722). Women's Herbs (754, 760)

EMERGENCIES: (973-). FIRST AID: (990-)

food—especially vegetables, fruits, nuts, legumes, and beans. Drink fresh **carrot juice** everyday. Eat only **fresh foods** (not canned) for the rest of the week to cleanse the system. Slowly add back **whole grains** and vegetable protein (**beans**, etc.).

• Take 500 mg of **vitamin C** every 2 hours of the day until the sinus problem disappears.

• **NAC** (N-acetylcysteine) is a form of the amino acid cysteine. Taking 500 mg, twice a day, helps liquefy mucus so that it can drain.

• **Do not eat meat, dairy products, white-flour foods, sugar, coffee, alcohol, spices, or tobacco**. Avoid **cigarette smoke**. **Milk products** clog the sinuses and make the situation worse.

• Drinking **hot liquids** help the sinuses flow out their contents.

HERBS

• Helpful herbs to reduce sinus congestion include **comfrey, slippery elm, fenugreek, mullein, aloe vera, yerba santa, red clover, and white oak bark**.

• **Garlic** contains a chemical which makes mucus less sticky. **Horseradish** has it also. **Cayenne** acts in a somewhat similar manner. **Peppermint** tea also helps open up the sinus passageways.

• Add crushed **garlic** cloves to 4 cups water and remove from the heat after coming to a boil. Cool and gradually drink. This will help clean out the sinuses and relieve stuffiness. Raw garlic is the most powerful remedy for sinusitis.

• Eat a healing vegetable soup, in which you add **garlic, onions, horseradish, cayenne, and ginger** to the vegetables.

• Take **echinacea** tea for a week and switch to **goldenseal** for the next week. Both are powerful antibiotics.

• Mix **eucalyptus oil** or **peppermint oil** with a few drops of vegetable oil and rub it on the forehead and temples to relieve sinusitis, but do not drink this.

• Place **peppermint leaves** over the painful area or apply a compress containing strong peppermint tea.

• Inhale **eucalyptus, peppermint, and sodium bicarbonate** for 20 minutes to remove the sinus secretions.

• **Oregano, ginkgo, and bromelain** also help clear the sinuses.

• Jethro Kloss suggests putting a tsp. of **bayberry bark** into a cup of boiling water, simmer 30 minutes, strain; and, when warm or cool, sniff it up the nose, one nostril at a time. It will cleanse and heal.

• An alternative is add ½ tsp. **sea salt** per cup of distilled water, taste it to see if it is half as salty as the ocean, then sniff it up your nose. Another alternative: Sniff up each nostril a tsp. of **goldenseal** or **mullein**.

OTHER HELPS

• Do not use **nose drops**. They aggravate the situation by stopping the drainage and hardening the mucus.

Decongestants also increase blood pressure.

• Placing **heat** on the sinuses helps relieve pain. This can be **compresses which are hot and wet, a heat lamp, a 60-watt light bulb, or a heating pad**.

• A variation of this is: Twice a day, lean over a pan of hot water with a towel draped over your head (or stand in a hot shower). **Inhale the vapors** as they waft up toward your nose. If you are at work, order a cup of something hot. And, leaning over, sniff up the moisture. An alternative: After the water has come to a boil, turn it off and add 15 drops of **eucalyptus** or **peppermint**. Then cover your head and inhale.

• Some prefer **cold applications** to the sinuses instead of hot ones. Put **crushed ice** in a plastic sack, wrap in a moist towel, and place over the sinus which hurts. At the same time, have the **feet in hot water**. This will help draw blood from the sinus area. However, the hot method is better for draining the sinuses.

• Mix 1 teaspoon of **salt** with 2 cups warm water. Pour it into a small glass. And, holding back your head, sniff it up into one nostril (as you pinch the other one closed). Repeat for the other side.

• **Rubbing** your sore sinuses brings a fresh supply of blood to the area. Press your thumbs firmly on either side of your nose and hold for 15-30 seconds.

• Pain relief was reported by 75% of a test group, after a mechanical vibrator was placed on the midline of the forehead or over the most tender area (45 minutes a day for as many days as needed).

• Sit with your **head down**, between your knees. Cough gently as though you were clearing your throat. Then hold your breath for a minute or so, as the mucus slowly drains. Then gently inhale. Be sure you are drinking enough fluids when you do this.

• **Twice a day**, apply a heating pad to your chest. Then lie with the top half of the body off the bed, using the forearms as support. This will help drainage of the lungs. Remain in this position 5-15 minutes, and cough and expectorate (spit) into a basin on the floor.

• **Walking** helps clear your sinuses.

• Each day, between meals, take six **charcoal** tablets with water. This will help remove toxins. Only do this during the crisis, or it can cause temporary constipation.

• It is better to **sniffle** than to blow your nose. If you must blow, only blow lightly and through one nostril at a time. **Wiping** the nose is better than blowing it.

• A **humidifier** will help keep sinuses moist indoors during the winter months. A humidity of 40%-50% increases sinus comfort.

• **Avoid cold, damp** living, working, and sleeping quarters.

ENCOURAGEMENT—Ask God to do for you those things which you cannot do for yourself. Tell Jesus everything. Lay open before Him the secrets of your heart;

for His eye reads it all. Surrender your life to Him. And let Him enable you to obey His Ten Commandment law. Ephesians 6:24.

How very thankful we are that, in all our problems, we have a kind heavenly Father we can turn to. He understands us better than we understand ourselves. He alone can provide the needed healing of heart and soul and body.

— HEAD AND THROAT —
2 - HAIR

BALDNESS AND HAIR LOSS
(Alopecia)

SYMPTOMS—It is hair on the head that we are concerned with here. There are several types of hair loss: baldness or loss of hair *(alopecia)*. Loss of all scalp hair *(alopecia totalis)*. Hair falling out in patches *(alopecia areata)*. Another type of hair loss is localized and caused by scarring.

Alopecia most frequently occurs in men, but occasionally in women. Most common of all is the standard male pattern of baldness and the female pattern of baldness.

A youthful scalp has 100,000-200,000 hairs. A single hair generally lasts 2-6 years and is then replaced by a new hair. When baldness begins, there is an excess of shorter, thinner hair—the kind babies have on their head.

Remember that it is normal to lose as much as 100 hairs a day. Once the hair follicle dies, it never again produces hair. Yet there are instances in which the follicle has not died, but only has stopped producing hair. Careful treatment restores hair growth.

CAUSES—**Heredity (especially in men), hormonal factors, aging, local or systemic disease.** Localized hair loss could also be caused by **scarring** following a wound or an operation.

Other factors include **poor circulation, high fever or other acute illness, surgery, radiation (x-ray therapy), medicinal drugs, anesthesia, drastic reducing diets, stress (depletes B vitamins), poor diet, skin disease, sudden weight loss, iron deficiency, thyroid disease, obesity, birth control pills, diabetes, or vitamin deficiency.** A nourishing diet should be eaten daily.

Significant causes of baldness include the use of **hair dyes, washing it daily,** or **hot-air dryers.** Hair pulled too tight in **ponytails** or **braids,** or set in **tight rollers,** can sometimes come out in patches.

Hair loss in women most often occurs after **menopause.** Some women lose some hair 2-3 months after childbirth because **hormonal changes,** during late term, tended to block normal hair loss. But this is

reversed within 6 months. **Hypothyroidism** can cause hair loss. Too little **vitamin A** can cause hair loss. And too much can do it also.

More than any other nation in the world, America has the greatest percentage of men with baldness. What is there about us, our diets, and our way of life that causes this?

NATURAL REMEDIES

• The circulation in the scalp (which is poorer in men than in women) needs to be improved. **Massaging the scalp** each day helps. **Keep the scalp and hair clean,** but **do not wash the hair too frequently. Avoid excess shampooing.**

• There should be **adequate protein** in the diet, especially **sesame seeds, pumpkin, sunflower seeds, almonds, and brewer's yeast.** But, as with everything, do not go overboard. People in the U.S. eat more protein than anyone else, yet they have the greatest hair loss.

NUTRITION

• Go on a **cleansing juice program,** for a couple days, and clean the bowels with an enema. Then only eat **nourishing food.** No more processed junk food. Eat a diet high in **fruits and vegetables and low in starch.**

• A variety of factors affect hair loss. **Minerals and vitamins** are important for hair growth. Take a good **supplement** at least twice a day. Drink **fresh vegetable juice** at least once a day. Take **vitamin A** (50,000 units daily for a short time). Several B vitamins especially affect hair growth (**biotin, inositol, niacin**) and color (**folic acid, pantothenic acid, and PABA**). Eat **Norwegian kelp or Nova Scotia dulse.**

• **Oatstraw** and **horsetail** teas are rich in silicon and trace minerals. **Rosemary** helps prevent premature baldness and stimulate head circulation. **Sage** is an astringent and helps stimulate growth. **Yarrow** helps liver activity.

• **Flaxseed oil** (2 Tbsp. daily), containing fatty acids, helps keep hair from thinning. **Black currant oil** (500-mg capsule twice a day) is even more powerful.

AVOID

• **Avoid salt, sugar, tobacco, and alcohol.** Overconsumption of salt and sugar increases dandruff and hair loss. Avoid large amounts of **vitamin A** (100,000 units daily over long periods). **Avoid crash diets** which are low in proper nutrients.

• Beware of the drug, **minoxidil.** Although given to restore scalp hair, it is high-priced and may cause heart damage. The hair it produces is of a poor quality and tends to fall out when the drug is terminated.

• Because **hair is fragile when wet,** do not comb it when wet because it can be easily broken. Avoid rubbing it too hard when it is wet. Better to squeeze out moisture with a towel and pat it dry. However, massaging your scalp (not your hair) is beneficial. **Do not blow- dry** your hair

• **Exposure to sunlight and seawater** is hard on hair.

HERBS

• Try rubbing the juice of a **quince** on the bald area everyday. Eat **flaxseed** and drink **sage** tea. Sage tea will stimulate hair growth. For falling hair, try wetting the scalp daily with strong **rosemary, sage, or white oak bark tea**.

• Dr. Christopher recommends making a strong tea of **bayberry** and rubbing it in well at night. Wash off in the morning, brush the hair thoroughly, and apply again. Possibly add a few drops of **lavender oil**. "This will quickly stop falling hair and remove dandruff."

• For centuries, men and women have massaged their scalps with **rosemary** herb in **olive oil** to maintain healthy hair.

• Eating **sesame seeds** is a Chinese remedy for preventing hair loss. Tincture of **stinging nettle** can also help prevent thinning hair.

• Make a paste of ½ tsp. **fenugreek** powder and ¾ cup unsweetened **coconut milk**. Then massage the scalp vigorously with it twice a week for 2 months.

• DHT *(dihydrotestosterone)* binds to hair follicles, shrinks them, and causes them to die and fall out. (It also causes prostate enlargement.) To eliminate this effect of DHT, take **saw palmetto** (160 mg) every morning and another dose every evening. (The product should be "concentrated and purified" and have 85%-95% fatty acids and sterols.) This herb works by preventing the conversion of *testosterone* (male sex hormone) into DHT. **Licorice** contains a compound which also blocks DHT. • The herb, **phygeum** (60-500 mg), also has this blocking action. And **nettle** (50-100 mg) enhances the effects of phygeum. **Zinc** (30 mg daily, for 6 months) helps keep DHT from getting to the hair follicles.

• Some people put a little **cayenne** pepper on their scalp. It surely will bring the blood and might even produce some hair! But it may get in the eyes! Most people are not prepared to deal with this extreme method.

• One woman had total hair loss by the age of 32. She restored it with the following formula. Using a wooden or plastic (not aluminum) utensil, mix the following essential oils in a glass bowl: 1 Tbsp. **jojoba oil**, 3 drops **rosemary oil**, 3 drops **lavender oil**, 1 drop **lemon balm**, and 1 drop **Atlas cedarwood oil**. Massage the mixture into your scalp and leave on for 30 minutes or overnight. Wash your hair, adding 1 drop of **rosemary oil** to each shampoo application. As a final rinse, add 1 drop each of **lavender oil** and **rosemary oil** to a quart of cool water and pour it over your head.

• To help hair grow, Kloss recommends **nettle, pepper grass, sage, marshmallow leaves, and burdock**.

OTHER HELPS

• There are others who **stand on their head** to bring the blood there! It is reported that this also helps. Do not do it at work, or folks will think you are crazy. (And, of course, too much of this might not be good for the brain.) A better alternative is to lie on a **slant board** for a time each day. Or **massage** your scalp in the sun.

• Never use **strong soaps or hair sprays**. Only use mild castile soaps.

• **Hats and wigs** are apt to cause hair to fall out faster, since they limit the air to the scalp.

• **Relaxing** a little more often and **reducing stress** helps women keep from losing their hair.

It is said that you must faithfully do your selected hair treatment for two months before you will begin to see results.

ENCOURAGEMENT—Happiness from earthly sources is constantly changeable. But Christ can give you peace and rest which is beyond compare. Let Him, by faith, dwell in your heart. 1 John 3:3.

DANDRUFF

SYMPTOMS—The greatest number of sebaceous (oil) glands are found on the face and scalp. Sebum, the oily secretion, lubricates the hair and scalp in order to keep both soft and pliable. Excess sebum may collect to form dandruff.

Dandruff is a covering of dead skin that prevents new hair from growing, because it cannot break through the dead skin. A scaling or flaking of scalp cells results. It may or may not be accompanied by itching.

CAUSES—A change in the surface cells of the scalp results in a scaling or flaking. This change is especially keyed to nutritional deficiencies. It often occurs in those with oily skin who are prone to develop superficial, acute, and chronic bacterial skin conditions.

There is generally excess secretion of oil in the sebaceous glands. It is this oil which binds the cells together on the scalp. Nutritional deficiencies can cause these abnormal secretions.

NATURAL REMEDIES

DIET

• **Biotin**, a B vitamin, is a major anti-dandruff compound. Take 6 mg daily. It treats both dandruff and the related seborrhea condition (overactivity of the sebaceous glands, resulting in an excessive amount of sebum). A handful of **soybeans** contains the 6 mg of biotin. **Garlic** is second in biotin content, followed by **oats, barley, avocado, alfalfa, sesame, and corn**.

• Often there are severe **B complex** deficiencies, as well as a lack of essential **unsaturated fatty acids and zinc**.

• Other important nutrients include selenium, sulfur, and lecithin.

• Cut out **excess fats, grease, and all fried foods** from the diet. Stop the use of **alcohol**. Check to see if you have **food allergies** (wheat, dairy products, citrus, or something else). **Avoid stress and poor elimination**. Do not use strong, **irritant shampoos or hair treatments**. **Avoid chocolate, sugar, white flour, and seafood**.

• Be sure the diet includes **flaxseed oil, vitamins E and A, PABA, Folic acid, B₆, and zinc**. If needed, take **digestive enzymes**. Also helpful are **kelp, biotin, and lecithin**. Eat 50%-75% **raw food**.

• A **short fast** is a good way to begin the program. Then begin eating only nutritious foods.

HAIR MASSAGE AND WASHING

• Massage **burdock root** oil into the scalp. Other herbs with anti-dandruff qualities are **comfrey, ginger, licorice, celandine, and plantain**. Make a tea of any, or several, and use them as hair rinses.

• Put 4 heaping tsp. dried **eucalyptus leaves** in a quart of boiling water. Stir. Then cover. Remove from heat and steep for an hour. Strain and pour the liquid into a squeeze bottle. Add 1 Tbsp. **apple-cider vinegar**. At the close of your shower, pour the rinse slowly over your head. For maximum effect, let it dry.

• The use of an **aloe vera shampoo**, once or twice a week, will control the dandruff.

• **Avoid** shampoos containing selenium sulfide. They can cause eye damage and hair loss.

• **Do not** put tar-based shampoos on your head if you have blonde hair. It will turn the hair brown.

• At bedtime, rub **aloe vera** gel on the scalp.

OTHER HELPS

• Kloss says that the leaves and bark of the **willow** tree, made into a tea, will cure dandruff.

• A little **sunlight** is good for your scalp and hair.

• Keep **calm and relaxed**. It will help your hair.

• **Walking outdoors** will help your hair and your entire body.

—*See Oily Hair (below).*

ENCOURAGEMENT—The peace of Christ is constant and enduring. We can find no rest apart from Him. Come, now, and make Him your own by faith.

OILY HAIR

SYMPTOMS—Excess amounts of oil in the hair. Redheads rarely have oily hair. Blondes tend to have it the most.

CAUSES—The sebaceous glands produce too much oil and there are nutritional aspects which need to be corrected. There are as many as 140,000 oil glands on the scalp. Oil wicks into fine, straight hair the easiest. Wiry hair tends to be the least oily.

Oil production tends to be increased by intense **heat and humidity. Hormonal changes and stress** can also affect it.

NATURAL REMEDIES

• **Only use clear shampoos**. They have less oil in them.

• Give yourself a **double shampoo**, with a rinse in between. After shampooing, feel your hair. Does it feel oily? This will help you know how well you are doing.

• Squeeze the juice of two **lemons** into a pint of water and use it as a finishing rinse. This helps remove soap residues which tend to weigh down the hair. Or use an apple cider **vinegar** rinse. After showering and blotting the hair dry, apply the rinse and massage it through the hair. Leave it on for 5 minutes. Then rinse with cool to tepid water.

• Or use a **horsetail** herb rinse. It strengthens the hair shafts and reduces oil on them.

• **Do not overbrush**, for this carries additional oil from the roots into the hair.

• **Avoid** too much fat in your diet. A diet of **fried foods, saturated fats, meat, and dairy products** triggers increased production of sebum. This results in an oily scalp and hair.

• Do not use a shampoo that contains *sodium lauryl sulfate* or NDELA *(nitrosodiethanolamine)*. Both are harsh and dry the scalp, perhaps causing flaking.

—*Many of the suggestions in Dandruff (above) should be considered.*

ENCOURAGEMENT—When you have asked for the things your soul needs, believe that God will give you the best, just what you need. It may not come in exactly the way you expected, but it will be just what is best. Psalm 31:24.

DRY HAIR

SYMPTOMS—Hair that is dry enough that it bothers you. It lacks luster and may be brittle. There may also be split ends.

CAUSES—A dry garden needs water. Dry hair does not need water, but it does need **natural oils**. You may be using **harsh shampoos** that remove all the oil from your scalp and hair. Lack of proper **nutrition** may be another cause.

NATURAL REMEDIES

• Include enough **unsaturated fatty acids** in your diet (unheated vegetables oils, such as **wheat germ, flaxseed, sesame, corn, or soy oil**). *See suggestions under Dry Skin (332).*

• **Do not use heat** to arrange your hair. Both curling irons and electric curlers produce heat that is too intense. Instead, women should use unheated plastic cylinder rollers.

• Dry hair tends to produce frayed ends. **Snip them off** about every 6 weeks or so.

• **Avoid whipping winds**. They also tend to fray your hair. Women do best not to swim bareheaded.

Use a **bathing cap**. It will protect the hair. For additional protection, rub on a little olive oil before putting on the cap.

• Shampoo with care, using only **mild shampoos**.

• **Avoid washing** the hair every night. **When washing hair**, only use warm, not hot water. **When rinsing** the hair, always use cool water. This increases circulation.

• Pour **sesame seed oil** on your hair and massage. Or apply **flaxseed oil**.

• Massage avocado into your hair. It provides both protein and oil to the hair shaft. In a bowl, mix 1 peeled **avocado**, 1 tsp. each of **jojoba oil** and **wheat germ oil**. After shampooing, rinsing, and drying your hair, apply the mixture, massaging it in. Then cover your hair with a plastic bag. Leave it on for 15-30 minutes. Then rinse thoroughly. Repeat once a week.

ENCOURAGEMENT—Accept His gifts with the whole heart. Jesus died that you might have the precious things of heaven as your own and, at last, find a home with the heavenly angels in the kingdom of God. Ephesians 6:24.

GRAY HAIR

SYMPTOMS—The hair is changing from its youthful color to a gray color.

CAUSES—A lack of three B complex vitamins is specific to this problem.

NATURAL REMEDIES

• To restore natural color to gray hair, the following vitamins have been reported to be successful for some people: **PABA** (para-aminobenzoic acid, 1,000 mg), **pantothenic acid** (1,000 mg), and **folic acid** (800 mcg), along with **brewer's yeast**, and **blackstrap molasses**. Also take a good **multi-vitamin / mineral** formula. Include some **kelp or dulse** in your diet.

HAIR RINSES

• Mix **nettles, sage, and rosemary;** and use it as a hair rinse to darken the hair.

• **Henna** is a natural, non-toxic coloring herb which has been used for centuries to make hair more blonde. It works best on thin, light, porous hair.

• **Chamomile and lemon** combined make a good rinse for blonde hair.

• **Rosemary and sage** rinse will help shine dark hair.

• **Cider vinegar** rinse helps balance hair pH.

• **Kelp or seawater** adds mineral body to hair.

• Apply **joboba** to damaged, brittle, and over-processed hair.

ENCOURAGEMENT—While self is unsubdued, we can find no rest. But if you will find time and voice to pray, God will find time and voice to answer.

INGROWN HAIR

SYMPTOMS—A hair, generally on the neck, grows down into the skin and causes irritation.

CAUSES—These tend to be caused by hairs which curl. Curly haired people are more likely to have this problem than others.

NATURAL REMEDIES

• The only practical solution is to **pull it out with tweezers**. Do not pull at just anything. Wait until you can actually see the hair. If necessary, place a warm compress on the area, for a time, to help it be seen better. Then use tweezers or a sterilized needle, followed by a dab of hydrogen peroxide on the area.

• People who find this too much of a problem might consider growing a **beard**. Once established, that generally solves the problem. If beards are frowned on at your work, have your physician write a note that it is a medical necessity for you to have one.

• Using an **electric shaver** is better than razors, because razors sharpen the hair end more, especially double track razors. If you do use a razor, try not to shave as close.

• If your neck hairs tend to be angled in different directions, train them to grow in only two directions, by only **shaving up and down** instead of crossways.

• Women should **shave their legs down**, not up. Shaving upward is far more likely to cause inward-growing hairs. This is because leg hairs grow downward.

ENCOURAGEMENT—However fierce the tempest, those who turn to Jesus will find deliverance. His providence will provide for their needs; and His grace will give power to resist temptation and sin.

If it were not for the continual help of our heavenly Father, we would be in terrible shape. He alone can provide the help we so much need, day by day. Trust in Him and He will never fail you, even though your immediate requests may not be fulfilled.

HAIR TONICS

• In order to cleanse your hair of soap, used apple cider **vinegar** as the rinse water.

• Drinking **nettle** juice cleanses the system and helps add sparkle to lackluster hair. Drinking **burdock** leaf tea also does this.

HEAD

• Make a strong **chamomile** tea and use it for a light hair rinse.

• Prepare a tea of **rhubarb** root and use it as a rinse to lighten light brown or faded blonde hair.

HAIR CONDITIONER

Your hair loses natural oils, due to too much sunlight, harsh chemical shampoos and dyes, hair preparations containing alcohol, or permanents. A hair conditioner replaces these natural oils. After a few weeks of applying one or another of the following conditioners, your hair should be softer to the touch and more attractive.

• Rub **olive oil** into your hair every 2-3 evenings before retiring.

• If you want an oil mixture that is sweet-smelling, mix the following formula and apply it to your hair every so often: 1 oz. **rosemary oil**, 3 oz. **sweet almond oil**, and 30 drops of **lavender oil**.

• Here is a formula which will help keep your hair in good condition: Add a little **oil of marjoram** to some **olive oil** and rub it into your hair. Every so often, mix a fresh batch and repeat.

• Here is a formula for an orange-scented oil for dry hair: Mix 1 oz. **rosemary oil**, 3 oz. of **sweet almond oil**, and 20 drops of **oil of orange**.

If you have naturally oily hair, only apply one of the above essential oils, and do it once a week at the most.

• If you have faded hair, mix 1 oz. **rosemary oil** and 1 oz. **coconut oil** with 3 oz. **oil of sweet almonds**. Rub a small amount gently into your scalp every other night.

HAIR FIXER

Commercial preparations, sold to keep your hair in place, frequently contain harsh chemicals, including alcohol. Here is a formula which will help keep the hair in place and tend to give it a beautiful sheen:

Squeeze a little **lemon juice** into a small bowl. Then apply it to your hair with a piece of cotton. Within a few minutes it will be dry.

— HEAD AND THROAT —
3 - EYES

Also: Sjögren's Syndrome (311)

WARNING - EYES !

• Do not lay compresses directly on the eyeball. The lids should always be closed.

CHART - 1043: Catagories of Eye diseases (387-404)

• Some natural therapists recommend placing hot compresses on the eyes, "as hot as possible." But there is great danger in doing that. A physician did that to the child, Fanny Crosby, and a scar-like film was permanently etched onto her eyes. In this book, only "very warm" eye compresses are mentioned, along with, at times, cold ones.

EYE PROBLEMS

SYMPTOMS—Various kinds of eye problems can develop (such as blurred vision, bulging, blood spots, dark circles, dryness, double vision, itching, lumps on the eyelids, redness, twitching, or watering).

Certain eye problems need specialized attention. But there are also general solutions to a wide variety of eye problems.

NATURAL REMEDIES

• The eyes and the brain use a lot of **oxygen**. Be sure to get enough.

NUTRITION

• Drink **carrot, celery, beet, and parsley juice**. You may need to go on a short **vegetable juice fast**.

• The mineral, **zinc** (20 mg daily), is important. Be sure it is included in your diet. **Vitamins A (500 IU), B complex, B_1 (25-50 mg), B_2 (25-50 mg), B_6 (25-56 mg), pantothenic acid (100 mg), niacinamide (50 mg), C (3,000-5,000 mg), E (400 IU), selenium**, are also important. Eat **fresh greens** everyday. The importance of vitamin A and **provitamin A- and B-carotene** on eyesight cannot be overemphasized. Eat fresh green and yellow vegetables for the carotenoids.

• Two days a week, drink **lemon water** instead of breakfast. Chinese healers say that this purifies the liver and helps the eyes.

• For blurred vision, eat dried, unripe **raspberries**.

• **Do not overeat**. Get plenty of **exercise** and **rest**.

AVOID

• **Poor nutrition** clogs tiny arteries, such as are found in the eyes. A gradual clogging of the veins in the eyes can lead to blindness. The tiny vessels within the eye become blocked with atherosclerosis, the result of a diet high in **fat** and **cholesterol**.

• Eliminate all **fried foods**. The free radicals in these greasy foods damage the eyes as well as other organs. Avoid **meat, eggs, refined grain products, sugar, dairy products, coffee, chocolate, and alcohol**.

• Avoid drinking fluids before bed. Avoid **salt**. Do not use **tobacco** and avoid **secondhand smoke**. Nicotine, **sugar**, and **caffeine** all weaken the eyes.

• **Margarine** and **vegetable shortening** are not good for the eyes.

• **Tinted sunglasses** often cause eyestrain. Only use **polarized sunglasses**, if you use them at all.

• A number of medicinal drugs are not good for the eyes. This would include **aspirin, ACTH,** anticoagulants, corticosteroids, diuretics, streptomycin, sulfa drugs, tetracycline, allopurinol, antihistamines, digitalis, haloperidol, anti-infection drugs, quinine, marijuana, and some others.

• Anti-infection drugs, including **diazepam (Valium), haloperidol (Haldol), some antidepressants, quinine, and sulfa drugs** can cause ocular abnormalities.

• Substances which are bad for your eyes: **chemical diuretics, cocaine, sulfa drugs, tetracycline, aspirin, nicotine, phenylalanine, liquor, and hydrocortisone**.

• Be very cautious about wearing **contact lenses**! They keep air from the eyeball surfaces which they cover. Infections can result. Leaving them in place more than 24 hours can produce ulcerative keratitis. The cells of the cornea are rubbed away by the contact lens, resulting in infection, scarring, and possible eventual blindness. Research shows that this danger applies equally to ordinary daily wear contact lenses or extended-wear lenses.

HERBS

• **Eyebright** is the master herb for eye problems, and has been used for this purpose for over 2000 years. Add one tablespoon of the herb to a cup of boiled water, strain, and let cool. Apply cool, fresh eyebright tea as an eye wash daily. It will strengthen the eyes and help reduce or eliminate many eye problems.

• **Goldenseal** and **red raspberry** teas all help the eyes. Eyebright is especially noted for what it can do for the eyes. People have used it for centuries.

• To strengthen the eyes, especially in weakness resulting from diabetes, use **chaparral** tea internally. Vitamin A is also important.

• Research studies have found that **bilberry** (European blueberry) contains flavonoid compounds *(anthocyanosides)* which improve the circulation of the eye and promote the formation of visual purple. In some studies, it was given along with vitamin E.

• **Dandelion** helps the liver detoxify. And seaweed (**Norway kelp or Nova Scotia dulse**) provides essential minerals.

• Blackfoot Indians made a tea of the leaves and flowers of **yarrow** and applied it as an eye wash. **Aloe vera** juice is another helpful eyewash.

• Drink strong **borage** tea, to strengthen the eyes, and eat young leaves in a salad.

• Add ½ tsp. **fennel** powder (made from crushed, blended fennel seeds) to 2½ oz. clear, cold water. Strain and apply to the eyes for eye problems.

• The ancient Greeks used fresh white **cabbage juice** with tiny amounts of **honey** added, to relieve sore, inflamed, moist, or running eyes. They also added **thyme** to food to help overcome dimness of sight.

• For runny eyes in infants, wash the eyes every half hour with **warm, clean water**. Bruise fresh **cabbage leaves** to a soft pulp and apply a cabbage pack to the closed eyes. This will increase the flow for a few days, but will eliminate the problem within a short time.

• For inflamed eyes, apply a lotion of **eyebright** or strained **chickweed** tea.

• Apply **witch hazel** compresses over closed eyes to relieve red, sore, strained, or inflamed eyes.

• Apply a compress of **tansy** tea for a sty or inflammation of the eye.

• *For dark circles* beneath your eyes, stop working so much, **get more sleep, and drink more liquids**. You may have lost weight too fast. This may be caused by iron deficiency, liver or kidney malfunction, or chronic allergies. Place **chamomile** tea bags over the closed eyes.

• Indians and Americans have been drinking **goldenseal** tea for the eyes, for over 200 years.

• Here is a tonic for poor and unhealthy vision. Mix equal parts of **eyebright, goldenseal root, bayberry root bark, red raspberry leaves**, along with a pinch of **cayenne**. Do not put on the eyes, but take 2-4 capsules of the powdered herbs daily. For acute problems, take 2-3 capsules, 3 times daily. The major effect is provided by the eyebright and goldenseal. The other herbs are antibiotics, astringents, and stimulants. This will help prevent cataracts and relieve eyes that are inflamed, stinging, weeping, or oversensitive to light.

OTHER HELPS

• Place a **washcloth, dipped in ice water**, over your eyes for 15 minutes, once or twice a day. Or **cold cucumber slices** can be put on your closed eyes. This will bring healing blood to your eyes and help strengthen them. This is good for pinkeye, sunburn, and eyestrain.

• For protection against ultraviolet rays, only wear **sunglasses** that block 99%-100% of UVA and UVB radiation. Any other sunglasses can damage your eyes. Eyes can get sunburned. UV radiation causes photokeratitis, in which the outer layer of cells is damaged. Treat sunburned eyes with cold compresses.

• **Palm your eyes** to rest them. Place the palm of your left hand over your left eye. Do the same with the right hand over the right eye. Both eyes are now covered, yet nothing is touching the eyes. This gives them a rest for a few moments. Do this several times a day, 10 seconds at a time.

—*See Eyestrain (next page), Computer Eyestrain (next page), and other eye topics in this chapter.*

ENCOURAGEMENT—Make God your entire dependence. When you find yourself starting to do otherwise, immediately call a halt—and run back to Him! Do not tarry. Do not wait. James 1:12. Remember the sweet promise: "The peace of God, which passeth all understanding, shall keep your hearts and minds, through Christ Jesus." Philippians 4:7. When we trust in His Inspired Writings—as found in the Holy Bible—we are on safe ground. Never forsake Him, and He will be with you to the end.

EYESTRAIN

SYMPTOMS—The eyes seem to be straining to see what they are trying to look at. After some time of doing this, you acquire a general feeling of eyestrain.

CAUSES AND TREATMENT—**Fatigue, poor diet, overwork, drugs, polluted air, city living**. Much of what is in our modern way of life is hard on the eyes.

NATURAL REMEDIES
• Is the area in which you do much of your eyework **properly lit**?
• **Flickering tubes** can bother the eyes. Try not to use **computers** too long at a time; do not watch **television** too long. Both are hard on your eyes. Keep the screen somewhat darkened. Shade your screen by placing a hood over the front.
• Every so often, **shut and rest your eyes**. Try "palming." To do this, place the palms of your hands across your open eyes, without touching them. This cuts out all light and enables you to momentarily rest them.
• Make sure you **blink** often enough. Each blink cleanses and refreshes them.
• **Refuse to strain** your eyes. Keep them relaxed at all times. If you cannot see the object clearly, then look at it relaxed unclearly!
• **Sunglasses** cause eyestrain for some people, but they help others. Only use Polaroid or approved anti-glare glasses.
• The **evening hours** are the worst time to read and use your eyes intensively for anything. The natural daylight is gone.
• Make sure you have adequate **illumination**. The best kind is a full-spectrum light or a combination of fluorescent and incandescent. Use a soft light that does not glare. Place the light so it does not reflect back into your eyes from the paper before you.
• Occasionally look off in the **distance**.
• **Blink** your eyes 400 times a day. This will massage, wash, and rest them.
• Go outside for the last 30 minutes before bedtime, **walk around, relax, breathe deep, and do not read anymore before you retire**.
• Get enough **rest** at night.
• You may need **reading glasses**. If your only eye problem is farsightedness, you can purchase eye glasses at your local pharmacy for $10 or $20. Always select the weakest, least powerful ones.
—*Also read Eye Problems (387) and Computer Eyestrain (next).*

ENCOURAGEMENT—By beholding Christ, we become changed. And this is what you want, is it not? Come, take the greatest prize of all. Let Christ come into your heart. He can give overcoming strength to resist sin and obey the Ten Commandments. Proverbs 8:17, 21.

COMPUTER EYESTRAIN

SYMPTOMS—Tired, dry, or burning sensation in the eyes after working before a computer monitor (screen) for several hours.

CAUSES—There are ways to continue in such work, without damaging your eyesight. Here are several suggestions to help you protect your eyesight as you work with computers:

NATURAL REMEDIES
• Try to keep the screen **two feet** from your eyes.
• Place the screen so that your **line of sight** is 10°-15° (about one third of a 45° angle) below the point on the screen where you tend to look at.
• Do not work with a screen which is dull, **blurred, or flickers**. Find the cause and eliminate it or call in a technician. Vibration from a nearby fan may cause the flickering. Move it farther away.
• The lower part (near view) of **bifocals** are located for looking down, not straight ahead. So you may need single (not bifocal) lenses for computer work.
• Reduce **glare**. Do not have overhead lights or windows reflecting into the screen.
• **Blink** often to keep your eyes from drying out.
• Try to arrange your **paperwork** so that it is set at an angle, nearly the same height as the screen and close to the same distance from your eyes as the screen.
• **Dust** the screen occasionally. Static electricity tends to coat it with dust.
• Take 5-10 minute **breaks** every hour.
• Use a glare-reduction **filter** approved by the American Optometric Association.
• An active-matrix LCD **flat display** is sharper and brighter than a CRT-based display screen.

ENCOURAGEMENT—We, too, are to walk with God. When we do this, our faces will be lighted up by the brightness of His presence; and, when we meet one another, we shall speak of His power and say Praise God. Good is the Lord, and good is the word of the Lord.

MUCUS IN EYE

SYMPTOMS—The eye seems be filled with mucus.

CAUSES—The cause may be a combination of an **inadequate diet, poor working conditions, and an airborne infection**.

NATURAL REMEDIES

390 **HEAD** **YELLOW EYES / PUFFY EYES / ITCHY** NATURAL REMEDIES ENCYCLOPEDIA
OVER 11,000 REMEDIES - OVER 730 DISEASES

HEAD

• **Improve the diet** and take a **vitamin / mineral supplement** twice a day. Obtain adequate **rest**. Work in a **clear and clean environment** that is not overly dusty.

• Wash each eye with **goldenseal** root tea. But do not use goldenseal in large amounts if pregnant.

ENCOURAGEMENT—He who receives Christ by living faith has a living connection with God. He carries with him the atmosphere of heaven, which is the grace of God and a treasure that the world cannot buy. Zephaniah 3:17.

YELLOW EYES
(Icterus, Jaundice)

SYMPTOMS—The whites of the eyes (sclera) have a yellow hue.

CAUSES—The **bile duct system** develops a blockage which may be caused by gallstones, tumors, or hepatitis. Red blood cells may also be destroyed in the process.

Those taking large amounts of carrot juice will develop a yellowish cast to their skin (which is in no way dangerous). But their sclera will not turn yellow, which is the sign of jaundice.

NATURAL REMEDIES
• The cause of the obstruction must be determined and treated. Treatment of jaundice includes **ultraviolet light exposure** in order to increase elimination and liver flush. For 3 days, drink **apple juice**, followed by a cup of **olive oil** and a cup of **lemon juice**. Also obtain **vitamins C, A, and E**. This large amount of olive oil dilates the bile ducts, so the stones can be ejected. This need only be done once to solve the problem.
—*Important: See Jaundice (448).*

ENCOURAGEMENT—Keep your mind on Jesus, and pride and the love of the world will vanish. Beside the loveliness of Christ, all earthly attractions will seem of little worth. Matthew 16:26.

PUFFY EYES
(Bags under Eyes)

SYMPTOMS—A small area beneath each eye appears puffy. It looks like there are bags under the eyes.

CAUSES—The **liver** and/or **kidneys** are being overworked and undernourished.

NATURAL REMEDIES
• Do not drink **liquor** or use **tobacco**.
• Limit **salt** intake. Avoid **monosodium glutamate**

(MSG).
• Improve your diet by switching to nutritious food: **fresh fruits, vegetables, whole grains, nuts, and legumes**.
• **Greasy, processed, and junk food** may seem to be nice because you can get it so quick. But the undernourishment it is causing is wearing out your body.
Caffeine products only whip the tired horse. Instead, get the proper rest you need each night.
• Avoid doing **work which requires you to bend over**. This intensifies the bags under your eyes. **Sleep on your back**.
• Wrap **ice cubes** in a cloth and apply to the area for quick relief.
• Avoid drinking **fluids** before bed.

ENCOURAGEMENT—Christ came to teach human beings what God desires them to know. In the heavens above, in the earth, in the broad waters of the ocean, we see the handiwork of God. All created things testify to His power, His wisdom, His love. But not from the stars or the ocean or the cataract can we learn of the personality of God as it is revealed in Christ.

ITCHY EYES

SYMPTOMS—The eyes seem tired and itchy.

CAUSES—**Enervation, poor diet, lack of rest, anxiety, eyestrain, or neglected eye problems**.

NATURAL REMEDIES
• **Do not overwork or overeat**. Eat a **nutritious diet**. Get enough **rest** at night.
• The diet should include the entire **B complex**, with an emphasis on **B$_6$**. Be sure your diet includes adequate **calcium**.
• **Do not strain** the eyes.
• **Eyebright** is a good herb for the eyes.
• **Do not rub** your eyes! Instead, apply **warm or cool compresses** to your closed eye to soothe the itch.
• **Do not share tissues, handkerchiefs, or towels** with anyone else.
• **Do not place a patch** over the itching eyes. Then bacteria can increase and cause even more serious problems.

ENCOURAGEMENT—The very first step in the path to life is to keep the mind stayed on God, to have His fear continually before the eyes. If you cannot take Jesus with you, do not go there. Do not watch it. Do not listen to it. Zechariah 10:12.

RED EYES
(Bloodshot Eyes)

DISEASES - List: 10-26 / Index: 1211-1224 / HERBS - Contents: 129- / Preparing: 132 / Using: 141-189 (dose: often 1 tsp. mixed herbs in 1 cup boiled water) / VITAMINS-MINERALS - Index: 100- / Dosages: 124 / HYDRO-THERAPY - Therapy index: 206- / Disease index: 263- / CARE OF SICK - 28-39 / EMERGENCIES - 973-, 990-

SYMPTOMS—Red lines in the whites of the eyes.

CAUSES—The sclera is the white of the eye, forming the outer coat of the eyeball. There are tiny blood vessels on the surface of the sclera, which can become congested with blood, due to an insufficient supply of oxygen. Causes include **eyestrain, fatigue, dust, pollen allergies, bright sunshine, cigarette smoke, other irritants, overwork, and staying up late at night**. **Drinking alcohol** is a special cause. Bloodshot eyes can also mean capillary fragility throughout the body. **High blood pressure** or a lack of certain **vitamins and amino acids** may be the cause of that.

People over 40 commonly experience this problem to some extent. But if it is excessive, or if you are younger, you may wish to give it closer attention.

NATURAL REMEDIES

• Improve your diet; take **vitamin A** (5,000 mg daily), **B₂** (100 mg), **B₆** (100 mg), and the three amino acids: **lysine, histidine, and phenylalanine**. If you are eating a nutritious diet of **fruits, vegetables, beans, and nuts**, you should be getting the needed vitamins and amino acids.

• Get more **rest** at night. Pause and rest a little more during the day.

• **Do not use "drops"** from the pharmacy. They have an agent in them that constricts the blood vessels. This may make your whites look whiter for awhile, but no problems have been solved. Do not tinker with your precious eyes! When the drops wear off in a couple hours, the redness generally appears redder than before.

• Lay a **cool, wet washcloth** over your closed eye. The cold constricts the blood vessels naturally and the moisture helps your eyes.

• Be sure and drink enough **water**, so you will have an adequate amount of fluid in your tear ducts.

• If the eyes are red when you wake up, the problem may be that you have a low-grade **infection of the eyelids**. Treat it by washing your eyes with warm water at night before retiring.

• Any problem in the eyes should be taken seriously. Infection can be treated with a small amount of **boric acid** mixed with sterile water.

• Helpful herbs include **eyebright, fennel, and cornflower**. Eyebright is remarkably helpful for a number of eye conditions.

ENCOURAGEMENT—There must be a constant, earnest struggling of the soul against the evil imaginings of the mind. There must be a steadfast resistance of temptation to sin in thought or act. But, in the strength of Christ, this can be done. In Him we can live clean, pure lives. Job 11:15-18.

BLACK EYE

SYMPTOMS—The area around the eye turns black, following a blow to it.

CAUSES—Blood tends to pool around the delicate eyeball, in order to hasten healing.

NATURAL REMEDIES

• Boxing trainers deal with black eyes all the time. They apply an extremely **cold piece of iron** (something like a small tire iron) to the area. This reduces the swelling. An alternative is to hold a clean, **cold soda can** against the cheek (but not against the eye itself) for several minutes. Do not place any pressure on the eye itself. Or, to constrict the swelling, apply **cold compresses** to the area.

• Do not take **aspirin**. Because it is an anticoagulant, the blood will not clot as well. Instead, the bleeding will continue longer.

• **Do not blow your nose!** If you received a severe strike, blowing your nose could cause blood vessels to burst beneath the skin in a much wider area! Sometimes the injury fractures the eye-socket bone. And blowing your nose could force air out of your sinus adjacent to the socket. The air is injected under the skin, making the eyelids swell even more. This can increase the likelihood of infection.

• There is always the danger that there may be internal bleeding. So you may want to visit an **ophthalmologist**.

ENCOURAGEMENT—Prayer takes hold upon Omnipotence and gains us the victory. And this is what we need! We must have God or perish. We must submit to Him and obey Him. By the grace of Christ, this can be done. Jeremiah 32:41.

CORNEAL ABRASION

SYMPTOMS—A scratch on the surface of the cornea, which is the transparent front part of the eye. Symptoms usually occur suddenly and may include blurry vision, redness, watering of the eye, severe pain in the eye, frequent blinking, and sensitivity to bright light.

CAUSES—The cause could be a scrape by the edge of a newspaper or by a foreign particle such as a speck of dirt. Those who wear soft contact lenses and rub their eyes excessively are particularly at risk of such damage, because tiny particles can become stuck behind the lenses and scratch the surface of the cornea.

The problem is generally not serious, unless the abrasion becomes infected and a corneal ulcer *(308)* may develop. A herpes simplex infection can cause that ulcer.

A corneal abrasion usually takes only a few days to heal, if the eye is closed and remained covered shut for 2 days.

NATURAL REMEDIES

• Improve your **diet**, take **vitamin C** (5,000 mg, 3 times a day). Drink **eyebright** tea. Take **echinacea** tea.

• If home remedies do not solve the problem within

a few days, visit an eye doctor.

ENCOURAGEMENT—Go to Jesus, just as you are; and He will open wide His arms and receive you as His child. There is no happiness equal to being with Him.

NEARSIGHTEDNESS
(Myopia)

SYMPTOMS—A person only clearly sees those things which are close up.

CAUSE—Light is focusing in front of the retina instead of on it. Only 2% of second grade children are nearsighted. By the end of high school, the figure is 40%. By the end of college, more than 60% of students are nearsighted. Heredity is another cause. There is both an occupational and nutritional cause for this problem.

NATURAL REMEDIES
• Every so often, rest your eyes by looking at something at a **distance** in the sky.
• **Vitamin D** (1,000 IU daily) **and calcium** are both important. Take **sunbaths** and **calcium citrate** tablets or powder. Take vitamin C (5,000 mg daily)
• **Do not strain** the eyes, thinking that will help you improve your eyesight! Doing so only weakens the delicate muscles and will result in still more vision problems. Ignore these "better sight without glasses" theories which tell you to strain your eyes in order to improve your vision!
—Also read Eye Problems (387), Eyestrain (389), and Computer Eyestrain (389).

ENCOURAGEMENT—Cry to God for help. Find in Him your all in all. He can help. He can satisfy your deepest soul desire. John 15:10.

FARSIGHTEDNESS
(Hyperopia)

SYMPTOMS—A person's distance vision is good, but his near vision is blurry.

CAUSES—The six **muscles** pulling on the eye do not function properly or the **eyeball** is abnormally short. As a result, light rays focus behind the back wall of the eyeball, which is the retina.

NATURAL REMEDIES
• Maintain a **nourishing diet** which includes a vitamin / mineral supplement. Be sure you are daily obtaining the entire **B complex, especially B$_6$. Calcium** is also important.
• **Do not strain** the eyes. If they seem tired or unable to focus properly, **rest them** from time to time.

Straining the eyes, hoping that will help you see better, only aggravates the problem.
—Read Eye Problems (387), Eyestrain (389), and Computer Eyestrain (389).

ENCOURAGEMENT—Heaven is not closed against the fervent prayers of God's little ones. The only reason for our lack of power with God is to be found in ourselves. Too many only offer a little hurried prayer and then rush off. Take time with God! You urgently need it. Hebrews 5:9.

NIGHT BLINDNESS

SYMPTOMS—You do not see as clearly in the dark as do others. When you go out into the dark, your eyes seem to adapt very slowly to it.

CAUSES—There are two types of light-sensitive cells in the retina: rods and cones. Up to 120 million rods are distributed throughout the retina. Although rods are sensitive to all visible light, they contain only one type of pigment and cannot distinguish colors. They are responsible mainly for night vision.

If you have this problem, you are not going blind. The primary problem is a lack of **vitamin A**, which the body uses to make visual purple and to help you see in the dark.

The lack of vitamin A in the system can be caused by an inferior diet. But it may also be traced to one of the following: The body has a **fat malabsorption syndrome** and does not properly absorb oil-soluble vitamins. A **zinc** deficiency will cause the liver to poorly convert carotene to vitamin A. **Cystic fibrosis, celiac disease, and various food allergies** can produce intestinal changes which would affect fat-soluble vitamin absorption.

NATURAL REMEDIES
• Make sure you are getting enough **vitamin A**. The therapeutic dose would be 25,000 IU daily for only a few days. Too much vitamin A can be dangerous.
• The safer form of vitamin A is **carotenoids**, such as beta or marine carotene (up to 100,000 IU daily). Drink 3 cups of **carrot juice** every day! Eat **green and yellow vegetables**.
• Take 15-20 mg of **zinc** daily.
• Some people wear a stronger prescription of **glasses** when they must drive at night. Keep the **headlights and windshield clean**. Do not wear **sunglasses** at dusk. **Drive slower** at night. Better yet, only drive during the day.
• Take **bilberry** extract capsules or liquid, **PCOs** from **grapeseed** or **white pine** (100 mg, 3 times daily), and **CoQ$_{10}$** (60 mg, 3 times daily).

ENCOURAGEMENT—By keeping our minds on

God and Bible themes, our faith and love will grow stronger. We will have a little heaven on earth. Those around us need our help so much. Psalm 31:24.

COLOR BLINDNESS

SYMPTOMS—The reduced ability to tell certain colors apart.

CAUSES—There are six million cones in each retina which provide detailed and color vision. There are three types of these cone cells, one is sensitive to blue light, another to green, and the third to red light. If one or more of these three types of cones are faulty, color blindness results. In one type of **inherited** color blindness, a color-blind father passes his recessive genes on to his daughters who are not color blind. But their sons may inherit color blindness. In another type, both males and females can inherit it equally.

The problem is more frequent in males than females. The most common type is red-green color blindness.

Other causes include **macular degeneration and several other eye disorder**s. The toxic effects of various **drugs**, including **chloroquine** (used for malaria) can also cause it. If the condition is caused by eye diseases or drugs, the color blindness can be alleviated to some extent.

NATURAL REMEDIES
• Take 5,000 units of **vitamin A** daily and 25,000 IU of **carotene**.

ENCOURAGEMENT—There are perils all about us. We must draw nearer to God. Cultivate the habit of talking with the Saviour. Let your heart be continually uplifted to Him in silent petition for help, for strength to obey, and for guidance. Let every breath be a prayer. 2 Corinthians 12:9.

AMBLYOPIA
(Inability to Focus Eyes)

SYMPTOMS—This condition exists when the eyes do not seem to focus clearly on anything, near or far. It can be serious enough to constitute a type of blindness.

CAUSES—This is blurry or absent vision in an eye that is structurally normal. It occurs in young children if the two eyes send different images to the brain. If the problem is not solved by the age of 5, later attempts to correct vision will fail. This is because the brain will disconnect the vision from one of the eyes.

Misalignment of the gaze of the eyes (strabismus, *309*) is the most common cause. Other causes include vision disorders in one eye, such as astigmatism (*see Eye Problems, 387*), farsightedness (*392*), and near-sightedness (*392*).

Certain nutritional and environmental problems are usually involved.

NATURAL REMEDIES
• Lack of **vitamins B$_1$ and B$_{12}$** appears to be a primary cause. **Smoke** from cigarettes and cigars is another important cause.
• Take **B$_{12}$** intermuscularly (1,000 mcg / day for a total of 20,000 mcg). This will often solve the problem, along with an adequate supply of **vitamin D** and **calcium**.
• Get **tobacco** out of your house and office.
—*Also read Eye Problems (387), Eyestrain (389), and Computer Eyestrain (389).*

ENCOURAGEMENT--Thank God that He is so near to help in time of need. Prayer and faith can do that which no earthly power can accomplish. Trust Him and obey His Written Word. And you will have the guidance you need. Isaiah 58:11.

KERATOMALACIA
(Xerophthalmia)

SYMPTOMS—The cornea is the domed clear bulge on the front of the eye. It becomes hazy and dry, and then ulcerated. The eyes feel extremely dry. Blinking increases, but does not seem to properly moisten them. Conjunctivitis and night blindness occurs.

Fat-like spots (Bitot's spots) appear on the sclera (white of the eye). These are white, foamy, elevated, and sharply outlined patches on the whites of the eyes.

CAUSES—"Xerophthalmia" means dryness of the eye. It occurs mainly in developing countries. The condition is caused by a dietary deficiency of **vitamin A**. Left untreated, it leads to chronic infection and the cornea (the transparent part of the front of the eye) may soften and perforate. If that happens, infection can spread inside the eye and blindness may result.

Not artificial tears, but large doses of vitamin A is the solution.

NATURAL REMEDIES
• Take **vitamin A** in the form of beta carotene (25,000 IU for children and at least 50,000 IU for adults) per day. Increase the amount of **zinc** and **protein** consumption, and improve the general **nutrition**. Take a **vitamin / mineral supplement** twice daily.
• Bitot's spots are caused by a vitamin A deficiency. **Vitamin D** and adequate protein are also needed.
• **Avoid eyestrain and smoke**-filled rooms.
—*Also see Dry Tear Ducts (below).*

ENCOURAGEMENT—We must be much in prayer if we would make progress in the spiritual life. Take time with God, and you will be blessed for it. He can give you strength to live a better life, a clean life, a new life in Christ. Matthew 4:4.

DRY TEAR DUCTS
(Dry eyes, Keratoconjunctivitis Sicca)

SYMPTOMS—The eyes seem dry all the time, due to insufficient production of tears.

CAUSES—There is a small tear duct (lacrimal gland) which keeps each eye moist; yet it does not seem to be working properly. In severe cases, corneal ulcers may develop. Dry eye affects more women than men and is more common over age 35.

NATURAL REMEDIES
• Take **vitamin A** (25,000 IU) for only several days. Eat lots of **green and yellow vegetables** and drink **carrot juice**. A lack of it causes small openings to close down.

• Include enough **essential fatty acids,** including **omega-3** in your diet (**flaxseed oil** is an outstanding source), along with more **calcium**.

• Do not eat **junk, sugar, saturated fat, or processed foods**.

• Increase **water** intake.

• Bathe the eye daily with **aloe vera juice**.

• Take a **B complex** supplement, with extra **B₂** and **zinc**.

—*See Sjögren's Disease (311). You may have it. Also see Keratomalacia (393), which is quite similar.*

ENCOURAGEMENT—Those who love God are changed from being rebels against the law of God into obedient servants and subjects of His kingdom. They live to help and bless others. Jeremiah 31:3.

STY
(Stye, Hordeolum)

SYMPTOMS—What appears to be a small pimple develops on the eyelid.

CAUSES—A sty is a bacterial infection (usually staphylococcal) of an eyelash follicle. It causes a pus-filled bump to form on either the inside or outside of the eyelid. An oil gland has become infected, inflaming the tissues of the eyelid. The pimple grows for a week or so and then usually subsides, sometimes rupturing spontaneously as it heals.

Some people never get sties. Other frequently get them. Adolescent girls get them from incomplete removal of **eye makeup**. Any eye cosmetics used before getting a sty should be discarded. Mascara that is kept longer than 3 months develops bacterial growth.

NATURAL REMEDIES
• Do not delay solving this problem. If it does not quickly heal, it may need to be drained by a professional. **Do not squeeze** the lump. This may spread the infection more widely. Sties can be dangerous. So do not be casual about them.

• Because you were not drinking enough **water**, eyelid secretions did not remain thin. Frequently **wash your hands** and keep them clean. **Do not rub your eyes** with dirty hands or fingers. Each person should have his own **towel and washcloth**. They should be washed daily if a person has a sty.

• Take adequate **vitamin A**. But take more, if you frequently have sties. Because too much vitamin A (from supplements) can cause problems, you would do well to get your vitamin A from **beta-carotene**. **Green and yellow vegetables and carrot juice** are rich in carotene.

Go on a 5-day **fruit fast**, plus **carrot and celery juice**. Keep the bowels clean with an enema every morning.

• Do not eat **refined, fried, and processed foods**. Also do not eat **meats, unsaturated oils, salt, alcohol, tobacco, dairy products, or white flour**.

• Carrots, which are chopped and diced, or mashed potatoes (raw or cooked) can be made into a **poultice** and applied over the area. They can be left on for an hour and repeated 3 times a day.

• Hot compresses on the area are sometimes recommended. —But keep in mind that it was a very hot compress which blinded young Fanny Crosby. Instead, hold a **warm, moist cloth** against the affected eye. This will hasten drainage.

• Very **warm compresses**, alternated with **cold**, will help draw the pus to a head and then break it open.

• Drink 3 cups of **goldenseal** tea or **eyebright** to help clean the liver. **Fennel** or **myrrh** may be substituted.

• Apply concentrated **thyme** tea directly to the sty with a cotton swab. Thyme is rich in *thymol*, an antiseptic.

• Take **echinacea** orally. It is a powerful antibiotic. It has anti-bacterial properties. Daniel Mowrey, Ph.D., says that just 6 mg of the active constituent (*echinacosides*) in echinacea is equivalent to one unit of penicillin.

• Varro Tyler, Ph.D., of Purdue University, recommends placing fresh scrapings from the inside of a **potato** onto a piece of clean cloth and then onto the sty. Replace once or twice with fresh scrapings. Within a couple hours, the swelling will be down and the sty improved. By evening it will be gone.

• A German treatment for sties is to place a very warm compress of **chamomile** tea on the sty.

• Swallow as much chopped **garlic** as you are able. It goes to work in the body to kill the staphylococci in the sty.

• If the eye itself becomes infected, add ½ tsp. salt to 8 oz. water and apply as an eyewash to the eye.

• After the sty drains, compresses should be continued until all drainage ceases.
—*See Chalazion (below).*

ENCOURAGEMENT—The Bible reveals the plan of salvation, and shows how sinful man may be reconciled to God and enabled to live a clean, godly life.

CHALAZION

SYMPTOMS—This appears to be a sty on the eyelid, but it is not. After several days, the swelling and pain disappears. But a slow growing pea-sized nodule remains on the lid.

CAUSES—A chalazion is the result of **plugged meibomian glands** in the eyelid, resulting from a **nutritional deficiency**.

NATURAL REMEDIES
• Take vitamin A in the form of **beta carotene** (at least 50,000 units per day) for many days. Also drink **carrot juice**, and eat **green and yellow vegetables**. Include a **zinc** supplement in the diet (15 mg, 3 times a day).
• Apply warm poultices of 3% **boric acid** on the closed lid. A boric acid ophthalmic ointment may be obtained without prescription from the pharmacy.
—*Also see Sty (394).*

ENCOURAGEMENT—When God gave His Son to our world, He endowed human beings with imperishable riches—with which nothing else can compare. Christ offers you all the love of God. Come, accept Him just now. James 2:5. "Light is sown for the righteous, and gladness for the upright in heart." Psalm 97:11. How very kind of our heavenly Father to provide us with such encouragement. He is always there when we call upon Him.

ULCERATED EYE AND LID
(Corneal Ulcer)

SYMPTOMS—The eye has become inflamed, resulting in an ulcer on the eyeball. The problem may then extend to the eyelid.

CAUSES—This occurred because the normal covering of the **eye was scratched or damaged** in some way, and then became infected The infection is generally caused by a **virus**. The ulcer can also be caused by blepharitis (400).

NATURAL REMEDIES
• Obtain **adequate rest, improve the diet, and take large doses of vitamin C** (2,000 mg, 3 times a day).
• Apply a warm **yellow dock** tea poultice to the eyelid. You can also drink it.

—*Also see Entropion (396).*

ENCOURAGEMENT—Everyday learn something new from the Scriptures. Search them as for hid treasures. They contain the words of eternal life.

XEROPHTHALMIA

SYMPTOMS—An inflammation of the cornea.

CAUSES—This is an infection of the cornea (the transparent part of the eye, through which light passes). The condition is caused by a lack of vitamin A.
If not treated, this disorder leads to chronic infection, night blindness (392), and / or Bitot's spots (below). The cornea may soften and perforate. Infection may then spread inside the eye, resulting in blindness.

NATURAL REMEDIES
• Very large doses of **vitamin A** are needed. Take 25,000 IU daily until the condition ends. Then reduce to 10,000 IU daily. If pregnant, do not take over 10,000 IU daily. Too much vitamin A can be a problem.
• Take **carotenoids** daily: 3 glasses of **carrot juice** daily, plus eating fresh **red and yellow vegetables**.
• Take **vitamin B$_2$** (100 mg), **vitamin B$_6$** (200 mg), **vitamin C** (1,000 mg), and **bioflavonoids** (50 mg),
• **Zinc** (20 mg daily) is also important.

ENCOURAGEMENT—Tender, compassionate, sympathetic, ever considerate of others, He represented the character of God. And He was constantly engaged in service for God and man. As Jesus was in human nature, so God means His followers to be. In His strength we are to live the life of purity and nobility which the Saviour lived.

BITOT'S SPOTS

SYMPTOMS—Elevated and quite distinct white patches on the conjunctiva.

CAUSES—The conjunctiva is the thin membrane which is on top of, and covers, the visible part of the eye. The usual cause is a severe vitamin A deficiency. But being in a smoke-filled room can aggravate the problem.

NATURAL REMEDIES
• Take 25,000 IU of vitamin A for 2 weeks. Then take 15,000 IU each day for a full month. After that, reduce to 10,000 IU daily. If pregnant, do not take over 10,000 IU daily. Use an emulsion form of the vitamin for improved assimilation. It is also safer at higher doses.
• Drink 2-3 cups of fresh carrot juice daily. Also eat lots of red and yellow vegetables.
• Do not remain in a smoky environment.
• Obtain enough rest, fresh air, and exercise.

ENCOURAGEMENT—Take the hand of Christ and hold it fast. His hand holds you much firmer than you can hold His hand. But you must choose to remain close to Him. He always gives you freedom of choice.

ENTROPION

SYMPTOMS—The eyelashes turn in, causing irritation to the eyeball. There may be pain in the eye area and a watery eye.

CAUSES—The eyelid turns inward; and the eyelashes rub against the cornea (the transparent front part of the eye) and the sclera (the white of the eye). Left untreated, the cornea may be damaged, ultimately leading to loss of vision.

The problem mainly affects older people in developing countries. Entropion most frequently follows trachoma, which formed scar tissue on the inner surface of the eyelids. Eventually, this shrinks, causing the eyelid to turn inward.

NATURAL REMEDIES
• Attach one end of a piece of **adhesive tape** to the skin beneath your lower lashes. Tape the other end to your cheek. Let it remain 3 days. Remove the tape and see if the condition has improved. If not, see an eye doctor immediately.
—*Also see Ulcerated Eye and Lid (395).*

ENCOURAGEMENT—Christ, who could not see human beings exposed to destruction without pouring out His soul unto death to save them from eternal ruin, will look with pity and compassion upon every soul who realizes that he can not save himself. How thankful we can be for God's blessings to us!

STRABISMUS
(Crossed Eyes, Squint)

SYMPTOMS—If mild, symptoms occur only when a child is tired. If severe, symptoms are present all the time and may include misalignment of the gaze of one of the eyes. Poor vision in one of the eyes is due to lack of use.

CAUSES—Only one eye points directly at the object being viewed. This abnormal alignment of the eyes causes the brain to receive conflicting images, which may result in double vision or, in children under the age of 8, suppression of the image from the misaligned eye.

The cause can be **inherited, nearsightedness** *(392)*, or **farsightedness** *(392)*. But the cause can be **structural differences** between the muscles controlling eye movements or **paralysis** of the eye muscles, due to a brain **tumor.** This is rarely caused by **cancer** of the eye.

A vision test can be performed and, if the problem suddenly developed, a CT scan may be done to look for a tumor.

NATURAL REMEDIES
• **Corrective glasses** can be given to the child to wear. Or he or she may wear an **eye patch** for a period of time each day, to force the weak eye to be used properly. These treatments are usually successful, although the problem can recur.

ENCOURAGEMENT—When the soul surrenders itself to Christ, a new power takes possession of the new heart. A change is wrought which man can never accomplish for himself. It is a supernatural work, bringing a supernatural element into human nature.

FLOATERS

SYMPTOMS—Small specks, known as floaters, that appear to float in the field of vision. They are especially seen in a well-lit room or outdoors on a bright day.

CAUSES—These are fragments of tissue in the jelly-like vitreous humor that fills the "ball" of the eye. They cast shadows on the retina. Any eye movement causes them to move rapidly. But, when the eyes are still, they drift slowly.

If they appear suddenly, or in large numbers, consult your eye doctor. This may indicate **separation of the retina** from its underlying tissue (retinal detachment) or a **leakage of blood** into the vitreous humor (vitreous hemorrhage). If you also see light flashes in the corners of your eyes, be sure and see an eye doctor.

Occasionally, floaters clump into long, stringy strands. If this occurs, the cause may be fibrillar degeneration of the vitreous, which results from excessive exposure to sunlight.

NATURAL REMEDIES
• Take **bioflavonoids** (500 mg, daily) and **vitamin K** (100 mcg, 2 times daily). **Vitamins A** (500 IU) and **E** (400 IU) will help remove lens particles. Also **pantothenic acid** (500 mg), B_6 (250 mg), and **vitamin C** (2,000 mg).
• Drink **carrot juice;** and eat **green and yellow vegetables.**
• Drink **dandelion** root tea and use as an eyewash.
—*Also see Scotoma (below).*

ENCOURAGEMENT— Christ knows every temptation that comes to man, and the capabilities of every human agent. He weighs his strength. He sees the present and the future, and presents before the mind the obligations that should be met, and urges that common, earthly things shall not be permitted to be so absorbing that eternal things shall be lost out of reckoning.

SCOTOMA

SYMPTOMS—The person seems to see one or more "spots" in front of the eyes.

CAUSES—An unnatural blind spot (scotoma), existing on the retina, is not transmitting any light through the optic nerve to the brain. When there is more than one blind spot, they are called scotomas.

NATURAL REMEDIES
• Increase the amount of **vitamin A** in the diet. And, of course, decidedly **improve the diet**. Throw out all **junk and processed food**. Obtain adequate **rest** at night.
—*Read Eye Problems (387) for more information. Also see Floaters (previous page).*

ENCOURAGEMENT—You cannot control your impulses or your emotions. But, in the strength of Christ, you can control the will. You can make an entire change in your life. Psalm 71:5.

DIMNESS OF VISION

SYMPTOMS—It is becoming more difficult to see. Less light seems to be entering the eyes.

CAUSES—Among the most common causes are cataracts *(398)*, glaucoma *(402)*, and diabetic retinopathy *(398)*. Less frequent causes include macular degeneration *(402)* and retinitis pigmentosa *(401)*.

Still another cause is retinal detachment *(397)*. A blood vessel which feeds the retina may be blocked by a blood clot. If this vessel is an artery, loss of vision is sudden. Usually only one eye is affected. An inflamed optic nerve is another possible cause, resulting from infection. This can cause loss of vision within a few days.

Toxic amblyopia *(right)* is another cause which produces a small hole, in vision, which gradually enlarges.

NATURAL REMEDIES
• Eat a good, nourishing diet of fresh **fruits, vegetables, whole grains, legumes, and nuts**, Take a full **multivitamin supplement**.
• **Avoid smoky air** from **tobacco, smoke stacks**, or living alongside a **highway**.
—*See the above-mentioned diseases for further information.*

ENCOURAGEMENT—The gifts of His grace through Christ are free to all. There is no election but one's own by which any may perish. God has set forth in His Word the conditions upon which every soul will be elected to eternal life—obedience, by the enabling grace of Christ, to God's commandments.

RETINAL DETACHMENT

SYMPTOMS—Flashing lights in the corner of the eye. Large numbers of dark spots in the field of vision *(see Floaters, 396)*. If a large area of the retina has become detached, you may see cloudy ring or a black area across your field of vision.

CAUSES—Separation of the light-sensitive retina at the back of the eye from the supporting tissues underneath occurs. In this disorder, part of the retina peels away from the underlying tissue. *Without rapid treatment, partial blindness can result.* See an ophthalmologist. This condition is more common over the age of 50. This sometimes runs in **families**. Participating in sports can cause a **blow to the eye**. Severe **nearsightedness** can also cause this condition.

A small tear occurs, permitting fluid to leak through and increase the separation.

NATURAL REMEDIES
• Contact an optometrist. He is able to test for retinal detachment.
• In some instances, there is only slight flashes of light in the corners of your eyes; yet the doctor may not see retinal detachment. In such instances, eat an extremely nourishing diet of fresh fruits, vegetables, whole grains, legumes, and nuts, plus a full multivitamin supplement; and the flashes of light may subside. But when in doubt, consult an optometrist for another checkup.

ENCOURAGEMENT—What an exalted position to be identified with one in whom is all perfection centered, who is indeed the Majesty of heaven, but who loved us (although fallen) so much that language cannot express it!

TOXIC AMBLYOPIA
(Tobacco Amblyopia)

SYMPTOMS—A small "hole" appears in the field of vision, which continues to enlarge over a period of time. Usually both eyes are affected. Blindness may eventually result.

CAUSES—This disorder primarily occurs in **people who smoke**, especially pipe smokers. Cigarette smokers tend to remove the cigarette from their face after taking a puff, whereas pipe smokers often leave the pipe in their mouth and the smoke drifts up into the eyes. But either form of tobacco smoking is dangerous to the eyes. The condition can also occur in individuals who drink **alcohol** or come in contact with **dangerous chemicals** (such as **lead, methanol, chloramphenicol, ethambutol, digitalis**, or certain others).

NATURAL REMEDIES

• Stop **smoking** immediately and do not linger in rooms where smoking is taking place.

• Stop using all **alcohol**.

• Dramatically improve your **diet**, as outlined elsewhere for eye problems. Get enough **rest, fresh air, and exercise**.

ENCOURAGEMENT—Though enduring most terrible temptations, Christ did not fail or become discouraged. He was fighting the battle in our behalf, and had He faltered, had He yielded to temptation, the human family would have been lost.

DIABETIC RETINOPATHY

SYMPTOMS—Symptoms may not be noticeable until damage to the retina is severe, although there may be areas of blurry vision. As the disease progresses, vision may suddenly be lost in one eye, due to rupture of one of the fragile new blood vessels in the retina.

CAUSES—If you have **diabetes mellitus** *(656)*, you have an increased risk of developing retinopathy. The diabetes can produce abnormalities in small blood vessels anywhere in the body—including in those in the retina.

At first, small blood vessels in the retina leak. Later, fragile new blood vessels may grow out into the jelly-like vitreous humor (in the center of the eyeball). If untreated, loss of vision can occur.

The longer a person has diabetes and the less it is controlled, the greater the risk. Only very few people with type 1 diabetes mellitus develop retinopathy within the first 10 years; yet once retinopathy begins, it usually progresses rapidly. By the time type 2 is diagnosed, it may already be present.

NATURAL REMEDIES

• Eat fresh **fruits, vegetables, whole grains, legumes, and nuts**. Take a full **multivitamin supplement**. Follow the recommendations in the section on Diabetes *(656)*.

• Take 25,000 IU of **vitamin A** daily. If pregnant, only take 10,000 IU. Also drink 3 cups **carrot juice** daily, and eat **red and yellow vegetables**.

ENCOURAGEMENT—Christ for our sakes laid aside His royal robe, stepped down from the throne of heaven, and condescended to clothe His divinity with humility and become like one of us except in sin, that His life and character should be a pattern for all to copy, that they might have the precious gift of eternal life.

CATARACTS

SYMPTOMS—The lens of the eye becomes clouded, so that the eye is unable to properly focus on objects. In advanced cases, the lens is becoming opaque, so that blindness is setting in. Only part of the eye is generally cloudy or opaque; but this can gradually extend to the entire eye.

CAUSES—Cataracts occur as a result of structural changes to protein fibers within the lens. These changes cause part or all of the lens to become cloudy. Cataracts usually develop in both eyes; but generally one eye is more severely affected. If it is in the central part of the lens or in the whole lens, total loss of clarity and detail in vision can result. But it will still be able to detect light and shade.

Congenital cataracts occur if the mother had **rubella** during the first three months of pregnancy or if the infant has **galactosemia**. This is an inherited inability to properly digest *galactose* (a type of milk sugar, called lactose). These cataracts generally do not get worse. Not using milk products at all can help prevent this in adults. **Smokers**, those who take **steroids**, and those who have **heavy metal poisoning** can get cataracts.

In one study, a group of women who smoked 30 cigarettes a day showed a 60% greater risk of developing cataracts.

Traumatic cataracts result from **blows** which rupture the anterior lens capsule, **harmful chemicals, intense infrared radiation, or X-rays**. **Radiation** causes free-radical damage in the eyes. This causes the lens to absorb aqueous humor. The lens becomes cloudy and must be removed in order to restore eyesight. People living closer to the South Pole (which has part of its **ozone** layer stripped away) are more likely to develop cataracts.

Other causes include **hypoparathyroidism, Down's Syndrome, and atopic dermatitis. High blood sugar** levels and **low calcium** levels can also bring it on. Higher blood sugar levels in **diabetics** and **hypoglycemics** causes the cells in the lens to absorb large amounts of glucose. This is converted into sorbitol, an insoluble form of sugar. This gradually crystallizes in the eye, forming a cataract. The longer one has diabetes, the greater the risk of cataracts.

Hair dye has been shown to cause cataracts. Only 23% of those not dying their hair get cataracts. Whereas 89% of those who dye their hair develop them.

Complications of **tumors, detached retina, iritis, glaucoma, and severe myopia** can also bring it on.

Other studies reveal that people with **stress, allergies**, or who eat **seafood** (thus ingesting methylmercury) are more likely to develop cataracts.

It is now known that a **lack of vitamins C or B$_2$** in the diet over an extended period of time can help produce cataracts.

Cataracts are the most common form of blindness

in older people, and should not be ignored when they are beginning to develop.

John D. Huff, M.D., a Texas ophthalmologist, says that 9 out of 10 patents in the early stages can reverse their cataracts with natural remedies. No single natural remedy can do it; but, when combined, good results can be obtained. Here is information which can help you:

NATURAL REMEDIES

• Obtain **adequate rest** at night. Do not sit up **watching television** till late at night! You are tiring your eyes and irradiating them with **X-rays** at the same time.

• Eat good "see foods": **fruits, vegetables**, and the nutrients listed below. Eat **whole grains, nuts, and legumes**. It is important that you eat a good **nutritious diet**! Get enough **vitamins E, C, B complex** (B_1 and B_2 is very important), **selenium, zinc, bioflavonoids, 1-glutamine, 1-arginine, 1-cysteine, and glutathione**. If diabetes is involved, add **chromium** supplementation. **Avoid excess cholesterol, sorbitol (artificial sweetener), unsaturated fatty acids, and mercury tooth fillings** (amalgam). Take a good high-potency **multivitamin**. It should include at least 50 mg of most of the **B vitamins**, 15 mg of **beta-carotene**, 30 mg of **zinc**, and 200 mcg of **selenium**. **Vitamin C** (1,500 mg daily) is extremely important. B_2 (200 mg) protects the crystalline lens of the eye. Also helpful: **copper** (3 mg) with **manganese** (5 mg) and flaxseed oil (1-2 Tbsp. daily).

• **MSM** (methylsulfonylmethane) is important for good vision. Take ½ tsp. of the powder, per 100 lbs. body weight once a day.

• The flavonoid, **quercetin**, is known to block sorbitol accumulation in the eye. **Lipoic acid** (15 mg daily) is also recommended by some.

• **Do not drink milk or eat cheese, ice cream, seafood, or grease**.

• Place a drop of **honey** in the corner of the eye at night. This will help absorb the crystals.

• **Antioxidants** prevent cataracts from forming. That which clouds the eye is damage for oxidation, caused by free radicals. Antioxidants neutralize free radicals.

• **Sources of antioxidants**: The best antioxidants are **vitamin A**, which you want to get from food in the form of carotenoids, like **beta-carotene. Green and yellow fruits and vegetables** are full of it. Other antioxidants include **vitamins C and E, flavonoids, and selenium**. Taking 1,000 mg of vitamin C daily definitely slows cataract formation. **Magnesium** and **manganese** are also important in helping antioxidants. One Harvard study found that getting 50 mg of carotenoids every other day will significantly reduce your risk of cancer, cardiovascular disease, and cataracts. Carrot juice is an excellent way to obtain carotenoids and antioxidants!

• **The mint herbs** are good antioxidant sources: **Catnip, peppermint, and rosemary.** Other sources include **ginger and turmeric.**

• Substances, such as **nicotine, heavy metal poisoning, insecticides**, etc., makes free radicals and destroy antioxidants in the body. **Saturated fats and fried foods** also have lots of free radicals. Steroid drugs can induce cataracts at any age. Avoid **aspirin, commercial antihistamines**, and **cortisone**.

• Certain foods contain *anthocyanosides*, which improve visual acuity: **blueberries, huckleberries, cranberries, blackberries, raspberries, grapes, plums, wild cherries, and bilberries**.

• Research studies found that taking **bilberry** (European blueberry) extract (80-165 mg daily, based on an *anthocyanidin* percentage of 25%) with **vitamin E** (400 IU daily) prevented cataract progression in some patients.

• **Papain** in **papaya** helps digest protein. If not digested properly, protein can concentrate in the lens.

• **Exercise** early in the morning and avoid long exposure to the sun. **Ultraviolet radiation** from sunlight can cause and worsen cataract problems. **Sunglasses** should be designated Z80.3. Prescription lenses should have a UV-protective film. **Tanning booths** intensify the risk.

• **Relaxing** at times during the day is good for your eyes. Alternate **hot and cold showers** stimulates circulation and proper hormonal balance.

ENCOURAGEMENT—Do not say that you cannot overcome your moral defects. In the strength of Christ, you can. He will empower you to do all that His Father asks of you. The impossibility is all in your will. If you will not, then you cannot. If you are willing, God will strengthen you to resist temptation. 1 Corinthians 10:13.

PHOTOPHOBIA
(Light Sensitivity)

SYMPTOMS—Light hurts the eyes.

CAUSES—This is the abnormal inability of the eyes to tolerate light. Looking at normally bright objects actually hurts the eyes.

This may occur occasionally or gradually increase. The cause is usually a lack of **vitamin A** in the diet. Other causes include acute **glaucoma** (402), **damage to the cornea**, or **uveitis**. If a child suddenly has this problem, it may be an early symptom of **measles** (743).

NATURAL REMEDIES

• If the problem is caused by a lack of **vitamin A**, take 25,000 IU daily for only a few days. More than that can be dangerous. If pregnant, do not take over 10,000 IU daily.

• Increase the intake of **beta-carotene** in the diet. The best way to do this is to eat more **green and yellow vegetables**. Drink 3 glasses of **carrot juice** daily.

ENCOURAGEMENT—All who have a sense of their deep soul poverty, who feel that they have nothing good in themselves, may find peace and strength by looking to Jesus. Thank God that He not only accepts us, but

He changes us. Matthew 7:24-25.

INFLAMED EYELIDS
(Blepharitis)

SYMPTOMS—Redness, swelling, burning, itching of the eyelids. Crusting and scales at the base of the eyelashes. It may feel as if there is something in the eye. Occasionally there is a discharge. In severe cases, there is so much swelling that it closes the eye. Swelling usually goes down within 1 or 2 days, with treatment.

CAUSES—There are two types: *seborrheic*, which produces oily or waxy scales that are easily removed, and *staphylococcal*, which has drier scales and more difficult to remove. Small children frequently have blepharitis. It may be caused by allergy or associated with eczema, dandruff, or seborrheic dermatitis.

Trachoma is the most frequent cause of blindness. Worldwide, 20 million have this.

NATURAL REMEDIES
• Careful, **daily cleaning** of the eyelid and increasing of the blood flow to the area are the best ways to deal with the problem. Clean each eye with a fresh swab (Q-tip) that has been dipped into a 50-50 solution of baby shampoo and water. Roll it against a clean swab to remove the excess liquid. And then carefully remove the crusts with a downward, outward motion to the tip of the eyelash. After this, thoroughly rinse off the shampoo with a fresh washcloth.

• Provide a **nutritious diet** which includes **no sweets, meat, spices, or processed foods**.

• Do not let water run over the eyes when washing the hair. Keep the **eyes and head clean**. Fingernails should be kept short. **Hands should be washed** frequently.

• Occasionally, **lice eggs** (nits) are the cause of the problem. If so, they must be removed.

—*Also see Conjunctivitis (below), which is similar.*

ENCOURAGEMENT—Christ wept at the grave of Lazarus, that He could not save every one whom Satan's power had laid low in death. When He raised Lazarus from the dead, He knew that for that life He must pay the ransom on the cross of Calvary. Every rescue made was to cause Him the deepest humiliation. He was to taste death for every man. Hebrews 2:9.

CONJUNCTIVITIS
(Pinkeye)

SYMPTOMS—The membrane lining of the inner part of the eyelid becomes inflamed. The eyes may appear swollen and bloodshot, and are often irritated and itchy. If there is pus, eyelids often stick together after being closed for a period of time. There may not be pain, but there may be a sensation of sand in the eye.

CAUSES—The conjunctiva is the delicate membrane which connects the eyeball and the inner eyelid. It is usually transparent; but, when irritated or inflamed, it turns a blood-red color.

There may be a discharge from the eye. The origin may be **viral** if the discharge is thin and watery. If it is white and stringy, the cause may be **allergenic**. If there is pus, it may be **bacterial** in origin.

Conjunctivitis is highly contagious when it is caused by a virus. The cause is generally viral or bacterial infection. But physical or chemical injury may be involved (such as **injury to the eye, bacterial infection, allergens, dust, animal danders, pollen, medications, contact lens solutions, fumes, smoke, chemicals, cosmetics, tobacco smoke, air pollution, or other foreign substances in the eye**). Be careful about **swimming pool water.** It can cause eye and ear infections. **Straining** one's eyes may also produce irritation or congestion of the conjunctiva. It typically occurs during a case of **measles**.

In chronic or persistent cases, conjunctivitis may be related to a lack of **vitamin A** or to toxicity due to **liver or kidney dysfunctions**.

When caused by allergens, the infection may reoccur at a certain time each year. In young children, "viral conjunctivitis" can occur from spring till fall and clear up in the winter.

Viral conjunctivitis is often found among groups of schoolchildren. Conjunctivitis is the most common form of eye infection in Western civilization.

Infants born at a hospital, and especially those who remain there for lengthy periods after birth, may be exposed to germs in the nursery. Those born at home are less likely to contract **newborn conjunctivitis**. **Chlamydial conjunctivitis** typically begins 5-12 days after birth. **Gonorrheal conjunctivitis** usually appears 2-4 days following birth. Both infections are transmitted from the mother during passage through the birth canal.

NATURAL REMEDIES
• Take **beta carotene** (10,000 IU, 3 times a day for 1 week; then 25,000 IU daily). This will provide needed vitamin A.

• Take 1 comprehensive **B complex** tablet daily. Also **vitamin C with bioflavonoids** (1,000-5,000 mg in divided daily doses). **Zinc** (25 mg daily).

• Apply warm poultices of 3% **boric acid** on the closed eye. A boric acid ophthalmic ointment may be obtained without prescription from the pharmacy.

• Apply **charcoal poultices** overnight. Mix enough water in to make a thick paste. And spread it over a piece of cloth larger than the inflamed area. Hold it in place with an ace bandage and leave on overnight. Use only enough pressure to hold it in place—but not so tight that pressure is placed on the lid or eyeball. To avoid spreading the infection, carefully dispose of the cloth in the morning. Do not save and use it again.

• During the day, slurry **charcoal water** can be applied: Add ¼ teaspoon of salt and 1 teaspoon of powdered charcoal to a cup of water, boil, let cool, and strain through several layers of cloth. With a dropper, put 4-5 drops of the clear fluid in the affected eye, by pulling back the lower eyelid and applying, every 2 hours. Wash hands carefully after each treatment.

• Do not place a patch on the eye. It can cause bacterial infection and weaken the eyelid, so it will later droop.

• **Ice-cold compresses** can be laid on the eye during the acute stage. The eye should always be closed when doing this. For half an hour, apply a wrung-out washcloth to the eye; change it every 2-3 minutes; stop for 30-60 minutes; and, then, repeat for another 30 minutes.

• **Very warm and cold applications** can be applied every 4 hours. But the water should never be too hot (hot compresses on the eyes are what blinded young Fanny Crosby). Apply a cloth wrung out of very warm water for 2 minutes, then a cold cloth for 30 seconds. Do this for 15 minutes.

• **Saline irrigations** are also good. Add 2 level-teaspoons of salt to 1 quart water, to rinse discharges out of the eyes.

• Bacteria causing this infection may be carried on towels, clothing, paper, toys, or hands. **Launder** bed and bathroom linens separately from those of other family members. All in the home should frequently **wash hands**. **Keep fingers away** from the face.

• Put a **chamomile** tea bag in warm (not hot) water for 2-3 minutes, squeeze out the excess liquid, place it over the infected eye for 2-3 minutes. Do this 3-4 times a day.

• Other good herbs for compresses and washes include **bilberry, aloe vera juice, chickweed, eyebright, fennel, catnip red raspberry leaf, or slippery elm**.

• Gauze pads saturated with **witch hazel** and placed over the closed eyes for 15 minutes may help relieve irritation.

• Children prone to conjunctivitis should be **protected from chilling;** because, when chilled, the person cannot resist bacteria as well.

• If you wear **contacts**, put them away for the several days that these treatments continue. Disinfect or, if necessary, replace contacts.

• Stop using **eye cosmetics**. They occasionally introduce infection into the eyes. Wash hands before using them.

• **Do not share** towels, washcloths, or cosmetics.

ALLERGENIC CONJUNCTIVITIS

• Take 1,000-3,000 mg **vitamin C** daily in divided doses.
• Take **quercetin** (1,000 mg daily and increase to 5,000 mg daily till symptoms are gone). It is one of the bioflav-onoids.

• **Cold compresses** are also good for this infection when caused by an allergy. Soak a washcloth in a dish with ice cubes and water. Squeeze out excess water, fold it, and place over both eyes. Keep it there till it warms. Repeat until the itching subsides.

GONORRHEAL CONJUNCTIVITIS IN NEWBORNS

• Gonococcal germs are quite sensitive to even slight heating or chilling. Therefore, flush the eyes with a slight **saline (salt) solution** (heated to 108° F.) for 1 full minute. Immediately afterward, apply an **ice water compress**, changed every 15 seconds. Continue for 5 minutes. Watch the infant for the next 5 days for signs of reoccurrence. Get a culture of secretions right away if gonorrhea is suspected.

PREVENTION—
• Avoid the problems noted under above *Causes*.
• When something gets in your eye, get it out. Grasping the eyelash and pulling the upper lid over the lower lid induces tears and helps wash out foreign bodies.

—*Also see Inflamed Eyes (Blepharitis, 400), which is similar.*

ENCOURAGEMENT—The heart of him who receives the grace of God overflows with love for God and for those whom Christ died. He becomes kind, thoughtful, humble, yet full of hope and encouragement to those around him. Isaiah 51:7-8.

RETINITUS PIGMENTOSA
(Tunnel Vision)

SYMPTOMS—The initial symptom is poor vision in dim light. Later, the outer edges of vision, known as peripheral vision, are lost. Eyesight deteriorates progressively inward until only a small area of central vision remains (narrow vision field). Full blindness rarely occurs. Dark patches of pigment form on the retina and vision deteriorates. Both eyes are equally affected.

CAUSES—A progressive degeneration of the rods and cones of the retina occurs. Tunnel vision can be inherited. This is progressive degeneration in the retina, the light-sensitive membrane at the back of the eye. The cells in the retina are gradually lost. The disorder is more common in men and is inherited. The disease is fairly rare, but begins in adolescence or young adulthood. The later stages occur after the age of 30, sometimes as late as the 80s.

NATURAL REMEDIES
There is no official cure for the problem. But, in the early stages, a careful diet can slow progression of the disorder. Read through other sections in this chapter on eye diseases; and carefully follow the suggested **diet** and **vitamin-mineral supplementation**.

• High doses of **vitamin A** (15,000 IU daily; but only 10,000 IU during pregnancy) may help slow the loss of remaining eyesight by about 20% a year. But another research study found that high doses of **vitamin E** might accelerate the loss of sight.

• **Flaxseed oil** (2 Tablespoons, two times daily).

• **Vitamin E** (400 IU 2 times daily), if retinitis is hemorrhagic.

• Take **bilberry** or **ginkgo biloba** extract. Research has found that both reduce this disease.

• Take **Coenzyme Q₁₀** (60 mg, 4 times daily). This is especially effective if the case is not severe.

• Also helpful: PCOs from **grapeseed** or **white pine** (100 mg, 3 times daily), **taurine** (500 mg daily), **zinc picolinate** (20 mg daily).

• **Special glasses** may help widen the field of vision if your visual loss becomes severe.

—Also see Macular Degeneration (below), which is a related disease. (Retinitis pigmentosa and macular degeneration are both retinopathy diseases.)

ENCOURAGEMENT—Christ is strong to deliver. Help has been laid on One that is mighty. He encircles man with His long human arm while, with His divine arm, He lays hold of Omnipotence.

MACULAR DEGENERATION

SYMPTOMS—Progressive visual loss occurs over several months. Symptoms may include increasing difficulty in reading, watching television, and recognizing faces. Distortion of vision so that objects appear larger or smaller than normal. Straight lines may appear wavy. However, the edges of vision (peripheral vision) remains clear. Usually both eyes are affected.

CAUSES—The macula is the most sensitive region of the light-sensitive retina at the back of the eye. Progressive loss of central and detailed vision occurs. So this disorder, which occurs more often in women, is the opposite of tunnel vision *(above)*.

Occurring most frequently after the age of 70, the risk of macular degeneration is increased by excessive exposure to sunlight and smoking.

There are two types of this disease: wet and dry. In the *wet form*, new blood vessels grow underneath the macula. If they leak or bleed, the macula is damaged, sometimes very suddenly. In the *dry form*, light-sensitive cells in and beneath the macula die gradually.

NATURAL REMEDIES

• Eat a **low-fat, nutritious diet**. **High cholesterol** levels are linked to macular degeneration. **Avoid processed foods and meat. Caffeine** in any form can intensify the disease. **Alcohol** damages the macula.

• Take **lutein** supplements. Regular intake of this nutrient, which is a pigment found in **leafy green vegetables** (kale, collards, etc.) can prevent macular

degeneration. For this purpose, eat five servings of leafy green vegetables each week. Otherwise, take lutein supplements.

• Animals given **antioxidants** have a much lower risk of macular degeneration. Avoid free radicals and eat antioxidants *(104)*. **Vitamins C** (1,000 mg), **vitamin E** (400-800 IU), **selenium, and zinc** are important antioxidants. Take flaxseed oil (1-2 Tbsp.).

• **Bilberry and lutein** can both be purchased. Take them in combination for better effect. **Taurine**, an amino acid which may help regenerate retinal tissues, may also be obtained at a health-food store. Take it in sublingual form or 500 mg tablets daily.

• **Do not smoke** or be in the same room with smokers. **Avoid smoke in the air** (wood, oil, tires, etc.).

• **Sunlight** can damage the eyes; so avoid looking into the sun or into **bright reflections** from it.

• Get regular exercise and practice relaxation. Drink at least 48 oz. water daily.

ENCOURAGEMENT—Christ came to earth that whosoever will believe in Him may be saved. It is beyond our power to conceive the blessings that are brought within our reach through Christ, if we will but unite our human effort with divine grace.

GLAUCOMA

SYMPTOMS—Early symptoms include eye pain or discomfort mainly in the morning, blurred vision, halos around sources of light, inability to adjust to darker conditions, and peripheral (side) vision loss (resulting in tunnel vision).

CAUSES—Fluid is continually produced in the eyeball. And, just as continuously, it is draining out. The balance is called intraocular pressure. Normal pressure is 15-20 millimeters of mercury; but glaucoma levels may reach 40 or more. The increased pressure, unless it is relieved, will damage the optic nerve and eventually produce blindness. Glaucoma is the second leading cause of blindness. There are several types of glaucoma.

It is more common in blacks than whites, tends to run in families, is more common in women than men, and especially affects people over age 40. Diabetics are more prone to glaucoma. About 3% of those over 65 have it. And about 60,000 Americans are legally blind from this disorder.

There appears to be no evidence that restoration of vision, lost through glaucoma-caused nerve degeneration, can be restored. Yet there are things which can be done to slow or stop the advance of this problem.

Nathan Pritikin says the cause of glaucoma is atherosclerotic plaque buildup within the eye, caused by eating too much **saturated fat**.

NATURAL REMEDIES

DIET

• Dietetic problems are among the most common causes of glaucoma. This includes **overeating, eating the wrong foods, and not eating the right ones**. It is important that one eat a **raw diet.** It should be rich in **vitamin C.** Studies reveal that vitamin C (2,000 mg or more daily) reduces intraocular pressure.

• The diet should include **betaine HCl, vitamin C, a good vitamin / mineral supplement, vitamin A, vitamin B$_2$, and nourishing, natural food**—but not too much of it.

• The diet should include **antioxidant foods** *(104).* These lower intraocular pressure. **Vitamin B$_{12}$** helps prevent the pressure from worsening. **Coenzyme Q$_{10}$** (3 mg daily) helps lower intraocular pressure. Take it with **vitamin E** (400 mg daily).

• **Omega-3 fatty acids** help unclog the eye's drainage system so the fluid can properly leak out, thus reducing pressure. For this purpose, take 2 Tbsp. **flaxseed oil** (1,000 mg) every day.

• **Alpha-lipoic acid** (150 mg daily), best taken with **magnesium** (500 mg daily), and **vitamin C** (1,500 mg daily) also helps lower the pressure.

• **Magnesium** dilates blood vessels. One research found that people given 245 mg per day experienced some improvement within 4 weeks.

• A research study found that 17 of 26 people who took the bioflavonoid, **rutin** (20 mg, 3 times per day), showed definite improvement.

• Less than 1 mg of **melatonin**, taken before retiring, helps reduce pressure increases while you sleep.

• Eat a diet rich of whole, unprocessed foods, especially fresh **fruits and vegetables**. Eat **whole grains, nuts, and legumes**.

• Do not eat **saturated fatty foods. This includes meat, dairy products, grease**, or most commercial **vegetable oils**. Use raw **flaxseed oil** or **wheat germ oil** instead.

• **Food "allergies"** (eating foods which do not agree with the system) can be a frequent cause of the disease. The most common ones in glaucoma patients are **milk, onions, eggs, and chocolate**.

• Do a pulse test and find out which foods may be causing your problems. In addition, a tonometer can be purchased, which you can use to immediately test your eyeball pressure in response to what you just ate.

• **Higher blood-sugar levels** increase pressure.

• **Avoid coffee, tea, tobacco, alcohol, and all junk and processed foods. Smoking** damages eyes which have glaucoma. Tobacco constricts eye blood vessels and increases intraocular pressure. Avoid **spicy foods**.

• **Avoid excessive fluid intake** (juice, water, milk, etc.) at any one time. Drink only small amounts, only an hour apart. But drink at least 48 oz. daily.

HERBS

• **Jaborandi** comes from a tropical tree in South America. It has been used for treating glaucoma for hundreds of years. The active ingredient is *pilocarpine,* which reduces intraocular pressure.

• **Oregano** is one of the richest herbs in antioxidants. 1-2 tsp. dried oregano in a cup of boiling water lower intraocular pressure.

• **Kaffir potato** contains *forskolin,* which lowers eye pressure. Taken in drops, it lowers it in just 1 hour, reaches its peak in 2 hours, and continues for 5 hours.

• **Pansy** flowers contain *rutin,* which lowers pressure.

• Warm **fennel** herb, alternated with **chamomile** and **eyebright**, is helpful. Apply as eyewash in an eyecup or three drops to each eye, 3 times a day.

• A Chinese herbal formula for glaucoma is this: Mix 1 oz. each of tinctures of **bilberry, dandelion, coleus, eyebright, milk thistle, and ginkgo** in a large bottle. Take 1 tsp. 2 times daily for 3-6 months.

• Research studies found that the root of **coleus forskohlii** contains *forskolin,* which reduces intraocular pressure. **Salvia mitiorrhiza** root also does this. Both are Chinese herbs.

• Avoid **bloodroot**. For it and its active ingredient, *sanguinarine* (which is used in toothpastes and mouthwashes), is known to increase intraocular pressure.

OTHER FACTORS

• **Moderate, daily outdoor exercise** helps reduce pressure.

• If anxiety seems to be a cause, increase the **B complex** intake. **Avoid stress, worry, fear, and anger.** Cultivate a tranquil, restful lifestyle. Great temperature changes (as found in northern areas) are a source of stress. It is extremely important that you avoid stress.

• **Avoid heavy lifting, pulling, etc.** Avoid **constipation**. Straining at the stool increases eye pressure (as does **diarrhea**). Maintain a slight, mild laxative effect. **Avoid sitting or standing still** for long periods. **Lying face down** significantly increases pressure. Standing on the hands dramatically increases pressure.

• Increased blood pressure brings increased pressure within the eyeball. Keep your **blood pressure** down!

• Fill a large basin with **ice-cold water**. Immerse both eyes in the water and rapidly blink eyes open and shut 5-10 times. Rest. Then repeat 2-3 times. Do this 2 times a day.

• Apply an **ice-cold moist, folded washcloth** (or towel) 2-3 minutes, rest 1 minute, and reapply 3-4 times. Repeat 2 times daily.

• Place a **very warm (not hot), folded towel** over both eyes for 3 minutes. Then apply an **ice-cold cloth** for 30 seconds. Repeat 3 times, ending with a cold cloth.

• **Do not use the eyes intensively for long periods** of time (TV viewing or excessive reading).

• **Motion sickness medication** patches increase eyeball pressure.

• Those with glaucoma do well to remain under the care of a professional. Every time the pressure increases, a little more eyesight is permanently lost.

ENCOURAGEMENT—No difficulty can hinder you, if you are determined to seek first the kingdom of God and His righteousness. Looking to Jesus, you will be willing to brave contempt and derision for His sake. Psalm 16:11. "Our help is in the name of the Lord, who made heaven and earth." Psalm 124:8. The more we trust to God and the less we trust to ourselves, the more help we receive.

THINNING EYELASHES

SYMPTOMS—The hairs in the eyelashes are getting thin and gradually fall out.

CAUSES—This disorder can have a variety of causes. A primary one is chemicals: **eye makeup, certain medicinal drugs,** and **environmental toxins** in the air. Other causes include **allergies, hypothyroidism, nutritional deficiencies** from a poor diet, **eye surgery,** and **injury**.

NATURAL REMEDIES
• Improve your diet. Eat fresh **fruits, vegetables, whole grains, legumes, and nuts,** Take a full **multivitamin supplement**.
• Take 25,000 IU of **vitamin A** daily for a month; then reduce to 10,000 IU. If pregnant, do not go over 10,000 IU daily.
• **Vitamin B$_2$** (200 mg) and **niacin** (2,000 mg) are also important.
• Take 2 Tbsp. **brewer's yeast** daily.
• **Vitamin E** applied to your eyelashes and eyelids at bedtime will help thicken the eyelashes. Put it on gently.

ENCOURAGEMENT—Amid the perplexities that will press upon the soul, there is only One who can help us out of all our difficulties and relieve all our disquietude. We are to cast all our care upon Jesus. We need to bear in mind that He is present and is directing us to commune with Him. 1 Peter 5:7.

— HEAD AND THROAT —
4 - NOSE

ANOSMIA
(Loss of Sense of Smell)

SYMPTOMS—One does not detect odors. This can occur either temporarily or regularly.

CAUSES—This occurs when one has a cold or rhinitis (nasal inflammation, resulting from colds or allergy).
But when it is chronic, it has one of several causes: a lack of **zinc** in the diet, an **injury, a tumor, or a stroke**. Zinc will not help in those cases.

NATURAL REMEDIES
• Take 30-60 (usually 50) mg of **zinc**, 3 times a day.

ENCOURAGEMENT—What love, what amazing love! That the King of glory would humble Himself to save fallen humanity! Come, fall before Him, just now, and give Him your life anew. Proverbs 15:29.

NASAL CATARRH
(Rhinitis. Runny, Stuffy Nose)

SYMPTOMS—The nose is runny or stuffed up.

CAUSES—Rhinitis is the inflammation of the nasal passages, producing nasal congestion and increased secretion of mucus. When a person drinks enough water, the nose may run. When not enough has been taken, the nose is stuffed and one has to breathe through the mouth. This condition accompanies a variety of problems, including the common cold. *Also see Allergic Rhinitis (578).*

NATURAL REMEDIES
• Go on a **cleansing fast** for a couple days, drinking lots of **liquids and fruit juice**.
• Obtain adequate **rest**, an adequate **fluid** intake, and a well-balanced **diet**. Increase the amount of **vitamin A**, as well as the other **vitamins**.
• **Eucalyptus oil** is an old-fashioned treatment, long in use. Other helps include **chamomile, scotch pine, and cayenne**.
• As a nose ointment, Dr. Christopher recommends this: Mix 1 part each of **oil of spearmint and oil of peppermint** in sufficient amount of vaseline and apply in the nose with a paintbrush.
• Another helpful formula is to mix powders of 1 oz. **witch hazel**, ½ oz. **wild cherry bark,** and ½ oz. **white oak bark**. Sniff the powder up the nose.
• If these herbs are not available, use powdered **witch hazel** alone. Sniff it up the nose or mix with vaseline. And paint your nose with a tiny paintbrush.
• **Do not blow hard**—and unintentionally force phlegm up the eustachian tubes. This can lead to ear infection.
• **Beware of decongestants**; they can hurt the nasal lining.

H
E
A
D

J.H. KELLOGG, M.D., PRESCRIPTIONS FOR NASAL CATARRH AND ITS COMPLICATIONS (how to give these water therapies: pp. 206-275 / list of treatments: pp. 206-207 / Hydrotherapy Disease Index: pp. 273-275)

(1) ACUTE Catarrh (Acute Coryza) —
GENERAL TREATMENT—Sweating bath at bedtime, followed by a short cold application: Wet Sheet Rub, Cold Douche, Hot Footbath with very hot compress to the face, Water Vapor Inhalation, and water drinking.

TO PREVENT—Cold Bath daily or twice a day and **outdoor life. Avoid excessively warm** clothing, warm living, or warm sleeping rooms in the winter. Wear linen next to the skin in summer and winter.

(2) CHRONIC CATARRH —
BASIC CONSIDERATIONS—Avoid taking cold. And when an acute catarrh is contracted, eliminate it as soon as possible.

INCREASE ACTIVITY AND TONE OF THE SKIN— Short sweating procedures, especially the Radiant Heat Bath and Wet Sheet Pack continued until the sweating stage. Follow by **short cold** applications. Wet Sheet Rub; Shallow Bath or Cold Douche; Neutral Bath at bedtime, 20-30 minutes, 3 times a week; daily Cold morning Bath; Cold Towel Rub; Cold Shower or shallow rubbing bath. All sweating baths ought, if possible, to be taken just before retiring at night.

IMPROVE NUTRITION AND LIFESTYLE—Avoid indigestible, spicy foods and meats. Eat simply of wholesome food. Obtain needed **outdoor exercise, sunbaths**, and swimming.

RELIEVE NASAL CONGESTION—Alternate Compress to the face, **Alternate Sponging** or Compresses to the upper spine, and **Cold Footbath** under running water if the extremities are cold.

GENERAL METHOD—Build up the general health by tonic measures, employing friction tonics, at least twice daily. Avoid hot baths and too warm clothing. Expose the body, as much as possible, to the open air. But use great care to avoid taking cold by undue exposures. Gradually train the body to the point of enduring exposure without injury. (Drink enough water to keep the mucus in the nose thin, so it can easily flow out without clogging the passageways. Do not blow your nose, lest mastoid infection occurs).

—*Also see Common Cold (289) and Catarrh (288).*

ENCOURAGEMENT—By yielding your will to Christ, He will hold you fast. You will have strength and determination to live a clean life and resist temptation to sin. Psalm 91:15.

NOSEBLEED
(Epistaxis)

SYMPTOMS—The nose bleeds. A tiny vein in the nose has been broken.

CAUSES—Nasal infection, injury to the nose, **scratching** with a fingernail, **blowing the nose hard**, a sudden **change in atmospheric pressure**, or a **foreign body** in the nose of children. It is more likely to occur during winter. **Excessive dryness** can cause nasal surfaces to crack and bleed.

Nosebleeds are common in children before puberty, but it usually stops by itself. They often follow upper respiratory tract infection. And the lining may have been affected by the blowing and wiping.

In people over 50, nosebleeds can be more serious. The small blood vessels in the nose can rupture more easily. It can also be caused by **drugs that prevent blood clotting; this** lasts longer if you have **high blood pressure**. Nosebleeds are common among **alcoholics**.

Most common is *anterior nosebleed*, which is bleeding in the nose itself. The other type is the *posterior nosebleed.* This occurs in the elderly. And it is caused by high blood pressure. The bleeding starts in the rear of the nose and runs down into the throat. The blood pressure must be lowered! Increase water intake and see a physician. If bleeding continues more than half an hour, see a physician.

NATURAL REMEDIES
ANTERIOR NOSEBLEEDS (from the nose itself)
• **Blow out the clots**, then **sit in a chair and lean forward** without tilting the head back. (If you lie down or lean backward, you will swallow blood.) **Put a small piece of wet cotton (or cloth) in the nose** and **pinch lightly** on it for 5 minutes. Then apply **cold washcloths or an ice pack** to the nose, cheek, and neck. (Another suggestion is to lightly **sniff cold water with a little salt or lemon juice** added.)

• Then apply **vitamin E oil** (or petroleum jelly) *gently* to the inside of the nose for 7-10 days, to keep the membranes moist. Lie back and **rest** for a time. If the nosebleeds are serious enough to warrant it, rest as much as you can for two days. The rupture in the blood vessel that caused the nosebleed requires 7-10 days to completely heal. When the bleeding stops, a clot forms and then becomes a scab. Do not pick it loose.

• **White oak bark and bayberry** are astringents. **Sniff** one of them up the nose before inserting the cotton.

• A little **cayenne** can be swallowed in some water. This will draw blood away from the head to the stomach.

• Here is Jethro Kloss' remedy for nosebleed: Add 1 tsp. **goldenseal** to 1 pint boiling water. Steep and let settle. When cold, pour a little into your palm and sniff it up your nose. Repeat several times a day. Or use tea made from **witch hazel leaves, wild alum root, and white oak bark**. Applying **cold or pressure to back of the neck** helps prevent free flow of blood to the head.

• Make sure you are getting enough **vitamin K** in the diet. It is found in all **dark greens**. Put **lactobacillus acidophilus** in the colon. It will synthesize, thus increasing the amount of, vitamin K in your body. (Frozen foods lack vitamin K.)

• Be sure to take enough **vitamin C. Calcium, magnesium, alfalfa, and vitamin E** are also important.

HEAD

• Along with vitamin C (1,000 mg), take 2 mg copper. It is essential for the formation of collagen and elastin, which helps eliminate nosebleeds.

• Eliminating **sugary sweets** tends to stop recurrent nosebleeds.

• When the nose dries out excessively, nosebleed can occur. Try increasing the **humidity** in the room. Consider purchasing a humidifier. **Smoking** dries out the nasal membranes.

• **Medicinal blood thinners** can cause nosebleeds. The active ingredient in D-Con rat poison is a blood thinner drug. Foods high in *salicylates* also tend to thin the blood. **Tea and coffee** are in this category.

POSTERIOR NOSEBLEED

• You need to **lower your blood pressure**. Read the section on high blood pressure *(526)*.

• Keep in mind that a posterior nosebleed is far better than having a blood vessel rupture from high blood pressure—inside the cranial cavity. Then you have a stroke! Whichever type of nosebleed may occur, here are additional suggestions:

• Those with frequent nosebleeds should **take extra iron**. It is needed to make hemoglobin. **Rutin** is also needed.

• **Avoid oral contraceptives**. Anything that changes estrogen levels can make you more prone to nosebleeds.

HYDROTHERAPY

Here are several treatments for nosebleeds, discussed in the *Hydrotherapy* section *(206-275)* of this *Encyclopedia:*

Contrast Bath to the hand and arm. Two very deep pails may be used. The hot water should be as hot as can be borne. A **hot footbath** can also be used to stop a nosebleed. A **cold water spray** to the bottom of the feet will also do it. Put an **ice bag** on the back of the neck. And, at the same time, place a **hot fomentation** over the face. Put **ice** to the hands; and, if necessary, **elevate the hand**s to a vertical position. Give a **hot footbath** or **Hot Leg Pack**.

ENCOURAGEMENT—If we are in Christ, we are heaven-bound. So we must not seem mournful to those around us. Rejoice. For every day is one day nearer heaven! Do all you can to be a blessing to those you come in contact with. Psalm 145:19.

NASAL CUTS
AND INFECTIONS

SYMPTOMS—Efforts to pick at the inside of the nose and clean it out will occasionally result in inside cuts which can become mildly infected for a time.

CAUSES—It is easy to get into a habit of picking at the nose, even when there is no reason to do so. People sometimes feel driven to pick at the nose, imagining they will somehow make it super clean. But unwashed fingers in the nose can result in cuts which infect for a day or two. Infection from contaminated hands is even more likely if you have a dog or cat in the house, or people who have them handle your doorknobs.

NATURAL REMEDIES

• The solution is simple enough: Routinely **rinse your nose** with water in the bathroom every morning. This only takes a few moments, but it will remove accumulated dust. The urge to afterward pick at the nose will be lessened.

• Teach yourself, whenever possible, to **leave your nose alone**. Or only put a **washed finger** in your nose.

• If an infection occurs in the nose, get extra rest and take antibiotic herbs *(297)* for a few days.

There is always danger when infection occurs on the face above the lips and below the eyes. For it can travel into the brain. If in doubt, see a physician.

ENCOURAGEMENT—All around us, souls are hungering for Christ and a knowledge of how to be saved. Do all you can to be a help to them. They need you to help lead them to God. In His strength, you can do it. Psalm 112:1.

NASAL POLYPS

SYMPTOMS—Symptoms often develop gradually over a period of months. Severity of symptoms depends on the number and size of the polyps. Symptoms may include decreased sense of smell, blocked nose due to obstruction by polyps, or a runny nose due to excess mucous secretion. Occasionally, they lead to recurrent sinusitis *(381)* and a loss of smell.

CAUSES—These are fleshy growths that develop in the mucus-secreting lining of the nose. They are more common in those with **asthma** *(714, 852)* or **rhinitis** *(404)*. Although they rarely develop in children, they sometimes occur in those who have inherited **cystic fibrosis** *(655)*.

Nasal polyps are always benign (non-cancerous)

NATURAL REMEDIES

• Eat a diet rich in **fruits and vegetables**. Eat **whole grains, nuts, and legumes**. **Avoid meat, dairy products, coffee, tobacco, and alcohol**. Avoid a **heavy protein diet** of any kind.

• Eliminate your **food allergies**. They cause a chronic swelling of the nasal lining and develop polyps.

—*See Colon Polyps (467) and Allergic Rhinitis (850).*

ENCOURAGEMENT—We are to keep our minds stayed upon God. In our weakness, He will be our strength. In our ignorance, He will be our wisdom. In our frailty, He will be our enduring might.

— HEAD AND THROAT —
5 - EARS

EARACHE AND EAR INFECTION, MASTOIDITIS
(Otitis Externa and Media)

SYMPTOMS—One or both ears ache. This is frequently accompanied by infection in the middle ear. The pain will be worse at night because the body is prone (flat) and it is more difficult for the eustachian tubes to drain out the phlegm.

Although not common, sometimes the ears will ache because there is trouble with the teeth (referred pain), not because of infection.

Symptoms of a ruptured eardrum: dizziness, ringing in the ears, bleeding or a bloody discharge, sudden pain, or a sudden lessening of pain, and/or hearing loss in one or both ears.

CAUSES—Infection of the outer or middle ear causes pressure to build up. This pressure on nerve endings causes pain. But, if there were no pain, there might be no warning that a serious ear problem existed.

Otitis externa is infection in the outer ear. The eardrum through the length of the eustachian tube becomes swollen and inflamed. There is a slight fever, discharge from the ear, pain (which increases when the ear is touched or pulled), and temporary loss of hearing.

Otitis media is infection in the middle ear. This is especially common in infants and children. The infection is located behind the eardrum, where the small ear bones are located. There is earache, fullness, pressure in the ear, and a fever as high as 103° F. or higher.

Here is an ear test: If you have an infection *lightly wiggle* your outer ear (the part you can see) if there is no pain, you probably have a middle ear infection. If there is pain, the infection is in the eustachian tube.

Another ear test: If you seem to have pain in the ear, *pull firmly* on the earlobe. If the pain increases, then you probably have an ear infection. If the pain does not increase, you may have a dental problem.

Going into **higher altitudes** can push phlegm, already in the eustachian tube, into the middle ear. Never sleep on your ear if you have a head cold and the vehicle is moving upward to a higher elevation! Chronic middle ear disease has increased since

the advent of **antibiotics**. They produce conditions favorable to that infection.

Swimming in public pools is a great way to get ear infections. If you go there, do not get the water in your ears—and do not dive! Bacteria go up the eustachian tubes. *(See Swimmer's Ear, 410.)*

Chronically enlarged **adenoids** may cause blockage of the eustachian tubes, leading to congestion and fluid buildup in the middle ear.

Otitis media is more frequent in **bottle-fed infants** than those that are breast-fed. Two reasons: Cow's milk produces inflammation and blockage of the infant's eustachian tubes; this leads to infection from outside. The immune globulin A in breast milk strengthens the infant's immune system. Allowing the child to feed with a bottle, while laying dow, will cause the problem.

Infection in the inner ear generally results from **meningitis** or from the spread of a middle-ear **infection**. Symptoms include loss of hearing, nausea, dizziness, vomiting, and fever.

Earache is a common childhood infection. Most children experience it (90% by the age of 6). It is easier for a child to have an ear infection, since his eustachian tubes are shorter than that of an adult. Causes include **childhood diseases, allergies, colds, and respiratory infections**.

If they are frequent, ear infections can lead to loss of hearing.

NATURAL REMEDIES
TREATMENT FOR INFECTION
• **Cut an onion in half. Wrap one of the halves in aluminum foil. Warm oven to 350° F. Put onion in oven and heat it until it becomes hot. Take from oven and remove foil. Place a dry washcloth over the round part of the onion (to retain heat), and hold it with hand. Place cut surface of the onion directly on the ear. To improve drainage of pus, lay on bed with infected ear down, as you continue to hold it in place. If there is pus, it may drain. Relief will come within 3-5 minutes. Remove onion. Ear problem is usually solved.**

• Keep the **ears warm** and the person **resting in bed**, preferably with his **head slightly elevated** and, perhaps also, his trunk (to assist natural drainage of the eustachian tubes). Surgical draining might be necessary. The fever increases the need for **vitamins A and C**. Keep the **feet warm. Heat applied to the feet** will draw blood from the head and improve circulation.

• **Sit up** when practical to do so, to decrease the swelling and start the tubes draining. **Swallowing** will help ease the pain. **Yawning** really helps open up the eustachian tubes.

• Only feed a child when he is **sitting up**.

• **Blow warm air** toward the ear, from a hair dryer 18-30 inches from it.

• Another way to reduce pain is to make a paste,

CHART - 1043: Catagories of Ear diseases (407-415)

using **onion powder** or **clay packs**. Then apply this to the outside of the ear.

• Bake a large **onion,** until it becomes soft, and tie it over the ear. This will often give great relief when pain is severe.

• Mix a tsp. of (or a drop of each tincture) **echinacea, goldeseal, and licorice root** (to add flavor) to a cup of boiling water. Drink this flavorful cup 3 times a day. Children will like it.

• Go on a brief **fruit and vegetable juice fast**.

• Take **vitamin C** (500 mg, 3 times a day), **vitamin A** (2,500 IU), **zinc** (15 mg), **vitamin E** (200-400 IU), and **B complex**.

DROPS IN THE EAR

IMPORTANT: Do not place liquid or oil in the ear if you think the drum has burst!

• Warm some **oil** to body temperature and place a **drop or two in the ear**. This will help lessen pain.

• A helpful method, used by many for a long time is this: Place a few drops of **garlic** juice in the ear. Then add a couple drops of **lobelia** oil. The garlic purifies and kills germs. The lobelia takes away the pain. To only take away pain: Place a little **olive oil** in the ear. Then add a drop or two of **lobelia** tincture.

• Place 2-3 drops of warm **mullein oil** in the ear 2-3 times daily. Mullein has been used to treat earaches for many years. Or add a few drops of **tea tree oil** to vegetable oil and place some in the ear. Never drink herb oils. *How to make your own mullein oil:* Gather fresh yellow mullein flowers and steep them in sunlight for 21 days. Strain out the oil. Or purchase the oil.

• Winnebago Indians steeped the whole **yarrow** plant and poured the liquid into the aching ear.

AVOID

• There is a tendency for people who have ear problems to be **heavy earwax** producers. To reduce the amount of earwax made, eat less saturated fatty acids. Unsaturated fatty acids are not a problem.

• A 1991 pediatric study of over 100 children with chronic otitis media revealed that 78% were **sensitive to foods**, such as corn, milk, peanuts, and wheat. By eliminating the allergenic foods, 86% were cleared of ear problems.

• **Avoid sugar, dairy products, meat, and heavy meals** until the crisis is past. Herb teas are helpful in assisting the healing process. This includes **peppermint, echinacea, goldenseal, pau d'arco, and slippery elm**.

• Because they increase sticky mucus in the body, **dairy products** increase ear infections. **Excessive sweets and starches** lower resistance and intensify ear problems.

• People with a tendency to ear infection should **avoid all cow's milk products**. But, in addition to producing so much mucus, it is reported that milk allergies can produce earaches (and even a burst eardrum), simulating otitis media—without an ear infection actually existing.

• Avoid **cigarette smoke**. For it can irritate the eardrum.

• Place drops of **hydrogen peroxide** in the ear, to help clean it out. Then rinse it out with water. Do not leave the peroxide there! It can sink through the eardrum and produce a fizzing sound which can last for several years.

• Dripping **garlic oil** directly into the ear canal has been shown to treat fungal infections as well as or better than drugs. It has powerful antibiotic properties.

• Take **garlic enemas**. These will help disinfect the body of higher levels of toxins that are building up from the infection. Signs of this are chills, fever, general aches, and pain increase.

TREATMENT FOR RUPTURE

What should you do if the eardrum ruptures? Causes can include a severe ear infection and sudden pressure inward on the ear which results from diving, slapping, a strong kiss to the ear, or a nearby explosion.

During an ear infection, pus builds up and causes pain in the ear. If this pus starts leaking to the outside, then the eardrum has ruptured. Sometimes a rupture brings a sudden reduction in pain, because the pressure has been lowered. A rupture causes hearing loss and a discharge of bloody fluid from the ear.

• In case the eardrum ruptures, **put nothing in the ear** until the eardrum is healed. A **fomentation** on the outside of the ear can be helpful.

• Once the infection increases to acute pain, you may need an antibiotic. **Echinacea** has both antibiotic and immune-boosting effects. Give a teaspoon of dried herb in tea, or a drop of the tincture in juice or tea. Drink either 3 times a day.

• An alternate method is this: When the eardrum has abscessed and broken, use **warm peroxide** to wash the ear out. The peroxide will loosen the putrefied matter and bring it out of the ear. This method is probably good for cleaning out the ear. But keep in mind that hydrogen peroxide is best used on outside body surfaces, where oxygen can cause it to fizz into harmlessness. When it gets inside sensitive body parts, it can continue there for quite some time. We know of one individual who had peroxide in his ear for several years thereafter. And, every so often, he could hear it lightly fizzing.

• Do not place a hot-water bottle over the infected ear and leave it there for a time. A suction effect can be caused which worsens the condition.

• Give a quick, **hot bath** of only a few minutes, Finish with **cold** water, dry quickly, rubbing briskly. Put into **bed** immediately and let him sleep.

—*Also see Swimmer's Ear (410).*

HYDROTHERAPY

Here are treatments mentioned in the *Hydrotherapy section (206-275)* of this *Encyclopedia*:

Irrigation of the Ear: A lean rubber tube is used to gently (gently!) introduce a flow of water onto the outer ear. The water is *never* applied with any pressure! It flows to the ear and out to the side. The temperature may be from 100° to 120° F., depending upon the effect desired. The source of water should be on a level with the top of the head (to maintain only a slight pressure). Never use force. Because perforation of the ear often exists, serious injury could result from introduction of water, with any degree of force, into the middle ear. The head should be inclined to the side as the water is applied.

The canal of the ear should afterward be carefully dried and covered with a cloth or a warm hand for a few minutes. In cold weather, the ear should not be exposed outdoors for at least an hour after warm ear irrigation is applied. Even after that, a small piece of cotton should be placed in the outer passageway.

This measure affords great relief in the pain of acute otitis media and earache due to other causes. In chronic suppurative disease of the ear, this measure is indispensable as a means of cleansing and disinfection.

Draining the middle ear: Applications should be made to the whole side of the head and face, diverting blood from the internal carotid and internal maxillary blood vessels. If the Hot Compress extends below the jaw, the common carotid artery will be dilated (enlarged), which you do not want. An ice bag should be placed below the jaw at the same time. This will increase the effect by contracting the carotid.

Draining the inner ear: The inner ear problem may be relieved, when congested, by warm applications to the arms and cold applications to the head and back of the neck, thus diverting the blood into the arms from the vertebral arteries by a proximal compress or an ice bag to the back of the neck.

Inflammation of ear: Fomentation over the affected part, derivative treatment to legs, Hot Leg Bath, Hot Footbath, Prolonged Leg Pack.

Inflammation of middle ear: Ice to throat of the same side, fomentation over ear.

Earache: Ice Bag to the neck of the same side. Fomentation over ear. Hot Ear Douche, if necessary. Protect the ear with warm cotton, to prevent chilling by evaporation after treatment.

Eustachian tube inflammation: The Heating Throat Compress is an application of a cold cloth, covered with flannel, which then heats up and results in improved circulation and a better flow of healing blood into, and out of, the afflicted area. Wring the cotton cloth from cold water and place it around the neck. This should be about 2-3 thicknesses about the neck. Cover it well with flannel (singly or doubly, depending on the thickness). Fit the flannel snugly, but not too tightly that it will be uncomfortable. Pin it securely.

Remove it the next morning. It should be entirely dry. In eustachian tube inflammation, the compress should extend upward about the lower part of the ear. You may need to hold up this part of the compress (the part by the lower part of the ear) with a bandage that is fastened to it and goes over the top part of the head and back down to it on the other side.

PREVENTION—Never dive below 3-4 feet below the surface of the water.

Never sleep in an airplane or vehicle when it is descending—or ascending. If you are in a car—climbing up or down the mountains—do not sleep, especially on your side. You do not swallow as often when you are asleep. And, if you have phlegm in your sinuses, it can go up into your ears.

Be careful when scuba diving. The greatest air pressure changes occur within the first 33 feet below the surface. Avoid earplugs and hoods which are too tight-fitting, so you cannot equalize air pressure in the ears.

Avoid the above three situations when your head is stuffy with phlegm.

Breast-feeding reduces a baby's chances of having ear trouble.

Do not smoke.

DR. WILLIAM L. McKIE'S PRESCRIPTIONS FOR EAR CONGESTION AND ITS COMPLICATIONS—This section deals with methods of reducing blood congestion in the middle ear and inner ear. It was taken, with slight adaptation, from Dr. William L. McKie's book, *Scientific Hydrotherapy,* page 55.

DRAINING THE MIDDLE EAR—Applications should be made to the whole side of the head and face, diverting blood from the internal carotid and internal maxillary blood vessels. **If the hot compress extends below the jaw, the common carotid will be dilated (enlarged), which you do not want. An Ice Bag should be placed below the jaw at the same time.** This will increase the effect, by contracting the carotid.

DRAINING THE INNER EAR—The internal ear, receiving its blood supply from the vertebral artery, a branch of the subclavian, is not affected by heat over the ear. But the inner ear problem may be relieved, when congested, by **warm applications to the arms and cold applications to the head and back of the neck,** thus diverting the blood into the arms from the vertebral arteries by a **proximal compress or an ice bag to the back of the neck**.

ENCOURAGEMENT—Christ will not be satisfied till the victory is complete in your life. He wants to change you into a full overcomer. Let Him empower you to obey the Ten Commandments. Romans 3:4.

EARWAX
(Wax Blockage)

SYMPTOMS—Hearing is becoming duller and the person suspects he may be losing his hearing. There may be a feeling of fullness or ringing in the ears (*see Tinnitus, 411*).

CAUSES—Earwax (cerumen) is secreted by glands in the outer ear. This cleanses and moisturizes the lining of the external canal, thus protecting the inner ear as a barrier against germs, moisture, dust, and insects.

The problem may be a hard plug of earwax (cerumen) in the ear canal. Some people have constant ear pain until the excess wax is cleaned out. If you do **not chew your food** thoroughly, earwax can build up. The chewing tends to break it down. **Saturated fats** contribute to excess production of earwax.

If there is not enough wax in the ear, it will be dry and itching. Dip a Q-tip in quality vegetable oil and place a little in the outer ear canal. *To relieve itchy ears*, insert a few drops of apple cider vinegar, wait 30 seconds, then tilt head and let it run out.

NATURAL REMEDIES

• **Never put anything sharp in the ear!** That includes bobby pins, paper clips, and pencil tips. They can puncture the eardrum.

• **Do not use cotton-tipped swabs** either, because they merely ram the wax down deeper and impact it the more.

• Place something in your ear which will soften it. This can be **hydrogen peroxide, mineral oil, or glycerin**. Add a drop or two of this to each ear. Let the excess run out. The liquid left inside will soften the wax. Do this for a couple days.

• Fill a bowl with body-temperature **water** and suck it into a rubber bulb syringe. Holding your head over the bowl, gently squirt the water into the ear. Use very, very little pressure. Turn your head and let the water run out.

• Do not rub the ears in order to dry them. Either use a **hair dryer** (18-20 inches away) or drop a little **alcohol** in each ear. Do not wash out the ears in this manner more often than every couple months. You need some earwax to protect your ears.

• There is a tendency for people who have ear problems to be heavy earwax producers. To reduce the amount of earwax made, eat **less saturated fatty acids**. Unsaturated fatty acids are not a problem. It is the over-balance of saturated fats which causes the earwax problem. Therefore, stop eating **junk foods**. Much of it is full of saturated fats. Instead, take **flax-seed oil** for its omega-3 and omega-6

• An alternate method of cleaning out the earwax is this: Using an eyedropper, place either a solution of 1 part **vinegar** to 1 part warm **water** or a few drops of **hydrogen peroxide** in your ear. Allow it to settle for a minute, then drain it. Do this 2-3 times a day. If the wax is hard and dry, apply **garlic oil** for a day or two, to soften it. Then wash out the ear with a steady stream of warm **water**, under no pressure. Patiently continue irrigating the ear canal, flushing with warm water. The wax buildup will come out.

• Yet another method is using **"ear candles,"** available at health-food stores. Someone will have to help you use them. Instructions come with the candles. Afterward, you may be bothered by the fact that an excess of wax has been eliminated. You may need to put cotton in each ear for a time. This method really works!

• If you take **vitamin C** (500 mg, 3 times a day) regularly, in 6 months your ears will no longer produce excess earwax.

ENCOURAGEMENT—One day alone is ours. During this day, we are to live for God. For this one day we are to place in the hand of Christ all our purposes and plans, casting all our care upon Him. For He careth for us. 1 Peter 5:7.

SWIMMER'S EAR

SYMPTOMS—An ache and/or infection in one or both ears, after swimming in a pond, creek, or public swimming pool. The outer ear canal becomes inflamed, swollen, and red. Tenderness and pain, discharge from the ear canal, difficulty hearing, itching. Touching the ear often causes pain. There may be a feeling of fullness in the ear. Symptoms usually appear over 1-2 days.

CAUSES—Swimmer's ear occurs when **pool water** remains in the outer ear canal too long. Bacteria or fungi in the water increases the chance of infection. When swimming in **contaminated water**, keep your head out of the water. The pool water, having repeatedly wet and softened the earwax, caused it to become an ideal place for bacteria to grow. **Chlorinated water** is more likely to cause swimmer's ear than saltwater.

But the most common cause is infection, from the nasal passages and throat, that has been pushed into the eustachian tubes when the **nose was blown** too hard.

Diving into water is remarkably unsafe.

Constant swimming throughout the summer can result in infestation of the external ear canal by **candida albicans** *(281)*. Constant dampness of the ear, in water not entirely clean, throughout the summer swimming season is thought to be the cause. A research report, issued in 1991, revealed that water can make earwax swell somewhat, partially plugging the ears. That effect is probably a protective device. **Hair dye**, entering the outer ear, can also cause infection as well as chemicals in some **commercial eardrops**.

People who wear hearing aids should remove them occasionally, so moisture in the ear can evaporate.

NATURAL REMEDIES
TREATMENT

• Experts say that 80% of the swimmer's ear problems can be cured by putting **alcohol-vinegar drops** in the ears 3 times a day, for two or three days after the swimmer's ear problem develops. *(See just below for the formula.)*

• *You may also want to read the extensive section on Earache and Infection (407).*

Contact a physician, if the drops cause burning or sharp pain, if symptoms persist for more than a few days, if fever develops, or there is a discharge from the ear.

PREVENTION

• The key to prevention is to **keep the ear clean and dry**. **Do not** let the children swim during periods of active disease. When swimming, keep water out of the ears or wear **soft earplugs** (firm ones may damage the ear lining).

• But, if water enters the ears, **shake your head** vigorously to remove as much water as possible from them. **Pull the ear** up and out, to straighten the ear canal so the water can get out easier.

• After leaving the swimming pool, apply **hydrogen peroxide** as eardrops to disinfect the ears. Or prepare this mixture: 1 oz. **rubbing (isopropyl) alcohol** and 1 oz. **apple cider vinegar** (5% ascetic acid). Then place a couple drops of this in each ear. This makes the water evaporate and, at same time, restores the acid balance of the skin, preventing itchy ears.

• Wear earplugs when bathing or shampooing the hair.

ENCOURAGEMENT—If you have given yourself to God, to do His work, you have no need to be anxious for tomorrow. He will take care of that. Instead (just for today) live for Him, obey Him, and be a blessing to all around you. 2 Timothy 2:11-12.

INSECT IN THE EAR

SYMPTOMS—An insect has gotten into your ear and is moving around and/or buzzing.

NATURAL REMEDIES

• Tilt your head toward the sun or, if you are in a darkened room, toward a flashlight. The little creature may head **toward the light** and leave.

• Place a piece of **ripe apple or peach** next to the ear to entice him to exit.

• The insect may be entrapped in the earwax or weakened, if your exploring finger pressed against him. Have someone pour a teaspoon of **warm vegetable oil** into that ear and keep it there briefly. He may come out when you tilt your head and let the oil out. As you tilt the ear, **pull the outer ear** backward and upward to straighten the canal so he can get out easier.

• If still no success, pour **warm water** into the up-tilted ear, so he can float out. As a last resort, contact a nurse or physician.

ENCOURAGEMENT—We may be assured that we need not go into the heavens to bring Jesus down to us, neither into the deep to bring Him up; for He is at our right hand, and His eye is ever upon us. We should ever seek to realize that the Lord is very near us, to be our counselor and guide. This is the only way in which we may have confidence toward God.

TINNITUS
(Ringing in the Ears)

SYMPTOMS—Sounds in the ear: ringing, whistling, roaring, hissing, chirping, buzzing, and whining cricket sounds—when there is no outside physical source for these sounds. At first, they come and go. The sound is constant. No one else hears them.

There are reported instances in which others have heard the sounds from as much as four feet from the person's ear. "Tinnitus," in Latin, means "to tinkle" or a "bell-like ring."

The frequency of tinnitus increases with age. The left ear seems to produce the sounds more often than the right ear. About 75% of deaf people report tinnitus.

CAUSES—There are several possible causes, including an **irritation of nerve endings** in the ear by loud noises. **Chemicals** and **drugs** can injure the internal ear. **Prescription drugs** can produce tinnitus or hearing loss (beware of **quinine** and **aspirin**). **Nicotine** constricts blood vessels and may be the cause. Other causes are **lead, aluminum, mercury poisoning, impacted wax, hormonal problems, high blood pressure, severe blows to the head, anemia, perforation of the tympanic membrane, fluid in the middle ear, epilepsy, migraine, food allergies, Ménière's disease, hypothyroidism, multiple sclerosis**, as well as repeated and prolonged exposure to **loud noises**. Whatever the cause, **stress** sometimes adds to it. Frequent food allergy causes include **milk, eggs, wheat, sugar, honey, and other sweeteners**.

Tinnitus is not a sign of a more serious problem or a precursor of any serious disease—unless it is associated with Ménière's Disease *(412).*

NATURAL REMEDIES

• Surgical success rates for this are very low. Beware of "tinnitus maskers." These products can cause hearing loss.

• Do the **pulse test** to check on problem foods. Have a **hair analysis** made. Find the cause and eliminate it. A 1981 medical study pointed to **coffee, tea, tonic water, red wine, grain-based spirits, chocolate, and cheese** as the most common dietary causes of tinnitus.

• Mix 1 teaspoon of **salt** and 1 teaspoon of **glycerin** in 1 pint warm water. Several times a day. Using a nasal sprayer, spray each nostril until it begins draining into the back of the throat. Also spray the throat.

• Eat a **nourishing diet**, which includes **trace minerals** (Norwegian kelp or Nova Scotia dulse), **vitamin A, calcium, magnesium, and betaine HCl**.

• A lack of **manganese** can cause deafness, dizziness, and ear noises. A lack of magnesium can produce nerve twitching and sensitivity to noise.

• Changing and correcting the diet, **reducing stress**, and getting more **exercise** outdoors has been helpful in dealing with tinnitus. Stress causes more adrenaline to be produced; this constricts blood vessels and keeps waste products from being as quickly eliminated. **Fatigue** increases this problem. Maintain a regular schedule of going to bed and arising. Make sure the colon is working well. An **enema** will help with this.

• Take **B complex** and higher levels of three of them: **thiamine** (100-500 mg daily), **B$_{12}$** (1,000 mcg daily for 6 months, then 100 mcg daily), and **niacin** (50 mg, 2 times a day). If there is no improvement after 2 weeks, increase the niacin by 50 mg every 2 weeks until you reach 500 mg twice a day. Also take **zinc** (15 mg, 2 times daily), and **magnesium** (400 mg daily). Manganese is also important.

• **Avoid loud noises** and noisy situations. **Alcohol** makes tinnitus worse. **Caffeine** is a common cause. **Marijuana** and **cocaine** intensify the problem. **Aspirin** is a known cause of tinnitus, as well as **blood pressure and arthritis drugs**. Also beware of **steroids, anticonvulsive medications, vasodilators, and anticholesterol drugs**. **Nicotine** damages the hearing.

• Avoid sugar, salt, and all fatty foods, including meat and dairy foods. Eat plenty of fiber: fresh **fruits and vegetables, whole grains, nuts, and legumes**.

• Over a dozen European studies have confirmed that taking **ginkgo** eliminates tinnitus in many, but not all cases. **Lesser periwinkle** (20 mg, 3 times daily) contains *vincamine*, which gives good results with tinnitus and Ménière's Syndrome (*below*). **Sesame seeds** helps reduce the effects of tinnitus.

• Other useful herbs include **bugleweed, garlic, gotu kola, cayenne, and prickly ash**.

• Do not take **wintergreen, meadowsweet, willowgreen**, or high doses of **aspirin**. They can cause ringing in the ears.

• Play some **music** softly at night, the time when the tinnitus is most noticeable. Actually, you can **train your mind** to ignore the tinnitus sounds and focus attention on other sounds.

• The cause may simply be **excess earwax**. *Read the section on Earwax (409).*

—*See Ménière's Disease (below) and Earwax (409).*

ENCOURAGEMENT—Christ desires to give you the riches of eternal life with Him. What can compare with that? Do not wait any longer. Come to Him right now. Kneel down alone and pray to Him right now. Hebrew 2:7, 2 Chronicles 7:14.

MÉNIÈRE'S SYNDROME

SYMPTOMS—This disease of the inner ear is characterized by recurring episodes of ringing in the ears (tinnitus, *411*), loss of balance, severe dizziness (vertigo, *550*), and nausea. There is progressive deafness (*413*) and a sensation of fullness in the ears. Sudden movement during an attack can induce nausea and vomiting. Sometimes there is an uncontrollable horizontal jerking of the eyeballs.

The condition may affect one or both ears. It generally occurs in adults (most often in women, 50-60 years old). The onset is sudden. It may last for hours or weeks and then return soon again, after years. In most instances, it is experienced only in one ear and can result in complete deafness in that ear.

Vertigo is the sensation that the world is turning around you. Ménière's Syndrome accounts for 10%-15% of all vertigo (and 5% of all dizziness).
—*See Vertigo (550).*

CAUSES—Ménière's Syndrome often results from a disturbed carbohydrate metabolism, such as is found in **hypoglycemia**.

Impaired blood flow to the brain may be a causative factor. Those experiencing Ménière's Syndrome often have a history of **vasomotor rhinitis, ear trouble, and allergies**.

Autopsies reveal an edema in the membranous labyrinth.

Most common causes include **allergies, viruses, infections,** and **hormonal intolerances**.

Symptoms exactly like Ménière's Syndrome can be caused by a **cholesteatoma**. This is a tumor-like growth in the middle ear, which gradually pushes on the central nervous system. Consulting with a specialist might be of help in diagnosing the cause.

In some instances, this disease is misdiagnosed. It is actually **salicylism**, from excessive self-medication of **aspirin**—which can also cause deafness, ringing in the ears, dizziness, headache, vomiting, confusion, and hyperventilation in the later stages. If that may be the cause, stop taking aspirin immediately.

Fluid retention in the semicircular canals might be putting pressure on the delicate nerves of the inner ear.

The majority of people with Ménière's Syndrome are **overweight** and have abnormal **carbohydrate metabolism**. At least half have **high-blood fats**. Ménière's generally first occurs after taking **antibiotics**, which destroy beneficial bacteria in the colon.

NATURAL REMEDIES

• A general cleansing routine is often met with excellent results. This would include **fasting** for 3-7 days on vegetable juices and repeating it every six weeks. In between juice fasts, a solid **nutritious diet** that is composed of lots of **vegetables, seaweed, seeds, nuts, beans**, etc., should be eaten.

• Ménière's patients are chronically deficient in B vitamins. **B complex** (1 comprehensive tablet daily), **B$_1$** and **B$_2$** (10-25 mg of each daily), **B$_6$** (50 mg, 4 times a day for 2 weeks), **niacin** (200 mg daily if pregnant, otherwise 50-250 mg before each meal). This may correct the disease in 2-4 weeks. **Niacinamide** may be substituted for half of the niacin. **Vitamin C,** plus **bioflavonoids** (1,500-5,000 mg, in divided doses) and **vitamin E** (400 IU). **Calcium** is also needed. A lack of **manganese** (5 mg daily) can cause deafness, dizziness, and ear noises. A lack of **magnesium** can produce nerve twitching and sensitivity to noise.

• Go on a **low-salt, low-fat, low-sugar diet**, with a reduction of **refined carbohydrates**. Drink enough **water**. Eliminate **white-flour products, white sugar, saturated fats, caffeine, nicotine, and alcohol**. An oil-free diet may improve circulation in the tiny capillaries. **Smoking** induces constriction and spasm of the blood vessels. In one study, 9 out of 10 patients improved, when placed on a **low-salt** diet. Take an **acidophilus product** to replace beneficial bacteria lost from taking antibiotics.

• Another research showed that **allergies to milk, eggs, corn, wheat, and yeast** caused Ménière's. Eliminating them essentially terminated the problem. Stop using all of these foods. Then gradually reintroduce one at a time and see which might be bothering you.

• Variations in **glucose levels** can prompt Ménière's. A New York study indicated that, when **insulin levels** are normal, the patient seldom has tinnitus, vertigo, fullness in the ear, or variable hearing loss.

• Gradually increase the amount of outdoor **exercise. Breathe deeply** as you do it. This will help the circulation in your head.

• Use one bowl for hot water and one for cold, once or twice a day, and take a **hot and cold head bath.** Immerse the head in the hot water for 30-60 seconds. And then plunge it into ice cold. (If elderly, weakened, or with a heart condition, begin with less extreme temperatures.)

• Herbs which may help include **cayenne, gotu kola, butcher's broom, ginkgo biloba, and ginger**.

• *At the time of an attack,* **lying quietly on the affected side, with eyes turned in the direction of the affected ear** may help reduce the immediate crisis.

• *If you are helping someone with this problem,* let him move about at his own rate. Avoid jarring him. When speaking to him, stand directly in front so he will not have to turn his head (which can add to the vertigo). —*Also see Vertigo (550) and Tinnitus (411).*

ENCOURAGEMENT—Do not try to manage your own life. You cannot do it as well as God can do it for you. Work with Him. Surrender your plans to Him, to be laid down or taken up as He sees best.

HEARING LOSS
(Increasing Deafness)

SYMPTOMS—One's sense of hearing is lessening.

CAUSES—It may be that the hearing is being lost. The most common cause is **aging**. But it also may be that the ear has too much impacted **earwax**. *See Earwax (409) for how to remove it.* If a pregnant mother has **Rubella** (German measles, *745*) or **syphilis** (*804*), her child may be deaf. **Premature birth, trauma, lack of oxygen at birth, or low birth weight** can damage the infant's hearing (usually only temporarily).

A **manganese** or **tin** deficiency in the diet can result in a hearing loss. Putting these back into the diet can reverse this and restore the hearing.

Other possible causes would include: **milk allergies, poor ear circulation, and vitamin A deficiency**.

The eardrums might be hardened with age. This generally accompanies **hardening of the arteries**.

Catarrhal deafness could be the problem. This starts when an acute infection (such as a cold or the flu) is suppressed and not allowed to run its course and be properly eliminated. A low level infection continues in the middle ear and gradually ruins the hearing. Temporary deafness can result from a **punctured eardrum** (*see Earache, 409*).

When acute diseases are treated with **aspirin or quinine**, partial or complete deafness can result. Other drugs which cause this effect are **aureomycin, streptomycin, barbiturates, cocaine, opium, and their derivatives**.

Smoking and **caffeine** cause spasms and narrowing of blood vessels. Smoking reduces the amount of oxygen reaching the delicate parts of the ear.

Other substances to avoid would include **lead, mercury, and cadmium**.

Excessive amounts of **noise** injures the fine structures in the inner ear and gradually produces deafness. If you cannot hear people talking to you, the surrounding noise is great enough to damage the hearing.

Some people have **occupational hazards** which eventually lead to deafness. This includes piloting **small planes** and running **chain saws** or **heavy equipment**.

Normal conversation is 50 dB (decibels). Vacuum cleaner or washing machine is 75 dB. Food blender, blow dryer, electric razor, or city traffic is 85. Power mowers or symphony orchestras is 90-105. Amplified rock concerts, car stereos or headsets, powerboats, stadium sporting events, air hammers, or rifle shots are 110-140. An increasing number of people are gradually losing their hearing.

H
E
A
D

If you seem to have pain in the ear, pull on the earlobe. If the pain increases, then you probably have an **ear infection**. If the pain does not increase, you may have a **dental problem**. Total deafness is rare. Deafness may be accompanied by tinnitus (ringing in the ears, 411) or *vertigo* (dizziness, *550*). In older folk who experience the most hearing problems, the hearing of high frequencies is first to be lost (called presbyacusis).

Nations with the highest **cholesterol** rates have the highest rates of deafness. And those with the lowest have almost no deafness, even in the aged.

NATURAL REMEDIES

• Consider the above factors and **make needed changes**. Some research studies show that hearing loss can be reversed, even in the elderly, by eating a proper diet and avoiding certain things. Other research reveals that reducing fat and cholesterol intake improves hearing.

• **Clean the ears**. Make sure **manganese** and **tin** are in the diet (take Nova Scotia dulse or Norwegian kelp). Take pulse tests and gradually eliminate **food allergies**. If milk is the problem, cut out all **milk products** from the diet. Avoid **medicinal drugs, chemicals, and loud noises**.

• Eat a **wholesome, nutritious diet** with **vitamin / mineral supplements**. Drink fresh **vegetable juices**.

• **Eliminate processed, sugared, and junk foods** from the diet.

• Each day take vitamin A in the form of **carotene** (25,000 IU), **B complex** (1 comprehensive tablet), **vitamin C** (1,000-5,000 mg, in divided doses), **vitamin E** (400 IU), and **magnesium** (750 mg). Loud noise reduces the amount of magnesium in the ears; and, without it, hearing impairment begins. Also needed for good hearing: **manganese, potassium,** and **zinc**.

• *In case there is an inflammation in the ear which causes the hearing loss:* **Mullein oil** can be put in the ear as ear drops. 2-4 drops of warm (not hot) **garlic oil** or liquid extract is also good. Do not use the same dropper in both ears, as it may spread the infection. Eat fresh **pineapple**. *(Read Earache and ear Infection, 407.)*

PREVENTION

If you lose your hearing from excessive noise, there is less likelihood that you will recover it.

• Always wear **ear protection** when using appliances or machinery which produce loud noises. This would include power tools, chain saws, lawn mowers, table or portable saws, and target practice. Use earplugs rated for at least twice as many decibels as you need to ensure protection.

• When listening to **music**, it should never be so loud you cannot hear the ring of the doorbell or the telephone. If you use **earphones**, no one else should be able to hear sounds from your earphones. If they can, you are playing the music too loud for the safety of your ears!

• The average **rock concert** or **stereo headset** at higher levels (100 decibels, plus) can damage your hearing in 30 minutes. Two hours in a **video game arcade** can do the same thing. By comparison, an air hammer is 120 decibels. Audiologists say 75 dB is the safe limit for extended periods. Ear protectors should be worn above 90 dB.

• Wear **earplugs** when swimming in public places.

• Reduce your **cholesterol** level. Those with high cholesterol have greater hearing loss as they age.

• Do not get **German measles** *(745)* while you are pregnant. If you are vaccinated for it, do not become pregnant for 3 months afterward. The ensuing birth defects to the child could include hearing loss.

• Beware of **medications** during pregnancy.

• Make sure your infant has good hearing. If not discovered, he or she will miss much instruction and a variety of speaking skills. Generally, you will be the first one to learn if such a problem exists, not the doctor.

ENCOURAGEMENT—The Bible reveals how we can be saved. From Eden lost to Eden restored, it tells the entire story of salvation in Christ. Read that precious book, and you will be blessed and be a blessing to others. Psalm 119:9-11.

PRESSURE PROBLEMS
(Barotrauma)

SYMPTOMS—A feeling of echo-like hearing, fullness, pain, and temporary ringing or buzzing in the ears when rapidly going upward or downward.

CAUSES—If the pressure on the outer side of the eardrum exceeds the pressure on the inner side, the middle ear may become painful or damaged. Changes in air pressure occur in **airplanes, when diving, parachuting, scuba diving, riding in a car at high altitudes, or riding in a fast elevator**.

An extreme pressure imbalance may lead to a ruptured eardrum (*Earache and Ear Infection, 407*), bleeding into the middle ear, or damage to the inner ear. This results in possible hearing loss (*413*) and vertigo (*550*).

NATURAL REMEDIES

• **Swallow** or **hold your nose, exhaling with your mouth closed**. The eustachian tubes that connect the ears to the nose and throat will usually open, allowing air into the middle ear and equalizing the pressure. When insufficient air enters the middle ear, barotrauma results.

• Other ways to equalize pressure: **Move the jaw from side to side, sip liquids, stay awake and sit upright during descent, suck on food or condiment, or yawn.**

• Here is the "popping" method (also called the Valsalva maneuver): **Pinch the nostrils** shut, take a **mouthful of air**, and **close the mouth**. Then either **puff out the cheeks**, or **use the cheek and throat muscles to force air** up into the back of the nose.

• Give a small child a **balloon** to blow on. Give babies a **bottle** of water or juice, so they will frequently swallow.

• Barotrauma is more likely to occur if the eustachian tubes are blocked, as a result of a cold or ear infection (earache, 407). If you have a cold or ear infection, avoid flying or diving.

ENCOURAGEMENT—The soul that is yielded to Christ becomes His own fortress, which He holds in a revolted world, and He intends that no authority shall be known in it but His own. A soul thus kept in possession by the heavenly agencies is impregnable to the assaults of Satan.

OUTER EAR INJURY

SYMPTOMS—The visible part of the ear is injured. This causes it to be swollen, painful, and distorted in shape.

CAUSES—Blood may collect (a hematoma) and cut off the supply of blood to the cartilage, which may be so damaged that scar tissue develops and permanent deformity occurs. Severe or repeated injuries can produce a "cauliflower ear." Boxers and athletes are most likely to have this problem.

NATURAL REMEDIES
• Reduce the discomfort and swelling by applying an **ice pack**. If the swelling is too extensive, a physician may need to drain a hematoma or apply a pressure bandage.

• When playing contact sports, wear **headgear** to protect your ears. Better yet, stop engaging in activities which cause ear injuries.

ENCOURAGEMENT— We need to educate and train the mind so that we shall have an intelligent faith, and have an understanding friendship with Jesus. Unless we continually cherish friendship between God and our souls, we shall separate from Him, and walk apart from Him.

— HEAD AND THROAT —
6 - THROAT
Also: Tonsillitis (740), Adenoids (742)

SORE THROAT

SYMPTOMS—The throat becomes sore and scratchy. This is often the first sign of an infection.

CAUSES—A variety of **bacterial or virus infections** can cause sore throat. Those which are of *Streptococcus Group A* origin tend to produce a higher fever than viral sources (**upper respiratory infections, cold viruses, flu**, etc.).

Anything irritating to the throat can initiate the problem (such as **chronic coughing** and **loud talking**). Other irritants include **smoke, dust, fumes, very hot foods or drinks, abrasions, tooth and gum infections. Smoking** is a major cause of sore throats. A continual throat tickle or cough could be an indication of a **food allergy**.

Bacteria on toothbrushes can cause sore throats. Buy a new toothbrush or boil the old one at least once a month. Between uses, store the toothbrush in hydrogen peroxide—but rinse it well before using.

A sore throat is a typical first symptom of colds. If a sore throat continues or recurs, it might be the onset of **mononucleosis** (especially if the sore throat lasts more than 2 weeks). *Do not dally. Go to bed and get well. A sore throat can be the first sign of something more serious:* a cold, the flu, mononucleosis, herpes simplex, Epstein-Barr virus. Also it might be one of several childhood diseases, such as chicken pox or the measles. Sometimes a sore throat can lead to chronic fatigue syndrome, gingivitis, epiglottitis, diphtheria, laryngeal cancer, or an abscess around the tonsils. A sore throat may be a symptom of *streptococcus*. If left untreated, it can result in kidney disease or rheumatic fever.

NATURAL REMEDIES
• Sip liquid **vitamin C**. Let it drip down the throat slowly (all the while trying to keep the acid C off the teeth, so it will not melt them). Coat the throat with **raw honey,** mixed with **lemon juice**.

• Drink plenty of fluids—**fruit and vegetable juices** and lots of **water. Go to bed, rest, trust in God, and get well**. Take **enemas**.

• Gargle with **saltwater** (½ tsp. sea salt in a cup of water). Or, every few hours, alternately gargle with **chlorophyll liquid** and **saltwater**.

• **Vitamin A** in the form of beta carotene (75,000 IU daily for 1 week, then 25,000 IU daily). **Vitamin C** (1,000-5,000 mg in divided daily doses).

• **Vitamin C** is powerful. Take a 250 mg tablet each hour, plus gargling each hour with 500 mg of powdered vitamin C, stirred in a glass of water. Doing this, plus going to bed and resting, may eliminate the sore throat by the second day.

HERBS
• The Germans use **eucalyptus** to treat sore throats. The aromatic oil has a cooling effect on inflamed tissue. And the tannins exert soothing astringent action. Add a few tsp. crushed leaf per cup of boiling water. Drink it.

• The Chinese use powdered, dried **honeysuckle flowers** to treat sore throat, colds, flu, bronchitis, tonsillitis, and pneumonia. It has over 20 antiseptic compounds. **Honeysuckle flower extract** is equally powerful.

• Both Europeans and Chinese use licorice to treat

sore throat. Add 5-7 tsp. **licorice root** pieces to 3 cups water. Bring it to a boil, simmer until half the water is boiled away. Then cool, and drink. It will also help you spit out the phlegm.

• **Garlic** is a powerful remedy for sore throat. It is both antiviral (for colds) and antibacterial (for strep throat). Make a tea and gargle with it.

• Both **goldenseal and echinacea** fight bacterial and viral infection. (But do not take goldenseal over a week at a time or during pregnancy.) Gargling with **fenugreek** tea will help relieve a sore throat. **Marshmallow root** tea soothes a scratchy, itchy throat. Hot **mullein** poultices soothe sore throats.

• Drink sage tea and inhale its hot vapors. It will help open nasal and head passages. A **vinegar compress** to the throat will relieve the most painful sore throat. Add a pinch of **cayenne** and a teaspoon of **wintergreen oil** to ½ cup **apple cider vinegar**. Soak strips of cloth, place around throat, with dry wool cloth over that.

• Mix **ginger with lemon juice and honey**. And gargle with it. Other powerful herbs for sore throats include: **marshmallow, agrimony, myrrh, plantain, slippery elm, German chamomile, and myrtle.**

• An old herb doctor makes these suggestions: Gargle the throat with **cayenne** tea, a half teaspoon to a cup. Put an **onion** poultice on the neck overnight, for 2-3 nights. Rub the outside of the neck and cover it with warm flannel.

HYDROTHERAPY

The following is from the *Hydrotherapy* section (225-226) of this *Encyclopedia*:

The **heating throat compress** is an application of a cold cloth, covered with flannel, which then heats up and results in improved circulation and a better flow of healing blood into, and out of, the afflicted area. Wring the cotton cloth from cold water and place it around the neck. This should be about 2-3 thicknesses around the neck. Cover it well with flannel (singly or doubly, depending on the thickness). Fit the flannel snugly, but not so tightly that it will be uncomfortable. Pin it securely. Remove it the next morning. It should be entirely dry, or you have failed to accomplish the desired objective. Give a **hot bath** or **steam bath**.

—See Flu (294), Pharyngitis (below), and Adenoids (742).

ENCOURAGEMENT—With the trusting faith of a little child, come to your heavenly Father. Tell Him all your needs. He is always ready to pardon and help. He can give you the guidance you need. He can give you strength to resist sin and obey His law. By His enabling grace, He can fulfill His will for you.

PHARYNGITIS

SYMPTOMS—Symptoms may include: sore throat, difficulty swallowing, pain in the ear (which may be worse when swallowing), and / or enlarged and tender lymph nodes in the neck.

CAUSES—The pharynx connects the back of the mouth and nose to the esophagus and larynx. Pharyngitis is usually the result of a viral infection, such as a **common cold** (289) or infectious **mononucleosis** (664). Other causes include **bacterial infections**, such as streptococcal bacteria, and **fungal infections**, such as **candidiasis** (281). Also **Smoking and alcohol. Straining the voice** can often lead to pharyngitis, when shouting.

—Pharyngitis (416) and tonsillitis (740) often occur together. Also see Sore Throat (415).

NATURAL REMEDIES

J.H. KELLOGG, M.D., PRESCRIPTIONS FOR PHARYNGITIS AND ITS COMPLICATIONS (how to give these water therapies: pp. 206-275 / list of treatments: pp. 206-207 / Hydrotherapy Disease Index: pp. 273-275)

(1) ACUTE FORM —

DIETARY FACTORS—Rest in bed, keep room at a uniform temperature. Eat a spare diet, consisting chiefly of fruits. Avoid meats of all sorts. Copious water drinking.

GENERAL CARE—Hot Blanket Pack. Sweating Wet Sheet Pack. Steam Bath. Radiant Heat Bath. Hot Full Bath. Follow this with Dry Pack or other sweating procedures, once daily, and by Cold Mitten Friction. Also cold Wet Sheet Rub or Cold Douche. Fomentation to the throat, 3 times daily. Cold Compress between, changed every 15-30 minutes. Enema, if bowels are inactive. Hot gargle every few minutes if throat is very sensitive. Ice Bag to throat if inflammation is intense. Inhalation of soothing vapors. Use of steam inhaler for 10-14 minutes, hourly or almost continuously. If the tonsil suppurates (it oozes pus), it should be lanced. See your doctor.

(2) CHRONIC FORM —

CLERGYMAN'S SORE THROAT DIETARY AND LIFE-STYLE—Aseptic dietary, outdoor life, open-air gymnastics, and swimming.

GENERAL CARE—Fomentations to the throat at bedtime, followed by throat pack (Cold Compress) during the night. Hot gargle, 3 times a day. Radiant Heat Bath. Sweating Wet Sheet Pack. Warm Vapor Inhalation or other sweating bath, 3 times weekly. Follow this with suitable cold application. Daily Cold Bath on rising. Moist Abdominal Bandage to be worn during the night. If necessary, remove tonsils and vegetations in throat or postnasal region.

ENCOURAGEMENT—Thank God every day of your life for all that He has given you and all that He means to you.

LARYNGITIS
(Hoarseness, Aphonia)

SYMPTOMS—A tickling, raw throat is the initial

symptom. The voice becomes hoarse, there is pain when speaking, the voice becomes weak, or it is lost entirely for a time (aphonia). The voice loss is frequently all that happens. No fever or infection accompanies it.

CAUSES—The larynx is located between the throat and trachea (windpipe) and contains the vocal cords. Laryngitis is rarely serious. It may be acute, lasting only a few days. But it may be chronic, persisting for months. It is usually caused by a **viral infection**, such as a **cold** *(289)*. But it may occur after **prolonged use of the voice**, especially in **loud speaking**. Chronic laryngitis may be caused by **smoking**. Drinking **liquor** aggravates laryngitis. Sometimes laryngitis is associated with **vocal cord nodules**. *"Hoarseness"* is when it is with difficulty that you can speak. *"Aphonia"* is when you have totally lost your voice.

NATURAL REMEDIES

• *Do not talk!* Try to avoid any speaking for a day or two. **Do not even whisper.** Just write notes. Put a **bell** by your bedside and ring it when you need help.

• Go on a short **fruit and vegetable juice fast**. This will help remove excess mucus.

• Drink lots of **liquids**, 8-10 glasses a day; but **do not drink cold** drinks or anything with ice in it.

• **Breathe through your nose**. This increases the humidity in your throat. Air in an airliner is very dry (because it is pressurized). So do not breathe through your mouth if you are on a plane.

• Put your head over a **hot bowl** of water for 5 minutes, twice a day.

• **Hot compresses** may be applied to the throat every 3 hours. A **heating compress** may be applied to the throat and chest at the same time.

• An **ice bag** may be applied to the throat. **Cold compresses** may be wrung out from ice water and placed on the throat. (Yes, both hot compresses and cold compresses help reduce laryngitis.)

• **Do not smoke**. Do not take **aspirin**. It increases clotting time, which can slow the healing process.

HERBS

• Helpful herbs include the following: **slippery elm, plus lemon and honey**. This is very soft and soothing on the throat, an outstanding help.

• **White oak bark** tea is excellent for the throat. Add 1 tsp. to 1 cup boiling water, strain, cool, and drink 4-6 times a day.

• Drink and gargle with herb teas of **wild cherry bark, mullein, and/or vervain**.

• Make a syrup out of **wild cherry bark** and take a little at a time.

• The "singer's plant" is **hedge mustard** *(sisymbrium officinale)*. Take it as a liquid extract.

• **Ginger, horehound, or mullein** (together or separately) are good for laryngitis. Add 1-2 tsp. dried herb per cup of boiling water. Cool and drink.

• **Marshmallow** soothes the throat. The mucilage in it soothes the throat and helps protect it from bacterial infection.

• Drink 1 cup of **eyebright** tea, 3-4 times a day.
• Gargle with **goldenseal** tea and drink some.
• Mix 2 tablespoons of **flaxseed** and 1 tablespoon of **horehound**. Boil in 1 pint of water for 10 minutes and strain. Squeeze 1 **lemon** into the tea and add a pinch of **ginger**. Take 1 tablespoon every half hour.
• Here are four herbs which the German government approves for treating laryngitis: **echinacea, plantain, knotgrass, and primrose**.

FUTURE PREVENTION

• **Learn to breathe and speak correctly**, without straining or being tense. Avoid loud speaking. Train yourself to speak softer. If you have something worth hearing, they will listen. Do not lose your temper and shout.

• When you feel the **slightest indication** of hoarseness coming on, cancel speaking engagements and get extra rest.

• **Watch your diet**. Eating mucus-forming foods (such as dairy products, meat, candy, and wheat) can produce hoarseness. Drinking liquids with a meal tends to do it also. Remember that **tobacco and alcohol** are hard on the voice. To strengthen your voice, gargle a quart of **cold water** everyday.

—Also see Sore Throat (415).

J.H. KELLOGG, M.D., PRESCRIPTIONS FOR LARYNGITIS AND ITS COMPLICATIONS *(how to give these water therapies: pp. 206-275 / list of treatments: pp. 206-207 / Hydrotherapy Disease Index: pp. 273-275)*

(1) ACUTE FORM —
GENERAL CARE—Steam Inhalation for 10 minutes, hourly, and **Heating Compress to throat** without plastic covering. Avoid use of voice while very hoarse.

(2) CHRONIC FORM —
INCREASE GENERAL VITAL RESISTANCE AND INVIGORATE THE SKIN—Graduated Cold Baths. Sweating baths or prolonged Neutral Bath at night, 2-3 times a week. Follow sweating procedure by any suitable **cold application**.
TO RELIEVE LOCAL CONGESTION—Warm Vapor Inhalation for 10 minutes, every 4 hours. **Fomentation** at night. Follow by well-protected **Cold Compress** to the neck, to be worn during the night. (It must warm up by morning!)
COUGH—See under Croup *(498)*.

ENCOURAGEMENT—The only safeguard against evil is surrender to Christ, studying the Bible, obeying it, and living to help others. Romans 8:35-37.

SNORING

SYMPTOMS—Wheezing, sighing noises made through the mouth while a person is sleeping. It drives everyone else to distraction, except the one making the noise. The tissue in the upper airway in the back of the throat relaxes during sleep; breathing in causes it to vibrate.

CAUSES—Snoring generally occurs while **sleeping on the back**. The mouth falls open and the singing begins. It is the sound made by the vibration of the soft palate which is the rear of the roof of the mouth.

Men snore more frequently (71%) than women (51%). Most snorers are overweight men between the ages of 30 and 50. But children snore at times (usually because of enlarged **adenoids** *(742)* or **tonsils** *(740).*

• Snoring can develop as a result of **allergies** *(848),* during or following **hay fever time** *(850),* or **after colds** *(289).*

NATURAL REMEDIES

• **Sleep on your side**, not on your back. One method which works fine is to **sew a tennis ball** into the middle of the back of your pajamas. When you roll onto it in your sleep, you will quickly roll off again—and there will be no snoring.

• **Do not sleep on a pillow**. They tend to elevate your head and increase snoring.

• Put blocks under the front legs of your bed and **elevate the upper part** of your body (head and trunk). This will reduce snoring.

• **Losing weight** tends to lessen snoring. The more overweight a person is, the more likely he or she will snore.

• Drinking **alcohol** or taking **sleeping pills** tends to increase snoring, by excessively relaxing the tissues of the soft palate, which narrows the nasopharynx. **Smoking** causes the soft palate (not to relax) to swell, also narrowing the nasopharynx.

• Tell your spouse to **shake you awake** when you snore. That will wake you enough that you will stop.

• Buy your spouse **earplugs** to wear at night.

ENCOURAGEMENT—We must not allow coldness to chill our love for our Redeemer. If we have fellowship with Him, we must ever set the Lord before us and treat Him as an honored Friend, giving Him the first place in our affections. We should speak of His matchless charms and constantly cultivate the desire to have a better knowledge of Jesus Christ. Then His Spirit will have a controlling power upon our life and character.

More Encouragement

"Those who are true to their calling as messengers for God will not seek honor for themselves. Love for self will be swallowed up in love for Christ. No rivalry will mar the precious cause of the gospel. They will recognize that it is their work to proclaim, as did John the Baptist,

" 'Behold the Lamb of God, which taketh away the sin of the world.' John 1:29. They will lift up Jesus, and with Him humanity will be lifted up. 'Thus saith the high and lofty One that inhabiteth eternity, whose name is Holy; I dwell in the high and holy place, with him also that is of a contrite and humble spirit, to revive the spirit of the humble, and to revive the heart of the contrite ones.' Isaiah 57:15.

"The soul of the prophet, emptied of self, was filled with the light of the divine. As he witnessed to the Saviour's glory, his [John the Baptist's] words were almost a counterpart of those that Christ Himself had spoken in His interview with Nicodemus. . . So with the followers of Christ. We can receive of heaven's light only as we are willing to be emptied of self. We cannot discern the character of God, or accept Christ by faith, unless we consent to the bringing into captivity of every thought to the obedience of Christ. To all who do this the Holy Spirit is given without measure. In Christ 'dwelleth all the fullness of the Godhead bodily, and in Him ye are made full.' Colossians 2:9-10."

—Desire of Ages, 179-181

Two editions of Desire of Ages, the classic (and best) book on the life of Christ are available from us.

The Natural Remedies Encyclopedia

- Disease Section 5 - Gastro-Intestinal

 # = Information, not a disease

Digestive System: Physiology 1015-1017 / Pictures 1038

GASTRO

— **Concluded on next page**

G
A
S
T
R
O

"There is forgiveness with Thee, that Thou mayest be feared . . He shall redeem Israel from all his iniquities." —Psalm 130:4, 8

"Who is among you that feareth the Lord, that obeyeth the voice of His servant, that walketh in darkness, and hath no light? Let him trust in the name of the Lord, and stay upon his God." —Isaiah 50:10

"Surely He shall deliver thee from the snare of the fowler, and from the noisome pestilence . . Thou shalt not be afraid for the terror by night; nor for the arrow that flieth by day; nor for the pestilence that walketh in darkness; nor for the destruction that wasteth at noonday." —Psalm 91:3, 5-6

"Cast thy burden upon the Lord, and He shall sustain thee. He shall never suffer the righteous to be moved." —Psalm 55:22

FOR MORE NATURAL REMEDIES:

HERBS: Herb Contents (pp. 129-130) will help you locate the 126 most important herbs and the diseases each one can treat. How to prepare herbs (132). How to use them (141-189)

HYDROTHERAPY: Therapy Contents (pp. 206-207) and its Disease Index (263-265) will lead you to over 100 water therapies and many more remedies. DIS. INDEX: 1211- / GEN. INDEX: 1221-

VITAMINS AND MINERALS: Contents (100-101). Using 101-124. Dosages (124). Others (117-)

CARING FOR THE SICK: Home care for a sick person (28-36). The healing crisis (36-39)

WOMEN'S SECTIONS: Female Organs (672) Pregnancy (701). Childbirth (765). Infancy, Childhood (722). Women's Herbs (754, 760)

EMERGENCIES: (973-). FIRST AID: (990-)

Section 5 - Gastro-Intestinal

GASTRO-INTESTINAL -
1 - TEETH AND GUMS

BRUXISM
(Teeth Grinding)

SYMPTOMS—Unconscious grinding of the teeth together, often while asleep.

CAUSES—Bruxism can wear down the teeth, loosen them, and even contribute to receding gums. So it is a condition you want to stop.

The experts tell us it is caused by **stress, anxiety, anger**, sensitivity of the teeth to heat and cold, and fluctuations in blood sugar levels. So **hypoglycemia** can be a factor. When a person has low blood sugar, he is more likely to clench and grind his teeth.

In reality, bruxism and gum chewing produce stress. Neither reduces it.

Another major cause is the habit of **idly chewing on something** during the day, when you are not eating.

Some people find it necessary to wear a splint while sleeping.

NATURAL REMEDIES

• You may find that the solution is simply to stop chewing during the day when you do not need to. **Do not chew gum**. Do not **chew bits of food** after the meal is ended. When you are not chewing something so you can swallow it, do not chew. This simple rule has totally eliminated the bruxism problem for many people. It can do it for you also. Actually, chewing, as a leisure time activity, is *not relaxing*. It actually makes one nervous. Having developed the habit of unnecessarily chewing during the day, it will tend to be repeated at night when asleep.

• **Keep your mouth relaxed** during the day. Do not clamp your teeth together. Do not grind. If you control yourself during the day, you will soon automatically do it throughout the night.

• Several times a day, slowly **shrug** each shoulder, then shrug both together.

• Take a **vitamin-mineral** supplement. To reduce stress reactions, take **vitamin C** (3,000-5,000 mg in divided doses), **zinc** (30 mg), **pantothenic acid** (500 mg), and **calcium** (2,000 mg). Eliminate **caffeine, candy, fast foods, meat, and white-flour products**.

Do not drink **alcoholic** beverages. They contribute to tooth grinding. Eat nothing **sweet** within 6 hours of going to bed. Do not eat **supper** an hour or less before bedtime. **Food allergies** *(848)* are sometimes the cause. Try to locate yours.

• **Just before bedtime**, do nothing stressful for 30 minutes. Instead, go for a pleasant walk outside and breathe deeply of the fresh air.

• Four times a day, **say each vowel**, A, E, I, O, U, out loud, exaggerating the muscle movements. This will relax your mouth. Reduce **television** viewing time.

• **Valerian, skullcap, hops, and chamomile** teas will relax you and provide deeper sleep.

—*See Temporomandibular Joint Syndrome (631)*. If bruxism is not eliminated, it can lead to TMJ. And you do not want that to happen!

ENCOURAGEMENT—With the trusting faith of a little child, we can come to our heavenly Father and tell Him of all our needs. He will not turn us away, but will hear and help. Matthew 5:11-12.

CALCULUS
(Tartar, Stained Teeth)

SYMPTOMS—The teeth are darker and more yellow than they should be.

CAUSES—The actual color of teeth is not white, but light yellow. However, as one ages, the teeth tend to become somewhat darker and more yellow.

Coffee and **cigarettes** are a primary cause of tooth staining. Stop using them both and you will look better. You will feel better, too.

NATURAL REMEDIES

• **Rinse** the food from your mouth after each meal. **Clean** your teeth after every meal. Brush with fresh **strawberries**. Place a strawberry on the toothbrush and brush as usual.

• Brush with **charcoal** powder. Polish them with **baking soda**. Many of the stains are acid in nature. And the soda neutralizes and removes them. An **electric toothbrush** removes more plaque than regular brushing. Keep in mind that hard brushing can scratch your tooth enamel. The super-whitening **tooth abrasives** in toothpaste take off even more. Be careful. You want white teeth, but you also want teeth.

• Since we are on the subject of ruining your teeth, an excellent way to melt your teeth is to drink cola drinks. They contain phosphoric acid, which

CHART - 1045: Digestive (419-484)

GASTRO

has a double whammy effect on your poor teeth! The acid melts your alkaline teeth. And the phosphorus immediately locks into the melted off calcium and carries it away. Place a tooth in Coca Cola, and it will be gone in a short time.

ENCOURAGEMENT—We need to come into the audience chamber of the Most High and ask forgiveness for our sins. He will hear, He will forgive, and He will give us enabling strength to resist sin. It all depends on our choice. But we must not waver in our loyalty to Him. Hebrews 11:26.

TOOTH SENSITIVITY

SYMPTOMS—The teeth feel extremely sensitive to heat and cold.

CAUSES—Some of the protective enamel has been worn away. The cause is too-vigorous brushing, an imbalance in your bite, the habit of chewing on pencils, tooth grinding *(see Bruxism, 421),* or inadequate nutrition.

NATURAL REMEDIES
• **Vitamin B₁** (thiamine) will reduce your sensitivity to pain. Take 100 mg daily.
• **Calcium hydroxyapatite** is a form of calcium which will help restore tooth enamel, making your teeth less sensitive.
• Mix ¼ tsp. **clove** powder with a few drops of water. Put a little on the sensitive tooth after each meal.
• Mix equal parts of liquid extracts of **fennel, white oak bark, and horsetail** herbs. Put 7 drops on sensitive teeth (but not on those that are cracked). Also use the mixture as a rinse each morning and evening. The fennel soothes the nerves. The white oak bark tightens and cleans gums. And the horsetail decreases bleeding.
—*Also see Receding Gums (425).*

ENCOURAGEMENT—If ever there was a time when men needed the presence of Christ at their right hand, it is now. We need the Captain of our salvation continually by our side.

TOOTHACHE

SYMPTOMS—One of your teeth hurts badly.

CAUSES—The primary cause is the "civilized" diet that we eat today. About 50 years ago, a dentist traveled around the world, visiting primitive people groups which never tasted our **Western diet.** And he found that they had strong teeth and no cavities.

NATURAL REMEDIES
To stop a toothache, until you can see a dentist, here are several suggestions:
• **Rinse** your mouth vigorously with a mouthful of lukewarm water. If the pain is from food caught between the teeth, this may flush it out. Try **flossing** gently between the teeth.
• Stir 1 teaspoon of salt into a glassful of water, at body temperature. Swish warm **saltwater** in your mouth and spit it out. Do this after every meal and before retiring at night.
• Somewhat warm **saltwater**, held in the mouth, will bring relief.
• Oil of clove contains *eugenol*; this anesthetic, an antiseptic, is a powerful toothache reliever. Apply 1-2 drops of **oil of cloves** to the affected tooth with a cotton swab. If the oil seems too strong, dilute it with **olive oil**. Put the clove oil on the tooth. But do not swallow it.
• Both **ginger** and **cayenne** act as counter-irritants, so the pain is not felt. Make a paste, dip a small cotton ball into it, wring it out, and apply the ball to the tooth without letting it touch your gum.
• Sprinkle a little **cayenne** in **vinegar**, swish it around in the mouth, and then spit it out. Or soak heavy brown paper in **vinegar**, place it outside the mouth on the cheek next to the affected area, and leave overnight.
• Put a **charcoal** tablet in your mouth and, with your tongue and cheek, press it against the swollen gum at the base of the problem tooth.
• Drink 1-2 cups of **mullein** tea or chew **catnip** herb.
• **Chamomile and hops** tea will help relax the body.
• Mash up the root of **plantain** and put it on the cheek near the tooth.
• Crushed **garlic** or grated fresh **horseradish** can be placed on the tooth.
• **Chaparral** has been used as a folk remedy for toothache. It contains nordihydroguarietic acid, a strong antiseptic. Swish chaparral tea in the mouth. Then spit it out.
• **Sesame** contains 7 pain-relieving compounds. Add 1 part sesame to 2 parts water, boil till half the liquid is gone. Apply to the tooth. An old Chinese remedy.
• Hold double-strength **sage** tea in the mouth for 30 seconds; then swallow it.
• **Myrrh** helps control mouth infections.
• For a temporary relief, mix **clove** oil with **zinc** oxide powder to form a paste. This will protect the cavity from food.
• Chew **willow bark**. The *salicin* in it relieves pain.

• Keep **heat** away from the tooth and nearby cheek. If it is an infection, the heat will draw it to the outside of the jaw and make the situation worse.

• With your fingers rub an **ice cube** until one side is shaped into a V-shape. Then press it gently against the tender place, pushing it back and forth over the area for 5-7 minutes. The effect of rubbing tends to cancel out the pain signal, which must travel along the same nerve route as the rubbing signal.

• Put **ice** on the nearby cheek for 15 minutes, 3-4 times a day.

• Avoid **biting** on that area of the teeth.

• To reduce infection in a tooth, put a few drops of **goldenseal** extract on a piece of cotton and apply it to the swollen area at night. Do this for 3 consecutive nights.

• Some individuals have found that, when a toothache begins, they quickly **skip a meal, rest,** take **vitamin C**, get **extra rest**, and live very **temperately** over the next several days—and the infection in the tooth is overcome by the body.

—Also see Tooth Decay (below).

ENCOURAGEMENT—The Lord has fullness of grace to bestow on every one that will receive the heavenly gift. The Holy Spirit will bring the God-entrusted capabilities into Christ's service. He will mold and fashion the human agent according to the divine Pattern, in proportion as the human agent shall earnestly desire the transformation.

TOOTH DECAY
(Dental Caries)

SYMPTOMS—A cavity or hole develops in a tooth, but may not be noticed until it begins to be painful.

CAUSES—The outer part of the tooth (the very hard enamel) erodes; then the body of the tooth beneath it (the dentin) also begins eroding. This is called tooth decay. An estimated 98% of Americans have dental cavities. Yet foreign groups which have never eaten Western food have none.

It is thought that **plaque** buildup (a sticky mass on the surface of the tooth) provides a place for bacteria to grow and feed on sugars in the mouth. The acid they produce digs holes in the teeth. If not stopped, the erosion enters the lower, center part of the tooth, called the pulp, where the nerve is. Then the pain begins.

However, certain things help produce tooth decay. These include **sugary foods, sticky foods, and acid foods**.

Cola drinks do an excellent job of melting teeth. Coca Cola, and similar cola beverages, contain phosphoric acid and lots of sugar. Frankly, the fluid is so terribly acid that it would be intolerable without lots of sugar to mask the acidity. Acid, sugar, and phosphorus are very dangerous when combined. The powerful acid melts part of the teeth. And the phosphorus chemically locks with the melted calcium and quickly carries it off. All of that sugar does its part to ruin the teeth also. It helps the bacteria to jump in and start still more trouble. Drop a tooth into a glass of Coke, and then time the number of hours it takes for the tooth to totally disappear.

NATURAL PREVENTIVES

• Do not drink **cola drinks**. Do not eat **sticky foods**. Do not eat **white sugar products**. Do not chew up **vitamin C tablets**! The acid in them will melt your teeth.

• **Rinse** out your mouth after eating or finish a fruit meal by eating an apple.

• **Goldenseal** extract, that is alcohol-free, can be used as an antibacterial mouthwash.

• Eat plenty of **raw fruits and vegetables. Leafy green vegetables, raw carrots, parsley, turnip greens, and garbanzo beans** help prevent tooth decay. Eat **whole grains, nuts, and legumes**.

• **Rhubarb, poke, and spinach** are extremely high in oxolic acid, which inhibits calcium formation; so do not eat them (especially rhubarb and poke!).

• Avoid all **toothpastes and powders**. The detergents in them are harmful to teeth and gums.

• It is vital that you take **calcium** supplements in order to maintain good tooth and bone structure. As you get older, you need even more calcium.

• **Massage your gums** with your finger once a day.

• **Bloodroot** helps reduce plaque on teeth. Bay leaf has a chemical (cineole) which kills dental bacteria. Licorice contains glycyrrhizin and indole, which kill bacteria on the teeth. Wild bergamot contains thymol and geraniol, which is a tooth decay preventive.

• Avoid soft, gooey foods, dairy products, especially soft cheeses.

• Strawberries are a good tooth cleanser. Rub strawberry halves on your teeth.

• To remove tartar, mix equal parts cream of tartar and sea salt, or baking soda and sea salt, and clean the teeth.

—Also see Toothache (422).

FLUORIDE TREATMENTS—Even more books have been written about **fluoride**! This deadly poison should be avoided at all costs. If it is added to your public drinking water supply, then you should buy bottled water (or buy a home distiller, to process your faucet water). If your dentist offers to give you fluoride treatments, you would do well to politely decline the opportunity.

AIR ABRASION TECHNOLOGY—Air abrasion dental work is the latest hi-tech method of drilling teeth. It is said to painlessly remove tooth decay without drilling, permit the dentist to make smaller fillings, and save a larger percentage of the tooth.

ENCOURAGEMENT—In the Bible, the will of God is revealed. He who makes these truths a part of his life becomes, in every sense, a new creature. God can do for you what you never could do for yourself. But it requires total submission and obedience to His Written Word. Ezekiel 36:26.

MERCURY FILLING SYNDROME
(Poisonous Dental Fillings) SPEC. REPORT 949

SYMPTOMS—Possible symptoms include dizziness, arthritis, colitis, multiple sclerosis, loss of mental acuity, psychosis, Alzheimer's, Parkinson's, and other degenerative illnesses of the nervous system.

CAUSES—Mercury is a deadly poison. Yet fully half of the amalgam fillings in your mouth are mercury. The rest is silver, copper, zinc, and tin. Mercury changes into a gas and evaporates. Mercury tends to evaporate slowly over a period of time. It is a scientifically proven fact that mercury fillings "outgas." With each meal or drink, a small amount of the mercury in the amalgam escapes in the form of a vapor and is swallowed with your food. Over 85% of the American public have amalgam fillings. Each year over 200 million cavities are filled, most of them with amalgam.

About 3,000 out of 150,000 U.S. dentists have stopped using amalgams entirely. Yet none of them dare ask to remove those already in place, or they will lose their dental licenses. But if you ask that it be done, they will do it gladly.

SOLUTIONS—Alternatives are ceramic-based materials, gold, or platinum-type metals. They are more expensive, but less harmful. It is best that you ask that replacements not include aluminum, barium, or other metals. Composite fillings, generally made of plastics, are the best. Plastic molecules are too large to be absorbed by the mouth or intestinal tract. If composites are placed correctly, they last as well as amalgam fillings. But they require careful placement, which many dentists do not know how to do.

Here are organizations which can help you find a qualified dentist for this task:

DAMS Newsletter (Defense Against Mercury Syndrome), 725-9 Tramway Lane NE, Albuquerque, NM 87122.

The International Academy of Oral Medicine and Technology (Michael Ziff, D.D.S., director), Box 808010 Orlando, FL 32860-5831.

Queen and Company Health Communications, Box 49308, Colorado Springs, CO 80949-9308.

ENCOURAGEMENT—While you have one desire to resist the devil and sincerely pray, Deliver me from temptation, you will have strength for your day. It is the work of the heavenly angels to come close to the tried, the tempted, the suffering ones. Psalm 34:7-8.

AVULSED TOOTH

SYMPTOMS—A tooth that has been partly or completely knocked out of its socket, as a result of a powerful impact to the jaw.

CAUSES—Through **accidents**, children frequently lose teeth; but an avulsed tooth is a problem only if a secondary (adult) tooth is lost. This is because primary (baby) teeth are eventually replaced by adult teeth.

Among teenagers and adults, avulsed teeth are more common in men because they play more **contact sports**. It is usually front teeth that are involved.

NATURAL REMEDIES
• *If a tooth is dislodged,* but still partly in the socket, **go to a dentist or emergency room** immediately.
• *If the tooth is knocked out completely,* quickly **put it back into the socket**, if possible. If this cannot be done, put it into a glass of milk or saltwater, or wrap it in a clean, damp cloth. Then rush to a dentist or emergency room. The tooth will reattach itself to the jaw 90% of the time, if it is reset in the socket within 30 minutes after being knocked out.
• The dentist will set the tooth back in place and, to keep it immovable, splint it to other teeth for 10-14 days.
• But if it has been fully knocked out, he may have to do a root canal, because the pulp (containing the nerves and blood vessels) have been killed. Sometimes, an artificial tooth has to be put in its place.
• In some instances, a lost tooth is swallowed. In such cases, an X-ray should be taken to make sure it was not inhaled into the lungs.

ENCOURAGEMENT—The law of love being the foundation of the government of God, the happiness of all intelligent beings depends upon their perfect accord with its great principles of righteousness.

DRY SOCKET
(Post-extraction Alveolitis)

SYMPTOMS—Severe throbbing pain that often radiates to the ear 2-4 days after extraction of a tooth. A bad taste in the mouth and bad breath. After a tooth is extracted, the hollow place (tooth socket) will not heal.

CAUSES—After a tooth is extracted, the tooth socket fills with blood and clots. Gradually, this clot fills in with flesh. But if the clot is washed away by premature rinsing, or if the clot becomes infected, the bony lining of the socket can become inflamed.

This is called "dry socket" and only happens once in every 25 tooth extractions. It occurs most frequently following a difficult extraction of a lower jaw molar, in those who smoke or in a woman taking oral contraceptives.

NATURAL REMEDIES

Return to your dentist.

• Take analgesic **herbs** and apply **water therapy** to lessen the pain *(see Toothache, 422)*.

• Take **vitamin C** (2,000-5,000 mg, in divided doses, daily) and apply **herbal antibiotics** *(298)*.

—*See Gingivitis (bellow) and Tooth Decay (423) for more information.*

The dentist will wash out the tooth socket with warm saltwater or a diluted antiseptic solution. Next, he will pack the socket with antiseptic paste. This will be repeated every 2-3 days until the tooth socket begins to heal. He may also suggest that you use hot saltwater mouthwashes at home to help reduce the inflammation. Healing should begin within a few days and be completed in a month or so.

ENCOURAGEMENT—It is today that the sweet voice of mercy is falling upon your ears. It is today that the heavenly invitation comes to you. Today, in Heaven, Christ invites us, "Come." Matthew 11:28:30.

GUM BOIL

SYMPTOMS—A bubble develops on the side of the gum, close to the teeth.

CAUSES—An infection in the base of a tooth is bursting out the side in a bubble. The tooth may, or may not, hurt.

NATURAL REMEDIES

• Give **antibiotic herbs** *(298)*.

• **Fig or other plant poultices** may be applied in order to hasten the ripening of the abscess or boil. Soak fresh or dried figs in water. Then apply them directly over the boil. This will promote healing of the abscess.

• **Improve the diet, brush your teeth** regularly, **avoid** the use of sticky and sugary foods.

—*Also see Toothache (422) and Tooth Decay (423).*

ENCOURAGEMENT—The more one sees of the character of God, the more humble he becomes, and the lower his estimation is of himself. This indeed is the evidence that he beholds God, that he is in union with Jesus Christ. Unless we are meek and lowly, we cannot in truth claim that we have any conception of the character of God.

GINGIVITIS
(Swollen Gums, Bleeding Gums, Gingival Hyperplasia)

SYMPTOMS—The gums swell and get red. Cleaning the teeth makes them bleed.

CAUSES—The gums enlarge and swell. This is an early sign of periodontal disease *(see pyorrhea, 426)*.

Gingival hyperplasia can also be a side effect of some **drugs**, such as hypertensives, anticonvulsants, and certain immunosuppressants. The condition may occur during **pregnancy** because of hormonal changes (which should clear up after childbirth). Rarer cases include **scurvy** (lack of vitamin C, *479*) and **acute leukemia** *(795)*.

NATURAL REMEDIES

• Begin taking more **calcium**. Get more **sunshine** or take supplemental **vitamin D**. Building the bones from within is the best way. If your teeth are having trouble, the other bones in your body, although hidden, probably are also. You do not want a fractured hip later.

• Eat a nourishing diet. Include raw **fruit and vegetables**. They help exercise your teeth and gums. They also help clean your teeth.

• Stop using **nicotine** and **alcohol**. They remove vitamins and minerals from your body.

• Fill a clean ear syringe (a rubber bulb with a long nose) with water and **hose out your mouth**.

Massage the gums at least once a day. Better yet, massage after every meal when you brush your teeth.

• Massage the **gumline** with a little **baking soda** on your finger, dipped in water.

• **Brush the teeth** carefully after each meal. Use a soft toothbrush and do it gently. Otherwise you will make scratches on the enamel. Move the toothbrush from the root to the top of the tooth. Brush carefully at the gumline.

• Alternate between **two toothbrushes**, so each one can dry out before it is used again. Soak the toothbrushes in **hydrogen peroxide** once a week. This kills bacteria buildup.

• An electric toothbrush is said to eliminate 98% of the plaque. Whereas a regular toothbrush is said to remove only 48%.

• **Floss** your teeth faithfully as needed.

—*See Receding Gums (below), Tooth Decay (423), Pyorrhea (426), and Mouth and Gum Infections (427) for more information.*

ENCOURAGEMENT—Thousands have drawn from the well of life. Yet there is no diminishing supply. In the Bible will be found the help you need, day by day. 2 Timothy 1:9.

RECEDING GUMS

SYMPTOMS—The gums are withdrawing away from the teeth, exposing part of the roots. The roots of the teeth may become overly sensitive to hot, cold, or sweet substances.

CAUSES—Normal, healthy gums form a tight seal around the base of the teeth. But when the gums recede, the teeth are not as solidly connected with the socket in the jaw. One or more teeth may eventually become loose. In extreme cases, tooth extractions may have to be made. Because the roots are softer than the enamel on the crown of the tooth, they are also more subject to decay.

The cause is poor oral hygiene, a buildup of plaque (deposits of food particles, bacteria feeding on them, and mucus), calculus (hardened plaque) between the base of the gum and the teeth, and poor diet. If the situation is not corrected, the gums eventually become inflamed. Also the results are gingivitis *(425)* and periodontal disease *(see Pyorrhea, below)*.

NATURAL REMEDIES

• Begin **brushing** and **flossing** your teeth well. **Massage** your gums daily.

• Improve your diet by only eating nourishing food: **fruits and vegetables, whole grains, nuts, and legumes** instead of junk food that is **candy, processed, or greasy**. Avoid **meat**.

• Obtain more **rest**.

• Take **vitamin C** (2,000-5,000 mg in divided doses daily) until the situation clears.

—See Gingivitis (425), Tooth Decay (423), and Pyorrhea (below) for more information.

ENCOURAGEMENT—There is not a moral precept found in any part of the Bible which is not engraved with the finger of God in His holy law, the ten commandments, on the two tables of stone.

PYORRHEA
(Periodontal Disease, Gum Disease)

SYMPTOMS—The gums become inflamed and extend to the ligaments and bones that hold the teeth in place. Eventually the teeth may loosen and fall out.

CAUSES—Periodontal means "located around a tooth" and refers to any problems in the gums or other supporting structures of the teeth. It includes pyorrhea, gum disease. Gingivitis *(425)* is inflammation of the gums, an early stage of periodontal disease. Receding gums *(425 & above)* is when the gums shrink and pull away from the teeth. All of these problems are closely related and have the same underlying causes. It especially affects people over age 55 and is a major cause of tooth loss.

Plaque (sticky deposits of mucus, food particles, and bacteria) adheres to the teeth and gradually accumulates. This plaque causes the gums to become infected and swollen. That infection (called gingivitis), leads to pyorrhea (also called periodontitis) in which the bone underlying the teeth is eroded away by the infection.

Other causal factors are an inadequate intake of **calcium, copper, vitamins D and C** (by the eating of **processed and junk food**), and dental erosion by

acids placed in the mouth. **Smoking and stress** are other crucial factors. **Diabetes** and certain **blood disorders** put a person at greater risk of developing periodontal disease.

NATURAL REMEDIES

• It is known that **inadequate nutrition, wrong foods, consumption of sugar, high phosphorous foods, smoking, drugs, excessive alcohol, chronic illness, and hormonal disorders** make an individual more susceptible to periodontal disease. **Smokers** have twice the risk of gum disease. Laboratory animals given **high-sugar diets** revealed a decrease in bone volume. These problems should, if possible, be corrected.

• **Calcium** (2,000 mg), **copper** (4 mg), **vitamin D** (1,000 mg), and **vitamin C** (2,000 mg) are needed for good strong teeth. **Folic acid** (5 mg), **niacin** (2,000 mg), **bioflavonoids** (100 mg) are also needed. As a rule, take care of the teeth, and the gums will take care of themselves. Give the teeth the nourishment they need. As you do that, you are also strengthening the bones throughout your entire body.

• Emotional stress is known to decrease the body's ability to resist gum disease. **Exercise** neutralizes stress and encourages the maintenance of healthy gums.

• If gum inflammation is present, **soften the toothbrush** by running very hot water over it before using it.

• Open a capsule of **vitamin E** and rub the oil on inflamed gums, to aid in healing.

• A powerful aid in stopping gum infection is to brush the teeth twice a day with powdered **charcoal**.

• Put **goldenseal** powder in the mouth to help eliminate the infection. But do not take goldenseal internally for more than a week at a time. (Too much can harm lactobacillus in the bowel.) Do not use it during pregnancy.

• Make a poultice of **goldenseal** and **myrrh** powder and place directly on the gums.

• Take **coenzyme Q$_{10}$** (60 mg, 2 times daily) for almost immediate relief.

• Take **quercetin** with **bromelain** for inflammation, plus **lysine**.

Note: Sores under the tongue can be an early sign of mouth cancer. But if you do not smoke or chew tobacco, you are unlikely to ever have that problem.

—See Receding Gums (425), Tooth Decay (423), Gingivitis (425), and Mouth and Gum Infections (427) for more information.

ENCOURAGEMENT—The Lord is soon coming. Talk it, pray it, sing it. Tell others to get their lives ready to meet their Lord. But it is now, before probation closes, that we must, by faith in Christ, put sin away from our lives. Matthew 24:30-31.

DENTURE PROBLEMS

SYMPTOMS—Loose-fitting dentures, dentures which may hurt the gums when chewing, dentures which cause difficulty in speaking properly.

CAUSES—Dentures are false teeth. The professional explanation for the problem is that the wearers do not take proper care of them and that the gums periodically change shape, etc.

There is another, less-known, reason: When the decision is made to extract teeth and fit an individual for dentures, the teeth are pulled out and the molds prepared for the false teeth. The entire process is frequently done quickly, so teeth will appear to be in the mouth as soon as possible. In addition, it is a convenience to the dentist to take the molds the same day that the extractions were done.

But when the extractions are made, the gums understandably swell! A number of sizeable wounds have been made in the mouth; and the gums are swollen and inflamed. That is not the time to take the molds.

Instead, the person should wait at least 10 days for the gums to heal and readjust into new positionings. Only at that time should the molds be made.

If your dentist tells you that you need all your teeth pulled out, discuss the matter with him and perhaps check with another dentist or two. Very often only certain teeth need be removed and a bridge can be put in, which locks onto the teeth which remain. This is far better than wearing dentures. Do all you can to keep your teeth.

But the solution for some individuals, with a mouthful of mercury fillings, is to get rid of those teeth entirely rather than to gradually replace mercury fillings with safer ones.

Retaining several lower teeth, so only a partial denture is needed, will help hold the lower denture in place. The upper denture tends to remain in place by itself.

LIVING WITH DENTURES—
• **Practice speaking**. Read aloud from books and learn how to articulate vowels, consonants, and various combinations.
• **Remove the dentures** at certain times, so the gums can rest.
• **Begin chewing** by eating soft foods. And gradually get used to chewing coarser foods with dentures.
• After each meal, **scrub the dentures** with soap and lukewarm water. **Wash your gums** gently with a soft toothbrush, to remove the plaque, and carefully **clean any remaining teeth**.
• **Massage your gums** everyday. Place your index finger over the outside of the gums, another finger over the inside portion, and rub back and forth. Or brush them with the toothbrush.

• **Rinse your mouth** each day with warm water mixed with a teaspoon of salt.

ENCOURAGEMENT—When the servants of Christ take the shield of faith for their defense and the sword of the Spirit for war, there is danger in the enemy's camp. Give your life fully to God, so He can use it for His glory and the advancement of His kingdom. Hebrews 4:12. "That by two immutable things, in which it was impossible for God to lie, we might have a strong consolation, who have fled for refuge to lay hold upon the hope set before us; which hope we have as an anchor of the soul, both sure and steadfast, and which entereth into that within the veil." Hebrews 6:18-19. A sweet promise, just for you.

GASTRO-INTESTINAL - 2 - MOUTH
Also: Cold Sores (Fever Blisters) (322),
Canker Sores (Aphthous Ulcers) (321),
Cleft Palate - see Birth Defects (725),
Cleft Lip - see Birth Defects (725)

MOUTH AND GUM INFECTIONS

SYMPTOMS—Ulcers and infections in the mouth and gums.

CAUSES—Infections in the mouth sometimes involve infections in the gums.
For much more information, see Gingivitis (425) and Pyorrhea (426).

NATURAL REMEDIES
• Eat a **nutritious diet** and take **vitamin-mineral** supplements. Also stop eating **fried, processed, sugary, and greasy foods**. Avoid **meat** products. Do not use **tobacco**—including chewing **snuff**. Do not drink **liquor**. Obtain adequate **rest** at night.
• For burning sensations in the mouth, take a B complex tablet, plus **vitamin B$_6$** (100 mg) and **vitamin B$_2$** (200 mg) daily.

MOUTHWASHES
Select from among the following mouthwashes, to help soothe and heal the mouth and gums during the time that remedial care is being given to them. However, they cannot take the place of brushing, flossing, proper diet, and keeping the mouth clean.

• Rinse your mouth with **saltwater** whenever you feel the first signs of a gum infection.
• For ulcerations in the mouth, mix **comfrey** with **burdock** root, add 1 tsp. to a cup of boiling water, steep, let cool, swish in the mouth several times a day.
• For a sore mouth, mix together 1 oz. **bayberry** root bark, ½ oz. each of **blue cohosh** root, **witch hazel** bark, and **goldenseal**. Steep the herbs 30 minutes in 1 pint boiling water, strain, sweeten as desired.

Gargle with it.

• A dilute tea of **St. John's wort** will promote healing.

• For mouth infections, rinse out the mouth 3 times a day (without swallowing it) with hot, **peach pit** tea.

• Rinse the mouth with a decoction of the ground rhizome of **bistort**. It is astringent and will give strength to weak, bleeding gums.

• Warm **chamomile** tea may be used as a soothing mouthwash after each brushing. Do not add sugar or milk to the tea.

• **Gotu kola** extract is good for gum healing.

• **Tea tree oil** is an anti-infective mouthwash. **Witch hazel**, and **calendula** extract are also good.

• Rinse with **white oak bark** tea. It is astringent; and it will reduce inflammation and cleanse the gums.

• Mix **aloe vera** juice with **myrrh** and apply to the gums.

• Drink 3 tsp. **chlorophyll** liquid, daily, and apply directly to the gums.

• Brush the teeth with **black poplar** powder, mixed with **charcoal**. The mixture absorbs residues and plaque. It also makes the teeth whiter.

• Prick capsules of **vitamin E** oil (400 IU) and rub the oil directly on gums. Or combine with **vitamin A** oil (500 IU) and place on gums.

• Use **folic acid** solution as a mouthwash.

• To control pain and soothe inflammation, massage gums with diluted **clove** oil, diluted **eucalyptus** oil, or **lobelia** extract.

• Put 4-5 drops **tea tree** oil or **grapefruit seed extract** in a water pick and use daily for recurring gum infections.

—*See Receding Gums (425), Tooth Decay (423), Gingivitis (425), and Pyorrhea (426) for more information.*

ENCOURAGEMENT—The ten commandments, "Thou shalt" and "Thou shalt not," are ten promises assured to us if we render obedience to the law governing the universe.

SALIVA PROBLEMS

SYMPTOMS—Not enough saliva, causing a dry-mouth condition. Or, perhaps, there is too much saliva.

CAUSES—Without proper saliva, you cannot absorb your food properly; for digestion begins in the mouth. Causes include **inadequate diet**, not drinking enough **fluids**, lack of **vitamin A** and other **nutrients**. Excessive salivation may be indicative of a **food allergy**.

NATURAL REMEDIES

• Drink at least two glasses of warm **water** 15-30 minutes before each meal.

• If you have a dry mouth, take a little **lemon juice** or **honey** before the meal, to stimulate the flow of saliva.

• If you are not obtaining enough **vitamin A** (5,000 IU or in the form of carotene in carrot juice, and green and yellow vegetables), your saliva flow may be inadequate.

• If you seem to have too much saliva, drink a tea of one of the following: **white oak bark, goldenseal root, or bayberry**.

• If you produce too much saliva, check to see if you have food allergies (848).

• **Chew your food** well, especially carbohydrate ("starchy") foods. They need partial digestion in the mouth before being swallowed. This includes such things as bread, all-grain products, potatoes, etc.

• The **chewing gum habit** is not good. It overworks your salivary glands when they should be resting.

—*Important: You may have Sjögren's Syndrome (241).*

ENCOURAGEMENT—Thank God everyday for temporal blessings and whatever comforts He bestows upon us in this life. He has a bright future for us; and, if we will but cooperate with His plans, our future is very bright. 2 Corinthians 1:22.

HALITOSIS
(Bad Breath)

SYMPTOMS—The breath has an unpleasant odor.

CAUSES—Touch the back of your hand with your tongue; then smell it. This is a simple test which may tell you something you need to know.

Not caring for your teeth properly, **not brushing them** can be a primary cause. But **tooth decay** (423), **indigestion, improper diet, gum disease** (426), **constipation** (456, 712), **inadequate digestion of proteins, infection in the nose or throat** (415-417), **poorly functioning liver** (446-449), **stress** (555-556), **heavy metal buildup** (868), or **mouth sores** can also be major problems. Bad breath may be a sign of an underlying **health problem**.

NATURAL REMEDIES

• **Brush your teeth** after each meal. Use dental **floss**.

• **Brush the tongue** carefully. It often has food particles and bacteria; it needs cleaning. Many people throughout the world rely on washing the tongue to get rid of bad breath.

• Drink more **water**. Dehydration often causes bad breath, especially first thing in the morning. Saliva does not flow during sleep, so no mouth cleaning occurs at night. Water is the best liquid for your body. The more water you drink, the more your mouth will stay clean.

• Go on a five-day **raw food diet**; during this time

50% of what you eat is raw. This will help clean out your system.

• **Garlic, onions, and curry** contain aromatic compounds that are exhaled as offensive breath for up to 24 hours. But, although **garlic** can be a temporary problem, it is such a powerful antibiotic that you may need to take it anyway.

• Eat **parsley**. Other **chlorophyll-containing foods** are also good for your breath. Include **acidophilus lactobacillus** in your diet to recondition your large bowel.

• Take a **B complex** supplement daily, plus **B$_6$** (50 mg). Also take **zinc** (30 mg).

• Take **charcoal** by mouth. Let it dissolve slowly in the mouth. This will help clean both your mouth and stomach.

• **Apples, carrots, celery**, etc., are excellent for cleaning out your mouth at the close of a meal. They remove odor-causing bacteria from the mouth.

• When you get up in the morning, take 3 **chlorophyll** capsules or tablets on an empty stomach.

• **Outdoor exercise** will bring more oxygen into the lungs and help clean out the system, reducing bad breath.

• **Gum disease** is a frequent cause of bad breath. *See Gingivitis (425) and Periodontal Disease (426).* Place **goldenseal** over the infected gums or mouth sores. Do this for 3 days, to help heal the gums.

• Although very unlikely, **mouth breathing** may cause bad breath. Yet, for many, the advantages of mouth breathing (obtaining more oxygen than otherwise could be done) outweighs the possible disadvantages.

• **Sinus infection** produces a discharge with a bad odor. If you have sinus trouble *(381),* this may be the cause of your bad breath.

• Use **myrrh, rosemary, or peppermint** to brush your teeth and rinse your mouth.

• In cases of bad breath caused by stomach problems, **thyme** tea can be helpful.

• Dr. Christopher especially recommends taking a little **myrrh** tea internally to eliminate bad breath.

• Chew **fennel** or **anise** seeds after eating an odorous meal.

• **Ginger, coriander, cumin, and fennel** are four herbs that can deodorize your intestinal tract. Chew **anise, cardamom, dill, or fennel** seeds.

AVOID

• **Alcohol, coffee, nicotine, and meat eating** are four of the worst offenders.

• Avoid bad teeth! **Unclean teeth, decayed teeth, or space beneath caps** (dental crowns) where food can lodge and rot can be significant causes of bad breath.

• Do not eat **spicy foods. Meat eating** can produce bad breath, both because of the particles left in the mouth and because of later indigestion. **Cheese** and **fish** both cause bad breath. Drinking **coffee, beer, wine, or whiskey** are excellent ways to have bad breath. Many **street drugs,** so disrupting to the body, also produce bad breath.

• Avoid foods that are likely to cause tooth decay (such as **meat, candies, and sticky sweets**). Avoid **foods that get stuck** between the teeth too easily.

• Other "bad breath foods" include Roquefort, Camembert, blue **cheeses**, canned **tuna** on pizza, and spicy deli **meats**.

• Do not use **commercial mouthwashes**. They irritate the mouth more than they solve any problems. All they have is alcohol, dye, and flavoring.

• Instances have been reported of **food allergies** *(848)* causing bad breath. Search out the foods you are allergic to and avoid them.

• Avoid **constipation** *(456, 712).*

• Once a week, rinse your toothbrush in **hydrogen peroxide**, soak it overnight, or boil it each month. Occasionally buy a new one. Bacteria grow on the toothbrush.

—*See Gingivitis (425) and Periodontal Disease (426).*

ENCOURAGEMENT—Give the Word of God, the Bible, the honored place as the guide in your home; you and your family will be blessed for it. The Bible presents a perfect standard of character; and its divine Author can give us the grace to obey it fully.

CHEILOSIS
(Angular Stomatitis, Geographic Tongue)

SYMPTOMS—Cracks appear in the corners of the mouth and in the (nasolabial) corners of the nose.

The top and sides of the tongue are irregular, denuded areas that appear very smooth. Geographic tongue is not painful; and the sense of taste may, or may not, be affected.

CAUSES—This is a nutritional problem, as explained below.

NATURAL REMEDIES

• The cracks are directly caused by a vitamin **B$_2$** (riboflavin) deficiency. Take 500 mg daily.

• The geographic tongue means you are not absorbing **vitamins B$_3$** (200 mg), **B$_6$** (200 mg), **B$_5$** (2,000 mg), **B$_{12}$** (1,000 mg), **folic acid** (5 mg), **or zinc** (30 mg) properly. The cause is frequently malabsorption from **celiac disease**-like *(474)* changes in the small intestine.

• Do a series of **pulse tests** *(847),* to determine the foods you may be allergic to. Avoid those allergens. You may need to take **betaine HCl** (hydrochloric acid) before each meal.

ENCOURAGEMENT—By firm principle and unwavering trust in God, we can live clean, honest lives that will be a blessing to all around us. This is the will of God for us. 2 Corinthians 7:6.

LOSS OF SENSE OF TASTE

GASTRO

SYMPTOMS—The ability to taste things seems to be disappearing or totally gone.

CAUSES—There are about 10,000 taste buds on the upper surface of the tongue. Each bud contains about 25 sensory receptor cells; these tiny taste hairs are exposed to drink and food dissolved in saliva. They sense four basic tastes: sweet, sour, salty, and bitter.

This condition may be caused by **allergies, infections, aging, nasal polyps, nerve damage,** or **deficiencies of B vitamins and zinc**. The cause may be certain **drug medications**.

NATURAL REMEDIES

• Switch to a **nutritious diet** of fruits and vegetables. Take a complete **B vitamin supplement**, plus added **zinc** (30 mg daily). After several weeks, reduce the zinc dosage to 15 mg.

ENCOURAGEMENT—Although you will have trials, yet these trials, well borne, only make the way more precious, if you are trusting in Jesus and humbly seeking to do His will.

DRY MOUTH
(Xerostomia)

SYMPTOMS—The mouth seems to be dry all the time.

CAUSES—An estimated 25% of older Americans have dry mouth syndrome. It is common among public speakers.

NATURAL REMEDIES

• Dry mouth is a side effect of more than 400 medicinal **drugs**, including many prescribed for **high blood pressure and depression.** In addition, avoid **antihistamines, diuretics, and tranquilizers.**

• **Hypoglycemics** and **diabetics** often have a dry mouth, due to blood sugar imbalance. They should drink enough **water**.

• **Breathe through your nose,** to avoid stress-induced dry mouth. (However, mouth breathing helps you take in much more air; you may do best not to stop the practice.)

• Sip **water** frequently. It is good for you. Or drink a glassful every hour or so between meals. It is an intriguing fact that those who rely on **coffee, soft drinks, or liquor** for their fluids tend to not get enough liquids. Instead, only drink **water and fruit juices**, and you will have lots of fluid in your body.

• Add a dropperful of **echinacea** tincture to juice, or chew the root of a fresh plant.

• Rinse the mouth with **goldenseal** mouthwash before bedtime. It will keep your mouth moist and relieve inflamed gums.

• Take **coenzyme Q$_{10}$** (10-30 mg) daily.

• **Jaborandi** (various species of Pilocarpus) is a Brazilian plant which increases salivation as much as tenfold. The active ingredient is *pilocarpine*.

• **Aloe vera** gel can relieve tender, burning, inflamed gum tissue. Do not eat for an hour afterward.

• In China, they simmer 2-4 tsp. dried **multiflora rose** per cup of boiling water to make a tea for dry mouth.

• **Cayenne** stimulates salivation.

• **Vitamin C** (2,000 mg) will help repair the damage to mouth cells which are too dry. Also take a complete **B complex**.

• You may have **Sjögren's syndrome** *(311)*. This causes dry eyes, dry mouth, and painful joints.

ENCOURAGEMENT— The truest, the most exalted, knowledge is found in the Word of God, the Bible. In its simplicity there is eloquence. It is the path to eternal life.

LEUKOPLAKIA

SYMPTOMS—White, painless patches on the tongue or lining of the mouth.

CAUSES—These patches frequently follow radiation treatment or long-term antibiotic drug therapy. But they may also be caused by pipe smoking, rubbing by a rough tooth, or thickening of tissues in the elderly.

Leukoplakia is closely related to candidiasis (281), which you may have.

NATURAL REMEDIES

• The patches often disappear when a B complex tablet and acidophilus capsules are taken with each meal.

• Rinse the mouth with **aloe vera** juice or a mixture of 2 tablespoons each of apple cider **vinegar** and **water**, plus a pinch of **cayenne**.

• Make a tea of **white oak bark, myrrh, goldenseal, and red raspberry**, and swish it in the mouth.

• Wipe the patches with a cloth dipped in a solution of **borax**, mixed with **water** or **honey**.

ENCOURAGEMENT—Present your petitions to the Lord in humility and real soul hunger for the blessing of God, without boasting of superior attainments. Come to Him as His little child, asking for help.

ORAL THRUSH

SYMPTOMS—Creamy-looking white patches form on the tongue and the mucous membranes of the mouth. If the patches are scraped off, bleeding

DISEASES - List: 10-26 / Index: 1211-1224 / **HERBS** - Contents: 129- / **Preparing: 132** / **Using: 141-189 (dose:
often 1 tsp. mixed herbs in 1 cup boiled water) / VITAMINS-MINERALS** - Index: 100- / **Dosages: 124** / **HYDRO-
THERAPY** - Therapy index: 206- / **Disease index: 263-** / **CARE OF SICK** - **28-39** / **EMERGENCIES** - **973-, 990-**

GASTRO

may result.

CAUSES—This is a fungal infection; and it is most common in those with compromised immune systems.

NATURAL REMEDIES

NUTRITION

• Eat a nourishing diet of **fruits, vegetables, whole grains, legumes, and nuts**. While treating the infection, a diet primarily of **raw food** is best.

• Avoid **tobacco, alcohol, caffeine**. Do not eat **meat or dairy products**. Avoid **sugary, fried, and processed foods**. Eat nothing **greasy**.

HERBS

• **Goldenseal** contains *berberine*, which destroys fungi. It can be used against every type of fungus infection. It can be applied both topically and as a drink. Only use goldenseal for a week; then switch for a time to another fungicide herb.

• **Pau d'arco** is strongly antifungal. Drink 3 cups daily.

• **Bloodroot** also contains *berberine*; and it has been shown to be quite effective as a fungicide.

• **Yellowroot, barberry, and Oregon grape** also contain *berberine*.

• **Tea tree** oil is excellent when applied externally; but do not drink it. Apply it several times a day to the affected area, either full strength or diluted with a little distilled water or cold-pressed oil. **Black walnut** extract can also be used.

• A powerful antifungicide is **wild oregano oil**. The most resistant forms of fungus infection can generally be eliminated by it.

• The **pepper tree** (horopito) is a New Zealand shrub which contains *polygodial*, which is useful against both fungi and bacteria. Another antifungal herb is the ***Licaria puchuri-major***, a Brazilian plant.

ENCOURAGEMENT—Genuine faith is the faith that works by love and purifies the soul. A living faith will be a working faith.

RED, CRACKING LIPS
(Chelitis, Perléche)

SYMPTOMS—Redness and tenderness on one or both lips, with inflammation, a burning sensation, and scaling. Sometimes cracks on the lips and often in the corners of the mouth.

CAUSES—**Nutritional deficiencies** and **allergic reactions** to toothpaste or mouthwash may be the cause. The problem might be due to skin conditions such as **seborrheic dermatitis** *(346)* or **psoriasis** *(351)*. In adults, the cause may be poorly fitted **dentures**. In small children, excessive **lip licking** or **drooling** (possibly caused by mouth breathing which keeps the mouth open, or injury from **dental braces**). Excessive **sun or wind exposure** can intensify the problem.

NATURAL REMEDIES

• Read the above paragraph carefully and make needed changes.

• Eat a nutritious diet of **fruits, vegetables, whole grains, nuts, and legumes,** plus a full **vitamin-mineral supplement**. Obtain adequate **rest** and **exercise**.

ENCOURAGEMENT—When the divine law is set aside, the greatest misery will result to families and to society. Our only hope of better things is to be found in a faithful adherence to the precepts of God.

LIP BALM

Here are a formula for a lip balm you can prepare in your own home. In this way, you can be sure there are no dangerous additives in the balm.

Warm 1 cup almond oil in a double-boiler. Stir continually. Add 1 Tbsp. beeswax. Add 1 tsp. of each of the following: vanilla extract, honey, vitamin E oil, aloe vera gel. While hot, stir as you pour it into a wide-mouth jar. Close tightly. The lip balm, which will soon harden, is very nourishing for the lips.

ENCOURAGEMENT—God never lets go one who commits the keeping of the soul to His care. Having loved them because of their love of Jesus, He loves them to the end.

GASTRO-INTESTINAL -
3 - GAS AND VOMITING

HICCUPS
(Hiccoughs, Singultis)

SYMPTOMS—Hiccups that you want to have stopped. This is a sudden inspiration of air caused by spasmodic contractions of the diaphragm. An irritation of the phrenic nerve causes the contraction of the diaphragm.

CAUSES—Charles Osborne of Anthon, Iowa, started hiccuping in 1922 and hiccuped for the next 65 years. After 430 million hiccups, he passed away.

Almost all hiccups are one-sided; that is, only one side of the diaphragm contracts. **Overeating** or **excessive drinking** is the most common cause. It causes the stomach to extend downward and press against the diaphragm—which then starts its hiccuppy motions. Other causes include **overeating, eating too fast, irregular times for eating, carbonated beverages, stomach inflammation due to fermentation, stress or excitement, cold showers, sudden temperature changes, smoking, drinking alcohol**. Nursing infants which **swallow air**.

A hiccup is a repeated involuntary spasmodic contraction of the diaphragm, immediately followed by a sudden closure of the glottis.

But that information does not help solve the

problem. Here is advice that may. All of the following methods really work for some people. Find what is best for you. (You will notice that these techniques are frequently based on diverting attention, changing the ongoing physical hiccup pattern, and getting the body to do something different for a few moments.)

NATURAL REMEDIES

• A high blood carbon-dioxide level is known to stifle hiccups. A well-known procedure is to **breathe into a paper bag**. Blow in and out exactly 10 times; and do it very hard until you are red in the face. You must do it fast; and you must form a good seal around the bag so no air gets in.

• **Hold your breath** as long as you can; then **swallow** when you think a hiccup is coming. Do that 2-3 times. Then take a deep breath and begin again.

• **Hold your breath** in for as long as possible; then **exhale and hold** that as long as possible.

• **Blow air out** in a slow, steady stream.

• Hold your breath while **extending your head as far backward** as you can.

• Swallow a teaspoonful of **dry sugar**. It often stops the hiccups in minutes. The sugar in the mouth probably sends different signals along the nerve routes, interfering with the hiccups.

• Close your mouth, hold your **nose and ears closed** with your fingers and thumbs, and **swallow** 3 times before you let go. This creates a slight vacuum and changes the rhythm of the diaphragm enough to bring relief.

• Chew gently, and swallow **ice,** for 10-15 minutes.

• Stand behind the person as he sits on a chair. Grasp the neck gently with your fingers and, with the thumbs, slowly **massage** down each side of the spine.

• Fill a glass of water, bend over forward, and **drink the water upside down**.

• Apply pressure with the flat of the hand, just **below the breastbone**.

• Take a deep breath and drink 10 **swallows** of water while not breathing.

• Put **ice** on the neck.

• Drink **catnip** tea.

• Place light fingertip pressure on each **side of the neck**, for about a minute.

• Take exactly 10 **sips** of water in rapid succession.

• A **sneeze** sometimes stops the hiccups.

Chew activated **charcoal** tablets, fresh **mint** leaves, or **dill** seeds.

• Drink **lemon and lime** juice.

• Hiccups are generally caused by **overloading food or drink** into the stomach. Relaxation is the most important thing. Often they can be stopped merely by bending over, with the head downward, and tipping a glass of liquid to drink it while upside-down. A few drops of **antispasmodic tincture** taken internally and rubbed on the chest area will often bring relief, as will a teaspoon of **onion juice**, a **cayenne poultice** on the chest area, **black cohosh tea, blue cohosh, or wild carrot flowers or seeds**.

• Have someone pull outward on your **tongue** for a few minutes.

• Drink a glass of water while **clenching a pencil** with the back teeth.

• Lie on the **left side** for 10-15 minutes.

• Stand **on your head**.

• **Shout or sing** as loudly as possible.

• **Bend over**, placing the head lower than the diaphragm, then drink a glass of cold water through a straw. Then remain in that position for several minutes.

• **Do Deep breathing**.

• A sudden, **loud noise** will startle an end to the hiccups; but make sure the person has no heart trouble.

• **Tickle** the soft section in the back of the roof of the mouth with a cotton-tipped swab.

• Have someone **massage your feet**.

• Drink a half glassful of fresh **orange juice**.

• Take a **hot bath** for 15 minutes.

• Place an **ice bag** to the pit of the stomach.

• **Soak both feet** in water for 15 minutes.

• Bend at the waist, **touch the toes**, and hold this position for about 60 seconds. This method is useful for both adults and children.

• When children run around and play, sometimes one ends up with the hiccups. When that happens, try **tickling** him while he holds his breath; and tell him to try real hard not to laugh. He will forget about the hiccups.

• When you are eating, just **be quiet and eat**; and you are not likely to get hiccups.

• Do not use **alcohol, caffeine, tobacco, cold or carbonated water**.

• In case you have hiccups which will not stop, go on a **3-day complete fast**, drinking only juices.

ENCOURAGEMENT—The work of conquering evil is to be done through faith. Those who go into the battlefield will find that they must put on the whole armor of God. The shield of faith must be their defense. God will give them the victory over temptation and sin. In Him they can be victorious. Psalm 119:105, 130.

BELCHING
(Eructation, Aerophagia)

SYMPTOMS—Burping up air from the stomach.

CAUSES—Belching is most frequently caused by bringing up air that was **swallowed with the food and drink** taken in. This is called eructation. When belching occurs repeatedly, all day long, it is called aerophagia, which is caused by unconscious, **repeated swallowing of air**.

We normally have about a cupful of air in our stomach all the time. Each day, we swallow air and make some in our stomach (about 10 cupfuls in 24 hours). Because this is 9 cupfuls too many, we belch occasionally.

NATURAL REMEDIES

• Make a habit of **not gulping down air** as you eat. Just thinking about being more careful will help a lot.

• **Chew with your mouth closed**, and **do not talk** while you are eating.

• Do not eat **foods which produce gas**, such as beans, carbonated drinks, and beer.

• **Do not drink in odd ways**: out of cans, bottles, or through a straw.

• Avoid **foods with high air** content. This includes ice cream, beer, omelets, and whipped cream.

• **Ginger** stimulates digestion and is good both for relieving and preventing belching. Take 1-2 550 mg capsules of powdered ginger before each meal. Or drink a cup of ginger tea with the meal.

• Eat **nutritious food** and take **vitamin-mineral supplements**, so you will make enough digestive enzymes.

• Add 1 tsp. **cardamom** to 8 oz. water, boil for 10 minutes, drink it hot. The herb helps reduce muscle spasms in the stomach, which cause the belching.
—*Also see Bloating (below).*

ENCOURAGEMENT—If we would give more expression to our faith and rejoice more in the blessings we know we have, we could have more faith and greater joy. If you will cooperate with His plan, as given in the Bible, He will give you eternal life.

FLATULENCE
(Gas, Bloating)

SYMPTOMS—There is an excess of gas in the stomach. The stomach (or intestines) seems to be too full.

CAUSES—Bloating is the accumulation of gas in the stomach, intestines, or bowels. Normally the stomach is sterile because of the acid environment. But when it does not contain enough **hydrochloric acid** (*achlorhydria, 351*), bacteria from the small intestine migrates up into the stomach. Arriving there, it ferments the carbohydrates and sugars. This produces gas or, what is called, bloat.

Flatus (which is gas or air in the gastrointestinal canal) is the result of poor digestion. The food becomes fermented and sour in the stomach, due to an acid condition. This is caused by wrong food combinations, drinking with meals, hasty eating, or poor mastication.

NATURAL REMEDIES

• You may wish to take 1 ounce of oral **hydrogen peroxide** (20 drops / ounce) twice a day, along with colloidal minerals, betaine HCl (hydrochloride), and pancreatic enzymes (75-200 mg, three times a day). Take this 15 minutes before mealtime. Be sure you take it through a straw and it does not get on your teeth! (The acid can melt them.)

• Instead take **lemon juice and water** before each meal. In your stomach, the lemon juice will act similarly to that of HCl.

• A **low-fat diet** helps reduce carbon-dioxide production in the top (duodenal) area of the small intestines.

• Drink enough **water**. A dry mouth encourages swallowing.

• Eat more **slowly**. **Chew** your food well. **Relax** when you eat.

• Eat **lactobacillus** to restore the bacteria needed to stop bloating in the bowel.

• Eat **digestive enzymes** at the close of the meal.

• Take **chlorophyll** to reduce gas and odor.

• Do not postpone **bowel movements**.

• **To reduce gas-causing sulfur** compounds in beans (garbanzo, pinto, navy, etc.), use the following tactic involves a lengthy soaking, and was developed some years ago by the California Dry Bean Advisory Board. For each pound of dried beans, use ten or more cups of boiling water. Boil for two to three minutes, cover, and set the beans aside overnight. This initial boiling breaks down the cell membranes of the beans, releasing the oligosaccharides so they can dissolve into the soaking water. Just make sure you discard the soaking water!

• An old Appalachian method: Cook **beans** with a small, whole **carrot**.

• Sprouting your beans first can also eliminate the gas-causing sulfur compounds.

• Try adding epazote (1 tablespoon to a large pot of chili, beans, or soup). Epazote is the leaf of a wild herb, prized for its gas-reducing abilities.

TO ELIMINATE AIR

• Take **charcoal** to help reduce the gas. The charcoal will adsorb it and carry it off. Activated charcoal is best.

• If you are going to a social gathering and must not produce gas, take 1-2 200-500 mg **charcoal tablets** before going there. Do not do this over 2 weeks at a time.

• **Walking** helps break down bubbles, so they can be more quickly expelled.

• Rock in a **rocking chair** vigorously with feet on the floor.

• When bloating occurs, this can be done: If it is in the stomach, seat the person upright, **apply heat over the stomach**. Have him **sip hot water**.

• If the bloating is in the intestines, have him **lie down** for a half hour, before and after meals. Give **no fluids with meals**, but hot water may be sipped afterward. If needed, give an **enema**.

• To expel excess air, rock back and forth in the knee-chest position.

• There are a number of herbs that will help relieve gas. Some of the best are **wild yam, celery seed tea, and peppermint or spearmint teas**. **Carminative teas** are specifics for the stomach area to soothe the flatulent condition and to correct the digestive functions. **Goldenseal with myrrh** is an excellent stomach tonic.

• Carminative herbs expel gas and bloat. Mix equal parts **balm, chamomile, and peppermint**. Steep 1 tsp. in ½ cup boiling-hot water. Take unsweetened in mouthful doses.

• Mix 3 parts **spearmint** and 1 part **ginger**. Add 1 tsp. to each cup of hot water. Drink the clear tea and leave the sediment.

• Mix equal parts of **German Chamomile, anise, caraway, fennel seed, and balm leaves**. Steep 1 tsp. in ½ cup boiling-hot water. Take ½-1 cup a day.

• Other carminative herbs include **allspice, cloves, cornmint, dill, horsebalm, sage, and thyme**.

• A little **ginger tea** is good for infant colic or flatulence.

AVOID

• Avoid **drinking with meals**.

• Avoid **gas-producing foods**, such as beans, cabbage, other members of the cabbage family, and whole wheat-flour products.

• You may have trouble digesting **milk sugar** (lactose). Try stopping all milk products for a week or two and see if that helps. Dairy foods can produce gas in the large bowels.

• It is possible to eat too much **fiber** at a time. This can induce some bloating.

• **Artificial sweeteners** produce gas.

• **Carbonated drinks** (beer, champagne, soft drinks) and foods with whipped air cause more air to be ingested.

• Avoid **fried food, hydrogenated fat, sugar, refined carbohydrates, junk food, ice-cold drinks, and poor food combinations**.

• Avoid drinking at **water fountains**. You can hardly drink at one without gulping down air.

• Both **chewing gum** and **smoking** increase the swallowing of air.

• Do not **sigh**. People who sigh often swallow air.

• Avoid **tight belts** and **tight-fitting clothes**. Those who do not wear belts and girdles have less indigestion.

• Avoid **repetitive belching**; for you tend to swallow more air than you release.

J.H. KELLOGG, M.D., PRESCRIPTIONS FOR GASEOUS STOMACH DISTENSION AND ITS COMPLICATIONS (how to give these water therapies: pp. 206-275 / list of treatments: pp. 206-207 / Hydrotherapy Disease Index: pp. 273-275)

COMBAT IT—Cold Compress over stomach without plastic covering, changed every 4 hours. Cold Fan Douche over stomach, twice daily.

INCREASE GENERAL VITAL RESISTANCE, COMBAT AUTOINTOXICATION—short sweating baths, such as the Radiant Heat Bath, Sweating Wet Sheet Pack, Hot Full Bath (4-6 minutes, at 1050 F.), Hot Blanket Pack, Hot Enema. Follow each hot bath with a **Tonic Friction** application.

PYROSIS—Hot water drinking before retiring at night. **Fomentation** over stomach at bedtime, with **Hot Abdominal Pack** overnight, and sipping half a glass of very hot water, when rising in the morning. A few ounces of orange juice or other natural, unsweetened fruit juice half an hour before eating is important.

CONSTIPATION—Graduated Cold Enema. Cold Douche to abdomen. **Hot Abdominal Pack. Regularity** of bowel habits.

PAIN—Fomentation over the abdomen, followed by a **Heating Compress** that is protected only by flannel.

—Also see Belching (432), Achlorhydria (439), Dyspepsia (437), and Colic in Children (735) and Infants (728).

ENCOURAGEMENT—Living faith and obedience, by faith in Christ, can give us the victory over every besetment and sin. He can enable us to stand firm to the end. 1 John 5:4.

HEARTBURN
(Acidosis, Overacid Stomach, Gastroesophageal Reflux Disease)

SYMPTOMS—A burning sensation in the stomach or chest. Or a burning sensation or gnawing pain in the area of the chest over the heart (precordium) or beneath the sternum and near the heart, usually a symptom of indigestion or esophageal spasm. Generally this comes from gastric pyrosis, a stomach problem characterized by belching (eructations) an acid, irritating fluid.

CAUSES—Heartburn is a sense of burning in the stomach. In most instances, some of the stomach digestive juices have backed up out of the stomach into the esophagus (the food tube between the mouth and the stomach). This backing-up action is called *reflux*. These juices include hydrochloric acid, which is a rather powerful acid. A heavier concentration is used in industry to clean metal. When it comes in contact with the esophagus, it burns the wall. Normally, the esophageal sphincter muscle shuts and prevents stomach acids from pushing upward.

Chronic heartburn can scar the esophagus. The acids make their way into the lungs, and asthma-like conditions can result. Chronic heartburn is now officially known as GERD (gastroesophageal reflux disease).

Heartburn can be caused by **excessive consumption of fatty or fried foods, alcohol, coffee,** spicy foods, chocolate, or just having **too much food** in the stomach. **Citrus fruits** or **tomato-based foods** cause it in a few people.

Other contributing factors are hiatal hernia *(436)*, allergies *(848)*, stress *(555-576)*, gallbladder problems *(451-453)*, and enzyme deficiencies *(120)*.

Having **too little stomach acid** *(439)* can cause a similar condition. People over 50 often have a deficiency; and the discomfort is nearly identical to having too much. Proper digestion does not occur; this causes bloating, belching, and other symptoms of heartburn. If this is your problem, you need to take lemon juice and water with your meal. If symptoms continue after taking the lemon juice, then your stomach is making **too much** acid.

NATURAL REMEDIES

IMMEDIATELY

• Drink a large glass of **water**. This will help wash the HCl back down and dilute it as well. Or drink some raw **potato juice**. Whiz up an unpeeled potato and drink it down.

• Do not lie down. Remain **upright**, so gravity can help push the HCl down and keep it down.

• Lose weight. The pressure of extra weight causes heartburn more frequently.

• Do not wear tight clothing around the waist. Loosen your belt; better yet, **wear suspenders**.

• Eat more **raw vegetables**, **chew your food** well, take small mouthfuls, and **eat slowly**.

• Prompt and temporary relief may be given for heartburn with **cramp bark, ginger, wild yam**, etc. Massaging tincture of **lobelia** externally into the area and internally taking two or three drops regularly is often sufficient.

HERBS

• **Peppermint** is excellent for heartburn. Make a tea and drink it. Lemon balm, basil, and oregano are also good.

• Chewing **licorice** protects the lining of the esophagus, which can be damaged by chronic heartburn. For best results, use deglycerinated licorice, which is a chewable form. Take 1-2 chewable tablets 3 times daily on an empty stomach. It can help protect against stomach ulcers from an excess of stomach acid.

• Two natural antacids are "**bitters**" (bitter herbs) and **ginger** root. Bitters includes **goldenseal, gentian root**, and **wormwood**. Take a small amount before the meal to prevent heartburn. Take 2 capsules ginger root at the end of the meal to prevent heartburn.

• **Papaya** and **pineapple** contain *bromelain*, which is a digestive enzyme.

• Drink a cup of **aloe vera** to stop heartburn symptoms rather quickly. It helps protect the lining of the esophagus.

• **Dill** has been used to soothe the digestive tract and treat heartburn for centuries. Crush a few seeds and make a tea of it. (If pregnant, do not use dill.) **Fennel** is another favorite for treating heartburn.

• **Slippery Elm** helps relieve the symptoms of acid indigestion by healing the mucous membranes.

• **Cardamom** help eliminate gas.

• **Angelica** is good for heartburn in adults and colic and gas in children.

• A cup of **gentian**, taken 30 minutes before a meal, prevents heartburn. Simmer 1 tsp. in a cup of water for 30 minutes, then add a sprinkle of **cayenne** and **ginger**, and drink it.

• Because heartburn is an acid condition of the system, it is necessary to go on a **complete cleansing program,** to clean out the system. **Proper foods, proper eating habits, and effective elimination** are very important. A cure is effected only with a complete change of living habits.

AVOID

• **Avoid bending over**; if you must lift something, bend at the knees. You do not want to compress your stomach when you have heartburn. Do not lift heavy objects.

• **Do not eat** 2-3 hours before bedtime or lie down after a meal. Acid can more easily flow into the esophagus; and, by doing so, it can also bring on a heart attack. Do not use **extra pillows** under your head; you do not want your body to bend at the waist. It is best to sleep on your **left side**; doing so helps prevent stomach acid from flowing up into the esophagus. Temporarily **elevate** the bed at the head by 4-6 inches.

• Do not eat **big meals**. Do not eat **high-fat foods**. Do not eat **spices, chocolate,** or **mints**.

• **Avoid foods** which upset you.

• Do not drink anything **caffeinated**; for it will irritate the esophagus even more. Caffeine relaxes the sphincter, so stomach contents can move on up. **Estrogens** relax it also. **Smoking** weakens your esophageal muscle.

• Drinking **milk** may feel good going down; but it encourages the stomach to secrete more acid.

• **Drinks with (carbonated) fizz** in them expand the stomach and make it more likely that HCl will come up the food pipe. So no colas or beer.

• **Greasy, fried, and fatty foods** sit in the stomach for a long time and increase HCl production. Avoid **meat** and **dairy** products.

• **Antidepressants and sedatives** aggravate heartburn. **Aspirin** and **ibuprofen** cause heartburn.

Antacids only mask the symptoms. They also contain aluminum, which is a cause of Alzheimer's disease *(587)*. Antacids interfere with the body's ability to digest and absorb food.

WARNING

Angina *(521)* and **heart attack** *(513-523)* are both very dangerous conditions. Among the earliest symptoms of both is, what appears to be, an "acid stomach." Beware. You are wise to eat so that you do not have heartburn. Then if major heart trouble sends a warning message that seems like heartburn, you will not ignore a crucial first signal of terrible trouble.

Heartburn usually occurs during, or shortly after, a meal and produces pain or burning in the chest. *Heart attack* and *angina* can strike at any time. The pain often radiates from the chest up under the jaw or along an arm, producing faintness and sweating. If in doubt, call 911 and describe your symptoms.

—*Read everything under Hiatal Hernia (below), Excess Hydrochloric Acid (440).*

ENCOURAGEMENT—Even on earth we may have joy as a wellspring, never failing, because it is fed by the streams that flow from the throne of God. All this is ours as we study the Bible and, in Christ's strength, obey it. 1 Peter 4:12.

HIATAL HERNIA
(Hiatus Hernia)

SYMPTOMS—Heartburn and belching. There may be difficulty in swallowing. Material from the stomach may suddenly return into the throat or mouth, causing a burning sensation. It may feel as if there is a lump in the throat or that food is sticking somewhere in the throat. Sometimes bloody mucus is coughed up.

CAUSES—A small portion of the stomach slips (pushes or herniates) through an opening (hiatus) in the diaphragm, causing the stomach to come up into the chest cavity (the thorax). A weakness in the diaphragm as it leaves the esophagus may enlarge the opening, where the esophagus (food pipe) enters the stomach. This enables the stomach to slide up somewhat.

The weakness is often caused by increased pressure upward, from what is in or near the abdominal cavity: **obesity, pregnancy, tumors, heavy lifting, overeating, straining at the stool, or tight clothing**.

It is said that nearly half the people over 40, in the U.S., have hiatal hernias. But most are unaware of it, since these hernias are often quite small and are hardly noticed. They occur in women four times as often as in men, perhaps due to tight clothing. They generally first occur after the age of 40.

The acid material that comes up into the food pipe, from the larger hernias, frequently causes ulceration in the esophageal wall.

But ulcers can also occur in the duodenum, which is the top part of the small intestine, just below the stomach. People with this condition have a tendency to have **overacid stomachs**.

Between the esophagus and stomach is the esophageal sphincter. This is a circular valve which can open and close. But its strength is damaged by **drugs, tobacco (smoked or chewed), or certain foods**. This weakening allows food and acid to go back up into the food pipe.

Those problem foods include **coffee and chocolate** (because of the methylxanthines in them), **spicy foods, tomato, alcohol, peppermint, spearmint, and citrus juices**. **Tobacco and coffee** are especially bad. **Whole milk** can also be a problem. Weakening of the sphincter occurs within 30 minutes after drinking coffee. One puff of a cigarette can lower sphincter pressure to zero; the result is called "smoker's heartburn."

NATURAL REMEDIES

After you eat, sit in a chair for awhile. Do not stoop or bend over.

• Eat **nourishing food**, plus **vitamin / mineral supplements**. Several **small meals** are best. **Avoid overeating**; it only intensifies the problem. If eaten at all, **supper should be light** and 2-3 hours before bedtime. Food in the stomach, after you are in bed, is more likely to flow back up into the food pipe. Stop eating supper entirely, and you are more likely to have success in overcoming hiatal hernias.

• Include extra **fiber** in your diet; this helps soak up some of the acid.

• **Do not drink liquids** immediately before, during, or up to 30 minutes after meals, so digestive enzymes work better. But, as soon as you sense heartburn coming on, drink 1-2 large glasses of **water**. This tends to wash the acid back down into the stomach.

• **Avoid fried food and fats**; they slow down the digestion process in the stomach. Do not take **tea, coffee, colas, alcohol, or tobacco**. Avoid **refined foods**, including **white-flour products and sugar**. Avoid **coffee, chocolate, spicy foods, alcohol, tomatoes, mint foods, whole milk,** and possibly **citrus juices**.

• Eat your meals on a **regular schedule** and do not eat between meals. Eating between meals causes the stomach to stop partway through and start all over again—still with everything from the previous meal in it.

• Even when not thirsty, drink a large glass of water every so often throughout the day.

• **Avoid heavy lifting** and **do not bend over** more than you have to. Wait till 2 hours after a meal before starting heavy exertion. Bend from the knees, not from the waist, to avoid upward pressure on the stomach.

• Daily outdoor **exercise** will strengthen the muscles.

• Avoid **stress** and stressful situations.

• Avoid **tight clothing** (corsets, girdles, belts, etc.).

• You may need to raise the head of the bed 4-8 inches to avoid reflux of food upward at night.

—*Read everything in Heartburn (434) and Excess Hydrochloric Acid (440). Also see Hernia (641) and Umbilical Hernia (642).*

ENCOURAGEMENT—We all need a guide through the many difficult places of life. But if we will cling to

God and His Written Word, the Bible, we can have the victory at each step. Zechariah 13:9. "Faithful is He that calleth you, who also will do it." 1 Thessalonians 5:24. Trust in your kind heavenly Father, and He will care for you.

VOMITING
(Emesis)

SYMPTOMS—The person vomits.

CAUSES—Vomiting is the return of the stomach contents through the mouth. Most cases of vomiting are not due to severe illness.

The cause is often **overeating**, eating the **wrong food, poor combinations**, or excessive **alcohol** consumption. But it can also be caused by **food allergies, poisoning, food poisoning, or infection** (flu, Epstein-Barr syndrome, candida, etc.). If the vomitus (that which comes up) looks like "coffee grounds," it includes large amounts of blood from a bleeding ulcer or stomach cancer—*and that is an emergency*; for extensive internal bleeding can result in death. Take him to the emergency room.

This may be either a voluntary body activity or it may be induced when it is necessary, to cleanse the stomach of undigested food poison and excess body waste.

If it occurs in infants, accompanied by fever and the child is unresponsive, it could indicate **meningitis**. Call a physician immediately. *See Meningitis (578).*

But it might be that you need to induce more vomiting, because someone has just eaten a poisonous plant, rat poison, etc.

NATURAL REMEDIES

TO HELP VOMITING OCCUR
• If you have eaten something poisonous or are having a gallbladder attack, an emetic will help. Drink an **emetic** herb tea. **Lobelia** is probably the best. When giving lobelia tea, give the full dose all at once or you will not induce vomiting. Add 1 ounce of lobelia to a quart of boiling water; let it steep for 5-10 minutes if you are in a hurry (15-20 minutes is better). Then give a cup or two of the liquid (not hot), and let him vomit.

• Other emetic herbs include **bayberry bark, myrica, white willow, peach leaves, and ragwort**.

• **Enemas**, **fasting**, mild **herbal laxatives** will cleanse the stomach. The nerve action of fear or panic sometimes induces vomiting.

• Use some type of herb to calm the stomach area. This may be simply done by taking teas of **peach, peppermint, or raspberry leaves**, or by simply chewing cloves. For the more difficult advanced cases, **turkey rhubarb** will do a thorough job.

TO STOP VOMITING
• Give *very small doses* of **lobelia**; they will relax the person and the vomiting will cease. Use a teaspoon of boiling water, steep, and take only a teaspoonful of this every 15 minutes until relief is obtained. A cup of hot **peppermint** or **spearmint** tea, taken after the stomach has been cleaned out, will also help settle it. **Catnip** or **sweet balm** is also useful. A hot **fomentation** over the stomach, or a **hot-water bottle** with a moist towel under it, will help settle the stomach.

• Old-fashioned remedies to control incessant vomiting: Hold half a peeled, **raw onion** under each armpit. Or place an **ice pack** against the back of the neck.

AFTER VOMITING
• Do not eat for several hours, but carefully take **fluids**, as you are able. You lose a lot of fluid when you vomit. Be sure to replace it. Drink water, do not become dehydrated. The fluids should be clear: **water, weak tea, or fruit juices**. Milk and heavy soups may be too much for the stomach just then.

• Drink small amounts of **peppermint tea**.

• Vomiting also flushes out minerals. These need to be replaced with electrolyte drinks, **clear soups, apple or cranberry juice**. If only water, add a couple pinches of sugar and salt to it. After vomiting, it is **best to sip** the fluids; pause, then sip a little more. Do not gulp them down.

• Sip plain **hot water** or **hot broth** with some **cayenne** in it. Give herbal teas of **chamomile, comfrey, cloves, basil, licorice root, or yarrow**.

• **Ginger** is unusually powerful. It can stop vomiting, motion sickness, altitude sickness, and nausea.

• Do not drink **cold** fluids; it is a shock to the weakened stomach. Do not drink **carbonated** products at this time.

• When you are ready to eat, start back with a **small carbohydrate meal**, such as rice soup. Avoid **fatty** substances; for they remain in the tired stomach too long.

—*Also see Vomiting in Children (735).*

ENCOURAGEMENT—God bids us to fill the mind with great thoughts, pure thoughts. He desires us to think upon His love and mercy to us; study, in the Bible, the plan He has to save us through faith in Jesus Christ. Matthew 7:7-8, 11.

INDIGESTION
(Poor Digestion, Dyspepsia)

SYMPTOMS—Disturbed or deranged digestion, sour stomach, acid stomach, indigestion, poor assimilation.

SYMPTOMS—Dyspepsia is a hyperacidity condition in the body, where certain cooked and secondary substances cannot be digested. The problem may also be with the liver or the gallbladder. This is caused by eating **processed and devitalized foods**.

Indigestion is poor assimilation or difficulty

in processing the food properly in order to get the proper value from it. The whole body must be toned up and the diet changed. The use of aluminum-based digestive tablets that are sold on the market give only temporary relief; and aluminum poisoning is a side effect, or aftereffect. Eat proper foods and use the Lower Bowel Tonic which is prescribed in the cleansing program.

NATURAL REMEDIES

• Instead of using those aids which are highly advertised and are high in **aluminum**, which cause aluminum poisoning, use the **herbs for the nerves, stomach, and bowels. Carminative herbs** will assist the stomach herbs to improve elimination. **Alternative herbs** will cleanse the blood and tone up other excretory organs. **Stimulant-diuretic herbs** will help eliminate waste matter that may be causing the problem. **Demulcents or emollients** will soothe the irritated stomach lining.

• A good digestive tonic, such as **sarsaparillas** or **ginseng,** may be taken fifteen or twenty minutes before eating. **Lemon juice** sweetened with honey may be taken before meals.

J.H. KELLOGG, M.D., PRESCRIPTIONS FOR NERVOUS DYSPEPSIA AND ITS COMPLICATIONS (how to give these water therapies: pp. 207-275 / list of treatments: pp. 206-207 / Hydrotherapy Disease Index: pp. 273-275)

IRRITATION OF SOLAR PLEXUS AND ABDOMINAL SYMPATHETIC NERVE—Fomentation twice a day; during interval between, apply **Heating Compress** and change every 4 hours, except during sleep. **Abdominal Compress** during the night, dry bandage during the day, and abdominal supporter when enteroptosis exists.

GENERAL WEAKNESS—Graduated Cold Baths, twice daily; Cool or Cold Percussion Douche (spray) to spine.

HEARTBURN—Dry aseptic **dietary**; gastric **Fomentation**, followed by **Heating Compress.**

ERUCTATIONS AND REGURGITATIONS OF FOOD— Fomentation over the stomach, twice daily. Continuous **Heating Compress** during the interval between, but without impervious covering, renewing every 4 hours.

SPINAL IRRITATION—Fomentation in the evening. Follow by a **Heating Compress** over the spine, to be worn during the night. **Hot Abdominal Pack.**

COLD EXTREMITIES—Revulsive Douche, running **Cold Footbath, Leg Pack**, massage

HEADACHE—Hot and Cold Compress to the head; **Alternate Sponging** to the spine; **Cool Compress**, if congestion is present. And massage the head and neck.

ANOREXIA—Ice Bag over stomach, half an hour before eating. Cold Douche (spray) over spine, **cold-air bath, outdoor life**, and small **Cold Enema** before breakfast.

ABDOMINAL WEIGHT AND TENDERNESS—Abdominal supporter; Hot fan Douche to the abdomen; **Hot Footbath**; **Revulsive Sitz Bath**; **Fomentation** twice daily,

followed by **Heating Compress**.

EXCESSIVE PERISTALSIS—Hot and Cold Compress to Abdomen; **Fomentation** over abdomen, twice daily. Follow by **Hot Abdominal Pack**, protected by plastic covering.

ASTHMA—Nervous or reflex asthma is commonly associated with dilated or prolapsed stomach and irritable lumbar sympathetic ganglia. The most important palliative measures are the **Hot and Cold Trunk Pack**; **Fomentation** over the abdomen, twice daily. Follow by **Heating Compress**, to be worn during the interval between. **Hot Enema, Hot Full Bath**, general set of **Tonic Friction** treatments, Revulsive Douche to legs.

GENERAL METHOD—The general method consists in improving the nerve tone, allaying general nervous irritability, lessening gastric irritation, and improving the general nutrition by the appropriate measures (as indicated above).

—Also see Dyspepsia (437),

ENCOURAGEMENT—The Father appreciates every soul whom His Son has purchased by the gift of His life. Every provision has been made for us to receive divine power, which will enable us to overcome temptations. Through obedience and Christ's enabling grace to all God's requirements, the soul is preserved unto eternal life. Psalm 5:12.

GASTRO-INTESTINAL - 4 - STOMACH

GRIPING

SYMPTOMS—An intense spasmodic pain in the lower bowels.

CAUSE—Overloading the stomach or bowel may cause the peristaltic area to cease functioning. This can be very painful; and it is generally caused by malnutrition, poor assimilation, by gorging, and by improper types of food. The overuse of corn which is not chewed properly or eating too many green apples are good examples of causes of bowel griping. Do not permit such unhealthful self-indulgence.

NATURAL REMEDIES

• Use hot packs of **mullein** or **slippery elm** with one-fourth part **lobelia** on the afflicted area; or, if tincture of **lobelia** is used, rub it into the specific area and over the spine area controlling the affected part. Taking a few drops of tincture of **lobelia** in warm water will stop the griping immediately. The use of a hot **castor oil pack** with a hot water bottle over it on the area will often stop the pain. If the griping is low in the bowel, use a **catnip tea enema**.

• Useful herbs include **anise seed, balm, bay leaves, caraway seed, catnip, coriander, ginger, pennyroyal, nutmeg, and thyme**.

ENLARGED STOMACH

SYMPTOMS—Although the person is eating far more than he needs, yet he is hungry and ready to eat still more.

CAUSES—The stomach changes in size, according to whether a person consistently eats small meals or large ones. Many people eat far more than they need.

NATURAL REMEDIES
• Step One: Go on a 3-day fruit and vegetable juice fast.
• Step Two: Carefully plan that you will no longer eat or drink (other than water) anything except that which is solidly nourishing: **fruits, vegetables, beans, nuts, vitamin-mineral supplements, uncooked flaxseed or wheat germ oil**.
You will take **small bites** and **chew everything** very well. Do not talk much while doing this, or you will forget and eat too much. You will not be rushed when you eat.
Henceforth, **no junk food, processed foods, greasy foods, or sugary foods** will pass your lips. No **carbonated beverages, coffee, tobacco, or alcohol**. Doing this clears your mind and body so you can regain simple tastes for worthwhile food.
• Step Three: Persistently, determinedly choose to eat smaller meals; and **leave the table** as soon as you are done. This is an exercise in will power, but you can do it. Others have done it.

J.H. KELLOGG, M.D., PRESCRIPTIONS FOR ENLARGED STOMACH (how to give these water therapies: pp. 207-275 / list of treatments: pp. 206-207 / Hydrotherapy Disease Index: pp. 273-275)
DIETARY FACTORS—Aseptic diet; avoid overeating, frequent eating, and gas-forming foods. Give very **simple dry dietary of well-cooked cereals or a liquid diet**, such as purees or gruels prepared from nut creams.

ENCOURAGEMENT—We cannot overestimate the value of simple faith and unquestioning obedience. It is by following in the path of obedience in simple faith that the character obtains perfection. Matthew 5:48.

ACHLORHYDRIA
(Insufficient stomach acid)

SYMPTOMS—Burping, belching, and bloating.

CAUSES—Gastric (stomach) acid is necessary for digestion, although most of its components are later reabsorbed in the intestine. The stomach begins losing its ability to produce hydrochloric acid (HCl) at the age of 35. Of those over the age of 50, 75% do not produce enough HCl. Yet, without it, protein foods cannot be properly digested.
When the stomach does not have enough HCl,

intestinal bacteria and yeast (candida albicans) are able to enter it and ferment high carbohydrate foods (juice, fruit, breads, etc.).
Continued low HCl production results in B12, calcium, and protein deficiencies. New food allergies can begin, because large fragments of food pass through the gastro-intestinal tract undigested. Bloated stomach and even anemia can result.

NATURAL REMEDIES
• Take **lemon juice**, diluted with water (or totally undiluted) at the beginning of each meal.
• Take English **bitters** (Gentiana lutea) before each meal. These are bitter herbs which have helped people's digestion for hundreds of years.
• Take **betaine HCl** (75-250 mg) 15 minutes before each meal.
• Do not take **antacids**; they neutralize stomach acids and make the problem worse. In addition, many of them contain aluminum and other harmful ingredients, including calcium carbonate which will cause the stomach to produce even more HCl than before. Magnesium compounds lead to diarrhea; and sodium bicarbonate can result in gas and bloating.
• **Gum chewing** keeps stomach acids flowing and weakens the stomach.
• Drinking lots of **fluids with a meal** dilutes the stomach juices.
• Due to their bitter qualities, **gentian** and **milfoil** increase stomach juice secretion.
• **Angelica, St. Benedict thistle,** or **sweet flag** increases secretion of gastric juice. **Pineapple** substitutes for it.

J.H. KELLOGG, M.D., PRESCRIPTIONS FOR INADEQUATE HYDROCHLORIC ACID AND ITS COMPLICATIONS (how to give these water therapies: pp. 207-275/ list of treatments: pp. 206-207 / Hydrotherapy Disease Index: pp. 273-275)
INCREASE GENERAL VITAL RESISTANCE—Graduated tonic hydrotherapy treatment (**Tonic Frictions**), twice daily; **outdoor life**; swimming.
INCREASE ACTIVITY OF GASTRIC GLANDS—Cold Fan **Douche (spray) over Stomach**, Cold Percussion Douche to Dorsal spine, general Cold Douche or other cold procedure, **Hot Abdominal Pack**. Drink a third of a glass of **cold water, half an hour before eating**.
INCREASE MOTILITY—Cold **Gastric Douche**, 3 hours after meals. Small **Cold Enema**, retained, 3-4 hours after eating. And abdominal massage.
INDIGESTION, BILIOUSNESS—Hydrochloric acid being absent, flesh foods must be withheld. **Aseptic diet; avoid fried foods, rich gravies, and animal fats**. These lessen the secretion of HCl (hydrochloric acid). **Eat no meat!** Also **avoid cane sugar and concentrated sweets**. Apply **hot applications** over the stomach, an hour after eating.
LOSS OF APPETITE—Ice Bag over the stomach, half an hour before each meal. **Cold Mitten Friction** before breakfast; repeat before dinner if necessary. Small **Cold Enema** or Cold Colonic before breakfast.

ENCOURAGEMENT—You need not go to the end of the earth for wisdom and help. God can help you just where you are. Give Him your life and all you are or hope to be. As you trust and obey, He alone can keep you kind and pure. Matthew 21:22.

EXCESS HYDROCHLORIC ACID

SYMPTOMS—Burning sensations in the stomach, acidosis. Possibly heartburn and reflux disease.

CAUSES—Most people, especially older ones, do not produce enough hydrochloric acid (HCl); but some produce an excess of it.

NATURAL REMEDIES
• Begin the meal with a few **nuts**, which you chew well before swallowing. They will soak up some of the stomach juice, giving it something to work on while you continue your meal.
• Eat a **nourishing diet**; but avoid very **acid foods** (such as citrus, vinegar, cranberries, or plums).
• Take a full **vitamin-mineral** supplement.
• Consistently eat **smaller**, highly nourishing meals; and the stomach will gradually adapt itself to producing less HCl. Make sure you are eating enough **protein**.

J.H. KELLOGG, M.D., PRESCRIPTIONS FOR EXCESSIVE HYDROCHLORIC ACID AND ITS COMPLICATIONS (how to give these water therapies: pp. 207-275/ list of treatments: pp. 206-207 / Hydrotherapy Disease Index: pp. 273-275)
DIETARY CONSIDERATIONS—Avoid irritating food: mustard, pepper, spices, condiments of all sorts, all kinds of flesh foods, excess of proteins, hot foods, farinaceous and sweet desserts, and frequent meals.
INCREASE GENERAL VITAL RESISTANCE—Graduated **Tonic Frictions**, twice daily.
COMBAT IRRITATION OF GASTRIC GLANDS, OR HYPERSECRETION—**Revulsive Compress** twice daily, an hour before meals; continuous **Heating Compress** without plastic covering during the interval between. Avoid Cold Douche over stomach and spine opposite the stomach, and also Prolonged Cold Baths. Hot Douche or **Fomentation** over stomach and spine opposite the stomach, 3-4 times daily. **Hot immersion Bath**, at 105° F., for 15 minutes or Radiant Heat Bath for 10 minutes, half an hour before dinner. Follow by **Cold Mitten Friction**. Sip half a glass of **hot water**, a half hour before eating.
COMBAT TOXEMIA—Sweating procedures: Radiant Heat Bath, Sweating Wet Sheet Pack, Warm Vapor Inhalation, Prolonged Neutral Bath. Follow hot baths by **short cold** applications (such as a Wet Sheet Rub, Cold Towel Rub, Cold Shower, Spray Douche, **Water** drinking. Also **an Enema** daily for a week or two, at 70° F., and injecting a second portion to be retained).
FLATULENCE OF STOMACH AND BOWELS—Cold

Compress over abdomen, changed every 4 hours. Following **fomentation** with **Cold Enema** for 15 minutes, twice a day.
PAINFUL DIGESTION—Hot **Fomentation** an hour after eating, for 15 minutes. Follow by **Heating Compress** to be worn until next meal.
GASTRIC IRRITATION WITH VOMITING AFTER EATING—Hot and Cold **Compress** over stomach or hot and cold **Trunk Pack,** applied half an hour before eating and continued for 2 hours.
CONTRAINDICATIONS—Avoid Cold Douche over stomach, Cold Shower, and prolonged cold baths of all kinds.

ENCOURAGEMENT—The tender mercies of God are unmeasured; and those who appreciate the love of Christ will be renewed in true holiness and brought into Christ, their living Head. They will be followers of God as dear children.
Kind words are as dew and gentle showers to the soul. The Scripture says of Christ that grace was poured into His lips, that He might "know how to speak a word in season to him that is weary." And the Lord bids us, "Let your speech be alway with grace," "that it may minister grace unto the hearers." When the heart is pure, rich treasure of wisdom will flow forth.

GASTROENTERITIS
(Acute Gastritis, Stomach Flu, Inflammation of the Stomach)

SYMPTOMS—Nausea, vomiting, fever, diarrhea, abdominal pain, loss of appetite, and muscle aches. Acute symptoms generally last only 24-72 hours.

CAUSES—Gastroenteritis is an inflammation of the gastrointestinal tract. This includes both the stomach and intestines.
It is usually caused by **viral (sometimes bacterial) infection, allergies, stress, chemical irritation, or medicinal drugs**. **Antibiotics** are a frequent cause; they weaken the body so a virus can attack.
It may be caused by excessive **alcohol, food poisoning, or a bacterial infection**. An attack can be triggered by **drugs**, such as **aspirin** or **antiarthritic medications**.
This disease is contagious; so be careful. Wash hands frequently, sterilize cloths, etc.

NATURAL REMEDIES
• Begin by giving the person activated **charcoal**: Each dose should be 4 capsules, 8 tablets, or 1-2 tablespoons of powder stirred into a glass of water. Give a dose each time there is vomiting or diarrheal stools.
• Keep him in **bed** and give a clear **liquid diet** during the acute stage while there is nausea and vomiting.

Throughout the day give small amounts of water, fruit juices, or ice chips to help restore lost fluid.

• When the vomiting and diarrhea cease, give small amounts of non-irritating food, such as **cooked rice, plain cooked potatoes, cooked carrots, bananas, or apple sauce**.

• Do not be quick to let him get out of **bed**; for the vomiting and loss of fluids may have weakened him.

• In small children and infants especially, watch for **signs of dehydration**. These signs include drowsiness, rapid respiration, and dry skin and mucous membranes. This is important.

• Mix 1 teaspoon of **catnip tea** leaves in a cup of water, steep for 15 minutes, and drink while warm. This is very soothing to the digestive system. If it is vomited up, give again immediately; it is more likely to be accepted and kept down the second time.

• If fluids cannot be kept down, then give small **saline enemas**, to replace lost body fluids. Using 1 level teaspoon of salt per pint of water, inject 1-2 ounces of the solution into the rectum (using a small rubber bulb syringe). Then hold the buttocks together for several minutes. Do this every 1-2 hours until improvement is seen and he is able to take fluids by mouth.

AVOID

• Do not give junk beverages (**colas, black tea, coffee, or alcohol**); for they will only irritate and intensify the symptoms. Caffeine inflames the stomach.

• Avoid **processed and greasy foods**; avoid **milk** and **high-roughage** foods. Avoid all irritants: **salt, pepper, strong spices, and very acidic foods**.

• Do not **smoke** or be near those who smoke.

• Search out **offending foods** and stop using them.
—*Also read Chronic Gastritis (below).*

HERBS

• Here is an herbal formula by Dr. Christopher for this condition: Mix 1 oz. each of **flaxseed, slippery elm, boneset,** and 1 stick **licorice**. Simmer herbs 20 minutes in 1 quart water. Strain, add 1 pint lemon juice, and sweeten. When cool, bottle and keep in a very cool place. Give 1 Tbsp. 2-3 times daily.

NATURAL REMEDIES

J.H. KELLOGG, M.D., PRESCRIPTIONS FOR GASTRIC CATARRH AND ITS COMPLICATIONS (*how to give these water therapies: pp. 207-275/ list of treatments: pp. 206-207 / Hydrotherapy Disease Index: pp. 273-275*)

REST—Withhold food if necessary, giving food and water by enema for several days.

COMBAT LOCAL INFLAMMATION—Fomentation for 15 minutes over stomach and bowels, every 2 hours. During the intervals between, apply **Heating Compress** at 60° F., changing every 30 minutes. **Hot Footbath**; Hot Leg Pack.

VOMITING—Ice Bag to epigastrium; **Hot and Cold Compress** over stomach; **Hot and Cold Trunk Pack**; ice to spine opposite the stomach.

PAIN—Revulsive Compress to area of pain, 10 minutes every hour. **Heating Compress** during interval between.

FEVER—Hot Blanket Pack, 20 minutes, followed by **Cold Half Pack**. Prolonged Neutral Bath, Cooling Wet Sheet Pack, following a **Fomentation** over stomach.

CONTRAINDICATIONS—Avoid Cold Full Baths and general Cold Douche.

ENCOURAGEMENT—God has a heaven full of blessings that He wants to bestow on those who are earnestly seeking for that help. Proverbs 10:22.

CHRONIC GASTRITIS

SYMPTOMS—Unlike acute gastritis *(above)*, which generally lasts only 24-72 hours, the symptoms of chronic gastritis can continue for an extended period.

SOLUTIONS—This disease is usually the sign of some underlying disorder, such as gastric or duodenal **ulcers** *(442)*, iron deficiency **anemia** *(537-541, 713, 761)*, or other diseases involving the stomach. It can also be related to a decrease in **stomach acid** *(439)* or **vitamin B$_{12}$ deficiency** *(479)*. There may be an invasion of **bacteria** which has infected the stomach lining.

NATURAL REMEDIES

• Stop smoking or using alcohol. Figure out which medicinal drugs may be causing the problem.

• The following herbs are helpful: calendula tea and aloe vera juice will help heal the stomach walls.

• **Chamomile, ginger, or turmeric** will help reduce the inflammation.

• **Marshmallow or slippery elm** will soothe the stomach.

• *Read Gastroenteritis (440).*

J.H. KELLOGG, M.D., PRESCRIPTIONS FOR CHRONIC GASTRITIS AND ITS COMPLICATIONS (*how to give these water therapies: pp. 207-275/ list of treatments: pp. 206-207 / Hydrotherapy Disease Index: pp. 273-275*)

AVOID CAUSES—such as **mustard, pepper, vinegar, strong acids, even acid fruits, sugar, preserves, cheese, alcoholic beverages, tea and coffee, all indigestible and irritating substances, coarse vegetables, pickles, confectionery, and hasty eating**.

PHYSIOLOGICAL REST—Avoid the use of fish, fowl, game, and **all flesh foods;** these excite the secretion of HCl (hydrochloric acid) and remain long in the stomach. **Coarse vegetables, fried foods, fats** (except in a natural emulsified condition), **large meals, tea, coffee, wines, and all liquors** are to be avoided.

INCREASE GENERAL VITAL RESISTANCE—Graduated Cold Baths, twice daily.

COMBAT LOCAL CONGESTION—Fomentation over stomach area, 3 times daily, 15 minutes at a time. During intervals between, apply **Heating Compress** over it. **Hot Leg Pack**, followed by **Heating Compress** to the legs, Revulsive Douche to the legs, **Hot Leg Bath**, followed by **Cold Friction** to legs. In acute stages, withhold all food and rest in bed.

MUCOUS VOMITING IN THE MORNING—Omit the evening meal. **Fomentation** over stomach in evening.

Followed by **Heating Compress**, to be worn during the night.

VOMITING SOON AFTER EATING—Hot and Cold Compress over stomach or apply a **Hot Trunk Pack** half an hour before eating, to be retained for 2 hours. Eat dry food in small quantities and rest in bed after eating; **Use Ice Bag** to spine after eating.

GASEOUS ERUCTATIONS—Dry diet of well-cooked grains, **Cold Compress**. **Use Heating Compress** over stomach at 60° F., changing every 4 hours. Massage for half an hour, 2 hours after eating, if local irritation or tenderness does not contraindicate. Drink a pint of **hot water** half an hour before eating. Avoid use of vegetables or of vegetables and fruits at same meal.

ABDOMINAL TYMPANITES—Heating Compress to Abdomen at 60° F., changed every 4 hours. **Colonic** 2-3 times a week, at 70° F.

CONSTIPATION—Graduated Cold Enema at 70° F., daily. Abdominal massage. **Hot Abdominal Pack**. Cold Fan Douche to abdomen for 20 seconds. **Cold Rubbing Sitz Bath**.

LIVER CONGESTION—Fomentation over liver, twice daily. During the interval between, apply a continuous **Heating Compress**.

EMACIATION—Rest in bed, mild and carefully graduated **Tonic Frictions**. **Ice Bag** over stomach, half an hour before eating.

PAIN IN STOMACH—Revulsive Compress over stomach and intestines; repeat several times daily if necessary. **Avoid acid fruits, very hot foods, very cold foods, and concentrated sweets**, if they cause pain.

—Also see Acute Gastritis (440) and Gastroenteritis (440).

ENCOURAGEMENT—The divine law requires us to love God supremely and our neighbor as ourselves. Without the exercise of this love, the highest profession of faith is mere hypocrisy.

PEPTIC ULCER
(Gastric Ulcer, Stomach Ulcer, Duodenal Ulcer)

SYMPTOMS—Chronic burning or gnawing stomach pain which often begins 45-60 minutes after finishing a meal or at night. Drinking a large glass of water or eating food relieves it. Vomiting or swallowing something quite alkaline also does. The pain sometimes awakens the person at 1 or 2 a.m.

Pain just beneath the breastbone is a frequent symptom of an ulcer. Sometimes it radiates to the back. The pain is often considered to be heartburn or an empty stomach.

Other symptoms may include headaches, a choking sensation, lower-back pain, itching, and possible vomiting.

CAUSES—*Gastric ulcers* are peptic ulcers occurring in the stomach. *Duodenal ulcers* are peptic ulcers

CHART 1054: Comparing different kinds of ulcers - Stomach 442-443 / Skin 321

occurring in the top part of the small intestine. However causes and treatment are essentially the same.

These ulcers can be caused by wrong food or too much food. They can also be induced by severe nervous and mental stress.

The walls of the stomach pour a powerful acid into the stomach (hydrochloric acid, or HCl). This powerful fluid is needed to digest protein. Although the walls of the stomach are protein, they are not normally disturbed by the fluid. But when there are problems with people or with the food—then trouble can begin.

Two problems bring trouble when stomach acids begin digesting the walls of the stomach, because too much HCl is being produced, or protective mucus, in order to protect the walls, is not being produced.

These ulcers can occur in the esophagus, but generally occur in the stomach or small intestine.

Gastric ulcers (peptic ulcers in the stomach) occur 2½ times more often in men than in women, most frequently in the 40-55 age group.

Duodenal ulcers (peptic ulcers in the small intestine) occur in the first 11 inches of the small intestine and are caused by excess HCl from the stomach. These ulcers are found in men 4 times as often as in women, and most frequently between 25 and 40 years of age. Duodenal ulcers occur 10 times more often than gastric ulcers.

As much as 15% of the U.S. population have ulcers, but only about half are diagnosed. Some are not discovered until the person begins vomiting blood. Ulcers especially occur during the spring and fall, and tend to run in families.

Many factors affect stomach-acid secretion. **Stress and anxiety** increase it. **Aspirin, steroids, anti-inflammatory drugs, and smoking**—all increase HCl production.

When you have stomach pain, drink some lemon juice. If the pain gets worse, you have too much acid in your stomach.

Hypoglycemics tend to produce too much HCl and are in danger of eventually having a peptic ulcer.

If you vomit blood or have "coffee-ground" stools, then the ulcer is bleeding. You are in danger of bleeding to death—go to a hospital immediately.

Is your stomach pain caused by an ulcer? Here is how to find out: When you have the pain, swallow 1 Tbsp. apple cider or lemon juice. If the pain disappears, you do not have enough HCl; if it makes it worse, you have an excessively acid stomach.

NATURAL REMEDIES

TREATMENT—

• For rapid pain relief, drink a large glass of **water**. It dilutes the stomach acids and flushes them out.

DIET

• Eat several **small** meals.

• **Potatoes** are very helpful. They are soothing and have an alkaline reaction.

• **Vitamin U** is the anti-ulcer vitamin. It is a specific for peptic ulcers. Raw cabbage juice and alfalfa have the most. Boiling destroys this anti-ulcer factor, and wilted cabbage contains less vitamin U. Drink fresh, raw cabbage juice immediately after juicing. Drink a quart daily. Carrot juice can be added to improve the flavor.

• Eat plenty of dark green **leafy vegetables**. If symptoms are severe, eat **soft foods** (potatoes, squash, **bananas, yams**, etc.). Put other vegetables through a **blender**. If you have a bleeding ulcer, add some **psyllium seed** to the food.

• Well-cooked **white rice** and **millet** are good.

• **Fiber** in the diet keeps food in the stomach longer, and reduces the likelihood of duodenal ulcers.

• In earlier years the recommended treatment included frequent feedings, milk intake, and a bland diet. But this approach is being discarded:

• It is now known that the **calcium in milk** stimulates acid production rather than decreasing it, as was taught for years. (Milk does initially neutralize HCl; but the calcium triggers gastrin, which causes the walls to excrete more HCl.) In addition, it is now known that sipping milk and cream can lead to myocardial infarcts (heart attacks). The problem seems to be the butter fat in the sippy diet.

• The **bland diet** approach is also being discarded because those foods neither relieve pain nor speed healing. So, instead, eat whatever good food works best for you.

• Doctors in India use dried **banana** powder to treat ulcers. Fresh bananas are also good.

• Take **vitamin A** (2,000 IU), **zinc** (15 mg), and **copper** (1 mg). **Glutamine** (500 mg), an amino acid, is the principal source of energy for stomach and intestinal wall cells.

AVOID

• Avoid all situations resulting in **tension, stress, irritability, nervous strain, anger, or fear**. Complete rest and relaxation from pressing problems and worries is needed.

• Do not eat **fried foods, tea, caffeine products, salt, chocolate, animal fats, strong spices, or drink soft drinks**. Do not drink **cow's milk**. Do not **smoke** (if you do, do not expect the ulcer to heal properly) or be around those that do.

• **Salt** is a stomach and intestinal irritant. High-salt intake increases stomach (but not duodenal) ulcers.

• A diet high in **sugar** increases HCl production. **White bread** also causes more HCl to be made. Those with ulcers tend to eat more sugar; and sugar increases HCl production.

• **Do not eat between meals**. Doing so slows emptying of the stomach, and thereby increases HCl amounts in the stomach.

• Do not take **antacids or pain killers**, such as **aspirin**. That increases the problem. The calcium carbonate in the antacids doubles the amount of HCl production. Most antacids contain aluminum, which can cause Alzheimer's. The aspirin causes the stomach to bleed!

• Do not use **medicinal drugs**.

• Exposure to **allergies** can cause stomach bleeding.

OTHER HELPS

• **Chew food** slowly and properly.

• **Exercise** neutralizes stress. Maintain a daily program of outdoor exercise.

• Make sure the **bowels** move daily or take cleansing enemas.

• For peptic ulcer pain, apply an **ice bag** to the abdomen just above the navel. Or place it on the spine between the shoulder blades.

• Do not chew **gum**. The digestive process starts when chewing. This prompts the body to secrete enzymes in the gastrointestinal tract. If there is no food in the stomach for the enzymes to digest, trouble begins.

HERBS

• Some bioflavonoids (including quercetin, catechin, and apigenin) inhibit the growth of the bacteria (Helicobacter pylori) which causes the ulcers. **Chamomile** contains those bioflavonoids.

• **Licorice** has been used for centuries to soothe inflamed and injured portions of the intestinal tract. It increases *mucin* and fights *H. pylori*. Best to take it in the form of **DGL** (deglycerinated licorice), which will not increase blood pressure or cause water retention. Take 1-2 chewable tablets of DGL 1-2 hours before bedtime. Also extremely good: **marshmallow root**.

• **St. John's wort** and **malva** both calm the stomach and reduce intestinal irritation.

• Also helpful are **bilberry, flax, catnip, goldenseal, bayberry, and myrrh**. **Aloe vera** accelerates healing.

• **Hops, skullcap, and valerian** will help you sleep.

—*Also see Gastroesophageal Reflux Disease (GERD) (434), which has very similar symptoms.*

J.H. KELLOGG, M.D., PRESCRIPTIONS FOR PEPTIC ULCERS AND THEIR COMPLICATIONS *(how to give these water therapies: pp. 206-275 / list of treatments: pp. 206-207 / Hydrotherapy Disease Index: pp. 273-275)*

DIETETIC CONSIDERATIONS—Rest in bed; **rectal feeding** for 2 weeks if necessary, repeating after a few days if needed. **Bland aseptic liquid diet**. Avoid solid food, condiments, flesh foods.

GENERAL CARE—Revulsive Compress, 3 times a day; **Heating Compress** during intervals between; hot **Fomentation** or Hot Douche to spine.

PAIN—Revulsive Compress, Fomentation over stomach, heat to spine, **Hot Blanket Pack** to hips and legs.

VOMITING—Ice pills, distilled water.

HEMORRHAGE—Rest in bed, **Ice Bag** over stomach, **Hot Hip and Leg Pack**. Withhold foods and drink from stomach by administering water and food by Enema.

ENCOURAGEMENT—God fixes no limit to the advancement His children can make, if they will but surrender their lives to His guidance and study and obey His Inspired Writings. Matthew 21:22.

STOMACH ACID SELF-TEST

STOMACH ACID TEST—Is your hydrochloric acid (HCl) production low or high? You have a stomachache; but is it caused by too little HCl or too much?

1 - When you have the stomach pain, take a tablespoon of **lemon juice**. If this makes the pain leave, you probably have too little stomach acid, not too much. If it makes your symptoms worse, then you have an overacid stomach.

2 - Do you crave **sour foods**, such as **citrus**? Do you like **grapefruit juice**? If you do, and they set well on your stomach, then you are underacid. If you do not like acid foods, then you may be overacid. If it does not matter, you are probably normal.

ENCOURAGEMENT—Those who make God their strength, realize their own weakness—and God supplies them daily with the help they need. This help is for you, as you come to Him. John 15:7.

STOMACH TONIC

HERBS FOR THE STOMACH—Here are several herbal formulas prepared especially as stomach tonics:

• Mix ¾ tsp. **wormwood**, ½ tsp. **peppermint**, ¼ tsp. **garden sage**. Steep in 1 cup boiled water, strain, cool, take 1 tsp. in water ½ hour before meals.

• Mix ¾ tsp. **European centaury**, ½ tsp. **buckbean**, and ¼ tsp. **juniper berries**. Infuse them in 1 pint water. Take 1 tsp. in water ½ hour before meals.

• Here is a stomach tonic by Potter, a well-known herbalist of many years ago: Mix 1 part each **buckbean, centaury, germander, and blessed thistle**. Infuse at a rate of 1 tsp. of combined herbs to a cup of boiling water. Take 1-2 Tbsp. between meals.

— *Also see # Tonic Herbs (284).*

ENCOURAGEMENT—The law of God, which is perfect holiness, is the only true standard of character. Love is expressed in obedience; and perfect love casteth out all fear.

GASTRO-INTESTINAL - 5 -
PANCREAS
Also: Pancreas (444-450, 655-659)

PANCREATITIS

SYMPTOMS—*Acute cases:* A sudden attack of severe burning or stabbing pain in the upper abdo-

men, possibly accompanied by nausea and vomiting. The pain may spread to the back. It is made worse by moving. Food, alcohol, and vomiting may worsen the pain.

Chronic cases: The pain is milder; and pain attacks do not come on suddenly. There is excessive gas, muscle aches, and fever. Because the constant inflammation can produce fibrosis in that organ, permanent damage to the pancreas can occur. The chronic state results in irreversible changes in the gallbladder.

Other symptoms of pancreatitis include abdominal swelling and distension, hypertension, sweating, and abnormal fatty stools.

Diabetes, digestive problems, and cancer can result. Also hearing, respiratory, and kidney failure.

CAUSES—Pancreatitis is inflammation of the pancreas. Normal cells are replaced with scar tissue and calcium deposits. It frequently produces mild diabetes.

The most frequent causes of pancreatitis are drinking **alcohol, viral infection, and diseases of the bile ducts or gallbladder**. A **diet rich in fats and meat** lays a solid foundation for pancreatitis to occur. Other causes include **surgical procedures, diagnostic procedures**, and a considerable variety of **prescribed medications. Oral contraceptives, steroids, estrogen, and ACTH** can also do it.

To this list should be added **abdominal injury, obesity, poor nutrition, and electric shock**.

Certain diseases can induce it: **hepatitis, mumps,** and possibly **anorexia nervosa**.

The pancreas produces two important hormones: insulin and glucagon; both of these regulate blood sugar levels and aid digestion. As a result, pancreatitis can produce glucose intolerance and diabetes.

With only supportive care, the acute symptoms will fade. But some will continue to have chronic symptoms arising every so often, for months or years. This is called *chronic relapsing pancreatitis.*

It is wise to do everything possible to avoid the chronic condition or, if it is has begun, try to clear it up as much as possible.

Pancreatitis can lead to pancreatic cancer, the fourth leading cancer killer in America.

NATURAL REMEDIES
• **Fast** and take only water until the acute symptoms subside. Food in the stomach triggers the pancreas to start working, and this you do not want just now.

• Give **slippery elm enemas**. Cut the slippery elm bark into very small pieces, and put a large handful in 4 quarts of water. Simmer for 1-15 minutes, stirring frequently. Then cover and let it set 30 minutes. Strain and use it warm. Drink it and use in enemas.

• Place a heaping teaspoonful of **lobelia** in a cup of boiling water and let it steep for a half hour. Add a tablespoon of this lobelia tea to each cup of **slippery elm** tea, and drink. Also drink a cup an hour before each meal and before retiring. This will both relax and cleanse the digestive tract.

• In case of a very serious acute crisis, give frequent **hot steam pack fomentations** to the abdomen. Give **charcoal** internally; and apply it as a poultice over the affected area. Place the person on a strict program of what he eats and drinks.

HERBS

• The following herbs increase the flow of pancreatic juice, which is needed for digestion: **Nettle** (an infusion of fresh juice), **Papaya tree** (an infusion of the leaves), and **St. Benedict thistle** (an infusion or decoction of the leaves).

• **Echinacea, gentian root, goldenseal, and cedar berries** strengthen the pancreas. But do not take goldenseal or echinacea for more than a week at a time.

• **Licorice root** helps all glandular functions.

• **Red clover, burdock root, and milk thistle** help the liver, which is a help to the pancreas.

AVOID

• Avoid **overeating**. This overworks the pancreas.

• After coming off the fast because the acute phase is over, eat a **low calorie, low-fat diet**. In chronic pancreatitis, that organ often no longer produces lipase normally. Without it, fats cannot be properly handled by the body. So eat a low-fat diet *for the rest of your life.*

• Go on a **low sugar diet**. A heavy diet of refined carbohydrates can cause pancreatitis.

• Say good-bye to all **alcoholic** beverages, and also to **caffeine**.

• **Smoking** weakens the pancreas and can directly cause chronic pancreatitis. Avoid secondhand smoke.

• Do not eat **meat** products. Eat beans and nuts.

OTHER

• There are no medications which can solve this problem. Indeed, it was medications which may have led to it; continuing to take them may only intensify the disease.

• Even though total pancreatomy may be recommended, avoid surgery if possible. It will probably only worsen the condition.

—*Also see Pancreas (444-450, 655-659), Nutrition of the Liver (below).*

ENCOURAGEMENT—The sinner may become a child of God, an heir of heaven. If he will cling to Christ and obey His Word, he will be enabled to fulfill God's plan for His life. John 16:23-24.

GASTRO-INTESTINAL - 6 - LIVER

NUTRITION OF THE LIVER

CARING FOR YOUR LIVER—There are few organs in your body as vital as the liver. It not only is the largest organ, it also performs more different functions than any other organ in your body.

Only God could make the liver. That relatively small structure (it only weighs four pounds) does literally thousands of different things; all of them are quite complicated and involve complex chemical changes. The liver is truly a special gift from God.

NATURAL REMEDIES
There are six fundamental things which tend to damage the liver:

1 - **Overeating**. This is an excellent way to ruin your liver. Just eat all you want, and you will wear it out.

2 - Eating and drinking the **wrong things**. Here are some of those items which your liver does not wish to face: **refined white-flour products, processed foods, junk foods, white sugar products, imitation foods**. Beware of **potato chips and corn chips**.

What is an **imitation food**? It is a food made to appear like the original, yet which has been stripped of vitamins, minerals, enzymes, and most everything else that might be worthwhile. **White carbohydrates, sugar, fats, protein, synthetic colors, flavors, and odors** are there to give the appearance and taste of real food.

3 - A **low-protein, high-carbohydrate and fat diet**. To make it even worse, make sure it is full of **saturated or hydrogenated fats**. All kinds of **snacks** in the stores consist of this. **Fried foods** may be a devilish delight, but they only add to the eventual misery.

4 - Eat the **specialty food poisons: alcohol, tobacco, caffeine, theobromine, and hard drugs**.

5 - Take **medicinal drugs**. Select from over-the-counter items or those which are prescribed. They will provide you with a real witch's brew of physical horror, much of it not known and realized until later. With hardly an exception, medicinal drugs are poisons. The liver has to work overtime in order to try to excrete these dangerous chemicals.

Some substances which are called "drugs," such as charcoal, are not drugs. They are natural substances which help your body. It is true there are some poisonous herbs, but these (such as digitalis from foxglove) are readily found in the drugstore. The rest, found in the meadow and forest, are for the healing of the nations.

6 - Have **insecticides, preservatives**, and **other cumulative poisons** where you can breathe or eat it. Some poisons directly damage the liver (**alcohol, oral contraceptives, caffeine**, etc.); others damage organs which the liver relies on for help (the pancreas, kidneys, etc.).

Here are several dietary suggestions:

• Make sure you obtain **foods high in potassium**. This includes **rice, bananas, blackstrap molasses, wheat bran, almonds, seeds, kelp and dulse, brewer's yeast, prunes, and raisins**.

• Drink lots of **water**; and, if at all possible, drink only pure water. Drink a little every hour.

• Emphasize **raw foods** in your diet.

• Drink **fresh vegetable juices**, especially **carrot and**

G
A
S
T
R
O

beet. Only eat **raw nuts and seeds**. They must be fresh, not stale!

• Use only cold-pressed **vegetable oils** (**flaxseed oil** and **wheat germ oil**, taken raw and not added to your cooking). Use no other type of oils—and **no grease** (**margarine, butter, shortening, or meat fat**).

• **Vitamin K** (140 mcg) is important, to help prevent cirrhosis of the liver. **Vitamin A** helps protect the liver (taken in the form of carotene in fresh carrot juice and leafy vegetables). **Zinc** (30 mg) builds resistance to many liver disorders.

• The **lemon** and the liver are sweethearts. The lemon is one of the best friends that the liver has.

• **Coenzyme Q₁₀** helps supply oxygen to the liver.

• **Lecithin** helps prevent fatty buildup in the liver.

• When taking **supplements**, either chew them up well or take them with a glassful of water.

• **Dandelion** is an excellent food for the liver. **Beet juice** slowly cleanses the liver. Eating fresh **apples** stimulates the liver into action. **Celery** is good for the liver. The root and leaves of **chicory** stimulate the liver. **Asparagus** roots and shoots stimulate kidneys and liver. **Prune whip** before breakfast cleanses the liver. Japanese use the active ingredient in **licorice** (*glycyrrhizin*) to inhibit liver cell injury caused by many chemicals. **Ginger** contains eight liver-protecting compounds. **Turmeric** also protects the liver. **Rosemary** tea stimulates a sluggish liver.

• Use **celandine and silymarin** (which is milk thistle extract) each day to help maintain good liver function. But do not use celandine during pregnancy.

AVOID

• Do not use **nicotine, alcohol, caffeine, fish, fowl, meat, salt, soft drinks, sugar foods, tea, or fried foods**.

• Avoid **constipating foods**. When there is a backup in the large colon, toxins are reabsorbed into the system and the liver labors to eliminate them. **Regular bowel movements** are vital to the health of the liver!

• Do not take too much **vitamin A**. For the same reason, do not eat **fish** more than twice a week. Avoid **cod liver oil**. Better yet, stop eating fish. **Meat** eating is also harmful to the liver. Anyone taking over 50,000 IU of **vitamin A** for over a year should either reduce intake or switch to natural beta-carotene, which is safe.

• Do not drink **milk** or eat **pastries, stimulants, white rice, black or white pepper, fried or fatty foods, cheese, and refined or processed foods**.

• Never eat raw or undercooked fish, meat, or poultry. There is a serious risk of infection from doing this. **Meat eating** is a major source of bacteria, parasites, viruses, and various malignancies.

• Take no **drugs** if you want your future years to be happy ones. Avoid taking **iron** supplements.

OTHER

• In addition to taking care of your liver, treat your **kidneys** well also. Poor kidney function results in damage to the liver. Drink water! *See Kidney Problems (489-595).*

• Do not use **harsh laxatives**. But do keep the colon clean.

Be good to your liver; and it will help you in years to come. It is a well-known fact, among natural healers, that, if the liver is all right, cancer can be eliminated. But if the liver is too degenerated, the hoped-for solution may not be achieved.

—Also see Liver Flush (450).

ENCOURAGEMENT—The knowledge of God is as high as heaven; yet He can reveal to you all you need, just for today, if you will but give your life daily into His hands. Matthew 6:33.

HEPATITIS

SYMPTOMS—Weakness, nausea, headache, vomiting, fever, muscle aches, loss of appetite, drowsiness, dark urine, joint stiffness and pains, abdominal discomfort, diarrhea, constipation, light-colored stools, and often jaundice (a yellowing of the skin, which will first be noticed in the eyes and mucous membranes). Skin rashes and itching may occur; the latter is caused by excess bile salts under the skin.

CAUSES—Hepatitis is an inflammation of the liver; it may be caused by a **virus, bacterium, or toxic substance**. But, in most instances, the cause is viral. There are actually several main types of hepatitis:

Hepatitis A (infectious hepatitis, HVA), also known as *infectious hepatitis,* can cause acute liver disease. In most cases, however, the liver heals within a few months. Hepatitis A can develop without sudden signs or symptoms. It is easily spread through person-to-person contact, fecal contamination of food or water, and raw shellfish taken from polluted water. It is contagious between two to three weeks before, and one week after, jaundice appears.

Transmitted by **contaminated water, milk, or food**, it has an incubation period of 15-45 days. The contagion is highest just before illness begins; so **food workers** can transmit the disease. Hepatitis A is contagious between one to two weeks before the illness starts. It is easily spread by **person-to-person contact** and through **contact with food, clothing, linens**, etc. It can be transmitted from **animals**. Eating **shellfish** is a good way to get it, even if the waters they live in pass national standards. Recovery generally occurs within 4 weeks. Chronic cases are less likely to occur.

Hepatitis B virus (serum hepatitis, HVB) is spread through contact with infected blood from adults to children living together in close contact, through sexual activity, and through blood transfusions (for example, from mother to child at birth or through the use of contaminated syringes, needles, and transfused blood). Most people (85 percent) recover from hepatitis B; although 15 percent go on to develop cirrhosis or cancer of the liver.

It is found throughout the world and spread as in the same manner HIV is—through contact with **infected blood (contaminated needles, syringes, blood transfusions) and sexual contact.** Six cases have been traced to **contaminated acupuncture needles**. About 5% of all Americans and 85% of gay men have it. Hepatitis B is very serious. It has an incubation period of 28-160 days (2-6 months); and recovery may require 6 months. Throughout that time, it can be passed from one person to another. In increasing numbers, cases are reverting to *chronic active hepatitis*, which can result in liver cirrhosis and death. Hepatitis B is the ninth major killer in the United States.

Hepatitis C (HVC) and Hepatitis C virus (HCV), the most serious forms of hepatitis, account for approximately 10,000 deaths a year in America. It is estimated that 4 million Americans are infected with HCV, 3 million of them chronically. Hepatitis C is the primary reason for liver transplants in this country. Hepatitis C is four times more prevalent than AIDS and twenty times easier to catch. About 85 percent of infections lead to chronic liver disease. Currently, more than 99 percent of people with HCV survive. The virus problems slowly progress; but, ultimately, the damage to the liver is devastating. In addition, people with hepatitis C virus often have elevated levels of iron in the liver. This also can cause liver damage. Tests can detect HCV antibodies in donated blood. But an infected individual may take up to six months to develop the antibodies; so it is still impossible to identify all infected blood. The U.S. Food and Drug Administration (FDA) maintains that only 7 percent of current hepatitis C cases were acquired as a result of blood transfusions, and that the risk of contacting the virus from a unit of blood is about 1 in 100,000. The incidence of hepatitis C infection from blood transfusions or the use of blood products has decreased since 1992, when screening was introduced. But there is always a risk; and the lack of testing before 1992 has left a huge legacy of HVC-infected people.

In the same manner as HIV and hepatitis B, hepatitis C may take 6 months to produce symptoms; yet all that time it can be **spread from one person to another**. Between 20%-40% of all hepatitis cases are of this type. It accounts for 90%-95% of all the hepatitis that is transmitted by **blood donations**. About 85% of infections lead to chronic liver disease.

You may be at risk for hepatitis C if you have:

• Had a blood transfusion prior to 1992, when screening for HCV antibodies started.

• Shared needles for intravenous (IV) drug use (even one incident, years ago).

• Shared straws for inhaling cocaine.

• Had body piercing or tattoos with nonsterile equipment. Had hemodialysis (used a kidney machine).

• Had frequent exposure to blood products (due to hemophilia, chronic renal failure, chemotherapy, organ transplantation, or any other reason).

• Had a needle-sticking incident (health care workers are at high risk).

• Used an infected person's toothbrush, razor, or other item that had blood on it.

Hepatitis E, hepatitis non-A, and hepatitis non-B also exist, but are of lesser significance in North America. Hepatitis E is found worldwide; it is in epidemic proportions in India, Mexico, Africa and Asia. It is generally contracted from **drinking sewage-contaminated water**. Such water should be boiled before using.

Toxic hepatitis: All of the above are primarily viral forms of hepatitis. But this one is caused by toxic chemicals. The degree to which the liver was exposed to the **poisonous chemicals, fumes, drugs**, etc., determines the amount of damage to that organ. Absorption of the poison can occur through the skin.

Overall, there are 40,000-70,000 reported new cases of various forms of hepatitis each year in America. But the experts suspect that there are probably ten times that many which go unreported. Hepatitis most often occurs in young adults; it is highest in teenage girls.

Hepatitis A is decreasing, and hepatitis B is rapidly increasing. It is fourth among the 30 leading communicable diseases.

In China, 10% of the population have hepatitis at any one time. That is 100 million new cases each year. As one might expect, the rate of liver cancer is quite high there.

A word to the wise: Gay men often take jobs working in restaurants; yet they have a high rate of hepatitis B and C infections which do not reveal symptoms for weeks or months. During this time they can, and do, transmit the infection to customers through the food they handle. Something to think about the next time you feel like eating in a restaurant or café.

NATURAL REMEDIES

• Give the patient the type of care you would give for any infectious disease; but remember that some of these hepatitis cases can be highly contagious.

• Give hot fomentations over the liver area for 15 minutes, followed by a **cold sponging** and concluded by a **shower**. Do this 4 times each day. Most cases of hepatitis are self-limiting and will heal with rest and supportive care.

• He should have **bedrest** until the acute stage is past; also he should have **initial liquid fasting**, followed by a **light diet**. He often has a poor appetite and does not feel like eating, even though he should. Glass of **lemon juice** and water every morning. **Fruit juice**. Every other day a glass of **carrot, beet, cucumber juice**.

• **Avoid sugar, fat, and alcohol**. Do not use **tobacco** or other poisons.

• Vitamin B12 (1,000 mcg) and vitamin C (2,000 mg or more, to bowel tolerance) are important. Also needed are vitamin A (5,000 IU) and B complex,

• Clinical studies reveal that two amino acids,

G
A
S
T
R
O

L-cysteine and L-methionine (500 mg twice daily of each), **unsaturated fatty acids** (2 tsp. **flaxseed oil**), and **choline** (1-3 grams) help speed recovery from hepatitis.

• Take **grapefruit seed extract** (10 drops 3 times daily for 1 month in juice).

• Robert Cathcart, M.D., says hepatitis is one of the easiest diseases for **ascorbic acid** (vitamin C) to cure. He gives very high levels (40-100 grams) intravenously; and great improvement occurs within 2-4 days.

• Drink plenty of **water** (preferably distilled water) and **bathe** frequently,

• Fresh or cooked **garlic**, or in capsule form.

• Avoid **constipation;** and **wash** hands with soap after every bowel movement. The toilet seat should also be washed after each usage.

• He should **not prepare food** for others; and his own **utensils** should be sterilized after each of his meals. His **linen and clothes** should be washed separately.

• Avoid **drugs** which greatly irritate the liver, including **tranquilizers, aspirin, certain tetracyclines, antidepressants, and antibiotics**. **Tylenol** (acetaminophen) and **iron** supplements are very toxic to the liver.

• Eating **meat and fish**, especially when undercooked, can cause infection from bacteria and viruses.

• **Activities** should be restricted for several months after recovery has occurred. Avoid strenuous sports.

HERBS

• Here are several herbs which would help the liver at this time: **St. John's wort** (300 mg capsule 2 times daily) and **Shiitake** (1,500-2,000 mg 2 times daily with meals).

• For an excellent liver tonic, combine equal parts **Oregon grape, dandelion, pipsissewa, fennel seed, and blessed thistle**. Take 3 cups daily.

• **Barberry** is one of the mildest and best liver tonics. Take 10-30 drops of the tincture daily.

• **Milk thistle** contains *silymarin*, which stimulates protein production from amino acids in the liver. This helps the liver regenerate itself. Take two 150 mg tablets or capsules of milk thistle extract, 3-4 times daily; or 15-30 drops of the tincture in water, twice daily for 2 weeks. It is important that you take this!

• Add 1 tsp. dried or fresh **lemon balm** to 1 cup boiling water. Steep 15 minutes, strain, drink 2-3 cups a day.

• **Goldenseal** tea may be taken 1-3 times a day.

HYDROTHERAPY

• To relieve discomfort, place **castor oil packs** over the liver area and keep warm. **Burdock leaf packs** are good on an inflamed liver.

• Make a strong tea of **peppermint** leaves, add a pinch of **cayenne**, and place as a poultice over the area.

• To strengthen the liver in its battle against infection, apply **alternate hot and cold compresses** over the liver area.

• A **hot half bath** (sitting in a partly full tub) may be given to raise the body temperature, assisting the body to fight the virus by strengthening the immune system. Give him plenty of fluids while in the bath.

—Also see Cirrhosis (450), Jaundice (bellow), Neonatal Jaundice (731), Infectious Juandice (449), Nutrition of the Liver (445), and Liver Flush (450).

ENCOURAGEMENT—Only those who read the Scriptures, as the voice of God speaking to them, are the true learners. They tremble at the Word of God; for to them, it is a living reality. 2 Peter 1:8. In order to receive God's help, we must cry to Him and surrender all that separates us from Him.

JAUNDICE

SYMPTOMS—The whites of the eyes yellow, then the mucous membranes, and then the skin generally.

CAUSES—When, for various reasons, the liver cannot handle the load placed upon it, bilirubin builds up. This is a yellow-brown substance which results from the breakdown of old red blood cells. The liver must constantly remove bilirubin from the blood; and, if this is not done, bilirubin begins collecting in tissues all over the body. The urine is darker and the stools are lighter because the bilirubin, usually contained, is not present.

But red blood cell destruction can also cause it. Blood tests identify whether the problem is obstruction or RBC destruction.

Jaundice is not itself a disease, but rather a symptom of one. It can point to **pernicious anemia, hepatitis, cirrhosis of the liver, and hemolysis** (which is an abnormal destruction of red blood cells). Jaundice can also be caused by a **blockage of the bile ducts** in the liver, because of **gallstones** or a **tumor**. More rarely, it is caused by a parasitic infestation, such as **tapeworm, hookworm, a flea, or mosquito** carrying a viral infection.

The problem arises from an improper diet that results in a derangement of the function of stomach, liver, and bowels. The liver is the main seat of the problem. The bile does not excrete properly and is passed off into the bloodstream and body tissues, causing a toxic condition (called cholemia) with indigestion, sluggishness, fatigue, constipation, upset stomach, chills, vomiting, and fever. The stools become a light clay or chalky color, the skin takes on a gold cast, yellow shows in the whites of the eyes, and bile deposits in the skin causes itching.

NATURAL REMEDIES

• Take a hot, high **herb enema** twice a day. Use **white oak bark** or **bayberry bark** tea.

• As long as fever continues, drink a glass of water with **lemon juice** every hour.

• Give **fruit juices** to begin with. Take 1 cup **goldenseal** or **echinacea** 1 hour before meals, 3 times daily.

• Eat only **raw fruits and vegetables** for a week. Then eat 75% raw foods for a month. Take fresh **lemons** daily during that time.

• Drink fresh **vegetable juices**.

• Treatment includes exposure to **ultra violet light** in order to speed up elimination; **vitamin C**, to bowel tolerance; and **vitamins A, E, and selenium**.

• **Silymarin**, extracted from the milk thistle, helps repair damage to the liver. It is well-worth taking.

• Go on a **liver flush** *(450)*. This is done by drinking **apple juice** alone for 3 days, followed by drinking a cup of **olive oil** and a cup of **lemon** juice. This is a good remedy which cleans out the bile ducts.

• **Carrot juice** will bring the skin from clear to yellow (as the liver clears) and then back to normal, which is a sign that the bile is now cleared and flowing properly into the intestinal tract. Helpful tonics for the liver are **barberry, carrot juice, blueberry bark, cranesbill (crow foot) root, red raspberry root, and white oak bark**. Proceed with caution; since rapid unloading of toxic bile may upset the body and induce vomiting as well as turn the skin extremely yellow. Take **goldenseal** and drink **fruit juice,** to help cleanse the body. Other excellent herbs for this liver problem are **agrimony, dandelion, mandrake root, self-heal, and yarrow**. **Unsweetened fresh lemonade** is also good.

• Helpful herbs include **burdock root, agrimony, celandine, red clover, licorice, dandelion, and chionanthus**.

• Jaundice often produces itching of the skin. Wash with hot **boric acid** water to reduce this.

• For jaundice, Dr. Christopher recommends 4 oz. **ginger** syrup, and 1 oz. each of fluid extracts of **butternut** and **boneset**. Give 1 teaspoon 3-4 times daily.

• Both **alcohol and tobacco** are very hard on the liver.

—*Also see Infectious Jaundice (449), Hepatitis (446), Neonatal Jaundice (731), Nutrition of Liver (445).*

J.H. KELLOGG, M.D., PRESCRIPTIONS FOR JAUNDICE AND ITS COMPLICATIONS *(how to give these water therapies: pp. 206-275 / list of treatments: pp. 206-207 / Hydrotherapy Disease Index: pp. 273-275)*

GENERAL—Cold Mitten Friction, **Cold Towel Rub**, **rest** in bed, **aseptic diet**.

PAIN—**Fomentation** over stomach and liver for 15 minutes every 2-3 hours; during interval between, **Heating Compress** at 60° F., renewed every 30 minutes. Copious **Hot Enema** at 110° F., twice a day. After discharge of hot water, an enema of one pint water, at 70° F. **Hot Trunk Pack**. Hot Full Bath, at 104° F., for 10 minutes. **Cold Towel Rub** or Wet Sheet Rub.

FEVER—Sweating **Wet Sheet Pack**, warm vapor Bath, Radiant Heat Bath, copious **water** drinking.

HEADACHE—**Hot and Cold Compress** to head, evaporating Compress to head, Cold Compress to head, **Hot Sponging** on back of neck.

ITCHING—**Neutral salt bath**, Hot Sponging.

CHILL—Hot **Water** drinking, **Dry Pack**.

ENCOURAGEMENT—All knowledge gained in this life, which will fit us to live with the angels in heaven, is knowledge worth gaining. Live to be a blessing to others. "I have blotted out, as a thick cloud, thy transgressions, and, as a cloud, thy sins: return unto Me; for I have redeemed thee." Isaiah 44:22.

INFECTIOUS JAUNDICE
(Weil's Disease, Leptospirosis, Spirochetal Jaundice)

SYMPTOMS—Sudden fever, chills, anemia, jaundice, sometimes abdominal pains, and occasionally aseptic meningitis.

Within a few hours, fever, extreme thirst, and severe aching of the limbs develop. Blood vessels in the eyeballs are markedly enlarged. Jaundice appears in about half the cases. In locations where the disease is common, mortality is about 10%-20%.

This disease can easily be diagnosed as something else. It is important to determine the true nature of the infection early.

CAUSES—This is an infectious disease caused by the *leptospira icterohaemorrhagiae*, a spirochete bacteria. **Rats, dogs, and various wild animals** carry it. People are infected when **urine-contaminated water (generally from rats)** penetrates cuts on their fingers or during butchering and skinning of infected animals. The rats are not harmed by the disease.

Leptospire is a parasite which travels to the liver and greatly multiplies there, but can also be found in the blood (in the early stages) and in the urine (later). Blood tests or urine cultures are necessary for diagnosis.

NATURAL REMEDIES

• Give him **bedrest** and keep his bowels open, using daily **enemas** if necessary.

• If he can take food, give him a **liquid diet**. Plenty of **water** is also needed.

• Go on a **liver flush** (450).

• Carefully **dispose** of all his discharges, so as not to contaminate anything.

• Do everything possible to **exterminate rats**.

• Avoid swimming in, or contact with, water that may be contaminated with **animal waste**.

—*Also see Jaundice (390), Hepatitis (446), Neonatal Jaundice (731), Nutrition of the Liver (445).*

ENCOURAGEMENT—Christ has a treasure-house full of precious gifts for every soul willing to receive it. But only by dedication, submission, and obedience in Christ's strength—can we have it.

CIRRHOSIS OF THE LIVER

SYMPTOMS—Upset stomach, fever, constipation or diarrhea, weakness, weight loss, poor appetite, vomiting, enlarged liver, and red palms. Fluid collects in the abdomen. Possible mild jaundice. Large veins often seen over the abdomen, especially about the navel and near the diaphragm. Enlarged veins in the rectum, intestines, stomach, and esophagus.

In the later stages, there is anemia, edema, and easy bruising, due to bleeding beneath the skin.

CAUSES—Cirrhosis is a hardening of the liver, because of too much connective tissue and a degeneration of the active liver cells.

It can be caused by certain poisons, chiefly **alcohol**. Certain infectious diseases can cause special types of liver cirrhosis; **viral hepatitis** is outstanding (446). This is especially true of **syphilis** (804), which produces nodes in the liver. **Malnutrition**, caused by **lack of food** or **eating junk food**, can also lead to cirrhosis.

The liver cells harden and scar, causing them to no longer function normally, due to the scarred tissue. This prevents the blood from passing properly through the liver.

NATURAL REMEDIES

• Eat a good, **nourishing diet.** And go off all **meat, tea, coffee, and spices**.

• Internal bleeding frequently occurs, so take **vitamin K** (140 mcg).

• **Silymarin** (200 mg 3 times daily) helps the liver.

• Drink ¼ cup **aloe vera** each morning.

• Do not eat **meat or fish**.

• Helpful herbs include **burdock, celandine, barberry, echinacea, goldenseal, fennel, red clover, milk thistle, and thyme**.

• Follow the program for **hepatitis** (447-448) and **jaundice** (390),

—*Also see Neonatal Jaundice (731), Infectious Juandice (449), Nutrition of Liver (445), Liver Flush (450).*

J.H. KELLOGG, M.D., PRESCRIPTIONS FOR CIRRHOSIS OF THE LIVER AND ITS COMPLICATIONS (how to give these water therapies: pp. 206-275 / list of treatments: pp. 206-207 / Hydrotherapy Disease Index: pp. 273-275)

DIETARY CONSIDERATIONS—Avoid tea, coffee, tobacco, alcohol, condiments. Use an **aseptic diet**.

ORGANIC CHANGES IN LIVER—Local applications to liver: Alternate Douche, Alternate Compress, Revulsive Douche, flannel-covered Heating Compress. Follow these local applications by a general Douche or a Wet Sheet Rub.

PAIN—Fomentation, Revulsive Compress or Revulsive Douche, with **Hot Leg Bath** or Hot Leg Pack. Follow by **Compress over liver**, twice daily.

JAUNDICE—Wet Sheet Pack, followed by **Wet Sheet Rub**. Radiant Heat Bath, followed by **Graduated Shower** or Wet Sheet Rub.

DROPSY—Revulsive Douche to legs and abdomen. **Trunk Pack**.

GENERAL WEAKNESS—Carefully **graduated tonic baths** (Tonic Frictions), Neutral Bath, Sunbaths, and outdoor life.

CONTRAINDICATIONS—Avoid Cold Full Baths and very cold general or prolonged Cold Douche.

ENCOURAGEMENT—God has provided abundant means for successful warfare against the evil that is in the world. The Bible is the armory where we may equip for the struggle. The shield of faith must be in our hand and the helmet of salvation on our brow. Proverbs 12:21.

LIVER FLUSH

WHAT IT IS—The liver filters the blood and excretes much of that waste through the bile, which it sends into the gallbladder. When some oil or fat is in a meal, its presence signals the gallbladder to contract and squeeze out some bile, which helps prepare those oils and fats to be properly absorbed by the body.

A liver flush occurs when much of the bile is flushed out of the gallbladder. However, there is the possibility that gallstones may be in the bladder. So phase one of the liver flush is to melt down those stones; and then, in the concluding phase, the bile and the stones are jolted out of the gallbladder into the small intestine.

NATURAL REMEDIES

HOW TO DO IT—There are several ways this can be done:

1 - This method is used for the purpose of flushing out gallstones, after first softening them. It is a three-day pattern for effectively flushing gallstones:

• Go on a liver flush by drinking **apple juice** alone for 3 days. On the third day, the juice is followed by drinking a cup of **olive oil** and a cup of **lemon juice**.

2 - This method is used for cleaning out the liver and gallbladder rather than eliminating stones:

• To cleanse the liver and gallbladder, drink as much pure **apple juice** as possible for 5 days. Add **pear juice** occasionally. **Beet juice** also cleanses the liver.

3 - This is a still more involved regime for restoring the functioning capacity of the liver and gallbladder. Slightly different than #2, above, it should not be used on anyone below the age of 25 or who has large gallstones:

• On Tuesday through Sunday noon, drink as much **apple juice** as you are able, in addition to your regular **meals**.

• At noon on Sunday, eat a normal **lunch**.

• Three hours later, dissolve 2 teaspoons of **magnesium phosphate** (Epsom salts) in an ounce of hot water and drink it. It may not taste good, so follow it with a little freshly squeezed **grapefruit juice**.

• Two hours later, repeat the drinking of the **disodium phosphate** and the **grapefruit juice**.

• That evening, only take **citrus juice** for supper.

• At bedtime: Either (1) drink a half cup of unrefined **olive oil**, followed by a small glass of **grapefruit juice,** or (2) drink a half cup of warm, unrefined **olive oil** blended with a half cup of lemon juice.

• Go immediately to bed and lie on your right side, with your right knee pulled up close to your chest for 30 minutes.

• The next morning, one hour before breakfast, drink 2 teaspoons of **disodium phosphate**, dissolved in 2 ounces of hot water.

• Eat your meals as usual. The cleansing regime of the liver and gallbladder is completed.

• In case there is slight to moderate nausea when taking the olive oil and citrus juice, this should be gone by the time you go to sleep.

• But if the oil induces vomiting (which only happens rarely), you need not repeat the procedure at this time. Drink a cup of strong **peppermint** tea, to help relieve the nausea.

• You may find small gallstones in the stool the following day. They are light green to dark green, very irregular in shape, the size of grape seeds to cherry seeds, and feel like gelatin. If there are a large number of them, repeat the liver flush in two weeks. —See Gallstones (452).

ENCOURAGEMENT—We see in the Word of God warnings and promises, with God behind them all. We are invited to search this Word for aid when brought into difficult places. If we place God and the Bible first, we will have divine help in meeting all our problems. Deuteronomy 28:7.

GASTRO-INTESTINAL -
7 - GALLBLADDER

GALLBLADDER INFLAMMATION
(Cholecystitis)

SYMPTOMS—Severe pain in the upper right abdomen, accompanied by fever, nausea, and vomiting. The abdomen may be rigid and is usually tender to pressure at, or below, the lower edge of the ribs on the right side.

CAUSES—The gallbladder becomes inflamed. When this happens, it must be cared for immediately. If not, you could die.

An acute infection of the gallbladder may be only catarrhal in nature; and recovery will come in a few days. But, in more severe cases, the gallbladder fills with pus. Be very careful; immediately treat this condition. In case of pus in the gallbladder, there may be (and may not be) chills and fever. Therefore be alert, if chills and fever occur.

The presence of gallstones tends to irritate the lining of the gallbladder. Bacteria in the bile are then able to invade the wall and cause inflammation.

Inflammation of the bile ducts (cholangitis) produces similar symptoms to inflammation of the gallbladder (plus jaundice); but the treatment is the same.

NATURAL REMEDIES

• **Stop all eating**. Take nothing but **water** for 2-3 days until the acute condition is past. Drink only distilled water.

• Then go on **juices** for several more days. **Pear, beet, and apple juice** are very helpful.

• Then add solid food, such as shredded **raw beets** with 2 tablespoons of **olive oil, fresh lemon juice**, and freshly blended (uncooked) **applesauce. Pears** should be eaten generously; they are very healing to the gallbladder.

• **Oil** is necessary in the diet, to stimulate the production and elimination of gall and the fat-digesting enzyme, lipase. Using only high quality vegetable oil helps keep gallstones from forming.

• Avoid all **meat, grease, processed fats and oils** (including **margarine and butter**).

HERBS

• It is crucial that you **not overeat!** Only eat **small meals**.

• To treat the gallbladder and increase bile flow, mix equal parts **pansy, St. Benedict thistle, milfoil, and buckthorn bark**. Soak 1 Tbsp. in ½ cup cold water for 8 hours; then bring to a boil. Take 1-1½ cups a day in mouthful doses.

—For more information, see Gallstones (below) and Liver Flush (450).

ENCOURAGEMENT—No man or woman can be good or great who has not learned to yield his will to God and to obey with alacrity. Those who learn to obey are the only ones who will be fitted to command. Luke 7:50.

GALLSTONES
(Cholelithiasis)

SYMPTOMS—Bloating, gas, discomfort, or indigestion after a heavy meal of rich, fatty food. There may be constant pain, below the breastbone, that shoots into the right or left shoulder area and radiates into the back. The pain can last 30 minutes to several hours.

A gallstone attack (caused by bile duct blockage): nausea, vomiting, and pain in the upper right abdominal region.

When a gallstone passes (a "gallbladder attack"), the pain can be very severe and last a few seconds or minutes, and recur frequently for hours or days. Chills and fever may accompany the attack. The symptoms often occur after the person has eaten fried or fatty foods.

Inflammation of the gallbladder. Severe pain in the upper right abdomen and possibly across the chest. Fever, nausea, and vomiting may occur.

CAUSES—The formation of gallstones *(cholelithiasis)* may lead to gallbladder infection *(cholecystitis)*. Gallstones may form in the gallbladder or (more rarely) in the bile ducts of the liver. They may form in the gallbladder as a result of infection or inflammation of the gallbladder wall.

They occur more often in women than men; they occur more often in women who have given birth to children, especially several of them. They are more frequent in obese women, and occur more often after the age of 40. In the United States, about 10%-20% of the population have gallstones.

Persons with diabetes, migraines, cancer of the gallbladder, cirrhosis, and pancreatitis are more likely to have gallstones.

Gallstones are formed from bile, a brown digestive fluid produced by the liver; these are 80% cholesterol (a blood protein) and 20% bile. But they do not look like regular "stones." Kidney stones are sharp and crystalline. But gallstones are smooth, soft, and gelatinous. They feel like dense fat. Often persons with them have no symptoms. An attack usually occurs in the evening.

When they block the exits of the liver or gallbladder, they produce nausea, vomiting, and pain (as described above).

Try to avoid having an operation on your gallbladder. The operation consists of removing it entirely; but you really need it. However, in a crisis, you may need to go through with the operation. Recent studies at the University of Pittsburg found that removing the gallbladder (cholecystectomy) doubled the risk of colon cancer.

NATURAL REMEDIES

To relieve pain, give a 15 minutes **hot fomentation** over the gallbladder area, followed by an **ice rub**. Repeat the process 3 times. This will reduce the swelling, inflammation, and pain.

• For information on how to flush stones out of the gallbladder, *read Liver Flush (450-451).*

NUTRIENTS

• Each day, take **beta carotene** (15-30 mg), 1 **B complex** tablet, **vitamin B$_6$** (2 mg), **vitamin C** (100 mg), and **vitamin E** (200 IU).

HERBS

• **Turmeric**, in tea and food, prevents and treats gallstones. It contains *curcumin*; this is shown, in research studies, to eliminate them. It increases the solubility of bile.

• **Milk thistle** contains *silymarin*, which protects the liver, but also increases bile solubility.

• To treat a gallstone attack, mix together as many **mints** as you can (**peppermint, spearmint, catnip**, etc.) with **cardamom**. Make a tea and drink it.

• **Chamomile** or **dandelion** tea helps dissolve gallstones.

PREVENTING GALLSTONES—Here are several points to keep in mind:

• Eating **omega-3 fatty acids** (**flaxseed oil** is rich in them) makes gallstones soluble. **Olive oil** is good.

• Taking 2 tablespoons of **lecithin** each day immediately results in increased phospholipid concentration in the bile. This directly lowers and disperses gallstones.

• Drinking **water** helps prevent gallstone formation. It has been discovered that those with gallstones do not drink enough water. Drinking a pint of water causes the gallbladder to empty about 10-20 minutes later. This is the way to keep the gallbladder cleaned out and in fairly good condition; that is, if you do not eat any fats of animal origin.

• **Lack of exercise** increases the likelihood of gallstone formation. Cholesterol is excreted more rapidly by the liver and bladder with more exercise. The truth is that everything works better when you exercise regularly.

• It is an interesting fact that people who never eat meat, dairy products, or eggs rarely have gallstone attacks. **Animal fat** tends to form gallstones.

• Do not **overeat**. This is very important. Do not eat **processed, fried, sugared, spicy, or junk foods**.

Eating too much **sugar** inflames the gallbladder ducts.

• Do not use **alcohol, caffeine, or tobacco**.

• **Animal protein** in the diet increases stone formation; vegetable protein tends to reduce the size of the stones.

• Eating **eggs** greatly increases the likelihood of stone formation. A diet low in **vitamin C** also does.

• Eating lots of **refined carbohydrates** increases stone formation. Not including enough **fiber** in the diet does also.

• Keep your **weight** down. Overweight women over 40 and who have had several children have the most gallstones.

• **Oral contraceptives** (and other drugs containing **estrogen**) increase cholesterol saturation of bile.

• **After the stones have passed, eat lots of** figs, pears, prunes, oranges, pineapple, grated apples, and melons. Eat lots of vegetables that stimulate the liver (including broccoli, brussels sprouts, cabbage, kohlrabi, and cauliflower). Eat dandelion greens, beets and tops, carrot juice, celery, garlic, onions, and tomatoes.

—*Also see Liver Flush (450) and Gallbladder Inflammation (451).*

ENCOURAGEMENT—The strength of Christ was in prayer. He went alone and pled with His Father for guidance and help. Through Christ's enabling grace, we are to do the same. And we can receive help as Christ did. James 5:15-16.

BILIARY COLIC

SYMPTOMS—Intense pain felt in the right upper quadrant of the abdomen from infection of a gallstone in the cystic or hepatic ducts or the ampulla of Vater. In common language, that means a gallstone from the gallbladder gets stuck in one of the tubes leading out of the gallbladder. This produces intense pain.

CAUSES—Biliary colic occurs when the gallbladder tries to expel a stone or calculus, but the stone has gotten stuck and cannot get out. This is an acute disorder which may last several days, with spasmodic contractions of the gallbladder and of the ducts through which the bile flows into the small intestine. The result is sporadic pain, nausea, vomiting, and general discomfort.

NATURAL REMEDIES

• For extensive coverage, *see Gallstones (452), Gallbladder Inflammation (451), and Liver Flush (450).*

J.H. KELLOGG, M.D., PRESCRIPTIONS FOR BILIARY COLIC AND ITS COMPLICATIONS (*how to give these water therapies: pp. 207-275 / list of treatments: pp. 206-207 / Hydrotherapy Disease Index: pp. 273-275*)

GENERAL—Fruit diet, water drinking, liquid aseptic dietary.

PAIN—Revulsive Compress, every 2 hours. Continuous hot applications to area of liver. Hot Colonic or Hot Enema,

every 2 hours. Hot Full bath.

FEVER—Prolonged Neutral Bath. Hot Blanket Pack. Follow by Wet Sheet Pack. Cold Mitten Friction or Cold Towel Rub.

AFTERWARD—After acute attack subsides, give treatment for Gastro-intestinal Catarrh.

ENCOURAGEMENT—While the Lord has not promised His people exemption from trials, He has promised that which is far better. He has said, "As thy days, so shall thy strength be." If you are called to go through the fiery furnace for His sake, Jesus will be by your side, even as He was with the faithful three in Babylon.

GASTRO-INTESTINAL -
8 - INTESTINES, APPENDIX

INTESTINAL CRAMPS
(Food Cramps)

SYMPTOMS—Intense pain in the intestines.

CAUSES—This is a spasm of the muscles covering the intestines. It tends to accompany gastroenteritis *(440)*, colitis *(463)*, irritable bowel syndrome *(462)*, spastic constipation *(456)*, and other intestinal problems.

NATURAL REMEDIES

HERBS

Here are herbs which relax the intestinal walls and stop excessive movement of the digestive tract:

• An infusion of **catnip flowers** and leaves calms diarrhea and the colic spasm usually associated with it.

• **Flaxseed, tormentil, passion flower, and rue** calm colic pain and spasm in the intestines.

• An infusion of the flower heads of **German chamomile** has an antispasmodic effect on the bowels.

These herbs reduce intestinal fermentation:

• **Bilberry, alfalfa, angelica, anise, thyme, and eucalyptus**.

These herbs reduce intestinal gas:

• **Peppermint, cumin, tarragon, black poplar, fennel, caraway, and garlic**.

• Dr. Coffin's formula for treating colic and stoppage of the bowels: Mix 1 tsp. each **lobelia and cayenne**, ½ tsp. each **myrrh gum and valerian root**. Make a strong infusion of raspberry leaves; then add the other herbs, mix, let stand tightly covered ½ hour, and strain. Inject 1/3 into the bowels at body temperature; repeat in 4 hours and the remainder in 4 more hours. This will produce copious and frequent bowel discharges for the next 8 hours. Give astringent and tonic herbs orally for the next several days, as the patient is able to retain them.

• The first thing to do is to locate the condition and then **cleanse the bowel**, if that is what is needed. Use **cramp bark** herb. For *stomach cramps*, take a little tincture of **rhubarb** in water. For *uterine cramping*, use **cramp bark, squaw vine, or wild yam**. Many times when a cramp comes on, all that is needed is one-half teaspoon of **ginger** in a cup of hot water.

— *Also see Cramps, Muscular (635).*

ENCOURAGEMENT—Here is the only safeguard for individual integrity, for the purity of the home, the well-being of society, or the stability of the nation. Amidst all life's perplexities and dangers and conflicting claims, the one safe and sure rule is to do what God says.

MALABSORPTION

SYMPTOMS—The most common symptoms include: bulky, pale, foul-smelling feces. Flatulence and abdominal bloating. Weight loss. Diarrhea. Abdominal pain with cramps. Fatigue and weakness.

CAUSES—Malabsorption occurs when the small intestine cannot absorb nutrients from food passing through it. If the problem is not solved, certain nutritional deficiencies may develop, which can result in anemia *(440, 723)*, lack of B_{12} and **iron,** or nerve damage *(nutritional neuropathies, 555)*.

Digestive enzymes or juices may be inadequate or missing. This may be due to **chronic pancreatitis** *(444)* and **cystic fibrosis** *(655)*. Those with **lactose intolerance** *(475)* lack an enzyme needed to break down the sugar from milk.

Other causes include **celiac disease** *(473-474)*, **Crohn's disease** *(464-465)*, and particular **infections** (such as **giardiasis,** *863)*.

NATURAL REMEDIES
• Stop eating **processed, fried, white-floured, sugared, and junk foods**.
• Eat a **nourishing diet of fruits, vegetables, whole grains, nuts, and legumes**. Take a broad-spectrum **vitamin-mineral supplement**.
• Obtain adequate **rest** and outdoor **exercise**.

ENCOURAGEMENT—God desires from all His creatures the service of love—service that springs from an appreciation of His character. He takes no pleasure in a forced obedience; and to all He grants freedom of will, that they may render Him voluntary service.

DUMPING SYNDROME

SYMPTOMS—The food entering the stomach is suddenly dumped into the small intestine instead of remaining in the stomach, to be initially digested.

CAUSES—The dumping syndrome is a common side effect of **stomach surgery**. It can continue for quite some time.

Because proteins are not properly digested, the small intestine becomes very acid; yet it requires an alkaline environment in which to function properly. Anemia and osteoporosis are frequent secondary results of the dumping syndrome.

The best plan is to refuse a stomach operation.

NATURAL REMEDIES
• Take **English bitters**, along with **folic acid** and **pectin**. Eat as carefully as you can. Take full **vitamin /mineral supplementation**.
• **Lie down** for half an hour after each meal.
• Eat **small meals**, which consist of very **nourishing food**.

ENCOURAGEMENT—That heart is the happiest that has Christ as an abiding guest. In this world there is neither comfort nor happiness without Jesus. Oh, may we so live, during this brief period of probationary life, that we shall be with Him throughout the ages to come. Luke 18:7-8.

ILEOCECAL VALVE SYNDROME

SYMPTOMS—Diarrhea, fatigue, constipation, irregular bowel movements, lower right bowel tenderness, acne, migraines, duodenal ulcers.

CAUSES—The stomach empties into the small intestine, which in turn empties into the large colon. The ileocecal valve is a sphincter (circular) muscle that closes the illeum, so that matter in the large colon cannot flow back into the small intestine. This valve also keeps the digested material in the small intestine until all the nutrients have been absorbed. Then bile is released, mixed with the residue, and the valve opens; so it all can pass into the large bowel.

The problem occurs when the valve opens—letting material flow back into the small intestine.

NATURAL REMEDIES
• **Fasting** on juices for 2-3 days will help speed healing of the intestinal tract. Take **aloe vera gel** and **slippery elm**.
• Eat a diet high in **fiber**, including whole grains.
• Emphasize **fresh fruits** and **vegetables**. Eat **stewed prunes, figs, and raisins** for breakfast.
• Include **antioxidants** *(104)* in the diet, along with **beta carotene** (carrot juice and green and yellow vegetables), **B complex**, **vitamin C** (1,000 mg), **bioflavonoids** (100 mg), **calcium** (2,000 mg), **magnesium** (1,000 mg), essential fatty acids (1 Tbsp.

flaxseed oil), and possibly plant digestive enzymes (**bromelain**, **papain**).

• **Avoid** constipating foods, such as **dairy products, meat, cheese, soft bread, processed starchy foods**.

• Stop eating **meat**. It ferments before it reaches the large bowel. (Predators, such as dogs, tigers, etc., eat meat and have a short bowel. But we have a long one.)

ENCOURAGEMENT— In keeping God's commandments there is great reward, even in this life. Our conscience does not condemn us. Our hearts are not at enmity with God, but at peace with Him.

APPENDICITIS, ACUTE

SYMPTOMS—Pain and tenderness in the lower right area of the abdomen, vomiting, and low-grade fever. In children, the fever can be quite high.

The first symptom usually is pain. There may be tenderness with pressure. Quickly the pain becomes severe. But sometimes the pain is first felt all over the abdomen; it may be especially strong over the navel.

But pain and tenderness with pressure are not enough symptoms to determine appendicitis. There will also be rigidity and tenderness of the muscles of the abdominal wall, especially on the right side, a little below the level of the navel. Coughing and deep breathing make the pain worse.

The attack may, or may not, begin with a chill; but generally some, or much, fever is present from the beginning—along with constipation, vomiting, loss of appetite, nausea, and a tendency while lying in bed to draw up the right leg to relieve tension on the sore side.

CAUSES—The appendix is located on the right side of the abdomen, about halfway between the point of the hipbone and the navel.

Causes of appendicitis include **constipation and overeating. And eating rich, complicated foods and foods low in fiber**. The resulting fermentation and digestive upset can produce appendicitis.

Older people are less likely to experience appendicitis; but if they do, the danger of rupture is more likely.

IF THE APPENDIX RUPTURES, the infection will spill into the abdominal cavity, causing peritonitis. Take him to a hospital immediately, so he does not die!

NATURAL REMEDIES

• Do not wait. Call a physician.

• The inflammation may subside if the person is put to bed and the infected tissues are kept quiet and not irritated.

• Do not give a cathartic; that is, do not swallow **laxatives or laxative herbs**, to flush out the gastro-intestinal tract !! This can cause the appendix to

rupture!

• Undertake a **water fast** immediately. Drink small amounts every so often. Take 2 **myrrh / goldenseal** capsules every 2 hours. Take **echinacea** 4 times a day.

• Immediately give a colonic or **high enema**, but only in this way:

1 - Give an enema of the lower bowel (the **descending colon** on the left side of his body). As you do this, massage that part of the colon *downward* toward the rectum.

2 - Then, always gently, slowly, and carefully, go up *higher* into the ascending colon and massage it toward the rectum.

3 - Then gently massage the **transverse colon** (horizontal part of the large bowel) toward his left and down the descending colon toward the rectum.

• Then slowly massage upward on the *upper part (only)* of the **ascending colon**. Then very lightly, *partway down* the ascending colon, gently massage *upward*. **Each time, continue the massage all the way across the transverse colon and down the descending colon**.

• Constantly be on the alert for indications that the appendix may have burst!!! **If there is a most terrible pain, rush the person to the hospital at once.** If you wait beyond that point, he may die.

• When the attack phase of appendicitis is past, and all is better, break the water fast by going on a **fruit diet** for 2 days.

• Take liquid supplements, including beta carotene (25,000 IU, 4 times daily, with liquid chlorophyll in water 3 times daily). Carrot juice is excellent. Vitamin E (400 IU 2 times daily), zinc picolinate (30 mg daily).

• Then go on a cleansing, building diet of **nourishing food**. Do not eat too much at a time. Include one teaspoon of psyllium in juice or water, 3 times a day, for 2 weeks after the appendicitis has ceased. That will help soften everything and help it slide past the appendix.

HYDRO—The following hydrotherapy information will be found in the *Hydrotherapy* section *(206-275)* of this *Encyclopedia*:

The objective is to draw the inflammation away from the appendix. There are two ways to do this. Start both immediately when the appendix attack occurs:

The first application is based on the reflex principle. Water applications, placed on certain areas of the body, will affect other areas. The navel affects the appendix. So place an **ice cap or ice bag**, about one-half full of finely chopped ice, on the navel. This will draw inflammation away from the appendix.

The second application is based on the derivation principle. You can draw blood away from one area, by placing hot packs on a distant area. A hot **Hip-and-Leg Pack** is applied, plus placing an **ice bag** on the area of the appendix *(see Hydrotherapy chapter, 206-275).*

Many cases of appendicitis heal without need for

an operation to remove the appendix. *But you must be very careful! Contact a physician.*

—Also see Appendicitis, Chronic (below).

One of the false theories, dreamed up by evolutionists nearly a century ago, was the idea that many organs in the human body are useless and only relics given us by our ancestors. But, in recent decades, all of these supposedly "useless" organs (including the thyroid) have been found to have important functions. The tonsils protect the gastro-intestinal tract where it begins and the appendix guards it where the small intestines end. The appendix is a lymphatic structure.

ENCOURAGEMENT—Let your confidence in the enabling power of Christ increase daily. He alone can enable you to resist temptation. He alone can give you the guidance you need throughout the day. In His strength, you can be an overcomer.

APPENDICITIS, CHRONIC

SYMPTOMS—Pain and tenderness in the lower right area of the abdomen, vomiting. This occurs every so often.

CAUSES—This is NOT acute appendicitis, but chronic appendicitis. Relatively few individuals have ongoing problems with their appendix, which do not come into the acute phase. But some do.

Chronic appendicitis is an on again, off again, type of problem. For such individuals, it might be best to have the appendix removed rather than to suffer with it as the months pass.

NATURAL REMEDIES

*If used at all, the following applications may be used only for ongoing chronic appendicitis, **NOT** for the acute phase (455), when a person experiences a sudden attack!!*

The following method requires the placing of heat over the appendix area. This would NOT be done for acute appendicitis:

• Prepare a **castor oil pack** in this manner: Place a folded wool flannel in a Pyrex glass or enamel baking pan. Pour castor oil over the cloth until it is saturated. Heat it in the oven, but get it no hotter than you can touch. It will be heated in 5-10 minutes.

• Or, instead of heating it in the oven, put the neutral (room temperature) pack on the appendix area and place a heating pad over it. Next put a waterproof covering over the pack. Over this, place a hot-water bottle half filled with hot water. Wrap a bath towel around the body, to secure the water bottle and pack. Cover everything with a heavy blanket or sleeping bag, to hold in the warmth.

• Remove it 1-2 hours later. In order to avoid a rash, clean the oil off the skin with a solution of 2 teaspoons of baking soda to 1 quart water. Do it gently. Do not try to wash the castor oil out of the pack or any cloth involved; castor oil cannot be washed out. You can use the same pack again later, by adding some more castor oil and reheating. It can be reused for 6 weeks. Do not spill the castor oil on anything valuable.

• Use the pack for 3-4 nights and then not use it for 3 nights. Then begin again.

• Aloe vera juice can help relieve symptoms. Slippery elm tea is very soothing.

• Stop eating **processed, fried, and junk foods**. Stop eating all **meat products**.

—For more information on appendicitis, see Appendicitis, Acute (455).

ENCOURAGEMENT—We can have a daily living experience in the power of Christ and His willingness to save to the uttermost all that come unto God by Him. Let Him be the center of your affections. He is the best friend you could ever have. Ephesians 2:8.

GASTRO-INTESTINAL - **9** - **BOWEL**

CONSTIPATION

SYMPTOMS—Stools are hard, dry, and infrequent. It is difficult to have a bowel movement.

Other symptoms may include abdominal discomfort, lack of energy, dull headache, poor appetite, and low back pain.

CAUSES—"Constipation" comes from the Latin; and it means "crowded together."

The bowels should move daily, ideally, after each meal. When this does not happen, waste material moves too slowly through the large bowel. Elimination becomes painful, and toxins are reabsorbed by the system, placing an overload on the liver and kidneys. All waste in the body should be expelled within 18-24 hours.

A number of different physical problems are partially caused by constipation: bad breath, body odor, depression, appendicitis, fatigue, gas, headaches, hernia, indigestion, the malabsorption syndrome, varicose veins, obesity, insomnia, and the coated tongue.

Toxins, reabsorbed from a constipated bowel, can also result in migraines, chronic gas and bloating, thyroid problems, meningitis, and myasthenia gravis.

Constipation tends to be common during pregnancy.

Older people often have constipation because they are not drinking enough water.

Persons with spinal injuries may have problems with constipation, due to damage to certain nerves.

There is always the possibility that, if constipation occurs too frequently, that cancer or some other obstruction of the bowel may be involved. Other symptoms of colon cancer include severe cramping, blood in the stool, a tender and distended abdomen, and very narrowed feces. But cancer can be present without these symptoms occurring.

Alternate diarrhea and constipation may point to irritable bowel syndrome (462).

NATURAL REMEDIES

• First and foremost, include enough **fiber** in your diet each day; drink enough **water**. Get enough **exercise**, especially outdoors, so you get enough **fresh air**. Avoid **poisonous substances** and **emotional tension**. **Relax**. **Be thankful** to God for your blessings; and take time to be a blessing to others. Follow the advice in this paragraph, and many of your problems will vanish.

• As soon as you awake, start drinking **warm water**, a little at a time. By the time you are ready for breakfast, you should have taken at least a quart. Faithfully follow this regime, and you will develop regularity in your morning bowel movement. This plan nicely starts the day off right.

• Then, after breakfast and every other meal, go outside and **walk** a little or a lot. **Breathe** deeply.

• The larger the amount of **fiber** in the diet, the larger and softer will be the stools.

• Squeeze a **lemon** into an 8-oz. glass of warm (or very warm) water and drink it first thing in the morning.

• Eat **smaller amounts** of food at each meal.

• Eat **prunes or figs**. Drink **prune juice. Flaxseed meal** (best freshly ground) is helpful. Both will soften stools. **Psyllium seed** is also good; but take it quickly with a full glassful of water (before it solidifies).

• **Beta carotene** (25,000 IU) or carrot juice will maintain the health of the intestinal lining. **Acidophilus** (2 capsules with each meal) will keep the large bowel healthy.

• Nursing babies are seldom constipated, if their mothers are taking enough bulk (**fiber**) in their diet. **Licorice** tea is good for constipation in babies.

• High doses of **vitamin C** powder are a quick-acting laxative.

• Weak **chamomile** tea can be used for constipation. **Fennel** seed powder will relieve the griping action of stronger cathartics, such as senna.

• Stimulant laxatives are high in *anthraquinones*, which stimulate bowel muscle contraction. The most frequently used are **senna leaves** and **cascara segrada** bark. Cascara is the milder of the two. Senna can induce the laxative habit; so do not use it over 10 days.

• **Senna** is powerful and is likely to cause intestinal pains. Add a pinch of **ginger** or **fennel** to reduce them.

• When necessary, take cleansing **enemas** to relieve the load on the bowel. But the solution is better living, not reliance on enemas.

• If you have taken laxatives, take **acidophilus** to replace the friendly bacteria in your colon.

• A **small, *cold*** enema helps eliminate the enema habit. *See Enema Habit, how to overcome (469).*

• When nature calls, obey and have a **bowel movement**.

• For quick relief, drink a large glass of good **water** every 30 minutes until you have a bowel movement.

• You may get quick, temporary relief by using an **herbal laxative** to clear the lower bowel tract, but only the lower bowel tonics will get at the cause. If one needs a quick herbal laxative, any of the following herbs may be used: **agar, or seaweed, boneset, bran, butternut bark, California bark berry root, and Chinese Rhubarb root, Culver's root, Indian sennal leaves, mandrake root, psyllium seed, sacred bark, senna, turtle bloom leaves, Virginia snake root.** One should be wary of an incorrect use of laxatives and purgatives, because liquefied fecal matter is immediately absorbed by the intestinal villi into the bloodstream, and if there be excess, some of it will be thrown out of the bloodstream into the lungs, skin, kidneys, or other organs, producing a chronic toxemia thus laying the foundation for chronic disease.

• The proper procedure is to build up the body, to cleanse it, and see that the bowels work freely. Often **prune juice or fruits** will give relief and start the peristaltic motion coming again with ease. The afflicted person can assist in restoring natural bowel action by drinking copious amounts of **water** between meals (one-half hour before and two hours after eating) and by eating **proper foods** at regular intervals, especially bulky foods (those with fiber). Avoid any inorganic or concentrated foods.

AVOID

• Avoid **concentrated foods**, such as **meats, sugar, and cheese**. They produce constipation.

• **Dairy foods, soft drinks, white flour, salt, coffee, alcohol, highly processed foods, and sugary foods** should not be used, if you want to solve this problem.

• **Iron supplements** cause constipation. So do **painkillers** and **antidepressants**.

• All **decongestants** and **antihistamines** are drying agents; they may cause the stool to become dryer than it should.

• Do not use **cloves** in herb teas if you are prone to constipation.

• Constipation is sometimes caused by food sensitivity. The problem may be **milk, eggs, chocolate, meat, nuts, wheat, corn, or citrus**. Some people become constipated by drinking large quantities of **milk**.

• If you have a tendency to constipation, do not use **aluminum cookware** or too much **salt**.

• Eating a **mono diet** (just milk or greens, etc.) can be constipating.

• Do not take **mineral oil** products to relieve constipation. They absorb fat-soluble vitamins. Do not take **Epsom salts, milk of magnesia, and citrate of magnesia**. They wash minerals out of the body.

• Do not take **laxative herbs** (or even prune juice) all the time for a laxative effect. Only use them when you really need to. After taking them for a week or

G
A
S
T
R
O

two, reduce dosage by one-half each week thereafter.

J.H. KELLOGG, M.D., PRESCRIPTIONS FOR CONSTIPATION AND ITS COMPLICATIONS (*how to give these water therapies: pp. 206-275 / list of treatments: pp. 206-207 / Hydrotherapy Disease Index: pp. 273-275*)
INCREASE PERISTALTIC ACTIVITY—Drink half a pint to a pint of **cold water** before breakfast, preferably distilled water. **Increase the bulk** of food, with free use of fruit (especially apples, oranges, and figs, and bran cakes instead of so much smooth nonfibrous food). Small **Cold Enema**. Graduated Enema. Fomentation over liver twice daily, followed by Heating Compress during interval between. **Hot Abdominal pack** at night, **Abdominal massage**, Cold Fan Douche to abdomen, Cold Percussion Douche to spine, Cold Plantar Douche (bottom of feet) for 1-3 minutes, **Cold Rubbing Sitz Bath** at 70°-75° F. for 5-20 minutes. Avoid complete emptying of colon, using small **Cold Enema** instead of a large quantity of warm water, except when necessary, to relieve autointoxication or remove hardened, impacted feces. If necessary, introduce into rectum (as high as possible) a small pledget of cotton saturated with raw linseed oil or with glycerin. Do this at night or before breakfast, to be retained till the next bowel movement.

INCREASE ACTIVITY OF INTESTINAL GLANDS—Half a pint to a pint of **water** in an enema at bedtime, to be retained overnight. **Abdominal message** and **Hot Abdominal Pack**, without plastic covering.

REMOVE ACCUMULATED FECAL MATTER—Large **Hot Enema** or Hot Colonic, **Neutral Enema**, **oil retention** (oil enema to be retained throughout the night). Repeat the application till bowel is thoroughly emptied; then inject a pint of water at 75°-70° F., to tone the bowel.

DILATION OF THE COLON—**Graduated enema**, Cold Fan Douche to abdomen and spine opposite the stomach, running **Cold Footbath**, Cold Rubbing Sitz Bath. Hot Abdominal Pack, without plastic covering, changing every 4 hours.

INCREASE STRENGTH OF ABDOMINAL MUSCLES—Cold Fan Douche (spray), Cold Plantar Douche, Percussion Abdominal Douche. **Cold Compress to abdomen**, renewed every 4 hours without impervious covering. Massage and **special exercises**, particularly head raising and leg raising while lying on one's back.

ENTEROPTOSIS—Restore prolapsed bowels to position, **strengthen abdominal muscles** as indicated above, **correct normal sitting position**, abdominal supporter.

HEMORRHOIDS—Long **Cold Sitz Bath**, Cool Anal Douche, **Cold Compress** to anal area, small **Cold Enema**. If inflamed, rest in bed. **Fomentations** over the nates, followed by cold compress. Repeat Fomentations every 3 hours.

PAIN—(1) If due to a fissure: **hot applications**, sitting over steam [hot vapor, not actual "steam"]. (2) If due to irritable rectum: **hot colonic**. (3) If due to pain in abdomen: **Revulsive Compress**, Revulsive Douche. **Hot Enema** at 110° F., followed by small **cool Enema** and Revulsive Sitz Bath.

RELIEVE SPASM OF SPHINCTER ANI MUSCLE—Prolonged **Neutral or Hot Sitz Bath**, **Warm Colonic**, Hot Colonic, **and Fomentations** over the nates (the "nates" are the fleshy prominences formed by the gluteal muscles—the area where a child is spanked).

RESTORE SENSIBILITY OF RECTUM—Alternate Hot and Cold Colonic, Cold Douche to lower spine and nates. **Shallow Cold Sitz**, Cold Anal Douche, Alternate Anal Douche.

CONTRAINDICATIONS—Strictly avoid Sweating Baths that sometimes induce constipation. Also strictly avoid abuse of the Fomentation and the habitual use of the Warm Enema. If the Enema is used daily, the temperature, at least at the conclusion of the enema, should be 65°-75° F.; so that a tonic effect may be secured.

GENERAL METHOD—Each case must be carefully studied, with reference to the leading cause or causes which are operative in the individual case. Most important of these are the following: aparalytic or atonic condition of the intestine through disturbed or defective enervation, diminished intestinal secretion, or an abnormal absorption of intestinal secretion which results in unusually dry and solid fecal mass, dilatation of the colon that gives rise to accumulation, relaxation and weakness of the abdominal muscles with lowered intra-abdominal tension, hemorrhoids and other diseases of the rectum, prolapse of the colon and abdominal viscera, loss of normal sensibility of the rectum, and spasm of the anal sphincter muscle.

ENCOURAGEMENT—The fallen world is the battlefield for the greatest conflict the heavenly universe and earthly powers have ever witnessed. It is fought anew in the life of every person born into this world. Both Christ and Satan want to have the control of your life. The choice is yours; which shall it be? Deuteronomy 31:8.

DIARRHEA

SYMPTOMS—Frequent and loose watery bowel movements. This is often accompanied by cramping, abdominal pain, thirst, sudden need to eliminate, vomiting, and possible fever.

CAUSES—Severe diarrhea can produce a loss of essential electrolytes, such as potassium, and result in pale pallor, listlessness, and dark circles under the eyes.

Diarrhea in infants is serious. Something must be done right away. If the child has five or more watery stools a day, consider it diarrhea.

Possible causes include **overeating, food poisoning, stress, incomplete digestion of food, taking certain drugs, flu, intestinal parasites, caffeine, contaminated water, infection (viral or bacterial), eating certain foods (such as unripe fruit, spoiled protein, or rancid fats)**, eating **soap** (from improperly rinsed dishes), ingesting **certain chemicals, inflammatory bowel disease (Crohn's disease** *[465]*, **ulcerative colitis** *[463]*, etc.)**, cancer, traveling to foreign countries** (*Turista, 461*)**, poor digestion,** or lactose intolerance from milk products. **Sorbitol,** the synthetic sweetener found in diet products, can cause diarrhea.

Giardia lamblia *(863),* a microscopic parasite, is the most common form of water-borne infestation in the United States.

A **rich meal** of wine, lobster, creamy desserts, and all the trimmings is a good start toward diarrhea. It is all too much for the body to handle. The body rejects the whole thing and sends it all out.

Dysentery *(460)* is diarrhea which is caused either by a disease organism of some kind or overeating of rich food. The symptoms are the same as diarrhea, but may be longer lasting.

Breast-fed babies are less likely to develop diarrhea than those which are bottle-fed.

NATURAL REMEDIES
• Treatment and prevention require **clean food sources, careful food storage and preparation, self-discipline, and cleanliness.**

• Because of the ongoing diarrhea, as much as 30% more **protein** than normal is needed, as well as an increased intake of **minerals** and **trace elements.**

• Avoid xanthine-containing foods such as **chocolate, tea, coffee, and spicy foods.** Also avoid **drugs, cold liquids, and carbonated beverages.** All these may produce diarrhea.

• **Milk** may also induce diarrhea. Lactose intolerance and virus are leading causes of diarrhea.

• In case of chronic diarrhea, electrolyte and trace mineral deficiencies are likely. **Rice water, lime water, potato broth, and fruit** will help restore lost electrolytes.

• Use **fiber (bran and pectin) foods** in order to tighten the bowels and stop the diarrhea. **Garlic** is helpful in purifying the gastro-intestinal tract.

• **Carob** powder is high in protein and helps stop diarrhea. It is rich in tannins, which helps the bowel wall resist diarrhea. It is good for young children and infants with diarrhea. Give 15 grams of carob powder with applesauce for children.

• Keep **liquid consumption** high in order to replace lost fluids. But it is recommended that no raw fruit juices be given until the acute stage is past.

• **Antacids** are the most common cause of drug-related diarrhea. **Antibiotics** and a number of other medicinal drugs cause it also.

• While you have diarrhea, **do not prepare food** for others; and **wash your hands** carefully.

• Apple pulp is rich in pectin. **Apples** and **applesauce** are centuries-old remedies for diarrhea. (Apple pectin also treats constipation by softening the stool.) **Psyllium** also helps diarrhea.

• Helpful herbs include **white oak bark,** an astringent which stops diarrhea. Also useful are **American blackberry, barley, clove root, whortleberry, black currant, burdock, and echinacea.**

• Here are more substances which work to eliminate diarrhea: **Agrimony** (stems, leaves, or flowers) is very good. Dried fruits of **bilberry and blueberry,** **blackberry** (bark or roots), **carob powder, cooked carrots, fenugreek seeds. Peppermint** tea will allay spasms, diarrhea, or digestive disturbances. **Cooked rice** controls irritable diarrhea.

• **Slippery elm** tea provides soothing relief. Open 2-3 370-mg capsules and mix with water into a paste. Take a Tbsp. of the paste. Or mix it with mashed **banana** or **applesauce** (both of which help reduce diarrhea). Bananas restore lost potassium and add fiber.

• One comprehensive **B complex** tablet daily, plus **folic acid** (400 mcg), **pantothenic acid** (100 mg), and **niacinamide** (100 mg). This combination produces rapid improvement in acute attacks and has cleared some long-standing cases of diarrhea.

• Diarrhea depletes the body of vitamins and minerals in the food; so **supplements** are helpful.

• **Brewer's yeast** has been shown to alter the immune system or the flora living in the intestine and may relieve infectious diarrhea.

• **Betaine hydrochloride** (supplemental hydrochloric acid) helps some people with diarrhea.

Should you immediately stop the diarrhea?
• Some say to use bran and pectin foods in order to tighten the bowels and stop the diarrhea; others say to let it run its course in order to rid the problem foods, etc., out of the system. But, generally, it is considered best to use fiber foods to get the diarrhea stopped. When increasing fiber intake, also increase fluid intake.

• The deciding factor is whether the diarrhea was caused by a bacteria or virus. If caused by either, you want the body to throw it off through the bowels, if this will happen fairly rapidly.

• If the diarrhea is caused by food poisoning, give **activated charcoal** (4-6 250-mg capsules every 2 hours until symptoms are relieved).

—Also see Dysentery (460), Chronic Diarrhea (below), and Diarrhea in Infants (729). Also see Turista (461) for more on preventing and terminating diarrhea.

ENCOURAGEMENT—If Christ abides in your heart, you will be happy and full of praise and joy. The crises of life are as nothing compared to the bright future God has in store for you. Stand true to Him; and soon heaven will be yours. John 14:18.

CHRONIC DIARRHEA
(Chronic Intestinal Catarrh)

NATURAL REMEDIES
• Read the section on Diarrhea *(458-459).* Obtain enough **fiber** in your diet, drink enough **water,** and avoid **problem foods.** Recurrent diarrhea may be due to a virus or bacteria.

J.H. KELLOGG, M.D., PRESCRIPTIONS FOR CHRONIC DIARRHEA AND ITS COMPLICATIONS *(how to give these water therapies: pp. 206-275 / list of treatments: pp. 206-207 / Hydrotherapy Disease Index: pp.*

273-275)

TO LESSEN CONGESTION—**Rest** in bed. **Enema**, 95° F., after each bowel movement. Follow by half a pint of cold water. **Fomentation** to abdomen twice daily, 15 minutes. During interval between, apply **Heating Compress** over abdomen, renewed every 2 hours. This heating compress should be covered with flannel only (not protected).

TO DISCOURAGE BACTERIAL GROWTH—Aseptic dietary (especially **fruit juices, purees, and well-cooked cereals**). Daily cleanse colon by large **Hot Enema**.

TO COMBAT WEAKNESS AND AUTOINTOXICATION— Short **Sweating Baths**, 3-8 minutes, and **Graduated Cold Baths**.

PAIN IN ABDOMEN WITH TENDERNESS—**Fomentation** to abdomen every 2-3 hours. **Hot Enema** at 100° F., after each bowel movement. **Heating Compress** over abdomen after each hot application, to be changed once an hour until the next hot application is made.

MUCOUS STOOLS—Large **Hot Enema** at 95° F. Follow by small **Cold Enema**. **Cold Compress** to abdomen, changed every hour. **Revulsive Sitz Bath** or Revulsive Compress to abdomen. Revulsive Fan Douche to abdomen.

FREQUENT STOOLS—**Abdominal compress**, as above. Prolong **Cool Sitz Bath** at 75° F., 15 minutes. Follow by short **Hot Pail Pour to spine** and **Wet Sheet Rub**.

ALTERNATING CONSTIPATION AND DIARRHEA—Large Warm (980 F.) **Enema** or Colonic, once or twice a week. Follow with a small **Cold Enema** and Hot Abdominal Pack.

CONTRAINDICATIONS—Avoid Cold Douche, protected Heating Compress, prolonged Fomentations.

GENERAL METHOD—Increase the general vital resistance and improve stomach conditions, regulating the diet so as to render the intestine an unfavorable place for bacteria which constitute the chief cause of this disease. Remove bacteria and masses of mucus by Neutral Enemas.

ENCOURAGEMENT—The happiness of man is found in obedience to the laws of God. In obedience to God's law he is surrounded as with a hedge and kept from the evil.

DYSENTERY

SYMPTOMS—Sudden loose watery bowel movements, often with blood and mucus. It is characterized by pain, tenesmus, fever, and dehydration. Tenesmus is not being able to defecate; yet there is an urgent desire to do so.

CAUSES—The cause of this diarrhea-like disease may be *Entamoeba histolytica* (amebic dysentery), *Shigella dyseneia* (bacillary dysentery), or about six other germs or parasites.

• The cause is **improper diet, liquids with meals, overeating, wrong food combinations, impure water, use of liquor, tobacco, coffee, tea, eating fruits or vegetables that have begun to decompose**

or **chronic constipation**.

NATURAL REMEDIES

• Bleeding from the bowels is quickly healed by **mullein in milk**. Give a warm, very high **enema** with an astringent such as **white oak bark, bayberry bark, wild alum root**, etc. Use fomentation of **lobelia, castor oil**, etc., placed on the abdomen and spine, followed by a liniment application of **wormwood oil**. The patient should be nurtured with a diet of **alkaline forming foods** and **mucilage herbs, such as slippery elm and Irish moss, barley or oatmeal water**.

• Carefully read everything in *Diarrhea (458-459) and Chronic Diarrhea (above)*.

J.H. KELLOGG, M.D., PRESCRIPTIONS FOR DYSENTERY AND ITS COMPLICATIONS (*how to give these water therapies: pp. 206-275 / list of treatments: pp. 206-207 / Hydrotherapy Disease Index: pp. 273-275*)

DYSENTERY (ACUTE), COLITIS —

DIETARY NEEDS—Free **water** drinking, a simple dietary with **no animal broths or meat preparations. Brown rice, fresh buttermilk, fresh ripe fruit, and fruit juices with well-cooked cereals**.

TO COMBAT VISCERAL INFLAMMATION—Hot **Blanket Pack**, with **Hot Hip and Leg Pack**. Follow by **Heating Compress** to abdomen at 60° F., changed every 20-40 minutes. **Ice** suppositories if the inflammation extends into the rectum. **Cold Sitz Bath** at 75° F., 15-30 minutes, with **Hot Footbath**. Cold Colonic and **Rest** in bed.

TO RELIEVE PAIN—Very **Hot Pack** over pelvis, with **Hot Footbath**. Very **Hot Enema** at 100° F. Follow by **Cold Colonic**. Repeat hourly if needed.

DYSENTERY (CHRONIC), COLITIS (CHRONIC) —

GENERAL CARE—**Rest** in bed, careful diet, **Graduated Cold Baths** (twice daily), **Cold Rubbing Sitz Bath**. Hot Revulsive Sitz Bath 6-10 minutes daily, immediately preceded by a Hot Enema.

PAIN—If much pain is present, give a **Revulsive Sitz Bath** once or twice a day. **Moist Abdominal Bandage**.

ENCOURAGEMENT—Christ calls our attention to their natural loveliness; He assures us that the most gorgeous array of the greatest king that ever wielded an earthly scepter was not equal to that worn by the humblest flower.

TURISTA
(Traveler's Diarrhea)

SYMPTOMS—Diarrhea caused by traveling in foreign countries.

CAUSES—**Hygienic conditions** and **bacterial flora** are different in other countries. The nationals are used to it; but, arriving in that strange land, it can be too much for your intestinal tract.

One problem is **foreign versions of the *esche-**

GASTRO

richia coli bacteria. Foreign versions produce a toxin that prevents your intestines from absorbing the water you ingest in food and drink. The result is diarrhea.

Salmonella and shigella bacteria can also produce turista, which is actually dysentery *(460)*; and a smaller number of cases are caused by rotavirus or the **giardia** *(863)* parasite.

Up to 50% of turista cases are unexplained; but suspicion is pointed to **fatigue, changes in diet, jet lag, and altitude sickness**.

Seasoned travelers say that there is a 50% chance you will get diarrhea if you visit overseas, even if you take the recommended precautions. Here is what you should do:

NATURAL REMEDIES

• American travelers are often given Entero-Vioform tablets, which they are instructed to take several times a day. But those medications are forbidden in Japan and Sweden, because they can cause severe nerve and eye damage.

• Instead, take **betaine hydrochloride** (betaine HCl) tablets with you when you travel; and swallow two tablets after each meal. The hydrochloric acid will kill bacteria in the stomach and help prevent infection.

• Straight **lemon juice or lime juice**, taken on an empty stomach, also has an sterilizing effect.

• To make the situation even better, eat some **raw garlic** with your meals.

• In cases of non-bacterial diarrhea, 3 tablespoons of raw, unprocessed **wheat bran** daily, taken in fruit juice, has been found to give relief.

Here are more ideas for preventing turista from happening to you:

• Drink **acidic drinks**, such as **fruit juice** or whatever else you can get overseas. If you cannot do better, drink carbonated beverages sealed in bottles or cans.

• Try to make sure the dishes and **eating utensils** have been cleaned in purified water and, hopefully, rinsed in very hot water.

• Avoid **uncooked vegetables**. This includes salads, **fruits** you cannot peel, **ice cubes**, and anything in which there is unpurified water.

• **Boil water** for 3-5 minutes to purify it. **Iodine** liquid or tablets purifies it also.

ADDITIONAL HELPS

• Take **dried blueberries** with you. They tend to constipate and thus eliminate the diarrhea. **Blackberry root** is equally good. Make it into a tea and drink it.

• **Plantain** is strongly astringent, so is **white oak bark**.

• Cook down **apple peels** and drink it. The pectin in it helps eliminate diarrhea.

• Tannic acid is in **acorns** and **oak bark**. Both are powerful astringents and will stop the muscular contractions of the intestines.

• Not only **charcoal**, but **clay** is also useful in stopping diarrhea. Many commercial antidiarrheal preparations contain clay.

WARNING SIGNS

When traveling overseas (or even if you remain at home), there is danger that diarrhea may indicate something more serious:

• **Abdominal bloating, vomiting, and pain** can point to colitis, appendicitis, or an intestinal obstruction. **Black or red stools** can indicate bleeding or a parasitic infection. **White or pale stools** can signify disease of the liver. If **fever** occurs with the diarrhea, then a serious infection may be involved.

• Amoebic dysentery is a serious problem in Mexico, Central America, and a number of other places. If you contract it, **garlic, goldenseal, colchicum, peppermint, and ginger** have been used successfully against it. A friend, traveling in Mexico, burned a wooden box and swallowed the **charcoal** with water.

—Also see Diarrhea and Dysentery (458-461).

ENCOURAGEMENT—Happy is the man who has discovered for himself that the Word of God is a light to his feet and a lamp to his path. It is a light shining in a dark place. It is heaven's guidebook for mankind. Isaiah 65:13-14.

SPRUE
(Psilosis)

SYMPTOMS—Mild morning loose bowels for many days. Later: sore mouth, indigestion with bloating, and diarrhea. Dark or muddy complexion, emaciation, anemic, weak, irritable, loss of memory, inability to concentrate. Tongue completely smooth, eroded at edges and beneath, and fissured in center. Mouth extremely tender and painful.

CAUSES—Early cases, properly treated, recover. Those over 50 and those who refuse to adhere to a careful diet may die.

Sprue most frequently occurs in tropical countries. Visitors there are in danger of contracting it.

NATURAL REMEDIES

• **Bedrest** is very important. Protect from chilling.

• Keep him **warm**. Give him a warm room, warm clothing, and avoid cold baths.

• Daily take **sunbaths** or UV treatments.

• Moderately heavy **massage** of the muscles, daily; and avoid the abdomen (unless he is constipated).

• **High protein, high vitamin, and low-fat** diet.

• Only **small meals** should be eaten.

• Take **brewer's yeast** (2 oz.), **rice polishings** (1 oz.), **vitamin D** (2,000 IU), or **folic acid** (10 mg) daily.

• Give **mouthwash** daily *(see Gum and Mouth Disease, 427)*. Control diarrhea *(459)* and constipation *(456, 712)* in some later cases. And treat anemia

(537-541, 713). He may develop pernicious anemia.

• As soon as he is able to travel, he should leave the tropics and never return.

ENCOURAGEMENT—Parents should teach their children to love God and to obey His law. This is the greatest and most important work that fathers and mothers can do.

IRRITABLE BOWEL SYNDROME
(Mucous Colitis, Spastic Colitis, Intestinal Neurosis)

SYMPTOMS—There are three basic patterns: (1) constipation and pain; (2) alternating constipation and diarrhea; (3) painless diarrhea with mucus.

Diarrhea frequently occurs upon arising and, again, following breakfast. For the remainder of the day, he may be constipated. Diarrhea at night is rare. Instead of diarrhea, stools sometimes are pasty and very narrow.

Also present may be gas, nausea, bad breath, heartburn, severe headaches, bloating, lack of appetite, weakness, faintness, backache, and heart palpitations.

Pain is often triggered by eating; it may be relieved by a bowel movement.

A fifth of those with this problem also experience rectal bleeding.

CAUSES—Irritable bowel syndrome (IBS) is the most common digestive problem which patients see their doctor about. About one-fifth of Americans have the problem. Primarily occurring between the ages of 20 and 50, women have it twice as often as men. It is said that three-fourths of the population experience it at some time in their lives. Yet IBS is comparatively unknown in cultures where people eat simply, and not too much.

The fundamental problem is that the muscles of the small and large intestines contract in spasms rather than regularly. Something in the food bothers the gastro-intestinal (GI) tract—probably the totality of the strange things Westerners eat: **processed, greasy, fried, sugared, chemicaled, synthetic, drugged, preserved food; plus eating hurriedly and at irregular times**.

These spasms cause the food to pass through the GI tract either too fast or too slow. When too slowly, too much water is absorbed, causing hard, dry stools; when too fast, too little water is absorbed and the stools are watery.

Although irritable bowel syndrome is a nuisance, it is not life-threatening. But be aware that symptoms of IBS may indicate more serious problems, which sometimes are related by IBS: **arthritis, diabetes melitis, gallbladder disease, malabsorption disorders, candidiasis, pancreatic insufficiency, skin disorders, ulcers, colon cancer, and parasitic infections (such as amoebiasis and giardiasis)**.

Several diseases have similar symptoms, including diverticulitis *(465-466)*, Crohn's disease *(465)*, ulcerative colitis *(463)*, and lactose intolerance *(475)*.

NATURAL REMEDIES

• To relieve gastro-intestinal pain and expel the gas, take an **enema**. Use a **heating pad, hot-water bottle, hot fomentations** to the abdomen, lukewarm **enemas**—given slowly. **Moist heat** will be more effective than dry heat, since it penetrates better. If the pain is severe: Apply the heat for an hour, remove for an hour, and then apply again for an hour until relief comes.

• Take **charcoal** tablets to relieve gas and bloating. But do not use it daily, or it will cause constipation.

• The person may think he has too much **gas**; but studies reveal only that the normal amount of gas in his intestines bothers him more than it bothers other people. It would still be wise to **avoid gas-forming foods**. *See Bloating (433) and "Belching (432).*

• Avoid **swallowing air**. Do not chew **gum, smoke,** or drink **carbonated beverages.**

• Eat additional **bran** (oat bran, etc.), and it will produce more normal bowel movements. Coarse bran works better than fine bran. A **high fiber diet** is particularly important in solving IBS. But drink additional **water**.

• Add crushed **psyllium** seed to your diet. Drink 1 Tbsp. **blackstrap molasses** in a cup of hot water.

• Drink enough **water**. Eat **acidophilus** twice weekly.

• Eat on a **regular schedule**. Do not skip meals or eat between meals. Let your digestive system rest before the next meal. **Five hours between meals** is a good rule.

• Do not eat before going to bed.

• Search for your **food allergies**. Keep written records and take the **pulse test**. *See Allergies (848)* and *Pulse Test (847).*

• Because of the ongoing diarrhea, people with IBS require as much as 30% more **protein** than normal, as well as an increased intake of **minerals** and **trace elements**. *See Diarrhea (458).*

• Regular outdoor **exercise** is needed in order to maintain good bowel health. Do **deep breathing**.

• When your intestines upset you, temporarily go on a **bland diet**. Put vegetables and nonacidic fruits through a blender. But be sure to include some protein and fiber, if you are on a soft diet. A **low-fat diet** is important.

• Wear **loose-fitting clothing**.

• **Peppermint** (3 or more cups per day) soothes the entire intestinal tract. **Chamomile** tea does also. **Peppermint oil** relaxes intestinal muscles.

• Each day, take a high-potency **multiple supplement**, vitamin **C** (1,000 mg 3 times), **vitamin E** (400 IU), **flaxseed oil** (2 Tbsp.), and **dietary fiber** (3-6 grams).

AVOID

• An attack of pain may be sharply increased by drinking **cold liquids** and eating **food**. It is now known that the pain is generally associated with constipation. *See Constipation (456).*

• Avoid **stress, worry, and rush**. Avoid **tobacco, tea, coffee, soft drinks, alcohol, and drugs**. Caffeine can trigger or heighten IBS. Liquor makes symptoms worse.

• Research shows that refined **sugar** needs to be avoided if you want to return to normal living.

• Do not use **sugar substitutes** (sorbitol, etc.).

• Do not take **antacids** or **laxatives**.

• Avoid **animal fats, butter, fried foods, and dairy products**.

• Studies of patients revealed that 70% of those with IBS had a **lactose-intolerance** problem. They had to stop drinking **milk** in order to partially, or wholly, solve the problem.

• If you want success, stay totally away from **cigarette smoke**.

• Do not use medicinal or street **drugs** if you want improvement.

—*Also see Colitis (below).*

ENCOURAGEMENT—There is a great work to be done in our world; and God has a plan just for you. He has a place for you to work; and, though it seems to be ever so insignificant, if you will do it to the best of your ability (ever trusting in Him for help), He will approve. Psalm 146:9.

COLITIS
(Ulcerative Colitis)

SYMPTOMS—Bloody diarrhea, bloody mucus, gas, pain, bloating, incomplete elimination of the bowels, weakness, weight loss, indigestion, headaches, and sometimes hard stools. Diverticula are often produced.

CAUSES—Colitis is a disease of the large intestine. Ulcerative colitis is a more severe variation of it. The symptoms and treatment of both are about the same.

Colitis is a chronic infection of the lower bowel. The mucous membrane wall becomes irritated as a result of fecal matter which has accumulated, due to constipation. In other words, the person **did not have regular bowel movements**; and so the bowel wall became infected as a result.

Over-the-counter laxatives, cooking in aluminum utensils, overeating of refined carbohydrates, too much sugar in the diet, and food allergies are other causes.

Constipation causes the person to strain. This produces diverticula *(465-466),* small pockets which fill with waste matter and toxins.

Low-fiber diets, wrong food combinations, and poor bowel habits—all work together to cause trouble. Toxic bacteria multiply quickly when retained in the lower bowel too long.

Nervous tension and emotional stress intensify the problem. **Antibiotics** change the intestinal flora; and that can also produce colitis.

It is important that you try to find the underlying cause of the colitis; otherwise it will be difficult to eliminate it.

More rarely, the intestinal wall weakens, balloons out, and could possibly rupture. This is called toxic megacolon.

• This is caused by **faulty diet, too many food mixtures irritating the stomach and bowels, hasty eating** (insufficient mastication and saliva), taking **liquids while eating**, excessive use of **cathartics**, and **foods cooked in aluminum**.

NATURAL REMEDIES

• **High-fiber foods** are very important; also drinking lots of **water**. But, for the first few days, you may need to not have too many high-fiber foods. To begin with, boil grains with plenty of water so the cereal is wet, like soupy porridge. After the diarrhea has eased off, bring back the fiber foods.

• To begin with, do not eat raw greens, carrots, or peanuts. Eat **cooked or steamed green leafy vegetables, cooked white potatoes, multigrain bread, and well-cooked oat bran, brown rice, millet, sweet potatoes, bananas, cooked carrots, squash, and avocados**.

• Drink fresh, raw **cabbage, carrot, celery, and parsley juices** to help heal the colitis.

• Do not eat **fruit** on an empty stomach; but, eat at the end of the meal until the colitis is gone.

• Avoid **milk** products; for they irritate the colon. Wheat products may do it also. Avoid **carbonated beverages** and **iced drinks**. Avoid very **hot foods**.

• Eat a **bland diet**. Practice **relaxing**. Add **pectin** to your diet; it reduces the colitis.

• Poorly digested roughage can be the problem. **Eat slowly** and **chew your food** well. Your intestines need fiber, but not chunks of food.

• Undigested cereals and carbohydrates are another cause. Take **digestive enzymes** and **smaller, more frequent meals**.

• Drink lots of **water**. Colitis is frequently reduced by **distilled water**.

• Use the **pulse test**, to ascertain whether allergic foods are being eaten. *See Pulse Test (847).*

• When no open peptic or intestinal ulcers are present, take 2-3 tablets of **betaine hydrochloride** (betaine HCl) after each meal with a glass of water.

This will help the stomach digest proteins and carbohydrates.

• **Slippery elm** is very soothing and healing to the bowel. Mix one teaspoon of powdered slippery elm with one pint of boiling water, blend well, add something for flavoring, and drink slowly. **Peppermint, catnip, goldenseal, and alfalfa** are also good.

• **Alfalfa, garlic, and papaya** are also useful. Helpful herbs include **aloe vera, myrrh, and pau d'arco**.

• **Beta carotene** (25,000 IU) to help prevent infection and aid tissue repair. **Vitamin C** (2,000 mg) with bioflavonoids to help eliminate irritating bowel toxins. **Vitamin E** (400 IU), **flaxseed oil** (2 tsp.), and **Calcium** (800 mg).

• Herbal aids include any of the following herbs used as a **high enema** are very beneficial and soothing: **alum root, bayberry, burdock, golden seal, myrrh, or yellow dock**. This irritation can be soothed by drinking teas of **cayenne, comfrey, marshmallow root, mullein leaves, or slippery elm**. The lower bowel tonic is excellent. Alleviate irritation of the bowels by **pureeing foods** until some healing takes place and normal food roughage can be handled.

• Use **hot fomentations** to the abdomen for 20 minutes once a day. Take 8 oz. freshly prepared **cabbage juice** immediately before each meal.

• If **charcoal** is used, take a heaping tsp. with each loose stool. It is a very effective remedy.

• Build health with daily outdoor **exercise**. Avoid **competitive sports**; for they cause tension and stress.

—*Also see Crohn's Disease (below) for additional information on ulcerative colitis. See Irritable Bowel Syndrome (462) for more on colitis.*

ENCOURAGEMENT—We are to love God with all our mind, soul, and body. Give Him your life; and let Him use you to be a blessing to all those around you. There is no other way to be genuinely happy. John 10:28-29.

CROHN'S DISEASE
(Regional Enteritis, Ulcerative Colitis, Inflammatory Bowel Disease)

SYMPTOMS—Loss of energy, appetite, and weight. Chronic diarrhea, fever, chronic rectal bleeding, malabsorption, pain in the entire abdomen, excess fat in the stool (resulting in pale, bulky stools that float). Malnutrition results.

CAUSES—Crohn's disease is also known as regional enteritis. Ulcerative colitis is a different disorder, but similar enough in symptoms and treatment that we will list them together.

The difference is that ulcerative colitis only involves the first two layers of the intestinal wall (the mucosa and submucosa); whereas Crohn's disease also affects the next two layers below that (the connective tissue and the wall muscles).

SUGGESTED DIET FOR COLITIS

Ulcerative colitis can be an extremely painful condition. Your diet is the most significant factor in eliminating this problem, and making certain it does not return. Here are several suggestions:

• Keep a daily record of everything you eat and the symptoms you experience. This will teach you a lot. Some people are sensitive only to certain foods, such as yeast products, wheat products, or dairy products. By checking your daily record, you can see which food or foods have caused flare-ups or made you feel better.

• Eat a low-carbohydrate, high-vegetable-protein diet. It should include alfalfa or barley. A few nuts are an excellent source of protein.

• Eat lots of vegetables. If you are not able to digest raw vegetables, steam them.

• Eat a high-fiber diet. Oat bran, brown rice. barley and other whole grains, lentils. and related products such as rice cakes are good. Be sure the grains are well cooked.

• Keep fats and oils out of your diet, and stay away from high-fat milk and cheeses. Fats and oils exacerbate the diarrhea that comes with colitis. The exception would a teaspoonful of flaxseed oil each day.

• Include garlic in the diet for its healing and antibiotic properties.

• Cooked foods can be broiled or baked, but not fried or sautéed. Avoid sauces made with butter.

• Totally avoid carbonated soft drinks, spicy foods, and everything containing caffeine. These substances can irritate the colon.

• Avoid meat, sugar, and processed foods.

• Try soy-based cheese instead of dairy cheese; try soymilk or rice milk instead of cow's milk. If you do eat dairy foods, use nonfat types. Try lactose-free milk if you have a lactose intolerance. Many lactose-intolerant people can tolerate low-fat yogurt.

• Drink plenty of liquids—at least ten 8-ounce glasses of water daily to make up for the fluid lost with diarrhea. Carrot and cabbage juices and "green drinks" are also good. Or, add chlorophyll liquid to juices.

• Eat nothing between meals. Only eat fruit and a little zweiback (twice-baked bread) or whole wheat crackers for the evening meal.

• Avoid acidic fruits such as oranges and grapefruit. Fruit juices should be diluted with water and taken during meals.

Crohn's disease is a chronic ulceration of one or more sections of the digestive tract. Three special facts about Crohn's disease are these: (1) The ulceration reaches into all layers of the gastro-intestinal (GI) wall. (2) The entire GI tract can be involved, from mouth to the anus, and (3) it is usually a long-lasting condition.

As the inflamed portions heal, scar tissue remains, which keeps narrowing the channel.

Many puzzles still surround this condition. The origin is not clearly understood; and certain racial groups contract it more than others

Yet certain facts stand out:

Food allergies may help it start; and identifying and avoiding them helps reduce it.

A **lack of vitamins C and E** in the diet aggravates the problem.

People in Europe and North America have it far more than those living elsewhere in the world.

Jews in America have it much more than Jews in Israel. Caucasians have it less often than Jews, but more often than other races.

Therefore it is likely that the modern **Western diet** is a significant factor. Eating simple, nourishing food is an important aspect of dealing with this problem.

Rarely does the disease strike once and go away. Most of the time it keeps recurring for years. When this happens, the ongoing scarring keeps reducing bowel functions.

If ignored, eventually Crohn's disease can lead to cancer.

No definite cure is known; but certain things tend to alleviate the problem.

It is believed that Crohn's disease is an **autoimmune** problem; that is, the GI tract has become so toxic from years of mistreatment, that the immune system becomes confused and begins attacking the part of the body that houses the toxic food.

NATURAL REMEDIES

• A **fat-free diet** helps. It is known that those with Crohn's disease cannot absorb fats well and do not tolerate high-fat diets.

• Drink plenty of liquids, such as **distilled water and fresh juices**.

• **Cabbage juice** contains vitamin U, the anti-ulcer vitamin, which is good for the walls of the GI tract.

• Eat **high-fiber, unrefined carbohydrates (whole grains)**. However, gradually increase the fiber content, all the while **chewing well**, so as not to irritate the GI tract. If you cannot chew well, then blend the food.

• Individuals who contracted Crohn's disease were found to have eaten few **raw fruits and vegetables** prior to developing the condition.

• Mainly eat nonacidic fresh or cooked vegetables, (such as **broccoli, cabbage, carrots, celery, kale, garlic, and Brussels sprouts**). **Never fry** anything.

• The amino acid, **glutamine**, helps heal the bowel.

• Regularly obtain **sunshine** and **fresh air**.

• **Charcoal** will help control the diarrhea. Take 4-6 tablets, 2-3 times a day between meals. If the charcoal irritates the colon, stir the charcoal into water; let the charcoal settle to the bottom and only drink the apparently clear top part.

• Make sure the **bowels move daily**.

• Helpful herbs are **black walnut, burdock, goldenseal, pau d'arco, psyllium, saffron, aloe vera, fenugreek, valerian, slippery elm, and white oak bark**.

• **Boswellia** and **turmeric** help the bowel wall.

AVOID

• Do not use **spices** (such as **mustard, vinegar, pepper, and horseradish**).

• Eat no **junk food** or use **tobacco, caffeine, alcohol**, or useless food and drink.

• Eliminate all **food additives**. Do not use sugar or sugar foods. One study revealed that patients contracting Crohn's disease had previously been eating more **sugar** than the average population.

• **Avoid overeating**, in order to reduce the inflammation of the GI wall.

• **Gluten** tends to make the problem worse. So **avoid gluten-containing grains (which are wheat, oats, rye, barley, and buckwheat)**. Remarkable results can be obtained; but the gluten-free diet must be strictly adhered to. Not even tiny amounts in the diet may be permitted.

• Lactose intolerance is frequent. Avoid all **milk products**.

• Eliminate all possible **food allergies** and other allergies. Crohn's patients tend to have allergic conditions, such as hay fever and eczema.

• **Avoid stress**, anxiety, and worry. Keep calm and relaxed. Avoid exciting, competitive games.

• Avoid **surgery, antidiarrheal drugs, and corticosteroids**. They worsen the condition rather than improving it. A full 50% of those who undergo surgery report a rapid increase in symptoms afterward.

—*Also see Ulcerative Colitis (463).*

ENCOURAGEMENT—There is a mighty power in prayer. Our great adversary is constantly seeking to keep us away from God. But the humblest soul can, through earnest prayer, penetrate the clouds and lay hold on the arm of God in heaven. John 14:23.

DIVERTICULITIS
(Diverticulosis)

SYMPTOMS—No symptoms appear until this becomes infected or inflamed, resulting in chills, fever, and pain. The pain may be localized in the left lower quadrant of the abdomen and may be constant. Sometimes there is a brief period of diarrhea.

If you are over 40 and have periodic abdominal cramps, gas, and diarrhea alternating with constipation, you may have diverticulitis.

GASTRO

CAUSES—*Diverticula* are small pouch-like sacs on the inside of the large bowel, generally in the descending colon. *Diverticulosis* is a disorder in which these pouches are present. *Diverticulitis* is when they become infected and inflamed.

When a person is **constipated**, he tends to push too hard. The air pressure exerted by this muscular squeeze on the bowel muscles can force small pockets to form in the walls of the lower colon.

Once they form, diverticula never go away. Of themselves, they provide no symptoms. The problem is that fecal matter can collect in them and eventually attract bacteria. This results in infection or inflammation and produces the fever, chills, and pain.

Diverticulosis occurs when the diverticula are inflamed or infected; then the unfortunate symptoms reveal themselves.

This is another disease caused by "civilized" **refined and junk foods**. It is practically unknown in Third World nations, where people eat **high-fiber diets**.

More than half of those over 60 in America have this problem.

NATURAL REMEDIES

• In order to avoid the formation of those little pouches, always **avoid constipation**.

This is done by including enough **roughage** in your diet (**fresh fruit and vegetables, bran**, and other sources of fiber), drinking enough **water**, etc. *See Constipation (456) for more information.*

• **Do not delay** bowel movements. Have them when you sense you ought to. Do not wait.

• Obtain adequate **exercise**, especially outdoors. A research study showed that men who exercised little were 2½ times more likely to have diverticulitis.

• **Prunes, pureed fruit juices, and herb teas** are very helpful. **Carrot, beet, celery, and green juices** are excellent. Of the fruit juices, **papaya, apple, pineapple, and lemon** are outstanding for your purposes.

• **Chew nuts, seeds, and popcorn well,** so they will be less likely to enter the diverticula.

• Eat **smaller meals**. **Garlic** heals and detoxifies.

• Rats placed on **high-fat diets**, for 90 weeks, all developed colon diverticula. Adding more fiber lowers the internal pressure, reducing or eliminating symptoms.

• Avoid **caffeine** products. They all tend to irritate the colon.

• Do not eat a lot of **sugar**.

• **Smoking** and **stress** make the symptoms worse.

• **Girdles, belts, and tight bands** around the waist tend to increase abdominal pressure on the colon.

• The German government recommends taking 1-3 Tbsp. crushed **flaxseed** 2-3 times a day *with lots of water* to treat diverticulitis. **Psyllium seed** can also

be used, but it does not agree with some people (1 tsp. mixed with 8-oz. glass of water or juice, taken at mealtime). Either one softens stools. **Slippery elm** does also.

• The fibrous bark of **slippery elm** soothes the bowel and keeps things moving. **Prunes** and **prune juice** contain lots of fiber and have been used for constipation for centuries. **Chamomile** tea (2 tsp. dried chamomile per cup boiling water, steep 5-10 minutes) has an anti-inflammatory action which soothes the digestive system. **Pau d'arco** (2 cups daily) kills bacteria and heals.

• Here is a winning formula: Mix 2 parts **wild yam**, 1 part **valerian**, 1 part **black haw**, and 1 part **peppermint**.

• Other beneficial herbs include **aloe vera, goldenseal, cayenne, yarrow, papaya, and red clover**.

• **B complex**, plus **acidophilus** to reinforce beneficial intestinal bacteria. **Beta carotene** (25,000 IU daily), to protect and heal the colon lining. **Vitamin E** (600 IU) protects the bowel lining. **Vitamin C** with **bioflavonoids** (2,000 mg in divided doses), to reduce inflammation.

DURING AN ATTACK—As soon as an attack begins, give yourself a cleansing **enema** (2 quarts of water and the juice of a fresh **lemon**). Take 4 **charcoal** tablets with a large glass of water.

In case of pain or spasm in the colon, apply a **heating pad** over the abdomen.

During the acute phase of an attack, it may be best to eat a low-**fiber** diet for a very short time. Then return to the high-fiber regime.

If the attack is severe, temporarily **blend** your food. Drink **carrot, cabbage, and green juices**.

To relieve pain, **massage** the abdomen on the left side. Stand up and **stretch**.

Try to have bowel movements on **schedule**. Take **fiber** first thing in the morning, and down a quart of **water** before breakfast.

Check your stools daily. If they are black, this means blood is present; take a sample to a physician.

ENCOURAGEMENT—Christ's followers are to be more than a light in the midst of men. They are to be *the* light of the world. God calls you to be His representative, to minister to the needs of those around you. As you do this, your life will become marvelously fulfilled. Matthew 5:14-16.

COLON POLYPS

SYMPTOMS—Intestinal polyps usually cause no symptoms. But if they occur, they include: diarrhea, blood in the feces, or bleeding from the anus (sometimes with mucus). Occasionally, anemia may develop due to blood loss, causing fatigue and shortness of breath. Rarely, a polyp protrudes through the anus.

CAUSES—Polyps are slow-developing growths that protrude inward from the lining of the large intestine. Some are small and spherical and are attached directly to the intestinal wall; others are over an inch long and attached to the wall by a stalk. They can occur singly or in groups. Those which are larger than ½ in diameter may become cancerous.

They are very common in developed countries, where at least 1 in 3 people over age 60 may be affected. Chemicals in the air, water, soil, and food are causal factors. Others include excessive eating and eating junk food. So much useless excess and harmful material enters the body that some of it is stored in polyps.

NATURAL REMEDIES
• Eat a small amount of nourishing food, consisting of fresh **fruits, vegetables, legumes, and nuts**. Eat a **high-fiber diet** which includes **no animal fats**. Fiber in the diet is important. Eating simply of high-fiber, nourishing food, and avoiding living in areas where **chemical pollution** exists can help one avoid the development of polyps. Increase **water** intake as you increase fiber consumption.
• Avoid **processed, fried, and junk food**. Do not use **caffeine, tobacco, or alcohol**.
• Take a **multivitamin supplement**, plus **vitamin A** (10,000 IU), **carotene** (in the form of **carrot juice** and **red and yellow vegetables**), **vitamin C** (1,000 mg), and **vitamin E** (400 mg).
• Keep the colon clean by occasionally taking a low enema when needed. Do not strain during bowel movements.
—*Also see Nasal Polyps (406), Diverticulitis (465-466).*

ENCOURAGEMENT—If you are willing to learn meekness and lowliness of heart in Christ's school, He will surely give you rest and peace. It is a terribly hard struggle to give up your own will and your own way. But this lesson learned, you will find rest and peace.

LEAKY GUT SYNDROME

SYMPTOMS—Recurring pain in the intestinal tract, resulting in a variety of complications.

CAUSES—This is a common, seldom recognized, problem in which the intestinal lining becomes hyperpermeable. Large spaces develop between the cells of the intestinal wall; and bacteria, toxins, and food leak through. Toxic materials (including bacteria, fungi, parasites, and fats) enter the bloodstream. This strains the liver's ability to detoxify the blood. Various gastro-intenstinal disorders can result, including Crohn's disease, colitis, migraines, eczema, and immune problems.

The causes of leaky gut syndrome include: **poor diet, antibiotics, alcohol, caffeine, NSAIDS (non-steroidal anti-inflammatory drugs), chemicals,** **molds and fungi (from grains and fruits), enzyme deficiencies, parasite infection, fatigue, low-grade fever, frequent colds, flue, infections, food intolerances, and skin rashes.**

Causative diseases include: **AIDS, liver disease, cystic fibrosis, asthma, rheumatoid arthritis, celiac disease, lupus, chronic fatigue syndrome, fibromyalgia, and autism**.

NATURAL REMEDIES
• The following vegetable juice combinations will help rid the body of leaky gut syndrome: **Carrot, parsley, and cabbage. Carrot, celery, and endive. Ginger, parsley, garlic, carrots, and celery.** Fast on these juices 2-3 days a week.
• **Cook grains in a thermos** jar. This slow-cooking helps heal the digestive tract. The grains are rich in enzymes, vitamins, minerals, and proteins. No enzymes are lost.
• Drink plenty of liquids: **pure water, fruit juices, almond milk**. Almond milk can be added to fruit juices.
• **Buckwheat and millet** can be eaten for breakfast. They are nourishing and easily digested. Eat **raw and steamed vegetables, also fruit**. Eat **whole grains, nuts, and legumes**.
• Take **acidophilus, plant digestive enzymes (papain and bromelain), beta carotene, B complex, vitamin C, antioxidants, calcium, magnesium**, essential fatty acids (**flaxseed oil and wheat germ oil** are the best), **seaweed**.
• Helpful herbs include **aloe vera juice, grapeseed extract, paul d'arco, cat's claw, licorice, slippery elm, comfrey, goldenseal**.

ENCOURAGEMENT— The character of God is righteousness and truth; such is the nature of His ten commandment law. Says the psalmist, "Thy law is the truth"; "all thy commandments are righteousness." Such a law, being an expression of the mind and will of God, must be as enduring as its Author.

HERBAL LAXATIVES

In the following herbal lists, you will notice some overlap. This is because some herbs fit more than one category. That is why they are repeated.

HERBAL LAXATIVES
Herbal laxatives promote bowel activity with mild purgation. They are used when there is constipation, insufficient fiber in the diet, blood toxicity, gallstones, hypertension, a skin condition caused by insufficient elimination, or an infection in which cleansing of the bowel is needed.

The most frequently used laxative herb is **cascara sagrada**. **Senna**, the second most-frequently used one, is actually a purgative (see below); it is stronger and harsher (only 1 cup of the tea daily).

Other laxatives include **aloe vera, licorice root,**

psyllium seed, wahoo bark, and dandelion root (when there is liver involvement). They can be combined or taken individually. Some, like **cascara and senna**, operate by purging the bowels; others (such as **psyllium seed, flaxseed, and agar agar**) provide a soft gel-like bulk that slides it out (see demulcents, below).

During fevers, these laxative herbs help cool the system by eliminating heat from the intestines.

Here is a list of herbs that promotes bowel action: **buckthorn bark, cleavers, agar agar, boneset, flaxseed, licorice root, cascara sagrada, elder, mandrake, motherwort, Oregon grape root, goldenseal, senna, safflower, yellow dock, and peach bark**.

DEMULCENTS

Demulcent herbs bathe and lubricate the intestines and help expel contents, especially when the fecal matter in the bowel is dry. The best ones are **psyllium seed, flaxseed, slippery elm, and agar agar. Here are several other demulcents: fenugreek, licorice root, comfrey root, aloe vera, and mullein**.

HERBAL ENEMA

Instead of a laxative, an herbal enema can be taken. A **peppermint tea enema** is one of the best.

PURGATIVES

Purgatives are fast-acting herbs which are best avoided. They deplete the energy of the body and should not be used during hemorrhoids, bleeding intestines, dryness of the bowels, or prolapse of the bladder, uterus, or intestines. Do not use them when the body is chilled or there are skin infections.

Purgatives are so powerful that they work within 8-24 hours; and only robust, strong individuals should take them. The most frequently used purgative herbs are **senna, castor oil, buckthorn bark, jalap, and American mandrake root**.

CARMINATIVES

Purgative herbs should be combined with carminative herbs, to lessen griping. Carminatives contain volatile oils which stimulate the expulsion of flatus (gas) from the bowels and peristalsis. The best is **peppermint**. Here are several other carminatives: **angelica, anise, caraway, catnip, celery, chamomile, coriander, cumin, dill, fennel, garlic, ginger, myrrh, peppermint, sassafras, thyme, and valerian**.

Here is a different categorizations of laxatives:
There are four basic types of laxatives: bulk-forming agents. stool softeners, osmotic agents, and stimulants. The following are basic descriptions of the way the different laxatives work to achieve their effects:

• **Bulk-forming agents** increase the bulk and water content of the stools. **They are the only type of laxatives that can be safe to take on a daily basis.** Examples include **bran** (both in foods and in supplement form), **psyllium**, and **methylcellulose**.

• **Stool softeners**, such as **mineral oil and docusate sodium**, soften fecal matter so that it passes through the intestines more easily. They should not be used on a regular basis because they can have other negative effects on the body. **Mineral oil can damage the lungs if inhaled, and it reduces the absorption of fat-soluble vitamins.** *Drugs:* Docusate sodium (found in Colace and Dialose) may increase the toxicity of other drugs taken at the same time, and may **cause liver damage** to occur.

• **Osmotic agents** contain **salts or carbohydrates** that promote secretion of water into the colon and initiate bowel movement. **They are among the safest laxatives for occasional use. But, if they are used more than occasionally, dependency can result.** Examples include **sorbitol** (which is cheaper than lactulose but just as effective), **milk of magnesia, citrate of magnesia, Epsom salts,** and *Drugs:* lactulose (a prescription medication sold under the brand names of Cephulac and Chronulac); lactulose is both expensive and harmful to the body.

• **Stimulant laxatives** irritate the intestinal wall and stimulate peristalsis. **They can damage the bowels with habitual use, and can lead to dependency.** Examples include **cascara sagrada, castor oil**, and **senna** (Perdiem, Senokot). *Also Drugs:* bisacodyl (found in Dulcolax), casanthranol (Peri-Colace), phenolphthalein (Dialose Plus). Not one of these are safe for the body.

ENCOURAGEMENT—God can help you as you commit the keeping of your soul unto the Lord as unto a faithful Creator. To learn the lessons Christ teaches is the greatest treasure you can find. Rest comes in the consciousness that you are trying to please the Lord.

OVERCOMING THE ENEMA AND LAXATIVE HABIT

PROBLEM—Having taken enemas for a long time, you find you cannot have a bowel movement without taking another. Or, because you have the cathartic habit, you need to take laxatives to have a bowel movement.

NATURAL REMEDIES

• A **small, cold enema** is especially useful in retraining the colon to evacuate normally by itself. Cold water has a bracing, strengthening, enlivening effect. In hydrotherapy, the enema is considered cold if the temperature is **55°-70° F.**; whereas it is only cool if it is 70°-80° F. The cold enema is a powerful stimulant to bowel movements and should be more generally used for this purpose instead of the warm enema. Use the cold enema to overcome both the enema habit and the cathartic habit.

How to do it: Obtain an ear irrigation syringe, from the drugstore, and inject one syringeful of cold water into the rectum. Hold it 1 minute; then expel. A bowel movement will generally follow. Use this treatment at the same time each day, to establish regularity.

BULK AIDS VS. LAXATIVE AGENTS

1 - Bulk-forming agents: **bran, psyllium, and raw fruits and vegetables** are not referred to as "laxatives." Their use is an ideal way to promote bowel movements; and they are safe to use on a long-term basis.

2 - Laxatives are supposed to promote bowel movements, but some only hinder it. They are also poisonous. **Mineral oil** and **docusate sodium** are stool softening agents. If used at all, they should only be used temporarily. The mineral oil can damage the lungs, if inhaled; it absorbs fat-soluble vitamins in the digestive tract. Docusate sodium increases toxicity of other drugs and may cause liver damage.

Salts are osmotic agents which draw water into the bowel for a flush. These are safe if used only occasionally; but, otherwise, they can initiate dependency. In addition, some people dare not take extra salts into their body (edema, pleurisy, etc.). Examples include **milk of magnesia, Epsom salt, and table salt**.

3 - Stimulant agents cause a laxative effect by irritating the intestinal walls and inducing peristalsis. But they can result in dependency and damage the bowels. Examples include various drugstore items, **castor oil, senna,** and laxative herbs (such as **cascara sagrada**).

ENCOURAGEMENT—Friendship with God. What privilege can be greater? Study His Word, pray often, and tell others how wonderful He is. Tell them that God is love. This can give them the peace and rest they so much want. Hosea 10:12.

GASTRO-INTESTINAL - 10 - ANUS

HEMORRHOIDS
(Piles)

SYMPTOMS—Burning, pain, itching, inflammation, swelling, irritation, seepage, and bleeding.

CAUSES—Hemorrhoids are enlarged varicose veins, which are found in the anus and rectum.

Those occurring below the internal sphincter (a circular muscle which closes the rectum) are called external hemorrhoids. Those above that sphincter are called internal hemorrhoids.

Internal hemorrhoids are generally painless, but often bleed. When they do, the blood is bright red.

External hemorrhoids are also called piles. Sometimes they protrude from the anus. Because they enlarge and lose their elasticity, they often form little sacs which protrude into the anal canal. The skin above them turns blue or purple and can be extremely painful.

A *prolapsed hemorrhoid* is an internal one which is protruding outside the anus. Often there is a mucous discharge and heavy bleeding. They can be extremely painful.

When they bleed, a fair amount of blood can issue forth. Yet it does not indicate a serious disease.

Older people are more likely to have them. **Pregnant women**, and **women who have had children**, tend to have hemorrhoids more often than other younger people.

Circulatory weakness of the veins, along with constipation, are primary causes of hemorrhoids. Liver congestion can also be a factor.

Any condition which increases pressure on that area or reduces the flow of blood through those veins can induce hemorrhoids.

Hemorrhoids are common in folk who live on **junk food diets, low-fiber diets, lack of exercise, sit while working (especially sitting when tense and nervous), do heavy lifting, are obese or pregnant, strain at the stool, do heavy coughing, frequently sneeze, have prolonged use of laxatives or enemas, have elevated pressure on the portal vein of the liver (as occurs in cirrhosis of the liver), and sit on something cold**.

NATURAL REMEDIES

• To whatever degree you are able, take corrective actions as indicated in the above two paragraphs.

• Avoid **spicy, highly seasoned foods**; for they irritate the inflamed area.

• Avoid **sitting or standing** for long periods of time.

• **When lifting**, bend your knees and not your back. Do not hold your breath as you lift. Instead, take a deep breath and exhale at the moment of lifting. Avoid heavy lifting as much as possible.

• Do not **sit on things** which do not warm up (a rock, steel, the ground, or deep foam) for periods of time. Sit on a soft cushion, but not on a doughnut-shaped one.

• A **high-fiber diet**, which is **nourishing**, is crucial to success in avoiding or managing this problem. **Fresh fruits and vegetables** are full of fiber.

• Use soft **toilet paper** and only dab with it. Use only non-perfumed, white toilet paper.

• Do not **scratch** the area.

• Avoid **diarrhea** *(458-459)*; it intensifies the problem. For the same reason, avoid **constipation** *(456, 712)*.

• **Sitz (sitting) baths** soothe inflamed tissues and relax spasms of the rectal and anal muscles.

• In severe cases, take an alternating **hot and cold sitz (sitting) bath**. Use two large galvanized washtubs, propped up at one end, to make sitting in them more comfortable. Fold a large towel and place it in the bottom and sides, for comfort. Fill one with

G A S T R O

hot water (100° F.), the other with tap water. Sit in the hot, for 5 minutes, and in the cold for 30 seconds. Spread the buttocks, as you do this, so the temperature changes will have the best effect on the desired area. Do this 3 times. You can come back later and do it again as needed.

• An alternate method, for less severe cases, is to **sit in a bathtub** with 10-12 inches of hot water. Do this 3-5 times a day.

• **Take B complex, beta carotene** (25,000 IU), **vitamin E** (400 IU), **vitamin C** (2,000 IU in divided doses), **calcium** (800 mg), and **magnesium** (1,200 mg).

• For hemorrhoids which are extruded or prolapsed, take supplements containing glycosaminoglycans.

HERBS

• Apply cold **witch hazel** tea to help shrink them.
• **Cranberry** poultices are helpful. Blend a handful of cranberries, wrap a tablespoonful in cloth, and lay against the area. Change an hour later and repeat when you wish.
• Dab **lecithin** on the area, as you would Vaseline.
• An **ice pack** to that area may also bring relief.
• Peel a **garlic** bulb and scrape it to get the juice to flow. Then insert it. It will be expelled the next day during elimination. Do this 3 times a week.
• Cut a piece of aloe vera, about 2½ inches in length, peel, and insert.
• Applications of **white oak bark** tea or **witch hazel** to the area will, through astringent action, tend to shrink the hemorrhoids.
• Apply **goldenseal** as an anal antiseptic.
• In a research study, 84% of those receiving a **psyllium** preparation reported improvement: less pain, itching, bleeding, and discomfort when defecating. **Psyllium** and **flaxseed** absorb water, expand, and soften stools.
• Very good poultices for this problem include **butcher's broom, horse chestnut,** and **plaintain**.
• Mix equal parts **witch hazel, slippery elm, mullein, wild alum,** and **goldenseal**. Internally, take 2-4 capsules daily. Externally, mix with vasoline and apply to area.
• Apply **ginger tea** or **yarrow extract**.
• Melt 2 oz. **cocoa butter** on top of a double boiler. Stir in 2 Tbsp. finely powdered **witch hazel, bayberry, or yellow dock** (all astringent). When pliable, roll into cigar-shaped inserts (suppositories). Harden them in refrigerator. Insert. Cocoa butter melts at room temperature.
• **Flavonoids** (found in fresh fruits and vegetables) strengthen the anal veins so hemorrhoids are less likely to occur.
• **Stone root** strengthens hemorrhoidal veins (2 capsules between meals twice daily during acute attacks; otherwise, use once a day).

OTHER INFORMATION

• Medicinal **drugs** generally contain local anesthetics; but these often irritate the area and delay healing.
• A 1976 report stated that there was no evidence that any of the ingredients in *Preparation H* could reduce inflammation or shrink hemorrhoids.
• Aspirin will intensify the bleeding.
• Prolapsed hemorrhoids can become *thrombosed*; that is, they can form clots inside them which prevent their receding. Severe, increased pain indicates this has occurred. Go to a physician to remove the clot. This is not the same as a hemorrhoidectomy and is a simple, rapid treatment.
• In case of persistent, severe problems, some may choose to have hemorrhoidectomy done. Find a physician who has done this and adequately knows what to do.

J.H. KELLOGG, M.D., PRESCRIPTIONS FOR HEMORRHOIDS AND ITS COMPLICATIONS (how to give these water therapies: pp. 206-275 / list of treatments: pp. 206-207 / Hydrotherapy Disease Index: pp. 273-275)
PORTAL CONGESTION—Cold Footbath, in running water. **Hot Footbath** or Hot Foot and Leg Bath, **Hot Leg Pack**, Revulsive Douche to feet and legs, **Hot Abdominal Pack**.
IRREDUCIBLE PROLAPSE—Rest in bed, lying on the face in knee-chest position, if required. **Ice Compress**, daily bathing parts with ice water. Small **Cold Enema** after stool. Relieve bowels while lying in horizontal position; avoid straining. Need abdominal supporter. In many cases, surgical measures are necessary.
INFLAMED HEMORRHOIDS—Rest in bed with feet and hips elevated; knee-chest position, if necessary. **Ice Cold Compress**, pressed firmly against anus. Ice suppositories (ice placed in rectum). Very shallow **Ice-cold Sitz Bath**.
PAIN—If due to inflammation, short **hot Fomentation** followed by **cold compress** applied to the anus and nates, with **Hot Footbath** at the same time; repeat **Fomentation** hourly or every 2 hours. Prolonged **tepid Sitz Bath**, at 85°-90° F. **Hot Hip and Leg Pack**, followed by **Cold Compress** over nates, perineum, and lower back.

ENCOURAGEMENT—Bible religion is to be interwoven into everything we do and say. Let others see Jesus in you. Make His honor first. Show others that the Ten Commandments are the best commands to be kept in the whole world. 2 Chronicles 13:12. Surrender your heart and life anew to Him.

RECTAL FISSURES
(Rectal Abscesses)

SYMPTOMS—After passing a larger-diameter bowel movement, there is burning, stinging, and possible bleeding on the rectum. Painful red swelling or sore at, or near, the anal opening.

CAUSES—Hemorrhoids are swollen veins in the

anus and rectum area. Fissures are ulcers or breaks in the skin which just happen to occur in the same area.

The margins where the skin meets the mucous membrane can have small tears. This occurs sometimes at the corners of the mouth. Fissures on the rectum are somewhat similar. A common cause is the passing of a **large, hard stool**.

NATURAL REMEDIES

• A research study revealed that patients given **sitz baths** and a **high-fiber, non-constipating diet** recovered the most quickly.

• Avoid **constipation**. Be sure to include enough **fiber** in the diet and drink enough **water** each day (at least 6-8 glasses). The two, combined, will produce soft stools. Eat more **fruits and vegetables**.

• Do not **scratch** the area. Wipe yourself gently.

• Avoid **diarrhea**. An ongoing case of it can soften rectal tissue, so it is more likely to tear.

• Sit on something soft. A special **pillow** can be purchased in the drugstore.

• Fairly **hot water** on the area will relax and soothe it. This can be a **sitz** (sitting) bath, with astringent plants which will dry and heal (such as **white oak bark** tea).

• Outstanding healing herbs for this purpose: Rhatany (use in sitz baths), Mother of thyme (antiseptic and cleansing), psyllium (soothing, anti-inflammatory, relieves discomfort).

• If needed, to keep it dry, place **cornstarch** on the area after each bath. Do not use **talcum powder** for this—or any other purpose. It can cause cancer. Talcum powder is rock dust and should not enter body openings or be inhaled.

• These swellings may be **opened** with a blade or by **soaking** them in hot sitz baths of 3% boric acid. A poultice of **echinacea** may be applied directly to the abscess, to disinfect and help bring it to a pointed shape, so it can be opened. Flush the opened abscess with 3% **hydrogen peroxide**, to clean it out and disinfect the wound.

• Infants with this problem should be taken off **cow's milk**, since it is constipating.

ENCOURAGEMENT—If Christ is dwelling in the heart, it is impossible to conceal the light of His presence. Let Him use you to be a blessing to others, which they so much need. Psalm 41:1.

"I will lift up mine eyes unto the hills, from whence cometh my help. My help cometh from the Lord, which made heaven and earth." Psalm 121:1-2. Claim this promise as yours. Plead with Him for help and determine to be His obedient child. He wants to help you in all your need.

RECTAL ITCHING
(Pruritis Ani, Anus Itch)

SYMPTOMS—Itching around the anus.

CAUSES—Causes include **infection, parasites, poor hygiene, diabetes, estrogen deficiency, or liver disease**. Skin diseases, such as **psoriasis, seborrheic dermatitis, and eczema** can also cause it. Another possible cause is **contact dermatitis**, due to **perfumed or dyed toilet tissue, deodorants, soap, or underclothing**. **Food allergies** are thought to be another cause.

Rectal itching is a symptom of a problem rather than a disease. Resolving the basic problem is essential to eliminating the itching.

NATURAL REMEDIES

• Take **pulse tests** to determine food allergies. *See Pulse Test (847).*

• Take **beta carotene** (carrot juice, green and yellow vegetables) and **flaxseed oil** (2 tsp.) orally.

• Use **wet tissue** to clean the area after a bowel movement, but do not leave the area wet.

• Eliminating **moisture** from the area is a key factor. Moisture, leakage, and fecal soiling are frequently primary causes.

• After a bowel movement, it will help to **wash** the area with a syringe of water. Dry thoroughly afterward.

• Take a hot **sitz bath** daily. After the bath, apply **lemon juice** to the area with a piece of cotton. Or rub **wheat germ oil** on all affected parts after washing and drying well.

• A warm (not hot) tea bag of **goldenseal** may be applied to the area for up to a half hour, to relieve itching.

• Avoid using **soap** in the area; for soap is highly alkaline.

• Avoid **tight clothing** of any type in the abdominal area.

• Avoid **drugs**; many irritate the colon, leading to rectal itching.

Pinworms are frequently the cause in children, but rarely in adults. *See Pinworms (863).*

AVOID

• Several foods have been found to cause allergies, leading to itching: **beer, wine, hard liquor, coffee, milk, cola drinks, tea, citrus, chocolate, tomatoes, popcorn, nuts, and spicy food**.

• Avoid **gas-forming foods**.

• Avoid **stressful situations**. High-strung individuals tend to have this problem more than others. Their nerves are on edge.

• Do not use **anesthetic medications** with "caine" in the name. They produce strong allergic reactions, making the condition worse. They also tend to keep moisture on the area.

—Also see pinworms under "Worms" (861).

ENCOURAGEMENT—Resolve that, not in your own strength, but in the strength and grace given of God, that you will consecrate to Him now every power and ability of your life. Psalm 18:27-28.

ANAL ECZEMA

SYMPTOMS—Itching, reddening, and irritation on the anal mucosa.

CAUSES—An eczema infection was transferred to the anal area, probably by unwashed hands.

NATURAL REMEDIES

• Mallow helps heal superficial skin and mucosa irritation. Use the herb tea in compresses with an infusion or decoction of flowers and/or leaves.

• For additional treatment information, *see Rectal Fissures (471), Rectal Itching (471), and Eczema (345)*.

ENCOURAGEMENT— Since the law of God is "holy, and just, and good," a transcript of the divine perfection, it follows that a character formed by obedience to that law will be holy. Christ is the perfect example of such a character.

GASTRO-INTESTINAL - 11 - DIGESTIVE

ANOREXIA NERVOSA

SYMPTOMS—Thin people who try to keep losing more weight. Special indications of the problem: Persistent, intense fear of gaining weight. Continuous dieting, to the point of self-starvation. Refusal to eat, except small portions. Abnormal weight loss. Irregular or stoppage of menstruation.

CAUSES—Both anorexia nervosa and bulimia are obsessive eating disorders; but they are not the same.

Anorexia describes people who, although thin and often weak, are certain that they need to lose additional weight. **They fear food and weight gain**, and will hardly eat.

Bulimia describes people who try to eat less, then go on eating binges because they feel starved. Each one is concluded by purging (induced vomiting) in order to bring up the food eaten. *See Bulimia (473)*.

Believing they are overweight, and terrified of putting on more pounds, these individuals rather consistently try to keep themselves starved. They tend to have **low self-esteem**, and often are **depressed**. Certain that they look terrible, and sure that eating still less might solve the problem, they have a thinking pattern which is difficult to change.

In some cases, **drug and/or alcohol abuse** is also involved.

Lack of proper nutrition tends to intensify the feelings and attitudes.

Almost all anorexics are women, typically between the ages of 12 to 18.

The word, "anorexia," means "appetite loss" and technically could apply to anyone who has an ongoing disinclination to eat food. This can be caused by stress, malnutrition, shock, or injury. But, today, the term is generally applied only to those who have anorexia nervosa; and this article only applies to this latter definition.

Some consider anorexia nervosa to be a psychiatric illness. Others believe that reaction to a strong, underlying collection of **allergenic foods** is the problem. The often repeated phrase, "I always feel better when I don't eat and feel bad when I do" can apply to both viewpoints.

About a third of those with this problem prematurely die from starvation, infections, heart disorders, or suicide.

The underlying cause must be dealt with. Love and understanding is needed. Help from someone outside the family may be needed. However, there is danger in consulting professional counselors or psychologists, since they have been trained in hypnotic procedures; a growing number of instances are occurring where so-called "repressed memories" are implanted in the counselee. —And that only adds to the problems!

About 30% of those with this problem tend to have it all their lives.

NATURAL REMEDIES

• **Pray with the person and help her find peace in God**. **We must accept ourselves as we are**, physically, and go on from there.

• **Perk up the appetite**. Give **betaine hydrochloride** and **pancreatic enzymes (papain and bromelain)**.

• Give herbs which help stimulate the appetite: **sweet flag, calamus, yellow gentian, buckbean, gotu kola, ginger, peppermint, or marsh trefoil**. Give these herbs before meals.

• **St. John's wort** will aid in preventing depression.

• A **good nutritional program**, along with **vitamin / mineral supplementation**, is urgently needed. The delicate problem is getting the individual to eat enough food, so that normal balances can be regained. If extremely nourishing food is eaten, a person can maintain good health on less food. And "less food" means less calories and less weight gain.

• Take a full **vitamin-mineral supplementation**. This, along with certain herbs (such as **ginseng**), will provide vibrant energy without weight gain. The very minerals (**potassium** and **iodine**) which girls lose through vomiting are the ones that help them control their weight. (Do not use ginseng if there is high blood pressure.)

• Try to locate **food allergies** (848). Research studies have disclosed that, because certain foods are undesirable to eat, anorexics decide to reject almost all food.

• Avoid **sugar foods, processed foods, white-flour products, and food additives**.

• Obtain mild **exercise** every day. It not only builds lung, heart, and muscle, but it makes a person more confident. The exercise should not be excessive, unless the girl is eating enough food.

• Help her cultivate **relationships** with girls who have positive outlooks on life.

• Get her into a project where she is **helping** others. It is impossible to be happy when we only think about ourself and our own appearance.

—Also see Bulimia (below).

ENCOURAGEMENT—No one can remain neutral in the conflict. Everyone must decide whether he will stand under the banner of Satan or the ensign of Christ. Everyday we are deciding where we will stand in this battle. "Choose you this day whom you will serve." Joshua 24:15.

BULIMIA
(Bulimia Nervosa, Binge Eating Disorder)

SYMPTOMS—The people appear normal; and the symptoms occur in secret.

CAUSES—Bulimia describes people who try to eat less to keep their weight down; then, every so often, they go on a eating binge. This is followed by purging (induced vomiting) or the taking of laxatives, so the food will be eliminated without being properly digested. Also see Anorexia Nervosa (472).

Bulimia can result in serious physical problems, including hypoglycemia, internal bleeding, ulcers, erratic heartbeat, kidney damage, menstrual cessation, low pulse rate and blood pressure, and glandular damage.

Some bulimics overdo on exercise, in order to better manage weight.

Professions requiring a beautiful appearance are where we are most likely to find bulimics (models, actors, dancers, ballet dancers). By her own admission, Princess Diana was a bulimic. Thinness is equated with beauty by many people.

Oddly enough, while anorexics tend to be overly thin, bulimics are generally just right—not too heavy or too thin.

But their way of life may produce hair loss, yellow skin, premature wrinkles, muscle fatigue, dizziness, and extreme weakness.

The primary physical signs are those which are caused by sessions of induced vomiting: swollen salivary glands, constant sore throat, hiatal hernia, esophageal inflammation, erosion of the enamel of the back teeth, swollen glands in the face and neck, and broken blood vessels in the face.

If laxative abuse is done, then rectal bleeding, bowel damage, and chronic diarrhea may result. Excessive laxative use removes an excess of potassium and sodium, leading to muscle spasms, dehydration, and eventual cardiac arrest.

Bulimics tend to have low levels of serotonin, which can lead to increased cravings for simple carbohydrates (sugars). Yet it is likely that the binges produced those chronically low levels.

NATURAL REMEDIES

• Follow the suggestions for anorexia (472). The person should expect to experience temporary anxiety, depression, insomnia, and possible irritation, as he or she attempts to break with the old way of life. But the rewards are outstanding and well-worth the effort.

• Do not eat any **sugar or sugary food**s. Avoid all junk food and white-flour products.

• A **simple diet of the most nourishing food** is urgently needed in order to restore the needed balance in life. Take a complete **vitamin-mineral supplementation**.

• CCK (cholecystokinin-pancreozymin) is a hormone, found in the small intestine and brain, which signals a satisfied feeling and that it is time to stop eating. When a person gets into a pattern of overeating, that hormone is not properly produced. So the person only feels satisfied after heavily overeating a meal. The only solution is to **rigorously eat just so much**, even though it does not seem like enough. Eventually, the hormone will start being produced again in the proper amount at the proper time.

• **Marjoram, valerian, and prickly lettuce** are sedative, ease anxiety, and calm nervous excitation. **Fucus and kelp** (both types of seaweed) produce a sensation of being full and decrease appetite.

• Take a **small plate** of the **most nourishing food**, take **small bites**, **chew your food** very slow, and **eat slowly**. Do not eat **complicated mixtures or meat**.

—Also see Anorexia Nervosa (472).

ENCOURAGEMENT—For Christ's sake, we are to endure trials. We are not engaged in mimic battles. Satan wants to have you. But, pleading with God for help, you can choose to cast in your lot with Christ. And you will have angels to help you win the battle.

CELIAC DISEASE
(Celiac Sprue, Gluten Intolerance)

SYMPTOMS—Diarrhea, weight loss, and nutritional deficiencies (such as anemia). Other symptoms include frequently pale and/or light-yellow, foul-smelling stools that float. Fatigue, depression, abdominal swelling, muscle cramps, wasting, and bone and/or joint pain. Diarrhea is the most commonly observed symptom.

Infants and children may show vomiting, stunted growth, intense burning sensation of the skin, and a red itchy skin rash. Ulcers may develop in the mouth. The child may look anemic and undernourished.

Some children develop blisters and sores all over their body from celiac disease. Symptoms vary, but can include fatigue, irritability, and/or behavior changes.

Babies may lose weight or gain it more slowly, and do not seem to be thriving well. The disease can begin in the first few months of life.

CAUSES—Celiac disease affects the small intestine. There are abnormalities in the intestinal lining, due to a permanent **intolerance to gluten**. Gluten is in **wheat, rye, barley, and oats**. (Corn, rice, millet, soybeans, quinoa, and amaranth do not contain gluten. There seems to be a little uncertainty about buckwheat.) The protein, **gliadin**, is thought to be the toxic part of the gluten. It interacts with the lining of the intestines, causing the tiny absorptive fingers which jut from it (the villi) to flatten and atrophy. As a result, nutrients are not absorbed (including vitamins A, D, and K) and the disease symptoms appear.

Unfortunately, many physicians and the food industries recommend that grains be introduced into the diet of the infant when they are less than a year old. This can prompt celiac disease to first appear then or even decades later.

This is important! Tell every expectant mother not to feed her child grains until it is at least a year old.

Celiac disease tends to start between 9 and 18 months, immediately after wheat, rye, barley, and/or oats is given to the child. Those are often the first solid foods given to infants. (Breast-fed infants first show the symptoms at 16 months while the bottle-fed ones first develop them at 10 months.) The disorder is rare in blacks and Asians, and tends to run in families.

Removing gluten from the diet of a celiac produces a marked change; whether an infant, child, or adult, the person starts feeling better again. But he must not return to gluten foods.

Some infants do not tolerate **cow's milk protein**; they react to it with celiac symptoms, even before gluten is given to them. So remove that also from them.

Celiac disease is often misdiagnosed as spastic colon, irritable bowel syndrome *(462)*, or something else which affects the intestines.

Yet, if left untreated, celiac disease can be quite serious. It can lead to pancreatic disease, infertility, miscarriages, internal hemorrhaging, bone disease, gynecological disorders, nervous system damage, intestinal lymphoma, and many more problems. For example, anemia is common, due to poor absorption of folic acid, iron, and vitamins B_{12} and K.

Scarring of the intestinal lining can progress so far that, by the ages of 45 to 50, 90% of the intestine can be damaged, resulting in a significant reduction (as much as 70%) of the absorptive surfaces.

But there is evidence that partial repair to those walls can be made within several months—if you permanently part company with the offending foods.

NATURAL REMEDIES

AVOID

• You will want to avoid *gluten foods*, which are **wheat, oats, rye, and barley**.

• Do not eat products containing **cow's milk**. Breast-feed the child, to avoid using cow's milk.

• Some celiacs must also exclude **soybean** products. **Eggs** are also a problem for some.

• Do not overeat **sugar or white-flour products**.

• Avoid **processed, fried, and junk food**. Do not eat **sugary foods, chocolate, and processed foods**. Do not eat **meat**. Avoid **tobacco, tea, coffee, and alcohol**.

• Read the **labels** and watch for "hidden" gluten or cow's milk ingredients in bottles and packages. Some of these are malt, modified food starch, some soy sauces, grain vinegars, binders, fillers, excipients, and "natural flavorings." Almost all commercial breads, bread mixes, crackers, cereals, pastas, and processed foods contain gluten. It is often found in commercially prepared puddings, candies, cookies, cakes, ice cream, salad dressings, luncheon meats, non-dairy creamer, beer, bouillon cubes, chocolate, frankfurters, canned chili, macaroni, noodles, spaghetti, bread stuffings, and anything thickened with flour (soups, vegetables, bottled meat sauces, gravies, flavoring syrups, sauces, bottled salad dressing, cocoa mixes, curry powder or seasonings, or mustard.

GOOD FOODS

• The follow grains do not have gluten: **corn, millet, and rice**. Soybeans, quinoa, potato starch, and **amaranth** are also okay. Breads and cereals made from any of these do well. **Buckwheat** is all right for some celiacs, but not for others. **Oats** should be okay, but some oat preparations include gluten.

• All grains fed to babies or adults should be **cooked for 2-3 hours**, if the preparation is done by boiling at 212° F.

• Eat a nourishing diet, including **fresh fruit, vegetables, and fresh vegetable juices**. **Fiber** is important in the diet of celiacs.

• Take a complete **vitamin-mineral supplement**. But everything should be **wheat-free, yeast-free, and hypoallergenic**.

• *Allisatin*, found in **garlic**, is said to help treat celiac disease.

• Ripe **bananas** are tolerated well and help control the diarrhea. Only eat **homemade desserts**.

• Frozen, fresh, canned **vegetables and vegetable juices** are all right.

• A **lactose intolerance** *(bellow)* frequently exists, requiring that milk products be excluded. **Vitamin K** deficiency frequently occurs. Therefore, be sure to include **acidophilus** in the diet.

• Helpful herbs include **aloe vera, burdock, pau d'arco, psyllium, saffron, slippery elm, and alfalfa**.

• **Infections** and **stress** worsen the symptoms; **sunlight** and **garlic** (raw or cooked) tend to improve them.

—Also see Lactose Intolerance (below). Lactose Intolerance and Crohn's Disease (464-465) have some similar symptoms and problems.

ENCOURAGEMENT—You may at times hesitate. Should you choose the right? But the command of God is "Go forward!" Do what is right, regardless of the consequences; and the angels of God will be by your side. Psalm 107:19.

LACTOSE INTOLERANCE

SYMPTOMS—Diarrhea, gas, and abdominal cramps. Symptoms generally begin 30 minutes to 2 hours after eating dairy products. Symptoms are similar to those of celiac disease *(473-474)*.

In infants, symptoms include foamy diarrhea with diaper rash, slow weight gain and development, as well as vomiting.

CAUSES—Lactose intolerance is inability to digest milk sugar. The intestinal wall is not able to make the digestive enzyme, *lactase*, which is needed to split lactose into *glucose* and *galactose*. When the lactose is not split, it remains undigested in the intestinal tract. It retains fluid and ferments in the colon, producing gas, diarrhea, and abdominal cramping. It can cause blood loss from gastrointestinal bleeding. It can inhibit the absorption of iron. (Milk also contains saturated fat, which is not good for the heart and blood vessels.)

Although it can cause digestive disruption and discomfort, lactose intolerance will not produce dangerous results. Fortunately, it can easily be controlled through careful diet.

Very few adults throughout the world can digest milk sugar after the age of 20. The exceptions are most caucasians of northern European origin. Milk is one of the two or three most common food allergens in Western diets. But most of the symptoms do not show up right away; so milk is not always suspected as the cause.

The following infections can result in lactose intolerance: irritable bowel syndrome, regional enteritis, and ulcerative colitis. It can cause allergic symptoms such as diarrhea, asthma, ear infections, rashes, and hives.

Although less common in infants and children, it can occur after a severe attack of gastroenteritis and injure the intestinal wall.

If you are pregnant and there is lactose intolerance in your family, plan to breast-feed your child or give him a nondairy formula (such as soy milk). But, if you do, give him added calcium gluconate powder, since soy milk does not contain enough calcium.

Lactose intolerance is different than milk allergy. A person with lactose intolerance cannot digest milk sugar; one with milk allergy can digest milk, but his immune system is antagonistic to one or more of its components.

SENSITIVITY TEST

To find out if you are sensitive to milk, cut out all diary products for 10 days and see how you feel. If your symptoms disappear during those 10 days, and then return when you start drinking it again, you probably have a milk sensitivity. During the test, it is best that you only eat food you have prepared yourself at home.

NATURAL REMEDIES

• Avoid all **milk and dairy products**. This includes **ice cream, frozen yogurt, powdered milk, whipped cream, creamed soups**.

• Beware of products which contain small amounts of **added milk ingredients**, such as "milk solids." Lactose is added to many processed foods, including **cookies, pancake mixes, breads, canned and powdered soups, flavored coffee, powdered drink mixes, processed meats, hot dogs, milk chocolate, non-dairy creamers, protein powder drinks, biscuits, candies, snacks, and ranch dressing**.

• Many **pharmaceutical drugs** contain lactose as a filler.

• Since you cannot drink milk, eat foods which are rich in **calcium**. This includes **broccoli, dried figs, apricots, blackstrap molasses, collards, turnip greens, cabbage, carrots, parsley, romaine lettuce, summer squash, and other vegetable greens**.

• Do not eat **spinach or rhubarb**, for they contain a chemical (oxalic acid) which blocks absorption of calcium.

• Take **supplemental calcium** powder (calcium citrate, calcium gluconate; but *do not take* calcium lactate). *See Strengthening the Bones (608) for much more information.* Osteoporosis *(612)* affects 1 out of every 4 women over age 50.

• During a **lactose attack** of diarrhea, do not eat any solid food. Just drink lots of good water and replace lost minerals.

• **Acidophilus milk** does not help the person with lactose intolerance; for the acidophilus works to improve conditions in the colon. And the problems with lactose occur in the small intestine.

GASTRO

• Milk-containing foods one eats or drinks **hot** are often better tolerated than are cold ones.

• Acceptable **milk substitutes** include soy milk, rice milk, almond milk, or a milk product which contains the lactose-digesting enzyme, lactase.

• Take a **lactose supplement** (in drops, capsules, or tablets) along with a milk product at a meal, to help digest that milk. When several drops of the enzyme in the supplement are mixed with a quart of milk and then refrigerated for 24 hours, about 70% of the lactose in the milk will have been predigested before you drink it. To speed up the process, heat the milk to 90o F. before the enzyme is added. Because the lactose has been changed to sweeter sugars (glucose and galactose), it may be best for diabetics not to use it.

• Some with lactose intolerance are still able to eat small amounts of **plain yogurt, goat's milk, or fat-free milk**. They have smaller amounts of lactose and allergy-causing components of whole milk.

• Never drink milk alone; take it with solid food (such as whole-grain cereal). This will slow digestion and help the lactose digest more of the milk.

• If you are pregnant and have a family history of problems with digesting milk, then you do well to **breast-feed your child** instead of giving him cow's milk.

—Also see Celiac Disease (473-474). Celiac Disease and Lactose Intolerance (475) have some similar symptoms and problems.

ENCOURAGEMENT—The victory can be gained; for nothing is impossible with God. Give Him your heart, and you have given Him the best gift you can. Is it not worth it? He offers you Christ and eternal life in heaven.

GLUTEN INTOLERANCE

SYMPTOMS—Indigestion, often severe, after eating a food containing gluten.

CAUSES—Gluten is a protein which is found in wheat, oats, barley, rye, and malt. It is in many processed foods. Gluten is not found in millet, rice, or corn.

NATURAL REMEDIES

• Do not eat wheat, oats, barley, rye, malt, or foods containing them. Here are these gluten foods:

Breads made from oats, barley, rye, or malt flavoring. Cakes, cookies, ice cream, pastries, pies, puddings, sherbert made with stabilizers. Cream, commercial salad dressings. Fried potatoes, potato chips, hominy, macaroni, noodles, spaghetti. Many soups, candy, jam, and marmalade. Chocolate, gravy, malt extract, pickles, white sauce, spices. Alcoholic beverages, cereal coffee substitutes, or beverages made with chocolate or malted milk.

• There are many, many foods which are not included in the above list.

ENCOURAGEMENT—Obedience to the Ten Commandments was the only condition upon which ancient Israel was to receive the fulfillment of the promises that made them the highly favored people of God; and obedience to that law, by the enabling grace of Christ, will bring as great blessings to individuals and nations now as it would have brought to the Hebrews.

WILSON'S DISEASE
(Copper Disease)

SYMPTOMS—There is a pigmented ring (the Kayser-Fleischer ring) at the outer margin of the cornea of the eye. This is called the "fissure sign."

Later symptoms include bloody vomit, drooling, an enlarged spleen, jaundice, loss of coordination, progressive fatigue, weakness, intellectual impairment, personality changes, bizarre behavior, spasms, tremors, rigidity of the muscles, fluid accumulation, swelling in the abdomen, weight loss. Also difficulty in speaking, swallowing, and/or walking.

Although the disease begins at birth, symptoms generally do not appear until the age of six or more often in the teens or later.

CAUSES—Wilson's disease is rare and inherited. The body is not able to metabolize the trace mineral copper, although it is still absorbed by the small intestine into the bloodstream.

The result is an excess of copper in the various organs (liver, kidneys, brain, and corneas of the eyes). If not cared for, Wilson's disease will result in serious damage to the liver and brain and, ultimately, death.

Early detection and treatment can minimize the damage. If you have a family history of this disease, have diagnostic tests made of you and your children. Early detection is important. The following is a treatment for one with this disease; it should not be used by those who do not have Wilson's disease:

NATURAL REMEDIES

• A lifetime must be spent **avoiding things which have copper** and **taking substances which remove it** from the body.

• Check your **drinking water**, to make sure it has no copper. If it has more than 1 part per million of copper, drink bottled water.

• Make sure your vitamin / mineral **supplements** do not include copper. Maintain a high intake of **vitamin C**, since copper in the body tends to destroy it.

• Onions and garlic contain **sulfur**, which **helps rid the body of copper**. But do not take flowers of sulfur (the chemical sulfur); they will give you boils.

• Eliminate from the diet those **foods which are high in copper**. This includes **chocolate, molasses, nuts, organ meats, shellfish, broccoli, mushrooms, avocados, legumes, oats, egg yolks, soybeans, raisins, and whole grains**.

• Avoid **exposure to metal**. Do not use copper cooking utensils or cookware.

• Grains are important; and so are nuts, legumes, and broccoli. All of these are high in copper. But by taking zinc supplementation (below), you may be able to eat them.

• **Zinc** is able to reduce copper absorption by the body, and has been used successfully in alleviating this disease. Take 50 mg 3 times per day. (One person with Wilson's disease, who took too much zinc [480 mg], experienced a copper deficiency!) Taking more than 300 mg of zinc per day may weaken immune function. Some research indicates that those with Alzheimer's should avoid zinc supplementation. Zinc destroys copper by locking with it; that is why you have to keep taking zinc. Zinc is nontoxic.

• **Hair analysis** reveals whether normal people have been exposed to too much copper. But, oddly enough, it does not show excess copper in those with Wilson's.

• The standard **drugs** for Wilson's disease destroy vitamin B6 and iron, which can produce extremely serious side effects (including kidney disease, damaged blood cells, bleeding of the lungs, and kidney failure).

ENCOURAGEMENT—The true man or woman is the one who will stand by principle, even though all others may be compromising. Obedience to the commandments of God, by enabling faith in Christ, is what is needed. Jeremiah 31:12.

COPPER DEFICIENCY

SYMPTOMS—Diarrhea, stunted growth, inadequate utilization of iron and protein. In babies: impaired development of bones, nerves, and lung tissue.

CAUSES—In contrast with Wilson's Disease (above), in which there is too much copper in the body, this is a disorder in which there is not enough.

Not enough red blood cells are made. White blood cells cannot fight infection. Iron is not absorbed. Copper-deficiency anemia results. Mental and emotional problems develop. It may be a factor causing anorexia nervosa *(472)*. It is one of several causal factors, resulting in sprue *(461)* and kidney disease *(489-595),*

Without enough zinc, copper cannot be absorbed and used. Without copper, iron cannot be absorbed and used.

NATURAL REMEDIES

• Take 5 mg of **copper** daily for 1 month; then reduce to 3 mg daily.

• Take 30 mg of **zinc** daily, but do not exceed this amount. Do not take too much zinc; for it will reduce copper absorption.

• Take the equivalent of 100 mg of **iron** daily. It is best not to take tablet supplements; but, instead, obtain it from a natural source. Each day take 1 tsp. **blackstrap molasses**, the richest source.

• Take a multivitamin supplement daily.

• Babies fed only **cow's milk** are more likely to develop copper deficiency.

ENCOURAGEMENT—Those who think themselves the strongest may become the weakest unless they depend on Christ as their efficiency, their worthiness. This is the Rock upon which we may successfully build.

GASTRO-INTESTINAL -
12 - NUTRITIONAL

EMACIATION

SYMPTOMS—Extreme thinness and gauntness.

CAUSES—Lack of proper nourishment, which is caused by **under-eating** and eating almost totally of **junk foods**. **Alcoholics** and those addicted to **street drugs** do not always obtain adequate nourishment. Decided changes need to be made.

Extreme cases of emaciation demand immediate attention. Here is Dr. John Harvey Kellogg's prescription:

NATURAL REMEDIES

J.H. KELLOGG, M.D., PRESCRIPTIONS FOR EMACIATION AND ITS SEVERAL COMPLICATIONS *(how to give these water therapies: pp. 206-275 / list of treatments: pp. 206-207 / Hydrotherapy Disease Index: pp. 273-275)*

BASIC FACTORS—Rest in bed, also **fattening diet** that will build tissue and blood. This should include dairy products, well-cooked cereals, malted or predigested cereals, a graduated program of tonic treatments (the Tonic Frictions). **Fomentation** over the stomach twice daily, followed by **Hot Abdominal Pack**.

GASTRIC ULCER—Withhold food by mouth. Do rectal feeding, **Fomentation** over stomach twice daily, well-protected **Heating Compress** during the interval between. **Graduated Tonic Frictions**.

CHRONIC GASTRITIS—Rest in bed. Abdominal **Fomentations** 2-3 times daily. Protected **Heating Compress** during intervals.

INTESTINAL CATARRH—Enema at 95° F. after each bowel movement. During the interval between, apply a **Heating Compress** at 60° F., changing it every 30 minutes.

HYPOPEPSIA—Graduated tonic treatment (**Tonic Frictions**). **Ice Bag** over stomach half an hour before each meal.

CONTRAINDICATIONS—Avoid prolonged Hot Baths and Cold Full Baths.

GENERAL METHOD—The general plan of treatment

G
A
S
T
R
O

must be such as to secure increased income of tissue-building material with a diminished outflow; hence the diet must be very simple, easily assimilable, and taken in as large a quantity as possible. Exercise must be diminished or, in grave cases, suspended altogether. Moderate exercise may be allowed, if necessary, to maintain the appetite. Special attention must be given to increase of the appetite and improvement of digestion by suitable hydrotherapy applications. Cold applications must be very short and intense, so as to produce strong nervous impressions upon the nerve centers without removing animal heat (to any considerable degree) or increasing oxidation.

ENCOURAGEMENT—The strength of every soul is in God and not in man. Quietness and confidence is to be the strength of all who give their hearts to God.

PICA
(craves dirt)

SYMPTOMS—The child keeps eating dirt.

CAUSES—Children eat dirt because they crave minerals they are not obtaining in the foods served them. Sometimes they eat paint chips from the walls. But paint often contains lead or cadmium, both of which are quite toxic. Lead can produce brain damage.

During pregnancy, the expectant mother may crave substances other than food, such as coal, dirt, ice, starch, or hair. These are signs of nutritional deficiency.

—*See Lead Poisoning (873) and Anemia (537-541).*

NATURAL REMEDIES

Supplement the child's diet with extra **vitamins and minerals**. Provide him with a nourishing diet of **fresh fruits, vegetables, beans, and nuts**.

Include Nova Scotia **dulse** or Norwegian **kelp** in his diet. This will supply trace minerals. If you live near the ocean, use a little ocean water to help salt the food.

Do **pulse tests** to determine if a celiac type of disease exists. *See Pulse Test (847) and Celiac Disease (473-474).*

Do a **hair analysis** test, to determine which minerals are needed and whether he may have ingested toxic minerals.

ENCOURAGEMENT—The temptations of Satan are greater now than ever before; for he knows that his time is short and that very soon every case will be decided, either for life or for death. It is no time to sink beneath discouragement or give up the battle. Cling to Jesus and, by His grace, live the life of an overcomer. John 17:3.

MALABSORPTION SYNDROME

SYMPTOMS—Anemia, diarrhea, and weight loss are frequent. Sometimes there is weight gain instead of weight loss. Nausea, vomiting, abdominal pain.

Other causes may include dry skin, fatigue, abdominal bloating, gas, constipation, diarrhea, PMS, thinning hair, tendency to bruise easily, depression, or inability to concentrate. There may also be vision problems (especially impaired night vision) and bulky, pale, and fatty stools (known as steatorrhea).

CAUSES—This disorder appears to be a waste-basket category. Whenever nutrients, in general, cannot be properly absorbed by the gastro-intestinal (GI) tract, the problem is dubbed "malabsorption syndrome."

Possible causes include an **impoverished diet, primarily junk food**. The body may not be producing enough **digestive enzymes**. Vitamin **B complex** may not be in the diet or is not being properly absorbed. **Diseases of the gallbladder, liver, bile ducts, or pancreas** may exist. There may be **food allergies**.

Other causes include **damaged intestinal walls** (caused by irritable bowel syndrome), **lactose intolerance, Crohn's disease, diverticulitis, celiac disease, colitis, or parasitic infestation**. Other causes include excessive consumption of **antacids, alcohol, or laxatives**. **Chronic constipation or diarrhea** can have a similar result.

Radiation therapy, sugary foods, or digitalis treatment can reduce the absorptive area of the intestines. An overgrowth of **candida** in the digestive tract or **obstructions in the lymphatic system** can have a similar effect.

Too rapid intestinal transit time causes nutrients to pass out of the body as waste.

AIDS and cancer can produce many of these symptoms.

There are a number of other possible causes, including a variety of **drug medications**.

Premature aging can be caused by a decline in secretions of stomach acid and digestive enzymes.

NATURAL REMEDIES

• Try to identify which of the above causal factors applies and apply solutions, as given elsewhere in this book. A great need is to cleanse the body and, then, rebuild it with a good healthy program.

• A good **nourishing diet of fresh fruits and vegetables. Include well-cooked brown rice or whole-wheat cereal.** Eat **smaller meals** and **chew thoroughly.**

• Omit all **fats and oils**, except 2 tsp. **flaxseed oil** daily. Do not eat **meat products, coffee, or alcohol; do not use tobacco**. Drink 8 glasses of pure **water** daily.

• Obtain adequate **rest, outdoor exercise, fresh air, and sunlight.**

• **Oregon grape** root is healing and improves digestion. **Chamomile** calms the nervous stomach. **Peppermint** and **parsley** are also healing.

• Make sure the **bowels** are kept open and working properly. This reduces toxins in the intestinal tract and digestive organs.

• Freedom from **worry and tension**.

• Do not use **drugs** which interfere with nutrient absorption (which includes antibiotics, sulfasalazine, corticosteroids).

ENCOURAGEMENT—God is love and He cares for us. "Like as a father pitieth His children, so the Lord pitieth them that fear Him." Trust and obey your sweet heavenly Father. You will never be sorry that you did. John 15:2, 5.

BERIBERI
(B₁ Vitamin Deficiency)

SYMPTOMS—In children: mental confusion, muscle wasting, impaired growth, convulsions, nausea, vomiting, stomach and intestinal problems, diarrhea, and constipation.

In adults: weight loss, diarrhea, edema, fatigue.

CAUSES—Beriberi is a nutritional disease, caused by a **deficiency of thiamine (vitamin B₁)**, but also all **the other B complex vitamins** as well.

Beriberi is not common in the West. In the East, where many subsist primarily on polished (stripped of it hull) rice, it is endemic. The rice bran contains the vitamins; and the polished kernel only contains starch and protein.

In America, beriberi occurs as a result of **alcoholism, hypothyroidism, pregnancy, infections, or stress**.

NATURAL REMEDIES

• Eat **brown rice, raw fruits and vegetables, seeds, nuts, legumes, and whole grains**.

• Take **vitamin-mineral supplements**.

• Do not drink **liquids** with your meals; for this washes away water-soluble vitamins.

ENCOURAGEMENT—All who give themselves to the service of Christ will follow the example of Christ and will be perfect overcomers. In His strength, you can stand firm amid the pollutions of this degenerate age. Psalm 91:14.

PELLAGRA
(Vitamin B Deficiency)

SYMPTOMS—Depression, anxiety, dizziness, headaches, diarrhea, loss of appetite, red tongue that is sore and inflamed, weakness, weight loss, dementia, and itchy skin on the hands and neck.

It is sometimes diagnosed as mental illness.

CAUSES—Pellagra is a deficiency disease, caused by a severe lack of several vitamins. It is rare in the United States at this time; but, when it does occur, it is caused by diseases which heavily deplete those vitamins.

The primary vitamins involved are **niacin (vitamin B₃)** and, secondarily, **thiamine (B₁)** and **riboflavin (B₂)**. Also needed is **folic acid** and **vitamin B₁₂**.

NATURAL REMEDIES

• Eat plenty of **foods high in the B vitamins** and take **nutritional supplements**.

• Worthwhile foods include **potatoes, legumes, broccoli, collards, bananas, figs, nuts, seeds, peanut butter, tomatoes, prunes, whole-grain breads, and cereals**.

ENCOURAGEMENT—All power to do good is God-given. His grace is sufficient for all our trials. If we trust wholly in God, we can overcome every temptation and, through His grace, come off victorious.

Christ has not a casual interest in us, but an interest stronger than a mother for her child. Our Saviour has purchased us by human suffering and sorrow, by insult, reproach, abuse, mockery, rejection and death. He is watching over you, trembling child of God. He will make you secure under His protection. Our weakness in human nature will not bar our access to the heavenly Father; for Christ died to make intercession for us.

—*Also see Pernicious Anemia (540) and Megaloblastic Anemia (540).*

SCURVY
(Vitamin C Deficiency)

SYMPTOMS—Swelling and bleeding of the gums, tenderness of joints and muscles, poor healing of wounds, and increased susceptibility to bruising and infection. Rough, dry, discolored skin. Scurvy may occur concurrently with gingivitis *(425)*.

An infant with scurvy is comfortable only when lying on his back with his knees partially bent and his thighs turned outward. His bones are less capable of retaining calcium and phosphorus, causing them to become weak and eventually brittle.

CAUSES—Scurvy is a malnutrition disease, caused by a diet that is deficient in **vitamin C**.

NATURAL REMEDIES

• Scurvy responds, in as little as 2-3 days, to a daily intake of 100-200 mg of vitamin C. Gradually increase the dosage, as the patient is able to do so, to 1,000-3,000 mg for 30 days.

• **Fresh fruits and green leafy vegetables** are also rich in vitamin C.

• In order to promote blood and bone repair from

damage caused by scurvy, a **well-balanced diet that is high in protein and iron** is also needed.

• Supply **bioflavonoids** (vitamin P), which work closely with vitamin C. These will be found in foods with vitamin C.

ENCOURAGEMENT—When temptations and trials rush in upon us, let us go to God and agonize with Him in prayer. He will not turn us away empty, but will give us grace and strength to overcome and break the power of the enemy. 2 Peter 1:2-3.

KWASHIORKOR
(Protein Starvation)

SYMPTOMS—Retarded growth, changes in skin and hair, diarrhea, loss of appetite, edema, and nervous irritability.

CAUSES—Kwashiorkor *(kwash-uh-OR-kor)* is a serious nutritional disease. Adequate carbohydrates are provided, but **not enough protein**.

This condition generally occurs in children, between the ages of one and five, who have been weaned from milk to **a diet primarily of starches and sugars**.

Low-blood protein levels cannot hold water in the blood vessels; water just goes into the cells and produces a distended, bloated belly and edema.

There are 22 amino acids which children need and 20 which adults need. Complete protein meals should be the objective.

NATURAL REMEDIES

• Add **protein** to the diet. In underdeveloped countries, a **skim milk formula** is usually first given, because the child's fat-absorption ability has been damaged. Other foods are gradually added until he can handle a **balanced diet**.

• Correct all **vitamin-mineral** deficiencies which may exist.

ENCOURAGEMENT—To obey the commandments of God is the only way to obtain His favor. "Go forward" should be the Christian's watchword. Let God lead you by His Written Word, and you will not take missteps. Psalm 46:11. "If . . we suffer with Him . . we may be also glorified together." Romans 8:17.

GASTRO-INTESTINAL - 13 - WEIGHT

OVERWEIGHT

SYMPTOMS—The person is heavier by at least 20% than the average for his height and weight.

CHART 1068: Recommended Weight Tables, by ages for men and women Obesity (480, 899)

CAUSES—Obesity is an excess of body fat; too much is being stored. It is also consuming more calories than one can use.

The average human body has 30-40 million fat cells. That is too many for some of us. It has been said that when a person makes an extra fat cell, in order to store some extra fat, he will keep that extra cell for the rest of his life—even though he may remove the fat from it.

Poor diet, fatty foods, and a lack of exercise are common causes of overweight. Other factors include **diabetes** *(656)*, **hypoglycemia** *(653)*, and **endocrine glands** *(1058)* which do not function properly. **Boredom, tension, and love of food** are other causes. Another factor is **inadequate intake or absorption of key nutrients**, which causes fat to be stored instead of used.

Each year in America, over $30 billion is spent on foods or equipment to help lose weight.

Obesity can be involved with hormonal imbalances in the **hypothalamus, pituitary, pineal, thyroid, adrenals, or pancreas**.

Obese people tend to store fat, not only in regular fat cells, but also in muscle tissue. Then, when they try to lose weight (via a weight loss diet), they lose both fat from the fat cells and protein from the muscles—before they lose fat from the muscles. The best solution is to keep fit, so you do not store fat in your muscle tissue.

It is said that 90% of obese people overeat and binge because they are eating **meals with too many empty calories**, which do not supply enough minerals (especially trace minerals) and vitamins.

SPECIAL HEALTH RISKS—Here are the health risks associated with excessive overweight:

(1) *High risks:* Diabetes melitius, Insulin resitance, High blood pressure, High blood fat levels (including cholesterol), Gallstones, Sleep apnea, Decreased physical fitness, Kidney disease.

(2) *Moderate risks:* Arthritis, Fibromyalgia, Heart disease, Lower back pain, Medical complications with surgery, Peripheral viascular disease, Stroke.

(3) *Low risks:* Accidents, Breast cancer, Colon cancer, Congenital defects in offspring, Depression, Hormone disorders, Infertility, Uterine cancer.

NATURAL REMEDIES

FOOD AND NUTRITION

People try to cut down on the calories, when they should make sure they steadily obtain **good basic nutrition, day after day**. Without adequate nourishment, they will generally binge or go off their special diets. It is now known that steady eating is better than losing weight and regaining it, losing it and regaining it. The up and down program damages the body and makes it more susceptible to disease. The 14-year Framingham Study established that repeated crash diets increase the risk of heart disease.

• To maintain **a program of weight loss** (that is, an ongoing program of gradually losing a little weight), calculate how many calories you need each day, in this way: **Multiply your weight by 10. Then add 30% (about a third) to the total.** This total is the amount of calories you can consume daily, without gaining the weight back which you have already lost. Assuming that you are moderately active, eating anything less than that total amount should cause you to lose weight. (*Example:* 150 lb. x 10 = 1,500 + 30% (450) = 1,950 calories.)

• **Crash diets** are useless. Quick weight loss tends to come back quickly, resulting in elevated cholesterol.

• Test for **food allergies** and eliminate them. *See Food Allergies (848) and Pulse Test (847).*

• Consistently eat a **lighter, but more nourishing, diet**. Do not eat food for fun; eat for health.

• Avoid **junk food, fatty food, fried food, processed food, caffeine, nicotine, and soft drinks**. Do not drink **alcohol** in any form. It has calories without giving nourishment. It inhibits the burning of fat deposits.

• Drink at least 8-10 glasses of **water** each day.

• **Do not skip breakfast and lunch**. Make breakfast the largest, lunch a moderate meal, and supper the lightest. Or skip the evening meal entirely. Do not eat before bedtime or at night. Best: Eat nothing after 3 p.m.

• Include Nova Scotia **dulse** or Norwegian **kelp** in your diet, to supply trace minerals.

• Include a good **vitamin-mineral supplement**. Be sure to obtain enough **fiber** in your diet. It fills you up, without adding body weight. **Phenylalanine**, an amino acid, helps in reducing weight because of its effect on the thyroid. It increases endorphins in the brain.

• Powdered **barley malt** sweetener is quite sweet, yet contains fewer calories than other sweets. Use it to sweeten your food. Do not end a meal with sweets.

• Here is an **all-in-one food drink** which, because it is so nourishing, can help you lose weight—if you will let it be your only nourishment at a meal. It is filled with nutrition! Mix the following ingredients in a blender and drink: 1 cup rice milk, 1 cup soy milk, 1 cup fruit juice (apple, orange, or other), 1 banana, 4 fresh strawberries (if available), 1 tsp. blackstrap molasses, 1 Tbsp. black cherry concentrate, 1 Tbsp. powdered "green" (Barley Green, etc.), 1-2 Tbsp. powdered nutritional yeast, and 1 Tbsp. flaxseed oil. Drink it slowly, leave the table, and eat nothing more till the next meal.

A BASIC DIET

Go on a good basic diet and stay on it. Here is an example of one:

• Eat moderate amounts of **raw citrus and sub-** acid fruits, but no sweet fruits (such as grapes or dried fruits). **No fruit juices, except diluted grape juice** taken a half hour before the meal, to reduce appetite. No bananas.

• Eat as much **raw vegetables** as you want. The only cooked ones should be **fresh and conservatively cooked vegetables**. Do not use frozen, fried, or canned vegetables.

• Primarily eat vegetarian protein foods with some moderation: **beans, sprouted beans, seeds, nuts**, etc.

• All **refined carbohydrates** are forbidden. This includes **sugar, alcohol, white-flour products, quick oats, most packaged cereals, and processed starch**.

• Eat only well-cooked, unrefined **brown rice, barley, rye, millet, buckwheat, wheat berries, bulgur, corn**, and other whole grains. Do not grind them, but cook and eat them in their natural state.

• Use **cold-pressed unsaturated oils**, plus **lemon juice**, and possibly some herbs for flavoring. **Flaxseed oil** (2 tsp. daily) will help you burn excess calories. Use no other oil. Put the raw oil on your food at the table.

• Eat **spirulina** 30 minutes before meals. It is very nourishing, adds energy, and will reduce your appetite.

ADDITIONAL SUGGESTIONS

• **Do not overeat**, ever. It is a very, very bad habit to get into. But it is a habit which can be stopped.

• When you end a meal, make a determined habit to **eat nothing until the next meal**.

• When eating, concentrate on **quietly eating and thinking about when you should stop**. Do not just relax, talk, socialize, and eat and eat. Do not listen to the radio, read a book, or watch television. Stick to your work of eating lightly of nourishing food, and quitting when you should.

• **You will not be harmed** by finishing the meal a little hungry. Keep that in mind. Frankly, you will be greatly helped; for your stomach will gradually shrink to the size it ought to be.

• People who are overweight do best to eat as much **food raw** as much as possible rather than cooked food. If cooked, the food should be baked, steamed, or boiled; never fried.

• Go on a cleansing **juice fast** once a week.

• A regular exercise program is needed. Aerobic exercises are better than other kinds. This simply means **exercise done out in the open air**. It helps lose weight and build strength. It strengthens the heart, arteries, and veins. It also invigorates the vital organs and endocrine glands.

• **Walking** uses up to 120 calories per hour while actual jogging burns 440 calories per hour. But walking remains the best exercise.

• **Swimming** is usually done in cold water; and this triggers the body to store extra fat as protection against the cold. So swimming does not help one lose weight.

• Regular **bowel movements** are important. Reduce **salt** intake. **Gum chewing** gets the stomach moving and makes you hungry.

• **Do not overfeed children** with an excess of starches and cow's milk. Most infants receive starches by four months; but that is far too early and only leads to later allergies or celiac disease *(473-474)*. Children who are overweight by the age of 2 turn into fat adults more frequently than others.

• If you are only moderately overweight, do not worry about the comments of your thin friends; they probably wish they could gain a little.

HERBS

• Take 3 grams of **plaintain** leaves (or 3 grams of **psyllium**, the seed of that plant) in water 30 minutes before meals. In an Italian research study, women who were 60% over their proper weight did this; and they lost more weight than another group of women who ate less. What to do? Simply mix 1 tsp. **psyllium seed** with juice or water and eat it before each meal. (But some are allergic to psyllium; if so, stop using it.)

• **Astragalus** improves nutrient absorption, thus adding energy. **Green tea** helps you reduce weight.

• Adding fresh **chickweed** (a common weed) to your salad each day will help you lose weight. Eating one whole, fresh **pineapple** daily also helps do it.

• **Ginger** and **butcher's broom** improves fat metabolism. **Fenugreek** helps dissolve fat in the liver.

• A study of 25,000 Seventh-day Adventists found that those who ate the most **nuts** were the slimmest. Nuts are rich in serotonin, which helps make us feel full. Adventists are vegetarians. But **Meat eaters** would have a harder time losing weight, since their diet is heavy in grease and saturated fat.

J.H. KELLOGG, M.D., PRESCRIPTIONS FOR OVERWEIGHT AND ITS COMPLICATIONS *(how to give these water therapies: pp. 206-275 / list of treatments: pp. 206-207 / Hydrotherapy Disease Index: pp. 273-275)*
INCREASE OXIDATION OF HYDROCARBONS—Moderately prolonged cold baths, especially **Wet Sheet Pack. Shallow Bath, Cold Shower**, Dripping Sheet Rub, Plunge Bath, and **moderate exercise** several times daily. The Cold Bath may be advantageously preceded by the Radiant Heat Bath or some other form of **sweating bath** that is not too prolonged. Exercise should always be preceded by a cold bath of sufficient duration to lower the temperature a few tenths of a degree.
CARDIAC WEAKNESS—Cold Compress over the heart (except in fatty degeneration of the heart) 15-30 minutes, 3 times daily; **graduated exercises outdoors** when possible.
CONTRAINDICATIONS—Avoid prolonged Hot Baths unless immediately followed by a cold bath.
GENERAL METHOD—The general plan of treatment must be prolonged cold baths and vigorous exercise while reducing the daily ration of food to the lowest point consistent with the maintenance of his strength. The treatment must never be conducted in such a way as to diminish his muscular or nervous energy. If he complains of feeling weak

or debilitated, the vigor of the treatment must be diminished. There should be a steady gain in muscular strength accompanying the loss of flesh. His strength should be tested weekly. Do not use Hot Baths; for they are especially debilitating.

ENCOURAGEMENT—Victories are not gained by ceremonies or display, but by simple obedience to the Lord God of heaven. He who trusts in this Leader will never know defeat. Proverbs 3:5-10.

UNDERWEIGHT
(Thinness)

SYMPTOMS—The person weighs at least 10% less than an average person of his height and weight.

In addition to thinness, symptoms may include hunger, dizziness, fatigue, weakness, sensitivity to cold, and loss of ambition.

CAUSES—For some, being underweight is seen as a problem; for others it is no problem at all. Actually, as one ages, being unusually slim can be an advantage in a number of ways. If a person is in good health, as the years pass, there is less and less reason to gain weight. Thinner people live longer and are in less danger from heart disease.

But underweight is sometimes associated with health problems. This especially should be a cause for concern if unintended, sudden weight loss has occurred.

REASONS FOR SUDDEN WEIGHT LOSS—Try, if possible, to ascertain the cause of the unplanned weight loss or inability to gain weight. Here is a list of several possible causes:

• Unplanned-for weight loss may be caused by **an inability by the gastro-intestinal tract to digest and absorb food** properly, resulting from **ulcerative colitis** *(463)*, **diverticulitis** *(466)*, etc.

• It may be caused by **intestinal parasites** *(861)*, or **problems with the liver** *(445-451)* or **pancreas** *(444-445, 655-659)*.

• It may be caused by **digestive enzyme deficiency, allergy, or food sensitivity**.

• It may be caused by endocrine imbalances, such as **diabetes** *(656)*, **hyperthyroidism** *(661)*, or (sometimes) **hypothyroidism** *(659)*. If you are both underweight and feel cold all the time, you may be hypothyroid. Problems in the **thyroid, pancreas** *(444-445, 655-659)*, **or adrenals** *(653-655)* can make weight gain impossible. **Hypoglycemics** *(653)* and **diabetics** *(656)* have an especially hard time maintaining proper weight.

• It may be caused by a **chronic illness, surgery, stress** *(555)*, **or emotional trauma** (such as the death of a loved one). It may be caused by **smoking** *(880)*.

• It may be caused by **surgery, chemotherapy**

(876), **radiation therapy** *(876)*, **medicinal or street drugs** *(953-963)*, or **AIDS** *(806)*.

• In addition, there may be **an eating disorder**: The person eats too little (anorexia, *472*) or, in some cases, eats too much (bulimia, *473*).

• **Zinc deficiency** and some **wasting diseases**, such as **cancer** *(782, 792-796)*, can reduce appetite.

A valuable diagnostic aid is the consistency of the bowel movement and a check for undigested foods.

In infants and children, the cause may be **not enough food**; in old people, it may result from **disinterest in eating** or **poverty**.

You should especially be concerned about an infant or small child who suddenly seems to stop gaining weight normally. This may be caused by **celiac disease** *(473-474)* or something else.

The problem is usually that, for one reason or another, thin people have a harder time digesting and absorbing food than those who can easily gain weight.

NATURAL REMEDIES

Your body is having a hard time meeting the challenges of life and needs help. The recommendations are simple enough:

• Eat a **nourishing diet**, such as is repeatedly outlined in this book. For some people, it should include **more calories and protein** than should normally be eaten. But for many who are habitually underweight, the solution is to continue eating moderate-sized meals—while only eating the most **nourishing food** (no junk or processed food). Adequate and complete proteins are essential.

• If you want to go on a careful **weight-gain program**, try to eat 2,500 to 3,000 calories a day, including 100 grams of protein and 300 grams of complex carbohydrates. Eat only nourishing food; nothing processed, no "foodless food." Be sure and correct **vitamin and mineral deficiencies**. You may need to take **digestive enzymes** and/or supplemental **hydrochloric acid** (betaine HCl).

• Obtain moderate outdoor **exercise** each day. This will help your system digest the food. Take a walk after every meal.

• Obtain adequate **rest** at night; and **try to lie down and rest 15, 30, or 60 minutes before each meal**. This is important and will strengthen your body for the challenge of coping successfully with another meal.

• Avoid **stress** of various kinds.

• Eat in relaxed surroundings. **Do not eat when you are nervous or upset**.

• Try to **maintain regularity** in all your habits and activities, including when you eat.

• You may have a **food allergy**, such as wheat, cow's milk, etc. *See Allergies (848-860) and Pulse Test (847)*.

• It is extremely important that you not eat **fried food, junk food or drink, and processed food**. Avoid **caffeine, tobacco, and alcohol.** If you are able to do so, do not take **medicinal drugs.**

• For infants, **mashed bananas** are more easily digested than some other foods.

Last but not least: If you are normally thin, but feel good, ignore the comments of others who say you need to gain weight. Some of them wish they could be thinner.

If you are determined to add more pounds, the experts tell us that, for adults, weight should not be gained at the rate of more than a pound a week.

ENCOURAGEMENT—If you will maintain a meek and quiet spirit, which is always obedient to God's Word, you will be spared many of the troubles in our world. Let Christ live in you and help others through you. Matthew 6:25, 30-32.

POOR APPETITE

SYMPTOMS—Day after day, a person does not want to eat hardly anything. He picks at his food and has little interest in eating.

CAUSES—A poor appetite may trace back to one or another of several possible causes. A medicinal **drug** he is taking may be the reason. Or he could be using too much **alcohol, tobacco, or street drugs**. It could be heavy **metal poisoning, nutritional deficiencies, depression, stress, or an injury**.

NATURAL REMEDIES

• In order to stimulate the appetite, the **food** should look good, taste good, and nourish the system. Eat **whole grains, fruits, vegetables, nuts, and legumes**.

• Do not drink **liquids** immediately before or during the meal. They fill the stomach so it does not want anything else.

• Eat **smaller meals** and more of them. Eat a **small amount** of quality food and nothing more till the next meal.

• Decide that you are going to **enjoy the food** and that you want to eat it. Be thankful that you have food to eat.

• Immediately after the meal, and at other times during the day, **get outside and walk**, work in the garden, or do something worthwhile.

• Forget yourself and **find someone else to help**. All around you are people who need encouragement.

• Stop **smoking**, drinking **liquor**, taking **hard drugs**, or doing anything that is damaging your health and interest in life.

ENCOURAGEMENT—The law of God is simple, and easily understood. If the children of men would, to the best of their ability, obey this law, they would gain strength of mind and power of discernment to comprehend still more of God's purposes and plans.

CELLULITE
(Lumpy Fat)

SYMPTOMS—Lumpy pockets of fat on the thighs,

insides of upper arms, and gluteus maximus.

CAUSES—With the passing of years, strands of fibrous tissue anchor to the skin. As they do this, they pull the skin inward. This causes fat cells to push upward. Women especially tend to have this problem in the buttocks, hips, and thighs.

NATURAL REMEDIES

There is no known cure, but there are suggestions you may wish to try:

• **Lose weight**. This will help reduce the protruding pockets of fat. Go on a cleansing **juice fast** once a week.

• Eat plenty of **fresh fruits and vegetables**, including plenty of **leafy greens**. These are both nourishing and lower in calories. Improve your general pattern of diet and take **vitamin / mineral supplements**. Eat **whole grains, nuts, and legumes**.

• Keep the channels of elimination open, so excess fluids and fat can be more easily removed from the body. Drink plenty of **water**, keep the **bowels** open,

maintain **regularity**, and avoid constipation.

• Avoid all **refined, fried, fatty, or canned foods**. Do not use carbonated drinks or liquor. Salty foods make your problem worse. Do not use **caffeine** or **tobacco**. Both constrict your blood vessels and make the cellulite more prominent.

• **Exercise** out in the fresh air and **breathe** deeply. The oxygen helps burn fat; and the better ventilation helps empty carbon dioxide from body cells. Do muscle-toning **exercises**. Take a vigorous, arm-swinging **walk** after every meal. Obtain adequate **rest** at night.

• To whatever degree you can, avoid **stress, tension, and time schedules**. Cellulite builds up when muscles become tense; and muscles tense when you are agitated.

• Hawthorn extract helps reduce blood fat levels.

ENCOURAGEMENT—The Lord has honored us by choosing us as His soldiers. Let us fight bravely for Him, maintaining the right in every transaction. Stand for the right though the heavens fall. God will help you. Psalm 71:3.

More Encouragement

"Those who are true to their calling as messengers for God will not seek honor for themselves. Love for self will be swallowed up in love for Christ. No rivalry will mar the precious cause of the gospel. They will recognize that it is their work to proclaim, as did John the Baptist, 'Behold the Lamb of God, which taketh away the sin of the world.' John 1:29. They will lift up Jesus, and with Him humanity will be lifted up. 'Thus saith the high and lofty One that inhabiteth eternity, whose name is Holy; I dwell in the high and holy place, with him also that is of a contrite and humble spirit, to revive the spirit of the humble, and to revive the heart of the contrite ones.' Isaiah 57:15."

—Desire of Ages, 179-180

"Our Redeemer thirsts for recognition. He hungers for the sympathy and love of those whom He has purchased with His own blood. He longs with inexpressible desire that they should come to Him and have life. As the mother watches for the smile of recognition from her little child, which tells of the dawning of intelligence, so does Christ watch for the expression of grateful love, which shows that spiritual life is begun in the soul."

—Desire of Ages, 191

"In all who are under the training of God is to be revealed a life that is not in harmony with the world, its customs, or its practices; and everyone needs to have a personal experience in obtaining a knowledge of the will of God. We must individually hear Him speaking to the heart. When every other voice is hushed, and in quietness we wait before Him, the silence of the soul makes more distinct the voice of God."

—Desire of Ages, 363

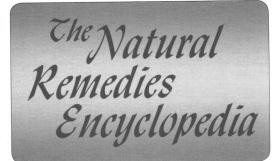

The Natural Remedies Encyclopedia

- Disease Section 6 -
Urinary

Urinary System: Physiology 1018 / Pictures 1040

U
R
I
N

"Ye shall serve the Lord your God . . and I will take away sickness from the midst of thee."   —*Exodus 23:25*

"If thou wilt diligently hearken to the voice of the Lord thy God, and wilt do that which is right in His sight, and wilt give ear to His commandments, and keep all His statutes, I will put none of these diseases upon thee, which I have brought upon the Egyptians: for I am the Lord that healeth thee."

—Exodus 15:26

"In God I will praise His Word, in God I have put my trust; I will not fear what flesh can do unto me."

—Psalm 56:4

"The name of the Lord is a strong tower: the righteous runneth into it, and is safe."   *—Proverbs 18:10*

FOR MORE NATURAL REMEDIES:
HERBS: Herb Contents (pp. 129-130) will help you locate the 126 most important herbs and the diseases each one can treat. How to prepare herbs (132). How to use them (141-189)
HYDROTHERAPY: Therapy Contents (pp. 206-207) and its Disease Index (263-265) will lead you to over 100 water therapies and many more remedies. DIS. INDEX: 1211- / GEN. INDEX: 1221-

VITAMINS AND MINERALS: Contents (100-101). Using 101-124. Dosages (124). Others (117-)
CARING FOR THE SICK: Home care for a sick person (28-36). The healing crisis (36-39)
WOMEN'S SECTIONS: Female Organs (672) Pregnancy (701). Childbirth (765). Infancy, Childhood (722). Women's Herbs (754, 760)
EMERGENCIES: (973-). FIRST AID: (990-)

Section 6 - Urinary

URINE PROBLEMS

NATURAL REMEDIES

WATER THERAPY

Here are a number of hydrotherapy treatments for several different urine difficulties. This brief summary is taken from the *Hydrotherapy* section of this *Encyclopedia (206-275)*, which will provide many more details on how to give the treatments:

Albumin in urine (Albuminuria): **Hot Blanket Pack** and **other sweating measures** to maintain cutaneous activity, repeated every 2-4 hours *(245)*.

Incontinence: **Percussion Douche** to spine, **Neutral Sitz Bath** for 15-30 minutes.

Urine too acid: Free use of **fruit** and **water drinking** in the forenoon.

Urinary suppression: **Hot Blanket Pack** *(245)*, followed by **Dry Chest Pack** *(229)*.

Nocturia: **Revulsive Sitz Bath**. Begin at 100° and increase rapidly to 106°-115° F. (with a **footbath** at 110°-112° F.) for 3-8 minutes. Keep the head cool with cold cloths over forehead or around back of neck. Finish with a cold (55°-65° F.) **pail pour** to hips *(254)*.

DIURETIC HERBS

These are herbs which increase the flow of urine. Whatever the problem may be with the kidneys, a major part of the solution is to increase the flow of urine. This is how the kidneys clean themselves out. For this purpose, you need to drink a large amount of liquids (either good water or fruit juices; no junk beverages), and take diuretic herbs.

• **Corn silk** tea is generally considered the best diuretic herb. *Go to p. 127 to learn how to use it.*

• **Celery seeds** act on the kidneys. Eat crushed **parsley**. Eat **grapes** freely to induce a free flow of urine. **Juniper berries** eaten in dried form produce a powerful diuretic action. Add raw **onions** to food to increase urine flow. Make a **salad** of raw tomato, onion, garlic, lemon juice, and oil.

• To improve the excretion of fluids, mix equal parts of **fennel root, celery root, parsley root, and asparagus root**. Steep 1 tsp. in ½ cup boiling hot water. Take ½-1 cup daily, unsweetened, in mouthful doses.

• Here is a powerful diuretic combination: Add ½ tsp. each of **juniper berries, dandelion root, and broom tops** (the herb, not your kitchen broom) to

1 pint water. Boil on a low flame till it is down to ½ pint. Strain, put in a jar, drink 2 Tbsp. 3 times daily.

• *Here are a few of the best known of over a hundred diuretic herbs:* You will find most of them listed in our chapter on herbs *(its index is on pp. 107-108)*. **Agrimony, asparagus, balm of Gilead, barberry, bayberry, bistort, black cohosh, blue cohosh, boneset, buchu, buckthorn, bugleweed, burdock, chamomile, catnip, celery, chaparral, chicory, cleavers, corn silk, dandelion, elecampane, elder, fennel, fleabane, juniper berry, kava kava, lady's slipper, marshmallow, mugwort, mullein, onion, Oregon grape, Peruvian barik, pipsissewa, plantain, pleurisy root, prickly ash, pumpkin seeds, purslane, radish, sarsaparilla, sassafras, saw palmetto, selfheal, shave grass, sheep sorrel, shepherd's purse, smartweed, sorrel, squaw vine, tansy, uva ursa, valerian, vervain, watermelon seeds, white oak, wild yam, wood sorrel, yarrow,**

ENCOURAGEMENT—The one who had revolted in heaven offered Christ the kingdoms of this world, if He would pay homage to the principles of evil; but He would not be bought. When Satan comes to you, answer him, "It is written"; and, in Christ's strength, stand true for God. Zechariah 13:9.

"This poor man cried, and the Lord heard him, and saved him out of all his troubles . . The eyes of the Lord are upon the righteous, and His ears are open unto their cry." Psalm 34:6, 15

ENURESIS
(Bed-Wetting)

SYMPTOMS—Bed-wetting during the night and sometimes during the day; this is usually after the age of 3 for girls and 4 for boys.

A slight loss of urine during the day by adults.

CAUSES—There can be a bladder infection that releases the urine. The infection in boys can be a residual effect of fecal contamination from earlier times when diapers were used. In girls, it can be the result of improper cleaning after urination. (They need to wipe from the front to back, not back to front.) Another cause can be stress from tensions in the home.

In adults, the cause can be the pressure at the office or shop to keep working and not promptly answer the urge to go to the restroom.

CHART - 1055: Uremia [Toxic substances in urine] (486)

CHARTS 1052-1053: Urine characteristics in 9 diseases / Urine pH causesS

NATURAL REMEDIES

• Teach correct hygiene methods to the child. Identify the pathogenic bacteria by means of a urine culture. Begin providing an antibacterial remedy. Cranberry juice is both a natural diuretic, and its acidity helps purify the bladder. Garlic, echinacea, and burdock root tea are also very helpful.

• Train yourself to pay attention to the slightest beginning of the urge to urinate. By responding to it promptly, you can regain control in this matter.

—*Also see Bed-wetting in the childhood section (486, 734).*

URINE RETENTION

SYMPTOMS—Flow of urine is lessening. Great pain is felt in the bladder; and the odor of urine is on the body. Almost total suppression can produce extreme pain in the back and bladder, and even convulsions. There is always a great desire to urinate.

CAUSES—There can be a blockage of some type. *See Urine Problems (486), Kidney Problems (489), Bladder Problems (495, 712), and other topics in this Urinary section.*

Urine retention is generally caused by **inflammation** and **swelling** in the bladder and its outlet. **Excess urine** in it causes the bladder to enlarge and can cause great pain. It can be caused by an obstruction, inflammation, and swelling at the bladder outlet, or along the prostate.

NATURAL REMEDIES

• In case of a serious stoppage, the first need is for a catheter to be placed through the urethra in order to allow the urine to flow. Attention can then be given to removing the cause of the obstruction.

• *Important:* See Diuretic Herbs in Urine Problems (486).

• *Poor urine flow:* Take a **cold sitz bath** (cold partial bath, as you sit in the bathtub). Stop using **salt**. Drink 2 quarts a day of 50-50 **orange juice and water**.

• *Alternate method:* Take a **hot sitz bath** repeatedly, followed by a **short cold bath**. If bedridden, **apply hot, followed by short cold**, over bladder, genital area, and entire length of spine.

• **Drink more water and take herbs which increase urine flow. Corn silk** tea is the best; others include **juniper berries, carrot tops, comfrey, plantain, cleavers, chickweed**. *See list under Urinary Problems (486).*

• Give a high **enema** of catnip tea. This is important in helping the urine to again begin flowing.

• Steep the following in a quart of boiling water: 1 teaspoon **goldenseal** and a half teaspoon each of **boric acid** and **myrrh**. Strain through a fine cloth and inject through a fountain syringe. Retain as long as possible. You can moisten the tip with slippery elm tea. Slippery elm is slippery!

• A **cold shower** often helps.

STOPPED URINE FLOW

• Almost total urine suppression generally points to the kidneys as the problem. There is a blockage.

If the urine has not been secreted for several days, there will be severe symptoms (such as convulsions, extreme pain the back and bladder, and a great desire to urinate).

Put the person to **bed** and give him **quiet**; give him a very warm high **enema** of catnip tea. This will bring great relief. Also apply hot **fomentations**, wrung out of **smartweed** tea, to the bladder and lumbar region (small of back). Give 2-3 hot **sitz baths** in a bathtub each day.

• An especially helpful remedy is a strong (hot as can be taken) tea of **catnip**, given as an **enema**. Drink it freely.

• Steep a heaping tsp. of **yarrow** in a cup of boiled water for 20 minutes. Drink a cup cold before each meal and before retiring.

• Insert a soft **catheter** and draw out the urine.

—*Also see the kidney and bladder diseases in this Urinary section.*

ENCOURAGEMENT—Christ's victory over Satan was as complete as had been Adam's failure. So we may resist temptation and force Satan to depart from us. It is in totally yielding ourselves to God that, in His strength, we can have power to resist the devil and come off more than conquerors. Psalm 41:1-3.

INCONTINENCE
(Urinary Stress Incontinence)

SYMPTOMS—Occasional dribbling. An involuntary loss of urine (in very small amounts) accompanies coughing, sneezing, laughing, walking, running, lifting, or any sudden shock or strain.

CAUSES—Incontinence tends to occur in women more than men, although older men may also have it.

The most common cause of urinary incontinence in women is a loss of muscle tone in the perineal area, due to multiple births. The second most frequent cause in women is chronic bladder infection.

Possible causes include **repeated births, poor pelvic floor tone, damage to pelvic floor** by the physician at time of delivery, **visceroptosis, overweight, poor abdominal tone, failure to do prenatal and postnatal exercises**.

A wide variety of other causes can be involved—including **food allergies, hypoglycemia, multiple dystrophy, multiple sclerosis, cancer, stroke, injuries, and surgical damage.**

It may follow a **prolonged labor** during childbirth, resulting from the stretching of the pelvic floor. If postpartum exercises are not done, this problem (which may disappear for years) can later return.

Incontinence is far less likely in the nullipara (women who have never delivered a child).

Urinary incontinence can occur in men as a result of **prostate surgery**.

URIN

NATURAL REMEDIES

EXERCISES

• The best pelvic floor exercises are variations of the **Kegel exercise**; these should begin early in pregnancy, or before, and continue on for at least 3 months after childbirth. These exercises strengthen certain muscles.

• Using your **urinary sphincter muscle**, slow urine flow and eventually stop it. Doing this helps you recognize the muscles involved. Later practice stopping the urine flow, by holding for 1-2 seconds and repeating 6-8 times, as you urinate. You should eventually be able to stop urine flow completely with no leakage. Learn to slowly relax pelvic floor muscles in stages from full contraction to full relaxation.

• Practice tightening these muscles at various other times during the day. Repeat 6-8 times each session and 50-100 times a day. Hold each contraction for 2-5 seconds; then relax. These are called "Kegel exercises."

• When doing these exercises, do not hold your breath. Bear down; that is, push down on the pelvic floor or contract the buttocks, inner thighs, or abdominal muscles. When beginning, do not exhaust the pelvic muscles. Whenever contractions weaken, discontinue at that time. Build muscle strength slowly; there is no rush.

HERBS

When this disorder is not caused by some other disease (such as gout, palsy, or kidney stones), do this:

• Mix equal parts of **white poplar bark, bistort root, valerian, sumach berries, and white pond lily**. Steep a heaping tsp. in a cup of boiling water. Drink 1 cup 1 hour before each meal and on retiring (at least 4 cups a day). Or take **plantain** tea by itself for similar effects. Increase the dose if necessary.

OTHER THINGS TO DO

• Drink cranberry juice. Avoid **alcohol, caffeine, tobacco, and grapefruit juice**. Use **cranberry juice** instead.

• Reduce general **fluid** intake, but not too much.

• Avoid **constipation**. Lose **weight**.

• **Go** when you have to; do not wait, or you weaken bladder control. And involuntary dribbling will afterward begin. This is very important.

• **Double voiding** is helpful: After voiding, stand up and sit down again. Lean forward slightly at the knees and try again.

• Sleep either on the side or face.

J.H. KELLOGG, M.D., PRESCRIPTIONS FOR INCONTINENCE AND ITS COMPLICATIONS (*how to give these water therapies: pp. 207-272 / list of treatments: pp. 206-207 / Hydrotherapy Disease Index: pp. 273-275*)

TO INCREASE ENERGY OF BLADDER—Cold Plantar (bottom of foot) Douche for 1-2 minutes. **Cold Footbath**, using running water over the feet. **Cold Percussion Douche**

to hips and legs at 60°-65° F. **Cold Douche** to lower back. Cold Fan Douche, at 65° F., over bladder. **Cold rubbing Sitz Bath**. **Colonic**, begin at 100° and lower 1° daily to 80° F.

RELIEVE VESICAL IRRITATION—Revulsive Sitz Bath. **Hot Pack** to pelvis. Prolonged **Neutral Sitz Bath**, following **Revulsive Sitz Bath**. **Neutral Douche** to lower spine. **Revulsive Douche** to feet and legs.

IMPROVE GENERAL NERVE TONE—Cold Mitten Friction or **Cold Towel Rub**, **Cold Pack** to pelvis, general Cold Douche, Shallow Bath, **Wet Sheet Rub**.

—*For incontinence in children, see Bed-wetting (486, 734).*

ENCOURAGEMENT—The gift of God to mankind was immense. It could not be said that anything was withheld. God gave all in Christ. Accept Him and you become a child of God, known and loved by Him. Matthew 10:42.

The truths of the Bible, received, will uplift the mind from its earthliness and debasement. If the Word of God were appreciated as it should be, both young and old would possess an inward strength of character, an indomitableness of principle, that would enable them to resist temptation.

HEMATURIA
(Blood in Urine)

SYMPTOMS—Blood appears in the urine. This blood shows a smoky sediment, and is reddish brown. Urine may be slightly smoky, reddish, or very red.

CAUSES—Red, or reddish, urine may be due to blood in the urine, known as hematuria, or to senna or rhubarb, which may color the urine either brown or orange. The urine should never contain blood, protein, or sugar.

If the blood is well-mixed with the urine, it is probably from the kidneys. If it is clotted in tubular casts of ureters, it is from the kidneys or urethra. If it is passed at the beginning of urination, it is from the urethra; if at the end, it is from the bladder.

Bleeding from the kidneys produces smoky urine, which may be bright red. Bleeding from the urethra is always bright red and precedes urination. Bleeding from the urine vesicle produces bright red urine, which is not uniform.

Other causes of blood in urine can be a **lesion of the urinary tract, contamination during menstruation, prostatic disease, tumors, poisoning (especially carbolic acid and cantharides), malaria, toxemias, and calculus (kidney stones), and bladder infection**.

NATURAL REMEDIES

• Apply a very **cold water spray** to the perineum.

• Read the other sections, elsewhere in this urinary section on urine, kidneys, and bladder.

CHARTS 1052-1053: Urine characteristics in 9 diseases / Urine pH causeS

• Drink herb teas which have hemostatic and astringent properties, and act on the urinary organs that bleed. Such herbs would include **horseweed**. Make an infusion or decoction of dry leaves. It is hemostatic and reduces kidney inflammation. Another herb is **smartweed**. Make an infusion of its powdered, dry leaves. This stops hemmorrhage.

• Dr. Christopher prescribes drinking a tea made from powdered **acorns** or powdered **cups** they are formed within.

ENCOURAGEMENT—When a soul receives Christ, he receives power to live the life of Christ. He becomes a new man in Christ. He can obey the Ten Commandments and resist sin; for he has God's help.

SCALDING URINE

SYMPTOMS—The urine seems to burn as it is ejected.

CAUSES—There is an excess of uric acid and other acids in the system.

NATURAL REMEDIES
• Cleanse the system by taking the following herbs, and the scalding urine will be eliminated. Mix equal parts of **fennel, burdock, slippery elm**. Steep 1 tsp. 20 minutes in a cup of boiled water. Drink 1 cold cupful before each meal and on retiring. A tea of **cubeb** berries is also excellent, prepared and used in the same way.

• **Change your diet. Meat eating** is a major cause of excess acids in the system. It fills the body with purines and other strong acids which settle in the joints, causing arthritis and other painful conditions. **Soft drinks, liquor, junk food, sugar, and processed foods** all contain harmful substances.

ENCOURAGEMENT—"Weeping may endure for a night, but joy cometh in the morning." Psalm 30:5. If faithful, soon we will see Jesus when He returns for His children; and what a happy day that will be! Oh, my friend, we must be ready every day! Trust Him and obey all His Word. He will not fail His promises to you.

URINARY - 2 - KIDNEY

KIDNEY PROBLEMS

PROBLEMS AND CAUSES—In addition to other conditions mentioned in this section on the kidneys, there are less known diseases which can be just as serious. These include:

Renal tubular acidosis: The kidneys fail to reabsorb bicarbonate properly, resulting in inadequate ammonia production and acid excretion. This leads to a severe lack of fluid and potassium

in the body, and an excess of acid. The bones can become deranged.

Hydronephrosis: The kidneys and bladder become filled with urine, due to obstruction of the flow.

Glomerulonephritis: This is an inflammation of the tiny kidney filtering units, sometimes resulting from a bacterial infection in the body.

Uremia: A toxic waste buildup in the blood, due to kidney malfunction.

In all of these conditions, a basic need is to cleanse the kidneys, increase urine flow, and restore proper function.

Kidney trouble is caused by a local infection.

NATURAL REMEDIES
• Eat **75% raw foods** (including **garlic, parsley, potatoes, celery, cucumbers, and bananas**). **Green vegetables** are especially important.

• Drink 6-8 ounces of distilled **water** every hour.

HERBS
• Corn-silk tea is the best single herb for increasing urine flow and restoring the kidneys. **Watermelon-seed tea, pumpkin seeds**, and **celery and parsley seeds** are also diuretic in function.

• **Cranberries** help acidify the urine, destroying bacteria and restoring the bladder.

• The greatest aids for this problem are **juniper berries, marshmallow root, parsley, and watermelon seeds**.

AVOID
• **Stop eating meat**. An excess of protein is part of your problem; and meat also has a variety of waste products, plus bacteria, purines, and uric acid.

• Avoid **dairy products**, except yogurt. Do not eat **chocolate, cocoa, or fish**.

• Do not eat much **phosphorous**. For this reason, **avoid beet greens, spinach, rhubarb, and Swiss chard**; they contain oxylic acid.

• **Lead, other metals**, **pain relieving drugs** (Advil, Nuprin, etc.), and **infectious diseases** (scarlet fever, measles, etc.) can damage the kidneys. **Spirulina** is known to reduce kidney poisoning that is caused by **mercury** and drugs.

ENCOURAGEMENT—Only those who receive Christ as their Saviour are given the power to become sons and daughters of God. The sinner cannot, by any power of his own, rid himself of sin. But Christ can give the needed strength to come off victor in the battle with Satan. Romans 8:37.

KIDNEY STONES
(Nephrocalcinosis, Lithemia, Uric-acid Diathesis)

SYMPTOMS—Initially an intermittent, dull, dragging pain radiating from the upper back to the lower abdomen, usually increased by motion.

There is bleeding and renal colic (strong kidney pain) when the stone enters the ureters. These sharp pains may last hours or days. There is increased urination with pus and blood, pallor, nausea, and vomiting. Sometimes there are fevers and chills.

When you have bloody urine and sharp pain in the bladder or kidneys (a pain stronger than those of childbirth), it is very likely kidney stones.

CAUSES—Kidney stones (also called bladder stones or cystic calculi) are an abnormal accumulation of mineral salts (primarily calcium oxalate [70%-80%], uric acid crystals [10%], and/or calcium phosphate, magnesium ammonium phosphate, uric acid, or cystine). They form in the kidneys and, during passage down the ureters, may lodge in them or in the bladder. Kidney stones primarily affect middle-aged and older men. (In contrast, women mainly have gallstones.)

Oddly enough, a key factor in the production of kidney stones is a **calcium and/or magnesium deficiency** often the result of drinking sodas instead of water. The minerals in the stones come from your own bones!

Refined carbohydrates, especially sugar, prompts kidney stone formation. The amount of sugar in the pancreas increases; and it excretes additional insulin which, in turn, causes the kidneys to discharge more calcium in the urine.

Calcium is needed by the body. If there is not enough calcium is in the diet, the parathyroids will signal the body to extract calcium from the bones in order to keep the blood calcium at normal levels.

A **vitamin B₆ and magnesium deficiency** may also cause stone formation. A Swedish research group found that taking both daily stopped stone formation in 90% of their patients. Magnesium, like calcium, can bond with the oxalate. B_6 (10 mg a day) lowers the amount of oxalate in the urine.

In response to reduced blood calcium levels, the parathyroids trigger the body to draw it out of the bones.

It is vital that you obtain a **balanced diet of vitamins and minerals** every day.

Partial causes of kidney stone formation can include **dehydration** (not drinking enough water), **infections**, **prolonged periods of rest in bed**, and only rarely taking **vitamin D and calcium**.

Too much food, including **acid-forming foods— especially meat, along with white-flour products, sugar foods, tea, coffee, spices, and vinegar**—all help produce an excess of waste in the kidneys. Eventually it accumulates into gravel and stones.

If you are eating the **wrong kind of fatty acids** (the kind found in meat and junk food), it can combine with the calcium and be excreted in the stool. This keeps the oxalate in your food from combining with the calcium; so it passes into the kidneys and forms stones.

NATURAL REMEDIES

INCREASE WATER OUTPUT

• It is vital that you increase the amount of **water** you drink! Kidney health is keyed to an adequate fluid level in the blood. It is best to only use distilled water. Buy a distiller and you will not have to pay for bottles of it at the store. (In addition, those bottles are soft plastic; some of which is probably absorbed by the water.)

• Used in conjunction with more fluid intake, **corn-silk tea** increases urine output, a very necessary factor in purifying and detoxifying the kidneys.

• **Watermelon** provides additional water. Eat it alone and often; but do not eat it with other foods during meals.

• Drink **watermelon-seed tea**; steep in hot water for 15 minutes, strain, add a little honey, and drink.

NUTRIENTS

• A lack of **vitamin A** can lead to stone formation. It helps protect the lining of the urinary tract. A **vitamin B₆** and **magnesium** deficiency may also cause stone formation.

• A more **acid urine** prevents and dissolves kidney stones. Drink **cranberry juice** frequently. (One writer says that Ocean Spray brand is only 30% cranberry juice, plus sugar, etc.) All other fruit juices become alkaline in the system. A research study found that, in 10 patients, drinking cranberry juice reduced the stones in size by an average of 50%.

• Drink **potassium broth**. This is made from thick potato peelings. The outer portion is rich in potassium. Cook it with carrots, garlic, and celery. Simmer for 30-40 minutes, then strain and drink the liquid. Excess can be stored in the refrigerator for no more than 2 days.

AVOID THIS

• Oxalate, a key chemical in kidney stone formation, occurs naturally in various green vegetables, some more than others. **Rhubarb** has the highest oxalic acid content of anything eaten by man. Hardly any bug will touch it. People should never eat it. Also do not eat **spinach, chard, or beet tops**. About 60% of all stones are calcium oxalate in nature. Do not put vinegar into the body.

There may be an excess of purines. **Stop eating meat**. Meat-based proteins are a causal factor in producing kidney stones. Do not overeat on other proteins. In addition, calcium and magnesium are crucial, to stop the calcium loss from the bones. But meat supplies too much phosphorus, which keeps the calcium from being utilized.

• Do not use **soft drinks, caffeine, chocolate,**

cocoa, pepper, nuts, poppy seeds, or black tea.
• Reduce **salt** intake.
• A strict **macrobiotic diet** (lots of grains, and little fruits and vegetables) tends to concentrate the urine and may cause stones. This can be a significant cause of them.

HERBS
• Take **licorice**, to reduce swelling of the ureters, so the stone can pass.
• Hot compresses made with concentrated **ginger** tea help alleviate the pain of kidney stone attacks. The compresses act as counter irritants, taking the mind off the pain.
• **Horsetail** tea is recommended by the German government to increase urine output during a kidney stone attack.
* **Parsley** tea will help prevent and treat kidney stones. Use 1 tsp. dried root, steep for 10-15 minutes, strain, and drink 2-3 cups daily.
• Drink several cups daily of **stinging nettle** tea to prevent and treat kidney stones. (Use gloves when gathering them, but the stings are lost during cooking; the leaves are delicious.)
• Other helpful herbs include **dandelion, rup-turewort, and madder.**

TO DISSOLVE KIDNEY STONES
• To dissolve most kidney stones located in the renal pelvis, ureters, or in the bladder, drink 3 quarts to 1 gallon of hot water, along with lemon juice or cranberry juice, for 3 consecutive days. After this, on the 3rd day, drink 2 oz. **olive oil.** *For the complete formula for how to do this, see Gallstones (452).*
• An alternate formula is **apple juice** and **lemon juice** fasts, followed later by **olive oil.**
• To dissolve kidney stones, Dr. M. Tierra prescribes this: Make a decoction of 2 parts each of **parsley root, gravel root, marshmallow root,** ½ part of **lobelia and ginger root.** Simmer 2 oz. per quart of water for 1 hour or until the liquid is reduced to ½ quart. Add an equal volume of vegetable **glycerine** to preserve it. Take ½ cup, 3 times, daily. Or make a tincture of the above herbs and take 15 drops, 3 times daily.
• To help pass stones, Dr. J.B. Lust prescribes this: Mix equal parts of witch grass, birch leaves, speedwell, and chickory. Steep 1 tsp. in ½ cup boiled water. Take 1-1½ cups daily, unsweetened, in mouthful doses.
• Guillermo Asis, M.D., prescribes this to eliminate the pain, when passing the stones: Fill an 8-quart or larger pot with water, bring to a boil. Wrap a piece of fresh **ginger** (about the size of your palm) in a cloth, tie it with a string, put it in the boiling water 2-3 minutes. Immediately reduce the heat so boiling stops. Remove the cloth and squeeze it so the juice runs into the pot, Replace the bag in the pot. Remove the cloth and wring it out. It should be hot but not scalding. Place it on the lower back over the affected kidney. Put plastic on top and a dry towel over that. Repeat the applications every 5-10 minutes for 30-45 minutes. If it is still painful in 12 hours, do it again. This should eliminate all pain; and the heat should open the duct so the stones pass out. It can be done by heat, combined with pain-relieving ginger.

J.H. KELLOGG, M.D., PRESCRIPTIONS FOR KIDNEY STONES AND THEIR COMPLICATIONS *(how to give these water therapies: pp. 206-275 / list of treatments: pp. 206-207 / Hydrotherapy Disease Index: pp. 273-275)*
GENERAL DIET AND LIVING—A spare **aseptic diet**, especially avoiding beef tea, animal broths, meat, tea, coffee, and cocoa. Use fruits freely. In extreme cases, eat **a fruit diet** for a few days. **Outoor life, abundant exercise, dry and cool climate, daily cold bathing.**
INCREASE OXIDATION OF PROTEIN WASTES— **Hot Full Bath**, prolonged sufficiently to elevate body temperature 2º-4ºF. Sweating **Wet Sheet Pack**, Dry Pack, Steam Bath. Radiant Heat Bath or Hot Full Bath, followed by **Dry Pack**. Follow all hot baths by a **short, cold application** adapted to his condition: Cold Mitten Friction, Cold Towel Rub, Wet Sheet Rub, Dripping Sheet, Shallow Bath. Follow bath by **prolonged moderate exercise**, massage, and inhalation of oxygen.
ENCOURAGE ELIMINATION OF TISSUE WASTES— In addition to the above: **Water** drinking, free use of **fruit juices** and distilled water, Hot **Abdominal Pack** day and night. Cool **Colonic** daily, if bowels are sluggish.
INCREASE ALKALINITY OF BLOOD—Exercise, **cold baths**, cold air bath, **sweating baths**, and **fruit diet.**
SWOLLEN AND PAINFUL JOINTS—Fomentation 2-4 times daily. **Heating Compress** during intervals between, well-protected with plastic covering and cotton (or flannel) covering.
PAINFUL JOINTS, NOT SWOLLEN—Revulsive **Compress** 3 times a day, followed by deep massage of the limb above the joint and light circular friction of the joint. During intervals between, **Dry Pack** or cotton poultice to the joint.
STIFF AND ENLARGED JOINTS—Alternate Douche (jet or spray) or the **Alternate Compress**, applied twice daily and protected with **Heating Compress** during intervals between. Follow by thorough massage of the joint with **passive joint movements,**
GENERAL METHOD—Diminish the production of uric acid by regulation of diet and elimination of meat products. Increase the destruction of uric acid by exercise, Prolonged Hot Full Baths, followed by short cold applications. Increase elimination of uric acid by copious water drinking.
If any of the following related problems exist, check on them under their respective headings: Headache and Migraine, Neurasthenia, Neuralgia, Insomnia, Muscular pains, Gallstones, Renal colic, Irritable prostate, Arteriosclerosis, Bright's Disease.
—*See Renal Colic (492) and Kidney Problems (489-595).*

ENCOURAGEMENT—Christ, after having redeemed man from the condemnation of the law, could impart divine power to unite with human effort—in keeping that law. Galatians 3:14.

RENAL COLIC
(Kidney Pain Attack)

The following natural remedies, by Dr. Kellogg, were prescribed for any kind of kidney pain. You will find them very helpful.

NATURAL REMEDIES

J.H. KELLOGG, M.D., PRESCRIPTIONS FOR RENAL COLIC AND ITS COMPLICATIONS (*how to give these water therapies: pp. 206-275 / list of treatments: pp. 206-207 / Hydrotherapy Disease Index: pp. 273-275*)

DURING ATTACK—Rest in bed, diet of **fruit** and **buttermilk**, hot **water** drinking. Hot **Enema**, repeated every 2 hours. **Hot Full Bath** with cold to head and over heart, if bath is greatly prolonged. **Hot Trunk Pack** renewed hourly. **Revulsive Sitz Bath**. **Cold Compress** over heart, if it is weak or much excited.

TO PREVENT ATTACKS—Combat lithemia.

VOMITING—Ice pills, ice to throat.

URINARY SUPPRESSION—Hot Blanket Pack, followed by **Dry sweating Pack**.

—*See Kidney Stones (489).*

NEPHRITIS
(Kidney Infection, Glomerulonephritis)

SYMPTOMS—There may be no symptoms or they may include blood and/or albumin in the urine and lower back, abdominal pain, even chills, fatigue, facial edema, nausea and vomiting, frequent urge to urinate, and loss of appetite. Severe cases may include anemia and high blood pressure.

CAUSES—This is inflammation of one or both kidneys. Thousands of tiny cells in the kidneys filter fluids out of the blood in order to purify it. But the filter can become plugged with toxins and mucus. When these tiny cells become swollen and inflamed, infection soon follows.

This infection can be acute or chronic, and may require hospitalization.

Constipation causes toxic matter to be reabsorbed by the blood. This clogs the kidneys.

Overuse of **aspirin** and other **pain killers** weakens the kidneys; **beer** can cause their failure. **Environmental toxins, s**uch as **heavy metals**, add to the damage. **Anti-hypertensive drugs** are used to reduce blood circulation and therefore injure the kidneys.

Kidney infection can also be caused by **bacterial infection** in the bladder (*cystitis, 495*) which has traveled up the ureters to the kidneys.

NATURAL REMEDIES

• Drink plenty of pure **water**. Eat nourishing food, and avoid processed and junk food. Avoid **coffee, alcohol, and artificial drinks**.

• Drinking unsweetened **cranberry juice** and **apple juice** helps reduce bacterial growth in the kidneys. **Carrot, celery, and parsley juice** is also helpful.

• Include enough **vitamins C, A, and B complex** in the diet. **Potassium** deficiencies can encourage kidney problems.

• Go on a 3-day cleansing water-and-juice fast. Take enemas and rest. Keep the fluid level high.

• Helpful herbs include **garlic, echinacea, burdock, red clover, and goldenseal**. Also of value are herb teas made of **juniper berries, parsley, watermelon-seed, Buchu tea and/or marshmallow**.

• Used in conjunction with more fluid intake, **corn-silk tea** has been used for hundreds of years to increase urine output, a very necessary factor in purifying and detoxifying the kidneys.

— *Read the previous articles on kidney problems.*

J.H. KELLOGG, M.D., PRESCRIPTIONS FOR NEPHRITIS, BOTH ACUTE AND CHRONIC, AND THEIR COMPLICATIONS (*how to give these water therapies: pp. 206-275 / list of treatments: pp. 206-207 / Hydrotherapy Disease Index: pp. 273-275*)

KIDNEY INFECTION (ACUTE) —

RELIEVE CONGESTION OF KIDNEYS—Congest the skin by means of the **Hot Trunk Pack**, Hot Blanket Pack, or Hot Full Bath continued to perspiration, followed by **Friction**, avoiding deep massage procedures. Rubbing until vigorous perspiration is induced. Maintain active cutaneous circulation; **Fomentation** to loins for 30 minutes every 3-4 hours. **Heating Compress** over lower back during the interval between.

ENCOURAGE KIDNEY ACTIVITY—Ice Bag over lower third of sternum, **Hot Enema**, hot water drinking, Prolonged **Neutral Bath**.

ENCOURAGE ELIMINATION OF TOXINS—Hot or Cold Enema twice daily, Prolonged **Hot Blanket Pack**, Sweating Wet Sheet Pack, Radiant Heat Bath, Steam Bath, copious **water** drinking.

NAUSEA—Hot and Cold Compress over stomach, **Ice Bag** over stomach, and sipping very hot **water**.

DIET—Fruit juice, fruit purees, and buttermilk.

CARDIAC WEAKNESS—Ice Bag over heart for 15 minutes, every 2 hours. Cold Mitten Friction. **Cold Towel Rub**, 2-3 times daily.

CONTRAINDICATIONS—Avoid prolonged general cold applications, Cold Douche, and Cold Pail Pour.

GENERAL METHOD—Absolute rest in bed. Maintain a warm and active skin, even to the extent of perspiration. An aseptic, liquid dietary, to encourage free diuresis. Copious water drinking.

KIDNEY INFECTION (CHRONIC) —

GENERAL—Aseptic dietary. Especially avoid meats, condiments, buttermilk diet, or exclusive fruit diet during

(vertical text, right margin:) CHARTS 1052-1053: Urine characteristics in 9 diseases / Urine pH causesS

acute attack. Strictly avoid tea, coffee, tobacco, and alcoholic liquors.

MAINTAIN ACTIVITY OF THE SKIN—Warm **woolen clothing**. **Friction** given dry and applied daily. Cold Mitten Friction, followed by dry friction. Oil rubbing, carefully **graduated cold applications** (Tonic Frictions), Radiant Heat Bath, followed by cold Towel Rub. A **sweating bath** twice a week at bedtime, followed by **Cold Mitten Friction**.

ACUTE EXACERBATION—Apply treatment recommended for Bright's Disease, Acute.

DROPSY—Short Radiant **Heat Bath**, followed by **Cold Mitten Friction** or Cold Towel Rub. And **water** drinking, 1-2 pints twice daily.

CONTRAINDICATIONS—Avoid Cold Full Baths, frequently repeated and prolonged Cold Douches, or prolonged Hot Baths.

GENERAL METHOD—The essential features are a carefully regulated regimen adapted to his condition. This would include warm clothing, avoidance of chill, frequent Neutral Baths, very gentle tonic measures, copious water drinking, perfect digestion and bowel action, an aseptic dietary, outdoor life. Avoidance of exposure to cold and excesses of every description, especially sexual and dietetic excesses.

—*See Cystitis (495), which is infection of the bladder. The two are closely associated in health and in sickness. Also see Bright's Disease (this page), which is a variant form of nephritis.*

ENCOURAGEMENT—The love of Jesus is an active principle, uniting heart with heart in bonds of Christian fellowship. Everyone who enters heaven will, on earth, have been perfected in love. How thankful we can be for the enabling strength of Christ, by which we can fulfill God's will for our lives and obey His commandments.

NEPHROSIS

SYMPTOMS—Swelling of the kidneys with loss of protein in the urine.

CAUSES—An abnormal amount of proteins is excreted by the kidneys.

The condition may be worsened by eating **foods which a person is allergic to**. This can include **meat, wheat, junk food, greases, synthetic sugars**, etc. **Medicinal or street drugs** can also trigger this condition. **Overeating** and **eating too much protein** can worsen the condition.

NATURAL REMEDIES
See your physician.
• **Eliminate the causes**, listed above. Eat a **nutritious diet**. Drink lots of clean **water** and **fruit juices**. Take **diuretic herb teas** to increase urine output, so the kidneys can clean themselves.
— *Read the previous articles on kidney problems.*

ENCOURAGEMENT—Resist the devil, and he will flee from you. Draw nigh to God; and if you are desirous of taking the first upward step, you will find

His hand stretched out to help you. It remains with you, individually, as to whether you walk in the light of the Sun of Righteousness or in the darkness of error. The truth of God's Inspired Word can be a blessing to you only as you permit its influence to purify and refine your soul.

BRIGHT'S DISEASE

SYMPTOMS—Fever, chills, urgency and frequency of urination, loss of appetite, nausea, and vomiting. The urine is cloudy with pus and often bloody. Pain may be intense and sudden in the lower back, just above the waist, and running down the groin. An excessive amount of blood protein in the urine is a marked symptom of Bright's disease. It is usually accompanied by hypertension and edema, which is retention of water in the tissues.

CAUSES—Bright's disease involves a chronic inflammation of the kidneys, similar to Nephritis (*492*); but it is unique in the following respect: The kidneys cannot properly excrete salt and other wastes. The result is that salt and various wastes are stored by the blood in tissues throughout the body. This produces tissue swellings, edema, and high blood pressure. Excessive amounts of blood and protein are also in the urine.

Gradually the blood itself becomes contaminated with these waste products; and uremia (uremic poisoning) is the result.

Consuming **alcohol, tea, coffee, and spices** are excellent ways to ruin your kidneys. Do not use **aluminum** cooking ware.

NATURAL REMEDIES
See your physician.
• Take a high **enema** and a daily hot half-hour **tub bath**. Give 2-3 cups of **pleurisy** tea or **sage** tea while in the tub. Finish with a short **cold shower** or **cold towel rub**. Do not let him chill. Wrap him up well, put him in **bed**, and give him more **pleurisy** tea or **sage** tea to encourage perspiration. **Fomentations** over the lower back and the entire length of the spine will help alleviate pain. Do this also over the stomach, liver, and spleen.
• Begin with a **fruit juice diet** for several days, before eating other foods. **Soybean milk with whole wheat flakes** dissolved in it is easily digested and nourishing. Avoid **salt**. Do not mix fruits and vegetables at the same meal.
• Then begin eating **vegetable broths, cauliflower, asparagus, eggplant**, etc. All the food eaten should be **low in protein**. **No stimulating or heavy foods**.

HERBS
• Make a tea of **Juniper berries**. It is a stimulating diuretic and helps the kidneys excrete waste products. It is also a great healer to the kidneys' urinary passages and bladder. American Indians used it for this purpose. It is also good for reducing the edema

associated with Bright's disease.

• Mix 1 oz. each of **juniper berries and gravel root**, 2 oz. **ginger**. Steep in 2 cups boiled water, take 1 tsp. 4 times a day.

For other natural remedies which can help control urinary tract infection, see under Nephritis (492) and Cystitis (next page).

ENCOURAGEMENT—You do not know how much good you can do by always wearing a cheerful, sunny face and watching for opportunities to help others. You may not always be appreciated, but God understands; and your work will be rewarded. He will always care for His own—even unto the end. You are safe in His hands.

EDEMA
(Dropsy, Water Retention)

SYMPTOMS—Swelling of the hands, ankles, feet, face, abdomen, or other areas of the body. Swelling is most often seen in the hands, in the feet, or around the eyes. The bloating or swelling causes muscle aches and pains.

CAUSES—Edema is a fluid accumulation in the body. It can be caused by **poor kidney function, chronic kidney disease, congestive heart disease, varicose veins, phlebitis, protein or thiamine deficiency, sodium retention, or cancer**.

Other causal factors include **pregnancy, standing for lengthy periods** of time, **premenstrual tension**, the use of **oral contraceptives**. A **confining injury**, such as a sprain, allergic reactions, or a bee sting.

Fluid retention is sometimes caused by a **food allergy. Hypothyroidism, anemia, adrenal malfunction, constipation**, or **lack of exercise** can be causal factors. Also **deficiencies of potassium, vitamin B complex, or vitamins B_1, B_3, or B_6**.

As soon as edema is found to exist, it is well to obtain a clear diagnosis. Once **congestive heart disease, kidney disease, or liver disease** are ruled out, more subtle causes can more easily be dealt with.

If the skin indents, forming little pits, when the skin of the feet or ankles is pressed by a finger, the situation is worsening. Contact a physician.

• Heavy **salt** users often have dropsy as do diabetics. The general problem is that fluid does not eliminate properly through the kidneys and skin. Dr. Edward Shook had the following to say about dropsy: "When sulfuric acid is generated within the organism, it immediately unites with water and swells up. This action produces heat, which expands the capillaries. The osmotic pressure forces the serum through the walls of the blood vessels, producing inflammation and dropsy. Hence the using of inorganic matter is always poisonous to the human organism in spite of all the apparent evidence to the contrary." (*Advanced Treatise on Herbs, p. 132*)

TREATMENT—
If edema is caused by heart disease, then turn to that section. If it is caused by kidney failure or other causes, then read the following:

• If it is the result of **protein or thiamine** deficiency, the intake of either or both should be increased. Fluid can be retained in the belly cavity because the protein content of the blood is so low that fluid cannot be kept in the blood vessels.

• **Excess salt** in the diet is major part of the problem. A very restricted salt diet should be adhered to. (Too much salt in the body requires additional water to keep the salt diluted, so it will not damage living tissue.)

• Increasing the **vitamin B_6** intake will reduce the amount of fluid retention.

• Take the pulse test *(847)*, to determine certain foods which do not agree with you. Then avoid those foods.

• A 1-3 day **juice fast** will be helpful. *But if a protein deficiency is the problem*, then **nutrition** is needed, not cleansing. Take **hot baths** twice a week. Eat more **fruits and vegetables**, emphasizing the **raw foods**.

• Carry out a regular **daily exercise** program, outdoors. **Poor circulation** because of liver or heart disease is a common cause of edema. When at rest, elevate the legs.

Avoid **tight clothing, stress, processed and junk foods. Do not cross the legs**. Stop eating **meat**.

• Helpful herbs include **corn silk, dandelion, Scotch broom, alfalfa, Canadian fleabane, garlic, English hawthorn, juniper berries, lily of the valley, parsley, nettle, marshmallow, pau d'arco, and prickly ash**.

• Exceptional results have been attained with dropsy by the use of **parsley, parsley root, juniper berries, verde cactus, ginger, and chaparral**. Diet is the key to eliminating the cause. **Meats, pastries, salt**, etc., should be avoided. Eat **fruits (grapes and coconut** especially), **sprouts, leafy and green vegetables**, (do not mix fruits and vegetables). Use **vapor baths** and **diaphoretic herbs** to open the pores, stimulant herbss to increase and regulate circulation, diuretic herbs for kidneys, and be sure to treat the whole digestive system with tonic herbs. Also rub the body with cold water and be sure to keep the bowels cleaned.

ENCOURAGEMENT—"The righteous cry, and the Lord heareth, and delivereth them out of all their troubles." Psalm 34:17. With such a promise as this, how can we become disheartened? Thank God for the our precious Bibles!

URINARY - 3 - BLADDER

BLADDER PROBLEMS

NATURAL REMEDIES

HYDRO—Here are several hydrotherapy applications found in the *Hydrotherapy* section *(206-275)* of this *Encyclopedia:*

Bladder atony: **Ascending jet or spray** directed upward, in this case, against the perineum. In addition, a **spray** to the front of the abdomen only.

Bladder inflammation: Copious **water** drinking. **Revulsive Sitz Bath**, twice a day. **Hot Leg Packs**, followed by **dry heat** (Radiant Heat Bath) to legs. **Neutral Bath** for 20-40 minutes, 2-3 times a week. **Prolonged Neutral Sitz Bath**, **Cold Mitten Friction**, **Cold Towel Rub**, **Fomentation** over bladder, **Hot Enema**, **Hot Pelvic Pack**, **Aseptic Dietary.**

Irritable bladder: When inflammation is not present, give a **very hot Sitz Bath** for 5 minutes, followed by **Neutral Sitz Bath** for 10-20 minutes. **Hot pack** to pelvis, **Heating Compress** over perineum and genitals, **Revulsive Sitz**, and **Hot Colonic.**

Bladder insufficiency: **Spinal** (Dorsal) **Spray.** This is a hand-held hosing of water to the dorsal (upper and central) part of the spine. The stream should be allowed to play rapidly up and down, extending 3-4 inches on either side of the spine. Use tepid water for irritability of the bladder (when of spinal origin).

Bladder paresis (paralysis): Daily **colonic**, **Cold Plantar Spray** to bottom of feet.

Bladder retention: **Lumbar Revulsive spray.** This spray should be hot and then very brief cold; it will help alleviate urinary retention, due to spasm in the neck of the bladder.

ENCOURAGEMENT—As we cherish and obey the promptings of the Holy Spirit to obey God and help others, our hearts are enlarged to receive more and more of His power and to do more and better work. As we seek to help others, the angels work with us.

CYSTITIS
(Bladder and Urinary Tract Infection, Irritable Bladder)

SYMPTOMS—Pain in the lower abdomen and back. Frequent, urgent, and painful urination. Urine often has a strong, unpleasant odor and may appear cloudy (from pus). A desire to urinate even after the bladder has been emptied.

Children with this condition may experience a painful burning sensation when urinating.

CAUSES—Cystitis is an infection of the urinary bladder. It is the most frequent bacterial infection in women. About 10%-15% of them have recurrent bladder infections.

The cause is generally **bacteria which have ascended up from the urinary opening**; but, it is less frequently from **infected urine** sent down from the kidneys. The usual cause is ascended bacteria.

Cystitis most often occurs in females. The urinary outlet of the urethra is close to the vagina. Ways to avoid cross infection between the two are given in the concluding paragraph of this article.

Frequency and urgency of burning urine is the obvious symptom of cystitis; but a home test can also be done. Purchase "Dipstick" at a pharmacy and follow the directions. A positive nitrate test will reveal the presence of a large quantity of white blood cells, indicating infection in the urinary tract.

Women who frequently have bladder infections often have enlarged bladders from **trying to retain their urine**. In order to maintain good urinary tract health, it is important to drink water and urinate frequently.

In older men, the cause of the bladder problem might be **kidney stones** *(489).*

Blood in the urine could indicate a more serious problem. Consult a physician. *Also see Hematuria (488).*

Bladder infection in men may signal **prostate trouble** *(668).*

Cyclamate (an artificial sweetener found in synthetic sugar) causes bladder tumors.

NATURAL REMEDIES

• Increase the fluid intake—lots of **water**, especially distilled, is best. Drink a half pint every 20 minutes for 3 hours, then one cup every hour. This is important.

• Acidify the urine by drinking 1-2 quarts of **cranberry juice** per day, for the first day, and 1 quart a day thereafter while the crisis continues. It is the only fruit juice that remains acid until it reaches the kidneys. When you have this problem, citrus juice is not as good; since it tends to make the urine more alkaline, encouraging bacterial growth.

• Eat a **nourishing diet**; avoid the wrong foods. *See Nephritis (Kidney Infection, 492)* for much more information on the proper care and healing of the urinary tract. The bladder and kidneys are closely associated; whatever helps one helps the other.

• **Potassium deficiencies** can lead to renal (kidney) disorders. Prepare a **broth** with thick potato peelings, plus carrots, and other vegetables.

• The use of **aluminum** cookware is one of several causes of cystic symptoms. Avoid **zinc** and **iron** supplements until this problem is healed.

HERBS AND WATER THERAPY

• Helpful herbs include **juniper, lovage, parsley, uvi ursa, rupturewort, bearberry, birch, and prickly ash**. Of course, do not add sweetener or milk to the tea.

• Drink tea made from 2-3 crushed or blended **garlic** bulbs several times a day.

• To relieve the pain and encourage healing, take

U
R
I
N

hot sitz (sitting) baths twice a day, for 20 minutes. To one of those daily sitz baths, add 1 cup of vinegar. The next day, add 2 cloves crushed garlic or garlic juice to the water of one of the two baths.

• A hot-water bottle placed in direct contact to the urethral and vaginal openings may be extremely helpful in reducing pain. A heat lamp can also be used.

SPECIAL NOTE

• Women should especially avoid bacterial infection ascending into the bladder: The urinary outlet of the urethra is close to the vagina. Improper female hygiene is the most common cause of cystitis; she should start wiping from the front and go toward the back. When sexual intercourse is not done with clean hands or too frequently, germs are more likely to enter the urethra. Wipe from front to back following bowel movements. Urinate before and after intercourse. And wear cotton underclothing; it lets air through and absorbs moisture better. Avoid douches, hygiene sprays, bubble baths, soap in the bathwater, and nylon clothing. Wash carefully during the monthly, to avoid bacteria from going up the urethra. Do not use tampons if there are frequent urinary tract infections. Rinse underwear well, to get all the soap out. Boil panties in plain (not soapy) water. Shower after having bathed in a swimming pool. Dress to keep the extremities warm; cold extremities weaken the trunk organs, including the urinary tract. Birth control pills and spermaticides may cause cystitis.

J.H. KELLOGG, M.D., PRESCRIPTIONS FOR BLADDER AND URINARY TRACT INFECTION AND ITS COMPLICATIONS (how to give these water therapies: pp. 207-272 / list of treatments: pp. 206-207 / Hydrotherapy Disease Index: pp. 273-275)

INFLAMMATION—Copious water drinking. Revulsive Sitz Bath, twice a day. Hot Leg Packs, followed by dry heat (Radiant Heat bath) to legs. Neutral Bath for 20-40 minutes, 2-3 times a week. Prolonged Neutral Sitz Bath, Cold Mitten Friction, Cold Towel Rub, Fomentation over bladder, Hot Enema, Hot Pelvic Pack, Aseptic Dietary.

IRRITABLE BLADDER—With inflammation not present: Very Hot Sitz Bath for 5 minutes, followed by Neutral Sitz Bath for 10-20 minutes. Hot Pack to pelvis, Heating Compress over perineum and genitals, Revulsive Sitz, Hot Colonic.

CONTRAINDICATIONS—Do not apply Cold Sitz Bath, Cold Full Bath, Cold Douche, or Cold Footbath.

ENCOURAGEMENT—Christ was lifted upon the cross of Calvary, to draw all men unto Himself. What shall we do then with Jesus? Shall we accept Him or reject Him? Isaiah 42:16.

When God gave His Son to our world, He endowed human beings with imperishable riches—riches compared with which the treasured wealth of men since the world began is nothingness. Christ came to the earth and stood before the children of men with the hoarded love of eternity. And this is the treasure that, through our connection with Him, we are to receive, to reveal, and to impart.

Never was there a time when the Lord would manifest His grace unto His chosen ones more fully than in these last days when His law is made void

Thank God every day for the immense blessings He grants us. Draw close to Him and He will care for you each day.

More Encouragement

"The Saviour did not wait for congregations to assemble. Often He began His lessons with only a few gathered about Him, but one by one the passers-by paused to listen, until a multitude heard with wonder and awe the words of God through the heaven-sent Teacher. The worker for Christ should not feel that he cannot speak with the same earnestness to a few hearers as to a larger company. There may be only one to hear the message; but who can tell how far-reaching will be its influence? . .

"Every true disciple is born into the kingdom of God as a missionary. He who drinks of the living water becomes a fountain of life. The receiver becomes a giver. The grace of Christ in the soul is like a spring in the desert, welling up to refresh all, and making those who are ready to perish eager to drink of the water of life."
—Desire of Ages, 194, 195

Two editions of Desire of Ages, the classic (and best) book on the life of Christ are available from us.

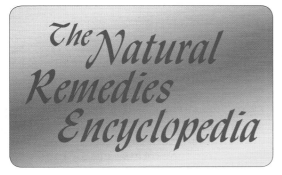

The Natural Remedies Encyclopedia

- Disease Section 7 -
Respiratory

Respiratory System: Physiology 1018 / Pictures 1039

"Many are the afflictions of the righteous: but the Lord delivereth him out of them all."   —*Psalm 34:19*

"Why art thou cast down, O my soul? and why art thou disquieted within me? hope thou in God: for I shall yet praise Him, who is the health of my countenance, and my God."

—*Psalm 42:11*

"Casting all your care upon Him; for He careth for you."
—*1 Peter 5:7*

"No good thing will He withhold from them that walk uprightly."   —*Psalm 84:11*

FOR MORE NATURAL REMEDIES:

HERBS: Herb Contents (pp. 129-130) will help you locate the 126 most important herbs and the diseases each one can treat. How to prepare herbs (132). How to use them (141-189)

HYDROTHERAPY: Therapy Contents (pp. 206-207) and its Disease Index (263-265) will lead you to over 100 water therapies and many more remedies. DIS. INDEX: 1211- / GEN. INDEX: 1221-

VITAMINS AND MINERALS: Contents (100-101). Using 101-124. Dosages (124). Others (117-)

CARING FOR THE SICK: Home care for a sick person (28-36). The healing crisis (36-39)

WOMEN'S SECTIONS: Female Organs (672) Pregnancy (701). Childbirth (765). Infancy, Childhood (722). Women's Herbs (754, 760)

EMERGENCIES: (973-). FIRST AID: (990-)

Section 7 - Respiratory

RESPIRATORY - 1 - BREATHING

POSTNASAL DRIP

SYMPTOMS—The back of the mouth drips fluid and runs down into the respiratory tract, starting a coughing attack, or into the voice box.

CAUSES—Most people only experience postnasal drip while they are sick with a bad cold or something similar. However, some have it when they are well. This article is for them. *See Common Cold (289) and similar articles in that section.*

Normally, these secretions from the sinuses flow down the back of the nose and throat and are swept away by cilia, which are small waving hair-like projections.

But sometimes the mucus dries out and the cilia no longer wiggle. Then the secretions pool in the back of the nose, thicken, and begin dripping into the bronchial tubes or into the voice box.

Postnasal drip may be due to **allergy**. **Spicy foods** are especially known to produce this symptom.

A primary cause is that **you never fully recovered from a sickness**. You may have never permitted yourself time to rest during a heavy cold; and, while all the other symptoms left, the nasal congestion became chronic.

Here are several suggestions; one or more of these may solve the problem for you at such times:

NATURAL REMEDIES
• **Blow** your nose regularly, but do it very gently.
• **Flush your nose** with saltwater and gargle with it. Place a half teaspoon of salt in about 8 ounces of warm water (the experts recommend only a third of a teaspoon if you have high blood pressure). Draw the water into an aspirator and put the tip into your nose. Then hold your head back, so you are looking up—and gently squeeze on the aspirator as you carefully suck it into your nostrils. Although this may, at first, seem uncomfortable, it can bring you a lot of relief. Conclude by **blowing** your nose gently, to get all the fluid out. Do this 3 times a day for 5 days. Next, **gargle** with the same ratio of salt in the water.
• Reduce the amount of **stress** you are under and stop drinking **milk**; but do drink lots of **water**

or nourishing fluids. An **herb tea** with some lemon and honey is helpful.
• A **humidifier** in the room can keep the air moist.
• **Avoid nasal decongestants, nose drops**, etc. In the long run, they will cause you more trouble than they are worth.
• If you want to really solve this chronic problem in the quickest and best way, go to **bed** for a couple days. Go on a **fruit juice fast**, take a few **enemas**, and by the third day you should be in perfect shape.

ENCOURAGEMENT—If you can exert a saving influence over one soul, remember there is joy in heaven over the one that repents. You may, by careful effort, be the means of bringing back the lost sheep into the fold of Jesus. It is wonderful to work with the angels. Psalm 34:7.

CROUP

SYMPTOMS—The larynx (vocal cords), or trachea, (windpipe) narrows. This is because of infection which causes the walls to swell inward. There is difficulty in breathing, hoarseness, tightness in the lungs. Also a harsh, barking cough and even a feeling of suffocation. Croup most often occurs in children, because their air pipes are smaller,

The special symptom of croup is a harsh, wheezing noise as air is breathed in through the narrowed windpipe and past the inflamed vocal cords, often accompanied by fits of coughing.

CAUSES—Very often the original cause is **overeating**. When the stomach is overloaded with food, it is easier to catch cold; and croup develops. The sickness may be either bacterial or viral. When caused by a bacteria, croup generally follows a cold or another mild respiratory infection. But when it is caused by a virus (as happens more often, especially in boys), more serious conditions, such as the flu, have occurred.

Croup most often occurs during the winter months; it most frequently affects children from 3 months to 3 years (9 to 18 months is the peak). It is most common in **areas with sudden changes in temperature**. Drinking cow's milk may be the cause. It is often associated with the third or fourth nights of **measles**.

In false croup, which is generally caused by stomach disorders and worms, there is less likelihood of

CHART - 1045: Respiratory (497-511)

fever; but, in true croup, there is often high fever. Work earnestly to help the child. The attacks are often worse at night.

NATURAL REMEDIES

• Maintain a good water intake, to help loosen secretions. Only drink **lukewarm water**. If the child is told to drink a glass of water after each coughing attack, the coughs will stop after the third or fourth glass. Water is the best cough medicine. It thins the mucus.

• Use a **vaporizer or humidifier** at night, or put a **pan of water** or teakettle on a hot plate. This will help keep the air moist for the child through the night.

• Try to have someone stay with the child. If he is too anxious, you may find it best to hold him for a time. This will reassure him.

• **Avoid sudden temperature changes**. Keep the child **warm, but avoid overheating**.

• During the day, you might wish to put a few drops of **eucalyptus oil** in a vaporizer; and, for a time, have him inhale the vapor.

• **Peppermint and honey** is good. A few drops of **lobelia** tincture **in catnip** tea **or peppermint** tea will relax the throat so he will not cough violently. Induce perspiration by giving the child warm **catnip** tea **or chamomile** tea. Give him a catnip tea **enema**.

• Teas made from **echinacea, fenugreek, goldenseal, and thyme** are helpful. Give the child very warm **ginger** herb baths. Then wrap him in a warm towel, put him in bed, and let him perspire

• Homemade **soups and broths** are good for the child. **Slippery elm gruel with oatmeal** is nourishing.

• **Fomentations** to the neck and upper chest region bring relief. After the acute phase, a **heating compress** may be applied to the chest.

• You can apply **hot onion packs** over the chest and back 3 times a day. Place sliced onions between cloths and cover with a heating pad.

• **Avoid steroids and antibiotics**; they are useless if this is a viral sickness. Do not use **cough medicines** and other colds preparations; for they tend to thicken the secretions (anti-congestants are always drying agents) and make it still harder to clear the throat.

• *When croup keeps reoccurring*, the cause may well be that the child is **allergic** to some type of food. Try to ascertain what it might be. *See Allergies (848).* Instead of using drug medications, carefully figure out the cause.

• Give a fruit diet for a few days, such as **pineapple juice, grape juice, orange juice, baked apples**. **Soybean milk with toast or whole wheat flakes** is easily digested. A **broth** of thick potato peelings, plus a few other vegetables, is good.

J.H. KELLOGG, M.D., PRESCRIPTIONS FOR CROUP AND ITS COMPLICATIONS (how to give these water therapies: pp. 206-275 / list of treatments: pp. 206-207 / Hydrotherapy Disease Index: pp. 273-275)

(1) ACUTE CATARRH OF LARYNX —
GENERAL TREATMENT—Hot Bath with **Cold Compress** to head. Hot **water** drinking. **Cold Mitten Friction**, every 3 hours. **Warm Vapor Inhalation**, inhalation of vapor from water with calcium in it. **Cold Compress** at 60° F. over throat, changed every 10-20 minutes. **Hot Blanket Pack**, every 3-4 hours for 15 minutes. Keep feet, legs, and arms warm.

ENCOURAGEMENT—When we accept Christ, we are adopted into His family. We have a nearness to Him and can hold sweet communion with Him. We learn what He is like; and we become changed into His likeness. 2 Corinthians 3:18.

FALSE CROUP
(Spasmodic Laryngitis)

SYMPTOMS—False croup is less serious than true croup, with generally no fever involved. But the coughing and difficulty in breathing are just as bad. Here are the Kellogg remedies for this problem.
—*Also see Croup (498).*

J.H. KELLOGG, M.D., PRESCRIPTIONS FOR FALSE CROUP AND ITS COMPLICATIONS (how to give these water therapies: pp. 206-275 / list of treatments: pp. 206-207 / Hydrotherapy Disease Index: pp. 273-275)

(2) FALSE CROUP, SPASMODIC LARYNGITIS —
PREVENT ATTACKS—Harden the skin with daily **Cold Bath. Remove nasal obstruction**, hypertrophies, or adenoid vegetation. Inhalations.
PREVENT CHILLING OF SHOULDERS—During sleep wear proper clothing, perhaps a **warm sleeping jacket**.
DEVELOP RESISTANCE—Graduated Tonic Frictions, outdoor life, careful regulation of **clothing**.
RELIEVE CONGESTION—If spasm is severe, relieve the congestion by Hot Blanket Pack or **Hot Full Bath**. Repeat every 3-6 hours. **Hot Half Bath with Cold Pail Pour** to head, back, and chest. Follow bath with **ice-cold Heating Compress** to neck, to be changed every 2-4 hours. **Fomentation** to cervical, upper, and middle spine for 15 minutes each time the ice compress is changed.
TO RELIEVE SPASM—Compress the phrenic nerve by pressure just above the sternal intersection of the sternocleidomastoid muscle; **percuss** (hit) the chest with the end of a cold wet towel or a dash of cold water over the chest and back.
BRONCHITIS—If present, relieve it with **Chest Pack**; repeat in 4-6 hours. **Cold Mitten Friction** twice a day. **Warm Vapor Inhalation** and copious **water** drinking when bronchial or laryngeal catarrh exists.

ASTHMA

SPECIAL NOTE: Asthma is a serious respiratory disorder. But, since 80% of asthma problems are caused by allergies, the large section dealing with it will be found in the allergy section. *Please turn to page 848.*

WHEEZING
(Whistling Breathing)

SYMPTOMS—A lightly audible sibilant, whistling or sighing sound produced in labored breathing, signaling an obstruction of air passages due to a spasm, edema, inflammation, a foreign body, tumor, or external pressure.

CAUSE—When there is wheezing, there is potentially serious trouble in the body which signals a need for immediate cleansing.

NATURAL REMEDIES
• **Lobelia** and **nervines** are generally used most effectively. Whenever there is heavy congestion in the lungs or bronchi, use **chickweed, lobelia, or mullein**.

• Other useful herbs include **antispasmodics, apple cider vinegar and honey, black walnut, catnip, chickweed, comfrey (preferably fresh, chewed or used as a vegetable), lobelia, marshmallow, mullein**.

DYSPNEA
(Difficult Breathing)

SYMPTOMS—Difficult breathing.

CAUSE—This usually arises from mucus in the air passages in the trachea, the nostrils, lungs, etc.

NATURAL REMEDIES
• Take a cup of **cayenne tea** and **antispasmodic tincture** internally and massaged on the chest area. With a breast-fed baby, the mother should take a tea of balm, hyssop, or pennyroyal. For the baby, where the problem is largely in the nose (sometimes referred to as snuffles), a mixture of **milk and olive oil** in the nose is good. The bowels may need to be relieved with a small injection of **lobelia**.

• Useful herbs include **almond (sweet), blue vervain, comfrey root, coriander, dandelion, hawthorn, imperial masterwort, garlic, lobelia, sarsaparillas** (German), **soapwort, veronica**.

SUFFOCATION

SYMPTOMS—The person is apparently suffocating.

NATURAL REMEDIES
• Immediate action must be taken. Quickly plunge him into cold water or **pour cold water** (the colder the better) on him. This simple procedure powerfully affects the breathing centers; and he may immediately begin taking deep breaths.

• Then begin other resuscitation treatments while someone calls for emergency help.

— *Turn to "How to Give **CPR**" in the Emergency Section of this Encyclopedia (991-995).*

ENCOURAGEMENT—When we love others as unselfishly as Christ loved us, then for us His mission is accomplished. We are fitted for heaven; for we have heaven in our hearts. Matthew 5:44-48.

RESPIRATORY -
2 - BRONCHIAL TUBES

ACUTE BRONCHITIS

SYMPTOMS—Coughing and mucus, pain in the chest (and possibly back), fever, sore throat, and difficult breathing. Sudden chills and shaking may occur.

CAUSES—There are two types of bronchitis: acute and chronic. *Acute bronchitis* very often occurs as an infection in the throat which moves on down toward the lungs. A cold or the flu, if not immediately given careful treatment, can spread into other areas (such as the bronchi or the eustachian tubes). If bronchitis is not carefully dealt with, the infection will move on into the lungs, resulting in pneumonia.

Chronic bronchitis is an ongoing infection in the bronchials, and will be dealt with in the next article *(below)*.

The bronchial tubes are the airways which lead into the lungs. The bronchi are two main branches of the trachea. They divide into many smaller bronchi, like tree roots. These, in turn, divide off into the grape-like maze, called the lungs.

Bronchitis is inflammation of the bronchi, and is frequently complicated by mucous obstruction of those passageways. When the bronchi are badly infected, the cause is often viral rather than bacterial. Irritating substances (or invading bacteria or viruses) cause the bronchi to produce an excess of mucus, which clogs the airways.

Acute bronchitis attacks occur most often in winter, among the elderly, smokers, infants, and those who have lung disease. Most are men over the age of 40.

NATURAL REMEDIES
• Take an **emetic**. Add ½ tsp. lobelia to a quart of boiled water, let steep. When lukewarm, strain, and drink as much of it as possible. Run your finger down your throat until you vomit. This will clear the stomach of mucus and phlegm. Then take a high **enema** (constipation is often a causal factor). Keep

the bowels open thereafter.

• Take a **full hot bath** or steam bath, followed by a short **cold shower** or brief **cold towel rub**. Put him in **bed** and give **hot fomentations** to the chest and spine, finishing with **cold**. This will do much to relieve congestion. **Hot footbaths** with a Tbsp. of **mustard** in the water brings good relief.

• Go on a **juice fast** for 1-2 days; then give a **light, nutritious diet** of fruit and vegetables.

• This is a condition from improper diet and results in bowel problems. Relieving the effects of the condition will not heal it. Bronchitis usually develops from a cold which settles in the lungs and develops into a chronic condition if not healed, eventually going into consumption or tuberculosis.

• Here is excellent help: **Comfrey and almond** are specifics for bronchitis. Since **constipation** is one of the chief causes of the problem, the bowels must be cleared and kept open with the lower **bowel tonic or herbal laxatives**. If one has shortness of breath and needs the throat cleared of mucus, he can use an emetic. **Cayenne** is very effective for cutting the phlegm, as are fruit juices such as **grapefruit, lemon, orange, or pineapple. Chickweed, comfrey, marshmallow or mullein** are the greatest cleansers to get the mucus out of the body. One can relax the throat, stomach, and bronchi rapidly with a very small amount of **lobelia**. Other useful aids for relief are a **hot vapor or steam bath** followed by a **cold shower or sponging**; also **hot fomentation of pleurisy root or mullein** (with **lobelia** in it) on the chest and spine. If you want to speed up any fomentation, add **cayenne** as a counterirritant.

—*Also read Acute Bronchitis (above) and Fevers (302-309).*

J.H. KELLOGG, M.D., PRESCRIPTIONS FOR ACUTE BRONCHITIS AND ITS COMPLICATIONS (*how to give these water therapies: pp. 206-275 / list of treatments: pp. 206-207 / Hydrotherapy Disease Index: pp. 273-275*)

INCREASE RESISTANCE—Graduated cold applications daily, **outdoor life**, daily air bath.

ELIMINATE TOXINS—Moderately prolonged **sweating procedures** followed by **cold applications**.

RELIEVE INTERNAL CONGESTION—Radiant Heat Bath for 10-20 minutes. **Sweating Wet Sheet Pack** for 1-2 hours or Steam Bath for 6-15 minutes, followed by Wet Sheet Rub or **Cold Douche** (spray). **Hot Full Bath** at bedtime for 6-10 minutes, followed by prolonged **Neutral Bath** for 2-40 minutes. Apply (daily or twice a day) **Hot Hip and Leg Pack**, followed by **Dry Towel Rub**.

COUGH—Heating Chest Pack, to be changed every 8 hours. If temperature is elevated, change Chest Pack every 2-4 hours. Copious **water** drinking, 2-3 pints daily.

IRRITABLE COUGH, WITHOUT EXPECTORATION—Sip very hot **water**, **gargle** hot water, **Warm Vapor Inhalations**. Avoid mouth breathing. Keep **air of room** warm (75°-80° F.) and moist with steam. Carefully **avoid exposure of the back of neck, chest, or shoulders** to drafts or to chill by evaporation during treatment.

COUGH WITH VISCID EXPECTORATION—Copious hot **water** drinking, **fluid diet**, **Fomentation** to chest every

(vertical text) **CHART 1051: Bronchial and Lung Problems: 500-507**

2 hours, followed by **Heating Compress**.

PAINFUL COUGH—Fomentation to chest every 2 hours. Tight bandage about the chest, to restrain movement, if necessary. **Revulsive Compress** for 15 minutes, every 2 hours, as often as needed. Dry cotton **Chest Pack** between applications.

ENCOURAGEMENT—God has built a hedge around about His subjects, to protect them. It is the Ten Commandments. By faith in Christ, we are empowered to obey the Father's law. Doing so preserves us from transgression. In requiring obedience to the laws of His kingdom, God gives His people health and happiness. Revelation 22:14.

CHRONIC BRONCHITIS

SYMPTOMS—There is almost continual coughing, which brings up quantities of mucus and phlegm. There is shortness of breath. The symptoms often become very severe.

CAUSES—Chronic bronchitis is an ongoing problem which results from repeated bouts of **acute bronchitis** or from something that is frequently **irritating the lungs**. This can be allergies, especially tobacco smoke. The only ones who gain from tobacco are the manufacturers. Interestingly enough, only 9% of bronchitis patients in the U.S. are non-smokers. Infants exposed to cigarette smoke are far more likely to come down with bronchitis.

Chronic bronchitis reduces the amount of oxygen to the lungs and the amount of carbon dioxide exhaled. This eventually can lead to enlargement of the heart, pulmonary hypertension, and finally heart failure. If it is not cured, it can go into tuberculosis of the lungs.

NATURAL REMEDIES

• Drink plenty of **fluids**: pure **water, soups, and herb teas**. Drink at least 2 quarts of liquid a day so the phlegm can easily be expelled. **No soft drinks, caffeine, or alcohol.**

• Take **vitamin C** to bowel tolerance.

• All kinds of **fruits and vegetables and their juices** are beneficial, if no allergic reactions occur.

• **Anise tea and almond milk** are helpful in bronchitis. Make the almond milk by blending 6 tablespoons of almonds in a pint of water.

• Swallowing a little **cayenne and lobelia** will help break up the congestion.

• If there is shortness of breath or gasping, clear the throat by giving a few drops of **lobelia tincture**. This will relax the throat and bronchi.

• Add moisture to the air with a **vaporizer** or **humidifier.** Or heat a pan of water on the stove.

• Remain in **bed** as long as fever is present. Bronchitis often hangs on because people think it is about over and begin going about their everyday duties. *Go to bed and get well!*

• **Breathe deeply**. Blow up a **balloon** several times everyday. This helps open up and enlarge the airways. Deep **breathing exercises** should be taken 3-4 times a day. Take a deep breath, hold it a few seconds, and exhale. Do this 10-20 times. This will help air out the infected area.

• Apply a **heating compress** at night.

• A **hot footbath** will help pull the blood away from the chest and reduce congestion.

• **Hot drinks** help you cough out the phlegm. Coughing is the only way the phlegm can come out. Do not use cough suppressants while you have bronchitis.

• Apply **warm, moist heat or a hot-water bottle** over the chest and back before bedtime. This will help relieve congestion and aid in sleep.

• Helpful herbs include **pau d'arco, chickweed, ginkgo biloba, burdock, lobelia, slippery elm bark, echinacea,** and **wild cherry bark**.

AVOID THIS
• **Stop smoking** and get tobacco out of the house. If you have chronic bronchitis, do not expect much improvement as long as tobacco smoke is in the home.

• Do not use **milk**; it produces a thick phlegm which complicates healing. **White-flour products** and **sugar** foods should not be used until bronchitis is past.

• **Avoid fatigue and chilling**. Do not walk **barefoot** on cold floors while you are trying to get well.

• **Avoid talking, laughing loudly, crying, or too much exertion**. They can trigger attacks.

BEWARE
• If the coughing gets worse, there is a high fever, wheezing sounds, lethargy, and weakness. And chest pains develop, along with very difficult breathing. — *Contact a health professional; the condition may be developing into pneumonia.*

• If the condition persists over too long a time, there is the possibility of tuberculosis or lung cancer.

• A professional can use bronchoscopy instruments to examine the bronchial tubes and to suction out phlegm. The problem is that, in recent years, such instruments are often contaminated.

• In recent years, a new type of bronchitis has arisen, which is contracted primarily by women. Difficult to treat, it often continues for 3 weeks to 5 months. Drinking goldenseal tea is helpful with this condition, as well as with other types of bronchitis.

J.H. KELLOGG, M.D., PRESCRIPTIONS FOR CHRONIC BRONCHITIS AND ITS COMPLICATIONS *(how to give these water therapies: pp. 206-275 / list of treatments: pp. 206-207 / Hydrotherapy Disease Index: pp. 273-275)*

IMPROVE GENERAL RESISTANCE—Graduated **cold treatment, aseptic dietary, warm dry climate, outdoor life**.

COUGH—**Heating Chest Pack**, protected by plastic covering. Copious **water** drinking (3-6 pints daily), and **Warm Vapor inhalation**.

NON-PRODUCTIVE COUGH—Increase expulsive power by rubbing or **percussion of the chest** with the hand dipped in ice water or slapping the chest with a cold, wet towel.

ASTHMA—Cold Fan **Spray** to back of chest, followed by **Heating Chest Pack**. **Revulsive Compress** to chest. Revulsive Douche to legs. **Hot Footbath** or Hot Leg Bath. Hot Leg Pack. **Hot Enema**. If sympathetic nerve is irritable, apply a **Hot Abdominal Pack**. Chest Pack that is well-protected.

EMPHYSEMA—**Alternate Compress** or Alternate Douche to spine, Cold Mitten Friction, **Cold Towel Rub**, Wet Sheet Rub. Hot Abdominal Pack, covered with flannel only. **Hot Leg Packs**. **Cold Compress** over heart for 5-30 minutes, 3 times a day.

GENERAL METHOD—The general method is the same as for "Intestinal Catarrh, Chronic."
See Acute Bronchitis (500).
—Also see Bronchiectasis (502).

ENCOURAGEMENT—Christ determined (in council with His Father) to spare nothing, however costly, that would rescue the poor sinner. He did all this for you. Kneel down and accept Him anew just now. Give Him your life and, by His enabling grace, obey His Ten Commandment law. Psalm 91:11-12.

BRONCHIECTASIS

SYMPTOMS—Chronic cough with sputum. He may cough up blood or bloodstained sputum and have inflammation of the lungs. In advanced cases, there may be shortness of breath when any exertion is made. The coughing is often worse with a change in position; and it may occur when the person lies down, rolls over, or sits up. Sometimes the coughing is severe enough to produce vomiting.

CAUSES—Bronchiectasis is permanent dilation and infection of one or more bronchi. It is a sac-like enlargement of the ends of the small bronchi, with a chronic inflammation. Some become partially or entirely blocked by mucus, scarring, or inflammation.

Causes can include **obstructions** in the bronchi, lung **infections**, breathing in of **foreign substances** or **vomitus**, enlarged **lymph nodes, pressure tumors, or dilated blood vessels**. It is often associated with **cystic fibrosis**. About 20% initially occur in children under 1 year of age. And 75% occurs before the child reaches 5.

If the condition lasts a long time, the child may develop an enlarged chest, anemia, clubbing of fingers, excessive fatigue, and may grow slowly.

NATURAL REMEDIES
• Determine to **cough slowly** by first breathing

slowly and deeply; then hold the breath for several seconds. Then give two short, forceful coughs with the mouth open. The first loosens the phlegm; the second brings it up. Hold the breath again; and then breathe in slowly, to avoid non-productive coughing.

• Drink lots of **fluid**, so the phlegm will be thinner and looser.

• Use a cool-air **vaporizer** each night. Try to maintain 30%-50% humidity in the house during the day.

• Outside in cold weather, wear a **scarf or mask** over the mouth and nose, to warm the air.

• **Do not use cough medicines** and **antihistamines**. They dry up the secretions, making them even harder to expel. Do not wear **belts**; the abdomen should be free to breathe and cough properly. Men should wear suspenders.

• There should be as much regular outdoor **exercise** as the condition permits.

• A simple **nourishing diet**, free of sugar and low in fats. No junk food. Extremely hot or cold foods should be avoided; for they can trigger coughing.
—*See Bronchitis (500) for much more.*

ENCOURAGEMENT—We are strangers and pilgrims in this world. We are to wait, watch, pray, and work. There are souls all around us who desperately need God. You can help them come to Him. Job 22:26.

RESPIRATORY - 3 - LUNGS

LUNG CONGESTION

NATURAL REMEDIES

J.H. KELLOGG, M.D., PRESCRIPTIONS FOR LUNG CONGESTION AND ITS COMPLICATIONS (*how to give these water therapies: pp. 206-275 / list of treatments: pp. 206-207 / Hydrotherapy Disease Index: pp. 273-275*)
ACTIVE CONGESTION—Fomentation to back, **Cold Compress** to chest with **Hot Leg Pack**, followed by **Cold Mitten Friction** and **dry heat to legs**, short cold applications to hands and arms, followed by Hot Packs to arms. Revulsive Douche to legs, Hot Leg Bath with very Cold Compress to the chest and to the back opposite the chest. Change compress as soon as it is warmed.
PASSIVE CONGESTION OF CHEST—Apply Fomentation over chest for 10 minutes every hour. During the interval between, apply a **Cold Compress**, renewing it every 15 minutes, rubbing the surface well at each change. This condition most frequently occurs with fevers. Prevent it by frequent change of position. Apply the same derivative measures as for active congestion (see just above).
PULMONARY HEMORRHAGE—Ice Pack to chest. Remove and **rub chest** with dry warm flannel, 1-2 minutes every 15 minutes. **Hot Leg Pack**, very **Hot Sponging** of the upper half of the spine. Place **hands in ice water** for 1-2 minutes; maintain skin circulation by **dry rubbing**. Keep him very quiet. *After hemorrhage ceases,* **graduated cold**

treatment to increase resistance and combat the disease causing the hemorrhage.
—*Also see Pneumonia (503) and Tuberculosis of the Lung (505).*

PNEUMONIA
(Lung Fever)

SYMPTOMS—Fever, chills, aching muscles, coughing, sore throat, bloody sputum, enlarged lymph nodes in the neck, pain in the chest. Rapid, difficult breathing and cyanosis (bluish skin and nails from lack of oxygen).

In bacterial pneumonia, the onset is sudden and the cough is dry at first; then a rust-colored sputum is produced, and breathing becomes rapid and labored. The viral form is more variable in seriousness, from the time it begins.

CAUSES—There is *lobar, bronchopneumonia,* or *interstitial* pneumonia, according to the area of the lungs involved. Pneumonia is a serious infection of the lungs and bronchial tubes. It can be caused by bacteria, viruses, fungi, or protozoa. The tiny sacs in the lungs (which look somewhat like grapes hanging from their stems) are where the oxygen and carbon dioxide exchange is made. These sacs become inflamed and filled with mucus and pus.

Generally an upper respiratory infection in the throat and the bronchial tubes (such as a cold, the flu, or perhaps the measles) occurs. Those under one year or over 60 are the most susceptible.

Bacterial pneumonia is more dangerous and severe than the viral type. There is also a fungal pneumonia; but those with HIV are most likely to contract it.

In children, the pain of pneumonia is frequently located in the abdomen; it causes others to think there is acute indigestion or appendicitis. Some 40,000 older Americans die of pneumonia every year. It is the fifth largest cause of death in the U.S.

If chills, high fever, rapid shallow respirations, cyanosis (blue color) of lips or skin, or delirium occurs, a physician should be contacted. If the treatment is early, careful, and vigorous, pneumonia can usually be successful controlled and eliminated. He will often have weakness for 4-6 weeks after the acute phase is past.

The use of antibiotics for minor infections, such as colds, can produce strong bacteria in the bronchials, which can later cause pneumonia.

NATURAL REMEDIES
• You will want to use essentially the **same treatment as outlined for bronchitis** (also see bronchial problems); except that, because the person's illness is so much more serious, he must be given much rest and intensified care.

• Getting enough **fluids** into the body is important;

for this will thin secretions in the lungs, making them easier to cough up. Increase air moisture in the room with a cool air vaporizer. As they become damp, change the bed clothing and linen to prevent chilling.

• **Rinse out the nose** with saltwater, gently taking it in and blowing it out. **Gargle** with saltwater. Then **repeat** the rinsing and gargling with a goldenseal and myrrh mixture. This will help keep a cold or flu from going down into the lungs.

• *If the lungs are already affected,* after giving the above treatment, give **hot footbaths** and a high **herb enema** at least once a day. Drink plenty of **water**. Take **laxative herbs**, to keep the bowels working properly. Every 2 hours give short, **hot fomentations** to the chest and upper back, with **short cold** between each hot application. Keep the heat on for 10-12 minutes; then sponge off vigorously with a cold cloth. Repeat the cycle 3 times in each series. **Dry** the chest. **Repeat** the series as often as every 2 hours. A **heating compress** may be used between other treatments and at night.

• The head should be kept cool with **washcloths** wrung from ice water if the temperature goes above 100°-101° F. by mouth (101°-102° F. by rectum).

• For those who are not very sick, give a **hot half bath**, followed by a **cold water pour** and vigorous **dry sponging**.

• A **heating pad or hot-water bottle** applied to the chest may ease chest pain; but some are better helped by an **ice bag**. **Coughing** is helpful in bringing up mucus; it should not be treated with medications to prevent it from occurring. Sneeze or cough into disposable tissues, which should be destroyed.

• Diet: Only give **liquids** the first few days. These should consist of **fruit juices** (diluted pineapple juice or orange juice) or **lemon and water** (without sugar), etc. Continue this until the high fever abates. Then give **strained vegetable broths, whole grains** (best in dry form, so they will be chewed well), fresh **carrot juice**.

• Numerous clinical trials show the effectiveness of the **dandelion** against pneumonia. **Echinacea** is also powerful; so is **garlic** and **goldenseal**. **Fenugreek** tea is very helpful in relieving the wracking cough. For small children, the easiest way to give garlic is liquid **Kyolic** (the Japanese preparation). Give a dropper to infants and a teaspoon 3 times daily to older children. **Astragalus** enhances the body's immune system. **Ginger** is a good antibiotic to fight fever.

• The **room** should be warm, but ventilated. Protect him from chilling.

—*See Lung Congestion (409), Bronchio-pneumonia (below), and Lobar Pneumonia (below). Also see Bronchitis (505), Bronchial Problems (504), and Pleurisy (510) for more.*

ENCOURAGEMENT—It is essential that every child of God obey His law. He never asks that you obey in your own strength. But, in Christ, you can be an overcomer, resisting all the wiles of the devil.

BRONCHIAL PNEUMONIA
(Bronchopneumonia)

SYMPTOMS—Cough that may produce rust-colored or bloody sputum. Chest pain that becomes worse when you inhale. Shortness of breath at rest. High fever, delirium, or confusion.

CAUSES—This is pneumonia which also extends into the bronchials. *Essentially treat it exactly like "Pneumonia" (503).*

NATURAL REMEDIES

J.H. KELLOGG, M.D., PRESCRIPTIONS FOR BRONCHIAL PNEUMONIA AND ITS COMPLICATIONS (how to give these water therapies: pp. 206-275 / list of treatments: pp. 206-207 / Hydrotherapy Disease Index: pp. 273-275)
GENERAL MEASURES—See Pneumonia (above).
BRONCHIAL IRRITATION—Warm Vapor Inhalation for 15 minutes every hour. **Fomentation** to chest every 2 hours for 15 minutes, followed by **Heating Compress**, Hot Blanket Pack.
CYANOSIS—Short **Hot Half Bath**. **Pour cold water** over head, spine, and chest (to induce cough, if cough is checked or inefficient while secretion is abundant). It is well to have him **sit in a tub** with a small amount of **hot** water while a **Cold Pail Pour** is given, followed by vigorous rubbing and wrapping in dry blankets in bed.
AFTER CONVALESCENCE BEGINS—Heating Chest **Pack** night and day. Graduated cold applications, to build up general resistance.
—*Also see Pneumonia (503, above).*

ENCOURAGEMENT— Thoughtful courtesies, that (commencing in our families) extend outside the family circle, help make up the sum of life's happiness. As we try to encourage and help others, we ourselves will be helped.

LOBAR PNEUMONIA

This is pneumonia in one or both lobes of the lungs, but without bronchial infection. *Treat it as "Pneumonia" (above).*

NATURAL REMEDIES

J.H. KELLOGG, M.D., PRESCRIPTIONS FOR LOBAR PNEUMONIA AND ITS COMPLICATIONS (how to give these water therapies: pp. 206-275 / list of treatments: pp. 206-207 / Hydrotherapy Disease Index: pp. 273-275)
GENERAL—Exercise special care to prevent lung congestion due to exposure of shoulders or chest to chill

by evaporation. Provide him with an abundance of pure **warm air**; have a supply of **oxygen** at hand for immediate use, if required.

MAINTAIN GENERAL VITAL RESISTANCE—Cold Mitten Friction or **Cold Towel Rub** 2-4 times daily, after some appropriate heating procedure, as a **Fomentation** to chest or back. **Hot Blanket Pack** or Sweating Wet Sheet Pack.

COMBAT LOCAL CONGESTION OF THE LUNGS AND INVASION OF THE SPECIFIC BACILLUS—Fomentation to the chest (both front and back) for 15 minutes every 3 hours. During the interval between, apply **Cold Compress** at 60° F., changing every 15 minutes or as soon as warmed. Lengthen the period between fomentations and change the compress less frequently as the temperature is lowered, the pain less, and the stage of the disease more advanced. Several **Ice Bags** may be used in place of the Cold Compress; but the bags should be removed at least every half hour and the chest should be rubbed until red and warm, to maintain surface circulation and skin reflexes. The skin must be kept warm.

ELIMINATION OF POISONS—Sweating Wet Sheet Packs, continued for 2-4 hours. Follow by **Cold Mitten Friction**, carefully administered. The Sweating Bath may be preceded by the short **Full Hot Bath**. Copious **water** drinking. **Neutral enema** twice daily.

COUGH—Fomentations every 3 hours. **Heating Compress**, changing every 15-30 minutes during the interval between. **Warm Vapor Inhalation** 15 minutes, every hour. Sip half a glass of hot **water** when inclined to cough. Carefully **protect neck and shoulders** from chilling by contact with wet bed clothing. Keep shoulders covered.

PAIN IN CHEST—Revulsive Compress covering the whole chest before and behind.

EXUDATION (ELIMINATION) OF PHLEGM—Alternate Compresses for 20 minutes, 3 times a day, with continuous well-protected **Heating Compress** during the intervals between and after convalescence begins. For unresolved exudation, Alternate Fan Douche or Alternate Spray.

CONSTIPATION—Daily **Cold Enema** or Cold Colonic.

DIARRHEA—Enema at 96° F. after each bowel movement. Cold Abdominal Bandage, renewing every half hour. **Fomentation** every 2-4 hours, if pain or tenderness is present.

TYMPANITES (gaseous distension of abdomen)—Hot **Enema** followed by small **Cool Enema**. Cold Colonic. **Cold Abdominal Compress**, changing hourly.

GASTRO-DUODENITIS—Fomentation over stomach and bowels or **Hot Trunk Pack** every 3 hours. During intervals between, **Cold Compress** at 60° F., changing every 30 minutes. **Neutral Enema** daily.

JAUNDICE—Large **Hot Colonic** at 105° F., followed by small **Cold Enema** twice daily. **Fomentation** over the liver and stomach every 2 hours. During the interval between, **Heating Compress**, changing every 30 minutes.

WEAK HEART, FEEBLE PULSE—Cold Compress or Ice Bag over the heart for 15 minutes every 2 hours. Cold Mitten Friction every 2 hours. Prolonged **Neutral Bath** with **Ice Bag** over heart, **Cold Pail Pour** to back of head and upper spine at the end of the bath.

CYANOSIS (BLUENESS)—Hot Blanket Pack for 15 minutes, followed by **Cold Mitten Friction**. Avoid exposure of the body to chill by evaporation.

HEADACHE—Ice Compress, or **Ice Cap**, to head. **Hot Pack to legs and hips**, or other derivative treatment. **Hot and Cold Head Compress**.

NOSEBLEED—Ice Bag to back of neck, short hot **Fomentations** to face.

DELIRIUM—Heating Wet Sheet Pack, **Ice Cap** to Head, Prolonged **Sweating Wet Sheet Pack**.

INSOMNIA—Neutral Wet Sheet Pack.

CEREBRAL CONGESTION—Hip and Leg Pack, Ice Cap to head.

FEVER—Prolonged **Neutral Bath**, Wet Sheet Pack, **Cooling Enema**.

SUBNORMAL TEMPERATURE—Dry Pack, **Hot Blanket Pack**, Hot **Enema**, and hot **water** drinking. Do not expose him during changing of application or after it.

PAIN IN ABDOMEN AND BACK—Hot **Blanket Pack** or large **Fomentations** over affected parts, followed by **Heating Compress**.

CAPILLARY BRONCHITIS—Hot **Blanket Pack** followed by Sweating **Wet Sheet Pack**. Hot **Enemas** followed by **Cold Friction**, carefully given. **Fomentation** to the chest followed by **Heating Compress** or Chest Pack, to remain in place an hour or until thoroughly warmed. Repeat bath when temperature rises to 102° F.

CONTRAINDICATIONS—Do not use Cold Full Baths or anything equivalent.

GENERAL METHOD—Maintain warmth and activity of the skin, taking special care to avoid chilling of the shoulders, which should be especially protected by a wrapping, closely applied. Combat pulmonary congestion by local applications made as directed above. Keep the temperature down by carefully managed hydrotherapy measures (such as the Heating Pack, the Hot Blanket Pack, followed by Cold Mitten Friction and like measures) rather than Cold Full Baths and Cooling Packs, which aggravate lung congestion by producing retrostasis. Promote vital resistance by frequently repeated partial Cold Frictions; and thus sustain the vital powers until opportunity has been afforded for the development of antitoxins and the suppression of the disease by the natural healing processes.

—*Also see Pneumonia (503).*

ENCOURAGEMENT—Let us, under all circumstances, preserve our confidence in Christ. He is to be everything to us—the first, the last, the best in everything. Then let us educate our tongues to speak forth His praise at all times, not only when we feel gladness and joy.

TUBERCULOSIS
(Consumption)

SYMPTOMS—Coughing, general fatigue, loss of appetite, chest pain, night sweats, and low-grade fever. The cough is at first not too productive; but, later, increasing amounts of phlegm are coughed up.

The person loses weight and the sputum becomes bloody.

CAUSES—In the 19th century, tuberculosis (TB) was called *consumption*; for the person seemed to waste away. It is caused by a highly contagious

RESP

bacteria, the Koch bacillus, called *Mycobacterium tuberculosis*. Although it generally affects the lungs, it can attack any part of the body: kidneys, bones, skin, intestines, spleen, and liver.

In adults, pleurisy is frequently a complication of tuberculosis. The sharp chest pain one may feel might be the pleurisy *(510)*.

It is spread by coughing. Tiny droplets are inhaled by others. The germ enters the lungs and remains there. As long as the person maintains a healthy lifestyle, the body encapsulates the germs; that is, a tiny calcium shell is placed around the TB germ, to render it harmless.

If the person continues to eat right, obtains enough calcium in his diet, gets adequate rest, exercises outdoors, and breathes vigorously to keep his lungs in good health—he will not develop TB, even though the germs are in his lungs. Remember that. Tuberculosis can progressively worsen at a slow pace; you do best to catch it in its early stages.

It is said that overweight people tend to have heart trouble and thin ones tend to have tuberculosis. So be extra careful if you are thin.

At the present time, tuberculosis is making a powerful comeback—and is once again becoming a modern plague. So be careful. It may be in the air of the next building you enter (especially buildings crowded with people). Live right everyday. Homeless shelters and prisons have the highest percentage of people with TB. It is estimated that, by 2020, there will be 200 million new cases throughout the world; and 70 million people will die from it.

NATURAL REMEDIES

• The treatment is obviously a matter of retracing one's steps—and doing what he should have done earlier. Initially, he must overcome the critical phase of the disease with **fasting, rest, and good food**, all the while having **fresh air** in his room.

• Maintain a moderate temperature, never too warm and always good ventilation. Avoid becoming chilled. The room should be sunny, airy, and dry. Stay outdoors, breathing deeply, as much as possible.

• If he is not too weak, clean the stomach out with an **emetic** (to induce vomiting). This will eliminate a large amount of mucus, which would otherwise be brought up in paroxysms of coughing; it contaminates the air for those helping him. To induce vomiting, drink some **lobelia** tea in warm water and run a finger down the throat. All **sputum** and discharges should be burned or buried.

• But later, he must take time each day to do something **outdoors** that will exercise his lungs, not only his body. Walking up a hill and **breathing deeply** is excellent. Maintain an erect posture, so you can breathe properly.

• *Remember the formula* to prevent and eliminate tuberculosis: adequate **rest**, good **diet** including

calcium, daily deep **breathing** outdoors.

• If you suspect you might be getting tuberculosis, here are excellent herbs for tuberculosis: **Echinacea**. Take two 450-mg capsules 3 times a day for a week; wait a week and do it again. **Garlic**: 1 garlic capsule a day or equivalent. **Licorice** has up to 33% antibacterial compounds on a dry-weight basis. The Chinese use licorice to treat TB. Add it to any herbal preparation you take for tuberculosis. Kloss suggests drinking at least 1 quart of **slippery elm** tea every day.

• To clean out the pus and accumulation, mix equal parts powdered **comfrey, marshmallow, chickweed, and slippery elm**. Add 4 oz. to 4 quarts water, boil down to 2 quarts. Strain and take ½ cup every 2 hours, either hot or cold.

• Give short, **hot fomentations** with **short cold** applied to chest and then to back. Also apply it the full length of the spine and over the stomach, liver, and spleen.

• In accordance with the strength of the patient, give **warm baths** followed by a **salt glow** and **massage**.

• *Take cough medicine*, especially after a coughing spell. Here are the best herbs for this purpose: **Ginger** has several chemicals with cough-suppressing, pain-relieving, and fever-reducing action. **Licorice** has a long history of use in treating coughs. **Slippery elm**, with its mucilage, is a throat soother and cough suppressant. **Marshmallow** and **mullein** have similar properties.

• Keep him warm with **warm clothing**, especially the feet, legs, and arms.

• Keep in mind that the *tubercle bacillus* remains in the lungs for the remainder of one's lifetime. So once you are on your feet again and appear to be well, you must continue a program of careful eating, living, and outdoor activity; all the while obtain adequate rest every night.

J.H. KELLOGG, M.D., PRESCRIPTIONS FOR TUBERCULOSIS AND ITS COMPLICATIONS *(how to give these water therapies: pp. 206-275 / list of treatments: pp. 206-207 / Hydrotherapy Disease Index: pp. 273-275)*

GENERAL—Destroy sputum (spit); avoid swallowing it again; live in the open air and sleep in cool, well-ventilated rooms.

INCREASE GENERAL VITAL RESISTANCE—Graduated **Cold Baths**, twice daily. **Fattening dietary**. Systematic **exercise**. **Outdoor life**. **Cool, dry, elevated climate**. Very brief Radiant Heat Bath, daily or 3 times a week.

ANEMIA—**Cold Bath** twice daily. Food rich in blood-making material. **Easily digested foods**, rich in protein.

INDIGESTION, ANOREXIA—**Dry aseptic dietary**, dry toast, malted cereals. Hot **Abdominal Pack**. **Ice Bag** over the stomach half an hour before meals.

CHILL—Rest in bed, **Dry Pack**, hot-water drinking.

COUGH—**Fomentation** to chest, followed by **Heating Chest Pack**. Sip hot water when inclined to cough.

PAIN—**Revulsive Compress** for 15 minutes, 2-3 times daily. During intervals between, apply well-protected

Heating Compress.
   PULMONARY (LUNG) HEMORRHAGE OR CONGES-TION—Very hot application to spine between shoulders, Ice to chest, ice to hands, Hot **Leg Pack**. Keep the extremities warm; elevate the chest and shoulders.
   FEVER—Neutral Pack for 15-20 minutes. Free **water** drinking. **Rest** in the horizontal position until the daily evening temperature becomes nearly normal.
   NIGHT SWEATS—Very **Hot Sponging** at bedtime.
   HYPOPEPSIA, ATONIC DYSPEPSIA—Daily, general **cold applications**. **Ice Bag** over stomach for half an hour before meals.
   DIARRHEA—Enema at 95° F., after each bowel movement, followed by Cold **Abdominal Compress** at 60° F., changing every half hour. **Rest** in bed till checked.
   CONTRAINDICATIONS—Avoid general cold baths when hemorrhage is threatened. This includes Cold Full Baths, Cold Pail Pours, Cold Sitz Baths. It also includes Steam Baths.
   GENERAL METHOD—The great object to be kept in mind, in the hydrotherapy treatment of this disease, is to build up his vital resistance by carefully graduated cold applications (the various Tonic Frictions), repeated 2-3 times a day. The intensity of the application should be steadily increased from day to day in order to secure good results. No one is too feeble to receive water therapy of some sort; and, by careful graduation, persons of feeble physique, but in whom the disease is not yet far advanced, may be trained to receive very vigorous cold applications with excellent effects. In making the cold applications, care must be taken to avoid chilling him; for this would immediately aggravate his cough.
   —*Follow the cleansing and healing program given to Bronchitis (500), Bronchial Problems and Pneumonia (500-503). Also see Pleurisy (510).*

   ENCOURAGEMENT—Day by day we are to live for God. Day by day, we are to help those around us. As we do this, angels work with us; and what a joy is ours! Matthew 18:10.

EMPHYSEMA

SYMPTOMS—It is only with great effort that the person can exhale air from his lungs. There is continual breathlessness. Most any exertion brings coughing. It is hard to breathe in, but worse to breathe out. The neck veins often stand out from the effort; and he breathes through the mouth in order to try to get enough air in and out. Breathing is usually rapid and short. He may breathe 25-30 times a minute; and he still does not get enough air.
   Eventually his chest becomes barrel-shaped, his face ruddy, and he speaks with short and broken phrases.

CAUSES—The word, "emphysema," comes from a Greek word meaning "to puff up with air." The walls of the lungs lose their elasticity; so air cannot be easily pushed in and out, as should normally happen. There is air in the lungs, but it is not moving in and out. As emphysema progresses and the obstruction to airflow increases, the lungs enlarge with trapped air.
   The most frequent cause is **smoking**; but **dust** and **air pollution** also receives some of the blame. Live in the country and do not have tobacco in your home; and you should be able to avoid this problem.
   Emphysema has become the most common modern lung infection in the Western world. Needing a continual exchange of air to survive, we use about a thousand cubic feet of air each day. It passes over lung surfaces which, if laid flat, would be as large as a tennis court. In emphysema, a large portion of the alveoli (the grape-like sacs where the air exchange occurs) are destroyed and the blood is not properly aerated.

NATURAL REMEDIES

TREATMENT: LIVING WITH THE PROBLEM—
• The person absolutely must **stop smoking**. **Tobacco smoke** should be banished from the home, car, and place of work. Also avoid **hair spray** and **other sprays**. Avoid **allergens** that you know of.
• Maintain a program of regular **exercise**. Walking outdoors is always the best. Try using 1- or 2-pound hand weights and work the muscles in the neck, upper shoulders, and chest. Those with chronic emphysema need strong muscles there more than others do.
• **Eat less** and a little **more often**. Prolonged digestion requires more oxygen and blood to the stomach, and away from other parts of the body which also need them. Maintain a **low-salt** diet. **Flaxseed oil** is rich in omega-3 fatty acids, which help to decrease lung inflammation and ease breathing.
• **Avoid gas-forming foods**, such as **legumes** and **cabbage**. These cause abdominal distention which can interfere with breathing. **Avoid hard-to-chew foods** and excessively hot or cold foods that may induce coughing. Do not eat when emotionally **upset** or angry.
• Drink enough **water**. The fluid intake is needed to keep the mucus, in the lungs, thin. Sip warm, clear liquids in the morning (such as herb teas), to help clear mucus from the airways.
• Maintain your ideal **body weight**. Some of those with this problem tend to put on weight and retain fluid. The closer you are to your ideal weight, the better for your lungs. Stay on a low-calorie diet. The thinner you are, the less flesh your lungs have to supply oxygen to. Obesity and **constipation** decrease the patient's resistance to respiratory infection.
• Learn to **breathe correctly**. The tendency is to breathe short and fast. But make yourself breathe steadily, from the diaphragm. Strengthen your respiration muscles by blowing out slowly through pursed lips for 30 minutes a day. Try to exhale twice as long as it took you to breathe in. Wear **loose clothing**; this helps you breathe better. Begin each morning by taking several deep breaths before rising.

R
E
S
P

• Learn to **cough properly**. Inhale slowly and deeply. Exhale through pursed lips and cough in short huffing bursts rather than vigorously.

• Learn when to **inhale and exhale** air. When working, lift while you exhale through pursed lips; inhale while you rest. When climbing steps, climb while exhaling; inhale when you stop to rest. **Pace yourself** in your work. Work steadily; it is not necessary to work fast.

• Go through the day **relaxed** instead of with a sense of alarm over your air problems.

• **Avoid** contact with anyone with a **respiratory infection**.

• **Avoid cough suppressant drugs**. They dry up secretions, which you do not want. Use only **essential and unscented soaps**.

• **Avoid perfumes, gas stoves, carpeting, curtains and draperies** which cannot easily be cleaned. Avoid **hot, humid climates**. Avoid **furry, feathered animals** in your home. Leave the house during major **housecleaning**; and stay away for two hours.

• Get plenty of **fresh air**. Use a **warm scarf or mask** over the mouth and nose when outdoors in cold weather. **Keep the body warm** at all times. Do not live in a **hot, humid climate**, unless you have central air conditioning.

• **Elevate the bed**. Place 3, 4, or 5-inch blocks under the foot of the bed. This will help prevent mucus from accumulating in the lower part of the lungs during the night. (But not too steep; for that would be hard on the heart.)

• **Hang** from the waist **over the edge of a bed** with a bowl placed at the head for easy expectoration. Apply a **hot, moist compress** to the back repeatedly for 5-10 minutes. Then have a friend **pound vigorously** on the back with open palms. As mucus is loosened, it should be **spit out**. Repeat 1-3 times a day.

• Alternate **hot and cold chest packs** to stimulate circulation, respiration, and mucus elimination. **Alternate hot and cold showers**.

• Herbs that can help thin mucus or clear it from the lungs are especially helpful. Here are some of the best: **mullein, licorice, peppermint, elecampane,** and **cayenne**.

TREATMENT: SOLVING THE PROBLEM—

The official pronouncement is that there is no cure for emphysema. But there is!

The suggestions above are typical of what you will find in most books. It is difficult to find remedial solutions, but here is one:

Several years ago, a Christian mother visited her neighbors and met a woman with emphysema. It was a small, stuffy house and the lady smoked. So the mother went back home and eventually found a treatment; it was a wet heating pack from Kneipp's book, written nearly two centuries ago. She gave the treatment to the woman, who got well within several weeks. This was the treatment:

• Place a **plastic sheet** on the bed, both above the bottom sheet and beneath the top sheet and covers. **Dip another sheet in very cold water, and wring it out somewhat**—quickly, to keep in the cold.

• Work quickly: **Wrap the sheet about the person**, who is standing unclothed. The sheet covers everything but the head and perhaps part of the neck. Than **wrap a dry blanket around him**. The person immediately gets into the bed, and is covered well with the top sheet and blankets. This is essentially something like a heating pack, but done only with a wet sheet. The effect is immediate freezing cold, which the body gradually warms and warms and warms. The person can remain like this all night.

In the years that followed, the mother mentioned the incident to a number of medical people and doctors who were astounded; for everyone says there is no cure for emphysema. Note: A more moderate treatment (with less intense cold to start) might have to be given to a very thin, frail person.

ENCOURAGEMENT—By both creation and redemption we are the Lord's property. We are required to obey His laws; but we are never asked to do it in our own strength. Christ helps us in all that we do.

LEGIONNAIRE'S DISEASE

SYMPTOMS—It initially appears to be the flu. There is headache, fatigue, achiness, and moderate fever. But then it develops into what seems more like pneumonia: a high fever (105° F.) with coughing, diarrhea, chills, disorientation, slow heart rate, dry cough, infection of the pleura, vomiting, severe chest pain, and shortness of breath. From lack of oxygen, the skin becomes bluish. The sputum that is coughed up eventually is gray or blood-streaked.

CAUSES—This is the strange disease which was first identified at the American Legion convention in 1976, which affected 182 partying in a hotel.

Those who **smoke, drink, have diabetes, emphysema, or kidney problems** are more likely to contract the disease. Younger people quickly recover; but the elderly can die from respiratory failure. **Immunosuppressed patients** (such as chemotherapy-treated cancer patients, **transplant patients**, and **AIDS patients**) are the most susceptible to contracting it.

The *Legionella pneumophila* bacteria are not directly transmitted from person to person, but through cool air-borne vapor droplets (primarily **heating and cooling systems**). That is how the Legionnaire's got it in that hotel. The bacteria have also been found in newly plowed soil and excavation sites.

NATURAL REMEDIES

• Essentially follow the regime listed under Pneumonia *(503)*, Bronchitis *(500)*, and Fever *(302-309)*. See your health-care provider. The present rate is that 80% of those contracting the disease die; so this disease is a very serious matter.

ENCOURAGEMENT—Copy the example of Christ: His love, tenderness, and obedience. Minister to the needs of everyone around you. They need the peace and happiness that you have found in Christ.

Q FEVER

SYMPTOMS—Some of the symptoms of Q fever are like those of typhus *(839)*; and some are like those of bronchopneumonia. See *Pneumonia (503)* and *"Bronchitis" (505)*. There is a sudden onset of fever, headache, weakness, and a pneumonia-like infection.

CAUSES—Q fever is quite rare in the Western world. The name comes from "query," because scientists initially questioned what it was. Caused by a rickettsial organism *(Coxiella burnetii)*, Q fever is worldwide in its coverage. First discovered in Australia, it is now known to even occur in the United States.

It is endemic in domestic animals. Sheep, goats, and cattle are the primary reservoirs for transference to humans. The disease is spread to humans by bites from an infected **tick** *(Dermacentor andersoni)* and from drinking **raw milk**.

NATURAL REMEDIES
• See your physician. Give this problem the care you would give to typhus *(839)*, bronchitis *(500)*, and pneumonia *(503)*.

ENCOURAGEMENT—There are many from whom hope has departed. Bring back the sunshine into their lives. You can do this as, prayerfully, you seek to bring a knowledge of Jesus into their lives.

HYPERSENSITIVITY PNEUMONITIS

SYMPTOMS—*Acute attack:* This resembles symptoms of influenza and usually develops within 4-8 hours after initial exposure. It may include fever and chills, coughing and wheezing, tightness in the chest, and sometimes shortness of breath. If exposure to the substance stops immediately, the symptoms usually clear up within 12-24 hours and often disappear completely within 48 hours.

Chronic attacks: If further exposure to the substance occurs, the problem becomes chronic with continuous symptoms: Coughing becomes progressively worse. Increasing shortness of breath. Loss of appetite and weight. Symptoms may continue even after exposure to the substance ends. Continued exposure can eventually lead to respiratory failure.

CAUSES—**Dust, fungal spores, chemicals, proteins, chemicals containing organic substances**.

Farmer's lung: The reaction is triggered by fungal spores from **moldy hay**. In *bird fancier's lung*, the cause is particles from **bird droppings**. Other causes include **cheese mold, coffee dust, mushroom soil, microorganisms in air-conditioning systems, humidifiers, certain chemicals used in manufacturing insulation, packing materials, or other materials**.

In reaction, the walls of the alveoli (the air sacs, or small airways, of the lungs) thicken and oxygen cannot get through the narrowed passageways.

NATURAL REMEDIES
• **Locate the source** of the problem. It may be your occupational work or a hobby. Instead of trying to take drugs to counteract the harmful effects of the substance, no longer be around the problem. **Switch jobs or change your hobbies**.
• Wearing a **protective mask** might work on a short-term basis; but you will still be breathing some of the substance. Make sure **air conditioners are cleaned** regularly.
—*See Occupational Lung Disease (below), which is concerned with mineral dusts. Also see Black Lung (510), which discusses coal-mining dust problems, and Silicosis (510), caused by silicon dust.*

ENCOURAGEMENT—As we associate together, we may be a blessing to one another. If we are Christ's, our sweetest thoughts will be of Him. We shall love to talk of Him; and as we speak to one another of His love, our hearts will be softened by divine influences. Beholding the beauty of His character, we shall be "changed into the same image from glory to glory."

OCCUPATIONAL LUNG DISEASE

SYMPTOMS—Coughing and wheezing, tightness in the chest, shortness of breath, fever, and chills. The coughing becomes progressively worse, with increasing shortness of breath. Asthma may begin.

CAUSES—**Small mineral particles and gases** are breathed into the lungs. Some **organic substances** may be included. The type and amount of particles determine the nature of the lung disease. Three primary ones are **coal** (causing black lung, *below*), **silicon** (causing silicosis, *510*), and **asbestos** (causing asbestosis, *510*).

Inflammation of the alveoli inside the lungs occurs. Asbestos can also cause thickening of the pleura (the two-layered membrane separating the lungs from the chest), and mesothelioma, a form of cancer of the pleura.

There is a growing list of substances which can cause this problem and an increasing number of cases each year.

Chemical factories, paper companies, oil firms, manufacturing plants (especially those burning coal) also cause problems by polluting the air in a wide area.

R E S P

NATURAL REMEDIES

• It is vital that you avoid the substances which are causing your problem; and you must do it as quickly as possible! **Change employment**. If the dust is in the air, **move to a different area**. There can be no other effective solution.

—*See Hypersensitivity Pneumonitis (509), which results from organic dusts. Also see Black Lung (below), which discusses coal-mining dust problems, and Silicosis (bellow), caused by silicon dust.*

ENCOURAGEMENT—Jesus is bending over you in love. He wants you to live in His presence forever. Accept Him just now as your Saviour.

BLACK LUNG
(Coal workers' Pneumoconiosis)

SYMPTOMS—Coughing up black sputum. Shortness of breath with exertion that becomes progressively worse.

CAUSES—The cause is inhaling **coal dust**. It gradually built up, produced scar tissue in the lungs over many years, and led to progressive and disabling shortness of breath. If the coal dust contains silicon, the effects are even worse.

NATURAL REMEDIES

• **Quit your job**; and, **if there is dust in the air, move** to a different locality.
—*See Occupational Lung Disease (509), which is concerned with mineral dusts. Also see Silicosis (below), caused by silicon dust, and Hypersensitivity Pneumonitis (509), which results from organic dusts.*

ENCOURAGEMENT—It would be well for us to spend a thoughtful hour each day in contemplation of the life of Christ. We should take it point by point, and let the imagination grasp each scene, especially the closing ones. As we thus dwell upon His great sacrifice for us, our confidence in Him will be more constant.

SILICOSIS, ASBESTOSIS

SYMPTOMS—Coughing up sputum, shortness of breath with exertion and tightness of the chest. Tuberculosis can later result.

CAUSES—This disease can affect those who work with **sandstone, granite, slate, or coal**. It can also injure **potters, foundry workers, sandblasters, and those who work in asbestos factories or handle asbestos** material. Between 1.2 to 3 million U.S. workers have been exposed to silica dust. The chronic form usually develops after 20-30 years of exposure. But only a few months of exposure to lots

of the dust can lead to sudden death. More than most dusts, silica causes a strong inflammatory response in the lungs. Thickening and scarring of the lungs occur and less oxygen is available to the body. The problem is intensified in those who **smoke tobacco**.

NATURAL REMEDIES

• **Stop smoking, change jobs, and (if necessary) move** out of the area.

ENCOURAGEMENT—The Lord Jesus loves you. If you doubt His love, look to Calvary. The light reflected from the cross shows you the magnitude of that love which no tongue can tell.

SWIMMING POOL SYNDROME

SYMPTOMS—Headaches and grogginess after swimming in an indoor swimming pool.

CAUSES—Public swimming pools are heavily chlorinated. The chlorine continually vaporizes into the air; and those working in those buildings or swimming in the water breathe that contaminated air. In addition, swimmers occasionally accidentally swallow some of the water. Because chlorine is bleach, those who inhale it are taking diluted bleach into their lungs. The chlorides especially affect the lungs and brain.

NATURAL REMEDIES

• Avoid public swimming pools which are enclosed. Open air pools are less dangerous, but still a problem.
• After swimming, shower off; then walk outside for a time, inhaling and exhaling a lot. Even city water has less chlorine than swimming pools.

ENCOURAGEMENT—By beholding we become changed. As we look in faith to Jesus, His image is engraven on the heart. We are transformed in character. He enables us by His grace to obey His ten commandment law and live pure lives. This is the only way to truly live a happy life: Living for Jesus, and doing all we can to help and encourage others.

RESPIRATORY - 4 - PLEURA

PLEURISY

SYMPTOMS—The pleural membranes become swollen and inflamed; they at first rub together with each breath, causing severe pain and sound that can be heard by a physician using his stethoscope. The pain suddenly becomes more severe if the person attempts to take a quick deep breath, cough, or sneeze.

Fluid may form in the space between the lung and the chest wall. When that happens, the rubbing sound disappears, as well as most or all of the pain. There may only be a little fluid or it may fill half the chest cavity, compressing the lung.

Pleurisy can also appear on the surface of the diaphragm. In this case, the pain is in the abdomen, at the pit of the stomach, or can even be referred pain to the shoulder.

In children, both the pain of pleurisy and that of pneumonia are frequently located in the abdomen, causing others to think the problem is acute indigestion or appendicitis.

CAUSES—The lungs are enclosed within a sacklike covering. Since the lungs are constantly in motion, they must be able to slip against this covering without harming themselves or the pleura. Pleurisy occurs when this sack becomes inflamed. The cause is generally the *tubercle bacillus* (the cause of tuberculosis), *pneumococcus*, or *streptococcus*. The two later germs are present in pneumonia.

Some pleurisy is always present in lobar pneumonia (*see Pneumonia, 509*); and, in adults, pleurisy is frequently a complication of tuberculosis (*505*).

But the underlying cause is **not eating right, getting enough sleep, or not avoiding stress and overwork**.

Damaged kidneys, caused by drugs or eating and drinking the wrong things, can also be a factor. One individual who contracted pleurisy regularly poured a couple spoonfuls (literally) of cayenne on his food, so that only the red color could be seen. Although small amounts of **cayenne** are excellent as a remedy, large amounts, week after week, weaken and injure the kidneys. This can result in an edemic condition affecting the pleural membrane, causing it to fill with water.

NATURAL REMEDIES

• Put him to **bed** and keep him **warm**. Give a high **enema**; and apply **fomentations** to the chest and upper back. Continue this for 1-2 hours, let the patient rest; then repeat. Keep doing this until the pain has ceased.

• Maintain hot **fomentations**; this will disperse the water in the lungs and keep the pain from returning. The fomentations should be large, thick, and hot, and changed frequently. Do about 5 changes; and do not follow with any cold treatment. This is important. Use a **hot-water bottle** on the chest following the fomentations. It may be kept there nearly all the time. If his chest is allowed to become chilled, the pleurisy

will become worse!

• Give hot **herb teas of pleurisy root, yarrow, valerian, and buckthorn bark**. Add **skullcap** if the pain is severe.

• Use of pleurisy root (a specific), slippery elm, comfrey root, hyssop, and vervain.

• An excellent herb tea is a tablespoon each of **pleurisy root and yarrow**, and a pinch of **cayenne**. Put it in water brought to a boil. Let it steep; and then drink a large swallow of the warm tea every hour.

• Only give **fruits, oatmeal water, vegetables, and grains**. Allow no meat, milk, alcohol, or junk food.

• Do not jar the patient. Move him carefully, gently. **Jars and quick motions** make the pleurisy worse and greatly increase the pain.

• He, of course, needs **fluid**; but do not give him too much during the crisis.

J.H. KELLOGG, M.D., PRESCRIPTIONS FOR ACUTE PLEURISY AND ITS COMPLICATIONS (*how to give these water therapies: pp. 206-275 / list of treatments: pp. 206-207 / Hydrotherapy Disease Index: pp. 273-275*)

(1) ACUTE FORM —
GENERAL—Improve general resistance by **cold applications**, 2-3 times daily. **Hot Leg Bath**, if extremities are cold. **Water** drinking. **Aseptic diet**.

PAIN—Very hot **Fomentation** for 10 minutes over the affected side. **Revulsive Compress**. Limit movement of lung by tight bandage to the chest. Repeat every 2 hours. During interval, apply either Cold compress or **Heating Compress** as best suits the case.

AFTER CONVALESCENCE—Alternate Chest Douche or **Alternate Compress**, if necessary to absorb exudation. Apply, 3 times a day, a continuous **Heating Compress** with plastic covering during the interval between.

EXUDATION—Alternate Compress or Alternate spray Douche 3 times a day, graduated general tonic applications. Prolonged **Neutral Bath**, half an hour to an hour daily.

(2) CHRONIC FORM —
GENERAL TREATMENT—Neutral Bath at night, 3 times a week, of 20-30 minutes duration. Graduated **cold applications** daily. **Fomentation** to chest, 3 times a day, or Revulsive spray Douche. Well-protected **Heating Compress** during the interval between.

TUBERCULAR PLEURISY—Short **Revulsive Compress** for 5 minutes for relief of pain, 3-4 times a day or as often as necessary. Flannel **Heating Compress** during the intervals between; graduated **Tonic Frictions**.

ENCOURAGEMENT—**Christ, the Majesty of heaven, became poor; that we, though His poverty, might become rich. What kind of riches? The riches of clean living, health, happiness, and eternity with Christ to look forward to. Job 22:26.**

"In whom we have boldness and access with confidence, by faith of Him."
—Ephesians 3:12

"A just man falleth seven times, and riseth up again."   —Proverbs 24:16

"The Lord is good unto them that wait for Him, to the soul that seeketh Him."
—Lamentations 3:25

The Natural Remedies Encyclopedia

- Disease Section 8 - Cardiovascular

C
A
R
D

= Information, not a disease   **Circulatory System: Physiology 1013-1015 / Pictures 1034**

FOR INFORMATION ON PREVENTING AND LIVING WITH HEART AND CIRCULATORY PROBLEMS:
READ EVERYTHING IN THE SECTION ON "HEART" (419-427) AND "CIRCULATORY" (427-439).

"Be of good courage, and He shall strengthen your heart,
all ye that hope in the Lord."   —*Psalm 31:24*

"A new heart also will I give you, and a new spirit will I put
within you."   —*Ezekiel 36:26*

FOR MORE NATURAL REMEDIES:

HERBS: Herb Contents (pp. 129-130) will help you
locate the 126 most important herbs and the
diseases each one can treat. How to prepare
herbs (132). How to use them (141-189).
HYDROTHERAPY: Therapy Contents (pp. 206-207)
and its Disease Index (263-265) will lead you to
over 100 water therapies and many more remedies. DIS. INDEX: 1211- / GEN. INDEX: 1221-

VITAMINS AND MINERALS: Contents (100-101).
Using 101-124. Dosages (124). Others (117-)
CARING FOR THE SICK: Home care for a sick
person (28-36). The healing crisis (36-39)
WOMEN'S SECTIONS: Female Organs (672)
Pregnancy (701). Childbirth (765). Infancy,
Childhood (722). Women's Herbs (754, 760)
EMERGENCIES: (973-). FIRST AID: (990-)

Section 8 - Cardiovascular

CARDIOVASCULAR - 1 - HEART

HEART ATTACK - EMERGENCY !!
(THREATENED CARDIAC FAILURE)

WHAT YOU SHOULD IMMEDIATELY DO IF YOU HAVE A HEART ATTACK

Since many people are alone when they suffer a heart attack, this suggestion may save a life. Even if someone is with them, the friend may not be able to do anything more than phone 911.

If, upon experiencing a sudden heart attack and being alone, you will not receive immediate help. You will begin to feel faint because your heart is no longer beating properly. You only have about 10 seconds left before losing consciousness. However, **you can help yourself by coughing repeatedly and very vigorously.** *Here is how to do it:*

• **Take a deep breath before each cough**.

• **The cough must be deep and prolonged**, as when producing sputum from deep inside the chest.

• **A breath and a cough must be repeated about every two seconds, without letup**, until help arrives or until the heart is beating normally again.

These deep breaths get oxygen into the lungs; and the coughing movement squeezes the heart and keeps the blood circulating. The squeezing pressure on the heart also helps it regain normal rhythm. In this way, heart attack victims are more likely to survive the trip to the hospital. Tell as many other people as possible about this. It could save their lives.

An Austrian study found that this coughing vigorously (called "cough CPR") until help arrives can help to save the lives of people experiencing heart attack or cardiac arrest.

• Also extremely helpful: If a heart attack is threatening and about to occur, *take half a teaspoon of* **cayenne pepper** (red pepper, not black or white pepper) *in some water and swallow it.* Just placing some cayenne in the mouth, with or without water, will help. It will nicely strengthen and speed up heart action.

• Here is another life-saving help: If you think you could have a heart attack, purchase some **arnica** and have it ready to take. It is said to be an immediate remedy for a heart attack.

NATURAL REMEDIES

J.H. KELLOGG, M.D., PRESCRIPTIONS FOR

COMPARATIVE CHART -1051: Coronary Thrombosis (530) vs. Angina Pictoris (521)

THREATENED CARDIAC FAILURE (*how to give these water therapies: pp. 206-275 / list of treatments: pp. 206-207 / Hydrotherapy Disease Index: pp. 273-275*)

THREATENED CARDIAC FAILURE—Cold bag (ice pack) over heart for 15 minutes every hour. **Cold Mitten Friction** every 2 hours. **Hot Blanket Pack** for 10 minutes, followed by **Cold Towel Rub**. **Hot Enema**, followed by **Cold Enema**. Artificial respiration.

These are all very grave conditions and must receive immediate attention. Immediately call your physician and begin water treatments.

—*Also see Heart Attack Signals (513-523), How to Give CPR (991-995), How to Do Rescue Breathing (when unconscious, see Emergency First Aid).*

—*Also see Heat Exhaustion (286), Heat Stroke (286), Sunstroke (286), Heart Problems (below), Arteriosclerosis (523), and Hypertension (526), Special Report (815-817).*

ENCOURAGEMENT—There is joy and consolation for the truehearted, faithful Christian, that the world knows not of. To them it is a mystery. The Christian's hope is big with immortality and full of glory. It reaches to that within the veil; and it is as an anchor to the soul, both sure and steadfast. And when the storm of God's wrath shall come upon the ungodly, this hope will not fail them; but they are hid as in the secret of His pavilion.

HEART PROBLEMS
(Cardiac Problems)

INTRODUCTION—Heart disease is the number one killer in civilized nations.

There are so many aspects to this, that it seems well to combine them all in one article rather than divide them into several.

Part of the confusion is that everything is so interrelated: diet, high blood pressure, arteriosclerosis, atherosclerosis, angina, and other degenerative heart changes.

In order to fully utilize the data in this article, you should also carefully read the companion articles in the first two parts of this chapter (*Heart, 513-523 and Circulatory, 523-536*).

The underlying cause of most heart disease is atherosclerosis (*523*). This is brought on by high blood cholesterol levels which are themselves caused by a diet low in antioxidants and high in animal fat, butter, and hydrogenated vegetable fats.

The principle cause of heart trouble is a wrong diet which causes the system to become sluggish with waste products which collect in the bloodstream.

C A R D

Because of lack of exercise, the circulation becomes poor and the blood supply to the extremities becomes congested and overburdens the digestive organs and the heart. Sometimes the heart valves become tired and weak from malnutrition and poor tone. Often the heart is slowed down because of cholesterol which restricts the walls and makes it difficult for the life-giving fluid to flow without causing high blood pressure which is very tiring to the heart muscles and eventually stops the heart completely. If the blood is not in good condition, a clot may form in the heart.

SYMPTOMS OF A HEART ATTACK—*Signs of a soon-coming heart attack* may include nausea, sweating, shortness of breath, dizziness, fainting, feelings of anxiety, difficulty in swallowing, vomiting, sudden ringing in the ears, and loss of speech.

The medical term for heart attack is *angina.*

The heart attack itself may feel as a band of intense pressure to the heart. A powerful pain is produced, which may last for several minutes. It often extends to the shoulder, arm, neck, or jaw.

But it may be a small attack, producing relatively little discomfort. Sometimes it is mistaken as indigestion. Sometimes there are no symptoms at all. This is termed a "silent heart attack."

An *angina pectoris* shows itself as recurrent pain beneath the sternum. It lasts 30-60 seconds. It is a severe constricting pain in the chest, often radiating from the heart to the left shoulder and down the arm.

SYMPTOMS OF HEART FAILURE—Shortness of breath, poor color, fatigue, accumulation of fluids, especially around the ankles (edema).

WHAT BRINGS ON A HEART ATTACK—What is a heart attack? What leads up to it? This article will provide you with an overview of the problem, along with several specific suggestions.

The *cardiovascular system* starts with the *heart,* which is a blood pump. The blood is sent through *arteries* and *veins* throughout the body.

Cardiovascular disease is the name given to several problems which can stop the heart and can lead to death.

1 - A *coronary* is one type of cardiovascular disease. The arteries which nourish the heart muscle itself are the coronary arteries. But if these arteries become narrowed, not enough oxygen and nutrients are supplied to the heart; and not enough carbon dioxide and waste products are carried off. This oxygen deprivation causes a tight, heavy chest pain, usually following some exertion or after a meal. There is a sharp, debilitating pain in the center of the chest. It is called *angina pectoris* (or simply *angina*). The pain generally recedes when the person rests. But it is a forewarning of events to come.

An angina attack may be precipitated by **stress,**

CHART - 1043: Catagories of Cardiovascular diseases (4512-545)

exertion, **a large meal (especially late in the evening), extreme cold, emotion,** or other factors. Average life expectancy after the first onset of angina is 5-7 years.

2 - If that blood flow through the coronaries becomes entirely blocked or limited enough, so that it does not reach part of the heart, then a *heart attack* or *myocardial infarction* occurs. This refers to the formation of *infarcts* (areas of local tissue decay or death) in the *myocardium* (heart muscle). A heart attack does not always kill. But, whether it is mild or severe, a heart attack always produces some irreparable damage to the heart.

3 - The problem may not be in the heart, but in the arteries which nourish it. The arteries have hardened (called *arteriosclerosis*); and, when cholesterol and other materials flow through them, a clot (also called a *thrombus*) occurs. The hardened walls do not flex to let the blob pass on through. Arteriosclerosis is responsible for most of the deaths due to heart attack.

4 - Lack of oxygen and nutrients can also cause *spasm of the coronary arteries,* resulting in a heart attack.

5 - Then there is *high blood pressure* (called *hypertension*). This is another form of cardiovascular disease, which also prepares the way for a heart attack. When the heart pumps blood, the blood shoots through the body at a fairly rapid speed. The muscular contractions of the heart produce a certain amount of pressure which produces this pumping action throughout the body. But sometimes the pressure builds up too high. This also is not the fault of the heart.

Here are some of the things which produce high blood pressure:

• **Hardening of the arteries** (*arteriosclerosis*) is a primary cause. Earlier, the flexing of the walls kept the pressure lower.

• **Clogged arteries:** A second major cause of hypertension is a reduction in the size (interior dimension) of the arteries. They come to look like old water pipes, with congealed stuff sticking to the walls. For years, certain foods had been eaten which caused this problem (**meat fat, grease, saturated fats, hydrogenated vegetables oils, margarine, butter, corn chips, etc.**).

• Too much sodium in the diet, eaten for too long a time, is another cause of hypertension. The solution should have been to earlier stop eating **sodium (salty) foods**.

• Other causes include **stress, enzyme imbalances, certain drugs (including oral contraceptives), and nutritional deficiencies**.

• There are still more factors which could be involved: **hyperthyroidism, kidney disease, adrenal or pituitary disorders, and heredity**.

PROCEDURES FOR
COMMON HEART PROBLEMS

If either you or a loved one has heart trouble, you can better understand and participate in treatment if you familiarize yourself with the following medical terms that may be used by your physician:

• **Aneurysm.** A spot in a blood vessel where the wall becomes thin and bulges outward as blood presses against it. If it ruptures, circulation is disrupted. Depending on the location of the aneurysm, the consequences of this can be grave. If detected in time, aneurysms can be repaired surgically in many cases.

• **Angina pectoris.** Pain or heavy pressure in the chest that is caused by an insufficient supply of oxygen to the heart tissue. This chest pain may be severe or mild and is usually associated with physical exertion and relieved by rest. It can be a warning sign of impending heart attack.

• **Angiogram.** A diagnostic picture produced by injecting into the heart and/or blood vessels a type of dye that is visible on x-ray. It may be done to diagnose valvular disease, blood vessel blockage, and other conditions.

• **Angioplasty.** A procedure in which a small balloon is inserted into a blocked or partially blocked artery and then inflated. This compresses the plaque on the vessel wall, widening the artery and allowing more blood to flow through it.

• **Aorta.** The main channel for arterial circulation; the large artery into which oxygenated blood is pumped by the heart.

• **Aortic atherosclerosis.** A systemic disease involving the heart, brain, aorta, and peripheral arteries. Blood tests have not traditionally been used to diagnose or to assess risk. Transesophageal echocardiography, a type of ultra-sound test, and **MRI** (magnetic resonance imaging) have been used to identify plaque buildup. A recent blood test for the presence of C-reactive protein may be helpful. The C- reactive protein is a systemic biomarker for inflammation.

• **Aortic stenosis (AS).** A condition in which the aortic valve is narrowed, restricting blood flow from the heart into the aorta. It can result from congenital malformation of the valve or from damage, such as from rheumatic fever. Symptoms, which may begin in early childhood, include fainting, chest pain, and shortness of breath, especially with exertion.

• **Arrhythmia.** Disruption in the natural rhythm of the heartbeat caused by improper functioning of electrical system cells in the heart. There are different kinds of arrhythmias. Palpitations is a term that refers to the feeling of a pounding heartbeat, whether regular or irregular. Tachycardia is an abnormal increase in the resting heart rate; bradycardia is the opposite, an abnormally slow heart rate. Ectopic beats are premature beats (often felt as "skipped" beats). Flutter and fibrillation are situations in which the normal steady beating of the heart are converted by electrical error into a rapid twitching of the heart muscle. This ineffective functioning results in an insufficient supply of blood being carried to the body's tissues.

• **Cardiac arrest.** Cardiac arrest occurs when the heart stops beating. When this happens, the blood supply to the brain is cut off and the person loses consciousness. A person in apparent good health who experiences cardiac arrest usually has unsuspected coronary artery disease.

• **Cardiomegaly.** The medical term for enlargement of the heart. If the heart is unable to function effectively, as in heart failure, or if there is too much resistance to the normal pumping of blood through the blood vessels, as in high blood pressure, the body attempts to increase the strength of the heart by increasing its size. Cardiomegaly is characteristic of a number of different heart disorders. It is also known as cardiac hypertrophy.

• **Cardiomyopathy.** Any of a group of diseases of the heart muscle that result in impaired heart function and, ultimately. heart failure. Cardiomyopathies are classified according to characteristic physical changes in the heart, such as enlargement of the heart, dilation of one or more of the heart's chambers, or rigidity of the heart muscle. These disorders may be related to inherited defects or may be caused by any of a number of different diseases. Often, the cause is unknown.

• **Cardioversion.** A procedure used to correct arrhythmia, in which electrical current is applied to the heart to restore normal rhythm.

• **Carditis.** Inflammation of the heart muscle. This can result from infection or from an inflammatory response, as in rheumatic fever; and it can lead to permanent heart damage if not treated.

• **Carotid artery.** The major artery to the brain.

• **Catheterization.** A procedure sometimes used to diagnose the condition of the heart and/or circulatory system and, in some cases, to treat cardiovascular disease. A hollow, flexible tube, called a catheter, is inserted by means of a very fine flexible wire into a blood vessel somewhere in the body (usually the arm, neck, or leg); and, from there, it is threaded through the blood vessel to the heart or other location being investigated. Catheterization can be used to detect (and in some cases to treat) arterial blockage, to discover malformations of the heart, and to study the electrical conduction in the heart, among other things.

• **Claudication.** Cramp-like pains in the legs as a result of poor circulation to the leg muscle. This usually occurs as a result of atherosclerosis.

• **Congenital heart defect.** A heart defect that is present at birth, though not necessarily inherited.

• **Congestive heart failure.** A condition of chronic heart failure that results in fluid accumulation in the lungs, labored breathing after even mild exertion, and edema (swelling) in the ankles and feet.

C
A
R
D

Unfortunately, there is no pain as the hardening and clogging of arteries (both of which produce hypertension) progresses. So people keep living and eating the wrong way until one day the crisis comes.

HEART FAILURE—So far, we have only discussed heart attack, which is an interruption in blood flow to the heart. But there is also *heart failure*, which is inadequate blood flow from the heart. It is not providing enough blood to supply the needs of the body. Heart failure can either be acute (short-term) or chronic.

Here are some of the problems which, over a period of time, can occur in the heart:

1 - *Arrhythmia.* The heart does not beat right. The natural rhythms are more irregular. This is caused by problems in the cells in the heart which send out electrical signals to do the pumping sequences.

2 - *Palpitations* occur when the heart seems to pound, whether regular or irregular.

3 - *Tachycardia* occurs when the heart beats too fast when it is resting.

4 - *Bradycardia* occurs when the heart beats too slowly.

5 - *Ectopic beats* (also called skipped beats) are beats which are premature, producing longer rests between some beats than between others.

6 - *Fibrillation* and *flutter* are a little different. An electrical error occurs, which sends some beat signals to the heart muscle, causing it to twitch instead of carrying out its normal blood pumping action.

7 - *Valvular disease* is the name for problems in the heart valves, so they do not open and/or shut properly. Sometimes this is **congenital**; at other times it is caused by **rheumatic fever** or **endocarditis** (infection of the heart muscle).

OTHER HEART PROBLEMS—There are a variety of problems which trace their cause to coronary problems, artery problems, or heart muscle problems. Here are some of them:

1 - *Cardiomegaly (cardiac hypertrophy)* occurs when the heart can no longer function normally. It works so hard that it enlarges. But this only weakens it. Causes of an enlarged heart include too much resistance from blood flow through the arteries.

2 - *Congestive heart failure* is a chronic condition that results in fluids accumulating in the heart and edema in the feet and ankles. There is labored breathing after mild exertion.

3 - *Cardiac arrest* occurs when the heart just stops beating. Because fresh blood is no longer reaching the brain, the person falls unconscious. Coronary artery problems are often the cause.

There are other problems which can occur in the heart, which can also weaken it. But these do not trace their causes to coronary or artery problems.

1 - *Carditis* is an infection in the heart muscle, sometimes caused by rheumatic fever. It can lead to permanent heart damage.

2 - *Endocarditis* is an infection of the endocardium. This is the sac-like membrane which surrounds the heart. People with **damaged immune systems** (from **HIV**, etc.) can acquire it. It can also be caused by **surgery,** to replace defective heart valves. Permanent heart damage occurs.

3 - *Cardiomyopathy* summarizes several heart problems, including enlargement of one or more heart chambers, heart muscle rigidity, etc. Causes include inherited defects and certain diseases.

Here are some of the risk factors which can lead to cardiovasular disease:

High blood pressure, Heart disease. especially a type of arrhythmia (irregular heartbeat) called atrial fibrillation (AF), Smoking, Diabetes, High blood cholesterol, Obesity/poor diet.

Here are some of the warning signs of the approach of present or possible future cardiovascular problems, including stroke:

Numbness or weakness in face, arm, or leg, Difficulty speaking, Severe dizziness, loss of balance or coordination, Sudden dimness, loss of vision, Sudden intense headache, Brief loss of consciousness.

NATURAL REMEDIES

Cardiovascular disease (which includes heart attack, stroke, and other disorders of the heart and blood vessel system) is the leading health problem in the Western world. Over 50 million Americans have heart and blood vessel disease; many do not realize it, since symptoms have not appeared yet. Here is a brief overview of some facts you need to know, if you would avoid a later buildup of conditions leading to a heart attack:

DIET

• Refrain from harmful **mucus-forming foods and drinks**. Take **cayenne** regularly. The best herb for this problem is **hawberries**. The heart valves can be toned up with the use of **cayenne, heart tonic herbs, and wheat germ oil**. For irregular beating, a tea of **black cohosh, lobelia, skullcap, and valerian** (with a little **cayenne** added) is excellent; and **lily of the valley** is especially good for quieting the heart.

• Be sure to drink enough **water** everyday, and frequently throughout the day! *This cannot be stressed too much.* Sludged blood is a very real cause of heart and vessel problems. If you sense your heart is bothering you, immediately drink two glasses of water!

• Do not eat **meat**. Fat is in all meat. Do not eat meat and you will have a longer life. It is well-known that vegetarians live longer than others. They have less coronary disease, fewer heart attacks, and less heart failure.

• Eat **smaller meals**.

• Do not use **refined, processed, fried, white flour, or junk foods**.

• Do not eat any type of **grease or oil (fatty foods, meat, margarine, butter, peanut butter, hydrogenated oil)**, saturated fats (animal fats), **hydrogenated vegetable oils**, or **overheated or oxidized vegetable oils**. Dean Ornish says: "Only a diet almost entirely free of animal fat, oil and cholesterol will significantly lower blood cholesterol levels reliably in just about everyone." Do that which will keep you from having **elevated cholesterol, triglyceride, and uric acid levels**.

• **Vegetables, fruits, grains, and beans** are low in the heart-hurting saturated fat found in meat and dairy products. But they are high in heart-healing fiber, and loaded with heart-nourishing vitamins and minerals. Avoid an excess of **carbohydrates (especially refined ones) and sugar**. Sugar increases triglyceride levels, platelet adhesiveness, uric acid levels, and blood pressure.

• **Garlic** lowers LDL cholesterol and raises HDL (the "good cholesterol").

• Use **cold-pressed vegetable oil**. See *Cholesterol, Reducing (532) for more information*. Take 1-2 tablespoons daily of uncooked **flaxseed oil**. It contains *omega-3* and *omega-6* fatty acids, which reduce the stickiness of platelets, blood components that can bunch together and form the kind of clot that lodges in an artery and causes a heart attack. You want a **high HDL-to-cholesterol ratio**, in order to avoid cholesterol deposits in your blood vessels. (This is later explained in detail in this article.)

• Be sure to include **natural fat emulsifiers (especially lecithin)** in your diet.

• Eat a **high-fiber diet**, using **whole grains, brown rice, beans, and fresh fruit and vegetables**. A 6-year Harvard study of more than 40,000 men showed that those who ate the most fiber had only one-third the risk of heart attacks.

• Do not eat many **peanuts**; but, when you do, leave the papery red skins on them because they contain the heart-protective compounds called *oligomeric procyanidins* (OPCs). OPCs are potent antioxidants that help prevent, not only heart attacks but also, cancer and stroke. OPCs are also in a number of other vegetables, including grape skins.

• Do not use **MSG** (monosodium glutamate).

• Locate your **food allergies** and eliminate them *(see Pulse Test, 847)*.

NUTRIENTS

• Through **nourishing food and supplements**, obtain all the vitamins and minerals you need. **Calcium, magnesium, and potassium** are important; so are the **vitamins (A, B complex, C, and E)**. Eat **Nova Scotia dulse or Norwegian kelp** for trace minerals.

• Helpful antioxidants include **wheat germ oil**, which raises oxygen levels 30%. Also good: **vitamin E** (400 IU) with **selenium**, **pycnogenol**, **Coenzyme Q_{10}** (30 mg), **ginkgo biloba** extract, and **rosemary**.

• Three B vitamins (**folic acid, B_6, and B_{12}**) help convert the amino acid, *homocysteine* to two other amino acids which do not injure your coronary arteries (by scarring them so arterial plaque can stick). As much as 30% of heart problems are partly due to high homocysteine levels. Each day take 800-1,000 g of folic acid, 400 mcg B12, and 50 mg B6.

• Heart attacks were reduced 40% in nurses who took **vitamin E** supplements. In another study, the arteries of men who had undergone bypass surgery were examined; and those who had taken vitamin E for the two previous years were found to have smaller lesions.

• If you are an adult, avoid very much **vitamin D** intake (from meat, milk, eggs, or sunlight). Taking over 3,000 units a day adds to the plaque development and hardening of atherosclerosis. It can result in calcification of the coronary arteries. But **carotene** (pro-vitamin A) in the diet, from orange and yellow vegetables and fruits, will not cause this problem.

HERBS

• Tonic herbs which help strengthen the heart include **hawthorn extract, cayenne, ginger, garlic, and Siberian ginseng extract**.

THE HEALTHIEST FOODS FOR YOUR HEART

1 - *Fresh fruit*. Fruit contains fiber, antioxidants, vitamins, and minerals.

2 - *Beans and legumes*. Beans and legumes contain fiber, and plant proteins that help to lower LDL ("bad") cho-lesterol levels.

3 - *Flaxseed oil*. The omega-3 fatty acids in flax-seed oil helps to lower LDL levels.

4 - *Dark leafy greens*. Spinach, mesclun, swiss chard, ar-gula, and other greens help to reduce levels of a blood enzyme implicated in heart disease.

5 - *Avocados*. Avocados are rich in potassium, which helps to regulate heart rhythm and blood pressure, and mo-nounsaturated fats, which lower LDL levels.

6 - *Whole grains*. Fiber and B vitamins are their greatest assets.

7 - *Nuts*. A good source of monounsaturated fats and min-erals.

8 - *Soy foods*. These are useful in keeping cor-rect blood fat levels and are rich in phytoestrogens.

9 - *Spices and herbs*. Fat is better digested with the help of the antioxidants and phytochemicals avail-able in many herbs.

10 - *Wheat germ and flax meal*. These are good for boosting your intake of fiber, vitamin E, and omega-3 fatty acids.

• *L-carnitine* helps dissolve fat deposits around the heart. **CoQ$_{10}$** and **germanium** strengthen veins and provide oxygen to the blood and cells.

• In Europe, people use **hawthorn** (as a syrup, extract, or fresh juice) as a heart tonic. The berry, leaves, and flowering tops contain *proyanidin* flavonoids which help patients with cardiac insufficiency. American herbalists also strongly recommend this.

Hawthorn has been used for thousands of years as an herbal medicine to strengthen the heart. It has been studied scientifically since the 19th century. The flowers mainly (with lesser amounts in its fruits) contain *flavonic glycosides (polyphenols)*, which is known for its action on the heart and circulatory system. Several other chemicals enhance its cardiotonic effect. It blocks the destruction of ATP, thus providing more energy in the cells and increasing the contractile strength of the heart. It is good for coronary insufficiency (weak heart) and arrhythmia (heartbeat disorders). It reduces angina pectoris by increasing the amount of blood in the coronary arteries and reducing their spasms. Like garlic, hawthorn has a balancing effect on blood pressure, decreasing it in those with high blood pressure.

• **Rosemary** tea is a quieting tonic and helps the kidneys reduce edema caused by a malfunctioning heart.

• **Grapeseed extract** contains *oligomeric proanthocyanidins* (OPCs); and it tends to lower high blood pressure, which can cause heart disease.

OTHER THINGS

• Do not put much **salt** and other **sodium products** (look at the labels!) into your body. Do not drink **chemically softened water**. Water softeners have sodium in them.

• Do not use **coffee**. Caffeine blocks the breakdown of adrenaline, resulting in the same response as heavy stress. Heavy caffeine consumption doubles the risk of coronary heart disease.

• Do not use **alcohol**.

• Do not use **tobacco**. The dangers of tobacco in producing heart attacks and other heart problems are well-documented.

• Do not use **drugs**.

• Make sure you are getting enough **exercise**. Sedentary living can kill you. Go outdoors and do something. Doing this is extremely important! All the nutrition in the world cannot help you, if you sit all the time. Regular exercise helps control weight, brings down high blood pressure, lowers blood sugar, increases HDL (the good cholesterol), reduces emotional stress, and helps reverse heart disease. Exercise outside 4-6 times a week. But if you have already had a heart attack, you will have to exercise more cautiously—but you must still exercise.

• Hot and cold showers are a good way to increase circulation.

• Keep your **weight** down. *See Overweight (480).*

• If you have **high blood pressure**, use natural ways to reduce it. *See Hypertension (526).*

• Research studies by the Chinese reveal that **constipation** *(456, 712)* is a significant factor in many heart attacks.

• Special problems: **Diabetes** *(656)* **or gout** *(627).* **Taking birth control pills. Heavy metal poisoning** *(868).* **A family history of heart trouble, living under heavy stress** *(555)*, **having a type-A personality**.

• If you tend to experience angina attacks at night, place 3-4-inch **blocks under the head of your bed**. This will reduce the attacks. More blood pools in the legs, and not so much tries to crowd in through the narrowed arteries into the heart.

Do everything in the above list that you can, and you will live a lot longer.

How to check your heartbeat:
• Check your heartbeat every so often. The best way to begin the day is to check your pulse when you wake up in the morning. If it is under 60 beats per minute, you are doing all right. But if your resting heart rate is above 80, that is not so good; it indicates that you may be developing hypertension or already have it. An estimated 25% of those who have heart attacks experienced no previous symptoms. So, right now, start eating right and living right.

An easy way to check your heartbeat: Place your finger on the side of your neck; and, looking at your watch, count the pulse for 15 seconds. Multiply that by four. A count of 15 means you are doing very well; you have a pulse of 60. A count of 20 means you are not: you have a pulse of 80. Immediately after jogging, it should not go above 30, which translates to a pulse of 120.

Sodium is a problem which must be dealt with; since it can increase the likelihood of heart disease. Here are items to omit from the diet:
• Table salt. Use a small amount of Nova Scotia dulse or Norwegian kelp instead. That will supply some salt, plus many vital trace minerals.

• MSG (monosodium glutamate), which is an accent flavor enhancer.

• Diet soft drinks.
• Canned vegetables.
• Commercially prepared food.
• Baking soda.
• Foods with preservatives.
• Meat tenderizers.
• Softened water.
• Saccharin products.
• Foods with mold inhibitors.
• Foods with preservatives.
• Some medical drugs.

• Some toothpastes.
• If you have any kind of heart problem, see your physician. Prevention—living right and eating right ahead of time—is the best key to success.

Specific help for specific problems:
• *Heart disease:* Eat no **fried foods**. Avoid **vitamin D**. Instead, obtain essential fatty acids; the best is cold-pressed **flaxseed oil or wheat germ oil**. Also take **selenium, vitamin E**, 5-10 **alfalfa tablets** daily. And, if needed, supplementary **hydrochloric acid**. Take a 30-minute **walk** outside every day. Keep a 30-minute **oxygen tank** in your house, ready for use when you need it.
• *Palpitations:* Do not eat **MSG, caffeine, sugar, or processed foods**. Avoid **food allergens** (foods that bother you). Obtain **vitamins B$_1$, B$_3$, C, selenium, and potassium**.
• *Cardiac arrhythmia:* Avoid **food allergens** and **MSG**. Add **selenium, chromium, magnesium, potassium**, and **CoQ$_{10}$** to your diet. **Hypoglycemia** (chronic low blood sugar) can be a cause.
• *Nervous heart:* Causes can include **anemia** and **low stomach acid**. Obtain **B$_1$, B$_{12}$, and iron**.
• *Angina:* If you survive, take **calcium, magnesium, essential fatty acids, and extra vitamins and minerals**. **Exercise** for 30 minutes everyday. Reduce **vitamin D** intake from all sources (meat, fish, dairy products, etc.). Avoid **caffeine, sugar, and cigarette smoke**.
• *Congestive heart failure:* Causes can include **lung disease** and **high blood pressure**. Obtain **vitamin B$_1$ and selenium**.
• *Myocardial infarction:* Rebuilding afterward (if you are still alive) should include **vitamin C** to bowel tolerance, **vitamin E, selenium**, vitamin A (in the form of **beta carotene**). Use supplementary **hydrochloric acid**.

Here is information about fats and oils:
Animal flesh contains fat. Do not eat animals. Doing so increases blood cholesterol. Some vegetable oils are also a problem: those that are **refined, heat-treated, and partly (or completely) hydrogenated oils**.
Heating the oil changes it from the *cis* form to the *trans* form (also called a trans-fat), which is abnormal and can cause heart diseases, just as animal fats do. Only use cold-pressed vegetable oils, and not too much of them.

Then there is the LDL and HDL story. It is also important, if you want to live longer. In order to better understand the following facts, also read the articles: *Lowering Triglycerides (531)* and *High Cholesterol (435)*. Much more information will be found there.
All kinds of fats (both the grease and oil forms) are carried in the blood in a protein-fat molecule, called a *lipoprotein*. There are two primary kinds: the *low-density lipoproteins (LDLs)*, which are large cholesterol-laden molecules, and the *high-density*

lipoproteins (HDLs), which are smaller molecules with more protein and less cholesterol and triglycerides.
High levels of LDLs in the blood increase the risk of coronary heart disease. But high levels of HDLs actually reduce the risk of heart disease. For this reason, the *cholesterol-to-HDL ratio* is very important. Physicians even use it to estimate how likely it is that you will have a heart attack. The HDLs get rid of excess cholesterol in your bloodstream! They carry cholesterol from the blood to the liver, so it can be converted into bile and eliminated from the body. Here are nutritional facts which have been found since the importance of HDLs was discovered:

How to make your blood vessels more youthful, so you can live longer:
• **Eat bran fiber.** It reduces blood cholesterol and triglycerides. It increases HDL and lowers LDL. It also helps prevent the recycling of bile from the bowel back to the liver. So bran fiber in your diet does three very important things.
• **Vitamin C** helps increase HDL levels and lower LDL levels. It also activates conversion of cholesterol into bile salts. Taking 1-2 grams a day can produce a 30% reduction in cholesterol levels (which are 400 or above). Vitamin C also lowers triglyceride levels.
• **Vitamin E** helps dissolve blood clots, dilate blood vessels, and conserve oxygen so the heart does not have to work as hard. Because of its antioxidant function, it also prevents fatty acids from becoming toxic.
• **Vitamin B complex** helps keep cholesterol from collecting as plaque in the blood vessels.
• **Flaxseed oil** (and to a lesser extent, wheat germ oil) is rich in Omega 3. It decreases platelet adhesion, reduces blood cholesterol, and increases HDLs.
• **Lecithin** is essential for utilizing fat and cholesterol in the body; and it significantly lowers blood cholesterol levels.
• **Brewer's yeast and chromium** reduce LDL levels and cause atherosclerotic plaques to recede.
• **Garlic** lowers blood cholesterol and reduces platelet adhesiveness, as well as lowering triglycerides and increasing HDLs. In addition, it also helps normalize blood pressure.
• **Alfalfa meal** (from ground seeds) contains *saponins*, which prevent bile-like substances from recirculating to the liver.
• **Soy protein** lowers blood cholesterol.

• It should be noted that *coronary bypass surgery* has failed to prevent second heart attacks or extend life. It is not the "cure" for coronary atherosclerosis and severe angina that it is said to be. Bypass operations are not the solution. They are only emergency repair jobs which do not remove the cause—which, unless properly corrected, will only return. It is a known fact that, unless changes are made in one's diet and way of life, the bypasses eventually clog up months or years later. $9 billion is spent each year on bypasses (300,000 each year, at a cost of $30,000 on each one).

• Fortunately, even the most advanced cases of heart disease can be helped by the discoveries provided by nutritional research.

• We will conclude this summary of ways to avoid heart attacks with this story: Dean Ornish, M.D., tells about genetically identical rabbits which were all fed the same diet; yet half of them had 60% fewer heart attacks. What was the difference? Half the rabbits were in upper cages and half in lower cages. The man who fed them all liked rabbits and would take time to reach in and pet the lower ones, the only ones he could reach.

—Also see Lowering Triglycerides (531), High Cholesterol (532); Hypertension (526), Stroke (529), Arteriosclerosis (523), and Atherosclerosis (523), Special Report (815-817).

ENCOURAGEMENT—Today Jesus is in heaven preparing mansions for those who love Him; yes, more than mansions, it is a kingdom which is to be ours. But all who shall inherit these blessings must be partakers of the self-denial and self-sacrifice of Christ. Obey the Ten Commandments, and live to help others.

PERICARDITIS, ENDOCARDITIS

SYMPTOMS—The symptoms of endocarditis are often generalized and unrelated to heart damage. They may include fatigue, fever, night sweats, aching joints, or weight loss.

The symptoms of acute pericarditis develop over a few hours and last for about 7 days. They include pain in the center of the chest; this worsens when taking a deep breath and is relieved by sitting forward. Pain in the neck and shoulders. Fever. In the chronic stage, the heart may become unable to properly pump blood.

CAUSES—Infective endocarditis is an inflammation of the lining of the heart, particularly affecting the heart valves. It is caused by an infection.

Pericarditis is an inflammation of the pericardium, the double-layered membrane that envelops the heart.

Both problems are caused by the kind of factors described under Heart Trouble *(513)*.

NATURAL REMEDIES

J.H. KELLOGG, M.D., PRESCRIPTIONS FOR PERICARDITIS OR ENDOCARDITIS AND THEIR COMPLICATIONS *(how to give these water therapies: pp. 206-275 / list of treatments: pp. 206-207 / Hydrotherapy Disease Index: pp. 273-275)*

TO COMBAT INFLAMMATION—Continuous **Ice Bag** over heart or **Cold Compress** over heart area at 600 F., changed every 15 minutes. **Rub chest** with dry flannel until skin is red.

TO ENERGIZE HEART AND MAINTAIN VITAL RESISTANCE—Cold Mitten Friction, **Cold Towel Rub** twice a day.

FEVER—Prolonged **Neutral Bath**, Neutral **Wet Sheet Pack**.

PAIN—**Fomentation** for 1-3 minutes every half hour. **Cold Compress,** changed every 15 minutes during the interval between.

MYOCARDITIS—Employ all the means recommended above, except avoid Ice Bag over the heart.

—Also see Heart Problems (513)

ENCOURAGEMENT—Talk of heavenly things. Talk of Jesus, His loveliness and glory, and of His undying love for you; and let your heart flow out in love and gratitude to Him, who died to save you.

CARDIOMYOPATHY
(Keshan Disease, Muscular Dystrophy of the Heart)

SYMPTOMS—In many cases of mild dilated cardiomyopathy, there are no symptoms. If they do occur, they usually develop over a number of years and may include fatigue, shortness of breath during exertion, palpitations (an irregular or abnormally rapid heartbeat), and swelling of the ankles. As the disorder progresses, the heart's pumping efficiency decreases, which worsens the symptoms.

CAUSES—The word means "heart muscle disease." This is a disease of the myocardium, which is the heart muscle itself. It is a damaged heart muscle, which leads to enlargement of the heart.

NATURAL REMEDIES

The World Health Organization recognizes that cardiomyopathy is a **selenium** deficiency disease.

J.D. Wallach, in his book, *Let's Play Doctor,* makes this statement:

"This is the type of heart disease that makes individuals a candidate for heart transplant . . It is typical that $1 per month in selenium supplement would prevent this disease and the need for a $250,000 procedure that carries a 20% mortality rate. This disease is also found in cystic fibrosis patients . . Veterinarians have eliminated this disease [cardiomyopathy] in animals with selenium injections and oral supplementation of diets."

ENCOURAGEMENT—Only Christ can satisfy the wants of the soul. If Christ is abiding in us, our hearts will be full of divine sympathy. We will do all we can to help and encourage others. Revelation 22:14.

CARDIAC ARRHYTHMIA

SYMPTOMS—Symptoms do not always develop; but, if they do, their onset is usually sudden and may include palpitations (irregular heartbeats). Other symptoms include light-headedness, sometimes leading to loss of consciousness, shortness of breath, pain in the chest or neck. Stroke and heart failure are possible complications.

CAUSES—These are abnormal rates in the rhythm of the heartbeat. In the more common palpitations, the heart occasionally seems to skip a beat or two. They are often minor and self-correcting. But cardiac arrhythmia is not. They generally do not normalize by themselves; and they can lead to a potentially fatal heart attack. Arrhythmia usually occur in people over 50. The following suggestions are for arrhythmia. But you might have a different type of heart problem.

NATURAL REMEDIES

• **Hawthorn** helps prevent heart problems by gently strengthening the heart muscle, improving blood circulation through the heart, and reducing the heart's need for oxygen. It also helps the heart circulate blood with less effort. It is best to take standardized extracts. If the extract is standardized to 18 percent OPCs, the recommended dosage is 240-480 mg once a day.

• **Coenzyme Q$_{10}$** is normally found in the body, where it helps manufacture energy. It can help stabilize the body's electrical system, thus helping to prevent arrhythmia. It is especially effective in preventing premature ventricular contractions (PVCs), which feel like skipped heartbeats. Those with this problem should take 120-240 mg daily.

• **Taurine** is an amino acid which can help stop your nerves from overstimulating your heart. This is necessary in order to control heart arrhythmia.

• **Magnesium** is the mineral which relaxes your heart. Too little magnesium jangles the electricity that controls muscles and nerves, possibly leading to arrhythmia. Taking enough can help keep the electricity stable and your heart calm. For mild arrhythmia, take 250 mg, 4 times daily, or 500 mg twice a day with food. Continue taking this for about 2 months; then lower the dose to 500-800 mg a day.

• **Angelica** contains at least 14 anti-arrhythmic compounds. You can blend it with raw vegetables, garlic, some water, and a little honey to improve the taste.

• **Astragalus** is an immune stimulant; and **Barberry** is an herbal antibiotic. Both are also heart tonics that help prevent and treat arrhythmia.

• **Motherwort** (*Leonurus cardiaca*), as its scientific name indicates, helps heart problems. The Chinese discovered that it slows a rapid heartbeat, improving cardiac activity. It also calms the nervous system.

• **Valerian** has been used for arrhythmia and palpitations as far back as Roman times. It also lowers blood pressure, increases blood flow to the heart, and improves its pumping action.

• Sometimes the problem is overstimulated adrenal glands. When you are stressed, these glands pump out hormones that can irritate and overstimulate your heart so that it races or flutters. Make fists of your

hands; put your **fists** behind the small of your back (on either side of your spine), and then gently rub your hands up and down. Do this 2-3 minutes daily.

—*Also see Heart Attack and Heart Problems (513), Arteriosclerosis (523), and Hypertension (526).*

ENCOURAGEMENT—When Christ returns, at His Second Advent, the redeemed will shine forth in the glory of the Father and His Son. The angels of heaven, touching their golden harps, will welcome the King and those who are the trophies of His victory,—those who have been washed and made white in the blood of the Lamb. A song of triumph will peal forth, filling all heaven. Christ has conquered. He enters the heavenly courts accompanied by His redeemed ones, the witnesses that His mission of suffering and self-sacrifice has not been in vain.

ANGINA PECTORIS

SYMPTOMS—A pain in the chest, usually brought on by exertion and quickly relieved by rest. The pain varies from mild to severe. It usually starts during mild exertion and is relieved after a short rest. There is a dull, heavy, constricting sensation in the center of the chest; a discomfort spreads into the throat and down one or both arms, more often the left arm.

CAUSES—The pain is due to an inadequate supply of blood to the heart muscle. It is less common in women before the age of 60, because estrogen protects against it. The most common cause of angina is coronary artery disease, which is a narrowing of the arteries that supply the heart muscle. The originating cause is eating meat, fat, etc. *See Heart Problems (419) and Atherosclerosis (523).*

NATURAL REMEDIES

• Eat fresh **vegetables, fruit, whole grains, nuts, and legumes**.

• Eat more **fiber** to lower cholesterol and improve bowel function. **Garlic** lowers LDL cholesterol and raises HDL (the "good cholesterol").

• Each day, take **vitamin C** (500 mg), **E** (200 mg), and **beta-carotene** to reduce the incidence and severity of angina. Also take **choline** (in lecithin).

• Eliminate all **animal fats** to avoid saturated fat and cholesterol. Reduce blood cholesterol to below 180 mg per deciliter (mg / dL) of blood.

Refined **sugar** increases triglycerides (blood fat) that cause platelet adhesiveness, thus increasing the frequency of angina attacks. Stop using **coffee** and **alcohol**, which interfere with calcium absorption. Stop all use of **nicotine**.

• Obtain mild but regular **exercise**. Walking is best. Begin with mild, stretching exercises; then walk, slowly at first. If angina pain occurs, stop and rest.

• Outstanding herbs include **hawthorn, angelica, ginger, garlic, bilberry, and purslane**.

ENCOURAGEMENT—Every action of ours in

COMPARATIVE CHART -1051: Coronary Thrombosis (530) vs. Angina Pictoris (521)

helping and encouraging others will be rewarded.

CONGESTIVE HEART FAILURE

SYMPTOMS—There is breathlessness, labored breathing after mild exertion. Also there is fatigue and accumulation of fluid in the lungs and/or the veins (primarily in the legs, ankles, and feet).

CAUSES—When you have a **heart attack**, part of the heart muscle is destroyed and the remainder tries to do the work. This is called congestive heart failure. Another cause is **high blood pressure. Lung disease** can intensify the problem.

In this chronic condition, the heart muscle is unable to pump blood as quickly as is needed. Too much exercise can be very dangerous to those with Congestive Heart Failure.

NATURAL REMEDIES
• The vitamin-like **coenzyme Q$_{10}$** stimulates the body to form ATP, a key chemical for producing energy in every cell. Take 30 mg 3 times daily. You may not feel the good effects for several months. However, do not stop taking it suddenly, lest your heart not be able to compensate for its loss.

• Because of Congestive Heart Failure, the cells of the body are not receiving enough oxygen. But this problem can partially be reduced by taking **carnitine** (500 mg 2-3 times daily), which is a natural substance made from two amino acids (lysine and methionine). Those who have Congestive Heart Failure tend to be low in carnitine.

• People with Congestive Heart Failure are often given drugs which deplete both magnesium and potassium. In those with Congestive Heart Failure, this depletion of magnesium and potassium often leads to heart arrhythmia. So take supplementary **magnesium** (300 mg per day). Eat thick, white potato peeling soup for **potassium**. Fruit and vegetables also contain it. (But be cautious: Some drugs given to treat Congestive Heart Failure actually cause a *retention* of potassium.) Those with kidney disease should not take extra magnesium.

• Those with Congestive Heart Failure have an inadequate flow of blood through the body. The amino acid, **arginine**, is used by the body to make nitric oxide, which increases blood flow. Arginine has been experimentally given to patients in doses of 5.6-12.6 g daily with good results.

• **Taurine** is an amino acid which helps the heart carry on its pumping action. Research has found that taurine (6 g daily) definitely helps those with Congestive Heart Failure. But if you have a tendency to any kind of herpes, do not take taurine.

• As discussed in the article on Heart Problems *(419)*, be sure to also take an extract of *Hawthorn*. This invaluable herb heals early-stage Congestive Heart Failure by increasing blood flow to the heart, increasing the strength of heart contractions, reducing resistance to blood flow in the extremities, and acting as an antioxidant. Take 80-300 mg, 2 times per day, or a tincture of 4-5 ml. 3 times daily.

• Also important are **vitamin B$_1$ and selenium**.
—*Also see Heart Attack and Heart Problems (513), Arteriosclerosis (523), and Hypertension (526).*

ENCOURAGEMENT—In view of so many encouraging promises in the Bible, how earnestly should we strive (by the enabling grace of Christ) to perfect a character that will enable us to be His obedient children and stand before the Son of God, when He returns in the clouds of heaven (at His Second Advent) for His people!

HEART PALPITATIONS

SYMPTOMS—Abnormally fast or irregular heartbeats.

CAUSES—Palpitations are most often caused by stimulants, such as **caffeine (in coffee, tea, and cola), nicotine**, and by **anxiety**. They may also occur as a side effect of medicinal **drugs** or because of a **heart disorder. Hyperthyroidism** or an overdose of a drug for hypothyroidism is a possibility.

Weak heart valves having poor tone may be the cause. Fever and excitement from **panic** can add to the problem. The fluttering of the heart is due to weakness within the entire body system, but more specifically in the heart area. **High cholesterol** and **dense mucoid stoppage** can cause sluggishness of the blood flow.

NATURAL REMEDIES
• Use tea made from **wild cherry bark** or wild cherry syrup added to a tea, to help nervous palpitations of the heart. This tea can also be used for a spasmodic cough.

• **Lemon juice plus water** has sedative action and can help sedate nervous palpitations.

• Jethro Kloss, who cured himself of a weak heart, recommended the following herbs: Make a tea of **tansy** for heart palpitation (1 heaping tsp. to a cup boiling water, taken 3-4 cups daily). For a weak heart or irregular beat, mix 1 tsp. each of **black cohosh, valerian, skullcap, lobelia, and a pinch of cayenne.** Add 1 heaping tsp. to 1 cup boiling water and steep ½ hour. Drink 4 cups daily or take a swallow every 2 hours. For heart palpitation, take **lily of the valley**. Also good: **angelica, blue cohosh, borage, cayenne, goldenseal, wood betony, valerian, and vervain.**

• Here is an herbal formula for a nervous heart: Mix equal parts **valerian root, lavender flowers, chamomile, and fennel.** Steep 2 tsp. in ½ cup boiling-hot water. Take 1-1½ cups a day, in mouthful doses.

• Take **cayenne, wheat germ oil, and hawberry tonic. Motherwort** is another specific

—*Also see Heart Attack and Heart Problems (513), Arteriosclerosis (523), and Hypertension (526).*

ENCOURAGEMENT—The only hope of any man lies through Jesus Christ. We must prepare now for what is ahead. How thankful we can be that Jesus will provide us with all the help we need, to live good, clean lives and encourage and help all those around us.

CARDIOVASCULAR - 2 -
CIRCULATORY
Also: Raynaud's Disease (368)

ARTERIOSCLEROSIS
(Hardening of the Arteries)
and
ATHEROSCLEROSIS
(Plaque Development and Hardening)

SYMPTOMS—Early warning symptoms are intermittent claudication *(530)*. These are pains in the legs and possibly feet, which leave upon resting. High blood pressure *(see Hypertension, 526)*, which produces the chest pains of angina *(521)*, and heart attack.

CAUSES—Arteriosclerosis and atherosclerosis are two separate, major diseases; yet they are here discussed together because the problems, effects, and solutions are so similar.

Arteriosclerosis is hardening of the walls of the arteries; atherosclerosis is the hardening of plaque on the walls, which causes the walls to harden. (The full explanation is somewhat more complicated.)

Hardened walls produce higher blood pressure; but plaque-hardened blood vessels, which narrow them, do it also. The end result of both is a heart attack.

The main difference between the two is that arteriosclerosis is primarily the hardened walls themselves (primarily produced by the plaque) and atherosclerosis is the thickening of that plaque in the arteries, so that the amount of space in which the blood flows keeps narrowing.

In arteriosclerosis, these deposits are primarily composed of calcium; in atherosclerosis, the deposits consist of fatty substances, primarily cholesterol (a blood protein). But, much of the time, an odd assortment of both, along with lipoproteins, fatty acids, and blood clump together, along with fibrous scar tissue.

Both conditions have essentially the same effect on circulation, both cause hardening of the artery walls, both cause high blood pressure, and both eventually lead to one or more of the same things: angina (chest pain following exertion), heart attack (the heart muscle can no longer bear the lack of blood supply to it), and stroke (when the blood supply to part of the brain is cut off). Death may or may not follow. The problem is that a clot of this plaque breaks loose, flows through the arteries, and gets stuck in a narrower artery. When this occurs in the heart muscle, angina and a heart attack may result; if in the brain, a stroke occurs.

To complicate the matter further, not only can arteriosclerosis and atherosclerosis cause high blood pressure, but high blood pressure intensifies them both. Therefore you should also read the article on *Hypertension (526)*.

Causes include **elevated cholesterol or triglyceride levels, eating high cholesterol foods (such as meat, eggs, whole milk, or milk products).**

Other causes include **smoking, hypertension (high blood pressure), obesity, diabetes, emotional stress, lack of exercise, or a family history of the disease.** Advancing age increases the risk factor.

LOWER LIMB ATHEROSCLEROSIS
Atherosclerosis is the most common form of arterial disease in the U.S. and most frequently occurs in the lower limbs (which is called peripheral atherosclerosis). It is the primary cause of death over the age of 65. Over 50% of those between 65 and 70 will die of some form of this.

Here are the earliest symptoms: pain in the legs (usually in the calf, but sometimes in the feet or elsewhere in the legs); this increases when walking but stops as soon as one rests, is intermittent claudication *(637)*, an early warning of blood vessel hardening and/or plaque development in them. There may also be weakness, numbness, and a heavy feeling in the legs. This is a symptom of atherosclerosis in the limbs (peripheral atherosclerosis). There can also, but less often, be pain in the arms.

There is a home test you can do to help determine if this is beginning to occur: Test the pulse in your legs and foot. There are three places where this can be done: Apply light pressure on the *top* of the foot, the *inner hollow* of the ankle, and *in the hollow* behind the knee. If you feel no pulse, then the artery may be narrowing.

Autopsies on U.S. soldiers killed in World War II showed little or no signs of arteriosclerosis; but autopsies on those young men killed in the Korea and Vietnam wars revealed that 77% had some form of it.

NATURAL REMEDIES
DIET
• Drink enough **liquids**! Drink **distilled water**.
• A strict **vegetarian diet** (without milk and eggs) is a good way to avoid artery problems. **Broccoli, Brussels sprouts, carrots, pumpkin, sweet potatoes, and cantaloupe** are considered especially beneficial for healthy arteries. All fresh **vegetable and fruit juices**.
• Eat **high-fiber foods** that are **low in fat and cholesterol**. Primarily eat **fruits, vegetables, and grains. Dark green leafy vegetables** are important.

Wheat bran, and other particulate fibers are not as effective as those in fruits, vegetables, and legumes.

• Eat foods rich in **vitamin E**. This includes **nuts, seeds, and whole grains**.

• Only use **cold-pressed vegetable oils** (soy, corn, wheat germ, flaxseed). Never heat these oils; place them on your food at the table.

• **Garlic** eaten with cholesterol foods tends to reduce the likelihood that cholesterol will clog the arteries. It lowers cholesterol, raises HDL, and prevents blood from forming clots. Many research studies support this.

• **Eggplant** tends to lower cholesterol levels.

• **Chromium** (found in brewer's yeast, whole grains, and supplements) added to the diet lowers cholesterol.

• Vitamin supplements include vitamin A in the form of **beta-carotene** (15,000-50,000 IU), **B complex** tablet (including B_6, B_{12}, **niacin, and folic acid**), **vitamin C** (500-5,000 mg), **bioflavonoids** (300-600 mg), **vitamin E** (400 IU).

• In addition to its antioxidant capability, **vitamin E** helps clear arterial scars, helps dissolve pre-existing blood clots, and reduces (by 80%) the ability of blood platelets to stick to artery wall plaque.

• **B vitamins** help metabolize fat. **Niacin** dilates small arteries and lowers cholesterol. **Vitamin C and bioflavonoids** protect the vessel walls. **Selenium** helps C and E protect against arterial plaque. **Lecithin** emulsifies fats in the blood so they can be used. It breaks up existing plaques.

• Other supplements you will need are **calcium** (500-1,500 mg), **magnesium** (300-750 mg), **selenium** (100-200 mcg), **zinc** (10-30 mg), **lecithin** (1-2 Tbsp.). All are important, along with the vitamins listed above.

• **Alfalfa** is rich in saponins, which are able to bind to cholesterol in the bowel and prevent absorption.

AVOID

• Avoid **refined sugar**. It has been shown to increase serum cholesterol levels, leading to atherosclerosis.

• Do not eat **animal protein**; there is a definite connection between eating meat and cardiovascular disease.

• Do not eat **processed, junk, dairy, white flour, spiced, or fried foods**. Avoid **pies, ice cream, salt, egg yolks, sugar, coffee, colas, nicotine, and alcohol**.

• If you know you are moving toward artery problems, eat no **free oils**.

• Eat no **animal fat, hydrogenated oils, trans-fat oils, butter, or margarine**. Both **peanut oil** and **coconut oil** increase atherosclerosis.

• Research at the University of Wisconsin disclosed that **skim milk** did not lower blood cholesterol.

• **Glucose intolerance** can produce a 100% increased risk of atherosclerosis. Keep your blood sugar

levels normal. Do not binge on **sweets**, etc.

• Too much **vitamin D** can elevate blood cholesterol.

• Reduce **stress** and avoid situations causing it.

• **Overweight** people should reduce. Even 20% or more above ideal weight carries a significantly increased risk of atherosclerosis. What is your ideal weight? Assume 100 pounds for the first five feet; add to this five pounds for each inch over that, for women; add seven pounds per inch over that, for men.

• Do not smoke or use **nicotine** in any other form. Avoid secondhand smoke.

• Do not take **shark cartilage**. It may inhibit production of new blood vessels needed to increase blood circulation.

• Eliminate all environmental sources of **metal poisoning (such as aluminum or copper cooking utensils, copper or lead plumbing, lead-glazed ceramics, contaminated water**, etc.). Toxic metals are known to be deposited, among other places, on artery walls.

• **X-rays** make premature arteriosclerosis more likely.

• Do not eat **big evening meals**. Best: Only eat plain fruit and plain bread for supper; and do this several hours before bedtime.

• Do not wear **constrictive clothing** (belts, garters, girdles, tight hosiery, etc.)

• Avoid **constipation.** This weakens the liver and kidneys, and sludges the blood. The Chinese treat stroke by treating constipation.

• All **alcohol** not immediately used for energy is changed into saturated fat, as are excess amounts of **sugar** and **refined carbohydrates**. So avoid them.

• Do not drink **caffeine**-containing beverages.

MORE INFORMATION

• Get regular moderate **exercise**. Walking every day is the best. Build up slowly; but keep at it. Do not do strenuous exercise until the cholesterol is lowered.

• Keep the **extremities warm**, to maintain good circulation in them.

• Periodically **check your blood pressure**. Buy a blood pressure set so it can be done in your own home.

• Chelation therapy (869) can greatly help reduce atherosclerosis and other circulatory problems.

HERBS

• Useful herbs include **Asian ginseng, bilberry, butcher's broom, fenugreek, fo-ti, garlic, ginger, hawthorn, psyllium, and turmeric.**

Hawthorn (80-200 mg daily) contains flavonoids that prevent blood vessels from constricting, thereby preventing angina pain. It lowers cholesterol and helps to reverse atherosclerosis.

• **Bilberry** reduces platelet clumping. **Bromelain** (in pineapple) inhibits platelet aggregation, reduces angina, and lowers constriction of vessels. **Curcumin** (the yellow pigment in **turmeric**) reduces cholesterol levels and inhibits clumping. **Fenugreek** lowers blood lipids. Ginger inhibits clumping.

• Here is an herbal formula for artherosclerosis: Mix 4 parts each of **European mistletoe** and **hawthorn** with 1 part each of **valerian root** and **shave grass**. Soak 1 Tbsp. of the mixture in ½ cup cold water for 8 hours. Drink ½ cup daily, spaced out in 3-4 doses.

—Also see Lowering Triglycerides (531), High Cholesterol (532), Stroke (529), Heart Problems and Heart Attacks (513), Arteriosclerosis (523), and Hypertension (526), Special Report (815-817).

ENCOURAGEMENT—He whose life consists in ever receiving and never giving soon loses the blessings he has. We must constantly seek to help others. Only in this way can God bless us. Jeremiah 7:23.

HYPOTENSION
(Low Blood Pressure)

SYMPTOMS—There are generally few symptoms which will tend to alert you to the problem. There may be headache, shortness of breath, dizziness, inability to concentrate, or digestive disturbances. There can be low energy and dizzy feelings when you stand up fast from a lying down or sitting position, fainting, blurred vision, palpitations, inability to solve simple problems, and slurring of speech.

CAUSES—The pressure at which the blood travels through the arteries is lower than normal, which means the blood is not circulating through the body as efficiently as it should.

This is one "disease" which many people are thankful to have! High blood pressure can be a killer; low blood pressure is generally just something to live with. Blood pressure readings below the average range of 110/70 to 140/90 are normal for some healthy people and are often considered a blessing.

One researcher who investigated the strange death of Pope John Paul I (who had low blood pressure and few other physical problems) asked 30 physicians and specialists whether low blood pressure would shorten life. Each one said it would tend to lengthen, rather than shorten, life expectancy.

For this reason, you will find that medical guides say relatively little about hypotension. But the risk of heart attack increases if *high* blood pressure is forced down by drugs to a diastolic reading (the lower figure) of 85 or less.

However, low blood pressure can become a problem when blood flow to the brain is reduced to the extent that dizziness or fainting spells are experienced.

In some instances, low blood pressure is due to an **impoverished diet**, the existence of some **chronic wasting disease**, or some other condition that needs treatment on its own account. Also it can be a symptom of a different problem (such as hypothyroidism, *549*).

Hypotension can be caused by **prescribed drugs,** **kidney disease, anemia, low blood sugar, food allergies, dehydration, adrenal exhaustion, malnutrition, underactive thyroid, diabetic nerve damage that disrupts blood pressure-controlling reflexes, or a debilitating disease**. Continuing to take **diuretics** (to increase urination) when no longer needed can initiate low blood pressure symptoms.

Acute hypotension (sudden drop in blood pressure) results from injuries with **heavy blood loss** or physiological **shock,** such as a **heart attack**.

Hypotension is usually diagnosed in this way: Blood pressure is checked while lying down. Then, after standing 1 minute, it is checked again—and a 20-point drop in the systolic pressure (the upper figure) is registered.

Low blood pressure and high blood are both due to malfunction of the circulatory system. High blood pressure in many cases works just like low blood pressure. **Cholesterol** must be eliminated from the system in order to get the blood flowing more freely. The condition is brought about by **improper diet, insufficient rest and exercise, and a lack of vitality** within the system.

NATURAL REMEDIES
• Treatment, if needed, should be aimed at locating and eliminating the problem of the symptom of hypotension.

• Drink one 6-oz. glass of **beet juice** and eat one serving of beets, 3 times a week to enliven lagging blood pressure. Other favorites for raising blood pressure include **dandelion greens, dandelion tea, ginger root,** or skullcap tea with a pinch of **cayenne**.

• Take **vitamin C** (1,000-3,000 mg), to bowel tolerance, and eight glasses of **water** each day. Also **vitamin B$_{12}$. Vitamin E** is important (100 IU, gradually increased to 600 IU).

• Eat **garlic**; it tends to normalize blood pressure. Raw garlic is a good friend, whether you have high or low blood pressure.

• **Ginger** tea helps those with low blood pressure. **Ginseng** helps normalize blood pressure, both high and low. **Sage** invigorates and stimulates suprarenal glands. **Rosemary** is a general invigorator. **Thyme** invigorates and helps recovery from physical exhaustion. **Winter savory** is a nervous system invigorator. **Hawthorn** normalizes blood pressure. **Lily of the valley** is a heart invigorator. **Camphor tree** stimulates respiratory and cardiac activity nervous centers.

• More **oxygen** is needed to correct this condition. **Garlic** is a good oxygen carrier. One of the greatest aids for low or high blood pressure, because of oxygen starvation, is **deep breathing**; this serves as a catalyst and helps the herbs react more rapidly. An immediate increase in circulation may be obtained by the use of **cayenne** and **nonmucus-forming foods. Grape juice,** as well as other juices, rebuild and give endurance to the system.

• Obtain adequate **rest** at night.
• You may want to do the morning **temperature test** to determine whether you are hypothyroid. *See*

C
A
R
D

Hypothyroidism (659).

ENCOURAGEMENT—Those who are filled with the love of Christ will not seek to hide their connection with Him. They will openly rejoice in all He has done and tell others how He can answer their needs also. Jeremiah 24:7.

HYPERTENSION
(High Blood Pressure)

SYMPTOMS—There may be no symptoms; but, if they occur, they may include headache, difficulty in breathing, blurred vision, rapid pulse, or a feeling of dizziness.

Overweight, a ruddy complexion, and apparently robust health may be the only outward manifestations in a man 50 or 60, who may have systolic pressure as high as 200 or more.

Hypertension is called the "silent killer" because it rarely reveals early symptoms.

CAUSES—High blood pressure is just that: The pressure of blood flow through the arteries is higher than it should be; and that pressure consistently remains higher.

Excessive pressure is exerted on the valves and the pumping muscles of the heart. A pressure is also exerted on the functioning lifelines in the body— the arteries, the capillaries, etc. This condition is characterized by a red or flushed complexion, excess weight, discomfort, and sometimes skin pallor. High blood pressure is the result of improper living habits which cause a run-down condition in the body.

A blood pressure gauge (sphygmomanometer) registers two readings: The first and higher one is the *systolic*; the second and lower one is the *diastolic*.

The *diastolic* pressure occurs just before the heart beats, and is less important for determining blood pressure. But the *systolic* pressure reveals the pressure built up as the heart pumps blood out of the heart into the aorta (and thence through the arteries). High systolic pressure indicates that the cell walls are hardened and/or plaques are forming in the arteries, which are narrowing the passageways.

Average normal systolic blood pressure in an adult varies between 120 and 150 millimeters of mercury, and tends to increase with age. The arteries of older people tend to harden and thicken with age; and this produces the higher readings in later life.

The age, in relation to the figures, tells a lot: Systolic readings of 140-150 at 55 to 70 years of age need not be considered high; but, occurring in a man of 30, it points to a definite problem which needs attention.

Normal blood pressure readings for adults vary from 110/70 to 140/90 while readings of 140/90 to 160/90 or 160/95 indicate borderline hypertension. Any reading over 180/115 is far too elevated.

The hardening and clogging produce changes in the arteries, resulting in hypertension that is caused by **aging, emotional stress, food, overeating, and heredity. Tobacco** is another cause of hypertension, as is the taking of **oral contraceptives**. Drinking **coffee or tea, drug abuse, and high sodium intake** are other causes.

Hypertension can result in coronary artery disease, enlargement of the heart, or strokes. The acute infections (such as tonsillitis, scarlet fever, and typhoid fever) or focal infections from tonsils or teeth sometimes lead to Bright's disease (a kidney disease), which is accompanied by high blood pressure. Sudden attacks of convulsions in pregnant women (eclampsia), and other kidney diseases of pregnancy, usually cause high blood pressure.

Primary hypertension (about 90% of the cases) is not caused by other diseases. Diet is an extremely important factor in producing high blood pressure. Sixty million Americans have this disease. At any one time, about 10% of the people in America have primary hypertension. It affects over half of all people in the U.S. over 65. African-Americans have it over a third more often than whites; and those 18-44 have it 18 times more frequently than whites. Women have hypertension less often than men until menopause is over; then, soon after, they have it as often.

Heavy snorers are more likely to have high blood pressure than silent sleepers.

Julian Whitaker, M.D. (Newport Beach, CA), says, "Volumes of scientific research show that dietary changes can eliminate high blood pressure in most patients,"

NATURAL REMEDIES

DIET

• Only drink **distilled water**. Another quote from Dr. Whitaker: "Drink 15 glasses of water a day. Almost all the blood pressure medications mimic the effects of increased water intake." They usually do that by thinning the blood. Drink water and it will do it naturally.

• Eat a **high-fiber diet of vegetables, fruits, nuts, and whole grains**. Eat oat bran; it appears to be the very best type for the purposes you have in mind. For oil, take 2 tablespoons **flaxseed oil** daily.

• Eat a diet rich in **potassium** (mostly fresh fruits and vegetables) because it helps the body get rid of excess sodium. Eat potato peeling soup (the potassium is richest just under the peeling of the white potato). Only eat **unsalted natural foods**.

• Raw **Garlic** is a vasodilator and normalizes blood pressure, whether it be too high or too low. If you take a commercial garlic preparation, make sure it has a dosage equivalent to 4,000 mg of fresh garlic.

• Include supplemental **calcium** in your diet.

• **Grapeseed extract** contains *oligomeric proanthocyanidins* (OPCs) and tends to lower high blood pressure, which can cause heart disease.

• **Tomatoes** contain the compound gamma-amino butyric acid (GABA), which reduces blood pressure and helps strengthen the heart muscle. There are a number of other vegetables (including **garlic, onions, and celery**) which also contain GABA. (The herb, **valerian**, contains *valerenic acid* which inhibits an enzyme that destroys GABA in the body. So also drink this herb.)

• Eating 4 stalks of **celery** has been shown to lower blood pressure measurably.

• **Broccoli** has 6 chemicals that reduce blood pressure. **Carrots** contain 8 compounds that lower it.

• Antioxidants help prevent artery-clogging plaque from being deposited on coronary artery walls. Foods with it include **asparagus, broccoli, cabbage, cauliflower, potatoes, tomatoes, oranges, grapefruit, and peaches**. The National Research Council urges Americans to "strive for five"; that is, get at least five servings of fruits and vegetables each day. Many nutritionists say eight or nine servings is even better. (Only 10% of Americans get even five.)

• **Apple pectin** tends to lower blood pressure.

NUTRIENTS

• Antioxidant-rich vitamins include **C, E, folic acid, and the carotenoids**. Many studies have shown that, as consumption of these nutrients increases, risk of heart attack falls by up to 40% (and cancer risk drops 50%).

• **Vitamin C with bioflavonoids** (1,000-5,000 mg) to maintain the health of blood vessels and improve the potassium ratio by helping to excrete sodium.

• **Vitamin E** (gradually increase monthly to 400 IU) to decrease the need for oxygen, thus improving heart function.

• **Lecithin** is rich in the B vitamins choline and inositol, which decrease blood pressure, by dilating blood vessels and preventing fatty deposits in the arteries.

• Too little **vitamin D** may contribute to high blood pressure. A 10-year study of patents 40-60 years of age showed a connection between low blood levels of the vitamin and higher blood pressures. Each day take 400 IU.

• **Coenzyme Q_{10}** is frequently deficient in those with hypertension. When they take supplements of CoQ_{10} (50 mg twice a day), blood pressure goes down significantly.

• **Taurine**, an amino acid, has been used to lower blood pressure (at 6 g per day).

AVOID

• **Habitual overeating**, even of good food, will lead to hypertension. A person does not tend to overeat on healthfully prepared natural foods.

• **Excessive protein food, sweets, rich pastry, and desserts** must be omitted; but the reduction in quantity of all foods is especially important.

• Do not use **salt**! Stopping it is essential for lowering blood pressure. Read the labels. Many foods contain **sodium**. Look for "salt," "sodium," "soda," or "Na" on the label. Also avoid **MSG** (monosodium glutamate), **baking soda, saccharin, soy sauce, diet soft drinks, preservatives, meat tenderizers, and softened water**. Excess sodium causes fluid retention, which exerts pressure on blood vessel walls and thus increases hypertension.

• Do not eat **meat**; and do not eat **canned vegetables**. Eliminate all **dairy products**; for they are high in sodium.

• Do not eat any **animal fat, grease, unsaturated fat, butter, margarine**, or any product containing them. Avoiding all of them will also lower hypertension.

• Do not eat **chocolate, alcohol, avocados, aged cheeses, or yogurt**.

• Avoid more than 400 units of **vitamin D** daily. Do not take supplements containing the amino acids **tyrosine** or **phenylalanine**.

• Do not take **antihistamines**.

• **No late meals**. Do not eat later than several hours before bedtime.

• **Stress, fear, anger, and pain** increase blood pressure. **Exercise** helps reduce the effects of stress.

• Noise raises blood pressure. Eliminate loud and sudden noises.

• Smoking is dangerous. Chemicals in **tobacco** can tighten your arteries, raising your pressure; it can also damage your lungs and other organs.

• Do a **pulse test** in order to ascertain offending foods you are allergic to (*see Pulse Test, 847*).

HERBS

• **Hawthorn** extract can dilate (widen) blood vessels, especially the coronary arteries. It has been used as a heart tonic for centuries. Make a tea from 1 tsp. of the dried hawthorn herb, per cup of boiling water, and drink up to 2 cups daily.

• Research studies also show that **kudzu** contains *puerarin*, which decreases blood pressure 15% in lab animals and in humans. Puerarin has 100 times the antioxidant activity of vitamin E, and helps prevent heart disease and cancer.

• **Saffron** contains *crocetin*, which lowers blood pressure. Make a tea of it or use it in your cooking.

• **Fennel** contains 10 compounds that lower blood pressure. **Oregano** has 7; **basil** and **tarrago** have 6.

• To reduce blood pressure, make a tea from either the seed or herb of **yellow dock** and drink it.

• Research findings reveal that **black cohosh** tends to lower blood pressure. **Cayenne** also lowers it.

• Dozens of studies, especially in Germany and Russia, have found that the major constituents of **valerian root**, the *valepotriates*, is the cause of its lowering of blood pressure. Unlike many other herbs, valerian root has no side effects, even at rather high doses.

• Here is a formula for high blood pressure: Mix 2 parts each of **chamomile and peppermint**.

C
A
R
D

Combine with 1 part each of **fennel, anise, caraway, and milfoil**. Steep 1 tsp. in ½ cup boiling-hot water. Take 1-1½ cups daily, in mouthful doses.

Dr. Shook was a famous Canadian herbalist. Here is his high blood pressure formula: Mix 15 tsp. **buckthorn** and 6 tsp. **Indian senna fruit** with 1½ tsp. each of **black cohosh, poke root, cassia bark, Indian senna fruit, European goldenrod, and sassafras bark**. Use 1 tsp. per cup of boiling hot water, simmer 2-3 minutes, then steep 10 minutes. Strain, sweeten to taste with honey, cool, bottle, and leave in a cool place. Drink 1 cup 3 times daily, before or after meals.

• There is a thickening of the blood from catarrhal and excess glutinous and fibrinous matters loading the circulatory system. Generally there is a clogging of the bowel with putrid body waste, making it necessary to cleanse the excretory systems in order to purify the blood. Herbal aids: With high blood pressure, cholesterol and mucus form a sludge within the body. Avoid the **mucus-forming foods** and take herbs that act as a solvent by liquefying impurities, such as **cayenne, garlic, or sassafras**. Take cayenne, working up to a teaspoon three times a day. This increases the power of the heart and corrects the circulation problems. **Garlic,** in copious amounts, will bring down high blood pressure. Pure **tomato juic**e is very good as a nutritional and a medicinal herb. **Wheat germ oil** is excellent for feeding the heart. It helps cut the cholesterol and smoothens its removal from the area. **Avoid** the use of **liquor and tobacco**, do not keep **late hours**, and avoid **over-tiredness and worry**. There is an intricate inter-relationship between one's living habits and his body condition.

OTHER HELPS

• You urgently need daily **outdoor exercise**. (Those who maintain their physical fitness are 34% less likely to develop hypertension.)

• Obtain sufficient **rest** at night.

• **Check your blood pressure** regularly, especially if you have a blood pressure problem or are pregnant.

• Keep your **weight** down! Loss of weight lowers blood pressure. If you are overweight and have high blood pressure, you would do well to fast one or two days a week.

IN ADVANCED CASES

When the situation is critical, special care must be given to produce successful recovery. **Adequate rest**, both physical and mental, is needed. Even the visits of friends and relatives may have to be restricted or prohibited for a time.

• Gradually start **mild exercise**. Walk outdoors and gradually (slowly!) build up the amount of time spent in outdoor walking.

• All blood pressure **medications** tend to have negative effects. **Moderate exercise, rest, sleep, and proper diet** will provide better help than drugging yourself.

• No vigorous or tonic hydrotherapy, or even massage, should be used. The **neutral bath** and complete bed rest are needed.

• One recommended program is **fruit and brown rice**, alone, for 1-2 weeks.

—Also see Lowering Triglycerides (531), High Cholesterol (532), Hypertension (526), Stroke (529), and Heart Problems (513), Special Report (815-818).

ENCOURAGEMENT—God can help you overcome the sins which so easily beset you. He can give you enabling grace to obey His Ten Commandments and remain true to Him, in spite of the compromise and wickedness in our world. Jeremiah 3:12, 22.

FACTS ABOUT BLOOD PRESSURE

Because it is so important and affects so many people adversely, here are several facts about blood pressure which you should be aware of:

Undetected and uncontrolled hypertension (high blood pressure) can lead to heart attacks *(419)*, heart failure *(419)*, strokes *(529)*, and renal (kidney) failure *(400, 533)*. Most individuals with hypertension do not have symptoms indicating they have the problem. It is a blood pressure check that reveals the difficulty and its extent. Early recognition and management are essential in preventing permanent damage, especially to the brain, eye, heart, or kidney.

There is a direct correlation between an increase in blood pressure and the rate at which arteriosclerosis *(523)* and atherosclerosis *(523)* develop.

A blood pressure reading involves the obtaining of two numbers. The first is the systolic (the systolic arterial blood pressure) and is always the higher number. This is the pressure existing in the large arteries at the height of the pulse wave. It is also called the systolic intra-arterial pressure.

Systolic pressure is the highest point caused by the contraction of the heart (generally 120 to 145 mm [millimeters of mercury]).

The second is the diastolic, which reveals the lowest point that the arterial pressure drops between beats. Diastolic pressure is the lowest point between beats (60 to 90 mm average in adults).

Blood pressure, which is the amount of pressure exerted by the blood on vessel walls, reaches its highest values in the left ventricle during systolic. It is successively lower in the left arteries, capillaries, and veins. The systolic arterial blood pressure normally rises during activity, or excitement, and then falls during sleep.

Normal blood pressure would be something like this: It should show a high systolic pressure of about 145 mm, with less for women. Normal diastolic pressure would be 60 mm to 90 mm.

At the age of 20, normal diastolic would be 120 mm, with ½ mm for each year after that age; this would give 135 mm as normal systolic pressure for a man of about 50.

With exceptions keyed to age differences, in general, the following conditions are considered abnormal: a systolic pressure persistently above 150 and a diastolic pressure persistently above 100.

Blood pressure is lower in childhood and in women. It is higher in men, during stress, and with advancing age.

A blood pressure reading of 160 mm systolic is generally thought to be the beginning of the high blood pressure. It may run well-above 200—or even as high as 250. Persistent high blood pressure can result in heart failure.

Hypertension is one of the most prevalent chronic physical problems receiving treatment in the Western world. People between 30 and 70 have it the most; and blacks have it more than whites.

All of the following are considered to have a part in causing high blood pressure: Overweight. Birth control pills. Estrogen supplements. Medications with sodium-retaining properties. Eating animal grease or saturated oils. Too much salt (table salt) in the diet. The use of tobacco. Lack of physical activity. Inadequate rest. Caffeine intake. Stress and tension. Genetic factors. Nitrites, nitrates, cadmium, or copper in drinking water. "Soft" water and chlorinated water tend to raise blood pressure.

ENCOURAGEMENT—In order to gain the victory over every besetment of the enemy, we must lay hold on a power that is out of and beyond ourselves. We must maintain a constant, living connection with Christ, who has power to give victory to every soul that will maintain an attitude of faith and humility.

STROKE
(Apoplexy)

SYMPTOMS—Light headedness, fainting, stumbling, blurring of vision, slurred or loss of speech or memory, numbness or paralysis of part of the body, difficulty swallowing, a coma for short or long periods. Symptoms may take minutes, hours, or days to develop. This could be a sudden, severe seizure or attack, often termed apoplexy. Apoplexy is generally accompanied by a stroke. A stroke does not necessarily mean apoplexy; because a stroke can come without heat prostration, which occurs in apoplexy.

CAUSES—A stroke is not a heart attack, but a brain attack. An artery to the brain is obstructed or small blood vessels inside the brain burst. Only heart disease and cancer kill more Americans than stroke. The incidence rises steeply with age and is higher in men than in women.

There is a calcium deficiency in the body, where the organic calcium has been burned out by a former fever or by an inheritance to an inorganic calcium, which is devoid of life and does not sustain the muscle, nerve, and bone structure. This causes weakness and inability to use the organ involved.

Strokes are caused by atherosclerosis (cholesterol plaques clogging the arteries of the neck and brain) or high blood pressure, which causes blood vessels in the brain to burst. There are four possible patterns which can result in a stroke:

An *embolism* is a clot that breaks loose and travels on up toward the brain, where the clot gets stuck in a smaller artery leading to the brain. This briefly cuts off blood flow to a portion of the brain.

A *thrombus* is a clot inside the brain which blocks the flow of blood to the brain.

An *aneurysm* is a portion of an artery that balloons outward. Filled with blood, this weak spot bursts.

A *hemorrhage* is a damaged artery within the brain which bursts.

A *tumor:* Sometimes a tumor, not a clot, is blocking an artery supplying the brain.

Whatever the cause, the result is local brain tissue death from lack of oxygen and food. Of all strokes, 40%-50% are caused by a thrombus, 30%-35% by an embolus, and 20%-25% by a rupture of a blood vessel.

If the damaged area is small enough, the brain will reroute the affected brain functions to other areas of the brain, as a period of relearning and compensation occurs. Surgery will be required for existing aneurysms.

About a third of all strokes are small or tiny strokes (transient ischemic attacks) which generally result in a full recovery within 24 hours. Another third cause weakness and paralysis (hemiplegia). The final third are fatal. Of the 4 million stroke survivors in the U.S., many suffer from speech problems, paralysis, and diminished mental capacity. Second strokes are very common. The inactivity following a stroke might lead to osteoporosis, a loss of calcium from the bones.

NATURAL REMEDIES

A STROKE OCCURS

• **HOW TO RECOGNIZE A STROKE:** How to **immediately** recognize if the person has just had a stroke: (1) Ask him to smile. (2) Ask him to raise both arms. (3) Ask him to speak a simple sentence. —*If he has difficulty with **any** of these tasks, **he has had a stroke!***

• Call 911 or have someone take you to the nearest hospital emergency room, if you experience the following symptoms: numbness or weakness on one side of your body (face, arm, or leg), vision problems, dizziness or loss of balance, confusion or trouble speaking, severe headaches that come on for no apparent reason.

Call 9-1-1. Give him ½ tsp. cayenne pepper, stirred in a small amount of water, and help him swallow it. Do other things suggested under "Stroke" (pp. 529).

Your heart attack risk (127) / How to tell if he is about to have a stroke (529) / What to do if you have a heart attack (513)

• The suddenness with which apoplexy comes necessitates the fastest therapeutic action. **Cayenne** pepper (one teaspoon to the cup) may be administered quickly; tincture of **lobelia** (three drops to one-half teaspoon, according to the size and age of the individual) should be given regularly; the **antispasmodic tincture** is excellent.

• Cayenne is known to have relieved the paralyzed condition of strokes, even though the person has been in a wheelchair for years. Through the use of cayenne and the cleansing herbs, many have been able to walk again.

• Here are several other useful herbs: Black cohosh, blue cohosh, burdock, catnip, lavender, lily of the valley, rosemary, skullcap, soapwort, vervain, ginger (bath or tea, especially for throat), sassafras.

• Assuming you are nowhere near a physician or hospital, here are three additional herbal treatments for stroke:

• Place ½ tsp. cayenne powder and ½ tsp. mustard powder in hot bathwater. Let the person soak in bath water as hot as possible, until he sweats profusely. Watch him so that he does not faint and his head slips down into the water.

• Mix 1 oz. each of fluid extract of black cohosh and wood betony, and 1 tsp. cayenne tincture. Give 1 teaspoon every 30 minutes, until patient improves; then continue every 1-2 hours as his condition warrants.

• Give him a footbath in hot water with mustard and cayenne. Ring out a piece of flannel soaked in hot water, with mustard and cayenne. Wrap this around a hot-water bottle and place it on his feet. To help equalize his circulation and remove pressure from the brain, give him an enema of the following: ¼ tsp. each of tinctures of lobelia, skullcap, and cayenne in ¾ pint warm water. If the enema does not evacuate the bowel, repeat it. He should perspire freely.

PREVENTION

• The best way to prevent a stroke is to **lower blood pressure** and fat intake in the diet.

• **Alpha-linolenic acid** is one of the group of omega-3 fatty acids. It helps to lower the risk of strokes in middle-aged men who are at high risk for cardiovascular disease. It does this by lessening the likelihood of clot formation. Walnuts and soybeans are sources; but the best is **flaxseed oil**. Total fat intake should be 30% of calories or less.

• **Bromelain** (a digestive enzyme in pineapple) can help dissolve a blood clot, preventing a second stroke. Starting no sooner than one day after the stroke, before meals take 1,500 mg 3 times a day. (If taken sooner, it could cause mild bleeding in the brain.)

• **Ginkgo** can help you recover from a stroke and prevent a second one by improving blood flow to the brain. Take 180-240 mg daily of a standardized 24%

extract of the herb.

• By helping to open and repair arteries and strengthening the heart, daily amounts of certain nutrients help reduce the probability of a second stroke: **Vitamin C** (3,000 mg), **vitamin E** (400-600 IU), **Omega-3** (1 Tbsp. flaxseed oil). **Coenzyme Q_{10}** (30-100 mg).

• So many toxins flow into the bloodstream when the bowel is constipated, that Chinese medical practitioners prevent strokes and also treat them by eliminating **constipation** (see *Constipation, 456*).

• Aneurysms are often caused by **copper** deficiency which results in weakened elastic fibers. Once the damage occurs, supplementation with copper cannot repair it; but the copper (2-4 mg/day) can help prevent aneurysms from occurring.

• **Oxygen** is powerful. Breathe deeply as much and as often as you can. An alternative is a hyperbaric oxygen chamber, in which the atmospheric pressure is artificially raised and you are breathing pure oxygen. This can help with stroke recovery. There are areas of the brain which are not dead, but only sleeping. The oxygen can awaken them and increase the speed of repair.

• The varied causes and suggested treatments of clots, artery problems, high blood pressure, and related problems resulting in strokes are explained in some detail in the following articles: *Lowering Triglycerides (531), High Cholesterol (532), Hypertension (526), and Heart Problems (513), Special Report (815-818).*

J.H. KELLOGG, M.D., PRESCRIPTIONS FOR STROKE AND ITS COMPLICATIONS *(how to give these water therapies: pp. 207-272 / list of treatments: pp. 206-207 / Hydrotherapy Disease Index: pp. 209-211)*

DURING ATTACK—Rest, with head and shoulders raised, **Cold Compress** to head, Tepid **Enema**, warm extremities by Hot-Water Bottles or **Hot Pack**. **Ice Collar**.

AFTER ATTACK—Cold Mitten Friction twice daily, well- protected **Hot Abdominal Pack** night and day, carefully graduated **Cold Baths**, prolonged **Neutral Bath**, **Wet Sheet Pack**. Later, carefully begin graduated **exercises**, massage, and Cold or **Alternate Douche** to affected muscles.

ENCOURAGEMENT—Be faithful, and God will give you a crown of life. Study the Bible, obey it, and do all in your power to be an encouragement and help to others. 2 Corinthians 6:16.

THROMBOSIS

SYMPTOMS—Symptoms vary, depending on which blood vessel is blocked. If blockage affects blood supply to the legs, symptoms may develop within a few hours and may be more severe if there

COMPARATIVE CHART -1051: Coronary Thrombosis (530) vs. Angina Pictoris (521)

is already a chronic reduction of blood to this region. Symptoms include pain in the legs (even at rest), pale and cold feet.

If the arteries supplying the intestines are affected, symptoms may include severe abdominal pain, vomiting, fever.

CAUSES—Obstruction of blood flow in a vessel with a blockage that has formed in that vessel or has traveled from elsewhere in the body.

Risk factors are primarily smoking, a high-fat diet, lack of exercise, and excess weight. Thrombosis is more likely to occur when there is an increase in the natural tendency of the blood to clot. Oral contraceptives can increase that tendency.

This can be a potentially fatal condition. Left untreated, the reduction in blood supply may eventually result in tissue death and may be life-threatening. The affected area will change color over several days, eventually becoming black.

NATURAL REMEDIES

Immediately go to the hospital.

• Certain herbs enhance blood circulation and make it more fluid, thus exerting a possible preventive action on this disorder: **garlic, mistletoe, lemon tree, sesame, linden**.

• Herbs and remedies which lower cholesterol levels are also useful in the prevention of thrombosis. *See High Cholesterol (532).*

—*For much more, see Heart Attack and Heart Problems (513), Arteriosclerosis (532), and Hypertension (526), Special Report (815-818).*

ENCOURAGEMENT—As those who hope to receive the overcomer's reward, we must press forward in the Christian warfare, though at every advance we meet with opposition. As overcomers, we are to reign with Christ in the heavenly courts, and we are to overcome through the blood of the Lamb and the word of our testimony. "Him that overcometh will I make a pillar in the temple of my God."

LOWERING TRIGLYCERIDES

PROBLEMS—The two major sources of fat in your bloodstream are cholesterol *(532)* and triglycerides. Both are necessary. Cholesterol helps build strong cells; and triglycerides provide energy.

But if either is too high, problems develop.

High cholesterol levels clog arteries. High tri-glycerides also cause vascular disease, if they are associated with low levels of HDL cholesterol (the good cholesterol). You then have fat particles in your blood which can ultimately be bad for your heart. The condition is called hypertriglyceridemia.

Triglycerides (TGs) are composed of three fatty chains linked together. People with **diabetes** *(656)* often have elevated TG levels. Successfully dealing with diabetes will often reduce TGs. The second

primary cause of high TGs is drinking **alcohol. Sugar** also increases them. **Smoking or chewing tobacco** is another significant cause. **Obesity** also causes it.

NATURAL REMEDIES

You can control your triglyceride level; and you want to keep it below 150. Here are several ways to do it:

DIET

• Reduce **the amount of fat** in the food you eat each day. Reduce total fat intake to less than 30% of daily calories; but, even better, reduce it to 20%. Reduce saturated fats to 10%. This can only be effectively done when you stop eating meat and dairy products.

• Eat a lot of **complex carbohydrates**. Racial groups doing this do not have a triglyceride problem. Cook rice, beans, and other grains **without including fat** in the cooking or the serving.

• Do not eat **candy, sweets, and sugar**. Eating such simple carbohydrates in the diet is a significant factor in raising the triglyceride levels very high.

• Include **fiber** in the diet. A low fiber, high sweet diet is even worse than high sweets alone. Water-soluble fibers, such as *pectin* in **fruit** and *beta-glucan* in **oats,** are especially helpful in lowering triglycerides. **Psyllium seed** also lowers triglycerides.

• **Omega-3** fatty acid (richest in raw **flaxseed oil**) lowers triglycerides. Take 3,000 mg per day. Do not take **cod liver oil**; for it contains too much vitamins A and D.

• Taking **garlic** also lowers triglycerides. Taken over a 1-4 month period, garlic can reduce them by 8%-27%. Garlic tablets, standardized for *allicin* content, can be taken in the amount of 900 mg daily (providing 5,000 mcg allicin). **Carnitine** is another supplement which has lowered triglycerides.

• Go on a **brown rice diet** for a couple days. In 1944, Dr. Walter Kempner discovered that a rice diet would dramatically lower triglycerides. This is a diet of **rice and fruit alone**, and no other food, for 2-3 days or as long as you can stand to remain on it. The diet is not appetizing; but it really works. One patient went down from 1,000 mg/dl to 117 mg/dl in a couple of months. In just 2-3 days, triglycerides will go down a fair amount. You can do it again later for another couple of days. By the way, when you do this, you will lose some weight also. The rice / fruit diet is practically fat-free. But do not remain on a rice diet! It does not provide adequate nutriments when eaten alone.

OTHER HELPS

• Lose **weight**. Even losing 10 pounds can reduce triglycerides in those who are 20%-30% overweight. Ultimately, try to maintain a weight that is not over 5%-10% above what is normal for your age-weight range.

• Do not drink **alcohol**; it decidedly increases triglycerides. Using **tobacco** does also.

• **Exercise** is very helpful in lowering triglyceride levels. Studies reveal that it does this even when weight is not lowered in the process.

• Herbs which reduce triglycerides include **wild yam, fenugreek, and reishi** (a type of mushroom).
—*Also see High Cholesterol (below).*

ENCOURAGEMENT—Do not dwell on your difficulties, so they get bigger and bigger. Instead, think on the love of Christ and plead with Him for the help you need. Be trustful and obedient, and He will give you the best answers. Hosea 14:4.

HIGH CHOLESTEROL

SYMPTOMS—High cholesterol is an invisible risk; because it has no direct, outward symptoms. The symptoms would be those of atherosclerosis *(523)* and hypertension *(526).*

CAUSE—Cholesterol is a fatty, wax-like substance found naturally in all body cells. It is used to build cells, make hormones, and aids in food digestion. Your liver can manufacture all you need. But it is also found in animal foods (including dairy products), lard, and hydrogenated oils. Excess cholesterol collects in fatty deposits along the inner linings of the arteries. These slowly build, along with clotted blood and scar tissue, to form fibrous plaque. The result is atherosclerosis.

Here are some facts about cholesterol, to help you understand the situation:

Dietary cholesterol is in the food you eat. Most of it is found in eggs and meat. One egg has 275 mg and an apple has none.

Serum cholesterol is in your bloodstream. This is what your physician measures. Ideally, it should be under 200. There are two types of serum cholesterol:

HDL (high-density lipoprotein) cholesterol cleans the arteries and is good for you. The higher it is, the better.

LDL (low-density lipoprotein) cholesterol clogs the arteries and is bad for you. The lower it is, the better.

There are several natural ways to lower the amount of LDL cholesterol in your blood.

For every 1% drop in cholesterol levels, there is a 2% decrease in heart attack risk. The total cholesterol level of the average American is above 200 mg per deciliter (mg / dl) of blood. Heart attack risk rises sharply above that level. So most people in our nation are in danger of an eventual heart attack. Yet the problem can be solved.

The ideal cholesterol range is 170-190 mg/dl. Below 150, there is an increased risk of death from other causes, including liver cancer, lung disease, and certain kinds of strokes.

Cholesterol and Blood Pressure Levels

Two important measurements used in assessing cardiovascular health are blood fat (including cholesterol and triglycerides) levels and blood pressure. The tables below are approximate guides to both cholesterol and blood pressure levels. Keep in mind that both levels vary from person to person, so it is always wise to have your blood pressure and cholesterol level checked by your physician on a regular basis. Also note that the values here reflect recent revisions in desirable levels:

Total cholesterol—*Good:* 200 or less. *Borderline:* 200-239, *High:* 240 and above.

LDL ("bad") cholesterol—*Good:* 130 or less. *Borderline:* 130-159. High: 160 and above.

Triglycerides—*Good:* 150 or less. *Borderline:* 150-199. *High:* 200 and above.

Blood Pressure Levels for those without heart disease. In the following listing, HT stands for hypertension;

Systolic (when the heart contracts and pumps blood out)—*Normal:* 120 or less. *Pre-HT:* 120-139. *Stage 1 HT:* 140-159. *Stage 2 HT:* 160 and higher.

Diastolic (between beats, your heart fills with blood again)—*Normal:* 80 or less. *Pre-HT:* 80-89. *Stage 1 HT:* 90-99. *Stage 2 HT:* 100 and higher.

NATURAL REMEDIES

DIET

• Do not eat **saturated fat**. This is the kind in **meat, butter, cheese, and hydrogenated oil**—which is the worst kind of oil or fat, since it raises blood cholesterol the most.

• Only include **polyunsaturated fat** in your meals. It lowers blood cholesterol. This kind is only found in certain vegetable oils, such as **corn oil, soy oil, wheat germ oil, and flaxseed oil**. Only buy cold-pressed oil—never, never use hydrogenated oil (even partially hydrogenated oil). The kind of vegetable oils in most stores are often hydrogenated. Never put **cottonseed oil** into your body.

• Eating **large meals** stimulates the production of an enzyme which increases the liver's output of cholesterol. Eat smaller meals.

• Eat nothing that is **fried**. Even worse, eat nothing **fried in fat** (which is most frying). Beware of fast-food restaurants.

• Drink at least 8 glasses of **water or juice** daily. It is needed to keep cholesterol-absorbing fiber flowing through the body.

• **Lecithin** is outstanding for emulsifying fats and cholesterol so they can be utilized by the body or flushed out. Take some (in the form of granules) every day. Each day put 1-3 Tbsp. on your cereal.

• The very best oils for your health are **wheat germ oil and flaxseed oil**. Prepare your meals without oil, fat, or grease. Then add a spoonful or two of wheat germ oil or flaxseed oil to the food after it has been dished onto your plate. In this way, you can carefully measure how much you get; and you ensure that the oil was not cooked.

• It is safe to use **monounsaturated oils**. It is now known that they also lower blood cholesterol. These include **olive oil** and certain other foods, such as **nuts, avocados, and peanut oil**. (There are questions about canola oil, so it is not recommended in this *Encyclopedia*.) Monounsaturated oils lower cholesterol faster than low-fat diets do; and the type they selectively lower is the bad LDL. **Avocado** is one of the highest fat foods; yet it tends to lower cholesterol!

• **Nuts** reduce cholesterol somewhat, especially **walnuts**. **Soybeans** and other **beans** are also good.

• Do not eat **fried food, fatty food, meat, or vegetable loaves**, etc. Do not eat **processed or junk food**. Do not eat **regular peanut butter**. The peanut oil has been taken out; and cheap, hydrogenated oils (sometimes lard) are put in its place. Only buy peanut butter from a health-food store. You can open the lid and smell the difference. Learn how to smell good food. Do not eat **corn chips, crackers, and other snack foods**.

• **Eggs** contain a lot of cholesterol (275 mg per egg); yet studies reveal that, in most people, they do not appreciably raise cholesterol levels. This is because egg yolk is rich both in cholesterol and the lecithin needed to dissolve it.

• Eat more **fruit and beans**. Both have pectin, which surrounds cholesterol and takes it out of the body. Pectin is in all kinds of beans and fruit. **Carrots** also help lower cholesterol, because of their pectin content. **Cabbage, broccoli, and onions** have calcium pectate.

• You need 6 grams of water-soluble **fiber** every day. **This kind of fiber is found in fruits, vegetables, whole grains, legumes, and nuts. Corn, rice, and oat bran** helps lower LDLs, without reducing helpful HDLs. **Wheat bran**'s insoluble fiber protects against colon cancer, but does not lower cholesterol. **Oat bran** lowers cholesterol in the same way that pectin does it. Make oat bran muffins; and eat one or two every day. **Oatmeal** is good.

• Fresh **garlic** lowers cholesterol (and also high blood pressure), but not cooked or deodorized garlic. It is said that Kyolic may lower cholesterol. The essential oil found in both **garlic and onions** are reported by researchers as lowering serum cholesterol levels and stimulating fibrinolytic activity. Taking 600-900 mg of **garlic powder** capsules every day for 3-4 months lowered cholesterol levels by 14%-20%, and triglycerides by 18%-24%.

• **Psyllium seed** lowers cholesterol. **Celery juice** significantly lowers it.

• All plants contain *phytosterols*, which reduce cholesterol. **Sesame seed** has the most. Other foods with high amounts include **sunflower seeds, lettuce, asparagus, okra, cauliflower, figs, strawberries, onions, squash, apricots, tomatoes, and celery**.

• **Vitamins C, E, and niacin** also lower cholesterol, along with **calcium**.

• **Vitamin C** (1,000-4,000 mg) reduces the oxidation of LDL and prevents heart disease. Also good for this purpose is **vitamin E** (800 IU) and **selenium** (200 mcg). **Zinc** (30 mg) and **copper** (1-2 mg) increases HDL and reduces LDL.

• Taking 30 mg of B_{15} (pangamic acid) 3 times a day for 20 days reduced cholesterol levels for 90% of those tested. **Niacin** (1,500 mg in the form of niacinamide) lowers LDL cholesterol; but you must be careful and not take too much of it.

OTHER THINGS

• **Exercise** also lowers bad cholesterol. Vigorous exercise raises HDL and lowers LDL levels.

• Do not use **coffee, tobacco, or liquor**. They increase the harmful LDLs. Carbon monoxide damages artery walls, so plaque can build up. Avoid **drugs** of all kinds.

• **Guggul** is an herb from India which lowers cholesterol so well that you should only take 3 doses totalling 900 mg daily. After your levels are normal, reduce it to 300 mg per day.

• Here are other things found to lower cholesterol: **ginger, fenugreek, barley, spirulina, and lemongrass oil.**

• When taken with a low-fat diet, **psyllium** (a soluble fiber from the seed husks of plantain) raises HDLs and lowers LDLs. One experiment (1 tsp. in 8 oz. water, 3 times a day) resulted in a 35% drop in total cholesterol in 6 months.

• **Activated charcoal** will powerfully lower LDL levels (40%) and raise HDLs (8%), when ¼ oz. is taken 3 times a day, an hour before or after meals. But it absorbs other things as well!

• **Sunlight** helps your body control cholesterol.

—*Also see Triglycerides (531), Heart Problems (513), and Atherosclerosis (523), Special Report (815-817).*

ENCOURAGEMENT—We are to love God, not only with mind and heart but, with the strength also. We are to treat our bodies carefully; for we belong to God. Jeremiah 30:22.

PHLEBITIS AND THROMBOPHLEBITIS
(Milk Leg, Phlegmasia Alba dolens)

SYMPTOMS—*Phlebitis:* Reddening and cord-like swelling of the vein, increased pulse rate, slight fever, and pain accompanying movement of the afflicted area.

Superficial thrombophlebitis: The affected vein can be felt; it feels harder than normal veins. It may appear as a reddish line under the skin, possibly accompanied by pain, localized swelling, and tender to the touch.

Deep thrombophlebitis: Pain, warmth, and

swelling, with possible bluish discoloration of the skin of the limb it is in. Sometimes there is fever and chills. The pain frequently feels like a deep soreness that intensifies when standing or walking; and it lessens when sitting or, especially, when the legs are elevated. Very often the deep vein in the thigh is involved.

CAUSES—*Phlebitis* is the inflammation of a vein wall. It usually occurs in the legs and more often in women than men. It can be a complication of **varicose veins** *(535)* or caused by **childbirth, infections resulting from injuries to the veins, and operations**. Infections in the legs, feet, and toes must be given immediate attention (especially if a fungal origin is involved). If the inflammation is associated with the formation of a blood clot (called a *thrombus*) in the vein, the condition is called thrombophebitis.

There are two types of *thrombophlebitis*. The first is *superficial thrombophlebitis*, which affects a subcutaneous vein near the surface of the skin. This is generally not serious; and many experience it. But if there is widespread vein involvement; the lymphatic vessels may also become inflamed and fluids may collect.

The superficial type can result from **infection, lack of exercise, standing for long periods, and intravenous drug use**.

Obesity, varicose veins, pregnancy, allergies, environmental chemicals, injury, and smoking can increase the risk.

Deep thrombophlebitis, also known as deep venous thrombosis (DVT), is more serious. It affects muscular veins far below the surface, which are much larger. This can occur after confinement. The reduced blood flow can produce chronic venous insufficiency, evinced by pigmentation, skin rash, or ulceration. But sometimes there are no symptoms. The risk of DVT rapidly increases after the age of 40; it triples with the passing of each decade after it.

Even though the person remains in bed until the swelling subsides, it will return slightly when he gets out of bed. Very little standing or exercise should be permitted while any swelling persists.

If the opening in the vein, in the thigh, is narrowed too much by the phlebitis (and nearly always if it is entirely clogged), varicose veins will appear lower down on the leg.

Blood Clots: Blood clots can be very dangerous. The origin of a clot is generally unknown. But it can form following an injury to the inside lining of a blood vessel. This initiates clotting, which is part of the repair process. Blood platelets clump together to protect the injured area. Fibrogen arrives and entraps blood cells, plasma, and more platelets; this process makes a blood clot to protect the weakened wall.

If a clot forms, it can break off and travel to a vital organ. Massage or rubbing may cause part of the clot to be dislodged and pass to other parts of the body, especially the lungs, causing serious damage or death. If there is any possibility that the person might have blood clots, he should not receive massage.

NATURAL REMEDIES

If a swollen, painful vein does not disappear within 2 weeks, consult a physician.

DIET

• Include **niacin** in the diet. This B vitamin helps prevent clotting. **Vitamin C** helps strengthen the walls of veins and arteries. **Vitamin E** (two 400 IU daily) dilates and strengthens blood vessels, reducing the formation of varicose veins and phlebitis.

• Eat a good nourishing diet of **fruits, vegetables, raw nuts, seeds, legumes, and whole grains**.

• Include enough **fiber** in the diet, so you do not have to strain at the stool. Straining increases venous pressure on the legs.

• Maintain a **low-fat diet** and drink enough **water**.

• Drink fresh **carrot juice** daily.

Mix **lecithin granules and brewer's yeast**; and take 2 Tbsp. daily.

• It is now known that **food allergies** can be involved. Search them out and eliminate them.

FOODS TO AVOID

• Do not eat **fried, salty, processed food, dairy products, or hydrogenated vegetable oils**. Do not eat **meat**.

• Avoid a **high-protein diet**; for it increases blood-clotting factors.

OTHER HELPS

• Superficial phlebitis inflammation generally is reduced within 7-10 days; but it may take 3-6 weeks for the problem to be entirely gone. It can be treated by **elevating the leg** and applying **warm, moist heat** to the area. It is not necessary to rest in bed; but, every so often, rest with the leg 6-10 inches above the heart. This speeds the healing process.

• Get regular moderate **exercise**. This is important. Walking is the best. Regular exercise increases the body's ability to dissolve clots.

• Avoid **dangling the feet**. Pressure against the popliteal vessels may cause obstruction of blood flow. Do not cross your legs.

• **Deep breathing or singing** helps empty out the large veins, thus increasing venous circulation.

• Quit **tobacco**. If you smoke, and seem to keep having recurring phlebitis, you may have Buerger's Disease *(370)*. Its symptoms are severe pain and blood clots, usually in the legs (and can lead to amputations!). Smoking constricts the blood vessels.

• Take alternating **hot and cold sitz baths** or apply alternating **hot and cold compresses**.

• Lie on a **slant board** with your feet higher than your head for 15 minutes a day, especially if you stand on your feet a lot.

• **Wear nothing tight** about the waist. Also do not wear bands on the legs.

• When traveling a distance by car, **stop and walk around** every so often. Do not let the circulation become sluggish. When it enters a low-flow state, that can lead to a clot. Beware of "economy class syndrome." A remarkable number of people who fly in the cramped economy class seats of jets develop thromboplebitis. You are confined to your seat more on planes than in cars or boats. So request an aisle seat and get up every 30 minutes and walk up and down the aisles.

• Wherever you may be, **do not sit more than an hour at a time**, without getting up and walking around.

• Better yet, **every hour exercise the legs** for 2 minutes, as if you are riding a bike (lifting the legs), and breathe deeply, in and out, 15 times.

• **Walking barefoot** improves venous blood flow.

• If they help you feel better, use **elastic stockings** (anti-embolism stockings).

• **Do not squat** (sit back on your heels), except momentarily.

• If you have a history of phlebitis or blood clots, do not take **birth control pills**. They will increase the likelihood of deep vein thrombophlebitis by 3-4 times.

• **Fasting** decreases blood coagulation. It can be beneficial when needed.

• If you have to lie in bed for a time, **move your legs** every so often, to increase circulation. **Elevate the foot of your bed** several inches, to reduce venous pressure in your legs. This also reduces edema and pain. Do not use **pillows** under the legs; for doing so elevates the knee above the digestive organs and reduces circulation, unless head is raised above the knees.

• The herb **gotu kola** helps restore normal elasticity to veins.

• **Butcher's broom** and **bilberry** are also veno-tonics; that is, they help strengthen veins and reduce inflammation. To prevent a recurrence of phlebitis, take 100 mg butcher's broom, once a day, and two 80 mg capsules of bilberry 3 times a day.

• Apply herbal compresses of **yarrow, calendula flowers, or St. John's wort** to the legs.

• Should you **massage a leg** with phlebitis? Yes and no. If you are certain there are no blood clots in the leg, you can gently but firmly knead each leg from your ankle to your mid-thigh once or twice a day. But no, if there is any possibility of clots, *do not do it!* It can result in paralysis or a stroke.

TENDING TO THE LIVER

The weakness in the veins that causes phlebitis is a sign that the liver has not been working properly. If the liver is clogged with toxins, the veins cannot flow as easily into it. The result is a backup of blood, which dilates the veins in the legs and weakens them.

• Turn to the **section on the liver** for ways to improve its function (445-451).

• Lie on your back on the floor and **put your feet and lower legs on the seat of a chair**. This will help move blood out of the veins into your liver. Do this once a day, staying in the position for 5-10 minutes.

Once you have had phlebitis, or clots of any type, you can have it again. Surgery or prolonged bed rests increase the likelihood that you will have another attack. Keep that in mind when you consider elective surgery.

—*Also see Varicose Veins (below).*

ENCOURAGEMENT—Thank God everyday for the many blessings you have. Determine that you will remain true to Him. By His enabling grace, resist temptations and obey His moral law. Leviticus 26:12.

VARICOSE VEINS
(Varicosities)

SYMPTOMS—Visibly distended veins, especially in the calves and inner thighs of the legs. They are enlarged, bulging, bluish, and lumpy. Small ones can appear red and spidery. There may be aching or tiredness, a feeling of fullness in the limbs. The skin may have a tense or burning sensation. Muscle cramps may occur, especially at night. Hemorrhage under the skin may cause the skin to discolor (light brown to bluish). Veins may be abnormally large, bulging, and lumpy looking.

CAUSES—The valves of the veins no longer function properly. They have become stretched from excess pressure. The valves in the veins that prevent blood from flowing backward do not work properly. The deep veins are surrounded by muscles which keep them in shape. It is those close to the surface (saphenous veins) which develop these problems. So much blood collects that it leaks out into surrounding tissue.

Contraceptive medications can induce varicose veins, as well as **hormonal vasodilation** just prior to menstruation. They can occur during **pregnancy** (especially during the first 3 months). **Overweight** individuals are at the greatest risk. **Heavy lifting** is another causal factor. About 15% of Americans experience the problem; most of these are women.

When varicose veins occur in and around the anus, they are called hemorrhoids. **Straining** at the stool, because of a lack of dietary fiber, causes constipation and can result in varicose veins, diverticulosis (466), hemorrhoids (469), phlebitis (533), and hiatus hernia (436).

Spider veins are unsightly, but cause no problems.

NATURAL REMEDIES

• Important: Follow the lengthy suggestions given under *Phlebitis and Thrombophlebitis (533)*.

HERBS

• An herbal wash that relieves varicose veins: Mix equal parts **sweet flag root, thyme leaves, nettle leaves, horse chestnut leaves, and fruit**. Add 3 Tbsp. to 1 quart cold water, bring to a boil. Add ½ tsp. salt and bathe the legs with the tea.

• **Horse chestnut seeds** have been used to treat varicose veins and hemorrhoids for years in Germany. The active ingredient, *aescin*, strengthens capillaries and reduces fluid leakage. Use the standardized extract.

• **Witch hazel** is an outstanding herbal wash. It is a soothing astringent which strengthens blood vessels. **White oak bark** is another useful astringent herb.

• Applying **aloe vera** gel is soothing to the veins.

• Apply fresh **wood sorrel** leaves to the area with extended veins. Cover with large **cabbage leaves**, and fasten with an ace bandage.

• Taking **bromelain** reduces risk of clot formation.

• Here are more useful substances: **Lemon peel** contains flavonoids, including rutin, which reduce blood vessel permeability. **Bilberry** stimulates new capillary formation. **Ginkgo** improves circulation.

• Both **violet and pansy flowers** contain rutin and are safe to eat. Add them to your salads.

• Drinking **dandelion** or **corn silk** tea helps the kidneys eliminate excess fluid, thus reducing tissue swelling.

• Dr. Christopher recommends making a tea of **sassafras,** drinking it, and using it to wash the legs.

• Apply hot applications of **tansy** tea on large veins. Replace when they become cool. Cover with wool or plastic to keep them wet and hot.

DIET

• Drink at least 48 oz. of water daily.

• Take **vitamin C** (500-1,000 mg 3 times daily), **vitamin E** (200-400 IU daily), **flaxseed oil** (1 Tbsp. daily).

• Include enough **fiber** in your diet, which should be **low in fat and refined starches**. Eat lots of fresh **fruits and vegetables**. Avoid **animal products**. Eat **whole grains, nuts, and legumes**.

• If you are **overweight**, you need to reduce.

OTHER HELPS

• Avoid wearing **garments** which constrict blood flow. But moderate pressure on the veins (**elastic stockings**) is helpful.

• **Never cross your legs**. It adds pressure to the veins.

• **Elevate your feet** while reading or watching TV. At least once a day, elevate your legs above your heart for 20 minutes.

• **Walking** is the best exercise for your legs.

• On lengthy trips, **walk around** every so often.

• **Do not stand in one place** too long. If you have

to do so, rise up on your toes occasionally, wiggle your toes, and move a little from time to time.

• **Sleep with your feet raised** slightly above the level of the heart. But do not do this if you have heart problems.

• If you are confined to a bed, **move your extremities** frequently to improve general circulation.

• In the morning, go out and **walk barefoot** on the cool, wet grass. Quickly dry and put on socks and shoes.

• Do not scratch the itchy skin above varicose veins. Doing so can lead to bleeding and surface ulcers.

ENCOURAGEMENT—God does not accept men because of their capabilities, but because they seek His face, desiring His help. God sees not as man sees. He judges not from appearances; but He searches the heart. Only with His help can you have purity of life; and this you must do. Leviticus 26:12.

"I will look unto the Lord, I will wait for the God of my salvation; my God will hear me." Micah 7:7.

"He that putteth his trust in Me shall possess the land, and shall inherit My holy mountain." Isaiah 57:13.

"The Lord redeemeth the soul of His servants, and none of them that trust in Him shall be desolate." Psalm 34:22.

With such promises as these, what need is there to fear in this earthly life?

CARDIOVASCULAR - 3 - BLOOD

POOR CIRCULATION AND CHILLS

SYMPTOMS—Cold fingers, hands, and feet. Also numb tingling fingers and toes. A general sense of chilliness when others are warm. Frequent bruising, infection, numbness in joints and digits.

CAUSES—Poor circulation can be caused by **cardiovascular disease, low thyroid, vitamin E deficiency, or low blood pressure**. Other causes include a **high-fat and high-cholesterol diet, atherosclerosis, cigarette smoking, lengthy periods of standing or sitting, lack of exercise, poor posture, diabetes mellitus, high blood pressure, prolonged muscle tension, inflammation, or being inadequately clothed**.

In some instances, poor circulation can lead to claudication *(637)*, gangrene *(367)*, blindness, senility *(589)*, heart attack *(513)*, and stroke *(529)*. Using nicotine can result in Raynaud's disease *(368)* and eventual amputation. Alcohol *(820, 881)* also restricts blood flow.

NATURAL REMEDIES

DIET

• Take 800-1,200 IU of **vitamin E** daily. Take **vitamin C** to bowel tolerance. Also needed: **niacin, RNA**, and **folic acid**.

• Purifying the bloodstream will help in restoring proper circulation. This would include **enemas** or colonics, **juice fasting** for a day or two, followed by a **nourishing diet**.

• **Do not eat meat, cheese. No fatty, processed, or junk foods.** Avoid **cold foods, sweets, ice cream**. Do not use **nicotine, alcohol, or caffeine**.

• Foods which increase the circulation include **lentils, beets, buckwheat, citrus peel, soybeans**. **Cayenne** is especially helpful; but only take in moderate amounts (or you can damage your kidneys).

OTHER HELPS

• Take **cool morning showers** or **alternating hot and cold showers** for 5 to 15 minutes, morning and evening. **Exercise afterward** and make sure you are warm. If you are not warm afterward, you did not gain.

• **Exercise** outdoors and practice **deep breathing**.

• Drink **red clover, sassafras, and burdock** teas in order to clean the blood.

• Other helpful herbs include **ginkgo, hawthorn, lily-of-the-valley, lavender, rosemary, scotch pine, and cayenne**.

• *In an emergency*, swallow some **cayenne** in water to warm a person up. **Goldenseal** is also helpful. Take 1 part each of **cayenne, skullcap**, and ½ part **goldenseal**.

• *Kloss recommends the following:* A high **enema**. Breathing exercises every day. **Cold towel rub** every morning followed by **rubbing with a dry, coarse towel**. Lots of **outdoor exercise** while breathing deeply.

—Also see Chills (293). If you are chronically cold, you are likely to have hypothyroidism (659).

ENCOURAGEMENT—No sooner does a child of God approach the mercy seat in the Sanctuary in heaven, where Jesus is, than he is received. Pray, earnestly; pray for the help that you so much need. God loves you and will answer your prayers in the very best way. How very thankful we can be that God not only shows us what He wants us to do, but (by the grace of Christ) gives us the power to do it. Hebrews 8:10.

CHLOROSIS
(Green Sickness, Chloremia)

SYMPTOMS—The person has a greenish cast to his or her skin, plus indications of continual fatigue.

CAUSES—This condition is characterized by a great reduction in hemoglobin, which is much greater than the decreased number of red blood cells. It is a type of chronic hypochromic microcytic (iron deficiency) anemia. Women, from puberty to the third decade of life, are the ones who primarily have this problem. The cause is **a diet deficient in iron and protein**.

Other names for this condition include chlorotic or asiderotic anemia, chloremia, chloroanemia, and green sickness.

—See Anemia (below)

NATURAL REMEDIES

• The diet needs to be improved. Instead of snacking on junk food and soft drinks, eat nourishing meals of **fruits and vegetables, plus whole grains, nuts, and legumes**.

• Eat at least 1 tablespoon of **blackstrap molasses** each day (1 teaspoon for a child).

• *For additional information on the richest foods and herbs in iron, read Anemia (above).*

J.H. KELLOGG, M.D., PRESCRIPTIONS FOR CHLOROSIS AND ITS COMPLICATIONS *(how to give these water therapies: pp. 206-275 / list of treatments: pp. 206-207 / Hydrotherapy Disease Index: pp. 273-275)*

Chlorosis is a form of anemia in adolescent girls, generally due to faulty diet during puberty. It is also called "green sickness."

CORRECT ENTEROPTOSIS—Abdominal supporter, abdominal massage, **corrective exercises**, Cold Douche to abdomen.

INCREASE VITAL RESISTANCE—General **graduated cold procedures** (Tonic Frictions) twice daily.

COMBAT AUTOINTOXICATION—**Aseptic diet**, sweating bath (**Hot Full Bath**) to begin perspiration, Radiant Heat Bath or **sunbath**, followed by **short cold** application.

VASOMOTOR SPASM—General **Revulsive Douche**. Alternate **Full Bath** at 105⁰-110⁰F., 30 seconds, and then into one at 80⁰-90⁰ F., for 15 seconds. Simultaneous **Revulsive Douche**.

VISCERAL ANEMIAS—**Douches** to visceral (trunk) areas. Alternate Douche or Revulsive Douche, with short percussion for either; **Alternate Compress** over the afflicted part, followed by a well-protected **Heating Compress**. Protected (plastic covered) Hot **Abdominal Pack** at night. Cool **Enema** at 75⁰-68⁰ F., 1-3 pints, daily.

ENCOURAGEMENT—By studying with greater earnestness and care the life of Christ, you may see the victories which you have to gain that you may win the precious white robe of a spotless character, and stand at last without fault before the throne of God. As you plead for help, Christ's empowering grace will enable you do all that God requires of you.

ANEMIA
(Simple Anemia, Iron Anemia)

SYMPTOMS—Easy tiring, dizziness, headache, rapid heart rate, shortness of breath or exertion. Pale skin, nails, and lips. A sensitivity to cold. Poor appetite and cravings for clay, ice, or starch.

Other symptoms include white or coated tongue, pale tissue beneath fingernails, and white skin inside the lower eyelid (when it is pulled down).

CAUSES—There are several types of anemia (simple, pernicious, sickle-cell, folic acid, copper). This article will deal only with simple anemia, which is by far the most common.

Millions of people are anemic. The cause is usually a reduction in the number of red blood cells or the amount of hemoglobin in the blood. In either case, not enough oxygen is carried throughout the body.

Iron deficiency anemia is the most common type of anemia; and it occurs when there is not enough **iron** in the body.

This can occur when the body is **not absorbing enough iron from the food, during chronic blood loss, pregnancy, menstruation, hemorrhoids or ulcers, diverticular disease, liver damage, surgery, repeated pregnancies, periods of rapid growth, and aging. Infections, hemorrhage, and nutritional deficiencies** can also cause it.

Infants and young children on a **milk diet, without minerals and essential fatty acids**, are prone to anemia. Others include the elderly who eat narrowed diets and pregnant women because of their increased nutritional needs.

Red blood cells (RBCs) are called *erythrocytes*; they are tiny discs which are concave on both sides. These cells contain hemoglobin, which is bright red because of the iron in it. About 60%-70% of the iron in your body is in the hemoglobin of your blood. (About 30%-35% of the iron is stored in the liver.) The percentage of RBCs in the blood is called the *hematocrit*. The primary function of the RBCs is to carry oxygen to the cells.

Following birth, the bone marrow of the infant, child, and adult makes the red blood cells. Aging causes RBC formation to lessen. An average RBC wears out in 120 days or less, so your body must keep making more.

Those who are anemic tend to have sore mouths or tongues, generally have poor blood circulation, and are cold. They need special care in regard to these matters. Of those suffering with anemia, 20% are women and 50% are children.

Peek incidence of anemia in children occurs between 6 months to 2 years, then declines, and rises again during adolescence (especially in girls). Low birthrate infants are at a greater risk for anemia. Some children are allergic to cow's milk and develop gastric bleeding which, over a period of time, results in the loss of considerable blood. The American Academy of Pediatrics recommends that children under the age of 1 year *not* (!) drink cow's milk. Milk can cause anemia by interfering with iron absorption and pos-

sibly causing internal bleeding.

Some children have a pallor of face and dark shadows under the eyes, which is caused, not by anemia but, by food allergies (especially, free fats of margarine, mayonnaise, fried foods, cooking fats).

Women with **menorrhagia** (*682*, heavy or prolonged menstrual bleeding), or who use intrauterine devices for contraception are at higher risk of blood loss. Anyone who takes aspirin or ibuprofen are also at risk, because they cause blood loss through the walls of the digestive tract.

NATURAL REMEDIES

THESE INCREASE IRON ABSORPTION

• Eat at least 1 tablespoon of **blackstrap molasses** each day (1 teaspoon for a child). This is, by far, the richest source of food iron. And it is a safe iron. Much of the iron in supplements is not safe.

• **Broccoli, lettuce, and tomatoes** help iron regeneration.

• **Avoid spicy foods, tea, or coffee**. They decrease absorption. **Do not smoke;** and avoid secondhand smoke.

• **Whole-wheat flour and oatmeal** are effective in increasing hemoglobin regeneration. **Yeast and wheat germ** are high in iron. Also good are **beets, beet greens, cabbage, whole grains, barley, peas, seeds, nuts, celery, parsley, cherries, dates, figs, and pears**. Good sources are **sesame seeds, sunflower seeds, pistachios, pecans, almonds**. Also vegetables, such as **Swiss chard and kale**. Others include **blueberries, carrots, celery, cranberries, grapes, and prunes**.

• Herbs rich in iron include **alfalfa, comfrey, dandelion, fenugreek, mullein, nettle, Chamomile, and red raspberry. Garlic extract** has been shown effective in treating anemia.

• There should be **sufficient stomach acid** to absorb the minerals. If there is not, take some **lemon juice.** Squeeze the juice of half a lemon, put it into a glass of water, and drink it before meals. An alternative is taking 1,000-2,000 mg **vitamin C** with each meal. (Vitamin C is also very acid.)

• **Orange juice** increases iron absorption.

• Do not take **calcium, vitamin E, or zinc** at the same time as iron supplements. They interfere with each other's absorption.

• Use a diet high in **fresh, raw fruits and vegetables** which are high in **vitamin C** (which is necessary for iron absorption). These include **citrus fruits, leafy green vegetables, and broccoli**.

• Each day drink ¼ cup **beet juice**, added to some **carrot juice**. The juice of fresh beets has been a successful remedy for anemia for many years.

• **Bananas** are moderately helpful in increasing iron absorption.

• Raw or lightly steamed **greens (or cooked as-**

paragus, **beets, broccoli, or brussels sprouts**) supply the folic acid needed for the absorption of iron.

Increase your intake of calcium-rich foods (**leafy green vegetables, beans, peas, soybeans, and sesame seeds**) to make up for the lack of milk (see below).

• **Cooking acidic food (tomatoes, apple sauce, etc.) in iron pots** increases the iron content of the food.

• Those with poor blood-making organs may need eggs in the diet (MH320; CDF 365).

• Water from **deep wells** has more iron than city water.

• **Exercise** stimulates the production of blood.

• **Short, cold baths** *powerfully* increase blood production and circulation.

• A **cold mitten friction** is a useful way to increase metabolism and blood production.

• Men need 10 mg of iron daily. Women of child-bearing age, who lose blood each month, should get 15 mg. After menopause, they only need 10 mg. (To reduce heavy flow in menorrhagia *(682)*, take **shepherd's purse**, which aids blood clotting. **Goldenseal** contains *berberine*, which helps calm the uterine muscles.)

• To strengthen the liver, so it can absorb iron better, take **yellow dock, turmeric, or milk thistle**. A healthy liver breaks down estrogen, which is important in preventing anemia; since excess estrogen can cause heavy bleeding.

THESE REDUCE YOUR IRON

• **Avoid milk and other dairy products**; since these decrease iron absorption from other foods.

• Avoid foods **high in oxalic acid foods**. The worst is **poke and rhubarb**. The others include **spinach, sorrel, Swiss chard, chocolate, cocoa, cashews, and soda**.

• **Avoid bran** as a source of fiber. It tends to link with iron and carry it out in the stool. (However, you may need bran to prevent other physical problems far worse than a mild case of simple anemia.) *Phytates* in **high-fiber foods** bind with some of the iron so the body cannot absorb it.

• *Phosphate* additives in **bakery goods, soft drinks, candy, beer, ice cream, and many packaged foods** reduce iron absorption, as does the *cadmium* in **tobacco**.

• *Polyphenols* in **coffee** and *tannins* in **black tea** reduce the amount of iron assimilated from foods by 70%.

• Many **medicinal drugs** destroy vitamin E and cause anemia. Some **insecticides** destroy bone marrow, so new blood cells cannot be made.

• Do not use **food additives** or **artificial sweeteners**.

• **Alcoholic beverages**, as well as **sugar**, deplete the body of B-complex vitamins and some minerals, which can intensify anemia.

• Caffeine products (**coffee, black tea, soft drinks, chocolate, etc.**) make it more difficult for the body to absorb iron.

• Taking aspirin tablets causes bleeding from the stomach and the loss of iron.

• It is true that **raw liver** contains iron; but it also contains large amounts of waste products that was about to be excreted before that animal was slaughtered.

IRON SUPPLEMENTS

• Have a complete blood test taken, so you will be certain whether or not you have iron anemia. **Too much iron can damage** the heart, liver, pancreas, and immune cells' activity. It has also been linked to cancer.

• If you do not need them, **avoid iron supplements. Ferric sulfate, ferrous sulfate,** and **other iron compounds** are often given to reduce anemia; but they definitely have toxic effects which you should be aware of: They destroy carotene and vitamins A, C, and E. They increase the need of the body for oxygen and damage unsaturated fatty acids. They also damage the liver, especially when the person has a poor appetite and is not eating very much. **Ferrous sulfate** also irritates the stomach and lymphatic system. Yet it is the kind of iron in most multi-vitamin food supplements. Liquid iron supplements stain the teeth. Iron compounds cause damage to the liver, miscarriages, premature birth, or prolonged pregnancy. Some suggest they may cause birth defects. Too much iron stored in the body leads to increased risk of cancer.

• In contrast, **ferrous gluconate, iron gluconate, and iron picolinate** are easy for the body to digest and absorb. They are less likely to irritate the stomach. Unfortunately, many labels of most food supplements only list "iron," without telling what kind it is.

• **Iron salts** taken during pregnancy are especially dangerous! They can increase the fetus' need for oxygen and induce miscarriage or premature and postmature births. Some infants have malformations or mental deficiencies because their mothers took iron supplements before birth. Young women, beware!

• Normal people do not need iron supplementation; for there is lots of iron in most real food. The iron in unrefined food is *never* toxic. *Nearly all* iron supplements cause stomach or intestinal irritation.

J.H. KELLOGG, M.D., PRESCRIPTIONS FOR SIMPLE ANEMIA AND ITS COMPLICATIONS *(how to give these water therapies: pp. 206-275 / list of treatments: pp. 206-207 / Hydrotherapy Disease Index: pp. 273-275)*

INCREASE BLOOD-MAKING PROCESS—Graduated **cold applications**. The Radiant Heat Bath is especially valuable as a means of heating before giving the general cold applications. **Have aseptic dietary** (a nourishing diet), **rest** in bed (if he is emaciated), **outdoor life**, cold-air baths, **sunbaths**, sea bathing, massage, oxygen inhalation.

GENERAL METHOD—Cold water is the most valuable of all measures in treating anemia. Apply twice daily, graduating carefully. Autointoxication, arising from dilation, prolapse of the stomach, or chronic constipation, is often an important factor.

—Also see Chlorosis (537) and Pernicious Anemia (below). Also see Poor Circulation and Chills (536).

ENCOURAGEMENT—We are to have a spirit of pity and compassion toward those who have trespassed against us. Pray for them, that they may come to Jesus. Unselfish ministry is the hallmark of the genuine Christian. Matthew 26:33, 1 Kings 8:50.

PERNICIOUS ANEMIA

SYMPTOMS—Weakness, slight yellowing of the skin, tingling of the extremities, and gastrointestinal disturbances causing a sore tongue. There can be partial loss of coordination of the fingers, feet, and legs. Some nerve deterioration may occur. Diarrhea and loss of appetite may also be present.

CAUSES—Pernicious anemia is caused by a **deficiency of vitamin B_{12}**. This is a severe form of anemia in which the bone marrow fails to produce mature red blood cells. Other causes include eating **junk food**, **malabsorption** problems, **Crohn's disease** *(465)*, **gastric surgery**, **drugs** which have destroyed the ability of the large bowel to produce B_{12}.

The stomach has to be able to produce, what is known as, *"intrinsic factor"* in order for vitamin B_{12} to be absorbed by the intestines. Pernicious anemia rarely occurs under the age of 30; but it becomes more common afterward. Without treatment, pernicious anemia may be fatal.

In some instances, B_{12} deficiency can be diagnosed by a physician who uses a Schilling test, a special blood test which evaluates B_{12} absorption.

NATURAL REMEDIES

• Persons with pernicious anemia must take B_{12} sublingually (dissolved under the tongue), by injection, or by a retention enema. Take 50-100 mcg injections of **vitamin B_{12}** daily. Unless the underlying cause can somehow be corrected, this treatment must be continued for the rest of your life.

• Here is a second recommendation: Take methylcobalamin (active vitamin B_{12}, 1,000 mg twice daily for at least 1 month, followed by a daily intake of 1,000 mcg).

• Eat a highly **nutritious diet** that is rich in **protein, calcium, vitamins C and E, and iron**.

• Take supplements of the entire **B complex**, to aid in B_{12} absorption.

• (Important exception: Folic acid should not be taken in amounts greater than 0.1 mg daily.) Folic acid has the effect of concealing the symptoms of pernicious anemia and permitting the unseen destruction of the nervous system to continue until irreparable damage has occurred.

• There should be sufficient **stomach acid** to absorb the minerals. If there is not, take some lemon juice *See Achlorhydria (439).*

—Also p. 25. Also see Anemia (537-541, 713) and Megaloblastic Anemia (below).

ENCOURAGEMENT—A lamp, however small, if kept steadily burning, may be the means of lighting many other lamps. Our sphere of influence may seem narrow, our ability small, our opportunities few; yet God can work through us to help many others.

MEGALOBLASTIC ANEMIA
(Folic Acid and B_{12} Anemia)

SYMPTOMS—The initial symptoms are fatigue and a feeling of faintness, pale skin, shortness of breath on mild exertion. Symptoms may worsen over a period of time.

CAUSES—Megaloblastic anemia occurs when large, abnormal red blood cells (megaloblasts) are produced by the bone marrow and the production of normal red blood cells is reduced. The blood gradually becomes unable to carry enough oxygen to the cells.

The cause is deficiency of two important B vitamins: **B_{12}** and **folic acid**.

Folic acid deficiency is usually due to a poor diet. Drinking alcohol intensifies the problem, because alcohol interferes with absorption of folic acid. Pregnant women have a higher risk, because their folic acid needs are greater. Taking certain drugs (such as anticonvulsants and anti-cancer drugs) can also cause it.

Lack of folic acid does not produce any other symptoms than those listed above.

B12 deficiency may be due to a lack of B_{12} in the diet or an autoimmune disorder may be the problem. Antibodies are produced which damage the stomach lining and prevent it from forming *"intrinsic factor"*; this is needed for absorption of B_{12}. Intestinal disorders, or surgery on the stomach or intestines, can also interfere with B_{12} absorption.

Lack of B_{12} can later result in more severe symptoms, which are tingling in the hands and feet, weakness and loss of balance, loss of memory and confusion. *—For more on B12 anemia, see Pernicious Anemia (539).*

NATURAL REMEDIES

• When external cuts are bleeding, cover the cut with cayenne powder.

• Take 400 mcg of **folic acid**, twice a day. Folic acid should not be taken in amounts greater than 0.1 mg daily. *See Pernicious Anemia (539) for explanation.*

• Take 50-100 mcg injections of **vitamin B₁₂**.
—*For other principles, see Pernicious Anemia (539) and the large section on Anemia (537-541, 713).*

ENCOURAGEMENT—We may have joy in the Lord only if, through the strengthening grace of Christ, we keep His commandments and do that which is pleasing in His sight. If we indeed have our citizenship above, and a title to an immortal inheritance, an eternal substance, we have that faith which works by love and purifies the soul. We are members of the heavenly family, children of the heavenly King, heirs of God, and joint heirs with Christ. At His coming we shall have the crown of life that fadeth not away.

THALASSEMIA

SYMPTOMS—Mild symptoms occur in most people; but, if the disease was inherited from both parents, they can be more severe and appear between 4-6 months of age. Symptoms may include pale skin, shortness of breath on mild exertion, swelling of the abdomen due to an enlarged spleen and liver. Affected children have slow growth, sexual development is delayed, the bones of the skull and face may thicken.

CAUSES—An **inherited genetic defect** prevents the normal formation of hemoglobin. The body tries to compensate by producing additional red blood cells, which causes a thickening of the bones (and may include those of the skull and face). The liver and spleen may become enlarged. Thalassemia primarily occurs in people from the Mediterranean, Middle East, Southeast Asia, and Africa. Those with mild symptoms can lead a fairly normal life.

NATURAL REMEDIES
• Blood tests can confirm whether a person has this problem. He should remain on a **nourishing diet**, which should include **folic acid** supplements.

ENCOURAGEMENT—The Monarch of heaven would have you possess and enjoy all that can ennoble, expand and exalt your being, and fit you to dwell with Him forever—your existence measuring with the life of God. What a prospect is the life which is to come! What charms it possesses! How broad and deep and measureless is the love of God manifested to man!

SICKLE-CELL ANEMIA

SYMPTOMS—Symptoms are highly variable, even within the same family. In children and adults, they may include those common to all anemias: fatigue and a feeling of faintness, pale skin, shortness of breath on mild exertion. There are also "sickle-cell crises," which are explained below.

CAUSES—The amount of hemoglobin within the red blood cell (RBC) becomes smaller. This causes the RBC to become distorted into a curved sickle shape.

This deprives the body of oxygen. Those with this problem are more susceptible to serious infections, such as pneumonia. Other effects include gallbladder problems, leg ulcers, kidney damage, stroke, and miscarriage.

"Sickle-cell crises" occur from time to time, in which the oddly shaped blood cells clump together inside small blood vessels, causing blocking of the blood supply to body tissues. These crises may be triggered by infection, dehydration, strenuous exercise, or high altitudes. The symptoms of a crisis are severe pain and swelling around the bones and joints, especially in the hands and feet of children. Also abdominal pain, chest pain, and shortness of breath. A severe crisis can be fatal; so you may want to contact a physician.

This is a genetic problem, occurring most frequently in persons of African ancestry; it is less common in people from countries around the Mediterranean.

NATURAL REMEDIES
• Folic **acid** is necessary for the production of RBCs. Take **folic acid** (800 mcg), **vitamin B₆** (100 mg 2 times daily), **zinc** (20 mg daily), and **vitamin E** (400 IU 2 times daily).
• It is vital that you **keep drinking enough water**, in order to avoid a crisis. The blood must be able to flow easily through your capillaries.
—*For more information on general nutrition and ways to avoid anemic problems, see Anemia (537-541, 713).*

ENCOURAGEMENT—The privileges granted to the humble, obedient children of God are without limit: To be connected with Jesus Christ, who, throughout the universe of heaven and worlds that have not fallen, is adored by every heart, and His praises sung by every tongue; to be children of God. To bear His name. To become a member of the royal family. To be ranged under the banner of Prince Immanuel, the King of kings and Lord of lords!

BLEEDING (EXTERNAL)

SYMPTOMS—Bleeding from a surface wound.

CAUSES—When a blood vessel is cut, bleeding (external bleeding) or hemorrhage (internal bleeding) begins. If an artery is cut, the blood spurts and flows fast; it is usually bright red. If a vein is cut, the blood is darker and flows more constantly and slowly.

NATURAL REMEDIES

HERBS
• When external cuts are bleeding, cover the cut with powdered **cayenne**; and it will stop the bleeding immediately. When an artery or vein is severed, apply powdered cayenne immediately. Then apply direct pressure, seek a physician, or go to a hospital. Cayenne powder or tea is also a good drink for internal bleeding. Cayenne has astounding styptic (blood stop-

page) action. A tiny amount on a cut will stop bleeding. A very small amount (1/8 tsp. in a large glass of water) will tend to stop internal bleeding—bleeding occurring inside your body.

• Although it will sting, squeezing **lemon juice** on a wound will immediately stop the bleeding, even when ice and other herbs have failed. In earlier times, midwives used diluted lemon juice to stop uterine hemorrhage after delivery.

• If outdoors, mash green **juniper berries** on the bleeding wound.

• Dampen **plantain** (powder or leaf) and apply to the wound. Or use **marigold**.

• Make a tea of the whole plant of **shepherd's purse**, a common weed. Drink it and apply it to the wound as a poultice. Or add it to bathwater.

• Other hemostatic (stop bleeding) herbs include **goldenseal, hazelnut, smartweed, burnet, grapevine, milfoil, horsetail, pau d' arco, bilberry, comfrey root, turmeric, and bistort. White oak bark** and **witch hazel** are especially good.

• Drink **red raspberry** leaf tea during pregnancy and at the time of delivery, to avoid bleeding.

• **Cayenne** will take care of most bleeding problems, external or internal, by the time you can count to ten. For bleeding of the lower bowel (commonly called dysentery), use **mullein** (preferably in milk). In the urinary tract, **marshmallow** (preferably in milk) is generally faster. Other excellent herbs; **comfrey root, European goldenrod, self-heal, shavegrass, shepherd's purse, and wild alum root** may be used. In bleeding of the nose, raise the arms above the head and administer **cayenne** dissolved in hot water; or the extract of **witch hazel** may be sniffed in the nostrils. A decoction of equal parts of **bistort root, cranesbill root, avens, or raspberry** taken internally works well.

• Other useful herbs include:

• Herbs for bleeding from the nose (epistaxis): **Alumroot** (snuffed)**, bethroot, calamine, cancer root, cayenne, forget-me-not leaves, gall oak powder** (on cotton)**, globe thistle, groundsel, nettle leaves** (snuffed)**, onion juice in vinegar** (snuffed in the nose)**, shavegrass, walnut leaves, willow bark and sprouts**. The bark is to be used on the nose and the sprouts in the nose.

• Useful **herbs for bleeding from the lungs:** Bethroot, black cohosh, bloodroot, bugleweed, comfrey root, cranesbill root, cypress tree, hound's-tongue, kidney liver leaf, lungwort, mullein, nettle leaves, oak bark, shavegrass, shepherd's purse, St. John's wort, succory, witch hazel, whortleberry, yarrow.

• Herbs for bleeding in the stomach: **Bethroot, cayenne** (one of the fastest healers of bleeding ulcers)**, geranium root, groundsel, lady's mantle, mullein, oak bark, shavegrass, shepherd's purse, tormentil, whortleberry, witch hazel, and yarrow.

• Herbs for bleeding in the bowels: **Adder's tongue (expressed juices), bethroot, geranium root, groundsel, lady's mantle, mullein, oak, redroot, shavegrass, shepherd's purse, tormentil, witch hazel, whortleberry, yarrow.

• Herbs for buchu, calendula (tincture), chervil, comfrey, European goldenrod, false sweet flag, garden daisy, garlic, ground ivy, groundsel, herb Robert, lungwort, marshmallow, mayflower, nettle leaves, oak bark, peach leaves, plantain, sanicle, shavegrass, veronica, vervain, and yarrow.

OTHER HELPS

• Put **citrus peel** directly on the wound. Sprinkle **alum** powder on the wound.

• As a preventive, take 100 mcg of **vitamin K,** 3 times daily.

• If the wound is on the **arm, hold it up** over your head. If the wound is serious enough, and you do not know what else to do, **apply direct pressure** to a vein or artery. Use **cold cloths or ice packs**. Sprinkle **alum powder** on the wound. Get to a physician and treat for shock.

• If you are at risk for internal hemorrhaging, **do not use aspirin** or other blood-thinning drugs (such as Heparin).

—*Also see Wounds (1007-1008), Hemorrhage (below), # Water Therapies which Control Bleeding (543).*

ENCOURAGEMENT—True happiness does not consist in the possession of wealth or position, but in the possession of a pure, clean heart, cleansed by obedience to the Word of God. How thankful we can be that God can enable us to obey His laws and resist temptation to sin. Isaiah 41:10.

HEMORRHAGE
(Internal Bleeding)

SYMPTOMS AND CAUSES—*Bleeding in the stool,* which indicates stomach ulcers (black blood stool), ulcerative colitis (bloody mucus in stool), colon cancer (bloody mucus in the stool), and hemorrhoids (bright red blood). *Coughing blood* indicates lung cancer or tuberculosis.

This can also be a discharge or escape of blood from the blood vessels, either by passage of blood cells through the intact and unruptured walls (diapedesis) or by flow through the ruptured walls.

NATURAL REMEDIES

• Hemorrhage throws many people into shock and can bring on death very rapidly. If the wound is small, the blood usually coagulates and the area seals itself, but if the rupture is large, some herbal aid is needed. The first thing one should think about is **cayenne** as quickly as possible. Using one teaspoon to the cup, as hot as can be taken without scalding. *This will stop* *any hemorrhage, internal or external, by the time a person can count to ten.* If the rupture is external and cayenne is not available, **comfrey** placed over the wound will stop bleeding quickly.

• External bleeding *(541)* is bleeding from surface wounds. Hemorrhage is bleeding inside the body. Natural healers today use one or a combination of four methods to stop hemorrhage: very **hot applications**, very **cold applications**, **cayenne**, or **astringent herbs**.

• *Hemorrhage of the lungs*—Tell him to cough as little as possible. Give a **hot footbath**. Give him a pinch of **cayenne** to swallow. It will stop the bleeding almost immediately. Also good: a tea made from **white oak bark** or **witch hazel**.

• *Hemorrhage of the stomach*—Briefly apply ice over the stomach. Have him swallow small bits of ice rapidly for a short time. Give him a cupful of **shepherd's purse** tea. A tea made from **white oak bark** or **witch hazel** is equally good. Other herbs which stanch internal bleeding include **red raspberry, bistort root, wild alum root, yarrow, or sumach**. How to make the tea: Steep a tsp. of the herb in a cup of boiling water 30 minutes, strain, and drink it.

• *Hemorrhage from the uterus*—Have patient lie down and elevate the feet. Give a hot douch of herb tea. It can be **bayberry bark, bistort root**, or one of the above-mentioned herbs. Steep 1 Tbsp. of the powder in a quart of boiling water for 10 minutes. If the herb is granulated, use 2 Tbsp. to 1 quart boiling water; steep 20 minutes. Let settle, strain, and apply as hot as possible.

• *Hemorrhage of the bowels*—Patient should lie down. Inject a tea made of one, or a mixture of several, of the **astringent herbs** (such as **red raspberry, white oak bark or wild alum root**). Inject 2-3 oz. with a small syringe. Retain as long as possible; then repeat. Have him drink the same tea.

• *Hemorrhage of the nose*—See *Nosebleed (711)*.

• It is of interest that, for all of the above internal bleeding problems, R.T. Trall, M.D., used **cold applications (water and ice)** alone to stop the bleeding.

• For chronic hemorrhage, Dr. Christopher recommends the following formula: Prepare an infusion of hops tea. Stir 1 tsp. **tormentil** root powder into 1 cup of the **hops** infusion. Drink 1 cup 4 times daily.

• For hemorrhage, he recommends giving 2 fl. oz. of **tormentil** tea as an infusion every ½ hour until the excessive discharges are checked.

—*Important: see # Water Therapies which Control Internal Bleeding (below) and External Bleeding (541).*

—*Also see Peptic Ulcers (442), Colitis (463), Cancer (792-796), Hemorrhoids (469), Tuberculosis (505), Nosebleed (711), Menstrual Disorders (678).*

ENCOURAGEMENT—The consciousness that you are doing those things which God can approve will make you strong in His strength; and, by copying Christ the great Pattern, you can be the blessing He intends for you to be in this world. Romans 5:10, 17.

WATER THERAPIES WHICH CONTROL BLEEDING

NATURAL REMEDIES

Hemostatic effects (stopping of bleeding) may be obtained either directly by application to the bleeding area or indirectly through **applications to a reflex area**.

To obtain direct effects, either very hot (110°-115° F.) or very cold (32°-40° F.) applications must be used. The most valuable hot application is the **hot compress**. A **jet of hot vapor** has also been used successfully. Here are some examples of hot applications: **hot nasal spray** and **sponging the face with very hot water** for nose bleed, **hot vaginal douche** for menorrhagia, **hot uterine irrigation** in metrorrhagia and postpartum hemorrhage.

The most convenient cold applications are **ice and ice compresses**. These should be applied directly to the bleeding area or (as a proximal compress) across the trunk of a main artery supplying the bleeding part. An example of this would be an **ice collar** (ice cravat) for nosebleed.

ENCOURAGEMENT—In place of the tinsel of the world, God wants to give you (for a life of obedience by faith in Christ) the kingdom under the whole heavens. He will give you an eternal weight of glory and a life that is as enduring as eternity.

HEMOPHILIA

SYMPTOMS—When a wound occurs, blood does not clot normally.

Early warning signs of internal bleeding include a bubbling or tingling sensation, a feeling of warmth, tightness, or stiffness in the hemorrhaging area.

Headache, confusion, drowsiness, or a blow to the head may indicate bleeding in the head.

If your hemophiliac child cries for no apparent reason, refuses to walk, use his arm or leg, or seems to have a swelling or unusual bruising, go to an emergency room.

CAUSES—Hemophilia is **hereditary**. It primarily affects males and is passed down through females (who are carriers). Children of carriers have a 50% chance of inheriting the defective gene. If they inherit it, the boys will be hemophiliacs and the girls will be carriers. The sons of hemophiliacs will not give the problem to their sons; but the daughters will always be carriers.

As many as two-thirds of all hemophiliacs in America have HIV. They contracted it from contaminated blood transfusion sources in the early 1980s. About 450 babies are born with hemophilia each year.

The blood of hemophiliacs does not clot properly; yet minor bleeding is not serious. It is the internal bleeding that can be fatal, if not treated.

Bleeding frequently occurs in the knees, which

causes painful swelling. Repeated swelling destroys the knee cartilage and results in a permanently stiff knee (called hemophiliac arthritis). Other joints and body parts, including the brain, can also be affected by internal bleeding.

The hemophiliac is periodically given blood transfusions to provide the missing blood factors.

Wear a bracelet which gives your name, address, phone number, and the fact that you are a hemophiliac. Be continually on the alert to possible signs that internal bleeding has started.

NATURAL REMEDIES

• Eat a diet high in **vitamin K**. Foods rich in K and other essential clotting factors include **alfalfa, broccoli, egg yolks, kale, and all green leafy vegetables**.

• Drink **green drinks**, consisting of pineapple juice and one or more of the above green vegetables. Take **vitamin K** (300 mcg daily).

• Other nutrients essential for clotting include the **B complex**, extra **niacin or niacinamide**, **vitamin C** (3,000 mg daily), **calcium** (1,500 mg daily), and **magnesium** (1,000 mg daily).

• Never take **blood-thinning drugs**, such as **aspirin** or **warfarin**. They eliminate clotting factors in the blood, and thus intensify the problem.

ENCOURAGEMENT—To go forward without stumbling, we must have the assurance that an all-powerful hand will hold us up and an infinite pity be exercised toward us if we fall. God alone can, at all times, hear our cry for help. Isaiah 63:9.

BLOOD POISONING
(Septicemia)

SYMPTOMS—Swelling, severe localized pain and discoloration. Red streaks from the wound which extend up the veins toward the heart. Sores which do not heal. High fever, chills, and violent shivering.

If not treated immediately, the bacteria can produce toxins which damage blood vessels, causing a drop in blood pressure and tissue damage. This is called septic shock; the symptoms are faintness, cold and pale hands and feet, restlessness and irritability, rapid and shallow breathing. Soon this leads to delirium and loss of consciousness.

Whenever a sore, cut, or abrasion becomes red and infected, it could produce blood poisoning.

CAUSES—Septicemia is a potentially fatal condition in which bacteria multiply rapidly in the bloodstream. They are normally killed by the white blood cells; but sometimes there are so many bacteria from a major source of infection (such as kidney infection), they threaten to overwhelm the body's defenses. Septicemia can develop as a complication of almost all types of serious infectious diseases.

People with reduced natural immunity are the most susceptible. This includes those who have diabetes mellitus, HIV, chemotherapy, or immunosuppressant drugs. Young children, the elderly, and intravenous drug users are also more susceptible.

NATURAL REMEDIES

• Contact a physician.

• Apply two **hot fomentations** and then place a **cold towel** over the affected area. Continue this alternate application until the red lines disappear.

• Apply a poultice of **lemons** or **charcoal**. Or crush one or more of the **herbs** listed later in this article.

• Take a high **enema**.

• Drink as many cups of **echinacea** tea a day as possible.

• Keep the temperature in the room evenly warm, have enough air, and give a little **cayenne** in water when he feels chilly.

• Drink **charcoal** water.

• If there is a wound, wash it thoroughly with **boric** solution. If the discharge from the wound is thin, apply powdered 50-50 **myrrh and goldenseal** directly to the wound.

• Go on a cleansing program of **juice fasting** for a time, followed by rebuilding on a good, **nourishing diet**.

• Drink a tea of **chickweed, plantain, goldenseal, and myrrh**.

• For blood poisoning, Dr. Christopher recommends mixing 4 parts **bayberry root bark**, 2 parts each of **cayenne** and **cloves**, 1 part each of **ginger** and **pinus bark** (or **hemlock spruce**). Put 1 Tbsp. of the mixture in 1 pint boiling hot water, cover and steep until cool, strain. Drink 2 Tbsp. or more 3 times daily.

ENCOURAGEMENT—It is a solemn thought that the removal of one safeguard from the conscience, the failure to fulfill one duty, the formation of one wrong habit may result in the ruin of another, not only in our own ruin. James 1:22-27.

BLOOD PURIFIER

Here are three herbal formulas for purifying the blood:

• Mix 4 Tbsp. each of yellow dock and burdock root, and 1 Tbsp. of blood root. Put them in 1½ quarts boiling water. Simmer and reduce to 1 quart. Strain, sweeten with honey and 1 pint of glycerine. Mix well. When cool, bottle and keep in a cool place. Take 2 fl. oz. 3-4 times daily.

• Mix ½ oz. each of red clover, yellow dock, burdock root, blue flag. Combine with ¾ oz. sarsaparilla and 1 tsp. wild giner or Canada snake root. Simmer the herbs in 3 pints of water until it reduces to 2 pints.

Strain, sweeten with honey, let cool, bottle and store in a cool place. Take 3 Tbsp 3 times daily.

Mix 1 oz. each of licorice root, cleavers, burdock root, sarsaparilla root, fumitory, and guaiac chips. Pour 3½ quarts of boiling-hot water over the herbs and simmer down to 2 quarts. Strain, sweeten with honey, allow to cool, then bottle and store in a cool place. Take ½ cup 3-4 times daily before meals.

ENCOURAGEMENT—All who resolutely cling to Christ will stand before Him as chosen and faithful and true. Satan has no power to pluck them out of the hand of the Saviour. Not one soul who in penitence and faith has claimed His protection will Christ permit to pass under the enemy's power.

More Encouragement

"The wind is heard among the branches of the trees, rustling the leaves and flowers; yet it is invisible, and no man knows whence it comes or whither it goes. So with the work of the Holy Spirit upon the heart. It can no more be explained than can the movements of the wind. A person may not be able to tell the exact time or place, or to trace all the circumstances in the process of conversion; but this does not prove him to be unconverted. By an agency as unseen as the wind, Christ is constantly working upon the heart. Little by little, perhaps unconsciously to the receiver, impressions are made that tend to draw the soul to Christ. These may be received through meditating upon Him, through reading the Scriptures, or through hearing the Word from the living preacher. Suddenly, as the Spirit comes with more direct appeal, the soul gladly surrenders itself to Jesus. By many this is called sudden conversion; but it is the result of long wooing by the Spirit of God,—a patient, protracted process.

"While the wind is itself invisible, it produces effects that are seen and felt. So the work of the Spirit upon the soul will reveal itself in every act of him who has felt its saving power. When the Spirit of God takes possession of the heart, it transforms the life. Sinful thoughts are put away, evil deeds are renounced; love, humility, and peace take the place of anger, envy, and strife. Joy takes the place of sadness, and the countenance reflects the light of heaven. No one sees the hand that lifts the burden, or beholds the light descend from the courts above. The blessing comes when by faith the soul surrenders itself to God. Then that power which no human eye can see creates a new being in the image of God.

" It is impossible for finite minds to comprehend the work of redemption. Its mystery exceeds human knowledge; yet he who passes from death to life realizes that it is a divine reality. The beginning of redemption we may know here through a personal experience. Its results reach through the eternal ages."
—Desire of Ages, 172-173

Two editions of Desire of Ages, the classic (and best) book on the life of Christ are available from us.

C
A
R
D

The Natural Remedies Encyclopedia

- Disease Section 9 -
Neuro-Mental

Nervous System: Physiology 1019 / Pictures 1036
Special Senses: Physiology 1023 / Pictures 1036-1037

 # = Information, not a disease

NERV

Section 9 - Neuro-Mental

NEURO-MENTAL - 1 - MISCELLANEOUS

INSOMNIA
(Sleeplessness)

SYMPTOMS—Inability to get to sleep, night after night.

CAUSES—If it only happens once in a while, it is sleeplessness; if it happens for weeks or months, it is insomnia. It is said that, to one degree or another, 100 million Americans have insomnia and take 600 tons of sleeping pills each year to avoid it. About seven times as many women as men experience the problem. Sleeping pills are second only to aspirin sales in the U.S.

Side effects from sleeping pills include anxiety, depression, skin rashes, irritability, loss of appetite, poor coordination, digestive disturbances, difficulty with vision, confusion, dizziness, high blood pressure, circulatory and respiration disorders, breakdown of parts of the blood (such as the white blood cells which fight infection), damage to the central nervous system, memory problems, and liver and kidney damage.

The experts tell us that if you go to bed on time, have a current of fresh air in the room, and lie there quietly—you will get enough rest even though you do not seem to fall asleep as quickly as you might wish. Many people who report not getting to sleep at night actually slept quite a bit without realizing it.

Many people have a hard time getting to sleep at night because of *restless leg syndrome (634).* These people are awakened by **legs which twitch** or kick.

Overeating, eating too close to bedtime, and eating bad food can produce sleeplessness or insomnia. Systemic **disorders in the heart, liver, kidneys, pancreas, lungs, digestive organs, endocrines, and brain** can all affect sleep.

NATURAL REMEDIES

DIET

• Eat **nutritious food**, and let breakfast and lunch be your main meals. Only **eat lightly in the evening**, several hours before bedtime.

• Foods with the amino acid, **tryptophan**, promote sleep. These include figs, dates, and whole grain crackers.

• Take **calcium** (2,000 mg) and **magnesium** (250 mg). A lack of them can cause you to wake up after a few hours and be unable to return to sleep.

• Take **B complex, vitamin B$_6$** (50 mg), **pantothenic acid** (100 mg), **niacinamide** (500 mg), **inositol** (600 mg), and **vitamin C** (1,000 mg in divided doses)

• Avoid **complicated and indigestible foods (including meat)** before bedtime. Better yet, keep those junk foods entirely out of your diet. Do not eat **eggplant, potatoes, sugar, spinach, or tomatoes** before retiring. They contain tyramine, which increases the release of *norepinephrine*, a brain stimulant.

• Other foods which keep people awake include **fatty foods, sugar, white flour, salt, monosodium glutamate (MSG), chemical preservatives, additives, and allergenic foods**.

• Stop eating **cheese, bacon, chocolate, ham, sausage, and wine.**

• **Alcohol, barbiturates, and hypnotics** do not solve the sleep problem, but only worsen it. Alcohol disrupts sleep later in the night. Nicotine appears to be calming, but it is actually a neuro-stimulant.

• The following substances, taken during the day, excite the brain and prevent good sleep at night: **caffeine, alcohol, tobacco, and aspartame** (NutraSweet). **Meat** eaten for supper will keep you awake.

• Do not take **nasal decongestants and other cold medications**. They stimulate many people and keep them from getting to sleep.

• The following **drugs** will keep you awake at night: Anacin, Exedrin, Triaminic, antidepressant drugs, some birth-control pills, many asthma drugs, Dopar (for Parkinson's), steroids, chemotherapy, tranquilizers, drugs for high blood pressure, and amphetamines.

FOR MORE NATURAL REMEDIES:

HERBS: Herb Contents (pp. 129-130) will help you locate the 126 most important herbs and the diseases each one can treat. How to prepare herbs (132). How to use them (141-189)

HYDROTHERAPY: Therapy Contents (pp. 206-207) and its Disease Index (263-265) will lead you to over 100 water therapies and many more remedies. DIS. INDEX: 1211- / GEN. INDEX: 1221-

VITAMINS AND MINERALS: Contents (100-101). Using 101-124. Dosages (124). Others (117-)

CARING FOR THE SICK: Home care for a sick person (28-36). The healing crisis (36-39)

WOMEN'S SECTIONS: Female Organs (672) Pregnancy (701). Childbirth (765). Infancy, Childhood (722). Women's Herbs (754, 760)

EMERGENCIES: (973-). FIRST AID: (990-)

• **Sunlight** during the day helps you sleep at night. Upon awakening, open the shades and let the sunlight in. Eat breakfast near a sunlit window. Avoid dark glasses in the morning and late in the day.

• Studies reveal that, in countries where people regularly **nap during the day**, there are fewer accidents and productivity is higher. The important factor here is consistency. Be regular in your hours for sleep at night. If you nap during the day, be regular in that. Naps before meals are better than naps afterward.

• If you are wakeful one night: **Do not nap the next day**, and you will be more likely to go right to sleep that night. If you find yourself very sleepy, go to bed early.

BEFORE BEDTIME

• Take a **hot bath** (instead of a shower) an hour or two before bedtime.

• Before bedtime **go outside and walk** around quietly in the fresh air for 30 to 45 minutes.

• Some people need to have the bedroom **quiet**. Others need some sound to mask background noise. In such cases, having a **fan** turned on works well.

• Trust in God. He promises to give His beloved rest.

• For some people, **daytime naps** make it more difficult to sleep at night. But, for some older people, a little rest before mealtime during the day helps them; so that any sleeplessness at night never fatigues them.

• Some take **melatonin or calcium** to help them go to sleep. Both promote sleep. Taking melatonin products continually can stop production of your own melatonin!

• Do not take **sleeping pills**. They contain pain relievers, such as bromides, antihistamines, and/or scopolamine. These are ineffective. They produce unpleasant side effects and interfere with normal brain functioning, causing poor-quality sleep. They can produce a hangover, so you cannot work as well the next day. The brain quickly adapts to the drug; so, after 4-6 weeks they are no longer effective, unless you take more. The easiest way to overcome the habit of taking sleeping pills is go on herb teas at the same time.

HERBS BEFORE BEDTIME

• Excellent herbal teas which help increase sleepiness include **hops, catnip, and skullcap**. But do not rely on herb tea to help get you to sleep every night. Lemon balm is both a sedative and stomach soother.

• Drink **valerian** tea (1-2 tsp. per cup of water or 150-300 mg of the valerian extract) about 30 minutes before bedtime. In Britain, it works so well; over 80 drugstore valerian preparations for sleeplessness are sold. **Passionflower** tea works equally well.

• Another English remedy: Hospitals put **lavender oil** in the evening bathwater or sprinkle it on the sheets. (Never drink any essential oil.)

• One old remedy to help a nervous person sleep is placing compresses of **wormwood, balm, chamomile, and lavender** on the head.

• Herbal teas to help you go to sleep: Mix 3 parts **hops** and 2 parts **valerian**, Steep 1 tsp. in ½ cup boiling water. Take ½-1 cup a day, unsweetened, in mouthful doses. Do not take it for more than 2 weeks, without interruption.

• An outstanding herb tea: Mix equal parts **valerian** root, **hops**, **skullcap**, and **passionflower**. Put the dried herb mixture into capsules. Take 2 one hour before retiring, and another 2 upon retiring.

DURING THE NIGHT

• **Regularity** in your habits is important. This is vital to good sleep. Always go to bed at the same time and get up at a definite time. The body has normal rhythmic cycles. People with regular habits have faster reaction time and are happier than those with irregular sleeping times. Getting up each morning at the right time will help you go to sleep at the right time each night. Sleeping in, on weekends, disrupts the biological clock. If you want sleep problems, stay up late every so often.

• The **bedroom temperature** should be 60°-65° F. If the room is too warm, you are likely to move about more and awaken frequently. The problem is a lack of air.

• If you want a restful night's sleep, make sure a little **current of air** is passing through the room, even in winter. You cannot sleep well when it is stuffy.

• If you cannot sleep, you can **just lie there, relax, and rest**. This is nearly as good as sleep.

• In the **middle of the night**, you can get up and do something quietly and calmly for a short time—and then go back to bed and to sleep. One excellent method is to go outside and breathe the fresh air, look up at the stars, breathe some more fresh air. Be thankful for your blessings—and then go back to bed and sleep.

• *Restless leg syndrome (634)* at night can be a problem. **Calcium** (2,000 mg), **magnesium** (250 mg), **potassium** (5,000 mg), **and zinc** (30 mg) supplements help eliminate that problem. In addition, make sure you are not anemic. *See anemia (537-541, 713).*

OTHER HELPS

• Obtain enough **exercise** during the day, with some of it being outside. Exercise regularly in the late afternoon or early evening, but not right before retiring.

• Make sure you have a **good mattress** on which to sleep.

MAINTAINING YOUR MELATONIN LEVEL

• Melatonin is a hormone, so it is best to live in

such a way as that you will not need to take a melatonin supplement from animal sources.

As darkness falls at the end of each day, melatonin production rises. In the morning, when daylight hits the retina. neural impulses cause production of the hormone to slow. Clearly, **light and darkness** are the primary factors that set the rhythms of melatonin production. However, they are not the only factors involved. In fact, it has been found that a variety of regular daily routines can strengthen the rhythm of melatonin production. *Here are several helpful suggestions in which you can help your body maintain high levels of this important hormone:*

• Eat **regular meals**. The rhythm of melatonin production is strengthened by regular daily routines. Keep your mealtimes as regular as possible in order to keep your body in sync with the rhythms of the day.

• **Several hours before bedtime, eat a small, light meal**. When melatonin production begins after nightfall, the digestive process is slowed. Thus, any heavy foods eaten close to bedtime may lead to digestive problems, which can make it difficult to sleep.

• **Avoid stimulants**. Stimulants such as coffee, tea, and caffeine-containing medications and soft drinks can interfere with melatonin production by interfering with your sleep. As much as possible, eliminate these stimulants from your diet and lifestyle.

• **Avoid exercising late at night**. Vigorous activity delays melatonin secretion. If you exercise in the morning, you will reinforce healthful sleeping habits that lead to regular melatonin production. For best results, do your morning exercise outdoors, in the morning light.

• **Keep your thoughts heavenward**, and you will find it much easier to go to sleep at night.
—*Also see Sleep Apnea (550).*

J.H. KELLOGG, M.D., PRESCRIPTIONS FOR INSOMNIA AND ITS COMPLICATIONS (*how to give these water therapies: pp. 206-275 / list of treatments: pp. 206-207 / Hydrotherapy Disease Index: pp. 273-275*)
TO RELIEVE BRAIN CONGESTION—Neutral **Douche**, 3-5 minutes at bedtime. **Cold Douche. Hot Leg Bath.** Footbath under running water. Heating **Wet Sheet Pack**, followed by **Wet Sheet Rub. Hot Abdominal Pack**, warmly covered and protected with plastic. **Heating Leg Pack.** Dry heat to the legs and feet. **Hot Leg Pack.** Follow with **Cold Mitten Friction** to the legs. **Heating Compress** to legs or Leg Pack at bedtime, to be prolonged during the night. **Hot Abdominal Pack** and **Leg Pack** through the night. Revulsive Douche to the legs at 102° F. for 2 minutes; then 60° F. for 15 seconds. **Neutral Douche**, 3-5 minutes. Downward stroking of head and neck [to eliminate phlegm and aid lymph flow].
RELIEVE IRRITABILITY OF THE BRAIN CELLS—Prolonged **Neutral Bath** at bedtime. **Neutral Wet Sheet Pack. Enema**, if constipation or flatulence is present.
IRRITABILITY OF SOLAR PLEXUS OR LOWER BACK NERVES—Abdominal **Fomentation.** Follow by abdominal **Heating Compress**, changing every 6 hours. Avoid eating anything but fruits after 4 p.m. Copious **water** drinking. **Colonic**, especially if the bowels are inactive. Constipation

is a frequent cause of insomnia by producing irritation of the abdominal sympathetic nerves.
EXCESSIVE CARDIAC ACTIVITY—Ice Bag over heart.
FIDGETINESS OR RESTLESSNESS—Warm Pail Pour to spine, at 95°-98° F. **Tepid Sponging** with rubbing of limbs, rubbing of spine, and massage of head.
GENERAL IRRITABILITY—Neutral **Wet Sheet Pack**. Neutral **Full Bath**. Neutral Fan Douche or Shower, for 2-4 minutes.
GENERAL METHOD—There may be said to be three forms of insomnia: Sleeplessness may be due to (1) congestion of the brain, (2) irritability of the brain cells, or (3) a combination of these two conditions. Here is how to go to sleep: (1) Come to God; and, in peace of heart, trust in Him. (2) Relax and let your mind rest; do not try to problem-solve, you just gave them all to Jesus. (3) Check the temperature and air; it is more difficult to go to sleep in a room that is too hot, too cold, too drafty, or one lacking fresh air. (4) With your nerves and muscles relaxed and cheerful in the thought of Jesus' love, concentrate on breathing slightly deeper and go to sleep.

ENCOURAGEMENT—Every faculty with which the Creator has endowed us should be cultivated to the highest degree of perfection, that we may be able to do the greatest amount of good of which we are capable. Matthew 25:14-29.

NARCOLEPSY
(Chronic Sleeping Disorder)

SYMPTOMS—A person can suddenly fall asleep, with almost no advance warning, as often as eight or more times a day. The deep sleep may continue for an hour or two. Although refreshed upon awakening, the person may fall asleep again soon afterward. While sleeping, they can be easily awakened. During the sleep, the person may experience complete loss of muscle control. Symptoms vary.

CAUSES—A chronic neurological sleep disorder involving sleep-wake mechanisms in the brain. There are two main types: dopamine dependent depression (DDD) and a type involving a deficiency of vitamin B_6 in the dopaminergic system. Also there is poor use of body oxygen.

NATURAL REMEDIES
• Obtain **an excess of rest. Lay down and rest before or after meals, and at other times through the day**. Retire early at night, even though you do not seem to be fatigued. Just lay there and rest.
• Eat only the most **nourishing food**. Take **vitamin-mineral supplements**.
• The diet should be low in **saturated fats** and **clogging foods**, including **dairy** products and **animal protein**. Search out your **allergenic foods**.
• **Avoid stressful situations**; and, when you feel tired, **stop and rest**. Maintain **strict regularity** in your hours for rest. **Never stay up late** at night.

• Do not use **tobacco, alcohol, caffeine, or any drugs** you can avoid.

• Make sure your **workplace is well lit**, preferably by full spectrum lighting. The brain makes melatonin to help you go to sleep; but bright light suppresses the production of that chemical.

ENCOURAGEMENT—Thank God every day of your life that, through the enabling grace of Jesus Christ your Lord and Saviour, you can do all that God asks.

SLEEP APNEA

SYMPTOMS—Frequent and abnormal cessations of breathing occur during sleep. They are followed by brief awakenings as the sleeper gasps for air.

The first obvious symptom is loud snoring. If it is so loud that it awakens anyone else in the room or elsewhere, and is interrupted by pauses and then gasps for air, sleep apnea is probably the cause. Frequent daytime drowsiness is another indication. Depression, forgetfulness, irritability, anxiousness, or difficulty in concentrating are other signs.

CAUSES—The word, apnea, means "interrupted breathing." While sleeping, the person intermittently stops breathing. He is usually unaware that his rest has been disturbed, but it has. Each apnea episode lasts about 20 seconds; but as many as 400-500 can occur during a single night. So he spends more time awake than asleep. But unaware of what has happened, the person cannot understand why he is so tired out after sleeping all night. He tends to be overweight.

Sleep apnea is also a risk factor for heart attacks, stroke, high blood pressure, right-and-left ventricular heart dysfunction, and heart failure. Sudden death sometimes occurs.

These people also have a higher incidence of emotional and psychotic problems.

NATURAL REMEDIES

• **Lose weight**. Excess weight is linked to this disorder. Even a 10% weight loss will produce decided improvement in the number of nightly episodes.

• **Sleep on your side** to avoid snoring. The gasping episodes are associated with snoring.

• **Alcohol, tobacco, and sleeping pills** cause the airway to more easily collapse during sleep, making each episode longer in duration.

• Special mouth guards can be worn at night, which prevent gasping episodes.

—*Also see Insomnia (547, 709).*

ENCOURAGEMENT—We will hide in Jesus Christ. We will trust in His love. We will believe day by day that He loves us with a love that is infinite. Let

nothing, nothing discourage you, and make you sad. Think of the goodness of God. Recount His favors and blessings.

VERTIGO
(Dizziness)

SYMPTOMS—Dizziness, faintness, or light-headedness. The person may feel that he is falling or sinking or that the room is moving around him, sometimes even spinning. There may be ringing in the ears. This sensation is usually accompanied by nausea, vomiting, perspiration, headache, or hearing loss.

CAUSES—Vertigo is caused by an **impaired sense of balance and equilibrium**, and is generally due to an **inner ear disorder** (labyrinthitis). Older people have it more often than those younger. *See Mèniére's Syndrome (412).*

If the original cause is **concussion, skull fracture, or injury to the inner ear**, the dizziness may occur long after the injury supposedly healed.

Other causes are **anemia, brain tumors, high or low blood pressure, psychological stress, lack of oxygen or glucose in the blood, nutritional deficiencies, viral infection, fever, changes in atmospheric pressure, the use of certain drugs, middle-ear infections, excess wax in the ear, or blockage of the ear canal or eustachian tube**.

Lower **oxygen levels at higher altitudes** can also cause it, as well as **vitamin B$_6$ and niacin deficiency**.

You can expect that you may temporarily experience it if you engage in certain activities, such as **amusement park rides, sailing, or virtual reality games**.

WARNING: Be aware that dizziness can be *a warning sign of a coming heart attack or stroke*. It can also indicate that a **concussion or brain damage** has just occurred.

Dizziness is not always the same as vertigo. From time to time, anyone can experience some dizziness or faintness. Those with **low-blood pressure** will frequently experience this when standing up suddenly.

Chronic vertigo can be caused by **atherosclerosis** *(523)* or **high blood pressure** *(526);* and it may recur frequently. *Senile vertigo* can result from **atherosclerosis** *(523)*.

NATURAL REMEDIES

• Immediately, **sit in a chair with your feet flat on the floor** and **stare at a fixed object** for a few minutes.

• When an attack occurs, **restrict your head movement** and keep your eyes fixed on a stationary object a great distance from you. Or **lie down, with your unaffected ear against the floor, and look in the direction of the affected ear**.

• If the cause is an inner ear disorder, the underlying disorder needs to be treated.

• But, if the cause is *low blood pressure*, **lower your head** while the blood gets up there.

• Eat a nutritious diet which includes the entire **B complex. Especially niacin, B_6** (200 mg), **B_1** (200 mg), **B_2** (200 mg), **and pantothenic acid** (50 mg). **Vitamin C** (1,000 mg), **vitamin E** (400 IU), and **lecithin** (1 tsp. per meal) are also needed.

• Do not take over 2,000 mg of total **sodium** per day. Too much sodium disrupts the operation of the inner ear.

• Avoid **nicotine, caffeine, alcohol, and fried foods**.

• The problem may be *low blood sugar*, not enough glucose. Solve this by increasing intake of **fiber** and decreasing simple carbohydrates (**white sugar and white flour**). Drink a glass of **orange juice** to overcome brief dizziness. But snacking on **refined carbohydrates or candies** may intensify it.

• A calorie-reduced diet **low in sugar and fat** can eliminate repeated dizziness. Sometimes **low-protein** diets cause the problem.

• If vertigo begins after taking some new **drug**, stop using it immediately.

• If vertigo seems to be *chronic*, **search out the causes**. You may need professional help.

HERBS

• In Europe, **ginkgo** (60-240 mg daily) is prescribed for vertigo. In one French study, people with chronic vertigo showed 47% improvement.

• For thousands of years, sailors on the open sea chewed **ginger** for seasickness. Research by the U.S. Navy found it reduced dizziness by 38%. Swallow 2 capsules 30 minutes before departure; and swallow another 1-2 capsules when symptoms begin. In another study, 1 gram of ginger relieved vertigo better than the standard drug.

• The Chinese use **celery seed** for dizziness.

• Dizziness, caused by low blood pressure, can be relieved by **licorice**.

• **Catnip** tea will help.

• **Black cohosh** or **garlic** will lower blood pressure.

—*Also see Mèniére's Disease (412) and Motion Sickness (287).*

ENCOURAGEMENT—When you live a life dedicated to helping others, yours is a life full of satisfaction and happiness. This is the will of God for you, even your sanctification. Obey God's laws. Find ways to bless others, and you will best fulfill your earthly probationary life. Thank God every day for the gift of His Son, Jesus Christ, who, by His grace, enables us to obey the ten commandments and live good, clean lives. 2 Corinthians 4:6-18.

NEURASTHENIA
(Nervous Exhaustion)

SYMPTOMS—The symptoms vary greatly. Most frequently there is easy fatigue, a sense of great weariness after slight exertion, or inability to perform a normal amount of mental or physical labor.

There may be mental depression, impaired memory, and inability to concentrate. There may be a sense of fullness, pressure, or pain in the head. Pains in the neck, shoulders, back, and limbs. Tender spots on the spine. Dizziness, ringing in the ears, attacks of palpitation and distress about the heart. Cold feet, clammy hands, hot flashes about the head. There is generally constipation, a disturbed digestion, and sleeplessness.

SYMPTOMS—There are at least 100 different problems that can include vertigo. There are also different types of vertigo. Among the most common are these:

• *Chronic vertigo* can occur as a result of hypertension or atherosclerosis. This type of vertigo either does not go away completely or recurs frequently.

• *Senile vertigo* can be caused by atherosclerosis, chronic eye disease, or a syndrome called benign paroxysmal positional vertigo (BPPV). However, it is worth checking to see if side effects or interactions might be causing the problem.

• *Juvenile vertigo* is usually caused by anxiety or hyperventilation.

• *Positional vertigo* is, as it states, an attack of vertigo that occurs when you assume a particular position. BPPV is an example of positional vertigo. It is thought to be caused by damage to the body's balance mechanisms in the inner ear. The structures in the middle ear might be dislodged by injury or infection, or as a result of old age, causing all the symptoms of vertigo when you move your head.

• *Sudden-onset vertigo* is, as the name implies, vertigo that strikes suddenly and may last for minutes or hours. It can be caused by motion sickness, Meniere's disease, or insufficient oxygen supply to the brain. Low blood sugar can also cause dizziness similar to vertigo.

Because of the effects of aging on the body, older people are more prone than others to vertigo. The body maintains a sense of balance through a complex mechanism involving the semicircular canals close to the ears.

NATURAL REMEDIES

• A variety of causes may, and probably are, involved. For example, the person may be hypothyroid and fears to exert himself. Yet **vigorous outdoor activity** is probably what he needs, along with **fresh air and sunlight**.

• The orthodox approach is to prescribe rest and quiet. But it may be that **getting outside and walking around** is a better solution during part of the day. **Find someone else who needs help** and help them.

• Start taking on small challenges, and then expand them. Begin by washing the dishes and sweeping the floor. Do something useful, and thank God that you can.

• Eat **nourishing food**—and nothing else. Include **niacin** and the entire **B complex**. Do not eat between meals. Chew your food well. Do not overeat. Do not go on binges.

• Stop consuming all **fried, processed, junk foods and drinks**. Stop **alcohol, tobacco, caffeine, and hard medicinal drugs**. Avoid **chemicals** in the food, air, and water.

• Take a **cool shower**; jump out and dry off in the cooler air.

• Run down the road a few yards. Go in and **lie down and rest. Go outside and run again**. Within good reason, keep pushing yourself; get yourself built up.

• Avoid **enervation and practices that cause it**. Think positive. Be thankful for what you have and what you can do.

—*Also see Debility (278), Emotional Fatigue Syndrome (278), Chronic Fatigue (279), and Epstein-Barr Syndrome (280).*

J.H. KELLOGG, M.D., PRESCRIPTIONS FOR NEUR-ASTHENIA AND ITS COMPLICATIONS (*how to give these water therapies: pp. 206-275 / list of treatments: pp. 206-207 / Hydrotherapy Disease Index: pp. 273-275*)

NOTE—Neurasthenia (nervous exhaustion) is not a distinct pathological entity, but a group of symptoms due to various etiological influences and connected with various morbid states.

BASIC ASPECTS—Rest cure for those who have been overworked, nervously and physically, and for those who are mentally and nervously tired.

COMBAT AUTOINTOXICATION—Aseptic diet. **Fruit diet**. Daily **Neutral Baths**, 1-3 hours. **Sweating procedures** of short duration (3-6 minutes), followed by suitable **cold applications**. Hot **Enema** daily. Copious **water** drinking. **Outdoor life**.

COMBAT EXHAUSTION—Rest for the overworked. **Improve digestion** by proper diet; in cases of starved dyspeptics, by appropriate measures. Tonic **cold applications** carefully graduated—especially Percussion Douche to spine.

CHECK EXHAUSTING DISCHARGES—Apply appropriate measures. See under "Menorrhagia," "Leukorrhea," and "Spermatorrhea."

RELIEVE REFLEX IRRITATION—If sexual, rectal, prostatic, or urethral irritation: Employ Revulsive **Sitz Bath**, Prolonged Neutral Sitz Bath, **Hot Footbath**, **Hot Pack** over pelvis. For ovarian irritation, in addition to above, hot vaginal irrigation for 15-20 minutes.

IRRITATION OF SOLAR PLEXUS AND SYMPATHETIC NERVES—Fomentation over abdomen, 3 times daily. During intervals, **Heating Compress**. Abdominal supporter.

IMPROVE GENERAL NERVE TONE—Graduated **cold applications**. The Cold Percussion Douche to spine is the most efficient of all measures. General Cold Douche. Very Hot Douche at 110° F. for 30 seconds, followed by

Graduated or Cold Douche.

HEADACHE—Hot and Cold Compress. Revulsive Compress. To spinal area, give **Alternate Compress** or Sponging. **Hot Footbath**. Footbath under running water.

FRONTAL HEADACHE—Revulsive Compress to forehead and eyes. **Hot and Cold Trunk Pack**. Derivative applications to feet and legs.

CONGESTIVE HEADACHE—Ice Bag to back of head and **Cold Compress** to face. Ice Collar, **Hot and Cold Compress** to head, Hot Footbath, **Hot Leg Pack**, **Heating Compress** to legs, **Cold Footbath** under running water, **Alternate Footbath**, and **wear felt shoes**.

OCCIPITAL HEADACHE [on back of head]—Hot Compress or Sponging to upper spine and occipital region. **Revulsive Compress**, **Hot and Cold Compress** to head. [The occipital region is the area around the bump on the back of your head).

NERVOUS HEADACHE—Fomentation to seat of pain, with simultaneous **Hot Footbath**. Daily **Cold Enema**, to relieve constipation if present. Special attention to the diet. A **dry aseptic diet** is indicated, avoiding milk.

SENSATION OF BAND AROUND HEAD—Hot Sponging or **Hot Compress**, **Alternate Sponging** of neck and upper spine, massage to head.

SENSATION OF PRESSURE AT VERTEX [top of head]—**Hot Footbath**, **Cold Compress** to head, **Ice Collar**, sleep with head elevated, heat to feet and legs if cold.

PAIN IN EYES. INTOLERANCE TO, OR USE OF, LIGHT IN READING—Light, warm (not hot!) **Fomentation** over eyes and forehead, but never over naked eyeball. Close eyelids and lay gauze or thin, dry cotton cloth over it, beneath the Fomentation. Protect eyes from bright light. Facial massage and massage to eye. An oculist should be consulted; for eyeglasses may be needed, temporarily or permanently.

BACKACHE—Fomentation to abdomen, **Hot Abdominal Pack**, abdominal supporter, Alternate Spinal Sponging or **Alternate Compress**, Revulsive Douche to spine, **Revulsive Sitz Bath**.

VERTIGO—Fomentation to stomach, followed by **Hot Abdominal Pack**. Bathe face or top of head with very hot water or Hot Compress for 2 minutes. Follow by **Cool Compress** for 15 seconds. Heat to back of neck in anemia of the brain.

ANOREXIA—Hot-Water Bottle (containing hot water) over stomach for half an hour before meals with Cold Compress or **Cold-Water Bottle** (containing cold water) to area, front and back, and opposite stomach. Cold Mitten Friction or **Cold Towel Rub**.

MUSCULAR WEAKNESS, ESPECIALLY IN LEGS—Cold Percussion Douche to spine. **Alternate Douche** to legs.

MENTAL DEPRESSION—Sweating Bath, followed by short general **Cold Douche**. **Neutral Bath** for 1 hour daily. Neutral Pack. **Cold Percussion Douche** to spine. **Alternate Sponging** to spine or Alternate Douche to spine.

FIDGETINESS—Fomentation to abdomen, followed by **Hot Abdominal Pack**. Empty colon, if loaded, by Enema. Abdominal supporter, **Revulsive Sitz Bath**, **Neutral Pail Pour** to spine.

DREAMS—Neutral Bath for half an hour before going to bed. **Hot Abdominal Pack**. Evaporating head cap. Elevate head of bed. Avoid eating after 4 p.m., except fruit.

COLD EXTREMITIES—Revulsive Douche to legs and feet, followed by standing Shallow Bath. **Fomentation** to abdomen twice daily, followed by heating compress during the intervals between. **Alternate Footbath**, massage to feet and legs, **Cold Mitten Friction**.

GENERAL METHOD—While not recognizable as a distinct malady, it is convenient from a practical standpoint to consider neurasthenia (general exhaustion) as a disease. The tonic effects of cold water are essential in the treatment of neurasthenic conditions. The management of cold applications in such a way as to secure the desirable tonic effects without aggravating any of his symptoms is a problem which taxes, to the utmost, the skill and experience of the hydrotherapist. Special attention must be given to the digestion, improvement of nutrition, regulation of the bowels, and the relief of prominent and distressing symptoms by suitable palliative measures.

CHOREA
(St. Vitus' Dance, Sydenham's Chorea, Nervous Twitching)

SYMPTOMS—For a few days before an attack, the patient is irritable in the daytime and sleeps poorly. Then irregular jerky movements begin, usually in one hand and arm; but they soon spread to the other hand and arm, the face, and the lower limbs. The jerky movements are constant during the waking hours, cannot be controlled by the person, and are increased by excitement or embarrassment; but, they usually cease during sleep. He shrugs his shoulders, makes faces, and may not be able to feed himself. In severe cases there is marked weakness and fever. Speech is disturbed, jerky, or impossible; and there is difficulty walking.

CAUSES—Chorea is an acute infectious disease; but it is not contagious. Its most prominent symptoms are those which concern the nervous system. It is common from 5 to 15 years of age, and most likely to occur in high-strung, nervous children, especially girls.

Chorea is a complication of **acute endocarditis and acute rheumatic fever**, or from **inflammation of the meninges from a steptococcal infection** that usually begins in the throat (and could spread to the heart (causing endocarditis and/or acute rheumatic disease). Acute disease of the heart is often present, resulting in inflammatory growths on the edges of the heart valves, followed by scarring, distortion, and leakage when healing occurs.

Most attacks last 1-6 months; but artificial fever treatments materially shorten the course. The person nearly always recovers; but the disease may recur. And the damage to the heart valves is liable to be permanent. The disease is more severe in pregnant women than in anyone else.

A variant form is Huntington's Chorea, which is a rare hereditary disease appearing in middle life and continuing for 10-15 years; it usually ends fatally.

NATURAL REMEDIES
• **Apply colloidal silver, echinacea, goldenseal, and garlic** for 30 days (alternating every 7 days between echinacea and goldenseal). The earlier you begin, the better.

J.H. KELLOGG, M.D., PRESCRIPTIONS FOR CHOREA AND ITS COMPLICATIONS (how to give these water therapies: pp. 206-275 / list of treatments: pp. 206-207 / Hydrotherapy Disease Index: pp. 273-275) **BASIC FACTORS**—Combat anemia and improve general nutrition by **graduated tonic applications** (Tonic Frictions), copious **water** drinking, large **Enema** or Colonic, **Fomentation** to abdomen morning and night, **Heating Compress** during intervals between. Secure mental quiet by isolation, if necessary. He should be kept in the open air as much as possible. **Outdoor life** and rhythmical **gymnastics** are especially useful.

INSOMNIA—Prolonged Neutral Bath or Neutral Douche, **Hot Abdominal Pack**.

AGITATION—Neutral Pail Pour to spine, **Wet Sheet Pack**.

IRREGULAR MOVEMENTS—Neutral Pail Pour to spine daily, prolonged **Neutral Bath**, special exercises.

ENDOCARDITIS—Ice Bags over the heart.

GENERAL METHOD—Improve the nerve tone by tonic measures and careful attention to nutrition. Train him to better mental and moral control and to combat choreic movements by systematic gymnastic training.

ENCOURAGEMENT—God gives us strength and time to build characters which He can improve. By the enabling grace of Christ, put away sin from your life and live to bless others. 2 Kings 17:39.

SHOCK

SYMPTOMS—Shock may not develop until hours after the injury or illness. But, as soon as blood pressure falls, the symptoms suddenly develop. These may include cold, clammy skin and sweating. There is contusion or agitation, rapid and shallow breathing, fast heartbeat, and loss of consciousness.

CAUSES—Shock is a state of profound depression of the vital processes from various causes; it could be from emotional trauma to injury which reduces the blood pressure and venous return, thus impairing circulation which may cause irreversible circulatory failure and eventually death. It is a severe reduction in blood pressure, causing poor blood supply to major organs. This cold, pale, collapsed state may develop as a result of **any situation in which the heart cannot pump blood effectively or in which there is too little blood for the heart to pump**. The usual cause is serious injury or illness.

It is a potentially life-threatening condition that necessitates immediate medical attention.

N
E
R
V

(This condition is not the mental or emotional distress, commonly called "shock," which follows a startling experience.)

It may result from **serious blood loss, such as bleeding from the digestive tract or from a serious injury**. The blood volume may also be reduced by **fluid loss due to severe burns or profuse diarrhea**.

An **allergic reaction** *(Anaphylaxis, 846)* or serious **blood infection** *(Septicemia, 544)* may cause the blood vessels in the body to widen, resulting in a severe drop in blood pressure and shock.

Bad news or an automobile accident will bring on shock sufficient to weaken the body and bring on the problem. With perfect body function, a shock would not have this effect. It could cause a disquieting moment, but the body system would not undergo the extreme shock. The shock is greater when the person is not well.

NATURAL REMEDIES

Take him to the emergency room immediately. Once the cause is ascertained, they will provide suitable treatment.

• For emergency measures which can be done until medical help arrives, turn to the section on Emergencies: *Shock (553), Heart Attack Signals, How to Do Rescue Breathing (991-995).*

• When a person goes into shock, the administration of medicinal aids orally will often be difficult or impossible. In this case, an anus injection (or enema) which will cause relaxation is applicable. Use one cup (to a pint maximum) of **catnip, peppermint, skullcap, spearmint, or valerian. Massage the abdomen and parts of the spine with lobelia,** externally, and make sure that the patient gets **undisturbed rest. Cayenne** should be taken internally, to equalize the blood pressure and insure that the internal functions will remain stabilized during the intense systemic distress.

Useful herbs include catnip, cayenne, hops, lady's slipper, lobelia, mistletoe, peppermint, skullcap, spearmint, and valerian.

ENCOURAGEMENT—All who have a sense of their deep soul poverty, who feel that they have nothing good in themselves, may find righteousness and strength by looking unto Jesus.

TRANSIENT ISCHEMIC ATTACKS

SYMPTOMS—Loss of vision in one eye or blurry vision in both. Feeling of unsteadiness and general loss of balance. Slurred speech. Difficult finding the right words. Problems understanding what other people are saying. Numbness on one side of the body. Weakness or paralysis on one side of the body, affecting one or both limbs. Loss of consciousness.

CAUSES—Transient ischemic attacks (TIA) consists of episodes of temporary loss of function in one area of the brain, resulting from a reduced blood supply to the brain.

Part of the brain suddenly and briefly fails to function properly because it is temporarily deprived of oxygen by blockage of its blood supply. This can last 1 second to 1 hour and has no aftereffects. If the symptoms last longer than an hour, it is called a stroke *(529)*.

In the U.S., about 1 in 600 people after the age of 45 has a TIA. Attacks are three times more likely in men. If the underlying problem is not solved, about 1 in 3 later has a stroke. So a TIA should not be ignored!

A thrombus usually forms in blood vessels that are affected by **atherosclerosis** *(523)*, a condition in which fatty deposits build up in blood-vessel walls. Those at increased risk are **smokers** and those on a **high-fat diet**. Other risk factors are **diabetes mellitus** *(656)*, **high blood pressure** *(526)*, and **sickle-cell anemia** *(541)*.

NATURAL REMEDIES

• When a TIA is identified, it is urgent that the person immediately stop eating all **meat products, saturated fats, and foods** containing meat or saturated fats. Stop eating all **white-flour and white sugar** products. Stop using all forms of **tobacco, alcohol, and caffeine**.

• Turn to the sections which apply to your case, and make needed changes: **Atherosclerosis** *(523)*, **Tobacco Withdrawal** *(880)*, **Diabetes Mellitus** *(656)*, **High Blood Pressure** *(526)*, and **Sickle-Cell Anemia** *(541)*.

ENCOURAGEMENT—If you will come to Jesus just as you are, weak, helpless, and despairing, our compassionate Saviour will meet you a great way off and will throw about you His arms of love and His robe of righteousness.

WERNICKE-KORSAKOFF SYNDROME

SYMPTOMS—Symptoms may start slowly or suddenly, sometimes after heavy drinking, and are frequently mistaken for a drunken stupor. Symptoms include unsteadiness when walking, confusion and restlessness, and abnormal movements of the eyes which often result in double vision.

CAUSES—This condition (WKS) is a brain disorder caused by severe **vitamin B$_1$ deficiency**; it is usually the result of chronic drinking of **alcohol**.

NATURAL REMEDIES

• The medical treatment is to immediately give him intravenous **injections of vitamin B$_1$**. Once treated, many of the symptoms may be reversed within days; but memory loss may persist. If untreated, the condition is fatal.

• Stop drinking **alcohol**. Begin eating an extremely **nourishing diet**, including the entire **B complex**, plus 3,000 mg of B_1 for 5 weeks, followed by 500 mg. daily.

• Stop all habits which tend toward alcoholism, including **spices, soft drinks, caffeine, and hard drugs**.

—*Also see Alcohol Withdrawal (881) and Delirium Tremens (881)*.

ENCOURAGEMENT—When God gave His Son to our world, He endowed human beings with imperishable riches—riches compared with which the treasured wealth of men since the world began is nothingness.

NUTRITIONAL NEUROPATHIES

SYMPTOMS—The tips of the fingers and toes are affected first. Symptoms appear gradually over several months or years, slowly progressing up the limbs to the trunk. Symptoms may include sensation usually referred to as "pins and needles" or loss of sensation. Pain in the feet and/or hands. Walking may be clumsy as a result of loss of sensation in the feet and legs.

CAUSES—The peripheral nerves, which branch from the brain and spinal cord, are damaged by deficiencies of essential nutrients, especially those of the vitamin B complex.

In developing countries, the cause is generally lack of proper nutrients; in developed countries, alcoholism is usually the cause. Not only do alcoholics not eat as well, but alcohol can directly damage the peripheral nerves. The risk increases greatly in those who have been drinking for 10 years or more.

Other causes include anorexia nervosa *(472)* and intestinal malabsorption problems *(454)*.

NATURAL REMEDIES

• Stop eating **processed and junk food**; only eat nutritious foods consisting of **fresh fruits and vegetables, whole grains, nuts, and legumes**.

• Take full-spectrum **vitamin-mineral supplementation**, including **B vitamins** and B_1 (1,000 mg).

• Stop drinking all **alcohol** products. Stop using **tobacco, caffeine, and hard drugs**.

—*Also see Alcohol Withdrawal (881)*.

ENCOURAGEMENT—If we lose everything else, we should keep conscience pure and sensitive. When asked to go where there is the least danger of offending God, doing that which you cannot do with a pure conscience, do not fear or hesitate. Look the tempter firmly in the face and say, "No, I will not imperil my soul for any worldly attraction. I love and fear God. I will not venture to dishonor or disobey Him for the riches of the world or the love and favor of a host of worldly relatives. I love Jesus who died for me. He has bought me. I will be true to Him."

NEURO-MENTAL - 2 - STRESS, ANXIETY, PAIN
Also: Claudication (637), Intestinal Cramps (453), Muscular Cramps (635)

STRESS AND ANXIETY
(Nervousness)

SYMPTOMS—Depression, anxiety, irritability, chronic fatigue, low-stress tolerance, nervous exhaustion, unable to cope, insomnia, panic attacks, unable to relax, or diseases caused by immune problems.

Tightening of stomach muscles which causes nausea or digestive problems. Increases in blood pressure, sweaty palms, nervous twitches, tooth grinding, trembling when not cold. Tense muscles, especially shoulder muscles.

Poor concentration, cannot retain information, negative thoughts, loss of sense of humor, demanding attitude, critical attitude, or becoming withdrawn.

CAUSES—Here are a few of the many causes: **deadlines, pressures, problems at home or work, special occasions, crowds, noise, pain, traffic, temperature extremes, overwork, lack of sleep, smoking, alcohol, a worrywart attitude**.

Researchers estimate that stress is significant in 80% of all major illnesses, including cancer, back problems, endocrine, cardiovascular, skin, and infectious diseases.

The adrenals especially suffer from stress. This results in a lowering of the immune system's ability to protect you from infection and cancer. It also disrupts the function of your entire endocrine system.

Everyone experiences stress from time to time. But frequent stress is more serious; and long-term stress wears out the body.

Some people can handle stress better than others. Some individuals work in hospital emergency rooms and thoroughly enjoy the excitement and challenge of every new crisis which comes along. Others burn out and have to transfer within a year.

NATURAL REMEDIES
BASICS
• **Find out what your ongoing problems are and solve them**. Problems are like a wall; you can go through them, go over them, or go around them. You go through a problem when you eliminate it. You surmount an immediate problem when you figure out a way to sidestep it and still do what is needed. You go around it when you learn to live with an ongoing situation you cannot solve. You stop worrying about it or letting it bother you, and turn your attention to other things.

N
E
R
V

Here are several basic suggestions:

• **Think positive** in every situation. See a good side to this; and learn to make the best of it. See it as an interesting challenge to solve difficulties. Trust in God to help you weather every crisis and carry on through to the end.

Think about something else for a time. That will help your brain to rest and your emotions to calm down. Gradually answers will come to mind.

• **Counsel with a good friend**. If it is a problem with your husband, counsel with a woman, not with a man. The same holds true for a man.

• The primary problems in a person's life are employment, spouse, money, children, deadlines, and guilt.

• Sometimes you need to **temporarily leave** a threatening situation, get away, and calm down. Take time to pray and rest your mind.

• **Avoid situations** which bring tension.

• **Learn to laugh** at some problems. **Learn to cry** over others. Both can relieve tension.

• **Stretching your muscles** can help move a circulation made sluggish by the situation, so you can think better. Massage muscles which have tensed up. Drop your jaw and move it left to right. This helps relax the jaw muscle.

• Take a relaxing **hot bath**, so you can start thinking constructively again.

• **Go outside and walk** in the open air. Hold your head up, breathe deeply, and relax.

• **Deep breathing**, wherever you are, refreshes the mind and helps you through a crisis.

• Get **extra rest**. It can help strengthen your mind and nerves to handle the problems you must deal with.

• Many times the underlying need is to **go to God and ask forgiveness**, obey His Ten Commandment law, and start living a clean life. **Make things right** with those you have wronged.

• Believe that, with God's help, the situation can be dealt with. **Keep trusting Him** as a little child trusts his parent to lead him by the hand across a busy street.

• A **change in diet** is needed to help restore a sickly immune system. **Fresh fruit and vegetables**, especially raw vegetables. Eating a diet of 60%-70% raw fruits and vegetables will really help you. Kelp or dulse and raw seeds or nuts. Be sure to take enough **vitamin C** (500 mg), as well as a full range of supplementary vitamins and minerals. **Calcium** (1,000 mg) and **magnesium** (500 mg) will help relax your muscles. The **B complex** vitamins nourish the nerves.

• Do not eat high carbohydrates (**white-flour and sugar products**) and **saturated fats**. Indulging in them can hasten burnout. Instead, eat the slower burning **proteins** and quality oils (**flaxseed oil**). Avoid **coffee, chocolate, strong spices, artificial sweeteners, MSG** (monosodium glutamate), **tobacco, and liquor.**

HERBS

• The following **herbs** are helpful: **ginkgo, echinacea, dong quai, gotu kola, bilberry, milk thistle, catnip, chamomile, hops, skullcap, and valerian**. Take them separately or mix 2-3 together; and take as a tea.

• Once in a while, but not too often, take a little **valerian** tea. This powerful remedy will relieve nervous attacks. Add bruised **cloves**, or very small amounts of **cumin oil**, to any tea to relieve nervous irritability.

• To reduce tension and calm anxiety, mix equal amounts of **valerian root, wood betony, black cohosh root, hops, skullcap, passionflower, and ginger root**. Take 2-3 capsules every four hours, as needed.

• Drink **chamomile** during the day and at bedtime to reduce fatigue and nervousness. This gentle tea can be used even for infants.

• Linden flower tea quiets the nerves and promotes sleep. Siberian ginseng helps the body cope better with stress, by strengthening adrenal function.

ENCOURAGEMENT—If you would find happiness and peace in all you do, you must do everything in reference to the glory of God. Seek earnestly to imitate the life of Christ, so others will be helped toward the pathway to heaven. Proverbs 16:7.

HEADACHE
(Nervous Headaches, Cluster Headaches)

SYMPTOMS—A pain or ache in any portion of the head. (Symptoms of 12 different kinds of headaches are listed on pp. 558.)

Cluster headaches: Often occur as a one-sided headache which comes on suddenly, causes debilitating pain, and comes and goes in severity.

CAUSES—Over 45 million Americans repeatedly have headaches. About 18 million have migraines.

Common causes of headaches include **eyestrain, tension, poor ventilation (lack of fresh air), sinus pressure, constipation, allergies (food, pollens, chemicals, etc.), stress, anxiety, muscle tension, infection, anemia, hunger, fever, hormonal imbalances, trauma to the head, nutritional deficiencies, sinusitis, alcohol, drugs, tobacco, spinal misalignment, temporomandibular joint syndrome, airborne pollutants, and chemicals (perfume, industrial fumes, etc.).** Other causal factors include **diseases of the eyes, nose, or throat. Nutritional deficiencies (niacin, pantothenic acid, B vitamins)** or an **overdose of vitamin A. Disturbances of the digestive or circulatory system. Birth control pills** cause headaches by causing a vitamin B_6 deficiency.

The headache may be caused by a reaction to a certain food, such as **chocolate, wheat, sugar, monosodium glutamate (MSG), dairy products, hot dogs, luncheon meats, citric acid, vinegar, or marinated foods. Sulfites**, found in certain foods, can do it. **Fermented foods, such as sour cream, yogurt, and cheeses** can do it also.

Headaches can be caused by **nitrites in hot dogs, sausages, and other processed meats.** They can be caused by too much **salt** in a meal, **ice cream** (chilling the roof of the mouth), **hunger**, and **cleaning fluids**.

Headache is often the result of a disturbance in some other part of the body, such as digestive disorders in the stomach, liver or bowel; problems in the abdominal area; menstrual irregularities, impingements in the cervical; concussion, eye strain, nervous excitement, fatigue, etc. The headache is a mechanism which signals some serious problem elsewhere. The common headache is due to **faulty elimination**, and the waste matter causes problems until the toxic wastes reach the stomach nerves and affects them. Sometimes headaches are caused from **panic, fear, or worrying** about the unknown. Headaches of this type are the hardest to relieve, generally requiring something strong like a heavy nervine tea with **lobelia** in it to diminish the nervous excitement. A nerve tea such as **valerian or skullcap** with a few drops of tincture of **lobelia** to a cup will give relief.

TYPES OF HEADACHES—There are two important subtypes of headaches. Emotional stress is an important cause in all of them:

Nervous headaches. These are muscle contraction headaches. The experts tell us that 90% of all headaches are caused by **tension, worry about problems, conflicts with others**, etc. Nervousness causes the muscles to tighten up.

Cluster headaches. These are severe, recurring headaches. Called histamine headaches, they are related to **allergic reactions. Inhalant allergens** may be a cause (including **perfume, house dust, cigarette smoke**, etc.). They may occur by themselves or be associated with other problems and diseases, including chronic fatigue syndrome *(280, 281)*. Keep a diet diary. Ninety percent of those with cluster headaches are men.

NATURAL REMEDIES

• Consider the causal factors, above, and see what you can change.

• Sometimes repeated headaches are a symptom of a serious disorder. If any of the following symptoms occur with the headache, the situation may be more serious and you may want to consult a professional: fever and stiffness in the neck, sensitivity to light, loss of speech or confusion, throbbing of the head and temples, pounding heartbeat, pressure in the facial sinus area, visual color changes, or a feeling that your head may explode.

• The treatment for headache depends on the underlying cause. Headaches caused by a certain problem frequently return. So identify what is causing them and many future headaches can be staved off.

• What are sometimes thought to be sinus headaches are actually tension headaches, migraines, or cluster headaches. When the headache is recurring, it is probably not sinus trouble.

HYDROTHERAPY

• When a headache comes, apply **cold compresses** to the place where the pain seems to be originating. This reduces muscle spasms and constricts blood vessels. Leave a damp washcloth in the refrigerator for 10 minutes or dip the cloth in water with ice cubes, wring it out, and apply. Also take an **enema**.

• Place a **heating pad, hot towel, or hot-water bottle** on the shoulder muscles, and possibly on the neck. Do that which helps you best.

• Take a neutral temperature **full bath** to get rid of a headache. Try taking a hot **footbath**. For more on water therapy, turn to *pp. 206-275.*

DIET

• **Do not overeat**. Include enough **fiber** in your meals and take an **enema** weekly.

• Make sure you are taking enough **B vitamins**, especially **niacin** (2,000 mg) and **pantothenic acid** (50 mg). **Vitamin A** (get beta-carotene in green and yellow vegetables) and **iron** are also important (but be sure to get your iron from food, such as **blackstrap molasses**, not from chemical supplements).

• People with regular **magnesium** deficiency tend to have tension headaches. Take 600 mg daily.

• **Eat on time** and do not eat **problem foods**.

• Do not use much **salt**.

• If you think that **something you just ate** might bring on a terrible headache, take 5 charcoal tablets within an hour; and, as soon as you can, take an **enema**. (But do not take charcoal tablets daily.)

OTHER HELPS

• Regular **exercise** can help prevent tension headaches. Exercise when it occurs, but do not exercise if it is severe.

• Get enough **sleep**; but do not oversleep.

• **Stand tall; sit tall**.

• **Breathe** deeply.

• **Bright light** can cause squinting, eyestrain, and headaches.

• Do not **chew gum**. The repetitive chewing can bring on a tension headache.

• Do not **overdo**. Learn to live within your limits.

• When you have to face **high altitudes**, take additional vitamin C (plus ginger), to avoid a high-altitude headache.

• Keeping a **diary** will help you determine the cause of the headaches. Note date, time of day, where the pain is felt, and any comments about what you think might be possible causes.

HERBS FOR HEADACHES

• Helpful **herbs** include valerian, feverfew, balm, fleabane, cowslip, lavender, and white willow.

• **Evening primrose** contains *phenylalanine*, a pain-relieving compound. **Ginkgo** increases blood flow, which reduces a headache. Rub diluted **peppermint oil** or **lavender oil** on the temples to alleviate a headache.

• Any of the **willows** will help reduce headache pain. They, along with **cayenne**, contain *salicylates*, which help stop headaches.

• **Turmeric** and **ginger** (combined or separate) are good for headaches.

• Drink a capsule of **hops** with water. **Skullcap** is antispasmodic and helps relax your nerves. **Periwinkle** increases the flow of oxygen in the brain.

• For severe headaches, fast with **juice and green drinks**, and take herb laxatives (**cascara sagrada or senna**).

• If the problem is in the stomach area, use any of the following stomach herbs: **angelica, black alder, elecampane, gentian root, raspberry leaves, rhubarb, strawberry leaves, wild cherry, wormwood**. Use **ginger** for a menstrual problem. To relieve the local headache pain, two or three drops of tincture of **lobelia** in a little water three times a day or up to every hour, if required, will often give temporary relief. If the contents of the stomach causes the problem, empty that area with an emetic. Where the nerves are raw, the following herbs are excellent: **catnip, peppermint (hot), rosemary herb, skullcap, spearmint, wood betony**. And, since plenty of rest is needed, any of the foregoing herbs, along with hops tea, is very soothing and will produce sleep.

TWENTY-FIVE TYPES OF HEADACHES

There are many types of headaches. Here are suggestions for 25 of them. Remedies for an additional 28 are listed by J.H. Kellogg, M.D. on the next page.

• *Nervous tension headaches:* Continual pain in one area or many, with sore muscles in neck and upper back, plus lightheadedness and dizziness. Treatment of this most common of headaches includes application of **ice packs** on neck and upper back. Take extra **vitamin C and bioflavonoids. Avoid sugar, caffeine, food allergens, stress.** Get enough **exercise**.

• *Cluster headaches:* Strong, throbbing pain on one side of head, tearing of eyes, flushing of face, congestion of nose. May occur 1-3 times a day for weeks or months. Take enough **protein**, avoid **inhalant allergens**, and keep a diet **diary**.

• *Hangover headache:* This headache has throbbing pain; it is caused by drinking liquor. Put **ice** on the neck and drink lots of **water and fruit juices**. Stop drinking **alcohol**.

• *Exertion headache:* This headache is caused by physical exertion or sexual excess. Apply **ice packs** to the point of pain, improve the **diet**, and stop the **excesses**.

• *Caffeine headache:* It is a throbbing pain that happens when you try to quit your **coffee** addiction too fast. Drink a small amount of coffee, to stop the headache; and then gradually reduce the amount and frequency, to get away from this addiction.

• *Sinus headache:* A nagging pain to the right and left of the nose and over it. Apply **moist heat**, to reduce sinus trouble *(381)*, and take more **vitamin C**.

• *Bilious headache:* The temples throb, and there is a dull headache in the forehead. It is caused by **overeating, wrong eating, and inactivity**. Take an **enema**; then change your **diet** and get more **exercise**.

• *Menstrual headache:* A headache which feels like a migraine *(560)*; it occurs at menstruation or during ovulation. Take **potassium, magnesium, and vitamin B$_6$**.

• *Hunger headache:* A general headache which occurs just before mealtime, and is caused by skipping meals or excessive dieting. Eat **better meals**, which include **complex carbohydrates and protein**, to help carry you to the next meal.

• *Eyestrain headache:* Pain in the frontal lobes, just behind the eyes. Many think this is caused by uncorrected vision problems; but it can also be caused by too much brain work at late hours. **Change** your way of life; perhaps you need a change in eyeglasses.

• *Arthritis headache:* Pain at the back of the head or neck, which increases with movement. **Feverfew** herb teas are recommended, but not during pregnancy.

• *Hypertension headache:* A dull pain over much of the head, increased by movement. You need to reduce your **blood pressure**.

• *Eyestrain headache:* Frontal pain on both sides, which is unusual, may be caused by **overuse of the eyes; eye muscle imbalance; uncorrected vision; astigmatism. Check your vision and correct if need**.

• *Fever headache:* Headache develops with fever, due to inflammation of the blood vessels of the head. **Reduce fever; apply ice packs**.

• *Migraine, classic:* Similar to the common migraine; but it is preceded by auras—such as visual disturbances, numbness in arms or legs, smelling of strange odors, or hallucinations. It is caused by excessive dilation or contraction of blood vessels in the brain.

• *Migraine, common:* Severe throbbing pain, often on one side of the head; nausea; vomiting; cold hands; dizziness; and sensitivity to light and sounds. This is caused by excessive dilation or contraction of blood vessels of the brain. —*See Migraine Headaches.*

• *Sinus headache:* Gnawing, nagging pain over nasal/sinus area, often increasing in severity as the day goes by. Fever and discolored mucus may be present.

Allergies, infection, nasal polyps, food allergies. Often caused by blocked sinus ducts or acute sinus infection. Increase intake of **vitamins A and C**; use **moist heat** to help get sinuses to drain.

• *Temporal headache:* Jabbing, burning, boring pain; pain in the temple or around the ear when chewing; weight loss; flu-like symptoms; problems with eyesight. Usually seen in people over fifty-five. Untreated, can lead to blindness, stroke, heart attack, or a tear in the aorta. Caused by inflammation of temporal arteries. Apply **cold cloth**; get more **rest**.

• *Bilious headache:* Dull pain in the forehead and throbbing temples. **May be caused by indigestion; overeating; lack of exercise. Colon cleansing** can help.

• *Temporomandibular joint (TMJ) headache:* Temporal, above-ear, or facial pain; muscle temple pain upon awakening. Caused by **stress**, contraction of one side of face; clicking or malocclusion (**poor popping of jaw; neck or upper back pain; bite**), jaw clenching. gum chewing. **Reduce stress; use relaxation techniques, biofeedback, nutritional supplements, ice packs**.

• *Tension headache:* Constant pain, in one area or all over the head; sore muscles with trigger points in neck and upper back; light-headedness; and dizziness. *The most common type of headache.* Caused by **emotional stress, anxiety, worry, depression, anger, food allergies, poor posture, or too-shallow breathing**. Apply **ice packs on neck and upper back**; take supplements of **vitamin C** with **bioflavonoids, bromelain, magnesium, primrose oil, and ginger** for relief of muscle spasms.

• *Tic douloureux:* Short, jabbing pains around the mouth, jaw, or forehead. More common in women over fifty-five years old. Take **nutritional supplements**.

• *Tumor headaches:* Progressively worsening pain; projectile problems with vision, speech, and equilibrium; personality changes. Treat as for cancer.

• *Vascular headaches:* Throbbing on one side of the head, sensitivity to light and often nausea. Related to cluster headaches and migraines. Caused by disturbances in the blood vessels. **Lie down** and keep your **blood pressure** under control.

• *Aneurysm-associated headache:* Early symptoms mimic those of cluster headaches and migraines. If an aneurysm ruptures, it can cause sudden extreme pain, double vision, rigid neck, and stroke leading to unconsciousness. A balloon-like bulge or weak spot on a blood vessel wall; or **high blood pressure**. Keep blood pressure low.

—*Also see Migraine (560) for more information.*

J.H. KELLOGG, M.D., PRESCRIPTIONS FOR 28 DIFFERENT HEADACHES (how to give these water therapies: pp. 206-275 / Hydrotherapy Disease Index: pp. 273-275)

NOTE—The following grouping of headaches is made for practical convenience. Because each type has a different cause, it has a different treatment.

HYPEREMIC HEADACHE (caused by excess of blood in the head)—**Rest**, head and shoulders elevated; heat to feet and legs by means of a **Footbath**, Leg Bath, Leg Pack, Revulsive Douche. **Cold** to head and neck, accompanied by **Neutral Enema** at 102° F. **Hot Abdominal Pack**, with well-protected plastic covering. **Wet Sheet Pack**. Neutral spray Douche, given for 24 minutes.

ANEMIC HEADACHE (caused by a lack of blood in the brain)—**Hot-Water Bottle** to back of neck, **Fomentation** over painful part, rest in bed with head low. General treatment for Anemia.

HIGH PRESSURE HEADACHE (head will feel as though it has a great pressure within it)—Abstemious **aseptic diet**. Prolonged **Warm or Neutral Bath** daily, with **Cool Compress** to head. Hot Footbath or, better, **Hot Leg Bath**. Revulsive Douche to legs, **Heating Compress** over heart.

DYSPEPTIC HEADACHE (a headache more directly traceable to indigestion)—(1) The immediate pain: **Hot and Cold Compress** to head; avoid sleeping soon after eating, though a very brief nap is sometimes beneficial. (2) If it keeps repeating, use an **enema** if constipated. **Dry aseptic diet, two meals a day** or only fruit at night.

HEADACHE DUE TO PROLAPSE (of the intestinal or abdominal organs)—(1) The immediate pain: **Alternate Sponging to spine** or Alternate Compress over spine, **Hot and Cold Compress** to head. (2) If it keeps repeating: **Abdomi**nal supporter, **Hot Abdominal Pack** at night, abdominal massage, **Cold Douche** to abdomen.

TOXIC HEADACHE (caused by an excess of uric acid, oxalic acid, urea and other wastes, or as a result of decomposed products absorbed through the alimentary canal)—**Sweating baths**, followed by a Cold Douche, **Wet Sheet Rub**, or Shallow Bath. Copious **water** drinking. **Enema** or Colonic daily or three times weekly. **Outdoor life. Aseptic diet.**

PERIODIC HEADACHE, NERVOUS HEADACHE, BILIOUS HEADACHE, MIGRAINE, OR LACK-OF-AIR HEADACHE—Dry, abstemious, **aseptic diet. Outdoor life**, air bath, large **Enema** the day before the attack is due, **Tonic Frictions** to build up the body, **Hot Abdominal Pack**. Abdominal supporter, if a prolapsed condition exists.

RHEUMATOID HEADACHE (a headache related to the presence of rheumatism)—**Sweating bath** daily, Hot Footbath or Hot Leg Pack, **Fomentation** to the painful part for 10-15 minutes, followed by **Heating Compress** (see also "Uric Acid Diathesis)."

NEURASTHENIC HEADACHE (caused by nervous exhaustion)—**Hot and Cold Compress**, Revulsive Compress, Alternate Compress to spine or Sponging to spine, **Hot Footbath**, Footbath under running water.

FRONTAL HEADACHE (often related to fatigue of the eyes or brain)—**Revulsive Compress** to forehead and eyes, **Hot and Cold Trunk Pack**, derivative applications to feet and legs (such as Hot Footbath or, better, **Hot Leg Bath**).

CONGESTIVE HEADACHE—Ice Bag to back of head, with a **Cold Compress** to the face. Ice Collar, **Hot and Cold Compress to the head, Hot Footbath**, Hot Leg Pack, **Heating Compress** to the legs, **Cold Footbath** in flowing water, Alternate Footbath.

OCCIPITAL HEADACHE (a headache centered on or near the bump at back of the head)—**Hot Compress** or Hot Sponging to the upper spine and, at the same time, to the area around the occipital region. **Revulsive Compress, Hot and Cold Compress** to the head.

NERVOUS HEADACHE (a form of headache accompanied by a feeling of nervous tension)—**Fomentation** to the seat of the pain, with simultaneous **Hot Footbath** and daily **Cold Enema,** to relieve constipation, if present. Special attention to the diet. A **dry aseptic diet** is advocated. Avoid milk.

BAND-AROUND-THE-HEAD HEADACHE (a form of an anemic headache)—Hot Sponging or **Hot Compress** to head, **Alternate Sponging** on neck and upper spine, **massage** to head.

VERTEX HEADACHE (a headache characterized by a pain at the top of the head)—**Hot Footbath**, **Cold Compress** to head, Ice Collar, sleep with the head elevated. Heat to the feet and legs, if they are cold.

EYE HEADACHE (pain in or near eyes, made worse by light)—Gentle (not hot!) **Fomentation** over eyes and forehead. **Protect eyes** from bright light, facial massage, and massage to eyes. Consult an optometrist; for eyeglasses may be needed, temporarily or permanently.

CLAVUS HEADACHE (This headache feels like the sharp pain of a nail being driven into the head.)—Very **Hot Footbath**, with **Fomentation** over painful point for 10 minutes, repeated every 2 hours. **Heating Compress** at night. Protect him from the cold during the day. Begin a series of carefully **graduated Cool Baths**, to build him up.

RENAL HEADACHE (This headache is caused by a kidney problem.)—Copious **water** drinking, **Enema**, **Hot Bath**. **Ice Bag** over lower sternum, with **Hot and Cold Compress** to head (see Nephritis, 492).

HEPATIC HEADACHE (a headache due to a weakened liver)—(1) For the immediate pain: **Revulsive Compress** to the head, **Hot and Cold Compress** to the head, with derivative applications to the legs (Hot Leg Bath, etc.). **Graduated Tonic Frictions**. (2) If it keeps repeating, need aseptic diet, **fruit diet, water** drinking, graduated **Enema**. **Fomentation** over liver twice a day for 15 minutes, with **Heating Compress** over it during the intervals between. **Outdoor exercise**, air bath, **breathing** exercises, massage to abdomen.

ORGANIC HEADACHES (caused by tumors, inflammation, abscesses, trauma, general paralysis, syphilis)—Very hot and frequently repeated derivative applications to legs (Hot Footbath or, better, **Hot Foot and Leg Bath**) with short, often repeated **Revulsive Compress** to the head. Follow by **Cold or Heating Compress** to the head.

INFECTION HEADACHE (headache caused by infection or disease of the eye, ear, nose, or teeth)—(1) For the immediate pain: **Hot Footbath** or Hot Leg Bath, with **Revulsive Compress** over the painful parts. (2) Longer term care: The problem causing these headaches should receive proper attention.

VARYING HEADACHE (with a sense of coldness, numbness, pressure, band sensation, etc.)—(1) For the immediate pain: **Massage** the head and neck. **Revulsive Compress** to the spine, head, and face. **Hot and Cold Compress** to the head. (2) Longer term care: Improve tone of the nerves by **Tonic Frictions** (see also "Neurasthenia," 551).

SUPRA-ORBITAL HEADACHE (This is a headache felt as a strong pain above the eyebrow.)—(1) For the immediate pain: **Hot Footbath** with **Revulsive Compress** above the eyebrow,

but not covering the eye. Avoid exposure to cold. Rest the eyes, protecting them from the light. **Hot Footbath** or Hot Leg Bath. (2) Longer term care: Begin a series of carefully **graduated Tonic Frictions**.

TEMPORAL HEADACHE (This is a pain over the side of the head, to the right and left of the forehead.)—(1) For the immediate pain: **Fomentation** over side of head, face, and ear for ten minutes. Follow by warm **dry Compress**, repeated every 2 hours. **Massage** to the area of the pain. (2) Longer term care: Between attacks give **Tonic Frictions**, to build the body so that the headaches will stop repeating. A nourishing, strengthening diet that **avoids all meat** is needed. Also see Lithemia (489). (Lithemia is an excess of uric acid in the blood.)

MASTOID, OR POST-AURICULAR, HEADACHE (This is a headache felt as a pain just below the ear.)—**Fomentation** for 10 minutes to side of head followed by cotton poultice or well-covered **Heating Compress**, repeated every 2 hours. Pain in the mastoid process must be given immediate attention or major ear infection can result! If pain does not subside fairly quickly, see your doctor.

CERVICO-OCCIPITAL HEADACHE (This is a headache showing itself in a pain extending from the back of the neck, on up to the occipital bump on the back of the head.)—**Revulsive Compress** to the back of the head and neck. **Fomentation** over the painful area for 10 minutes. Follow by a **warm, dry Compress** over it.

—Also see Neurasthenia (551) for more additional help in building up the nervously exhausted body.

UTERINE HEADACHE (This is a pain or pressure at the very top of the head, caused by uterine problems.)—(1) For the immediate pain: **Hot and Cold Compress** to the head, massage of the head. (2) Longer term care: **Revulsive Sitz Bath**, abdominal supporter, **Hot Abdominal Pack**. Correct any ovarian or uterine disease that is present.

FEVER HEADACHE (a headache caused by a raised body temperature or fevered condition)—(1) For the head pain: Ice Cap or **Cold Compress** to the head. Ice Collar. (2) To lower the fever: **Ice Bag** to the heart. **Cooling Wet Sheet Pack**, **Prolonged Neutral Bath**. See also under the specific disease causing the fever.

—See Migraine (below) for more information.

ENCOURAGEMENT—True happiness comes from an entire surrender of the will to God. It is living by every word that proceeds from the mouth of God. It is doing the will of our heavenly Father. It is trusting God in trial and in darkness as well as in light. It is relying on God with unquestioning confidence. It is resting in His love. 1 Peter 1:5-7.

MIGRAINE

SYMPTOMS—Generalized or one-sided head pain and possibly nausea, vomiting, and visual disturbances (light sensitivity, bright spots and patterns before the eyes). It might last for days. The first sign is frequent flashes of light or tingling. There may be nausea, vomiting, diarrhea, and cyanosis (blueness) of the fingers from lack of circulation and oxygen. The pain is most common in the temple, but may occur anywhere on the head, face, or neck. The pain is frequently on one side; but it may change to the opposite side, alternate sides, or be on both sides.

IS IT A MIGRAINE?—*Migraines* will tend to be on one or both sides of the head, last 4-72 hours, and usually be severe (but may be mild)

In contrast, *tension headaches* will be on both sides of the head, only last 2 hours to a day or so, and only have mild or moderate pain. *Cluster headaches* will only be on one side of the head, and last 30-90 minutes at a time (yet they can recur many times during the day).

Migraines will be accompanied by nausea and sensitivity to sound, light, or smells; this will produce red and/or and watery eyes or runny nose. These symptoms will not appear in tension or cluster headaches.

CAUSES—These are caused by a disturbance in the blood circulation. The name comes from the Greek word, *hemikrania*, or "half the head"; this describes the location of most migraines (around the forehead, temple, ear, jaw, or eye). There is **alternating constriction and dilation of the blood vessels in the brain**; it occurs between the ages of 10-30, more often in women (70%) than men. **Food allergies** are frequently the cause. Search them out. Here are six of the most common causes: **food allergy, low blood sugar, tension, depression, water retention, menstruation, changes in barometric pressure, liver malfunction, too much or too little sleep, emotional changes, hormonal changes, sun glare, flashing lights, lack of exercise, dental problems, low blood sugar**. There often are no migraines during the second and third trimester of pregnancy or after menopause is past.

Migraines can disappear for years and then reappear. They usually decrease after middle age.

Over 50% of those with migraines report that one or both parents also had the problem.

NATURAL REMEDIES

EARLY WARNINGS

• Know the early signs of a coming attack, so you can take immediate measures to avoid or lessen it:

1 - A day earlier, there may be problems with memory, the five senses, or your mood.

2 - Just before it begins, you may see flashes or patterns of light, or feel numbness in hands or mouth. These indications are called an "aura."

AVOIDING AND REDUCING THEM

• Exposure to **sunlight** triggers migraines in some people. They cannot take the bright light in their eyes. Staying in the shade on bright days greatly helps them.

• Resting **in a darkened room with an ice cap** or **ice compress** to the head is helpful. There may first be an increase of pain; but, within three minutes, the symptoms may disappear, except for a mild

headache. To increase the effect, take a **hot footbath** at the same time. This will help abort a migraine at its first indication.

• As soon as one begins, if possible, take an **enema**. This will help stop the attack.

• When an attack begins, try wrapping something **tight about the head**.

• When it is a throbbing pain, place **light pressure on the arteries of the neck** for a few seconds at a time.

• Vigorous daily **outdoor exercise** helps decrease attacks. Do not do vigorous exercise during an attack.

• Maintain a **regular schedule. Too much sleep, too little sleep, missed meals**, etc., may trigger an attack. Do not sleep in late. Some people must avoid naps during the day.

• Exposure to **smoking** increases the attacks; so does taking **birth control pills**.

• **Chills** can induce migraines. **Tiredness, anxiety, or eating late** also can. Other causes include **antibiotics, odors and inhalants, caffeine, emotional stress and resentment, and allergy shots**.

• Do not sleep in cramped, awkward positions. Even sleeping on your stomach can tighten and contract neck muscles. Learn to **sleep on your back**.

DIET

• Eat foods which will help you **keep your blood sugar stabilized**. This would be **fresh fruits and vegetables, whole grains, nuts, and legumes**. Stay away from fast-acting carbohydrates: **sugary foods and drinks, all white-flour products and processed foods**.

• Take 1 comprehensive **B complex** tablet daily, **vitamin C** (2,000-6,000 mg in divided doses), **rutin** (200 mg of this bioflavonoid), **calcium** (2,000 mg), and **magnesium** (1,000 mg).

• Migraine sufferers have lower levels of **magnesium** than other people. Magnesium helps calcium (which relaxes and reduces pain) do its work. In research studies, intravenous magnesium injections have relieved some migraines within minutes. Taking as little as 350 mg of magnesium daily decreases attacks. Better yet, take 1,000 mg when the problem gets worse.

• Also important are high doses of **calcium** (1,000-2,000 mg daily). Calcium and **vitamin D** (400 IU daily) have been found to reduce migraine attacks.

• A research study found that high daily amounts of **vitamin B$_2$** (400 mg) helped most patients.

• It is thought that 25% of migraines trace their cause to **food allergies**. *See Allergies (848).* Various studies have identified the following as possible causes: **cola drinks, chocolate, pork, corn, onion, garlic, eggs, tea, citrus, wheat, coffee, cane sugar, yeast, beef, alcohol, cheese, fried foods, seafood, mushrooms, peas, high-salt diet, caffeine, refined carbohydrates, fatty fried foods, and tobacco smoke**.

• Eliminate **tyramine** foods. The amino acid, **tyrosine**, produces a breakdown product, called *tyramine*. Tyramine is a significant cause of migraine headaches.

N
E
R
V

It does this by releasing *norepinephrine* from brain tissue, which causes constriction of scalp and brain blood vessels. Any substance which has undergone bacterial decomposition has high levels of tyramine. Such foods include **plums, oranges, bananas, raspberries, avocados, ripened or aged cheese, beef and chicken livers, sour cream, eggplant, salami, meat tenderizers, chocolate, wine, caffeine products, and soy sauce**.

• **Tryptophan**, another amino acid found in protein-rich foods, is converted to serotonin, a substance which might make some migraines worse. For this reason, **low-protein diets** have been used, with some success, to reduce the frequency of migraine attacks.

• Eliminate any **suspected food** from your diet, for five days, and see if that helps solve the problem.

• Stop using all **alcoholic** beverages and MSG (monosodium glutamate) foods; these trigger attacks.

• **Cured meats** contain **nitrates** and other preservatives which dilate blood vessels and give a headache.

• If you wake up in the morning to a headache, it may be **low blood sugar**. Drink a glass of **lemon or fruit juice** on arising. Schedule smaller, more frequent meals. Avoid **sugar** and **processed starchy foods**. Studies show that blood sugar levels are low during a migraine attack; the lower the level, the worse the attack.

HERBS

• **Bay, feverfew**, and **tansy** contain *parthenolides* which help prevent migraines.

• **Feverfew** is widely used in England, to reduce migraines. Take 3-9 grams; but do not use when the migraine results from a weak, deficient condition.

• **Ginger** is used in Asia to prevent migraines.

• Steep **fenugreek** 5-15 minutes; take 1 cup during the day, hot or cold.

• **Garlic** and **onions** help prevent migraines.

• **Lemon Balm** is another herb used to treat migraines.

• **Chamomile** tea is extremely soothing to ease pressures that trigger headaches. It helps take the sense of tightness out of your head.

• Take **peppermint** in fluid extract form, ½-2 tsp., 3 times daily. In infusion form, steep 5-15 minutes; take 6 oz. 3 times daily.

• Dilute 1 part **rosemary oil** in 10 parts vegetable oil; rub on forehead and temples. Also use as a nasal vapor inhalation. You can also steep the **powdered** herb 5-15 minutes; take 2 oz. 3 times daily.

• A combination of **valerian-lavender** tea is soothing and eases stress accompanying migraine. Relaxes vascular contractions.

J.H. KELLOGG, M.D., PRESCRIPTIONS FOR MIGRAINE AND ITS COMPLICATIONS (how to give these water therapies: pp. 206-275 / Hydrotherapy Disease Index: pp. 273-275)

PREVENT FORMATION OF URIC ACID—Avoid use of meats, tea and coffee. Aseptic dietary and outdoor life is important.

ELIMINATE URIC ACID—Hot Baths, especially moderately **prolonged sweating baths**. Follow by **short Cold Baths**, Radiant Heat Bath, Wet Sheet Pack, Steam Bath, **prolonged Neutral Bath, water** drinking.

LOWER ARTERIAL TENSION—Hot Full Bath at 102° F., for 5-10 minutes. Hot Leg Bath or Hot Leg Pack. **Hot Enema**. Rest in bed in a darkened room.

PAIN—Hot Footbath, **Alternate Compress** to spine or sponging of spine, **Revulsive Compress** to seat of pain, local application of Ice Bag in some cases, **Hot Leg Pack. Protect the eyes** from light.

NAUSEA AND VOMITING—Ice pills, **ice to stomach and the spine** opposite the stomach.

CONSTIPATION—Colonic.

TO PREVENT ATTACK—Fruit diet, large **colonic, water** drinking.

TO RELIEVE HYPERESTHESIA OF LOWER BACK NERVES—Fomentation over abdomen, twice daily. Continuous **Heating Compress** during the interval between. Abdominal supporter.

GENERAL METHOD—Every case is curable by sufficiently prolonged treatment, carefully managed. The general nervous system must be built up by measures essentially the same as those indicated for neurasthenia and other conditions requiring tonic treatment. The causes must be removed, especially autointoxication and morbid reflex influences arising from dilation of the stomach, enteroptosis, and indigestion.

—*Also see Headache (556).*

ENCOURAGEMENT—We must take hold of divine power; and, with determination, we must resist the temptations of Satan. Through the enabling strength which Christ provides, we can be more than conquerors in the battle with evil. Jude 24.

NECK PAIN
(Stiff Neck)

SYMPTOMS—A pain in the neck.

CAUSES—Working in a hunched-over position for long hours is a frequent cause. Working so that you must lean your head forward, to better see what you are doing. But an injury may also have occurred. A common cause is stress, insomnia, or arthritis.

NATURAL REMEDIES
IMMEDIATE

• Place an **ice pack** on the back of the neck or apply ice, wrapped in a towel.

• Then place **heat** on the painful area. This can be a **heating pad** or a **hot shower**.

• Wrap a rolled-up **towel** around your neck and

fasten it snugly with a safety pin. It will support your head and reduce painful movements.

PREVENTIVES

• Do **neck exercises** each day, to stretch your neck muscles and strengthen them.

• To **stretch those muscles**, slowly tilt your head forward, back, and from side to side.

• To **strengthen muscles**, put your hand on the side of your head and push. Then do the other side, and then the back and front. Hold light weights (3-5 pounds) in your hands, keeping your arms straight while shrugging your shoulders.

• Or do this: Lift your **shoulders** easily and let them flop down a couple times. Do not push them down.

• **Sit in chairs** which give you good back support.

• **Sit up**, not forward. Keep your **head level** and pull in your chin. Arrange your work so you can **look forward**, and not downward, most of the time. Do not sit in any one position too long.

• Stop every so often and **take a break**. Get up, stretch, and do a few simple neck exercises.

• Your **car seat** should be high enough so you can comfortably look forward.

• Do not compensate for your **height**. If short, do not lift your shin up; if tall, do not slump.

• Do not sit with most of your weight on the back of your neck.

• Always **carefully lift** heavy things with the legs and not the back.

• Sleep on a **firm** (orthopedic) **mattress**.

• **Sleeping position** is important. Do not sleep on your stomach, but on your side or (best) on your back.

• Keep your **neck warm** when you are outside in the cold. Avoid letting a **draft** chill it while sleeping.

• You may do better with a smaller **pillow** or no pillow at all. Do not sleep on thick, hard pillows.

• Avoid talking on the **phone**. It develops neck tension, because you tend to tilt your head to the phone instead of keeping the head balanced and upright.

• When you **brush** your hair, keep your head straight; do not bend it to the comb.

If there is numbness in your hands, arms, or legs, consult a physician.

ENCOURAGEMENT—Thank God that there is hope for each one of us! In Christ we can have the victory over every temptation and come off more than conquerors. Trust in Him and He will carefully guide you step by step. 2 Peter 1:10.

PAIN CONTROL

Here are hydrotherapy prescriptions for reducing levels of pain in various parts of the body:

WATER THERAPIES WHICH RELIEVE PAIN AND NERVOUS IRRITABILITY - Hydrotherapy applications can greatly help also (*how to give these water therapies: pp. 206-275 / Hydrotherapy Disease Index: pp. 273-275*)

The general **neutral bath** is very effective in relieving nervous irritability, inducing sleep in insomnia, delirium, and even acute fevers. **Moist abdominal bandage**. Cool **head cap**. **Heating spinal compress**, in certain cases. For relieving localized pain and irritability, the hot **Fomentation** and the **heating compress** are both good. The **cold compress** and **ice compress** are both valuable in those instances in which the pain is in superficial (near the surface) parts and the applications can be made directly to the area of pain.

ENCOURAGEMENT—The love of God in our hearts is manifested in kindness, gentleness, forbearance, and long-suffering. The countenance is changed. Christ abiding in the heart shines out in the faces of those who love Him and keep His commandments.

NEURALGIA
(Neuropathy)

SYMPTOMS—Pain which comes on suddenly, followed by intervals of freedom from pain. The pains are severe and seem to shoot along the course of the affected nerves. The nerve trunks become tender to pressure. In severe cases, there is twitching of the muscles of the affected part, with burning and tingling sensations in the skin. The attacks are rarely on both sides of the body at the same time. They generally continue from a few minutes to a few days, and may occur frequently for months. As time passes, the attacks tend to become more severe.

CAUSES—Neuralgia is nerve pain; whereas neuritis *(568)* is nerve inflammation.

Neuralgia is an irritation of a nerve which can be caused by many factors, including **trauma, herpes, shingles, diabetes, multiple sclerosis, or alcoholism**.

Another cause is **nutritional deficiencies;** these include the **B complex (especially B_1, B_6, folic acid, pantothenic acid, and B_{12})**.

Other causes include **decayed teeth, wrong diet, constipation, tension, insomnia, fatigue, exposure, lack of exercise, sinus infections, and eye strain**.

A frequent cause of the problem is **chilling of part of the body** over a period of time while the rest of the body is relatively warm. This may occur in the winter months, when you are in bed sleeping. A current of cold air is passing across your face or shoulder and the rest of your body is tucked under covers. The result is tic douloureux or Bell's Palsy (565) on the face or neck. If the shoulders are uncovered, for instance, there is neuralgia of the shoulder.

The cause can also occur as a result of regular commute driving. A window is kept open slightly to provide fresh air; but a slight chilling breeze blows on the face for a lengthy period of time.

The formula for trouble is (1) a chilling draft to

part of the body while the rest is warm (2) over a lengthy period of time, (3) day after day.

NATURAL REMEDIES

• Give attention to the causal factors mentioned above and try to solve them. Give close attention to the conditions you place your body under each day. You will learn some interesting facts. Avoid unnecessary **drafts** on part of your body while other parts are warm.

• Give a high **catnip** herb enema. It should be as warm as can be taken.

• Put alternate **hot and cold** applications over the painful area. The cold should be very short! This can be done for several hours at a time.

• **Fomentations** wrung out of **mullein, lobelia, or chamomile** tea are also helpful.

• Place the hand and arm (which are on the opposite side of the body from where the head and neck pain are located) in very **hot water** for 20 minutes.

• Make sure the diet includes **lecithin** (1 tsp.) and enough **calcium** (1,000 mg) and **magnesium** (500 mg).

• Get **sunshine, fresh air, and exercise**.

• Helpful herbs include **mullein, sage, hops, plantain, valerian root, skullcap, nettle, lobelia, black cohosh, poplar bark, and mint**.

• The Chinese rub fresh, sliced **lemon** on neuralgic areas to relieve pain.

• Crush **juniper** berries and place them to the area in pain, and you will obtain relief.

• **Bilberry** contains flavonoid compounds (*anthocyanosides*) which relieve pain when applied. Use a bilberry extract dosage of 160-480 mg daily

• Place powdered **chamomile** in several small bags. Steep them in ½ cup boiling water; and apply them as hot as possible to the area in pain.

• *Capsaicin* in **cayenne**, when applied to the painful area, stimulates and then blocks small-diameter pain fibers. Many research studies have supported this.

• Scrape **horseradish** and apply the scrapings directly to the affected area.

• **Ginkgo biloba**, when given to patients, significantly decreased pain and sensitivity in the painful area.

• Dried **coltsfoot** can be soaked in boiling water. When cooler, dip a cloth in the hot water and place it on neuralgic pains.

—*Also see Bell's Palsy (565), Neuritis (568), and Brachial Neuralgia (567).*

J.H. KELLOGG, M.D., PRESCRIPTIONS FOR NEURALGIA AND ITS COMPLICATIONS (*how to give these water therapies: pp. 206-275 / Hydrotherapy Disease Index: pp. 273-275*)

COMBAT TOXEMIA WHEN PRESENT—Sweating bath followed by appropriate general **Cold Bath**, 3 times a week. The Radiant Heat Bath, Steam Bath, and **sweating Wet Sheet Pack** are especially helpful. Copious **water** drinking, **aseptic dietary**, **dry friction** of skin or oil rubbing daily after short **sweating bath**. Follow by **tonic cold** application.

COMBAT ANEMIA AND GENERAL WEAKNESS—Graduated cold applications. Avoid the increasing pain preceding or accompanying the Cold Bath by a hot application to the affected part; cover or avoid the part during the cold application.

PAIN—Fomentation or Revulsive Compress to the seat of pain. **Revulsive Douche** or Alternate Douche; **Ice Bag** is sometimes more effective than heat. This is often the case when the parts are congested as shown by redness of the skin, throbbing sensation, and when the nerves are extremely superficial.

REFLEX NEURALGIAS—Fomentation to abdomen, twice daily. **Hot Abdominal Pack** during intervals between, abdominal supporter. After baths, avoid chilling and general prolonged **cold applications** (such as Full Baths, Shallow Baths, and Wet Sheet Packs).

NEURALGIA OF THE HEAD—Employ derivative measure (such as **Hot Sitz Bath**, Hot Leg Bath, Hot Pack to legs, **Hot Footbath, Cold Footbath** under running water, Heating **Wet Sheet Pack**, Fan Douche to head, **Hot and Cold Compress** to head, heat over primary area of pain). **Fomentation** to the abdomen twice daily. Follow by **Heating Compress** and very hot application to forearm of opposite side.

SPINAL NEURALGIA AND LUMBAGO—Fomentation to spine, 2-3 times a day. During interval between, apply **Heating Compress**, Hot and Cold Pack to spine, Alternate Compress, Revulsive Douche, **Hot Trunk Pack**, Hot Half Blanket Pack, **Fomentation** to spine with **Hot Leg Bath**, **rest**.

GENERAL NEURALGIC PAIN—Hot Full Bath 4-5 minutes. Follow by Prolonged **Neutral Bath** at 95° F. **Hot Blanket Pack**, Radiant Heat Bath, Steam Bath or Sweating Wet Sheet Pack. Follow by **Dry Pack**.

NEURALGIA DUE TO CHRONIC NEURITIS—Alternate Compress and/or Alternate Douche. Revulsive Douche for persistent nerve stretching in sciatica.

NEURALGIC AFFECTIONS OF OVARIES, UTERUS, RECTUM, BLADDER, AND COCCYX—Revulsive Sitz Bath, Hot **Pack** to pelvis. Follow by **Cold Mitten Friction, Hot Enema, Hot and Cold Pelvic Pack**, hot vaginal irrigation, **Revulsive Compresses** over affected parts.

GASTRALGIA—Very hot **Fomentation** over stomach and abdomen. **Hot Trunk Pack**. **Revulsive Compress** for 10-30 minutes over stomach, repeated every 2 hours or as often as needed. **Hot Leg Pack**, hot **water** drinking, **Hot Enema**. Withhold food until pain is relieved. Aseptic diet. If necessary, **liquid diet** for a few days.

ENTERALGIA—Abdominal **Fomentation** for 15 minutes every hour. **Hot Enema**. **Heating Compress** applied at 60° F. during interval between. **Graduated Tonic Frictions**.

ERYTHRO-MELALGIA (RED NEURALGIA)—Rest and elevation of the affected part. **Cold Compress** changed every 20-30 minutes. Graduated **Tonic Frictions**.

HERPES ZOSTER—During eruption, **need Dry cotton**

Pack several times daily; but do after **Revulsive Compress**. **Heating Compress** during the interval between.

CONTRAINDICATIONS—Cold applications increase pain unless very carefully graduated, but are usually necessary for permanent results.

—*Also see the three most common forms of neuralgia: "Bell's Palsy" (bellow), "Sciatica" (566, 626, 645, 713), and "Tic Douloureux" (also called trigeminal neuralgia, this page).*

ENCOURAGEMENT—There is no happiness to be gained from living in indulgence for self. Your happiness will be found in helping those around you and obeying the Word of God. Here, alone, you will find true happiness. Acts 2:39.

BELL'S PALSY
(Facial Palsy)

SYMPTOMS—There is pain in the temples and/ or neck. Only one side is usually affected. There is weakness, pain, and a sensation of pricking, tingling, or creeping on the skin. One side of the face can droop.

Partial or complete paralysis of the muscles on one side of the face. Pain behind the ear on the affected side. Drooping of the corner of the mouth, sometimes with drooling. Inability to close the eyelid on the paralyzed side, plus watering of the eye. Impairment of taste.

CAUSES—Bell's palsy is a type of paralysis on one side of the face, characterized by distortion of the face, due to a lesion of the facial nerve.

It is usually the result of a **viral infection** that attacks the facial nerve (forehead, cheek, eye, and mouth). It may be caused by **injury, irritation of a sensory nerve or nerve root**. A **decayed tooth** may be the cause. **Chilling** of the face at night while one is sleeping can also produce it; the blood has been chilled back from the area. Sometimes Bell's palsy follows a **respiratory infection**. **Meat-eaters** are far more likely to develop this problem; vegetarians seldom do.

Bell's palsy is often mistaken for a stroke, because it comes on suddenly and results in numbness and partial, or total, loss of muscular control on the affected side. Yet it is not a stroke.

Treated properly, there can be as much as 80% chance of significant recovery. All those with partial palsy, and three fourths of those with complete palsy, recover with no treatment of any kind. Because most of those with this problem recover spontaneously, they should not be given drugs or surgery.

But severe taste impairment and/or reduced tearing of the eyes are bad signs, especially in older people, that the condition may continue.

Bell's palsy can occur in anyone at any age; but it most frequently occurs between 20 and 40, often in the summer months (especially August). The younger the person is, the more likely he will have a full recovery. With appropriate treatment, facial palsy usually improves in about 2 weeks. However, full recovery may take up to 3 months. Some people are left with weakness; and facial palsy may then recur.

NATURAL REMEDIES
• *See Neuralgia (563) for detailed information.*
• Take **B$_{12}$** (1,000 mcg per day) for a total of 20,000 mcg. Also **calcium** (2,000 mg per day), **magnesium** (800 mg per day), and essential fatty acids (2 Tbsp. **flaxseed** daily).
• Make sure, when he goes to bed at night, that a decided current of **cold air** is not blowing across his uncovered face while the rest of his body is under the blankets. When this happens, the chilled part does not receive adequate rest. A nerve in the face or neck can become chilled and cause problems.
• Apply **warm, wet washcloths** twice a day, for 20 minutes at a time, to relieve pain and tenderness. Follow with gentle massage, both backward and upward.
• *If an eye is affected,* apply pure **water** to the affected eye 4 times a day, to keep it moist and free from dust. Wearing **sunglasses** will reduce evaporation from that eye. Occasionally **close that eye** with a finger, to rest it. Wear an **eye patch** at night to protect it.
• Later, as the muscles begin functioning again, he should **exercise** his facial muscles: Standing before a mirror, wrinkle the forehead, close the affected eye, purse the lips, move the mouth to one side and then the other, blow out the cheeks, and try to whistle.
• Until the problem clears up, place **charcoal** poultices over the weakened nerve area at night and maintain a low-salt diet. This will help eliminate fluid released by the nerve.
• Prednisone is a drug often given; but it has negative side effects.
—*Bell's palsy is a form of neuralgia; see Neuralgia (563) for additional helpful information.*

ENCOURAGEMENT—Through defects in the character, Satan works to gain control of the whole mind; and he knows, that if these defects are cherished, he will succeed. It is urgent that you cling to Christ, plead for help, and earnestly seek to do that which is pleasing in His sight. Isaiah 54:13.

TIC DOULOUREUX
(Trigeminal Neuralgia)

SYMPTOMS—There is sudden darting pain which is severe. This is accompanied by spasms of the muscles of the face, with tingling and burning of the skin. A slight redness and swelling of the affected side will be seen, along with an increased flow of saliva and tears.

The affected nerves and skin become very tender; and movements of the face, speaking, and chewing may provoke violent pain.

CAUSES—Tic douloureux is a common form of neuralgia. It generally occurs in winter.

There are three divisions of the sensory nerve of the face most likely to be affected. The first is in the eyeball and over the forehead. The second is in the side of the face, the cheekbone, and the upper teeth. The third is inside the mouth and in the lower teeth.

The cause of the problem is **chilling of the face** over a period of time, when the rest of the body is relatively warm. The formula for trouble is (1) chilling draft to part of the body while the rest is warm (2) over a period of several hours, (3) day after day. *For more on tics, see 736; also see Neuralgia (563).*

NATURAL REMEDIES

• Keep the affected area **warm**. Immediately apply **hot Fomentations** to it. **Bed rest** is helpful, depending on the severity of the problem. Later apply **warm Fomentations** (or warm **whole baths**) several times a day.

• A cleansing **fruit juice fast** for several days will enable the body to more efficiently solve the problem. But keep in mind that a nerve was damaged by chilling over a lengthy period of time; so healing may not always come immediately.

• Eliminate **chilling drafts** on parts of the body.

The medical route is to operate on the face and destroy a nerve. This eliminates the pain and also permanently numbs part of the face. Some operations result in paralyzing part of the face; you cannot know, in advance, what the operation may do to you.

ENCOURAGEMENT—Upon obedience depends life, happiness, health, and joy in this brief probationary life. God alone can answer your problems and give you that which is for your best good. Trust Him, and you will be safe. Acts 16:31.

SCIATICA

SYMPTOMS—Pain is noted down the back of the thigh, the outer side of the calf. Perhaps it is along the outer side of the foot, on the top of the foot that is in line with the big toe. The person compensates by placing more weight on the other leg and foot. The pain is often worse at night. Coughing, walking, heavy labor, or sneezing increases both the pain in the back and in the sciatic nerve.

Later still, the area, where the pain may be felt, may feel numb when the hand is rubbed over it.

Still later, a wasting of the muscles of the calf and a weakness in running and even walking may be noticed.

CAUSES—The sciatic nerve is the largest nerve in the body. This nerve comes out of the spine. A branch of this runs down each leg, along the back of the thigh

of each leg, and down the inside of the leg to the ankle.

There are two primary causes of sciatica:

The first is **chilling the thigh** over a lengthy period of time. Sciatica usually begins as a neuralgia of the sciatic nerve. If you **sit on cold surfaces** a lot (steel-folding chairs in cool rooms, steel-tree chairs while hunting, or steel-boat seats while fishing, etc.) for lengthy periods of time, you can irritate the sciatic nerve and produce sciatica. A less recognized example is sitting on deep foam cushions, which never sufficiently warm up, for hours while watching exciting television dramas that cause you to be tense.

Fortunately, this form of sciatica is rather easy to solve: Apply neuralgia-type treatments; and only sit on warm surfaces or surfaces your body can heat relatively easily. Do not use chairs with foam that are too deep to easily warm up within a short time (say, 8 inches).

On your favorite chairs, place a folded, wool blanket or a piled thinner blanket. That is something you can warm up. Experiment and see what works best for you. If your body does not begin warming it up in a few minutes, lay something down that will.

Unfortunately, there is a second, and much more serious, cause:

The second cause of sciatica is **damage to the lower spine**. There may be a history of an **accident**, a **fall**, the **lifting** of a heavy weight, or a twist under some tension. Some men derange their lower back by the simple method of always carrying a **thick wallet** in one of the back pockets of their pants. The mechanical **vibration** of long hours behind the wheel of a car or truck, or work requiring repetitive **lifting,** may bring on sciatic attacks.

It is significant that *the pain is first felt in the lower back*. Later (weeks or even years later) pain begins to be felt at one or more places along the entire course of the sciatic nerve—back of the thigh, outer side of the calf, or in the top of the foot to the big toe.

One of the cartilaginous plates (disks, also spelled discs) in the lumbar region of the lower back has been damaged. The cartilage bulges and later breaks, creating pressure backward against a nerve root. (It is also possible for a tumor to develop and press against the sciatic nerve; but this is far less likely.)

Other important facts are these: (1) The person probably was not maintaining a **nourishing diet**, with supplemental **calcium, magnesium, vitamin D**, and other bone-building factors. (2) He may have been overworking his body in running, weight lifting, etc. (3) He was not lifting objects properly. (4) He was working at an occupation such as lifting heavy patients in a nursing home, which can be hazardous.

In older people who do not obtain enough bone-building materials in their diet, degenerative problems can occur in newly formed spicules, or ridges, of bone. These may press on a nerve root.

NATURAL REMEDIES
• Read again the above causal factors and try to correct those which apply to you.
• **Rest the painful limb** in as comfortable a position as possible.

HYDROTHERAPY
• *For pain in the leg from the sciatica:* Apply **hot, wet applications** to the affected leg, for the relief of pain and inflammation.
• *For pain in the back:* At the onset of a back attack, apply an application of **ice** for 10-20 minutes. This will deaden pain, relieve spasms, and minimize swelling.
• For the sciatica in the leg, give prolonged applications of **dry heat** in any form (**hot-water bottles, radiant heat, or electric heating pads**).
• Apply heat in the form of **hot Fomentations**, 3 times a day, omitting any use of ice or cold water.
• After each application of heat, **rub the limb** to increase circulation.
• Add 2 cups of **salt** to a boiling quart of water. When quite warm, apply with a cloth to the affected area until relief comes.

STRETCHING EXERCISES
• *Carefully* apply **stretching exercises**; *but always stop before there is pain or it becomes too uncomfortable.* Do each exercise 3 times, 2-3 times a day, increasing the number as improvement occurs:
• **Pull the knees up** as close to the chin as possible. You will feel a pulling sensation in the lower back.
• Sitting in a chair, **reach down** under it as far, as possible, and bend from the hip only.
• While lying on the back, the **leg is raised** with the knee straight. Someone else raises the leg, bending it from the hip only. This stretches the sciatic nerve and the hamstring muscles.

OTHER HELPS
• If the attack of pain lasts so long that the leg muscles have lost considerable strength, **massage and a daily hot and cold leg bath** (cold after the painful period is over) will help to restore circulation and strength.
• There are times when a **back adjustment** helps. If the back is out of adjustment, pain can occur. You will want to weigh this possibility carefully before doing it.
• **Fast** one day a week and eat only **raw food** for a month.
• Have a good **foot massage** every 3 days and especially around the Achilles tendons, up the back of the ankles.
• Get **fresh air, sunlight**, and (if possible) moderate **exercise**.
• Low-impact activities, like **swimming and walking**, are good for the back. But jogging, jumping, or twisting can damage bones and muscles. Gradually build stronger muscles and bones, but without pain.

HERBS
• **Dang quai**, the herb that is so helpful for female problems, is also good for sciatica.
• **Willow bark** contains *salicin*, which effectively relieves pain. Begin with a low dose of ½ tsp. of dried herb; and gradually increase it until you have effective pain relief. But long-term use can cause stomach distress and even ulcers.
• Take **wintergreen** internally, and apply it externally to the painful area. It contains *methyl salicylate* (similar to *salicin*, above).
• Mix 2 Tbsp. grated **ginger** with 3 Tbsp. **sesame oil** and 1 tsp. **lemon** juice. Rub this into the painful area. This remedy has been used in Egypt for centuries.
• Compresses of **Mistletoe** leaves alleviate sciatic pains.

OTHER HELPS
If you identify the problem early on, there is greater likelihood of eliminating it.
• Taking vitamin **B complex** is very important for healthy nerves. Take supplemental **calcium** (1,000 mg), **magnesium** (500 mg), **vitamin D** (1,000 IU), **vitamin E** (400 IU), **zinc** (30 mg), and **vitamin B$_{12}$** (1,500 mcg.).
• **Be careful** of your back when you work! Do not attempt something you know you should not do. Avoid accidents and falling.

If no improvement results from home treatments, you may wish to consult a specialist. He is likely to tell you that an **operation** is necessary. Should you have an operation on your spine? *Carefully read the article, Backache (645-648) and Strengthening the Bones (608) for additional information on the entire subject.*
—*Also read Neuralgia (563); because sciatica is a form of it.*

ENCOURAGEMENT—The Saviour overcame, to show man how he may overcome. Christ met all the temptations of Satan with the Word of God. By trusting in God's promises, He received power to obey God's commandments. So it is to be with us.

BRACHIAL NEURALGIA
(Thoracic Outlet Syndrome)

SYMPTOMS—There is a sense of pins, needles, numbness, and pain in one or both hands, 1-3 hours after falling asleep. The discomfort generally awakens the person. There may be wasting in the small muscles in the hands, as well as coldness or swelling. It generally occurs among adults, not children.

The symptoms can eventually include the lower arm, upper arm, and even the shoulder. This is generally worse after a day of heavy lifting.

During the day few symptoms are present, unless heavy lifting occurs.

CAUSES—Neuralgia is caused by irritation of the nervous system and by heavy mucus throughout the body. An acid condition is also a factor.

This is to the shoulder what sciatica is to the leg. A nerve, leading to the shoulder, is **pinched** in the spine. But it can also be caused by **overworking** of the

NERV

arms, carrying excessively **heavy weights, poor posture**, and letting the **arms and hands get cold** at night. More rarely, there may be an abnormality in the seventh cervical rib.

The lower branch of the brachial plexus of nerves exits from the lower cervical vertebrae, then passes underneath the clavicle and on into the arm. If this somehow experiences compression, the nerves to the arm and hand will be affected.

It is best to eliminate this disorder; otherwise it is likely to keep getting worse.

A similar affliction is called the *cervical rib syndrome*. But it occurs more often in younger people; and it produces pain or numbness soon after heavy lifting, wearing a heavy coat, etc. The symptoms occur in the day, not at night.

NATURAL REMEDIES

• **Back adjustments** by a competent chiropractor may be the solution.

• Keep the **hands and arms warm** at night, especially if there is a cool draft on the body.

• Improve the diet. A good, nourishing diet which will build the nerves and bones is important. **Raw green vegetables are needed,** along with daily **vitamin / mineral supplements**. A diet similar to that used in treating arthritis *(618)* is helpful.

• The sharp, excruciating pains can generally be relieved by placing a poultice or fomentation of **mullein and cayenne** over the area. Relief may also be obtained by applying a liniment of equal parts **cayenne and prickly ash** tincture. To remove the cause, rebuild the body with tonics, change the diet, and improve the person's general health.

• Maintain an ongoing **exercise** program, to strengthen the muscles of the shoulders and arms and improve the posture: **arm lifts, neck exercises, shoulder shrugs, horizontal upper trunk push-ups,** etc.

• Avoid heavy **lifting**. When you have to lift, first take several deep breaths to strengthen your muscles, shrug your shoulders, and remain in a semi-shrugged position while you lift. This will ward off nerve compression.

—Also see Sciatica (566,626,645,713), Neuralgia (563), Bell's Palsy (565), Neuritis (bellow).

ENCOURAGEMENT—The rainbow of promise encircling the throne on high is an everlasting testimony that God loves you. He will never forsake His people in their struggle with evil. We have the assurance of strength and protection. But we can always choose to leave Him; and therein lies our danger.

NEURITIS

SYMPTOMS—There may be pain, tenderness,

tingling, and loss of the sensation of touch in the affected nerve area along with redness and swelling. Pain is not always a prominent symptom of true neuritis. But the numbness, burning, tingling, crawling, with possible pain, tends to occur in spells. Weakness, and even paralysis and loss of sensation, are common. In serious cases, convulsions may occur. The affected muscles may shrink in size.

CAUSES—The symptoms can vary with the cause, which can include an **injury to a nerve, infection involving a nerve, or a disease** (gout, diabetes, leukemia, etc.). **Poisons inhaled or swallowed (mercury, methyl alcohol, or lead)** can cause nerve trouble. A lack of the vitamin **B complex**, especially **thiamine** in the diet. A **degenerative illness** can produce neuritis as a side effect.

Men between the ages of 30 and 50 are the most likely to experience neuritis.

Foot-drop, due to **sitting with knees crossed**, occurs when ankle or foot muscles weaken, causing the toes to drag as one walks. Wrist-drop is caused by pressure in the armpit from a **crutch** or other support. Optic neuritis occurs when inflammation affects the optic nerve in the eye. This can produce gradual, or sudden, blurring and loss of vision. Blindness can occur in severe cases. However, it is usually temporary if prompt treatment is given.

There is mucus in the system. Mucus causes an upset in the specific area conducting nerves into the spinal column and throws out a vertebrae, causing even more irritation. The nerves must be rebuilt, and the acid condition of the nerves and the worn sheath around the nerves must be replaced by taking nervines. Besides using the cleansing program, rebuild the entire nervous system and use the cleansing program.

NATURAL REMEDIES

• A **well-balanced diet**, including a full spectrum of **vitamins and minerals,** is vital. The entire **B complex** is very important. If the problem is not too far advanced, administration of enough B complex and **thiamine** (200 mg) can bring great improvement within 3-4 days.

• If **poisoning** is a factor, the source of contamination must be avoided and eliminated. Obtain an abundance of **fresh air**.

• Treatment for neuritis includes **rest** and **good diet**; and, after the pain subsides, do **massage** and careful **exercise**. Identify the cause and solve it.

• A **fruit and vegetable juice fast** for a day or two may help eliminate toxins and thus strengthen the body to more rapidly heal the affected nerves.

• **St. John's wort** helps regenerate nerve tissue. **Hawthorn** strengthens circulation.

• Dr. John Christopher recommends the following formula for neuritis: 1 oz. each of **Lady's slipper** and **skullcap**, ½ oz. each of **wild yam, ginger, and damiana**.

Pour 1 quart boiling hot water over the herbs, cover tightly, let stand until cool. Strain, sweeten to taste, and drink 2 fluid oz. every 3-4 hours.

• Neuritis is frightening because of the pain. Use **nervines and antispasmodic herbs** to correct the cause. Ease the pain with **fomentations, poultices and the green drinks**.

• Avoid **caffeine, tobacco, alcohol, and drugs**.

J.H. KELLOGG, M.D., PRESCRIPTIONS FOR NEURITIS AND ITS COMPLICATIONS (*how to give these water therapies: pp. 206-275 / list of treatments: pp. 206-207 / Hydrotherapy Disease Index: pp. 273-275*)

IMMEDIATE—Rest of the affected parts until the acute stage is over.

COMBAT TOXEMIA—Sweating bath 2-3 times a week, preferably the Radiant Heat Bath. Follow sweating bath by a suitable **cold application**.

COMBAT INFLAMMATION—Local **Revulsive Compress** for 15 minutes every 2-4 hours. Follow by **Heating Compress** during intervals between. Suitable derivative applications.

PAIN—Revulsive Douche (spray). Steam Bath. Follow by graduated **Fan Douche**, gradually lowering from 100° to 80° F. Protect by Dry cotton Pack or **Heating Compress** that is covered with plastic.

PARALYSIS—Alternate Compress, Alternate Douche, **Percussion Douche** to spine and affected parts.

—*Also see Multiple Neuritis and Strengthening the Nerves (bellow).*

ENCOURAGEMENT—Where can we find a surer guide than the only true God? Where is a safer path than that in which the Eternal leads the way? When we follow Him, we have powerful guidance. The path of obedience to God is the path of virtue, of health, and happiness. Proverbs 3:5-10.

"Receiving the end of your faith, even the salvation of your souls . . Gird up the loins of your mind, be sober, and hope to the end of the grace that is to be brought unto you at the revelation of Jesus Christ." 1 Peter 1:9, 13. Thank God for such sweet promises. They are such a comfort to our souls!

MULTIPLE NEURITIS

SYMPTOMS—Symptoms will be like those for neuritis, except that the pain is felt in several locations.

CAUSES—Multiple neuritis is indicated by pain occurring in two or more locations instead of just one. It is inflammation of more than one nerve at the same time. *See Neuritis (568) for much more information.*

NATURAL REMEDIES

J.H. KELLOGG, M.D., PRESCRIPTIONS FOR MULTIPLE NEURITIS AND ITS COMPLICATIONS (*how to give these water therapies: pp. 206-275 / list of treatments: pp. 206-207 / Hydrotherapy Disease Index: pp. 273-275*)

BASIC—Rest in bed while the disease is rapidly progressing.

COMBAT TOXEMIA—Prolonged Neutral Bath 1-2 hours, daily. **Aseptic dietary**. Avoidance of tea, coffee, tobacco,

alcoholic liquors, and all excesses. **Sweating**, especially by Radiant Heat Bath, 10-20 minutes. Follow by **Cold Mitten Friction**.

COMBAT LOCAL INFLAMMATIONS—Revulsive Compresses, then **Heating Compress** or packing in dry cotton (Dry Pack). **Fomentations** to spine. Follow with **Heating Compress**. When affecting the lower extremities, **Hot Footbath** or Hot Leg Bath. Hot Leg Pack, complete rest of the affected part.

IMPROVE THE GENERAL NUTRITION—by **Graduated Cold Baths**, massage; **outdoor air** with careful protection, **sunbaths**, **aseptic diet**.

ATROPHY—Alternate Douche, massage.

CONTRAINDICATIONS—During acute stage, carefully avoid cold applications unless very short and preceded by heat. Avoid percussion applications, when tenderness exists; that is, all forms of the Douche. Avoid especially Cold Full Baths and very prolonged Hot Baths.

—*Also see Neuritis (568).*

ENCOURAGEMENT—The followers of Christ are to become like Him—by the grace of God to form characters in harmony with the principles of His holy law. This is Bible sanctification.

STRENGTHENING THE NERVES

NATURAL REMEDIES

BUILDING UP THE NERVES—Good blood, healthy nerves, and strong bones and joints are needed for outstanding health. Brain cells cannot properly function without proper nutrients and a healthful way of life.

Here are several suggestions to help you strengthen your nerves. This is a building program:

NUTRIENTS

• The vitamin **B complex** (100 mg per day; best taken as 50 mg twice a day) is especially important in maintaining good nerve action and response. Deficiencies of the B complex are common among people eating modern, devitalized, processed, and assorted junk foods. Take a good **vitamin / mineral supplement** at least twice a day. It should include all the B vitamins.

• **Vitamin B$_1$**, also called thiamine (100 mg, twice a day), is especially needed for neuritis.

• **Vitamin B$_3$** (niacin, 50 mg twice a day). Do not take more than 100 mg of niacin a day. **Niacinamide** is equivalent to niacin and does not produce the flushed face which niacin does.

• **Vitamin B$_{12}$** (2,000 mcg, twice a day).

• **Vitamin B$_6$** (250-500 mg, 1-2 times a day), especially for carpal tunnel syndrome.

• **Folic acid** (400-800 mcg, daily).

• **Inositol** (1,000 mg, 1-2 times a day), especially for diabetic neuropathy.

• In addition to the above B vitamins, also take **vitamin C** (3,000-6,000 mg daily, when you have a nerve crisis) with **bioflavonoids** (100 mg daily).

• **Vitamin E** (400 IU, 2-3 times a day), especially

with post-herpes syndrome.

• **Vitamin A**. It is best to take vitamin A in the form of beta-carotene (in carrot juice and fresh green and yellow fruits and vegetables).

• Minerals include **calcium** (400 mg, 2-3 times daily), **magnesium** (200 mg, 2-3 times a day), **zinc** (30 mg daily, not to exceed 100 mg daily from all supplements), and **iodine**.

• **Essential fatty acids**, obtained from 1-2 Tbsp. cold-pressed oils daily. Never put it into your cooking; instead, put it on your food after the plate is served. **Flaxseed oil** and **wheat germ oil** are the best sources.

• **Fresh and steamed vegetables** are rich in minerals which are needed for the nervous system and brain. Eat **whole grains, nuts, and legumes**.

• **Brewer's yeast, kelp or dulse, and lecithin** are very helpful. Eat regularly, chew slowly, and do not overeat.

• *Octocosanol* is found in **wheat germ oil**. It helps the neuron membranes.

OTHER HELPS

• Increase your **fluid** intake.

• Obtain enough **rest** at night and avoid sexual **enervation**. Medical professionals know that such enervation is one of the quickest ways to produce weakened, degenerate, and diseased nerve tissue.

• A good balance between **exercise and rest** has a powerful effect in building the body, if a **nutritious diet** is maintained.

• Avoid **stimulants** and **all processed, refined, and junk foods**.

• Cool and cold **water treatments** will help tone and strengthen the nerves.

• The nervine herbs include **skullcap, hops, chamomile, valerian, dong quai, wood betony, passionflower, lady's slipper, mistletoe,** and small amounts of **lobelia**.

Here is additional information about the close relationship of nutrients to the brain and nerves:

ADDITIONAL FACTS ABOUT NUTRIENTS

• Deficiencies of the **B complex** and **vitamin C** decrease the metabolic rate of the brain. Lack of **niacin** can produce deep depression, often seen in psychosis. Symptoms of a severe **vitamin B_6** deficiency are headache, irritability, dizziness, extreme nervousness, and inability to concentrate. A **thiamine** deficiency results in a lack of energy, constant fatigue, loss of appetite, and irritability; if this continues too long, there are emotional upsets and overreaction to normal stress. **Pantothenic acid** (a B vitamin) is needed to handle stressful situations. Lack of **vitamin C** leads to irritability.

• Vitamin **B complex** (especially **B_3, B_6, B_{12},** and **folic acid**) reduces excess estrogen from the liver and prevents it from causing mental troubles.

• It is vital to obtain enough **oxygen**, if you want a clear mind which functions properly. **Vitamin E** helps the brain obtain enough oxygen, from the amount supplied to the lungs.

• Adequate **calcium** in the diet is vital. See *Strengthening the Bones (608)* for ways to maintain enough calcium in the body. Inadequate calcium results in insomnia, tenseness, and fatigue.

• **Calcium** works with **magnesium** to protect the nerves from damage.

• A person with a **magnesium** deficiency tends to be uncooperative, withdraws, is apathetic or belligerent.

• Too much **copper** in the body occurs in schizophrenia; it can be reduced by dietary intake of **zinc** and **manganese**. **Vitamin C** deficiency can cause copper retention which accumulates in the brain and liver.

• Many of the schizophrenias, autism, abnormal behaviors, and subsequent learning disorders are caused by too much **lead or copper** in the body. Check your plumbing pipes. Plastic water pipes are the safest.

ADDITIONAL FACTS ABOUT FOODS

• There is a direct relation between the **transverse colon** and the brain. When the colon is clogged, mental illness is triggered in some and an attack of epilepsy *(574)* in others. Eliminate the "**glue foods**"; these tend to clog the colon, produce a buildup of mucus and toxins in it, and lead to mental problems. Such foods include **white flour, sugar, eggs, meat, peanuts, and dairy products**.

• A **whole grain diet** stimulates the amount of tryptophan in the brain and produces a calming, peaceful feeling.

ADDITIONAL FACTS ABOUT HORMONES

• A lack of **thyroxine**, the hormone from the thyroid, results in a slowing of physical and mental functions. Hyperthyroidism is related to emotional disturbance, forgetfulness, slow thought processes, and irritability.

• When the **adrenals** do not function properly, depression and other forms of mental illness may result.

• **Exercise** (especially outdoors in the **fresh air**) combined with **relaxation** helps rejuvenate the body and mind.

• In addition to some other herbs, **ginkgo biloba** improves brain function and cerebral circulation and enhances memory.

ENCOURAGEMENT—We have been bought with the precious blood of Christ as of a lamb without blemish. What a price has been paid for us! Now Christ invites you to come and accept the salvation which He alone can work out in your life. He can strengthen you to obey all that He asks of you.

SEASONAL AFFECTIVE DISORDER (SAD)

SYMPTOMS—Withdrawal, social isolation, depression, cravings, weight gain, loss of energy, oversleep, decreased sexual desire.

CAUSES—This condition, also called the "winter blues," is caused by several factors:

The **winter months** bring **dark and dreary overcast days**; this emotionally bothers some people more than others.

The winter months have **shorter hours of daylight** and more overcast skies during the daytime, resulting in less light entering the eyes. This light deficiency sends signals to the pineal, pituitary, and hypothalamus glands; and they do not function as fully as usual.

There is often more **stress** and greater **nutritional deficiency** in the winter. Less fresh fruit and vegetables may be available.

All this combines, in some, to produce seasonal affective syndrome. In our waking hours, we need sunlight every so often. We have a friend who, moving to Labrador, on the eastern Canadian coast, could not tolerate the incessant dreary fog and moved away within a year.

Women have this problem 4 times as often as men.

NATURAL REMEDIES

• In most cases, an **improvement in diet** will greatly help. Foods rich in the **B complex** are needed, along with **fresh fruit and vegetables**. The nervous system needs to be built up with better food.

• Negative attitudes are also powerful. Train your mind to **be thankful** for the blessings you have.

• If possible, obtain a **full-spectrum light** for your dining room, living room, and work area.

• Spend more time **outdoors** on sunny or bright days.

• Build a **"light box."** It is about 2 feet long and 1½ feet high, with white fluorescent bulbs behind a plastic screen. It should deliver 2,500-10,000 lux (a measurement of intensity of light). Ten minutes a day in front of the light box may be all you need at the beginning of winter, but 45 minutes daily may be needed in the heart of winter. Sit 1-3 feet from it, facing it, and looking down. Read, do writing, do paperwork. Or just sit (without looking directly at the light) and listen to music. If you are getting headaches or eyestrain, reduce the time before it.

• **St. John's wort** is a helpful antidepressant. Take 300 mg, 3 times a day.

• Take the bioflavonoid, **quercetin** (100 mg), and **bromelain** (500 mg). Take **calcium** (1,000 mg), **magnesium** (500 mg), and **zinc** (30 mg).

• Each morning and evening, take a **hot and cold shower** and do gentle **muscle stretches**. Each day, go outside, **breathe deeply,** and **walk vigorously** for awhile.

ENCOURAGEMENT—To those who love God, it will be the highest delight to keep His commandments and to do those things that are pleasing in His sight. Isaiah 30:18, 1 John 5:23.

TENNIS ELBOW

SYMPTOMS—Tenderness and pain in the elbow, weakness in the hand.

CAUSES—Tennis elbow is an occupational and recreational problem. Those who do a lot of **hand-gripping** can have this disorder. This would include **golfers, carpenters, factory workers, housewives,** and even **politicians** who shake hands a lot.

The weakness occurs when gripping an object; it is not a true muscle weakness. The tendons are involved. This is a form of neuritis.

NATURAL REMEDIES

• For 3-4 days, **do not do those activities** which cause the pain.

• Apply **cold or hot to the affected area**, according to that which helps you best. Apply **ice** on the affected area for 30-90 minutes each day; the more the pain, the longer the application. Or apply **heat**, especially after the first few days.

• Careful **exercise** is also needed, to eliminate tennis elbow; **rest** is not enough. The tendons and the muscles supporting them need to be strengthened. Purchase a hand gripper at a sporting goods store and slowly increase your usage of it until you are using it 5-10 minutes, 4 times a day. When you use it, the elbow should be straight and the wrist bent. This will stretch the extensor tendons and help strengthen the fibrous tendons.

• **Other exercises** are also helpful. Place your forearm on a table (palm down) and grip a 3-pound dumbbell. Flex the wrist upward slightly, hold for 5 seconds, lower, and rest for 3 seconds. When you can easily do this 15 times, increase the weight by 1 pound. Over a period of 4-6 weeks of doing this everyday, you may be able to lift up to 8-10 pounds without pain. Fourteen of 18 patients, on a four-week program with this exercise, obtained complete pain relief.

• Athletes sometimes place a **band** several inches wide around the forearm near the elbow and another just above the wrist. Be sure they are not too tight.

• Avoid **cortisone** injections; for these can produce tendon atrophy or even dissolve the tendon! —Also see Carpal Tunnel Syndrome (572).

ENCOURAGEMENT—Satan and his evil angels are watching at every avenue leading to the human heart, seeking to force souls to accept evil suggestions. He presents us with bribes as he bribed Christ, pretending that he will give us the world if we will obey him. But, in the strength of Christ, we can resist him. Luke 1:77-79.

CARPAL TUNNEL SYNDROME

SYMPTOMS—Mild numbness and faint tingling, maybe excruciating pain; but there is generally only burning, tingling, or numbness in the thumb and first three fingers. Crippling atrophy of the thumb can result.

Symptoms are often worse at night or in the morning. The pain may eventually spread to the arm and shoulder. Symptoms normally affect only one hand, but may be present in both.

CAUSES—Carpal tunnel syndrome (CTS) is a cumulative trauma disorder that develops over time, due to **repeated stressful movements of the hands and wrist.** It affects 23,000 workers a year. The median nerve in the wrist is compressed or damaged. This nerve controls the thumb muscles and sensation in the thumb, palm, and first three fingers. The median nerve passes through a very small opening, about a quarter inch below the top of the wrist.

Either **compression or injury to this nerve** can cause problems: pressure from **bone spurs, inflammatory arthritis or tendonitis, swelling due to pregnancy or water retention.**

Other causes include **repeated stressful motions, such as writing, typing, or hammering. Bookkeepers and checkout clerks can develop it; so can hairstylists, musicians, writers, drivers, athletes, restaurant servers, and jack hammer and chainsaw operators.** The occurrence of CTS has greatly increased since the 1980s, when personal computers came into use. The **tendons swell and compress the median nerve** that runs to your hand, causing great pain. A common pattern is **rapid and continuous use of the fingers,** producing a **repetitive wrist motion injury.** Women between 29 and 62 experience CTS more often than anyone else.

Raynaud's disease, pregnancy, hypothyroidism, diabetes, and menopause increase the risk of developing CTS.

Other disorders, especially arthritis in the neck, have similar symptoms. But, *if the first three fingers in one or both hands are affected* by the pain, then it is probably CTS.

NATURAL REMEDIES

HAND EXERCISES

• As soon as the tingling begins, begin doing some gentle hand exercises. **Rotate the wrist in a circle** for 2 minutes. This exercises all the muscles of the wrist, restores circulation, and gets your wrist out of the position that usually causes the trouble.

• Raise your hands above your head and **rotate your arms** while rotating your wrists at the same time. Also do some **neck turns**; look over your right, then left, shoulder. Learn to exercise and relax as you work.

DIET

• **Vitamin B₆** (100 mg, twice a day) is especially important in solving this problem! In one study, two thirds of those taking B_6 reported improvement. Do not take larger dosages.

• Eat part of a fresh **pineapple** daily, for 1-3 weeks. The bromelain in it will reduce swelling and pain. **Niacinamide** (2,000 mg) will increase circulation.

• **Vitamin C** (500-1,000 mg, 3 times daily), **vitamin E** (400 IU daily), and **flaxseed oil** (2 tsp. daily).

• Eat only moderate amounts of **oxalic acid foods** (beets, beet greens, sorrel, Swiss chard, Rhubarb with 860 mg. per 100 grams, cabbage family, parsley, asparagus.). Avoid spinach, and especially rhubarb. Oxalic acid blocks calcium absorption.

• Avoid **salt** and all sodium foods; for they promote water retention.

HERBS

• **Aloe vera, yarrow, and yucca** help restore flexibility and reduce inflammation. **Skullcap** relieves muscle spasms and pain. **Wintergreen oil** reduces pain and aids circulation to the muscles. **Turmeric** contains *curcumin*, a potent anti-inflammatory chemical. **Cumin** contains anti-inflammatory, pain-relieving, and anti-swelling chemicals. **Ginkgo biloba** extract (2-3 times daily) will increase circulation.

Willow contains *salicylates* which relieve pain and reduce inflammation. Steep 1-2 tsp. dried, powdered bark or 5 tsp. fresh bark for 10 minutes, strain, add lemonade (to mask the bitter taste), and drink 2-3 cups a day.

OTHER HELPS

• Place an **ice pack** on your wrists to reduce pain. Do not use heat; for that will increase the swelling.

• Try to **reduce the impact** of repetitive mechanical tasks on your wrists and hands. If possible, stop all such movements for several days and see if improvement occurs. If so, try to do these functions less frequently. If possible, rotate your duties, so you do not do those repetitive tasks daily. It is repeatedly flexing your wrists under the pressure of pushing or pounding that causes CTS.

• Keep your **weight** down. Extra weight puts more pressure on the carpal tunnel.

• Keep your **arms close** to your body and your **wrists straight** while sleeping. For example, if you let your hand drop over the side of the bed while you are sleeping, the pressure on the median nerve is increased.

• You might wish to temporarily wear a **wrist splint** at night. This helps to keep the wrist straight.

• **Do not wrap** your wrist in an Ace bandage. This

could cut off the circulation.

• If you have to **carry** something, make sure the handle is the right size. If it is too small or large, it could hurt your wrist.

PREVENTION

• Carpal tunnel syndrome is an increasing problem in our time. Here are several suggestions for avoiding its occurrence:

• Use a **tool** instead of flexing your wrists forcibly.

• Keep your **wrists** essentially straight (your forearms and hands are on the same plane) when you exert force with the hand.

• Use your **whole hand** and all your fingers when you grip an object.

• In doing a task, use your **whole arm**, not just your wrist. For example, when hammering, swing your arm rather than just your wrist.

• Select a **pair of scissors** with angled blades. **Do not wring** wet laundry by hand. **Musicians** (especially piano players) should not have a chair that is too low, so their wrists are crooked.

WHEN TYPING

• When typing, writing, or working with papers at a desk, maintain good **posture** and keep your **elbows bent**.

• Typing is the special problem. What is **the ideal position**? Cock your wrist back slightly, so that your thumb is parallel to your forearm. Your hand should be in approximately the same position as if it were holding a pen. This position keeps the carpal tunnel as open as possible. Place a wrist pad on the table, just in front of the keyboard.

• In order to do this, the **height** of your chair and the height of the desk (with your keyboard and mouse on top of it)—are both very important.

• Ideally, the **mouse** should be located very close to your body, so you do not have to reach for it. Carefully plan your **desk** arrangement. If necessary, ask the boss if you can bring in your own desk. Then have one made to exactly fit your specifications.

• Make sure the office **chair** is the right height. Use a chair with **armrests**. When your arm is on the armrest, the hands can rest; then lift off the armrests a little, with wrists straight, to work the keyboard.

• When operating the **mouse**, your arm can rest again on the armrest and the hand can reach a few inches to the front and side to the mouse while the wrist remains straight. (That is how the author is typing right now.) The key to avoiding CTS while typing is keeping the wrists straight.

• The computer **screen** should be about 2 feet away, and just below your line of sight.

• **Before starting** handwork, **exercise** the fingers and wrists for a couple of minutes, to warm them up. **Take a break** from handwork every hour. **Shake out** your hands every so often throughout the day.

—*Also see Tennis Elbow (571).*

ENCOURAGEMENT—The wrath of God will not fall upon one soul that seeks refuge in Him. God cares for His children who trust in Him. They may have

CHART - 1055: Cerebral Compression (573) Brain Concussion (573)

trials in this life, but their life is secure; they will live with their Maker in heaven. John 1:12.

NEURO-MENTAL - 3 - CONVULSIONS

CONVULSIONS
(Spasms, Seizures, Fits)

SYMPTOMS—A sudden, involuntary, and unnatural muscular contraction. Such paroxysms of involuntary muscular contractions and relaxations occur most frequently in children.

CAUSES—Convulsions are uncontrolled body movements set off by an electrical malfunction of the brain.

Convulsions can be caused by **epilepsy, meningitis, tetanus, uremia, hysteria, or eclampsia**. They can also be induced by **poisoning from camphor, cyanide, strychnine, santonin, brucine, or aspidium**.

In children the cause is often **wrong diet, rickets, syphilis, malaria, toxemias, or acute infectious diseases**. **High fevers** of 104°-105° F. are often a cause of convulsions in children.

In adults, the cause is often **epilepsy, heat cramps, strychnine, or food poisoning**. Spasms may also arise from **calcium deficiency, panic, fear, or overeating**.

Convulsions, due to tetanus and hydrophobia, are easily distinguished and, for the most part, involve a small portion of the voluntary muscles. Strychnine poisoning causes spasms which involve the whole body.

NATURAL REMEDIES

• Know the cause before administering any herbal remedy. If convulsions are caused by poisons taken into the body through the stomach, then **emetics** must be used quickly; so he will vomit. If they are from fright or fear, an antispasmodic tincture with **cayenne** will usually stop the attack at once. If the convulsions are caused from an impacted bowel, **catnip** injection into the colon will relieve the constipation and soothe the nervous system. Often the individual is in no condition to take oral aids. In such cases, give an enema or an injection of antispasmodic, nervine, or catnip; this will ease and soothe the convulsive condition.

• Loosen the **clothing** and give plenty of **fresh air**. If the cause is undetermined, keep him from injuring himself. Some place a **soft pad** between the teeth—but he could choke on it!

• If an infant, put him in a **bath** of 95° F. or in **mustard and water bath** at 85° F. **Cold** should be applied to the head. The cause must first be found, or injury may result from the bath. *If fever* is present, it should be a **tepid or cool bath**.

• Produce **vomiting** by placing the finger down the

NERV

throat. *If gums are hot and swollen*, give **cold water** and **rub gums** with a cloth that has been held on ice.

• The bowels should be emptied immediately with an **enema**. Take some **laxative herbs**, to clean out the small intestine. **Fast** on fruit juices, water, or nervine herb teas (listed below) until all symptoms subside. Keep the body **warm**. **Lobelia** tincture should be rubbed well into the neck, chest, and between the shoulders. It is extremely relaxing.

• If the spasm is in a muscle and easy to reach, a good nervine (especially **wormwood oil**), as a liniment massaged into the problem area, will give quick relief. For internal spasms (such as in the stomach area), give a few drops of **lobelia** tincture each half hour.

• Helpful herbs include **catnip, skullcap, and peony**. Two cups of **valerian** root may be taken every 2 hours after the convulsions. **Antispasmodic tincture** *(576)* is best and works faster.

• Other useful herbs include **rue, black cohosh, valerian, vervain, peppermint, chamomile, wild cherry bark, goldenseal, and a little cayenne**.

• Give weak **chamomile** tea in small doses several times a day. Give a warm chamomile tea enema.

• After this, **rest** absolutely quiet in bed; give careful diagnosis without disturbing him.

• One successful method of therapy has been the injection in 1 large dose of 600,000 IU of **vitamin D**. This helps the utilization of calcium, which relaxes the muscles.

• Take **calcium** (2,000 mg, daily) and **magnesium** (1,000 mg, daily) supplements. Also B_6 (100 mg, twice a day) and **chromium** (75-100 mcg, 3 times a day).

Advice from a reader who is an expert, having had them since childhood: "Move anything out of the way that might injure him. Turn the person on his side so anything coming out of his mouth might run out. If the head is bouncing off the floor, put something soft under it. Never put anything in his mouth; he may choke on it! Don't take time to cause him to vomit, but put him in bed to rest, because he is exhausted."

SPECIAL PROBLEMS

• *Parasites and constipation:* Parasites are the primary cause; constipation is less frequently a cause. Most frequently occurs in countries the most heavily infested with parasites, and there is poor personal cleanliness. Put the person on a cleansing and building program (**fresh fruits and vegetables, whole grains, nuts, and legumes**), discarding all **meat eating** and requiring that he never return to it (so he will not again become infested with worms).

• *If parasites* are the cause, use **garlic** enemas, plus eating garlic. *See Worms (861) for more information.*

• If the child or adult is *constipated*, immediately give a warm **catnip tea enema**.

• There is a definite possibility, especially in children, that a *food allergy* is involved—very possibly accompanied by malnutrition (maybe partially caused

(vertical text) CHART - 1055: Epilepsy (574)

by being fed too much junk food and soft drinks). After the convulsion is past, begin testing with pulse tests for food allergies. *See Pulse Test (847).*

• If it should be a spasm of *asthma*, take 8 drops of **antispasmodic tincture** *(576)* or inhale eucalyptus oil.

• If it is a *muscle spasm*, wring a **towel** out of hot water and lay it on the area.

• A *coughing spasm* can be relieved by the **antispasmodic tincture** or an **emetic**.

—Also see Antispasmodic Tincture (576) and Epilepsy (below).

ENCOURAGEMENT—The psalmist says, "The law of the Lord is perfect." How wonderful, in its simplicity and comprehensiveness, are the Ten Commandments! In Christ's strength we can obey them; whereas, apart from Him, we cannot. John 15:4-5.

EPILEPSY

SYMPTOMS—There are several types of, what are called, seizures:

Absence (petit mal): A blank stare lasting about half a minute and the person is unaware of his surroundings. Most often in children.

Complex partial (temporal lobe): A blank stare, random activity, and a chewing motion. No memory of this seizure afterward. An aura, or warning indication, may occur before. It may be a certain odor, sound, thought, etc. No after memory of the seizure.

Myoclonia: Brief, but massive, muscle jerks.

Simple partial (Jacksonian): Jerking begins in the fingers and toes, and progresses throughout the body. The person remains conscious.

Simple partial (sensory): Things that do not exist are seen, heard, or sensed. A general seizure may follow.

CAUSES—Epilepsy is defined as an episodic disturbance of consciousness, during which generalized convulsions may occur. There are recurring seizures, generally one of seven patterns (listed above). This is caused by electrical disturbances in the nerve cells, in a portion of the brain.

Electroencephalographic studies reveal a direct relationship between changes in electrical brain potentials and the occurrence of seizures.

Epilepsy is the most common form of seizures, also called convulsions or fits. Epilepsy can be caused by **injury to the head, neck, or spinal cord** (especially before or during birth). **High fevers** during early childhood or **infectious diseases** can also cause it. Heredity can be involved. **Oxygen deprivation** at birth or a later **head injury** may be causal factors.

A variety of factors may trigger the onset of a seizure. Oddly enough, an important one is **constipation in the transverse colon**. Eating bread, especially **soft bread**, is known to lead to seizures among epileptics.

An improperly functioning **ileocecal valve** is a possible cause. This permits powerful toxins to return into the small intestine and enter the bloodstream, affecting the delicate nervous system and brain.

During a seizure, the person may fall during the attack, often injuring himself; he may bite his tongue, pass urine, and awake to realize that, because of muscular soreness, something has happened.

There is a tendency to sleep following the attack. Sometimes attacks occur only during sleep.

Some seizures take the form of antisocial or unnatural conduct.

On recovery, amnesia is generally complete, so no effort is made to hide what happened. The epileptic may gradually deteriorate.

NATURAL REMEDIES

IMMEDIATE TREATMENT
• During the attack, arrange the **head** to facilitate breathing. Prevent the **tongue** from being bitten or from obstructing the windpipe. Place a **pad** between the teeth during the attack. Afterward allow him to **sleep**.

• Here is an herbal formula, used for over a hundred years. Prepare the following powdered herbs in advance, for use when an attack occurs: Mix 2 oz. **skullcap**; 1 oz. **valerian** root, and ¼ oz. each of **cayenne** and **lobelia**. Sift the herbs. When an attack occurs, give 1 tsp. in a cup of hot water, every hour if necessary.

See Convulsions (573-576) for more information on dealing with them.

DIET
• Maintain a well-balanced, **nutritious diet. Do not overeat!** Do not eat **excessive amounts** of food or fluid at one time.

• Do not eat **soft bread**; better yet, do not eat any bread. You may find that you should not eat mush either.

• Drink fresh **fruit and vegetable juices**.

• Include **raw vegetables** in your diet.

• **Check your diet** with pulse and other tests, to see which foods are a problem. Use rotation diets to this objective. *See Allergies (848) and Pulse Test (847).*

• **Vitamin B**$_6$ deficiency has been linked as a factor in some cases of epilepsy. When given to some babies in their formula, the epilepsy ceased.

• Do not be deficient in **vitamin A** (in the form of carotenes: carrot juice and yellow and orange fruits and vegetables), **vitamin D** (1,000 mg), **folic acid** (5 mg), **zinc** (30 mg), **and aurine** (an amino acid).

• Take **manganese** supplementation (25 mg). A lack of it can produce epilepsy. Women who lack it can give birth to epileptic children.

• **Magnesium** (1,000 mg) deficiency may cause muscle tremors and convulsive seizures. Epileptics have a lower than normal amount of this mineral. Infants with excess calcium intake had a magnesium loss. Yet other studies revealed that calcium was also important.

AVOID
• Avoid **white sugar and white-flour** products. Avoid **fried foods, animal protein, and artificial sweeteners**.

• Avoid **alcohol, caffeine, pesticides, and aluminum cookware**. High levels of aluminum have been found in the brains of those with epilepsy. Aluminum is a conductor of electricity; and trace amounts in the brain may trigger seizures.

• **Toxic metals (lead, copper, mercury, and aluminum)** are known to cause seizures. **Lead** is in old water pipes and wall paint. **Mercury** is in amalgam dental fillings. *See Lead Poisoning (873), Copper Poisoning (872), Mercury Poisoning (874), Aluminum Poisoning (871), and Heavy Metal Poisoning (868).*

• The artificial sweetener, **aspartame** (Nutra-Sweet), has been linked to seizures, as well as other disorders.

• Avoid the herb, **sage**. This herb should not be used by anyone with a tendency to seizures.

• **Allergies** cause seizures in some. This includes **chemicals, pesticides, food additives, or common foods such as peanuts**.

• **Folic acid** is important (!), but doses in excess of 15 mg per day, might trigger seizures.

OTHER HELPS
• Keep the **colon** clean. Take enemas or colonics weekly if necessary. Pressure from a clogged colon can press against the ileocecal valve and release toxins which are absorbed by the bloodstream.

• If the bowels do not move each day, take a **lemon enema** (juice of 2 lemons in 2 quarts water) before going to bed that night.

• **Hypoglycemia** is linked to convulsions. Serum glucose levels fall just before a seizure.

• Have a **hair analysis** done, to see if metal toxicity could be involved as a causal factor.

• In some instances, a **ketogentic diet** is prescribed; but, if used, it should be under the guidance of someone who understands how to apply it. This diet is keyed to restricting protein and carbohydrate intake, increasing fat intake, and producing acid levels in the bloodstream which act to inhibit brain stimulation of seizures.

J.H. KELLOGG, M.D., PRESCRIPTIONS FOR EPILEPSY AND ITS COMPLICATIONS *(how to give these water therapies: pp. 206-275 / list of treatments: pp. 206-207 / Hydrotherapy Disease Index: pp. 273-275)*

BASIC FACTORS—Abstemious, **dry, aseptic dietary**. Chiefly fruits and grains. Daily do **vigorous outdoor exercise** to the extent of fatigue. Prolonged **Neutral Bath,** daily. **Sweating process,** 2-3 times a week. Graduated **cold procedures** (Tonic Frictions), avoiding prolonged and intense applications. [**Avoid constipation in the transverse colon**: This is a key factor in avoiding attacks. Avoid doughy foods that tend to constipation.]

WHEN ATTACK IS THREATENED—**Colonic** twice daily, copious **water** drinking, **Neutral Pack, ice** to head, **rest** in bed. Seizure may sometimes be averted by placing the person in cold water.

AFTER ATTACK—Rest, **cold to head,** Cold Mitten Friction or **Cold Towel Rub, Half Bath, Revulsive Douche** (spray) to legs, and **Percussion Douche** to spine.

N
E
R
V

GENERAL METHOD—Train him to a vigorous regimen, a simple abstemious dietary, abundance of outdoor exercise, the daily employment of the Prolonged Neutral Bath. Follow by short, moderate cold applications. Copious water drinking, regulation of all the vital functions, avoiding all sources of nervous irritation and exhaustion.

—See Convulsions (573-576) and Antispasmodic Tincture (576).

ENCOURAGEMENT—Unless we depend on a power outside of ourselves, Satan will succeed in accomplishing our ruin. In looking to Jesus and obeying His Word, you will be safe. How thankful we can be, every day of our lives, for the love of God in Christ! Proverbs 20:13.

ANTISPASMODIC TINCTURE

It is best to use herb teas; but they have to be made fresh at the time. However, there are times when emergency help is needed fast, because a person is having another attack. At such times, an herbal tincture is superior, because it is instantly available.

A tincture is an extract made from herbs by soaking them in vinegar or alcohol. (Only grain alcohol should be used for internal use; wood alcohol, such as rubbing alcohol, will cause blindness.) The resultant mixture does not spoil.

When a spasm occurs, an extremely small amount of the antispasmodic tincture is given to the person (often a few drops), and he usually pulls out of the crisis quickly.

Antispasmodic tincture is used for all spasms or attacks such as those of the heart, asthma, cough, epilepsy, or shock.

The formula for this preparation, originally given by Jethro Kloss, is the one described here. This formula has been used for decades by veteran naturopaths with great success. Here is the formula:

ANTISPASMODIC TINCTURE
One-half ounce **cayenne** and 1 ounce of each of the following herbs: **skullcap**, **skunk cabbage** root or seed, **gum myrrh, lobelia** seed (or the plant if the seed is not obtainable), and **black cohosh** root.

Mix each of the above together while dry and put into a large-mouth jar. Add 1 pint pure grain alcohol of 70-100 proof. Eighty proof Vodka works fine because it is tasteless. (An alternative to alcohol is, instead, to use 1 pint of apple cider vinegar. Store in the same manner.) (Never drink isopropyl alcohol, rubbing alcohol, for it will cause blindness.)

Let this stand for 10-14 days, tightly covered, and shake well. Also shake this well everyday.

At the end of that time, strain it through a very fine cloth and squeeze out all the sediment that you can. Store most of it in a tightly capped bottle. But put some into a small dropper bottle.

In a crisis, it is given in 8-10 drop doses. It can be squirted into the mouth or taken in a tablespoon of water. (If stored in vinegar, give in teaspoonful doses, not drops. Its effects will not be quite as rapid.)

Jethro Kloss mentions a man who was released from clenched **lockjaw** by a small application of antispasmodic tincture.

When the case is severe, especially with an infant, the tincture can be rubbed onto the chest, neck, and between the shoulders. Place 2-3 drops in the mouth, and wash down with teaspoon doses of warm water while the person is kept in bed. If necessary, repeat every 1-2 hours.

There are six herbs in the formula. The **lobelia** is the active agent in relaxing the muscles and normalizing breathing. The **cayenne** warms, stimulates, and reduces inflammation. The **skullcap** and **valerian** soothe the nerves and keep small vessels from rupturing. The **skunk cabbage** and **gum myrrh** aid in reducing infection. *—Go to p. 312-313 for more on Tincture.*

COUGH SYRUP
As a cough syrup for children, prepare it in this way: Pour 1 quart water over the **herbs** mentioned above, in the same amounts. (No vinegar or alcohol is added.) Let it stand for 1 hour, then strain. Add 1 pint **honey**. Place it over low heat and let it evaporate to the equivalent of 3 cupfuls. Pour this hot syrup into hot baby-food jars and seal for future use. Give it in teaspoonful doses for **cough, asthma, convulsions, or insomnia**.

ENCOURAGEMENT—Our Lord is pleading for us in the presence of the Father, at the throne of grace in heaven. He is our only hope. Our faith looks up and grasps Him as the One able to save to the uttermost; and we are accepted by the Father. Psalm 18:30.

NEURO-MENTAL - 4 - PARALYSIS

PARALYSIS

SYMPTOMS—A rapid or partial loss of muscle function and motion or of sensation because of nerve injury or neuron destruction. A slight loss of function is called "palsy."

CAUSES—Most cases of paralysis are caused by **calcium deficiency**. Paralysis is generally classified as incurable; but no disease is incurable. The problem is due to toxic wastes in the body; and it becomes essential to cleanse the body and give it tone and a positive regeneration in order to correct the paralysis.

NATURAL REMEDIES

• Paralysis can be cleared with **cayenne** alone. Correct the cause with a **cleansing program** and the **regenerative diet**. Use **nerve tonics and antispasmodic tincture** (xxx).

Useful herbs include black cohosh, catnip, cayenne, dandelion root, ginger, goldenseal, hydrangeas, lady's slipper, pokeroot (bowels), poplar bark, prickly ash berries, red clover, red pepper, rosemary, skullcap, valerian root, vervain, wild cherry bark, and yellow dock.

Paralysis of throat: As an aid, chew ginger root often.

LOU GEHRIG'S DISEASE
(Amyotrophic Lateral Sclerosis)

SYMPTOMS—Progressive muscular weakness and atrophy, weakened respiratory muscles (which can result in pneumonia), difficulty chewing and swallowing, stiffness, cramping, and involuntary quivering of small muscles.

CAUSES—Amyotrophic lateral sclerosis (ALS) is the most common motor neuron disease, resulting in muscular atrophy.

Causes include **heredity** (10% of the cases) or **strenuous physical work** in one's occupation, combined with **nutritional deficiencies** (especially **vitamins B complex, E, F, and C**). Other factors include **viral infections, physical exhaustion, and trauma**.

Heavy metals, ingested or inhaled, can also induce damage to the nervous system.

NATURAL REMEDIES

• A nourishing diet, which includes **complete vitamin / mineral supplementation, plus fresh fruits, vegetables, and vegetable juices**.

• A **vitamin E** (800 IU) deficiency is a special factor inducing ALS.

• **Calcium** (2,000 mg), **magnesium** (1,000 mg), and **potassium** (5,500 mg) are also needed.

• **Flaxseed** (or, secondarily, wheat germ oil) is essential.

• Avoid **dairy products, meat, sugar, and white-flour products**. Doing so will accelerate healing.

— *Also see Convulsions (573-576), Strengthening the Nerves (569), Antispasmodic Tincture (576).*

J.H. KELLOGG, M.D., PRESCRIPTIONS FOR AMYOTROPHIC LATERAL SCLEROSIS AND ITS COMPLICATIONS (how to give these water therapies: pp. 206-275 / Hydrotherapy Disease Index: pp. 273-275)

BASIC APPLICATIONS—Prolonged Neutral Baths, 1-3 hours, daily. And massage.

GENERAL METHOD—Build up the general health by gentle **tonic measures** which are slowly increased in intensity, suppressing the formation of toxic substances and promoting their elimination by a suitable **dietary**, improvement of digestion, and the employment of the other measures indicated above.

By the suppression of the active causes of the disease and the adoption of better means for the **improvement of general nutrition—and especially of the nutrition of the spinal cord**—it is usually possible to arrest the disease; and, not infrequently, a considerable degree of improvement may be secured. Therapeutic measures must be most thoroughly and perseveringly employed. The progress of the disease may be delayed, even when it cannot be altogether arrested.

ENCOURAGEMENT—God's Ten Commandment law is so brief that we can easily memorize it; yet so far-reaching as to express the whole will of God for our lives. Thank God that there is a moral standard in our world, whether men like it or not. Psalm 19:7-14.

LOCOMOTOR ATAXIA
(Tabes Dorsalis)

SYMPTOMS—This is a type of brain damage in which a person cannot seem to move, or his arm or leg may be placed in a certain position and he is unable to move it.

CAUSES—Locomotor ataxia is a progressive damage to the rear portions of the spinal column. This condition is caused by earlier diseases, primarily syphilis. A man, perhaps in the prime of life, begins to have abdominal pains which he cannot account for. They increase in severity, resembling a girdle-like constriction about the trunk. Excruciating pains shoot through his legs and body. He soon finds that he cannot walk well in the dark. He loses control of his legs. He cannot control the discharges from his bladder and bowels. He becomes a helpless invalid for the rest of his life. Yet he may live on for years.

NATURAL REMEDIES

J.H. KELLOGG, M.D., PRESCRIPTIONS FOR LOCOMOTOR ATAXIA AND ITS COMPLICATIONS (how to give these water therapies: pp. 206-275 / Hydrotherapy Disease Index: pp. 273-275)

IMPROVE GENERAL NUTRITION—Careful Cold Mitten Friction or **Cold Towel Rub**. Very carefully **apply Graduated Cold Baths** and **Wet Sheet Pack**, protecting the spine by a dry towel. Follow by **Cold Mitten Friction** and Pail Pour or **Half Bath** at 85°F.

COMBAT TOXEMIA by **short sweating baths**, followed by appropriate **Graduated Cold Baths**. **Prolonged Neutral Bath**, beginning at 96°F. and daily lowering the temperature to 90°F. Increase duration from 30 minutes to 2-3 hours, daily. Copious **water** drinking and **colonic** daily.

IMPROVE NUTRITION OF SPINAL CORD—Fomentation to the spine at 110°-120°F., twice daily, with **Heating Compress** during the interval between. Thorough massage of the back, suspension or spine-stretching by flexion of the trunk upon the thighs or flexion of the thighs upon the trunk.

ATAXIC MOVEMENTS—Special exercises in small movements of each of the affected muscular groups.

LIGHTNING PAIN—Prolonged **Warm Fan Douche** to spine at 95°-100°F., 2-3 times a day (with pressure at 2-5 pounds).

N
E
R
V

GASTRIC CRISES—Very hot **Fomentation** to the abdomen several times a day, followed by **Heating Compress** when nerves of lower back are sensitive. Continue for several weeks. **Revulsive Compress** to stomach.

LOCAL PAINS—**Revulsive Compress** and Revulsive Douche, followed by **Heating Compress**.

RECTAL PAIN—Very hot **Anal Douche** at 115°-122°F., with little pressure. **Revulsive Sitz Bath**, **Fomentation** over buttocks, Hot **Colonic**.

PARESIS OF BLADDER—Daily **Colonic**. Cold **Plantar** (bottom of foot) **Douche**.

TROPHIC CHANGES - CHARCOT'S JOINTS—**Fomentation** to the parts when painful, 3 times a day, with **Heating Compress** during the intervals between. Apply mechanical support when necessary.

CONTRAINDICATIONS—Cold baths, cold applications to spine, general cold douche, very hot applications.

GENERAL METHOD—Build up his general health by gentle tonic measures, carefully avoiding such applications of cold water as are found to increase pain or aggravate other symptoms; combat the local morbid process in the spine by the above indicated measures. And restore the power of co-ordinated movement in the affected muscular groups by special gymnastic training.

ENCOURAGEMENT—Difficulties will be powerless to hinder him who is determined to seek first the kingdom of God and His righteousness. Looking to Jesus, the believer will willingly brave contempt and derision.

MENINGITIS

SYMPTOMS—Symptoms vary considerably, but usually include a sore throat, fever, headache, stiff neck, and vomiting. Children and adults can become critically ill in 6-24 hours after the first appearance of the symptoms. *This condition requires rapid diagnosis and initiation of treatment.* Take him to the emergency room immediately! Demand immediate help!

Symptoms include sore throat, red or purple skin rash, fever, chills, malaise, headaches, vomiting, sensitivity to light, nausea, delirium, stiff neck, and convulsions.

In infants: vomiting, fever, difficult feeding, irritability, a high-pitched cry, a bulging fontanel (soft spot on top of the head). Changes in temperament and extreme sleepiness indicate dangerous changes in cerebrospinal fluid.

Warning: A child with this condition can be injured when he is picked up.

CAUSES—The meninges are three membranes that cover the brain, separating it from the skull. Other membranes cover the spinal column. Meningitis is an inflammation of either one or both of them (cerebral meningitis and spinal meningitis). It is a contagious disease.

Causes include several different **viruses** (including those causing **polio, measles, rubella, fungi, yeast infection**) and several types of **bacteria**.

Infection can spread from the nose and throat to the meninges. A depleted **immune system** (along with **nose and throat trouble**) can cause it to enter the bloodstream and go to the brain.

If not properly treated, a case of **flu (an ear, nose, and throat infection)** can develop into meningitis.

Eating **heavy meals or taking drugs while sick** can cause an infection to drive deeper into the system and enter the brain area.

Other factors aiding in the development of meningitis are **alcoholism, brain surgery, brain cancer, exposure to chemical agents, head injury, pneumonia, Lyme disease, syphilis, tuberculosis**, or anything that weakens the immune system (**chemotherapy, radiation treatment, steroid therapy, HIV infection, and certain types of cancer**).

Of the three main types of meningitis, *viral infection* is more common and produces milder symptoms, such as malaise and headache, which generally clears up on its own in a week or two.

But the *bacterial type* requires prompt, aggressive treatment—or brain damage or death can result. (Any time a bacterial infection in the head or throat occurs [such as **strep throat or an ear infection**], eliminate it; do not ignore the problem.)

Fungal meningitis progresses more slowly, but also requires medical care.

Do not guess! Call a physician!

Meningitis is more common in children than adults.

If there are no complications, recovery usually takes three weeks under a physician's care.

Remember: Meningitis is contagious. Those caring for a person with this disease must be very careful to be sure to obtain adequate rest.

NATURAL REMEDIES

Meningitis can progress quickly and become life threatening in 24 hours for adults, and even quicker for children. Call a physician. If untreated, permanent brain damage and possible paralysis can result.

• *If cerebral meningitis:* Immerse back of head in warm **epsom salts solution** several times daily to draw out inflammation. Alternate **hot and cold packs** on the neck and back of the head to stimulate circulation to the area, plus Fomentations to the liver and abdomen.

• *If spinal meningitis:* Give Fomentations to the spine, liver, and abdomen.

• **Rest** in bed (with a very **dim light, at the most) in a well-ventilated** room, with no visitors. Drink plenty of clean **liquids**.

• **High enemas** are very important. The bowels must move 2-3 times a day. Use an herbal laxative if necessary. *See Herbal Laxatives (468).*

• If there is fever, take **cool sponge baths**. Use **catnip tea enemas** to reduce fever. The tea can also be sipped.

• Thorough **massage** will do a great deal to hasten recovery.

• Get some fresh **air** and early morning **sunshine** each day. Get plenty of **rest** during healing.

• **Goldenseal** and **Echinacea** are both antibiotics. But do not take either one for more than a week; you can shift from one to the other. Take 6-8 **garlic** tablets daily. *See Antibiotic Herbs (297).*

• To strengthen the nerves, take **skullcap** tea and **gotu kola**.

DIET

• It is best **not to eat food** during the acute phase. Eating food stops the elimination of toxins from the tissues, so that digestion of the food can take place. This causes toxins to be thrown still deeper into the system.

• Drink **citrus juices**, from lemons, oranges, and limes.

• When the acute phase is ended and recovery is beginning, eat a **nourishing diet of fresh fruits, vegetables, whole grains, nuts, and legumes**. Fresh **pineapple** helps reduce the infection.

• **Niacinamide** (100-500 mg daily), **vitamin A** (400 IU for children; 5,000 IU for adults), **B complex**, **vitamin B$_6$** (100 mg), vitamin B$_{12}$ (2,000 mcg.), **choline** (500 mg). **Vitamin C** (½ tsp. every hour during acute phase; reduce by ½ for maintenance until remission).

• Avoid **meat, dairy products, caffeine, and salt.** Avoid **processed, sugared, and white-flour foods**.

• Avoid **aluminum** cookware, deodorants, and other alum-containing products.

J.H. KELLOGG, M.D., PRESCRIPTIONS FOR MENINGITIS AND ITS COMPLICATIONS (*how to give these water therapies: pp. 206-275 / list of treatments: pp. 206-207 / Hydrotherapy Disease Index: pp. 273-275*)

GENERAL—Careful Cold Mitten Friction, 2-4 times daily.

COMBAT CONGESTION OF THE BRAIN AND SPINAL CORD—Ice Cap, Ice Collar, **Cooling Compress to the head**, **Ice Bag to the spine**, general derivative treatments (such as **Hot Hip Packs and Hot Leg Packs**), Hot Blanket Pack, **Hot Full Bath** at 102° F. The head should be protected by the **Ice Cap** or Ice Collar during all hot applications. **Fomentation to the spine** every 2 hours. **Spinal Ice Bag** during intervals between. Vigorous skin circulation must be maintained, with **Cold Mitten Friction**.

PREVENT BRONCHITIS—**Fomentation to the chest**, twice daily. Well-protected Heating Compress during interval between. Keep shoulders dry and well-protected while in bed. In Cold Bath, see that the water covers the shoulders. The Chest Compress must cover the shoulders.

HEADACHE—**Fomentation** to the back of the neck, **Ice Compress** to head and neck, Hot and Cold Head Compress.

PAIN IN BACK AND LEGS—**Fomentation** to back. **Hot Hip Pack**. Repeat every 4 hours or more often. Heating Compress or Ice Bag during interval between.

VOMITING—**Ice Bag** over stomach. **Hot and Cold Trunk Pack**.

DIARRHEA—**Enema** at 95°F. after each movement. During interval between, give **Cold Abdominal Compress** at 60° F., renewed every 15 minutes with **Fomentations** to the abdomen for 15 minutes, every 2 hours.

MUSCULAR RIGIDITY—**Hot Blanket Pack. Hot Full Bath**. Hot Fomentation, followed by well-protected **Heating Compress**.

HYPERESTHESIA—**Neutral Bath** at 94°-96°F.

DELIRIUM OR MANIA—Prolonged **Wet Sheet Pack**, Ice cap, or Ice Collar.

MUSCULAR SPASM—**Hot Full Bath** at 102° F. for 15-30 minutes, with Ice Cap and Ice Collar. Prolonged **Neutral Bath**. Heating Spinal Compress.

CONTRAINDICATIONS—Do not use Cold Full Baths and other general cold procedures.

GENERAL METHOD—The object to be sought, by treatment, is to relieve congestion of the brain and spinal cord by diverting as much blood as possible into the skin; hence the skin must be kept constantly warm. General cold procedures, such as the Cold Full Bath and the Cooling Pack must be avoided. Undue excitement of the brain and spinal cord during hot applications is prevented by protecting these parts by Ice Compresses and the application of an Ice Bag over the heart. Partial cold applications, as Cold Mitten Friction, should be administered several times daily to maintain vital resistance. Care should be taken to maintain surface warmth by the application of heat to the spine, legs, or other parts during the treatment so as to avoid retrostasis.

ENCOURAGEMENT—Christ calls to you, "Choose you this day whom ye will serve." There is necessity for a decided choice; for Jesus said, "You cannot serve God and mammon." We cannot have divided service, part for God and part for the devil. Give your life to God. Matthew 6:24.

MENINGOCELE
(Spina Bifida)

SYMPTOMS—A severe birth defect.

CAUSES—Technically, this is a protrusion of the membranes of the brain or spinal cord through a defect in the skull or spinal column. This severe birth defect results in exposure of the brain or spinal cord and its coverings (meninges) because of the improper formation of the vertebrae. In simple words, this means that part of the brain (or spinal cord) tissue is sticking through an opening that should not be there in the skull (or spinal column).

Death may result. Medical treatment is limited to surgery.

We cannot provide you with solutions once this has occurred. We can only tell you what would have prevented it.

N
E
R
V

NATURAL REMEDIES

PREVENTION—This birth defect is **caused by a deficiency of folic acid, B₁₂, zinc, or vitamin A** during early pregnancy.

These deficiencies may be the result of poor and inadequate nutrition or intestinal malabsorption problems in the mother.

Millions of dollars are spent on advertising junk food while the government keeps telling people they can get all the nutrients they need from the food they eat.

ENCOURAGEMENT—Christ's glory is concerned in our success. When (by faith in Him) we live for Him and obey Him, we honor and glorify Him. What a thought is this! He is our sympathizing Saviour. Yield Him your life. Psalm 147:7-8.

MENKES' SYNDROME

SYMPTOMS—Kinky, sparse, and brittle hair. Loss of hair color, arterial aneurysms, scurvy-like bone disease (ostosis), and progressive brain degeneration.

CAUSES—The current theory is that it is a genetic disease; but it is actually a malabsorption problem in early infancy.

NATURAL REMEDIES

• Give this vital trace mineral, **copper**, to the child (copper IV, at 200 ug /kg / day).

• In addition, deal with the malabsorption problems by **taking the infant or child off wheat, cow's milk, and soy milk**.

• Give **copper** orally at 1-2 mg per day, after elimination of symptoms.

Celiac disease can produce a copper deficiency, along with other deficiencies. Celiac disease is primarily caused by feeding the infant wheat products (cereal, etc.) at too early an age. *See Celiac Disease (473).*

ENCOURAGEMENT—If the sinner's heart is filled with love for Christ, it will be shown that He is stronger than the passions which have ruled him in the past, whose indulgence undermined noble impulses and left the soul to the mercy of Satan's temptations. When the heart of the sinner is touched, he yields his will to God's will. 2 Thessalonians 3:16.

MULTIPLE SCLEROSIS

SYMPTOMS—Earlier stages: occasional dizziness, mood swings or depression, numbness in the fingers and feet, weakness in the hands and feet, loss of balance, nausea and vomiting, muscular stiffness, tremors, slurred speech, and difficult breathing.

Later stages: difficulty in walking, a staggering gait. Later still: spastic movements, paralysis, extreme fatigue, and bowel and bladder incontinence.

Symptoms flare up and then nearly disappear for a time. Yet the problem keeps worsening, over a matter of weeks, but sometimes slowly over decades.

CAUSES—Multiple sclerosis (MS) is a progressive, degenerative disorder of the central nervous system. The nerves are covered with a coating called myelin. MS destroys this covering, leaving scar tissue (called *plaques*) in its place. Eventually the nerves themselves become sclerotic (hardened) and stop functioning.

Possible causes include an **autoimmune** attack on the white blood cells of the myelin sheaths, **malnutrition or poor diet, stress, possible food allergies (dairy products or gluten), metal poisoning (lead, mercury, etc.), chemicals (industrial chemicals, pesticides, etc.), toxins from bacteria and fungi in the body, and vaccinations**.

Diet appears to be a primary factor: heavy consumption of **meat, sugar, refined grains, and rancid oils**.

Overwork, emotional stress, fatigue, pregnancy, acute respiratory infections, chemical poisoning, and poor diet are known to precede the onset.

MS usually begins between 25 and 40; it is twice as often in women more than men. In America alone, 350,000 people have MS. It is the most common acquired disease of the nervous system in young adults.

There is no known cure; but suggestions, below, will help retard (and possibly halt) the progress of the disorder.

NATURAL REMEDIES

• Give attention to solving as many of the above possible dietetic and environmental causes as possible.

• Eat a **nourishing diet** with supplemental **vitamins and minerals. Fruit and vegetable juices** are important.

• Each day take **beta-carotene** (15-30 mg), **thiamine** (1.5 mg), **riboflavin** (1.8 mg), **vitamin B₆** (2-10 mg), **vitamin C** (100-500 mg), and **vitamin E** (400 IU).

• Avoid **meat, milk, eggs, dairy products, and caffeine**. Do not drink **alcohol**.

• Avoid **sugar, excess fat, white-flour, rancid oils, fried foods**—all of these destroy nerve cells.

• The **mercury fillings** in your teeth may be a factor. The levels of mercury in people with MS are seven times higher than those in other people. Get rid of your mercury fillings, if you have any symptoms of MS.

• **Massage** and regular **exercise** are helpful. Keep **mentally active**.

• Avoid emotional **stress, anxiety, and excessive fatigue**; they can bring on attacks. Avoid **smoking** and secondhand smoke. You need oxygen.

• Short **fasts** are helpful.

SPECIAL HELPS

• Roy Swank, M.D., spent 20 years studying the problem and found that a **high-saturated fat diet** makes the problem worse. It is important you only maintain a low-fat, unsaturated fat diet (2 Tbsp. daily of raw **flaxseed oil**, and no other oil). Also take 1 tsp. granulated **lecithin** daily.

• Take **magnesium** (375 mg daily). **Purslane** is the herb richest in magnesium (2% on dry weight basis), followed by **poppy seeds** and **cowpeas**. Steam purslane or eat it raw in salads.

• **Black currant oil** contains *gamma-linolenic acid* GLA), useful in treating MS. GLA is good for all autoimmune disease *(857)*. GLA is also in **borage** and **evening primrose oil**. Evening primrose oil is very good for MS.

• **Blueberries** contain *oligomeric procyanidins* (OPCs), which help prevent myelin sheath destruction. They also relieve anti-inflammatory activity in MS.

• **Pineapple** contains *pancreatin* and *bromelain*, two enzymes which break up protein molecules in the stomach so they can be digested better. These enzymes also reduce *circulating immune complexes* (CICs), which occur in several autoimmune diseases. The CICs activate the immune system to attack the body.

• **Ginkgo biloba** contains several unique terpene molecules *(ginkgolides)* which reduce MS, inflammation, and allergic processes in autoimmune diseases. Take ginkgo biloba extract (24% concentrate; 40-80 mg. 3 times daily).

• **Chelation therapy** *(869)* may be able to help multiple sclerosis.

• **Hyperbaric oxygen therapy** has been used successfully in some other countries (outside the U.S.).

• Here is folk medicine which has helped many people: They find **stinging nettle** plants and, handling them with gloves, slap it against exposed skin. This places the tiny, hair-like stingers into the skin and gives microinjections of several beneficial chemicals, including histamine (the chemical that often induces allergies such as hay fever). Another method is to get stung by **honey bees**. Both methods include similar helpful chemicals which can help the condition, but will not cure it. The nettles keep regenerating new leaves.

• Take **sunbaths** and **vitamin D**. The disease occurs more frequently in localities farther away from the equator (northern Europe has more cases than southern Europe).

• Other helpful herbs include **ginkgo, suma, gotu kola, kelp, hops, chamomile, skullcap, and valerian**.

• Some researchers believe **mercury** poisoning is a significant cause of MS. Get rid of your **amalgam** dental fillings.

ENCOURAGEMENT—There is no mystery in the law of God. All can comprehend the great truths which it embodies. Everyone can grasp its rules. Obedience to the law is essential for our own happiness and the happiness of all with whom we are connected, not only for our salvation. But only in Christ's enabling strength can we render that obedience.

MUSCULAR DYSTROPHY

SYMPTOMS—Weakness of the muscles, scoliosis (curvature of the spine), enlargement of certain muscle groups (calves, trapezius, etc.) to compensate for loss of major muscle groups. The muscles gradually shrivel and weaken. The muscles in the trunk are especially affected. All muscles eventually become involved.

CAUSES—Muscular dystrophy (MD) produces a weakening and wasting of muscle tissue which is not noticed (because of replacement of muscle tissue with fat and fibrous scar tissue) until there is substantial damage.

Animals given a **vitamin E**-deficient diet develop muscular dystrophy. It is believed that MD could be wiped out if vitamin E were given to all expectant mothers and bottle-fed babies. **Mother's milk** has six times as much vitamin E as cow's milk; and this is almost twice as much **selenium**.

There may be a hereditary factor; but diet is still the crucial issue.

NATURAL REMEDIES

• **Vitamin E** and **selenium** should be given orally, intramuscularly, and intravenously at the very outset of the disorder in order to arrest it. Vitamin E: intramuscularly at 80 mg per day; orally at 800-1,200 daily. Selenium: orally, intravenously, and intramuscularly at 50-1,000 mcg per day, based on weight.

• **Essential fatty acids** are needed (5 gm daily; 2 Tbsp. flaxseed oil). Also **choline** or soy **lecithin**, at 10-20 gm per day.

• Avoid **food allergens** and **excessive fats**; no more than 20% of daily calories should be in fat.

• Avoid **exercise** for one month during initial treatment period, to avoid undue injury to already weakened muscles.

—Also see Birth Defects (724-727).

ENCOURAGEMENT—Battles are to be fought everyday. A great warfare is going on over every soul, between the prince of darkness and the Prince of life. And you and I are in the middle of it. We must stand true to God; and we do this by continually choosing to remain submissive to His will. No one but your own choice can remove you from Christ's protection.

MYASTHENIA GRAVIS

SYMPTOMS—Muscular weakness, fatigue, emotional stress, and droopy eyelids. Difficulty in breathing, swallowing, and speaking.

The onset is gradual; and the symptoms are worse in the evening. The person complains of difficulty in chewing, swallowing, and talking.

CAUSES—Myasthenia gravis is a disease characterized by great muscular weakness (without atrophy) and progressive fatigability. The name means "muscle weakness."

Adolescents and young adults, especially women, are the most likely to have this problem. But it sometimes occurs in newborn infants and adults over 40. In the latter case, a **tumor in the thymus** is involved. It rarely occurs past 50.

The muscles of the face and neck are primarily involved; but those in the trunk and extremities may also be involved. Some cases are mild; others rapidly become fatal. When the respiratory system is involved, death is much more likely to result from this disease. Progress of the disorder is variable; and prolonged remission may occur.

It is thought to be an autoimmune disease that causes malfunctioning of an enzyme (*acetylcholine*) which is responsible for inducing muscles to contract. (It is conjectured that there may also be an excess of *cholinesterase* at the myoneural junction, causing nerve impulses to fail to induce normal muscle contractions; but this is less likely.)

There is a failure in transmission of nerve impulses at the neuromuscular junction. Either the acetylcholine release is not adequate or the muscle response to the acetylcholine is not sufficient. An autoimmune factor may be involved (*i.e.*, there are so many toxins in the body, that the system interferes with normal functions.)

Autointoxication may thus be a primary cause. **Toxins** accumulate in the bloodstream from **chemicals, chronic constipation, etc**. They destroy the muscular system or trigger other body systems to do so.

Chronic **constipation** can cause the cecum to press against the ileocecal valve, releasing poisons of the colon back into the small intestine. This is a dangerous situation, since toxins in the small intestine are absorbed into the blood far more quickly than when they are in the colon.

NATURAL REMEDIES

• Clean out the colon, by means of **colonics or high enemas**. Go on a **fruit / vegetable juice fast** for several days.

• Begin eating a **nourishing diet, not overeating**, and always including an abundant amount of roughage (to aid in preventing constipation). Drink enough **fluids**.

• A deficiency in **vitamin A** can produce muscular and spinal cord degeneration. It is best taken in the form of carotenes (carrot juice, and green and yellow vegetables). Also important for the nerves and muscles are vitamin B complex, vitamin C (1,000 mg), vitamin E (400 IU), Calcium (2,000 mg), magnesium (1,000 mg), potassium (5,500 mg), manganese (50 mg), and zinc (30 mg).

• **Lecithin** is very important for good nerves, as well as chlorophyll.

• Good foods include **buckwheat, millet, rye, and red potato peeling broth**.

• Avoid the solanaceous crops; for they contain *solanine*, which interferes with the neurotransmitter, *acetylcholine*. These foods include **tomatoes, white potatoes, green and red peppers, eggplants, and tobacco**.

• Avoid the glue foods, such as **white flour and dairy products**. Stay away from **fried foods, meat, all animal fats, cheese, and eggs**.

• **Do not overwork**. Learn to relax; learn to work at a more moderate pace and stop more frequently to rest.

• **Walk** a little outdoors and gradually build up. But do not overdo. A little walking is good; too much of any exercise might not be.

• Helpful herbs include **slippery elm, comfrey, oatstraw, and the nervine herbs: skullcap, hops, chamomile, valerian, dong quai, wood betony,** and small amounts of **lobelia**.

—*Also see Parkinson's Disease (below)*.

ENCOURAGEMENT—The world that Satan has claimed and has ruled over with cruel tyranny, the son of God has, by one vast achievement, encircled in His love and connected again with the throne of God. Thank your heavenly Father for what He offers you! And accept it now, right now. Colossians 3:15.

PARKINSON'S DISEASE
(Shaking Palsy, Paralysis Agitans, and Parkinsonism)

SYMPTOMS—Initially: mild to moderate tremor of the hand or hands while at rest, a feeling of being slow and heavy, tendency to tire more easily, muscular stiffness, loss of skill in the fingers and thumb (writing, buttoning and unbuttoning, playing the piano, etc.)

Later: depression, loss of appetite, muscular rigidity, permanent rigid stoop, shuffling gait, drooling, tremors, fixed facial expression, and impaired speech. Ability to maintain balance may be affected.

The body gradually becomes rigid as limbs stiffen. Dementia may occur.

Principal signs are tremor at rest, muscle rigidity, and slow or retarded movement. Tremors and slowness generally begin in one limb, then progress to the other limb on the same side; later still to the other side. Usually the hands are affected before the feet.

CAUSES—Parkinson's disease is a gradual degeneration of the nervous system. The nerve cells in the basal ganglion of the brain are gradually destroyed.

Parkinson's disease is one of the most common debilitating diseases in the United States (over 450,000 have it). But actual disability usually does not occur for 10-15 years after onset of symptoms. Most of those with it are over 60. More men have it than women.

Although the underlying cause is not known, symptoms appear when there is a lack of *dopamine* in the brain. Dopamine is made by the body; it carries messages from one nerve cell to another. Normally, another neurotransmitter, *acetylcholine*, is made, to keep dopamine in balance. When there is not enough acetylcholine, myasthenia gravis *(582)* occurs; when there is not enough dopamine, the result is Parkinson's disease.

In Parkinson's, the problem generally is destruction of the cells which make dopamine. But sometimes the cause is blockage of the dopamine receptors in the brain.

One possible cause of this disorder is that too many **toxins** have been released in the body for the blood to filter out through the liver. An excess of **chemicals, drugs, toxins in meat eating**, etc., are thought to be involved. It is known that one of the chemicals in **heroin** directly destroys the key brain cells which prevent Parkinson's. A **chronic poor diet**, over many years, is also considered to be a significant factor.

NATURAL REMEDIES

• It is very important that the person afflicted with Parkinson's disease **keep active**. Muscles which are not used atrophy more quickly. The person's own determination and faithfulness in an **exercise program** will forestall the progress of the disease better than almost anything else. Every exercise keeps the muscles more useful. Use a wide variety of simple exercises! Buy a book on weight lifting; but, of course, use much smaller weights. Swing the arms forcefully when walking. Exercises involving **joint movements** (including the neck) are very important.

• Keep the feet a distance apart, when **walking**, and take short steps when turning.

• **Typing, writing, working with clay**, etc., helps the fingers.

• **Breathe deeply** in and out.

• Take frequent **rest** periods.

• **Read aloud**, to keep the mouth muscles in good condition.

• **Any act difficult to perform** should be done daily.

• **Overweight** is a problem; take the extra off.

• **Chelation therapy** *(869)* may be able to help Parkinson's.

DIET

• A **nutritious diet**, adequate rest, exercise in the open air, enough **fluids**, and **sunlight** help slow the effects of Parkinson's disease.

• *Octocosanol* is found in **wheat germ oil**. It helps the neuron membranes.

• Eat foods and take supplements containing **antioxidants** *(921)*. The most important of these is **vitamin E** (3,200 IU daily!) and **vitamin C** (3,000 mg daily!). This can slow the progression of Parkinson's disease by 2-3 years! Theoretically, a person who takes significant dosage levels will never contract Parkinson's disease in the first place. It appears that free-radical damage may be a major cause of damage in dopamine-producing brain cells.

• Take **coenzyme Q$_{10}$** (200 mg), **thiamine** (5,000 mg), **zinc** (30 mg), and **vitamin B$_{12}$** (100 mcg).

• **Iron** supplementation seems to help in some cases. The production of tyrosine, an enzyme involved in *dopa* production (the precursor of dopamine), is stimulated by iron supplementation in the diet.

• Here are some additional helps and dosages of worthwhile natural substances: **octocosanol** (300 mcg, three times a day), **Neuro-Gen leucine** (10 gm / day), l-methionine (5 gm / day), **essential fatty acids** (1 Tbsp, twice a day), **l-tyrosine** (100 mg / day), **dl-phenoalanine** (100 mg, three times a day), **vitamin B$_1$** (200 mg, 3 times a day), **vitamin B$_6$** (100 mg, 3 times a day), **betaine HCl** (75-200 mg, 3 times a day before meals).

• **Fava beans** *(vicia faba)* have more natural L-dopa than any other plant food. It takes about a 16-oz. can of fava beans to provide enough L-dopa to have a physiological effect on Parkinson's. It has recently been discovered that **fava bean sprouts** contain ten times more L-dopa than the unsprouted beans. Begin eating them at the earliest stages of the disease!

• **Velvet beans** (*Mucuna*, various species) also contain large amounts of L-dopa.

HERBS

• **Ginkgo biloba** is widely used in treating Alzheimer's, stroke recovery, and also useful for Parkinson's.

• **St. John's wort** inhibits an enzyme which interferes with the release of dopamine in the brain. Take 20-30 drops St. John's Wort tincture daily.

• **Passionflower** contains two reportedly effective anti-parkinson's compounds: harmaline and harmine alkaloids. Take 10-30 drops 3 times daily of the standardized tincture.

• **Evening primrose oil** (EPO) improved Parkinson's-induced tremors in 55% of those who took 2 tsp. a day for several months.

• Put 20 grams of **Larkspur** in 4 cups boiling water. Drink mouthfuls at a time, but not over 3 cups daily.

• **Lady's slipper** reduces tremors and depression. Take 3-9 grams of the tincture. Combine **skullcap** with lady's slipper for better results.

• Ingestion of **aluminum** is a factor in Alzheimer's

disease; and it may also be involved in Parkinson's disease. Do not use **aluminum cookware** or **deodorants** containing it (**alum** is aluminum). Also avoid **lead**. Some people with Parkinson's disease have high levels of lead in their brains.

• Avoid **processed food, coffee, caffeinated tea, sugar, and tobacco.**

L-dopa *(L-dihydroxyphenylalanine)*, in the form of the drug brand, Levodopa, is a synthetic dopamine which is given to patients to supply the missing dopamine. Intriguingly enough, actual dopamine (from animal sources) cannot be given, because there is a blood-brain barrier rejecting it. So Levodopa is given, which is accepted (through conversion to dopamine in the basal ganglion). But two facts should be noted: (1) **Vitamin B₆** reverses the effects of Levodopa, so efforts must be made to eliminate B₆ from the diet. (Eat in moderation bananas, oatmeal, peanuts, whole grains, potatoes, meat, and fish; and only eat protein foods in the evening.) (2) Levodopa usually produces side effects, such as nausea, vomiting, insomnia, mental confusion, and agitation, as well as liver and kidney damage. L-dopa and carbidopa can aggravate and speed up the progress of Parkinson's disease in many cases; they are said to have little beneficial effect in over half the cases.

ENCOURAGEMENT—Man's happiness must always be guarded by the law of God. That law is the hedge which God has placed about His vineyard. By it those who obey are protected from evil. But only through Christ's enabling merits can you be empowered to obey the Ten Commandments. John 14:27.

POLIO
(Poliomyelitis, Infantile Paralysis)

SYMPTOMS—Fever, nausea, diarrhea, headache, and irritability.

Incubation is generally 2-7 days; and the onset is often abrupt. There may be digestive disturbance, plus a slight elevation of temperature, usually for not more than 3 days. Then paralysis may, or may not, develop.

Bend the person's neck forward, down toward the chest. If it aches, polio may be coming on.

CAUSES—Poliomyelitis means "gray marrow," and is inflammation of the gray matter of the spinal cord. The condition is not confined to infancy, nor is paralysis always involved. Polio is a viral infection of the spinal cord which destroys the nerves controlling muscular movement, often resulting in paralysis of certain muscles.

The first of two stages of polio is the infectious stage, when the virus is active. The second is the noninfectious stage, when recovery may occur.

Paralysis may be confined to a small part of the body—or much, or nearly all of it. But muscle atrophy may also occur. Death generally occurs only in bulbar and respiratory cases. Aside from bronchopneumonia, other complications are relatively few.

Epidemics, when they occur, usually reach their peak during the warmest months (July and August).

In the late 1940s, Benjamin Sandler, M.D., was interviewed on the radio in the spring, just before the summer polio season. He declared that if **sugar foods**—and especially **cola drinks and other soft drinks**—were avoided, polio would not be contracted. This went into the newspapers; and the East Coast area covered by the announcement had very little polio that summer. Later, Sandler wrote a book detailing his concept.

Sugar injures the nerves. Calcium is needed by the nerves; but highly **acid** substances remove calcium. **Phosphorous** locks with calcium and carries it off, making it unavailable. **Coca Cola-type drinks** combine all these special qualities! The liquid in Coke is more acid than vinegar; yet it is not noticed because of the very high sugar content. Coke is phosphoric acid. So the sugar and acid eat away the calcium; and the phosphorus immediately locks into it. A tooth, dropped in a glass of Coke, will entirely melt away in a matter of hours.

Another factor is being **cold**. People drink Cokes and other soft drinks at swimming pools, then jump in and vigorously swim in the cold water. Because many people contract polio at swimming pools in the summer, it is suspected that there must be something in the pool water. But the problem is the soft drinks, not contaminated pool water. The body is adapted to the intense heat of mid-summer; but poor diet plus soft drinks weaken it, then the cold plunge intensifies the effects.

Franklin D. Roosevelt was very athletic. He fought a forest fire near his home, ate some junk food, and jumped in an ice-cold river to cool off. He then came down with polio.

Because it was so dangerous to the health, Coca Cola was banned from interstate commerce by the original Food and Drug Administration early in the 20th century. That is why, to this day, Cokes and Pepsi's are made in local bottling plants. Only the syrup is shipped interstate. At the local plant the syrup and water are poured into bottles.

PREVENTIVES

• Do not drink cola drinks. Do not drink other soft drinks. Avoid sugar foods. Only eat nutritious food. Do not become chilled when fatigued from work or play.

• Medical history reveals that people who rarely contracted polio were vegetarians, did not eat junk foods, drink soft drinks, avoided polio vaccines, and lived clean lives.

NATURAL REMEDIES

• As soon as a person comes down with polio, the standard medical routine is to place him in bed and observe him to see if polio develops. —But, what should be done is to **place him immediately in a warm, full bathtub**, or better, give him the **"Kenny packs."**

• Nurse Kenny (called Sister Kenny, because nurses in Australia are called "sister") applied **hot packs** to polio patients (covering parts, or all, of their bodies), and eliminated polio with few or no aftereffects. But this water therapy method was not permitted in America. Only the medical association knows why.

Other factors:

• During the infectious stage, **keep the diet high in protein and potassium**, to replace that which is lost because of tissue destruction.

• **Fluid, caloric, and sodium intake** should also be increased because of the fever. Additional **B vitamins** are needed, along with **vitamin A (carrot juice** and/or 5,000 IU vitamin A), and **vitamin C** (2,000-5,000 or more mg.)

• Give antispasmodic tincture *(242)* doses (according to age) of 8-15 drops in ¼ glass of hot water.

• Helpful herbs include **prickly ash berries, wild cherry bark, valerian root, skullcap, goldenseal, black cohosh, red clover, catnip, and yellow dock**.

• Dr. Salk, himself (developer of injectable polio vaccine), warned against the serious dangers in taking oral polio vaccine! **Beware of oral polio vaccine!** In the latter part of the 20th century, oral polio vaccine has produced more cases of polio than any other agency.

• In addition, there is extreme danger in handling the bowel movement of an infant who has received the oral polio vaccine! You can get crippling polio from doing so.

ENCOURAGEMENT—The way of salvation has been opened to the fallen race on Planet Earth. That salvation is offered to you, right now. It is yours to claim as you accept Christ and let Him strengthen you, to obey the precepts in the Bible. Psalm 86:5, 7.

POST-POLIO SYNDROME

SYMPTOMS—Difficulty in swallowing, which could produce a risk of choking. A progressive muscle weakness.

CAUSES—More than 125,000 Americans have post-polio syndrome.

NATURAL REMEDIES

• A **cleansing diet**, followed by a **rebuilding, nourishing diet**. Avoid all the junk foods.

• Eat foods high in **fiber** and **vitamin / mineral** supplementation. **Calcium** (2,000 mg), **magnesium** (1,000 mg), **potassium** (5,500 mg) are important. **Selenium** (500 mg) **and zinc** (30 mg), **along with vitamins A** (5,000 mg), **C** (2,000 mg), **D** (1,000 IU), **and E** (400-600 IU) are antioxidants. The **B complex**

is important for strengthening the nerves.

• A regular **exercise** program.

—*Also see Polio (584) and Strengthening the Nerves (569).*

ENCOURAGEMENT—There are many battles to be fought, but our part is to cling to Christ as little children, pleading for His help. He will enable you to come off more than conqueror in the battles with temptation and sin. Trusting in Him, we can do all things through Christ who strengthens us. Matthew 6:26.

CREUTZFELDT-JACOB DISEASE
(Mad Cow Disease, Kuru)

SYMPTOMS—Ataxia (balance problems) and decreased coordination progressing to paralysis, dementia, slurring of speech, and visual disturbances.

CAUSE AND PREVENTION—Creutzfeldt-Jacob Disease (CJD or Kuru) is a slow, progressive, fatal viral infection of the central nervous system. The incubation period may be 7 to 30 years; but death usually occurs within months of the onset of symptoms. This is also called Mad Cow Disease.

There are only four classes of people who contract kuru: (1) cannibals, particularly in the central New Guinea highlands. (2) Those who submit to **transplant surgery**. (3) Those who take **raw hormones or glandulars**. And (4) **those that eat beef, pork, chicken, or fish which has been fed regular animal feed** (which contains dead, diseased animals and/or animal blood). **IMPORTANT:** *Read page 747. The problem is that livestock in America, Britain, and some other nations, are regularly fed rations containing dead, diseased animals—thus causing the cows, etc., to become cannibals. We eat them and the prions (cause of Kuru) are passed on to us.*

The condition is frequently (erroneously) diagnosed as being Alzheimer's Disease, so a reading of that disorder *(587)* will provide you additional symptoms. —*See Mad Cow Disease (585, 813, 816) for much more information. Also see the author's book, International Meat Crisis, for extensive facts.* Once contracted, there is no cure for this condition.

ENCOURAGEMENT—We owe to Christ all that makes life desirable; and He asks of us the affections of the heart and the obedience of the life. His precepts, if obeyed, will bring happiness into the home life, happiness to every individual. John 17:15.

NEURO-MENTAL -
5 - MEMORY PROBLEMS

MEMORY IMPROVEMENT

NERV

NATURAL REMEDIES

IMPROVING YOUR MEMORY

Here are several suggestions to help you remember (if you can remember them long enough to try them):

• The **attitude** toward remembering is important. As we get older, it is easier to become lazy about trying to learn.

• **Pay attention** to what you want to remember. Sometimes we are too busy or indolent to really give our attention to what we need to remember.

• An outstanding way to remember something is to **say it out aloud** to yourself. When you do this, you both speak it and hear it. If it is written down and you do this—you see it, speak it, and hear it.

• An equally outstanding way to memorize something (or teach it to children) is to **say it over several times**. Saying it, speaking it, hearing it, and repetition are powerful ways to learn math tables and other things.

Here are additional suggestions:

• **Categorize the items** you want to remember. List what you need to remember under their logical categories, and you will be more likely to remember the main points and the subsidiary ones.

• When you set your glasses down on a table where you do not usually place them, **take a good look at them and think** about what you have done.

• As you walk away from your car in a mall parking lot, **say (out loud to yourself) aspects of the location**, so you can return to it.

• When trying to remember someone's name, **take a good look at their face** as you think of, or **speak, their name**.

• When trying to remember numbers, **put them into units or chunks**. It is harder to remember 6-8-7-2-5-0-9 than it is to recall 687-2509.

• If you are trying to memorize a new word (or how to spell it), **learn the meaning** of the word and make it part of your everyday vocabulary. Or **write it down** several times.

• **Associate** a new word or name with a similar word or an object.

• **Select** the most important things to remember and skip the rest.

• **Quiz** yourself on what you are supposed to remember before you come to the time when you have to use that knowledge.

• **Avoid stress**. When you are under tension or in a time schedule, it is harder to remember things.

• Of course, you can also **jot down lists** on paper. Some people quickly write notes on the palm of their hand.

• And, of course, make sure you are eating a **good diet**, skipping the **junk food**, getting **fresh air** and **exercise** everyday, and getting enough **rest** at night.

• **Ginkgo** is the best single herb for improving memory and safeguarding brain power. **Blue cohosh,**

gotu kola, ginseng, blessed thistle, and mullein oil also increase brain and memory function.

• **Valerian** (taken at bedtime) improves sleep. **Melatonin** (taken 2 hours or less before bedtime) also does.

• There are other nutrition and lifestyle factors which also affect your memory. *See Strengthening the Nerves (569) and Memory Problems (below).*

ENCOURAGEMENT—How much should those rejoice who are the objects of such amazing love! Christ loved you, or He would not have died to forgive your sins and enable you to obey His Father's law. Accept His great salvation for you; and rejoice that your name is written in heaven. Ephesians 2:18.

"He became the author of eternal salvation unto all them that obey Him." Hebrews 5:9. Those who obey the Word of God will inherit eternal life.

MEMORY PROBLEMS
(Forgetfulness)

SYMPTOMS—You find you are forgetting too many things.

CAUSES—People fear memory problems, because it might indicate the onset of Alzheimer's disease *(587)*. Alzheimer's generally begins gradually in the mid-40s, and is fairly common among many older people; so folk have reason to be concerned.

But two facts stand out: Some memory loss does not have to mean Alzheimer's; it is possible to keep the mind in good shape, even into advanced age.

Alcoholism, aging, candidiasis, stress, allergies, thyroid problems, hypoglycemia, diabetes, and poor circulation are factors in memory loss. Others are cited below.

• Memory loss can also be caused by senile dementia *(589)*, Korsakoff's Syndrome *(587)*, Alzheimer's disease *(587)*, allergies *(848)*, or alcoholism *(821-823)*.

NATURAL REMEDIES

• Avoid the problems listed above.

DIET

• Eat a **nourishing, balanced diet** and skip all the **junk, processed, and fried foods**. Good food is needed to nourish the brain.

• Nutritional deficiencies, especially of the **B complex** and **amino acids**, add to memory loss. Obtain your protein from **brewer's yeast, brown rice, millet, nuts, soy, and whole grains** rather than from meat sources.

• Maintain an even amount of blood sugar. This is best done by eating **complex carbohydrates** (cereals and bread instead of sugar foods) at mealtime. And **no food between meals**.

• Avoid **greasy and high-cholesterol foods**; both

interfere with passage of food through the blood to the brain.

• Avoid **free radicals** in the diet; these can greatly damage brain memory. *See Antioxidants (921).*

• Avoid **refined sugars**; these reduce brain power.

• For some people, **dairy and wheat products** cause memory reduction. Try cutting them out for a month and see if there is improvement.

• Drink enough **water**. Get enough **rest** at night. **Exercise** regularly.

• Stop using **liquor, drugs, caffeine, and tobacco**. Alcohol does an excellent job of destroying the brain.

HERBS

• **Ginkgo biloba** increases blood flow to the brain. Other helpful herbs include **ginseng, anise, and blue cohosh**.

• **Boron** (3 mg daily) improves memory function. **Pycnogenol** (60 mg, 3 times daily) and **selenium** (200 mcg daily) protect brain cells from free-radical damage. **Melatonin** (2-3 mg daily, taken 2 hours or less before bedtime) improves sleep and brain function.

—*Also see Memory Improvement (586), Korsakoff's Syndrome (below), and Alzheimer's Disease (below).*

ENCOURAGEMENT—We owe to Christ all that we have. In requiring obedience to the laws of His kingdom, God gives His people health, happiness, peace, and joy. The more fully we obey, through faith in Christ, the happier we shall be. Galatians 6:14.

KORSAKOFF'S SYNDROME
(Recent Memory Loss, False Alzheimer's Disease)

SYMPTOMS—Inability to keep new events or facts in the memory, although earlier data already in the memory is still there.

CAUSES—This is a type of "amnesia" which can result from **chronic alcoholism, a blow to the head, or vitamin B$_1$ deficiency**.

Because of embarrassment, people with this problem tend to make up stories and invent "facts," to satisfy others.

If caused by a blow to the head, recovery is much easier; but the problem is less likely to be reversed if **alcoholism** or **B$_1$ deficiency** is the cause.

Memory loss can also be caused by senile dementia *(589)*, Alzheimer's disease *(below)*, allergies *(848)*, or alcoholism *(23, 170, 608, 775-777)*.

NATURAL REMEDIES

• Three times a day, take **vitamin B$_1$** (100 mg), lecithin (2,500 mg), **chromium / vanadium** (50-200 mcg), **selenium** (200-1,000 mcg), and **betaine HCl**.

• Obtain adequate **rest, exercise, water, and fresh air**.

• Do **pulse tests** *(575)*, to determine allergies. Avoid **sugar and alcohol**.

ENCOURAGEMENT—Christ will be with you in the daily battle with self, that you may be true to principle. The appetites and passions may be controlled as you rely on Him for help. Jesus has been over the ground; and He knows the temptations you must meet. He knows how to guide you through them.

ALZHEIMER'S DISEASE

SYMPTOMS—Disoriented perceptions of space and time, inability to concentrate or communicate, and memory loss.

This produces depression, agitation, withdrawal, insomnia, irritability, memory loss, personality changes, severe mood swings, and senility.

An intriguing early warning sign has been discovered at the San Diego Medical Center: As much as 2 years before mental decline, those with Alzheimer's begin to lose their sense of smell. The rate at which the ability to distinguish strong odors is an indicator of how rapidly an individual will lose mental functioning. (But smokers have already lost part of their sense smell; so the diagnostic test does not work as well when applied to them.)

CAUSES—Alzheimer's disease is a progressive mental deterioration. Memory and thought processes are weakened and disoriented. First described by Alois Alzheimer in 1906, it is a condition of gradual deterioration of the ability to think. It is a slow, progressive wasting of the brain. It gradually shuts off production of vital neurotransmitters such as acetylcholine, serotonin, dopamine, GABA, noradrenalin and glutamate.

Nerve fibers, leading into, and out of, the hippocampus in the brain become tangled and short circuited. As a result, information is no longer carried to, and from, the brain. New memories cannot be gained and old memories cannot be retrieved.

In addition, plaques of a certain protein *(beta-amyloid)* build up in the brain, damaging nerve cells.

One form of Alzheimer's occurs between 36 and 45; it is quite rapid. The more gradual form develops in those who are 65 or 70. Alzheimer's strikes about 5% of those who reach 65 and over 20% of those who reach 85.

Simple forgetfulness is not Alzheimer's. If you do not remember your wife's name, that is forgetfulness; if you forget you have a wife, that is dementia (of which Alzheimer's is a form).

There are other disorders which produce similar symptoms: a series of minor strokes *(529)*, hypothyroidism *(659)*, advanced syphilis *(804)*. Arteriosclerosis *(523, hardening of the arteries)* slowly reduces blood flow to the brain. Some of those with **Down's Syndrome** *(726)*, who live to be in their 30s or 40s, develop Alzheimer's.

NATURAL REMEDIES

The following suggestions deal with ways to prevent Alzheimer's, which will also help retard its

NERV

development:

• Many elderly people are taking 8 or 10 **medicinal drugs**. This drugging will surely affect the brain. You can see the effects in nursing homes across the continent. Added to this is a devitalized diet of **fried, processed, and junk foods**.

DIET

• **Folic acid** (5 mg daily) helps control homocysteine levels (which become too high in Alzheimer's).

• Adequate intake of **calcium** (1,500 mg daily) reduces aluminum absorption. **Magnesium** (800 mg daily) works with calcium. Include plenty of **fiber**.

• **Vitamins A and E** are antioxidant vitamins which are also important. In addition to shielding neurons from free radicals, **vitamin E** (400-800 IU) also regenerates areas on neurons where neurotransmitters enter. (*Neurotransmitters* are chemicals that relay messages from one neuron to another.) Vitamin C (500-1,000 mg daily) and Flaxseed oil (1 Tbsp. daily) is needed.

• Those with Alzheimer's have low levels of **vitamin B_{12}** and **zinc** (30 mg) in their bodies. All the **B complex** vitamins are important. Take thiamine (3-8 grams daily).

• Those who undergo a trial of intensive **nutritional therapy**, especially **B_{12} injections**, may ward off the developing problem.

• **Coenzyme Q_{10}** (200 mg daily) is vital for producing energy in neurons and throughout the body.

• Those with Alzheimer's tend to have a strong craving for **sweets**. But such a craving is frequently an indication of a food hunger for **vitamins and minerals, especially calcium**.

• **Free radicals** are another factor. Avoid foods which contain them.

HEAVY METALS

• Other causes include **heavy metals** in the body. One in particular stands out: When you hear the words, "Alzheimer's disease," think of it as "**aluminum disease**"; for this is what it often is. Autopsies on persons who died with Alzheimer's reveal accumulations of up to 10 times the normal amount of aluminum in the nerve cells of the brain (up to 50 times in certain parts). Significantly, especially high concentrations are in, and around, the hippocampus. Rats given aluminum develop identical symptoms to Alzheimer's. *See Aluminum Poisoning (871) for more information.*

• Do not use **aluminum cookware**! Use stainless steel or glass. Do not use **aluminum foil** on food. Do not take **buffered aspirin and certain antacids**; both are extremely high in aluminum! Drink **distilled water** instead of tap water (which may contain aluminum).

• But those with Alzheimer's also have high levels of **mercury** in their brain. Beware of **amalgam** dental fillings. Mercury from the fillings gradually passes into the body and, over a period of time, accumulates in the brain.

• **Zinc** may be another problem mineral. Recent lab research indicates that zinc, alone of 26 metals tested, made human proteins clump together and form *amyloid*, the destructive substance that builds up in the brains of Alzheimer's patients.

OTHER POINTS

• Stop using **alcohol, tobacco, and nicotine**. Smoking doubles the risk of getting Alzheimer's.

• Women with Alzheimer's have lower **estrogen** levels than normal.

• **Docosahexaenoic acid** (DHA) is a fat which helps retain brain function. (Do not mistake it for DHEA, a hormone.) Take 100 mg of DHA (which is manufactured from microalgae) daily.

• **Chelation therapy** (869) may be able to help Alzheimer's patients.

HERBS

• **Ginkgo biloba** is one of the best herbs for preserving memory. *See Memory Improvement (592) and Memory Problems (586).* Many studies have been done on ginkgo biloba extract. It helps delay mental deterioration in the early stages of Alzheimer's; but, in later stages, it has been found to be of little value.

• The Chinese use **Asian ginseng** (100-200 mg daily of the standardized extract), **Siberian ginseng** (2-3 grams daily of the dried root or 300-400 mg of solid extract), and **astragalus** (2-3 500 mg capsules, 3 times a day) for maintaining memory functions.

• **St. John's wort** helps calm people who anger easily, which sometimes occurs in later stages of Alzheimer's.

*—Also see Memory Problems (586) and Senility (589). **Also Special Report (815-817)***

ACETYLCHOLINE

In the early 1990s, it was discovered that Alzheimer's can be slowed if a chemical, *acetylcholine* (normally in the brain) is kept from being destroyed. This chemical is a neurotransmitter important for memory in the brain. The drug used to preserve that chemical damages the liver. But several herbs help protect acetylcholine.

• **Rosemary** not only contains several compounds which attack free radicals, but also some which prevent the breakdown of acetylcholine. Rosemary has, for a long time, been used as a "memory enhancing" herb.

• The Chinese herb, **club moss**, contains *huperzine A*, which blocks the breakdown of acetylcholine.

• **Horsebalm** (*Monarda, various species*) contains carvacrol, which helps keep acetylcholine in the brain. In addition to swallowing it, some recommend rubbing it on the scalp.

• **Choline**, a B vitamin, is one of several important building blocks for acetylcholine. The richest sources of choline are **blackstrap molasses** and **lecithin**. Levels of **choline** and **ethanolamine** are lower in those with Alzheimer's.

IMPORTANT !! —There is now evidence that eating **beef, pork, chicken, or fish which have been fed regular animal feed** (which contains dead, diseased animals) can produce *Creutzfeldt-Jakob disease,* the symptoms of which are *essentially identical* to those of Alzheimer's. **IMPORTANT:** *Read pages 585, 813.*

LIVING WITH ALZHEIMERS

• Maintain simple routines. Avoid unscheduled changes. Frequently reassure him that everything is all right and of your concern for him. Be calm, patient, and understanding. Provide him with a safe environment. Your touch, smile, tone of voice, and frequent eye contact reassures him, even when he cannot understand your words. Do not show anger. Express only one idea at a time, and in simple sentences. Speak in a clear, low-pitched voice. If he does not grasp it, speak the same simple words again. Demonstrate what you want (gesture toward the street he should go to, etc.). Be punctual, so he doesn't wait. If he is doing something inappropriate, distract him with a different activity. In case he may wander off, sew name and address labels in his clothing. If a person is developing Alzheimer's, he should be told early on, so he can prepare for the future and settle his affairs.

ENCOURAGEMENT—How can we be in doubt and uncertainty, and feel that we are orphans? God gave all heaven in Christ; and, as we come and claim the great Gift, heaven begins here. Rejoice, rejoice. If you will cling to Christ, your future is very bright.

SENILITY
(Senile Dementia, Cerebrovascular Disease)

SYMPTOMS—Memory loss and an inability to reason properly (in the older years) interferes with the home and employment. It also causes depression.

CAUSES—Also called Dementia, this occurs in old age; yet it is not widespread. Most older people do not have this problem. Many people in advanced age are quite clear in their thought processes.

There are actually two types of dementia: *Primary dementia* comes on gradually, without apparent cause. *Secondary dementia* comes on suddenly from brain injury, operation, drugs, or diabetic coma; it is usually reversible. Senility and Alzheimer's are examples of primary dementia.

Common causes of senility include **poor blood circulation** to (and in) the brain, **cerebral arteriosclerosis, heavy metal toxicity, prolonged nutritional deficiency, prolonged use of medicinal drugs, and lack of exercise and fresh air**.

Calcification and fatty cholesterol deposits in the middle cerebral artery reduces the main blood supply to the brain, resulting in a poor oxygen supply to it. This produces a loss of memory and typical "senile" changes.

The experts tell us that, over a matter of years, wearing **uncomfortable collars and neckties** tend to cause eddies in the carotid arteries, contributing to the deposition of cholesterol.

Many of those diagnosed as senile are actually suffering from the effects of **medicinal drugs**. If you want a happy old age, avoid drugs throughout your life. **Hearing, thyroid, liver, or kidney problems** can also produce apparent memory loss. There is the possibility of **brain tumors**, as well as **stroke**, and various problems with the nervous system.

A combination of **nutritional deficiencies** is often the underlying cause.

NATURAL REMEDIES

• Try to eliminate **causal factors**, mentioned above.

• Reduce **vitamin D** intake to a maximum of 400 units a day; because an excess works with cholesterol to cause blood vessel problems. Vitamin D is angiotoxic; that is, toxic to blood vessels.

• Each day, taking both **Choline** (500 mg) and **lecithin** (1 tsp.) is important. Also take **vitamin C** (1,000 mg) to bowel tolerance, as well as **vitamin E** (400-800 mg). The **B complex** vitamins are important for the nervous system and brain. **Flaxseed oil** (1 Tbsp.).

• A New England hospital successfully treated senility by giving **niacin** (2,000 mg) and a high-potency vitamin supplement. This opened up the narrowed blood vessels. Niacin has a vasodilatory effect on the body. That is why, when taken, it temporarily causes the face to flush.

• Eat lightly of **nutritious food**. Mainly eat **raw or slowly cooked foods**. **Raw seeds and nuts** help the brain, but eat in moderation. **Millet and buckwheat** are good. Eat **garlic** every day (or take capsules).

• Increase intake of **fiber**-rich foods (**fruits, vegetables, grains, legumes, raw nuts, and seeds**).

• Avoid **fatty foods, fried foods, and saturated fats**.

• **Ginkgo** may help prevent further deterioration of mental capacities; it is the best single herb for this. **Blue cohosh, gotu kola, ginseng, blessed thistle, and mullein oil** increase brain and memory function.

• **Valerian** (taken at bedtime) improves sleep. **Melatonin** (taken 2 hours or less before bedtime) also does.

• Here is a special formula for avoiding senility: Mix equal amounts of powdered **peppermint, skullcap, Siberian ginseng, wood betony, gotu kola, and kelp**. Adults, take up to 12 capsules per day. For acute conditions, 3-4 capsules, 3 times daily.

• Daily **exercising**, to the point of breathlessness, is vital to good circulation. But do not overdo! Only go up to the point of breathlessness, not beyond. Too much can lead to a heart attack. Achieve ideal body **weight**.

• Avoid **constipation**.

• **Heavy metals** must be avoided. Never use **aluminum cookware** or other aluminum products. Do not use **canned goods** any more than necessary.

• Do not **smoke**, or drink **alcohol** or **coffee**.

—Also see *Organic Brain Disorder (590), Aging (312), Alzheimer's Disease (587), Memory Problems (586).*

NERV

ENCOURAGEMENT—The spirit of unselfish labor for others gives depth, stability, and Christ-like loveliness to the character. It brings peace and happiness to its possessor. Every duty performed, every sacrifice made in the name of Jesus, brings an exceeding great reward. Galatians 1:4.

"I will rejoice over them to do them good, and I will plant them in this land assuredly with My whole heart and with My whole soul." Jeremiah 32:41. God's plan for all of us, regardless of age, is the same: eternal life to those who will accept Him as Lord and God.

ORGANIC BRAIN DISORDER
(Chronic Brain Syndrome)

SYMPTOMS—Errors in judgment, lack of reasoning ability, short-term memory loss, disorientation, poor intellectual function, neglect of personal hygiene.

Severe symptoms include hallucinations, incoherent speech, agitation, and restlessness.

CAUSES—**Malnutrition** can induce the symptoms of organic brain syndrome. **Chemicals** and **other toxins** can influence it also, as well as **food allergens**.

NATURAL REMEDIES
• Eat a **nutritious, balanced diet**.
• **Niacin** (2,000 mg), **vitamin B$_1$** (200 mg), **vitamin B$_{12}$** (1,000 mcg), **folic acid** (5 mg), **chromium** (50 mg), and **zinc** (30 mg). Essential fatty acids are also needed. **Vitamin E** (400 IU) repairs brain damage. **Manganese** (1,000 mg) improves memory. The brain also needs **calcium** (2,000 mg) and **magnesium** (1,000 mg). **Lecithin** (1 tsp.) helps clean plaques from the arteries.
• Include enough **fiber** in the diet. A congested colon weakens the blood supply to the brain.
• **Avoid overcooking** and too many cooked foods.
• Avoid **alcohol, lead poisoning, and mercury** poisoning (found in dental amalgam).
• Do a **pulse test**, to determine if food allergens are part of the problem.
• Do a six-hour **glucose tolerance test**, to see if diabetes or hypoglycemia is involved.
• **Hydrochloric acid** (Betaine HCl) supplementation may be needed, to increase food absorption.
• Herbs which help include **capsicum, burdock, echinacea, garlic, ginkgo, psyllium, and gotu kola**.

ENCOURAGEMENT—He who has given His precious life, because He loves you and wants you to be happy, will be a Captain who will always be mindful of your interests. By faith in Christ and obedience to Him, in the very act of fulfilling your duties, God will bring you a blessing. Jesus does not release us from the necessity of effort; but He teaches that we are to make Him first and last and best in everything.

How thankful we can be that, in the enabling strength of Christ, we can fulfill God's will for our lives, and live forever with Him in heaven!

ATTENTION DEFICIT DISORDER (ADD)

SYMPTOMS—Some of the following: Learning disabilities. Lack of concentration. Easily distracted. Procrastination. Lack of goals. Cannot concentrate. Difficulty in solving problems. Impulsive and sloppy workmanship. Cannot manage time. Cannot remember sequences or events. Mood swings. Forgetfulness. Sleep disturbances. Loses things easily. Lack of goals. Absentmindedness.

CAUSES—Attention Deficit Disorder (ADD) and Attention Deficit Hyperactivity Disorder (ADHD, *the next disorder, 489*) are closely related. The difference is that ADD is a general foggy mindedness; whereas ADHD may or may not be foggy minded; but it is hyperactive and possibly disturbing to others. They have had multiple labels in the past, including hyperactivity and learning disability. Residual attention deficit disorder (RADD) is the name given to individuals, 18 or older, who have ADD. Boys are far more likely than girls to be classified as ADD or ADHD.

Many child experts believe there is no such thing as ADD or ADHD; and that both "disorders" were invented to provide more employment to psychologists and psychiatrists.

Because so many parents are frightened over the possibility that their child may have ADD or ADHD, when they take them in for a checkup, they are frequently told that the child has a terrible disorder, called ADD or ADHD; and he needs to take drugs. Some of those drugs are dangerous.

Well then, what are the real causes of these problems? *First*, the symptoms for ADD and ADHD would apply to nearly every child in the world! Actually, according to the symptoms, we all have ADD or ADHD! Should we then all start taking powerful mind-altering drugs?

Second, a frequent reason that many children today are overactive or absent-minded is our present "civilized" way of life. They eat lots of **processed foods** at home and lots of **junk foods** away from home. They ride **long hours on school buses** and sit in **classrooms** where teachers are not allowed to discipline. So children run wild, are not permitted to learn how to **work** (because of "child labor laws"), grow up on vicious **television dramas**, and then go outside and learn about **street drugs**. In addition, many of them live in **quarreling** homes, **alcoholic** or **street drug** homes, or **one-parent** homes with no one home much of the time. Little wonder that the symptoms of ADD and ADHD are becoming epidemic.

The drug, prescribed by the physician or psychiatrist for ADD or ADHD, is generally *methylphenidate* (sold under the brand name, Ritalin). This powerful chemical compound is so nearly identical to cocaine that the two are used interchangeably in medical research. Ritalin helps the child focus—by turning him into a narrow-brained robot. The drug destroys his curiosity, imagination, sociability, and vitality.

NATURAL REMEDIES

BASIC
• Many of the symptoms will be reduced when the child is given a **nourishing diet, loving care, proper rest at night, and opportunity to do worthwhile and appreciated work assignments, especially those that help someone else**.
• **Believe in the child, listen to him, do things with him. Take time to be with him**.
• Feed the child a very nourishing diet of **fresh fruits and vegetables,** plus **vitamin-mineral supplements** and **carrot juice**.
• There should be an **orderly routine** in the home, with **duties he is in charge of** (and warmly thanked for) each day. This imparts a sense of security and self-respect.

OTHER POINTS
• Instead of Ritalin, each day give the child **high-B complex, thiamine** (25 mg), **vitamin B$_6$** (100 mg), **pantothenic acid** (50 mg), **folic acid** (400 mcg), **bata-carotene (in carrot juice), vitamin C** (1,000 mg), **vitamin E** (400 IU), **calcium,** (500-1,000 mg), **magnesium** (100-400 mg), **and zinc** (15 mg). The calcium and magnesium will help calm him.
• A diet of **unsaturated fatty acids** reduces ADD and ADHD. Give him 4 tsp. of **flaxseed oil,** daily .
• Give him complex carbohydrates (whole grains) instead of simple sugar foods.
• He might have a milk (or some other) **food allergy**. If a food makes him excitable, cut back on it awhile and see if that helps.
• Eliminate all **junk, sugary, processed, and fried foods** from his diet. No more **soft drinks** or **coffee**.
• **Valerian** root extract produces good results.
• ADD and ADHD children often have an excess of **heavy metals** in their body. *See Heavy Metal Poisoning (868).* Take steps to identify and eliminate them.
• "I refer parents to Dr. William Crook's book, *Help for the Hyperactive Child* (Professional Books) or any of the excellent books on ADD and hyperactivity written by Dr. Doris Rapp. Also Meridian Valley Clinical Laboratory (206-859-8700) and National Biotech Laboratory (800-846-6285) offer a food allergy test that measures both IgE and IgC antibodies, tests for over 100 different foods which come with

detailed dietary instructions and is reasonably priced at about $20."—*Michael T. Murray, Encyclopedia of Nutritional Supplements, p. 427.*

—See Memory Improvement (592) and Memory Problems (586) for additional suggestions. Also see Hyperactivity (bellow), Dyslexia (592).

ENCOURAGEMENT—The blessing comes when by faith the soul surrenders itself to God. Then that power which no human eye can see creates a new being in the image of God.

ATTENTION DEFICIT HYPERACTIVITY DISORDER (ADHD)

SYMPTOMS—Some of the following: A tendency to disturb other children. Impatience. Difficulty waiting. Not able to sit still very long. Difficulty in adapting to new things. Easily frustrated. Impulsive, unpredictable, or daring. Self-destructive behavior. Temper tantrums. Clumsy or awkward. Talks too much. Blurts out answers before hearing the entire question. Disruptive in the classroom. Low stress tolerance. Failure in school in spite of normal intelligence.

CAUSES—Carefully read the article on ADD, *just above*.

NATURAL REMEDIES
• The natural remedies for ADD *(590)* apply equally to ADHD.
—Also see Hyperactivity (bellow), Attention Deficit Disorder (590), Dyslexia (592).

ENCOURAGEMENT—What love! What amazing condescension: that Christ would die on Calvary to save us from sin and enable to obey the laws of God.

NEURO-MENTAL - 6 - EMOTIONAL, MENTAL

HYPERACTIVITY
(Hyperkinesis)

SYMPTOMS—Cannot sit still, short attention span, impulsive acts before one thinks, runs rather than walks, forgets easily, moody, temper tantrums, irritated and indifferent when disciplined, determined to get his own way.

Sleep disturbances, clumsiness, head-knocking, bothers other children, speech and hearing disorders, extreme distractibility, absent-mindedness, unable to follow a series of instructions.

Not all symptoms are found in any one child. The

symptoms are not limited to children, but are also found in some adults.

Keep in mind that most children display some hyperactive symptoms at times.

CAUSES—Hyperactivity primarily occurs in children; it produces a variety of learning and behavior problems. It is closely related to Attention Deficit Disorder *(488)* and Attention Deficit Hyperactivity Disorder *(489)*.

NATURAL REMEDIES

Some of the above symptoms can be alleviated or eliminated through other methods. Some other causes which can be corrected include:

• Provide the child with a **nourishing diet**, as discussed elsewhere in this book. This is important.

• **Foods that irritate the stomach or inflame the nerves** must be removed from the child's diet. Avoid all **refined, sugary, fried, and junk foods** from the diet. This includes **soft drinks**. Eliminate **artificial flavorings, colorings, and preservatives**. Do not attempt to only change the diet partway. Nourishing food, and only nourishing food, must become a way of life. It will help all in the home. It will be easier for the child to accept the new regime if the mother (and hopefully, father) does also.

• **Food allergies** to milk, wheat, chocolate, yeast, food additives, oranges, and antibiotics. Locate and eliminate food allergies. *See Allergies (848) and Pulse Test (847).*

• **Lead poisoning** can be a significant factor.

• Eating too much **sugar or sugary foods.**

• Artificial **food additives, preservatives,** and foods containing **salicylates**.

• A diet that is too low in **protein**.

• **Emotional problems** and inadequate, inconsistent, or ineffective **discipline** in the home. Hyperactive children often control the situation in the home more than the parents. Because parents are too yielding, children find they can scream their way to dominance and become uncontrollable. When spoiled children enter school, they sometimes try to use overactivity to control their new environment.

• The parent must learn to control the situation, by training the child to obedience and self-control. This is vital. Teaching the child to obey you causes him to learn to control himself. This enables him to organize, and better manage, his mental discipline and his entire life.

• Regularity in rising, eating, bedtime, and other daily schedules is important.

• Hyperactive children often have **learning disabilities**.

• Certain types of **fluorescent lights** are overstimulating. Research studies reveal that children sitting beneath the end of those lights receives X-rays.

• Overstimulation from **television, competitive games, violent TV programs,** and **nutritional deficiencies** are major factors.

• Children from **broken homes** are more likely to have this problem. A strong link has been established between learning disabilities and juvenile crime. Try to solve the problems early.

• **Smoking during pregnancy, oxygen deprivation at birth, prenatal trauma**. Mothers who smoke are more likely to give birth to brain-damaged or hyperactive children.

—*Also see Dyslexia (below).*

ENCOURAGEMENT—A strong, helpful grasp of the hand of a true friend is worth more than gold or silver. Christ has been such a friend to you. He asks that you be such a friend to others. Rejoice in all that He is to you! 1 John 3:2.

DYSLEXIA
(a disturbance of the ability to read)

SYMPTOMS—Difficulty in reading as a result of a brain lesion. Similarly shaped letters cause the victim to transpose ("pot" for "top") or reverse ("b" for "d").

CAUSES—Dyslexia is sometimes called hyperactivity *(591)*; but there is a partial difference. Dyslexia is a complex syndrome rather than a simple disorder.

In some instances, a true organic or biochemical brain injury has occurred. But most of the time, the problem is more easily treatable.

Food allergies are often a key problem.

NATURAL REMEDIES

• **Food allergies** should be located and eliminated. Food sensitivities can produce learning disabilities which may appear to have organic origin. Especially beware of **sugar, wheat,** possibly certain other grains, **milk products, and meat**. One or more (often several) of these may be the problem. Carry out the *pulse test (847),* to determine possible causes and eliminate offending foods. *See Food Allergies (848).*

• Sometimes, taking **hydrochloric acid** (betaine HCl) and **digestive enzymes** may be necessary for awhile.

ENCOURAGEMENT—In all His dealings with His creatures, God has maintained the principles of righteousness by revealing sin in its true character. It is obvious that the wages of sin is misery and death. The unconditional pardon of sin never has been and never will be. God saves us from sin, not in sin.

NIGHTMARES

SYMPTOMS—Unpleasant dreams while sleeping.

CAUSES—In most cases, nightmares can be solved. They sometimes occur because of illness, excessive fatigue, or stress. A sudden, loud noise may initiate one. Some medications are known to induce them. The simple remedies, listed below, clarify many of the causes.

NATURAL REMEDIES

• The primary cause of nightmares is eating a meal that is not digested before retiring for the night. **Do not eat** less than 4 hours **before bedtime**. Eat a **light supper** of fruit and toast.

• **Food allergies** are another prime cause. Search them out and eliminate them. *See Allergies (848) and Pulse Test (847).*

• **Hypoglycemia** is another significant cause. The low point of low blood sugar level occurs at 4 to 4½ hours after food is eaten, especially sugar foods and drinks (cookies and milk, etc.).

• Include **chromium** in the diet.

• Avoid **caffeine**.

• **Liquor** drinking and **hard drugs** induce nightmares.

• Sometimes the problem is **emotional**; a parent that is mean to the child, a terrifying incident that a person has had, etc. Go to God with these problems; only He can bring peace of heart.

• Before bedtime, go outdoors and **walk in the cool night air, breathe deeply, and relax**.

• Some take a whole, **warm bath** before bedtime, to relax.

• Avoid **enervation** of any kind. Do not **overwork**.

• To prevent nightmares, mix equal parts **anise** and fragrant **valerian** root. Simmer 1 tsp. of the mixture in ½ cup water for 15 minutes. Let cool, strain, add enough water to return it to ½ cup of fluid. Drink before bedtime.

• **Sleeping on the back** is said to be the cause of nightmares.

CHILDREN

Children can have nightmares as early as the age of two. In order to avoid them, there should be vigorous outdoor activities during the day.

The evening meal should be light and several hours before bedtime. Evening activities should be calm and non-stimulating. Avoid exciting television. Better yet, throw it away and teach your child Bible stories and lessons drawn from them. There is very little morality in television.

A regular bedtime routine should be followed. This may include a 20-minute warm or neutral bath, story time, bedtime prayers, and tucking in by the parent.

If the child awakens in the night from a nightmare, comfort him in his own bed. Remain calm and softly reassure him you are there to protect him and the nightmare is not real. *Also see Night Terrors (738).*

ENCOURAGEMENT—It would fill the unfallen worlds with consternation if God were to take men, who love and revel in sin, to heaven. Thank God, there is power in the blood, to cleanse from sin and defilement. There is strength in the atonement, to enable man to fulfill the will of God in his life.

PHOBIAS AND PANIC ATTACKS
(Irrational Fears, Agoraphobia, Claustrophobia, etc.)

SYMPTOMS—An irrational fear of something, by which ordinary people are not bothered. The experts call it an irrational, involuntary, inappropriate fear reaction that generally leads to an avoidance of common everyday places, objects, or situations.

Symptoms include attacks of tension, panic, dizziness, tightening of the throat, inability to swallow, muscle twitching, sweating, depression, nausea, and obsessions. Feeling of being outside the body.

The heart starts beating faster; the person feels nauseous, shaky, as if about to faint.

CAUSES—There are three types of *phobias*: *simple phobias, social phobias,* and *agoraphobia.*

Those with simple phobias dread a certain situation, place, or object.

Social phobics are those who do not like to be in public situations, such as a party. They fear doing something which may embarrass themselves.

Agoraphobics fear being alone, being in public places, or being in strange places. It is a fear of being away from a safe person or place. This is the phobia that people most frequently talk to professional counselors about. Most agoraphobics are women who develop it between 15 and 35.

Panic attacks are closely related to phobias and strongly held anxieties.

The body has a natural fight-or-flight mechanism. When more adrenaline is produced, it causes the body to increase metabolism of proteins, carbohydrates, and fats, so the body will have more immediate energy. Muscles become tense; heartbeat and breathing become more rapid.

But when this mechanism occurs without a reasonable cause, the result is a panic attack.

The problem often develops suddenly after a major problem, such as a severe illness, accident, or mental depression.

The attack may occur suddenly, perhaps while standing in line at the checkout counter. The worst thing such people can do is to go home and stay there, in order to avoid facing the problematic situation. This prevents the formation of coping skills and only intensifies the problem.

Some people can only go outdoors if they have a

certain friend or trusted dog with them. Some can move freely about in a feared area only if it is dark (or light).

Hot weather, fatigue, or illness often makes the symptoms worse. **Post-menstrual syndrome** is another cause. It is now known that people with **inner ear problems** (where the sense of balance is located) tend to have phobias and panic attacks.

NATURAL REMEDIES

DIET

• Panic attacks and **calcium** deficiencies go hand in hand. Calcium protects the nerves and prevents toxins from irritating them. Calcium, **magnesium**, and **potassium** are depleted by stress. The **B vitamins** are also important in resisting stress. **Selenium** elevates mood and decreases anxiety.

• Take **chromium** (200-300 mcg, daily), B_6 (100 mg, 3 times each day), B_3 (450 mg, 3 times each day), B_1, B_2, B_5 (50 mg, 3 times each day), **tryptophan** (10 gr, 3 times each day), **calcium** (2,000 mg daily), **magnesium** (800 mg daily), **potassium** (5,500 mg), and **selenium** (500 mg).

• Eat a rounded balance of **amino acids**; but, of course, do not consume too much protein.

AVOID

• Phobics often eat lots of **sweets**. They should be eliminated from the diet.

• **White flour** should also be eliminated. Only eat whole grains.

• Avoid **caffeine** in every form (including **chocolate**) if you have panic attacks. Do not drink **alcohol**. **Medicinal drugs** can be a cause.

• **Food allergies** can be the cause (cow's milk, corn, etc.). Keep a food diary and gradually, over a period of time, determine which foods are bothering you. Do pulse tests *(847).*

• Rebound anxiety and panic attacks can occur when **Valium, Xanix, or Prozac** is taken to ward them off. Xanix can be addictive!

• **Chemical fumes** (such as formaldehyde from newly purchased clothes or carpets) can induce panic attack feelings.

OTHER HELPS

• A severe hypoglycemic **(low blood sugar) reaction**. Professionals call this a "crash and burn" curve because the down slope on the glucose curve is almost vertical. **Diabetes** can be involved here. *See Diabetes (656, 714).* Do a six-hour glucose tolerance test.

• Get regular **exercise** outdoors. Adequate **rest** is important.

• When you have a problem, **have a friend** you can talk it over with.

• Avoiding your fear keeps you from overcoming it. **Face your fear** and, slowly, reason with yourself

that it is nothing to be worried about. One individual feared allowing a small bird on, or near, her. She overcame it by slowly placing her finger near a tame canary in a cage, which hopped on it and sat quietly. After doing this for several days, the fear was overcome.

• **Think** to yourself, "That person (object, place) cannot hurt me." It is the truth; and keep telling it to yourself. Shift, from negative thoughts toward it, to positive thoughts.

• **Recognize** the attacks for what they are. You have had them before; so you know you are not going to die. You have left the house before, and you know you can do it again. You can do it.

• Be easy on yourself, but keep pushing forward. Even if an attack comes on, tell yourself how you succeeded and keep at it. **Do not give up.**

• **Start out slowly**; and expose yourself to the unpleasant environment a little every week. Set goals for yourself: one-week goals, 8-week goals, etc. Push forward and accomplish them.

• You will notice that sometimes the fear is stronger than at other times. **Determine what causes it to increase**: a dietary problem, not enough rest, etc.

• When an attack comes on, you have an excess of adrenaline. So do not sit still. Instead, **move about** and do something; this will help use it up. Walk around or exercise during the attack. If the situation is such that you cannot move about (you are standing in line, etc.), then play a game at alternatively tightening and loosening various muscles in your body. Tighten the large muscles in your upper legs, then release them.

• When an attack seems to be coming on, **breathe deeply**. Take repeated deep breaths. This relaxes the mind and helps the whole system brace against the intruding fear. When an attack begins, phobics tend to take short, rapid breaths. The body is not receiving enough oxygen and is losing too much carbon dioxide, the heart begins beating faster, and there is a sense of air hunger. Instead, breathe slowly and deeply.

• Women who wear **tight-fitting clothes** tend to become chest breathers and are more likely to have panic attacks. Men should wear suspenders. It is important to be able to easily inhale and exhale enough air.

• Maintain good **posture**. Practice **deep breathing** every so often.

• When an attack begins to occur, or if even the thought of the feared item begins to come to mind, **tell yourself "stop!"** If necessary, say "Stop!" out loud. Then consciously **change your thoughts** to something else, something pleasant. Keep doing this. By doing "thought-stopping," you will see excellent progress in as little as four weeks.

• When you are completely relaxed and in a pleasant environment, **think casually** about the feared item. Candidly tell yourself that it does not amount to anything. Then change the thought to something else.

• **"Flooding"** occurs when the person goes into the feared situation (such as a shopping mall) and stays there until the fears leave. This generally takes 8 to 12 hours.

• **Reinforcement** takes place when you write the shopping list until it no longer bothers you. Then you put on your coat and go to the door. Then you go outside to the car. Then, when this no longer bothers you, go to the store and walk up to the door. Later, you go on in and buy the groceries. You keep doing the feared thing until it becomes commonplace.

• **Pray to God for help.** He can give you the strength you need to meet your needs. Thousands have come to Him and obtained the help needed to win great victories in their lives. It is a sweet experience to have peace with God.

• Herbs to help strengthen the body include **dong quai, gotu kola, kelp, ginkgo, passionflower, slippery elm, suma, valerian, and lady's slipper**.
—*Also see Anxiety Disorder (595), Post-Traumatic Stress Disorder (595), Hyperventilation (596), and Strengthening the Nerves (569).*

ENCOURAGEMENT—God is the lifegiver. From the beginning, all His laws were ordained to life. But sin broke in upon the order that God had established, and discord followed. It is only because the Redeemer died on our behalf, that we can be enabled to return obedience to the King of the universe. Psalm 31:19.

ANXIETY DISORDER

SYMPTOMS—Heartbeat and breathing become more rapid, as more adrenaline is produced. There is a continued state of worry and stress. There can be shortness of breath, dizziness, hot flashes, chills, trembling, sweating, or nausea.

CAUSES—This is a complex, involuntary physiological response in which the body prepares itself to deal with an emergency situation—when none may actually exist. Stress causes the body to produce more adrenal hormones, especially adrenaline. Muscles tense up and metabolism increases, so the body can resist a crisis or threat of some kind. A tendency to anxiety disorder may, to some extent, be hereditary.

NATURAL REMEDIES
Each day, take these nutrients:
• Take **calcium** (2,000 mg) daily, along with **magnesium** (1,000 mg). A **multivitamin supplement** is important.
• The **B vitamins** are needed for healthy nerve and brain activity. **Vitamin B$_1$** (200 mg) helps reduce anxiety and calm the nerves. **Vitamin B$_2$** (200 mg) works closely with it; it reduces anxiety and energizes the system. **Niacinamide** (300 mg) helps in the production of needed brain chemicals. Do not take niacin in large doses.
• **Vitamin C** (1,000 mg) strengthens proper functioning of the adrenals, so they do not wear out. In large doses (2,000-5,000 mg in divided daily amounts), it has a calming effect on the system.
• **Vitamin E** (400-800 IU) helps transport oxygen

to the brain and nerve cells, protecting them from free-radical damage.
• **Zinc** (30 mg) calms the nerves. Do not take over 100 mg daily.
• **Flaxseed oil** (2 tsp.) for proper brain functioning.
• Relaxing herb teas include **catnip, hops, skullcap, chamomile, St. John's wort**, and **motherwort**.
—*Also see Phobias and Panic Attacks (593).*

ENCOURAGEMENT—We must put on the whole armor of righteousness. We must resist the devil. And we have the sure promise that, if we will humbly plead with God for help, Satan will be put to flight.

POST-TRAUMATIC STRESS DISORDER

SYMPTOMS—A set of emotional problems after experiencing an extremely difficult situation. Here are typical symptoms: flashbacks, in the form of frequent thoughts, feelings, or memories of the traumatic event. Physical problems such as difficulty digesting food. Depression which causes the person to feel numb and uninterested in life. Hypervigilance is when he is anxious. He is continuously alert, especially near things or places reminding him of the event.

CAUSES—An example of this is the person who accidentally drives off the side of the road and hurtles down a steep bank. Afterward, even though he may not be injured, he has a difficult time readjusting.
After undergoing an extremely difficult situation, if you find you are experiencing any of the above symptoms, then start working to ease and gradually eliminate them.

NATURAL REMEDIES
• Carefully read the section on phobias and panic attacks *(593)*. It is full of helpful suggestions.
• Sit down with someone you trust and discuss the matter with him. **Talking it out** is very helpful. Discussing the matter with someone who has also experienced a difficult event is extremely helpful; for he can be even more understanding.
• Maintain **daily, careful routines**. Doing so brings reassurance that you are in control of the situation. Eat your meals on time. Go to bed on time. Get enough sleep at night.
• **Be cheerful and thankful** to God for your blessings.
• **Find someone you can help**. We forget our own problems as we help others.

HERBS
• Take **chamomile** (350 mg capsules, 2 times daily) or steep a heaping Tbsp. of chamomile flowers in a cup of water for 10 minutes. Drink a cup 3 times a day.
• Take powdered **valerian** root extract (150 mg capsule, 2 times daily). Take 400 mg at bedtime. Do

not take valerian during the day if it causes you to become sleepy.

A calming herb can lose its effectiveness after several weeks, as the body becomes adapted to it.

ENCOURAGEMENT—Not one soul who in penitence and faith, pleads for His protection will Christ permit to pass under the enemy's power.

HYPERVENTILATION

SYMPTOMS—Pounding heart, fingers which are tingling, and palms which are sweaty.

CAUSES—Hyperventilation is **excessive breathing** (also called overbreathing). It can be induced by stress. When some people are frightened, they start breathing very fast—both rapidly and deeply, even though they do not need the extra oxygen. This causes them to exhale a lot of carbon dioxide, which in turn causes the blood to become somewhat alkaline. That results in the symptoms of a panic attack (593).

Episodes of hyperventilation can last for hours, but generally for only 20-30 minutes. But, for the one going through it, the experience can be quite difficult.

NATURAL REMEDIES

• When this happens, people often go to the emergency room of the hospital. And what do those experienced nurses do? They may hand the sufferer a **paper sack and ask him to breathe into it** for a short time. This replenishes the carbon dioxide in the body and brings him back to normal. People who know they might experience hyperventilation attacks, from time to time, sometimes carry a paper sack with them.

But there is a danger here: The person might be having, not a hyperventilation problem, but a real heart attack (513-523). In this article, we will assume that heart trouble is not the problem. But you may want to check our various sections under heart problems (513-523).

• **Exercise** also helps. It not only reduces anxiety, but exercise requires more oxygen—so faster breathing just then is just fine.

• Do not **smoke**. This only adds to the problem; for nicotine is a stimulant and can aid in triggering attacks. Caffeine is another stimulant to avoid.

• **Practice** calm, relaxed breathing. The average you should strive for is one moderate breath every 6 seconds or 10 every minute. Ordinary people need never concern themselves with how often they breathe; but, if you have this special problem, you may want to practice doing it the right way every so often.

• The more tense you are, the faster you will breathe; so be calm and **think** about breathing slower.

• **Think about someone else** beside yourself; and do something to help them. We can focus on our fears so much that they become magnified out of proportion.

• **Avoid situations** which tend to make you overly nervous. For example, for some people this occurs when they are required to stand in crowds.

—*Also see Phobias and Panic Attacks (593).*

ENCOURAGEMENT—Christ says, "Ye are the salt of the earth: but if the salt has lost his savour, wherewith shall it be salted?" How careful we must be that we live like Jesus, so we do not become worthless salt. Matthew 5:13-14, Psalm 25:14.

"Thou wilt shew me the path of life: in Thy presence is fulness of joy; at Thy right hand there are pleasures for evermore." Psalm 16:11.

"Blessed is the man that feareth the Lord, that delighteth greatly in His commandments." Psalm 112:1. Thank the Lord every day for the gift of His Son, Jesus Christ, our only hope of help and salvation."

DEPRESSION

SYMPTOMS—Decreased energy and appetite, chronic fatigue, sleep disturbances, headaches, backaches, weight loss, slowed movement, purposeless thinking, irritability, quickness to temper, and feeling like doing nothing.

CAUSES—Depression may be caused by the **loss of a loved one or a job, food allergies, hypoglycemia, environmental problems, or post-menstrual syndrome**. It could be anything that disrupts a person's sense of worth, stability, security, or effectiveness.

Forty percent of those with this problem have one or both of their parents who suffered it also.

Depression during the dark, dreary winter months is called seasonal affective disorder (571).

Individuals with **severe viral illness, hepatitis, endocrine problems, or stroke** can have it.

An alternate type is bipolar depression (manic depression), in which a person varies between episodes of depression and mania (over-excitedness). *See Manic Depression (597).*

Depression is twice as common in women as in men.

NATURAL REMEDIES

DIET

• **Eat meals on a regular schedule**; and only eat **nourishing food**.

• **Low blood sugar** induces depression. And eating a **high-sugar diet** also produces depression. Learn to eat nourishing **fruits, vegetables, whole grains, nuts, and legumes**. All are fiber-rich foods which help reduce depression. They are also filled with nutrients.

• Eating **complex carbohydrates** increases the amount of the amino acid, tryptophan, that is ingested. This, in turn, increases the amount of serotonin made by the brain, which calms and relaxes the whole system. (In contrast, high-protein foods promote the production of dopamine and norepinephrine, which increases alertness.)

• Increase intake of fiber-rich foods.
• **Omega-3** helps reduce depression. The richest plant source is flaxseed oil (2-4 tsp. daily).
• Each day take **vitamin C** (1,000 mg), **vitamin E** (400 IU), and **calcium** (1,000 mg).
• Take **vitamin B$_{12}$** (1,000 mcg). Deficiencies can produce depression, even in the absence of macrocytic anemia. B$_{12}$ injections by a physician may be needed, prior to going on a daily taking of the B$_{12}$ dosage.
• Take **folic acid** (5 mg daily). Many depressed people are low on folic acid. Make sure you are also taking adequate amounts of vitamin B$_{12}$.
• **Niacinamide** (2,000 mg daily), a form of vitamin B$_3$ (niacin), also helps reduce depression.
• **Vitamin B$_6$** (20 mg, twice a day) helps reduce depression.

AVOID

• Avoid **processed and junk foods**; they are a great source of emotional depression.
• **Caffeine and tobacco** both are known to induce depression.
• **Food allergies** are very significant. Locate and eliminate them. *See Allergies (848) and Pulse Test (847).*
• Over 200 different **medicinal drugs** are reported to cause depression! You might consider throwing out your medicine chest.
• Beware of **antidepressant drugs**! They lead to a wide variety of physical and mental damage!
• Beware of **eating or shopping binges**, to help you feel better. Neither accomplish the intended purpose.
• Avoid the following drugs: **Birth-control pills** cause a wide variety of mood responses, including depression. **Corticosteroids**, especially **steroids**, can produce severe depression. They are used to treat rheumatoid arthritis, lupus, and severe asthma. **Diet pills** initially boost mood, but later depress it.

OTHER HELPS

• **Gotu kola** reduces mental fatigue, which is common in depression.
• **Ginseng** stimulates the entire body, counteracting depression.
• **St. John's wort**, taken regularly (in capsules, tablets, or tincture) will usually improve sleep, appetite, energy levels, and physical well-being within a week. By the end of the second week, anxiety and stress levels should reduce. Start with 300 mg a day; a few days later, increase to 600 mg. A few days later, increase to the maximum of 900 mg daily. Always divide the doses into thirds, taking them morning, noon, and night.
• **Ginkgo** biloba helps strengthen the mind.
• **Valerian** root reduces depression caused by anxiety; but it can make you sleepy.
• **Siberian ginseng** consistently increases a sense of well-being during depression and neurosis.

• The supplement **5-hydroxytryptophan** (5-HTP) increases levels of serotonin, a brain chemical which fights depression. Othniel Seiden, M.D., recommends this: Start with 100 mg at bedtime. If you are not feeling better in 3 days, increase it to 100 mg in the morning and 100 mg at night. If still depressed after 3 more days, increase it to 200 mg in the morning and 200 mg at night. If still depressed, stop taking it entirely; for it will not help you. If you are being helped, continue the dosage for several weeks; then taper off gradually and stop taking it. (Tryptophan, an amino acid, helps produce serotonin, a neurotransmitter which helps you feel more positive. A diet rich in corn and low in other protein sources will increase depression in some people. This is because corn is extremely low in tryptophan.)
• **Tyrosine**, an amino acid, also significantly reduces depression. Take 7 grams daily for 12 weeks. It converts into *norepinephrine*, a neurotransmitter that affects mood. Women taking oral contraceptives have lower levels of tyrosine.
• **L-phenylalanine**, another amino acid, converts to positive mood-affecting substances. Take 3-4 grams per day for one month. Even low dosages (75-200 mg) are helpful.
• **Go to bed on time** at night and maintain **regularity** in your daily schedule.
• Maintain a regular **exercise** program in order to increase feelings of well-being and cheerfulness. Purposeful outdoor exercise, such as gardening, is ideal. Practice **deep breathing outdoors**, twice a day. This reduces a sense of gloom.
• **Sunlight** is beneficial for depression; since it suppresses melatonin production.
• Keep your weight down; and, if you are overweight, go on a gradual **weight reduction** program.
• Do something active. Forget yourself and find happiness in **purposeful activity**. Do something worthwhile that helps others. It may be washing the dishes; it may be going out and helping a sick person.
• **Talk it out**; you may find that many of your problems really do not amount to much.
• Have a good cry. **Crying** releases tension and worry.
• **Be respectful and kind** to others. Making others miserable will only add to your own misery. Being kind to others helps you feel better yourself.
—*See Manic Depression (below), Strengthening the Nerves (468), and Chronic Fatigue Syndrome (279-281).*

ENCOURAGEMENT—If you would have broad views, noble thoughts and aspirations, choose associations that will strengthen right principles. Let every thought and the purpose of every action bend to the securing of the future life, with the eternal happiness it will bring you. Psalm 103:11.

MANIC DEPRESSION
(Bipolar Disorder)

SYMPTOMS—Extreme pessimism, withdrawal from society, changes in sleep patterns. A sudden loss of interest and failure to complete projects started with enthusiasm. There is chronic irritability, sudden attacks of rage when crossed, and loss of inhibition. More symptoms are given below.

CAUSES—Mania is a mental state characterized by excessive excitement. Depression is a mental state characterized by dejection, lack of hope, and absence of cheerfulness.

Both of these qualities are strikingly observed in manic depression. Manic depression is cyclic, a circular affective psychosis in which there are alternating moods of depression and mania. Ordinarily there is a series of periods of psychotic depression or excessive well-being, appearing in any sequence and alternating with longer periods of relative normalcy.

Though intensity may vary greatly, the manic shows an elevated though unstable mood, a flight of ideas, and great physical activity. The case of primary depression finds one thinking that all exertion is exhausting. There is difficulty in thinking or acting and the person is very unhappy.

Manic-depressive disorder is also called bipolar disorder. It typically begins as depression and then develops into alternating periods of depression and mania.

Both mania and depression can vary in intensity and length of the cycles (a few days to many months). During the depression phase, some do nothing while others go through the motions of everyday work while always feeling depressed.

Hypomania is a burst of energy and activity; but full-blown manic psychosis includes delusions of grandeur, invincibility, or persecution, and may result in day and night activity without sleep.

Factors inducing manic depression include an overgrowth of **yeast** in the intestinal tract (281) and certain diseases: **hypothyroidism** (659), **hyperthyroidism** (661), **diabetes** (656), **Alzheimer's** (587), **multiple sclerosis** (580), **Parkinson's disease** (582), **food allergies** (848), **environmental toxicity** (870), **hypoglycemia and hyperglycemia** are major causes.

NATURAL REMEDIES
• A good **nourishing diet** is very important, omitting all **junk foods**.
• Avoid **processed, sugary, and fried foods**.
• Locate **allergy foods** and eliminate them. *See Allergies (848) and Pulse Test (847).* Foods which are common offenders include **cow's milk, corn, wheat, rye, soy, and sugar**. Solving the manic-depressive problem can require weeks of careful diet and elimination of offending factors.
• But also consider **house dust, perfume, formaldehyde, and cosmetics** as allergenic factors to be avoided.

• To test for glycemia, take a 6-hour **glucose tolerance test**. During the test, someone must stay with the person and record his emotions and events. (Is he on an up, down, or both?)
• **Folic acid** supplement improves the effects of lithium in treating manic-depressives.
• To normalize and strengthen nerve function, high doses of **B-complex** are important. The **minerals** found in nourishing food are also needed.
• **Chromium** and **vanadium** (500 mcg, 4 times a day), essential **fatty acids** (5 gm, 3 times a day), **niacin** (450 mg, 4 times a day), **vitamin B$_1$** (200 mg), **vitamin B$_5$** (50 mg), **vitamin B$_6$** (200 mg).
• Avoid the amino acids, **ornithine**, and **arginine**. Some say these and **choline** may make symptoms worse. Others say that choline is needed. Still others say that choline should only be taken in normal amounts with other B vitamin supplements. Researchers at Massachusetts Institute of Technology found that choline helped reduce manic depression. So do as you think best regarding choline.
• Obtaining sufficient amounts of balanced amino acids, especially **tyrosine** and **taurine**, are important.
—*Also see Depression (596), Strengthening the Nerves (569), and Mania (below).*

ENCOURAGEMENT—We must accept Christ as our personal Saviour; and, as we do, He imputes to us the righteousness of God. He enables us to obey the Bible. "Herein is love, not that we loved God, but that He loved us, and sent His Son to be the propitiation for our sins." 1 John 4:10, Psalm 26:1.

MANIA

SYMPTOMS—This psychosis is characterized by excessive excitement, exalted feelings, delusions of grandeur, elevation of mood, and psychomotor overactivity.

CAUSES—Causes include taking of **medicinal or street drugs, guilt** from wrongdoing, **bad diet** for years, and **alcoholism**.

NATURAL REMEDIES
J.H. KELLOGG, M.D., PRESCRIPTIONS FOR MANIA AND ITS COMPLICATIONS (*how to give these water therapies: pp. 206-275 / list of treatments: pp. 206-207 / Hydrotherapy Disease Index: pp. 273-275*)
FOR MALNUTRITION—Graduated Tonic Baths and generous **aseptic diet**.
TO INCREASE BLOOD PRESSURE—Hot Baths. Radiant Heat Bath. Hot Full Bath, at 100°-102° F., for 8-15 minutes. Hot Leg Bath or Hot Sitz Bath (either one at 108°-115° F. for 8-12 minutes). Follow by **Shallow Bath** (68°-74° F.), Pail Pour (75°-70° F.), or Percussion Douche (60°-50° F.) with duration of 20-40 seconds. **Ice bag** over heart for 15 minutes, every two hours.

TO DIMINISH CEREBRAL HYPEREMIA—Short **Hot Full Bath** or Shower, followed by **Douche** at 70°-60° F., 20-40 seconds; **Ice Bag** over heart for 15 minutes every 2 hours.

FOR AUTOINTOXICATION—**Aseptic diet**. If necessary, fruit diet. **Colonic** daily, for a few days. Long **Neutral Bath**, 30-60 minutes.

TO RELIEVE OR PREVENT EXHAUSTION—**Rest** in bed. **Tonic Friction,** twice daily.

FOR FEVER—Local fever-reducing measures, as may be indicated. **Neutral Bath. Cooling Pack.**

CONTRAINDICATIONS—Avoid very hot or prolonged cold baths; avoid cold to head when face is pale.

ENCOURAGEMENT—There is absolutely no safeguard against evil but truth. No man can stand firm for right in whose heart the truth does not abide. There is only one power that can make and keep us steadfast—the power of God, imparted to us through the grace of Christ.

HYSTERIA

SYMPTOMS—There are a great variety of possible symptoms: The mental attitude (when not excited) is calm and somewhat aloof. There may be easy laughing, crying, and episodes of emotionalism (possibly without any apparent explanation) even occurring in sleep. The problem may, or may not, be psychotic in nature.

In some cases, fugues occur. These are episodes when the person takes on a different personality, name, etc., and leaves and goes somewhere else for a time. When the primary personality returns, there is a forgetting of the secondary state. But this problem is not the same as the psychotic condition, known as schizophrenia—in which there is a splitting in personality, incongruities, and confusion co-existing in a person at the same time.

CAUSES—There may be an emotional instability, various sensory disturbances, and a marked craving for sympathy which sometimes leads to unusual words, actions, and activities.

Hysteria can result from **post-menstrual syndrome, food allergies, hypoglycemia, prescribed or illegal drugs, or alcoholism**.

• Hysteria is considered to be due to mental causes— such as autosuggestion, dissociation, or repressed emotion. This condition only occurs while a person is awake and is therefore a willed emotional release to obtain sympathy, to frighten, etc., if another person is involved. This type of person suffers much anxiety and fear.

NATURAL REMEDIES

• Place the person on a **nourishing diet**, avoiding all junk foods.

• Test for **allergies**; see Allergies (848) and Pulse Test (847).

• Give a 6-hour **glucose tolerance test**.

• Keep a daily diary, to test for **PMS**. Look in a Physician's Desk Reference, to locate **drugs** which might be causing problems.

• Take the **vitamins and minerals** needed to build strong nerves. See Strengthening the Nerves (569).

• Place the person in a **quiet place**, devoid of spectators. Give **cold applications to the head, face, and neck**. Quiet, firm suggestions are important.

• For immediate relief, give a nervine tea such as an infusion of lady's slipper, skullcap, ginger, raspberry leaves, poplar bark, balmony, colombo root, cayenne, or antispasmodic herbs to relax the nerve tension. Add a little tincture of lobelia to the nervine as an antispasmodic. If it is impossible to administer these aids orally, the same tea in the form of an enema will ease the condition very quickly. Rest and cheerful surroundings are needed. The digestive system needs to be toned up properly.

J.H. KELLOGG, M.D., PRESCRIPTIONS FOR HYSTERIA AND ITS COMPLICATIONS (how to give these water therapies: pp. 206-275 / list of treatments: pp. 206-207 / Hydrotherapy Disease Index: pp. 273-275)

DIETARY AND LIFESTYLE—Tonic, reconstructive, and restful measures. **Graduated cold applications** (Tonic Frictions) are of the first importance and must be carefully managed at first; need short and intense application, twice daily. **Prolonged Neutral Bath,** in cases due to autointoxication. Also need **outdoor life, generous aseptic diet**, suitable moral and mental surroundings.

CONVULSIONS—**Neutral Bath**, Neutral Pack, Hot Blanket Pack, **Hot and Cold Compress** to spine or Sponging, **Hot Enema, Hot Half Bath** with **Tepid Pail Pour** to head and spine, **Heating Compress** to spine.

COMA—**Alternate Compress** or Sponging to spine, **Cold Mitten Friction**, Hot Half Bath, Cold or Hot **Compress** to head.

VOMITING—**Hot and Cold Compress** over stomach area. Dry diet. Rectal feeding. If necessary, ice to the area above the stomach. Ice pills.

ANOREXIA—**Ice Bag** over stomach half an hour before meals. **Alternate Compress** over stomach, twice daily. **Cold Douche** to spine and epigastrium.

COUGH—**Fomentation** to spine, sipping hot water, **Chest Pack, Cold Compress** to the throat, **gargling** hot water several times daily.

MUSCULAR PARALYSIS—**Alternate Pail Pour** or Alternate Douche, Alternate Compress, Cold Pail Pour, Cold Douche, massage.

CONTRACTIONS—**Fomentations** to affected parts. Follow with **Heating Compress** and **Revulsive Douche**.

TREMBLING—**Neutral Pail Pour** to spine at 92°-96° F., for 15 minutes.

INCONTINENCE OF URINE—**Percussion Douche** to spine. **Neutral Sitz Bath** for 15-30 minutes.

RETENTION OF URINE—**Hot Sitz Bath**. 5 minutes, Follow by **Cold Plantar Douche**, Cold Perineal Douche. Cold Douche to the lower back area, front and back, opposite the intestines and pelvic organs. **Cold Rubbing Sitz Bath**.

PARESTHESIA—Alternate Douche or **Alternate Compress**. Cold Percussion Douche to spine. Cold Hand Rub or Cold Mitten Friction to affected area. Do this after a hot **Fomentation** for 5-10 minutes.

HYPERESTHESIA (PAIN)—Hot Fan Douche, **Fomentation** followed by **Heating Compress**. Revulsive Compress. Cold Douche to the symmetrical part of the opposite side,

VISCERAL NEURALGIA—Very hot **Fomentation** over the affected part for 20 minutes, twice a day. Follow with **Heating Compress** during the interval between. Revulsive Compress, Revulsive Fan Douche.

MOTOR PARALYSIS—Alternate Douche, **Cold percussion Douche**.

HICCUP (also Hiccough)—**Hot Trunk Pack**, **Heating Compress** over stomach, sipping ice-cold water.

SYNCOPE—Heat to neck, **short cold application** to chest and face, **Alternate Compress** to spine, percussion of the chest with the hands dipped in cold water or with the end of a cold towel, vigorous centripetal friction, rhythmical traction of the tongue.

SPINAL IRRITATION—**Fomentation** to the spine twice a day, followed by continuous **Heating Compress** during the intervals between. Revulsive Fan Douche. **Fomentation.** Follow by **Pail Pour** for 5 minutes, 80°-85°F.

ANAL SPASM—Hot Anal Douche or **hot Shallow Sitz Bath** at 102°-106° F. General applications of massage and regular gymnastics.

APHONIA—**Ice Bag** to the throat with general **Cold Douche**.

GENERAL METHOD—Improve his general health by vigorous tonic measures continued during many months or even years. Improve the general nutrition by a nutritious, simple, unstimulating dietary. Combat special symptoms by the hydrotherapy measures indicated above, together with suitable mental and moral treatment.

—*Also see Melancholia (bellow).*

ENCOURAGEMENT—It is because of the love of God that the treasures of the grace of Christ have been offered to men. What love is this! What unfathomable love, that Christ would die for us while we were still sinners! Look at the cross of Calvary. It is a standing pledge of the boundless love, the measureless mercy of the heavenly Father. Proverbs 13:25.

"For His great love wherewith He loved us." Ephesians 2:4. "Heirs of the kingdom, which He hath promised to them that love Him." James 2:5.

MELANCHOLIA

SYMPTOMS—A mental state characterized by marked depression, physical and mental apathy, brooding, mournful and doleful notions, and inhibition of activity.

CAUSES—Melancholia is a form of chronic depression which, at times, can switch to strong excitement and even hysteria.

Hysteria can result from **food allergies, hypoglycemia, prescribed or illegal drugs, post-menstrual syndrome, extremely impoverished diet for years, or alcoholism**.

NATURAL REMEDIES

J.H. KELLOGG, M.D., PRESCRIPTIONS FOR MEL-

ANCHOLIA AND ITS COMPLICATIONS *(how to give these water therapies: pp. 206-275 / list of treatments: pp. 206-207 / Hydrotherapy Disease Index: pp. 273-275)*

FOR ANEMIA AND MALNUTRITION—**Fomentation** to abdomen. Followed by **Cold Mitten Friction,** twice daily. **Aseptic diet**, **water** drinking, air bath, Radiant Heat Bath, sunbaths, **rest** in bed, **massage**.

FOR CEREBRAL ANEMIA (which is usually present)—**Warm compress** at 98°-100° F. to back of neck for 15 minutes, 3 times daily.

TO DIMINISH BLOOD PRESSURE (which is usually excessive)—**Warm Full Bath**, 98°-100° F., 10-20 minutes, twice daily. **Heating Wet Sheet Pack**. Heating Trunk Pack, 30 minutes, twice daily. **Neutral Douche**, 94° F., pressure 10-20 pounds, duration 2-4 minutes.

CONSTIPATION—**Laxative diet**, **fruit**, **malted cereals**; Cool **Enema**.

MENTAL AND NERVOUS IRRITABILITY—Neutral Bath at 94°-96° F., 30 minutes to 2 hours. **Heating Wet Sheet Pack**, Hot Abdominal Pack, Heating Compress to spine.

CONTRAINDICATIONS—Avoid cold immersions and all very cold general applications which, by raising blood pressure and exciting the irritable cerebral structures, aggravate the condition.

GENERAL METHOD—A person suffering from melancholia requires essentially the same therapeutic measures as the neurasthenic, with the special moral treatment and control indicated.

ENCOURAGEMENT—Everyone who enters the pearly gates of the city of God will enter there as a conqueror; and his greatest conquest will, through the enabling grace of Christ, have been the conquest of self.

In Christ, God offers us all the best treasures of heaven. By faith in His enabling grace, we can obey all the law of God and live good, clean lives.

MÜNCHAUSEN SYNDROME

SYMPTOMS—Dramatic presentation of symptoms and their history. Highly emotional and argumentative behavior toward medical staff. Wide knowledge of medical terms and medical procedures.

CAUSES—Münchausen Syndrome is a rare condition in which a person claims to have symptoms of illness and may repeatedly need treatment from a number of different hospitals. Medical care is sought for nonexistent or self-induced symptoms.

Common symptoms that he complains of include abdominal pain, blackouts, and fever. It is thought that this is done as an attempt to escape from everyday life and be cared for and protected. The syndrome usually begins in early adulthood and is more common in men. Those affected often have had previous experience working in a medical-related profession. For this reason, their bogus claims may not be detected until shown by test results or exploratory surgery. Multiple surgical scars may be present.

A related problem is called Münchausen Syndrome by proxy; maybe it is a parent. Often the mother repeatedly claims her child is ill and in need of treatment.

Sometimes the cause is an addiction and the person wants narcotics.

As soon as the medical staff realizes the true nature of the situation, the person leaves and goes to another hospital or physician.

NATURAL REMEDIES

• The only practical solution is to make friends with the person and try to calmly discuss the matter with him. Lead him to Christ, the only one who can help us.

ENCOURAGEMENT— The work of conquering evil is to be done through faith. Those who go into the battlefield will find that they must put on the whole armor of God. The shield of faith will be their defense and will enable them to be more than conquerors. Nothing else will avail but this—faith in the Lord of hosts and obedience to His orders. Ephesians 6:11-12, 16.

PHENYLKETONURIA (PKU)

SYMPTOMS—This is a rare disease. Lack of a certain enzyme results in a buildup of *phenylalanine* in the body. Over a period of time this can lead to mental retardation; organ damage; abnormal posture; and, sometimes, severely compromised pregnancy. Symptoms in affected infants include drowsiness, lethargy, difficulty feeding, light eyes, as well as light pigmentation in skin and hair. A rash similar to exzema may develop.

If not properly treated, PKU can develop into severe mental retardation and neurological symptoms—such as seizures, hyperactivity, clumsy walking, unusual posture, aggressive behavior, or psychiatric disturbances.

Fortunately, the problem is detectable through blood tests within the first days of life. Screening for PKU is part of routine testing for newborns in many states.

CAUSES—PKU is an inherited error of the metabolism, caused by a deficiency of the enzyme, *phenylalanine hydroxylase;* this is responsible for processing the essential amino acid, *phenylalanine.*

NATURAL REMEDIES

• If treated properly with a carefully controlled diet which does not have the amino acid *phenylalanine* in it, mental retardation can be prevented.

• First and foremost, a healthful diet must be eaten, which totally excludes the artificial sweetener, aspartame (which is found in Equal, NutraSweet, and many processed food products). Therefore, eat no processed foods of any kind!

• In addition, follow the other information given throughout this *Encyclopedia* about nutrition, water, herbs, rest, sunshine, outdoor exercise, and all the rest.

MENTAL ILLNESS

SYMPTOMS—Depression, anxiety, delusions, nervousness, loss of interest in school or work, sleep pattern changes, irritability, withdrawal from society, sudden rages, lack of enthusiasm, and panic attacks.

CAUSES—It is important that we note that this article includes both neurotic and psychotic syndromes. Just because a person has one or more of the symptoms noted here—does not mean he is crazy. He may just be having a hard time dealing with life.

The experts divide mental illness into two main varieties: mood disorders and schizophrenia *(602)*. Elsewhere in this *Encyclopedia*, you will find discussion of several episodic mood disorders: Depression *(596)*, Manic Depression *(597)*, Phobias *(593)*, and Hysteria *(599)*. Individuals with episodic problems generally return to normal between spells.

In this article, we shall overview a few primary factors in all mental illness. An important related article is *"Strengthening the Nerves" (569)*.

A person is no longer able to cope effectively with emotional or physical stresses, which others are normally able to handle. Women are twice as likely to experience mental illness.

NATURAL REMEDIES

• There may be heredity factors; but the **environmental factors and lifestyle** are very important! **Nutritional deficiencies** have a strong effect on mental health.

• **Autointoxication** and **constipation** are contributing factors in mental illness. Eliminating them can reduce symptoms ranging from mental sluggishness to hallucinations. Even schizophrenia *(602)* can be greatly lessened.

• There is a direct relation between the **transverse colon** and the brain. When the colon is clogged, mental illness is triggered in some and an attack of epilepsy *(574)* in others.

• Eliminate the "glue foods"; these tend to clog the colon, produce a buildup of mucus and toxins in it, and lead to mental problems. Such foods include **white flour, sugar, eggs, meat, peanuts, and dairy products**.

• Brain cells cannot function properly without proper nutrients. *See Strengthening the Nerves (569).* It is known that many cases of mental illness are solved when a **simple nourishing diet**, including sufficient **fiber** and adequate **vitamins and minerals**, is given and the colon is cleaned out with **enemas** or colonics.

• **Food allergies** may produce edema (swelling) of certain areas of the brain, which can change the personality, reflexes, motor activity, or the function of the central nervous system. Allergy specialists successfully treat individuals with mental illness by isolating foods and chemicals in the environment which induce the mental problems. Allergic reactions may be a factor in criminal behavior. In some cases, the offending food does not cause mental reactions until hours after being eaten. This is called "masked food allergy." Do not under-rate the allergy factor! *See Allergies (848) and Pulse Test (847).*

• A **whole grain** diet stimulates the amount of tryptophan in the brain; this produces a calming, peaceful feeling.

• **Exercise**, especially outdoors in the fresh air, combined with relaxation helps to rejuvenate the body and mind.

• Many persons with schizophrenia, autism, abnormal behavior, and subsequent learning disorders are caused by too much **lead** or **copper** in the body. Check your plumbing pipes. Plastic water pipes are the safest.

• Herbs which calm the brain and nerves include **hops, chamomile, skullcap, valerian, and wood betony**.

—*Also see Schizophrenia (602) and Strengthening the Nerves (569).*

ENCOURAGEMENT—There is a God in Israel, who can bring deliverance to all that are oppressed. He will draw near to you, right where you are, and minister to your needs. All you need to do is ask Him—just now. Psalm 37:6.

INSANITIES
(Post-Febrile, Post-Operative, Puerperal Confusional)

SYMPTOMS—Any mental disorder or psychosis, characterized by inability to distinguish between right and wrong, possession of delusions or hallucinations which prevent an individual from looking after his own affairs with ordinary prudence or which render him a menace to others, actions resulting from impulses of such intensity that they cannot be resisted.

NATURAL REMEDIES

Dr. John Harvey Kellogg recognized that a basic treatment could be applied to a number of insane conditions. Here are his recommendations:

J.H. KELLOGG, M.D., PRESCRIPTIONS FOR SEVERAL INSANITIES AND THEIR COMPLICATIONS (*how to give these water therapies: pp. 206-275 / list of treatments: pp. 206-207 / Hydrotherapy Disease Index: pp. 273-275*)

MALNUTRITION—Rest, careful **Tonic Frictions**.

AUTOINTOXICATION—**Aseptic dietary**, **fruit diet** for 3-4 days, **warm Baths**, Radiant Heat Bath, **Sweating Wet Sheet Pack**. Follow by **short cold applications**, Wet Sheet Rub or brief Cold Douche, copious **water** drinking, **Colonic** daily for a week or two.

PUERPERAL LESIONS OR COMPLICATIONS—Hot **vaginal irrigation**, Neutral or tonic **Sitz Bath**.

FEVER—Absolute **rest** in bed. Prolonged **Tepid Bath** at 88°-92° F., for 30-60 minutes. Cooling **Enemas**, **Cold**

Compress to head, copious **water** drinking.

ALCOHOLISM—**Withdraw alcohol** at once. **Withhold food for 3 days**. **Nutritive enemas**. Copious **water** drinking. Neutral **Colonic** daily for a week.

UREMIA—See under "Nephritis, Acute."

CONTRAINDICATIONS—The same as those of mania, when conditions coincide. Especially avoid all intensely exciting procedures.

GENERAL METHOD—In most cases essentially the same as for mania, giving special attention to the particular causal element which may be a prominent factor in the case. In certain cases, the symptoms are those of Melancholia; and the treatment must be modified accordingly.

ENCOURAGEMENT—It is a part of God's plan to grant us, in answer to the prayer of faith, that which He would not bestow did we not thus ask. Oh, please, my friend, believe and know that God is your best Friend!

SCHIZOPHRENIA
(Paranoiac, Catatonic, Hebephrenic, Dementia Precox)

SYMPTOMS—Principal signs are moodiness, solitary habits, stupor and excitement, delusions and hallucinations.

Hallucinations are common, especially of hearing. Loss of emotion or, if shown, it is out of place. Actions are absent or inappropriate. There may be impulsive destructive acts and negativism. Extremities tend to be cold, blue, and edematous (puffy with fluids). Conscious, but takes little cognizance of what is going on about him. Delusions frequent but absurd, often of grandeur and persecution. May have attacks of tears or laughter. There may be excited activity. May remain in a stupor. Grimaces and mannerisms are frequent. Symptoms sometimes change form.

Schizophrenia affects about 3% of the population at some time in their lives.

CAUSES—This is the most important of the psychoses, and is characterized by a loss of contact with the environment and a disintegration of personality. The earlier name for it was dementia precox.

There are four primary types. A vague sense of being two personalities and "changed" occurs in all types:

1 - Simple schizophrenia: The person becomes dull emotionally, loses ambition, and tends to withdraw. Yet there is no serious intellectual impairment.

2 - Paranoid schizophrenia: The person develops extensive delusions of persecution. He believes people are plotting against him.

3 - Catatonic schizophrenia: The person may show stereotyped excitement or simulate a stupor.

But, if he recovers later, he will clearly remember it.

4 - Hebephrenic schizophrenia: There are mannerisms, speech anomalies, hysteroid symptoms, delusions, hallucinations, and often a dreamy, ineffectual reaction.

Some believe schizophrenia is **hereditary**; others think that only **attitudinal, dietetic, and external factors** lead to it (**head injuries, complications during birth, reaction to a virus or medicinal drug, environmental poisons**).

A wide range of **medicinal drugs** can produce schizoid symptoms. It is known that many schizophrenics had **birth complications** or a **head injury in childhood**.

Being born in the winter in cities is more likely to produce schizophrenia. The lack of good nutrition of the mother and child is the likely cause.

NATURAL REMEDIES

When using orthodox psychiatric treatment, complete recovery is rare. The orthodox methods use various tranquilizers, all with severe side effects. These include electroconvulsive shock therapy and psychotherapy. Orthodox remedial substances deplete many essential vitamins, are highly toxic, damage brain tissue, and should be avoided.

Solutions are more likely when using natural remedies.

MINERALS AND HEAVY METAL POISONING

• Schizophrenia is linked to an **excess of copper** in the body. High copper levels cause vitamin C and zinc levels to drop. *See Copper Poisoning (872).*

• It is believed that a **zinc deficiency** may be a key factor inducing schizophrenia. A full 80% of those with this disorder have a deficiency of zinc and an excess of copper and iron in their body tissues. Supplementation of **zinc** (30 mg) **and manganese** (25 mg) are needed to correct this. Zinc deficiencies occur more frequently in the winter; and this is when this disorder frequently begins. It is now known that some individuals, who later in life are schizophrenic, had a prenatal zinc deficiency from their mother's diet and way of life. The pineal gland in the brain normally has high levels of zinc; and weakening of this endocrine gland may be a factor.

• **Magnesium deficiency** may also be involved, since schizophrenics have lower magnesium levels in their blood; and, when they recover from it, their magnesium levels are higher.

• An excess of **lead** or **mercury** in the body can also induce schizophrenic symptoms. *See Lead Poisoning (873), Mercury Poisoning (874), Heavy Metal Poisoning (868).*

DIET AND NUTRIENTS

• Eat a high-fiber diet, including plenty of fresh raw vegetables and quality protein. Complex carbohydrates in the diet are important for a normal blood sugar level.

• **High-quality food** should be eaten. **Mineral and trace mineral imbalances** exist in schizophrenics. A **nourishing diet**, along with **vitamin / mineral supplementation** is needed.

• Severe **vitamin B$_3$ (niacin) deficiency** (pellagra), with its characteristics such as nervousness, loss of memory, confusion, paranoia, insomnia, depression, and hallucinations—resembles schizophrenia so closely, that the two disorders probably are the same. Here is an interesting fact: When experiments were made on prisoners who were given no niacin for extended periods of time before they were again given normal diets, it required 60 times as much niacin to return them to normal in order to prevent pellagra.

• Go on a **fruit and vegetable juice diet** for a time. This will provide vitamins and minerals while keeping the blood sugar normal during the fast. Repeat short juice fasts or one longer juice fast for 4-6 weeks. Overly sweet fruit juices should be avoided or diluted 50-50 with water.

• During this fasting time, give massive doses of niacin in the form of **niacinamide** (1,000-3,000 mg with each meal; often as much as 25,000-30,000 mg per day). An equal amount of vitamin C, B vitamins (especially pantothenic acid), and 3-5 Tbsp. of brewer's yeast should be given. Repeat: Do not give massive doses of niacin; instead, give niacinamide.

• After recovery, a large daily dose of niacinamide will have to be continued indefinitely.

• Severe deficiencies of other B complex vitamins can also produce schizoid symptoms. Severe **B$_{12}$ deficiency** caused difficulty in concentration, poor memory, agitation, hallucinations, and manic or paranoid behavior.

• **Biotin deficiency** causes depression, lassitude, panic attacks, and hallucinations.

• Faulty **essential fatty acid deficiency** or metabolism is another factor leading to schizophrenia. The remedy is 2-6 Tbsp. of **flaxseed oil** in divided doses, given daily. Wheat germ oil or sunflower seed oil works just as effectively.

• **Hypoglycemia** appears to be frequently involved in schizophrenia. A good blood sugar level is vital, if oxygen is going to be regularly provided to the brain. Yet it is believed that an undersupply of oxygen is a key factor inducing the disorder.

AVOID

• Avoid all **processed, junk, and fried foods**. Do not use **white flour or sugary foods**. Stop eating **meat**. Avoid **alcohol, tobacco, and caffeine**.

• Schizophrenia is rare in areas of the world where little or no **cereal grains** are used; but it is more frequent where **wheat, rye, or barley** are common. Celiac disease *(473-474)* is especially caused by infants being fed wheat before six months of age. Schizophrenia is more common in celiacs. When a **gluten-free diet** brought improvement to celiac symptoms, the mental problems improved also (gluten is wheat protein). **Milk protein** (lactose) increases the deleterious effects of wheat gluten in some celiacs. In one study, schizophrenics placed on a **milk- and cereal-free diet** were released from the hospital in half the time. Gluten was found to be the key factor.

• A 1982 study noted that 80% of schizophrenics were allergic to **eggs**.

• **Caffeine** worsens symptoms of schizophrenia.
—*See Mental Illness (601) and Strengthening the Nerves (569) for additional information. Also see the vitamin dosage section of this book for high dosage amounts.*

ENCOURAGEMENT—Serving Christ will place upon you no restriction that will not increase your happiness. In complying with His requirements, you will find a peace, contentment, and enjoyment that you can never have in the path of sin. Psalm 31:20.

AUTISM

SYMPTOMS—Symptoms are very obvious before the age of three: A marked unresponsiveness to people and surroundings, indifference to affection, and withdrawn into oneself.

Sometimes strange actions, such as pounding feet while sitting, continual rocking back and forth, silent sitting for long periods of time, bursts of hyperactivity while he bites or pounds on his body.

Key early symptoms: Does not babble at 1 year of age. Begins developing language, then stops abruptly. Does not respond to his name, but has normal hearing. Does not point to things to direct his mother's attention. Avoids eye contact and cuddling.

CAUSES—There are about 100,000 autistic children in America. They look normal in appearance; but they have weak contact with reality. In addition to the above symptoms, they have learning disabilities and are often mentally disabled. A rare few have astounding abilities in mathematics or music.

Nutritional improvement appears to be the best route for natural treatment.

In some instances, autistic children have recovered, usually during adolescence. Some progress well; but later they might lose what was gained.

According to the *National Institute of Neurological Disorders and Stroke*, the criteria used to diagnose autism include the following:

Absence or impairment of imaginative and social play. Impaired ability to make friends with peers. Impaired ability to initiate or sustain a conversation. Stereotyped, repetitive, or unusual use of language. Restricted patterns of interests that are abnormal in in-tensity or focus. Apparent inflexibility with regard to changes in routine or rituals. Preoccupation with parts of objects.

NATURAL REMEDIES

• This high-fiber diet should be 50%-75% raw fruits and vegetables.
• No junk, processed, sugar, dairy, wheat, or white-flour foods of any kind should be given. Avoid fried and fatty foods and meat of any kind.

• Dr. Bernard Rimland, a research psychologist in San Diego, found that 50% of his patients improved when placed on a **megavitamin therapy**. If you have an autistic child, give him a **high B-complex supplementation**, plus other nutritional factors.

• In research studies, the vitamins which especially helped the autistic child were niacin (use the **niacinamide** form), **pantothenic acid, vitamin B$_6$, and vitamin C.** When improvement did not occur, additional B$_6$ was given, along with **magnesium**, to offset the B$_6$; then improvement was seen. *See the vitamin dosage section of this book for high dosage amounts.* As a result of vitamin therapy, there was a reduction in tantrums, improved speech, better sleep patterns, increased alertness, and greater sociability. As soon as the vitamin therapy ceased, the symptoms returned.

• Some researchers found that adding **magnesium** (10-15 mg per 2.2 pounds of body weight) to **vitamin B$_6$** (3.5 mg to 100 mg per every 2.2 pounds of body weight) worked better than taking B$_6$ alone. The amounts of B$_6$ and magnesium used for treating autism are very high, and have the potential for toxicity.

• Allan Cott, M.D., a New York psychiatrist, gave 200 mg of **pangamic acid** (vitamin B$_{15}$) to autistic children and decided improvement frequently occurred.

• Use an elimination diet, to test for **food allergies**. *See Allergies (848) and Pulse Test (847).*

• Regular, moderate **exercise** is important.

SPECIAL NOTE: AUTISM AND VACCINATIONS

The author's book, *The Vaccination Crisis is* available from the publishers of this *Encyclopedia* and contains important information about the relationship of MMR vaccinations, given to infants and children, and the stupendous increase in autism. The evidence is overwhelming: MMR vaccines are the primary cause of autism!

"Serious problems can occur when children, especially small children, are vaccinated. Of these, the rubella (German measles) vaccine is especially dangerous. It is a standard part of the MMR (measles, mumps, and rubella) combination vaccine.

"A 1998 research study, published in the British medical journal, *Lancet*, reveals that the MMR vaccine could be a cause of that terrible condition, known as *autism.*"—*The Vaccination Crisis, p. 139.*

"One of the earliest vaccines introduced for general use in the U.S. was the pertussis vaccine for whooping cough in the 1940s. Autism, a form of childhood schizophrenia, characterized by mental retardation, muteness (inability to speak), and a lack of responsiveness to human contact, was not known or described until 1943, about the same time that vaccinations were introduced. Here are some of the latest facts on this:

"The Wakefield / Walker-Smith Study. In a 1998 study of twelve children in Britain, all twelve had intestinal problems and had suddenly lost language skills; and nine were diagnosed as definitely autistic. The significant part is that, in the case of eight of the children, parents or a doctor noticed the problems developed shortly after the child had received the measles, mumps, *and rubella (MMR) vaccine!"—pp. 138-139.*

"The Wakefield / O'Leary Study: In a separate British study in the summer of 2001, scientists uncovered additional evidence that the MMR vaccine is primarily responsible for autism."—*Vaccination Crisis, p. 141.*

"The Singh Report on MMR and Autism: In late September 2002, scientists at the Department of Biology and Biotechnology Center, Utah State University, Logan, Utah, reported finding a strong association between the MMR vaccine and the autoimmune reaction believed to pay an important role in autism."—*Vaccination Crisis, p. 141.*

"273% increase in autism in California. On April 17, 1999, the California State Department of Developmental Services (DDS) issued a special report to the state legislature. The report, entitled, *"Changes in the Population of Persons with Autism and Pervasive Developmental Disorders in California's Developmental Services System, 1987-1998,* revealed a shocking increase in the number of children with autism . .

"In the past 10 years, California has had a 247% increase in the number of children with autism who enter the developmental services system, 1,685 new cases last year alone. What is generally considered a rare condition is increasing faster here than any other developmental disabilities . . The complete report is available from the California State Department of Developmental Services, in Sacramento.

"While the increase in other child disability problems has been 50%, for autism it has been 273%. This figure does not include data for the more than 13,000 children in the early start program, for 0 to 3 year olds.

"In 1987, there were 2,778 cases of autism in California; in 1998, it was 10,360. That is a 272.93% increase."—*Vaccination Crisis, pp. 144-145.*

Do not let your child be vaccinated! Our book, *Vaccination Crisis,* tells you how, in most states, you can avoid it.

ENCOURAGEMENT—The Lord has not changed. He is true, merciful, compassionate, and faithful to do what He says. Trust your life to Him! You will not be sorry. The future He offers you is a marvelous one.

DEMON POSSESSION

SYMPTOMS—The person will frequently babble, or talk nonsense; he frequently says vulgar words. He will display superhuman strength and endurance, and may go without food or drink for days. He appears frightened, angry, or disturbed, with no interest in his appearance.

CAUSES—He has attended a spiritist sceance, had a hypnotic encounter, been reading occult (witchcraft) literature, played with a ouija board, attended a church of Satan, or been prayed over by a witch doctor.

NATURAL REMEDIES

• **Concerned family members and friends should take turns reading the Bible aloud in the presence of the devil-possessed person and alternate with ongoing prayer. Those participating in this must confess to God all known sins and plead for forgiveness.** The evil spirit may cry out and complain; but he will always tremble when the name of Jesus Christ is mentioned. This prescription will cause the evil spirit to leave the person.

When that occurs, all should kneel and praise God for his deliverance and plead for the Holy Spirit of God to fill the life of the person, so the evil spirit will not return.

That person must also be told to go and sin no more; and he should intend to change his way of life and never again dabble in satanism.

ENCOURAGEMENT—The faces of men and women who walk and work with God express the peace of heaven. They are surrounded with the atmosphere of heaven. For these souls, the kingdom of God has begun.

"In God I will praise His word . . in God I have put my trust; I will not fear what man can do unto me."
                                                    —Psalm 56:10-11

"Believe in the Lord your God, so shall ye be established; believe His prophets, so shall ye prosper."
                                                    —2 Chronicles 20:20

"Be perfect, be of good comfort, be of one mind, live in peace; and the God of love and peace shall be with you."
                                                    —2 Corinthians 13:11

"Ye shall serve the Lord your God . . and I will take away sickness from the midst of thee."
                                                    —Exodus 23:25

S
K
E
L
M
U
S

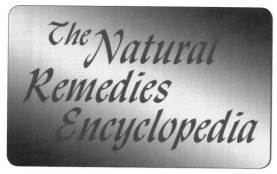

Disease Section 10 - Skeletal-Muscular

Bones and Muscles: Physiology 1011-1013 / Pictures 1026-1032

"The Lord is nigh unto them that are of a broken heart; and saveth such as be of a contrite spirit."—*Psalm 34:18.*

FOR MORE NATURAL REMEDIES:
HERBS: Herb Contents (pp. 129-130) will help you locate the 126 most important herbs and the diseases each one can treat. How to prepare herbs (132). How to use them (141-189)
HYDROTHERAPY: Therapy Contents (pp. 206-207) and its Disease Index (263-265) will lead you to over 100 water therapies and many more remedies. DIS. INDEX: 1211- / GEN.

INDEX: 1221-
VITAMINS AND MINERALS: Contents (100-101). Using 101-124. Dosages (124). Others (117-)
CARING FOR THE SICK: Home care for a sick person (28-36). The healing crisis (36-39)
WOMEN'S SECTIONS: Female Organs (672) Pregnancy (701). Childbirth (765). Infancy, Childhood (722). Women's Herbs (754, 760)
EMERGENCIES: (973-). **FIRST AID:** (990-)

Section 10 - Skeletal-Muscular

SKELETAL-MUSCULAR - 1 - BONES

FRACTURE
(Broken Bone)

SYMPTOMS—There may be extreme pain and tenderness in the injured area, a protruding bone, blood under the skin, or swelling. There may be tingling, numbness, weakness, or paralysis below the fracture.

A digit, or limb, may be at an abnormal angle or there may be pain at a specific place on a bone.

A major fracture can cause a loss of pulse below the fracture, weakness, and inability to bear weight.

CAUSES—A fracture is a crack or break in a bone. If the skin over the bone remains intact, it is a closed or simple fracture; if the bone breaks the skin, it is a compound fracture.

Accidents are a common cause of broken bones; but the bone can also be weakened from **osteoporosis, bone tumors, or metabolic disease**. A weakened bone can break much more easily—even from a slip of the foot, a slight fall, or knocking against something.

Malnutrition can also be involved. There can be a **deficiency of calcium and/or magnesium**, or there may be an **improper calcium / phosphorus ratio**.

Oddly enough, although phosphorus is needed for good bone formation, you will find, below, that it is important that you avoid phosphorous foods if you want strong bones. This is due to the fact that phosphorus is the one mineral which is abundantly found in food. Yet too much of it in a meal locks into the calcium and removes it from the body.

Older people do not absorb calcium and other minerals as well. This begins at 40, increases at 50, and very much so beyond 60. It is believed that 200,000 hip fractures occur in people over 65 every year. Very often, this results from **osteoporosis**. The bone has somewhat hollowed out and the break more easily occurred.

Older people who take **tranquilizers** have 70% more hip fractures than other people their age.

When a break occurs, protein fibers form a bridgework between the two parts. Then calcium, phosphorus, and silica are deposited between the

CHART - 1045: Skeletal-Muscular (606-651)

protein fibers.

First aid includes covering any wound and immobilizing, or splinting, the broken part in the position it was found (so the problem will not worsen during transport). Take the person to a physician or the hospital, depending on the seriousness of the problem. Medical treatment involves placing the bones in their proper position and keeping them there while healing occurs.

A vibrating tuning fork can be placed against the area; if it causes pain, there is a fracture. X-rays will confirm whether it is a fracture.

It is important that the bone be properly set; otherwise it may thereafter be deformed and not function as well.

NATURAL REMEDIES

DIET

• Obtain a **nourishing diet**. *(See Strengthening the Bones, 608.)*

• Take 1,000 mg of **calcium** daily. Bone breaks in lab animals given **silicon** healed in 17 days. Take 1 mg daily. **Magnesium** works with calcium to build bones. Take 250-500 mg daily. Also important are **boron** (2 mg) and **manganese** (10 mg) daily.

• An alternative to taking silicon is the herb, **called horsetail**. Pour 1 cup water over 2 tsp. dried (not powdered) herb in a pan and boil for 5 minutes; then steep for 10-15 minutes.

• Foods rich in calcium and magnesium include dark green leafy vegetables, broccoli, and parsley. Eat at least 1 serving daily.

• Take 400 IU of **vitamin D** for the first 4 weeks after your injury. It will help your body absorb calcium. In addition, get out in the direct sun for 15-30 minutes a day. That will help your body make its own vitamin D.

• **Pineapple** contains bromelain, an enzyme which acts to reduce swelling and inflammation. Eat half a fresh (not canned or processed) pineapple daily, until the fracture heals. Canned pineapple or pineapple juice may contain aluminum salts, pulled by the acid from the wall of the can by the very acid liquid.

• *Lactobacillus acidophilus* and *Bifidobacterium bifidum* are two kinds of **intestinal bacteria** that make vitamin K in your bowel. That vitamin helps your body produce *osteocalcin*, a protein that aids in building bone. You can find supplements contain-

S
K
E
L
M
U
S

ing these bacteria in most health-food stores. Look for a brand that must be refrigerated. The usual dose is 1 tsp. of powder.

• During healing, the diet should include enough **calories** in order to provide the energy necessary for new bone-cell formation.

• **Coffee** blocks calcium absorption. **Excess phosphorus** locks with calcium so your body cannot absorb it. **Meat** and the **preservatives** in processed food are rich in phosphorus. **Soft drinks** (Coke, etc.) contain large amounts of phosphoric acid, which is worst of all. The acid melts your bones, and the phosphorus locks with the calcium and carries it out of the body.

OTHER HELPS

• You may use **clay poultices** to alleviate bruising and swelling. Other helpful herbs include **comfrey, alfalfa, plantain, and mistletoe. Turmeric** paste can also be applied to the surface to reduce swelling.

• To speed healing and reduce pain and swelling, place **comfrey** over the site of the fracture.

• Too much **calcium** supplementation, during bone healing, can induce kidney stone formation during the immobile period while the cast is on. The problem is that the person is not active enough at that time.

PREVENTION

• Try to eliminate slippery floors and throw rugs in your home. Put handrails on stairs. Have enough light where you walk and keep the path clear. Do not have pets that keep getting in your way. Shoes and slippers should have rubber soles. Avoid drugs which weaken your sense of balance.

—*For detailed information on rebuilding the bones, see Strengthening the Bones, just below.*

ENCOURAGEMENT—The grace of Christ and the law of God are inseparable. In Jesus, mercy and truth are met together. By His death and mediation, Jesus can forgive our sins; He can enable us to resist temptation and live clean, godly lives. 1 Corinthians 10:13..

STRENGTHENING THE BONES

It is important that you maintain strong bones, especially as you grow older. People 85 years old are 15 times more likely to break a hip than those who are 65. Unfortunately, enzymatic action and nutrient absorption continue to be reduced from the mid-40s onward. This problem accelerates after 60. Yet there are things everyone, at any age, can do to improve the quality of his or her bone structure.

NATURAL REMEDIES

You cannot succeed in life without good bones. The bones most likely to be damaged by lack of care include the jawbone, teeth, spine, hip, legs, and joints—all very important.

The objective is to achieve the highest possible bone mass before old age, and then to maintain it as long as possible. The following recommendations will help you fulfill these objectives:

DIET

• Eat plenty of **vegetables**, raw and steamed.

• Those with dentures tend to find vegetables difficult to eat. This results in a magnesium and calcium deficiency. They should have **vegetable soups, potassium broth (made of thick, white potato peelings), and raw vegetable juices** daily.

• Calcium and minerals are found abundantly in natural foods such as **green leafy vegetables, carrot juice, and broccoli**. All three are outstanding. Along with them ranks **sesame seeds**. They have the best ratio of high calcium and low phosphorus of any food. (You want a two-to-one ratio of calcium to phosphorus.)

• Other foods high in calcium include **brown rice, kale, turnip greens, pinto beans, spirulina, collard greens**.

• **Millet** is rich in calcium and magnesium. **Almonds** are high in calcium. The grains, **amaranth and quinoa**, are rich in minerals.

• **Do not just eat fruit**. Fruitarians (people who only eat fruit) do not get enough calcium or the magnesium needed to help the calcium be utilized.

• Seaweed (**Nova Scotia dulse or Norwegian kelp**) is a good source of many major minerals, and an outstanding source of the trace minerals.

• **Kelp, dulse, blue-green algae, hijiki, and kombu** are rich in minerals. **Wheat grass juice, green drink, and liquid chlorophyll** are also.

• **Garlic and onions** contain sulfur, which is needed for healthy bones.

• Eating **flaxseed oil** helps the body produce hormones needed for good bone development.

• **Chew your food** well, so it will be properly absorbed.

• **Distilled water** is an excellent way to obtain pure water. But keep in mind that you must also include proper minerals in your diet, including some kelp or dulse, to replace the minerals lost by drinking distilled water. (Distilled water is chemically hungry; it locks onto some minerals in your body when you drink it.) However, if you are eating a good diet, distilled water is the best to drink.

MINERALS

• The body requires **calcium** for many things, although bones are the most obvious need. For example, there has to be a certain amount of calcium in the blood all the time. But when, for one reason or another, the intake of certain minerals is not adequate, calcium is reabsorbed out of the bones in order to supply other needs elsewhere. (One of these needs is providing calcium to a growing fetus during pregnancy.) The bones become porous and "honeycombed," so fragile that breaks can more easily occur.

• A major cause is a lack of **calcium intake** over

a period of years. Other causes include inability to absorb calcium as well, a calcium-phosphorus imbalance (caused by **too much phosphorus** in the diet), **lack of exercise**, or **lack of certain hormones**. *For much more information on Calcium, see p. 110. For information on Vitamin D, see p. 106.*

• Obtaining enough nutrients, through diet and supplements, is important to maintaining strong bones. Foods high in calcium include **sesame seeds, spirulina, almonds, and parsley.**

• **Calcium** at 2,000 mg a day, **magnesium** at 1,000 mg per day, along with plant-derived **colloidal minerals** are needed. Those under the age of 50 need at least 1,000 mg of calcium daily; those over 50 need a minimum of 1,500 mg per day.

• *Calcium supplements:* The calcium molecule combines with another substance, such as carbonate, citrate, gluconate, lactate, or phosphate before being absorbed into the body. Here are the absorption rates of the five basic types of calcium supplements: (1) **Calcium carbonate** (41% calcium) is very poorly absorbed (5%). (2) **Calcium citrate** (21% calcium is better absorbed (40%). (3) **Calcium gluconate** (9% calcium) contains little calcium and may cause diarrhea or nausea. (4) **Calcium lactate** (13% calcium) is easily absorbed by some people. (5) **Calcium phosphate** should be avoided! Do not use it! The phosphate blocks absorption of the calcium. *Therefore, the two best are calcium citrate and calcium lactate.* The powdered form is best, not the tablets.

• *How to test your calcium supplement:* Put a tablet in a cup of vinegar, stir every few minutes. If it is not completely dissolved in 30 minutes, it will not dissolve in your stomach!

• Lack of **hydrochloric acid** (HCl) can be a cause of poor calcium (and other mineral) absorption. Adequate HCl is needed in the stomach in order for the body to absorb minerals.

• It is important that there be sufficient **acid in the stomach** in order to absorb the calcium and other minerals from the food. An increasing lack of this acid, with age, is part of the reason why older people do not absorb minerals as well and have poor bone structure. If necessary, take supplemental hydrochloric acid (betaine HCl) or lemon juice before each meal.

• **Digestive aids** may be needed to help absorb this and other minerals. Especially important is sufficient acid in the stomach. Either **betaine HCl** (hydrochloric acid supplement) or **lemon juice** can be taken. Or take 1-3 10-grain capsules (tablets may be too hard to digest) of **betaine hydrochloride** with the first few bites of every meal. (Only do this if you have low stomach acid. If you experience heartburn or stomach ulcers, do not take HCl in any form.)

• An **excess of calcium** supplementation, during bone healing (when in bed or confined to a chair while recovering from a fracture, etc.), can induce kidney stone formation during the immobile period while the cast is on. The problem is that the person is not active enough at that time.

• **Potassium** is needed for cell formation; and **vitamin C** is necessary for the maintenance and development of bones. Vitamin C is called "cell cement"; it not only fights infection, but also holds your body together!

• **Manganese** helps prevent osteoporosis (loss of bone mass). Rats on a low manganese diet developed porous bones.

• Trace amounts of **fluorides** are also needed for bone development; but get it out of food—not from additives, fluoridated water, toothpaste, etc. But beware of fluoridated drinking water. More on that below.

• A summary of minerals which are needed includes **silicon, boron, zinc, manganese, and copper**, along with **calcium**. (The body also needs phosphorus and **magnesium**; but beware of taking too much of either one. Too much of either one inhibits the body from absorbing calcium. These minerals tend to compete with calcium for absorption in the blood and bone marrow. In the case of magnesium, though, normal supplementation should not be a problem.)

VITAMINS

• **Vitamin D** is necessary (400-1,000 IU daily) for calcium absorption and repair. You need a basic 400 IU daily. Sunlight will help you get part of what you need. It is estimated that, on the average, only 10% of our daily requirement comes from sunlight; so other sources are also needed. People over 65 may need 800 units daily. But excess doses of vitamin D, taken repeatedly, caused bone deterioration.

• In one study, the more **sunlight** that was obtained by the test group, the less likelihood of osteoporosis developing.

• **Vitamin A** helps increase the rate of bone growth. It is needed for proper digestion and assimilation of nutrients.

• **Vitamin B** complex helps bone mass formation. B_6 increases connective tissue strength in bones.

• **Vitamin K** (found in **alfalfa, greens, and other chlorophyll foods**) is needed to help the body synthesize *osteocalcin,* a special protein matrix which attracts calcium to the bones.

• **Folic acid** works to prevent the formation of toxic *homocysteine* from the essential amino acid, methionine. The presence of *homocysteine* is involved in producing osteoporosis. (**Alcohol, tobacco, and oral contraceptives** increase folic acid deficiency.)

• The **acidophilus bacillus** in the large bowel is needed for the digestion of food. The bacilli make **vitamins B_6, B_{12}, and folic acid**, all of which are needed by the body for bone mass. **Lactic acid foods** (including acidophilus products, or plain yogurt) are very helpful; for they make the colon more acid and feed the helpful acid-loving acidophilus (lactic acid is a type of sugar) and reduce the amount of harmful bacteria (which dislikes an acid colon).

HERBS

• Horsetail extract is a good source of **silica**, a vital mineral in the formation of bones. **Horsetail**, along with **oat straw**, is consistently recommended as the best supplemental sources for absorbable silica. **Boron** and silica, both needed for good bone formation, are found in horsetail and oat straw. When your friends come over to visit, invite them to have some savory oat straw tea with you!

• **Alfalfa, comfrey, and slippery elm** also help build strong bones.

• Supplementing your diet with two herbs, **suma and dong quai**, will help regulate hormonal imbalances. Suma contains *sitosterol*. This increases natural estrogen production without stimulating an oversupply.

FOODS TO AVOID

• The following substances remove calcium and other minerals from the food before it is digested or leach it from the bones: **white-sugar products, chocolate, caffeine products, and alcohol**. Each of these are harmful to the bones.

• **Vinegar** and **meat acids** also diminish bone mass. This is because most other dietetic acids are later changed to alkaline forms after they leave the stomach, but not vinegar or meat acid (purines, uric acid, etc.).

• It is well-known among medical professionals that **sugar, coffee, caffeine, a high-meat diet, and smoking** produce osteoporosis and similar bone problems. One study of middle-aged men and women with symptomatic osteoporosis were almost exclusively heavy smokers.

• Do not eat **meat** if you want strong, healthy joints. A diet high in animal protein tends to cause the body to excrete increased amounts of protein. Beef, for example, contains 25 times as much phosphorus as calcium! A high-meat diet will invariably lead to calcium deficiencies. A study, conducted by *The Journal of Clinical Nutrition*, reported that vegetarian women have significantly less bone loss than women who eat meat.

• The amount of protein a man eats may influence the level of calcium in his body. Tests at Wisconsin University, confirmed by other studies, revealed that a **high-protein diet** causes calcium loss. Eskimos, on their high-protein diets, had lower bone mineral levels than Americans. In the 60-90 age bracket, bone loss in meat eaters was 35%; in vegetarians it was 18%.

• Excessive **fat intake** reduces bone mass. On test animals, the daily loss of calcium on the high-fat diet was more than four times as much as on the low-fat diet.

• The **harder the fat** was, prior to being eaten, the more calcium loss it caused.

• Avoid **large meals** and **overeating**.

• A **high-sugar diet** causes calcium to be excreted in the urine. Excess **sodium** does this also.

• **White-flour products** contain chlorine, which is harmful to the bones. Try to avoid drinking **chlorinated water**.

• Women who drink **coffee and soft drinks** are more likely to have osteoporosis.

• **High phosphorous foods** tend to compete with calcium and also combine with it, locking it out. Such foods include **soft drinks, high-protein animal foods, and yeast products**. Do not use foods with **preservatives**, because of their phosphorous content.

• **Cola drinks** are especially harmful in this respect. Cola drinks, frankly, are a terrible concoction: (1) They contain an acid which is more acid than vinegar! (2) The acidity is masked by an excessive amount of sugar which also leaches calcium from bones. (3) Cola drinks are basically phosphoric acid, or a strong acid in a phosphorous medium. Phosphorus locks directly onto calcium, and carries it out of the system, making it unavailable to the body. A tooth placed in a glass of cola drink will entirely melt away within a few hours.

• A dietary **calcium / phosphorus ratio of 2:1** is ideal; yet it can only be attained by taking calcium supplements. Here are some samples of this ratio of calcium to phosphorus in several foods: grain - 1:8; red meat - 1:12; organ meat (liver, kidney) - 1:44; fish - 1:12; carbonated drinks - 1:8. Those who eat meat and/or drink various colas and sodas obtain an immense amount of phosphorus.

• Certain foods contain **oxalic acid** in moderate amounts (the cabbage family, which includes kale, collards, and asparagus). Some contain it in still larger amounts (chard and, especially, spinach), and some in extremely large amounts (rhubarb, poke). Avoid **chard, spinach, rhubarb, and poke** if you want strong bones in your old age.

• **Chocolate** contains oxalic acid and prevents the absorption of calcium.

• Some foods contain the calcium inhibitor, *solanine*. These include **tomatoes, eggplant, bell peppers, tobacco**, and greenness (when it occurs on the outside of **white potatoes**).

• **Whole grains** contain *phytin*, a substance which tends to bind with calcium and prevent its absorption and use by the system. Some suggest that you take calcium supplements at different times than grains, to ensure its absorption. Those who desperately need additional calcium will want to take this advice. They can take calcium powder near bedtime, when it is best absorbed. Calcium also aids in sleeping; for it tends to relax the muscles.

OTHER THINGS TO AVOID

• Avoid **chilling**. Rats exposed to cold stress developed bone mass which was less dense.

• The use of **sodium fluoride**, once thought to help treat osteoporosis, is now known to do the opposite. While it does increase bone mass in the spine, the bone is inferior in quality. Woman receiving the compound were three times more likely to fracture an arm, leg, or hip than if they took a placebo. As little as 16 mg of sodium fluoride a day produces abnormal bone marrow cells. Adequate natural fluoride is easily obtained in all food and non-fluoridated water sources.

• **Drugs**, such as **diuretics**, inhibit calcium assimilation.

• Do not take **estrogen** alone because it also places the user at high risk for cancer, even though it does increase bone mass somewhat. Estrogen therapy initially increases bone formation; but it eventually leads to decreased bone mass and lack of response to the parathyroid hormone. Taking estrogen alone also increases the risk of breast cancer, stroke, and myocardial infarction (heart attack).

• If you take the **thyroid hormone** or an **anticoagulant drug**, increase the amount of calcium you take by 25%-50%.

• Older people who take **tranquilizers** have 70% more hip fractures.

EXERCISE

• For both men and women, most experts recommend an aerobic, **weight-bearing workout** three to five times per week for 35 to 45 minutes. There are lots of exercise options out there, but brisk walking is best. However, if it is not weight-bearing, it does not strengthen bones; so swimming, while it does burn calories and boost aerobic capacity, is not as helpful. Whether your exercise is social or solo, start slowly and check with your doctor or other health practitioner before taking up a new routine. Injuries, even minor ones, can derail good habits before they're ingrained.

• **Exercise** strengthens the bones. It causes the body to strengthen the insides of the bones, by increasing the webbing connections within them. Exercise definitely increases bone density. The body must have regular weight-bearing exercise, such as walking. When this occurs, more minerals are laid down in the bones, to strengthen them—especially where you need it the most: the bones of the legs, hips, and spine. Conversely, a lack of exercise accelerates the loss of bone mass. It is believed that **lack of activity** in old age is a factor in the increased levels of bone loss in those years.

Daily exercise outdoors provides vitamin D and stimulates osteoblastic cells. Exercise increases muscle tone, strengthens muscles, prevents disuse atrophy and further demineralization of the bones.

NASA research experts say the best activity for maintaining bone mass is **gravitational exercise**: walking or jogging. When you are not pushing against gravity very much (because you are sitting in a chair or lying in bed), you are tending to lose bony material. Try to walk outdoors at least 20 minutes a day.

• **"Strain changes"** are important in building and maintaining bone mass. How often you do it is more important than the intensity when it is done. Try to maintain the bounce of earlier years: Keep that spring in your step; put a little strain on your body and muscles every so often. Do this more moderately as you age, but keep it up.

• **Bed rest** tends to cause a negative calcium balance. Bones placed in **plaster casts** develop localized osteoporosis, regardless of the diet, hormonal balance, etc. It is called "disuse osteoporosis." Exercise is vital to healthy bones.

—*See "Fracture" (607) and "Osteoporosis" (612) for additional information on factors affecting bone formation and loss. Also see Lactose Intolerance (475).*

ENCOURAGEMENT—God's faithful ones are in the majority. They have all heaven on their side, in the battle to fulfill God's will for their lives and resist temptation to sin. Go to Jesus and surrender to Him. He can give you all the help you need. Psalm 4:3.

BROKEN RIB

SYMPTOMS—A sharp pain, which often starts a day or two after the blow to the rib.

CAUSES—Frequently the rib is not broken, but only has, what is known as, a green splint. This is a hairline crack. Yet it is still very painful!

If you are not able to go to a physician or emergency room, and the break is more than hairline, you may wish to use the following treatment:

NATURAL REMEDIES

• **Apply some cold water** to the bruised area, so it will not swell too much.

• When the water applications have been removed and the skin carefully dried, **place six tapes to hold the ribs in proper position**. Here is how to do it: Cut about six pieces of 1½" or 2" adhesive tape. Each piece should be 8"-10" long. Check the ribs, making sure the ends are properly together. Center the first piece of tape over the break; stretch firmly and apply to the skin. Repeat with the second piece, but at a right angle to the first piece. Continue until you have 6 tapes radiating from the center outward in all directions from where the break occurred.

• Try to **leave this on for about a month**, so it will heal well. A skin rash may develop; but it will be far less a problem than caring for the break.

—*For detailed information on rebuilding the bones, see Strengthening the Bones (608).*

ENCOURAGEMENT—Come into the presence of God with praise for the blessings you have, and you will be helped all the more as you present your requests for help. Psalm 50:15.

BONE SPUR
(Heel Spur)

SYMPTOMS—Possible pain at a place where the bone seems to protrude out from the body more than it should. Heel spurs can cause severe pain with the first step in the morning and after sitting awhile.

CAUSES—A bone spur is a pointed growth on a bone. Occurring most frequently on the heel, the bone sticks out and occasionally strikes against something, causing pain. Or there may be ongoing pain at the site.

Bone spurs can cause the formation of tiny, painful tumors at the end of some of the nerves in that area.

Those with problems with the heel are generally **overweight** or **middle-aged**. But they are also common in those who have **tendonitis, neuritis, arthritis, or alkalosis**. Other causal factors may include **gout, lupus, walking, or excessive standing**.

If bone pain is felt at an unusual bumpy and protruding place, X-rays will confirm whether the problem is arthritis, fracture, bone spur, or possibly primary metastic bone cancer.

NATURAL REMEDIES
DIET
• Give **vitamin C** to bowel tolerance, along with vitamin E and magnesium.
• Correct the calcium / phosphorus ratio by taking 2,000 mg of **calcium** a day.
• Research indicates that **plant-derived colloidal minerals** tend to reverse spurs and calcium deposits, without surgery, by remodeling the bones.
• The *bromelain* in fresh **pineapple** helps reduce pain. **Turmeric** also does. Do not use canned pineapple or its juice, because of the aluminum content.
• A 1-2 week **raw food fast** can be helpful.
• Only drink **distilled water**.
• Do not eat **meat, coffee, sugar, and alcohol**. These upset the mineral balance in the body and retard healing. Temporarily avoid **citrus fruit**.

OTHER HELPS
• For heel spurs, apply **hot and cold footbaths**. Rubbing the bottom of the feet with **ice** will help draw healing blood to the area. In the early morning, **walk barefoot outside** on the wet grass. Then come in and dry off; make sure your feet are warm afterward.
• If the shoes are not comfortable, this can make the pain feel worse. Wear **rubber heels** on your shoes, not leather. Adding **heel cushions** to your shoes may reduce pain.
• Avoid walking on **hard surfaces**.
• If you usually walk or jog for exercise, try cycling or swimming instead. Use **stretching exercises**. Deep massage around the painful area may help.
• In some cases, applying **night splints** provides a constant stretching across the sole of the foot during sleep.

ENCOURAGEMENT—Do not be enticed by seeming advantages or the advice of friends, to do wrong. Cling to God and obey His Written Word, and you will have the help that He sees is best for you.

OSTEOPOROSIS
(Brittle Bones)

SYMPTOMS—There is skeletal pain (especially in the hip and back), deformities (such as a hump in the upper back), a stooping and rounding of the shoulders, increased susceptibility to fractures, and a reduction in height. Do you find that your clothes are getting bigger? Unfortunately, symptoms are frequently not very obvious until the bones are quite weak.

There is lower back pain, loss of height (up to several inches), stooped posture, and increased risk of fractures, especially of the hip.

CAUSES—Osteoporosis is a reduction in the total mass of bone, so that the remaining bone is fragile or "brittle." This weakening continues to increase. The bones actually become thinner. This loss of bone mass occurs because bone formation is slowed; and bone reabsorption increases. "Bone reabsorption" means that the body is removing calcium and other minerals from the bones, in order to use them elsewhere.

About 25%-30% of all white females in the U.S. reveal symptoms of this condition, especially after menopause. Older men, above 50, also have it, but to a lesser degree than women. Osteoporosis is rare in black men, but somewhat more common in black women.

White women in America tend to lose 30%-40% of their bone mass between ages 55-70.

But younger women should be careful; research indicates that osteoporosis often begins early in life rather than just after menopause. (However, bone loss definitely accelerates after that time, due to a drop in estrogen levels.)

People with larger and denser bones tend to have less trouble with osteoporosis later in life. They started out with a more bony structure.

A major cause is a **lack of adequate calcium intake** over a period of years. Other causes include **inability to absorb calcium** as well, a calcium-phosphorus imbalance (**too much phosphorus** in the diet), **lack of exercise**, or **lack of certain hormones**.

Still other factors include **late puberty, early menopause** (natural or artificially induced), **chronic liver or kidney disease**, and the **long-term use of anticoagulants, corticosteroids, and antiseizure medications**. **Smoking** is an excellent way to damage your bones.

Compression fractures in the vertebrae occur as bone loss advances. This causes a loss in height and crowds the nerves, resulting in pain. Nerve damage is possible. Older women often have a hump in the upper back as a result.

Osteoporosis can also result in loose teeth which fall out, because the jawbone has weakened.

There are two types of this disease:

Osteoporosis, Type I, is thought to be caused by hormonal changes, especially a loss of estrogen.

Osteoporosis, Type II, traces its cause to dietary factors (lack of calcium, vitamin D, etc.), poor absorption and intake of foods which block absorption.

NATURAL REMEDIES

• Sleep on a **firm bed** to give support to the spine.
• **Do not lift heavy objects**. When you do lift, do it carefully and properly.
• **Avoid fatigue**.
• Look around your house and yard and **make necessary changes, so you will be less likely to fall** (placement of lights, rugs, treads on stairways, etc.).
• Take 1,000-1,500 mg of **calcium** daily.
• Eat a **diet rich in bone-forming minerals and vitamins**.
• **Folic acid**. This water-soluble vitamin plays an important role in supporting healthy tissues and bones it's important in the breakdown and metabolism of proteins; it also inhibits the action of an enzyme responsible for the production of uric acid. *Typical dosage:* 200 to 400 micrograms per day.
• **Higher uric acid levels promote bone health.** They are strongly associated with increased bone mineral density (BMD) in older men and, according to new research studies. Uric acid levels were also positively associated with serum calcium, parathyroid hormone and 25-hydroxy-vitamin D levels.
• **Cherries** (especially **black cherries**), **blueberries**, and **strawberries** have proven their ability to reduce levels of uric acid in research studies. Black cherry juice is probably the most effective. Therefore use them in moderation.
• **Alpha lipoic acid** (ALA), **vitamin E, and selenium**. This terrific trio helps to suppress the production of *leukotrienes*, chemicals that play a role in joint inflammation. ALA and selenium help vitamin E fight damaging free radicals more effectively. *Typical dosage:* 50 to 800 milligrams of ALA per day; 200 to 400 IU of vitamin E per day; and 200 micrograms of selenium per day.
• **Omega-3 and omega-6** fatty acids. You can get these in **flaxseed oil** or **evening primrose oil**, but the source doesn't matter. What matters is that these fatty acids inhibit the production of the inflammatory agents released in gout in several ways. *Typical dosage:* 1,200-2,000 mg of omega-3 per day (flaxseed oil); 500 to 1,500 milligrams of omega-6 fatty acids per day (sunflower, olive, or soy oil).
• **Bromelain**. This enzyme is found in the **pineapple** plant also functions as an effective anti-inflammatory. *Typical dosage:* 500 to 1,500 GDUs (gelatin digestion units) per day; or just eat plenty of fresh pineapple.
• **Percussion** builds bone mass. This is a massage technique called "tapotement," a light tapping on the body that mimics the bone-building stimulation from exercise. Bring the fingers of each hand together so there's no space between them (as if you were about to take a swimming stroke). Next, bend the palm and fingers to make a cup shape. Then, using the tips of your fingers and bottom of your palms, tap very lightly over your hips, ribs, and (with one hand at a time) your forearms. These are the three areas commonly weakened by osteoporosis.
• *See Strengthening the Bones (608) for a vast amount of information!*

Also see osteomalacia under Rickets (614), which is sometimes misdiagnosed as osteoporosis.

AVOIDING

• *Who gets osteoporosis?* There are several risk factors that suggest a significantly greater likelihood of developing brittle bones. **Women** with any of the following risk factors may want to begin watching their bone density while still in their forties.
• **Smokers** are 40% to 50% more likely than nonsmokers to experience osteoporosis-related hip fractures. Even if you've smoked for a long time, quitting can improve your health.
• **Caucasian and Asian women** are at greater risk for osteoporosis than Hispanic or African-American women.
• **Small-statured, thin-boned women**, regardless of race, are more likely to develop osteoporosis than other women.
• Having a **mother or grandmother with osteoporosis** increases your risk.
• Taking **drugs** that contribute to loss of bone mass and density raises risk. The most damaging are **glucocorticoids or corticosteroids; cortisone**, prescribed for inflammatory diseases; rheumatoid arthritis; asthma; or certain lung diseases.
• Those who have had diseases that interfere with digestion or the absorption of nutrients are more susceptible to osteoporosis. Such disorders include **Cushing's disease, diabetes, anorexia nervosa, bulimia, Crohn's disease, irritable bowel syndrome, hyperthyroidism, hyperparathyroidism, liver disease, multiple myeloma, and kidney failure**.

ENCOURAGEMENT—Do unto others as you would have them do unto you, and you will be greatly

S
K
E
L
M
U
S

blessed. Live like Jesus, and you will be sunshine in the lives of others. Deuteronomy 7:13.

RICKETS
(Osteomalacia in Children)

SYMPTOMS—Early symptoms include nervousness, numbness in the extremities, leg cramps, painful muscle spasms, restlessness, irritability, and profuse sweating.

Later indications include knock-knee, bowleg, narrow rib cage, protruding breastbone, or scoliosis (abnormal curvature of the spine). There may be delayed walking, tetany, bony beads along the ribs, and decaying teeth. Swelling and tenderness at the growing ends of the bones.

Left untreated, bowleg or knock-knee may develop in affected children.

In adults, in addition to the above symptoms, aching joints and generalized weakness may also occur. *See Osteomalacia, below.*

CAUSES—Rickets is caused by a deficiency of vitamin D in children. When it occurs in adults, it is called osteomalacia *(see below).*

It can result either from not obtaining enough **vitamin D** in the food or from not getting enough **sunlight**.

When sunlight strikes the skin, oils on it are irradiated, vitamin D is synthesized in the skin. Those oils are then reabsorbed into the bloodstream and carried to the liver, where it is stored and, as needed, sent throughout the body to strengthen the bones. Without this vitamin, the body cannot absorb calcium and phosphorus; and the bones cannot retain calcium. As a result, they become soft. This results in deformities when the bones are required to support weight. Yet weight gain and growth will usually be normal. But growth is sometimes retarded.

Normal **liver and kidney function** is needed for production and utilization of vitamin D in the body. Damage to either organ can cause rickets.

Oils on the skin do not make pro-vitamin D quite as well if the children have dark skin and/or lack sunlight exposure. Vegetarians must obtain adequate sunlight on the skin. Research studies found that Muslim women who are entirely covered in black cloth, when outside their homes, could obtain adequate sunlight by exposing their bare feet to the sunlight for a relatively short time each week.

A deficiency of **vitamin C** can make the bones less able to retain bone-building minerals. Rickets is worsened by inadequate **calcium** in the diet.

Certain disorders can interfere with absorption of nutrients: **asthma, bronchitis, colon problems, severe allergies, or celiac disease**. Intestinal surgery and drugs used to treat epilepsy can also interfere.

Osteomalacia is often misdiagnosed as osteoporosis (*612*).

After treatment with proper nutrition and sunlight, most people make a full recovery; although early deformities may be permanent in children.

NATURAL REMEDIES

• Eat a diet rich in calcium. This includes green-leafy vegetables, broccoli, and raw fruits, nuts, and seeds. Avoid processed, junk, or sugar foods. Do not drink soft drinks, which pull calcium out of the bones. *See Strengthening the Bones (608).*

• In order to avoid rickets, the National Institutes of Health recommends the following **vitamin D supplementation**: 400 mg until 6 months of age, 600 mg for ages 6-12 months, 800 mg for 1 year through age 5, 800-1,200 mg for ages 6-10. The safe adult dose is 400 IU per day. More than 1,000 IU daily for long periods of time can lead to headaches, weight loss, kidney stones. In rare cases, there is deafness, blindness, and death.

—See Strengthening the Bones (608) for additional information on how to make the bones strong.

ENCOURAGEMENT—You can safely choose only those who love God for your close friends. But, whatever your lot in life, determine that you will do all you can to help and encourage all with whom you come in contact. Psalm 42:8.

OSTEOMALACIA
(Rickets in Adults)

SYMPTOMS—Painful, tender bones. This is most often in the ribs, hips, and bones of the legs. There is difficulty in climbing stairs, getting up from a squatting position, and bone fractures after a minor injury.

CAUSES—This is the adult form of Rickets; and all the information listed under Rickets applies to osteomalacia.

The adult form of rickets, osteomalacia, generally occurs during **pregnancy or breast-feeding**. But it may also be caused by a **kidney disease or defect, calcium deficiency, a lack of vitamin D**, or inability to utilize the vitamin D. It can also occur in those who do not obtain enough sunshine or whose bodies are so low in fat that they cannot produce the bile needed to absorb the vitamin D in the food.

In addition, certain disorders can interfere with absorption of nutrients: **asthma, bronchitis, colon problems, severe allergies, or celiac disease**. Intestinal surgery and drugs used to treat epilepsy can also interfere.

—See Rickets (above) for how to eliminate osteomalacia. Also see Strengthening the Bones (608) for additional information.

ENCOURAGEMENT—God's gift of Christ to us is a pledge of His great love for us. How thankful we can be that God loves us so!

PAGET'S DISEASE OF THE BONE

SYMPTOMS—At first, there are no symptoms other than possibly mild pain in the affected bones (generally at night or when working). There may be joint pain in nearby joints.

In one area, one or more of the bones are deformed. There is bone pain and degeneration, arthritis, obvious bony deformities, and an increased tendency to fractures. Bone deformities may include bowleg, bent spine, barrel-shaped chest, or enlarged forehead.

The bones most frequently affected are those of the spine, thighs, pelvis, skull, hips, shins, and upper arms.

Long-standing Paget's disease may also lead to numbness, tingling, or weakness in the affected area if the bone presses on adjacent nerves. It may cause ringing in the ears or hearing loss if abnormal growth of bone compresses nerves to the ear.

CAUSES—In a healthy person, bone is continually being broken down and replaced by new bone, to maintain the normal bone structure. However, Paget's Disease is an ongoing deterioration of certain parts of the skeleton. At those locations, the bone degenerates at the same time that new bone is made, which is deficient in calcium and therefore fragile. The result is larger bony areas which are deformed.

Because it produces few symptoms, the disease is often first diagnosed when a chance X-ray discovers it.

The cause is unknown; but a viral condition may be involved. Those who live in rural settings, eat wholesome diets, and have outdoor activities are less likely to contract this disease.

NATURAL REMEDIES
• Eat a **nutritious diet**! This is extremely important. The likelihood is that toxic substances in the food or environment, along with an impoverished diet of junk food, are causative factors.
• **Garlic, echinacea, goldenseal, and other antibiotic herbs** are helpful. *See Antibiotic Herbs (297) and cautions concerning them in the chapter on herbs (129-189).*
• *Read the sections on Strengthening the Bones (608), Rickets (614), and Fractures (607).*
• **Heat therapy**, such as hot compresses, heat lamps, etc., can alleviate pain. See the chapter on *Hydrotherapy (206-275).*

ENCOURAGEMENT—Darkness and discouragement will sometimes come upon the soul and threaten to overwhelm us, but we should not cast away our confidence. We must keep the eye fixed on Jesus, feeling or no feeling. We should seek to faithfully perform every known duty, and then calmly rest in the promises of God. Trusting in Christ, we can move steadily forward, obeying God's holy book, the Bible.

SKELETAL-MUSCULAR - 2 - JOINTS
Also: Sciatica (566, 626, 645, 713), Neuritis (568), Neuralgia (563), Lumbago (648)

KNEE PAIN

SYMPTOMS—Pain in, or close to, the knee. In severe cases, it may be difficult to bend the knee.

CAUSES—The problem is generally inflammation of the bursa in front of the kneecap. The tendons of the knees may also be injured. Obvious causes include **running, jumping, climbing stairs, scrubbing floors, sports, bumping against a hard object, poor posture, leaning against a ladder**.

NATURAL REMEDIES
• Putting **ice on the knee** is a soothing natural remedy. Keep ice in the freezer and fill an ice bag (ice cap). Fill some paper cups with water and freeze them. Keep water-soaked Ace bandages in the freezer. Rub ice on the knee until it is numb. Put cold packs on the knee.
• After applying the ice, **stretch the stiff or sore muscle** to restore the range of motion. The stretching should be gradual and not jerky. Gently stretch them.
• Put **ice on an inflamed knee** for 20 minutes at a time, 3-4 times a day, for the first 48 hours. Thereafter, **apply heat** (moist heat is best, or even a hot shower) for 15 minute intervals 3 times a day.
• **Lose extra weight**. It will take a lot of pressure off your knees.
• *If you have to kneel*, wear protective **knee pads**.
• *If you have to work below your waist*, **sit** on a stool or on the floor.
• *When kneeling* (as in gardening), put a **foam cushion under your knees**. Keep shifting your weight and changing leg positions.
• *When sitting for a long time*, keep shifting your position. **Get up and walk around** every 35-40 minutes.
• *If you do fast walking*, do not over-extend the knees, or a pain will develop in the tendons in back.
• *For normal walking or running*, keep the knees slightly bent.
• Do not wear thin-soled or high-heeled shoes. **Walking shoes** should be well-cushioned, especially at the heels.
• *If pain starts*, stop what you are doing. RICE:

CHART 1056: Diseases of the Joints 615-633

Rest the knee by sitting or laying down. Put **ice** on the knee. **Compress** or wrap the knee gently. **Elevate** the leg. But a very effective alternative is alternate hot and cold to the area.

• Minimize squatting or excessive stair climbing. The stress between kneecap and thigh can be more than 2,000 pounds when you stand up.

• Begin **massage** of the area 24 hours after the injury. Put oil on the top, sides, and back of your knee, so your hand will easily slide over the skin. *If there is swelling,* then stroke all around it, always gliding in the direction of the heart. Use light to moderate pressure.

If there is little or no swelling, stroke with deep circular friction. Press on the skin and move it in circles; then move to a nearby area and begin again. Use firm, not painful pressure. Never apply pressure behind the knee between the two cord-like tendons (because large nerves are there). Repeat the circular friction all over. Do this once a day.

• *Danger signs:* If you feel numbness or tingling in your feet or toes, when your knee is swollen, and especially if you feel something moving inside your knee. If you heard a "pop" in your knee when the injury occurred.

ENCOURAGEMENT—Make your requests known to your Maker. Never is one repulsed who comes to Him with a contrite heart.

OSGOOD-SCHLATTER'S SYNDROME

SYMPTOMS—Knee pain and stiffness. There may be swelling about the knee and tenderness, when it is touched. Pain is often worse when jumping, running, or climbing stairs. The knee is usually sore to pressure at the point where the large tendon from the kneecap attaches to the prominence below.

CAUSES—The patellar tendon, which normally attaches to the tibial tuberosity, has been strained by the powerful quadriceps muscles. This tearing (avulsion) can be extremely painful and is sometimes disabling. Teenagers (especially boys) experience this problem more frequently than others; and it often occurs during or shortly after a growth spurt. It is common in those engaged in sports. Osgood-Schlatter's Syndrome may occur in both knees at the same time.

The problem tends to occur during the ages of 10 to 15, in boys, and 8 to 13 in girls. It generally lessens over a two-year period as the youth grows. The bone overgrowth may cause a protuberance.

Children with Osgood-Schlatter's Syndrome were formerly restricted from physical activity. Now most orthopedic physicians let the child decide his own level of activity.

NATURAL REMEDIES

• It has been found that **vitamin E** (400 U daily) and **selenium** (50 mcg, 3 times daily) has been very helpful in improving the situation in 2-6 weeks.

• If you experience pain, try to **avoid or restrict the activity** causing it. But you need **exercise**; for it is part of the healing process. Activities, such as running and climbing, may need to be reduced or stopped for a time. Do quadriceps **stretching exercises** during a warm-up period prior to active exercise.

• Daily **gentle massage** improves blood flow in the knee area. An **ice pack** over the knee may reduce pain.

• **Exercises** which strengthen the quadriceps are helpful after the pain subsides; for they improve muscle strength.

Pain medications are sometimes prescribed; although they eliminate pain, the youth may overdo and injure the knee even more, resulting in permanent injury.

Treat the knee right, and the problem tends to eventually subside and disappear.

ENCOURAGEMENT—When in discouragement, let the eye of faith see Jesus in heaven. He is preparing a home for His faithful children.

CHONDROMALACIA
(Patellofemoral Pain Syndrome)

SYMPTOMS—Symptoms vary in severity in different persons; but they may include pain in the knee when the leg is bent and straightened (as in going up and down stairs), stiffness after prolonged sitting, and crepitus (a crackling noise) during knee movement. The problem usually, but not always, occurs in only one knee.

CAUSES—The cartilage surface of the back of the patella (kneecap) has been damaged. This can be caused by **strenuous exercise** or **repeated knee injuries**. In teenagers, it can be caused by **increased weight bearing** on the knee joint during growth spurts. But a **misaligned or recurrently dislocated patella**, or **muscle weakness in the upper leg**, may be part or all of the cause.

To identify whether pain in your knee is caused by chondromalacia, press down on the knee cap and see if the symptoms worsen.

NATURAL REMEDIES

• Recovery can usually occur within several months **if strenuous exercise is not resumed** prematurely. Eat a **nourishing diet**. If you are not careful, there is increased risk that in later life you may develop osteoarthritis (622).

—Also see Strengthening the Bones (608).

ENCOURAGEMENT—By faith grasp the hand of Christ, and trust Him as fully in the darkness as in the light.

TYPES OF ARTHRITIS

There are several types of arthritis. **A usual symptom is swollen, painful joints.** Here are several distinguishing symptoms of the four leading kinds:

The largest number of Americans (over 15 million) have *osteoarthritis (622)*. This begins after 40; and there is pain and stiffness when a joint is moved. It usually begins gradually over many years. Inflammation does not develop until later.

Rheumatoid arthritis (623) affects 3 million; it begins between 25 and 50. Joint stiffness occurs for the first hour or so upon awakening. There will be swelling in and around a certain finger or wrist joints. There may, or may not, be pain. The condition may worsen or remain the same.

Gout (627) affects 1.5 million (mostly men), and is a rapid onset of extreme pain and swelling of one or more joints, usually the big toe.

Ankylosing spondylitis (629), along with several related disorders, affects 2.5 million; it usually begins between 20 and 40. There is pain, stiffness, inflammation in the spine, along with postural changes.

Here is still more information on 13 types of arthritic conditions: Swollen, painful joints can have a variety of causes. The particular symptoms make different arthritic and related conditions distinguishable from one another.

Juvenile Arthritis: This is a general term for all types of arthritis that occur in children. Juvenile rheumatoid arthritis is the most prevalent form in children; and there are three major types: *polyarticular* (affecting many joints), *pauciarticular* (affecting a few joints), and *systemic* (affecting the entire body). The signs and symptoms of juvenile rheumatoid arthritis vary from child to child. There is no single test that establishes conclusively a diagnosis of juvenile arthritis; and the condition must be present consistently for six or more consecutive weeks before a correct diagnosis can be made. Heredity is thought to play some part in the development of juvenile arthritis. However, the inherited trait alone does not cause the illness. Researchers think this trait, along with some other unknown factor (probably in the environment), triggers the disease. The *Arthritis Foundation* says that juvenile arthritis is even more prevalent than juvenile diabetes and cerebral palsy.

Gout: This is a disease that causes sudden, severe attacks of pain, tenderness, redness, warmth, and swelling in some joints. It usually affects one joint at a time, especially the joint of the big toe. Needle-shaped uric acid crystals that precipitate out of the blood are deposited in the joint to cause the pain and swelling associated with gout. In people with gout, the body does not produce enough of the digestive enzyme, uricase, which oxidizes relatively insoluble uric acid into a highly soluble compound. Factors leading to increased levels of uric acid, and then gout, include obesity, improper diet. overeating. stress, surgery,

joint injury, excessive alcohol intake, hypertension, kidney disease. and certain drugs. —*See Gout.*

Ankylosing Spondylitis: This is a chronic inflammatory disease of the spine that can fuse the vertebrae, to produce a rigid spine. Spondylitis is a result of inflammation that usually starts in the tissue outside the joint. The most common early symptoms of spondylitis are low back pain and stiffness that continues for months. Although the cause of spondylitis is unknown, scientists have discovered a strong genetic or family link, according to the *Arthritis Foundation*. Most people with spondylitis have a genetic marker, known as HLA-B27. (Genetic markers are protein molecules located on the surface of white blood cells that act as a "name tag.") Having this genetic marker does not mean a person will develop spondylitis, but people with the marker are more likely to develop the disease. Ankylosing spondylitis usually affects men between the ages of sixteen and thirty-five, but it also affects women. Other joints besides the spine can be involved.

Systemic Lupus Erythematosus: This is an autoimmune disease that can involve the skin, kidneys, blood vessels, joints, nervous system, heart, and other internal organs. Symptoms vary among those affected; but there may be a skin rash. arthritis, fever, anemia, hair loss, ulcers in the mouth, and kidney sediment or function abnormalities. In most cases. the symptoms first appear in women of childbearing age: however, lupus can occur in young children or in older people. Studies suggest there is an inherited tendency to get lupus and lupus affects women about nine to ten times as often as men. It is also more common in African-American women.

Bursitis, Tendinitis, and Myofascial Pain: These are localized, nonsystemic (not affecting the entire body) painful conditions. Bursitis is inflammation of the sac surrounding any joint that contains a lubricating fluid. Tendinitis is inflammation of a tendon; and myofascial pain is a problem that results from the strain or improper use of a muscle. These conditions may start suddenly and usually stop within a matter of days or weeks.

Carpal Tunnel Syndrome: This is a condition in which pressure on the median nerve at the wrist causes tingling and numbness in the fingers. It can begin suddenly or gradually and can be associated with another disease, such as rheumatoid arthritis; or it may be unrelated to any other condition. If untreated, it can result in permanent nerve and muscle damage. With early diagnosis and treatment, there is an excellent chance of complete recovery.

Fibromyalgia Syndrome: This is a condition characterized by generalized muscular pain, fatigue, and poor sleep. It is believed to affect approximately 2 percent of the U.S. population, or about 5 million people. The name, *fibromyalgia*, means "pain in the muscles, ligaments, and tendons!' The condition

SKEL MUS

mainly affects muscles and their attachments to bones. Although it may feel like a joint disease, the Arthritis Foundation says it is not a true form of arthritis and it does not cause deformities of the joints. It is, instead, a form of soft tissue and muscular rheumatism.

Infectious Arthritis: This is a form of joint inflammation that is caused by a bacterial, viral, or fungal infection. The diagnosis is made by culturing the organism from the joint. Infectious arthritis can be cured using antibiotic medications.

Osteoarthritis (OA): This rarely develops before the age of forty, but it affects nearly everyone past the age of sixty. Nearly three times as many women as men have it and; at present, over 20 million people are affected. Previously known as "degenerative joint disease," osteoarthritis results from the "wear and tear" of life. Other risk factors include joint trauma, obesity, and repetitive joint use. The simple effect of gravity causes physical damage to the joints and surrounding tissues, leading to pain, tenderness, swelling, and decreased function. Initially, osteoarthritis is noninflammatory; and it may be so mild that a person is unaware of it until it appears on an x-ray. Usually, only one or two joints are affected, most often the knee, hip, and hand. Pain is the earliest symptom, usually exacerbated by repetitive use. —*See Osteoarthritis.*

Psoriatic Arthritis: This condition is similar to rheumatoid arthritis. About 5 percent of people with psoriasis, a chronic skin disease, also develop psoriatic arthritis. With psoriatic arthritis, there is joint inflammation and sometimes inflammation of the spine. Fewer joints may be involved than in rheumatoid arthritis; and there is no rheumatoid factor in the blood.

Reiter's Syndrome: involves inflammation in the joints, and sometimes at the location where tendons attach to bones. This form of arthritis usually develops following an intestinal or a genital/urinary tract infection. People with Reiter's Syndrome have arthritis and one or more of the following: urethritis, prostatitis, cervicitis, cystitis. eye problems, or skin sores.

Rheumatoid Arthritis (RA): This type of inflammatory arthritis is an autoimmune disorder that occurs when the body's own immune system mistakenly attacks the synovium (the cell lining inside the joint). An overactive immune system can be just as harmful as a weak one. As with other autoimmune disorders, rheumatoid arthritis is a "self-attacking-self" disease. In this case, the body's immune system improperly identifies the synovial membrane as *foreign.* The synovium becomes inflamed and thickened. Inflammation damages cartilage and tissues in and around the joints. Often, the bone surfaces are destroyed as well because inflammation in the joints triggers the production of enzymes that slowly digest adjacent tissue. The body replaces this damaged tissue with scar tissue, forcing normal spaces within the joints to become narrow and the bones to fuse together. Rheumatoid arthritis creates stiffness, swelling, fatigue, anemia, weight loss, fever, and often crip-

pling pain. Rheumatoid arthritis frequently occurs in people under forty years of age. Currently, 2.1 million Americans have this disabling disorder, 75 percent of them female. Juvenile arthritis is a form of rheumatoid arthritis that strikes children under the age of sixteen. It affects 71,000 young Americans, again most of them female. The onset of rheumatoid arthritis is associated with physical or emotional stress, poor nutrition, and bacterial infection. Rheumatologists have discovered that the blood of many people with rheumatoid arthritis contains antibodies, called *rheumatoid factors,* a finding that can aid in the diagnosis of the condition. While osteoarthritis affects individual joints, rheumatoid arthritis affects all of the body's synovial joints. —*See Rheumatoid Arthritis.*

Scleroderma: This is a disease of the body's connective tissue that causes thickening and hardening of the skin. It can also affect joints, blood vessels, and internal organs. There are two types of scleroderma: localized and generalized.

ENCOURAGEMENT—If we would permit our minds to dwell more upon Christ and the heavenly world, we should find a powerful stimulus and support in fighting the battles of the Lord. Beside the loveliness of Christ, all earthly attractions will seem of little worth. Philippians 4:8.

ARTHRITIS

SYMPTOMS—Swelling in one or more joints. Body stiffness and pain in joints, especially during damp weather, in the morning, or after strenuous activity. There may be a sharp burning or grinding pain or it may feel like a toothache. There may be stiffness and/or pain when moving a joint. Recurring pain or tenderness in any joint. Inability to move a joint normally. Obvious redness and warmth in a joint. Unexplained weight loss, fever, or weakness combined with joint pain. Symptoms such as these that last for more than two weeks.

CAUSES—Arthritis is the inflammation of one or more joints. The word, "arthritis," covers a number of disorders, some of which are covered in this present article—which deals the most completely with the problem.

The most common forms are Osteoarthritis *(622),* Rheumatoid Arthritis *(623),* Gout *(627),* and Ankylosing Spondylitis *(629).* Other diseases which also infect the joints include Lupus *(310),* Lyme Disease *(813, 840),* Psoriatic Arthritis, Sjögren's Syndrome *(310),* and Reiter's Syndrome. Untreated Lyme disease can lead to chronic arthritis.

The various types of arthritis affect the synovial (movable) joints. These are the fingers, toes, wrists, elbows, hips, and knees. There are also joints between the bones of the spine. Each joint has cartilage covering over the end of the bone; it is continually bathed in synovial fluid in a capsule.

CHART 1056: Diseases of the Joints 615-633

Osteoarthritis: Cartilage is a smooth, soft, pearly tissue. Among other places, it is found on the ends of the long bones; it provides a smooth surface for the bones in the joints to slide against.

As a result of years of wear and improper diet, this cartilage becomes pitted, thin, and may even disappear. There is pain and stiffness. Older people experience this most often; and it generally occurs in the weight-bearing joints (hips and knees).

The connecting ligaments and muscles, which hold the joint together, become weaker. The joint may become deformed. There may be pain, but usually no swelling. Bony outgrowths may later develop.

Osteoarthritis rarely occurs before 40; but it affects most people after 60. Sometimes it is so mild as to be unnoticed. Women have it three times as often as men.

For information on rheumatoid arthritis (623), bursitis (629), and gout (627), turn to their respective articles.

Here is a brief comparative overview:

In *osteoarthritis (622)*, the cartilage at the end of bones wears down and produces rough, hard edges of bone which causes trouble. This generally begins after 40; 16 million persons in the U.S. have it.

In *rheumatoid arthritis (623)*, the cartilage at the end of bones is destroyed; and it is replaced with scar tissue. Then swelling occurs and the joints may eventually fuse together. While osteoarthritis only affects individual joints, rheumatoid arthritis ultimately affects all synovial joints in a person's body. This problem usually begins between 25 and 50; 3 million in the U.S. are afflicted with it.

Gout (627) produces extreme pain, usually starting in a big toe (or other smaller toe or finger joint). This generally does not begin until 40 or after; 1.5 million experience it. Over 90% are men.

The *spondyloarthropathies* affect the spine, causing pain, stiffness, joint fusion, and changes in posture. The most common is ankylosing spondylitis *(629)*. These difficulties generally start between 20 and 40, afflicting a total of 2.5 million. Men have it over twice as often.

Infectious arthritis is the result of viral, bacterial, or fungal infection within a joint; it is most frequently bacteria or fungi, especially from candida *(281)*. The infection can come from injury, surgery, or disease. There are body aches, chills, and fever, along with throbbing pain in the affected joint. The pain and infection may spread to other joints. It may strike at any age; 100,000 in the U.S. have it.

The following suggestions will help one deal with a variety of arthritic conditions:

NATURAL REMEDIES
DIET

Arthritis is the result of a complex of nutritional deficiencies.

• European clinics have treated arthritis with a diet of **raw food and fresh juices** for over 75 years. Drink 1-2 glasses daily of any combination of **raw juices of beets, carrots, celery, parsley, or alfalfa**.

• A dietary **calcium / phosphorus ratio of 2:1** is ideal; yet it can only be attained by taking calcium supplements *(see Strengthening the Bones, 608)*. **Meat** is especially bad; it has a ratio of 1:12. Organ meats, such as liver and kidney, are even worse: 1:44. So the more meat you eat, the more calcium you need. It is as simple as that. To really help solve the problem, stop eating all types of meat!

• In addition to the calcium problem, meat is also heavy in purines and uric acid, both of which are extremely acid. Eventually this hodgepodge of acids collects in the joints to such a degree that the bone is eaten away, the bursa becomes inflamed, etc.

• The sulfur-containing foods (**asparagus, garlic, and onions**) help repair bone, cartilage, and connective tissue. They also aid in the absorption of calcium.

• Eat **green leafy vegetables, whole grains, oatmeal, and brown rice**. These supply vitamin K,

• Eat **fresh pineapple** frequently. The *bromelain* in it is good for reducing inflammation. It must be fresh, since freezing or canning destroys the enzyme. Canned pineapple contains aluminum, which can lead to Alzheimer's. An alternative is to take 6-8 **bromelain tablets**. Research studies found that bromelain reduced or eliminated swelling and inflammation in the soft tissues and the joints affected by rheumatoid arthritis.

• The most beneficial vegetables include **celery, parsley, alfalfa, wheat grass, garlic, comfrey, and endive**.

• The most beneficial fruits include **bananas, pineapples, sour apples, and sour cherries**.

• Foods containing the amino acid, *histidine*, include **wheat, rye, and rice**. Histidine helps remove metals; and many arthritics have high levels of copper and iron in their bodies.

• Eat some form of fiber (such as **oat bran, rice bran, flaxseed**, etc.) Take 1 Tbsp. **flaxseed oil** daily. It is a good source of omega-3 fatty acid, which helps alleviate arthritic problems.

• **Vegetable juice therapy** is especially helpful for arthritics, especially those with rheumatoid arthritis.

• **Repeated juice fasts** of 4-6 weeks are recommended, along with about 2 months of an extremely nourishing diet. The alkaline action of raw juices and vegetable broth dissolves the accumulation of deposits around the joints and in other tissues. Underweight people should not fast as long.

• Daily **green juice, mixed with carrot, celery, red beet juice, and vegetable broths** are specifics for arthritis and other rheumatic diseases.

• Drink **raw potato juice**. Slice a potato with the

skin on, cut it into thin slices, and place in a large glass. Fill the glass with cold water and let it stand overnight. Drink the water the next morning on an empty stomach.

• **Potato juice** can also be made in an electric juicer. Make it fresh, dilute it 50-50 with water, and drink first thing in the morning.

• People who are low in the antioxidant compound, *glutathione*, are more likely to have arthritis. Vegetables rich in glutathione include **asparagus, cabbage, cauliflower, potatoes, and purslane**.

• Once a day, drink 1 Tbsp. **blackstrap molasses** in ½ cup **apple juice** or **grape juice**.

• **Milk, wheat, eggs, corn, pork and soda drinks** have been shown to produce arthritic symptoms.

• **Vitamin C** is necessary, to prevent the capillary walls in the joints from breaking down and causing bleeding, swelling, and pain. Vitamin C is vital to joint health.

• **Folic acid, vitamin B$_{12}$, and iron** in food help treat the anemia which frequently accompanies arthritis.

• A British research study revealed that arthritic patients had a low **pantothenic acid** level in their blood. This important B vitamin should be included in the diet.

• Treatment of arthritis should include **calcium** (2,000 mg per day, assuming no meat is eaten), **vitamin C** (to bowel tolerance), **B$_6$** (100 mg, twice a day), **B$_3$** (450 mg, twice a day), **vitamin E** (1,000 IU daily), **copper** (2 mg per day), **selenium** (300 mcg per day), and **zinc** (30 mg, three times a day).

• **DMSO** (dimethyl sulfoxide) is a by-product of the wood industry. It can be applied to the skin above the affected area—to relieve pain, reduce swelling, and promote healing. Obtain it from a health-food store.

• Take a **free-form amino acid complex** regularly, to help repair tissue damage.

• Arthritic patients frequently have liver disorders. This can deter the conversion of carotene into vitamin A. Therefore additional **carotene-rich foods** should be eaten.

• The Rheumatoid Disease Foundation suggests taking 3 mg **of boron** (a trace mineral) daily, to treat osteoarthritis and rheumatoid arthritis.

• **Histidine** (an amino acid) is useful for its anti-inflammatory effect in rheumatoid arthritis. **Proline** is an amino acid used in treating arthritis.

• Arthritis is caused by acids and waste matter in the body, which eventually become solidified and lock the joint. This condition is caused and aggravated by improper diet. Some of the worst intakes are **eggs, bread, milk, meat, salt, sugar**, etc. because they cause arthritic calcification. The use of extremely hard water (generally of twelve or more grains in hardness) will often accentuate an arthritic condition, but softer water will help relieve it. Sometimes an individual with a good inherent structure can throw off the hardest water without arthritic effect. The weaker person may drink water that is not very hard and absorb, from it, relatively larger quantities of the inorganic minerals.

• For eliminating toxic substances from the bowels, one may use a high enema of slippery elm or white oak bark tea. The system should be cleansed by a daily sweat bath with **pleurisy root;** massage (except the inflamed joints) with **angelica, black cohosh, buckthorn bark, gentian root, skullcap, or valerian root**. One may use poultices—such as **cayenne, lobelia, mullein, slippery elm** for relieving pain of the swollen joints. Liniments of oils are also good with **cayenne, coconut, lobelia**.

• Other useful herbs include: **Bear's-foot, bitterroot, blackberry, black cohosh, buckthorn bark, burdock, hydrangeas, Irish moss, saw palmetto berries, skullcap, wintergreen, yellow dock.**

AVOID

• Reduce the amount of **fat** in your diet. Avoid dairy products and fatty foods. You must also avoid **hydrogenated oils**.

• **Do not eat meat**. The purines and uric acid in it inflame arthritic conditions. If the blood is too acidic, the cartilage in the joints can dissolve. Stop the meat diet!

• Avoid **salt, caffeine, tobacco, paprika, and citrus fruits**.

• Do not eat anything with **added sugar**.

• A **high-protein diet** induced arthritis in research on pigs. The first symptoms occurred within a week.

• Some arthritics are sensitive to foods in the nightshade *(solanaceous)* family. This includes **eggplant, white potato** (only when it has green on the skin), **bell pepper, tomato, and tobacco**. These foods contain *solanine*, which interferes with muscle activity. In one research study, 85% of arthritics were benefited when they stopped using those foods. Unfortunately, such items are sometimes included in other foods as "natural ingredients." One research study found that 28% of those avoiding nightshade plants, but were unknowingly eating foods that had these ingredients (labeled as "natural ingredients"), had a "marked positive response" and another 44% had a "positive response." So not eating those foods helped 68% of those who did it.

• **Chocolate, tea, coffee**, and **cortisone injections** may also cause problems.

• Do not use **iron supplements** or vitamin / mineral supplements that contain iron. Get your iron from food (blackstrap molasses, broccoli, etc.).

• Reduce your **body weight**, and you will reduce the amount of pain in your spine, knees, hips, ankles, and feet.

HERBS

• Helpful herbs include **black cohosh, parsley, slippery elm, alfalfa, peppermint, buckthorn bark, ragwort, burdock root, and chaparral**.

• Researchers in India gave 1½-3½ tsp. **ginger** to patients with osteoarthritis and rheumatoid arthritis. More than 75% experienced some—or a lot—of relief from pain and swelling. None showed any ill effects after taking these high doses for 2 years.

• **Cayenne** interferes with pain perception, when

placed on the extremities or trunk. It triggers the body to release *endorphins*, which reduce the pain. But do not get it in your eyes. Some people are too sensitive to cayenne to put it on their skin.

• **Turmeric** is a yellow spice from India. It works as well as a pain medication, to reduce arthritic pain and inflammation; and it does not have side effects.

• **Kombucha tea** has nutrients needed to strengthen connective tissue; so it tends to relieve pain, increase energy, and improve mobility in arthritics.

• **Chaparral**, according to Indian folklore, it has anti-rheumatoid properties. They used it extensively. The primary constituent, NDGA *(nordihydroquaiaretic acid)*, possesses analgesic (pain relieving) properties.

• **Sarsaparilla** has been found to be an effective treatment for rheumatism. This is due to the *saponins* in it.

• In 1958, British researchers discovered that **licorice root** has anti-inflammatory properties useful in treating arthritis. It is the *glycyrrhizin* in it that does this.

• Here is an a good **tea for arthritis**: Mix equal parts black cohosh, chamomile, bearberry leaves, cascara sagrada, pokeweed root, and sassafras. Steep 1½ tsp. mixture in 1 cup boiling-hot water for 10 minutes. Take 1 cup in the morning and evening. Sweeten with honey, if desired.

• Here is an alternate **tea for arthritis**: Substitute parsley, yerba buena, and yerba santa for the above herbs, and prepare in the same way. Drink 2 cups a day in mouthful doses.

• The following **poultice** has been used with good results on swollen joints: Take 3 Tbsp. of granulated slippery elm bark, 1 Tbsp. of lobelia, 2 Tbsp. of mullein, 1 tsp. of cayenne, and mix it all in a bowl. Add hot water to make a paste. Spread it on a cloth and cover the swollen joints. Over it, wrap a plastic sheet and then a dry towel. Leave it on for ½ to 1 hour or less, if burning sensation becomes unbearable.

• A second **poultice** for swollen joints: Mix 9 parts slippery elm bark, 6 parts mullein leaves, 3 parts lobelia, and 1 part cayenne. Add 3 oz. of the mixture to boiling-hot water, to make a paste. Spread it on a cloth and apply to the affected area.

• **To promote circulation**: Mix 2 parts ginger root, 1 part cayenne, and ½ part lobelia. Make a paste (as described above). Apply either as a poultice, Fomentation, or liniment. Also use this for rheumatism.

• Mix **eucalyptus oil** with water and rub on the affected area. Wrap the joint in plastic wrap, and apply moist heat with hot towels.

• Apply packs of warmed **castor oil, moistened comfrey tea leaves, or grated raw potato** to the affected area.

• Here is an odd treatment which has been used with partial success for thousands of years: Go find some stinging **nettle plant** *(urticadioica)* or grow it in your backyard. Whenever your arthritis gives you too much trouble, pick some stinging nettle with a gloved hand, and then hit it against the arthritic hand, etc. This is called "urtication," and will greatly improve the situation. It can bring considerable relief and sometimes reduce the swelling within minutes. What happens: The stings bring blood to the area, which provides temporary healing. An application of **cayenne pepper**, mixed with some water in a paste, would have much the same effect. However, the experts say that the tiny stingers of the plant inject several chemicals that produce an anti-inflammatory action. Stinging nettle is a common weed on most continents.

• Take 3 **yucca** tablets with each meal or 2 **primrose oil** capsules twice daily.

• Here are other herbal remedies to reduce inflammation and pain, and stimulate circulation. Try any of them: **white willow bark** or **meadowsweet** (2 capsules or 1 cup of tea, as needed to reduce pain). **Hawthorn** (2 capsules or 1 cup of tea). **Devil's claw** or **wild yam** (3 capsules, 3 times daily).

• **Feverfew** (2 capsules of freeze-dried herb, 3 times daily) has a long history of usage as an anti-arthritic herb.

• **Boswellia serrata** is a large branching tree native to India. It produces an exudative gum resin, known as *salai guggul*, and has been used for centuries to treat arthritic problems. Take the 150 mg capsules or apply it, in cream form, to the area.

• The Polynesians, in the South Pacific Islands, have used **noni** to treat arthritis for hundreds of years.

• Those living in the Mediterranean have used **olive leaf** extract for centuries for the same purpose. It contains *oleuropein*, which is so helpful.

• **Burdock root** has been used for years, both internally and externally, to treat painful joints.

HYDROTHERAPY

• If you are unable to exercise your joints because the pain is too great, do the **exercise program in a tub of warm water** (93°-98° F.).

• Place **cold gel packs** on inflamed joints, to relieve pain. Alternate with applications of heat.

• **Charcoal poultices** may be applied to affected joints.

• **Hot packs** applied to stiff joints tend to decrease morning stiffness.

• **Hot tub baths** also provide relief.

• In the morning, take a **hot shower**, to help relieve morning stiffness.

OTHER HELPS

• **Exercise** is very important in both preventing and treating arthritis. Joints which are not used tend to stiffen. Practice bending all your joints (not merely the affected ones) in different positions, 5-10 times, twice a day.

S
K
E
L
M
U
S

• **Swimming** is an ideal exercise for maintaining joint flexibility and stamina. Since the water supports your body, muscles can be exercised without straining your joints.

• Good **posture** is also important. Poor posture does not distribute weight evenly and can intensify the problem.

• Sleeping in a sleeping bag often reduces stiffness and pain in the morning. An electric blanket may also help. **Keeping the body evenly warm at night** is important.

• **Hot castor oil packs** are very useful. Heat castor oil in a pan, but do not boil it. Dip white cotton cloth into it until saturated. Apply to the affected area and cover with a piece of plastic which is larger than the cloth. Place a **heating pad** over the area and keep it warm for 1½ to 2 hours.

• An **arthritis liniment** may be made in this way: Mix 1 pint alcohol, 1/4 ounce menthol, and ½ ounce camphor. Rub it on the affected joints, twice a day.

• A 50-50 mix of **mineral oil and alcohol** is another formula. You can add 1 Tbsp. of wintergreen oil to the mixture, if you wish.

• **Chelation therapy** (869) can decidedly help alleviate certain arthritic conditions.

OTHER FACTORS
• **Reduce stress** in your life. Worry, anger, and similar emotions weaken your body and help induce arthritic problems.

• **Chlamydia** (804) has been linked to a form of arthritis that affects young women. In one study, half the women with unexplained arthritis were found to have chlamydia.

• **Overweight** (480) increases strain on the joints. Arthritics should try to keep their weight slightly below average.

• Avoid **immunizations**. Various immunizations have brought on arthritis.

• **Food allergies** can cause neck and shoulder pain, imitative of arthritis.

• Silicone gel **breast implants** can cause arthritic-like symptoms; it also induces lupus and scleroderma. Antibodies develop which attack collagen.

• In its early stages, **ulcerative colitis** (463, 465) can produce arthritic-like symptoms.

• **Lyme disease** (840) can appear to be arthritis.

• **Lupus** (310), an autoimmune disease, can produce arthritic-like symptoms.

—See Rheumatoid Arthritis (623), Acute Articular Rheumatism (624), Acute Muscular Rheumatism (626), and Chronic Rheumatism (626).

J.H. KELLOGG, M.D., PRESCRIPTIONS FOR ARTHRITIS AND RHEUMATOID GOUT AND THEIR COMPLICATIONS (how to give these water therapies: pp. 206-275 / list of treatments: pp. 206-207 / Hydrotherapy Disease Index: pp. 273-275)

DIET AND LIFESTYLE—The diet must be especially nourishing and digestible. A warm, rather dry, and uniform climate is most desirable.

GENERAL MEASURES—Carefully **graduated cold applications**, preceded by very **short hot applications**. **Fomentation** to spine or the Radiant Heat Bath for 3-5 minutes. Also the **sunbath**, followed by **Cold Mitten Friction** are especially suitable. Massage. **Hot Abdominal Pack**.

FEVER—Prolonged Neutral Bath at 92° F., **Fomentation** to spine followed by Cold Mitten Friction or **Wet Towel Rub**.

FREQUENT PULSE—Cold Compress or Ice Bag over heart for 15-20 minutes, 3 times a day.

PAIN IN JOINTS—Revulsive Compresses followed by **cotton poultice** and **vapor bath** to the area.

NEURALGIA OF HANDS—Hot Hand Bath followed by **cotton poultice** (to keep it warm).

RADIATING PAINS—Fomentation to spine, 3 times a day, with well-protected (plastic covered) **Heating Compress** during the interval between; **Revulsive Compress** to spine.

NUMBNESS AND TINGLING OF HANDS AND FEET—Fomentation to spine and **Hot or Alternate Sponging** of limbs, repeated 3 times a day.

MUSCULAR CRAMPS— Fomentation or hot immersion of affected parts, two or more times daily; during interval between, **Hot Sponging** and **firm bandaging**. Protect him from chills.

JOINT DEFORMITIES—For thickening of synovial membranes, or accumulation of fluid in joints or bursa, apply Alternate Douche and **Alternate Compress**. Apply, to joint, a dry flannel bandage or **cotton poultice**.

CAUTIONS—To painful joints, avoid cold douches, long sweating processes, and prolonged general applications.

METHOD—Improve the general health by using general tonic measures, especially using carefully Graduated Cold Baths and massage.

ENCOURAGEMENT—Think back over the past and recall to mind all the ways God has helped you through the years. Praise Him for what He has done and continues to do for you. Stay close to Him and trust the future to Him. He will not fail you, even though you may not understand all the workings of providence. He will guide and help you, as you trust in Him. Isaiah 61:1-3.

OSTEOARTHRITIS

SYMPTOMS—Morning joint stiffness is often the first symptom. Later, there is pain on motion of that joint, that is made worse by prolonged activity and relieved by rest. Inflammation is generally not present.

Pain and tenderness that worsen with activity and are relieved by rest. Swelling around the joint. Stiffness lasting a short time after a period of inactivity. Restricted joint movement. Enlarged, distorted finger joints, if the hands are affected. Crackling noise (called crepitus) on moving the affected joint.

CAUSES—Osteoarthritis is a degenerative joint disease; it is the most common form of arthritis—especially in the elderly (80% of those over 50 have it). Under 45, it is more common in men; over 45, it is 10 times more common in women than men.

There is gradual degeneration of the cartilage covering the bone ends within joints. It most often affects the hands and the weight-bearing joints (such as the knees and hips). Wear occurs most often in joints that have been damaged by repeated strenuous activity or by repeated minor injuries.

NATURAL REMEDIES

• *See Arthritis (618) for a rather complete list of natural remedies.*

ENCOURAGEMENT—Through Christ we may present our petitions at the throne of grace. Through Him, unworthy as we are, we may obtain all spiritual blessings. Hebrews 4:16.

RHEUMATISM

SYMPTOMS—Pain, muscle stiffness, and tenderness in soft-tissue structures. Afflictions of muscle tendon, joint, bone, or nerve that results in discomfort and disability from stiffness of the joints or muscles, pain on motion, etc. This category often includes rheumatoid arthritis, degenerative joint diseases, spondylitis, bursitis, fibrositis, myositis, neuritis, lumbago, sciatica, and gout.

CAUSES—Excess acid settles in the joints, causing pain and inflammation. Poor elimination causes rheumatism, due to toxic matter becoming stagnated in various parts of the body. Thomas Deschauer explains it thus: "Urea should be daily expelled from our body, an ounce every day. Urea, as you might know, is completely changed waste matter and is easily expelled. Now if the process of turning the dead tissues into urea is incomplete, it forms uric acid. Certain foods and drinks cause the urea to be left unfinished. Or if the urea is hindered or stopped in trying to be expelled, it also returns into the system and forms uric acid. This can be done by stopping perspiration, by cooling off quickly, by neglect of proper bathing, changing of underclothing, inhaling urea at night while sleeping in an ill-ventilated room, etc. Avoid all these things if you want to get well. Some persons have what is known as the uric acid habit; that is, the waste matter does not break down completely. This tendency is due to an extremely abnormal and diseased condition of the blood."

See Rheumatoid Arthritis (below) for much more information.

NATURAL REMEDIES

• Drink parsley and/or juniper berry tea, along with lots of organic cranberry juice, to eliminate uric acid crystals in the joints.

• Rheumatism can be relieved rapidly by a **cleansing program** and by the use of **burdock root tea**, with the **burdock root and leaf fomentation** on

CHART 1050: Acute Rheumatism 623 / Rheumatoid Arthritis 623 / Osteoarthritis 622 / Gout 627

the painful areas. Use **lemon juice and honey** to cut the toxic wastes loose and expel them from the body. Use **chaparral tea** (three times a day, a teaspoon to the cup). The **bowels and urethral tract** should be kept open. A stimulant diuretic (**corn silk tea**) for the kidneys will aid in waste elimination and a diaphoretic (**blue vervain tea**) should be used to assist in eliminating through the skin.

— *See Rheumatoid Arthritis for much more information (below). Also see Arthritis (618) for even more.*

ENCOURAGEMENT—Confess your secret sins alone before your God. Acknowledge your heart wanderings to Him who knows perfectly how to treat your case.

RHEUMATOID ARTHRITIS

SYMPTOMS—Vague pain, stiffness, weight loss, numbness, and tingling of the hands and feet may precede its onset.

Swelling, stiffness, redness, and often crippling pain in joints, which eventually may fuse together. There is fatigue, anemia, weight loss, and fever.

Affected joints sound like crinkling cellophane. In contrast, osteoarthritis joints sound like popping, clicking, or banging. Joints of the hands, elbows, knees, and ankles are most commonly involved.

Upon awakening in the morning, there may be a joint stiffness which lasts an hour or longer. Swelling will occur in a specific finger, wrist joints, and also around other joints. Pain may, or may not, be present.

The condition can worsen or remain the same for years and later worsen again.

A chronic arthritis affecting multiple joints and resulting in debility, weakness, and loss of weight. There is painful limitation of motion, often with deformity, and sometimes a complete fusion of a joint (bony ankylosis). Rheumatism, arthritis, and gout are very similar; although the basic cause may be the same.

CAUSES—Rheumatoid arthritis (RA) is an inflammatory arthritis. It is an autoimmune disorder. So many acids, purines, etc., have collected in the joints; and the calcium supply has been so low for so long, that the body gets "confused"—and begins attacking the synovial membranes in the joints. Cartilage, nearby tissues, and even the bone surfaces are destroyed.

This damaged area is then replaced with scar tissue, which tends to fuse together the joints—making them immovable.

Oddly enough, this form of arthritis most commonly occurs between the ages of 35 and 45, but may occur at any age. It also occurs even in children. Two-thirds of the 3 million Americans who have RA are women. Among those under 18, about 70,000 have it; most of them are girls.

Causes include poor nutrition, bacterial infection, and/or physical or emotional stress. Stress seems to be the active agent which initially brings it on. Exposure, overwork, or acute infections can also do it.

Unlike osteoarthritis (622), which only affects joints here or there, RA affects all the synovial joints in the body.

In the first year after the disorder appears, 75% improve without any treatment at all. Therefore natural treatments should help the situation even more. Keep in mind that 10% of those with RA become disfigured in one way or another. So this is a problem which is worth taking the time and effort to reduce or eliminate.

The likelihood of remission is greater early in the course of the disease. Each attack seems to be worse than those preceding it.

Improper diet consisting of unwholesome, denatured, and processed foods.

NATURAL REMEDIES

NUTRITION

• **Fasting** brings temporary relief to RA; but the pain, swelling, and stiffness tend to return a few days after the fast is ended. Some recommendations require a longer vegetable juice and vegetable broth fast of two or more weeks as having more lasting effects.

• People with RA were found to have lower blood levels of **folic acid, protein, and zinc** than other people.

• Each day take **calcium, magnesium, selenium, copper, vitamin B$_6$, histidine, and bromelain**. *See Arthritis (618) for much more information.*

• Taper off of the "secondary" and inorganic-type foods—such as **eggs, starches, and carbohydrates**. Eat the regenerative organic foods (**fresh fruits and vegetables**) as much as possible. **Chaparral** (creosote bush) is one of the best herbal remedies. Another fine remedy which is excellent internally as a decoction and externally as a liniment is the following combination of herbs: **black cohosh, capsicum, lobelia, mullein and prickly ash**. The daily use of **lemon juice and honey** will do wonders.

• Other herbs are the same as for gout (627) and arthritis (618).

AVOID

• **Do not take iron supplements** (such as ferrous sulfate, which is commonly given for anemia). These will intensify RA and arthritis.

• **Food allergies** can be involved. One study showed that 86% of a group of rheumatoid arthritics could trace the onset of their problem to allergies; most common were **soy products, milk, eggs, coffee, and sugar foods**. Try avoiding all those foods. *See Arthritis (618) for other helpful and problem foods. Also see Alergies (846-860).*

• One research study noted that people who use large quantities of **wheat, rye, and oats** tend to have high rates of RA.

CHART 1056: Diseases of the Joints 615-633

OTHER HELPS

• **Lose weight**, to reduce the strain on your joints.

• **Keep your hands warm** at night. Stretch nylon gloves, worn at night, do this. Better yet, keep your arms and hands under the covers at night.

• **Deep breathing exercises,** done outdoors, helps those with RA.

• Alternating **hot and cold baths** help. Give 6 minutes for the hot and 4 minutes for the cold, to increase blood flow to the area. The healing is in the blood which is brought to the area, and then recharged as more arrives.

• **Aloe vera gel**, placed on the area, helps relieve pain.

—For extensive information: See Arthritis (618) Osteoarthritis (622), Acute Articular Rheumatism (624), Acute Muscular Rheumatism (626), and Chronic Rheumatism (626).

There is also a Juvenile Rheumatoid Arthritis (751), which is different; it affects children from 6 months of age to the age of 12.

ENCOURAGEMENT—By His life and His death, Christ proved that God's justice did not destroy His mercy; but that sin could be forgiven and that the law is righteous. With Christ's help, His law can be perfectly obeyed. Proverbs 11:3, 6, 20.

ACUTE ARTICULAR RHEUMATISM

NATURAL REMEDIES

J.H. KELLOGG, M.D., PRESCRIPTIONS FOR ACUTE ARTICULAR RHEUMATISM AND ITS COMPLICATIONS (how to give these water therapies: pp. 206-275 / list of treatments: pp. 206-207 / Hydrotherapy Disease Index: pp. 273-275)

GENERAL—Absolute **rest** in bed. **Abstinence** from all solid food for a few days, allowing only ripe fruits, fruit juices, well-dextrinized (well-cooked) cereals, and malted foods. Avoid meats, animal broths, beef tea or extracts, eggs, oysters, cheese, and all foods rich in proteins.

COMBAT INFLAMMATORY PROCESS IN JOINTS—Secure active cutaneous circulation by **Hot Blanket Pack** and **Sweating Wet Sheet Pack**, hot **Fomentations** to the joints, followed by **Heating Compress**. Keep him sweating until acute pain ceases and temperature falls.

PREVENT EXTENSION OF THE DISEASE TO THE HEART, LUNGS, PLEURA, AND MENINGES—by promoting activity of the skin and kidneys, building up the general vital resistance, and by carefully administered cold applications. The **Hot Blanket Pack**, Hot Enemas, Hot Trunk Pack, following each hot application by **Cold Mitten Friction**. Administered carefully to all portions of the body that are free from local inflammation.

ENCOURAGE ELIMINATION—The prolonged **sweating bath** (given by means of the **Hot Blanket Pack)** should be continued for several hours; this is a most valuable measure. He should not be taken out of the pack suddenly, but gradually; **Cold Mitten Friction** should be applied to each part until good reaction occurs before uncovering another portion. After rubbing, the surface should be carefully protected by **flannel blankets**. Free **water** drinking and large **Enema** twice daily.

PAINS IN JOINTS—Hot Blanket Pack. Follow by dry wrapping (Dry Pack). **Fomentation** to joints, repeated every 2 hours. During the interval in between, a well-protected **Heating Compress** applied as soon as the **Fomentation** is removed. Smear joints with **Vaseline** daily.

FEVER—Hot Blanket Pack continued to full sweating, followed by a **Sweating Wet Sheet Pack** that is prolonged for several hours is the best means of lowering the temperature. When the temperature is very high, the **Neutral Bath**, at 92°-95° F., may be employed. **Ice Compress** to head and neck. Cold Mitten Friction or **Cold Towel Rub** may be given after the **Sweating Wet Sheet Pack** or the Hot Blanket Pack, 2-3 times daily.

PROFUSE PERSPIRATION—Do not check during the early stage; simply wipe him with a dry cloth. If the temperature is very high (104°-105° F.), the **Graduated Bath** may be given; the temperature should not be lowered below 85° F. As the temperature is lowered, he should be rubbed with sufficient vigor, to prevent chill. The **Cool Enema** may also be used in connection with the Fomentation to the back. Be careful not to check perspiration suddenly, at least until all until acute symptoms (of pain, high temperature, etc.) subside.

DURING CONVALESCENCE—Encourage blood making by **Graduated Cold Baths**, especially Cold Mitten Friction.

HYPERPYREXIA (ELEVATION OF SYSTEMIC TEMPERATURE ABOVE 104°-106° F.)—(1) Prevent it by Ice Cap, **Cold Mitten Friction** at 50°-40° F., or Cold Towel Rub at 60°-50° F., 2-3 times a day, when temperature rises above 101.5° F. May precede cold application by **very Hot Sponging**. (2) Combat it when temperature rises above 101.5° F. by **Cold Mitten Friction** at 60° F., given every 2 hours and continuing until temperature falls to 101° F. Continue application to each part until reddened, so as to prevent retrostasis. **Graduated Baths** (102°-85° F.) may be resorted to in obstinate cases, also the **Cool Enema**. In all cases apply **Ice Cap and Ice Collar**, to offset cerebral congestion and coma.

ENDOCARDITIS, PERICARDITIS (INFECTION OF HEART MEMBRANES)—The hot **Fomentation** (and it should not be very hot) should be applied over the heart for half a minute at intervals of 1 hour. This should be followed by the **Ice bag or Cold Compress** above the heart.

CEREBRAL RHEUMATISM—Ice to head. **Prolonged Neutral Baths** at 92° F. Colonics at 80° F., 3 times a day. Ice to head and neck. **Cooling Wet Sheet Pack**. **Sweating Wet Sheet Pack**, repeating 2-3 times a day.

TO PREVENT PERMANENT DAMAGE OF JOINTS— Simple **flexions** (movements) of the joints as soon as the fever declines. Short applications of **Alternate Compress** or Alternate Douche, 2-3 times daily, after convalescence begins, with a well-protected **Heating Compress** during the interval in between.

ARTICULAR AFFUSIONS—Alternate Compress or Alternate Douche, 3 times a day. Well-protected **Heating Compress** during the interval in between. Massage. Bandaging.

NODOSITIES—Revulsive Douche or **Fomentations**, 3 times a day. **Heating Compress** during interval in between until tenderness is removed. Then **Alternate Douche**, 3 times a day. Follow by well-protected **Heating Compress** and **massage**.

ARTHRITIS AND PHLEBITIS—Fomentation over affected part every 2-3 hours for 20 minutes; **Heating Compress** during interval in between, wrung very dry and protected with plastic covering.

NEURALGIA—Revulsive Compress. Follow by dry cotton poultice; renew every hour or two.

NEURITIS—Complete **rest** of part; **Fomentation** every 2-3 hours, followed by well-protected **Heating Compress**.

TACHYCARDIA (RAPID HEART BEAT)—Cold Compress over heart for 15 minutes every hour; avoid hot food and drinks. **Ice Bag** over heart during hot applications to joints and other parts.

DIARRHEA—Neutral Enema at 95° F., after each bowel movement. Cold **Abdominal Compress** at 60° F., during intervals in between, changed every hour.

GASTRALGIA—Hot and Cold Compress over stomach, heat to area above stomach, cold to spine, hot **water** drinking; **dry diet** of well-dextrinized (well-cooked) cereals.

PERIOSTATIS and **OSTEITIS**—Very hot **Fomentations** for 15 minutes every 2 hours. **Heating Compress** during intervals in between, well-wrung and well-protected with flannel and covered with plastic. If suppuration (pussing) occurs, open it with a knife.

URTICARIA—Sponging with very hot water, hot salt or alkaline Sponge; **Prolonged Neutral Bath**.

CONTRAINDICATIONS—Avoid Cold Full Baths and Cold Douche.

GENERAL METHOD—Aid the elimination of acids by promoting activity of the skin. This is also the best means of relieving the articular pains. He should be drenched with water through both the stomach and rectum, to encourage profuse perspiration and prevent undue increase in the specific gravity of the blood. Tonic and fever-lowering measures must be used with great care; these must be so managed as to avoid retrostasis (a retrograding of his condition). Chilling him will increase the pain. The cold rubbings (frictions), applied to maintain general vital resistance, must be accompanied by hot applications to the joints; and, if necessary, use more extensive hot applications to the spine or legs, to prevent chilling of the surface. The most efficient hydrotherapy measures aid heat elimination by dilating the surface vessels rather than by lowering the temperature of the skin.

Also see Acute Muscular Rheumatism (626), Chronic Rheumatism (626), Rheumatoid Arthritis (623), and Juvenile Rheumatoid Arthritis (751).

ENCOURAGEMENT—While the Lord has not promised His people exemption from trials, He has promised that which is far better. He has said, "As thy days, so shall thy strength be" (Deut. 33:25).

S
K
E
L
M
U
S

ACUTE MUSCULAR RHEUMATISM

NATURAL REMEDIES

J.H. KELLOGG, M.D., PRESCRIPTIONS FOR ACUTE MUSCULAR RHEUMATISM AND ITS COMPLICATIONS *(how to give these water therapies: pp. 206-275 / list of treatments: pp. 206-207 / Hydrotherapy Disease Index: pp. 273-275)*

NUTRITION—A **nourishing dietary** that excludes meats. Avoid fruits and vegetables at the same meal, all indigestible foods and dishes, tea, coffee, condiments, excess salts. Carefully Graduated **Cold Full Baths** daily.

INCREASE GENERAL VITAL RESISTANCE—This is the most important indication in this disease, as in malarial infection, in acute rheumatism, and other infectious diseases. Short sweating procedures of any sort (**Full Hot Baths**, Steam Baths, etc.), followed by short and graduated cold applications, are the most important general measures.

SWELLING OF JOINTS—**Fomentation,** 3 times a day. And, during the intervals in between, apply **Heating Compress,** wrung dry and well-protected by plastic. Also derivative measures.

PAIN—**Revulsive Fan Douche**, other pain-relieving measures.

STIFFNESS OF JOINTS—**Fomentation,** 3 times a day. Well-protected **Heating Compress** during intervals in-between. **Alternate Articular Douche** [alternate hot and cold spray to afflicted joints], massage of joints and muscles, **Prolonged Neutral Bath**.

DRY SKIN—**Sweating Wet Sheet Pack**, oil rubbing on skin, Cold Mitten Friction, **Cold Towel Rub**, Wet Sheet Rub, Steam Bath, hot-air bath, electric-light bath [heating from electric lights or electric heater], sunbath.

CONTRAINDICATIONS—Do not give very Cold Baths, especially Cold Full Baths.

Also see Acute Articular Rheumatism (624), Chronic Rheumatism (626), Fibromyalgia (639), Rheumatoid Arthritis (623), and Juvenile Rheumatoid Arthritis (751).

ENCOURAGEMENT—The first step toward salvation is to respond to the drawing of the love of Christ. Christ draws men through the manifestation of His love in order that they may understand the joy of forgiveness and the peace of God. If they respond to His drawing, yielding their hearts to His grace, He will lead them on (step by step) to a full knowledge of Himself; this is life eternal.

CHRONIC RHEUMATISM

NATURAL REMEDIES

J.H. KELLOGG, M.D., PRESCRIPTIONS FOR CHRONIC RHEUMATISM AND ITS COMPLICATIONS *(how to give these water therapies: pp. 206-275 / list of treatments: pp. 206-207 / Hydrotherapy Disease Index: pp. 273-275)*

RHEUMATISM (CHRONIC) GENERAL CARE—The same as for "Acute Rheumatism," except that the local applications are made to the muscles instead of to the joints. **Sweating baths**, especially the Radiant Heat Bath and the Steam Bath. Long **Neutral Baths**, **Fomentation** over painful parts. Follow with well-protected **Heating Compress**. **Water** drinking and **aseptic diet**.

Also see Acute Articular Rheumatism (624), Acute Muscular Rheumatism (626), Rheumatoid Arthritis (623), and Juvenile Rheumatoid Arthritis (751).

ENCOURAGEMENT—As we approach God through the virtue of the Redeemer's merits, Christ places us close by His side, encircling us with His human arm, while, with His divine arm, He grasps the throne of the Infinite.

SCIATICA

SYMPTOMS—The sciatic nerve is the largest nerve in the body, and is close the bottom of each leg. Sciatica is neuralgic pain along the course of the sciatica nerve, which runs down the back of the thigh. It is supposed to be due to inflammation or injury to the nerve that results in pain, numbness, tingling, and tenderness along the course of the nerve and eventual wasting away of the muscles that are enervated by the malady. With inflammation of the sciatic nerve, there is extreme pain around the hip region and in the lumbar muscles.

CAUSES—Crippling pain of the lower extremities has long been blamed on the sciatic nerve; but, actually, it is not a nerve problem at all. But it is due to toxic poison from the sigmoid section of the bowel (which is the area going from the descending colon over to the rectal area). This important small section of the intestines is subject to kinks or pockets which cause toxic poisons in the area and in the leg area, which in turn irritate the sciatic nerve, dislocating the sacroiliac. When the affected part of the bowel is cleaned out with the lower bowel tonic and cleansing program, the poisons no longer affect the nerve area.

NATURAL REMEDIES

• The best remedy is to **empty the bowel** and **cleanse the sigmoid**; then give organic aid as fast as possible. The best herb for this problem is **chaparral** supplemented with **burdock root** tea. **Sassafras** and **Brigham tea** may also be added. This combination makes a delicious drink when sweetened with honey. Do not drink it with **chaparral** (creosote bush) tea. Bathing the feet in hot apple-cider vinegar will help; and, if you wish faster action, place the right foot into a pan of chopped **garlic** (with the bare foot on the garlic) and the left foot in hot apple-cider vinegar. This will start a circulatory movement which will give quick relief. The internal use of **lemon juice and honey** (a tablespoonful of each, three times a day) will speed the cleansing. For external fomentation or poultices, use **burdock root or crushed burdock leaves**, with one-fourth part **lobelia** added.

Other helpful herbs are **chaparral, broom, burdock, rue, sassafras, tansy, wintergreen**.

GOUT

SYMPTOMS—Sudden attack, often in the middle of the night, of extreme pain and swelling of a joint in the fingers or toes (usually the big toe). But it can affect the ankles, knees, hands, elbows, and wrists. Motion or pressure greatly increases the pain. After the swelling subsides, the skin tends to itch and peel.

During attacks, there often is loss of appetite, stomach and intestinal problems, fever, and decreased urine output.

CAUSES—Gout is an acute type of inflammatory arthritis; it occurs most often in people who eat rich foods (such as meat, gravies, spices, and alcohol). Frequently, those individuals are also overweight.

Gout is caused by a buildup of uric acid in the blood. When levels rise beyond a certain point beyond which the kidneys cannot excrete it, uric acid crystals form and collect in the affected joint or joints, causing excruciating pain. They can also form in major body organs and do great damage.

The body cannot handle all the purines and other acids in the meat; and so these products settle in the body. Uric acid is the end-product of the breakdown of purine compounds.

Gout typically attacks the smaller joints of the feet and hands, especially the big toe. Uric acid salts crystallize in the joint and produce swelling, redness, and a sensation of heat and extreme pain.

Unlike most forms of arthritis, gout affects men over 30 in 90% of the cases. It generally does not begin until after 35 years of age; peak age of onset is 45. Women who have it are generally post-menopausal.

This condition is caused from overloading the system with improper foods. If the general living habit is not changed, the condition that starts on the great toe will go into various parts of the foot and ankle and sometimes into other parts of the body. Babies may be born with gout or rheumatoid arthritis, although it is usually caused by improper diet. Gout is always rheumatoid arthritis; but rheumatoid arthritis is not always recognized as being gout because, at times, it comes to different parts of the body instead of just the foot.

NATURAL REMEDIES

NUTRITION

• **Dietetic changes, water drinking, and weight control** are all very important. *See Arthritis (618).* The amount of urates in the blood is keyed to dietary intake and the amount of body weight.

• Those with this disorder need to **reduce to 10%-15% below calculated normal weight**. However, weight reduction must be done gradually, so as not to stir up more urates and temporarily increase the number of gout attacks.

• Drink at least 2 quarts of **water** a day between gout attacks in order to rid the body of uric acid and reduce the likelihood of kidney damage and kidney stones. Those with gout tend to have kidney stones. One physician says to drink a gallon of water daily to wash out the acids. Make sure it is clean, good water.

• **Vitamin B$_{12}$** helps distribute water in the body to keep the tissues loaded with water, thus helping the prevent uric acid concentration into crystals. **Magnesium** aids in the absorption of B$_{12}$.

• **B complex** (1-3 tablets daily) and 500 mg **pantothenic acid** assist the body's conversion of uric acid into harmless compounds.

• To lower serum uric acid, take 1,000 mg of **vitamin C** per hour at the onset of an attack, and then gradually lower it to 500-8,000 mg daily.

• Take 100 IU of **vitamin E** and gradually increase it to 600-800 IU daily, to reduce uric acid buildup.

• A **high-carbohydrate diet** tends to increase uric acid excretion. In contrast, a **high-fat diet** decreases excretion and may bring on a gout attack (even though they may be unsaturated fats). Keep your diet **low in protein and fat**.

• Natural therapists have found that they can eliminate all gout with diet, by eliminating all **meat, eggs and cheese**.

• Eat **high-potassium foods**, which includes most vegetables. Put thick, **white potato peelings** into your pot of vegetables or soup; it is rich in potassium.

• Eating **cherries** is very helpful. The uric acid level in the blood decreases and the attacks tend to stop. They can be any type of cherries, either fresh or canned (½ pound per day). One or two Tbsp. of **cherry concentrate** can be taken instead. If canned cherries are used, only use water-packed ones; most have too much sugar and additives. Estimates as to how much to eat vary from ½ cup to 1 pound (about 70 cherries). Some pit them and blend them to make juice. One research study found that store-bought cherry juice has been pasteurized, which removed the active ingredient, *anthocyanin*. Wild or black cherries work best.

• **Celery extracts** (2-4 tablets daily) help eliminate uric acid.

• Japanese researchers have found that compounds in **chiso**, an Asiatic plant, relieve gout. Chiso contains four *xanthine oxidase inhibitors*, which helps prevent uric acid synthesis. Licorice also contains those inhibitors.

• The *curcumin* in **turmeric** stimulates the adrenal glands to release the body's own cortisone, a potent reliever of inflammation and the pain it often causes.

• Mix **cayenne** with enough **wintergreen oil** to make a paste. Put in on the area to relieve pain and inflammation.

• Here are useful herb teas: **yarrow, peppermint, chamomile, devil's claw, juniper, and birch**.

• The eliminative organs must be improved. Drink **lemon juice with honey** and bathe the area in hot **apple cider vinegar**. Herbal teas work well to relieve pain. **Lobelia** on the afflicted parts is very good. A good herb combination is equal parts of **skullcap, valerian, and yarrow** taken in tea form, to assist in freeing the toxic waste from the tissues and to eliminate the waste through the various excretory organs.

—For more on foods and herbs which will reduce the inflammation and pain, see Arthritis (618-622).

AVOID

• **Do not fast** when you have gout. Doing so greatly increases the amount of uric acids in the blood.

• Avoid excessive **food yeast**.

• **Overeating** tends toward gout.

• A vegetarian diet is the best program for a person with gout. **Stop eating all types of meat**.

• Here are foods which are very high in purines: **liver, brains, kidneys, heart, anchovies, sardines, meat extract, herring, consommé, mussels, and sweet breads**.

• Here are foods of lesser purine content: **fowl, fish (except those listed above), other seafoods, and other meats**.

• Here are foods of moderate amounts: **whole-grain cereals, lentils, peas, beans, asparagus, mushrooms, oatmeal, cauliflower, and spinach**.

• (Here are the foods which have only negligible amounts of purines and do not cause gout: **vegetables, fruits, and cereal products**.) There are cases in which drinking large amounts of **milk** or eating lots of **tomatoes** produced gout.)

• Avoid **rich foods such as cakes and pies**. Drop **white flour and sugar products** from your diet.

• Do not take any alcoholic beverage. All kinds of beverage **alcohol** increase uric acid production and reduces excretion of urates. It triggers the body to produce uric acid.

• **Direct injury to a joint**, tending toward gout, can bring on an acute attack.

OTHER HELPS

• It is known that the skin can excrete uric acid; so **baths** are very helpful.

• During acute attacks, **keep the affected joint elevated and at rest**.

• **Hot fomentations** for 15 minutes every 3 hours, to help relieve pain. But, to reduce pain, some do better using **cold applications**.

• **Mud packs**, applied to the affected area, will absorb a fair amount of the uric acid.

• **Charcoal** is very helpful. Take it by mouth (12-16 tablets daily) and also put a poultice of **charcoal** on the area.

• A compress of **comfrey root or leaves**, blended with water, helps relieve gout pain. Apply for two hours

or more or overnight.

• **Burdock** will help clean uric acid deposits from the joints and other areas. **Kelp, red clover, and yucca** help eliminate uric acid and other toxins.

• Apply **plantain, ginger,** or **fresh comfrey** compresses to the inflamed area.

Colchicine is the primary drug medication for gout. But it causes nausea, vomiting, diarrhea, cramping, hair loss, anemia, liver damage, and decreased leukocytes and platelets. Natural remedies can do the job better.

A number of drugs increase uric acid levels; so it is best to avoid drugs. Diuretic drugs are especially bad.

J.H. KELLOGG, M.D., PRESCRIPTIONS FOR ACUTE GOUT AND ITS COMPLICATIONS *(how to give these water therapies: pp. 206-275 / list of treatments: pp. 206-207 / Hydrotherapy Disease Index: pp. 273-275)*

DIET AND LIFESTYLE—Avoid meats, tea, coffee, tobacco, milk, and eggs. Take daily sufficient **exercise** in the open air, to cause perspiration. Follow by **short Cool Full Bath** for cooling purposes. Diet would include **fruits, well-cooked cereals, and nuts**.

ENCOURAGE TISSUE CHANGE, ESPECIALLY OXIDATION OF PROTEIN WASTES—Prolonged Sweating Baths, Steam Bath, Radiant Heat Bath, Sweating Wet Sheet Pack, Dry Pack, Hot Blanket Pack. Follow by daily **Graduated Cold Bath**, carefully given and nicely graduated. **Outdoor life**.

MAINTAIN NORMAL ALKALINITY OF THE BLOOD—Tonic graduated cold applications and free use of **fruits**. **Avoid** flesh foods, tea, coffee, and alcohol.

GOUT (ACUTE) —

HEADACHE—Water drinking. **Enema. Hot and Cold Head Compress**, with **Hot Footbath** or Hot Leg Bath.

MIGRAINE—Revulsive Compress to the area, where the pain is located. **Hot Leg Bath** or Hot Foot Bath, **Enema**, Hot Enema, **Fomentation** over stomach, Fomentation over spine, **Alternate Compress** over spine.

HEMORRHOIDS—If inflamed, hot **Fomentations** to relieve pain. Follow with **Cold Compress** to anal region and buttocks. Also **Cool Enema**.

PRURITUS ANI—Very Hot Anal Douche.

PAIN AND SWELLING OF JOINTS—Elevate limb. **Cooling Compress**, change as soon as warm.

FEVER—Hot Blanket Pack, followed by **Prolonged Neutral Bath**.

SCANTY URINE—Water drinking (distilled water). **Enema**, twice daily.

RETROCEDENT GOUT—For coma or delirium, cold to head and neck. Large **Enema. Hot Blanket Pack. Hot Full Bath**.

CARDIAC COMPLICATIONS, SYNCOPE—Hot Enema, Alternate Compress to spine.

GASTRO-INTESTINAL DISTURBANCE BY RETRO-CESSION—Fomentation over stomach. **Hot Trunk Pack**. Hot Full Bath or Hot Blanket Pack, with **Heating Compress** during the interval between.

CONTRAINDICATIONS—Avoid cold baths of any kind, and avoid immersion of affected parts in cold water.

J.H. KELLOGG, M.D., PRESCRIPTIONS FOR

CHRONIC GOUT AND ITS COMPLICATIONS (*how to give these water therapies: pp. 206-275 / list of treatments: pp. 206-207 / Hydrotherapy Disease Index: pp. 273-275*)

GOUT (CHRONIC) —

GENERAL MEASURES—Use the general measures given in the two sections, just above.

INCREASE CIRCULATION in affected parts by hot Fomentations. Follow by Dry cotton Pack or Heating Compress. Massage, at first derivative only (applied elsewhere to draw blood away from afflicted part) and later to the joint itself.

CONSTIPATION—Relaxing diet, Hot Abdominal Pack, cold water drinking, abdominal massage.

HEPATIC CONGESTION—Revulsive Compress over the liver every 3 hours, Heating Compress to it during the interval between.

GRAVEL—Copious water drinking and large Enema daily.

MELANCHOLY—Vigorous Sweating Baths. Follow by short Cold Douche, given with percussion to spine.

ASTHMA—Revulsive Douche to legs, large Enema, Prolonged Neutral Bath, Fomentation to chest. Follow by the Chest Pack.

ANGINA PECTORIS—Fomentation over heart for 1 minute. Follow by Cool Compress for 10 minutes; repeat. Hot Footbath or Hot Leg Pack, Ice Bag to spine, rest in bed, keep extremities very warm.

GENERAL METHODS—The general methods to be pursued in this disease are essentially the same as those applicable in the Uric Acid Diathesis or Lithemia section.

If any of the following related problems exist, look them up under their respective headings: Bronchitis, Epilepsy.

—*Also see also Gout (627), Arthritis (618), and Rheumatoid Arthritis (623).*

ENCOURAGEMENT—Could the curtain be rolled back, you would see the entire universe intently watching what is occurring on earth. During these few years of your earthly probation, you can choose to stand resolutely for God. He will help you do this.

BURSITIS

SYMPTOMS—Swelling, tenderness, and possible redness. A dull, persistent ache that increases with movement. Immense pain in the affected area, which frequently limits motion.

It most often occurs in shoulder joint; it is less often in the hip joint, the elbows, or feet.

CAUSES—Bursitis is the inflammation of the liquid-filled sac, called a *bursa* (*bursae is* plural), found within joints, muscles, tendons, and bones. These sacs normally help muscular movement occur.

Overstimulation of the bursae causes the synovial membrane to produce excess fluid. This distends the bursa, which causes the discomfort.

Injury to the area is a common cause; but chilling of the area during the day, especially at night, can also lead to it. Bursitis can also be caused by **calcium deposits** in the bursa wall, **reactions to certain foods** or **airborne allergies**. In some instances, **suddenly working tight muscles** can do it; it is called a *stretched muscle*.

Chronic overuse of a body part is a common cause. According to where it is centered, bursitis has many names: housemaid's knee, tennis elbow, policeman's heel, frozen shoulder, or beat knee.

The lowly bunion (caused by **friction in tight shoes**) is also a form of bursitis. A bursa sac on the joint of the big toe becomes inflamed.

Athletes and older people are most likely to get bursitis; but it can happen to anyone at any age.

What is the difference between bursitis and tendonitis? Both produce pain in the shoulder or other body parts.

Bursitis is an inflammation of the bursae, the fluid-filled sacs that lubricate the joints in places where muscles and tendons meet bone. Tendonitis is an inflammation of the tendons (the tough, elastic fibrous tissues that connect muscles to bones).

Bursitis generally exhibits a dull, persistent ache that increases with movement. Tendonitis causes a sharp pain during movement; it is most likely to be caused by over-reaching for something. But it can also be caused by calcium deposits pressing against a tendon. There is no swelling and fluid accumulation, as with bursitis. *See Tendonitis (633) for more on that problem.*

• The cause of bursitis is the same as arthritis and rheumatism: malnutrition and poor circulation. Generally, the problem of most bursitis in the shoulder and neck areas comes from a congested condition in the transverse colon. A toxic acid condition irritates a specific area, causing the specific inflammation.

• **Fomentations and liniments** will give very quick relief (but this is just giving relief and not healing). A **fomentation**, poultice, or tea of **burdock leaves** (three parts) and **lobelia** (one part) is good. **Wormwood** oil, in combination with other oils, is one of the fastest and most effective pain relievers. Cleanse the inflamed tissue of the toxic accumulations with the **cleansing program** and change to a **mucusless diet**.

• Helpful herbs include **chaparral, lobelia, mullein** (poultice), and **sassafras**.

NATURAL REMEDIES

• Initially give ice applications. Apply an **ice pack** for 30 minutes, every 2-3 hours.

• As pain decreases, **hot applications** can be given. Heat should be applied for 45-60 minutes at a time. It should be as intense as can be tolerated. Hot castor oil packs are useful. *See Arthritis (618) for* *information on how to prepare them.* Ten minutes of hot applications, followed by 10 minutes of cold, seems to work best.

• Follow this with a **range of motion exercises** at least once a day. *(Some are given later in this article.)*

• **Do not become chilled**.

• **Keep exercising**, so joints will not lock up.

• **Do not push yourself too hard** or too long during the day. If you are in pain, stop.

• **Sometimes rest and immobilization** of the joint is needed for a time.

NUTRITION

• **Vitamin E** (400-1,000 IU until the pain stops, then 400 IU thereafter). Beta carotene (up to 60,000 IU daily for 1 month, 50,000 IU for 2 weeks, then 25,000 IU each day). **B complex** (1 tablet daily, 1,000 mcg sublingual **B**$_{12}$ for 10 days, then every other day for 3 weeks). **B**$_1$ (50 mg). **Vitamin C** with **bioflavonoids** (1,000 mg every hour or 2 for several days, then 3,000 mg in divided doses daily for several weeks). **Vitamin D** (400 IU daily for only a few weeks).

• **Calcium** (1,500 mg) and **Magnesium** (750 mg). Both should be in divided daily doses.

• **Ginger** has been used for centuries, in Asia, in treating bursitis. Combine it with **pineapple** and a little **licorice** for a tasty treat, if you have recurring bursitis.

• **Licorice** is said to be as effective in treating bursitis as the drug hydrocortisone, without its side effects. Do not take over 3 cups of licorice tea a day.

• **Pineapple** has *bromelain*, which has anti-inflammatory properties. It reduces swelling, bruising, pain. And it speeds healing of joint and tendon injuries. **Papaya** has similar enzymes.

• *Curcumin*, a compound in **turmeric**, is as effective as cortisone in the treatment of certain kinds of inflammation, without the side effects. Here is another tasty treat with healing properties: Mix ripe **pineapple** with **turmeric** and toss in **papaya** and **ginger**. What a wonderful way to feel better!

• If you want to take the enzymes alone, take 250-500 mg of **curcumin** and 250 mg **bromelain,** 3 times a day, between meals.

• The *omega-3* fatty acids found in **flaxseed oil** decreases inflammation.

• **Magnesium** is an important mineral for muscles, bones, and connective tissues.

• **DMSO,** from a health-food, store will help. Apply it to the skin of the affected area.

AVOID

• **Do not eat meat**. Not only can the purines and uric acids in it eventually produce severe arthritic problems, but they can aggravate bursitis and tendonitis as well.

• Do not eat **processed or junk foods**. They only intensify the problem.

• Unlike flaxseed oil, the fatty acids in most **polyunsaturated vegetable oils** (including **corn** and **safflower**) and all **hydrogenated oils** (**margarine** and many **baked goods**) increases inflammation.

EXERCISES

• Clasp your hands behind your head, and **touch your elbows**. Then separate them as widely as possible. Gradually work up to ten repetitions at a time.

• A helpful exercise for bursitis of the shoulder: Stand in a corner and **"walk" the fingers up the wall** as high as possible without overstretching. Move away from the wall and **let your arm swing back and forth** like a pendulum, gradually increasing the arc. Gradually work up to 10 and 20 repetitions.

• **Touch your shoulder** with the same hand.

• While lying on a firm mat or bed, **lift one leg, knee bent, and bring it toward your chest**. Use your hands, holding it below the thigh, to help do this. Work up to 10 repetitions.

—*Also see Tendonitis (633) and Arthritis (618).*

ENCOURAGEMENT—When Jesus speaks of the new heart, He means the mind, the life, the whole being. To have a change of heart is to withdraw the affections from the world and fasten them upon Christ. To have a new heart is to have a new mind, new purposes, new motives. What is the sign of a new heart? It is a changed life. There is a daily, hourly dying to selfishness and pride. Those with whom Christ dwells will be surrounded with a divine atmosphere. Their faces will reflect light from His, brightening the path for stumbling and weary feet.

ANKYLOSING SPONDYLITIS
(Rheumatoid Spondylitis, Marie-Strümpell Disease)

SYMPTOMS—Weight loss, fatigue, malaise, low back pain, sacroiliac pain, back leg pain, stiffness in the back (especially early in the morning), aching and stiffness in the hips and shoulders.

CAUSES—Ankylosing spondylitis (AS) is an autoimmune disorder. It is a form of arthritis which causes inflammation along the spinal column, resulting in back pain and stiffness. The phrase means *ankylosing* (rigid), *spondy* (spine), and *itis* (inflammation). So many poisons have accumulated in the body (from **wrong eating, overwork, and stress)** that the immune system attacks the tissues lining the joints.

Uric acid toxins, a by-product of eating **meat**, accumulate in the joints. They form crystals, which result in inflammation and pain.

For some reason, **tension and stress** help bring on the pain and stiffness. Men develop AS 2.5 times more often than women; and 90% of the cases develop between the ages of 20 and 40.

Malnutrition can also be involved. When proper nutrients are lacking, toxins tend to accumulate in the body. A lack of **minerals** (especially **calcium, magnesium, and silicon**) can strengthen the problem.

The chronic inflammation can destroy the cartilage between the vertebrae. AS can also lead to bony growths that fuse the vertebrae and cause permanent spinal rigidity.

NATURAL REMEDIES

• **Eliminate meat** from the diet. **Reduce the tensions and rush**. Eliminate the anger, worry, and a feverish way of life.

• Go on a **3-day fast** of vegetable juices and green drinks. Clean out the bowels with enemas or colonics.

• **Improve the diet** to a simple, nourishing one, as discussed elsewhere in this book. A **low-calorie, vegetarian diet** helps alleviate the pain and inflammation of AS; it also eliminates the symptoms of a broad range of autoimmune diseases.

• **Avoid processed, sugar, and meat foods**.

• Include a **vitamin / mineral supplement**; and, very important, also include a **calcium** supplement. Essential fatty acids are important (**flaxseed oil** is the best). **Vitamins A, C, E, selenium, and zinc** are needed to rebuild the immune system.

• **Learn to relax** and appreciate the blessings of life which you have.

• *Proteolytic enzymes* help relieve inflammation. One is *zingibain*, which is in fresh **ginger root**. It is as powerful a proteolytic enzyme as the *bromelain* in **pineapple** or the *papain* in **papaya**. All are more effective than the nonsteroidal anti-inflammatory drugs (NSAIDs), which produce stomach ulcers. You can take any of these in capsule form, as a tea, or enjoy it as part of your food.

• In case your AS develops to the point that you have to wear a neck brace, apply cornstarch to eliminate the chaffing.

ENCOURAGEMENT—In this life, you will ever have disappointments; but know that Jesus is the living, risen, Saviour. He is your Redeemer; and He loves you deeply. Trust your life to Him, and you will be safe. Psalm 91:16.

TEMPOROMANDIBULAR JOINT SYNDROME
(TMJ)

SYMPTOMS—Pain in the muscles and joints of the jaws, which can radiate to the face and neck. There is a frequent clenching of the jaws.

Possible headaches, toothaches, dizziness, pain and ringing in the ears, and pressure behind the eyes.

When eating or yawning, there is a clicking, grinding, and popping noise; perhaps there is pain. There may be difficulty in opening and closing the jaws.

CAUSES—The temporomandibular joint connects the lower jaw to the skull. The bite is misaligned, either as a cause of the jaw problem or as an effect. The cartilage disc (disk) that cushions the joint becomes damaged. This causes the bones of the temporomandibular joint to rub against one another instead of gliding smoothly past each other. If the **tooth repair or replacements have not been done properly**, this can be a factor in causing the problem.

Stress, a poor bite, and bruxism are the most frequent causes. Some people develop the habit of clenching their teeth together during the day and/or at night. Called bruxism, this is very hard on the joint in the jaw. *See Bruxism (421).*

An **injury, poor dental work, osteoarthritis, bad posture, repeated or hard blows to the jaw or chin, whiplash, gum chewing, thumb sucking, chewing on only one side of the mouth, or holding the phone between the shoulder and jaw** can cause it.

Rheumatoid arthritis *(623)* can also cause jaw pain.

About 10 million Americans have this problem; yet it is estimated that 90% of all cases respond well to simple, inexpensive treatments.

Put your little fingers in your ears (to block outside noise) and slowly open and shut your jaw. If you hear any clicking or grinding sounds, your jaw may be out of alignment.

NATURAL REMEDIES

DIET

• It is important to have a diet that is rich in **B complex vitamins, calcium, magnesium, silicon, zinc, lecithin, and flaxseed oil**.

• **Fast** once a month, to give the body and jaws a rest, so rebuilding can take place.

• **Avoid sugar foods, which deplete calcium and other minerals**. Avoid **smoking**, and do not eat **meat**.

• Do not drink **caffeine beverage**s (including chocolate), because the caffeine increases muscle tension and sensitivity to pain. Avoid **salt**, salty foods, and sodium-containing foods. Do not use **alcohol**.

• You may need to eat **softer, easy-chew foods** for a time. Avoid **hard foods**. Do not bite your **fingernails**.

• **B complex** (1 tablet, plus 100 mg **pantothenic acid**) twice a day. At bedtime in order to help relieve anxiety and improve sleep, take **vitamin C** (2,000-5,000 mg in divided doses daily), **B₆** (50 mg), and **skullcap** tea.

• **Boswellia** and **ginger** herb teas of ginger or boswellia have anti-inflammatory effects. **Hops, catnip, skullcap,** or **valerian root** will help calm you. **Turmeric** will help reduce pain and inflammation.

OTHER HELPS

• **Hot and cold packs** (either together or separately) will help relieve pain in the neck and shoulders. A washcloth soaked in almost hot water makes a good compress. Place it against the aching TM joint.

• Learn to **relax** and **avoid stressful thinking or**

situations. Herb teas of **hops, skullcap, or valerian root** will help relax you.

• If you sit a lot, relax and **maintain good posture**. Do not hunch over and strain.

• **Do not sleep on your side** or lie on your side, with your head turned to the side. It is crucial that you sleep on your back. Place a bean bag on each side of your head, so you will stay on your back all night.

• **Do not prop your head at an angle** (especially in bed) when reading, talking, or watching television. Do not lean your **head on your hands** at any time.

• **Do not chew after eating**, either bits of food when the meal is over or chewing gum.

EXERCISES

• **This will greatly relieve jaw and head pain:** Put ice on the tense neck muscle and stretch it. First, place a washcloth partly around an ice cube; and then, 3-4 times, rub the ice directly down the side of your head and neck over the muscle. Then stretch that side of your neck by bending your head toward the other shoulder. Hold 10 seconds; then put your hand on the muscle to warm it up. And then work the muscle with your hand. Then repeat the procedure on the neck muscle on the other side. The cold blocks pain, so you stretch the painful muscles more than you otherwise could.

• **This exercise will help relieve neck pain:** Place your fingers on the muscle near where it ends on the back of the neck behind the ear. Place your thumb on the point above your collarbone, close to your Adam's apple, where that muscle ends. Then gently pull the two ends of the muscle together. This is a "reverse stretch." Do this whenever your neck is painful.

• **This exercise will help reduce pain in the facial muscles on the side of your jaw:** Wash your hands and hook the index finger of the right hand inside the corner of the right side of your mouth. Do the same on the left side. Both fingers, down to the middle knuckles, should be in your mouth. Next, gently push out your cheeks, stopping before you feel pain. Release and do this stretch 3-4 times, several times a day.

• **This exercise will help relieve pain and pressure deep behind the eyes:** The source of the pain is a spasm in the muscle that opens the jaw and moves it from side to side. If the pain is behind the right eye, put the end of your right index finger behind the upper right molar of your upper jaw, so the finger is pointed at the center of your skull, behind the eye. Press up 4-5 times, each time holding for 2-3 seconds. Whether left, right, or both eyes, this is the treatment to reduce pain.

• **To balance your jaw muscles:** Gently try to open your jaws with your hands while resisting with your jaws. Then gently try pushing the jaw sideways while resisting with your jaw. Repeat on the other side. Do each exercise for 30 seconds, 3-4 times a day. Another helpful exercise: When you feel a yawn coming, resist it with your hands under your jaw. At any rate, do not open your mouth too wide when you yawn.

• **How to stop grinding your teeth:** First, think that your jaw is relaxed. Will to do it. Do this whenever you begin tensing or clenching your teeth. Second, never chew any substance when you are not eating. This includes no more chewing of gum. Keep your teeth apart, lips together, tongue on the roof of your mouth.

—Along with tension, bruxism is usually an underlying cause. It is important that you also read Bruxism (421), as well as Rheumatoid arthritis (623). Also read Strengthening the Bones (608), to help maintain and rebuild strong bones.

ENCOURAGEMENT—Come daily to Jesus; He loves you. Open your heart to Him freely. In Him there is no disappointment. You will never find a better counselor, guide, and defense. Psalm 32:11.

GANGLION
(Ganglion Cyst)

SYMPTOMS—A hard bump which develops on the wrist or back of the hand, but sometimes on the foot. It varies in size from a small pea to a plum.

CAUSES—A cyst is an abnormal sac in the body which contains fluid. A ganglion is a cyst that develops under the skin near a joint. It is filled with a jelly-like fluid. The ganglion is usually an outgrowth from the capsule surrounding a joint or from the sheath of a tendon. Tendons are the fibrous cords which attach muscle to bone. The fluid inside the ganglion cyst is derived from the synovial fluid which lubricates both tendons and joints.

Ganglia are quite common and are generally painless. As mentioned above, they may be felt as a lump under the skin and may be present for several years without causing a problem. But some ganglia become very uncomfortable or even cause pain.

NATURAL REMEDIES

A ganglion may disappear spontaneously. It can be removed surgically under local anesthesia. Sometimes these cysts recur.

• A very nutritious diet of **fresh fruits, vegetables, whole grains, legumes, and nuts**, plus a wide-spectrum **of vitamin-mineral supplementation**, will help reduce its size. Do not **overeat**, even of good food. **Constipation** will make it more difficult to shrink the cysts.

• Maintaining outstanding health, through proper **rest, exercise, and outdoor walking** strengthens the body and helps it resolve this problem. Do not **overwork** with your hands while not obtaining enough rest.

• The cyst is a fluid enlargement, so astringent herb **compresses**, saturated with **witch hazel or white oak bark** tea, may help shrink them. It is easier to eliminate them while they are still small.

• In some instances, taking **antibiotic herbs** (297) have helped to reduce these cysts.

It is known that bone spurs (612), which in some

ways are similar, can be removed with **ultrasound**.

ENCOURAGEMENT—"Ask in my name," Christ says . . Christ is the connecting link between God and man. He has promised His personal intercession.

SKELETAL-MUSCULAR - 3 - TENDONS
Also: Gout (627)

SHINSPLINTS

SYMPTOMS—Pain in the shins of one or both legs. There may, or may not, be a specific area of tenderness; pain and aching will be felt in the front of the lower leg after, or during, activity.

CAUSES—The experts are not clear as what shinsplints are. They may be an irritation to the tendon which attaches the muscle to the bone. Or they may be a muscle irritation or the beginning of a stress fracture.

Active people have shinsplints. For example, 28% of **long distance runners** and 22% of **aerobic dancers** have them.

They are caused by **excessive walking, running, or jumping on a hard surface**. But other factors include **poor shoes, fallen arches, insufficient warm-up, poor posture, faulty walking and running techniques, overstraining, or pinched nerves**.

Sometimes the early stages of *stress fractures* are thought to be shinsplints or vice versa. But there is a difference: Stress fractures begin with pinpoint pain, about the size of a dime or quarter, around or on a bony area. A shinsplint is a generalized pain or aching discomfort up and down the whole shin. But, if the problem is not stopped, shinsplints can develop into stress fractures.

NATURAL REMEDIES

• Athletic trainers call it RICE: **rest, ice, compression, and elevation**. Do this for 20-30 minutes. Prop up the leg, wrap it with an Ace bandage, and place the ice pack on it for 20-30 minutes.

• An alternate method is a one-minute **contrast bath** of ice, followed by a minute of heat. Do this for at least 12 minutes. This is especially good for pain in the *inner* leg (rather than the front where the shinsplints occur).

• **Massage** the area near the shinsplint pain, but not on it. If you rub on it, the inflammation will worsen. Sit on the floor and lightly stroke on the sides several times. Then wrap your hands around the calf; and, with your finger tips, stroke deeply around on each side of the shin from ankle to knee. Do the entire area, pressing as deeply as possible.

• Try to **correct flat feet or very high arches**, if you can. They can also cause shinsplints.

• The nutritional supplement, **MSM** (methylsulfonylmethane), is a form of sulfur that can help reduce muscle soreness and inflammation. Take 1 gram daily.

• A podiatrist can give you shoe inserts which correct **problems with your gait** (orthotics).

PREVENTION

Try to avoid a lot of **hard activity on unyielding** surfaces, such as concrete. Even carpet on concrete can cause problems. Grass or dirt is better than asphalt; asphalt is better than concrete.

• Wear **good, comfortable shoes**; and, when they start wearing down, buy new ones.

• **Stretch your calves and Achilles tendon** frequently. This helps prevent shinsplints. Shortened calf muscles throw more weight and stress forward to the shins.

To stretch your calves, place your hands on a wall, extend one leg behind the other, and press the back heel slowly to the floor. Do this 20 times, and repeat on the other leg.

To stretch your Achilles tendons, have both feet flat on the ground, about 6 inches apart. Bend your ankles and knees forward while keeping the back straight. When you achieve tightness, hold it for 30 seconds. Repeat 10 times.

ENCOURAGEMENT—Only by following Christ's example can we have genuine happiness. He alone can strengthen us for the trials of life; He alone can guide us through them.

The Lord has not changed. He is true, merciful, and faithful to fulfill His Word. Determine that you will stand with Him in the battles of life. He is the best friend you will ever have; and He deserves your love and obedience. 2 Peter 1:11.

TENDONITIS AND TENOSYNOVITIS

SYMPTOMS—Pain in a tendon. Whereas simple muscle soreness soon goes away, tendon pain can continue for some time.

CAUSES—A tendon is used in the same repetitive motion while ignoring initial indications of tiredness. It occurs most frequently in the shoulders, hips, or Achilles tendons in the ankles.

Tendonitis is inflammation of a tendon, which is the fibrous cord that attaches a muscle to a bone. *Tenosynovitis* is inflammation of the sheath of tissues that surrounds a tendon. These two conditions usually occur together and are treated together.

Tendons around the shoulder, elbow, wrist, fingers, thigh, knee, or back of the heel are most commonly affected.

NATURAL REMEDIES

• When this occurs, you have to **stop the activity** for a time, even though that activity is your primary employment or sport (window washing, long-distance swimming, pitching, etc.).

• But **do not rest too long or too much**, or the muscle tends to atrophy. And while you are resting, you do not want absolute rest.

• Soak in a **warm bath** or a whirlpool bath. **Warming** the tendon before stressful activity decreases the soreness.

• Apply a **heating compress**. Place a warm, damp towel over the area (knee, etc.). Put plastic over that, a heating pad on top and, finally, a loose elastic bandage. Keep it in place for 2-6 hours, with the pad set on low. During this time, try to keep the injured part higher than your heart.

• An alternate method is to **wrap the painful area in an Ace bandage**, but not too tightly or kept on too long. Proper circulation must be maintained.

• **Raise the affected area**, to help control swelling.

PREVENTION

• Before a workout, **carefully warm up**. This is important. The tub bath, mentioned above, can precede the warming-up exercises out in the field.

• Before hard exercise, carefully **stretch your muscles**, to limber them up. Stretching helps prevent the shortening which accompanies exercise.

• **Ice** can be placed on the area after exercise, to reduce swelling and pain. But those with diabetes, heart disease, or problems with blood vessels should be cautious about using ice. The danger is that doing so can constrict blood vessels and loosen clots.

• If possible, **switch to a different exercise format** for a time. (Runners can switch to cycling, etc.)

• **Strengthen your muscles** generally.

• Whatever your activity, **take breaks** occasionally and walk around or do something different. This helps relax your body and improves circulation. **Breathe deeply** and enjoy life for a moment.

—*See Bursitis (629), Repetitive Strain Injury (636), and Arthritis (618) for more information.*

ENCOURAGEMENT—The temple of God is opened in heaven; and the threshold is flushed with His glory. He will help all who will surrender their lives to Him.

SKELETAL-MUSCULAR - **4 - MUSCLES**
Also: Hiatal Hernia (436)

RESTLESS LEG SYNDROME

SYMPTOMS—A chronic sensation of discomfort in the legs, generally between the knees and feet, which urges a person to move his legs. There may be twitching of the leg muscles or deep creeping, crawling sensations. Sometimes it feels like a pain, cramps, or aches.

It tends to occur shortly after retiring at night or after sitting still for quite some time. Sometimes this happens several times a night.

CAUSES—Restless leg syndrome is not a serious neurological disorder; and moving the legs or walking around a little terminates the sensation for a time.

Women and older people have the syndrome more often than men; and a full 5% of the U.S. population have experienced it. Yet the cause is not certain. Mild weakness of the legs may be present.

It seems to be related to **iron deficiency, exposure to cold, stress, heredity, and motion sickness**. It also seems to be related to **pulmonary disease, stomach operations, diabetes, and uremia**.

Very likely, there is a circulatory factor involved: **Blood circulation is impeded** in the legs or blood is being drawn away from the legs in excessive amounts, to care for a problem in the trunk.

People who have **food or other allergies** often have restless leg syndrome.

It is obvious that the solutions, listed below, are keyed to improving leg circulation and bettering the diet:

NATURAL REMEDIES
IMMEDIATE TREATMENT

• **Move your feet** back and forth for a few moments.

• **Rotate the feet** back and forth momentarily.

• **Get up and walk about** for a couple of minutes. This seems to work best at night, when you have been trying to sleep.

• **Change position in bed**. It has been noted that some people experience the problem more often when they sleep in certain positions.

• Some find using a **heating pad** helps; others do better by **soaking the feet in cold water**.

LONGER-TERM CARE

• Some studies have shown **folic acid** and **vitamin E** to be helpful.

• There may be a relationship between this problem and **iron** deficiency. But be sure your iron is from food, not chemical supplements; iron from chemical supplements can initiate other physical problems.

• It would be well to **improve your general diet** and take a **multivitamin supplement** daily.

• Some **sponge the legs with cold water**. Others take a **warm soaking bath** before bedtime. Do not let your bare feet touch the cold floor afterward.

• You may wish to wear **knee socks**.

• **Lie down** every so often to rest your legs.

• Get plenty of **rest**.

• **Walk before going to bed**. Better yet, walk outside in the fresh air. This will help you sleep better.

• Possibly **massage your legs** just before climbing into bed.

AVOID

• Drinking **caffeine products** is a special causal factor of this problem.

• Stop **smoking**. Studies reveal it is also a factor.

• Do not eat much **salt**.

• Never eat **big meals before bedtime**. This draws the blood to the stomach, so that you do not rest well. It can also lead to a nighttime heart attack.

• Do not take **drugs to induce sleep**. They only add another problem to your life.

• Reduce your overall **stress** level.

• Avoid prolonged **exposure to the cold**, which increases the need for additional healing blood to the legs.

• Avoid **overusing the legs**. Strenuous exercise seems to increase the problem.

• Avoid **narrow, pointed shoes** and also **high heels**.

• Sluggish venous blood flow may be a problem; so **do not cross your legs**.

—*See Varicose Veins (535) for more information.*

ENCOURAGEMENT—All heaven unites in praising God. Let us learn the song of the angels now, that we may later sing it when we join their shining ranks. Let us say with the psalmist, "While I live will I praise the Lord: I will sing praises unto my God while I have my being." Psalm 146:3 and 2 Corinthians 4:8-9.

MUSCLE CRAMPS
(Muscle Pain, Leg Cramps, Charley Horse)

SYMPTOMS—A pain in a body muscle, most often in the legs (especially the calf muscles) or feet.

CAUSES—Instead of relaxing and stretching out after contracting, a muscle contracts and remains that way, causing pain. It is an involuntary contraction of a muscle. Muscle cramps may occur at any age. Between the ages of 15 to 80, a full 50% of people will, at some time, have pain or cramps in the legs. Leg pains in children are frequent enough that they are called "growing pains."

Reduced blood supply to the legs is part of the problem. Another is an **imbalance in the levels of calcium and magnesium** in the body or a **deficiency of vitamin E**.

But other causes have also been noted: **arthritis, anemia, tobacco usage, inactivity, poor circulation, too much or too little exercise, muscle injury, allergy, fibromyalgia, arteriosclerosis, dehydration, hypothyroidism, heat stroke, and varicose veins. Diuretic drugs for heart problems or hypertension** can also induce cramps. Those who have had **part of the stomach removed** tend to have muscle cramps thereafter.

If cramping occurs *when walking* and stops when you cease, it may be impaired circulation and nothing more.

If leg cramps occur *during pregnancy*, they may be caused by hormone changes, fatigue, uterine pressure, chilling, or muscle tenseness.

A **calcium deficiency** can make the leg muscles trigger-happy; the contractions in the muscles are stronger.

Leg cramps in older people may be caused by **arteriosclerotic changes** in the circulatory system. Turn to the articles on heart and blood vessels, and see your physician.

NATURAL REMEDIES

IMMEDIATE TREATMENT

• Find the center of the cramp, where the pain is worst. With your thumb, fist, or heel of hand, **press into the center of the cramp**, exerting enough pressure to cause pain but not to the point of excruciation. Hold the pressure 8-12 seconds. The cramp will often vanish.

• If you get a calf cramp in the middle of the night, try **slipping that leg out of the covers**. As it gets cold, the cramp will go away. If you have a cramp that will not quit, put a **cold pack or ice pack** over the area for 20 minutes.

• **Massage** the muscles and use **heat** to relieve pain.

• A **heating pad** may be applied to the area. For some, alternate **hot and cold compresses** work better (heat for 6 minutes and cold for 30 seconds, with 4 changes).

• Drink **peppermint** tea; and apply it as an external compress.

• Rubbing **lobelia** extract on the painful area will relieve muscle spasms.

• **Pinch the upper lip** between the thumb and index finger; and hold it for 20-30 seconds till the cramping disappears.

• If you are pregnant and cramping occurs, **push the toes upward** while applying pressure to the knee, to flatten the affected part.

• Here is the strangest advice of all: The next day, **repeat the activity that made you sore**. Do it with much less intensity. This will help work out the soreness. Thereafter, follow this hard / easy routine; for it takes 48 hours for the muscle to properly recover. This is how serious athletes train.

• An alternate method is to **vary activities**, such as regular walking, with occasional biking or swimming instead.

• After hard exercise or physical work, **slow down** instead of stopping suddenly. The bloodstream is loaded with lactic acid; so slowly exercise at a relaxed pace while it drains off. (However, that will not protect you from soreness the next day, resulting from a torn muscle fiber.)

• Perhaps you need to change into **more comfortable shoes**, in order to improve your leg and foot problems.

• If you have "exercise cramps" during or after exercise, do this: **Stretch the affected muscle** before and after exercise, and **drink more water** to prevent muscle dehydration.

S
K
E
L
M
U
S

ONGOING CARE

The **blood circulation** needs to be improved and equalized:

• Drink enough **water** each day.

• A common mistake is to drink water and take salt tablets during heated exercise. Instead, you need a full range of **electrolytes**, not so much sodium chloride. Drink **fruit drinks**. At mealtime, eat lots of **fresh fruits and vegetables,** especially **dark-green leafy ones** such as **broccoli and kale.** Include **seaweed** in your diet. **Potassium broth** (from thick white potato peelings) is excellent. Eat **whole grains, nuts, and legumes**.

• A **fat-free, sugar-free, salt-free diet** improves the circulation.

• Eat an abundance of **green leafy vegetables**, in order to improve the quality of the blood and the mineral balance.

• **Alfalfa, brewer's yeast, and kelp** are important.

• A deficiency of **calcium** (80-500 mg), **potassium** (500 mg), **magnesium** (500-700 mg), **selenium, and vitamin E** (600-800 IU) exists. Low levels of **calcium, potassium, and magnesium**, especially, are factors in cramping.

• **Mineral imbalances** can produce cramping. Be sure you are getting enough **calcium** through supplementation. Otherwise the phosphorus in certain foods locks with it, so the calcium cannot be absorbed. *See Strengthening the Bones (608) for more information on solving the calcium-phosphorus problem.*

• Those with dentures, who find eating vegetables difficult, are especially prone to magnesium and calcium deficiency and leg cramps. They should have **vegetable soups, potassium broth, and raw vegetable juices** daily.

• Every 3 hours, drink a large glass of quality **water**; this helps clean the bloodstream, liver, kidneys, and bowels of stored toxins.

• Drink less **whole milk**.

• **Eat your meals slowly** and **chew well**.

AVOID

• Do not **smoke**. Nicotine greatly impedes blood circulation. Avoid secondhand smoke.

• If you are taking diuretic drugs, take supplemental potassium. Better yet, switch to **corn-silk tea** and other herbal diuretics; also drink more water. *See the several articles on kidneys and urine (485-496).*

• **Do not stand in one position** for hours without moving. Some motion or shifting of body weight is vital.

• Do not sit with **crossed legs**.

• **Stretch your legs** every so often, with the feet flexed up, not down.

• When sitting, try to **elevate your feet** every so often.

• Do not wear **garters** or any **binding clothes**.

• If you are **overweight**, reduce to normal range or slightly below.

OTHER HELPS

• **Get off your feet** for 5 minutes every hour. If possible, during that time, take your shoes off; massage your feet and wiggle your toes.

• Twice a day, **soak in a tub of warm water** (100°-110° F.). **Massage** the toes, feet, and calves.

• Rub **olive oil or flaxseed oil into your muscles** before and after strenuous exercise.

• At night, wear **roomy pajamas**.

• Keep the **bed covers loose** or use a foot cradle, to **keep bedding weight off the feet**. If you sleep on your stomach, extend your feet over the edge of the bed. Another method is to sleep on your side, with your legs bent and a pillow between your knees.

• If leg cramps are caused by *varicose veins or pregnancy*, **elevate the foot of the bed** 9 inches.

• If leg cramping occurs *during pregnancy*, take **frequent rest periods with the feet elevated**. Wear comfortable, **not tight, clothing**. Be sure you are getting enough **calcium**; this is important.

• Here is **an exercise** which really helps stop ongoing lower leg cramps for many people: Stand with shoes off, facing a wall 2-3 feet away. Lean forward, bracing against the wall with hands and arms, all the while keeping your heels on the floor. When a moderate pull is felt in the calves, hold that position for 10 seconds. Then stand straight for 5 seconds of rest, and lean forward and repeat. Do 3 stretching cycles.

• Here is **another way to relieve a cramp** in your calf: Sit on the floor or on the bed and draw the cramped leg toward your chest, bending it at the knee. Push your thumb gently into your calf, hold it, and breathe normally until you feel the cramp relax.

—Also see Claudication (637), which has the same leg symptoms—but some very special, dangerous causes. It also has additional information on improving the circulation of the legs. Also see Intestinal cramps (453).

ENCOURAGEMENT—In His service, God will place upon you no restriction that will not increase your happiness. In complying with His requirements, you will find a peace, contentment, and joy you can never have in the path of sin. Exodus 34:7.

REPETITIVE STRAIN INJURY
(RSI, Overuse Injury, Cumulative Trauma Disorder)

SYMPTOMS—The symptoms develop gradually; at first it may only occur while performing the repetitive activity. They may include pain, aching, tingling, and restricted movement in the affected area. In some cases, tissue swelling occurs in that area.

In the early stages, symptoms may disappear when the affected body part is rested. Later, symptoms may be present even at rest.

CAUSES—Repetitive strain injury (RSI) is caused by activities that involve prolonged, repeated movements of part of the body, especially if the movements are rapid and forceful. Examples of such activities include typing, using a computer mouse, sweeping bar codes over a laser at a checkout counter, cutting hair, playing a violin, or running the 100-yard dash. The problem most often occurs when using a keyboard or working on a production line. Musicians and athletes are also at risk. It can occur at any age, most often affecting muscles and tendons in the arm. The condition may be associated with stress in the workplace. RSI causes approximately 2 in 3 occupational injuries in the U.S.

The condition is more difficult to treat once it has become chronic. If the problem is recognized early enough, there can easily be a complete recovery. But some people wait too long to make needed changes; and the affected muscles and tendons cannot thereafter be used in a repetitive manner without discomfort.

Other disorders that cause pain in the muscles and tendons [such as Tendonitis *(633)* or Carpal Tunnel Syndrome *(572)* are sometimes classified as RSI. Many people are misdiagnosed and do not make needed changes until the problem has become chronic.

NATURAL REMEDIES
The body will usually heal naturally, if allowed to do so. Here are several pointers:

IMPORTANT MODIFICATIONS
• Stop or modify the activity that is causing the problem. Change your workstation. Use a headset instead of resting the phone on your shoulder.

• The keyboard and mouse should be as close to your body as possible. The monitor (screen) should be directly in front of you at eye level, so you do not have to look up or down. The screen typeface should be large enough, so you do not have to lean forward to see it.

• The papers you are typing from should be on a slant board or copy stand. Use a wrist rest when typing. Type with a gentle touch. You should only have to move the mouse 30° horizontally away from you. You might want to place the mouse pad on a board that tilts slightly upward away from you. Consider typing on a specially designed keyboard.

• *Here is an important point:* Your wrists should remain straight as you type! You should not have to bend your hand up or down when typing. If you keep doing it wrong—then welcome to Carpal Tunnel Syndrome! *(572).*

• If necessary, find someone who will sew a pair of cotton gloves which do not cover beyond the midpoint of your fingers. This will keep your hands warmer. Doing this will greatly increase the work "longevity" of your hands. Use those gloves whenever your fingers are cooler than your cheek.

• Maintain proper posture throughout the day. Sit in a chair with a proper-fitting back. You may need a lower back pillow.

• While driving, keep your hands low on the steering wheel in a secure, but relaxed, grip. On long trips, rest your forearms on a pillow on your lap.

• While sleeping, do not lie on your stomach with your head tilted, sleep with your arms overhead, or lie on the injured side. Instead of this, lie on the unaffected side, with one pillow under your head and another under the injured arm. Or lie on your back, possibly with one pillow under each arm up to the shoulders.

• When working, take a 1-2 minute break every half hour and stretch your wrists and neck a little. Roll your shoulders.

OTHER HELPS
• Drink 2-3 quarts of **water** every day. Also drink fresh **vegetable juices** daily.

• An extra 20-30 pounds of **weight** can quadruple your chances of RSI or Carpal Tunnel Syndrome nerve damage. All that extra fat in the wrist area squeezes against the median nerve. **Stop eating meat, fat, junk food, and starches**; and your weight will go down.

Do not use **caffeine** (it drains water out of the body), **nicotine** (it reduces blood flow to the extremities), or **alcohol** (it increases inflammation).

• Make sure you are taking **deeper breaths**, when working and not working. The oxygen recharges your body.

ENCOURAGEMENT—There is a remedy for the sin-sick soul. That remedy is in Jesus. Precious Saviour! His grace is sufficient for the weakest; and the strongest must also have His grace or perish.

CLAUDICATION
(Intermittent Claudication)

SYMPTOMS—Cramping pain, weakness, and tension in a limb (usually the calves) after muscular exercise. Upon resting, the pain always ceases. Typically, after a few moments of rest, the person can begin walking again.

CAUSES—Intermittent claudication (also simply called claudication) is often a symptom of something more serious: **arteriosclerosis** of the femoral and popliteal arteries. When cholesterol-laden plaques narrow the arteries in the heart muscle, the result is angina. When it happens in the leg, the result is claudication.

Other causes include **Buerger's disease** *(370)* or other occlusive arterial diseases of the limbs. **Diabetics** *(656)* tend to have claudication more than the average. **High blood pressure** (above 160 systolic or 90 diastolic) triples the risk of claudication *(see Hypertension, 526)*.

Diagnosis of claudication is done by a physician,

S
K
E
L
M
U
S

by taking the "pedal pulse." This is the pulse at the instep of each foot. These pulses should be strong and equal; but if one or both is weak or absent, then there is claudication.

NATURAL REMEDIES

• Maintain a **total vegetarian diet, free from grease and animal foods. Avoid most vegetable oils** also. Because of the connection between claudication and blood vessel diseases, the life you save may be your own. *See Arteriosclerosis (523) and related articles on the heart and blood vessels (513-523).*

• Take **vitamin C** (to bowel tolerance), **vitamin E, B$_6$, chromium**, and **selenium**.

• Using **nicotine** is ruinous to the health in several ways; choking off circulation to the limbs is one of them. Those who smoke are 6 times more likely to develop claudication *(also see Buerger's Disease, 370).*

• It appears that abnormally high blood viscosity can be a primary cause of poor blood flow. The solution is to drink lots of **water** and use a **diet low in fats, sugars, and concentrated foods**. Those are the foods which have a very low moisture content.

• **Stress** also reduces blood viscosity; so avoid stress.

• A regular **exercise** program is very helpful, especially for those who do it everyday. *See Muscle Cramps (635) for some sample exercises.* Ten repetitions of the exercises should be done at least once a day.

• Gentle exercise is appropriate for people with intermittent claudication, but not beyond the point of pain. If you begin hurting, *stop*—you've reached the point where tissue damage begins.

• In addition to other exercises, take a **daily walk**. Build up to a total of an hour, each morning and evening.

• For those who can take them, **hot baths** are helpful. Always keep the head cool with cool washcloths that are changed frequently.

SPECIAL HELPS

• In one 12-week study, a large number of people with claudication were given 800 mg of raw **garlic** daily. Most walked better by their fifth week. Their blood pressure and cholesterol levels were also lower.

• **Ginkgo** improves blood flow through the legs, just as it does through the heart and brain. It does this by dilating the arteries. In a research study, people who took 40 mg of ginkgo extract daily were able to go 75%-110% farther without pain. But you must take the standardized extract, not the leaf (Ginkgo sometimes produces side effects of abdominal distress, headache, or dizziness.)

• **Ginger** is another remarkable herb, which is almost as effective as garlic in preventing blood clots in the arteries.

• Taking **hawthorn** (120-240 mg of a standardized extract) improves blood flow and ability to walk painlessly.

• **Flaxseed oil** (1 Tbsp. twice a day) contains omega-3, which helps prevent cardiovascular disease. Or take 500-1,000 mg of **omega-3** supplement daily.

• **Carnitine** (2,000 mg, twice a day) is a protein component which helps blood cells work better, even when they are not obtaining enough oxygen.

• People who take 400 IU of **vitamin E** daily can walk farther without pain.

• **Niacin** (500 mg twice daily) widens the arteries, bringing more oxygen to the leg muscles.

• Intermittent claudication can be a **sign of general circulatory or cardiovascular problems**. A thorough medical exam is in order, to detect any problems before they become serious.

—*See Muscle Cramps (635) which, in the legs, have the same symptoms. Also see Arteriosclerosis (523) and related articles.*

ENCOURAGEMENT—Come apart and worship God. The everlasting assurance shall be yours, that you have a Friend that sticketh closer than a brother.

SIDE STITCHES
(Pain in the Side)

SYMPTOMS—A sharp, temporary pain in the side.

CAUSES—This pain is caused by a spasm in the diaphragm when this muscle, located between your chest and abdomen, does not receive enough oxygen.

Running is a common immediate cause. The dual pressure from the contracted belly muscles (caused by the raised knee during running) and the expanded lungs from above (caused by deeper breathing) can momentarily shut off blood flow to the diaphragm. This causes it to cramp.

Not breathing evenly can cause you to get these cramps, even when heavily laughing.

However, the pain can also come from trapped **gas** in the intestines.

If the pain is only on the right side, it may be due to temporary **lack of oxygen to the liver**.

NATURAL REMEDIES

• **Stop what you are doing** and let your muscles calm down. Exhale deeply and **take slow, deep breaths** in and out. You may wish to massage your side as you do this.

• **Learn to breathe more deeply.** Breathe from the diaphragm more, less from the chest. This is part of the problem.

• Do not do very **strenuous exercise** closer than 2 hours to a meal.

ENCOURAGEMENT—Though now He has ascended to the presence of God and shares the throne of the universe, Jesus has lost none of His compassionate nature. He wants to comfort and help you just now. Psalm 65:3, 111:3.

FIBROMYALGIA SYNDROME
(Chronic Muscle Pain Syndrome, Fibromyositis, Fibrositis, Tension Myalgia, Muscular Rheumatism)

SYMPTOMS—Anxiety, depression, tension, fatigue, chronic muscle aches and pain, joint swelling, headaches (sometimes migraine), irritable bowels, sleep disturbances, and stiffness.

The pain is described as burning, throbbing, shooting, and stabbing. Pain and stiffness are greatest in the morning.

Depression appears to be a key factor. Other symptoms include menstrual problems, palpitations, memory impairment, dizziness, dry eyes and mouth, frequent changes in eyeglasses, and impaired coordination. Lifting or climbing stairs seems hard to do.

As explained below, the existence of "tender points" is a distinctive symptom.

CAUSES—Fibromyalgia is more of a set of symptoms than a disease; and it is primarily caused by stress. Women have it more often than men.

Often mistaken for arthritis, rheumatism, or Epstein-Barr Syndrome, fibromyalgia causes the muscles and joints to tighten up when under stress. The emotions have a powerful effect on the body.

Those experiencing this problem frequently have shallow sleep. Muscle spasms and pain in various places may occur at night or during the day. *Also see Muscular Rheumatism (639).*

Then there are the so-called "tender points." These symptoms are unique to this disease, unlike any other disease. There are 10 pairs of specific points, where muscles are especially sensitive to the touch. Here are those 10 locations:

In the muscles at the base of skull, neck, upper back, or mid-back. On the side of the elbow, around the lower vertebra of the neck, at the insertion of the second rib, in the upper and outer muscles of the buttocks, around the upper part of the thigh bone, and at the middle of the knee joint.

Those with fibromyalgia experience so many sleep problems [insomnia *(547)*, bruxism *(421)*, restless leg syndrome *(634)*, etc.], that they often have chronic fatigue.

The symptoms frequently begin in young adulthood, develop gradually, and slowly increase in intensity until many become incapacitated by the problem.

Sometimes the syndrome disappears; at other times it is chronic. And, in some cases, it comes back in recurring flare-ups.

The cause is not really known; but Chronic Fatigue Syndrome *(280)* is similar to fibromyalgia, but less painful.

Prior infection by the **influenza** virus tends to pre-dispose humans to fibromyalgia at a later time.

Of the 3-6 million people with this problem, the majority are women, primarily 25 to 45 years of age.

Physicians prescribe antidepressants for fibromyalgia. These can cause side effects which are not helpful.

NATURAL REMEDIES
DIET
• Maintain a **well-balanced diet**.
• **Do not drink coffee, tea, cola drinks. Do not drink or eat chocolate. Do not take pain relievers**. Avoid all types of **drugs**; they only add to your problems. If you have been taking any of these, the symptoms may worsen for a time when you drop them; but persevere, and you will feel better for having done so.
• Poor absorption of food is involved with this problem. So **eat slowly** of good nourishing food; and **chew it well**. Be sure to take **vitamin / mineral supplementation**. **Magnesium** is important.
• Drink plenty of **liquids**, including quality water.
• Do not eat **meat, dairy products, white-flour products, processed foods**, or any food high in **saturated fats**.
• Avoid **wheat and brewer's yeast** until your symptoms fade.
• **Food and chemical allergies** may be involved. Try to search out the source of your allergies and avoid them.

OTHER HELPS
• Learn to rest and **be relaxed**. Be able to relax after work. Go out and walk in the fresh air and thank God for your blessings. Indeed, count them all, one by one, and thank Him for every one.
• Determine what your problems are and solve them. Know you are no longer being bothered by those problems because you are working toward solving them or learning to live with them.
• A fair amount of **muscular activity** helps relax a person mentally and emotionally. Enjoy **outdoor activities**, such as gardening or raising flowers. You need a regular amount of daily exercise, **not a hard workout** every so many days. Building up such a regular exercise program will do much to alleviate the problem.
• Take a **hot and cold shower** each morning, to stimulate circulation and help reduce morning stiffness. **Cold showers** are actually better than hot ones for reducing fibromyalgia pains.
• Put 4-6 oz. of **ginger** powder into a somewhat hot bath, to induce sweating and remove toxins. Drinking hot ginger tea has a similar effect.
• Helpful herbs include **comfrey, alfalfa, hops, skullcap, white willow bark, and valerian**.
• Jacob Teitelbaum, M.D. (Annapolis, MD), says that fibromyalgia is specifically caused by a long-term

S
K
E
L
M
U
S

lack of **deep sleep**. He has treated hundreds of patients, with over 85% cured or improved to the point that their symptoms are no longer a problem. He treats the problem as a malfunction of the **hypothalamus**, the master gland in the brain (endfatigue.com). He suggests using each of the following for six months: **Valerian** (160-480 mg) and **lemon balm** (80-240 mg) before bedtime. **Valerian** (100 mg, 3 times a day), for its calming effect. **Kava kava** (200-750 mg before bedtime), to relax the nerves. **Melatonin** (200-300 mcg before bedtime), to help you go to sleep. **Magnesium** (200 mg daily). **Deep massage**: Put three fingers on an area of muscle tension or tenderness; apply enough pressure so your fingers won't slide. Make 5-10 circular motions, rubbing just hard enough to produce mild discomfort only. Then move a hand-width away, to a new area, and begin again. He says to also take a high-potency **multi-vitamin supplement.**

Research studies have demonstrated each of the following:

• An early study found that **vitamin E** (100-300 IU daily) produced positive and sometimes dramatic results.

• Fibromyalgia patients are low in **vitamin B$_1$** and **thiamine**.

• **Cayenne**, applied topically, alleviates the pain.

• **Chlorella** also decreases the pain. All **deep green vegetables** also help do this as well.

• **Aloe vera** (taken orally), **olive leaf**, and **St. John's wort** each reduce the symptoms.

• Regular **exercise** provides positive, but short-term, benefits.

• **Melatonin** helps correct the impairment of Slow Wave Sleep (deep sleep) experienced by the patients.

• **Magnesium** deficiency within muscle fibers is believed to be a factor in causing fibromyalgia.

• Taking **malic acid** has caused significant improvement in the number of tender points. It binds and removes aluminum with iron (or just aluminum) from the brain and excretion of aluminum and iron from the body. The best single source of malic acid is **prunes**. The other good sources are **apples, limes, passion fruit, raspberry leaf, quinces, cherries, peaches, apricots, nectarines, plums, grapes, strawberries, pears, and tomato**. It is also in the herb, **fennel**.

• Malic acid and magnesium help muscles use glucose properly. Together, they may help reduce fibromyalgia symptoms. Researchers give 2,400 mg per day of malic acid, combined with 600 mg magnesium, in order to effect good results in patients. Malic acid is available from health-food stores in both tablet and capsule forms. (The two forms are calcium malate and magnesium malate.)

• Being happy helps fight pain and inflammatory conditions. **Cheerfulness and even laughter** stimulates the brain to produce *catecholamines* (known as "alertness hormones"); these trigger the release of *endorphins*, which are natural painkillers.

• In addition to the above, the following supplements are designed to nourish muscle cells and enable them to use energy more efficiently through better oxygenation. They also control inflammation and depression and promote more restful sleep.

• **NADH** (Nicotinamide adenine dinucleotide-hydrogen). This compound helps control pain and muscle spasms. *Typical dosage:* 5 to 10 mg each morning on an empty stomach; take with 6 to 8 ounces of water.

• **5-HTP** (5-Hydroxy-tryptophan). Studies have found this compound helps decrease the pain and insomnia of fibromyalgia by increasing serotonin levels. *Typical dosage:* 50 to 300 mg per day.

• **SAM-e** (S-adenosylmethionine). This new compound is being hailed as a natural antidepressant. But clinical studies show that it can also reduce fibromyalgia pain and elevate mood. Because depression can occur with fibromyalgia, this supplement may be worth a try. *Typical dosage:* 200 to 1,600 mg per day.

• **Coenzyme Q$_{10}$**. This enzyme helps boost oxygen supplies to muscle tissue, helping it to flush inflammatory chemicals more quickly. *Typical dosage:* 60 to 400 mg per day.

—See Acute Muscular Rheumatism (626), Chronic Fatigue Syndrome (280), and Depression (596).

ENCOURAGEMENT—Real happiness is found only in being good and doing good. The purest, highest, and most rewarding enjoyment comes to those who faithfully fulfill their appointed duties. Living for God is the best way to live. 1 Peter 1:8.

MYELITIS

SYMPTOMS—Moderate fever, loss of appetite, numbness, tingling, burning, "girdle pain" at level of the disease (pain encircling the trunk at the point where the disease is). Paralysis soon develops, and may become complete.

CAUSES—This is inflammation of the spinal cord. Here is Kellogg's remedial treatment for this crippling nerve infection:

NATURAL REMEDIES

J.H. KELLOGG, M.D., PRESCRIPTIONS FOR ACUTE AND CHRONIC MYELITIS AND THEIR COMPLICATIONS *(how to give these water therapies: pp. 206-275 / list of treatments: pp. 206-207 / Hydrotherapy Disease Index: pp. 273-275)*

MYELITIS (ACUTE) —

COMBAT INFLAMMATORY PROCESS IN SPINAL CORD—Ice Bag, continuously changing **Fomentations** for 5 minutes, every half hour. **Revulsive Compress** to the spine. **Fomentation** for 20 minutes every 3 hours, during intervals between. **Heating Compress** to spine at 60° F., renewed every 15 minutes.

AFTER ACUTE STAGE HAS SUBSIDED—Alternate Compress or Alternate Douche to spine, 3 times a day.

PAIN AND PARESTHESIA IN LEGS—Hot Leg Pack, Hot Footbath, Hot Half Bath, **Revulsive Compress** to spine several times daily, duration 15-60 minutes.

GIRDLE SENSATION—Hot Trunk Pack, followed by **Cold Mitten Friction**. **Hot Abdominal Pack** that is well-protected. **Fomentation** to spine, followed by **Heating Compress** to spine.

NEURALGIC SPINAL PAIN—Fomentation or Hot Sponging of spine, followed by **Heating Compress**.

PARAPLEGIA—Alternate Compress or Fan Douche to spine and legs, **massage**.

SENSORY PARALYSIS—Alternate Spray Douche, **Alternate Sponging**, Alternate Compress, Percussion Douche (twice daily).

MUSCULAR SPASM—Revulsive Compress to spine. **Fomentation** over irritated muscular groups. Follow by continuous **Heating Compress**, repeated twice daily or as often as necessary. **Heating Compress** to spine.

GASTRIC CRISES—Hot and Cold Trunk Pack, **Revulsive Gastric Compress, Fomentation** to spine, **Hot Footbath**, Hot Leg Pack, **Hot Full Bath** or Hot Sitz Bath.

CONTRAINDICATIONS—Avoid Cold Full Baths and other general cold applications. Carefully avoid burning or blistering him with hot applications.

MYELITIS (CHRONIC) —

GENERAL—Short sweating procedures, followed by **graduated cold applications** twice a day. **Revulsive Compress** or Fan Douche to Spine, temperature 120°-170° F.; Prolonged **Neutral Full Baths,** for 1-6 hours. **Heating Compress** to spine. Later stage: Alternate Douche or **Heating Compresses** to spine.

PRICKLING SENSATION IN LEGS—Revulsive Douche, Hot **Fomentations** or **Pail Pour** at 96° F. to spine and legs.

DURING EARLY STAGE AND EXACERBATIONS—Pail Pour to spine (96° F.), 2-10 minutes, 2-3 times daily. Absolute **rest** in bed and spinal **Fomentation** every 4 hours, **Heating Compress** during the intervals between.

CONTRAINDICATIONS—Avoid Cold Full Bath, very Cold Douche, Cold Pail Pour, and all prolonged cold applications.

ENCOURAGEMENT—Not one sincere prayer is lost. Amid the anthems of the celestial choir, God hears the cries of the weakest human being.

HERNIA
(Rupture, Abdominal Hernia, Femoral Hernia)

SYMPTOMS—Visual awareness of the problem. In the case of a strangulated hernia, there is pain, vomiting, and abdominal distention.

A weak spot develops in or around a muscle wall, usually as a result of straining while lifting heavy objects. An *abdominal hernia* occurs in the abdomen (lower belly), often in the lower left or lower right. A *femoral hernia* occurs in the femoral muscle of the upper front leg. The weak spot slowly enlarges and becomes an opening.

If it is in the abdomen, a loop of intestine may protrude from it at times. Unless corrected, such a condition will grow progressively worse. A *strangulated hernia* occurs when a loop of intestine is caught in the opening and becomes pinched, blocking the intestinal passage. Gangrene of the bowel, peritonitis, and death may result if a strangulated hernia is not given prompt surgical attention.

A hernia in a child is less serious; and the opening may repair itself if the protruding bowel loop is pushed back and held in place by a firm band or adhesive strap for a few months.

Hernias can also develop near the navel; these are called paraumbilical hernias. These are most common in women who are overweight or have had several pregnancies.

NATURAL REMEDIES

• First, a truss can be purchased and worn. This is not a very practical solution; but it may be necessary for a time if funds are not available for an operation.

• Second, a surgical operation can be performed. This is often the best solution, if done by a properly trained physician.

• Third, simple remedies may be applied which may, or may not, succeed. If they do not, then an operation can be performed.

Here are some suggestions:

• If you are overweight, it would be best to **go on a cleansing program, to lose some weight** and cleanse the system.

• Eat a **nourishing diet,** supplemented by **vitamins and minerals.** And **avoid all grease, meat, and junk foods.**

• Avoid **foods cooked by microwave.** Doing so increases the likelihood of developing a hernia.

• Begin a program of **exercises** each day to strengthen your muscles (abdominal or leg, according to where the hernia is). For example, push-ups from the knees will strengthen the abdominal muscles.

• You may wish to try an astringent tea. Make a very strong tea of **white oak bark**, consisting of one cup of finely broken bark to one quart of water. Boil it 2 minutes and let stand 2 hours. Strain and add 1 tsp. of **alum powder.** Wet a folded piece of cloth in the tea and place it over the hernia. Cover with plastic and hold in place with a truss, elastic bandage, or adhesive tape. Using a clean cloth, repeat this about 4 times a day for a month. The tannin in the bark and the alum will tend to pull together and thicken the area. This may, or may not, close the area.

• You may also try a poultice made of **comfrey leaves, bistort root, and giant Solomon's seal root.** Renew every 12 hours; keep it on continually for a month.

• A **shave grass tea compress** may also be used.

• Another possibility is, for a month, apply a **poultice** at night and a **compress** during the day.

—*Also see Hiatal Hernia (436) and Umbilical Hernia (642).*

ENCOURAGEMENT—Through all our trials, we have a never-failing Helper. He does not leave us alone to struggle with temptation and battle with evil. Give Him all your heart and hear Him say, "Fear not; I am with you." Luke 12:32.

UMBILICAL HERNIA
(Omphalocele, Navel Hernia)

SYMPTOMS—A grape- to basketball-sized skin sac in the belly button.

CAUSES—*"Omphalos"* means navel, and *"kele"* means hernia. Babies may be born with an umbilical hernia, which developed behind the navel due to a weakness in the abdominal wall.

This flaw, called a *hernial ring*, occurs more frequently than might be expected. The mother did not receive enough **vitamin A and/or zinc** during pregnancy.

NATURAL REMEDIES
• If the hernial ring is larger than your finger tip, **surgery** is needed to correct it.
• If the defect is about the size of the diameter of your finger tip, the following method has been used with good success, to heal it at home without surgery:
• Place a golf-ball size **of virgin wool** on the hernia and tape it firmly down to the level of the skin's surface. Three times a day, remove the wool ball. Make sure the fat is pushed back into the belly cavity; carefully use your finger to do this. At the same time, rub the hernial ring in a rotary fashion for several minutes, to irritate it. Over a period of several weeks or months, the defect will fill in and entirely heal; so no surgery will be needed.

—*Also see Hernia (641) and Hiatal Hernia (436).*

ENCOURAGEMENT—Educate the soul to cheerfulness and thankfulness to God for the great love which He has for you. Christian cheerfulness is the very beauty of holiness. Isaiah 55:12.

SKELETAL-MUSCULAR - 5 - SPRAINS

MUSCLE INJURIES
(Sprains and Strains)

SYMPTOMS—Bruised wrists, ankles, fingers, knees, back, hips, and sore or swollen muscles.

CAUSES—*Sprains* are a painful stretching of the ligaments of the joints beyond its own capacity; this can be caused by excessive lifting, sudden stops or turns, injuries, or falls.

Severe sprains involve torn ligaments and a torn joint capsule, with bleeding and swelling.

Muscle injuries can occur when **muscles are strained too much, used too long or hard, suddenly twisted, or hard falls occur**. Athletes frequently have such problems.

First degree: mild injury with little pain and little loss of movement. *Second degree:* moderate injury, sharp pain with motion, swelling, possible discoloration. *Third degree:* severe injury, extreme pain, swelling, spasmodic muscle contraction.

Note: A *bad bruise* on any part of the body can be treated as for a sprain or strain.

To prevent strains and sprains, do stretching exercises both before and after exercise. You are at the highest risk of such injury in contact sports.

NATURAL REMEDIES
IMMEDIATELY
• Immediately: Move the injured part until you find a position which hurts the sprained area the least. Leave it there for 2 minutes, all the while breathing deep and regular. Then slowly return it to its normal position. If it is a minor sprain, this may solve the problem.
• If there is still pain, feel for the tender point; and then lightly press it till it reaches the point of nearly unbearable pain. Hold it until the pain eases (about a minute). What you did was to reduce the maximum muscle contraction at that point. If the pain does not ease, then the sprain is too severe and perhaps you need to see a doctor.

Next, apply water therapy:

HYDROTHERAPY
• According to one view, sprains should be treated with **ice or very cold water**. Follow this by bandaging the injury with an Ace bandage. This is known as RICE: rest, ice, compression, and elevation.
• But, according to a different view, sprains should be initially treated with **alternate hot and cold applications**—especially if it is in the *wrist, elbow, or ankle*. This method works *better* than using cold alone! Here is how to do it:
• *If the injury is in the wrist, elbow, or ankle,* put the injured part in very **hot water**. And keep it there 20-30 minutes. Every few minutes take it out of the hot water and plunge it into **cold water** for about a minute, then back into the hot. Keep the hot water hot. This can continue for up to 2 hours with good results. Repeat this for several days; and, twice a day, **massage** around the area.

If you use the cold method alone on a sprain, you may not be able to walk on a sprained ankle for days; use the alternate hot and cold method, and you may be much better in half the time.
• (A third method calls for **cold** on strains to begin with, to reduce initial swelling, followed very

soon afterward by **alternate hot and cold**.)

• If the sprain or strain is *in the back or shoulder*, treat it with **hot fomentations, short cold, and massage**.

• While the area is hot from the hot water, **slowly move it about** without causing pain. If necessary, move it with your hand. But do not stretch or stress the joint beyond its comfortable limits.

• In addition to the above, very severe strains frequently require a **cast** similar to that used for a fracture, so the injured joint area can be immobilized for more complete rest.

• **DMSO** (dimethyl sulfoxide) is a liquid that can be applied externally to the injured area, to relieve pain, reduce swelling, and promote healing. But only buy it in a health-food store. Be sure your hands are clean when you apply the gel.

DIET

• Research studies found that taking **bromelain** (125-450 mg, 3 times daily on an empty stomach) speeds healing of contusions, sprains, ecchymoses, hematomas and other soft tissue injuries. (*Bromelain* is the active ingredient in pineapple.)

• Drink plenty of fresh, raw **vegetable juices**.

• Each day take **calcium** (1,500-2,000 mg), **magnesium** (750-1,000 mg), **maganese** (15 mg), and a **multivitamin** supplement.

HERBS

• Here is a liniment for sprains and bruises, recommended by Dr. Christopher: Mix 2 oz. each of **lobelia fluid extract and cayenne**. Combine with 1 tsp. each of **oil of spearmint, rosemary, and wormwood**. Apply as much as can be absorbed. To speed the action, place a hot-water bottle on the area.

• Here is Jethro Kloss' herbal formula: Mix equal amounts of **skullcap, gentian, buckthorn bark, valarian,** and add a pinch of **cayenne**. Put a heaping tsp. in boiling water. Take a tablespoon (or more) every hour.

• Here is the Kloss liniment: 2 oz. **myrrh**, 1 oz. **goldenseal**, and ½ oz. **cayenne**. Rub gently on the affected area.

• Make a poultice of **burdock** leaves or drink burdock tea. Towels can be wrung out of hot burdock or **catnip** tea and applied several times daily.

• Apply compresses of **yellow dock**.

• Bind **orange peel** (with white side next to skin) over the sprain to reduce swelling.

• Put **raw or roasted onions** in a poultice on the sprain.

• Apple cider **vinegar** compresses often relieve the sprain. Apply strips of newspaper, soaked in vinegar, then wrap this with airtight material.

• Add **ginger** tea to bathwater and soak in it.

• **Boswellia** or **goldenseal** can be applied to reduce inflammation.

• **Ginger** and/or **feverfew** will reduce pain and soreness.

• Mix **fenugreek and flaxseed** powder and apply as a poultice, to reduce swelling. Or apply a **mustard** poultice.

LATER EXERCISES

• *Do A to Z for ankle injuries:* While standing (holding onto something for support) or sitting, move your foot and trace every capital letter of the cursive (printed) alphabet. This works all the ligaments of the ankle, prevents adhesions, and improves healing.

• *Towel exercise for ankle injuries:* Stand, holding onto a table, and pick up a section of a towel with your toes; then drop it and pick up another section, etc. Do this once every morning and once every evening.

• *Thumb injury:* About a week after the injury, begin twiddling your thumb in a circle, clockwise, then counterclockwise. Then try to touch it against each of its companion fingers. Next, pick up a newspaper sheet, with the injured hand, and try to crumple it up into a ball.

• *Shoulder injury:* Bend over slightly so your arm is free; then swing it in a circle, in a pendulum, and in figure eights. This will reduce adhesions.

If there is significant swelling, you may need to see a physician.

RICE

• You can treat mild sprains and strains at home, starting with **RICE**—an acronym for **rest, ice, compression, and elevation**.

• **Rest** means just that. Sounds easy; but, if you must keep active, gently exercise the parts of your body that don't hurt. Swimming can often be tolerated.

• **Ice** is also simple—apply a plastic bag of cubed or crushed ice, a bag of frozen peas or corn, or a commercial cold pack. Protect your skin by covering it with a damp cloth. The day of the injury, ice the area for 20 to 30 minutes, three or four times per day. Continue ice compresses until a couple of days after the injury begins to feel better. Because heat increases swelling, some experts don't recommend using it within the first two weeks—unless the primary problem is tight muscles; in this case heat helps muscles relax. Others say you can alternate hot and cold applications as long as you end with cold.

• **Compression** entails wrapping the injured limb with an elastic bandage; but only do it snugly with a trouser sock. You don't want to cut off the circulation and increase swelling below the injury. Remove and rewrap the bandage at least twice a day.

• **Elevation** means raising the injured area above the heart—not just propping your ankle, if that's what you've hurt, on a footstool. Instead, lie flat and prop your leg or other injured area on pillows. This improves the return of blood and other fluids to the heart, to reduce swelling.

—*Also see Athletic Workouts (below).*

S
K
E
L
M
U
S

ENCOURAGEMENT—Those who put away iniquity from their hearts and stretch out their hands in earnest supplication unto God will have that help which God alone can give them. In His strength, you can fulfill His will for your life. Psalm 68:3.

ATHLETIC WORKOUTS (STRENGTHEN AND BUILD MUSCLES)

Protecting and strengthening muscles is an important part of physical conditioning, along with aerobic exercise. Muscle fibers are packed with thin protein filaments, that contract to allow movement. The strain of exercise creates tiny tears in muscle tissue. The body produces proteins to repair them. Over a period of time, the proteins accumulate, increasing the size of muscle fibers and producing larger, stronger muscles. However, maintaining a healthy body, by giving it proper nourishment and care is actually more important than merely building larger muscles.

Here are a few helpful suggestions for those engaged in ongoing athletic workouts or other heavy labor or activity:

NATURAL REMEDIES
• Maintain a **nutritious diet**, including **full vitamin / mineral supplementation**. Eat **salads, whole grains, seaweed, seeds, nuts, and drink vegetable juices**.
• Maintain strong bones. *See Strengthening the Bones (608)*. Include silica (**horsetail and oat straw herbs**), to help calcium strengthen the bones.
• **Vitamins A, D, E, C, zinc, and manganese** are needed.
• **Locate your allergies** and eliminate them. If you have food allergies, exercise may increase the absorption of the allergenic food, resulting in severe reactions. *See Allergies (848) and Pulse Test (847)*.
• **Glucose** is the main fuel for the muscles. It is stored in the liver and muscles in the form of glycogen. You can only work as long as you have stored glycogen ready to be changed into glucose. The best way to store up this glycogen is to eat **complex carbohydrates**.
• Although body fat can also be converted to energy, avoid eating much **fat**. Focus on getting carbohydrates, not fat, in your diet.

THE WORKOUT
• At **the meal before a workout**, do not eat much roughage, requiring energy to digest; it will make you sluggish. At that meal, avoid peaches, grapes, bananas, and celery.
• **Stretch and warm up** your muscles before exercising. Before doing this, muscles are about 98° F. and stiff. After a 5-minute warm-up, they are several degrees higher and ready for action.
• **Drink fluids** before, during, and after workouts. To prevent dehydration and cramping, do this whether or not you are thirsty.

• Be sure to obtain adequate **electrolytes**. A 50-50 mix of **fruit juice and water** will help supply this.
• **Proteins** are needed for muscles and tissues; they are not an energy source. The need for protein does not increase during a workout. Excess protein intake (at any time) increases urine elimination, which produces dehydration unless you are drinking enough water. Eating too much protein can damage the kidneys.
• **Do not use steroids** in order to increase muscle mass and athletic performance! You may see temporary gain, but you are injuring your body. In men, long-term use can lead to cancer, sterility, breast enlargement, shrinkage of the testicles, and osteoporosis (hollowing of the bones, leading to breakage). Once the steroid treatments are stopped, all the buildup is lost, and fat tends to infiltrate the tissue. In women, excess facial and body hair, breast cancer, shrinkage of the breasts may occur. Steroids tend to be psychologically addictive. The person feels dependent on taking them, until the physical damage becomes deeply ingrained. Anabolic steroids can produce heart attacks.
• **After a workout**, keep moving until you are rested. Do not take a shower until your body temperature has cooled down. This cooling-down wait will help you avoid cramping and even a heart attack.
• Do not lift weights if you have a heart problem. At the moment of the lift, breathing stops, circulation to the heart decreases, and great pressure is placed on the heart and lungs by surrounding muscles.

Quotation: "Although muscular work is the largest single factor in determining energy needs, it has no appreciable effect on the protein requirement . . Although there is no basis for the idea that a man requires extra meat because he is doing muscular work, he does require more fuel foods, in order to provide necessary energy . . The energy for muscular work usually comes chiefly from carbohydrates."—*L. Jean Bogart, Nutrition and Physical Fitness, p. 101.*

ENCOURAGEMENT—Real happiness is found only in being good and doing good. Live to bless others, and you will find your deepest satisfaction. Live only for yourself, and you will perish alone. John 15:11.

SKELETAL-MUSCULAR - 6 - SPINE

POSTURE, IMPROVING

SYMPTOMS—A round-shouldered appearance.

NATURAL REMEDIES
It is easy, over the years, to let your posture collapse. Here are several suggestions to get it back into shape:
• Relax and **practice standing up straight**. Put your back and head against a wall as you look forward. Hold it for a minute and get a feel for what the

ideal is like.

• Recognize that, as you go through the day, you will not always maintain this ideal. But it gives you something to work toward.

• The best place to practice good posture is when you are walking outside. **Try to walk erect**. Notice that doing so makes it easier to take full breaths of air, and you feel better.

• Then, when it is time to work or relax, do not worry about keeping a ramrod back when you are stooping over, writing, washing the dishes, etc. **Real living is not ramrod**; it is a variety of positions.

• But, when you take your outdoor exercise, return closer to that ideal of perfect posture.

Here are more ideas:

• When you stand, **keep both feet flat** on the floor. Resting on one leg leads to curvature of the back.

• **Adjust your chair height**, so that your thighs are parallel with the floor and your knees are level with, or slightly higher than, your hips. If not, they pull your body forward. Your back slumps; and you work harder, trying to keep your back upright.

• If you place a **small pillow** between the small of your back (the lumbar area) and the back of the chair, you will tend to sit straighter.

• As you are sitting, you ought to be able to feel the **bones in your buttocks** against the seat. If you cannot do so, wiggle around until you can. When you cannot feel them, you are slumping.

• When seated at a table and not working, **sit 6-8 inches away** from it. This will keep you from slumping over onto it. Only your wrists will be on the edge of the table before you. Maintain this same distance if you are working on a computer or typewriter.

Television news announcers use the following two methods, to make a better appearance when they talk while being seated:

• (1) Tend to **sit on the edge** of your chair; you will be less likely to slump back into it.

• (2) While sitting on the edge of your chair, curl **one foot under the chair** and stretch the other out for balance. This will help keep your back straight.

• **Do not cross your legs**. Doing so throws your body out of alignment. Keep your feet flat on the floor.

• In a car, **pull the seat toward the pedals** until your knees are bent and slightly higher than your hips and your thighs are parallel to the floor. Either place a **small cushion** behind the small of your back or use the seat adjustment available in some cars.

• **Get enough sleep** at night. You cannot stand or sit straight if you are exhausted.

• Sleep on a **firm mattress**. When you lie on your side, both hips and shoulders should sink in just a little.

• When sleeping, either **sleep on the side** (with a pillow under your head that is thick enough to keep your head untilted) **or sleep on your back** with only a thin pillow under your head and possibly a small pillow under your knees.

• Walk, run, cycle, or **do exercises and stretching**, to keep your muscles extended and in good condition.

• Here is a way to rest your back and improve your posture at the same time, either during break or at the end of the day: **Lie on the floor** for a few minutes with your legs on a low chair or stool.

ENCOURAGEMENT—A ransom has been paid for the souls of men; but we must individually surrender our lives to God, so that we may claim that ransom. God has a heaven full of blessings for you.

BACKACHE
(Low Back Pain, Lumbago, Sciatica, Slipped Disc, Lumbar Disc Herniation, Spinal Disc Prolapse)

SYMPTOMS—Pain in the back, frequently in the lower back.

If pain comes after lifting something heavy, after coughing, or after unusually heavy exercise, and the pain prevents you from moving or shoots down one leg, you may have a herniated disc.

CAUSES—Backache, or pain felt in the spinal column, is one of the most common reasons for hospitalization in the Western world. Your spinal column has a complicated interconnection of muscles, tendons, bones, and ligaments.

It is helpful to identify the various parts of the spine, also called the *vertebrae* (singular is *vertebra*): The top part of the spine, where the neck is located, is called the cervical spine (or *cervicals*); the shoulder and mid-part (which protrudes outward in an adult) is called the *thoracic*; the lower portion (called the hollow of the back) is the *lumbar*; and the bottom part (ending in the tailbone or *coccyx*) is the *sacrum*. The first cervical is the *atlas*. This enables your head to tilt up or down. The second is the *axis*; it permits your head to turn from side to side.

Aches and pains in the lower back can be a chronic problem. This pain can be in the spine or sacroiliac. The *sacroiliac joint* connects (*articulates* is the correct word) the spine to the pelvic bone. (There can also be pain in the *muscles* of the lower back; this is called *lumbago, 648*.)

A *subluxation* occurs when two vertebrae get out of proper alignment with one another. A chiropractor puts these back in place for relatively little cost.

Sciatica (566, 626, 645, 713) is chronic pain in the sciatic nerve, which is the largest nerve in the body. This nerve, which passes down through the upper leg, can experience *neuralgia (563)* or *neuritis (568)* as a result of a pinched nerve in the lumbar region. If the

SKEL MUS

problem is not solved, eventually the painful leg may no longer receive nerve signals from the brain or the central nervous system. When that happens, you can no longer lift it and walk.

The invertebral *discs* (also spelled *disks*) are made of cartilage and act as cushions between the vertebrae. Each disc has a tough, fibrous, outer layer surrounding a soft interior.

Lumbar disc *herniation* and lumbar disc *prolapse* occur when the disc herniates (ruptures or breaks) and some of this soft inner disc material pushes outward against the spinal cord to one degree or another. This may be very serious. As in sciatica, it can lead to muscle wasting, reduced nerve reflexes, and muscle weakness. Disc herniation and prolapse are often erroneously referred to as a *"slipped disc."*

Causes of lower-back pain include **wrenched or damaged muscles, bones, tendons, ligaments, kidney or bladder infection, prostate problems, female pelvic disorders**. **Overeating, overdrinking, eating the wrong kinds of food, and constipation** can also be involved. The spinal bones, and muscles attached to them, are weakened by wrong habits. Chronic conditions causing back pain include **arthritis, bone disease, or abnormal curvature of the spine** (*scoliosis, 649*).

Other causes of back pain are **poor posture, bad walking habits, improper shoes, lifting, straining, calcium deficiency, slouching when sitting, or soft mattresses**.

A common cause of lower back pain is emotional stress. **Feelings of fear, anger, or anxiety** increase muscle tension on the face, head, and spine. This crams joints together, overworks muscles, and increases pain. In addition, anger, anxiety, exhaustion, illness, or depression causes the brain to increase its sensitivity to pain.

There is a definite relationship between a smoker's cough and severe back pain. Injecting the **nicotine** equivalent of one cigarette decidedly reduced the measured blood flow in the vertebral body. It is also thought that using tobacco interferes with the elasticity of connective tissue.

Sometimes a serious case of **constipation** will cause an ache in the back, from **impacted stools or pressure from gas**.

(More rarely, back pain can result from **congenital abnormalities, metabolic disorders, cancer.**)

The back pain can also be the result of an **excess of lactic acid in the muscles**, following muscular exercise. Drinking enough water helps to lessen this problem.

The body twisting needed for **batting, golf, tennis, weight lifting, basketball, football, and bowling**—all put strains, often very severe, on the back.

Where can you go to get help with your bad back? There are lots of experts out there:

Chiropractors adjust the back by pushing and thrusting. They also recommend nutritional and lifestyle changes. In 1994, the U.S. Agency for Health Care Policy and Research issued a report that chiropractors generally provided the most effective treatments for acute back pain. They cost far less, do the job quicker, and do not give medicinal drugs (most drugs are usually poisonous). The *British Medical Journal* reported that chiropractic treatments proved more successful than hospital treatments in nearly every way.

X-rays are generally considered a routine part of back pain diagnosis; yet only a few back conditions show up on X-rays! If the pain is caused by muscle strain or a herniated disc, an X-ray will not reveal anything because muscles, discs, and ligaments are all soft tissues. Avoid unnecessary X-rays! Beware of X-rays if you are pregnant.

Orthopedic surgeons are another source of help. These are medical doctors who also do back surgery; they are very likely to recommend an operation—and that is something you want to avoid, if at all possible.

In addition to prescribing drugs, *osteopaths* can also do back surgery; but they are less likely to do so.

Physiatrists, also called doctors of physical medicine, are also medical doctors. They have a good record of helping to solve serious back problems (such as disc problems) without resorting to surgery (which they are not licensed to do). They recommend lifestyle changes, back braces, etc.

Physical therapists try to restore muscle strength and joint and spine mobility through a range of motion exercises, etc.

Bad backs cost the country a fortune: $16 billion a year in medical treatment, and $80 billion in lost wages and productivity. At some time in their lives, 80% of Americans experience back pain, usually lower back pain. About 45% will have repeated attacks.

Which back pains are the most serious?
Back pain that comes on suddenly, for no apparent reason.

Back pain that is accompanied by other symptoms (such as fever, stomach cramps, chest pain, or difficult breathing).

An acute attack of back pain that lasts more than 2-3 days, without any relief.

Chronic pain which lasts more than 2 weeks.

Pain in the back which radiates down the leg to the knee or foot.

Back pain plus higher temperature or weight loss could indicate **cancer or another trunk disease**. Pain in one side of the lower back could be **kidney infection** (or lack of water drinking). After an accident, a sudden loss of bowel or bladder control, pain or numbness in a leg, or pain after coughing indicates a **herniated disc**.

NATURAL REMEDIES
SIMPLE BACK PAIN
First, we will consider less serious back pain:
• The most common cause of backache is muscle strain. **Rest** will generally eliminate the problem. Bed rest for 24 hours may be needed.

• Soaking in **a tub of warm water** can be quite relaxing to a strained back. **Epsom salt baths** are relaxing and antispasmodic.

• For the first 72 hours after a back strain occurs, an 8-minute **ice massage** often helps. Use ice cubes (or frozen water in a paper cup or frozen fruit-juice can). Massage the area about 6-8 inches around it.

• After 72 hours, use **alternate hot and cold** applications. Apply a wrung-out hot towel for 30 seconds, followed by brief cold. Do this 4-5 times.

• **Ice packs** are especially helpful in relieving muscle spasms.

• **Moist heat** reduces local inflammation and increases blood flow to the area.

• **Avoid long bed rest**. Some people think that staying in bed for a week will help back pain. This is not true. If you remain in bed a week, it will take two weeks to rehabilitate.

• **Stretching** a sore back will tend to accelerate the healing process. Gently bring your knees up from the bed and to your chest. Once there, put a little pressure on your knees. Stretch, then relax. Do this again. Do not underestimate the value of this.

HERBS

• **Cayenne** contains *capsaicin*, which interferes with pain perception, while at the same time triggering production of endorphins. Mash a red pepper and place it on the painful area. Or sprinkle the powder in vegetable oil, mix it together and apply. If it irritates your skin too much, stop using it.

• **Peppermint** and **spearmint** contain menthol. Camphor is in **coriander, spike lavender,** and **hyssop**. All these herbs reduce pain, when applied to the back.

• Herbs containing essential oils relieve back pain. These include **thyme, rosemary, and sage**. They contain *thymol* and *carvacrol*, which help muscles relax. To use them, add a few drops to a teaspoon of vegetable oil and rub into the affected area.

• Herbs containing *borneol* and *bornyl-acetate* relieve back spasms. Such herbs include **sage, cardamom, and rosemary**. Mix with oil and rub them in.

• Here is one doctor's formula for reducing back pain: Mix 2 parts **uva ursi** and 1 part each of **dandelion root, marshmallow, ginger, and plantain**. Simmer 2 oz. of the mixture in 1 quart distilled water 10 minutes, covered tightly. Steep for 10 minutes; strain. Drink 1 cup, 3 times daily.

PREVENTING BACK INJURIES

Preventive measures that will help you, either before or after experiencing back problems:

• **Dietary principles: Reduce fat** in your diet. The greater the deposits of fatty plaque, the greater the degeneration of spinal discs. Your diet should be high in **minerals** and **vegetable proteins**. Vegetarians have stronger bone density. Uric acid increases back pain; so **stop eating meat**. Also stop **caffeine, tobacco, and alcohol**.

• Most people with back pain have a problem with short, tight, rigid back muscles. And it can be relieved by **improved posture while sitting, standing, working, regular aerobic exercise, stretching, and exercises that help strengthen the back muscles**.

• **Special helps**. Take frequent stand-up breaks throughout the day, if you are sitting too long. Carry smaller bundles; and divide the weight onto both arms. If you use a shoulder bag, frequently switch it to the other side. Make sure the computer screen is at eye level. Use a slanted bookstand to copy from.

• **Lifting instructions:** Be very careful when lifting something. Take several deep breaths, to increase muscle strength; and then squat and slowly lift with the legs, not the back, and hold the object close to your body. Do not lift from a bending forward position (opening windows, lifting things from deep in the car trunk). Only lift something in front of you, not off to the side.

• If you cannot manage a squat, put one knee on the floor, then use your arms to move the object onto your opposite thigh (which is horizontal). Then, with a firm grip on the object, simply stand up.

• **Be warm, not exhausted.** Keep the body warm and do not become overly fatigued. When the muscles are chilled or you are exhausted, it is easier to injure joints because the muscles are not able to do the work needed.

• **Not after hot baths**: Do not take a hot bath just before doing heavy exercise; for your muscles will be in a weaker condition.

• **Proper nutrition**, including adequate amounts of **calcium, minerals, vitamin D**, etc. *See Strengthening the Bones (608) for much more on this.*

• **Walking and rowing** are good for the back (walking is good for just about everything!).

BEDTIME

• When sleeping, either a **firm mattress** should be used or a ¾-inch thick ply board should be placed beneath the top mattress. If needed, place 1-2 **pillows** under the knees, to straighten the lumbar curve. *When lying on the side*, **flex the knees** and, if needed, place a **pillow** between them.

• **Do not sleep on the stomach**; it increases the swayback and twists the neck. This is due to the fact that the trunk, being heavier, sinks farther into the bed, causing the back to arch. (One expert says to sleep on your stomach if you have sciatica; but most do not recommend it because of the twist it puts in your neck.)

• It is reported that **water beds**, when they do not make a lot of waves, may help people with back trouble to sleep.

• *When you get out of bed*, roll out slowly and carefully. **Do not sit straight up** in bed.

• *If you have back pain*, slide to the edge of the bed. Then, keeping your back rigid, let your legs off the bed first. That will act as a springboard, lifting your upper body up and off the bed.

• **If your bed has a slight sag** in the middle, it can give you a low-back pain in the morning. Place a ¾-inch plyboard under your mattress, to level it out.

WHEN STANDING AND SITTING

• **Good posture** when sitting, standing, or walking should be the goal.

• **When sitting**: Sit in a straight chair with a firm back. The knees should be higher than the hips; if necessary, use a small footstool. Avoid soft sofas and stuffed chairs. Chair arms help support the shoulders and upper back. Get up and move about every so often.

• **When in a car**, push the car seat forward, to raise the knees higher than the hips. This lessens back and shoulder strain. Use safety belts. Look for a car with adjustable lumbar support; and adjust the support down as low as it goes. Then, if necessary, raise it a notch or two.

• **When standing**: Do not stand in one position for long periods. Do not lean against things. High-heeled shoes will bring trouble sooner or later. Women should wear low-heeled shoes if they want to protect their pelvic organs and spine.

EXERCISES

Exercises to build the muscles are very important if you would avoid back trouble. Here are several which will strengthen the back:

• **Do press-ups**. (These are half a push-up). Lie on the floor, on your stomach. Keep your pelvis flat on the floor and push up with your hands, arching your back as you lift your shoulders off the floor. This will help strengthen your lower back.

• **Do floor swimming**. Lie on your stomach on the floor. Raise your left arm and right leg. Hold for one second; then alternate with the right arm and left leg. Go back and forth. This extends and strengthens the lower back.

• **Do a crunch sit-up**. Lie on your back on the floor, with knees flexed and feet flat on the floor. Cross your arms with your hands on your shoulders. Raise your head and shoulders off the floor as high as you can while keeping your lower back on the floor. Hold for one second; then repeat.

• **Lean over exercise**. Sit in a chair and lean forward until pain is felt; breathe out and slowly lean farther, stretching muscles further.

• **Knee pulls**. Sit in a straight-backed chair. Lift your right knee, clasp it in both hands, and pull it as close to your chest as possible. Exhale deeply as you feel tension or mild pain in your back. Repeat with the left leg. Do several repetitions. / Do the same

exercise while lying on floor, but pulling both knees up at the same time.

• **Reverse ankle pull**. Stand behind a straight-backed chair. Bring your right ankle up behind you, grasp it with your right hand, and gently but firmly pull upward toward your back so your thigh muscles stretch. Exhale as you pull. Do the same with the other leg.

• **Know your limit when exercising**. If you feel fine 1-2 days after such exercises, then it is safe to continue them at the same intensity.

• **Give yourself a back rub**. With or without some oil on your hands, stroke gently along the tops of your shoulders and up and down your back. If you feel areas that are tight, rub around and press into those tight spots. This will relieve tension and stiffness in your lower back.

• *Spinal surgery:* Should you have a back operation? Sometimes the problem is so serious that a back operation is necessary. But, if at all possible, try to avoid having one. Not only are they expensive, but very frequently they do not solve your movement and pain problems. It is an intriguing fact that, according to U.S. government reports, only 1% of those with back pain obtain relief from back surgery. And there is always the possibility that the operation will only result in greater pain, more serious damage, and even less mobility. But, after weighing all the possibilities, you may still decide to undergo it. A full 80% of those who experience painful back trouble recover in four months without surgery. There are 20 times more back operations in America than in Canada or Europe.

—Also see Lumbago (below), Sciatica (566, 626, 645, 713), Neuritis (568), and Scoliosis (649).

ENCOURAGEMENT—Those who come frequently to the throne of grace and offer up sincere, earnest, prayers for God's help will not fail of fulfilling His plan for their lives. Revelation 21:6-8.

LUMBAGO
(LOWER BACK PAIN)

SYMPTOMS—Muscular stiffness, cramped tightness, shooting spasms.

CAUSES—Most low-back pain comes from **poor posture, wrong lifting and carrying, being hunched over a desk for long hours, standing on one's feet all day, carrying heavy briefcases, wearing high heels, being overly fatigued, and incorrect sleeping positions**. Another cause is **not keeping one's muscles strong**. A small percentage of lower-back pain may be linked to **flat feet**.

Lumbago is an inflammation of the lumbar muscles and is considered by many to be rheumatism of the lumbar muscles.

NATURAL REMEDIES

• Read *Backache (712).* It is filled with helpful suggestions, exercises, and much more for both upper and lower back problems.

• For acute lumbago, sciatica, or rheumatism, combine **juniper berries and gravel root**, and drink daily.

• Here is Dr. Christopher's formula for lumbago: Take 1 oz. each of **buchu, goldenrod, and uva ursi.** Combine ½ oz. each of **licorice root, Prince's pine**, and 1 tsp. **cayenne.** Simmer all the herbs but buchu and cayenne in 3 pints water. Then pour hot over the buchu and cayenne, steep covered till cool. Strain and drink 2 oz., 3 times daily. One hour before going to bed, drink 6-8 oz. of warmed tea.

• Lumbago is one of the most painful conditions. The use of **vapor baths** and the **cold sheet** treatment will bring relief. A massage with a tincture of **cayenne** and **prickly ash** liniment with **antispasmodic tincture** *(xxx)* will work very well. The eliminative functions should be corrected, especially the bowels which need to be cleaned during attacks. **Garlic** and **lobelia** enemas work well.

—*For much more specific help, see Backache (645).*

ENCOURAGEMENT—Pray with unshaken faith and trust. The Angel of the covenant, even our Lord Jesus Christ, is the Mediator who secures the acceptance of the prayers of His believing ones.

SCOLIOSIS
(Curvature of the Spine, Posterior Lateral Scoliosis)

SYMPTOMS—The spine is curved slightly to the left or right. There is back pain and abnormal gait. If severe, the rib cage may become deformed; sometimes this leads to heart and lung problems.

CAUSES—The spine naturally forms a straight, vertical line when viewed from the back. Scoliosis is an abnormal sideways curvature of the spine, most commonly affecting the spine in the chest area and the lower back region. Early diagnosis is important because, if left untreated, the deformity tends to become worse.

Scoliosis occurs 80% of the time in girls; this is primarily in preteen and teen years, during rapid growth spurts.

Diagnosis is made by having the person bend over, away from you. Look for lateral deviation (a leaning to the left or right).

The primary cause is that **one set of the spinal muscles (right side or left side) is stronger** than the other. This causes an "S" curve in the spine. Other causes include **one leg longer** than the other, **cerebral palsy,** or **polio**. Temporary scoliosis occurs as a result of muscle spasm following a spinal injury.

If not corrected, the result may be degeneration of muscles on one side. In some instances, muscles may be in the early stage of **muscular dystrophy**.

NATURAL REMEDIES

• In the early stages, scoliosis can be eliminated. But the person must be faithful in taking **mineral and vitamin supplements**. Failure to do so can result in serious damage, back braces, and surgery.

• **Avoid food allergies and eat a nourishing diet. Drop all junk foods, caffeine, alcohol, soft drinks, etc.**

• Each day take **vitamin E** (800-1,200 IU), **selenium** (500-1,000 mcg), **calcium** (2,000 mg), and **magnesium** (1,000 mg).

J.H. KELLOGG, M.D., PRESCRIPTIONS FOR SCOLIOSIS AND ITS COMPLICATIONS *(how to give these water therapies: pp. 206-275 / list of treatments: pp. 206-207 / Hydrotherapy Disease Index: pp. 273-275)*

TO IMPROVE GENERAL NUTRITION AND BLOOD MOVEMENT—Graduated **Tonic Friction baths**. Massage, carefully administered. **Nutritious dietary**. **Sweating baths**, especially the Radiant Heat Bath. Follow by **Cold Mitten Friction**, carefully given. Copious **water** drinking.

TO COMBAT LOCAL MORBID PROCESSES—**Fomentation** to the back twice daily, followed by **Heating Compress** to spine. The Heating Compress may be applied at night and retained until morning. **Hot Leg Bath** with **Fomentation** to the spine. Prolonged **Neutral Bath**, 1-4 hours daily.

TO RELIEVE COLONIC SPASM AND NERVOUS IRRITABILITY—**Warm Bath** at 96°-100° F. Prolonged **Neutral Pail Pour** to the spine at 93°-98° F., with **Heating Compress** at night. **Rest** in bed, when symptoms are progressing.

FOR MUSCULAR WEAKNESS OR PARALYSIS—**Massage**, **exercise** of muscles, special **gymnastics**.

CONTRAINDICATIONS—Avoid the Cold Douche and other general Cold Baths, prolonged Hot Baths, exercise to the extent of fatigue.

—*See Strengthening the Bones (608) and Backache (645) for much more information.*

ENCOURAGEMENT—No sin is small in God's sight; but, in His strength, we can resist all temptation to leave His side and run after the trinkets Satan offers us. Cling to Jesus; and, in spite of the disappointments of earth, you will have peace of heart.

"He will fulfil the desire of them that fear Him. He also will hear their cry, and will save them. Psalm 145:19. Sweet, sweet are the precious promises of Scripture! Read them often.

S
K
E
L
M
U
S

SKELETAL-MUSCULAR -
7 - ABDOMINAL CAVITY
Also: Pelvic Congestion (689) and Pelvic Pain (689)

PERITONITIS

SYMPTOMS—Inflammation of the peritoneum, the smooth, transparent membrane lining the interior of the abdominal cavity and surrounding the digestive organs and other internal organs (viscera)—such as the heart, liver, intestines, etc. Symptoms usually develop rapidly. Severe, constant pain in the abdomen, fever, abdominal swelling, nausea and vomiting. Rigidity of the abdominal muscles, rapid pulse, sunken eyes, and a pinched expression of the face. In severe cases, dehydration and shock may also occur.

CAUSES—Peritonitis is serious and frequently fatal. Take the person to the hospital.

The usual cause is bacterial infection that has spread from elsewhere in the abdomen, caused by blows, most often from stab wounds, gunshot wounds, complication of a surgical operation, appendicitis, childbirth, or ovarian disease. The bowel is often pierced and the contents have leaked out. Sometimes the cause is leakage of bile from an inflamed gallbladder into the abdominal cavity or leakage of digestive enzymes into the abdominal cavity, resulting from acute pancreatitis.

Less common is chronic peritonitis, also called tuberculosis peritonitis. This is tubercular in origin, and shows little pain or fever and few symptoms other than great emaciation, loss of strength, and fluid in the abdominal cavity.

If you have this problem, you will want to be admitted to the hospital immediately. If treated immediately, recovery is usually rapid; and long-term problems, such as adhesions, are less likely to occur.

Adhesions can develop, in which fibrous bands of scar tissue grow between loops of intestine, causing the loops to stick together. This can cause pain months after the attack of peritonitis.

NATURAL REMEDIES

After surgery, to clean out the area and sew up the organs, consider the following:

• **Tense the abdominal muscle** on a regular basis. This strengthens it and helps it rebuild.

• Use warm, whole **baths** or warm, wet **packs** over the abdomen. A **castor oil pack** is also good.

• If there is pain, take a **slippery elm** retention enema every morning.

• Go on a 3-day **carrot juice fast** or a diet of **oatmeal gruels, lentil and barley soup**, and other **potassium fruits and vegetables**.

• During the inflammatory stage, **avoid eating**. Instead, drink as much **slippery elm tea** as possible, sipping it continually.

• Helpful herb teas include **bryonia, pleurisy root, and aconite**.

• Once past the critical stage, drink **comfrey root** tea every 3-4 hours, along with **taking echinacea** tablets.

• Use **lobelia** in either tea or tincture form. Also use **garlic** (enema, tea, or tincture) and a diet of liquids and juices. **Castor oil fomentation** over the abdominal area will give relief.

• Useful herbs include **apple cider vinegar and honey, garlic, onion, blood purifiers** of a powerful nature (**chaparral, Brigham tea, burdock root and seed** in equal parts, **sassafras**), and **lobelia**.

• If it is tuberculosis peritonitis, the patient should be treated as if for tuberculosis (505).

J.H. KELLOGG, M.D., PRESCRIPTIONS FOR PERITONITIS AND ITS COMPLICATIONS (*how to give these water therapies: pp. 206-275 / list of treatments: pp. 206-207 / Hydrotherapy Disease Index: pp. 273-275*)

PERITONITIS (ACUTE) —
DIETETIC FACTORS—Rest in bed, **fluid diet, fruit juice** without sugar, **gruels** of dextrinized or malted cereals. Withhold food for 24-48 hours.

ALBUMIN IN URINE—Hot **Blanket Pack** and other sweating measures, to maintain cutaneous activity, repeated every 2-4 hours.

FEVER—Hot **Blanket Pack**, followed by **Cold Mitten Friction**, prolonged **Neutral Bath, Fomentation** to abdomen with Cooling **Wet Sheet Pack** at the same time.

GENERAL ASPECTS—Enema at 80° F. Repeat in order to remove gas. **Fomentation** every 2 hours for 15-20 minutes. During interval between, apply **Heating Compress** at 60° F., changing every 5 minutes while the body temperature is elevated, less frequently as temperature falls. Copious **water** drinking. Prolonged **Neutral Bath**. Cold **Compress** or **Ice Bag** over heart for 15 minutes, 2-3 times a day, for cardiac weakness.

PREVENT OBSTRUCTION—Large **enema**, 3 times a day from beginning, temperature 75° F.

CONTRAINDICATIONS—Same as chronic form, just below.

PERITONITIS (CHRONIC) —
GENERAL ASPECTS—Aseptic dietary, **liquid diet**. Hot **Enema**. Follow by **Fomentation** to abdomen for 20 minutes, 3 times daily. Well-protected **Heating Compress** during the interval between. Copious **water** drinking. **Graduated cold applications** (Tonic Frictions), twice daily. If temperature is elevated, **Neutral Bath** half an hour to an hour daily.

CONTRAINDICATIONS—Avoid Cold Full Baths, Prolonged Cold Douche, Cold Pail Pour, Cold Wet Sheet Rub, and Cold Sitz.

PERITONITIS (PELVIC), CELLULITIS —
BASIC CONSIDERATIONS—Surgical and puerperal asepsis, care to avoid exposures at menstrual periods, protection of feet and legs in damp and cold weather, proper clothing.

INCREASE RESISTANCE—Cold Mitten Friction or

Cold Towel Rub 2-4 times a day. Protect pelvic viscera by simultaneous **Hot Foot Pack,** Hot Foot and Leg Pack, or by hot-water bottle to sacrum and Cold Compress over stomach area.

COMBAT LOCAL INFLAMMATION—Hot Hip and Leg Pack 20 minutes every 2 hours. During intervals between, **Cold Compress** at 60° F. to area over stomach, pudendum and inner surfaces of thighs. Do this with heat to feet and legs or **ice bag** over seat of pain. Hot-water bottles or **Fomentations** to feet, hips and thighs. Hot and cold **pelvic compress** with **ice bag** over seat of pain; continue 20-40 minutes and repeat when needed. Hot **vaginal irrigation** at 110°-120° F., one gallon, every 4 hours.

ENCOURAGE RESOLUTION—After the acute stage has passed, apply **Alternate Compress** for 30 minutes, 3 times a day. During interval, **Heating Compresses**, changing every 2 hours or as soon as well-warmed. **Graduated Baths** for tonic purposes. Alternate **vaginal irrigation** (110°, 80° to 70° F.); later, pelvic massage.

PAIN—Fomentation or **Revulsive Compress** every 2-4 hours or oftener, if necessary.

CONSTIPATION—Large **Hot Enemas**, twice a day, during acute pain and inflammation. Later, give graduated **Cold Enema**.

CHILL—Anticipate chill by wrapping her / him in **warm blankets** with **hot bags** to trunk and limbs. Hot **water** drinking.

SEPTIC FEVER—Add to local measures, if fever is high, **Hot Blanket Pack** for 10-15 minutes. Follow by sweating **Wet Sheet Pack**, **Prolonged Neutral Bath**. If suppuration (pussing) occurs, surgical interference is generally indicated.

CAUTIONS—Avoid Cold Baths; instead use partial cold applications, such as the Cold Mitten Friction and the Cold Towel Rub.

—*Also see Appendicitis (455-456) and Tuberculosis (505).*

ENCOURAGEMENT—*Jesus cares for each one, as though there were not another in the whole world. You can trust your case with Him. He will not fail you. Your only danger is in leaving His side, to follow after the luring temptations Satan offers you.*

More Encouragement

"We are often led to seek Jesus by the desire for some earthly good; and upon the granting of our request we rest our confidence in His love.

"The Saviour longs to give us a greater blessing than we ask; and He delays the answer to our request that He may show us the evil of our own hearts, and our deep need of His grace. He desires us to renounce the selfishness that leads us to seek Him. Confessing our helplessness and bitter need, we are to trust ourselves wholly to His love.

"The nobleman wanted to see the fulfillment of his prayer before he should believe; but he had to accept the word of Jesus that his request was heard and the blessing granted. This lesson we also have to learn. Not because we see or feel that God hears us are we to believe. We are to trust in His promises. When we come to Him in faith, every petition enters the heart of God. When we have asked for His blessing, we should believe that we receive it, and thank Him that we have received it. Then we are to go about our duties, assured that the blessing will be realized when we need it most. When we have learned to do this, we shall know that our prayers are answered. God will do for us 'exceeding abundantly,' 'according to the riches of His glory,' and 'the working of His mighty power.' Ephesians 3:20, 16; 1:19."

—**Desire of Ages, 200**

Two editions of Desire of Ages, the classic (and best) book on the life of Christ are available from us.

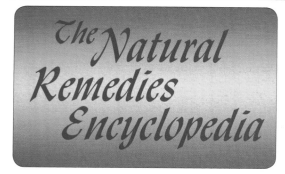

The Natural Remedies Encyclopedia

- Disease Section 11 - Endocrine

Endocrine System: Physiology 1020 / Pictures 1038

ENDO

"O bless our God, ye people, and make the voice of His praise to be heard: Which holdeth our soul in life, and suffereth not our feet to be moved."   —*Psalm 66:8-9.*

"I will strengthen them . . saith the Lord."   —*Zechariah 10:12*

"The Lord raiseth them that are bowed down."   —*Psalm 146:8*

"I will be glad and rejoice in Thy mercy: for Thou hast considered my trouble; Thou hast known my soul in adversities."   —*Psalm 31:7.*

"I will not leave you comfortless: I will come to you."   —*John 14:18.*

"He that putteth his trust in Me shall possess the land, and shall inherit My holy mountain."   —*Isaiah 57:13.*

FOR MORE NATURAL REMEDIES:
HERBS: Herb Contents (pp. 129-130) will help you locate the 126 most important herbs and the diseases each one can treat. How to prepare herbs (132). How to use them (141-189)
HYDROTHERAPY: Therapy Contents (pp. 206-207) and its Disease Index (263-265) will lead you to over 100 water therapies and many more remedies. DIS. INDEX: 1211- / GEN. INDEX: 1221-

VITAMINS AND MINERALS: Contents (100-101). Using 101-124. Dosages (124). Others (117-)
CARING FOR THE SICK: Home care for a sick person (28-36). The healing crisis (36-39)
WOMEN'S SECTIONS: Female Organs (672) Pregnancy (701). Childbirth (765). Infancy, Childhood (722). Women's Herbs (754, 760)
EMERGENCIES: (973-). **FIRST AID:** (990-)

Section 11 - Endocrine

ENDOCRINE - 1 - ADRENALS

STRENGTHENING THE GLANDS

This is the glandular balance formula which Dr. Christopher prescribes to strengthen glands:

Mix thoroughly 1 part each of fine powders of **black cohosh, licorice root, bladder wrack** (or another **seaweed**), **goldenseal, lobelia,** ½ part **ginger**; and ¼ part **cayenne**. Place in #0 capsules (each one equivalent to ¼ tsp.). Take 1-2 capsules (or ¼-½ tsp.) before noon each day.

HYPOGLYCEMIA
(Low Blood Sugar)

SYMPTOMS—Confusion, depression, nervousness, anxiety, antisocial behavior, emotional instability, exhaustion, headaches, impatience, inability to cope, fears, craving for sugar, faintness, dizziness.

Symptoms especially occur a few hours after eating sweets or fats. The more that is eaten and the longer the span before the symptoms occur, the worse they are.

CAUSES—The problem is **adrenal exhaustion**. The cause is too much **stress, worry**, and an excess of **undigested sugars, starches, proteins, and dairy products**. The hormone, *cortin*, is depleted; so food cannot be digested properly.

People consume **large quantities of sugars, caffeine, soft drinks, and alcohol**. These all contain simple sugars and **insufficient amounts of complex carbohydrates**. Add to this the **high stress levels**; and the two adrenal glands become exhausted.

Hypoglycemia can be **inherited**; but, more often, it is brought on by an **inadequate diet** (and is then called *functional hypoglycemia*). However, there are several other physical problems which can weaken adrenal function and help bring on hypoglycemia. These include weaknesses in the **thyroid, liver, kidneys, pituitary, and pancreas. Immune deficiency** and **candidiasis** can also lead to it. Other causes include **smoking** and large amounts of **caffeine**.

Hypoglycemia is sometimes mistakenly diagnosed

CHART 1061: Glycemic load and index 1053

CHART 1057: Diabetic (656) and Hypoglycemic (653) Coma

as asthma, allergies, fatigue syndrome, or weight problems. It is also said to be stomach or intestinal problems, perhaps a mental or nervous disorder.

Half the people over 50 who have hypoglycemia, are **hypothyroid**. A six-hour glucose tolerance test (GTT) is the most reliable method of diagnosis; having blood drawn while experiencing symptoms is an alternative. But, even with these tests, hypoglycemia is difficult to diagnose with certainty. Many cases are "subclinical"; in other words, the borderline levels of blood sugar may produce serious symptoms.

Living fast, worrying a lot, and eating wrong results in any one of the following: overproduction of insulin, damage to liver cells, insufficient secretion of adrenocortical hormones, and pituitary gland abnormalities. The result is low blood sugar.

The following conditions are linked to low blood sugar: migraine headaches, leg cramps, depression, premenstrual syndrome, aggressive and criminal behavior, angina.

NATURAL REMEDIES

AVOID
• **Refined starches, sugars, and a high-meat diet** wear out the adrenals. Too much **sugar** shocks the adrenal cortex; and the resulting physical reaction is to crave still more sugar.

• Stop eating or using **meat, nicotine, alcohol, chocolate, soft drinks, black tea, and sugared and fat foods. Caffeine, alcohol, and tobacco** produce wide swings in blood sugar levels.

• Read the labels at the grocery store. Avoid **dextrose, dextrin, lactose, maltose, sucrose, fructose, modified food starch, corn syrup, corn sweetener, cornstarch, and natural sweetener**. Also stay away from **sorbitol, hexanoyl, mannitol, aspartame, and glycol**.

• **Avoid stressful situations**. You may have a **milk allergy**, which often accompanies this disease.

PROPER DIET
• Eat **natural foods**, the ones you should have been eating to begin with. **Whole grains, raw and simply cooked vegetables, some fresh fruit**. But eat in moderation **starchy foods such as corn, noodles, pasta, brown rice, hominy, and yams**.

• Eat a **high-fiber diet** and **vegetables that are raw or steamed**. These foods are also good for you: **beans, lentils, brown rice, white potatoes, soy products, and fruits**.

E
N
D
O

• Useful fruits include **apricots, apples, bananas, grapefruit, lemons, cantaloupes, and persimmons**. For example, eat a raw apple instead of applesauce; for the **apple** has more fiber which will help keep blood sugar stabilized.

• Only use **honey** and **molasses;** and use them in small amounts. Too much **salt** exhausts the adrenals and causes a loss of potassium, leading to lower blood sugar.

• *During a blood sugar reaction*, eat something that has both fiber and protein, such as **rice or bran crackers with almond butter**. Fiber alone (**popcorn, rice, oat bran, crackers, ground flaxseed, and psyllium husks**) has the ability to slow down a hypoglycemic reaction. A half hour before each meal, eat some of this high fiber, to stabilize blood sugar. Protein, fiber-rich carbohydrates, and enough fat to slow digestion are the cornerstones of a hypoglycemia-control diet.

• Once a month, go on a **fresh vegetable juice fast** for a day. Take enemas with some added lemon juice at that time. If a reaction starts to occur, reach for the fiber, protein powder, or spirulina.

• Take **vitamin C** (1,000 mg), **bioflavonoids** (1,000 mg), **magnesium** (200 mg), **vitamin E** (400 IU), **chromium** (200-400 mcg), **zinc** (30 mg).

• Some forms of low blood sugar involve very low serum **potassium** levels. Make sure you are obtaining enough potassium.

• Do not skip meals or go on a water fast. The binge-purge eating scheme used, by those with bulimia to control weight, only adds to the problem.

HERBS

• **Licorice** acts like *cortin* and helps the blood sugar. It is the best single herb you can take. It increases the effectiveness of glucocorticoids (adrenal hormones) circulating in the liver and mimics the action of those hormones. Eating it helps prevent the destruction of the pancreas.

• Other helpful herbs: **bilberry** and **wild yam** help control insulin levels. **Cedar berries** help the pancreas. **Spirulina** tablets, taken between meals, help stabilize blood sugar. Standardized **milk thistle** extract (25-500 mg daily) contains *silymarin*, which helps your condition. **Ginger** root works indirectly to help increase the availability of dietary nutrients for digestion and metabolism.

ENCOURAGEMENT—Jesus cares for each individual as though there were not another person on the earth. He will help you also, as you earnestly seek Him with all your heart. Psalm 10:14, 18.

ADDISON'S DISEASE
(Adrenal Underactivity)

SYMPTOMS—Dizziness, fainting, nausea, loss of appetite, moodiness, decrease in body hair, inability to cope with stress. A slight darkening and discoloration of the skin, which is more noticeable when body parts are exposed to the sun. This would include forehead, knees, elbows, scars, skin folds and creases (on the palms, etc.). The mouth and freckles may appear darker. The hair becomes darker.

Bands of pigment run the length of the nails.

Reduced adrenal function (resulting either from Addison's or Cushing's Disease) can result in weakness, headaches, memory problems, dizziness, allergies, food cravings, and blood sugar disorders.

CAUSES—Both the adrenal underactivity of Addison's Disease and the overactivity of Cushing's Disease are caused by problems in the function of the adrenal glands.

Continued use of **cortisone drugs** for arthritis and asthma, etc., damage the adrenals. Those drugs cause them to shrink in size and not work properly. Yet, surprisingly enough, the shrunken glands can still overproduce and cause Cushing's Disease or underproduce and cause Addison's.

There is a way you can pinpoint whether or not your adrenals are functioning normally:

The systolic is the first number in a blood pressure reading; and the diastolic is the second number. For example, 120/80. The systolic should be 10 points higher when you are standing than when you are lying down.

Lie down and rest for 5 minutes; and then have someone take your blood pressure. Then stand up and have it immediately taken again. The blood pressure will probably be somewhat higher.

But if it is lower when standing than when lying flat, the adrenals are not working properly. The lower it is, the worse the condition of the adrenals.

You will want to contact a medical professional. Addison's is a chronic condition which needs to be continually worked with. You may moderate the problem; but it is never fully eliminated.

NATURAL REMEDIES

• Maintain a good **nourishing diet**. Include Nova Scotia **dulse** or Norwegian **kelp** for trace minerals. Greens (fresh, raw, and cooked) and **garlic** should be part of your regime. **Garlic** contains *germanium*, which stimulates the immune system. Include in your diet **brown rice, legumes, nuts, flaxseed oil, whole grains,** and **wheat germ.**

• Take a high-**B complex** daily, especially **pantothenic acid** (1,000 mg) and **brewer's yeast** (2 Tbsp.).

• Take licorice extract twice daily.

AVOID

• **Avoid tobacco, alcohol, caffeine, and soft drinks**. Do not use **sugar foods, fried foods, processed or junk foods**. Do not eat **meat**.

• Avoid **stress**! This is very important; for stress is hard on weak adrenals. Take time for prayer and the study of God's Word, the Bible. He can help you solve the problems you experience. Stress releases ACTH through the pituitary; this can raise blood pressure, store sodium, and excrete potassium. Water retention in the tissues is another result.

—*Compare the opposite of Addison's Disease, which is "Cushing's Disease" (655).*

ENCOURAGEMENT—All your habits are to be brought under the control of a mind that is itself under the control of God. We can fulfill God's will for our lives as we trust in the strength God imparts. Hebrews 11:16.

CUSHING'S DISEASE
(Adrenal overactivity)

SYMPTOMS—Rounded "moon" faces, heavy abdomen and buttocks, thin limbs. The muscles seem weak and wasting away. The eyelids may appear swollen and round; red spots may appear on the face. It is characterized by obesity in the stomach, face, and buttocks; but there is severe thinness in the limbs. There is poor wound healing and thinning of the skin, leading to stretch marks and bruising. Peptic ulcers, high blood pressure, mental instability, and diabetes may also occur. Women have Cushing's disease five times as often as men. There is scalp balding; yet there is excess body and facial hair, and brittle bones. Body hair grows faster; and women may grow mustaches and beards. Healing is more difficult and illnesses are more frequent.

Reduced adrenal function (resulting either from Addison's or Cushing's Disease) can result in weakness, headaches, memory problems, dizziness, allergies, food cravings, and blood sugar disorders.

An **overactive adrenal cortex** is the cause. This condition especially results from an overdose of corticosteroid drugs (especially those used to treat rheumatoid arthritis). It is also a metabolic disease that causes the formation of kidney stones.

CAUSES—There are two adrenal glands in your body. One is on top of each kidney. Each one is remarkably small, weighing only about one-fifth of an ounce.

The outer thick "rind" of each adrenal is the cortex. It produces cortisone. The inner portion is called the medulla; it secretes adrenaline (epinephrine) when stress occurs. *See Addison's Disease (654) for more information.*

NATURAL REMEDIES
• The objective is to **live better;** so the adrenals, whether working too fast or too slow, can normalize.
• Maintain a **vegetarian diet that is low in fat, sodium, and sugar.** Eat high **potassium** foods daily. Eat lots of **fresh greens, other vegetables, and fruits.** Make **green drinks** (whizzed green leaves and pineapple juice). Eat **whole grains, nuts, and legumes.**
• *Follow the directions given under Addison's Disease (654).*

ENCOURAGEMENT—We have not a high priest who is so high, so lifted up, that He cannot notice us or sympathize with us; but Jesus was in all points tempted like as we are, yet without sin. He can help you fulfill God's will for your life. As a child of God, fill your mind with the truths of the Bible. The more you do this, the more strength and clearness of mind you will have to fathom the deep things of God. You will become more earnest and vigorous, as the principles of truth are carried out in your daily life. Psalm 37:19.

ENDOCRINE - 2 - PANCREAS

CYSTIC FIBROSIS

SYMPTOMS—The symptoms are first seen in very small children. Large amounts of thick mucus develops in the lungs, blocking lung passages. This causes difficult breathing, chronic coughing and wheezing, and lung infections.

There are digestive problems, inadequate absorption of fats, after-meal stomach pain, and thinness. Body sweat will have very large amounts of sodium, potassium, and chloride salts. Any, or all, of these symptoms may occur.

CAUSES—In 1938, this physical problem was named "cystic fibrosis" because it was mistakenly thought that abnormal changes in the pancreas were true cysts (tiny pockets of fluid lined with normal tissue). But it was later discovered that those spots were just part of the **shrinking process of the pancreas**, as the disease worsened.

There are three views of the cause of cystic fibrosis (CF):

1 - CF is an inherited disease which the sufferer must learn to live with.

2 - CF is caused by inadequate absorption of selenium, zinc, essential fatty acids, and other minerals (including trace minerals) as a result of subclinical celiac disease. (Celiac disease is the inability to digest wheat and some other foods.)

3 - Dr. Joel Wallach was a veterinarian who, in 1978, was the first to diagnose CF in a laboratory animal, by noting characteristic CF changes in the pancreas and liver of baby monkeys. He says he was fired when it was discovered that he could reproduce those CF changes in the human body by giving or withholding the element, selenium. He had shown that CF was a nutritional problem which could be solved if caught early enough. (*See Let's Play Doctor, J.D. Wallach, D.V.M., N.D., pp. 109-110.*) Here is what he says:

"The prevention of CF has been accomplished in

ENDO

pet, farm, and laboratory animals by the veterinary profession, by assuring **adequate levels of selenium and essential fatty acid nutrition to the pregnant and nursing mother**. This is not as easy as it sounds because of malabsorption problems (*i.e.*, celiac disease and Crohn's disease) in a percentage of women. All things being normal, **a supplementation of 200 mcg selenium per day and 5 gm of flaxseed oil, three times a day [to the pregnant and nursing mother]**, would be adequate to prevent CF.

"Treatment of CF is very basic: **treat the infant as early as possible with selenium IM [given intramuscularly] at 10-25 mcg per day**."—*Op cit., p. 109.*

He adds that it is vital that it be determined **if the infant is allergic to wheat, cow's milk, or soy milk; so as to avoid what he is allergic to**.

We might conclude that all three theories are correct; in that, if you give the mother and infant proper supplementation, the disease can be eliminated at the beginning of the child's life.

But if this is not done, he will thereafter not be able to absorb nutrients properly, will exhibit the symptoms of CF, and will have to cope with the problem the rest of his life.

However, Wallach says that, even later, the person can lead a more normal life if he regularly receives **essential fatty acids, intravenously, and selenium intramuscularly**.

"The lungs of CF patients are normal at birth and only develop bronchiectasis after **chronic essential fatty acid and copper deficiencies** have taken their toll."—*Ibid.*

"CF . . is preventable, 100% curable in the early stages, and can be far better managed in chronic cases than it is currently managed by 'orthodox' medicine."—*Op. cit., p. 108.*

NATURAL REMEDIES

In addition to the above instructions, the CF patient should consider the following:

• Eat a **nourishing diet, high in raw fruits and vegetables** and with adequate amounts of **carbohydrates, protein, and vitamin / mineral supplements**. A problem is that those with CF do not absorb food properly. They need to eat more than other people, in order to absorb the needed nutrients. Eat **whole grains, nuts, and legumes**.

• Include **germanium** (found in garlic and onions), **selenium**, and **vitamin E**.

• Drink plenty of **liquids** and an adequate amount of **salt** in hot weather (but not too much).

• **Do not eat processed or junk food** of any type. Avoid **tobacco, alcohol**, etc.

• Helpful herbs include **echinacea, licorice root, ginger, yarrow, and peppermint. Cayenne** helps reduce inflammation. **Cayenne, garlic, and mullein** help clear congestion. **Garlic and tea tree oil** fight infection.

—*Also see Birth Defects (724-727) for more information on cystic fibrosis.*

CHART 1057: Diabetic (656) and Hypoglycemic (653) Coma CHART - 1055: Diabetes and Insulin (656)

DIABETES
(Diabetes Mellitus, Diabetes Insipidus)

SYMPTOMS—*Diabetes insipidus:* Extreme thirst and enormous quantities of urine, regardless of how much water is consumed.

Diabetes mellitus - Type I: (insulin-dependent, also known as juvenile diabetes): Excessive hunger, thirst, frequent urination, depression, weakness, blurred vision, dry mouth, and vomiting.

Diabetes mellitus - Type II: (maturity-onset diabetes): Unusual thirst, frequent urination, general weakness, obesity, skin disorders, boils, blurred vision, and dry mouth.

CAUSES—Diabetes is a major problem; entire books have been written on the subject. We can only touch on the subject here.

Of the two types of diabetes, *diabetes insipidus* is the more rare and is caused by an inadequately functioning pituitary hormone (*vasopressin*) or kidneys which somehow cannot respond properly to it.

Diabetes mellitus is the third largest killer in the U.S.; it is caused by a defect in the production of insulin by the pancreas. Without insulin, the body cannot utilize glucose, which is an important blood sugar. A blood glucose level above 180 mg percent causes excess sugar to spill over into the urine and make it sweet. (*Mellitus* means "sweet.") *Diabetes* comes from a Greek word for "flow through," since diabetics produce so much urine.

To summarize: In *diabetes mellitus (Type I, also known as insulin dependent diabetes)*, the pancreas cannot make the insulin needed to process glucose. This is *childhood-onset diabetes*.

In the rarer diabetes, *diabetes insipidus*, the cause is either a problem with the production of antidiuretic hormone (central diabetes insipidus) or kidney's response to antidiuretic hormone (nephrogenic diabetes insipidus).

Some people can develop diabetes mellitus as a result of **stress, obesity, or pregnancy**. Certain medicinal **drugs** can also cause it: **oral contraceptives, adrenal corticosteroids, phenytoin, or thiazide diuretics**. A diet high in **sugar** and **white flour** can lead to diabetes. **Hypothyroidism** or **Parasites** (especially in children) can also do it.

It is of interest that people who eat too much **sugar** eventually cannot taste it as well; so they pour on more sugar! But Type II diabetic sufferers also lack this sugar-tasting discernment. Leave off the sugar and learn to enjoy the natural flavors in your food.

Because the diabetic **cannot utilize glucose** for energy, he loses weight and is weakened by excess consumption of his protein and fat stores. Because of this, he may be very hungry and eat large amounts of food.

Diabetes can lead to poor wound healing, higher risk of infections, and many problems involving the eyes, kidneys, nerves, and heart.

STANDARDS AND GOALS—

Before breakfast (fasting)
With no diabetes: Less than 110 mg/dL
Goal for those with diabetes: 90-130 mg/dL
Before lunch, and dinner
With no diabetes: Less than 110 mg/dL
Goal for those with diabetes: 90-130 mg/dL
Two hours after meals
With no diabetes: Less than 140 mg/dL
Goal for those with diabetes: Less than 160 mg/dL
At bedtime
With no diabetes: Less than 120 mg/dL
Goal for those with diabetes: 110-150 mg/dL
Anytime (A1c hemoglobin)
With no diabetes: Less than 6 percent
Goal for those with diabetes: 7 percent

NATURAL REMEDIES

• Eat **smaller meals** (if necessary, eat them more frequently), and **chew the food** thoroughly. Do not eat late in the evening. **Overeating** can induce diabetes or, once contracted, increase it.

• **Vegetable broths** and **fresh fruit** are nourishing. A **high-carbohydrate, high-fiber diet** will reduce the need for insulin; it will also lower the amount of fat in the blood. (A low-fiber diet can bring on diabetes.) Get your protein from vegetable sources. A **fat-free diet** will help reduce blood sugar.

• **Onions and green beans** appear to lower blood sugar. A diet high in **raw food** is also helpful. One individual dropped his insulin dosage from 60 to 15 units per day, by increasing his raw food intake. Eat **raw garlic** every day. It will reduce your blood sugar.

• **Vitamin C** (1-3 grams daily) improves glucose tolerance and lowers *sorbitol* in diabetics. Sorbitol is a sugar which can accumulate and damage the eyes, nerves, and kidneys of diabetics. **Vitamin E** (900 IU) improves glucose tolerance, prevents damage to diabetic blood vessels, and protects against diabetic cataracts. **Vitamin B$_6$** (1,800 mg) improves glucose tolerance in women with diabetes caused by pregnancy or birth control pills. **Vitamin B$_{12}$** (500 mcg, 3 times daily) reduces nerve damage caused by diabetes. Those given 16 mg of **biotin** daily for 1 week had their fasting glucose levels drop 50%. It also reduces pain from diabetic nerve damage. **Chromium** (200-1,000 mcg) improves glucose tolerance. **Magnesium** (1,000 mg) leads to improved insulin production in elderly people and reduces eye damage. **Zinc** (15-25 mg) lowers blood sugar levels. **Coenzyme Q10** (120 mg) is needed for normal carbohydrate metabolism.

CHART - 1055: Diabetes and Insulin (656)

CHART 1061: Glycemic load and index 1053

Inositol (500 mg, 2 times daily) sometimes reverses nerve damage in some diabetics.

Note that one study found that diabetics should not take large amounts of **niacin** (vitamin B$_3$), **thiamine** (B$_1$), **PABA** (para-aminobenzoic acid, another B vitamin), or **vitamin C**. But they should take them regularly. Several studies found that high levels of **niacin** (B$_3$) impair glucose tolerance and should not be taken by diabetics.

• Diabetes is a forerunner for Bright's disease. Heavy users of insulin have been able to cut their intake rapidly by a number of herbal remedies such as **verde cactus and ginger; also chaparral**. Clean the colon area with a high enema of **burdock** root, **yellow dock** root, or **bayberry** bark. Assist nature in its elimination of sugars and body poisons through the skin by taking long **hot baths** and soaking in the bathtub. Accompany the baths by taking internally diaphoretic teas. Finish off with a **cold shower** or by sponging with **cold water**. Use the lower bowel tonic herbs to regulate elimination. He should avoid all **processed denatured foods and "secondary" foods—such as animal by-products—meat, milk, eggs, fish**, etc. Herbs, such as **Irish moss and slippery elm,** are nutritive mucilages that soothe while they feed the irritated digestive areas. In general, the diet for diabetes should consist of the **fresh fruits and tender greens and vegetables** from the garden, preferably raw or cooked at low heat. **Deep breathing** and plenty of vigorous **outdoor exercise** are also vital.

AVOID

• **Stop eating sugar, white-flour products, greasy food, meat, eggs, cheese, excess vegetable oil, as well as rancid nuts and seeds**. Totally avoid **tobacco** and those who use it. Because it restricts circulation, it will aggravate your condition. Do not drink **cow's milk**.

• Do not eat **fruits** and **melons** in large amounts. Do not eat **apples** or **bananas**. Do not eat **milk and sugar combinations**. **Coffee** can induce very high blood sugar levels. Avoid **gluten foods** (wheat, rye, oats, barley). Eat **buckwheat, rice, corn**, which have no gluten.

• Eat your meals at **regular times. Chew the food** and do not be in a rush to swallow the food. The quicker you eat, the higher goes the blood sugar.

OTHER INFORMATION

• Since obesity clearly contributes to the majority of chronic health problems experienced by people with diabetes, experts agree on the importance of maintaining a **healthy weight** and **monitoring your total percentage of body fat**. They recommend between 22 percent and 24 percent in women and 15 percent to 17 percent in men. The best method for doing so is a program of negular exercise.

• Get enough **exercise**; it will improve circulation,

E
N
D
O

which is always poor in diabetics. This will also lower blood sugar levels.

• **Fenugreek** contains six compounds which help regulate blood sugar levels. **Onions** have been used for centuries to treat diabetes in Europe and Asia. In India, the herb, **gurmar,** is used to treat diabetes.

• **Uva Ursi** contains a group of compounds, called *phenolic glycosides,* that help the kidneys excrete excess sugar. **Dandelion** root reduces blood sugar in experimental animals. It contains insulin-like chemicals and may actually substitute, on a limited basis, for insulin.

• **Huckleberry** helps promote insulin production. **Cedar berries** help the pancreas. Other helpful herbs include **black walnut, echinacea, burdock, buchu, dandelion root,** and **uva ursi.**

• James Duke, Ph.D., says that daily taking the tropical herb, ***Neurolaena lobata,*** helped a woman on the island of Trinidad to completely normalize her blood sugar.

• *In case of a hyperglycemic attack,* go to an emergency room. You must be given fluids, electrolytes, and possibly insulin.

• *In case hypoglycemia occurs,* in an emergency, immediately drink **fruit juice, soft drinks, or anything else that contains sugar**. If you are insulin dependent, carry a glucagon kit with you at all times.

• **Hot and cold packs** over the pancreas and kidneys will help insulin production and kidney elimination.

• Take good care of your **feet**; for they can become more easily infected than those of non-diabetics.

If your child has diabetes, tell his teacher the warning signs of hypoglycemia and hyperglycemia.

TYPE II DIABETES

Non-insulin dependent diabetics have high blood sugar. Here are several helps:

• Add more whole foods (such as **fruits, vegetables, grains, beans, nuts, and seeds**) to your diet. They are rich in fiber and nutritionally help stabilize blood sugar.

• Do not overindulge in **sweet, fatty foods**.

• Jonathan Wright, M.D., prescribes **chromium polynicotinate** because it is closest to the form of chromium found in the glucose tolerance factor, the body's internal regulator of blood sugar.

• **Exercise** twice a day, every day. Exercise is insulin's best friend. It moves sugar out of the bloodstream into the cells.

—*Also see p. 35; Also Diabetic Retinopathy (398).*

J.H. KELLOGG, M.D., PRESCRIPTIONS FOR DIABETES AND ITS COMPLICATIONS (*how to give these water therapies: pp. 207-272 / list of treatments: pp. 206-207 / Hydrotherapy Disease Index: pp. 273-275*)

INCREASE OXIDATION OF SUGAR—A large amount of moderate **outdoor exercise**, especially respiratory exercise (exercise that requires deeper breathing), and daily **Cold Baths**.

INCREASE ABSORPTION OF OXYGEN—Graduated **Cold Baths**, **outdoor exercise**, breathing exercises, oxygen inhalation.

IMPROVE INTESTINAL DIGESTION—Cold Douche (spray) with percussion to spine. Short Cold Fan Douche to abdomen. Hot **Abdominal Pack**, day and night. **Fomentation** to abdomen, twice daily. Abdominal massage.

DIABETIC DIET—Zwieback (twice-baked bread), **fruits**, etc.; but do not use dates and figs, green peas, strawberries, spinach, nuts, and nut products of all sorts except chestnuts. **No meats** of any kind.

SCIATICA—Hot **Leg Pack**, **Revulsive Douche**, **rest** in bed.

RHEUMATIC PAINS—Radiant Heat Bath or **Sweating Wet Sheet Pack** until he perspires for 5-8 minutes. Follow by a suitable **cold application**.

OBESITY—Vigorous **exercise**. **Monotonous diet** (which automatically lessens the desire to overeat). **Sweating baths**, 3 times a week. Vigorous **cold applications** daily. Dripping Wet Sheet Rubs, Half Bath, Cooling Wet Sheet Pack, Plunge Bath.

EMACIATION—**Rest** in bed, Cold Mitten Friction or **Cold Towel Rub**, **Massage**, a **fattening diet.**

BOILS—Prolonged **Neutral baths**. Wash boils with **shampoo** three times a week.

PRURITUS—Prolonged **Neutral baths** followed by **Cold Mitten Friction** to sound parts of skin, **Neutral Compress**.

SOMNOLENCE—Copious **water** drinking. Hot **Enema**, repeated every 3-4 hours. Prolonged **Neutral Bath**, with **Cold Pail Pour** at 60° F. to head and spine during intervals of every 15 minutes. **Hot Blanket Pack** for 15 minutes. Follow by **cold Friction** and **Dry Pack**.

CONSTIPATION—**Enema**, at 70° daily. Hot **Abdominal Pack**.

INSOMNIA—Prolonged **Neutral Bath** at bedtime. Neutral Pack, 30-40 minutes. Neutral **Spray Douche**, 3-4 minutes, at bedtime.

BRONCHITIS—Chest Pack, **Warm Vapor Inhalation**, **Revulsive Douche** to legs.

EDEMA OF LEGS—**Rest** in bed; **Cold Compress** over heart, 15-30 minutes, 3 times daily. **Revulsive Compress** or Revulsive Douche to legs, 3 times a day. Follow, during intervals, by **Heating Compress**.

CARDIAC DILATATION—**Cold Compress** over heart or **Ice Bag** over heart, 15 minutes, 3 times a day. Carefully increased moderate **exercises**.

THREATENED GANGRENE—**Alternate Compress** or alternate **Pail Pour** to affected part and large adjacent area, 3 times a day. Protected **Heating Compress** over it during the interval between.

CIRRHOSIS OF LIVER—**Alternate Compress** over liver or a Spray Douche to it twice daily. During the interval between, apply a well-protected **Heating Compress**.

ECZEMA—**Alkaline Bath** (using oatmeal, etc., in water) or a **Neutral Bath**, 30 minutes, twice daily.

THIRST—Frequent drinking of small quantities of cold **water**, half a glass every hour. Sipping very hot water.

DRY SKIN—Steam Bath or Prolonged **Neutral Bath**. Follow by oil rubbing daily or 2-3 times a week.

CONTRAINDICATIONS—If emaciated, avoid exercise and prolonged hot or cold baths.

GENERAL METHOD—The general plan of treatment in this disease is essentially the same as that required in the treatment of obesity, which this disease closely resembles. But, in cases of diabetes accompanied by emaciation, very cold procedures (especially cold immersions used in cases of obesity or in cases of diabetes in which he is fleshy) must be carefully avoided and the principal reliance must be placed upon short, cold procedures which build up his resistance while increasing oxidation of carbon to a moderate degree. Special attention must be given to improving the intestinal digestion.

If any of the following related problems exist, look them up under their respective headings: Pneumonia, Nephritis, Cystitis.

ENCOURAGEMENT—The love of God toward the fallen race is unfathomable. It is without a parallel. This love led Him to give His only begotten Son to die, that rebellious man might be brought back into harmony with the government of Heaven.

ENDOCRINE - 3 - THYROID

HYPOTHYROIDISM
(Underactive Thyroid, Goiter)

SYMPTOMS—Fatigue and inability to tolerate cold are the most common symptoms.

Others include loss of appetite, a slow heart rate, muscle weakness and possibly cramps, dry and scaly skin, recurrent infections, water retention (edema), overweight, brittle nails, constipation, depression, difficulty in concentrating, a yellow-orange coloration of the skin (especially on the palms of the hands). In women, there might be painful menstruations, a milky breast discharge, and fertility problems.

CAUSES—An underactive thyroid is the most common glandular problem in America. The thyroid gland is the body's thermostat. It tells the rest of the body when to produce more heat or less. *Thyroxine* is secreted by the thyroid (a butterfly-shaped gland in the front of your neck) and affects several body functions, including the general rate of metabolism. The pituitary, located in the center of the skull, sends out *TSH* (thyroid-stimulating hormone), to tell the thyroid to speed up or slow down. When a weak thyroid does not respond, TSH levels remain high—and you have hypothyroidism. The hormone, thyroxine, is almost pure iodine. Women are eight times more likely to have hypothyroidism than men.

First thing in the morning, place a thermometer under your arm for 15 minutes while keeping still. A temperature of 97.6° F. or lower may indicate an underactive thyroid. Write down the result for five days. (Others say that if the test is consistently below 98, you are low thyroid.)

A low thyroid condition generally does not produce goiter. It is produced when the thyroid gland enlarges.

It is thought that **Hashimoto's Disease** is the most common cause of an underactive thyroid. This occurs when the body becomes allergic to its own thyroxine! It is not clear why this happens.

In addition, the immune system can produce antibodies that invade and attack the thyroid, disrupting hormone production. This destruction of the thyroid, resulting in hypothyroidism, is called **myxedema**. It is actually a disease of the immune system. It is believed that **an excess of chemicals, poisonous fumes, medicinal drugs, tobacco smoke, impure living, etc.**, disrupts the immune system and starts it on such rampages.

Get away from the chemicals by moving to the **country**, live a **clean life**, **eat right**, use a distiller to make your own **pure water**, work outdoors part of the time—have peace with God, and you will feel better every day.

Myxedema coma can occur, but rarely. Someone with advanced hypothyroidism can go into a coma from overexposure to cold, during an illness, after an accident, or after taking sedatives or narcotics. Call a physician immediately. *Also see Iodine, p. 113.*

THYROID SUPPLEMENTATION
Medical treatment includes the taking of thyroxine from animals or a synthetic product (synthroid or levoxyl). This is generally 3-9 grains each morning. An excess will cause increase in heart rate and shaking of the extended arm. (Levoxyl tablets are standardized better than synthroid; therefore they are better for you.)

The active ingredient in synthetic thyroid medications, is *levothyroxine*. It can cause a loss of as much as 13 percent of bone mass. An estimated 19 million people in the U.S. take this drug for thyroid problems or thyroid cancer.

Thyroid supplementation can cause cardiac arrest in those whose hearts are not strong enough for the increased activity the thyroid dosage places upon it.

Thyroid medication can have a similar effect on the adrenals. They may be working poorly, as a result of years of low thyroxine. The medication can cause adrenal insufficiency. Diabetes can be made worse by the thyroid pill. Anticoagulants can be upsetting.

Thyroid supplementation also increases the need for insulin and some antidepressants; since this causes some people to become extremely agitated.

Thyroid medication can produce arrhythmia, angina, tachycardia, and hair loss.

After menopause, a smaller dose of thyroid medication is often needed by women.

In newborn infants, synostosis can occur if they are given thyroid. The skull bones close prematurely and the brain does not develop properly.

In cretins, who are born hypothyroid, try taking

them off the thyroid medication after three years of supplementation. Maybe their thyroid will start functioning on its own.

The human body needs less thyroid as it gets older; so older folk should try reducing their dose of an animal or synthetic thyroid supplement. To do this, try reducing the amount you take by one dose a week (example: 5 doses a week, then 4 doses the next week, etc.). When you encounter problems, stay with that amount for 4 weeks to see if the thyroid will adjust itself to this new amount. After a month, try reducing the dosage again, staying one month at each reduced level.

Take thyroid medications at a different time than other **drugs**, because they can interact. Do not take **iron supplements** with thyroid supplements. The iron binds with the thyroxine, rendering it insoluble. For the same reason, do not take **calcium** or **carbonate supplements** at the same time with thyroxine medications.

For some, thyroid problems can be corrected; but, for others, it is something to live with for a lifetime while doing that which may lessen the problem.

Some people may think they have a hypothyroid problem, when, instead, they have sugar intolerance, depression, or menopausal symptoms.

The thyroid problem is not a simple one. The *thyroid* in your neck sends out *thyroxine*, which is loaded with iodine, to cells throughout your body, telling them to get to work. But the thyroid is told what to do by hormones from the *pituitary* in the middle of your brain, which sends it *THS* (thyroid stimulating hormone). And the pituitary is told what to do by part of your brain: the *hypothalamus*. So all types of thyroid problems may not be caused by the thyroid gland at all, but by problems in the pituitary or hypothalamus.

NATURAL REMEDIES

IODINE

• You need iodine everyday, at every meal. But how do you obtain it? Extended use of thyroid medication can weaken the bones or result in breast cancer.

• Among the seaweeds, **Nova Scotia dulse** or **Norwegian kelp** are the best-balanced sources of trace minerals. Most other seaweed products also contain iodine; but they are not always as balanced in providing a wide spectrum of other trace minerals. California kelp is not as good.

• Here is an address for Nova Scotia dulse: Roland's Sea Vegetables, 174 Hill Road, Grand Manon, NB E5G4C4, Grand Manan, N.B. [New Brunswick], Canada. I let it dry, whiz the leaves, put them in jars, and sprinkle it on my food.

• Iodine is an element. You must not drink it; for it is poison. But you can purchase a **bottle of iodine** at the drugstore. Then paint a 3 inch by 3 inch area of the skin on your thigh or the top of your foot. If you need iodine, the iodine on your skin will totally disappear (because it has been absorbed) within 24 hours. This technique is also helpful if a nuclear blast

has occurred and you need to avoid Strontium 90. An alternative is taking potassium iodide in order to protect your thyroid from being damaged by radioactive fallout. —*See Radiation Poisoning (812).*

• Another source of iodine is **Lugol's solution**. This, of course, should be taken in extremely small doses. Unfortunately, it is difficult to obtain. Pharmacies have it; but they will not dispense it without a prescription.

• There is also **iodized salt**. The problem here is that aluminum is in store-bought salt (so it will not cake); and that can lead to Alzheimer's disease (587).

• Some use "**sea salt**"; but generally this is nothing more than regular salt, extracted from the ocean rather than from salt mines. It is just regular salt, probably with the added aluminum.

• Some use rock salt (from salt mines) and grind it up. But this lacks the iodine.

• There is a firm in France which produces **salt from the ocean** which does have all the natural trace minerals, including iodine: The U.S. address is Grain & Salt Society, P.O. Box DD, Magalia, CA 95954 / 916-872-5800. Of the three products (Light Grey, Fine Ground, and Flower of the Ocean), the Fine Ground seems to strike a balance between fine grain and low price. The salt is slightly moist; but this is natural. Dry, free-flowing salt has always been treated with chemicals. I prefer Nova Scotia dulse.

• Because **chlorine, fluoride**, and iodine are chemically related, an excess of the first two will block entrance of iodine into the thyroid. So avoid **chlorinated water and fluoridated water** or **toothpaste**.

• In addition to iodine, the amino acid, **tyrosine**, is another building block of thyroid hormones; you may want to try taking 250 to 500 mg per day.

DIET

• In addition to taking added iodine, eat a **nutritious diet**. The experts say to eat foods in the cabbage family in moderation (**broccoli, cabbage, kale, Brussels sprouts, mustard greens**); for they tend to suppress the thyroid function. The same is said to hold true for **peaches and pears**. Fresh **carrot juice** improves thyroid function slightly. Drink **green drinks** and **potassium broths** (thick, white potato peeling soup).

• **Mustard greens** contain the largest amount of *tyrosine* (1.9%) of any cooking greens. Tyrosine is a constituent of thyroid hormone. Various beans and seeds contain lesser amounts. **Radishes** have been used, in Russia, to treat both types of thyroid problems. One chemical in radishes, *raphanin*, is said to keep thyroxine levels in balance. Turks use walnuts to treat various glandular problems. In one study, the fresh juice of **green walnuts** (especially the **husks**) doubled levels of thyroxine. A decoction of green walnuts, made by boiling them 20 minutes, boosted thryoxine at least 30%.

• **Mother's milk** is a good treatment for hypothyroid babies; and it helps protect normal babies from developing the problem until weaning.

• **Vitamin A** is necessary for iodine to be properly

absorbed. The **B vitamins** work together, to nourish the thyroid. **B₆** helps the thyroid use its iodine effectively in hormone production. B_{12} helps the thyroid work properly. A thyroid deficiency can result from lack of **sunshine**.

• Remain on a **salt-free, oil-free, sugar-free diet** until the thyroid is under control. But, on the long term, you need a little salt and oil.

MORE HELP

• *To stimulate the thyroid:* Eat one serving each of **oats** and **bananas** daily, take a **cool shower** each morning and night, and **work** 3-5 hours outdoors everyday. Functions of the thyroid will be increased by more **exercise**; for it stimulates TSH production by the pituitary. T3 increases slowly in the blood during, and after, vigorous exercise.

AVOID

• A thyroid deficiency can result from eating free fats (**margarine, butter, mayonnaise, fried foods, cooking fats, salad oils, and** commercial **peanut butter**).

• The following foods are "goitrogens"; that is, they hinder the body's use of iodine: *raw* **cabbage, turnips, peanuts, mustard, pine nuts, millet, soy products**. *Cooking* these foods inactivates the goitrogen factor.

• Avoid **electric blankets** if you can.

• Avoid drinking **fluoridated water**.

• **Nitrates** are goitrogenic; that is, they stimulate goiter formation. Nitrates can be found in **hot dogs, sausages, luncheon meats, and variously prepared meat products**. Nitrates are also found in **well water, from fertilizer runoff**.

HERBS

Gentian provides bitter principles known to normalize the functioning of the thyroid. Take it alone or combine it with cayenne, kelp, and saw palmetto.

TO ELIMINATE SUPPLEMENTATION

• A natural healer in Central America recommends the following procedures: *To go off thyroid supplementation:* Go on a **fasting, cleansing program of fruit and vegetable juices**, followed by a building program of eating **simple, nourishing foods** (especially raw food). Do this for 2-4 weeks. Get back and neck **spinal adjustments**, and take one **kelp** tablet daily. He says this always works.

TO REDUCE A GOITER

• A goiter is an enlargement of the thyroid gland, which is in the front of the neck. To eliminate that enlargement, the above practitioner recommends this: Follow the above program; and then, after the 2-4 weeks, do one or more of the following four neck applications: (1) Put an **Epsom-salt compress** on the neck every night, leaving it on all night for 10 nights. (2) Use a compress of **white oak bark** tea over the

goiter for better results. (3) Put two **hot fomentations** around the neck, for 4 minutes each, and one cold compress for 4 minutes. Continue alternating this for an hour. Then spend 5-10 minutes doing **exercises** with the neck in various positions. (4) Put a poultice of ground-up **almonds** completely around the neck and leave it on all night, for 3-10 nights. This is especially good for harder, more fibrous goiters.

• To reduce a goiter, a different natural healer says to apply **black walnut** extract as paint on the throat. Take ½ dropperful of the extract, twice daily, and apply **the calendula** herb compresses twice a day for a month.

• For goiters, Dr. Christopher prescribes mixing **burdock root** powder with **olive oil** and applying externally over the affected gland.

NOTE

Many people with Parkinson's Disease *(582)* tend to have hypothyroidism.

Cancer of the thyroid has been linked to drinking highly fluoridated water.

ENCOURAGEMENT—The secret of happiness is to live a life wholly dedicated to God. You are the Lord's; for He created you. Give Him your heart and your plans, obey His Written Word, and He will wonderfully guide your life. Psalm 146:7.

HYPERTHYROIDISM
(Overactive Thyroid, Graves Disease)

SYMPTOMS—Fatigue, insomnia, intolerance, irritability, increased perspiration, constantly feeling hot, frequent bowel movements, hair and weight loss, nails separate from nail bed, change in skin thickness, hand tremors, intolerance of heat, rapid heartbeat, goiter. Sometimes the eyeballs protrude. In women, there may also be less frequent menstruation and decreased flow.

CAUSES—Hypothyroidism (spoken of in previous pages) is caused by an underactive thyroid, resulting in a slow metabolism and all it brings with it. Hyperthyroidism is the opposite: The **thyroid is overactive**. Metabolism is too fast; and that brings its own problems. The thyroid gland is producing too much thyroxine.

Sometimes called *thyrotoxicosis*, hyperthyroidism is not a simple problem to deal with. Graves' disease is the most common form of it, which 2.5 million Americans have.

A detailed discussion of the thyroid is found in our article on Hypothyroidism *(659)*, which is far more common. Both affect women more often than men. When the thyroid does not work properly, a variety of different physical problems can develop.

ENDO

In fact, the word, "hypochondriac," was coined in the 19th century to describe those strange people who have all kinds of things wrong with them when they apparently do not seem to have anything wrong with them. Surely, it must all be in their heads! Well, it was in their throats. We now know that those misunderstood people had under or overactive thyroids.

Infection of the thyroid or certain prescription drugs can temporarily produce hyperthyroidism.

The pituitary, parathyroids, and sexual functions work closely together and are affected by the thyroid. Problems in one area can affect them all.

Improving hypothyroidism will improve Parkinson's Disease in those who have both.

NATURAL REMEDIES
• Eat 75% fresh foods, including plenty of **vegetables**. Also need **brown rice, green drink, brewer's yeast, wheat germ, and lecithin**. Eat carefully of good food. Hyperthyroidism speeds up digestion, so you may not properly absorb nutrients.

• Eat the **cabbage** (cruciferous) family of foods (**broccoli, cabbage, kale, brussels sprouts, mustard greens**); for they tend to suppress the thyroid function. Eat as much as you can raw; for this increases the thyroxine-suppressing factor. They contain substances, called *isothiocyanates*, which help restrain the thyroid from producing too much thyroxine. Also eat **radishes**; it is in the same family and is the most powerful thyroxine suppressor of them all. **Rutabagas, soybeans, turnips, peaches, and pears** also slightly suppress the thyroid function.

• The eating of **kelp** helps every type of thyroid problem, including hyperthyroidism. Kelp is a rich source of iodine and thyroxine. The hormone produced by the thyroid is almost pure iodine. Genuine sea salt is another worthwhile source of iodine. *See Hypothyroidism (659)*.

• Deficiencies of **vitamins C and E** can result in overproduction of the thyroid hormone.

• Get some early morning **sunlight** on the body, whenever possible. If you are near the **ocean**, wade or swim in it every so often.

AVOID
• Cut down on **dairy products** and avoid **nicotine, alcohol, caffeine, soft drinks, and processed and junk foods**.

• **Radioactive sodium iodine** (iodine 131, also called I-131) may be recommended by a physician; but be aware of the fact that it can cause severe side effects.

• Do not be quick to try **surgery** on your thyroid. You have enough problems without doing that.

HERBS
• **Bugleweed** (*Lycopus*) has been used for a long time, to treat thyroid problems. It mildly (slightly) inhibits iodine metabolism and reduces the amount of hormone that is produced by cells within the thyroid. It is widely used in Europe for this purpose. **Lemon balm** is also used in Europe for the same purpose. Studies show that lemon balm causes a decrease in blood and pituitary levels of TSH after a single injection; thus thyroid hormone production is reduced. Other herbs with this property include **vervain** (*verbena*) and **self- heal**.

—*For much more, see Hypothyroidism (659)*.

ENCOURAGEMENT—In Christ, the family of earth and the family of heaven are bound together. Christ glorified is our brother. Go to Him with all your sorrows and cares. Isaiah 41:17.

"Thou wilt light my candle: the Lord my God will enlighten my darkness." Psalm 18:28.

"They cry unto the Lord in their trouble, and He saveth them out of their distresses." Psalm 107:19.

The work of conquering evil is to be done through faith. Those who go into the battlefield will find that they must put on the whole armor of God (Ephesians 6). The shield of faith will be their defense and will enable them to be more than conquerors.

"The Lord God is a sun and shield: the Lord will give grace and glory: no good thing will He withhold from them that walk uprightly." —Psalm 84:11

"The Lord preserveth the simple: I was brought low, and He helped me." —Psalm 116:6

"In God I will praise His Word . . in God I have put my trust; I will not fear what man can do unto me." —Psalm 56:10-11

"Believe in the Lord your God, so shall ye be established; believe His prophets, so shall ye prosper." —2 Chronicles 20:20

"Be perfect, be of good comfort, be of one mind, live in peace; and the God of love and peace shall be with you." —2 Corinthians 13:11

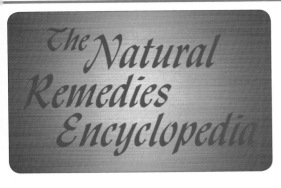

The Natural Remedies Encyclopedia

- Disease Section 12 - Lymphatic

Section 12 - Lymphatic

LYMPHATIC - 1 - LYMPH SYSTEM

SWOLLEN GLANDS
(Lymphadenitis)

SYMPTOMS—This generally refers to the swelling of lymph nodes (commonly referred to as "glands") on the sides of the neck, by the throat.

But it can also refer to enlargement of any other lymph glands, such as are under the armpits or in the groin.

There may also be heat, tenderness, and reddening of the overlying skin, as well as fever.

CAUSES—The lymph system filters out infections of various types, in order to rid them from the system. But an infection in the lymph nodes can occur. This can be a localized infection or an infection symptomatic of a more serious condition (such as **measles, chicken pox, mononucleosis, tuberculosis, syphilis, leukemia, or cancer**).

NATURAL REMEDIES
• The specific infection needs to be overcome through **fasting, bed rest, careful diet, keeping the bowels open, and not consuming improper foods or drink**.
• **Vitamins A, B complex, and C** are important.
• To reduce swellings, apply an herb tea wash of one or more of the following: **comfrey, plantain, apple cider vinegar, and witch hazel**. Also helpful are **carrot poultices, castor oil packs, lavender lotion or lavender water**. Bruised **parsley** poultice or parsley tea can also be used to reduce swellings. While **witch hazel** is outstanding, some of the other herbs provide additional healing.
• In India, **ginger** has been used for centuries to reduce swellings of various kinds, including glandular swellings. Take 2 oz. daily; results should be seen within 30 days. Do not take this during pregnancy. They also apply 2 parts **turmeric** and 1 part **salt** to the swollen area.
• Take 400-500 mg pure **pineapple compound** (from health-food store) 3 times a day on an empty stomach. It contains the proteolytic enzyme, *bromelain*.

L
Y
M
P

FOR MORE NATURAL REMEDIES:

HERBS: Herb Contents (pp. 129-130) will help you locate the **126 most important herbs** and the diseases each one can treat. How to prepare herbs (132). How to use them (141-189)

HYDROTHERAPY: Therapy Contents (pp. 206-207) and its Disease Index (263-265) will lead you to over 100 water therapies and many more remedies. DIS. INDEX: 1211- / GEN. INDEX: 1221-

VITAMINS AND MINERALS: Contents (100-101). Using 101-124. Dosages (124). Others (117-)

CARING FOR THE SICK: Home care for a sick person (28-36). The healing crisis (36-39)

WOMEN'S SECTIONS: Female Organs (672) Pregnancy (701). Childbirth (765). Infancy, Childhood (722). Women's Herbs (754, 760)

EMERGENCIES: (973-). FIRST AID: (990-)

• Dr. Christopher suggests applying a fomentation or compress of a strong decoction of **rue** tea to the area.

• Another helpful compress is 2 oz. **mullein**, ½ oz. **lobelia** powder, and 1 tsp. **cayenne**. Simmer in 2 quarts apple cider **vinegar**, cover for 15 minutes, strain, and apply when cool.

Note: **Cat scratch disease** *(739)* is thought to be the primary cause of one-sided lymphadenopathy, a disease affecting the lymph glands. Also see **Tonsillitis** *(740)*, another lymphatic disorder of the tonsils and adenoids affecting children.

—*See Fevers (302-309) and other topics in this section on the Lymphatics.*

ENCOURAGEMENT—Precious are the privileges of the soul who abides in Christ. In Christ's strength, we are able to meet whatever trials that life may bring. Psalm 103:3.

"In all these things we are more than conquerors through Him that loved us." Romans 8:37.

The promises are rich and full! Claim them!

LYMPHANGITIS
(Splenic Inflammation)

SYMPTOMS—This begins with a chill and high fever, with moderate swelling and pain of the lymphatic tissues. A severe pain develops in the left side and extends up to the shoulder. When the infection is in the deep layers of skin, there is a deep general flush with raised borders in the affected areas. The skin becomes hot and dry, and the person becomes very thirsty.

CAUSE AND TREATMENT—The most common cause is streptococcal pyogenes, although it can also be caused by the fungus Sporothrix schenckii.

NATURAL REMEDIES

• Provide a **fruit diet** for the first few days. Follow by a light, **nourishing diet**. Give the kind of care for one with a fever. Keep the **bowels** open, using laxative herbs. **Do not strain** at the stool; for this could injure a temporarily enlarged spleen. Give plenty of **fluids**, to help flush out the lymphatics.

• Apply **hot fomentations**, followed by short **cold**. This will greatly help to reduce pain and inflammation. Do this 2-3 times a day until the pain is relieved; then do this once a day.

• Kloss' liniment is excellent, when applied over the spleen. Mix 2 oz. powdered **myrrh**, 1 oz. powdered **goldenseal**, ½ oz. **cayenne**. Put into 1 quart 70% rubbing **alcohol**. Mix and let stand 7 days, shaking well each day. Put the upper fluid in covered bottles. This is good for all kinds of swellings and skin problems.

—*See Fevers (302-309).*

ENCOURAGEMENT—We must be living branches, connected closely to Christ, so that we may bear the fruit of unselfish kindness to all about us. By His grace this can be done. Isaiah 41:17.

MONONUCLEOSIS
(Mono, Infectious Mononucleosis)

SYMPTOMS—Depression, fatigue, fever, generalized aching, sore throat, swollen glands, headache, jaundice, with possible red rash in the form of raised bumps.

CAUSES—Mono is a contagious disease, primarily affecting the spleen and lymphatic system.

It can be transmitted by **kissing, sexual contact, or sharing food or utensils**. But it can also be spread through the air, **breathing** contaminated air exhaled by another. So it is not necessarily the "kissing disease" it is described to be. It is not highly contagious; for brothers and sisters of the infected person rarely contract it.

Most frequently contracted by children and teenagers, the incubation period is 10 days among children and 30-50 days among adults.

The symptoms are very similar to those of the flu; but those of mononucleosis continue for 2-4 weeks! Even after the other symptoms are gone, a general fatigue can continue for 3-8 weeks more. Some people continue to feel fatigued for months or years.

Individuals frequently say that they felt sick but continued working, thinking they would shake it off— and then came down with mono. So, if you feel like going to bed and getting well, do it before something worse happens to you.

The Epstein-Barr virus (EBV) or, more rarely, the cytomegalovirus (CMV), is the cause of this infection. Therefore, it cannot be treated with antibiotics. (Giving them can produce an allergic rash or worse.) Both EBV and CMV remain in the body throughout the rest of one's life; but the infection, carefully treated, generally seems to go away. Therefore, rest and care for yourself; so the outward symptoms will successfully go away!

Be alert to signs that a more serious splenic infection may be about to begin: a fever over 102° F., severe pain in the middle of your left side that lasts 5 minutes or more, breathing becomes difficult, or swallowing becomes difficult. If this happens, contact your physician. This occurs because you did not go to bed and properly care for yourself when the infection first started. As a result, the spleen ruptures and there is internal hemorrhage. Fever may reach 103°-104° F. and persist for 1-2 weeks. There may be chills; and sore throat may make eating difficult for several weeks.

NATURAL REMEDIES

• Go on a **light fast of fruit and vegetable juices** for a day or two.

• Eat a **nourishing diet**, emphasizing **vegetable soups, potato peeling broth, and brown rice**. Eat

small meals. Because of the sore throat, avoid acid juices, such as **citrus**. A **soft diet** is best if the patient is a child with a severe sore throat.

• Drink plenty of **distilled water**; and be sure your intake of **trace minerals** is adequate. Drinking cool water often soothes the throat. **Saltwater gargles** help this.

• Do not eat **processed or junk foods**. Do not eat **meat, sugary, fried foods. No coffee or soft drinks**.

• **Stay in bed** until the worst part is over. As long as the spleen is enlarged, you need lots of rest. However, it has been found that, after a few days, **mild activity** is all right. But excessive activity may lead to a relapse and injury to the spleen. It may require 6-8 weeks before the person can return to regular activities.

• **Do not strain** at the stool; for this could injure a temporarily enlarged spleen.

• Isolation of the ill person is not required. But no one else should use his glasses, cups, drinking straw, etc.

• **Dandelion** tea will protect the liver and **echinacea** will boost the immune system.

• An expert knows how to give 30 minutes of **fever therapy** daily for 3 days, maintaining the body temperature at 102°-103° F. This will successfully treat even the most advanced cases of infectious mononucleosis. Giving a **hot bath** (which induces a brief fever) produces as dramatic results as the use of corticosteroid drugs, with none of their drawbacks (these drugs impair immunologic function).

• Treat headaches with a **hot footbath**. Do not give **aspirin** to a child or youth; for it might cause Reye's Syndrome.

Several weeks of **rest in bed** is required to produce complete healing; but many young people do not want to do this. As a result, some develop a chronic mono fatigue for months or years afterward.

• There is a *"pseudomononucleosis,"* which produces an enlargement of the cervical lymphatic glands and fatigue. This condition may be due to **food allergies**; it often occurs in high school and college age students. This condition is treated with an **allergen-free diet** and completely eliminates the unusual fatigue.   —*See Allergies (848) and Lymphangitis (664).*

ENCOURAGEMENT—Jesus is your Counselor. It is your privilege to cast all your care upon Him; for He careth for you. We must exercise that living faith which will penetrate the clouds that, like a thick wall, separate us from heaven's light. We have heights of faith to reach, where all is peace and joy in the Lord. How thankful we can be for the love of God! John 15:11.

You can have the heart of a little child in its simplicity and unreserved obedience. Your soul will yearn after holiness, and more and more of the treasures of truth and grace will be revealed to you to be given to the world. God has a wonderful plan for your life; and, day by day, it will be fulfilled more and more as you trust and obey His Written Word.

SCROFULA
(Lymph TB)

HYDRO—Scrofula is a type of tuberculosis which affects the lymphatic organs.

SYMPTOMS—Tuberculosis of the cervical lymph nodes, particularly with enlargement and cheesy degeneration of the lymphatic glands of the neck.

CAUSES—Scrofula is caused from mucus accumulating into large lumps in specific areas of the lymphatic glands. This is basically a diet problem. The mucusless diet will decrease the mucus in the area. Poultices and cleansing will complete the process.

NATURAL REMEDIES

Use three parts **mullein** and one part **lobelia** as a fomentation or poultice over the area, to reduce swelling. The entire bloodstream must be purified and the whole body cleansed to effect a cure.

• Mix 2 oz. each of **Dandelion root, yellow dock root, bittersweet, and stillingia root** with 1 oz. each of **sassafras root bark, figwort root, and American ivy (or Virginia creeper bark or only its twigs)**. Simmer the ingredients in 3 quarts water and reduce to 2 quarts. Strain, sweeten to taste with **honey**, allow to cool, bottle and keep in a cool place. Take 1 Tbsp. 3 times daily.

• R.T. Trall, M.D., prescribes the following: Being out in the **sunshine** is extremely important. Eat only quality **fruits, vegetables, and cereals**. Drink **water** freely, especially before noon. Take 1-2 **full baths** (tepid, cool, or cold) daily. Whenever the body is feverish, constantly apply cool or cold **wet compresses** and the **wet sheet pack**, followed by the **dripping-sheet** or **half-bath** (sitting in a partly filled tub). At other times, apply them only 1-2 times weekly. When the patient has torpor or over-fullness, apply moderate **sweating in a dry blanket**. He says not to be surprised if boils, eruptions, and abscesses occur during active treatments. Toxins are being released.

• The following suggestions are from the *Hydrotherapy* section of this *Encyclopedia*:

• **Graduated cold applications, sunbaths, cold air baths,** and **outdoor exercise** and living.

• Eat a careful, **nutritious diet**, rich in protein.

• Live in an **elevated region**, not in an area of damp lowlands.

J.H. KELLOGG, M.D., PRESCRIPTIONS FOR

SCROFULA AND ITS COMPLICATIONS *(how to give these water therapies: pp. 206-275 / list of treatments: pp. 206-207 / Hydrotherapy Disease Index: pp. 273-275)*

    INCREASE GENERAL VITAL RESISTANCE—Graduated cold applications, **sunbaths**, cold air baths, **outdoor exercises and living**. **Aseptic diet** that is rich in protein. And live in an elevated region, not in the damp lowlands.

    GENERAL—Revulsive or Alternate Compress over swollen glands, twice a day. During intervals between, apply flannel-covered **Heating Compress**, renewed before it becomes dry.

    ENCOURAGEMENT—As the heart is opened to the entrance of God's Written Word, light from heaven shines upon the soul. Determine to make God first, best, and last in everything you say and do. Psalm 1:1.

More Encouragement

"Jesus does not ask this sufferer to exercise faith in Him. He simply says, 'Rise, take up thy bed, and walk.' But the man's faith takes hold upon that word. Every nerve and muscle thrills with new life, and healthful action comes to his crippled limbs. Without question he sets his will to obey the command of Christ, and all his muscles respond to his will. Springing to his feet, he finds himself an active man.

"Jesus had given him no assurance of divine help. The man might have stopped to doubt, and lost his one chance of healing. But he believed Christ's word, and in acting upon it he received strength.

"Through the same faith we may receive spiritual healing. By sin we have been severed from the life of God. Our souls are palsied. Of ourselves we are no more capable of living a holy life than was the impotent man capable of walking. There are many who realize their helplessness, and who long for that spiritual life which will bring them into harmony with God; they are vainly striving to obtain it. In despair they cry, 'O wretched man that I am! who shall deliver me from this body of death?' Romans 7:24, margin.

"Let these desponding, struggling ones look up. The Saviour is bending over the purchase of His blood, saying with inexpressible tenderness and pity, 'Wilt thou be made whole?' He bids you arise in health and peace. Do not wait to feel that you are made whole. Believe His Word, and it will be fulfilled. Put your will on the side of Christ.

"Will to serve Him, and in acting upon His word you will receive strength. Whatever may be the evil practice, the master passion which through long indulgence binds both soul and body, Christ is able and longs to deliver. He will impart life to the soul that is 'dead in trespasses.' Ephesians 2:1. He will set free the captive that is held by weakness and misfortune and the chains of sin."

—Desire of Ages, 202-203

Two editions of Desire of Ages, the classic (and best) book on the life of Christ are available from us.

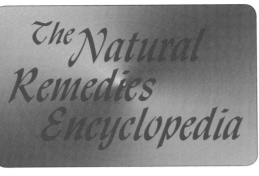

The Natural Remedies Encyclopedia

- Disease Section 13 -
Reproductive: Men

Reproductive: Physiology 1021-1023 / Pictures 1040

 # = Information, not a disease

R
E
P

M

"This God is our God for ever and ever; He will be our guide even unto death."   —*Psalm 48:14.*

"Blessed is the man that walketh not in the counsel of the ungodly, nor standeth in the way of sinners, nor sitteth in the seat of the scornful."   —*Psalm 1:1.*

"The Lord hath set apart him that is godly for Himself."
                                    —*Psalm 4:3*

"There is no want to them that fear Him . . They that seek the Lord shall not want any good thing."—Psalm 34:9-10.

"Though your sins be as scarlet, they shall be as white as snow; though they be red like crimson, they shall be as wool."   —*Isaiah 1:18*

"God is able to make all grace abound toward you; that ye, always having all sufficiency in all things, may abound to every good work."   —*2 Corinthians 9:8.*

Section 13 — Reproductive: Men

REPRODUCTIVE: MEN -
1 - MALE PELVIC ORGANS
Also: Male Infertility (704)

SPERMATORRHEA
(Nocturnal Emission)

SYMPTOMS—Involuntary loss of semen, without orgasm, often while asleep.

CAUSES AND TREATMENT—The male generative organs, the testes, must remain somewhat cooler than body temperature. When they become overheated (by taking a **hot tub bath**), a release of sperm will be made in the night; since that particular supply of sperm has become damaged and must be eliminated from the body.

If you sleep **too warmly at night**, due to an electric sleeping blanket set on high, the overheated testicles will eject sperm the next day.

Another cause is visual or thought **sexual stimulation**. A **poor diet** is another cause.

NATURAL REMEDIES
• A low-protein diet, free from the use of eggs, may prove of benefit.

J.H. KELLOGG, M.D., PRESCRIPTIONS FOR SPERMATORRHEA AND ITS COMPLICATIONS (*how to give these water therapies: pp. 298 / Hydrotherapy Disease Index: pp. 263*)
BASIC—Graduated cold applications to improve general conditions.
GENERAL NERVOUS IRRITABILITY—Prolonged **Neutral Bath** at night.
IRRITABLE PROSTATE, IRRITABLE URETHRA—Prolonged **Neutral Sitz Bath**, 30-60 minutes, at bedtime. **Revulsive Douche** to perineum with little pressure. Tepid **Colonic** at 80° F.
RELAXED EJACULATORY DUCTS—Rubbing Cold **Sitz Bath**. Cold or alternate hot and cold **Colonic**. Cold **Douche** to feet and legs, Cold **percussion Douche** to lower spine. Bowels must be kept regular by the Cool **Enema**, if necessary. And proper **diet**. An aseptic dietary is essential. Condiments must be strictly avoided.
CAUTION—When losses are frequent or parts irritable, avoid Cold Sitz Baths and prolonged Hot Baths.

ENCOURAGEMENT—Pray with unshaken faith and trust. The Angel of the covenant, even our Lord Jesus Christ, is the Mediator who secures the acceptance of the prayers of His believing ones. God can give you the help you need. Hebrews 11:6.

"Give diligence to make your calling and election sure: for if ye do these things, ye shall never fall." 2 Peter 1:10.
"The Son of man came . . to give His life a ransom for many." Mark 10:45.

ENLARGED PROSTATE
(Benign Prostatic Hypertrophy)

SYMPTOMS—Pain on urination, frequent urination, urine retention, often a fever. There may be a discharge. It becomes harder to urinate forcefully. The outstanding symptom is having to get up at night to urinate.

CAUSES—The prostate is a doughnut-shaped male reproductive gland. It is under the urinary bladder and surrounds the urinary tube (urethra).

Muscles located within the prostate squeeze prostatic fluid into the urethral tract during ejaculation. Most of the semen consists of this fluid, which provides nourishment and protection for the sperm.

Prostate enlargement is also called benign prostatic hypertrophy. The prostate gland gradually becomes bigger. This occurs in half of all men over 50 and three-fourths of men over 70. It is probably the most common infirmity of aging in the human male. More than 500,000 American men are afflicted each year.

It is believed that, with age, testosterone production and levels decrease and certain other hormones (prolactin and estradiol) increase. This results in more of a powerful form of testosterone, called dihydrotestosterone, in the body. This hormone causes an overproduction (hyperplasia) of prostate cells—which causes the prostate gland to become larger. As it does, it eventually tends to pinch the urethra and interfere with the flow of urine.

As a result, neither the bladder nor kidneys empty fully. This produces pressure which can damage them. Urination becomes more frequent; and the urine flows more slowly. There may be difficulty in starting and stopping the flow. Sometimes there is blood in the urine.

Here is how to check your own prostate:
The prostate can be felt (palpated) with the gloved finger. If you are going to do this effectively, you would need to examine it monthly. The normal prostate is firm like an orange and about the size of a walnut. You would reach into the rectum, to carry out this examination. The prostate is found at a depth in the rectum that is just comfortably in reach of the index finger. An acute case of enlargement may be hard while a chronic enlargement may be boggy. Tumors, either benign or malignant, tend to be irregular and nodular.

Prostatic cancer: Although this section is not about prostate cancer, it will be briefly mentioned here. *For a fuller discussion, go to Prostate Cancer (789).* An enlarged prostate can become cancerous; but, fortunately, it always proceeds very, very slowly. So slowly, in fact, that an operation to remove the prostate, because of cancer, is generally not needed. This is because, before the man is likely to die of prostate cancer, he is quite aged and dies of something else first. But, of course, you will want to consult your medical specialist. For more information on home care (in those instances in which cancer is present) *see Prostate Cancer (789).*

Vasectomy, for purposes of male sterilization, has been linked to prostate disorders and even cancer.

NATURAL REMEDIES

DIET

• Eat a **nourishing diet**, including **vitamin / mineral supplementation,** especially zinc.

• The diets of those who have prostate trouble are usually low in **essential fatty acids** (**flaxseed oil** and **wheat germ oil** are the best). Never heat these oils.

• Treat it with **zinc**, essential fatty acids (**flaxseed oil**, 1 tsp., three times a day), and a **high-fiber diet** which includes **pumpkin seeds** and **alfalfa**. Vitamin A (such as beta-carotene, 300,000 IU a day), **vitamin C** to bowel tolerance, **chlorophyll** (such as alfalfa), **selenium** (250 mcg, three times a day), **amino acids** (alanine, glycine, and glutamic acid; 5 grams each, daily for 90 days), and **cranberry juice** (2 pints a day).

• The prostate contains more **zinc** than any other organ in the body. Take 30 mg, 3 times daily, in the highly absorbable form of zinc picolinate or zinc citrate. Taper slowly to 60 mg daily; then taper down to 30 mg daily as symptoms recede. Also take 2 mg copper with every 30 mg (because zinc can cause a copper deficiency).

• Take high-lignan **flaxseed oil** (2 Tbsp.) twice daily, along with 400 IU **vitamin E**.

• Drinking **cranberry juice** can protect the urinary tract against infection.

OTHER HELPS

• Maintain optimal physical and emotional **health**.

• Regular **exercise** outdoors in the open air is important. **Walking** for an hour or two everyday is excellent.

• Increase **fluid intake**, in order to flush the kidneys and bladder of toxins and bacteria. Drink at least 48 oz. water daily, but no fluids after 7 p.m.

• Do not let the bladder become too full. **Urinate** as quickly as possible, when the urge comes. Try to completely empty the bladder each time.

• When there is an acute condition, take **hot sitz baths** daily and add **chamomile** tea to the water.

• **Sit** 15-30 minutes daily in a partly full tub of very hot water.

• Each day, 3 times, **spray** the lower abdomen and pelvic area with hot water for 3 minutes, alternating with 1 minute for cold.

• Also helpful is a **short cold bath**.

• A high **charcoal and water enema** helps the healing process. Use 1 cup of hot water to 1 teaspoon of powdered charcoal. Allow it to remain as long as possible.

• In order to increase circulation in the area, **lay flat on your back** on the floor. Then swing one leg across the other till the knee touches the floor and vice versa. Do this as many times as you can; eventually bring it up to 50 repetitions at a time.

• James Duke, Ph.D., recommends daily eating a special food mixture to keep the prostate from enlarging: Place a half-cup or so of fresh **pumpkin seeds** in a blender. Open 1 capsule of **saw palmetto** and pour it in. Add a few drops of **licorice extract**. Blend until smooth. (A few drops of **flaxseed oil** can be added to make it more spreadable.) Keep it refrigerated! Spread it on bread, eating a couple tablespoonfuls daily. Only mix small batches (enough for 2 days), so it will be fresh until eaten.

• **Saw palmetto** contains a compound which inhibits the action of the enzyme *(testosterone-5-alpha-reductase)* that turns testosterone into dihydrotestosterone—this preventing prostate enlargement. Saw palmetto is also a diuretic, increasing urine flow.

• **Pumpkin seeds** have been used for centuries to increase urine flow and help the prostate. The seeds contain *cucurbitacins*, which also helps prevent prostate enlargement. They also contain zinc, which is recommended for avoiding enlargement. In addition, pumpkin seeds contain large amounts of three special amino acids: glutamic acid, glycine, and alanine. Each of these has been found to reduce enlarged prostates (given in doses of 200 mg of each, daily). Or eat ¼ cup raw pumpkin seeds each day.

• **Licorice** contains a compound which also prevents the conversion of testosterone to dihydrotestosterone. (But eating it in large doses for years can produce headaches and other problems.)

• Two other herbs which researchers have found to reduce prostate enlargement are **pygeum** (50 mg of the bark extract, 2 times daily) and **stinging nettle** (2-3 tsp. of extract daily). Pygeum (pygeum aficanum) is an African evergreen tree; and extracts of the bark are used.

• Here is another formula for treating the prostate: Mix equal amounts of **cornsilk, buchu leaves, parsley, saw palmetto berries, kelp, and pumpkin seeds,** plus a pinch of **cayenne**.

• Other helpful herbs include **echinacea** and **goldenseal**, for bactericidal purposes. **Horsetail**, combined with **hydrangea**, helps contract the prostate. **Saw palmetto** and **cayenne** are also useful.

R
E
P

M

AVOID

• Do not eat **junk foods, fried foods, spices, chocolate, cashews, or caffeine products. Do not drink alcohol or use nicotine**.

• **Avoid sexual stimulation** without a natural conclusion (an orgasm). Continued stimulation leads to a prolonged engorgement. This is not good for the prostate. Keep your mind where it belongs. Do not look at anything hinting of a pornographical nature. Avoid everything that is sexually stimulating.

• **Avoiding sexual activity** as much as possible is the best way to care for your prostate in the older years.

• Avoid exposure to **dampness or cold**.

• Avoid **constipation**. This is important.

• **Riding bicycles, motorcycles, or horses** may injure the perineum, resulting in congestion of the prostate. Especially avoid riding bicycles.

• Do not sit for hours on **padded seats in cold places** (such as buses, trains, etc.). It keeps the healing blood from flowing in and out of your prostate.

• Avoid **deep foam chairs**. Whenever possible, sit on a hard chair. This reduces compression, which especially occurs when sitting in deep foam chairs.

• Many medicinal **drugs**, including pilocarpine, irritate the prostate.

—*Also see Prostatitis (below) and Prostate Cancer (789).*

ENCOURAGEMENT—Cling to God with all your heart, and He will guide you aright. You need His help every moment. Trust and obey His Written Word.

PROSTATITIS

SYMPTOMS—Pain during urination, fever, and a discharge from the penis.

Acute prostatitis: Pain around the base of the penis. Pain between the scrotum and rectum, Fever and chills. Lower back pain. Pain during bowel movements. Frequent, urgent, painful urination. There is urinary retention, a feeling of fullness in the bladder. Painful swelling behind the testis, the formation of an abscess in the prostate, frequent and burning urination, pus or blood in the urine.

Chronic prostatitis: The chronic form may not have any symptoms. If they appear, it occurs gradually: Frequent and burning urination, blood in the urine, lower back pain, pain on ejaculation. Blood in the semen. Eventually impotence (inability to copulate). Gradually urination becomes still more difficult. Pain and tenderness at the base of the penis and in the testes, groin, pelvis, or back.

CAUSES—Prostatitis is inflammation of the prostate gland. It may be acute or chronic. Acute prostatitis produces severe and sudden symptoms which clear up rapidly. Chronic prostatitis may cause mild symptoms for a long time; and it is difficult to treat. Both types are most common in men, aged 30-50, who are sexually active. It can be in men of all ages; it is the most frequent type of prostate problem.

The cause is often a **bacterial infection** which has spread from the urinary tract to the prostate gland. But it can also be caused by a **sexually transmitted disease** *(802-806).*

The inflammation tends to block off the urine flow (urine retention); and this causes bacteria to build up. Sometimes **hormonal changes**, from aging, may be a contributing factor.

When urine retention results, the bladder becomes distended, weak, tender, and liable to infection. Infection can easily pass up the ureters to the kidneys.

NATURAL REMEDIES

• Eat a nourishing diet of **fruits, vegetables, whole grains, legumes, and nuts.** Include cruciferous vegetables (**broccoli, brussels sprouts, cabbage**). Take **vitamin C** (2,000-5,000 mg), **vitamin E** (800 IU), and **flaxseed oil** (4 tbsp. daily). Also **selenium** (500 mg) and **zinc** (45-60 mg for 3 months, then 30 mg daily). Zinc is very important.

• Avoid **spicy foods, stress, smoking, and alcohol**. Do not eat **meat**. Do not eat **saturated fat**.

• Jay Cohen, M.D., had chronic nonbacterial prostatitis for five years. Having notice that his epididymis swelled and ached the more he was on his feet, he tried laying on his wife's **slantboard** (which raised his feet above his head at an angle of 30°) for 20 minutes, daily. Gradually, over a period of a year, the symptoms disappeared. Now he only feels the problem slightly when he has been on his feet for a long day. (But he suggests caution, if you have high blood pressure, cardiovascular distress, glaucoma, breathing difficulties, or intracranial problems.)

• **Cernilton** is a flower pollen extract which has been used successfully for decades in Europe.

• Identify and eliminate allergies.

—*Important: see Enlarged Prostate (668) for more information about the prostate which you can use. Also see Prostate Cancer (789).*

J.H. KELLOGG, M.D., PRESCRIPTIONS FOR PROSTATITIS AND ITS COMPLICATIONS *(how to give these water therapies: pp. 298 / Hydrotherapy Disease Index: pp. 263)*

BASIC APPLICATIONS—Revulsive **Sitz Bath**. Hot **Colonic**. Neutral **Sitz Bath**, for 30-60 seconds. **Cold Mitten Friction**.

PAIN—Revulsive **Sitz Bath**. **Fomentation** or the Revulsive Douche to perineum, with little pressure. **Colonic** in chronic cases. Hot **Enema**, when bowels are constipated.

CHRONIC ENLARGEMENT WITH INDURATION—Good results often follow the use of the following measures: alternate hot and cold **Colonic**. Shallow Cold Rubbing **Sitz Bath**, for 4-8 minutes. Cold **pelvic pack** (Wet Sheet Pack over pelvic area) with Hot **Leg Pack**. Massage of prostate. Graduated tonic baths. Ice bag to perineum, with Hot **Hip and Leg Pack** for 15-30 minutes.

CAUTIONS—When pain is present, avoid general cold baths, cold Sitz Baths, Cold Footbaths, and chilling of feet. Absolute sexual continence is essential.

ENCOURAGEMENT—When humanity depends wholly upon God, trusting in Christ and relying on His empowering grace, men may keep God's commandments and live clean, godly lives.

TESTICLE INFLAMMATION, ACUTE

SYMPTOMS—Pain in the testicles, which gradually becomes sharp and severe.

CAUSES—Bacterial infection of the testicles can be difficult to work with. Here are Dr. Kellogg's recommendations:

NATURAL REMEDIES

J.H. KELLOGG, M.D., PRESCRIPTIONS FOR ACUTE TESTICLE INFLAMMATION (how to give these water therapies: pp. 206-275 / list of treatments: pp. 206-207 / Hydrotherapy Disease Index: pp. 273-275)

BASIC POINTS—Rest in bed. Elevation of scrotum upon a tense broad band of cloth, placed about the thighs and close to hips. Hot Pelvic Pack or Hot Hip Pack with Cold Compress over genitals, every 3 hours. During intervals, Compress (at 60° F.) over perineum, genitals, and stomach (with heat to feet). Tepid Enema, twice daily. Cold Mitten Friction or Cold Towel Rub, twice a day. Prolonged Neutral Bath or Neutral Pack to control temperature, if necessary.

ENCOURAGEMENT—God is love, and He cares for us. "Like as a father pitieth his children, so the Lord pitieth them that fear Him." As in humility of heart, we bow in prayer, pleading for His mercy, God will forgive our sins, adopt us as His children, and enable us to fulfill His will as we seek to help and encourage those around us.

TESTICULAR ATROPHY

SYMPTOMS—Progressive wasting and shriveling of the testes.

CAUSES—This condition is not uncommon in aging men. It can also follow an episode of mumps.

Testicular atrophy may result in lessened sexual drive and possible feminization.

NATURAL REMEDIES

• Eat a nutritious diet, plus a full range of vitamin / mineral supplementation.

• Take zinc (30 mg, three times a day).

• Helpful herbs include saw palmetto and ginseng. —For much more helpful information, see Testicular Inflammation (above), Prostatitis (670), Enlarged Prostate (668).

ENCOURAGEMENT—Jesus says to ask God for the help you need. It is wonderful to be able to call on God. Do not neglect this privilege. He can do for you that which you can never do for yourself.

MALE MENOPAUSE

SYMPTOMS—Reduced energy, tendency to gain weight, less ambition, sore muscles, and less masculine drive.

CAUSES—Male menopause occurs with the gradual decline of the hormone, testosterone. Every system in a man is affected by this lessening of the male hormone. The circulatory system, muscles (including the heart), bones, nervous system, and brain are especially affected.

The following home remedies can help reverse this downward trend.

NATURAL REMEDIES

• Lose weight or regularly keep your weight down. Overweight men produce lower amounts of testosterone. That is due to the fact that the body, as it accumulates fat, makes less testosterone—while converting some of that testosterone into estrogen.

• As your muscular strength lessens, it becomes more difficult for you to burn excess fat. That only adds to the excess weight. This, in turn, causes even less testosterone and more estrogen. The solution is more exercise, and done on a regular basis. Three times every week, take a brisk walk for 20 minutes. As your weight drops, so will your estrogen. This will let your testosterone levels rise.

• Do not overeat. Only eat the most nutritious food, and not much of it. As you get older, you do not need much food.

• Take 25 mg of zinc, twice a day. The zinc enables your body to deactivate aromatase, an enzyme which converts testosterone to estrogen. It may take a couple months to see solid improvement; during this time, reduce your zinc intake to 30 mg once a day.

• Take vitamin C (1,000-3,000 mg) for 1-2 months; then lower it (to 1,000 mg). The vitamin C also reduces aromatase, raising testosterone.

• Take a complete multivitamin supplement daily.

• Drink carrot juice and eat broccoli, brussels sprouts, and cabbage. They are high in antioxidants. They also contain indoles, which help break down estrogen more efficiently. Do not eat grapefruit; for it blocks the body's elimination of estrogen.

• Soybeans contain isoflavones, which increase the liver's ability to eliminate estrogen.

• Do not smoke. Do not drink caffeine or alcohol. Alcohol decreases zinc levels.

ENCOURAGEMENT—God wants us to stand firm amid the pollutions of this degenerate age. He wants us to hold so fast to His divine strength, that we can overcome every temptation to wrongdoing. Trusting in Him and obeying His Written Word, we can be more than conquerors in the battle against temptation and sin. God wants you to live with Him forever in heaven.

The Natural Remedies Encyclopedia

SPECIAL SECTIONS FOR WOMEN - 1

Disease Section 14 - Reproductive: Women

Reproductive: Physiology 1021-1023 / Pictures 1040

 # = Information, not a disease

"This God is our God forever and ever; He will be our guide even unto death."—*Psalm 48:14.*

FOR MORE NATURAL REMEDIES:
HERBS: Herb Contents (pp. 129-130) will help
you locate the 126 most important herbs and
the diseases each one can treat. How to prepare herbs (132). How to use them (141-189)
HYDROTHERAPY: Therapy Contents (pp. 206-207)
and its Disease Index (263-265) will lead you
to over 100 water therapies and many more
remedies. DIS. INDEX: 1211- / GEN. INDEX:
1221-
VITAMINS AND MINERALS: Contents (100-101).
Using 101-124. Dosages (124). Others (117-)
CARING FOR THE SICK: Home care for a sick
person (28-36). The healing crisis (36-39)
WOMEN'S SECTIONS: Female Organs (672)
Pregnancy (701). Childbirth (765). Infancy,
Childhood (722). Women's Herbs (754, 760)
EMERGENCIES: (973-). FIRST AID: (990-)

Section 14 - Reproductive: Women

REPRODUCTIVE: WOMEN - 1 - BREAST
Also: Breast Cancer (788)
Tumors and Cancer (780-798)
Also: Pelvic Congestion (689)
Pelvic Pain (689)

BREAST DISCOMFORT
(Breast Tenderness)

SYMPTOMS—There is tenderness and discomfort in the breast.

CAUSES—Breast tenderness is a common characteristic of premenstrual syndrome (PMS) and early pregnancy. If caused by PMS, the tenderness may occur regularly every month; if associated with early pregnancy, missed periods and a positive home pregnancy test will reveal that.

The cause is generally the **natural cycles of the reproductive hormones**, which are estrogen and progesterone. They signal the milk-producing glands in the breast to grow and areas around them to expand with blood and other fluids to nourish the cells. This can result in stretched nerve fibers and a sense of pain.

Then there are fibrocystic changes which include lumps and cysts. *See Breast Cyst (674) for more information).*

NATURAL REMEDIES

• For breast tenderness, apply **vitamin E** on the area; and be sure to include enough essential fatty acids in the diet (1 tsp., 3 times a day). **Flaxseed oil, sunflower seed oil, or wheat germ oil** are best.

• **Selenium** is an antioxidant and helps prevent breast tenderness.

• Avoid **caffeine** products; they are linked to breast tenderness.

Discomfort and soreness in the breast is also a symptom of fibrocystic breast disease. *See Breast Cyst (674).*

ENCOURAGEMENT—Since Jesus came to dwell with us, we know that God is acquainted with our trials and sympathizes with our griefs. Obey God's Ten Commandment law by faith in Jesus Christ; and you will have a much happier, fulfilled life.

CHART - 1044; Reproductive - Women (672-700)

Those who accept Christ as their personal Saviour are not left as orphans to bear the trials of life alone. He receives them as members of the heavenly family; He bids them call His Father their Father. They are His "little ones," dear to the heart of God, bound to Him by the most tender and abiding ties. He has toward them an exceeding tenderness, far surpassing what our father or mother has felt toward us in our helplessness. The divine is superior to the human. Proverbs 1:23.

BREAST INFLAMMATION

SYMPTOMS—Painful and hard swelling in the breast. There is restlessness, throbbing, burning pain, and possible fever.

CAUSES—**Injury** or **improper diet** are among the causes of inflamed, swollen, caked breasts, or sore nipples.

NATURAL REMEDIES

• Soak a cloth in a mixture of 1 pint of **linseed oil** and 4 ounces of spirits of **camphor**, and cover the entire affected area. Apply as often as needed.

• **Hot and cold applications** of dry cloths help relieve the soreness and inflammation. Give these continually until relieved. Then apply the mixture again.

• When the breast is swollen, give a poultice of **slippery elm**, with a little **lobelia** added to it.

• Bathing an inflamed breast with **alder** tea will often relieve the inflammation and pain.

• Drink a tea of **goldenseal, black cohosh, and ginger**.

• Go on a short fruit and vegetable **juice fast**, and clean out the **bowels**.

—Also see Breast Discomfort (above) and Breast Cyst (below).

ENCOURAGEMENT—As the Son of man, Christ gave an example of obedience to God's holy law; as the Son of God, He gives us power to obey that law.

"God, who commanded the light to shine out of darkness, hath shined in our hearts, to give the light of the knowledge of the glory of God in the face of Jesus Christ." 2 Corinthians 4:6.

"Blessed are all they that wait for Him." Isaiah 30:18.

REP
W

BREAST CYST
(Fibrocystic Breast
Disease, Cystic Mastitis)

SYMPTOMS—Discomfort, soreness, tenderness, lumpiness, and possible felt lumps and cysts in the breast. These will be round lumps which move freely and are either firm or soft.

The symptoms are the most prominent before the monthly, and almost entirely absent during pregnancy.

CAUSES—This is the most common breast problem that women have; over 50% of adult females have it. It is most frequent in women of childbearing age; it primarily occurs between the ages of 30 and 50.

When there is too much fluid in the breast, instead of moving it out of the breast, the lymph system stores it in small spaces, here and there. Eventually, fibrous tissue surrounds them and thickens, forming cysts. These cysts frequently swell just before the monthly, causing pain.

These cysts may change in size; but, although tender, *they move freely*. In contrast, a cancerous growth generally does not move freely, is usually not tender, and does not leave.

It is important to regularly examine each breast for lumps and determine what kind they are. It is best to do this weekly. It is known that the risk of breast cancer is three times as great in women with cysts.

Breast cysts rarely appear after the age of 50, when estrogen levels are less.

Hormonal imbalance, abnormal production of breast milk (caused by high levels of estrogen), and an **underactive thyroid** can induce cysts.

Other causative agents are listed below. Here are suggestions to help you avoid problems with benign breast changes. It may take up to six months for these remedies to reduce the cysts:

NATURAL REMEDIES

DIET
• Eat a **low-fat, high-fiber diet**, including more **raw foods**. Emphasize **fruits, vegetables, and whole grains**. Stop eating **meat**. Reducing blood cholesterol (preferably to 170 mg or lower), by avoiding foods containing saturated fat and cholesterol will greatly help you. Fiber binds with estrogen in the intestine and eliminates it.
• The trace element, germanium, is important. It is found in **garlic** and **onions**.
• Research shows that milk and dairy products have high estrogen levels. It is best to avoid them; for the cyst problem can always lead to a cancerous condition.
• **Vitamin B₁** (25 mg), **vitamin B₂** (5 mg), **vitamin B₆** (200 mg), **vitamin C** (500-1,000 mg), vitamin E (400 mg), **calcium** (1,000 mg), magnesium (1,000 mg), **flaxseed oil** (2 tsp.). The **B vitamins, vitamin C, calcium, and magnesium** help regulate the production of *prostaglandin E*, which in turn slows down *prolactin* activity. Prolactin activates breast tissue.
• In animals, **iodine** deficiency causes fibrocystic disease. Eat Nova Scotia dulse or Norwegian kelp.
• Drink enough **water**, so it is easier for the blood and lymphatic system to care for the milk glands.

AVOID
• Avoid a diet high in **meat, eggs, butter, and cheese**. Do not eat **nuts** which have been heated.
• **White-flour products** should be avoided.
• Do not eat **animal products, cooked oils, fried foods, sugar, salt** or drink beverages with **alcohol** or **caffeine**. Do not use highly **salted foods**.
• Methylxanthines (which include caffeine, theophylline, and theobromine), found in **caffeine** and **chocolate** foods, have been found to induce breast disease. Cut out caffeine products entirely.
• Do not use **nicotine** products. They stimulate the growth of cysts.
• Do not use **diuretic drugs**. Instead, drink more water to help improve kidney function.

OTHER HELPS
• Keep the **weight** low. It is more difficult to locate tumors in larger breasts.
• Check for food allergies. See *Food Allergies (848-860)* and *Pulse Test (847)*.
• If you have an underactive **thyroid**, do what is needed to strengthen it; since hypothyroidism *(659)* has been linked to fibrocystic disease.
• Breast congestion can be caused by **padded bras**. Do not overheat the breasts; this can lead to breast cancer.
• Be aware that **birth control pills** increase estrogen levels and raise the possibility of breast disease. Have estrogen levels checked; then reduce them. A **low-fat diet** (especially eliminating all **saturated fat**) reduces estrogen levels.
• Excess **clothing** on the trunk, and not enough on the extremities, is a significant cause of female problems of various types. The body is not kept evenly warm; and blood pools in the trunk organs.
• Some find that applying **cold water** to the breasts helps when they are painful. But others find that alternating **very warm and cold** works better. This can be done via heating pads, cold cloths, showers, etc.
• Gentle **breast massage** will help move liquids out of the breast area into the lymph passages.
• Not using caffeine and applying **primrose oil** (3 grams daily) will help reduce the cysts. Primrose oil is especially good for fibrocystic breasts.
• **Dong quai** helps regulate hormonal levels. **Goldenseal** helps heal infections. **Red clover** cleans the blood. **Chlorophyll** helps clean the liver and prevents formation of cysts. **Germanium** and **CoQ₁₀** provide oxygen to the cells and prevent free-radical damage. **Flaxseed** oil helps prevent breast cancer. **Dandelion** tea cleanses the liver.
• **Red clover, pau d'arco, squaw vine, mullein, and curcumin** (turmeric) are useful in treating breast cysts.
• Women who **exercise** more have less breast tenderness.

—Also see Cancer (613).

ENCOURAGEMENT—When you open your eyes in the morning, thank God that He has kept you through the night. Thank Him for His blessings. Live your days in the presence of God. Revelation 22:17.

"Who are kept by the power of God, through faith, unto salvation." 1 Peter 1:5.

"Unto Him that is able to keep you from falling, and to present you faultless before the presence of His glory with exceeding joy." Jude 24.

"The promise is unto you and to your children." Acts 2:39.

BREAST ENLARGEMENT
(Gynecomastia)

SYMPTOMS—The breasts become excessively large.

CAUSES—Overweight is a primary cause.

NATURAL REMEDIES

• Eat only **nutritious food**; and **do not overeat** or eat between meals. Do not eat **saturated fats, meat products, mayonnaise, margarine, fried foods, cooking fats, or salad oils**. Your only oil should be 2 tsp. twice a day of **flaxseed oil** or **wheat germ oil**.

• **Obesity** can cause breast enlargement. All **milk and diary products** must be removed from the diet.

• **Estrogens**, fed to food animals, will tend to enlarge the breasts of those eating them (beef, pork, etc.).

• Women who take **fenugreek** tea, to help control diabetes, might have their breasts enlarge. It contains *diosgenin*.

ENCOURAGEMENT—We are to follow God as dear children, to be obedient to all His requirements and walking in love as Christ also hath loved us. We must follow the example set by Christ and make Him our pattern, until we shall have the same love for others as He has manifested for us.

ABNORMALLY SMALL BREASTS
(Increase breast size)

SYMPTOMS—Breasts are abnormally small.

NATURAL REMEDIES

• The seeds and sprouts of **fenugreek** have been used for centuries to increase the size of breasts. The seeds contain *diosgenin*. Drink the tea and gently massage powdered **fenugreek** into the breasts.

• **Fennel** is an estrogenic herb used to promote milk production. Do not use fennel oil; this can cause miscarriage in pregnant women. Doses of fennel larger than a teaspoonful can be toxic. Fennel contains phytoestrogens, which are plant chemicals similar to estrogen.

• Other herbs which contain phytoestrogens include **anise, basil, dill, caraway, licorice, marjoram, and lemon grass**. They could be mixed together with the other herbs listed here.

• **Wild yam** also contains *diosgenin*, but not as much as fenugreek. Shave off the outer bark of the root and make paste of the inner bark in a blender. Mix with oil or water and apply as a salve.

• **Cumin** and **black cumin** increase the number of mammary cells in test animals.

Birth control pills contain estrogen, which, as a side effect, cause the breasts to retain water. But this is not true breast enlargement.

• **Saw palmetto** is known to shrink mens enlarged prostate gland and increase the breast size of women.

ENCOURAGEMENT—God has given you life and all the rich blessings that make it enjoyable; and in return He has claims upon you for service, for gratitude, for love, for obedience to His law. These claims are of the first importance and cannot be lightly disregarded; but He requires nothing of you that will not make you happier, even in this life.

CERVICAL DYSPLASIA
(Abnormal pap smear)

SYMPTOMS—Normal cervical cells are regular in shape and size. Abnormal ones are distorted, indicating cervical dysplasia.

CAUSES—Cervical dysplasia is changes in the surface cells of the cervix which may become cancerous. A Pap smear is given to check cells from the cervix for any evidence of precancerous or cancerous changes. Because cancer of the cervix is fairly common and sometimes fatal, women are counseled by physicians to have periodic Pap smears. There are three grades of dysplasia: mild, moderate, and severe. Mild dysplasia may return to a normal state; but severe dysplasia may progress to cancer of the cervix if not treated. The most common cause is the presence of infection. Both the woman and her spouse must be treated.

Cells are collected from the cervix, using a spatula or brush, and are sent away to be examined under a microscope.

NATURAL REMEDIES

• **Licopene**, a carotenoid found in both fresh and cooked **tomatoes**, seems to pnotect against dysplasia. Of course, in any condition that challenges the immune system, the more chemical toxins you avoid the better;

so consider looking for organic tomatoes or growing your own. If you want lycopene as a supplement, take 1 to 5 mg daily.

• Often, women with cervical dysplasia are deficient in several nutrients. If you are at risk, check whether you're getting enough of the following daily nu-trients: **Vitamin A** (5,000 to 10,000 IU), **Ribofia-vin** (1.6 to 10 mg), **Vitamin C** (1,000 to 2,000 mg), **Folic acid** (400 to 600 mg), and **Vitamin E** (400 to 800 IU)

• Compared with healthy women, those with cervical dysplasia may have lower blood levels of **beta-carotene** and **vitamin E**. For beta-carotene, eat green and yellow vegetables. Take 400 IU of vitamin E daily.

• Low levels of **selenium** and low dietary intake of **vitamin C** are frequent in those with cervical dysplasia. Daily take 500 mcg (but not over 1,000 mcg) of selenium and 1,000 mg of vitamin C. If taking higher amounts of vitamin C, also include **copper** (4 mg).

• Women with a low intake of **vitamin A** are more likely to have an abnormal pap smear. If pregnant, or may become pregnant, do not take over 10,000 IU daily, to avoid birth defects.

• Large amounts of **folic acid** (10 mg daily) have been found to improve the abnormal pap smears of women who are taking birth control pills. Folic acid does not appear to improve the smears of women not taking oral contraceptives. But another study found that high blood levels of folic acid protected against cervical dysplasia. Along with the folic acid, take 1,000 mcg B_{12}.

• This **cervical dysplasia tea** can be stored in the refrigerator for up to three days; drink 2 to 3 cups per day before meals. Here is the formula: 2 teaspoons **vitex** berries, 1 teaspoon **burdock** root, 1 teaspoon **red clover**, 1 teaspoon **astragalus** root, ½ teaspoon **stevia** leaf (optional), ½-1 teaspoon **peppermint, spearmint, or wintergreen** (optional), 5 cups water. Bring herbs and water to a boil. Simmer gently for 5 minutes. Cover pot and let steep 20 more minutes. Strain out herbs.

ENCOURAGEMENT—There are many from whom hope has departed. Bring back the sunshine to them. Many have lost their courage. Pray for these souls. Bring them to Jesus. Tell them how He can help them.

REPRODUCTIVE: WOMEN -
2 - MENSTRUAL PROBLEMS

PREMENSTRUAL SYNDROME
(PMS)

SYMPTOMS—There are over 150 symptoms linked to PMS; the most common include abdominal bloating, anxiety, acne, backache, breast swelling and tenderness, swollen feet, depression, cramps, food cravings, fainting spells, headaches, fatigue, joint pain, insomnia, nervousness, impatience, drastic mood swings, angry outbursts.

Other symptoms include sluggishness, lethargy, delusions, indecisiveness, dizziness, constipation, hemorrhoids, skin eruptions, and migraines.

CAUSES—PMS affects many women during the one to two weeks prior to the onset of menstruation. It affects one-third to one-half of all American women between the ages of 20 and 50. As many as 75% have the problem at one time or another. About 5% are incapacitated by it; and about a third report symptoms severe enough to interfere with their daily life.

Bearing children or **being married** seems to increase the likelihood. The problem is a major cause of divorce.

Hormonal imbalance is part of the PMS problem. *See Menstrual Disorders (678).*

The liver regulates hormonal balance, by selectively filtering out of the blood and excreting unwanted excess hormones. One of these is *estradiol*, a type of estrogen which causes problems. If not eliminated, it can build up in the body.

Part of the hormonal imbalance problem is that there is **too much estrogen** in the body and **not enough progesterone**. Fluid retention is the result. This affects the circulation and impedes oxygen and nutrient flow to the brain and female organs.

Additional causative factors are mentioned below.

NATURAL REMEDIES
DIET
• Correct the diet. Compared with women without significant PMS problems, those that experience them eat 275% more **refined sugar**, 62% more **refined carbohydrates** (white-flour products), 75% more **dairy products**, 75% more **sodium** (salt), 53% less **iron**, 77% less **manganese**, and 52% less **zinc**.

• Typically, women with serious PMS problems tend to have high estrogen levels, had an early menarche (onset of periods, usually at 12 years of age or younger), and are on a **high fat / high cholesterol diet**. Fat cells produce estrogen, which disrupts the estrogen / progesterone balance. You will be greatly helped by significantly lowering your fat and cholesterol intake.

• Meals high in **complex carbohydrates** help one deal with stress. It is thought that they increase the production of serotonin, a brain chemical which counteracts depression.

• **High-fiber fruits, vegetables, and whole grains** help the body eliminate excess estrogen and prevent constipation.

• Take a full **vitamin / mineral supplementation**.

• An inadequate intake of **B complex vitamins** is another factor causing PMS. B vitamins and **magnesium** (1,000 mg) help the liver excrete unwanted estrogen. **Fried foods** block the absorption of magnesium.

• During the premenstrual period, the body wants

more sugar as fuel. Satisfying these cravings with lots of sweet foods (even good ones) causes blood sugar levels to shoot up and then plunge. This triggers much of the fatigue, mental fog, and emotional imbalance. Mildly **salty food** will tend to satisfy the cravings for sweets.

• Eating **smaller meals** of nourishing food and complex carbohydrates (whole grains) helps keep blood sugar levels stable and reduces sugar cravings.

• **Vitamin E** has been found useful in the treatment of PMS, with most improvement where benign breast disease was a major problem. Vitamin E is an antioxidant and helps prevent inflammatory reactions to dietary fats. It is possible that **vitamin A** and **zinc** also aid in this function.

• **Vitamin B$_6$** (50-3,000 mg daily), especially during the 10 days preceding menstruation, helps relieve premenstrual edema and soreness. It helps the liver eliminate excess estrogen.

• Adequate **calcium** (2,000-5,000 mg) intake during the monthly cycle is very important. Blood calcium drops 10 days before menstruation. A lack of it causes headaches, tension, nervousness, depression, insomnia.

• **Magnesium** (1,000 mg) and **vitamin D** (1,000 IU) help in calcium absorption. Adequate stomach acid is also needed.

• **Selenium** is an antioxidant and helps prevent menstrual cramps.

• **Daidzein** and **genistein** (two bioflavonoids in soybeans) help control excess estrogen. Take 1,000-2,000 mg daily.

• **Fast** for 1-3 days on **fruit and vegetable juices** before the onset of the period, to reduce problems.

• **Pycnogenol** (50 mg once or twice daily) can reduce bloating, fluid retention, and breast tenderness.

AVOID

• **Constipation** is a primary reason why the liver cannot get rid of excess estradiol. Eat **natural foods with sufficient bulk**. Avoid **processed and junk foods**. Estrogen is eliminated through the bowels. Fiber binds with it and carries it out.

• According to the *New England Journal of Medicine*, **vegetarian** women eliminate 2-3 times more estrogen in their feces than nonvegetarians. They eat diets low in fat and high in fiber.

• Eating **chocolate, caffeine, sugar, and excess sodium** are additional causative factors. Women who regularly consume caffeine are four times more likely to have severe PMS. Do not use **nicotine or alcohol. Alcohol, animal fats, and the lactose in milk** products can elevate already high estrogen levels and may contribute to overproduction of pre-period breast cells and other discomforts. The more caffeine consumed, the greater the PMS symptoms.

• It is important that you not eat foods (**meat and dairy products**) **which contain hormones**! They are fed to meat cattle, swine, cows, and chickens. Meat and dairy products help produce a hormonal imbalance—exactly the kind in PMS, excessive estrogen and inadequate progesterone.

• Another factor is unstable **blood sugar levels**. This can be caused by **hypoglycemia** or simply **poor eating habits**. Either way, eat complex carbohydrates and avoid the **sugar foods**.

• **Food allergies** are another factor. Search out the offending foods and stop eating them. *See Allergies (848) and Pulse Test (847).*

• Do not eat **synthetic sugars** (Aspartame, etc.).

OTHER HELPS

• Regular outdoor **exercise** is important. Walk at least half a mile a day. This increases oxygen intake, which in turn aids in nutrient absorption and elimination of toxins.

• Here are herbs which may help reduce the pain of cramps: **rosemary, black haw, cramp bark, red raspberry, and angelica**.

• Use **warm sitz baths, heating pad, or hot-water bottle** for cramps. This draws the healing blood and relaxes muscles.

• Some women with PMS are deficient in **melatonin**.

• When melatonin is low, women do not sleep well. When serotonin is low, they feel tense, depressed, and irritable. This can be interpreted as cravings for sugar, white bread, or alcohol. Exposure to **sunlight** boosts levels of both melatonin and serotonin. For the winter months, buy **full-spectrum light boxes or bulbs**.

• Not keeping the **legs and feet properly clothed** can cause uterine problems, due to pooled blood in the trunk organs.

HERBS

In addition to drinking at least a quart of **water** each day, drink a cup or two of any of the following herbal teas:

• **Wild yam** cream contains *diosgenin*, which helps many women. Rub the cream into the skin on the chest, inner arms, thighs, and abdomen just after ovulation. The active ingredient is absorbed through the skin.

• American Indian women chewed the seeds of the **evening primrose** for premenstrual and menstrual complaints. In Great Britain, **evening primrose oil** is an approved PMS treatment. The product is available commercially; and it is an excellent help.

• **Chinese angelica** (*Angelica sinensis*) is widely used in China to treat PMS and menstrual cramps. Take 2 tablets to help prevent PMS. Do not use if pregnant.

• **Chasteberry** (*Vitex agnus-castus*) is the small fruit of the chaste tree; it has been used for centuries for PMS, by balancing hormones. It increases

R E P

W

production of the luteinizing hormone and inhibits release of the follicle-stimulating hormone. This results in the production of less estrogen. But do not take it if you have significant depression. Chasteberry has proven superior to vitamin B_6 in treating PMS.

• **Skullcap** helps relieve nervous tension and irritability.

• **Raspberry** quiets an irritable uterus. Also used for PMS.

• **Ginger** tea substitutes for the emotional lift of chocolate. It also helps cure the fatigue of PMS.

• Herbs helpful in treating PMS include **dong quai, false unicorn root, fennel seed, squaw vine, blessed thistle, and sarsaparilla root**. They help balance the hormones.

• Take a capsule of **black cohosh, dandelion root, false unicorn root, or skullcap** daily for 10 days before the anticipated onset of menstruation and until 3 days after its cessation.

• Take valerian or chamomile.

• This **calming tea** helps ease premenstrual symptoms: 1 teaspoon **vitex berries**, 1 teaspoon **wild yam root**, ½ teaspoon **burdock root**, ½ teaspoon **dandelion root**, ½ teaspoon **feverfew leaves**, 1 teaspoon **orange peel**, **licorice root, or stevia** (optional), and 4 cups water. Combine the herbs and water. Bring to a boil; then turn off the heat and let steep for at least 20 minutes. Strain out the herbs. Drink at least 2 cups daily.

Discuss the problem with your spouse. This will help him understand the situation.
—*Also see Menstrual Disorders (below) and Breast Discomfort (673).*

ENCOURAGEMENT—The angels of God guard us every moment. Have we not reason to be thankful for the protection we are given? All through the day, thank God for His blessings.

MENSTRUAL DISORDERS
(Amenorrhea, Dysmenorrhea, Metrorrhagia, Oligomenorrhea)

NOTE: Separate articles on some of these topics immediately follow this one.

SYMPTOMS—Depression, tension, melancholia, breast tenderness, cramps, fainting, water retention, rapid heartbeat, and backache may occur.

CAUSES—The first menstruation is also called menarche. Women whose general health and resistance are good are less likely to have menstrual problems.

An irregular cycle often indicates the general state of a woman's health; it is usually the result of nutritional deficiencies or autointoxication caused by constipation, an organic malfunction, drugs, vitamin or mineral deficiency, and/or chemicals or stress.

Amenorrhea: Absence or suppression of menstruation.

Dysmenorrhea: Painful or difficult menstruation.
Metrorrhagia: Bleeding between periods.
Oligomenorrhea: Infrequent or scanty menstruation.

Periods tend to stop in athletes and in women who drop below 20% body fat.

There are two types of dysmenorrhea (painful menstruation):

Primary dysmenorrhea usually does not occur until several years after menstruation begins. The pain begins a few hours before or at the onset of bleeding. This may last from a few hours to 1-2 days; and it is generally worst the first day. At first, there is a scanty flow, which increases as the pain subsides.

Secondary dysmenorrhea may start 2-3 days before onset, with pain in the abdomen, small of back, and on down the legs. It is a more constant pain; but it includes sharp cramps and continues throughout the period. This type is often linked to a pelvic disorder (**inflammation, uterine malposition, endometriosis, tumors**, etc.), which needs to be eliminated in order to lessen or remove the pain.

Important: Because toxic shock *(663)* occurs most frequently during the menstrual period, the women who uses tampons should change them every 3-4 hours, during the day, and use pads during the night. But it is far better for the health not to use tampons at all.

Hormonal imbalance is usually involved. *See Premenstrual Syndrome (676).*

NATURAL REMEDIES
DIET

• The diet should contain an adequate, but not excessive, amount of high quality **proteins**; it, preferably, should be from nonmeat sources.

• Eat complex carbohydrates (**whole grains**), to avoid blood sugar drops. This is important. Low blood sugar is common during menstruation.

• **Avoid overeating**! This encourages abdominal congestion. Do not overeat on anything.

• Fresh, raw **beets, beet juice, or beet powder** is very helpful in regulating all menstrual problems.

• Include **B complex, especially B_{12} and B_6, along with vitamins C and E**. Take **brewer's yeast, kelp, and essential fatty acids**. B vitamins, especially B_6 and **folic acid**, help reduce some of the tensions associated with menstruation. Vitamin B_{12} helps restore normal menstrual cycles.

• Deficiencies of **essential fatty acids**, together with cyclic hormonal patterns, produce the classic symptoms of fragile emotions, irritability, etc.

• Take vitamin A as **beta-carotene** during the last 14 days of the cycle (**Carrot juice, orange and yellow vegetables**).

• **Iron** is vital because of the loss of blood each month. **Vitamin C** helps the body absorb iron. *Beware of supplemental iron tablets during pregnancy!* Iron-rich sources include **blackstrap molasses** (best single source), **apricots, and raisins. Iodine** is also needed, when there is a blood loss. Eat **kelp or dulse**.

• Cramping may be relieved by additional intake of **calcium and niacin**. Calcium supplementation is very important for avoiding painful cramps!

• **Manganese** is needed for normal reproduction and the mammary glands, and helps prevent osteoporosis.

• Limiting **salt and fluid intake** a short time before menstrual onset may help reduce edema in the legs and elsewhere in the body. A low-salt diet helps relieve bloating and water retention.

• **Food allergies** can be involved in painful menstruation. In one study, eight patients were freed of the problem when all foods they were allergic to were eliminated. *See Allergies (848) and Pulse Test (847)*.

• Allergenic foods most frequently listed are **wheat, milk, eggs, beef, chocolate, nuts, fish, beans, cauliflower, pepper, and cabbage**.

• Extreme diets (**strict fruitarianism, very low protein diets, or repeated strict weight loss regimens**) can produce amenorrhea.

• **B-complex vitamins**. These nutrients help to reduce water retention, combat fatigue, and prevent nervous and mental disorders. In fact, **vitamin B$_e$** injections have been used to reduce hot flashes and treat mood disorders. Take a good daily B-complex supplement that provides at least 25 to 50 mg of vitamin B$_6$, 50 to 100 mcg of **vitamin B$_{12}$**, and 400 to 1,000 mcg of **folic acid**.

• **Selenium**. This mineral helps to maintain normal hormone function; some research suggests it may also brighten moods and help fend off heart disease. *Typical dosage*: 200 mcg per day.

• **Acidophilus**: These beneficial bacteria work to prevent vaginitis, yeast infections, and cystitis; these are problems that can crop up more frequently after menopause. *Typical dosage*: 2 to 6 capsules daily or 1 teaspoon of liquid one to three times daily.

• **Evening primrose oil**. This oil contributes to estrogen production and works as a sedative and a diuretic. It has also helped some women control hot flashes. Using flaxseed oil with evening primrose oil can help you maintain a healthy cardiovascular system. *Typical dosage*: 800 to 1,200 mg standardized to 20 percent gamma-linolenic acid (GLA, omega-3), per day. To help your heart, supplement your evening primrose oil with 1 to 2 tablespoons of **flaxseed oil** per day.

OTHER HELPS

• Clinical studies have found that women who engage in **regular physical activity** are half as likely to experience menopausal hot flashes as women who don't. Exercise is also one of the most important weapons against the increased risk of osteoporosis

and heart disease that women are exposed to after menopause. And working up a sweat marshals *endorphins*, the body's own mood-menders and painkillers.

• Most experts recommend an aerobic, **weight-bearing workout** three to five times per week for 35 to 45 minutes. There are lots of exercise options out there, but brisk walking is best. But, if it is not weight-bearing, it does not strengthen bones; so swimming, while it does burn calories and boost aerobic capacity, is not as helpful. Whether your exercise is social or solo, start slowly and check with your doctor or other health practitioner before taking up a new routine. Injuries, even minor ones, can derail good habits before they're ingrained.

• Taking the **birth control pill** greatly upsets the entire hormonal system; and it does not recover, even after the pill is stopped for many months or years.

• Problems with the **pituitary, adrenals, or thyroid** may produce amenorrhea or abnormal bleeding cycles. **Stress** or the **birth control pill** can seriously affect the adrenals (which produce 20% of the total estrogen used by the body).

• **Poor posture** causes the female organs to move out of place; and this can affect menstruation. Proper posture tends to reduce cramping. Do not wear **high heels**; this throws the pelvic organs forward and cramps them.

• Those who have diaphragmatic (**abdominal**) **breathing** tend to have no menstrual pain. **Avoid belts and tight clothing** about the waist. No **corsets**.

• Adequate **exercise** is also needed.

• Avoiding **constipation** is very important.

• Avoid **overfatigue** just prior to the period. Maintain a **regular daily schedule** throughout the month.

• An excess of **stress** can also affect menstrual flow and attendant problems.

• **Sexual stimulation** at that time of the month increases abdominal congestion.

• Not keeping the **legs and feet properly clothed** can cause uterine problems, due to pooled blood in the trunk organs.

• If you are **overweight**, lose weight in order to reduce painful periods.

• Using **tobacco** aggravates menstrual disorders. Smoking induces painful menstruation.

• Here are several easy, noninvasive ways to ease menstrual difficulties:

• Get some sunlight. Some studies suggest that sunlight may help regulate the menstrual cycle. Plus, sunlight produces vitamin D in the body.

• Stay away from fried foods, potato chips, corn chips, crackers, baked goods, and anything that contains hydrogenated oils, including margarine; these may increase menstrual discomfort.

• Check your eating and exercise habits. If

R
E
P

W

excessive exercise, low body fat, or malnutrition is the likely cause of missed periods, increase your caloric intake and decrease the exercise.

• Reduce your sugar intake. To satisfy your sweet tooth, turn to fresh whole fruit in season, carob, nuts, and dried fruit. Eat several small meals per day. This strategy supports the immune system and reduces food cravings and emotional swings.

• Avoid caffeine. Reduce your intake of coffee, chocolate, and tea before and during menstruation.

• Adjust your nutrition. Before your period, increase whole grains in your diet, to help stabilize moodiness. Then, once your period starts, eat fewer whole grains. When it ends, consume more protein.

• Try ginger tea. Ginger tea can relieve nausea and abdominal discomfort (grate 1 to 3 teaspoons of fresh ginger root; add to 1 cup of hot water and steep for 10 to 15 minutes; strain). Drink 1 to 3 cups per day.

• Get regular aerobic exercise. Exercise releases endorphins, the body's natural pain relievers.

HYDROTHERAPY
• Take a daily **hot sitz bath**. If available, add **chamomile or juniper needles** to the water. A **hot sitz bath** (105°-115° F.) **with a hot footbath** (110°-117° F.) for 3-10 minutes is often helpful. Or take **two hot baths** each day at the beginning of menstruation. This draws blood from the over-congested uterus to the skin.

• A four-minute **back massage** to an area an inch to the right of the lumbar (small of the back) spine may bring relief from painful menstruation.

HERBS
• Drink **catnip** tea each morning and evening during the period.

• Helpful herbs include **yarrow, blue cohosh** (in mentrual difficulties), **wormwood, pennyroyal** (when there is painful menstruation). **Chamomile** relieves menstrual spasms. **Peppermint tea** eases the pain. **Desert tea** (*ephedra viridis*) is for delayed or difficult menstruation. Life root (when there is suppressed menstruation), **black cohosh** (when there is obstructed menstruation), **garlic** and **motherwort** (to promote menstrual flow), **amaranth** and **lady's mantle** (when there is excessive menstruation), **blazing star** (for low-ovarian function and lack of estrogen).

• **Red raspberry leaf** tea (1 cup) helps the entire reproductive system.

• Massage **chamomile** into lower abdomen and/or place in bath or in vaporizer.

• Taking **Vitex** (½ tsp. of tincture or 2 capsules, 3 times daily), especially during last two weeks of cycle (after ovulation occurs), helps stimulate progesterone production and normalize the estrogen / progesterone balance.

• This is the herbal formula recommended by Dr. Christopher for female disorders: Mix 4 parts **squaw vine** with 1 part each of **cramp bark, blue cohosh root, and false unicorn root (helonias)**. Add 1 tsp. per cup of water, simmer slowly 5 minutes, and drink 1 cup 3 times a day.

• The following are **emmenagogue plants**. They produce or ease menstruation. As a rule, they have a balancing and normalizing effect on the menstrual cycle. But do not use them during pregnancy, because they increase the risk of abortion: **Rowan, jalop, buck bean, European pennyroyal, laurel, saffron, tarragon, wormwood, basil, German chamomile, Roman chamomile, butterbur, Venus' hair, motherwort, sage, groundsel, wild betony, milfoil, aloe, birchwort, heliotrope, clary, sage, tansy, juniper, wild balm, parsley, madder, mugwort, calendula, rue**. It is fortunate that there are so many useful herbs.

• Pain may be quickly relieved with **squaw vine or bark**, or any emmenagogue. Stimulants should be given to equalize circulation; and **ginger** is excellent. **Pennyroyal and vapor baths** will relieve the colds and congestions.

WILD YAM
Contrary to popular claims, wild yam roots do not contain progesterone; they are not converted into progesterone or dehydroepiandrosterone (DHEA) in the body. But it has properties similar to those compounds. The saponins and similar constituents in wild yam are converted by pharmaceutical firms into progesterone, using a chemical conversion process. But this cannot be duplicated by the body. Wild yam also contains *diosgenin*, but not as much as fenugreek. Shave off the outer bark of the root and make paste of the inner bark in a blender. Mix with oil or water and apply as a salve. Rub it on the abdomen and it will greatly help reduce various symptoms. Wild yam works similarly to progesterone; but it does not contain true progesterone.

—*Also see Premenstrual Syndrome (676), Lack of Menstruation (681), Painful Menstruation (684), Profuse Menstruation (682), Menstrual Cramps (683), and Uterine Fibroids (692).*

ENCOURAGEMENT—All heaven is interested in the work going on in this world, to prepare people to live forever in heaven. It is important that we cooperate with God by accepting Christ as our Saviour and, by faith in Him, obeying His Ten Commandments. 2 Corinthians 9:8, 10.

IRREGULAR MENSTRUATION MENOMETRORRHAGIA

SYMPTOMS—A menstrual cycle that has wide variations in the length of time between periods.

CAUSES—Although the average menstrual cycle lasts 28 days, they may occur as often as every 24 days or as infrequently as every 34 days. After puberty, most women develop a regular cycle; but, for some, they remain irregular. Menstrual bleeding normally lasts 2-4 days, with the average length being 5 days. Wide variations are common at puberty, the first few months after childbirth, and as menopause approaches.

Variations are usually the result of a **temporary hormonal imbalance, stress, depression, severe or chronic illness, excessive exercise, and extreme weight loss**. Other possible causes include **disorders**

of the ovaries or uterus (especially **polycystic ovary syndrome**), in which there is an imbalance of the sex hormones. Or it might be **endometriosis** *(659)*, in which fragments of the tissue that normally lines the uterus are displaced and attached to other pelvic organs. Another cause is an **unsuspected pregnancy**. A single, late, heavy period may be due to a **miscarriage**.

NATURAL REMEDIES

• Raw **beets, beet juice, or beet powder** is very helpful in regulating all menstrual problems.

• **Diets that cause extreme weight loss** can disrupt periods, as can hypoglycemia, nutritional anemia, iodine deficiency, and hypothyroidism.

• **Dong quai** (½ tsp. of tincture or 2 capsules, 3 times daily), taken during the first two weeks of the menstrual cycle, helps regulate hormonal production, particularly estrogen. Do not take during menstruation or pregnancy, because it can stimulate bleeding.

• Gently simmer 1 Tbsp. **elecampane** root 10 minutes in a pint of water. Let cool, strain, drink 1-2 Tbsp. several times daily.

• To promote delayed menstruation, drink **angelica** root tea several times a day. Bruise 2 tsp. of root, simmer in 2 cups boiling water for 15 minutes, strain.

• **Evening primrose** balances the hormonal system. An infusion of **parsley** fruit stimulates and regulates menstruation.

• A decoction of **calendula** flowers helps regulate menstruation.

• An infusion of the flower clusters of **rue** contracts the uterus and helps regulate menstruation.

• An infusion of **mugwort** flowers or root helps regulate menstruation.

• Alternating **hot and cold sitz baths** stimulate pelvic circulation.

—*Also see Lack of Menstruation (below), Menstrual Disorders (above), and Scanty Menstruation (647).*

ENCOURAGEMENT—Godliness is an entire surrender of the will to God. It is living by every word that proceeds from the mouth of God. It is doing the will of our heavenly Father. It is trusting God in trial, in darkness as well as in light. It is walking by faith and not by sight. It is relying on God with unquestioning confidence and resting in His love.

LACK OF MENSTRUATION
(Amenorrhea)

SYMPTOMS—Absence of mentrual periods for at least 3 months in women who would otherwise be menstruating regularly.

CAUSES—There are two types of ammenorrhea. The primary kind refers to menstruation that has not started by the age of 16. If the condition later stops at any time, longer than 3 months, it is secondary.

A late menstrual period that is accompanied by severe abdominal pain should receive immediate medical attention—because it may be due to an ectopic pregnancy *(653; a pregnancy that develops outside the uterus, usually in one of the fallopian tubes)*.

A single, heavy period that is late may be due to a **miscarriage** *(678)*.

NATURAL REMEDIES

• Take **blazing star** tincture (10-30 drops, 3 times daily) for low ovarian function.

• **Pulsatilla** (10 drops of tincture, 3 times daily), especially when due to stress or emotional suppression.

• Simmer bruised **fennel seeds** for 5 minutes in boiling water, cool, strain, and drink frequently.

• **Life root** (10-30 drops tincture, 2-4 times daily) increases local circulation and is a uterine tonic.

J.H. KELLOGG, M.D., PRESCRIPTIONS FOR AMENORRHEA AND ITS COMPLICATIONS (*how to give these water therapies: pp. 206-275 / list of treatments: pp. 206-207 / Hydrotherapy Disease Index: pp. 273-275*)

BASIC APPLICATIONS—Tonic **Sitz Bath**. **Cold Pelvic Pack**. **Graduated Baths**, twice daily, for tonic purposes. Short very **cold Douche** to lower spine, over stomach, and to inner surfaces of thighs. Pelvic massage daily, especially when period is due.

SUPPRESSED MENSTRUATION—Short **Cold Douche** to spine, thighs, and over stomach, daily or twice a day. **Hot Footbath** or **Hot Blanket Pack** during the interval between the periods. **Hot Hip Pack**. Warm **vaginal irrigation** at 95°-100° F.

GENERAL METHOD—It is very necessary to seek for the problem and not merely to "treat a malady." Apply such measures as may be required for relief of anemia, chlorosis, indigestion, or any other disturbance of the nutritive functions.

—*Also see Irregular Menstruation (646), Menstrual Disorders (678), and Scanty Menstruation (below).*

SCANTY MENSTRUATION
(Oligomenorrhea)

SYMPTOMS—An extremely insufficient menstrual flow which is inadequate to provide thorough cleansing.

CAUSES—This problem may be caused by **stress, depression, hormonal imbalance, chronic or severe illness, too much exercise, or extreme weight loss**. Other possible causes include **disorders of the ovaries or uterus**.

NATURAL REMEDIES

• Take **blazing star** (tincture, 10-30 drops, 3 times daily).

R
E
P

W

• To increase flow and elimination, place a **hot-water bottle** over uterus during the period.

—*Also see Menstrual Disorders (678), Lack of Menstruation (681), and Irregular Menstruation (680).*

ENCOURAGEMENT—How thankful we can be that God, who loved us so much that He gave us His Son, is ever ready to help us.

PROFUSE MENSTRUATION
(Menorrhagia)

SYMPTOMS—Menstrual periods that are heavier than normal. There may be a dragging pain in the lower abdomen. Menstruation may also be irregular.

CAUSES—Some women have heavier flows than others. However, if the bleeding lasts longer than 7 days, cannot be controlled by napkins or tampons, or includes large blood clots, it is classed as menorrhagia.

General debility is a primary cause. The condition occurs more frequently in women with **kidney or liver disease**. **Marital excess** is another cause.

About 1 in 20 women have menorrhagia regularly. It is more common when **approaching menopause** *(685)*.

This condition may be caused by **uterine polyps** or **fibroids** *(692)*, or **cancer of the uterus**. *(See Tumors, 782).* It is also a well-known side effect of using an **intrauterine contraceptive device** (IUD). A single, heavy period that is late may be due to a **miscarriage** *(715)* or **ectopic pregnancy** *(688)*. The cause also may be a **hormonal disorder**, such as **hypothyroidism** *(659)*. The condition is more common in **overweight** women. If your periods have always been heavy, there may be no cause for concern. Yet there may be an underlying problem.

If not checked, profuse menstruation can lead to difficult urination, uterine prolapse *(693)*, or leukorrhea *(698)*. It can also produce iron deficiency anemia *(537-539, 713)*, causing lightheadedness and fatigue.

NATURAL REMEDIES

DIET
• Eat plenty of **leafy greens**, plus **trace minerals** (Nova Scotia dulse or Norwegian kelp), to help regulate metabolism.
• Eat omega-3 rich foods; the best is **flaxseed oil** (2 Tbsp. daily). Eat **garlic** for natural sulphur.
• Heavy blood loss can lead to **iron** (simple) anemia *(537-539)*. Iron deficiency can both result from, *and induce,* menorrhagia. Take 1-2 tsp. blackstrap molasses daily. *Do not take extra iron during pregnancy!* This is a must.
• Studies revealed that, taking 25,000 IU of **vitamin A** twice a day for 15 days, showed significant improvement, even to complete normalization of blood loss. But women who are, or could, become pregnant must not take more than 10,000 IU (3,000 mcg) per day. Birth defects could result from taking more.

• **Vitamin E** (100 IU daily for 2 weeks) was found to reduce excessive blood loss caused by the IUD (intrauterine device).
• **Vitamin C** and **bioflavonoids** protect capillaries (small blood vessels) from damage. In one study, 14 of 16 women improved when given 200 mg vitamin C and 200 mg bioflavonoids.
• Add a few grains of **cayenne** to any herbal tea of your choice. Cayenne is able to powerfully regulate bleeding, internally and externally, and may help the menstrual flow.
• Drink diluted **lemon juice** throughout the menstrual period. It will slightly help reduce the flow.
• Restrict intake of **animal products**. Reduce **fried and saturated fatty foods, sugars, and high cholesterol foods**. Avoid **caffeine foods, tobacco, and liquor**.

HERBS
• Here is a special formula to decrease excessive flow during menstruation: Mix equal parts **cranes bill root, red raspberry leaves, witch hazel leaves, uva-ursi leaves, shepherd's purse, papaya leaves, and black haw bark**. Drink it and apply externally in compresses. This formula can also be used for hemorrhoids.
• Make a strong tea of **red raspberry** leaves to control an excessive flow. Drink a half cup of strong **thyme** tea each morning and evening to control excessive flow. Also apply a compress of the tea to the pelvic area.
• Take **amaranth** (tincture, 15-25 drops, 3-4 times daily).
• Shepherd's purse is good at stopping hemorrhaging anywhere in the body. Drink 2 cups, 3 times daily. Also apply a compress, soaked in the tea, to the pelvic area during excessive flow.
• **Two other astringent teas are good: agrimony and cranes bill** (3 cups, 3 times daily).
• Hemostatic herbs which help regulate menstruation include **mistletoe** (infusion or cold extract of dry leaves), **hazelnut** (decoction of leaves and bark), and **nettle** (infusion of fresh juice of the leaves).
• **Horsetail** heals bleeding tissues; use a decoction of the plant. **Blind nettle** (an infusion of the leaves and flower clusters) stops excessive blood loss. **Calendula** (decoction of the flowers) is a menstrual regulator. **Knotweed** (decoction of the plant) increases capillary resistance.
• **Witch hazel** stops bleeding and strengthens venous and capillary walls. Use an infusion of leaves and/or bark.
• An infusion of fresh **smartweed** reduces too abundant menstruation. An infusion of **goldenseal** contracts the uterus and reduces bleeding.
• Blend this **tincture for too-heavy periods**, and keep it on hand for times when your menstrual flow is uncomfortably heavy: 1 teaspoon **shepherd's purse** tincture, 1 teaspoon **yarrow** tincture, ½ teaspoon **red raspberry** leaf tincture, and ½ teaspoon **vitex** tincture. Combine all of the ingredients in a dark glass jar with a tight seal. Take three dropperfuls every 15 to 30 minutes for very heavy bleeding or two dropperfuls

every hour for moderately heavy bleeding. (Try to purchase shepherd's purse tincture made from the fresh herb; it loses some of its strength when dried.)

• **B-complex vitamins**. These nutrients help to reduce water retention, combat fatigue, and prevent nervous and mental disorders. In fact, **vitamin B**$_e$ injections have been used to reduce hot flashes and treat mood disorders. Take a good daily B-complex supplement that provides at least 25 to 50 mg of vitamin B$_6$, 50 to 100 mcg of **vitamin B**$_{12}$, and 400 to 1,000 mcg of **folic acid**.

• **Selenium**. This mineral helps to maintain normal hormone function; some research suggests it may also brighten moods and help fend off heart disease. *Typical dosage: 200 mcg per day.*

• **Acidophilus**: These beneficial bacteria work to prevent vaginitis, yeast infections, and cystitis; these are problems that can crop up more frequently after menopause. *Typical dosage: 2 to 6 capsules daily or 1 teaspoon of liquid one to three times daily.*

• **Evening primrose oil**. This oil contributes to estrogen production and works as a sedative and a diuretic. It has also helped some women control hot flashes. Using flaxseed oil with evening primrose oil can help you maintain a healthy cardiovascular system. *Typical dosage: 800 to 1,200 mg standardized to 20 percent gamma-linolenic acid (GLA, omega-3), per day.* To help your heart, supplement your evening primrose oil with 1 to 2 tablespoons of **flaxseed oil** per day.

OTHER HELPS

• Not keeping the **legs and feet properly clothed** can cause uterine problems. Blood is chilled back from the extremities and pools in the trunk organs.

• Get extra **sleep** during that time. Avoid all **drugs**, including aspirin. Many inhibit vitamin K formation.

• For excessive bleeding or pain, apply an **ice pack** to the uterus, pubic, or sacral region. **Hot compresses** applied to the legs and feet will enhance the action of removing blood from the pelvic region.

• After the period is over, take a warm douche of **white oak bark, wild alum root, or bayberry bark**. Steep 1 heaping tsp. to a quart of boiling water, let steep while covered. Inject 4-5 times a day with a bulb syringe. In addition, drink the herb teas.

• If periods are extremely profuse, make small balls of absorbent cotton, immerse in a tea of equal parts **white oak bark** and **wild alum root**, plus a little **lobelia**. Tie a strong cord around the middle, long enough to extend to the outside. Press it against the vagina. Every 12 hours, remove the ball and wash with an herb douche.

—*Also see Menstrual Disorders (678), Uterine Bleeding (691), Vaginal Discharge (698), Uterine Fibroids (692).*

ENCOURAGEMENT—He who has given His precious life because He loved you, and wanted you to be happy, will always be mindful of your problems. He can provide you with encouragement and help, as no one else can.

MENSTRUAL CRAMPS

SYMPTOMS—Strong cramping sensations during menstruation. A cramping lower abdominal pain that comes in waves, radiating to the lower back and down the legs. Dragging pain in the pelvis.

CAUSES—This is a severe form of dysmenorrhea *(684).*

NATURAL REMEDIES

—*Also see Painful Menstruation (below).*

• The diet should be light and simple. Primarily eat **fresh fruits and vegetables. Do not overeat.**

• Omega-3 fatty acids (2-4 tsp. **flaxseed oil** daily) keeps prostaglandins trapped in cells, so they cannot enter muscle tissue and trigger spasms.

• Avoid *arachidonic acid* (a type of fatty acid), which is found in **meat, diary products, and palm kernel oil** (a common ingredient in processed foods). **Reduce salt intake. Food allergies** *(848)* are sometimes a cause.

• **Niacin** helps relieve cramps. Take 25-200 mg, beginning 7-10 days before menstruation begins.

• **Vitamin B**$_6$ helps convert fatty acids to a form which helps produce pain-relieving chemicals.

• **Vitamin C** helps strengthen the uterine intake of nutrients and discharge of toxins. Take 1,000-3,000 mg daily, especially when symptoms are experienced.

• **Magnesium** (1,000 mg) and **vitamin E** (800-1,000 IU daily) are also important. Studies show that taking this vitamin helps reduce menopausal symptoms.

• **Calcium** is a great wonder-worker, when it comes to relaxing muscles and reducing pain. Take 1,000-5,000 mg daily.

HYDROTHERAPY

One of any of the following hydrotherapy methods will probably help you greatly:

• Place an **ice pack** over the abdomen.

• Place a **heating pad or hot-water bottle** to the abdomen or back.

• With the first sign of pain, place a **heating pad** to the back from the waist to the end of the spine. Keep the heat high.

• Take a **warm bath**.

• Take a **hot sitz (sitting) bath** (105°-115° F.) with a hot footbath (110°-117° F.) for 3-10 minutes.

• Take a **cold sitz bath** (55°-75° F.) for 2-10 minutes while constantly rubbing the skin.

HERBS

• Women of several Indian tribes (Cherokee,

R
E
P

W

Delaware, Iroquois, Oklahoma, and Menominee) regularly took **squaw vine** tea for menstrual pain. They also used it to make childbirth easier and to treat sore nipples while nursing. Use it with red raspberry tea for better effect.

• According to a special German research team, **strawberry** leaf tea relieves menstrual cramping. Also recommended for this purpose is **yarrow** tea.

• **Chinese angelica** (also known as **dong-quai, or dang quai**) is one of the most widely used herbs in Chinese herbal medicine. Considered a female tonic, it is especially used for menstrual cramping.

• **Red raspberry** leaf tea is used by many women to reduce period cramping. It is also used to soothe uterine irritability during pregnancy.

• Here are several other very effective anti-cramping herbs used by women: **Bilberry** contains *anthocyanidins*, which relax muscles. **Ginger** contains 6 pain-relieving compounds and 6 anti-cramping compounds. **Red clover** has phytoestrogens, which reduce cramping by balancing hormones better. **Chasteberry** fruits are also good for reducing menstrual cramping.

• A combination of **ginger, valerian, black haw, and motherwort** is very helpful in relieving menstrual cramps. Black haw specifically relaxes the uterus.

• **Motherwort** alone can stop menstrual cramps. Take 5 drops of motherwort extract, keep increasing it until the cramps stop; then take that amount each time cramps begin.

OTHER HELPS

• Continue taking regular outdoor **exercise**. It has been proven that those who exercise have less pain. The best exercises are those which involve the pelvis and legs: **waist-bending,** and **leg exercises. Walk up 100 steps** and back down every day.

• If you are **overweight**, you need to reduce. This will significantly lessen painful periods.

• Maintain **regularity** in times for rising, sleeping, eating, and exercise.

• Improve your **posture**, and the pain will lessen. Women who do diaphragmatic (abdominal) breathing, experience less problems.

• Every so often, take a brief **rest** period, with your **feet elevated**. This will bring healing blood to the abdominal area.

—*Also see Painful Menstruation (below), Pelvic Pain (689), and Menstrual Disorders (678).*

ENCOURAGEMENT—Come daily to Jesus, who loves you. Open your heart to Him freely. In Him there is no disappointment. You will never find a better counselor, a safer guide, a more sure defense.

PAINFUL MENSTRUATION
(Dysmenorrhea)

SYMPTOMS—Lower abdominal pain and discomfort experienced just before or during menstruation. The pain may be accompanied by any of the symptoms of premenstrual syndrome *(676).* These symptoms can be headache, breast tenderness, and abdominal bloating.

CAUSES—Up to three-fourths of women have menstrual period pain. In about one-fifth of these women, the pain is severe enough to disrupt normal activities. The pain is usually experienced within the 24 hours before menstruation or the first few days of the period.

Primary dysmenorrhea occurs in the early teens. One to two years after periods begin, ovulation generally begins. An increase in *prostaglandins* occurs some days after ovulation and makes the uterine muscles contract. This contraction interferes with blood supply and causes pain. This type of pain lessens after the age of 25 and, generally, disappears by age 30. It becomes less severe after childbirth.

The *secondary* type occurs in women who previously had little menstrual pain. Affecting women, aged 20-40, it is often caused by **endometriosis** *(694)* or **uterine fibroids** *(692).* A **chronic infection** of the reproductive organs or the use of an **intrauterine contraceptive device** (IUD) are other causes.

NATURAL REMEDIES
—*Also see Menstrual Cramps (683).*
• Drink **catnip** tea each morning and evening during the period. Place 1 tsp. of the powder in a cup of boiling water. Let steep, cool, and drink.

• **Strawberry** leaf tea, taken over a number of months, will eventually help regulate the flow.

• **Chamomile** tea gently relieves painful spasms.

• **Peppermint** tea aids digestion and reduces bloat and pain.

• The following are **uterine antispasmodic herbs**. They relax the spasm of the uterine muscles, thus alleviating dysmenorrhea and many female pelvic pains caused by uterine spasms. These herbs also exert antispasmodic action, though not as specific, on other hollow organs (such as the intestines and urinary pathways): **calendula, rue, wild betony, cramp bark, venus' hair, buck bean, Roman chamomile, pasqueflower.**

J.H. KELLOGG, M.D., PRESCRIPTIONS FOR PAINFUL MENSTRUATION AND ITS COMPLICATIONS (*how to give these water therapies: pp. 207-272 / list of treatments: pp. 206-207 / Hydrotherapy Disease Index: pp. 273-275*)

BASIC—Rest in bed during period.

WHEN DUE TO OVARIAN DISEASE (beginning before flow)—Hot **Hip and Leg Pack**, Hot Blanket Pack, **Fomentation** over stomach, hot Pelvic Pack, **Revulsive Sitz**, hot **Colonic**. Follow with hot **Footbath** if flow is checked. Hot Douche at 99°-102° F. Also very Hot **Full Bath** (105°-110° F.) for 5-8 minutes.

WHEN DUE TO UTERINE DISEASE (beginning with, and accompanying, flow)—Hot **Hip Pack** with Hot **Footbath**, followed by Cold **Compress** to area above stomach and inner surfaces of thighs for 30-40 seconds.

WHEN DUE TO INFLAMMATORY DISEASE OF APPENDAGES—Hot **Enema**, hot **Fomentations**, Hot **Pelvic Pack**, Hot Blanket Pack.

GENERAL METHOD—In addition to the local measures for relief of pain which have been indicated above, it is, in most cases, necessary to combat some general disorder to which the local disease may be, more or less, directly related. See "Anemia," "Neurasthenia," "Hysteria." General tonic measures must be used between the menstrual periods. In chronic ovarian congestion, apply the stomach compress during the night. Also give a daily Revulsive Sitz Bath or Hot Pelvic Pack and the very hot vaginal irrigation, 115°-120° F., for 15 minutes. In cases of deficient development, as in infantile uterus or nerve spasm of the uterine vessels, employ the Revulsive Sitz Bath, alternate genito-urinary douche, tonic sitz bath, pelvic and general massage. Surgical measures are often required for permanent relief. But a surprisingly large number of cases are resolvable without surgery; hence water therapies should be perseveringly tried before resorting to surgical procedures.

—*Also see Menstrual Cramps (683), Pelvic Pain (689), Menstrual Disorders (678), and Uterine Fibroids (692).*

ENCOURAGEMENT—Disappointments you will have; but ever bear in mind that Jesus, the living and risen Saviour, is your Redeemer and your Restorer.

MENSTRUAL FLUID RETENTION

SYMPTOMS—Hands, and especially feet, tend to swell during menstruation.

CAUSES—Hormonal imbalances cause the tissues to take up an excess of water.

NATURAL REMEDIES

• Reduce **salt** intake. Read labels and avoid foods containing **sodium**. Take no salt, especially from a week before the period starts to the onset of the period. All dairy products are high in salt.

• Take **dandelion leaf tea** if there is water retention.

• **White birch tea** increases the volume of urine and reduces tissue swelling. Use an infusion of leaves and/or buds.

—*For much more information, see Edema (494, 714) and Menstrual Disorders (678).*

ENCOURAGEMENT—Through all your trials you can have a never-failing Friend who has said, "I am with you alway, even unto the end of the world."

MENOPAUSE
(Post-Menstrual Syndrome, Climacteric, Change of Life)

SYMPTOMS—Hot flashes, insomnia, disturbances in calcium metabolism, irritability, mental instability, dizziness, backaches, headaches, bladder problems, dryness and aging of the skin, shortness of breath, and heart palpitations. Some have almost no symptoms at all, other than absence of menses.

CAUSES—Menopause is the cessation of ovarian function, the stopping of the menstrual cycle, and the end of the reproductive years. Glandular changes cause this to happen. It is a natural event in a woman's life; and it usually occurs between 42 and 55. The average age is about 50; and the transition is generally up to 5 years.

While it is occurring, there tends to be a hormone starvation; since menopause usually results from a decreased production of female sex hormones.

The lessened supply of estrogen increases the possibility of cardiovascular disease *(513-545)*, osteoporosis *(612)*, and vaginal atrophy.

It is popular to take estrogen supplements, to prevent or postpone menopausal symptoms. But keep in mind that there is an increased risk of cancer when this is done unwisely. *See Hormone Replacement Therapy Disorder (687).* Some recommend that oral estrogens should not be accompanied by progesterone because they increase the risk of cancer, especially of the uterus or breast. Others disagree with that.

Keep in mind that synthetic, not natural, estrogens are given in hormone replacement therapy. These tend to accumulate in the body and can also cause metabolic changes in the liver. This can lead to high blood pressure, fluid retention, and blood clots. But natural estrogens are available. One is equine estrogen; this is extracted from the urine of pregnant mares. But it is very powerful and may also cause changes in the liver. Do not use it if you are obese, smoke, or have high blood pressure, high cholesterol, or varicose veins.

Somewhat safer estrogens are estropipate (Ogen) and estradiol (Estrace, Emcyt, and Estraderm); these are all metabolized more easily by your body. Be sure and use the smallest possible dose; and take it only every other day.

It is coming to be recognized that it is often more important to replace the lessened progesterone than the lessened estrogen. Natural progesterone-like creams (from the herb, **wild yam,** which contains *diosgenin*) provide a simplified way to do this. Many, many, have been helped by doing this! *(See the note on wild yam in Menstrual Disorders, 678.)*

When the menopause proceeds normally, the adrenals and liver increase their output of female hormones and make up the difference from the lost ovarian function.

Proper diet, nutritional supplements, exercise, and adequate rest can minimize the effects of menopause.

NATURAL REMEDIES
DIET

• Smart eating, begun in the years that precede menopause, may help to decrease unwanted

R
E
P

W

---

symptoms.

• Vegetables from the cruciferous family—**broccoli, Brussels sprouts, cabbage, cauliflower, kale, kohlrabi, rutabagas, and turnips**—may help the body make substances called *indoles*. These help protect women from the dangerous effects of excess estrogen, among them breast cancer. Plus they are all good sources of vitamins and fiber. If you eat them without cheese sauce, they're all low-fat.

• Here are more excellent foods: **Whole grains. Garlic. Sesame seeds. Whole grain pastas. Sunflower seeds. Flaxseed oil. Almonds. Dates. Fresh vegetables. Pomegranates. Fresh fruits.**

• Here are foods and substances to avoid: **Rich dairy products. Caffeine. Sugar. Alcohol. Fried foods. Cigarettes. Red meats. Nicotine.**

• **Raw fruit and vegetable juices, brewer's yeast, lecithin, kelp, and cold-pressed vegtable oils** are needed. The diet should be at least 50% **raw food**.

• Hypothyroidism *(659)* is common during menopause; this is responsible for a number of the symptoms. So be sure to take additional amounts of **Nova Scotia dulse or Norwegian kelp**.

• Mounting evidence suggests that getting enough of certain vitamins and other nutrients can make menopause a breeze.

• Vitamin E. Tests dramatically support its use for hot flashes and other symptoms of menopause. In some tests, vitamin E worked better than barbiturates to calm anxiety, cool hot flashes, protect against heart disease, and ease vaginal dryness. *Typical dosage:* 200 to 800 IU per day.

• Vitamin C with bioflavonoids. Clinical studies of women in menopause found that half experienced relief from discomfort by using vitamin C with the bioflavonoid hesperidin. Leg cramps, bruising, and hot flashes significantly decreased. *Typical dosage:* 500 to 5,000 milligrams per day.

• Calcium/magnesium. This dynamic duo of minerals helps prevent osteoporosis and ease mental stress and anxiety. In fact, adding supplemental calcium to the diet as early, as age 20, can increase bone density, which puts you ahead in the race against bone loss after menopause. Use absorbable forms—such as calcium citrate, gluconate, or carbonate. *Typical dosage:* 1,000 to 1,500 milligrams of calcium per day in a 2:1 ratio with magnesium. So if you take 1,000 milligrams of calcium, take 500 milligrams of magnesium, too.

• If estrogen (hormone replacement) therapy is begun, take **vitamin E** several hours earlier or later, not at the same time. Daily taking up to 1,200 IU of vitamin E is especially important during this time.

• In addition, generous amounts of vitamins **B_6** (500 mg), **C** (1,000 mg), **folic acid** (5 mg), **pantothenic acid** (200 mg), **PABA** (100 mg), and **B_{12}** (1,000 mg) will make the estrogen therapy more effective. **Vitamin C** works with bioflavonoids (100 mg) to maintain capillary strength. **Pantothenic** acid and **PABA** relieve nervous irritability.

• It is very important that sufficient **calcium** (4,000 mg) be taken, to maintain a proper calcium-phosphorus balance. After menopause begins, you will not have as much calcium in your body, due to the lessened estrogen; it is important that you henceforth supplement with calcium. Of the 250,000 hip fractures that occur in the U.S. every year, 80% are due to osteoporosis *(612)*.

• An increase in **protein** and reduction in **carbohydrates** is recommended at this time.

• Maintain an adequate intake of **vitamin D** (1,000 IU), **iron** (50 mg), and **magnesium** (1,000 mg).

• Eliminate all **processed, refined, and junk foods**. This includes **white sugar** and **white-flour products**.

• Avoid **animal products** and **dairy products**.

• Do not use **alcohol, caffeine, spicy foods, sugar, hot soups or drinks**. They make the emotional swings worse and the blood more acidic. This causes the bones to release extra calcium, to balance blood pH and weaken the bones if extra calcium is not taken.

• Substitute **garlic** and **onion** powder for salt. Consuming **salt** increases urinary excretion of calcium.

• Studies reveal that menopausal hot flashes and sweating are sometimes caused by **food, or other, allergies**. *See Allergies (848) and Pulse Test (847).*

OTHER HELPS

• Drink 2 quarts of **water** each day, to help prevent drying of skin and mucous membranes.

• Avoid mental / emotional **stress** and **worry**. Be happy with the blessings you have; and thank God for them.

• Get plenty of outdoor **exercise** and sufficient **rest**. Lie down and rest a little before lunch and supper. A lack of exercise weakens bone density.

• The body expels toxins during menstruation. When it ceases, the body may instead use hot flashes to eliminate them. In a research study, women who took a 20-minute **sauna or steam bath,** for 6 out of 7 days for a month, experienced almost total relief from hot flashes. (Instead of a steam bath, you can take a **hot bath** for 20 minutes a day.)

• Avoid **hot environments. Stay cool**. Dress in "layered" fashion, so you can take outer clothing on and off. Do not eat hot meals.

• Try to be **calm and relaxed**. Only do one thing at a time and avoid becoming anxious.

HERBS

• Here is a formula recommended by Dr. Christopher: Mix 2 parts each **squaw vine, rue, red raspberry leaves, white pond lily** with 1 part each of **ginger root, chamomile, spearmint, uva ursi leaves, and black cohosh root**. Add 1 tsp. to boiling water, cover tightly, and let cool. Drink 2 fl. oz. every 2 hours or as needed.

• In one study, 80% of women who used the natural progesterone hormone for 1 year reported improvement from hot flashes. Apply a cream, containing **wild yam**, to the pelvic area.

• **Black cohosh** (20 mg of tablets, twice daily) and **motherwort** (½-1 cup tea, 3 times daily) are extremely helpful herbs.

• **Sage** (½-1 cup tea, 3 times daily) tea is good for a woman having hot flashes throughout the day.

• **Siberian ginseng** (200-1,000 mg, in 3 divided doses, daily) helps restore energy and cool hot flashes.

• **St. John's wort** also helps reduce menopausal symptoms.

• Several research studies have been done on **black cohosh, dong quai, licorice root, and Chinese (or Korean) ginseng**. All were found to be very effective in treating menopausal symptoms.

—See Menstrual Disorders (678) for related information. Important: Also see Hormone Replacement Therapy (below) and Postmenopausal Bleeding (687).

ENCOURAGEMENT—All the instructions we need to obey God are found in the Bible. Read it everyday; and, accompanied by earnest prayer for help, you will receive the strength needed to fulfill God's will one day at a time. Psalm 34:9-10.

HORMONE REPLACEMENT THERAPY DISORDER

FACTS ABOUT HRT—Hormone Replacement Therapy (HRT) is given to help reduce problems during, and after, menopause. The female sex hormone, estrogen, relieves hot flashes, vaginal dryness, and other discomforts of menopause. Some research indicates that it may also increase a woman's risk of getting cancer of the breast or some other part of the reproductive system. Other research shows that including progesterone as part of the therapy reduces that risk somewhat.

HRT is associated with a dramatic increase in uterine cancer, along with a smaller but still significant increase in breast cancer. Progesterone is given to reduce the risk of uterine cancer; but it also reduces HDL cholesterol in the bloodstream, making women more at risk of heart disease and stroke.

HRT should be avoided if you have a personal or family history of cancer of the breast, ovaries, uterus, etc.

If you take HRT, also take a low dose of estrogen (1.25 mg daily, maximum). Never take HRT without progesterone for at least part of the monthly cycle.

Medical literature is filled with warnings both for and against using HRT. Physicians keep using it because it seems to accomplish good results.

It is true that HRT also reduces the risk of heart disease *(513)* and osteoporosis *(612)*. But a woman may wish to consider natural remedies to prevent them.

HRT can increase the size of uterine fibroids *(692)*.

NATURAL SOLUTIONS

• Eat **nourishing food, consisting of fruits, vegetables, whole grains, legumes, and nuts**. Hot flashes and other menopausal symptoms are rare among people groups which are vegetarian, especially those consuming lots of legumes (beans, especially soybeans). This is because beans and many other plants contain *phytoestrogens*, which produce a mild estrogenic activity in the body. These compounds include *lignans, saponins, isoflavones, and phytosterols. Phytoestrogens* reduce the risk of estrogen-linked cancers. One cup of soybeans, for example, contains the equivalent of 1 tablet of Premarin, a synthetic hormone used in estrogen replacement therapy.

HERBS
• A number of herbs are helpful. Wild yam contains *diosgenin*, similar to natural progesterone. Drink tea and rub salve on the pelvic area.

• **Red clover** contains 1-2.5% *isoflavones*. In one research study, postmenopausal women who ate **clover, flaxseed, and soy** for 2 weeks, had definitely higher estrogen levels; this declined when they left the diet.

• **Alfalfa, chasteberry, strawberry, and Chinese angelica** are also extremely good.

• In one study, menopausal women given **black cohosh** root extract, showed significant estrogenic activity. In another study, it reduced vaginal dryness.

• **Licorice** contains *glycyrrhizin*, which reduces estrogen levels in women, when too high; it also increases estrogen levels in women, when too low. Use licorice herb, not the candy. Many licorice products contain anise, which has anethole; this is less estrogenic.

—Also see Menopause (685) and Menstrual Disorders (678).

ENCOURAGEMENT—We must not study to have our own way, but God's way and His will. We suffer when we step out of the path that God has chosen for us to follow. The sure result is affliction, unrest, and sorrow which we might have avoided if we had submitted our will to God. Let us bow in humility before God and follow the path that He chooses for us. That is the only safe path.

POSTMENOPAUSAL BLEEDING

SYMPTOMS—Bleeding from the uterus, which occurs at least 6 months after menstruation has stopped.

CAUSES—Normally, menstruation ceases at the end of menopause. But there are instances in which this does not happen. Postmenopausal bleeding (PMB) should be normalized only with certain forms of hormone replacement therapy, which limits bleeding to once each month. Any other PMB which occurs indicates a serious disorder. Whatever the cause, PMB is

R
E
P

W

generally painless; it ranges from light spotting to a heavier flow of blood.

The most common and least serious cause of PMB is atrophic vaginitis; the vagina becomes inflamed, due to a decline in estrogen after menopause.

The cause could be a disorder of the cervix, such as cervical erosion or cancer of the cervix. In such instances, bleeding is more likely to occur after intercourse.

The cause of PMB could be a thickened endometrium (the lining of the uterus), cancerous growths, or non-cancerous growths in the uterus (see uterine polyps, 693).

You will want to consult your physician. If the cause is not serious, the use of astringent herb teas and douches can help eliminate the problem.

NATURAL REMEDIES

• A large collection of helps will be found in the section, *Profuse Menstruation (682)*, which explains ways to reduce uterine bleeding. Also see *Uterine Bleeding (691) and Uterine Fibroids (692)*.

ENCOURAGEMENT—A faithful fulfillment of home duties and filling the position you can occupy to the best advantage, be it ever so simple and humble, is truly elevating. In doing this, there is peace and sacred joy. It possesses healing power. It will secretly and insensibly soothe the wounds of the soul, and even the sufferings of the body. Humbly trusting in Jesus and doing the best you can to help those around you will bring great encouragement to your own heart.

VAGINAL DOUCHE

HOW TO DO IT—A douche is especially helpful if one has a history of discharges or infection (primarily vaginitis, 695). But do not use it otherwise.

• Retention douches are quite effective and are best done in a bathtub with the feet up on the sides, to aid in retaining the fluid for 10-15 minutes. Warm the douche to body temperature before taking. Possible douches include:

• Add 4-8 ounces of diluted **vinegar** to a pint of distilled water.

• Add 4-8 ounces of **hydrogen peroxide** and 1 ounce of **bayberry myrtle** (myrica cerifera) to 1 pint water.

• A replant of **lactobacillus acidophilus** may be needed, to normalize flora after vaginitis or antibiotic drug medications. Acidophilus capsules (6-8) from a health-food store) or 4 oz. of plain, unsweetened yogurt can be emptied into warm water (10-20 oz.).

• Routine douching is not necessary for personal hygiene. Douching is best reserved for therapy, in time of infection. Excessive douching may actually help promote infection.

• If herbal douches are used, they should be steeped for many minutes in water that has just been boiled; then store this preparation in a sterile environment until used.

• Mix equal parts of **chamomile, wintergreen,**

and sage. Add ½ cup to 2 cups boiling-hot water, let steep 10-20 minutes, strain. Add warm, sterile water to make up the full amount. Best to use immediately. This is used to soothe and heal; also for abnormal discharges.

Another herbal douche formula is equal parts of **peppermint, comfrey, spearmint, and wax myrtle**. Prepare in the same manner as the above formula.

WARNING—Douching may induce pelvic inflammatory disease (PID, 690). In one study, almost 90% of the women with PID were vigorous douchers, often since the age of 16 or 17. Very likely, infected fluid has been flushed up into the uterine cavity by the douche.

Regular douching can kill beneficial microorganisms and leave you open for invasion by the infection-causing variety of microorganisms.

ENCOURAGEMENT—Home is to be the center of the purest and most elevated affections. Through prayer and earnest effort, each person in the home is submitted to be molded by the Spirit of God. Home can become a little heaven. Isaiah 1:18.

ECTOPIC PREGNANCY

SYMPTOMS—**This specifically refers to a late menstrual period that is accompanied by severe abdominal pain. Because of this symptom, this disorder is placed here instead of in the section on Pregnancy.**

CAUSES—*If this symptom occurs, you should see a physician immediately.* You may have an ectopic pregnancy. This is a pregnancy that develops outside the uterus, usually in one of the two fallopian tubes.

Because of the seriousness of the situation, this topic is placed here along with menstrual problems, with cross-references to the pregnancy section (702-721).

About 1 in 100 pregnancies is ectopic. This means that the fertilized egg has become implanted in the tissues outside the uterus instead of in the lining of the uterus. Where it is implanted, the egg begins developing into an embryo. In most ectopic pregnancies, the fertilized egg lodges inside one of the two fallopian tubes. Much more rarely, the egg implants in the cervix or in the abdominal cavity. Unfortunately, a fetus which cannot grow normally, cannot survive. If the placenta develops inside a fallopian tube, the tube will eventually rupture (break open). This will immediately result in life-threatening bleeding into the mother's abdominal cavity. Such pregnancies need to be surgically removed as soon as possible.

Ectopic pregnancies are more common in women aged 20 to 29, primarily those exposed to sexually transmitted diseases (especially gonorrhea). Here are other causes: Previous **damage to one of the fallopian tubes** obstructs the passage of a fertilized egg to the uterus. This damage may be caused by an **unsuccessful sterilization procedure** ("tying the tubes"). But an ectopic pregnancy is also more common in women using **intrauterine contraceptive devices** (IUDs). This is due to the fact that these devices increase the risk of a pelvic infection, if the woman is exposed to sexually transmitted diseases. Another cause is Pelvic Inflammatory Disease *(655)*. You are especially at risk if you have had a previous ectopic pregnancy. Having one increases the risk of later having another.

A physician can measure levels of chronic gonadotropin (hCG), a hormone produced by the placenta which increases in quantity until the end of the first trimester. If it is not increasing, the next step is to do an ultrasound to locate where the fetus is growing.

ENCOURAGEMENT—A home where love dwells and where it finds expression in looks, in words, in acts, is a place where angels delight to dwell. Let the sunshine of love, cheer, and happy content enter your own hearts; and let its sweet influence pervade the home . . The atmosphere thus created will be to the children what air and sunshine are to the vegetable world, promoting health and vigor of mind and body.

While grief and anxiety cannot remedy a single evil, they can do great harm; but cheerfulness and hope, while they brighten the pathway of others, "are life unto those that find them and health to all their flesh." Trust in Jesus, and He will help you to the very end. He is faithful who hath promised.

REPRODUCTIVE: WOMEN -
3 - FEMALE PELVIC ORGANS

PELVIC CONGESTION

SYMPTOMS—A feeling of heaviness and discomfort in the pelvic area. It may result in fatigue or depression.

CAUSES—The preceding sections on menstrual problems cited a wide variety of possible causes, ranging from poor diet to hormonal imbalances. In this present section, we will consider a number of water therapies which were used a century ago by the world's leading hydrotherapy expert.
—*Also see Menstrual Disorders (678).*

NATURAL REMEDIES

J.H. KELLOGG, M.D., PRESCRIPTIONS FOR PELVIC CONGESTION AND ITS COMPLICATIONS *(how to give these water therapies: pp. 207-272 / list of treatments: pp. 206-207 / Hydrotherapy Disease Index: pp. 273-275)*
BASIC APPLICATIONS—Graduated cold applications. Hot **vaginal irrigation**, 10-15 minutes, twice daily.

Hot **Blanket Pack** to legs with cold pelvic pack (Wet Sheet Pack over pelvic area), continued to sweating stage. Follow with **cold friction** or Wet Sheet Rub.
PAIN—Prolonged Neutral **Sitz Bath** at 95°-97° F., for 15-20 minutes.
LEUKORRHEA—In addition to the above measures, antiseptic **vaginal irrigation** is recommended. In certain cases, cool irrigation, at 75°-65° F., produces better results than hot irrigation. Constipation and portal congestion must be relieved. Cervical catarrh and erosions often require the use of the curette [a spoon-shaped scraping instrument for scraping foreign matter from a cavity].
ACUTE INFLAMMATION—If attacks of inflammation occur, **rest** in bed; Hot **Hip or Leg Pack**; hot and cold **pelvic compress** or hot and cold pelvic pack.

PELVIC PAIN

SYMPTOMS—Pain in the pelvic area, the cause of which may or may not be due to problems in the female reproductive organs.

CAUSES—Pains in the pelvic region should be identified. The cause could be a problem in the uterus, ovaries, vagina, bowels, or anus. If the pain is on the left or right rear side, the problem is in the kidneys.
—*See Menstrual Cramps (683), Painful Menstruation (684), Menstrual Disorders (678), Pelvic Inflammatory Disease (690), Kidney Problems (489), Renal Colic (492), Colitis (463), and Hemorrhoids (469, 712).*

NATURAL REMEDIES

J.H. KELLOGG, M.D., PRESCRIPTIONS FOR PELVIC CONGESTION AND ITS COMPLICATIONS *(how to give these water therapies: pp. 207-272 / list of treatments: pp. 206-207 / Hydrotherapy Disease Index: pp. 273-275)*
BASIC FACTORS—Remove all known causes: tight bands around the waist, tight shoes, cold extremities, sexual excess.
GENERAL APPLICATIONS—Rest in a horizontal position, with proper general treatment for any existing general or local morbid condition (as anemia, neurasthenia, hysteria, enteroptosis, constipation, or any discoverable pelvic disease). If caused by neuralgia: Give hot **Hip and Leg Pack** or very hot **Revulsive Sitz**, 3 times a day. **Hot-water bottle** over seat of pain and **heat** to feet and legs. Very hot **vaginal irrigation**.
If due to chronic congestion in a pelvic organ: Hot **Hip and Leg Pack** every 2-4 hours, with abdominal **Heating Compress** and heating **leg packs** during the interval between.
If due to inflammation or acute congestion: Hot Hip and Leg Pack or Hot and Cold **Pelvic Pack** every 2-4 hours. Follow by continuous **heat** to legs with **cooling compress** to lower abdomen, external genitals, and inner surfaces of thighs. **Vaginal irrigation** at 105° F. for 15 minutes, every 3 hours. Apply **Ice Bag** over seat of pain during the hot

vaginal irrigation and Hot Hip and Leg Pack.

ENCOURAGEMENT—With the eye of faith, with child-like submission as obedient children, we must look to God, to follow His guidance; and difficulties will clear away. The promise is, "I will instruct thee and teach thee."

PELVIC INFLAMMATORY DISEASE (PID)

SYMPTOMS—Lack of appetite, nausea, fever, chills, generalized aching, fast heartbeat, and occasional vaginal bleeding. There is acute aching of both sides of the abdomen. Bowel movements may intensify the pain.

Frequently there is mild pain that is dismissed as "just cramps." There may be chills, fever, and a smelly vaginal discharge. Even walking may be extremely painful. Chronic PID can develop with a continual pain in the lower pelvis, which is especially severe during intercourse. Be alert to lower abdominal pain which increases with motion (walking).

CAUSES—Pelvic inflammatory disease is an infection of the fallopian tubes, ovaries, and surrounding structures; it results from an infected uterus. It occurs most often among sexually active women between the ages of 15 and 25; and is the most common gynocological reason for the hospitalization of women. However, most women with PID experience no complaints.

Although abortions can result in sterility, pelvic inflammatory disease causes sterility even more frequently. A single attack of this disease produces sterility about 15% of the time.

Other complications include recurring infections, ectopic pregnancy *(688)*.

It is believed that this disorder owes its origin to **unsanitary conditions**, especially during intercourse.

The use of **intrauterine devices** (IUD) is another cause. The disorder was over four times higher in IUD users. They may not have been sterile or may have been inserted by hands that had not been carefully washed.

Douching is yet a third cause of this problem *(see Vaginal Douch, 688)*. When it is not done carefully, bacteria can be flushed up into the uterus. In one study, 90% of the infected women regularly douched; they frequently did this since the ages of 16 or 17.

A fourth cause is **wiping** the wrong way after a bowel movement. Aways wipe from front to back, to avoid spreading germs from the rectum to the vagina. PID occurs when disease-causing organisms travel upward from the vagina and cervix into the reproductive organs.

—Also see Salingitis and Ovaritis (693), Menstrual Cramps (683), Painful Menstruation (684), Menstrual Disorders (678), Ectopic Pregnancy (688), Pelvic Pain (689), Kidney Problems (489), Renal Colic (492), Colitis (463), and Hemorrhoids (469, 712).

NATURAL REMEDIES
- Go on a **fruit and vegetable juice fast** for a time.
- When solid food is started, eat **nourishing food**, free of **sugar** and **oil**. Avoid **junk food**. Do not use **tobacco, caffeine, or alcohol**.
- For pain relief, apply **heat** to the lower back or abdomen. **Sitz baths** are also helpful.
- A **hot half bath** is useful in fighting the infection.
- Every 4 hours, take a **hot footbath** while **ice bags** are on the lower abdomen for 30 minutes, followed by 30 minutes' **rest** in bed. This will speed the healing process.

PREVENTION
- If vaginal **douches** are used, they must be done in a very sanitary manner. *See Vaginal Douche (688).*
- If feasible, avoid the use of **IUDs**.
- **Require** that, immediately prior to intercourse, your spouse carefully wash his hands with soap and water, cleaning beneath the fingernails; then hands should be dried on a clean towel. Also require that he carefully wash his male organ with soap and water. If he really loves you, he will be glad to do this. If this is not done, Pelvic Inflammatory Disease *(690)* or Kidney Infection *(492)* can easily result. It can take as little as a few weeks of PID to cause permanent sterility!
- Never have **unprotected sex** or **multiple sex partners**.

ENCOURAGEMENT—A great name among men is as letters traced in sand; but a spotless character will endure through all eternity. God stands ready to help all willing to surrender their lives, so He can help them live a better life. Galatians 3:28-29.

CHRONIC METRITIS
(Inflammation of Uterus)

SYMPTOMS—Severe pain in the uterine area.

CAUSES—Metritis is a severe infection in the uterus. It is designated as endometritis if the endometrium is involved. It is designated as myometritis if the uterine musculature (myometrium) is the part which is infected.

The following remedies are especially adapted to the chronic form of metritis.

—See Endometriosis (694); this is a problem with ovarian cysts.

NATURAL REMEDIES

J.H. KELLOGG, M.D., PRESCRIPTIONS FOR CHRONIC METRITIS AND ITS COMPLICATIONS *(how to give these water therapies: pp. 207-272 / list of treatments: pp. 206-207 / Hydrotherapy Disease Index: pp. 273-275)*

BASIC APPLICATIONS—Graduated cold applications. Hot **vaginal irrigation**, for 10-15 minutes, twice daily. Hot **Blanket Pack** to legs with cold **pelvic pack** (Wet Sheet Pack over pelvic area) that is continued to sweating stage. Follow with cold friction or **Wet Sheet Rub**.

PAIN—Prolonged Neutral **Sitz Bath** at 95°-97° F., for 15-20 minutes.

LEUKORRHEA—In addition to the above measures, use antiseptic **vaginal irrigation**. In certain cases, cool **irrigation**, at 75°-65° F., produces better results than hot irrigation. Constipation and portal congestion must be relieved. Cervical catarrh and erosions often require the use of the curette (a spoon-shaped scraping instrument for removing foreign matter from a cavity).

ACUTE INFLAMMATION—If attacks of inflammation occur, rest in bed. Hot Hip or Leg Pack. Hot and cold pelvic compress or hot and cold pelvic pack.

ENCOURAGEMENT—Trusting in Jesus and humbling submitting to His guidance will brighten and sweeten every detail of life with more than an earthly joy and a higher than earthly peace.

UTERINE BLEEDING
(Metrorrhagia)

SYMPTOMS—Excessive bleeding from the uterus.

CAUSES—This difficulty may be related to Profuse Menstruation *(682)* and Postmenstrual Bleeding *(687)*. You will also want to check those sections for possible causes and many other natural remedies.

Infection is a frequent cause of prolonged bleeding from the uterus.

NATURAL REMEDIES

• After the period is over, take a warm douche of **white oak bark, wild alum root, or bayberry bark**. Steep, while covered, 1 heaping tsp. to a quart of boiling water. Inject 4-5 times a day with a bulb syringe. In addition, drink the herb teas.

• Bleeding between periods or prolonged or excessive menstrual bleeding may indicate the presence of a uterine tumor. Bleeding after menopause is not normal; if this happens, contact your doctor for an evaluation.

—*See Profuse Menstruation (682), Postmenstrual Bleeding (687), Vaginal Discharge (698), and Uterine Fibroids (692).*

NATURAL REMEDIES

J.H. KELLOGG, M.D., PRESCRIPTIONS FOR UTERINE BLEEDING AND ITS COMPLICATIONS *(how to give these water therapies: pp. 207-272 / list of treatments: pp. 206-207 / Hydrotherapy Disease Index: pp. 273-275)*

BASIC APPLICATIONS—Hot **vaginal irrigation**, short **Hot Hip Pack**, **Hot Footbath**. Follow with **Cold Compress** over stomach and inner surfaces of thighs. In obstinate cases, cold **vaginal irrigation**. Moderately prolonged, very cold, Shallow **Sitz Bath** at 50°-65° F. for 5-15 minutes. Accompanied by Hot **Footbath** when other measures fail.

Hot **Douche** to lower spine area over stomach and inner surfaces of thighs, twice daily during intervals.

CAUTIONS—Avoid prolonged Hot **Sitz Bath**, Hot Douche, Hot Leg Bath, Hot **Footbath**, or Hot **Sitz Bath**. In some cases, even avoid **Fomentations** and hot **vaginal irrigation**. It is equally necessary to avoid short cold applications to the lower spine, abdomen, thighs, and feet, as the reflex effects of such applications increase pelvic and uterine congestion.

GENERAL METHOD—It is always highly important to inquire closely for all possible causes of the profuse flow. The cause may be simple anemia from defective nutrition, constipation, sexual excess, enteroptosis, uterine displacement, ovarian or tubal disease, uterine inflammation, or congestion. The most common cause is vegetation of the endometrium, which must be removed by surgical measures. The operation must be followed by treatment for chronic metritis. In many instances, several of these conditions may be combined. Good results generally follow water treatments.

AUTHOR'S NOTE—The following two paragraphs were typed as part of the "how to stop bleeding" section; but they have been placed here instead because they are lengthy, cover the subject of uterine bleeding well, and are not duplicated in this present section of Kellogg formulas.

For hemorrhage from the uterus, apply short, very hot **fomentations** (or the hot douche) to the thighs and spine while an **ice bag** is placed over the lower abdomen and a hot **vaginal douche** is given. Another very useful procedure for uterine hemorrhage is this: a very short hot **douche** to the lower back, the inner surfaces of the thighs, and the soles of the feet. Prolonged **cold applications** to the same surfaces produce like effects. These applications may be made either with or without a simultaneous use of the hot **uterine or vaginal douche**, according to the severity of the case.

Caution: Cold applications must not be used in cases of menorrhagia (excessive bleeding during menstruation, either in amount of loss or number of days), except with the utmost care and discretion, on account of the danger of producing hematoma or hematosalpinx through the sudden checking of the outflow of blood. Therefore, use only less strong measures during the first 24 or 36 hours of the period. Reserve the cold applications to a later time. During the first day, the hot vaginal douche is better and safer. "The danger of producing hematoma is very small after the first day." Kellogg then tells of a girl who had suffered for nearly a year without relief, although she had gone to many physicians. When brought to him, she was "placed at once in a **sitz bath** of about 50° F. for 15 minutes, the feet being placed in **cold** water at the same time, with the result that the hemorrhage ceased at once; and, by continued and repeated application of the cool **sitz bath** for a few weeks, the difficulty was relieved. The above measures will not solve the problem when the hemorrhage is due to vegetation, a uterine fibroid, or a malignant disease. In cases where the hemorrhage is accompanied by severe nerve pain or acute pelvic inflammation, use **very hot** rather than very cold applications to the inside of the thighs and lower back region.

R
E
P

W

This should be brief and the temperature sufficiently high to be somewhat painful; it is best done by **sponging** the parts with water at 140° F. or by applying, for 1-2 minutes, **cloths** wrung from 140° F. water.

ENCOURAGEMENT—Trust in the Lord and never forsake Him, regardless of what may happen.

UTERINE FIBROIDS
(Fibroids, Uterine Fibroma, Uterine Polyps)

SYMPTOMS—There are no symptoms, in half of the cases. But these growths can cause abnormally heavy and frequent menstrual periods; they even result in infertility. Other possible indications: anemia, fatigue, bleeding between periods, weakness from blood loss, increased vaginal discharge, bleeding after intercourse.

Most small fibroids (about half of them) produce no symptoms. The common symptoms of larger fibroids are prolonged menstrual bleeding, pain during menstrual periods, heavy flow during periods.

Depending on their location, fibroids can cause pain in the back, legs, and/or pelvis. They can exert pressure on the bladder or bowels; fibroids even block the flow of urine through the urethra.

CAUSES—Uterine fibroids are common noncancerous tumors that grow slowly within the muscular wall of the uterus. They vary in size from a millet seed to large enough to fill the entire abdominal cavity, and may be single or multiple. The tumors are completely covered by a fibrous connective tissue capsule. They may be as small as a pea or as large as a grapefruit. Larger ones may affect menstruation or case infertility.

Fibroids rarely cause symptoms before the age of 30; but they are common after that age, especially among blacks (3 times as likely). 20%-30% of women have them. They are the most common of tumors. The type of symptoms shown depends on where the fibroids are located. They can exert pressure and cause pain to the bladder, bowels, or even block the urethra (producing kidney obstruction).

When they produce no symptoms, *they should be left alone;* but they should be removed if unusually rapid growth occurs.

If the flow is far too heavy or rapid, you may have interfering fibroids.

Fibroids do not occur before puberty; and they usually stop growing after menopause. They increase in size at times when there are increased levels of estrogen in the body. This increased size can be caused by **pregnancy**, taking the **contraceptive pill**, or **hormone replacement therapy (HRT,** *687).*

NATURAL REMEDIES
• Taking **oral contraceptives** increases the likelihood of developing fibroids. If fibroids are found, do not take oral contraceptives with a high-estrogen content; the estrogen may make them enlarge faster.

• Over 30% of the **hysterectomies** done in the U.S. are for the purpose of removing fibroids. But, if possible, do not remove them. Fibroids generally shrink when menopause begins. This is due to the decreased amount of estrogen in the body from that time onward.

• An alternate surgery is a **myomectomy**, which removes the fibroids and leaves the uterus intact. It is true that there is a slightly higher possibility of complications with a myomectomy; the results are not always permanent (50% of the time, new fibroids will appear). But a hysterectomy works hovac with the hormonal system.

If you practice the following rules, you will be far less likely to develop fibroids, or have them enlarge.

• A simple, nourishing diet of **fruits, vegetables, whole grains, legumes, and nuts** (supplemented with **vitamins and minerals**) strengthens the body. Drink **carrot juice** daily. **Flaxseed oil** (2 tsp. daily) should be your only oil source. **Vitamin C** (1,000-2,000 mg) and **vitamin E** (400-800 IU) daily are important.

• Do not eat large amounts of food! **Do not overeat** on protein! Obtain adequate **rest** and get outdoor **exercise**.

• Avoid high-fat foods, including **full-fat dairy products**. They cause imbalanced estrogen levels, a clear cause of fibroids. **Obesity** from a high fat diet also increases the risk. Avoid **concentrated starches. Also avoid fried, sugary, and salty foods**.

• Avoid **caffeine** and caffeine-containing foods, such as **chocolate**. Avoid cooked **spinach, rhubarb** (both high in oxalic acid), and **carbonated sodas**.

• Avoid hormone-laden **meat**. Do not **smoke** or be around those who smoke.

• Do not take **drugs** (including HRT). **Do not overindulge** in sex.

• Obtain adequate **iodine** from seaweed. Iodine deficiency can be caused by **alcohol, refined sugars, and X-rays**.

• Do not take any **estrogen compounds**.

• This **tea** blend combines hormone-balancing herbs with those that ease cramps, and help with uterine fibroids: 2 teaspoons **vitex** berries, 1 teaspoon **black cohosh** root, ½ teaspoon **dandelion** root, ½ teaspoon **prickly ash** bark, 3/4 teaspoon **cramp** bark, ¼ teaspoon **cinnamon** bark, and 4 cups water.

Combine the herbs in the water and bring to a boil. Lower heat and allow the tea to simmer for a few minutes. Remove from the heat and steep for 20 minutes. Strain and drink at least 2 cups of tea per day for 3 to 4 months.

• Try these simple methods to ease the discomfort of uterine fibroids:

• **Hot sitz baths**, in water as hot as you can stand; so it will increase circulation in the pelvis, relax tight muscles, and relieve discomfort.

• **Essential oils**. Add several drops of rosemary, lavender, or juniper essential oils to the sitz bath in order to stimulate pelvic circulation.

• **Castor oil**. The skin absorbs the warm castor oil's active constituents, *lectins*, which stimulate the immune response to help shrink fibroids. Five drops of **lavender** essential oil added to a castor-oil pack encourages relaxation.

To make a pack, soak a clean cloth in castor oil; then place it on the abdomen or on any painful area. Cover the cloth with plastic wrap; then cover that with another clean cloth. Finally, apply a heat source—a hot-water bottle, a heating pad, or a cloth bag of lentils, corn, or rice that's been microwaved for a few minutes. Leave on for about an hour.

• *Also read Hysterectomy Problems (699).*

ENCOURAGEMENT—God wants us to be happy. He desires to put a new song on our lips, even praise to our God. He can give you overcoming strength. Walking with Him, you can have peace and assurance.

Speak of Jesus. Educate the tongue to speak of His mercy, to tell of His power, showing forth the praises of Him who hath called you out of darkness into His marvelous light.

Thank God every day of our life that, through the enabling grace of Christ, you can live a clean life in obedience to the ten commandments.

UTERINE PROLAPSE
(Prolapse of Uterus, Pelvic Floor Hernia)

SYMPTOMS—A feeling of fullness in the vagina. A dragging sensation or mild pain in the lower back. Increased frequency of urination. Difficulty urinating or defecating. A lump protruding into, or even out of, the vagina. Leakage of urine when laughing or coughing.

CAUSES—Prolapse of the uterus (which usually also prolapses the vagina) is a downward displacement of the uterus and/or wall of the vagina. Both are held in place by strong pelvic muscles and ligaments. If they become weakened or stretched (often as a result of **childbirth**), the displacement can occur. Women who have **given birth to several children** or have had a **difficult or prolonged labor** are more likely to have a prolapse.

It is after menopause that prolapse generally occurs, as a result of lessened amounts of estrogen. **Obesity**, a **chronic cough, asthma, diabetes, chronic bronchitis, or straining** during bowel movements are other causes. Prolapse is more common in white people; the reason is not known. Most prolapses occur before the age of 55.

When the uterus drops too far, a *cystocele* results (the bladder bulges into the front wall of the vagina or a *ureterocele*; a urethra that does the same).

NATURAL REMEDIES
• Eat a nourishing diet of **fruits, vegetables, whole grains, legumes, and nuts**. Include enough **fiber**.
• Take a multivitamin. **Vitamin C** (2,000 mg) and **bioflavonoids** (100 mg) lessen bladder infections.
• **Calcium** (1,200 mg) and **magnesium** (1,000 mg) provides needed minerals to strengthen uterine support.

• **Exercises** that strengthen the pelvic floor muscles can help treat a mild prolapse and prevent urinary incontinence. These are called **"Kegel exercises."** You can do them sitting, standing, or lying down. Do them as often as you can, at least once an hour throughout the day. To identify the proper muscle, imagine that you are urinating—and have to stop suddenly. The muscles which you feel tightening are the pelvic floor muscles that support the bladder, uterus, and rectum. Contract (tighten) these muscles and hold for 10 seconds. Relax slowly. Repeat 5-10 times, as often as you can.

• Rubbing **wild yam** cream on the pelvic area is good; it helps to strengthen the supporting tissues.

ENCOURAGEMENT—How thankful we can be for the enabling grace of Christ, which alone can give us the victory over sin.

SALPINGITIS AND OVARITIS
(Fallopian Tube Inflammation, Ovarian Inflammation)

SYMPTOMS—Tenderness of one or both fallopian tubes. In severe cases, there is pelvic pain, usually felt on both tubes. Vaginal discharge, swelling, fever, possible abscesses. Peritonitis may later occur. Peritonitis *(541)* is inflammation of the peritoneum, which is the membranous coat that lines the abdominal cavity.

CAUSES—*Salpingitis* is inflammation of the fallopian tubes. *Ovaritis* is inflammation of the ovaries. Ovaritis may involve the substance of the organ (*oophoritis*) or its surface (*perioophoritis*). This may be acute or chronic. These technical words are defined because it is easy to confuse ovaritis and oophoritis in the medical literature.

The fallopian tubes and ovaries are normally protected by the acidic vagina, the mucous plug of the cervix, and cilia in the uterus and fallopian tubes. But there are five situations, during which infection can more easily penetrate those delicate organs:

During **menstruation**, the vagina is alkaline, the plug is gone, and only a healthy flow protects the fallopian tubes and ovaries from infection. **Sexual intercourse with an infected individual who has a venereal disease** can result in these problems.

Activity, during a period, can introduce bacteria.
During and just after childbirth.
Following an abortion. It has been well-documented that abortion clinics tend to operate on a mass-production basis instead of the careful and sterile conditions one would find in a hospital operating room.

Use of an **IUD** (intrauterine device) is also a significant cause of infection.

General **enervation or local congestion** due to a variety of causes—ranging from **poor diet, overwork, constipation** *(456, 712)*, **pelvic infections**, etc.

Once salpingitis or oophoritis occurs, there is a 70% likelihood of sterility. *(See Female Infertility Problems, 666).*

NATURAL REMEDIES

Antibiotics are usually given; but they only work on a short-term basis. Frequently a chronic case of salpingitis follows. While it is being treated, scar tissue and other blockage can occur on the tubes. Whether or not antibiotics are used, it is highly recommended that natural methods also be used. The objective is to clear up the infection as soon as possible, to prevent possible sterility.

• **Vegetable juice fasting** for a time, followed by all **raw fruits and salads**. Follow this with a **nourishing vegetarian protein diet**. **Vitamins A** (in the form of beta-carotene: carrot juice and green and yellow vegetables). **Vitamins C** (2,000-5,000 mg), **E** (800 IU), **also zinc** (30 mg) are especially needed. But include a full **vitamin / mineral supplement**.

• These fasts will need to be continued until all acute symptoms are gone. If a chronic infection has already started, then alternate the fasts with nourishing food.

• Use **hot and cold contrast sitz baths**, to remove pelvic congestion and infection. Do this 3-4 times a day. The alternate hot and cold bath pumps healing blood throughout the affected area.

• Alternate 2-3 minutes **hot** and 2-3 minutes **ice-cold compresses** directly over the painful pelvic area.

• Helpful herbs include **echinacea, goldenseal, black cohosh, black haw, and bearberry**.

• Here is a douche for ovarian infection: Prepare a rosemary tea with 1 Tbsp. dried **rosemary** to 2 quarts boiling water. Steep, cool. Use for 7 days as a vaginal douche. Or use **red raspberry**, preparing it in the same manner.

—*Also see Pelvic Inflammatory Disease (690).*

J.H. KELLOGG, M.D., PRESCRIPTIONS FOR SALPINGITIS AND OVARITIS AND ITS COMPLICATIONS *(how to give these water therapies: pp. 207-272 / list of treatments: pp. 206-207 / Hydrotherapy Disease Index: pp. 273-275)*

(1) ACUTE FORM —
GENERAL CARE—Rest in bed. Hot **vaginal irrigation**, twice daily. Hot **pelvic pack**. Hot Leg Pack or Hot Footbath, twice daily. Follow by **cold friction**. If suppuration of tubes occurs, operation is usually necessary. During the first few days, **ice bag** over inflamed part. Interrupted, at intervals of 1-3 hours, by **Fomentation** for 15 minutes, or use hot and cold **pelvic compress** for 30 minutes. Heat the limbs.
CAUTIONS—Avoid general cold applications and cold applications to the feet.

(2) CHRONIC FORM —
BASIC APPLICATIONS—Hot **vaginal irrigation**, twice daily. Hot **rectal irrigation** once daily, if exudation in pelvis

is extensive. Pelvis **massage**. General **tonic applications**, general **massage**, **sunbaths**. **Outdoor exposure with proper protection**, carefully avoiding chill. Also nourishing and blood-building **diet**. If suppuration is present, give **drainage**. Removal of the diseased appendages is sometimes required; but, in most cases, this can be avoided by the proper application of water treatments at the outset.

ENCOURAGEMENT—You are the Lord's; He created you. You are His by redemption; He gave His life for you. Preserve every portion of the living machinery, so that you may use it for God. Psalm 16:5.

ENDOMETRIOSIS
(Ovarian Cysts)

SYMPTOMS—Abdominal pain, back pain, pelvic pain, constipation, bladder problems, bleeding between periods, very painful menstrual cramps, and the passing of large clots and shreds of tissue during the menses. In 30% of the cases, there are no symptoms. Iron deficiency anemia commonly occurs.

CAUSES—Tissue cells, which appear to be like those in the endometrium (the lining of the uterus), are able to grow elsewhere in the abdominal cavity: the ligaments, ovary, bladder, rectum, bowel, appendix, etc. They rarely occur outside the pelvic area. These tissue implants, wherever they settle in the body, will be affected by estrogen and will bleed during the monthly.

Endometriosis is generally diagnosed between 30 and 40 years of age. About 25%-30% of white women have it; but blacks rarely do have this. There is a **hereditary** factor, passing from mother to daughter.

The problem lessens during pregnancy and lactation; and it sometimes does not return. But, more often, it does return and continues **until menopause**; after which time, it becomes inactive, though scar tissue remains (unless **hormone replacement therapy** is done after menopause).

A frequent result of endometriosis is the inability to become pregnant. Many women who have the disorder have never been pregnant. *See Female infertility Problems (703).* **Tampons** reduce the internal flow and can increase the likelihood of developing or increasing the implants. They also increase pain and cramping. A hysterectomy will not solve the problem if implants have occurred elsewhere in the pelvic region.

When **internal fetal monitors** are placed in an expectant mother, the chances of later developing endometriosis are increased threefold.

Avoiding **sexual activity during menstruation** reduces the risk of developing this disorder.

NATURAL REMEDIES

DIET
• The **diet** must also be improved. A simple, nourishing diet of **fruits, vegetables, whole grains, legumes, and nuts** (supplemented with **vitamins and minerals**) strengthens the body. Eat much **raw food**;

it is high in **fiber**. Drink **carrot juice** daily. **Flaxseed oil** (2 tsp. daily) should be your only oil source.

• A **B-vitamin supplement, vitamin C** (1,000-2,000 mg), and **vitamin E** (400-800 IU) are important. Also needed is **calcium** (2,000 mg) **and magnesium** (1,000 mg; to reduce nervous tension), and **potassium** (5,500 mg).

• Do not use **caffeine** products; for this aggravates the pain. A diet that is high in **sugar** and **white-flour products** contributes to endometriosis.

• Eliminate foods containing **hormones and antibiotics**; since they upset the natural balance in the body and can lead to endometriosis. Such foods include **meat** and **dairy products** (including **eggs**).

• Hot and cold sitz baths, **for 20-30 minutes at a time, help reduce congestion. Another help is a** hot footbath **for 30 minutes. Conclude either treatment with a** cold mitten friction.

• **Hot fomentations** to the lower abdomen are helpful; and, it is reported, when this is done faithfully, there frequently is complete remission.

• An **ice bag, hot-water bottle, or heating pad** may be placed on the lower abdomen or back.

OTHER HELPS

• **Fast** for 3 days (on distilled water and fresh fruit and vegetable juices) each month before the anticipated beginning of the menstrual period.

• Helpful herbs include **black cohosh (to balance hormones), echinacea and goldenseal** (to eliminate infections), **cayenne** (to stop bleeding), and **burdock** (to cleanse the blood).

ENCOURAGEMENT—With the rich promises of the Bible before you, you can have assurance of God's love for you. As you read the promises, remember they are the expression of unutterable love and pity. He loves you. Revelation 21:4.

OVARIAN INSUFFICIENCY

SYMPTOMS—An inadequate amount of female sexual hormones are being released by ovaries.

CAUSES—The ovaries store and release eggs, which pass along the fallopian tubes into the uterus. But they also produce important female hormones: estrogen and progesterone. But secretion of these hormones is controlled by the follicle-stimulating hormone and the luteinize hormone, which are produced in the pituitary gland in the brain.

Causes of ovarian insufficiency may include **poor diet, lack of exercise, and overwork**.

NATURAL REMEDIES

• A nutritious diet of **fruits, vegetables, whole grains, legumes, and nuts** that is supplemented with **vitamins and minerals** strengthens the body. Drink

carrot juice daily. **Flaxseed oil** (2 tsp. daily) should be your only oil source. **Vitamins C** (1,000-2,000 mg) and **E** (400-800 IU) are also important.

• Obtain adequate **rest** and outdoor **exercise**.

• The seed oil of the **evening primrose** helps to balance the hormonal system.

• An infusion of **damiana** leaves regulates menstruation and stimulates ovary function.

• An extract of the plant and powdered root of the **pasqueflower** stimulates ovaries, calms menstrual pain, and regularizes menstruation.

ENCOURAGEMENT—Obedience to God's Word is our only safeguard against the evils that are sweeping the world to destruction.

VAGINITIS
(Vaginal Candidiasis, Yeast Vaginitis, Trichomoniasis, Atrophic Vaginitis, Bacterial Vaginosis)

SYMPTOMS—Vaginal pain or tenderness, itching, increased vaginal discharge, burning sensation, painful intercourse, and urination.

CAUSES—Vaginitis is an inflammatory infection of the vagina. There are four types:

1 - Yeast vaginitis, also called monilia or vaginal candida. The yeast infection causing it is *Candida albicans (see Candida, 281)*. It is more common in pregnant women and diabetics. Also as common are those on **antibiotics, oral contraceptives,** or **long-term steroid therapy. Changes in the vaginal pH** (caused by tap water, tub baths, certain additives to bathwater, and some commercial douches) permit the yeast to grow in the vagina. The discharge is moderate in amount; but it is thick yellowish, or white, and curd-like. It may cause severe itching of the external genitalia. *(See Candida, 281)*. Yeast vaginitis is the most common form of vaginitis.

2 - Trichomoniasis, caused by *Trichomonas vaginalis*. This is a protozoan which likes an alkaline environment. It may be **sexually transmitted** (so both should be treated at the same time). In the man, there are no symptoms; in the woman, there is a greenish white or heavy yellow, frothy discharge which may have a slight odor. The discharge causes itching, burning, and reddening of the skin. If it spreads to the urethra, there may be frequent burning urination. Flagyl, which is a medication for this, is known to cause cancer in animals. *See also page 805.*

3 - Bacterial vaginosis is the most common infectious cause of vaginitis, being twice as common as candidiasis *(281)*. The predominant vaginal lactobacillus flora is replaced by anaerobic bacteria that produces a "fishy" vaginal discharge, especially noticeable during intercourse.

DISEASES - List: 10-26 / Index: 1211-1224 / **HERBS** - Contents: 129- / **Preparing: 132 / Using: 141-189 (dose: often 1 tsp. mixed herbs in 1 cup boiled water) / VITAMINS-MINERALS** - Index: 100- / **Dosages: 124 / HYDRO-THERAPY** - Therapy index: 206- / **Disease index: 263- / CARE OF SICK - 28-39 / EMERGENCIES - 973-, 990-**

4 - Atrophic vaginitis occurs in postmenopausal women and those whose ovaries have been surgically removed. Adhesions form and there is a high susceptibility to infection. Symptoms include itching or burning, painful intercourse, and a thin watery discharge that is sometimes tinged with blood.

Vaginitis may have one or more of the following causes: **bacterial or fungal infection, intestinal worms, vitamin B deficiency, congestion of the pelvic organs, gonococci, chemical irritation (strong douches), mechanical irritation (tampons), drug medications, and deodorant sprays**.

Other contributing factors include **tight and nonporous clothing, diabetes,** and the use of **antibiotics**.

The **birth control pill** causes a B_6 deficiency and changes the vaginal pH.

Pregnancy makes the vaginal pH somewhat more alkaline and also contributes to its glycogen content. This is favorable to yeast infection.

Tight-fitting **synthetic underwear** provides poor ventilation and a warm, moist environment for yeast infection to occur.

Eating **excess sugar and refined carbohydrates** feed yeast infection. This is important! **Alcohol** also changes into sugar (glucose) in the body.

Normally, the pH of the vagina is acid; anything that alkalinizes it contributes to vaginitis. Causes include **diabetes** *(656)*, **menstrual period** *(676)*, **pregnancy** *(705-721)*, **and the time just after a miscarriage** *(715)* **or abortion**.

The most common aftereffect of **antibiotic therapy** in women is a vaginal yeast infection. About 5% of women given **tetracycline** for acne develop vaginitis.

Frequent **douching** upsets vaginal pH and flora.

Excessive sex or intercourse, without proper lubrication, irritates vaginal walls.

Intrauterine devices (IUDs) produce a favorable environment for yeast infection; since they reduce normal vaginal secretions.

Four primary factors are **antibiotics, oral contraceptives, diabetes, and pregnancy**.

If you have chronic or persistent vaginitis, you may have **diabetes**. If you have recurring vaginitis, you may be getting it from your **husband**.

One or another form of vaginitis accounts for about half of all gynecologic visits.

NATURAL REMEDIES

• All of the **above factors** should be carefully noted.

DOUCHES

• For yeast vaginitis, use a hot **soda-water douche** (1-3 teaspoons of soda to 1 quart water) twice a day for 7 days, then once a day for 30 days.

• If there is not clear and rapid improvement, a trichomonas may be the cause. If so, apply a **vinegar douche** (1-4 tablespoon of vinegar to 1 quart water) twice a day for 7 days, then once a day for 30 days.

• **Garlic-water douche** (1 clove into part of a quart of boiling water; add the remainder of the quart, let cool to 110° F. twice a day for 7 days, then once a

day for 30 days). Or blend a small clove of garlic with a pint of water and strain before using.

• For organisms other than yeast and trichomonas, a warm normal **saline douche** (1 teaspoon of salt per quart water) is useful.

• Do not use **sweet-smelling douches**. Plain acidophilus or a plain yogurt douche is much better. *Also see Douches (696, 688).*

• Douche with an herb tea of any of the following: **chaparral, goldenseal, white oak bark, or witch hazel**. A douche of **slippery elm tea** is an old remedy for irritated vaginal membranes.

• Make a tea of equal parts **goldenseal, chaparral, comfrey root, and slippery elm**. Use 1 oz. herb per pint of water, simmer gently for 30 minutes. Strain, cool and add 1 Tbsp. **vinegar** per pint. Use as a douche once a day for 1-3 days.

• Dr. Christopher recommends a douche of **bayberry**, as a cleansing to the membrane and toning of the tissues.

• Here is a yeast infection douche: Add 1 cup boiling **water** to 1 tsp. each of **chamomile flowers** and **goldenseal** powder. Steep 15 minutes. Strain out the flowers. Add 1 cup strained **comfrey leaf** or **comfrey root** tea. Steep. Mix 2 Tbsp. of apple cider **vinegar**, 1 tablet of **acidophilus** which is liquefied, 2 Tbsp. **of witch hazel** liquid, plus 2 quarts **water**. Douche every other day for a week. This is very effective and should help control the infection.

ALTERNATIVES TO DOUCHING

• Beware of regular **tub baths**, unless the tub has been sterilized! Take showers instead.

• **Hot sitz baths**, 2-3 times a day, will soothe local irritation; but it is important that the tub be sterilized first, lest bacteria be introduced into the vagina.

• An alternative to douching is the **sitz (sitting) bath**. Fill a shallow tub to the hip with warm water; then add salt (enough to make the water taste salty, about ½ cup) to match your body's natural saline state. Add ½ cup vinegar, to help rebalance the vaginal pH to 4.5. Then sit in the water, knees apart, until it gets cool. The bath will do the cleansing. Douching can be done with a similar mixture (4 teaspoons of vinegar to 1 pint of water). Vinegar has the same pH as a normal vagina.

• Another alternate to douching is to apply **garlic suppositories**. Peel a clove of garlic, with no nicks on it, and wrap it in a piece of sterile gauze, with a clean, unbleached string attached. Lubricate the suppository with pure organic vegetable oil and insert it in the vagina; yet keep a piece protruding outside. Insert a freshly prepared packet into the vagina each night for up to 6 consecutive nights. In many cases, this cures the infection.

• Add a tsp. of fresh **garlic juice** to a few tablespoons of yogurt. Either soak a tampon in it or use it as a douche (twice a day while symptoms persist). *Allicin* is the major compound in garlic which kills *Candida albicans*, the fungus causing yeast infections.

• **Tea tree oil** is good for vaginitis. Use creams,

suppositories, etc. The oil contains *terpinen-4-ol,* which is especially effective against candida. Research studies have found it to be as effective as medicinal drugs, but without the side effects.

• Mix 2-3 drops of **tea tree oil** in a Tbsp. of plain yogurt, soak a tampon in it. Insert it at night for up to 6 nights. But do not take tea tree oil (or any essential oil) internally; they can be poisonous.

• Cardmom also contains *terpinen-4-ol.* You can substitute it for tea tree oil.

• Apply an opened **vitamin E capsule** to the area, to reduce itching.

• For atrophic vaginitis, apply natural **progesterone cream** to the vagina. Prescription ointments for this condition contain estrogen. But they increase the need for **vitamin B$_6$** (500 mg). Vaginal absorption of estrogen may be dangerous.

HERBS

• **Aloe vera** is helpful for infections, including yeast infections. It can be taken internally or used as a douche.

• Also helpful are **bayberry, goldenseal, yarrow, marshmallow root, calendula, chamomile, pau d'arco, and dandelion.**

• Combine equal amounts of powdered **echinacea, chaparral, goldenseal, and squaw vine.** Fill gelatin capsules. Take 2 capsules, 3 times a day, before meals. Also take a tsp. of garlic oil with meals.

• **Goldenseal** is a broad-spectrum herbal antibiotic: it contains *berberine* and *hydrastine.* These compounds treat the trichomonal form of vaginitis, which is caused by an amoeba. Take it orally as a tea, capsule, or tincture.

• Combine **goldenseal** with **echinacea,** which is both antibiotic and immune-stimulating.

• Add 1 oz. each of **echinacea root, goldenseal root, ginseng root, yellow dock root,** and 2 oz. **echinacea root.** Either prepare as a tea to drink or put the mixture into gelatin capsules and take 2-3 a day.

DIET

• Adequate **rest, a healthful diet, and meticulous personal hygiene** with frequent **bathing** are important.

• According to the *New England Journal of Medicine,* **vegetarian** women eliminate 2-3 times more estrogen in their feces than nonvegetarians. They eat diets low in fat and high in fiber.

• Take a complete **multivitamin supplement,** which includes **vitamins A.**

• Include adequate **fiber** in the diet.

• To normalize vaginal flora, apply **acidophilus bacillus** (6-8 capsules, from a health-food store) or plain *yogurt* to the vagina.

• Eliminate coffee, alcohol, sugar and refined carbohydrates. Diets high in sugar can radically change the normal pH of the vagina.

• One research study showed that vaginitis may be due to **milk or pollen allergy.**

• Do not take **iron supplements** until the infection is reduced. Infectious bacteria require iron for growth.

OTHER HELPS

• **Other precautions include:** Dry thoroughly after the daily bath (with a hair dryer, if desired). Do not dust with cornstarch; this encourages yeast growth. (Talcum powder is powdered rock and can cause cancer.) Alternate cotton tampons with sanitary napkins, to permit natural vaginal flushing.

• Each time you use the bathroom, day or night, **wipe** from front to back, away from the vagina. While on the toilet, **pour a full cup** of hot or cold (not lukewarm) water through the pubic hair and let it run over the vaginal area. Blot dry with tissue. This will eliminate many cases of vaginitis accompanied by itching.

• The **vulva** must be kept as clean as possible and very dry, because infection spreads in moisture and heat. So dry well after a shower or bath.

• Thoroughly clean diaphragms.

AVOID

• Wear **cotton underpants** rather than close-meshed synthetic or silk. Candida survives normal laundering. To kill the yeast spores deposited on panties, either boil them, soak in bleach 24 hours, or press with a hot iron. Avoid **panty hose, girdles, or synthetic pants** or panties. **Tight-fitting clothing** increases moisture retention. Wear cotton clothing. Change from **bathing suits** soon after swimming. **Clothing** that comes in contact with your vulva must be washed between each wearing.

• Avoid **chemical deodorant sprays, colored toilet paper, harsh soaps or detergents.** Do not use commercial **sexual lubricants.**

• Avoid feminine hygiene **sprays or bubble baths.** The chemicals in them can induce vaginal problems.

• **Synthetic hormones,** including **birth control pills,** can alter the hormonal balance of the vagina.

• Avoid the use of dry **tampons.** They can injure the vaginal wall. If you must use them, alternate with pads part of the time.

• When **washing underwear,** do not wash it with socks and stockings, lest foot infections be transferred to the pelvic organs. Cotton underwear can be microwaved to destroy yeast. Wet it, wring it out well, and microwave on high for 30 seconds.

• Do not have **marital relations during menstruation, pelvic problems, or other infections** (if you can avoid it). At least wait before doing again, perhaps a few days immediately afterward.

• Always require that your **husband wash** his hands and genitals well before intercourse. If he really loves you, he will gladly do this.

• If you have vaginitis, **alert** your husband so he can be treated for candida also. Otherwise, he may reinfect you.

R
E
P

W

For more information on dealing with a yeast infection, see *Candida (281) and Athlete's Foot (377).*
—*Related articles include Chlamydia (804), Toxic Shock (699), Leukorrhea (698), Trachomoniasis (695), and Douches (688, 696).*

ENCOURAGEMENT—By sin, earth was cut off from heaven and alienated from its communion. But Jesus has connected it again with God's throne. His love has encircled man and opened the way, so you can find God anew and walk with Him every day.

VAGINAL DISCHARGE

SYMPTOMS—Irritation of vagina and vulva, redness, intense itching, odor, discharge of mucus, and pain during intercourse.

CAUSES—A mucous discharge from the vagina is normal during the childbearing years, especially as part of the menstrual cycle.

The discharge may be abnormal if it is excessive, yellow or green, odorous or offensive in smell, and causes irritation or itching. Vaginitis (inflammation of the vagina, *695*) is among the most common causes of vaginal discharge; it is often accompanied by itching of the vagina and vulva.

A normal discharge is used by the body to eliminate toxins. But this discharge can become abnormal when there is a **bad diet and lifestyle**. Because of the modern Western diet, discharge problems have been quite common.

The diet is loaded with **fat**, which stimulates fat cells throughout the body to produce estrogen. The lack of **fiber**, along with the excess estrogen, encourages the growth of intestinal bacteria (clostridia) which converts bile acids into additional estrogen-like hormones.

Using **birth control pills** affect the mucous membranes of the vagina, increasing or decreasing the discharge. They disrupt normal vaginal health by causing it to be become too alkaline. This condition encourages the growth of bacteria and the fungus known as *Candida albicans.*

Allergies are another cause of abnormal discharge. Foods, especially food additives and colorings, may be the source; or it may be soaps and bubble baths.

NATURAL REMEDIES

• Eat a simple, nourishing diet of **fruits, vegetables, whole grains, legumes, and nuts** (supplement with **vitamins and minerals**). Drink **carrot juice** daily. **Flaxseed oil** (2 tsp. daily) should be your only oil source. **Vitamin C** (1,000-2,000 mg) and **vitamin E** (400-800 IU) daily are also important.

• Do not **overeat**! Avoid high-fat foods, especially **animal fat** and **full-fat dairy products**. They cause imbalanced estrogen levels. **Obesity** increases the number of fat cells in your body. Avoid **concentrated** starches. **No fried, sugary, and salty foods**.

• Obtain adequate **rest** and get outdoor **exercise**.

• *Go to Vaginitis (695) for many more helps, including douches. Also see Leukorrhea (below), Profuse Menstruation (682), and Uterine Bleeding (691).*

ENCOURAGEMENT—There never was a more important time to study the Bible than now. Deceptive influences are on every side. We need the protection of God's angels every day. Do nothing that will separate you from Christ!

LEUKORRHEA

SYMPTOMS—A thick whitish vaginal discharge. Related symptoms may include burning and itching of the vulva.

CAUSES—Leukorrhea is a nonspecific vaginal discharge that contains mucus and white blood cells; sometimes it is tinged with blood. The amount of discharge increases when **estrogen levels** are heightened. If blood is present, a more serious disorder may be indicated.

It is often a symptom of vaginal infection. Infective causes include **candida** (*281*, also called yeast infection or monilia), **Trichomonas vaginalis** (*695*), **Vaginitis** (*695*), **chlamydia** (*804*), **hemophilus vaginitis**, **streptococcus or neisseria gonorrhea** (*803-804*). It can also be caused by **staphylococcus**; this is the bacteria which will cause **toxic shock syndrome** (*699*), when vaginal tampons are used incorrectly. Culture growth of bacteria and examination of discharge under a microscope is needed for specific diagnosis.

Other causes include a **vitamin B complex deficiency**, **excessive douching** (*douches, 696*), the use of **antibiotics or oral contraceptives**, or **intestinal worms** (*861*). A **hormonal imbalance**, due to poor diet or eating animal fat can be another cause.

Leukorrhea frequently occurs where there is **diabetes** (*656*) or **pregnancy**.

NATURAL REMEDIES

• The infective cause should be determined and then treated. See articles listed above.

• Wear white **cotton underwear**, so air can circulate freely. Keep the area clean and dry.

• To restore natural vaginal flora, douche with 6-8 **acidophilus** capsules or plain yogurt. Also douche with fresh **garlic** juice and water. *See Vaginitis (695) for much more on douches.*

• **Pau d'arco** tea is a natural antibiotic. Drink 3 cups daily.

• Use an injection of the distilled extract of **witch hazel** in warm water as a warm infusion.

• Mix equal parts **parsley root, uva ursi, burdock root, and parsley root**. Use 1 oz. per pint of water. Alternately, take 2 capsules of equal parts **echinacea, goldenseal, and myrrh**. Every 2 hours, alternately take first one, then the other, of the above two herbal compounds.

• Mix equal parts **shepherd's purse** and **blind nettle**. Steep 1 tsp. in ½ cup boiling-hot water. Take 1-1½ cups a day, unsweetened, in mouthful doses.

• Once each day, use a douche made of **white oak bark tea** or **bayberry bark tea**.

• Here are several other herbal douches which are effective: A decoction of **walnut** leaves and/or fruit green rind. **Myrtle** berries and leaves. **Pomegranate** flowers and bark. **Bistort** rhizome. **Rhatany** bark. **Great burnet**, **blind nettle**, **white willow**, **goldenseal**.

Also see Vaginal Discharge (698).

ENCOURAGEMENT—Let the peace of God reign in your soul. Then you will have strength to bear all suffering; and you will rejoice that you have grace to endure. God can give you help that no one else can.

TOXIC SHOCK SYNDROME

SYMPTOMS—Sudden onset of the condition: diarrhea, vomiting, headache, confusion, skin rash, and sore throat. *There can be rapid deterioration, and even death, within 48 hours*.

CAUSES—Prevention is far better than treatment. Aside from the name, this is an actual disease. Circumstances have permitted staphylococcus into the system, producing exotoxins faster than the body defenses can eliminate them.

Young women between 13-32 years of age contract 85% of this disease. In their case, the cause is usually the improper use of vaginal **tampons**. A single one is kept in place more than 4 hours. This produces an ideal environment for rapid staphylococcus growth with terrible consequences.

Another cause is **tight-fitting clothes, or synthetic or silk undergarments** which do not permit air to circulate to the vagina. A less frequent cause is **food poisoning** *(858)*, caused by poor food handling.

NATURAL REMEDIES

• *Immediately take the person to the emergency room*, at the hospital. *Do not let the staff make you wait* awhile! The person needs fluids and electrolytes by IV, along with penicillin.

—*Also see Leukorrhea (698).*

ENCOURAGEMENT—Praise the Lord. Talk of His goodness; tell of His power. He is the health of your countenance, your Saviour, and your God. Psalm 92:1-2.

HYSTERECTOMY
(Post-Hysterectomy)

SYMPTOMS—Depression, urinary tract problems, joint pain, headaches, dizziness, insomnia, fatigue, loss of bone mass, and increased likelihood of heart disease—resulting from a hysterectomy.

CAUSES—A hysterectomy is the surgical removal of the uterus; it is done to remove fibroids (30% of the time), endometriosis (20%), or uterine prolapse (18%).

There are three types of hysterectomies, each more complete than the preceding one:

1 - Partial hysterectomy: The uterus is removed; but the cervix and other female reproductive organs remain.

2 - Total hysterectomy: Both the uterus and cervix are removed.

3 - Panhysterectomy: The uterus, fallopian tubes, and ovaries are removed.

Certain difficulties lead to the decision to have a hysterectomy. These may include urinary tract problems, lengthy and heavy periods, a heavy and bloated feeling, abdominal swelling due to fibroids, infertility resulting from fibroids or endometriosis, or reactions to drugs given for endometriosis.

Yet the problems resulting from a hysterectomy are, if anything, more significant and sometimes devastating:

The hormones are suddenly stopped. This sends shock waves throughout the entire system.

Lack of those hormones can result in immense bone-mass loss, osteoporosis *(612)*, and greater likelihood of heart disease *(513-522)*, urinary tract problems *(486)*, dizziness *(550)*, insomnia *(547)*, headaches *(556)*, and general fatigue *(278-284)*.

Even those women who do not have their ovaries cut out still experience a drastic lessening of estrogen output. In addition, menopause begins years earlier for half the women who are spared their ovaries.

Depression *(596)* may also occur; however, reduced sexual desire frequently does occur. There is a 50% chance of a minor post-operative complication (such as fever, bleeding, or wound healing). One in a 1,000 die; and 10% require a blood transfusion.

It has been estimated that many of the 600,000 hysterectomies performed in America each year are totally unnecessary. No foreign country has even half that per-capita amount.

Once the operation has been performed, you are permanently sterile; and it cannot be reversed.

It is often recommended that the ovaries also be taken out, because they might later become cancerous. Yet statistics reveal that ovarian cancer is rare.

It is frequently recommended that a hysterectomy be performed to eliminate fibroids; since they might be malignant. But modern technology permits them to be examined, by ultrasound, for abnormalities. A myo-

R
E
P

W

mectomy should be performed to remove problematic fibroids, not a hysterectomy. *Also see Fibroids (692).*

Women who have hysterectomies have a higher incidence of cardiovascular disease *(513-522).*

If you decide to have a hysterectomy, ask that a horizontal incision be made, not a vertical one. The scar will thus be less noticeable afterward.

NATURAL REMEDIES

IF YOU HAVE HAD A HYSTERECTOMY

• Eat a **nutritious diet**, with **vitamin / mineral supplementation**. This will reduce the amount of estrogen deprivation, especially if you still have your ovaries.

• **Vitamin B complex, vitamin C** (1,000-3,000 mg; to bowel tolerance, without producing a slight diarrhea), **vitamin E, Calcium** (2,000 mg), **magnesium** (1,000 mg), **potassium** (100 mg), and **flaxseed oil** (2 Tbsp.) are important.

• Avoid **caffeine, dairy products, processed foods, meat, sugar, and fried foods**.

• *If you do use hormonal replacement therapy,* take the lowest dosage possible. Ask for a combined hormone that contains both estrogen and progesterone. That will help reduce the risk of cancer. Progesterone, not estrogen, is the hormone most needed in replacement therapy.

ENCOURAGEMENT—Keep your thoughts on Christ and the heavenly world, and you will have more strength for the trials of life. Talk His praise and rest in His love. Proverbs 16:3.

"Now the Lord of peace Himself give you peace always by all means." 2 Thessalonians 3:16.

Many who are sincerely seeking for holiness of heart and purity of life seem perplexed and discouraged. Darkness and discouragement will sometimes come upon the soul and threaten to overwhelm us; but we should not cast away our confidence. We must keep the eye fixed on Jesus, feeling or no feeling. We should seek to faithfully perform every known duty, in His enabling strength obey His Written Word (the Bible), and then calmly rest in the promises of God.

If we would permit our minds to dwell more upon Christ and the heavenly world, we should find a powerful stimulus and support in fighting the battles of the Lord. Beside the loveliness of Christ, all earthly attractions will seem of little worth.

How very thankful we can be that we can walk closely with Christ every day! You will draw strength from praising him! Rejoice in His saving grace. By His enabling strength, keep His Ten Commandment moral law (Exodus 20:3-17).

More Encouragement

"The words of Christ teach that we should regard ourselves as inseparably bound to our Father in heaven. Whatever our position, we are dependent upon God, who holds all destinies in His hands. He has appointed us our work, and has endowed us with faculties and means for that work. So long as we surrender the will to God, and trust in His strength and wisdom, we shall be guided in safe paths, to fulfill our appointed part in His great plan. But the one who depends upon his own wisdom and power is separating himself from God. Instead of working in unison with Christ, he is fulfilling the purpose of the enemy of God and man . . The dominion of evil is broken, and through faith the soul is kept from sin."
—Desire of Ages, 209, 210

"No man can succeed in the service of God unless his whole heart is in the work and he counts all things but loss for the excellency of the knowledge of Christ. No man who makes any reserve can be the disciple of Christ, much less can he be His colaborer. When men appreciate the great salvation, the self-sacrifice seen in Christ's life will be seen in theirs. Wherever He leads the way, they will rejoice to follow"
—Desire of Ages, 273

"As Jesus rested by faith in the Father's care, so we are to rest in the care of our Saviour. If the disciples had trusted in Him, they would have been kept in peace. Their fear in the time of danger revealed their unbelief."
—Desire of Ages, 336

SPECIAL SECTIONS FOR WOMEN - 2

- Disease Section 15 -
Pregnancy and Breast Feeding

 # = Information, not a disease

— Also see Herbs during Pregnancy (754-757, 760-763),
   Herbs at Childbirth (757-758, 763-764), Herbs for
   Nursing Mothers (720, 726), Herbs for Infant Care (758-
   759, 764)

P
R
E
G

FOR MORE NATURAL REMEDIES:
HERBS: Herb Contents (pp. 129-130) will help
  you locate the 126 most important herbs and
  the diseases each one can treat. How to prepare herbs (132). How to use them (141-189)
HYDROTHERAPY: Therapy Contents (pp. 206-
  207) and its Disease Index (263-265) will lead
  you to over 100 water therapies and many
  more remedies. DIS. INDEX: 1211- / GEN.

INDEX: 1221-
VITAMINS AND MINERALS: Contents (100-101).
  Using 101-124. Dosages (124). Others (117-)
CARING FOR THE SICK: Home care for a sick
  person (28-36). The healing crisis (36-39)
WOMEN'S SECTIONS: Female Organs (672)
  Pregnancy (701). Childbirth (765). Infancy,
  Childhood (722). Women's Herbs (754, 760)
EMERGENCIES: (973-). FIRST AID: (990-)

Section 15 - PREGNANCY AND BREAST-FEEDING

PREGNANCY AND BREAST-FEEDING -
1 - FERTILITY

FEMALE STRESS SYNDROME

SYMPTOMS—Allergies, frigidity, infertility, amenorrhea, anorexia, anxiety neurosis, menopausal melancholia, post-partum depression, premenstrual tension.

CAUSES—Women experience many stresses, because they have so many tasks: bearing children and raising them, caring for the husband, working in and around the house, perhaps working outside the home.

Increasing nutritional intake can help meet these stresses.

NATURAL REMEDIES

• **Fresh fruit and vegetable juice**, lots of **fresh fruits and vegetables, whole grains, nuts, and legumes. Flaxseed oil** and **lecithin** are also important.

• Adequate **vitamin and mineral supplementation**, especially **B complex, vitamin C** (1,000 mg), **vitamin E** (400 IU), **selenium** (40 mcg), **zinc** (30 mg), **calcium** (2,000 mg), **magnesium** (1,000 mg), **potassium** (5,500 mg), **and iron** (in the form of blackstrap molasses).

ENCOURAGEMENT—Do not forget the One who gives you all blessings. God alone can provide for your needs. Trust in Him. He can give you the peace of heart you so much need.

FRIGIDITY

SYMPTOMS—Absence of sexual desire, or an inability to find pleasure in sexual intercourse. Inability to have an orgasm.

CAUSES—Frigidity is generally of psychic, not organic, cause. There is guilt, fear, depression, a sense of inferiority or conflict with one's mate. Unfortunate experience and misinformation, received earlier in life, often lays the groundwork for the problem.

However, in some cases the woman may find intercourse painful because of inadequate stimulation, insufficient lubrication, or underlying infection or disease.

NATURAL REMEDIES

• Eat **eggs** fresh from the hen (not those in the stores which have been stored cold), **alfalfa, olive oil, pumpkin seeds and other seeds, nuts, soy oil, avocados, and wheat**.

• Avoid **meat** products.

• **Vitamin deficiencies** can result in lowered estrogen levels and thus poor lubrication. Especially take **B complex** and **vitamin E** (400 IU). Take **zinc** (30 mg) and **copper** (3 mg) daily.

• Helpful herbs include **wild yam**. This contains a natural steroid which may help. Take it for 2 weeks, stop for 2 weeks, and then back on again.

• **Damiana** contains alkaloids which, like testosterone, directly stimulates nerves. Place an eyedropperful under your tongue an hour or two before coming together. It may require several days before a desired effect will be noted.

• Extra **lubrication** may help reduce possible pain.

• Also helpful are **gotu kola, Siberian ginseng, saw palmetto, and sarsaparilla**.

ENCOURAGEMENT—Songs of praise to God will help you keep up your courage. Trust Him and know that He is the best Friend you can ever have. In His strength you can have the help you need. He will do for you that which is best.

FERTILITY TESTS

There are twelve fertility tests, six for men and six for women, that may be performed if conception does not occur. It is both easier and frequently more cost-effective to test the husband before testing the wife. Most of the following tests occur within a twelve-month period.

Tests Performed on Men

Endrocrine test—Blood tests are done to determine levels of the follicle-stimulating hormone (FSH), the luteinizing hormone (LH), and the thyroid hormones (T). LH levels are tested only if T levels are abnormal.

Postcoital test—The partners have sexual intercourse and the ejaculate is tested for surviving sperm.

Semen analysis—A sample of semen is examined no longer than one hour after ejaculation. It is tested for sperm motility (the percentage of sperm that are swimming) and morphology (the percentage that are normally shaped).

Sperm penetration test—Sperm is tested, to see if it has the ability to penetrate hamster egg cells. This indicates the sperm's ability to penetrate the spouse's egg.

Testicular biopsy—A sample of testicular tissue is examined under a microscope, to determine the condition of the sperm or to determine if sperm are being made.

X-ray—This test is done to check for damage to the ducts in the male responsible for transporting the sperm to the penis.

Tests Performed on Women

Endometrial—A tiny sample of the endometrium (the lining of the uterus) is taken in the later part of the menstrual cycle biopsy and tested to see if there is enough progesterone in the lining as it matures. If not, the condition is called luteal phase defect. It can be treated with hormone therapy.

FSH test—A blood sample is taken on day three of the menstrual cycle and tested for FSH. FSH levels increase as a woman reaches menopause. If there is a high FSH level, pregnancy is unlikely.

Hysterosalpingo gram (HSG)—Dye is inserted through the cervix into the fallopian tubes and uterus; and an x-ray is taken, to determine whether the tubes are open and if the uterus is a normal shape.

Laparoscopy—A surgical procedure in which a physician examines the reproductive organs by means of a tiny scope. If scar tissue or endometrial buildup is found, it can be removed by means of the scope as well.

Postcoital test (PCT, Sims-Huhner test)—The husband and wife have intercourse 2-8 hours before this test. A sample of cervical mucus and tissue is removed and examined, to determine whether the mucus or the cervix is prohibiting fertilization. Undergoing a PCT is much the same as having a Pap smear.

Transvaginal ultrasound—A probe is inserted into the vagina to look for fibroid tumors or ovarian cysts. This can also be done to track early pregnancies.

FEMALE INFERTILITY
(Female Fertility Problems)

SYMPTOMS—Seeming inability of a woman to become pregnant.

CAUSES—Infertility is generally defined as the failure to conceive after a year or more of regular sexual activity during the time of ovulation. Either the woman or the man may be the cause. *See Male Infertility (704).* The primary cause is generally low sperm count; but, in women, it is ovulatory dysfunction.

Infertility usually means that the problem can be reversed; sterility means that the situation is permanent. An estimated 20% of American couples experience infertility. Determining the exact cause can be difficult.

In general, 60% of couples conceive within 6 months; and 90% conceive within a year. If you both are under 28, and have no reason to think otherwise, you ought to have a baby within a year.

A frequent cause is a **deficiency** in one or more nutrients.

The problem may be that the woman is **not cycling and ovulating properly**. If she has less than 20% body fat, she may not.

Other causes include **inherited disorders, infections, venereal disease** (802, **mishandled abortions, bacterial organisms, drugs, plugged fallopian tubes, emotional trauma, or frigidity** (702).

If you are producing milk or have male-pattern hair growth on your breasts, upper lip, or chin, you may have a **hormonal imbalance**. There may be a **thyroid** problem.

You or your spouse may have had **chlamydia, gonorrhea**, or other sexually transmitted diseases which can destroy the fallopian tubes in women and inflame and scar the ductile system in men. Over 4,000 Americans contract these diseases yearly.

You may have had **pelvic infections, endometriosis** (694), **polycystic ovary disease, abdominal or urinary tract surgery, injuries to the perineum, excessively high fevers, the mumps or measles**. You may have used an **intrauterine device** (IUD). **Salpingitis and Ovaritis** (693) can cause sterility.

One of you may have been exposed to a harmful chemical, such as **lead** (873).

Kidney problems (489) can result in reproductive imbalances. Clean out the kidneys.

The more women **smoke**, the less likely they will conceive. In fact, women whose mothers smoked are only half as likely to conceive as those whose mothers were nonsmokers.

In rare instances, women develop **antibodies** to their partner's sperm.

In some cases, one or the other is only half-hearted about having a baby.

—Also see Male Infertility (704).

NATURAL REMEDIES

DIET

• Eat a **nourishing diet**; be sure to include sufficient **vitamins, minerals,** and (if necessary) **digestive aids**. A **high-protein diet, essential fatty acids** (flaxseed oil is best, 2-4 tsp.), **vitamin A** (in the form of carotenes), **B complex, zinc** (30 mg), **germanium** (100 mg), **and CoQ$_{10}$. Folic acid** (5 mg) helps female fertility.

• **Vitamin E** (400 IU) is very important if you wish to conceive. In women with irregular or absent periods, extra **vitamin B$_6$** can boost fertility (50 mg daily).

• In one study, taking over 1,000 mg of **vitamin C** daily can reduce fertility in a women (whereas, in men it increases it).

• A deficiency of **selenium** (500 mcg; not over 40

P
R
E
G

mcg if pregnant) can lead to infertility in women.

• **Para-aminobenzoic acid** (PABA) is a B vitamin which stimulates the pituitary gland and sometimes restores fertility to a woman (100 mg).

• Test for **food allergies**. *See Pulse Test (847) and Food Allergies (846-854).*

AVOID

• Avoid **fried, sugary, junk, and caffeine foods**. Do not eat **white flour or animal fats**.

• A **gluten-free diet** has enabled women, who previously were unable to conceive, to become pregnant.

• Stop **smoking** and do not be around cigarette smoke. Avoid **medicinal drugs**. Studies reveal that **caffeine** can prevent pregnancy from beginning. Just one drink a day can reduce your chances of becoming pregnant. (In addition, **decaffeinated coffee** has been linked to spontaneous abortion!) It is suspected that the cause is the tannic acid in coffee and **black tea**.

• Women who drink **alcohol** can prevent implantation of the fertilized egg in their womb.

• Avoid **stress**. Avoid **overweight**. The closer a woman's weight is to the ideal, the more likely she is to conceive.

• Do not **exercise** too much at that time of the monthly period. It can, in some, cause a skipped ovulation or increase infertility.

• Avoid **hot tubs and saunas**; for they may cause changes in ovulation.

• Do not **douche**. It can interfere with vaginal pH. Beware of commercial douches, lubrication agents, and jellies.

• Do not work so hard that you are **fatigued**. It is well-known that people who go on a vacation trip are more likely to conceive. They have more time to relax and rest up.

• There is the possibility that you have had **heavy metal poisoning** *(868)*.

HERBS

• Helpful herbs include **black cohosh, red clover, yellow dock, wild yam, chamomile, skullcap, dong quai**. **Black cohosh** balances hormones, **False unicorn, wild yam, and dong quai** help increase fertility.

• Add 2 Tbsp. each of **chasteberry, Chinese angelica** (dong quai), **and false unicorn root**, plus 1-2 tsp. **blessed thistle** to a quart of boiling water. Steep for 15 minutes. Drink 2-3 cups a day, 4-5 days a week.

• Here is one physician's formula for improving fertility in a woman: Mix equal amounts of **damiana leaves, Siberian ginseng, sarsaparillia root, saw palmetto berries, licorice root, and kelp**. Swallow the powder. Or make a tea and drink it.

• The use of natural **progesterone cream** has helped many women become pregnant. An excellent alternative is **wild yam**, which contains a progesterone-like compound. Rub it on the abdomen.

• If the infertility is due to elevated prolactin levels or ovarian insufficiency, **chasteberry** extract may help (175-225 mg daily). Several months may be needed

for the chasteberry to restore female balance.

OTHER HELPS

• Make sure you **time it** just right, in accordance with the monthly cycle.

• The woman should **remain lying down** for 20 minutes after ejaculation.

• If a woman has developed **antibodies** to her husband's sperm, avoid releasing sperm for a month (via a condom, etc.). This should cause the sperm antibodies to decrease.

There is always risk if you give consent for a physician to do fertility testing inside your body.

—*Also see Male Infertility (bellow).*

J.H. KELLOGG, M.D., PRESCRIPTIONS FOR FEMALE INFERTILITY AND ITS COMPLICATIONS *(how to give these water therapies: pp. 207-272 / Hydrotherapy Disease Index: pp. 273-275)*

GENERAL CARE—When not due to organic disease, this may be eliminated by a course of water treatments. A series of **graduated cold applications** (Tonic Frictions) is most useful. The **Cold Rubbing Sitz** is highly useful. Remove catarrhal conditions of uterus and vagina; also remove subinvolution by means of **hot vaginal irrigation**. Follow by **tonic (cool or cold) Sitz**.

—*Also see Male Infertility (below).*

ENCOURAGEMENT—Pray earnestly for help, and God will give you the very blessing that is best for you. Whatever path God chooses is the very best for us. Ecclesiastes 5:18-20.

MALE INFERTILITY
(Male Impotence Problems)

SYMPTOMS—Inability of a man to produce viable sperm which will unite with an ovum and result in conception.

CAUSES—There are more than 20 million sperm in a teaspoon. The most frequent cause of male infertility is **low sperm count** or an **anatomical abnormality**. Sperm factors account for 40% of all cases of infertility.

Factors affecting this include **excessive heat to the testes, exposure to toxins or radiation alcohol consumption, endocrine disorders, recent acute illness, or prolonged fever**. Any **viral illness** associated with a fever up to 3 months earlier. **Testicular mumps** is another cause.

A very common structural damage problem in men is a **varicocele**. This is a dilated vein of the spermatic duct.

If your sperm count is healthy, a **cold or flu** probably will not affect it. But if sperm count is borderline, an illness might render you infertile for a time.

Modern **pesticides** contain estrogenic materials, which cause animals to become infertile.

—*Also see Female Infertility (previous page).*

NATURAL REMEDIES

DIET

• Obtain an **adequate diet**; include enough **protein, essential fatty acids**, and (if necessary) **digestive aids**.

• Pay special attention to **selenium** (500 mcg) deficiency as a factor in male infertility. **Vitamin B$_6$** (200 mg) and **vitamin C** (500 mg, twice a day) increase male fertility. **Zinc** may be involved in male infertility (30 mg). Researchers found that choline (a B vitamin) increases male fertility in rats. Take 1,000 mg.

• **Arginine** (an amino acid) helps raise sperm counts. Take 4 grams daily (the amount in 2 oz. sunflower seeds, the richest source).

• Strictly adhering to a **gluten-free diet** has enabled some men, who previously thought they were sterile, to become fathers.

• Do not use **anabolic steroids**! They can shut down the pituitary gland and throw the body's hormonal system out of balance. Athletes often have fertility problems. Long-time use of steroids can permanently damage the testicles.

• Drinking **alcohol** reduces sperm count in men.

OTHER HELPS

• **Ginger** increases sperm count. **Ginseng, schisandra, and saw palmetto** may reduce male infertility. The Chinese herb, **cangzhu,** has been used for thousands of years to increase male fertility. **Ashwaganda** is used in India for the same purpose. Animal breeders add **red raspberry** leaf tea to animal feeds to increase male fertility. The Chinese herb, **astragalus,** improves sperm motility.

• Do not **overheat** the testes. If you do, they will produce sterile sperm for several hours or up to a day afterward. The testes must remain a half degree cooler than your core body temperature. **Fevers** to the body, **close-fitting underwear**, or **hot tub baths** can cause this. The scrotal sac is supposed to keep the testes at a temperature of 94°-96° F. If it rises above 96°, sperm production is greatly inhibited or completely stopped.

• Do not have **intercourse** for seven days prior to the special fertile time.

• **Tagamet and Zantac**, two ulcer medications, decrease sperm counts and may even produce impotence.

In some cases, sperm count is so low that the only means of fertilization is artificial insemination.

If a varicocele is the problem, it must be treated by surgery.

—*Also see Female Infertility (703) for additional factors. Much of that information also applies to the man.*

J.H. KELLOGG, M.D., PRESCRIPTIONS FOR MALE INFERTILITY AND ITS COMPLICATIONS (*how to give these water therapies: pp. 207-272* / *Hydrotherapy Disease Index: pp. 273-275*)

GENERAL TREATMENT—Graduated Cold Baths. Cold Douche to spine, especially the lower part. **Cold Rubbing Sitz Bath**, beginning at 80° F., lowering temperature 5° daily to 60° F. Duration of bath is 3-8 minutes, with vigorously rub, to prevent chilling. If urethral irritation is present, short **Revulsive Sitz Bath** (2-4 minutes). **Cooling Compress**, 5 minutes daily.

ENCOURAGEMENT—Christ could have spent His days in self-seeking and idleness; but He chose to come to earth and die, so you could have eternal life. Trust your life to Him, and you will not regret it. Isaiah 45:21-22. God can do far more for you than you could ever do for yourself.

PREGNANCY AND BREAST-FEEDING -
2 - PREGNANCY AND CHILDBIRTH

IMPORTANT: Other important chapters in this book: Herbs for Pregnancy (760-762), and The First Nine Months (774).

The section in this chapter, Pregnancy Problems (706), tells you what to do to avoid birth defects. Also read Birth Defects (725).

BIRTH CONTROL

Many ask this question: **When does the baby start existing?** Various theories have been proposed. The answer is simple enough: The baby begins existing as soon as growth begins. That is obvious. It is as soon as the baby begins growing. Growth begins as soon as the two cells (the sperm and the egg) unite. From that point onward, a new person exists.

Another important question is **How can we properly prevent this from occurring, without killing the child?** Here is how this is done:

The rhythm method of birth control consists simply of abstaining from intercourse during the "fertility period." This extends from about one week after the menstrual period ends, onward for another 10 days or so. At that point, it will be at least 5 days past ovulation. In summary, an interval of abstinence between the 10th and 18th of a 28-day cycle usually suffices for birth control.

A third question is **What is the best time in the monthly cycle to have a child?** If you are having an infertility problem, the wife may take her oral temperature early in the morning before rising or drinking fluids. At the time of ovulation, the morning temperature (called basal temperature) increases about 0.5° to 1° F. This change marks the day of ovulation. This is the time to have intercourse.

P
R
E
G

Another question: **How can we select the sex of the baby?** To have a baby boy, have intercourse only on the 16th day from the first day of the menstrual period. To have a baby girl, have intercourse on the 12th day instead. Either way, the couple should not have intercourse seven days before or after. Intercourse facing one another tends to produce girls; and with the man behind his wife tends to produce boys (because the semen initially is shot farther up the vagina).

PREDICTING THE BIRTH DATE

How you can tell the date when you are likely to give birth:

Start with the date the last menstrual period began, subtract three months, and add 7 days.

For example, suppose your last period began May 10.

May 10 minus 3 months is February 10.

Plus 7 days is February 17.

The baby is likely to be born around February 17.

BIRTH DATE CHART

The Birth Date Chart (below, left) was prepared by Frederick M. Rossiter, B.S., M.D., for his book, *Practical Guide to Health*. The paragraph immediately following the graph explains how to do it.

January	October	February	November	March	December	April	January	May	February	June	March	July	April	August	May	September	June	October	July	November	August	December	September
1	8	1	8	1	6	1	6	1	5	1	8	1	7	1	8	1	8	1	8	1	8	1	7
2	9	2	9	2	7	2	7	2	6	2	9	2	8	2	9	2	9	2	9	2	9	2	8
3	10	3	10	3	8	3	8	3	7	3	10	3	9	3	10	3	10	3	10	3	10	3	9
4	11	4	11	4	9	4	9	4	8	4	11	4	10	4	11	4	11	4	11	4	11	4	10
5	12	5	12	5	10	5	10	5	9	5	12	5	11	5	12	5	12	5	12	5	12	5	11
6	13	6	13	6	11	6	11	6	10	6	13	6	12	6	13	6	13	6	13	6	13	6	12
7	14	7	14	7	12	7	12	7	11	7	14	7	13	7	14	7	14	7	14	7	14	7	13
8	15	8	15	8	13	8	13	8	12	8	15	8	14	8	15	8	15	8	15	8	15	8	14
9	16	9	16	9	14	9	14	9	13	9	16	9	15	9	16	9	16	9	16	9	16	9	15
10	17	10	17	10	15	10	15	10	14	10	17	10	16	10	17	10	17	10	17	10	17	10	16
11	18	11	18	11	16	11	16	11	15	11	18	11	17	11	18	11	18	11	18	11	18	11	17
12	19	12	19	12	17	12	17	12	16	12	19	12	18	12	19	12	19	12	19	12	19	12	18
13	20	13	20	13	18	13	18	13	17	13	20	13	19	13	20	13	20	13	20	13	20	13	19
14	21	14	21	14	19	14	19	14	18	14	21	14	20	14	21	14	21	14	21	14	21	14	20
15	22	15	22	15	20	15	20	15	19	15	22	15	21	15	22	15	22	15	22	15	22	15	21
16	23	16	23	16	21	16	21	16	20	16	23	16	22	16	23	16	23	16	23	16	23	16	22
17	24	17	24	17	22	17	22	17	21	17	24	17	23	17	24	17	24	17	24	17	24	17	23
18	25	18	25	18	23	18	23	18	22	18	25	18	24	18	25	18	25	18	25	18	25	18	24
19	26	19	26	19	24	19	24	19	23	19	26	19	25	19	26	19	26	19	26	19	26	19	25
20	27	20	27	20	25	20	25	20	24	20	27	20	26	20	27	20	27	20	27	20	27	20	26
21	28	21	28	21	26	21	26	21	25	21	28	21	27	21	28	21	28	21	28	21	28	21	27
22	29	22	29	22	27	22	27	22	26	22	29	22	28	22	29	22	29	22	29	22	29	22	28
23	30	23	30	23	28	23	28	23	27	23	30	23	29	23	30	23	30	23	30	23	30	23	29
24	31	24	1	24	29	24	29	24	28	24	31	24	30	24	31	24	1	24	31	24	31	24	30
25	1	25	2	25	30	25	30	25	1	25	1	25	1	25	1	25	2	25	1	25	1	25	1
26	2	26	3	26	31	26	31	26	2	26	2	26	2	26	2	26	3	26	2	26	2	26	2
27	3	27	4	27	1	27	1	27	3	27	3	27	3	27	3	27	4	27	3	27	3	27	3
28	4	28	5	28	2	28	2	28	4	28	4	28	4	28	4	28	5	28	4	28	4	28	4
29	5			29	3	29	3	29	5	29	5	29	5	29	5	29	6	29	5	29	5	29	5
30	6			30	4	30	4	30	6	30	6	30	6	30	6	30	7	30	6	30	6	30	6
31	7			31	5			31	7			31	7	31	7			31	7			31	7
January	October	February	November	March	December	April	January	May	February	June	March	July	April	August	May	September	June	October	July	November	August	December	September

Normal labor occurs about 280 days from the beginning of the last menstrual period. The left-hand columns, below, list the last-menstrual dates for an entire year. In order to find the normal delivery date, look across to the date in the right-hand column. *Example:* If the last menstrual period began on January 2, then the baby would normally be born on October 9.

SIGNS OF PREGNANCY RISK

Signs of special risk that make it important that a doctor or skilled midwife attend the birth—if possible, in a hospital:

- If regular labor pains begin more than 3 weeks before the baby is expected.
- If the woman begins to bleed before labor.
- If there are signs of toxemia during pregnancy.
- If the woman is suffering from a chronic or acute illness.
- If the woman is very anemic or if her blood does not clot normally (when she cuts herself).
- If she is under 15, over 40, or over 35 at her first pregnancy.
- If she has had more than 5 or 6 babies.
- If she is especially short or has narrow hips.
- If she has had serious trouble or severe bleeding with other births.
- If she has diabetes or heart trouble.
- If she has a hernia.
- If it looks like she will have twins.
- If it seems the baby is not in a normal position in the womb.
- If the bag of waters breaks and labor does not begin within a few hours. (The danger is even greater if she has a fever.)
- If the baby is still not born within 2 weeks after 9 months of pregnancy.

PREGNANCY RELATED PROBLEMS

SYMPTOMS—A variety of problems can occur during pregnancy—ranging from backache, constipation, stretch marks, and gas to hemorrhoids, varicose veins, and miscarriage.

INTRODUCTION—Pregnancy is that special 40-week period between conception and birth, when the child grows and develops. A weight gain of 20-35 pounds is desirable and, in most cases, is in keeping with good health. But a number of problems can occur. Here are several of them. *For more information, see Morning Sickness (708), Premature Labor (715), and Miscarriage (715).*

Many of the problems occurring during pregnancy are related to hormonal changes, nutritional needs, or various expansion pressures as the fetus continues to grow.

NOTE: A late menstrual period that is accompanied by severe abdominal pain should receive immediate medical attention—because it may be due to an ectopic pregnancy (a pregnancy that develops outside the uterus, usually in one of the fallopian tubes). If the mother does not receive immediate attention, she may die. *See Ectopic pregnancy (688).*

NATURAL HELPS

DIET

NUTRITION—Proper nutrition is important. There is a 20% increase of blood volume during pregnancy. This requires additional complete **protein**.

• A healthy diet during this time would include **2 fruits a day, 7 vegetables (including salads, grains, and other worthwhile foods)**, etc. Complex carbohydrates, best obtained in **whole grains**, are important. Also **nuts, legumes, and seeds**.

• Do not eat junk food of any type. Avoid caffeine, alcohol, and tobacco. Also do not eat spicy, fried, or overly processed foods. If possible, avoid all drugs.

VITAMINS

• Complete **vitamin / mineral supplementation** is also important.

• *Vitamin A* protects the immune system and avoids **eye abnormalities, cleft lip, and cleft palate**. Do not let vitamin A intake go over 10,000 IU daily. Excessive intake of vitamin A is linked to **cleft palate, heart defects, and other congenital defects**. Foods rich in vitamin A (meat, milk, and eggs) may also cause problems. But foods with natural beta-carotene (green and yellow vegetables) are not harmful. (This is because carotene is only converted to vitamin A as it is needed.)

• All the *B complex* is important. They help prevent **leg, back, and joint pains** in the mother during pregnancy.

• *Vitamin B$_1$* (thiamine) prevents **stillbirths, low birth weight babies, and heart disorders**. In late pregnancy and post-delivery, B$_1$ requirements are greatly increased.

• *Vitamin B$_2$* (riboflavin) prevents **short limbs and cleft palate**.

• *Vitamin B$_3$* (niacin, niacinamide) prevents **irritability, depression, disorientation, fatigue, nervousness, and muscular weakness**.

• *Vitamin B$_6$* (pyridoxine) prevents several fetal abnormalities (including **seizures, cleft lip, and cleft palate**). Take 100 mg daily until birth, followed by only 50 mg daily. This is because an excess of B$_6$ after delivery can hinder the amount of **mother's milk** produced.

• *Folic acid* prevents **anemia and birth defects**. It is involved in cell growth and DNA production. But it is vital that this supplementation be started prior to conception. Take 400 mg daily. If there is not enough folic acid in the system during the first six weeks of pregnancy, **spina bifida** and **anencephaly** can result. But most women do not know they are pregnant until several weeks after conception has occurred. Therefore it is crucial that you be taking this vitamin regularly.

• *Vitamin C* prevents **infections** and the birth of **small babies**.

• *Vitamin D* works with **calcium**, to build strong **bones**.

• *Vitamin E* is the **anti-abortion** vitamin, and is needed in order to bring a baby to full term.

MINERALS

• *Magnesium* helps prevent **birth abnormalities and miscarriag**e.

• *Calcium* prevents **weak bones and teeth, premature births, and damaged nerves**.

• Although *phosphorus* is important, you always get enough in your food. Too much blocks **iron** and **calcium** absorption. Soft drinks eliminate calcium. *See Strengthening the Bones (608-611).*

• The *trace minerals* are also important. Nova Scotia dulse and Norwegian kelp are good sources.

• *Iodine* prevents thyroid problems, abnormal development, and certain types of mental retardation.

• *Zinc* prevents dwarfism and limb defects.

• *Manganese* prevents certain brain abnormalities.

• Inadequate *folic acid, manganese, zinc,* and *amino acid* imbalances have been linked to **mental retardation and deformities** in the fetus.

DO NOT DO THIS

• Do not use an **electric blanket**. Studies indicate it may increase risk of miscarriage and problems in development.

• **Aspirin** has been linked to fetal deformities, bleeding, and complications during pregnancy.

• Do not use **cinnamon** in large quantities during pregnancy.

• The drug, Etretinate (**Tegison**), is prescribed for psoriasis; but it can cause birth defects.

• **Avoid the following herbs** during pregnancy: **feverfew, goldenseal, black cohosh, tansy, angelica, bloodroot, celandine, dong quai, Oregon grape, rue, cat's claw, barberry, cottonwood bark, and pennyroyal**.

• Do not take anything containing **shark cartilage** during pregnancy. It reduces production of new blood vessels.

• Do not take supplements containing **phenylalanine**. This is an amino acid which can alter brain growth in the fetus. The sweetener, **Aspartame** (Equal, NutraSweet), contains high levels of phenylalanine.

• A drug prescribed for acne (Isotretinoin, under the trade name of **Accutane**) can cause birth defects.

• Avoid **mineral oil**; it inhibits the absorption of fat-soluble vitamins.

P
R
E
G

• Two medications, used to control seizures, increase by four times the risk of producing a baby with heart defects. These drugs are **phenobarbital and phenytoin** (Dilantin).

• Drinking large quantities of **coffee, cola drinks**, or other caffeine sources can result in birth defects.

• Certain chemicals in drugs can stunt fetal growth. These include acetaminophen (**Tylenol, Datril**, and others); antacids (**Pepto-Bismol, Alka-Seltzer, Rolaids, Tums, Di-Gel, Maalox, Gelusil**); as well as **aspirin, cough remedies, cold pill, antihistamines, estrogens, and decongestants**.

• Do not permit any **X-rays** to be taken of you—even of your teeth—during pregnancy.

DO THIS

• If at all possible, have your baby by **natural childbirth**—and with the help of a midwife.

• Be sure to **breast-feed** your baby for at least the first three months, and longer if possible (*see Breast-feeding, 716*).

• Keep yourself healthy; and keep eating an **adequate diet**. Avoid long fasts, cleansing diets, or strictly limited diets during pregnancy and lactation. *See Eclampsia (716)*.

—*Also see Pregnancy Herbs (760-762)*.

ENCOURAGEMENT—With the eye of faith and a child-like submission, trust your life to God; and He will wonderfully guide you. His promise is, "I will instruct thee and teach thee." Psalm 32:8.

MORNING SICKNESS
(Pregnancy Nausea)

SYMPTOMS—Nausea and vomiting by the mother between the sixth and twelfth weeks of pregnancy.

CAUSES—Although called morning sickness, it can occur at any time of the day. Morning sickness is caused by **rising progesterone levels**; this is quite normal.

Morning sickness is said to be a cleansing of the body, to prepare a clean environment in which the fetus can properly develop.

However, about 1 woman in 200 experiences an abnormal amount of vomiting and severe nausea. This can result in acidosis, malnutrition, dehydration, and significant weight loss.

Possible causes of this abnormal condition include **drug toxicity, vitamin deficiency (especially of B₆), pancreatitis, bile duct disease, and inflammatory bowel disorders**.

It can also be caused by the production of high levels of **human chorionic gonadotropin**, which is a hormone. **Cysts** in the uterus or multiple pregnancy can also be the cause.

Morning sickness generally does not continue beyond the first 13 weeks of pregnancy. If there is persistent vomiting or nausea later, consult with your health-care provider.

At its worst, morning sickness can degenerate into *hyperemesis gravidarum*. In this situation, the mother-to-be has far too much vomiting and nausea, is overly dehydrated, and not urinating properly. She cannot keep food, water, and juice down for over a period of 4-6 hours.

This condition can lead to pulse irregularities, electrolyte imbalance, and even kidney and liver damage. Ketones, produced by the breaking down of stored fat, can damage neurological development in the fetus.

How to avoid this danger? Do not stop eating and drinking fluids, even though you feel nauseated and vomit.

NATURAL REMEDIES

• Because morning sickness is caused by rising progesterone levels, you need a **complex carbohydrate** (or possibly **protein**) **snack** upon awakening in the morning. This will relieve much of the nausea.

• Keep **crackers or whole-wheat toast** near your bed and eat some as soon as you arise in the morning. Pop them in your mouth, chew well, and swallow; then place your feet on the floor.

• It helps to keep some food in the stomach all day long. Eat **small and frequent meals**; but do not overeat. When needed, snack on **whole-grain crackers**, possibly with a little **nut butter** (but not peanut butter).

• Another method is to carry some **raw almonds** with you, wherever you go. Make sure they are not old and stale.

• **Do not go without food or drink;** you must continue to have both—even though you feel nauseated and may vomit.

• **Vitamin B₆** and the entire **B complex** is important. **Essential fatty acids** and a complete line of nutritional supplements should be taken.

• Drink lots of fluids: **water, fruit or vegetable juice, broth**, or certain **herbal teas**. Drinking fluids at frequent intervals also helps neutralize the extra hydrochloric acid produced by the stomach at this time.

• **Avoid eating or smelling fried and fatty foods**. Do not use **caffeine** products.

• **Ginger** is extremely helpful in relieving morning sickness. But only drink 1 cup of this tea at a time. Too many cups can induce miscarriage.

• Helpful herbs for nausea include **peppermint, red raspberry leaf, catnip, or dandelion**.

• **Do not sit up** or get up out of bed too rapidly.

ENCOURAGEMENT—The Lord Jesus came to our world to save those who would come unto Him. But He can save no one against His will. In Him you can find the rest, courage, and peace of heart that you so much need. 2 Corinthians 6:18.

DIZZINESS IN PREGNANCY

SYMPTOMS—Dizziness when, during pregnancy, you suddenly stand.

CAUSES—So much is happening in your digestive and reproductive organs, that the blood tends to pool in them; this causes a lack of blood in the brain when you stand up suddenly.

In addition, especially during the second trimester, blood pressure drops as the uterus presses on major blood vessels.

NATURAL REMEDIES
• **Do not quickly arise or change positions**. Breathe deeper when you sense that you need to do so. —*Also see Dizziness (550, 708)*.

ENCOURAGEMENT—When temptations and trials rush in upon us, let us go to God and agonize with Him in prayer. He will not turn us away empty, but will give us grace and strength to overcome and to break the power of the enemy.

SWEATING IN PREGNANCY

SYMPTOMS—You are sweating more than previously, perhaps more than you want.

CAUSES—As your size increases, it becomes more difficult to walk, climb stairs, and do your daily chores. This increases the tendency to sweat. In addition, you body is primarily concerned with providing a correct temperature for your baby, but only secondarily for you. This can, at times, add to your warmth.

NATURAL REMEDIES
• **Do not overheat** your body. Do not take a **hot tub bath** during pregnancy; for doing so can overheat your baby. Do not **exercise** too strenuously.
• Wear **light-weight, loose clothing**, preferably of cotton or other porous natural fibers.

ENCOURAGEMENT—The gift of God to man is beyond all computation. Nothing was withheld. God would not permit it to be said that He could have done more or revealed to humanity a greater measure of love. He gave all heaven when He gave the gift of Christ.

INSOMNIA IN PREGNANCY

SYMPTOMS—During the final weeks of pregnancy, you are having an increasingly difficult time getting to sleep at night.

CAUSES—Difficulty in finding a comfortable position is a significant part of the problem. Lack of B vitamins can add to it. Emotional changes also affect it.

NATURAL REMEDIES
• Include more **B complex** vitamins in your diet. Take 500 mg **calcium** and 250 mg **magnesium** at bedtime to calm the nerves and muscles, and help you sleep. Calcium citrate or calcium lactate provides maximum absorption.
• Avoid **heavy meals** before bedtime. Do not use **stimulants** or **sedatives**; they affect your baby.
• Drink a cup of **hot herb tea** before retiring. Select from **lemon balm, marjoram, or passionflower**.
• Do not **sleep** until you feel like doing so. You may want to just **sit** in a very comfortable chair for a time before going to bed. **Walking outside** in the fresh night air, before retiring, can also be helpful.
• Place **pillows** behind or under your abdomen, to help you breathe better.
—*Also see Insomnia (547)*.

ENCOURAGEMENT—All who have been born into the heavenly family are in a special sense the brethren of our Lord. The love of Christ binds together the members of His family; and, wherever that love is manifest, there the divine relationship is revealed.

COUGHS AND COLDS IN PREGNANCY

SYMPTOMS—Coughs and colds are occurring more frequently; they seem to be harder to get rid of.

CAUSES—Your physical resources are being stretched at this time; since you are providing care for two people.

NATURAL REMEDIES
• For information on how to treat colds and coughs, *see under Colds and Coughs (288-292)*.
• To prevent these problems, maintain a **healthy, nutritious diet** of fresh fruits, vegetables, whole grains, legumes, and nuts. Take a **multivitamin-mineral** supplement. Maintain a program of **rest and light exercise**, without overworking.
—*Also see Colds and Coughs (288-292)*.

ENCOURAGEMENT—Every soul is cherished, because it has been purchased by the precious blood of Jesus Christ.

SKIN PROBLEMS IN PREGNANCY

SYMPTOMS—An increasing number of pimples, red marks, acne, and dark blotches on the face.

CAUSES—The dark blotches are called the "mask of pregnancy. During pregnancy, your body is undergoing great adaptations. It is a time when you want to give your body the best care; so it, in turn, can better care for your little one.

NATURAL REMEDIES
• Eat only wholesome, **nutritious food**; and take a **multivitamin** supplement. **Folic acid** (one of the B vitamins) is especially helpful.
• Do not eat **greasy, fried food**. Do not be around those who **smoke.**
• Keep your **skin clean** by showering twice a day.
• Avoid the use of **makeup** or only use water-based hypoallergenic cosmetics.
—*Also see Acne (328) and Oily Skin (338).*

ENCOURAGEMENT—The more we make known the rich treasures of God's blessings to others, the more blessings will be imparted to us.

STRETCH MARKS IN PREGNANCY

SYMPTOMS—Wavy stripes which (during pregnancy) appear on the breasts, abdomen, buttocks, and thighs. Initially reddish in color, they gradually turn white.

CAUSES—Rapid weight gains, which frequently occurs during pregnancy, is the cause. As the skin is stretched, fibers in the deeper layers tear, causing permanent marks which after childbirth usually become difficult to see.

NATURAL REMEDIES
• In order to avoid these stretch marks, apply **oil**, once a day, all over the areas where the marks are likely to appear. The formula includes ½ cup of **olive oil**, ¼ cup of **aloe vera** gel, 6 capsules of **vitamin E**, and 4 capsules of **vitamin A**. Cut open the capsules, mix it all together, and apply. If you make extra, store it in a closed jar in the refrigerator.

ENCOURAGEMENT—The Lord looks upon His redeemed heritage with pity. He is ready to pardon their sins if they will surrender and be loyal to Him.

VARICOSE VEINS IN PREGNANCY

SYMPTOMS—Enlarged veins close to the surface of the skin which are present during pregnancy.

CAUSES—These enlarged veins may disappear after childbirth.

NATURAL REMEDIES
• If possible, **walk** a mile a day in order to increase circulation. **Change positions** frequently; and never cross your legs. Sit with your **feet elevated**. If necessary, wear support hose. Do not wear bands on the legs.
• To improve blood flow from your legs to your upper body, do "**pelvic tilting**" during your second and third trimesters. Stand with feet shoulder-width apart and hands on hips. Slowly tip your pelvis for-

ward, then backward, gradually increasing speed until you are doing it somewhat vigorously. You can also roll and rock. Do this exercise 5-10 minutes a day.
—*Also see Varicose Veins (535).*

ENCOURAGEMENT—Shall we, sons and daughters of God, forget our royal birth? Shall we not rather honor our Lord and Saviour Jesus Christ? Shall we not show forth the praises of Him who has called us out of darkness into His marvelous light? How thankful we can be that, through the grace of Christ, we can be enabled to obey God's ten commandment law.

SORENESS IN RIB AREA DURING PREGNANCY

SYMPTOMS—Your ribs feel sore and hurt a little.

CAUSES—Pressure from the expanding womb is the cause of this. This pressure tends to stop when the baby drops down within the last six weeks of the pregnancy.

NATURAL REMEDIES
• **Change positions** frequently. **Sit or lay down** every so often and rest a little.

ENCOURAGEMENT—God does not accept men because of their capabilities, but because they seek His face and desire His help.

LEG CRAMPS IN PREGNANCY

SYMPTOMS—Leg cramps occur every so often.

CAUSES—Significant hormonal and physical adjustments are being made at this time. But there are solutions to the problem. The cramps are primarily due to lack of a nutritious diet, necessary vitamins and minerals, plus circulatory and positional factors.

NATURAL REMEDIES
• It is important that you correct nutritional deficiencies. **Calcium** (2,000 mg), **magnesium** (1,000 mg), and **potassium** (5,500 mg), are needed daily.
• Avoid too much **salt** in the diet.
• There is now extra **weight** on your legs. Walking about is important; but try not to stand in one place too long. When you must do so, frequently shift your weight from one leg to the other. **Flex your feet** every so often, with your toes pointed upward.
• **Elevate your legs** while sleeping; so they are higher than your heart. Apply a **heating pad** to the cramping area. **Massage** the area with your hands.
—*For much more, see Leg Cramps (372).*

ENCOURAGEMENT—Christ intercedes in behalf of those who have received Him. To them He gives power, by virtue of His own merits, to become members of the royal family, children of the heavenly King. And the Father demonstrates His infinite love for Christ, who paid our ransom with His blood, by receiving and welcoming Christ's friends as His friends. He is satisfied with the atonement made. He is glorified by the incarnation, the life, death, and mediation of His Son.

NOSEBLEEDS AND NASAL CONGESTION IN PREGNANCY

SYMPTOMS—Nosebleeds and nasal congestion become more frequent.

CAUSES—In order to provide for the needs of two of you, your bones are making an increasing volume of blood. This can cause pressure in the small capillaries of the nasal passages. When one ruptures, a nosebleed results. This problem will stop when the baby is born.

NATURAL REMEDIES
• **Vitamin C** (1,000 mg daily) and **bioflavonoids** (100 mg daily) are very important in preventing nosebleeds. Make sure you are eating enough **fresh fruits and vegetables**.
• You may need to reduce your intake of **dairy products** if you have nasal congestion; but make sure you have an adequate intake of **calcium** (2,000 mg), **magnesium** (1,000 mg), and **potassium** (5,500 mg).
• Avoid **nasal sprays**. Instead, spray a little warm water into your nose to moisten it. Or use a **humidifier**.

ENCOURAGEMENT—Christ declares to all who would follow Him: "My grace is sufficient for thee" (2 Cor. 12:9). Let none, then, regard their defects as incurable. God will give faith and grace to overcome them.

INDIGESTION IN PREGNANCY

SYMPTOMS—Food does not seem to be digesting as well.

CAUSES—During this special time, your body craves good quality food. You need to eat enough; but you should not overeat.

NATURAL REMEDIES
• Eat **smaller meals** and **chew** your food well. **Acidophilus, peppermint tea, ginger, and aloe vera** juice will help.
• Do not take **baking soda** to alleviate indigestion; because the sodium content will increase fluid retention.
Also see Indigestion (437).

ENCOURAGEMENT—As Christ intercedes in our behalf, the Father lays open all the treasures of His grace for our appropriation, to be enjoyed and to be communicated to others. "Ask in my name," Christ says; "I do not say that I will pray the Father for you; for

the Father Himself loveth you, because you have loved Me. Make use of My name. This will give your prayers efficiency, and the Father will give you the riches of His grace; wherefore, "ask and ye shall receive, that your joy may be full" (John 16:24).

HEARTBURN IN PREGNANCY

SYMPTOMS—Burning sensations in your stomach, especially in the upper part.

CAUSES—Because of the expanded size of the womb, there is a tendency for stomach fluids to be pushed up and reenter the esophagus (the food tube above your stomach). In addition, pregnancy hormones tend to soften the sphincter muscles of the stomach.

NATURAL REMEDIES
• Do not eat **fried, greasy, and spicy foods**. Avoid **baking soda, coffee, alcohol, and antacids**.
• For several hours after a meal, **do not bend over or lie flat**; remain active.
• When you feel heartburn, drink a glass of warm **rice milk** or **soymilk**.
• Take your daytime **naps before eating**, not immediately afterward. Do not eat **supper** close to bedtime.
• While in bed, place **pillows** under or behind your abdomen.
—*Also see Heartburn (434).*

ENCOURAGEMENT—By faith let us look upon the rainbow round about the throne, the cloud of sins confessed behind it. The rainbow of promise is an assurance to every humble, contrite, believing soul, that his life is one with Christ and that Christ is one with God.

FLATULENCE IN PREGNANCY

SYMPTOMS—Intestinal gas is more likely during pregnancy.

CAUSES—You experience significant hormonal changes at this time; and your nutritional needs are somewhat different.

NATURAL REMEDIES
• Try to determine which **foods** are causing the problem. You may need to eat fewer meals more often.
• Make sure you are obtaining enough **fresh fruit and vegetables**. Avoid foods which you know tend to disagree with you. **Chew** everything slowly and thoroughly. Drink as much **water** as you can.
• Walking helps alleviate bloating and gas.
—*See Flatulence (433) for more information.*

PREG

ENCOURAGEMENT—The slain lamb—Christ now alive in heaven—is our only hope. Our faith looks up to Him and grasps Him as the One who can save to the uttermost; and the fragrance of the all-sufficient offering is accepted of the Father. Christ's glory is concerned in our success. He has a common interest in all humanity. He is our sympathizing Saviour.

CONSTIPATION IN PREGNANCY

SYMPTOMS—Constipation tends to increase during pregnancy.

CAUSES—Higher progesterone levels relax the bowel muscles and make them less efficient. Normal rhythmic contractions are slowed. The result is constipation; this most frequently occurs in the third trimester. In addition, the baby increases pressure on the intestines, slowing the movement of feces.

Constipation can lead to high blood pressure, water retention, toxemia (toxic blood), and injure both the mother and baby. It can also produce leg cramps, backache, fatigue, and varicose veins.

NATURAL REMEDIES
• Do not eat **constipating food** (such as soft bread, hard cheese, etc.) Drink lots of **water**, beginning as soon as you arise in the morning.
• Increase the amount of **fiber** in your diet. Eat **fresh and dried fruit**, especially stewed **prunes**. **Bran** can also be taken; but, if so, accompany it with a lot of water—or it will constipate. These fiber-rich foods help soften stools and make elimination easier.
• Iron supplements can cause constipation; they may also induce a miscarriage. It is best to get the iron (which you need) from blackstrap molasses.
• Do not use over-the-counter laxatives.
• Do a lot of walking each day.
• Regularity is important. Try to set a certain time each day for bowel movements. Elevating your legs during each one will help relax your anal muscle.
—*Also see Constipation (456).*

ENCOURAGEMENT—The grace of Christ and the law of God are inseparable. In Jesus, mercy and truth are met together; and, by His grace, we are enabled to obey all that God asks of us in the Bible.

BLADDER PROBLEMS IN PREGNANCY

SYMPTOMS—Difficulty urinating, possibility of bladder infections.

CAUSES—The expanding uterus presses against the bowel and the bladder, compressing both. It becomes necessary to urinate more frequently. Because the bladder may not fully empty, it can become infected.

NATURAL REMEDIES

• **Do not reduce intake of liquids**, thinking this will solve the problem! Instead, increase your fluid intake. Drink quality water.
• Avoid **sugary foods**; for they feed wrong bacteria.
• Eating an **acidophilus** preparation daily will help maintain "friendly" bacteria in the system. Also eat **cranberries** (either sauce or juice) in order to maintain proper acidity in the bladder.
Wear **cotton** underwear. Do not wear anything tight, synthetic, or non-porous next to your skin.
• Do not **douche**; for that can lead to bladder infection.
—*Also see Kidney Problems (489) and Bladder Problems (495).*

ENCOURAGEMENT—Through the cross, man was drawn to God and God to man. Justice moved from its high and awful position. And the heavenly hosts, the armies of holiness, drew near to the cross, bowing with reverence; for, at the cross, justice was satisfied.

HEMORRHOIDS IN PREGNANCY

SYMPTOMS—Painful anal hemorrhoids.

CAUSES—Pressure by the womb on the anus can induce hemorrhoids if constipation is present.

NATURAL REMEDIES
• Drink more **water**. Increase intake of **roughage**. Eat lots of raw fruits and vegetables, plus dried fruits.
Keep **legs elevated** on a stool during elimination.
• Apply cold **witch hazel compresses** to help shrink hemorrhoids.
• Do not **strain** to have a bowel movement.
—*Also see Constipation (456) and Hemorrhoids (469).*

ENCOURAGEMENT—We need often to recount God's goodness and to praise Him for His wonderful works.

BACKACHE IN PREGNANCY

SYMPTOMS—The back hurts when sitting, standing, or walking.

CAUSES—Your entire center of gravity changes during pregnancy. The added weight and muscle-relaxing effects of progesterone are other causal factors.

NATURAL REMEDIES
• When your back hurts, soak a small **towel in cider vinegar**. Squeeze off the excess, lie down on your side, and place the towel across your back. Remain there relaxed for 15 minutes.
• It is important that you maintain **proper posture. Relax your shoulders** and stand tall, keeping your **head up and back straight. Avoid fatigue**. Be careful to lift correctly; so pressure is on the legs, not

on the back.

• Do not wear **high-heeled shoes;** and do not remain in **one position** too long. Wear flat or low-heeled shoes. You may need larger shoes during pregnancy.

• Get down on your **hands and knees** and gently round your back upward while holding in your abdominal muscles. Continue breathing and hold this position while you count 10. Relax your muscles by flattening your back (but do not let it become concave, curved downward toward the floor). Do this 12 times. Backaches can last long after childbirth; so continue it later if it is helping you.

• Gently **stretch** (without straining) for 2-3 minutes at a time. Have someone **massage** your back.

• Sleep on a **mattress** firm enough to support you, with a **pillow** supporting your back. Sleep on your **side**, not on your back.

—*Also see Backache (645-648).*

ENCOURAGEMENT—In every assembly of the saints, below, are angels of God; they listen to the testimonies, songs, and prayers. Let us remember that our praises are supplemented by the choirs of the angelic host above.

SCIATICA IN PREGNANCY

SYMPTOMS—Nerve pain in the back of one or both legs.

CAUSES—The sciatic nerve is the largest and longest nerve in your body. It comes out near the base of your spine and goes down through the back of each leg. Pressure from the uterus can irritate this nerve.

NATURAL REMEDIES

• A **back adjustment** by a chiropractor who is qualified to do this may be able to help alleviate this problem. A pelvic adjustment can reduce the pressure on that nerve.

—*Also see Sciatica (566, 626, 645).*

ENCOURAGEMENT—No sooner does the child of God approach the mercy seat than he becomes the client of the great Advocate. At his first utterance of penitence and appeal for pardon, Christ espouses his case and makes it His own; He presents the supplication before the Father as His own request.

GROIN SPASM OR PRESSURE IN PREGNANCY

SYMPTOMS—There is a "stitch" or pain on the right side. Later in pregnancy, lower groin pressure may develop.

CAUSES—The ligaments which connect the corners of the uterus to the pubic area sometimes kink. When this happens, they go into spasm and produce the side stitch. In later months, the weight of the womb presses down on the groin, causing pressure and discomfort.

NATURAL REMEDIES

• During a spasm, **breathe deeply and bend** toward the point of pain. Doing this permits the ligaments to relax. **Lie down** and **rest** until the pain leaves.

• Maintaining daily **exercise** will help avoid this.

ENCOURAGEMENT—If we are following Christ, His merits, imputed to us, come up before the Father as sweet odor. And the graces of our Saviour's character, implanted in our hearts, will shed around us a precious fragrance.

BLEEDING GUMS IN PREGNANCY

SYMPTOMS—The gums tend to swell and become softer. At times, they may bleed.

CAUSES—An increased estrogen output causes this swelling and softening. In addition, more blood is circulating throughout the body, including the gum area. Poor hygiene and infected gums are other causes.

NATURAL REMEDIES

• Give your teeth and gums special care. **Brush** your teeth after each meal. Increase your **calcium** (2,000 mg), **vitamin C** (1,000 mg), and **bioflavonoid** (100 mg) intake. Do not **smoke** or be around it! Nicotine destroys vitamin C.

• Eat a balanced, nutritious diet of **fresh fruits, vegetables, whole wheat, legumes, and nuts**. **Soy** products will help you obtain enough protein.

• Apply **aloe vera gel** to the gums.

ENCOURAGEMENT—Jesus cares for each one as though there were not another individual on the face of the earth. As Deity, He exerts mighty power in our behalf while, as our Elder Brother, He feels for all our woes.

ANEMIA IN PREGNANCY

SYMPTOMS—Paleness of skin and gums, fatigue, rapid heartbeat. There may be an increased craving for sweets or unusual foods (a sign of nutritional deficiency).

CAUSES—Blood volume greatly increases during pregnancy; but it is primarily an increase of plasma

P
R
E
G

(the liquid part of blood) rather than hemoglobin and the red blood cells it is in. Because of this, if you are not eating well, you can develop simple iron deficiency anemia. This is most likely to occur during the second trimester. Fortunately, the baby, itself, is unlikely to develop anemia.

NATURAL REMEDIES

It is important that you obtain enough **iron**—the right kind—so you can avoid simple anemia. Natural iron herbal formulas, which include **yellow dock and dandelion**, will build up the blood. **Chlorophyll, kelp, dulse, rice bran, whole grains, beans, dried apricots, and green leafy vegetables** are other sources. But the richest source of natural iron is **blackstrap molasses**.

• You should be aware of the fact that bottled **iron supplement** tablets frequently have the wrong kind of iron in them. Because it is not natural, it can block the absorption of vitamins E and A. Vitamin E is the anti-abortion vitamin; it is needed in order to bring a baby to full term. Do not take iron tablets during pregnancy!

• Take **folic acid** (5 mg), **vitamin B$_{12}$** (1,000 mcg), and a complete **B complex** supplement.

—*Also see Anemia (537-541).*

ENCOURAGEMENT—The love of the Father toward a fallen race is unfathomable, indescribable, without a parallel. This love led Him to consent to give His only begotten Son to die, that rebellious man might be brought into harmony with the government of Heaven and be saved from the penalty of his transgression.

EDEMA IN PREGNANCY

SYMPTOMS—Swelling develops in the hands and feet.

CAUSES—The increase of estrogen during pregnancy increases the tendency for the body to retain liquids. Some swelling of the hands and feet is normal.

But this must be carefully watched, because too much swelling is a symptom of pre-eclampsia *(716)*.

NATURAL REMEDIES

• Avoid salt and highly processed foods. Do not take diuretics (water pills). Try to walk at least a mile a day.

• Wear loose clothing and comfortable shoes. You may need a larger pair of shoes till the baby is delivered. When sitting, have your feet elevated.

• Remove finger rings early in the pregnancy, or they may have to be cut off later.

• If the swelling increases too much, see your physician. You may have pre-eclampsia *(716)*.

—*Also see Edema (494).*

ENCOURAGEMENT—Because Jesus came to dwell with us, we know that God is acquainted with our trials and sympathizes with our griefs. Every

son and daughter of Adam may understand that our Creator is the friend of sinners.

DIABETES IN PREGNANCY
(Gestational Diabetes)

SYMPTOMS—Frequent urination, excessive thirst, and increased fatigue. But possibly no symptoms at all. Identified by testing the woman's blood sugar levels around the 28th week of pregnancy.

CAUSES—This type of diabetes affects 3%-5% of pregnant women and only occurs during pregnancy. Because of hormonal secretions, not enough insulin is produced and blood sugar can become very high.

Although this condition does no permanent injury to the mother, the baby tends to gain weight and could be born with a low blood sugar level and excess weight. This could cause a difficult delivery. Fortunately, if fed sweet drinks, the baby's blood sugar can return to normal within hours after birth.

NATURAL REMEDIES

• Never miss meals, even if nauseated. Eat **small meals and frequently**. Do not eat **sugary** foods or too many **high-carbohydrate** foods.

• If the baby is determined to be too **large**, it may be best to deliver him early by cesarean section.

—*Also see Diabetes (656).*

ENCOURAGEMENT—In taking our nature, the Saviour has bound Himself to humanity by a tie that is never to be broken. He is linked with us throughout the eternal ages. "Unto us a child is born, unto us a son is given" (Isa. 9:6). God has adopted human nature in the person of His Son; He has carried the same into the highest heaven. It is the "Son of man" who shares the throne of the universe. In Christ, the family of earth and the family of heaven are bound together. Christ glorified is our brother. Heaven is enshrined in humanity; and humanity is enfolded in the bosom of Infinite Love.

ASTHMA IN PREGNANCY

SYMPTOMS—A pregnant woman has asthma.

CAUSES—For the sake of the child, it was previously thought best for women with asthma to stop taking any asthma medicine during pregnancy. It is now believed that the baby may be injured more by the mother's asthmatic attacks than by her taking the medicine. (Pregnancy usually reduces her asthmatic condition. If an attack occurs, take the medicine.)

NATURAL REMEDIES

• Avoid airborne pollutants. Purchase an air purifier for your bedroom, at least. Avoid anything that might trigger an asthma attack.

—*For an extensive coverage of these natural*

remedies, see Asthma (852).

ENCOURAGEMENT—We have not a high priest who is so high, so lifted up, that He cannot notice us or sympathize with us; but He was in all points tempted like as we are, yet without sin.

MISCARRIAGE
(Spontaneous Abortion)

SYMPTOMS—The fetus is ejected by the mother's body prior to the time that normal delivery should occur; this is usually before the 20th week.

CAUSES AND TREATMENT—Possible causes include cervical incompetence, ectopic pregnancy (implantation of the fertilized egg into a fallopian tube), *abruptio placentae* (placenta separates from the uterine wall), *placenta previa* (implantation of the placenta over the cervical opening). It can also be caused by chromosomal abnormality in the fetus or cervical incompetence (the cervix opens prematurely).

Other causes include emotional stress, general malaise, glandular disorders, and pregnancy-induced hypertension. But a frequent and often underlying cause is malnutrition.

Bleeding should always be taken seriously; for it may indicate that a miscarriage is about to begin. *See your physician.*

NATURAL REMEDIES

IMMEDIATE

• For a threatened abortion, have the woman lie very still and give a cup of false unicorn tea every ½ hour. As hemorrhaging decreases, give the tea every hour; then give it every 2 hours. Add 6 lobelia extract drops (no more) as a relaxer to the last cup.

• Every hour until bleeding is controlled, give a tea of wild yam, cranes bill, and comfrey.

• Take black haw tea in small doses throughout the danger period of habitual spontaneous abortion.

PREVENTION

• There can be deficiencies of **vitamins, trace minerals, and/or protein**. Vitamin A (taken in the form of **carotenes**, 5,000 IU), **folic acid** (5 mg), **zinc** (150 mg), and **complete amino acids** are especially important. **Vitamin E** (600-1,000 IU) is the "anti-abortion vitamin."

• Taking iron supplements can block the absorption of vitamin E, resulting in a miscarriage. Do not take iron tablets. Instead, take a little **blackstrap molasses** daily. It is the richest natural source of iron.

• It is vital that the mother-to-be take full **vitamin / mineral supplementation**, eat sufficient amounts of good **nourishing food** and avoid **junk food** of all types.

• **Ignore** the advice that you should eat whatever you want. If it is junk food, do not eat it! If it is real food and you crave it, then eat it. Getting enough **minerals** in your diet will help you avoid a craving for sweets, chocolate, etc. The cravings come because not enough vitamins, minerals, and complete proteins are being consumed.

• You may be eating certain foods which you, personally, ought to avoid because of malabsorption syndromes (such as **celiac disease**). Do **pulse tests** *(847)* to identify offending foods.

• In order to prevent another miscarriage, start on a fully nourishing diet six months before the planned conception.

• Do not **smoke** or be around it. Smokers are twice as likely to miscarry; and they have low birth-weight babies. Do not have **X-rays**, not even dental X-rays.

• Drinking **coffee** (either decaffeinated or regular) may induce miscarriage, especially during the first trimester.

• Take **red raspberry leaf tea** frequently, especially during the last few months of pregnancy. Or take **red raspberry leaf and catnip tea** throughout the pregnancy.

TESTING IF THE FETUS IS ALIVE

• To determine if the baby within you is alive, shake down a thermometer and place it by your bed. Upon awakening in the morning, move as little as possible, and take your temperature before arising. The fetus is alive if **your body temperature is 98.6 or above** (unless, due to hypothroidism, your normal temperature is lower).

ENCOURAGEMENT—Jesus understands. Go to Him and give Him all your heart. Trust your future to Him, and He will wonderfully guide.

PREMATURE LABOR

SYMPTOMS—The baby is born a number of weeks ahead of schedule.

CAUSES AND PREVENTION—Premature labor is the onset of rhythmic uterine contractions prior to fetal maturity; this is most likely to occur between the 20th and 37th weeks. About 5%-10% of infant deaths are premature.

For possible causes and prevention, *read Miscarriage above;* caution may avert this possibility.

ENCOURAGEMENT—The closer we are to God, the happier we are. Take time in prayer. Lay out before Him all your trials and sorrows, and He will provide the answers you need. Isaiah 32:18.

FALSE LABOR

SYMPTOMS—Strong contractions, which are close

together, begin coming—and then suddenly stop—hours or days before childbirth actually begins.

CAUSES—It is normal for a woman to have a few practice contractions weeks before labor begins. But sometimes she may have false labor, as described above.

NATURAL REMEDIES

• Sometimes **walking**, a **warm bath**, or **resting** will help calm the contractions, if they are false, or bring on childbirth if they are real. (Even if it is false labor, the contractions help to prepare the womb for actual labor later on.)

• An alternate method: Take 2 capsules each of **cayenne** and **bayberry**; and get to the hospital or call your midwife immediately.

ENCOURAGEMENT—God permitted His beloved Son, full of grace and truth, to come from a world of indescribable glory to a world marred and blighted with sin, under the shadow of death and the curse, in order to save us.

CHILDBIRTH

TO MAKE LABOR EASIER—Take earlier **training classes**. Later they will help you relax during contractions, reduce pains, help train the coach to assist, and explain how to recognize potential problems. Helpful herbs include **blue cohosh**.

TO STOP POST-PARTUM HEMORRHAGE—**Raspberry** tea can be used to stop post-partum hemorrhage. Give it either orally or intramuscularly).

TO STOP AFTER-BIRTH PAINS—**Wild yam, cramp bark, and black haw** are specific herbs which help reduce after-birth pains and cramping throughout the pelvic area. Rub **warming liniment** into the skin, followed by **hot fomentations** over the area

Warm whole baths help the pain subside. Make sure the bathtub is sterile beforehand. Fast on **vegetable juices and broths** until the pains are gone. Once the pain is relieved, apply a **castor oil pack** for an hour.

ENCOURAGEMENT—Let God's Word, the Bible, be a lamp to your feet and a light to your path. In Him you can find the help you need.

PRE-ECLAMPSIA, ECLAMPSIA
(Pregnancy Toxemia)

SYMPTOMS—*Pre-eclampsia:* Sudden weight gain, high blood pressure, albuminuria, headaches, dizziness, spots before the eyes, epigastric pain, edema (swelling) of the legs and feet.

Eclampsia: Symptoms of pre-eclampsia, plus convulsions and coma. The convulsions begin with fixation of the eyeballs and rolling of the eyes. There is also twitchings of the face, arms, and hands. Then coma with temperature at 103°-104° F. The person can die in the coma.

CAUSES—Beginning about the turn of the century, physicians have sometimes prescribed that women keep their weight down in order to have smaller babies (which are easier for the doctor to deliver).

But such **arbitrarily restricted diets—low in protein, salt, and water**—can lead to serious consequences.

The sudden weight gain occurs because of fluid retention, due to low blood protein, high blood pressure, and albuminuria.

If pre-eclampsia is not treated properly, it develops into eclampsia—an even worse form of the disorder.

Both forms of this disorder *occur after the 20th week* of pregnancy. The orthodox treatment is to place the woman in the hospital, wait until convulsions occur, and then give her barbiturates. But what she needs is nourishing food before then and during that time.

Diet, blood pressure, and weight must be watched—but proper nutrition and fluid intake is most important.

NATURAL REMEDIES

• A **balanced high-protein diet**. Do not restrict **salt**. Take **seaweed** products, for trace minerals, and a full **vitamin / mineral supplement**. *See Pregnancy-related Problems for a list of nutritional needs (706).*

• Take **vitamin B$_6$** (100 mg daily until birth; then only take 50 mg daily) and 10-12 glasses of **water or fruit juice** a day, especially in the hot months.

ENCOURAGEMENT—The old song says, "Trust and obey; for there is no other way to be happy in Jesus, but to trust and obey." And how very true that is. Ezekiel 36:25.

PREGNANCY AND BREAST-FEEDING -
3 - BREAST-FEEDING

BREAST-FEEDING
(Lactation, Nursing)

YOUR OWN NUTRITION

• Try to nurse your little one for at least nine months, if at all possible. It will have fewer allergies, respiratory diseases, hypoglycemia, obesity, and gastroenteritis. Both you and the child will be happier and bond together more fully. The infant will have increased health and adapt better to later physical and emotional situations which may develop. Breast-fed babies are less susceptible to SIDS (especially if they are not given infant vaccines!). *See SIDS (734).* Research studies reveal that the docosahexaenoic acid (DHA) in mother's milk improves intellectual development in the infant.

Formula-fed babies do not receive DHA.

• A high-**calcium** diet is very important in maintaining a good milk supply. *See Strengthening the Bones (505) for information on obtaining enough calcium.* Be sure and obtain enough **sunshine** on your skin, so it can be converted into vitamin D in your liver.

• A high-**protein** diet is very important. Take B complex, plus all the other vitamins and minerals, along with a sizeable amount of **brewer's yeast** at every meal. You need to stuff yourself on yeast and calcium foods in order to have enough milk for your baby.

• Drink lots of **lemon juice**. Avoid **sage tea**; for it dries up the milk. Do not eat **beans, onions, and cabbage;** for they will upset your baby.

• Keep your **bowels** open and clean with high-**fiber** foods.

• To increase milk supply, helpful herbs include **milkweed, caraway, goat's rue, and fenugreek.**

OTHER HELPS

• Keep yourself in good **health**; so you can continue eating an adequate diet while you are nursing your little one. You want to avoid long fasts, cleansing diets, or strictly limited diets during lactation.

• Avoid **mental depression** and **violent exercise**. They will also upset the baby.

• Do not **smoke** while nursing! Please, do not smoke at all! Avoid **caffeine, liquor, junk food, fried food, and drugs**.

• Be happy, rest often, and pray that God will help you raise a child who is dedicated to Him.

BREAST-FEEDING

• Sore, fissured, and possibly infected nipples will be avoided if certain principles are followed.

• Try to **wash your hands** before handling your breasts.

• **Position the baby** properly. His entire body should face you. His buttocks should be in one of your hands and his head in the bend of your elbow. The other hand is under the breast, with all four fingers supporting it. But do not place your fingers on the areola (the darker area around the nipple).

• **Prepare the nipple**. If—if—your hands are clean, you can rub the nipple lightly to firm it. Pinching it lightly flattens the nipple, to fit his mouth better. Do not try to toughen your nipples by vigorously rubbing them. This can damage them.

• **Bring the baby to the nipple**. As you tickle the baby's lower lip with your nipple, his mouth will open wide. When it is open wide, pull his body in quickly. His mouth should fix on the areola, and the nipple should be deep in his throat. At least an inch of the areola should be in his mouth. In this way, there is no movement of the nipple as the infant sucks.

• **Breaking the suction.** If you feel pain, do not delay; but immediately use your finger to break the suction and reposition him. Break the suction by placing a finger inside the corner of the infant's mouth to allow air to enter and break the vacuum. Do not, instead, just pull the nipple out of his mouth!

• La Leche (an organization advocating breast-feeding) says that 95% of the nipple soreness problems are caused by the way the baby sucks; and this can be corrected.

• **Leave him on a breast** as long as he is sucking effectively (swallowing every suck or two). If he begins pausing, burp him, wake him, switch sides, and let him nurse as long as he wants. Feeding time is usually 20-30 minutes.

• (But, for the first few days, it may be necessary to limit feeding periods to 5 minutes on each breast, before rotating to the other. It is very important that you work with the baby properly; so that you avoid fissures developing on, or near, the nipples.)

• Do not let him remain on the breast after he has finished actively feeding. *See Mastitis (674, 719) for why these precautions are given.*

• **The next time you start**, begin on the breast you ended with previously. Always have him nurse on both sides.

• You will find that the baby will want to nurse often—frequently 8-12 times a day in the early weeks. God designed that these frequent feedings would bond the infant to his mother.

• **After feeding**, empty the breasts manually or with a breast pump until supply and demand reach an equilibrium.

• Air-dry the breasts after each feeding, before covering them. (Exposing the breasts to the air for 20 minutes at a time, two or three times a day, is helpful.) A 40-watt bulb can be placed near them for 15 minutes at a time. Never use breast pads that might retain moisture (especially those with plastic in them). Do not wear bras with plastic liners. If needed, place a folded handkerchief there.

• **Nipple cleanliness** is important. But never use soap on the nipples; it dries them out. The milk contains its own oil and also a self-cleaning antiseptic. Leave a little on at the end of each feeding, to lubricate and soften the nipple.

• Baby saliva contains an enzyme which softens the skin. So, if possible, wash the nipples with clean water. (Water or alcohol applied to the nipple will toughen the skin and assist in preventing sore nipples.) Or, better yet, place some mother's milk on them.

• You will want to do that which will avoid each of the following problems: *Sore Nipple (718), Nipple Candida (720), Plugged Duct (719), Engorgement (718), and Mastitis (674, 719). See each section for more information.*

• **Other helps**. Clothing worn next to the breast should always be soft and non-irritating. Cotton is generally best.

• Feed the baby before the breasts become too full; then the infant will not have difficulty grasping the breast. Stasis of milk (when it is not flowing on out, but remaining in the breast too long) helps lead to mastitis *(674, 719)*. Also see Engorgement *(718)*.

• If the baby is fed before he is hungry, he will not suck the nipple too vigorously. Never allow him to chew the nipple.

• If a nipple is cracked, pierce a vitamin E capsule and apply the oil just after nursing. Do not use very much.

• Apply hot, wet compresses to the breast, if the baby is not taking as much milk as you are producing and you are getting too full. This will open up the ducts and increase the flow. Then nurse the baby more often and longer. Drink more fluids, so you can urinate every hour.

—Also see Mastitis (674, 719), for an explanation of prebirth preparation of the nipples.

ENCOURAGEMENT—Only the love that flows from the heart of Christ can heal. Only He can restore the wounded soul. Submit your life to Him everyday, obey His Written Word, claim His promises; and you will find the help you need.

SORE NIPPLE

SYMPTOMS—One or both nipples becomes sore.

CAUSES—Sore nipples are generally caused by one of the following: The baby is not being positioned properly on the nipple. The nursing schedule is irregular or not frequent enough. The baby is permitted to incorrectly suck on the nipple. The breast becomes engorged (overly filled) with milk. As a result of one or more of these, infection may have set in. The infection is usually the fungus *Candida albicans*. *See Nipple Candida (720)*.

NATURAL REMEDIES

• **Position** the baby so that his jaws are over the least tender parts of the nipple. Do not pull away when the infant is about to begin feeding. Relax and let him feed.

• Nurse on the breast that has the least soreness.

• If both breasts are sore, **hand-express** (with your hand or a breast pump) the milk until the "let-down" occurs (the milk is flowing well). Then put the baby to the breast so he can easily get it.

• **Frequently feed** the baby so he will not be hungry and bite down roughly on the nipple.

• **Position him** properly. His mouth should cover over as much of the areola (dark area of the nipple) as possible. He should not make slurping noises when feeding. Frequently change nursing positions, to rotate the pressure of his mouth on the nipple. Always cor-

rectly break the suction, instead of just pulling him off the nipple.

• Keep the **nipples dry** between feedings. Expose them to sunlight and air.

• Do not **wash** the nipples with soap, alcohol, or petroleum-based products. Put a little of the milk on the nipples and let them air-dry.

• If the nipples are cracked, as well as sore, apply fresh **aloe vera gel** or a paste form of **calendula**, **marshmallow**, or **slippery elm** to them. This will soothe them.

• In order to avoid engorgement *(718)*, **massage** your breasts from base to tip. Begin doing this in the final weeks of pregnancy; and continue doing it through to the time the baby begins nursing, and beyond.

• If a nipple becomes sore, put a little **milk** on it. Then let it air dry. The nipples should be checked daily; and, if they are sore or cracked, treatment should begin promptly. Do not wait. *See Mastitis (674, 719)*.

• For sore nipples, use **sunshine** or the light of a **light bulb** that is close enough to feel warm but not burn.

• Place some cold grocery-store **tea** (containing tannic acid) on a folded tissue and lay it on the area for 20 minutes; then dry and expose it to air for 20 minutes. Rinse it before the next nursing. The tannic acid will promote healing.

• Poultices of **comfrey** root or leaf may be used for sore nipples.

• If the condition continues, you may have a candida infection. *See Nipple Candida (720)*.

ENCOURAGEMENT—When we obey God's holy ten commandment law (through the enabling grace of Jesus Christ), our lives are ennobled and we live cleaner, happier lives.

ENGORGEMENT

SYMPTOMS—The tissues in the breast swell. They feel full, hard, tender, and tight. The skin of the breast is shiny, hot, and distended. You may have a low-grade fever.

CAUSES—Especially during the first two weeks, there is an increased blood supply to the breast; and newly produced milk is placing pressure on the breast.

NATURAL REMEDIES

• Until engorgement ends (usually within two weeks), give your baby short, frequent feedings every 1½-2 hours, day and night. Express (pump out) milk between feedings, to relieve pressure.

• Apply moist heat to the engorged breast (or breasts) for 30 minutes before each feeding. While the infant is nursing, massage the breast to help get the milk flowing.

• Feed your baby whenever he wants it. Do not delay doing this.

• Do not feed your baby anything else (except clean water) during this initial engorgement period.

Let him empty each breast completely at each feeding. According to the American Academy of Pediatrics, newborns should nurse 8-12 times every 24 hours; continue nursing each time until the baby is satisfied, which is usually 10-15 minutes on each side.

• Do not give him formula or sugary water.

• To reduce milk supply (or the pain of breast engorgement), the herb, **goldenrod**, is helpful. (But do not take it if you are allergic to that herb.)

• Research studies have found that, because of a stillbirth or neonatal death, the flow of breast milk was suppressed (reduced or stopped) by placing **jasmine flowers** on the area. They are held in place with tape. Each breast had 50 cm. of stringed flowers applied to it. This lowers serum prolactin levels.

ENCOURAGEMENT—God has given His holy law to man as His measure of character. By the enabling grace of Christ, you may see and overcome every defect in your character.

PLUGGED DUCT

SYMPTOMS—Soreness or a lump in one area of the breast. A place on the breast will feel hard and painful to the touch.

CAUSES—The breast is full of thousands of tiny milk ducts. They are the sources of the milk which is fed to your baby. But some of them can become plugged.

Causes include incomplete emptying of the breast in each feeding by the infant. If the milk does not come out, it begins drying in the duct and clogs it. Wearing a tight bra can also cause a plugged duct.

Binding clothes, fatigue, or prolonged periods without nursing can cause them. If not dealt with promptly, infection can begin.

If milk is left on the nipple after a feeding, so that it dries, that can also keep the milk from flowing out freely during the next feeding.

NATURAL REMEDIES

• After each feeding, carefully check each nipple, looking for tiny "dots" of dried milk. Gently wash them away. By doing this each time, plus emptying the breast fully at each feeding, will generally clear plugged ducts within 24 hours.

• Massage the breast, starting at the chest wall and working down with a circular motion. This stimulates milk flow. It is important that you let the baby nurse on that side frequently. The sucking clears out the duct better than anything else.

• Offer the child the affected breast first. This will ensure that he will fully empty it.

• You may need to alter the position of the infant on the nipple, so all the ducts are drained.

ENCOURAGEMENT—It is not necessary that anyone should yield to the temptations of Satan and thus violate his conscience and grieve the Holy Spirit.

MASTITIS

SYMPTOMS—Breast inflammation, redness, pain, fever, chills, hard swelling, malaise, headache, and possibly swollen cervical and/or axillary lymph nodes. Soreness and redness in the breast, fever, pus-like secretions from the nipple which are yellow, general tiredness, flu-like symptoms.

CAUSES—Mastitis generally occurs between the fifth day after childbirth to the second or third week. —It especially occurs to mothers nursing their first baby. Usually limited to one breast, it must be treated promptly or an abscess may develop. Treatment must be started within 12-18 hours after the first symptoms are noted.

The breast and milk duct system has become inflamed by staphylococci invading a fissured or cracked nipple.

Causes include **shallow grip on the nipple** by the infant, **incomplete emptying** during each feeding, **blocked duct, poor nipple care and hygiene, irritating clothing, engorged breast** (because of trying to wean the child off milk), or **lack of proper nipple preparation** prior to lactation. *See Breast-feeding (716), Engorgement (previous page), Plugged Duct (above), Sore Nipple (previous page).*

It is important that the infant completely empty the breast each time. If he is not properly positioned on the nipple, the infant can excessively suck it while trying to get milk. *See Breast-feeding (716).*

Most minor infections will heal by themselves within a week.

NATURAL REMEDIES

• **Do not stop nursing** the baby because you have mastitis! The milk is not infected, the baby needs it; and you must keep giving it for months to come. The milk gives the baby valuable antibodies. If you stop nursing, the mastitis could more easily lead to an abscess in the breast.

• **Go to bed, keep drinking lots of clear fluids, and nurse more frequently**.

• Air-dry the nipples after each nursing, to prevent cracking. (Bacteria enter through the cracks.) If they do crack, place breast milk on them. Then, when they dry, put fresh aloe vera gel on them.

• Apply heat to the breasts, to help heal the cracks and prevent infections. Place a 100-watt bulb about 12-18 inches from each breast. It should not be close enough to cause discomfort.

• Alternate **hot and cold compresses** are often

PREG

all the treatment required. Apply a hot compress for 3 minutes; then apply cold for 30 seconds. Do this 3 times and repeat the series 2-3 times each day.

• Sometimes, a continuous **cold application** is preferred. If so, give a **hot footbath** at the same time.

• Nurse the affected breast twice as often, but for shorter periods of time. Try to **keep it emptied**. Let no one tell you that you should stop nursing if you have mastitis! Keep nursing; you will recover more quickly and the baby will not be injured.

• Obtain plenty of **rest**, including frequent rest periods throughout the day.

• Always wash your hands before and after each breast-feeding. Always wash the breast and nipple afterward.

PREVENTION
• Prevention of mastitis begins prior to childbirth. For 2-3 months, the mother-to-be must get her nipples ready for lactation. She should **massage** the nipples daily with **chickweed** ointment. **Vitamin E** may also be used. Perform the "nipple pull" several times each day during a shower.

• During breast-feeding, **position the baby right**. Place the baby on the breast correctly, empty the breast fully, and break suction properly. This should be followed by **emptying the breast** with a hand pump, if necessary. Nipple **cleanliness** is also important. Proper **clothing** should be worn. *All this and more is explained in "Breast-feeding" (716).*
— *Also see Fibrocystic Breast Disease (674).*

ENCOURAGEMENT—There are many whose hearts are aching under a load of care. Go to God with your trials and problems, and find in Him the solutions you so much seek. Matthew 25:21.

BREAST ABSCESS

SYMPTOMS—The symptoms of mastitis have worsened into pus in the breast and breast milk.

CAUSES—In rare instances, a breast abscess develops—and the breast fills with pus. If this happens, milk should be hand-expressed (pumped by hand) and discarded. Drainage may be necessary; and this can be done in a physician's office. Breast-feeding should continue on the uninfected breast until the abscess in the other one has healed.

NIPPLE CANDIDA

SYMPTOMS—A reddened, itchy, area on the nipple. Or severe pain while feeding the infant.

CAUSES—This is a fungal infection. This condition can be further complicated if the baby develops oral thrush. Treat oral thrush essentially the same as for nipple candida.

NATURAL REMEDIES
NUTRITION
• Eat a nourishing diet of **fruits, vegetables, whole grains, legumes, and nuts**. While treating the infection, a diet primarily of **raw food** is best.

• Avoid **tobacco, alcohol, caffeine**. Do not eat **meat or dairy products**. Avoid **sugary, fried, and processed foods**. Eat nothing **greasy**.

HERBS
• **Goldenseal** contains *berberine*, which destroys fungi. It can be used against every type of fungus infection. It can be applied both topically and as a drink. Only use goldenseal for a week; then switch for a time to another fungicide herb.

• **Pau d'arco** is strongly antifungal. Drink 3 cups daily.

• **Bloodroot** also contains *berberine*; this has been shown to be quite effective as a fungicide.

• **Yellowroot, barberry, and Oregon grape** also contain *berberine*.

• **Tea tree** oil is excellent when applied externally; but do not drink it. Apply it several times a day to the affected area; it can be applied either full strength or diluted with a little distilled water or cold-pressed oil. **Black walnut** extract can also be used.

• A powerful antifungicide is **wild oregano oil**. The most resistent forms of fungus infection can generally be eliminated by it.

• The **pepper tree** (horopito) is a New Zealand shrub which contains *polygodial*; this is useful against both fungi and bacteria. Another antifungal herb is the *Licaria puchuri-major*, a Brazilian plant.

OTHER HELPS
• Keep the **nipples clean and dry**. Expose the affected area to air as much as possible. Your **clothing** should be kept clean.
—*Also see Candida (281).*

ENCOURAGEMENT—In the religious life of every soul who is finally victorious there will be scenes of terrible perplexity and trial; but his knowledge of the Scriptures will enable him to bring to mind the encouraging promises of God, which will comfort his heart and strengthen his faith in the power of the Mighty One.

PREGNANCY AND BREAST-FEEDING -
4 - EMOTIONAL PROBLEMS

BABY BLUES

SYMPTOMS—Symptoms start 3-10 days after giving birth. They are often worse about day 5 and include weeping, dramatic mood swings, fatigue and irritability, lack of concentration.

CAUSES—It is very common for a new mother to feel low or miserable during the first few days or weeks after childbirth. Major changes have to be made. Up to 8 in 10 women experience the "baby blues."

This condition is caused by the sudden fall in hormone levels (especially estrogen and progesterone) that occurs after a baby is born.

Baby blues generally clear up within a few weeks, as the mother obtains more rest and adapts to her new responsibilities.

NATURAL REMEDIES

• Obtain extra **rest**. Take time to **walk outdoors** in the fresh air. **Be thankful** to God for all your blessings; for they are many. **Set to work helping** your new baby. **Recognize the possibilities** of how much you will be able to help him now and in the coming years.

—*Also see Depression (596).*

ENCOURAGEMENT—Summon all your powers to look up, not down at your difficulties; then you will never faint by the way. You will soon see Jesus behind the cloud, reaching out His hand to help you; and all you have to do is to give Him your hand in simple faith and let Him lead you.

POST-PARTUM DEPRESSION

SYMPTOMS—Symptoms are like those of baby blues, but more severe; they begin any time within the first 6 months. The new mother constantly feels exhausted; she has little interest in the baby. There is a sense of anticlimax, feeling inadequate and overwhelmed by new responsibilities, difficulty sleeping, loss of appetite, and feelings of guilt.

CAUSES—This is more severe than baby blues; yet it is somewhat common in the first few weeks or months after childbirth. It affects about 1 woman in 10. Hormonal changes are involved.

Inadequacy, isolation, concerns about the new responsibilities can cause stress and lead to depression. There is also lack of sleep, exhaustion from a lengthy birth labor, painful wounds (vaginal tears or cesarean stitches).

Some women, who have post-partum depression, have had depression *(596)* prior to becoming pregnant. Some women have panic attacks which lead to post-partum depression.

The problem generally clears up within a few months or up to a year.

NATURAL REMEDIES

• Take time to rest, count your blessings, ask God for courage and strength for each day's new duties. And dedicate your life to serving others; right now, it especially includes your new child.

• Rest and take time to be around other mothers with their little ones. Make more friends and take time to talk to them. Find ways to help others. We forget ourselves when we are busy thinking about how to help someone who needs us.

—*Also see Depression (596).*

ENCOURAGEMENT—Jesus is always ready to help you in forming a strong, symmetrical character.

POST-PARTUM PSYCHOSIS

SYMPTOMS—Symptoms usually develop rapidly, about 2-5 weeks after childbirth, and include extreme mood swings from depression to mania, insomnia and overactivity, confusion, false beliefs of being disliked and persecuted by people, hallucinations.

CAUSES—About 1 woman in 1,000 develops a serious psychiatric condition, known as post-partum psychosis. It requires special care.

The woman usually has previously experienced episodes of severe depression *(596)*, alternating with mania *(598)*. Some of these women have close relatives who have a history of bipolar disorder (manic-depression, *597-598*) or severe depression.

NATURAL REMEDIES

• This person needs understanding friends. It is best that she not be left alone until she can feel happy caring for her baby.

— *Also see Mental Illness (601).*

ENCOURAGEMENT—**As you draw near to God with confession and repentance, He will draw near to you with mercy and forgiveness.**

Oh, how thankful we can be for the love of God in Christ Jesus our Lord! As we trust him and obey His ten commandment law, He ennobles our lives and enables us to prepare to live forever with Him in heaven.

PREG

"The Lord God is a sun and shield: the Lord will give grace and glory: no good thing will He withhold from them that walk uprightly."
—Psalm 84:11

"The Lord preserveth the simple: I was brought low, and He helped me."
—Psalm 116:6

"The Lord is good unto them that wait for Him, to the soul that seeketh Him."
—Lamentations 3:25

"Ye shall serve the Lord your God . . and I will take away sickness from the midst of thee."
—Exodus 23:25

SPECIAL SECTIONS FOR WOMEN - 3

The Natural Remedies Encyclopedia

- Disease Section 16 - Infancy and Childhood

— Concluded on the next page

CHILD

"The promise is unto you, and to your children."   —Acts 2:39

"Behold, I and the children whom the Lord hath given me."   —Isaiah 8:18

"Thus saith the Lord that made thee, and formed thee from the womb . . Fear not."   —Isaiah 44:2

"All thy children shall be taught of the Lord; and great shall be the peace of thy children."   —Isaiah 54:13

"Believe on the Lord Jesus Christ, and thou shalt be saved, and thy house."   —Acts 16:31

"Suffer the little children to come unto Me, and forbid them not: for of such is the kingdom of God . . And He took them up in His arms, put His hands upon them, and blessed them."   —Mark 10:14, 16

"Teach us what we shall do unto the child that shall be born."   —Judges 13:8

"Who are those with thee? And he said, 'The children which God hath graciously given thy servant.' "   —Genesis 33:5

"Children are an heritage of the Lord: and the fruit of the womb is His reward."   —Psalm 127:3

"The babe leaped in my womb for joy."   —Luke 1:44

"Suffer little children to come unto Me, and forbid them not."   —Matthew 19:14

"Thou knowest not what is the way of the spirit, nor how the bones do grow in the womb of her that is with child: even so thou knowest not the works of God who maketh all."   —Ecclesiastes 11:5

"Can a woman forget her sucking child, that she should not have compassion on the son of her womb? yea, they may forget, yet will I not forget thee."   —Isaiah 49:15

"And I will bless her, and give thee a son also of her."   —Genesis 17:16

"God Almighty bless thee, and make thee fruitful, and multiply thee."   —Genesis 28:3

"He maketh the barren woman to keep house, and to be a joyful mother of children. Praise ye the Lord."   —Psalm 113:9

"Whosoever shall not receive the kingdom of God as a little child, he shall not enter therein. And He took them up in His arms . . and blessed them."   —Mark 10:15-16

"In all thy ways acknowledge Him, and He shall direct thy paths."   —Proverbs 3:6

"Peace I leave with you, My peace I give unto you; not as the world giveth, give I unto you."   —John 14:27

C
H
I
L
D

Section 16 - Infancy and Childhood

INFANCY AND CHILDHOOD -
1 - INFANT NUTRITION

INFANT FEEDING

DOS AND DON'TS

From the beginning, give your baby a little **water**, gradually increasing the amount. Do not give **orange juice or tomato juice** until he is older. He is a precious gift; so you want to give him the best of care.

At 3 months, begin a little **blended food**. By 9 months, the baby should be eating a variety of carefully prepared natural foods. However, in order to avoid food allergies, many experts declare that breast-feeding alone, with nothing else for the first 6 months, is best.

Do not give the baby any grains (wheat, oats, rice, etc.) until he is 6 months old! When the baby is 6 months old, dilute 4 teaspoons of whole-wheat flakes in boiling water till entirely dissolved, put through a fine sieve, and add to the baby's bottle (if you are giving him a bottle by then). A little powdered oatmeal can also be added.

When the first teeth appear, begin feeding wholesome simple foods in puree form (such as **greens, vegetables, fruit juices, and gruels**).

Do not give the infant **cane sugar** in any form. This can lead to fever and various ailments. Use **malt sugar**. Do not give **honey** or **orange juice**.

Do not give the infant **meat**! Feeding an infant **meat, cane sugar, white-flour products, candies, or soft drinks** causes him to lose his taste for simple, natural foods; and it is responsible for rickets, scurvy, tonsil trouble, night terrors, anemia, and convulsions.

INFANCY AND CHILDHOOD -
2 - BIRTH DEFECTS

CONGENITAL INFECTIONS

SYMPTOMS—A variety of problems to the infant include miscarriage, preterm birth, illness at birth, or physical abnormalities.

CAUSES—Most infections contracted by a mother during pregnancy do not affect the fetus; but some cross the placenta and cause harm. These infections are often brief, minor illnesses for the mother; and she may be unaware of them. However, chronic infections such as HIV may also be passed on.

The effect on the baby depends on when the baby received it. In early pregnancy, the development of organs may be disrupted and a miscarriage *(715)* may occur. Infections in later pregnancy may result in premature labor *(715)* and a baby who is seriously ill at birth. Infections may also be transmitted as the baby passes through the birth canal.

First part of pregnancy: In the first 3 months, **rubella** can produce heart abnormalities (congenital heart disease), impaired hearing, and/or impaired vision. **Toxoplasmosis** (cat coccidia, *846*), or **cytomegalovirus** (CMV), can cause miscarriage or malformations, The first can cause damage to the retina; the second (CMV) is the leading cause of congenital deafness.

Later in the pregnancy: The above two diseases can result in preterm labor, stillbirth, and serious illness in the newborn. **Listeriosis** *(878)* may cause miscarriage.

Chronic viral infections: which may be transmitted include **HIV** *(806)*, **hepatitis** *(446)* **(either B or C)**, **syphilis** *(804)*, and **trichomoniasis** *(695, 805)*. These infections do not always produce symptoms at birth; but they may cause serious illness later in life. **Herpes simplex** and **bacterial streptococcal infections** (cause acute and sometimes fatal illness in the newborn. The risk of infection is greater if the mother's waters break prematurely.

NATURAL PREVENTIVES
• If people in your neighborhood are getting rubella (German measles), **avoid extensive contact** with others during the first three months of the pregnancy.
• To avoid toxoplasmosis, do not have a **cat** in the house; and **do not clean cat feces**!
• To avoid listeriosis, do not eat **soft cheese, pate, poorly cooked meat, or dairy products**.
• In order to avoid venereal diseases *(802)*, do not practice **unsafe sex**.
• Do what is needed to **avoid hepatitis** *(446)*.
• If you have HIV or active genital herpes, it is best to have delivery by **cesarean section**.

ENCOURAGEMENT—God can encourage your heart as no one on earth can. Go to Him with all your trials and problems. He alone can give you the peace of heart that you so much desire.

BIRTH DEFECTS

IMPORTANT: Be sure to read Pregnancy Problems *(706)*. **It tells you what to do to avoid birth defects.**

SYMPTOMS—A variety of partially, or wholly, incapacitating physical or mental defects which are present at birth.

CAUSES—More than 90% of birth defects are the result of **early pregnancy malnutrition** of the mother. Such defects include cleft palates, cleft lips, heart defects, limb defects, spina bifida, cystic fibrosis, muscular dystrophy, heart defects, brain defect, fetal hernia.

All of the above diseases have been eliminated from valuable livestock by the veterinary profession. This has been done by giving the animals excellent nutrition. Why is it that we feed animals better than we feed humans! Yet junk food (which leads to a variety of diseases in adults, children, and newborns) is sold—and no warnings are given to the public. Indeed, the official government message is that "you can get all your vitamins and minerals in the food you buy at the store."

It is well-known that **bearing a child after the age of 40** can cause problems. Yet teenagers have a greater percentage of children with birth defects than do women over 40, because of their generally poor eating habits and lack of vitamin / mineral supplementation. Many young people today live on junk food and have damaged offspring as a result.

As an example, let us consider **cystic fibrosis** *(655-656)*. It is a type of adrenal damage disorder; this is said to be the "most common genetic defect." Yet, in reality, cystic fibrosis is caused by a **selenium** *(114)* **and fatty acid deficiency** *(100-105)* in the fetus and/ or newborn breast-fed infant. If the mother has **celiac disease** *(473)*, this can impede her absorption of essential nutrients (such as selenium and even more).

In 1958, Dr. Kaus Schwartz reported in the NIH publication, *Federal Proceedings*, that selenium was an essential nutrient. The deficiency symptoms he reported all fit cystic fibrosis. But no one paid attention.

In 1972, Cornell University found that chicks hatched from selenium-deficient hens developed all the classical symptoms of cystic fibrosis of the pancreas. They found that chicks were totally cured from selenium difficiency within 21 days, if selenium was given within 30 days after hatching.

In 1978, J.D. Wallach, a veterinarian researcher, identified this problem in animals and birds as being "cystic fibrosis." But, when other researchers agreed with his findings, Wallach was fired within 24 hours from his government research laboratory.

Since that date, Wallach has treated over 450

CHART - 1044: Birth Defects (724-727)

cystic fibrosis patients with excellent results. He has cured three-month-old infants of the disorder. Wallach later did joint research with the Chinese government, in their hospitals, and helped thousands of their people.

Yet, in America, the people are told fibrosis is a "genetic defect" and nothing can be done, except expensive and time-consuming rehabilitation programs. Why does this cover-up continue?

Dr. Arthur F. Coco, inventor of the pulse test, made this statement: "I am a realist. As long as the profit is in the treatment of symptoms rather than a search for causes, that's where the medical profession will go for its harvest."

It is true that radiation is another cause of birth defects; yet only .1% of birth defects result from X-rays, etc. Most pregnant women realize that they should avoid them.

What is the solution to the problem? *It is to give women a good, nourishing diet. But it must begin a couple of years before conception!*

Prevention of birth defects requires more than "prenatal" vitamins after the second month of pregnancy, when the physician gives his pronouncement, "You are pregnant." By that time, the embryo has formed all organs and tissues—for better or worse! **Proper supplementation of vitamins and minerals, nourishing food, and avoidance of tobacco, alcohol, caffeine, drugs, and junk foods must have had its effect on the mother's body—before conception took place!**

Do a home pregnancy test as soon as you suspect the possibility of being pregnant; and immediately begin eating nourishing food and taking supplements.

Here is a vitamin you must be taking before you become pregnant: **Folic acid** *(105)*. This B vitamin helps prevent **brain and spinal column defects** in newborns. To prevent such defects, women should begin taking 400 mcg a day at least one month prior to conception—and continue for at least 3 months afterward. The only effective way that this can be done is for them to be taking it from the time they become able to bear children.

—A sample of such a birth defect is Cerebral Palsy (below). Also see Cystic Fibrosis (655).

ENCOURAGEMENT—Faith is needed in the world today, faith that will lay hold on the promises of God's Word and refuse to let go until Heaven hears.

CEREBRAL PALSY

SYMPTOMS—A form of paralysis caused by a prenatal brain defect, characterized by involuntary motions and difficulty in control of the voluntary muscles.

C
H
I
L
D

CAUSES—The cause of this disorder, which affects the fine motor coordination of the body, is a **deficiency of zinc and B$_6$** in the mother's diet prior to, and during, the formation of the brain of the fetus. It is possible that **celiac disease** *(473-474)* in the mother may also have been a factor in inducing this deficiency.

There is, at this time, no known treatment.

NATURAL REMEDIES
• As reported in *Annals of Allergy (August 1981, Abstract 28*, many victims of cerebral palsy experience an increase in the intensity of their symptoms because of allergies. Recognizing and removing these **allergies** may improve their quality of life.
—*Also see Birth Defects (725).*

ENCOURAGEMENT—Let the afflictions which pain us so grievously draw us closer to God. Find in Him the help that you need.

DOWN'S SYNDROME
(Mongolism)

SYMPTOMS—Slow physical development, moderate to severe mental retardation, and facial features which are somewhat flattened. Ears are set low, tongue is large and furrowed, hands are broad and short—and have a single (simian) crease across the palm.

CAUSES—Also called *trisomy 21*, Down's Syndrome occurs during fetal development; but it is not inherited. The problem is **an extra 21st chromosome**. It occurs in 1 out of 700 live births. The risk increases greatly after the age of 34.

People with Down's Syndrome can, with care, live to old age. But they are prone to Alzheimer's disease *(587)*, pneumonia *(503)*, and other lung diseases.

NATURAL REMEDIES
• A nourishing diet of fresh **fruits, vegetables, legumes, and nuts** is very important, plus proper rest. Avoid foods containing gluten (**wheat, oats, barley, and rye**). Avoid **sugars, refined foods, dairy products, tobacco smoke, and alcohol**. Give him **supplements** in liquid (not tablet or capsule) form. The entire **B complex** is important for brain development.
• **Exercise** is important, so oxygen gets to the brain. Carefully planned activities are needed at an early age, to provide exercises to improve his motor skills.
• Children with this problem tend to be very affectionate. **Hold your child** and show him love; and he will become even more kindly and affable. **Involve him** in whatever you are doing; encourage your other children to do the same.

NEW HELPS
There are several **new methods** that have been developed for helping children with this problem. The result can be a lengthening of life and an increase of mental ability. Details are lengthy; and here is where you can learn more about this. You can obtain real help from them:
• Nutri-Chem Labs, 1303 Richmond Road, Ottawa, Ontario K2B 764, Canada / 613-820-9065 or 613-829-2226. Ask about MSBPlus formula and anything else they have for Down's Syndrome. It has had fairly good success.
• Warner House, 1023 East Chapman Avenue, Fullerton CA 92631 / 714-441-2600. Their formula reduces infections in persons with this problem.
• The Registrar, Institutes for the Achievement of Human Potential, 8801 Stenton Avenue, Philadelphia, PA 19118 / 800-736-4663.

ENCOURAGEMENT—Rejoice that Jesus is soon to return and all the problems of life will be past. Then all who love God and, by faith in Christ, obey His Word will be with Him forever.

MITRAL VALVE PROLAPSE

SYMPTOMS—Possible palpitations or chest pain in some children; but most cases are undiscovered until a routine physical exam. Diagnosis can easily be made with a stethoscope. The heart sound is like a click; and sometimes a murmur is heard.

CAUSES—This is the most common heart abnormality in children and adolescents; it is usually first noticed in childhood. The mitral valve (which lets blood flow from the left atrium of the heart into the left ventricle) flops closed, making a "click." If the valve does not close tightly, some blood will leak back, causing a murmur sound. Neither the click nor the murmur generally causes much problem for the heart. Only 3.6% of those with this prolapse also have other medical problems.

NATURAL REMEDIES
• In nearly every case, **the child does not need to be especially protected** or have physical activity restricted. Unnecessary diagnostic procedures are not needed.
• For one who has this defect, **deep breathing** exercises will help relieve stress.
• Eat a **nutritious diet**, which is low in **salt and fat**. Do not **overeat**; and keep the **weight** down. Every extra pound requires an extra 5 miles of blood vessels. **Caffeine** will induce palpitations.

INFANCY AND CHILDHOOD -
3 - INFANT PROBLEMS

NORMAL DEVELOPMENT:
AGES 1-5

During their first 5 years, children learn the basic skills necessary for their future development. The four main areas are physical skills, manual (hand) dexterity, language, and social skills.

In the normal development of a child, the following ages indicate when the ability normally begins.

Can lift head to 45° - by 3 months.
Startled by loud sounds - till 2 months.
Can roll over - 1½-4½ months.
Can bear weight on legs - 1½-5 months.
Squeals - 1-4 months.
Smiles spontaneously - 1-5 months.
Looks at own hands - 1-4 months.
Holds hands together - 2-4 months.

Reaches out for a rattle - 3-6 months.
Makes cooing sounds - 3-5½ months.
Turns toward voice - 3½-6½ months.
Passes rattle from hand to hand - 5-8 months.
Can sit unsupported - 5½-8½ months.
Says "dada" and "mama" to *anyone* - 5½-9½ mo.

Can crawl - 6-10 months.
Can stand by hoisting up own weight - 6-10 months.
Plays with feet - 6-8 months.
Plays peekaboo - 6-10 months.
Can grasp object between finger and thumb - 7-11½.
Eats with fingers - 8-12 months.
Can stand without help - 9-14 months.
Can pick up a small object - 9-14 months.
Says "dada" and "mama" *to parents* - 9-13 months.
Can walk holding on to furniture - 9½-14½ months.
Can walk without help - 10-18½ months.
Can drink from a cup - 10-16½ months.

Likes to scribble - 12-24 months.
Starts to learn single words - 12-24 months.
Mimics housework - 12-19½ months.

Can walk up stairs without help - 14-21 months.
Can point to parts of the body - 14-24 months.
Can put two words together - 14-27 months.
Can eat with a *spoon* and fork - 14-27 months.
Can undress without help - 14½-27 months.
Can throw a ball - 16-24 months.
Can build a tower of 4 blocks - 16-27 months.
Stays dry in the day - 16½-38 months.
Can kick a ball - 18-24 months.

Can draw a straight line - 20-36 months.

Separates easily from parents - 23½-57 months.
Can pedal a tricycle - 24-36 months.
Knows first and last names - 24-32 months.

Can copy a circle - 29½-53 months.
Can balance on one foot for a second - 30-54 mo.
Can talk in full sentences - 30-42 months.
Can name a color - 32-46 months.
Can dress without help - 30-60 months.
Stays dry at night - 30-60 months, or beyond.

Can draw basic likeness of a person - 36-60 months.
Can eat with a *knife* and fork - 39-60 months.

Can catch a bounced ball - 42-60 months.

Can hop on one leg - 48-60 months.
Can copy a square - 48-60 months.
Can define seven words - 48-60 months.

DIAPER RASH
(Ammoniacal Dermatitis)

SYMPTOMS—A reddish rash affecting the diaper region, with or without secondary infection by fungi or bacteria. Redness, tenderness, thickening of skin, inflammation. If secondary yeast infection appears, the skin will be bright red with well-defined borders, frequently with distinct red papules.

CAUSES—The pelvic area is **covered and damp** (especially damp) too much of the time. About 50% of the rashes go away within a day. The rest can last 10 days or longer. Breast-fed babies have less diaper rash; and this resistance continues long after the baby has been weaned. When diaper rash is more prominent later, a **food allergy** may be the cause.

NATURAL REMEDIES
• The basic solution is to keep the diaper area **dry and warm**.
• **Change the diaper** frequently; wash the area with cool water and gently dab dry, using a soft cotton diaper. All urine and stool must be removed. Special attention should be given to skin folds. Avoid harsh soaps. Mineral oil may be used to remove stool.
• To dry the baby, use **cornstarch** (or ordinary flour) as a drying agent; never use talcum powder! It is a powdered rock dust; and it can cause cancer in anyone (infant or adult) that uses it. Do not apply alcohol. Research studies show that cornstarch or flour will not cause *Candida albicans*.
Try **blow-drying** the baby before re-diapering.
• The new **super-absorbent diapers** greatly help in solving the problem. They reduce skin wetness, but cause allergies.
• When **washing diapers**, add vinegar to the final rinse. This will help reduce the pH of the cloth. Add 1 oz. of vinegar to 1 gallon of water during the final rinse. Diapers should be sun-dried if possible. If machine dried, fabric softeners should be avoided

C
H
I
L
D

(they may cause allergic reactions).

• **Give air** to that region. Take the diaper off and lay the baby chest down, with his face turned to one side, on towels underlaid with a waterproof sheet. Keeping an eye on him, leave him that way for as long as practicable. If you do not watch him, problems could develop. Keep the child bare and exposed to air and sunlight as much as the climate will permit.

• Expose the infant to small daily doses of **sunlight**. Be careful not to burn him. No ocean bathing until the rash is gone. But fresh pool water or rainwater is all right.

• Giving 2-3 ounces of **cranberry juice** to older infants will make urine pH slightly more acid. This helps reduce irritation.

• For a **diaper rash ointment**, add ½ cup **cornstarch** to ¼ cup **vitamin E oil**, mix thoroughly, store in a refrigerator, apply with each diaper change. It will last a week.

• **Aloe vera gel** is also effective in healing an irritated diaper rash.

• Do not use **commercial diaper ointments**; some of these produce nerve damage.

• **Allergies** to cow's milk, citrus fruits, and wheat have all been associated with diaper rash.

• If the child is not drinking enough **fluids**, urine acidity increases. Also diaper rash comes along with it.

ENCOURAGEMENT—The majority may choose the wrong; yet you can choose the right. Stay on God's side of the battle, and you will have victory.

CRADLE CAP

(Infantile Seborrheic Dermatitis)
SYMPTOMS—Thin, whitish, flaky scales. Or thick, yellow, greasy crusts. Sometimes it spreads to the eyelids, external ear canal, and nose.

CAUSES—Cradle cap is the most common scalp disorder of infants. About 50% have it at some time. It can occur up to the age of 5. There is an overproduction of sebum; this is a waxy, oily substance that may plug the sebaceous glands, leading to inflammation and acne formation. The entire scalp can become covered with a thick mat of sebum and dead skin cells. It can spread to the eyelids, outer ear canal, and sides of the nose. Hair may temporarily be lost.

Possible causes include **food allergies**. Of 187 infants which had it, in later years 67% had an allergy (whereas 20% have allergies in the general population). A deficiency of **vitamin B$_6$ and zinc** may be involved.

NATURAL REMEDIES
• **Gently remove** the crusts. Shampoo 2-4 times a week with a mild soap. Massage the scalp gently; but do it firmly enough to remove the flakes. Do not break the inflamed skin underneath. Massage **vegetable oil** into still-adhering flake areas. Let it set for

a few minutes; then shampoo it off.

• Include **vitamin B$_6$** (10-25 mg daily) and **zinc** (15-25 mg daily) in the infant's diet.

• Check for **food allergies**. The problem most frequently develops within the first 3 months and usually 3-4 weeks after introduction of a new food. When that food was withdrawn, cradle cap cleared up. Most likely to cause problems: **milk, wheat, eggs, oranges, beans, peas,** and occasionally **oatmeal.**

• Avoid **strong shampoos and medications**; for they may be absorbed through the child's skin.
See Pulse Test (847) and Seborrhea (346).

ENCOURAGEMENT—There is an ornament that will never perish; this will promote the happiness of all around us in this life and will shine with undimmed luster in the immortal future. It is the adorning of a meek and quiet spirit.

COLIC IN INFANTS
(Infant Colic)

SYMPTOMS—Stomach or intestinal pain in an infant. There is abdominal pain, distension, insomnia, extreme fretfulness, or hysteria. The child cries out, pulls the knees up to the stomach, and has a distended stomach. The child may be red in the face and symptoms worsen at night.

CAUSES—Abnormal amounts of gas are passing upward or downward through the infant's stomach and intestines; this is causing pain. Infant colic usually begins around the 3rd or 4th week and clears up by the 12th week. It occurs in 1 in 10 babies. **Food allergies** are a frequent cause. Colic is rare in countries that subsist on regular food and do not use medicinal drugs. Mothers who are given **drugs during labor and delivery** are more likely to give birth to babies who have colic. **Milk formulas** which use pork skin to fortify the vitamin D is frequent cause of allergies and infant colic.

NATURAL REMEDIES
• You can immediately give the infant warm **catnip tea** in a bottle. A catnip tea **enema** will also help. Crying spells occur at regular intervals; so, if a very **warm bath** is given an hour before an expected attack, it may be prevented. Have catnip tea on hand to use in an emergency. In addition, a **hot footbath** or **hot fomentation** over the abdomen will relieve the baby.

• One or 2 oz. of **warm water** bring relief to some. Warm **anise, peppermint, chamomile, thyme, or catnip** tea may help him. Make 1 cup of the tea and give 1 Tbsp. at a time to the distressed baby.

• **Charcoal** will help relieve gas. Put a little powdered charcoal into a bottle of water and give it to him. Too much can constipate him; and it will blacken the stool.

• If the baby is *totally breast-fed*, the cause is in the **mother's diet**. Any food the mother eats may, through her milk, cause the baby to suffer infant colic.

Onions, cabbage, garlic, wheat, yeast, broccoli, and brussels sprouts are common offenders. Another major cause is **fried foods, junk foods, refined foods,** and all types of **confused food combinations**. Both the mother and the child need an excellent diet.

• Colic in a *formula-fed infant* points to the food given to the child. It may be the **milk, wheat, soy, or sugar** in the formula. If possible, substitute vitamin-enriched **goat's milk**. Also try to have the mother begin **breast-feeding** the baby. Even if she did not begin doing it after delivery, she can, with some effort, get the flow started later. This is done by frequent attempts to feed the baby over several months. The mother should eats lots of brewer's yeast! *See Breast-feeding (716-720).*

• If the infant is *bottle-fed*, for added nourishment at this time you might pour boiling water over **wheat flakes** to dissolve them. Put them through a sieve and add **soybean milk**, to bring it to a desired consistency. **Potassium broth** (soup made of thick white potato peelings) and **oatmeal gruel** are also helpful.

• If colic develops *after weaning* has begun, the **new food** is the problem. The infant must be given proper foods. Only one new food should be added at a time. This way the infant can be carefully monitored for colic, rashes, or other reactions.

• After weaning, helpful foods include sweet vegetable broths (of carrots, squash, parsnips, or sweet potato). Also good is cooked fruit, milled to be soft.

• **Wheat and dairy products** are especially suspect. When in doubt, eliminate them first. **Wheat and other grains** are often introduced far too early. And this can cause the child to later develop celiac disease, which will affect him throughout life. *See Celiac Disease (473).* The infant does not have the digestive enzymes to handle grains until he is 5-6 months old. Let grains be one of the last foods introduced; and do not give yeast bread until the baby is a year old.

• Give fresh, boiled **goat's milk**; it is far less of a problem.

• Keep **diet diaries** and do **pulse testing**, to ascertain offending foods. *See Pulse Test (847).*

• It may help to give **pancreatic enzymes** (75-200 mg three times a day) before meals (enzymes may be constipating), **flaxseed oil** (1-2 drops) after each meal, and **vitamin B$_6$** (10 mg, twice a day).

• **Discourage daytime sleep** in a child. Do not let him sleep more than 3 hours during the day. This will help him go to sleep at night. Keep him awake during the early evening hours.

• Feed him in an **upright position**; and **burp him** frequently during feedings. Never feed him while lying down. Never prop up his feeding bottle. If formula is given, it should be at body temperature. Feed him in a calm, quiet environment.

• Dr. J.H. Kellogg found that **cold feet** could give babies colic. Keep booties on him 24 hours a day if he is colicky. **Smoking** parents tend to have colicky babies. Babies given **iron**-fortified foods tend to have colic. Breast-feeding mothers should not take iron supplements. (Take blackstrap molasses instead.)
—*Also see Colic in Children (735).*

ENCOURAGEMENT—Speak words of hope and good cheer, and you will encourage all about you in the pathway of life. Ask God to help you be a blessing to others. Proverbs 8:35.

DIARRHEA IN INFANTS

SYMPTOMS—Abnormally frequent discharge of fecal matter and fluid.

CAUSES—Diarrhea is a common problem in young children; it is more of a symptom than a disease. Fortunately, in children it is often brief. It occurs as a way to **rid the body of toxins, viruses**, or other substances which are causing the bowel to be inflamed. It is best not to take drugs to stop it.

Acute diarrhea in a small child under one year may quickly cause dehydration, causing him to need more fluids.

The cause is generally **improper feeding** (especially of infected animal products). Very often it is **overfeeding**. Do not give an irritable or fussy child food or sugar drinks to soothe him. Overfeeding can also lead to vomiting.

A **food allergy** may be involved. Chronic diarrhea may be caused by intolerance to **cow's milk**. Other frequent causes are eating **eggs, chicken, and meat**.

Changing formulas may cause brief diarrhea. Too much **sugar** in the diet will produce soft, watery stools. **Honey** added to milk will also do it.

Infections, antibiotics, and other **medicinal drugs** will induce diarrhea. The body is trying to quickly cast off substances which should not be in it. Children in **day-care centers** are at greater risk of viral diarrhea. Inadequate hand washing between diaper changes readily spreads the infection. Blood may be in the diarrhea stool if the cause is a **gastro-intestinal infection, urinary tract infection** *(495)*, **Crohn's disease** *(465)*, or **ulcerative colitis** *(463,465)*.

If the cause is **food poisoning** *(858)*, there may also be nausea, abdominal pain, and vomiting.

The child swallows a lot of saliva during **teething**; and this sometimes causes slight diarrhea. Avoid feeding him **cold foods**.

Unusual **excitement or anxiety** can cause extremely brief diarrhea.

You will want to try to find possible causes. Each time it happens, take note of what happened that was special or different. Was a new food added? Was the daily scheduling different? Was there stress?

C
H
I
L
D

NATURAL REMEDIES

• Medicines are generally not needed. Give the child only **clear, warm** (not cold) **fluids** for 24-48 hours. **No milk** during that time. Fluids should be given in small amounts (a teaspoonful at a time) and frequently. If he vomits, give him another teaspoonful immediately.

• Diarrhea in infants can be checked by the use of thin, homemade, boiled **rice or barley water**. For an older child, use **oatmeal gruel**. This should be given until the looseness is checked.

• To restore electrolytes, add 1 level tsp. table **salt** (no more) and 4 heaping tsp. **sugar** to 1 quart boiled **water;** and give that to him. Do not give **soft drinks**.

• If the child wants solids, give him **mashed ripe banana, cooked carrots, beets, blended raw apple, or rice cereal**. Do not give him green or overly ripe (black) bananas. If he does not want solids, only give him fluids.

• Pull gently on the skin of his abdomen. If it stands up and stays there, he is getting dehydrated. Give him fluids! Other signs of dehydration: reduced urine output, sunken eyeballs, fever, rapid breathing, dry mouth.

• To eliminate the cause of diarrhea, give 1 Tbsp. **charcoal powder** in a little water, and let him suck it through a straw or drink from a baby bottle.

ENCOURAGEMENT—The plan of salvation, as revealed in the Bible, opens up a way for you to go to heaven. Do all you can to take that path. Work to save your family. Jude 24.

INFANT CRIES OFTEN

SYMPTOMS—The baby is crying a lot.

CAUSES AND TREATMENT—

• This is often due to a deficiency of **B complex vitamins**. But he could also be lacking other important **nutrients**, including **vitamins and minerals**.

• Undue **stress** in the home could be another problem.

• **Fatigue, constipation, or not enough sleep** may be involved.

• Helpful herbs include **hops** and **skullcap**.

ENCOURAGEMENT—In the heart of Jesus there is perfect peace. Trusting in Him, you can have that peace also. Philippians 4:19.

ROSEOLA
(Roseola Infantum)

SYMPTOMS—High fever, mild diarrhea, dry cough, swollen lymph nodes in the neck, earache. Symptoms occur in two stages: a high fever (occasionally with fever convulsions) of about 4 days, followed by a rash of tiny pink spots on the face and trunk which disappears in about 4 days.

CAUSES—This is a **viral infection**. It most com-

monly occurs between the ages of 6 months and 2 years; and it affects about 3 in 10 children in the U.S. It especially occurs in the spring and fall; and it is caused by strains of the herpes virus, from close contact with other children. One attack of the infection gives lifelong immunity.

NATURAL REMEDIES

• Give the child **rest**, a spare diet of **fluids** and **juices** during the fever, plus a little solid (best blended) food if he wants it. Within a few days, the fever will end; and, when the spots appear, he will feel better. But caution is needed if the child with a fever is under 6 months of age.

ENCOURAGEMENT—There is nothing so great and powerful as God's love for those who are His children.

TEETHING

SYMPTOMS—The baby's gums become swollen and tender; and he is irritable and restless. Teething has begun!

CAUSES—An infant's teeth begin developing months before birth. In fact, the buds begin appearing in the fetus by the fifth or sixth week of pregnancy!

All 20 teeth will begin coming through during the two and a half years following birth, beginning about 4-8 months of age.

NATURAL REMEDIES

• **Massage** the baby's gums, beginning before the teeth appear. Wrap a piece of clean gauze around your finger and gently rub the gums. This removes bacteria and gets him used to having your finger in his mouth.

• Place **teething rings** in the refrigerator; then, when cold, give them to him to mouth. This feels good on the gums. If the baby is 6 months old or older, a **clean, cold washcloth** does well.

• Wrap a piece of **cold apple** in a wet child-size washcloth, and let the infant bite on it to help his gums.

• Apply **clove** to the gum area.

ENCOURAGEMENT—True happiness is found in surrendering to Christ and, by His grace, obeying His Ten Commandment law. Galatians 3:26.

REGURGITATION

SYMPTOMS—Food comes up into the mouth from the stomach.

CAUSES—Regurgitation is not exactly the same as vomiting. A small mouthful of food comes back up out of the stomach. It is fairly common during early infancy. The cause is thought to be immaturity of the upper end of the stomach; it disappears as the child grows older. The problem usually disappears by the time the child has been walking for 3 months. In most children, it is totally gone by eight months of age. If the child is growing normally, there should be little reason to be concerned.

Some infants regurgitate for several hours after they are first born. The stomach is being emptied of blood, amniotic fluid, and other substances swallowed during delivery.

NATURAL REMEDIES

• **Do not overfeed** the child. If the stomach is full, regurgitation is more likely to occur. Only feed for 20 minutes or less, and not more often than every 2½ hours apart (4-5 hours is better). There should be longer intervals between feedings at night.

• While he is steadily sucking, do not interrupt him. But as soon as the baby pauses, **burp him**.

• The best food for the infant is **breast-feeding alone**, with nothing else (including water) for the first six months. When the child becomes older, **thickened feedings** will help reduce regurgitation. After the first 6 months, this can include cereal with some breast milk added to it.

• Try to keep the child **upright** for 30-45 minutes after each feeding. Hold him, carry him, or place him in his infant seat.

—*See Gastroesophageal Reflux in Infants (below).*

ENCOURAGEMENT—Parents are to look upon their children as entrusted to them of God to be educated for the family above. Train them in the fear and love of God; for "the fear of the Lord is the beginning of wisdom."

GASTROESOPHAGEAL REFLUX IN INFANTS (GRI)

SYMPTOMS—An extreme amount of regurgitation occurs in an infant. Larger amounts of milk or food come up. Coughing or wheezing may occur if the regurgitated milk is inhaled into the lungs.

CAUSES—If the mother is eating properly and breast-feeding her child, this should not happen; although normal regurgitation may regularly occur for a time. *See Regurgitation (above).* Gastroesophageal reflux is likely to occur if the breast-feeding mother is not eating properly. This can also happen if she is feeding the infant meat and/or junk foods.

GRI is more common in preterm babies and babies with cerebral palsy *(725)*. How can you tell whether this is normal regurgitation or GRI? If it is GRI, the baby will not be gaining weight. Severe GRI may also cause inflammation and bleeding of the lining of the esophagus (due to stomach acid brought up). This may make the vomit bloodstained. If milk is inhaled into the stomach, pneumonia *(503)* sometimes develops. Rarely, a baby stops breathing temporarily after inhaling milk. So watch to see if

the baby regularly regurgitates more than a dribble of milk after feeding or if the milk is bloodstained.

NATURAL REMEDIES

• Make corrections in your diet and the baby's diet. Follow the instructions given in Regurgitation *(730)*. If that does not solve the problem, contact a physician.

ENCOURAGEMENT—Those who are loyal to God will represent Him in the home life. They will look upon the training of their children as a sacred work, entrusted to them by the Most High.

COW'S MILK ALLERGY

SYMPTOMS—Diarrhea, with loose stools containing blood and/or mucus. Wheezing and coughing. Vomiting. Abdominal discomfort, causing the baby to cry and become irritable. Failure to gain weight.

CAUSES—This is an allergic reaction to the proteins present in **cow's milk and cow's milk products**. It occurs in over 1 in 25 babies. Reaction to the cow's milk causes inflammation of the digestive tract. This allergy rarely leads to anaphylaxis *(846)*. This problem also occurs when there is a deficiency of the lactose enzyme needed to digest milk (which occurs in 20% of Caucasian children).

Many children by the age of 3 no longer have this allergy; but some continue it through to adulthood.

NATURAL REMEDIES

• **Exclude cow's milk** from your diet, if you are breast-feeding the child. If the infant is eating other foods, exclude cow's milk from his diet.

• **Goat's milk** is generally better for a child; since the curds are smaller. In addition, goat milk tends to be healthier. A sick cow is given drugs; but a sick goat dies.

• **Soymilk** might be a partial solution. But make sure the child is getting enough vitamins, minerals, and calcium.

If the child's symptoms disappear while you (and the child) are not eating or drinking the cow's milk products, then that is the cause of the problem. As soon as the problem is resolved, the child quickly recovers and begins gaining weight.

ENCOURAGEMENT—By patient work, you can bring your little ones to the Saviour.

NEONATAL JAUNDICE

SYMPTOMS—A yellowing of the skin is seen in the infant, appearing first in the upper body and progressing downward toward the toes. *In a full-term normal infant*, it is first seen about the third day; and, by the fifth day, it is disappearing. *In a preterm infant,*

C
H
I
L
D

jaundice may appear later, but last longer.

CAUSES—Jaundice is probably the most common disorder in newborn babies. Old blood is broken down, by the liver, into bilirubin, a yellowish pigment. But when too much is made, the excess is dumped into the bloodstream and is deposited in tissues for temporary storage. To one extent or another, about a fifth of infants have this condition.

"Breast milk jaundice" occurs in only about 3% of infants. Peak levels of bilirubin do not occur until the tenth or fifteenth day; it may not return to normal for 12 weeks. But do not stop breast-feeding during this time.

If the baby has prolonged jaundice, have a thyroid check done; he may have a tendency toward hypothyroidism *(659)*.

Neonatal jaundice is more common in infants in one or more of **these conditions:** born at high altitudes, are males, have a brother or sister who had it, premature, low birth weight, firstborn child, or rapid weight loss after birth. Delivered by cesarean section, forceps, or vacuum extraction. Mothers had epidural anesthesia during delivery, have blood type O. Or she is older at the time of birth of this child.

Certain drugs given to the mother during pregnancy, labor, delivery, and/or breast-feeding can lead to neonatal jaundice. This includes **sulfonamides, hydrocortisone, Valium, Orinase, Gentamicin, thiazide diuretics, and oral contraceptives**.

NATURAL REMEDIES
• If the baby is **breast-fed more frequently**, the bowel movements will carry bilirubin out of the body faster. One research team found that the 3-4 hour feedings, recommended by many hospitals, is incorrect; the **feedings should be every 2 hours**, in order to reduce bilirubin levels.

• **Activated charcoal** is very helpful in lowering bilirubin levels. Stir 2-3 teaspoons powdered charcoal into a little water and give with a nipple. Beginning at 4 hours of age, give it every two hours for 120 hours in normal newborns and for 168 hours in premature infants (until bilirubin levels fall).

"Newborn babies who experience jaundice will usually be improved with activated charcoal. Bile secretion from the liver into the intestines is usually followed by an efficient reabsorption process. Charcoal binds this bile and carries the pigment out, reducing the risks from jaundice. Charcoal can be mingled with the baby's formula, or with breast milk expressed into a bottle, or be mixed with the mother's milk and given for several days until the neonatal jaundice clears."—*Richard A. Hansen, M.D., Get Well at Home, p. 260.*

• Exposure to **sunlight** helps reduce bilirubin levels. A little can fall on the infant through a window or he can be taken outside. Do not let direct sunlight enter his eyes; but let it fall on as much bare skin as possible. Of course, be careful and do not sunburn him.

—*Also see Jaundice (390,448), Infectious Jaundice (449), and Hepatitis (446).*

ENCOURAGEMENT—By yielding your life to Christ, you can experience a peace and contentment which will make life a joy rather than a burden. Children are a great blessing which the Lord gives us; as we prepare them for heaven, we are more likely to get there ourselves. John 15:11.

INFANT THRUSH
(Oral Thrush)

SYMPTOMS—White patches in the mouth which may look like milk curds. Although milk curds are easily rubbed off, thrush sticks to the oral tissues. When removed, it leaves a red, raw appearing area. Discomfort may hinder food intake in severe cases.

CAUSES—Infant thrush is an infection of the mucosa of the mouth by *Candida albicans*. Occurring in 4% of infants, it generally begins within 8-9 days after birth. Sources of infection are infected mothers who either have candida *(281* or vaginitis *(695)*; perhaps the infant was exposed in the newborn nursery. Infants of diabetic mothers are especially susceptible. Also susceptible are infants born with cleft palate or cleft lip.

NATURAL REMEDIES
TREATMENT
• Three or 4 times a day, swab the infected areas with a cotton-tipped applicator, saturated in a **baking soda** solution. Carefully clean all candida spots within reach.

• The mouth can also be swabbed several times a day with a **garlic** solution. Blend 1 peanut-size clove in 1 cup water till smooth. Garlic overpowers candida

• Simmer 5 **bay leaves** in 2 cups water for 20 minutes. Strain, let cool, and use the solution as a mouthwash. Apply it in a sterile dropper to the baby's mouth, twice a day. Store it in the refrigerator; and prepare a fresh solution every 2 days.

PREVENTION
• **Breast milk** contains substances which help the infant's immune system to resist the candida infection.

• **Pacifiers and bottle nipples** should be soaked in 130° F. water for 15 minutes between each use. (Candida spores are heat resistant). All other objects going into his mouth should be clean. Breast-feeding mothers should **wash** their nipples well with plain water after each feeding.

• Both mother and child should avoid **antibiotics**; and mothers should avoid **steroids**. They destroy natural, friendly bacteria; these help candida to grow.

• If the mother has no candida, swabbing the infant's mouth with some of her **saliva** will establish a flora that is unfavorable for the growth of candida.

Give plain water, to **cleanse the mouth** after every feeding. Inspect the mouth before each feeding; and begin treatment if thrush is seen.

—Also see Candida (281) and Vaginitis (695).

ENCOURAGEMENT—The judgment shall sit and the books shall be opened, when the "well done" of the great Judge is pronounced and the crown of immortal glory is placed upon the brow of the victor. At that time many will raise their crowns in sight of the assembled universe; and, pointing to their mother, they will say, "She made me all I am through the grace of God. Her instruction, her prayers, have been blessed to my eternal salvation."

ANAL FISTULA
(Fistula-in-Ano)

SYMPTOMS—Tenderness, swelling, redness, and painful bowel movements. Pus or mucous drainage may be present. Symptoms subside and recur again.

CAUSES—This is a type of perineal abscess that occurs most frequently during the first year of life; it is more frequent in males than in females.

NATURAL REMEDIES
• **Sitz baths** and a **nonconstipating diet** generally solves the problem within a short time.
• The child should **not strain** in order to have a bowel movement.
In some instances, surgery may be necessary.

ENCOURAGEMENT—Keep praying and keep working to help your children, and God will help you.

INFANT FLATFEET
(Pes Planus)

SYMPTOMS—The bare footprint of the child does not show where the inner arch is raised (producing no print mark).

CAUSES—Many young children appear to have flatfeet. But, by the age of 10, only 4% have it. Many children with "flatfeet" really have fat feet. Raise his big toe while you have him stand. If he has an arch, you will see it raise.
The child with true flatfeet walks on the inner or outer (usually inner) edge of his feet; and he wears down the edge of his shoe soles.

NATURAL REMEDIES
• Let the child run and play outdoors with **bare feet**. "Corrective shoes," often very costly, accomplish little. Letting him walk barefoot outside is better.
• While the child is laying on his back relaxed, with the knee straight and the heel turned slightly inward, the parent should **flex the foot**; this is done by moving the foot up toward his body and holding it for a count of 10. Relax and repeat 20 times, 3

times daily.
• An older child can do the same exercise, standing flat on the floor as he **leans into a wall** 12-18 inches away.
• Alternate **hot and cold footbaths**, using two basins, help some children with painful flatfeet. For 10 minutes, put both feet in the hot for 1 minute; then put both feet into the cold for 1 minute. Do this twice a day.

ENCOURAGEMENT—Heaven will be cheap enough if, in spite of all our prayers, tears, and suffering, we arrive there with our children.

INFANTILE CONVULSIONS

NATURAL REMEDIES
J.H. KELLOGG, M.D., PRESCRIPTIONS FOR INFANTILE CONVULSIONS AND THEIR COMPLICATIONS *(how to give these water therapies: pp. 207-272/ Hydrotherapy Disease Index: pp. 273-275)*
BASIC ASPECTS—Regulate **diet**, withholding meats and all indigestibles. Avoid cow's milk, if curds are present in the stools. Daily Cold Bath, Wet Hand Rub, or **Cold Towel Rub**.
GENERAL CARE—When due to autointoxication from intestinal irritation, give a large **Hot Enema**. For immediate relief, give a **Hot Blanket Pack** with **Warm Bath**, at 95°-98° F., for 1-2 minutes. If not quickly relieved, remove from bath and employ **Cold Pail Pour** to head and spine. **Alternate Hot and Cold Pail Pour**, if necessary. Apply **Hot Abdominal Pack**, changing every 4 hours.
—*Also see Convulsions (573-576).*

ENCOURAGEMENT—Help your children learn how to trust and obey God, and you will point them in the direction of the Holy City, where you want to live with them throughout all eternity.

CHOLERA INFANTUM
(Gastro-intestinal Catarrh in Children)

NATURAL REMEDIES
J.H. KELLOGG, M.D., PRESCRIPTIONS FOR INFANT CHOLERA AND ITS COMPLICATIONS *(how to give these water therapies: pp. 207-272 / Hydrotherapy Disease Index: pp. 273-275).*
GASTRO-INTESTINAL CATARRH IN CHILDREN (ACUTE) AND CHOLERA INFANTUM BASIC FACTORS—**Withdraw all food. Hot Blanket Pack** till skin is reddened. Follow by **Cold Mitten Friction or Cold Wet Hand Rub**. If his temperature is high, apply a **Heating Wet Sheet Pack**. Repeat if necessary. **Rest** in bed.
PERSISTENT VOMITING—Ice Bag to stomach.
FREQUENT BOWEL MOVEMENTS—Hot **Enema** at 105°- 110° F. after every bowel movement. **Fomentation** to abdomen every 3 hours. Follow by **Heating Compress**,

C
H
I
L
D

changing every 20 minutes.

PAIN IN ABDOMEN—Revulsive Compress over abdomen for 15-20 minutes every hour or two.

COLLAPSE—Hot Blanket Pack until warm. Follow with **Prolonged Neutral Bath** at 92°-95° F. Hot **water** drinking and large Warm **Enema**.

—*Also see Cholera (306).*

ENCOURAGEMENT—Amid all your suffering and grief, cry to God for help, and He will comfort and help you. He can do for you that which no one else can do.

SUDDEN INFANT DEATH SYNDROME
(SIDS)

SYMPTOMS—The infant suddenly dies.

CAUSES—There is no advance warning or symptom. This is what it is called "sudden infant death syndrome." The central nervous system is affected, which in turn suppresses the involuntary act of breathing.

Each year, in the United States, there are 10,000 deaths from this problem. SIDS primarily occurs in the winter and especially to underweight babies from poor families; the mothers are generally under 20.

Several possible causes have been traced:

It has been reported that there are high levels of **lead** in the blood of infants who die of SIDS.

Suffocation may be the cause. It has been found that infants who were **laid on their stomachs**, to go to sleep, are much more likely to suddenly die than infants who are laid on their backs.

Breast-fed babies are less susceptible to SIDS. In addition, they have less allergies, respiratory diseases, hypoglycemia, obesity, and gastroenteritis.

It is now known that SIDS can be caused by the **pertussis vaccine**, which is given to infants at 2, 4, and 6 months of age. The following quotation is from a book which can be purchased from the publisher of this *Encyclopedia*:

"Three research studies were made on **the relationship that the pertussis vaccine had to death**. Each one specifically examined DPT vaccinations; and each found a decided relationship. In Waler's case-control study, **the relative risk of the child having SIDS (sudden infant death syndrome) within 3 days after immunization was 7.3%!** Did you hear that? That is almost one child out of every ten vaccinated with DPT (the diphtheria-pertussis-typhoid vaccine, a standard vaccination given to schoolchildren). *(The three studies were: Baraff, et al., 1983, reported in Pediatric Infectious Disease Journal, 1983, Vol. 2, pp. 7-11; Torch, 1982, reported in Neurology, 1982, Vol. 32, p. A 169; Waler, et al., 1987, reported in American Journal of Public Health, 1987, Vol. 77, pp. 945-951)."—Vaccination Crisis, pp. 121-122.*

NATURAL REMEDIES

• Give careful attention to each one of the **above factors**.

• Both the mother and child should receive **nourishing food**. If the infant is breast-fed, the mother's diet should be excellent; if the baby is bottle-fed, then, if possible, fresh boiled goat's milk should be used. Mothers should nurse their babies, if at all possible.

• Locate **allergenic foods** and eliminate them.

• **The mother should avoid** chemicals, drugs, and junk foods during and after pregnancy. Even aspirin is not good; it interferes with blood clotting and could damage the fetus. Do not use caffeine, alcohol, or tobacco; they harm the unborn child, so it does not develop properly.

ENCOURAGEMENT—Heaven is very near to those who suffer for righteousness' sake. Christ identifies His interests with the interests of His faithful ones. Be His little child, and He will care for you. Galatians 4:4-5, 7.

INFANCY AND CHILDHOOD -
4 - CHILDHOOD PROBLEMS
Also: Fever (302-309), Worms (861), Hyperactivity (591-592)

BED-WETTING
(Enuresis)

SYMPTOMS—A child continues to wet the bed after infancy.

CAUSES—Bed wetters tend to have a small bladder capacity; this makes it difficult for them to go through the night without voiding. They also tend to urinate more frequently during the day.

Here are the frequency statistics: 50% wet by the age of 2, 10%-15% by 4 years of age, and 4% at 12 years old. Boys do it more frequently than girls; but girls can develop urinary tract infections from it.

A primary cause of bed-wetting is **allergy**. Their parents are more likely to have hives, hay fever, urinary tract infection, food allergies, or drug allergies.

Food allergies in the children are responsible for many cases. The most frequent problem foods were **cow's milk** (60% of the time), **chocolate, eggs, citrus fruits, wheat, grains, corn, chicken, meat, peanuts, and fish**. You would need to do pulse tests *(847)*, to determine the problem food. Removing milk from the diet reduced bed-wetting in 50% of a group being studied.

Hyperactive children tend to be bed wetters.

Constipation may at times be involved, by pressing on the bladder. Some children, especially older ones, continue to wet the bed because of **tensions** they live under in the home or at school.

Anemia, pinworms, upper respiratory tract **infections**, or any toxic condition can be contributing factors.

NATURAL REMEDIES
• Consider all the **above factors**.
• A common method used to solve the problem is to have the child **stop and start the flow** of urine each time he urinates. This causes him to acquire better mental control of the function. This may solve the problem in as little as six weeks.
• Spanking the child is not the solution! Do not praise and do not punish. The child does not do it on purpose; he is sorry. Just change the bed and do not say a word. —But keep working on possible solutions listed here. No child wants to do it.
• The child should be encouraged to have **vigorous outdoor exercise**. (It is known that bed wetters wet less during the summer months; and some who have stopped may return to it in the winter.)
• In children over 10 years old, **limit the amount of fluid intake after 5 p.m.**, until several months after bed-wetting ceases.
• Bed-wetting **alarms** can be purchased. They often wake up everyone at night; but it, many times, accomplishes the task within 60 days.

Victory is said to come with 21 days of consecutive dry nights.

J.H. KELLOGG, M.D., PRESCRIPTIONS FOR BED-WETTING AND THEIR COMPLICATIONS *(how to give these water therapies: pp. 207-272 / list of treatments: pp. 206-207 / Hydrotherapy Disease Index: pp. 273-275)*

IMPROVE GENERAL AND LOCAL NERVE TONE—Cold Pail Pour at 75° F. at bedtime. Follow by **Neutral Pail Pour** to spine, 2 minutes, 96° F. Sea bathing and swimming, if this is available. **Avoid water drinking for 2 hours before retiring**. Aseptic **dietary**. Meats and salts are especially to be avoided.

RELIEVE CONSTIPATION AND FLATULENCE WHEN PRESENT—by using Hot **Abdominal Pack** and **Graduated Enema**. If necessary, carefully Graduated **Cold Baths**, cool **Enema**, and proper diet.

DIMINISH ACIDITY OF URINE—by free use of **fruit** and **water** drinking in the forenoon.

—*For incontinence in adults, see Incontinence (487).*

ENCOURAGEMENT—While the Lord has not promised His people exemption from trials, He has promised that which is far better. He has said, "As thy days, so shall thy strength be." Deuteronomy 33:25. "My grace is sufficient for thee." 2 Corinthians 12:9.

COLIC IN CHILDREN

SYMPTOMS—The child cries out, pulls his knees up to his stomach, and has a distended stomach. His stomach and/or intestines hurt.

CAUSES—**Pressure from gas** moving upward or downward causes pain. The cause is usually **im-** proper food or constipation. **Indigestion** is the most frequent cause.

NATURAL REMEDIES
• Put him into bed and give him warm catnip tea in a bottle.
• Herbal treatment can include **wild yam, cramp bark, some nervines and antispasmodic tinctures** to relieve cramping. The bowels should be cleansed with a **catnip injection**. Hot **bran fomentation** over the stomach-abdominal area will give ease and comfort. For *gassy colic*, the following decoction is excellent: **dandelion root, fennel seeds, marshmallow root, sweet flag root (with cayenne and ginger** added as stimulant carriers). For *bilious colic*, use a decoction in equal parts of **agrimony, barberry bark, centaury, dandelion root**, or an infusion of a handful of fresh **parsley** will decoction in equal parts of **agrimony, barberry bark, centaury, dandelion root**, or an infusion of a handful of fresh **parsley** will do the job.
—*Also see Colic in Infants (728).*

ENCOURAGEMENT—True happiness is found in learning of Christ and living for Him. Those who take Christ at His Word and surrender their soul to His keeping will find peace and quietude. 2 Thessalonians 2:16-17.

VOMITING IN CHILDREN

SYMPTOMS—The child is vomiting, perhaps frequently.

CAUSES—Vomiting is a symptom rather than a disease. There are about 60 different things which can cause it; none of them are serious. However, continued vomiting is not good for the child.

If the child is growing, vigorous, gaining weight, and happy, occasional vomiting should not be a cause for concern. Primary causes of *infant vomiting* is **poor feeding techniques, immaturity of the stomach and intestines**, or a variety of other factors.

Young children often spit up a little food; but that is usually not serious. *See Regurgitation (730).* Some children repeatedly vomit *(cyclic vomiting)*. It is usually preceded by a mild headache. These children generally have an allergic disease (such as **asthma, hives, eczema, rhinitis, or allergic conjunctivitis**). Fatty or fried foods cause attacks in many of these children; but sometimes other foods are the problem, including oranges. Many of these children later develop **migraines**; there frequently is a family history of this problem. Cyclic vomiting usually begins late in infancy and ends by the age of 10.

Vomiting can be a sign of **Reye's Syndrome** *(750)*, which can occur after a viral illness, especially if aspirin was given to the child. This is very serious. A blow to the head, causing a **concussion**, can cause

C
H
I
L
D

vomiting.

NATURAL REMEDIES

• **Withhold all food and fluid** for 2 hours after the vomiting occurs. Give a teaspoon or two of **water or peppermint tea** every 20 minutes. Older children may be given **ice chips** and told to let them melt in the mouth before swallowing. If vomiting recurs, given nothing for another hour. If vomiting ceases, give a little fluid again. About 6 hours later, give **mashed banana, potato, applesauce, rice, or toast**. If this is accepted, about 24 hours later return to a regular diet; but this should be **without milk, greasy or fatty foods, or spices**.

• **Burp** the infant regularly and **do not overfeed** him. Be careful when giving him new foods. Avoid giving him any **spices, highly seasoned foods, or junk foods**. Maintain a **regular feeding schedule**.

• **If he has a cold**, clear his nasal passages before feeding him. Otherwise mucus in the back of his throat might cause him to vomit. Do not play vigorously with him for an hour or so after feeding. Avoid foods which cause him to vomit. **Cow's milk, eggs, or gluten (in wheat, rye, oats, and barley)** may be the problem.

• **After feeding**, place the infant on his right side, with a folded towel behind his back, or upright in an infant seat. Do not place him on his back, because he may inhale and choke on the vomitus.

• **Avoid dehydration**. Signs are if he cries without tears or has not passed urine in 8 hours. *See Diarrhea (458-459)*.

• **Charcoal** is an excellent help. Stir 1 heaping Tbsp. of the powder into ¼ cup water or juice; and let him drink it through a straw. Repeat each time he vomits. Caution: Too much charcoal can be constipating. For many children, a little **peppermint** tea is soothing.

ENCOURAGEMENT—You must make the Bible your guide if you would bring up your children in the nurture and admonition of the Lord. Let the life and character of Christ be presented as the pattern for them to copy.

GIGGLE MICTURITION

SYMPTOMS—Accidental leakage of urine while laughing.

CAUSES—More common in girls, it often disappears as the child gets older. But, in some instances, it continues until the age of 20. The child should not unnecessarily be subjected to urological examination.

NATURAL REMEDIES

• The child does not need reproof but **encouragement** to persevere in trying to stop the problem. **Reassure** the child that it will eventually be outgrown. It helps some to **sit down** while laughing.

• Have the child practice **starting and stopping the flow** of urine while urinating, in order to practice gaining control over that muscle.

ENCOURAGEMENT—If faithful, you will someday see your children in heaven, and what a glorious day that will be! Whatever our trials down here may have been, it will be worth it all.

NERVOUS TICS

SYMPTOMS—Rapid, uncontrolled eye blinking. Twitching of the muscles around the mouth. Shrugging of the shoulders or jerking movements of the neck. Involuntary contractions of the diaphragm, causing grunting or hiccups.

CAUSES—This uncontrolled muscle twitch is called a "tic." It only lasts a fraction of a second and is painless. The muscle contraction may occur repeatedly. Nervous tics occur because a muscle or group of muscles controlled by peripheral nerves contracts repeatedly and involuntarily. The condition usually affects the facial muscles; but sudden, uncontrolled movements of the limbs and sounds (such as grunts and throat clearing) can also occur.

Tics generally develop during childhood and occur more commonly in boys than girls. The cause is frequently unknown; but they may be associated with **stress**. This is more common in children who are tired or upset. When children are asleep, tics usually disappear. Sometimes the tics continue into adulthood.

If a **cool wind** blows on one side of a person's face when he is driving or sleeping, a muscle can be chilled and a tic can begin. *For more on tics, see 736*.

NATURAL REMEDIES

• Do not scold the child or ridicule him. Instead, try to improve his diet and way of life. Perhaps too much is expected of him. He should have time for exercise and also time to rest.

• The diet should be simple and non-stimulating. He should try to maintain a regular schedule. Deep breathing exercises will help him.

• The nerves are nourished by the entire **vitamin B complex, by lecithin, calcium, trace minerals,** and (to a lesser degree) by **other vitamins and minerals**. Set aside the processed, fried, and junk foods. And only eat nourishing food: **fresh fruits and vegetables**, plus **lecithin** and **flaxseed oil** (2 tsp.). Take **calcium** daily (2,000 mg); it is a specific for relaxing the muscles.

• Avoid **stress and pressure**. Choose to work relaxed. Do the best you can and be contented.

• Try to solve learning disabilities. These add to the problem. Take time to **study** at school **and do your homework. Learn to read, write, spell, and do basic math**. But also **get proper** outdoor **exercise**.

• Stand in front of a mirror and **try to repeat the tic**. Oddly enough, this is almost impossible to do; but, gradually, the attempt can help you gain control over the affected muscle.

• Try to **remain motionless** for as long as possible, gradually increasing the amount of time, until it can be done for 5 minutes.

ENCOURAGEMENT—"These things I have spoken unto you, that in Me ye might have peace. In the world ye shall have tribulation: but be of good cheer; I have overcome the world." John 16:23.

STUTTERING

SYMPTOMS—The child tends to stutter or have speech difficulties.

CAUSES—It is normal for children to have some difficulty with speaking. The child's speech abilities do not progress as fast as his thought processes. It is also normal for boys to be slower than girls in learning to speak without impediments. It is believed that only 1% of children really have a true stutter. In most children, speech problems are usually resolved by the age of six or seven. Most speech abnormalities disappear over two or three months, if properly handled.

NATURAL REMEDIES

• **Avoid calling attention** to the child's speech problems. They are normal and do not mention them. Calling the child's attention to it increases the risk that he will become concerned about it—and believe it is something he will always have.

• If the child mentions it to his parents, they should **tell him that it is a part of normal development**, which many children have.

• **Do not talk too fast** to a child. More important: Before the parent replies, the parent should **pause 2-3 seconds after the child speaks**

• This will help the child relax and feel he does not need to speak faster.

• **Spend time** each day with the child, doing things, conversing with him, reading to him and asking questions. This helps his speech development.

• **Do not correct his grammar** when he is having speech problems. He can learn grammar later.

• In some instances, removing **milk** from the diet will lessen stuttering by the child.

• Mothers who avoid **eye contact** when the child speaks, or **express displeasure** with his performance, lengthen the time he will stutter. At times, when she is working and cannot maintain eye contact, she should be pleasant and say "uh, huh," "yes," etc., which show she is carefully listening.

• **Do not supply a word** which the child is stumbling over. **Give him time** to say what he wants to say. Do not put him under **stress**.

For more information, go online to nspstutter.org, or stuttersfa.org.

ENCOURAGEMENT—Help your children to become like Jesus, and you will later be glad you did. Let them see Jesus in you.

BOW LEGS
(Genu Varum)

SYMPTOMS—The child's legs bow outward.

CAUSES—It is quite normal for young children to be bowlegged. This is due to their position before birth. In nearly every case, as the child grows older, his legs will straighten. Bowleg is most apparent between the age of one and two. Thick diapers tend to bow the legs; and after they are outgrown, the legs straighten—sometimes becoming knock-kneed. As the child nears his teen years, the legs straighten.

Rickets *(614)* is a cause of bowleg; but so much Western food is fortified with vitamin D that rickets is not usually the cause.

NATURAL REMEDIES

• If you are feeding your child a **nourishing diet**, and he is healthy, growing, gaining weight, and obtaining enough **sunlight** (for vitamin D), his legs will eventually straighten.

ENCOURAGEMENT—If you lack wisdom, go to God; He has promised to give liberally. Pray much, and fervently, for divine aid. One rule cannot be followed in every case. The exercise of sanctified judgment is now needed.

RECTAL PROLAPSE

SYMPTOMS—The bright red or dark inner part of the anus protrudes after a bowel movement. A discharge of mucus or blood may occur.

CAUSES—Protrusion of the rectal mucosa out of the anus. This condition primarily occurs in children under the age of 5. **Prolonged straining** at the stool and **inadequate nutrition** are the usual causes. But causes can include **chronic diarrhea, constipation, cystic fibrosis, or physical abnormalities**.

NATURAL REMEDIES

• Each bowel movement loosens the rectal tissue from the supporting wall a little more. Eventually the mother may have to replace it. Wrapping a piece of toilet paper around her finger, she should carefully **press the extended tissue back in**. Once it is inside the anus, she carefully pulls her finger out, leaving the toilet paper there. It will be expelled with the next bowel movement. (Trying to withdraw the finger, with the toilet paper still around it, would pull the tissue back out.) Instead of toilet paper, a finger lubricated with petroleum jelly could be used. Next, place a wad of cotton or cotton material against the area, and place tape across the hips to compress the region.

• Work steadily to avoid constipation in the child.

C
H
I
L
D

The section on constipation *(456, 712)* will provide guidance on this.

• Teach the child not to **strain** when having a bowel movement. Make sure he is drinking large amounts of **water**, obtaining sufficient **bulk** in his food, and not eating any **processed foods**.

• One method that has been used successfully is this: Insert a cone-shaped piece of ice into the rectum after the bowel movement. This will greatly strengthen the anal muscles.

ENCOURAGEMENT—Trust and obey; for there is no other way to be happy in Jesus, but to trust and obey.

NIGHT TERRORS
(Pavor Nocturnus)

SYMPTOMS—Vivid, terrifying experiences for the child (and his parents) in the middle of the night and sometimes during naps.

CAUSES—Night terrors occur in about 3% of children between the ages of one and twelve. These are not nightmares, which are bad dreams that one awakens from. Instead, the child partially awakens and sits up or runs around the room, thrashing and screaming. His eyes are open; but he does not recognize his parents or anyone else who comes into the room. His heart rate, breathing, and perspiration are rapid; and he cannot be comforted or really awakened.

These experiences may occur several times a week, many times a month; but they usually subside several months later. The child tends to have these experiences when he has a fever, has irregular hours for going to sleep, is very tired, or is frightened by a story or movie. A heavy meal before bed can induce them.

NATURAL REMEDIES

• **Do not try to awaken him**. Instead, let him fall back asleep. He will remember nothing the next morning. If you did manage to awaken him, he would be confused and have difficulty going back to sleep.

• **Protect him**. Remove sharp objects from the room and lock the doors and windows. Do not later mention it, and he will not remember it.

• Give the child **no supper** or only a very **light supper** until the night terrors cease. Eliminate all **frightening TV, movies, and bad stories**.

• He should **go to bed at the same time** every night, even on weekends. If he is very tired, let him **nap** during the day. Sleep deprivation increases night terrors.

• Do not bring him into your room for the rest of the night. If done, he may want to always sleep with you.

• Notice when the terrors occur and **awaken him 15 minutes ahead of time**. Doing this will usually cause them to stop within one week.

—*Also see Nightmares (593).*

ENCOURAGEMENT—Impatience in the parents excites impatience in the children. Kindly, patiently, lead them in the right way, the way that leads to heaven.

MALNUTRITION

SYMPTOMS—The child is thin and does not grow or gain weight properly.

CAUSES—Malnutrition occurs primarily among poor people, whose children do not get enough good food to eat. This problem is more common in developing countries.

Mild malnutrition is the most common form; but it is not always obvious. The child does not grow or gain weight as fast as a well-nourished child. Although he may appear rather small and thin, he usually does not look sick. But because he is **poorly nourished**, he may lack resistance to fight infections. So he tends to become seriously ill and takes longer to get well.

Such children are more liable to have diarrhea and colds. Their colds usually last longer and are more likely to turn into pneumonia. They are at higher risk of getting measles, tuberculosis, and many other infectious diseases. More of them die.

Here is the best test of whether a child is malnourished: After 1 year of age, any child whose middle upper arm measures less than 13½ cm. (5-5/16 in.) around is malnourished—no matter how "fat" his feet, hands, and face may look. If the arm measures less than 12½ cm. (4-15/16 in.), he is severely malnourished. Another helpful way to tell if a child is well or is poorly nourished is to weigh him regularly: once a month, in the first year and then once every 3 months thereafter. A healthy, well-nourished child gains weight regularly.

There are two types of *severe malnutrition*: Dry malnutrition (marasmus), in which the child does not get enough of any kind of food. He is starved. His body is small and thin; and he has a potbelly. Wet malnutrition is the same; except that his feet, hands, and face are swollen. This is caused by a lack of bodybuilding foods: proteins. Eating beans, lentils, or other foods that have been stored in a damp, moldy place can also be a cause.

Other types of malnutrition include night blindness (lack of vitamin A), rickets (lack of vitamin D), anemia (lack of iron), goiter (lack of iodine), various skin problems, sores on the lips and mouth, or bleeding gums as a result of the lack of enough fruits, vegetables, and other foods containing certain vitamins.

NATURAL REMEDIES

• In much of the world, most people eat one main low-cost food with almost every meal; it may be rice, maize, millet, wheat, cassava, potato, breadfruit, or banana. But other foods (called "protective foods") are also needed (such as **dark green-leafy vegetables, orange and yellow fruits and vegetables, nuts, beans, and peanuts**).

• If available to them, the children could also use a **multivitamin** tablet every day.

SPECIAL NOTE: This section was especially prepared for readers in developing countries. Severe malnourishment is far less likely in the Western world. Parents should not try to stuff children with food, just because they are slender. A certain percentage of the population are thin and will always be thin, even though their parents may be able to easily gain weight. Set before your child nourishing food. Let him eat what he wants while requiring that he eats a little of everything on his plate; but do not let him eat snacks or junk foods. Do not let him drink between meals. If you habitually let him eat junk foods and eat between meals, he is certain to have inadequate nourishment.

ENCOURAGEMENT—How lovingly the angels guard the steps of God-fearing, God-loving youth. Jesus knows them by name; and their example is helping other youth to do right. The youth who has hidden within his heart and mind a store of God's words of caution and encouragement, of His precious pearls of promise from which he can draw at any time, will be a living channel of light.

INFANCY AND CHILDHOOD -
5 - CHILDHOOD INFECTIONS
Also: Fever (302-309), Worms (861), Hyperactivity (591), Rickets (614), Impetigo (349), Ringworm (335), Croup (498), Bronchiectasis (502), Head Lice (860)

CHILDHOOD DISEASES

SYMPTOMS—Fevers, rashes, coughs, sore throat, weakness, etc.

CAUSES—The childhood diseases include *chicken pox (742), measles (744), mumps (743), German measles (rubella, 745), rheumatic fever (750), whooping cough (748), and scarlet fever (745).*

Many of these common childhood diseases are contracted by nearly all children. Some experience only mild cough or cold while others have serious cases. A few receive permanent damage.

NATURAL REMEDIES
PREVENTION
• If the child is receiving excellent **nutrition, exercise, rest, sunshine, fresh air**, etc., he is unlikely to experience serious difficulty with these diseases. Louis Pasteur, developer of the germ theory of disease, said, "The germ is nothing; it is the soil that matters." If the person is living a good life, the germ has a hard time obtaining a foothold.
• Avoid excess **milk and carbohydrates**, especially refined ones. Avoid **sugar, fried foods, and junk foods**.
• Include **vitamin-mineral supplements** in a diet. Eat **fresh fruits and vegetables, whole grains, nuts, and legumes**. A well-fed child will usually be strong enough to resist the onslaught of childhood diseases. He may contract them; but the case will not be serious, usually brief, and often mild.

TREATMENT
• Give a **liquid diet** in the acute stages, later followed by **fruits and vegetables**. Do not suppress the fever with drugs. Use **water therapy** treatments *(298)*, to help the body fight the infection. The bowels must be kept open by means of herbal **enemas** and, if needed, herbal **laxatives**.
• Treat the kidneys and bowels, so they can keep discharging toxins. Sweating therapy (hot packs) can be used to bring waste products out through the skin.
• **Garlic** is helpful, along with the **fruit and vegetable juices**, and **herb teas**.
• **Vitamins A and C**, with an abundant amount of **bioflavonoids,** are needed.
• Never, never, give **aspirin** to a child or youth who has a fever! It can lead to Reye's Syndrome *(750)*, which can cause irreversible coma or death. This is what happens: The child has a fever and aspirin is given. There is improvement for a day or two—then a sudden turn for the worst; and coma or death follows.

ENCOURAGEMENT—Worry is blind and cannot discern the future; but, trusting in Jesus, you need not fear. Take His hand, and He will lead you step by step. Malachi 4:2.

CAT SCRATCH DISEASE

SYMPTOMS—Infections from cuts and scratches, frequently on the arms. The scratched areas become enlarged and infected. The area may be swollen and red; and a slow-healing ulcer may form. Within 10-30 days, there is fever, headache, nausea, vomiting, loss of appetite, chills, abdominal pain, general aching, and enlargement of the lymph glands.

The low-grade fever may continue for months. Half the time, swelling of the lymph gland is the only symptom; but it can last 2 to 12 months. Usually only one lymph node is swollen.

CAUSES—The child may be scratched by a **cat, splinter, thorn, fishhook, pins, pet bird**, etc. The disease is thought to be carried by rodents and birds. When the cat gets this problem, it thereafter carries the infection on its claws for about 3 weeks. When a cat bites or licks the child, the disease can also be spread. Three-fourths of all cases occur in children and adolescents, usually in the fall or winter. It is estimated that only 10% of those scratched or bitten develop the disease.

Cat scratch disease is thought to be the primary cause of one-sided lymphadenopathy, a disease affecting the lymph glands; this primarily affects those glands under the arms and in the neck. Antibiotics are not effective and should not be given.

When an ulcer forms, it can heal very slowly.

NATURAL REMEDIES

• Give **warm, moist soaks** to the involved lymph glands, along with **bed rest** or very **little physical activity**. As long as those glands are swollen, vigorous activity should be avoided.

• Require the children to **immediately wash** any cuts or scratches. Do not allow the cat to **lick** any part of the skin. The child should **wash** his hands immediately after petting a cat. Teach him to **handle cats gently**, so he will not be scratched or bitten. (If you are tired of all the washings, you might try giving away the cat.)

—*Diseases which you can get from cats include Cat Coccidia (846), Poison Ivy and Oak (854), Pinworms (863), Lyme Disease (813, 840), and Toxoplasmosis (846, 864-865).*

ENCOURAGEMENT—The Saviour of the world loves to have children and youth give their hearts to Him.

TINEA CAPITIS
(ringworm of the sculp)

SYMPTOMS—Moist, possibly itchy, red patches on the scalp.

CAUSES—This is a fungal infection; it is most common in schoolchildren.

NATURAL REMEDIES

NUTRITION

• Eat a nourishing diet of **fruits, vegetables, whole grains, legumes, and nuts**. While treating the infection, a diet primarily of **raw food** is best.

• Avoid **tobacco, alcohol, caffeine**. Do not eat **meat or dairy products**. Avoid **sugary, fried, and processed foods**. Eat nothing **greasy**.

HERBS

• **Goldenseal** contains *berberine*, which destroys fungi. It can be used against every type of fungus infection. It can be applied both topically and as a drink. Only use goldenseal for a week; then switch for a time to another fungicide herb.

• **Pau d'arco** is strongly antifungal. Drink 3 cups daily.

• **Bloodroot** also contains *berberine*; it has been shown to be quite effective as a fungicide.

• **Yellowroot, barberry, and Oregon grape** also contain *berberine*.

• Place a compress of **goldenseal and pau d'arco** on the area.

• **Tea tree** oil is excellent when applied externally, but do not drink it. Apply it several times a day to the affected area, either full strength or diluted with a little distilled water or cold-pressed oil. **Black walnut** extract can also be used.

• A powerful antifungicide is **wild oregano oil**. The most resistent forms of fungus infection can generally be eliminated by it.

• The **pepper tree** (horopito) is a New Zealand shrub which contains *polygodial*, which is useful against both fungi and bacteria. Another antifungal herb is the ***Licaria puchuri-major***, a Brazilian plant.

OTHER HELPS

• Keep the **skin clean and dry**. Expose the affected area to air as much as possible. The **clothing** should be kept clean. The child should keep his hands clean.

—*Also see Candida (281).*

ENCOURAGEMENT—Jesus knows the needs of His children and He loves to listen to their prayers. Trusting in Him, obeying Him, they can grow up into strong Christian adults who are able to help many others.

TONSILLITIS, ADENITIS, STREP THROAT, AND QUINSY

SYMPTOMS—Inflammation and possible infection of the tonsils and adenoids. If streptococcal bacteria have caused the infection, it is called *strep throat*. There is a sore throat with fever, lack of appetite, chills, headache, muscle pain, nausea, vomiting, nasal obstruction and discharge. The lymph glands may become swollen. Symptoms continue for 24-72 hours; then they gradually subside over 7-10 days. The tonsils may look red and enlarged; and pus may be observed.

CAUSES—The tonsils and adenoids are glands containing lymphatic tissue, located in the upper throat. Both are part of the immune system; they protect the body, at the top of the gastrointestinal tract, against infection. Each tonsil contains 200 million lymphocytes. We will here primarily deal with tonsillitis; treatment for adenitis is essentially the same. Strep throat also has the same treatment.

When the **body's resistance is lowered**, viruses or bacteria (usually streptococcal) set to work. And a **diet of processed and junk foods, that is high in carbohydrates and low in protein**, can also bring on this condition.

If streptococcal infection (strep throat) is not present, then the throat condition is eliminated much quicker.

If not cared for properly, strep throat can be potentially dangerous and can lead to rheumatic fever or meningitis.

Food allergies weaken the body: usually **cow's milk, chocolate,** or too much **white flour** or **sugar** products. Cow's milk and **wheat** are the two primary allergens to beware of. **Antibiotics** weaken the body more.

The more frequently this infection occurs, the more difficult it is to eliminate. The tonsils become scarred from previous inflammations.

Quinsy is a peritonsillar abscess. It is an infection of the tonsil, between the tonsil and the pharyngeal constrictor muscle. The solution is not a tonsillectomy, but the care specified below.

• The cause is frequently sinus drainage with mucus coming down the eustachian tubes and causing irritation. The basic cause is a dirty transverse colon, which causes poison in the sinus and head areas, which, in turn, drains down into the throat.

NATURAL REMEDIES
• **Cold applications** to the throat may bring relief and shorten the high point of the infection. This could be an **ice collar** or **flannel** wrung out of cold water and frequently changed.

• Hot **saltwater gargles** will help. To increase blood circulation in the throat, do alternate hot and cold gargling.

• Gargle with **goldenseal** tea, drinking it as you do this (1 cup 3-4 times a day).

• **Colloidal silver** is an inexpensive and safe way treat sore throats.

• Place a **heating compress** on the throat at other times. Prepare a strip of cotton sheet (dipped and wrung out of cold water) in a strip of dry wool; and put this on the throat.

• Give a hot **footbath**, along with hot (5 minutes) and cold (5 minutes) **cloths** to the throat (2-3 times daily). Finish with a **cold mitten friction** to the whole body. Then immediately put him into a warm **bed** and let him rest.

• Drink plenty of **liquids**. *Fresh* juices are the best. Drink fruit and vegetable juices, green drink, and lots of water. Avoid **sugary, processed, and junk foods**. A cleansing **juice fast**, alternated with **vegetable broths**, for 3 days is helpful. **Lemon or lime juice** in warm water with **honey and ginger** will help the cleansing process. **Peppermint** tea will help settle the stomach.

• Maintain a high intake of **vitamin C**. It powerfully fights the infection and also produces interferon which does the same. Along with the light meals, include **vitamin A, selenium, and zinc**.

• Dissolve in the mouth a **charcoal** tablet several times a day. It will both soothe the throat and combine with toxins, absorbing them.

• **Catnip tea enemas** are good for fevers.

• **Goldenseal, echinacea, and garlic** act as antibiotics. **Tea tree oil** helps heal the throat infection. **Fenugreek** and **comfrey** loosens the mucus and carries it out of the body.

• ¼ tsp. of **lobelia** extract (swallowed every 2 hours) will help alleviate fever, pain, and swelling.

• Use an antispasmodic (such as **lobelia**) both internally and externally (wrapping the throat with a soaked fomentation). This can also be aided quickly by the use of a **bayberry gargle** (drinking several tablespoons every hour or so) or using **mullein** (three parts) and **lobelia** (one part) which should draw off the toxic poison into the blood stream and disperse it quickly. Use a **hot water bottle** and either a **poultice or a fomentation**.

• Avoid people who **smoke**. Children whose parents are smokers have very high rates of tonsil infections. *Also see p. 740.*

J.H. KELLOGG, M.D., PRESCRIPTIONS FOR TONSILLITIS AND ITS COMPLICATIONS *(how to give these water therapies: pp. 207-272 / Hydrotherapy Disease Index: pp. 273-275).*

(1) ACUTE FORM —
DIETARY FACTORS—Rest in bed. Keep room a uniform temperature. **Eat a spare diet** that consists chiefly of fruits. Avoid meats of all sorts. Copious water drinking.

GENERAL CARE—Hot **Blanket Pack**, sweating Wet Sheet Pack, Steam Bath, Radiant Heat Bath, Hot Full Bath. Follow with **Dry Pack** or other sweating procedures, once daily. Follow with **Cold Mitten Friction**, Cold Wet Sheet Rub, or Cold Douche. **Fomentation** to the throat, 3 times daily. **Cold Compress** during intervals, changed every 15-30 minutes. **Enema,** if bowels are inactive. Hot **gargle** every few minutes, if throat is very sensitive. **Ice Bag** to throat if inflammation is intense. **Inhalation** of soothing vapors. Use of steam inhaler 10-14 minutes hourly or almost continuously. If the tonsil suppurates (discharges pus), it should be lanced. See your doctor.

(2) CHRONIC FORM —
CLERGYMAN'S SORE THROAT DIETARY AND LIFESTYLE—Aseptic **dietary**, **outdoor life**, open air gymnastics, swimming.

GENERAL CARE—**Fomentation** to the throat at bedtime. Follow by **throat pack** (Cold Compress) during the night. And **gargle with hot water,** 3 times a day. Radiant Heat Bath, sweating **Wet Sheet Pack**. Steam Bath or other sweating bath, 3 times weekly. Follow by suitable **cold application**. Daily **Cold Bath** on rising. **Moist Abdominal Bandage,** to be worn during the night. If necessary, remove tonsils and vegetations in throat or postnasal region.

—Also see Adenoids below (742).

ENCOURAGEMENT—Strength for today, courage for tomorrow; trusting Christ and obeying Him. God can help us have all this. Psalm 138:8.

"I pray not that Thou shouldest take them out of the world, but that Thou shouldest keep them from the evil." John 17:15.

Surrender to Jesus and let Him guide your life.

ADENOIDS
(Adenoid Hypertrophy)

SYMPTOMS—It hurts at the back of the child's throat. When he opens his mouth, the area of the tonsils appears red and swollen.

CAUSES—What is commonly called adenoids is enlargement of the pharyngeal tonsil, which is a tissue close to the tonsils. This infection frequently occurs in children. *Also see Tonsillitis (740*

• Do a 3-5 day **fast** on diluted **citrus juices**. Follow this with a **careful diet**.

• Three times a day, give herb teas such as **red clover, sassafras,** and **burdock root**.

• **Gargle** several times a day with **goldenseal** tea. **Echinacea** and **myrrh** are very good for all glandular swellings.

—*See Tonsillitis (740) and Childhood Diseases (739-752).*

ENCOURAGEMENT—Jesus sees the end from the beginning. He can plan for you better than you can plan for yourself. Luke 3:79.

CHICKEN POX
(Varicella Zoster, Pox)

SYMPTOMS—Small, round pimples on the face and body, filled with fluid and appearing like water blisters. As the fluid leaks, it forms a crust.

CAUSES—Chicken pox is a viral disease which first manifests itself as a fever and headache, 7-21 days after exposure. The eruptions continue in cycles from 3-7 days; and the disease generally runs its course in 14 days. It is communicable for 1-2 days before the rash develops, until all the blister-like lesions have crusted (averaging 5-6 days).

Chicken pox mainly occurs between 2 and 8 years of age; *it is much more severe if not contracted until one is an adult*. If a pregnant mother has it in the first four months of pregnancy, birth defects are possible in the infant. Once you have had it, you generally have lifetime immunity. *This is why chicken pox vaccines are dangerous.* It is better to get the disease as a child, when it is relatively harmless, than to wait till adulthood to contract it.

Oddly enough, the same virus that causes chicken pox in children *(varicella zoster)* is the one which causes shingles *(350)* in adults.

Chicken pox is transmitted by **contact** and by **airborne droplets**. Epidemics tend to occur in the winter and spring.

NATURAL REMEDIES

• Drink freshly made **juices**, with added **protein** powder and **brewer's yeast**. Drink **vegetable broth**.

• When the fever drops and appetite returns, give **mashed bananas** and fresh, raw **applesauce**. Use a light, **fat-free, sugar-free diet**. You can give **vitamin C** to bowel tolerance.

• **Catnip** tea, with a little **molasses**, is good during the fever. If the child is over two, catnip tea enemas will help reduce the fever.

• The only real concern with childhood chicken pox is pock scarring. This may be minimized by several simple **baths** and **soaks** to the skin. And, of course, do not scratch.

• To avoid scratching the pocks, keep the child's **nails short**, to minimize spreading of the infection. Have the child wear **mittens or gloves**, to avoid scratching—especially at night. Instead of scratching, apply pressure to the area. Bathe him often.

• Relieve itching with **calamine lotion, moist baking soda, or starch baths**. **Vitamin E oil** can be applied directly to each papule.

• A deep, warm 15-minute **bath** at the onset of the disease will help the pox develop more rapidly. Keep the **head cool**; but do not let him become chilled.

• Each day give a **tepid bath**, followed by a change of clothes and linens. Protect against chilling while bathing and at other times. Chicken pox pneumonia can develop!

• **Oatmeal baths** are soothing because they are alkaline. Put 1 pound of uncooked oatmeal (or 1 heaping cup of uncooked rolled oats, ground fine, in a blender) in a bag made of 2 thicknesses of old sheeting. Soften it with hot water and then float it in the bathtub or hang it on the faucet. Water will flow through it. You can use the bag to gently sponge the body. Pat dry when finished; do not rub.

• If needed, mix 1 level teaspoon of **salt** with 1 pint (2 cups) of water and **gargle** with it.

• Avoid **constipation**.

• **Isolation**. Keep the infected child away from newborn infants, elderly people, and pregnant women. They may not have had chicken pox before. Do not send the child back to school until all the lesions have finished being crusted.

• **Antibiotics and corticosteroids** do not help in any way; and they should not be given. (Chicken pox is a virus.)

• **Do not give aspirin to children!** About 10% of Reye's Syndrome *(750)* cases occur after chicken pox as a result of aspirin dosages. Reye's can cause irreversible coma or death.

• *If you contract chicken pox as an adult*, go on a fasting program of **fresh fruit and vegetable juices**, interspersed with **light meals**.

ENCOURAGEMENT—Guard against the tendency to forget God. You dare not do this. He is the only one who can give you the extra help you need everyday. 2 James 1:22-24.

MUMPS

SYMPTOMS—Swelling of one or both salivary glands, fever (up to 104° F.), chills, headache, sore throat, and pain when swallowing or chewing. Swelling often occurs in one gland first; and then it begins in the other as swelling in the first subsides. But it may occur on only one side.

CAUSES—Mumps is an infection of the salivary (parotid) glands, located in front of, and below, each ear. It rarely occurs before 3 years of age or after 40. Either **direct contact or droplets** spread the disease.

Mumps is not as contagious as chicken pox or measles. But a person with the disease is still contagious 48 hours before symptoms develop to 6 days afterward. Incubation is 14 to 21 days.

If no complications occur, complete recovery generally results within about 10 days. One bout, and lifetime immunity generally follows.

If it is acquired after puberty, the ovaries or testes may become involved and sterility may result. Other complications can also occur; these affect the heart, kidneys, and brain.

Swollen salivary glands can also be caused by several other diseases: A partial list includes cirrhosis of the liver *(450)*, leukemia *(795)*, lupus *(310)*, and tuberculosis *(505)*. It also includes strep throat and taking of certain drugs. If it seems to be an isolated case of "mumps," it might actually be something else.

NATURAL REMEDIES

• Keep the **diet simple, fat-free, and sugar-free**. Eat mostly **raw fruits and vegetables** that are juiced or softened. Avoid foods that require **chewing** or might be irritating.

• Drink plenty of pure **water** and fresh **juices**. This will keep the body working well, help flush toxins, and render it less likely that complications may occur.

• Do not eat **junk food** of any type. Avoid **caffeine, tobacco, alcohol, soft drinks**, etc. Avoid **acidic foods**, such as pickles or citrus fruits.

• To relieve pain, **cold or warm compresses** (whichever feels best) may be placed on the neck and over the glands. But avoid hot or icy cold applications.

• **Do not give aspirin** to a child or youth with a fever; it may result in death! *See Reye's Syndrome (750).*

If nausea and/or pain on swallowing becomes so severe that the person becomes unable to eat, intravenous administration of dextrose and fluids may be needed.

J.H. KELLOGG, M.D., PRESCRIPTIONS FOR MUMPS AND ITS COMPLICATIONS *(how to give these water therapies: pp. 207-272 / Hydrotherapy Disease Index: pp. 273-275)*

GENERAL—Cold Mitten Friction or **Cold Towel Rub**, 24 times a day. **Neutral Bath** for one hour, daily. Copious water drinking.

TO COMBAT LOCAL INFLAMMATION—Hot Blanket **Pack**. Follow by **Heating or Sweating Wet Sheet Pack**, continued 1-2 hours. Repeat the application twice a day. **Fomentation** over the affected parts every 2 hours for 15 minutes. Follow by **Heating Compress** at 60°F., to be changed every 10 minutes or as soon as warm. **Ice Bag** over swollen glands until active inflammation is subdued. Remove ice every half hour and apply **Fomentation** for 5 minutes.

HEADACHE—Cool Compress.

NOSE BLEED—Ice to back of neck, **Hot Compress** over face. Ice to hands. Elevate hands to vertical position, if necessary. **Hot Footbath** or Hot Leg Pack. Very **Hot Nasal Douche**.

DIARRHEA—Enema at 95° F. after each bowel movement. **Abdominal Bandage** at 60° F., renewed every 15-30 minutes. If pain is present, **Fomentation** to abdomen for 15 minutes or until it is relieved; do this every 2 hours. Empty colon with a large Hot **Enema,** if due to fecal accumulation.

VOMITING—Ice over stomach or spine opposite the stomach. Or **Hot and Cold Compress** over stomach. Ice pills. Sipping very hot water.

EARACHE—Ice Bag to neck of the same side. **Fomentation** over ear. **Hot Ear Douche**, if necessary. Protect the ear with warm **cotton**, to prevent chilling by evaporation after treatment.

CONVULSIONS—Hot Blanket Pack or Hot Immersion at 105°-108° F., with cold to the head (**Cold Compress, Ice Bag, Ice Cap**, etc.).

INFLAMMATION OF THE BREAST—Fomentation over the breast for 15 minutes, every 3 hours. During interval between, apply a **Heating Compress** at 60° F.; this is renewed every 15-30 minutes. **Hot Pack** to arm of the same side. **Hot Hip and Leg Pack** for derivative effect if pain is severe.

INFLAMMATION OF TESTICLE—Ice Compress covering entire genitals and inner surfaces of thighs with simultaneous **Hot Hip and Leg Pack** for 30 minutes. Repeat every 4 hours. During interval between, apply **Heating Compress** at 60° F. in place of the **Ice Compress**, renewed every 15 minutes.

—*Also see Childhood Diseases (739).*

ENCOURAGEMENT—"What doth the Lord thy God require of thee, but to fear the Lord thy God, to walk in all His ways, and to love Him, and to serve the Lord thy God with all thy heart and with all thy soul."—Deuteronomy 10:12.

C
H
I
L
D

MEASLES
(Rubeola)

SYMPTOMS—First symptoms are fever, coughing, sneezing, runny nose, and inflammation of the eyes. The eyes may become red and sensitive to light. Within 24-48 hours, small red spots with white centers appear on the insides of the cheeks. A rash appears 3-5 days later on the sides of the neck, forehead, and ears; then it spreads over 5-7 days to the rest of the body. As it spreads, the fever subsides.

CAUSES—There are two types of measles: **common measles (rubeola)** and **German measles (rubella, 745)**. Common measles is highly contagious; it is **spread by droplets** from the nose, throat, and mouth. At the present time, adolescents and young adults are affected more often than children. If the person was previously healthy, the disease will pass within 10 days.

But it can be followed by one of several serious complications, including pneumonia, bronchitis, croup, middle-ear infection, meningitis, encephalitis, or injury to the nervous system.

Approximately 98% of the population have had common measles. Lifelong immunity follows this infection.

The best protection is to live right and eat right.

NATURAL REMEDIES

• He should be **isolated** in a room which is **well-ventilated**. If he is sensitive to light, **darken** the room. He should not read or watch television. Keep the lights dim.

• Drink plenty of **water** and **fruit and vegetable juices**, preferably fresh.

• Fevers increase the body's need for calories and **vitamins A and C**. He should be encouraged, but not forced, to eat. **Frequent small meals** of nourishing food may be best.

• Avoid **processed foods**.

• **Rest** until the rash and fever have disappeared.

• **Garlic** or **catnip** tea enemas help lower fever.

• If a cough is present, cool moisture from a **vaporizer** may help. But **water,** given copiously, is the best cough medicine.

• A **hot bath** may help reduce the fever. Place the child in a hot tub (105°-108° F.) for one minute for each year of his age. Keep the **head cool**. This may be repeated every 2 hours. Dress him warmly afterward, so chilling does not occur.

• This disease must be brought to the surface of the skin as rapidly as possible. Diaphoretic herbs, such as **yarrow and raspberry leaves,** are excellent. Use **vapor baths** (such as **ginger, mustard, and cayenne**) which bring the toxic wastes to a head quickly. Drinking **water** is required, or the organic calcium will turn into inorganic calcium, because of the feverish dry body heat, and cause further tissue damage. Rheumatic fever is often the aftermath of diseases,

such as chicken pox and measles. Take care of the eyes and the bronchial tubes in the lungs. **Avoid bright light;** since the eyes are weak at this time. The bowels should be kept open with the lower bowel tonic. A **catnip enema** is soothing and beneficial. **Ripe fruits** will assist in the cleansing process.

• Helpful herbs include **yarrow, pleurisy root, and marigold**.

COMPLICATIONS

• **Antibiotics** are useless against measles and do not decrease the likelihood of complications. But, in an emergency (if complications occur), they could be used.

• Complications can be serious; but they are unlikely in the developed nations. Most such problems stem from secondary bacterial infection, primarily middle-ear infection or pneumonia (503-504). But special care and vigorous use of simple, natural remedies can generally deal with them.

• *Bronchitis (500)* may occur; it can be treated with hot **fomentations** to the chest. Apply them twice a day, along with a **hot footbath**. A **heating compress** to the chest can be applied at night.

• *If there is itching of the skin,* bathe him with one of the following teas: **goldenseal root, yellow dock root, or burdock root**. Another formula: Mix 1 oz. **goldenseal** and 9 oz. **flaxseed oil**; and apply freely as needed.

• **Do not give aspirin** to a child or youth with a fever; it may result in death! *See Reye's Syndrome (750).*

J.H. KELLOGG, M.D., PRESCRIPTIONS FOR MEASLES AND ITS COMPLICATIONS (how to give these water therapies: pp. 207-272 / list of treatments: pp. 206-207 / Hydrotherapy Disease Index: pp. 273-275)

MAINTAIN GENERAL RESISTANCE—Wet Sheet Pack, Graduated Bath.

PREVENT LUNG COMPLICATIONS—Fomentation to chest, twice a day. **Chest Pack** during interval between.

NASO-PHARYNGEAL IRRITATION—Apply light, very Hot **Compresses** to the face. **Inhale** vapor of water, aromatic oils, and balsams. **Fomentation** to the throat every 2 hours. **Heating Compress** during the interval between, changing every 15 minutes at first, less frequently later.

INFLAMMATION OF MIDDLE EAR—Ice to throat of same side, **Fomentation** over ear.

HEMORRHAGIC FORM—Hot Blanket Pack or short Hot Full **Bath**, followed by **Heating Wet Sheet Pack**. Repeat every 3-4 Hours. Prolonged **Neutral Bath** at 93°-95° F.

BRONCHIAL CATARRH—Fomentation to chest, **Cold Towel Rub**, or **Cold Mitten Friction** (twice daily), **Heating Chest Pack** night and day.

LOBAR PNEUMONIA AND BRONCHO-PNEUMONIA—**Fomentation** for pain and irritable cough, repeated every 2-3 hours. **Cold Compress** during interval at 60° F., changing every 15-30 minutes. Hot **Hip and Leg Pack**, if the local inflammation is severe. *See Pneumonia (503-504).*

—For any of the following associated problems, see under their respective headings: *Cough (291), Nosebleed (711), Inflammation of the Eye (or eyelids, 400), Headache*

(556), Acute Nephritis (kidney inflammation, 492).
—*Also see German Measles (below) and Child-hood Diseases (739).*

ENCOURAGEMENT—In this life, we will encounter many difficulties and trials; but, if we will make God the center of our lives, He will wonderfully work to help us through our problems. He will guide, guard, and keep us from the evil one, if we will submit our lives to His control. Isaiah 11:4.

GERMAN MEASLES
(Rubella)

SYMPTOMS—Fatigue, coughing, headache, mild fever, muscle aches, and stiffness in the neck. A pink rash often develops 1-5 days later. It generally first appears on the face and neck; then it spreads to the rest of the body.

CAUSES—As we mentioned earlier, there are two types of measles: common measles and German measles:

Common measles (*rubeola, above*) is highly contagious and can have serious complications if cautions are not taken; but this usually passes within 10 days.
German measles (*rubella*) is different in several ways. It is usually a mild contagious illness with a rapid recovery period (5-7 days). But it is dangerous if a woman contracts it during the first trimester (first 3 months) of her pregnancy. If that happens, she might give birth to a child with heart defects, deafness, mental retardation, or blindness. Therefore, **a pregnant woman must guard against exposure to rubella.**

NATURAL REMEDIES
• Follow the **treatment** specified for common measles. *See Measles (745).*
• Drink plenty of fluids. This can be **water, fruit juices, and vegetable broths**.
• **Rest in bed** until the rash and fever have disappeared.
• If you need to lower the fever, **catnip tea** or **garlic enemas** will help. **Peppermint tea** is also good.
• The person with rubella should **avoid contact** with others, especially children and adolescents—*and especially women of childbearing age and their children until a full week after the rash disappears.*
• Do not give **antibiotics**; since they are ineffective against rubella, which is a virus.
• Do not give **aspirin** to a child or youth with a fever; it may result in his death! *See Reye's Syndrome (750).*
What precautions should a woman take?
• A pregnant woman must avoid exposure to German measles. The disease should be considered contagious from 1 week before the rash appears until 1 week after the rash fades. The rash usually lasts about 3 days.
• If she thinks she has been exposed to the disease, she can immediately see a physician and request that she be given a gamma-globulin injection. If given soon after exposure, it may reduce the severity of the disease or possibly prevent it from occurring.
• Immunity to German measles can be determined by a special blood test. She may wish to be vaccinated. If this is done, pregnancy must be avoided for 3 months following immunization. (A woman who previously has had rubella will give immunity to her child for 1 year.)
—*Also see Childhood Diseases (739).*

ENCOURAGEMENT—God has given, in the Bible, sufficient evidence that His Word is from Him. Study and obey it, and God will guide you day by day as you pray for help. Claim the power of its many, many promises. Psalm 22:26.

SCARLET FEVER
(Scarlatina)

SYMPTOMS—Symptoms appear 2-7 days after exposure. Vomiting, along with sore throat and headache. Within a day, high fever develops. The throat membrane is inflamed and the soft palate may show a fine light-red rash. The tongue is coated white; but, on the second day, reddened raised points show through, especially at the tip and sides.

The throat condition becomes more severe, with redness and enlargement of glands under the lower jaw.

The rash usually begins on the chest within 1-2 days after the first symptoms; it later extends to other parts of the body and limbs. But infection can occur without a rash occurring.

CAUSES—Scarlet fever is an acute contagious disease and is caused by one of several different streptococcal germs. Urine and discharges from nose, mouth, ears, and any abscesses are highly infectious. One attack generally brings lifelong immunity. Few contract it after the age of 15.

The fever usually does not remain high more than 4 days; and the rash fades within a week. The more intense the rash, the more scaling forms on the skin.

Inflammation of the ear is one of the most frequent complications of scarlet fever. The infection in the throat passes up the eustachian tube into the middle ear. *See Earache and Infection (407).* Children can become deaf as a result.

The infection may extend from the ear to the mastoid cells in the bone behind the ear or to the membranes covering the brain, or to both. This produces mastoiditis (*407*, brain abscess, or meningitis (*578*). These conditions are serious and often fatal.

C
H
I
L
D

Rheumatic fever (750) frequently follows scarlet fever; and this sometimes results in inflammation of the lining membranes and valves of the heart.

Enlargement of the lymph glands of the neck can turn into an abscess of these glands, as late as 5-6 weeks after the disease began.

In a child that is well-advanced toward recovery (especially in the third week), nephritis *(492)*, a kidney infection, can develop. So, this is another danger to be warded off by proper treatment.

Scarlet fever is not a matter to be taken lightly.

You do well to call a physician, if possible. He may need to lance the middle ear if infection develops. He will probably examine the heart daily, for indications of damage, and do frequent urinalysis for signs of nephritis.

NATURAL REMEDIES

• Put the child on a **fruit and vegetable juice fast**, followed by a simple diet of **fruits, vegetables, and broths** for a time.

• **Avoid** giving the child inadequate care, improper food, and too early physical activity. This is a **contagious** disease; so proper precautions must be taken.

• Keep him **in bed** at least 3 weeks, even though he feels well! Muscular activity too soon can result in kidney damage.

• *If the temperature* goes above 103° F., reduce it by means of **tepid sponge baths**. Lightly rub the face and upper body with a cloth wrung out of lukewarm water.

• *If there is a sore throat*, apply a hot **fomentation** twice a day to the area, followed by continuous heating compresses.

• *When the rash begins to appear*, help him to sweat. Give a long-continued hot **footbath**, along with hot **drinks**, all the while keeping him covered with **blankets**. The objective is to get him to sweat. But, afterward, guard against chilling!

• *To help prevent kidney damage*—when he goes back on food—**eliminate eggs, meat, meat broths, and legumes** from the diet. Give him only **milk, cereals, fruit juices, pureed vegetables, and** all the **water** he will drink.

• *To hasten the scaling of the skin*, and get it over with, give a **daily sponge** bath with warm water and mild soap. Follow by an **olive oil rub**.

• *If there is itching of the skin*, bathe him with teas of **goldenseal root, yellow dock root, or burdock root**. Another formula: Mix 1 oz. **goldenseal** and 9 oz. **flaxseed oil**; and apply freely as needed.

• Helpful herbs include **black rose, twinleaf, and bloodroot**.

J.H. KELLOGG, M.D., PRESCRIPTIONS FOR SCARLET FEVER AND ITS COMPLICATIONS (*how to give these water therapies: pp. 207-272 / list of treatments: pp. 206-207 / Hydrotherapy Disease Index: pp. 273-275*)

BUILD GENERAL RESISTANCE—**Hot Blanket Pack**, 3-8 minutes. Follow by **Cooling Wet Sheet Pack**. (The cold sheet should be well-heated by him before removing it.) Or, the Hot Blanket Pack may be followed by **Cold Towel Rub**, Wet Sheet Rub in bed, or Tepid Pail Pour at 85°-80° F. while he sits in a bathtub. Avoid giving him a **Cold Mitten Friction**.

ELIMINATE TOXINS—Copious drinking of **water, fruit juices**, fruit purees, etc.

REDUCE FEVER—Cooling Wet Sheet Pack. Hot Blanket Pack. Follow with **Cold towel Rub** or Wet Sheet Rub. Graduated Bath, copious **water** drinking, **Cooling Enema**.

IF ERUPTION IS DELAYED—**Wet Sheet Pack**, prolonged to heating stage.

DIARRHEA—75°-80° F. **Enema** after each bowel movement. **Fomentation,** for 15 minutes, over the abdomen every 2 hours. Follow with **Heating Compress**, changed every half hour. If most of his skin surface is cold, use the **Hot Full Bath** for 5 minutes. Follow with short **Cold Towel Rubbing**.

VOMITING—**Hot and Cold Trunk Pack. Ice Bag** over the stomach or spine opposite stomach.

CONVULSIONS—**Hot Blanket Pack** for 10 minutes. Follow by **Cold Wet Sheet Pack** with ice to the head. Hot Bath for 5 minutes. Follow with **Neutral Bath** at 92°-95° F. **Water** drinking. Large **Enema**.

PHARYNGITIS—**Fomentation** to throat 10 minutes every hour with **Ice Compress** during interval between. **Warm Vapor Inhalation** for 5-10 minutes every half hour. **Gargle** throat with very hot water, hourly. **Throat Compress** at 60° F., changed every 15 minutes. It should be protected by a **Heating Compress,** changed once in 3 hours.

DELIRIUM WITH INSOMNIA AND NERVOUS AGITATION OR CHOREA—**Ice Bag** to head, Hot **Fomentations** to spine, followed by Prolonged **Wet Sheet Pack**.

SCALING OF THE SKIN—Neutral (92°-95° F.) Alkaline **Bath** daily, for 15 minutes to 1 hour.

NEPHRITIS, OR SUPPRESSION OF THE URINE—Hot **Blanket Pack** for 20-30 minutes. Follow by **Heating Compress** to the loins. Copious **water** drinking. **Enema,** at 80°-90° F. twice daily.

PLEURISY—**Fomentation** to the chest for 15 minutes, every 2 hours, with **Heating Compress** during the interval. Tight muslin **bandage** about chest, if pain is intense.

RHEUMATISM—Sweating **Wet Sheet Pack**. Copious water drinking. **Fomentation** to joints every 3 hours, with **Heating Compress** during interval between.

PERICARDITIS OR ENDOCARDITIS—Ice Ball or **Cold Compress** over heart, to be removed for 5 minutes, every 15-20 minutes.

ENTERITIS—**Hot Trunk Heating Pack** with **Hot Footbath** or Hot Leg Pack, for 20 minutes. Follow by **Cold Abdominal Compress** at 60° F., to be changed every 30 minutes. **Enema** after each stool, at 95° F.

PNEUMONIA—**Fomentation** for 15 minutes, every 2-3 hours. **Cold Compress** at 60°F. during interval, changing every 10-20 minutes. **Hot Hip and Leg Pack** once or twice daily, to relieve congestion. Keep skin warm and active. **Hot Blanket Pack,** if he is chilly. Follow by heating **Wet Sheet Pack**.

ENLARGED SPLEEN OR LIVER—**Fomentation** over the afflicted body part, for 10-20 minutes, twice daily. Follow with **Ice Water Compress**, to be changed every 2 hours during the interval.

CONTRAINDICATIONS—**Avoid** short Cold Baths, prolonged Hot Baths, and all other measures which diminish heat elimination or increase heat production.

GENERAL METHOD—At the beginning, encourage eruption by hot-water drinking, very Hot Baths, Heating Pack. After eruption is fully developed, give Cooling Wet Sheet Pack, Graduated Bath, Cool Enema, and other fever-reducing measures. Copious water drinking is especially important. Give attention to the throat, to prevent infection of the ears. Warm Vapor Inhalation. Irrigation of the throat (gargling). Heating Compress. If albumin appears, the blood must be kept in the skin by Hot Packs and warm wrappings that are covered well with blankets. And the cold applications must be "partial" (such as Wet Hand Rub, Cold Mitten Friction, Cold Towel Rub). Prolonged chilling of the skin must be carefully avoided.

ENCOURAGEMENT—God has boundless love and mercy toward us. You can find in Him the help you need. Only He can protect you from the evil one. Romans 8:6.

DIPHTHERIA

SYMPTOMS—It begins with sore throat and fever. Frequently a dirty, white or grayish membrane forms in the throat or nose, or both. There are slight chills, possible vomiting and diarrhea, always fetid breath, difficulty in swallowing, and hoarseness.

Children first complain of feeling tired and sleepy. The tonsils appear inflamed, dark red, and unevenly swollen. White parchment-like patches appear on them. The glands in the neck usually swell. *If there are no white patches or developing membrane, it is not diphtheria.*

CAUSES—Diphtheria is an acute, contagious disease. It begins 3-8 days after exposure; and it primarily occurs between 1 and 10 years of age.

Part of the danger is the obstruction to breathing, due to the above-mentioned false membrane; this is partly due to the toxins carried by the diphtheria germs which—carried throughout the body—especially harm the heart muscles, nerves, and kidneys.

This is a serious disease. Diphtheria is transmitted by **clothing, contact, domestic animals and pets,** and sometimes by **raw milk.** Anything (dish, garment, etc.) coming in contact with the person must be disinfected.

Highly contagious: Individuals can carry the germs on them for several years and transmit them to still others. A carrier should be isolated until the germs can no longer be found in his throat, nose, or catarrhal discharge.

The membrane is tenacious and dangerous. If not checked, it will cover the air tube and the child will suffocate. It is generally whitish; but it may appear yellowish or greenish. When the child breathes harder and then has a frightened look, his air flow is narrowing.

When someone develops diphtheria, there must be no delay. Give him vigorous treatment. You will want to call a physician.

NATURAL REMEDIES
• Give the child all the **water** he can drink; and keep him in **bed**, in a well-ventilated room.
• **Avoid** chilling him. Too early exercise may overstrain the heart.
• **The diet** should be liquid. Fast on fresh **carrot juice or citrus juices**. If the child insists on eating something, give him **bananas, raisins, figs, and oranges**—and no other food. *It is best to give him only liquids (water and fresh juices) until he is cleaned out, the throat is clean, and the phlegm and false membrane are totally gone.*
• After the disease appears to be ended, give him no **meat** for quite some time. (It is better not to give it to him at all.)
• Give him **warm baths**.
• An **emetic** to make him vomit is usually needed to empty the stomach of putrefying matter; otherwise, high fevers will result. **Lobelia** in water can be given, but combined with **bayberry bark** is better. The vomiting must be repeated until the stomach and throat are entirely clean.
• As the disease progresses, **lobelia** and **bayberry bark** tea can be given at any time, to clean out the mucous membranes of the mouth and throat. Bayberry cleans the membrane and eliminates the odor. It is also healing and antiseptic. A very small amount of **cayenne** or **ginger** can be added as stimulants.
• *Problems can develop while the child is sleeping*—serious ones. Therefore, always give the **emetic** before he goes to sleep each time. Otherwise he might suffocate during sleep.
• Give him an **enema** every morning and evening. This helps clean out toxins from the diphtheria germs. An herb tea can be added, to detoxify the colon: **bayberry, white oak bark, or red raspberry**. There should be at least 3-4 bowel movements a day.
• **Bayberry** is excellent in all throat or stomach mucous conditions.
• *If the heart rate is rapid*, apply an **ice bag** over the heart.
• *In case of headache*, place cold compresses or ice bags to the head and neck.
• A gargle can be made of **goldenseal and myrrh**, with a pinch of **cayenne**. Use this every half hour. It will clean the mucus and germs out of the throat.
• Apply **hot and cold fomentations** over the liver, stomach, kidneys, and spine to keep the circulation normal. This stimulates the lymphatic system, to help clean out toxins.
• *If there is any danger of paralysis*, give **hot and cold applications** to the spine, stomach, and liver.
• Give 2 high **enemas** daily.
• If symptoms of heart failure appear, give a half

C
H
I
L
D

teaspoon of **cayenne** in hot water. Have him drink it all down immediately. Repeat if necessary.

• Each day, **clean all clothing and bed linens** by boiling them.

• As he begins to recuperate, he can be given **baked apples, potato peeling broth, fresh fruits, cooked vegetables, and soy milk**.

• If properly cared for, the disease will end within 7-10 days.

• Do not give **aspirin** to a child or youth with a fever; it may result in his death! *See Reye's Syndrome (750).*

• With diphtheria, the throat area should be cleared of the false mucous membrane, with a **bayberry and raspberry leaf** combination, or **garlic**. Take a few drops in a tea. Quick relief is given through **antispasmodic and cayenne fomentation** on the chest and the lung area. **Antispasmodic tincture and cayenne** can be taken internally. (This will also ward off the danger of paralysis). One should always give an **emetic** before allowing the patient to go to sleep; and the bowels should be cleaned of the poisons with high enemas accompanied with stimulant herbs. Any of the following may be used with the enemas: **bayberry bark, raspberry leaves, catnip, chickweed, white oak bark, shepherd's purse, wild alum root, echinacea, strawberry leaves, raspberry leaves**. A **hot vapor bath** is beneficial as is a **hot footbath of mustard and water**. Also apply **fomentation of mullein and ragwort** to the throat. Decoctions of **raspberry leaves, mullein, agrimony, bayberry bark or lemon juice** will relieve the soreness in the throat. Ample **fresh pineapple juice** is also very good.

J.H. KELLOGG, M.D., PRESCRIPTIONS FOR DIPHTHERIA AND ITS COMPLICATIONS *(how to give these water therapies: pp. 206-275 / list of treatments: pp. 206-207 / Hydrotherapy Disease Index: pp. 273-275)*

INCREASE AND MAINTAIN VITAL RESISTANCE—Hot Fomentation to the spine or short **Hot Bath**. Follow by **Cold Mitten Friction** or Cold Towel Rub, 2-3 times a day.

TO COMBAT LOCAL INFLAMMATION—Fomentation to throat for 15 minutes, every 2 hours. **Ice Compress** to throat during interval between. If inflammation becomes intense, and suppuration (pus flowing) or sloughing (separation of dead tissue from living tissue) is threatened, use the **Heating Compress** at 60° F., changing every hour. **Warm vapor Inhalation**, antiseptic lotions to throat, **hot-water gargle**.

COMBAT GENERAL TOXEMIA, RESULTING DEGENERATIONS, AND LOCALIZED INFLAMMATIONS—Copious enemas, twice daily. Copious **water** drinking, 3-6 pints daily. The free use of **fruit juices**. Hot **Fomentations** to the spine or short Hot **Full Bath**. Follow with Cold Mitten Friction or **Cold Towel Rub,** 2-3 times a day.

TO COMBAT LOCAL INFLAMMATION—Hot Blanket Pack. Follow with Sweating **Wet Sheet Pack**; repeat every 3-4 hours, if necessary. **Fomentation** to throat every 2-3 hours, for 15 minutes. **Ice Compress** to throat during interval. **Ice pills**. The **Heating Compress** at 60° F., changing every hour. Warm Vapor Inhalation. Antiseptic lotions.

FEVER—Hot **Blanket Pack**. Follow by **Wet Sheet Pack**. Prolonged **Neutral Bath,** when rectal temperature rises above 101° F. **Fomentation**. Follow by **Cold Towel Rub**. Cold **Enema** with simultaneous **Fomentation** to the back. Hot **Enema.** Follow by **Cold Towel Rub** or Cold Mitten Friction.

COMA OR COLLAPSE—Hot **Blanket Pack**. Colonic at 80° F. **Alternate Compress or Sponging** to spine. **Cold Mitten Friction. Hot and Cold Head Compress**, in case of collapse. Short Hot **Full Bath**. Follow by **Dry Blanket Pack**. Hot **Enema**. Follow by **Dry Blanket Pack**.

PARALYSIS—**Fomentation** to spine with **Cold Mitten Friction** or short Hot Blanket Pack. Follow by **Cold Mitten Friction**. **Hot and Cold Friction** over the affected part. Gymnastics, **massage**, and appropriate **exercise**.

NEURITIS—**Fomentation** over the course of the affected nerve for 15 minutes, every 2-4 hours. During the interval between, apply a well-protected **Heating Compress**. **Colonic** daily. Water drinking, 2-4 pints daily. **Aseptic diet**. **Rest** to the affected part.

CROUP—**Warm Vapor Inhalation**. **Fomentation** to throat for 15 minutes, every 2 hours. **Cold** (or very cold) **Compress**, changed every 15 minutes, during the interval. **Hot Blanket Pack**. Keep skin warm.

THREATENED SUFFOCATION—Put him in a **Neutral Full Bath** at 102°-105° F. And **pour cold water** over the chest and spine. **Cold Mitten Friction**.

—Also see Childhood Diseases (739).

ENCOURAGEMENT—Only in humble reliance upon God and obedience to all His commandments can we be secure. Trust your case to Him. He is the Great Physician.

The youth may have principles so firm that the most powerful temptations of Satan will not draw them away from their allegiance. How very important this is—at this time in history, when there is so much wickedness in the world. Psalm 119:165.

WHOOPING COUGH
(Pertussis)

SYMPTOMS—An infectious catarrhal inflammation of the air passage with violent convulsive coughs (paroxysms), consisting of several expirations followed by a loud, sonorous whooping inspiration. This is generally a children's disease and begins with spasmodic coughing spells. The face reddens and the eyes bulge. A sore throat, and often vomiting, may occur. Advanced cases develop into bronchopneumonia.

A week or two after exposure, the catarrhal stage begins. The eyes may be red and the child seems to have a cold in the head. There is sneezing and watering of the eyes. Then a persistent cough develops, especially bad at night. This coughing continues a week and keeps getting worse—this is the most significant indication that the problem may be whooping cough.

In about 2 weeks, the typical whoop begins. At first, only 1-2 times a day; it degrades to every time there is coughing. It is a deep breath at the end of a series of deep coughs. The child's face may be reddish or bluish from the effort and lack of air. Vomiting may also occur.

This whooping stage lasts 3-6 weeks; the cough may not entirely disappear for several months.

CAUSES—Whooping cough is a contagious bacterial disease, which usually attacks children between 6 months and 5 years of age. But infants and adults can also be affected. A person rarely has a second attack of this disease.

It is a rapid accumulation of mucus in the throat, which causes choking and will cause death if not cleared. Eliminate the mucus as fast as possible.

The disease is not highly contagious after the first few weeks. The most contagious phase is before a definite diagnosis is possible.

Whooping cough occurs more frequently, and seriously, in overcrowded and unhygienic quarters and cold weather. In very young, delicate, or undernourished children, it is more likely to develop into broncho-pneumonia—which is the principal cause of death in cases of whooping cough.

Complications include convulsions, bleeding from the nose into brain or area around the eyes. Broncho-pneumonia can also occur; death rarely occurs.

Whooping cough is an experience to frighten parents. There are three stages: (1) During the *catarrhal stage* (7-10 days), there are cold-like symptoms of runny, stuffy nose and sneezing. (2) During the *paroxysmal stage* (up to 2 days to 4 weeks), there are violent episodes of coughing which may last for several minutes. Each one may occur a few or many times each day. The child is gasping for air and his face may turn red; there may be vomiting and nosebleeds. The coughing gradually decreases. (3) During the *convalescent stage* (3-4 weeks), there is a chronic cough of less intensity than earlier.

You may choose to have the child vaccinated at an early age (2 months is recommended for the series). You should weigh the fact that *pertussis vaccine is one of the most dangerous of the shots* in its occasional side effects. *See Vaccination Poisoning (876-877).*

NATURAL REMEDIES

COUGHS

• Treat the cough—**When a cough first develops, treat that cough!** If you do so, the whooping cough phase can be entirely prevented! (Cough medicines, sedatives, expectorants, and antispasmodic drugs are useless.)

• In all kinds of coughs, first cleanse the system with high herb **enemas** and an herbal **laxative**.

• *When the cough is severe,* have him drink **warm water**, one cup after another; then stick your **finger** down his throat and have him vomit.

• **Wild cherry bark tea** is excellent. *Here are other herbs useful for coughs;* select from those you have on hand or can most easily obtain. They can be

mixed: **black cohosh, flaxseed, rosemary, comfrey, horehound, hyssop, myrrh, white pine, bloodroot, red sage, blue violet, ginseng, coltsfoot**. Prepare a tea and give a teaspoonful every hour until the cough is better.

• Thick **slippery elm** tea is very good in whooping cough; mix in a little lemon juice and drink it freely.

• David Reeder, M.D., used the following method for many years; and he never lost one patient to whooping cough. He would place a **poultice of garlic on the bottom of the child's feet**! This is the procedure: Remove the outer shells from the cloves and chop them finely enough to make a poultice about ¼ inch thick to cover the bottom of each foot. Spread it evenly on a piece of soft cloth. Place a thin piece of cloth over the garlic. Grease the bottoms of the feet with vasoline (because if the garlic is placed directly on the skin it will burn and blister). On each foot, place the poultice and bind with a cloth and tape. Then put an old sock on each foot. Prepare the two poultices in the evening, put them on the feet, and remove them carefully the next morning (because the same poultice may be used several times). You will smell garlic on the child's breath. Clean the feet, apply vasoline, and apply another set of poultices. With the poultices on, the child will have a sound sleep without coughing while the garlic works in his body to kill the infection.

• Be sure to include other worthwhile practices, such as partial or complete **fasting on fruit and vegetable juices** until the cough is past.

• To help him sleep at night (or any time), give him a **tepid bath** (99° F.) for 10-15 minutes, with the head or face kept cool with an ice pack or wet washcloth. This will give him great relief; and he will often sleep afterward. Coughing episodes seem to decrease.

DIET

• *As soon* as it is perceived that the problem is whooping cough, place him on a **full fruit-juice fast**. First, give citrus juices. This can be followed by other fruit juices, then carrot and other vegetable juices, and clear vegetable broth soup. Later still, fruit can be added. Give vitamins A and C in large doses.

• A **light diet** is essential. **Overfeeding** during the whooping cough prolongs the disease and leads to complications. In case it is a breast-fed infant, do not overfeed either. The child is thirsty, not hungry.

OTHER HELPS

• **Lobelia** herb or tincture used in **fomentation**, as well as a few drops internally every few minutes works well. To cut the phlegm, use a **bayberry tea** as a gargle (swallow after gargling). Use crushed **garlic** with **cayenne and honey** every few minutes, to help clear the throat.

• It is good to **soak the feet** in hot water, with a little **mustard** and **salt** added to it.

• A little **petroleum jelly** can be placed under his

C
H
I
L
D

nose and around the lips, to prevent skin irritation.

• As soon as the child finishes vomiting, **rinse his mouth** to get rid of hydrochloric acid, which could damage his teeth.

• **Warm vapor inhalations** are often very helpful. They can be given every 2-4 hours, according to the severity of the case. In his room, place a humidifier or a steam kettle on a hot plate.

• Keep his bedroom **well-ventilated,** day and night; but avoid drafts.

• If the weather is warm, sunny, and not too damp or dusty, keep him **outdoors** most of the day. But he should not exert himself in play or become chilled.

• When there is sunshine, air and sun his bedding every day.

• Keep him **isolated** from other children.

• Do not give **aspirin** to a child or youth with a fever; it may result in his death! *See Reye's Syndrome (750).*

J.H. KELLOGG, M.D., PRESCRIPTIONS FOR WHOOPING COUGH AND ITS COMPLICATIONS *(how to give these water therapies: pp. 207-272 / Hydrotherapy Disease Index: pp. 273-275)*
INCREASE VITAL RESISTANCE—Cold Mitten Friction or Cold Wet hand Rub, 3 times a day.
TO RELIEVE COUGH—Chest and neck **Heating Pack**, changing every 4 hours. Copious drinking of hot **water**, especially just before coughing paroxysm. He should drink 3-8 pints of water daily.
HELP KIDNEY ACTION—Neutral Bath daily for a half hour. Follow by **Cold Mitten Friction,** to promote activity of skin and kidneys.
GENERAL METHOD—The disease cannot be greatly shortened. But the strength may be maintained, suffering mitigated, convalescence facilitated, and grave effects prevented by the faithful employment of the above measures. The above measures should be continued for several weeks after the beginning of convalescence, not only during the active stage of the disease.
—Also see Childhood Diseases (739), Fever (302-309).

ENCOURAGEMENT—God is grieved with our griefs. He bends down in sympathy and tender love. Cry to Him for help, and He will give you that which is for the best. How thankful we can be for the love of God in Christ, our Lord and Saviour! Rejoice every day that you can be His humble, obedient child. 1 John 2:25.

RHEUMATIC FEVER

SYMPTOMS—Inflammation, and stiffness in a large joint (such as the knee). These initial symptoms are accompanied by pain.

The pain and swelling can travel from one joint to another. A skin rash may also appear.

CAUSES—Rheumatic fever is a streptococcal disease *(Streptococcus Group A);* it occurs between the ages of 4 and 18. It tends to follow a bout with tonsillitis, scarlet fever, strep throat, or an ear infection. Most

often it follows strep throat. *See Tonsillitis (740).* After the disease appears ended, it may recur again later.

Rheumatic fever affects one or several body organs or locations: joints (arthritis), brain (chorea), tissues (nodules), skin (erythema marginatum), or heart (carius). It may also result in residual heart disease, producing permanent damage to one or more heart valves. *See Arthritis (618) and Chorea (553).*

The residual heart valve damage is the most dangerous aspect of untreated rheumatic fever. Treatment early in the course of the disease will generally prevent the heart damage. But this treatment may require the help of a physician and a stay in the hospital. Here is supplementary information:

NATURAL REMEDIES
• Give a **nourishing diet**, restricting all **salt**. Give a **diet with water** and **fresh fruit and vegetable juice**. Eat no solid food until the fever subsides and joint pain is reduced. Then maintain a **light diet**, including **fresh fruits and vegetables, fruit juices**, etc. **Bioflavonoids** are especially valuable in preventing and treating rheumatic fever.
• Avoid **caffeine, fried foods, soft drinks, processed or refined foods, sugar, or salt**.
• **Bed rest** is very important.
• While *in bed*, **massage** and **mild exercise** is helpful. A planned exercise program should later be undertaken.
• **Catnip tea** (a nerve tonic) can be used as an enema to relax the child and reduce fever.
• Useful herbs include **bayberry bark, goldenseal, yellow dock, pau d'arco, and burdock root. Echinacea and dandelion** are also good.
• Do not give **aspirin** to a child or youth with a fever; it may result in his death! *See Reye's Syndrome (750).*

ENCOURAGEMENT—To many, as to Mary, Christ says, "Why weepest Thou? Whom seekest thou?" He is close beside us; but so often our tear-blinded eyes do not discern Him. Pray earnestly for help, and He will supply it. Psalm 147:14.

"O how great is Thy goodness, which Thou hast laid up for them that fear Thee." Psalm 31:19.

"For whosoever is born of God overcometh the world: and this is the victory that overcometh the world, even our faith." 1 John 5:4.

Trust in the Lord. His guidance is safe.

REYE'S SYNDROME

SYMPTOMS—A fever and vomiting suddenly occur. A rapid change in mental status to a deep depression, nausea, amnesia. Then pneumonia, coma, convulsions, fixed and dilated pupils, and death.

There can be confusion, drowsiness, memory lapses, lethargy, irritability, or unusual belligerence.

There may be weakness or paralysis in the limbs, speech impairment, hearing loss, double vision, etc.

CAUSES—Reye's Syndrome is a disaster worth avoiding. This disease affects many internal organs, especially the brain and liver.

It primarily strikes children between the ages of 4 and 15 (most frequently young teens) in the fall or winter months.

Not long ago, the death rate stood at 42%-80%; but, more recently, it has dropped to below 10%.

Most cases occur after a **viral infection**, such as the flu or chicken pox. Influenza B, Epstein-Barr virus, and viruses which primarily affect the gastro-intestinal tract (enteroviruses) can also occur prior to its onset.

It is known that giving **ASPIRIN** *to a child or youth who has a fever can lead to Reye's Disease and the likely possibility of death.* In the early 1980s, it was discovered that **a viral infection, plus the taking of aspirin**, dramatically increased the risk of developing Reye's Syndrome.

The cause of the disease may be consumption of aflatoxin, which is an exotoxin of the grain mold, *aspergillus flavus.*

A biopsy generally shows liver necrosis (the liver is dying). Yet, if the person survives, there will be a full recovery of the liver within 12 weeks.

If you see the above symptoms, just after your child has come out of a viral illness—do something quickly! Here are the key symptoms again:

Just after a virus infection, the child has:

(1) Agitation, disorientation, and delirium.

(2) Fatigue, lethargy, and lapses in memory.

(3) Prolonged and heavy vomiting, followed by drowsiness.

Call a physician! Phone 911 and send the child to a hospital!

NATURAL REMEDIES

DURING THE CRISIS

• It would be well for the child to be intravenously given **vitamin C** (5-10 gm per day). Intramuscularly, give him **B-complex, vitamin B$_{12}$** (1,000 mcg.), **and selenium** (250-500 mcg per day).

• If the child is in the hospital, and he receives an **IV solution** of glucose and electrolytes (mineral salts) within 12-24 hours after the heavy vomiting begins, his chances of recovery are very good.

AFTER THE CRISIS

During recovery, after the acute phase of the disease is successfully passed, give peppermint and ginger; this will relieve nausea. To strengthen and rebuild the liver, give hawthorn berry, wild yam, milk thistle, and/or pau d'arco.

PREVENTION

• Never give a child or youth **aspirin after any kind of fever**. The pattern of events is this: The child has a fever; then aspirin is given. There is improve-

ment for a day or two—then a sudden turn for the worse occurs; and coma or death follows. A Centers for Disease Control study revealed that 96% of the children contracting Reye's Syndrome had been given aspirin while they had a viral infection. It was also found that there was a direct correlation between the amount of aspirin given and the severity of the illness. Children's aspirins are banned in Britain because of this problem.

• The drug, **Tigan**, used in suppository form, to control vomiting and nausea, may also be a cause of Reye's.

• In an emergency, if you are determined to give him a drug pain reliever, give him acetaminophen (Tylenol, Datril, and others) or ibuprofen (Advil, Nuprin, and others) instead.

ENCOURAGEMENT—Often our trials are such that they seem almost unbearable. Go to Him just now; and find in Him the peace of heart you so much need. John 6:47.

JUVENILE RHEUMATOID ARTHRITIS

SYMPTOMS—Pain or tenderness on movement, limitation of motion, swelling and redness of the joint. If symptoms persist more than 6 weeks, other causes of joint pain (infection, cancer, rheumatic fever, connective tissue disorders) could not be the problem. It is only by ruling out other diseases as the cause, that physicians determine Juvenile Rheumatoid Arthritis is the disorder.

CAUSES—The juvenile form of rheumatoid arthritis (JRA) begins before the age of 16. Peak onset is between 1 to 3 years of age. It also occurs between 8 and 12; but children get this as early as 6 months of age.

Something (cause unknown) induces the immune system to begin making antibodies which attack the linings of the joints. Sometimes it starts after the child has had an infection.

There are three types of JRA: systemic, polyarticular, and pauciarticular.

Most people with *systemic JRA* will recover with little or no disability. The remaining 20% will have stunted growth. They have fever, lace-like rash, joint pain and stiffness, plus fever spikes which will reach 103°-105° F. Boys have this slightly more often; onset can be at any time during childhood.

Children with *polyarticular JRA* have symptoms in many joints (frequently the hand joints). Fever and rash are usually not present. More than five joints are usually involved; and the symptoms will last for long periods. Girls have this problem more than boys. This is the most common type of JRA. This type usually recovers the most fully.

Pauciarticular JRA is the third type; it affects few joints (*pauci* is Latin for "few"). More common in girls, symptoms generally appear before the age of 5. Some of these develop into the polyarticular form; and loss of vision can result if not treated early and properly.

NATURAL REMEDIES

• A woman who had the effects of this disease (into her 30s) was placed on a diet without **milk, butter, and cheese**—and eventually made a full recovery.

• There is a relationship between the nightshade family (**white potatoes, tomatoes, eggplant**, and tobacco) and all forms of arthritis. The physician who made that discovery (Norman Childers) also found that **milk** worsens symptoms of rheumatoid arthritis.

• **Wheat** has often been found to be a cause of rheumatoid arthritis

—*For much more information on the treatment of JRA, see Arthritis (618). Also see Autoimmune Diseases (857), Rheumatoid Arthritis (623), and Strengthening the Bones (608).*

ENCOURAGEMENT—If you are seeking to reflect the life and character of Christ, you will be true and obedient to your parents. You will show your love for them by your willing obedience.

INFANCY AND CHILDHOOD -
6 - LATER PROBLEMS
Also: Dyslexia (592) and Autism (604)

GROWING PAINS

SYMPTOMS—Pains in the joints, twitches in the legs, etc.

CAUSES—No, it is not a disease. Growing pains are a part of life in many homes, as the children grow toward adulthood.

But growing pains are not necessary. If good food and proper vitamin / mineral supplementation are provided, along with proper rest and an active exercise program, there is no need for "growing pains" to occur.

NATURAL REMEDIES

• Prevention of growing pains include a daily nutritional program that is rich in **calcium** (2,000 mg), **magnesium** (1,000 mg), **selenium** (500 mg), **vitamins A** (in the form of carotene from orange and yellow fruits and vegetables, and carrot juice), **B-complex, E** (400 IU), **and C** (1,000 mg).

ENCOURAGEMENT—Rejoice in the Lord always, and He will give you the courage you need. The more you praise Him, the more you will have to praise Him for. Psalm 138:8.

GROWTH PROBLEMS

SYMPTOMS—The child fails to grow properly in height.

CAUSES—The key to growth is the pituitary, the master gland, which is located in the center of the skull. When it does not function properly, normal growth does not occur.

The pituitary gland produces the growth hormone, *somatotropin*, and sends it throughout the body, to stimulate normal enlargement of bones and muscles in children.

Too little production of this hormone will produce dwarfism; too much results in abnormally enlarged hands, feet, jaw, and possible gigantism.

The **pituitary** may not be functioning properly because of a tumor growing in, or near, it. But the **thymus** gland may not be working properly; and that will affect a child's growth and increase the likelihood of infection.

Malabsorption disorders, such as **celiac disease** *(473-474)*, can also reduce growth somewhat.

Excess amounts of **lead** *(873)*, a toxic metal, can produce growth problems.

NATURAL REMEDIES

• Be sure to provide a well-balanced, **nourishing diet**. Omit **junk foods**.

• Adequate amounts of **protein** are important, especially the amino acid, **arginine**. Arginine is used to synthesize *ornithine*, an amino acid which prompts the pituitary to release its growth hormone. Sources of arginine include **coconut, oats, soybeans, walnuts, wheat, wheat germ, carob, and dairy products**. If a child's protein intake is reduced severely, he develops Kwashiorkor *(480)*, a protein-deficiency disease. This condition can occur in any nation, not just India.

Growth hormone therapy can be prescribed by a physician; but it is very expensive.

ENCOURAGEMENT—"The eye of the Lord is upon them that fear Him, upon them that hope in His mercy." Psalm 33:18. He gives His faithful children the help they need. So turn to His Word today! Isaiah 65:24.

VACCINATION PROBLEMS

SYMPTOMS—Physical problems resulting from a vaccination (including fevers, permanent brain damage, paralysis, autism, and/or death).

DISCUSSION—This is a wide-ranging subject, too large for discussion in detail here. See the author's book, *The Vaccination Crisis*, for detailed discussions of the various vaccines, their dangers, and how to avoid vaccination requirements. It is available from the publisher of this *Encyclopedia* (Harvestime Books).

The underlying problem is simple enough: Each person normally take substances into his body through his stomach, where harmful bacteria are generally destroyed.

But a vaccine is injected directly into a muscle or directly into the bloodstream, thus bypassing the normal protections. This is highly dangerous!

The problem is that it is impossible to purify the vaccines properly. To do so would require too much time and expense to try to examine every microscopic portion (identify every toxin, poison, and microbe) and eliminate the bad ones. It simply cannot be done.

So monkey pus, horse urine, raw animal hormones, and other substances are "purified" somewhat; then they are injected into your child.

In addition, the vaccines are frequently given to very small children who are especially susceptible to nerve damage.

The solution is to live right, eat right, and avoid vaccinations. See the author's book, *The Vaccination Crisis*, for further information on vaccinations.

—*See Vaccination Poisoning (876) for a list of a few of the harmful effects of various childhood vaccines.*

ENCOURAGEMENT—God can provide solutions, when earthly trials seem hard to bear. Go to Him and find in Him the courage and help you so much need. Psalm 89:15-16.

By learning the lessons of obedience, children are not only honoring their parents and lightening their burdens, but they are pleasing One higher in authority. "Honour thy father and thy mother" is a positive command. Children who treat their parents with disrespect, and disregard their wishes, not only dishonor them, but break the law of God. And none can hope for the love and blessing of God when they do not learn obedience to His commandments and stand up firmly against temptation.

"And Adam knew Eve his wife and she conceived, and bare Cain, and said, I have gotten a man from the Lord."   —Genesis 4:1

"Blessed are all they that wait for Him."   —Isaiah 30:18

"I have blessed him, and will make him fruitful, and will multiply him exceedingly."   —Genesis 17:20

"And she conceived again and bare a son, and she said, Now will I praise the Lord."   —Genesis 29:35

"The Lord gave her conception, and she bare a son."   —Ruth 4:13

"A father of the fatherless, and a judge of the widows, is God in His holy habitation."   —Psalm 68:5

"The Lord . . relieveth the fatherless and widow."   —Psalm 146:9

"Leave thy fatherless children; I will preserve them alive, and let thy widows trust in Me."   —Jeremiah 49:11

"In thee the fatherless findeth mercy."   —Hosea 14:3

"I will be a swift witness against . . those that oppress . . the widow, and the fatherless."   —Malachi 3:5

"Lo, children are an heritage of the Lord, and the fruit of the womb is His reward. As arrows are in the hand of a mighty man; so are children of the youth. Happy is the man that hath his quiver full of them: they shall not be ashamed, but they shall speak with the enemies in the gate."   —Psalm 127:3-5

"Children's children are the crown of old men; and the glory of children are their fathers."   —Proverbs 17:6

"Honor thy father and thy mother, that thy days may be long upon the land which the Lord thy God giveth thee."   —Exodus 20:12 [The Fifth Commandment]

SPECIAL SECTIONS FOR WOMEN - 4

The **Natural Remedies Encyclopedia**

- Disease Section 17 -
Basic Women's Herbs

— Also see Herbs during Pregnancy (754-757, 760-763), Herbs at Childbirth (757-758, 763-764), Herbs for Nursing Mothers (720, 726), Herbs for Infant Care (758, 764)

W
H
E
R
B

HOW TO USE HERBS

On pp. 107-152 of this *Natural Remedies Encyclopedia*, you will find a wealth of information on purchasing, gathering, storing, preparing, and using the 126 most important herbs in your own home.

In this present section, you will find an invaluable collection of information on herbs of particular importance to women. An attempt has been made to make it as complete as possible.

SOME SPECIAL HERBS

Ashwagandha (Winter cherry; *Withania omnifera)*

Root. In India, it is valued as a rejuvenative herb as highly as ginseng is in Chinese medicine. Among other properties, it helps weak, pregnant women and is said to stabilize the embryo. It acts as a tonic to the hormonal system and is recommended for sexual debility, infertility (in men and women), and promotes conception.

Bayberry *(Myrica cerifera)*

Root. Douche made with tea. / Prolapse of the uterus, excessive menstrual bleeding, vaginal infections, and leukorrhea.

Beth Root *(Trillium pendulum)*

Root. Tincture (1-2 tsp. 3 times daily) or fluid extract (½ tsp. 3 times daily). / Excessive uterine bleeding (menorrhagia and metrorrhagia). Controls excessive menstruation and vaginal discharges.

Black Cohosh *(Cimicifuga racemosa)*

FOR MORE NATURAL REMEDIES:

HERBS: Herb Contents (pp. 129-130) will help you locate the 126 most important herbs and the diseases each one can treat. How to prepare herbs (132). How to use them (141-189)

HYDROTHERAPY: Therapy Contents (pp. 206-207) and its Disease Index (263-265) will lead you to over 100 water therapies and many more remedies. DIS. INDEX: 1211- / GEN. INDEX: 1221-

VITAMINS AND MINERALS: Contents (100-101). Using 101-124. Dosages (124). Others (117-)

CARING FOR THE SICK: Home care for a sick person (28-36). The healing crisis (36-39)

WOMEN'S SECTIONS: Female Organs (672) Pregnancy (701). Childbirth (765). Infancy, Childhood (722). Women's Herbs (754, 760)

EMERGENCIES: (973-989). FIRST AID: (990-1009)

Rhizome. Tincture (½-1 tsp. 3 times daily) or fluid extract (5-30 drops 3 times daily). / American Indian women used it for all female complaints, pelvic conditions, uterine problems, cramps, and to relieve pain in childbirth and menstrual cycles. Helps induce menstrual flow that has been retarded by exposure to cold. *Warning:* An overdose will produce nausea and vomiting.

Black Haw *(Viburnum prunifolium)*

Bark of the root. Tincture (½-1 tsp. 3 times daily) or fluid extract (½-2 tsp. 3 times daily). / Afterbirth pains, cramps, dysmenorrhea, irregular menstrual flow, leukorrhea, uterine inflammation, congestion, scanty menstrual flow, and the threatening of miscarriage. It is a tonic and sedative to the female reproductive organs. Gives a good tonic effect during pregnancy.

Blue Cohosh *(Caulophyllum thalictroides)*

Rhizome. Tincture (½-1 tsp. 3 times daily) or fluid extract (10-30 drops 3-4 times daily). / American Indians used it to ease childbirth and relieve associated pains. Regulates menstrual flow, useful for suppressed menstruation. Warning: Pregnant women should not use except during last month of pregnancy.

Chamomile *(Matricaria chamomilla)*

Flowers. Tincture (30-60 drops [½-1 tsp.] 3 times daily) or fluid extract (½-1 tsp. 3 times daily). / Menstrual cramps (6 oz. infusion or 1-2 tsp. infusion at a time).

Chaste tree *(Vitex agnus-castus)*

Seeds. This Mediterranean shrub stimulates and balances the pituitary in relation to female hormones, by its effect on the follicle stimulating hormone (FSH) and luteinizing hormone (LH), produced by the anterior pituitary gland. It helps the work of producing hormones in the second half of the menstrual cycle. It appears to have a more progesteronic than estrogenic action, and makes a fine remedy for PMS and a range of menstrual and gynecologic problems that are related to hormone imbalance. It can be used effectively for irregular and painful periods, heavy bleeding, fibroids, and to re-establish hormone balance after stopping use of the contraceptive pill. It is a good remedy for menopausal problems and stimulates milk production in nursing mothers. Because it has a calming and relaxing effect, it can be used for any emotional distress associated with the reproductive system, such as PMS and menopausal depression.

Cramp bark *(Viburnum opulus)*

Bark. Tincture (½-1 tsp. 3-4 times daily) or fluid extract (½-2 tsp. 3-4 times daily). / Menstrual cramps, dysmenorrhea, menorrhagia nervous conditions during pregnancy, prevents miscarriage.

Dong qui (Dang gui; *Angelica sinensis)*

Root. This is the best Chinese herb for women, and is the most highly valued blood tonic in the East. It tones the reproductive system and maintains normal function of the sex organs. It regulates hormones, menstruation, brings on delayed or suppressed periods, relieves menstrual cramps, and can be used during menopause. Eaten raw or taken as a tincture, it relaxes the uterus; used with water, it tones the uterus, stimulates uterine contractions, increases circulation, and relieves congestion in the pelvic area. As a tonic, it is used in convalescence and to speed recovery and increase energy after childbirth. When cooked, it improves the circulation and helps speed tissue repair. Warning: Do not take during pregnancy.

False Unicorn *(Chamaeilirium luteum; Helonias)*

Root. Tincture (15-30 drops 3 times daily) or fluid extract (½-1 tsp. 3 times daily). / Amenorrhea female hormone imbalances, infertility, irregular menstruation, leukorrhea, menorrhagia, miscarriage, prolapse uterus, threatened abortion, uterine and ovarian problems, uterine displacement. False unicorn is a common herb for female infertility, impotence, and other problems. It can be taken for several months. Generally combined with cramp bark or black haw, but can be taken alone. During especially difficult situations, 15 drops of tincture or ½ tsp. of fluid extract can be taken each hour. Do not confuse with True Unicorn herb.

Motherwort *(Leonurus cardiaca)*

Tops. Tincture (30-60 drops [½-1 tsp.] 3-4 times daily) or fluid extract (½-1 tsp. 3-4 times daily). / Amenorrhea, suppressed menstruation, cramps, dysmenorrhea, uterine pains. For female cramping and suppressed menstrual flow, combine motherwort with cramp bark and squaw vine. To relieve cramps and pain during menstruation, use a hot fomentation made from strong tea.

Mugwort *(Artemisia vulgaris)*

Tops. Tincture (30-60 drops [½-1 tsp.] as needed) or fluid extract (1 tsp. as needed). / Menstrual cramps, menstrual obstruction, suppressed menstruation. Best combined with cramp bark, marigold, and black haw.

American Pennyroyal *(Mentha Pulegium)*

Tops. Tincture (30-60 drops or ½-1 tsp. frequently) or fluid extract (1 tsp. frequently). / Delayed or scanty menstruation, cramps, regulates menstrual flow. To induce menstrual flow, use hot footbaths of pennyroyal tea.

Pulsatilla (Pasque flower; *Anemone pulsatilla)*

Dried aerial parts (everything above ground). Best used in small doses: 1-2 ml of tincture or half a tsp. of herb to a cup of boiling water as tea, 3 times daily when necessary. / Helps debilitated women and children who feel depressed, irritable, and weep

W
H
E
R
B

easily. It promotes sleep and rest and thereby helps recuperation. It is particularly helpful for spasm, pain, and inflammation of the reproductive system. It relieves premenstrual tension, period pains, scanty or suppressed periods, uterine colic, and inflammation and pain in the ovaries. Its analgesic (pain-relieving) properties are useful during childbirth. Its properties promote and facilitate birth. It is good for sluggish, ineffectual and weak labor pains, and for peevishness and irritability in labor. After the birth, it is helpful for overexcitement, depression, and anxiety about the birth of the new baby. Warning: Never use this plant fresh, for it will be poisonous. Do not store it for more than a year.

Saw Palmetto (Serenoa serrulata)

Fruit. Tincture (15-60 drops 2-3 times daily) or fluid extract (10 drops 2-3 times daily). / Ovarian enlargement, dysmenorrhea, sterility. Very useful in the treatment of disease in the reproductive organs. Helps speed recovery afterward. It also increases milk flow in nursing mothers. It helps relieve painful periods, regulate the menstrual cycle, and for inflammatory conditions such as salpingitis and ovarian pain.

Shatavari (Tian men dong; Asparagus racemosus)

Root. This is one of the most important herbs for women in India. Its main action is on the female reproductive system. Use it for sexual debility, infertility, and to balance hormones. It increases milk production in nursing mothers and is excellent during menopause, as it supplies many steroidal precursors (building blocks for production of sex hormones). It nourishes and strengthens the reproductive system. It is so valued in India that its name (shatavari) means "who possesses a hundred husbands."

Squaw Vine (Mitchella repens)

Whole plant. Tincture (15-60 drops 3-4 times daily) or fluid extract (½-1 tsp. 3-4 times daily). / Leukorrhea, painful menstruation, uterine and ovarian pains, cramping and pains before and during labor in childbirth. American Indian women used squaw vine as a tea or infusion throughout pregnancy in order to produce a safe, easy delivery and help proper lactation. Relieves congestion of the uterus and ovaries. Very good for painful or absent menstruation. Good combined with raspberry leaf during pregnancy. Crush the berries and add to a tincture of myrrh, allow to steep for three days and strain; then use as a fomentation for sore nipples. Combined with witch hazel, it makes a very good injection for leukorrhea.

Tormentil Root (Potentilla tormentilla)

Root. Tincture (15-30 drops 3 times daily, 5-10 drops in water every hour) or fluid extract (½-1 tsp. 3 times daily). / Prolapsed uterus, leukorrhea,

White Oak Bark (Quercus alba)

Bark. Tincture (15-30 drops as needed) or fluid extract (½-1 tsp. as needed). / This is one of the best astringent herbs known. Outstanding for stopping bleeding. Also good for vaginal infections, leukorrhea, prolapsed uterus.

Witch hasel (Hamamelis virginiana)

Bark. Tincture (15-60 drops as needed) or fluid extract (½ tsp. as needed). / Leukorrhea, prolapsed uterus, stops uterine bleeding. A powerful astringent. Excellent for stopping excessive menstruation, hemorrhage from the uterus. Use as a retention douche in leukorrhea; as a fomentation or salve for sore breasts; as an injection for vaginal discharges and infections.

Wild Yam (Dioscorea villosa)

Root. Tincture (10-40 drops 3-4 times daily) or fluid extract (1 tsp. 3-4 times daily); 5 to 10 #0 capsules (30-60 grains) 3-4 times daily. / Cramps, morning sickness, nausea, neuralgic dysmenorrhea, ovarian neuralgia. Wild yam contains a steroid-like substance, and is used in many gland-balancing formulas. An excellent antispasmodic, it is used for abdominal cramps and menstrual cramps. To prevent miscarriage, combine 1 tsp. wild yam with ½ tsp. powdered ginger. Also helpful: Add 1 tsp. red raspberry to that formula, strain, and take a mouthful every half hour in times of danger of miscarriage. For afterbirth pains, use 10 drops of tincture in cold water. Do not use hot; for it may overly relax uterus and cause hemorrhage.

The wild yam is so unusual that it deserves special attention. It is a perennial twining vine. The heart-shaped leaves have conspicuous, deep-set veins and are hairy beneath. The leaves are arranged in an alternating pattern, with the lower ones in whorls of 3 to 8. The flowers are green and not showy. It grows from May to August in wet woods from Connecticut to Tennessee, and from Minnesota to Texas.

American Indians used tea made from this root, to relieve labor pains. Fresh dried root, made into a tea, is good for morning sickness.

Wild yam contains diosgenin, a chemical used by scientists to manufacture progesterone and other steroid drugs. Wild yam does NOT contain progesterone; yet it has a beneficial progesterone-like effect on the human body.

A majority of the steroid harmones used in modern drug medication, especially those in contraceptives, have been developed from elaborately processed chemical components which are derived from yams.

Drugs made with yam-derived components (diosgenins) are used to relieve asthma, arthritis, and eczema. They also regulate metabolism and control fertility. Synthetic products manufactured from diosgenins include human sex hormones (contraceptives), drugs to treat menopause, dysmenorrhea, premenstrual syndrome, testicular deficiency, impotency, prostate hypertrophy, and psychosexual problems, as well as high blood pressure, arterial spasms, migraines, and other ailments. Cortisones and hydrocortisones are other products from the wild yam. They are used for

Addison's disease, some allergies, bursitis, contact dermatitis, psoriasis, rheumatoid arthritis, sciatica, brown recluse spider bites, insect stings, and a number of other diseases. But ignore claims that wild yam is a plant "source" of estrogen or progesterone, for it does not contain human sex hormones.

With all this in mind, women would do well to make use of the wild yam herb. But do not use the fresh plant, for it may induce vomiting and other undesirable effects. Only use the dried root.

HERBS DURING PREGNANCY

For much more information on Pregnancy, turn to Section 18 - **Pregnancy and Breast-Feeding** *(701-721).*

Just below, you will find additional helpful information on pregnancy.

Anemia—Pregnant women need extra iron. *Yellow dock* herb is said to contain nearly 50% iron. *Blackstrap molasses* is the richest source of iron you can purchase.

Constipation—Bulk laxatives, such as *psyllium seed*, can be used for a long time. One lower bowel formula is *cascara sagrada bark, bayberry root bark, goldenseal root, red raspberry leaves, fennel seed*. Use one or several together, but do not take them too long. Avoid a laxative habit. Do not use mineral oil!

False labor—Drink *catnip tea* in small amounts. *Blue cohosh* is another very helpful herb in relaxing the uterus.

Gas—*Papaya tablets* and small amounts of *ginger*.

Heartburn—*Papaya tablets, comfrey,* and *pepsin* are useful.

Insomnia—Additional *calcium* in the diet. Drink teas of equal parts of *hops* and *chamomile* before retiring. Another formula is equal parts of the following and make an infusion. Drink one cup before bed or when needed: *wood betony, chamomile, valerian, peppermint, catnip*.

Morning sickness—*Red raspberry* tea is excellent. *Catnip* tea is another good one. A little *ginger* is useful.

Miscarriage—*Red raspberry* tea is very helpful in avoiding miscarriage. This is a good formula: *Wild yam, false unicorn, squaw vine, cramp bark*. Also helpful: A tiny amount of *lobelia* will help relax the uterus. *Catnip* and *bayberry* also help prevent miscarriage.

Toxemia—*Raspberry, alfalfa,* and *comfrey tea* provides a nourishing, cleansing effect.

Last three months before delivery—Here is an excellent pelvic tonic; use equal parts: partridge berry, cramp bark, blue cohosh, false unicorn root.

Last six or seven weeks before delivery—Here are three formulas, each of which will help the delivery and make labor easier: (1) *Squaw vine, black cohosh,* *false unicorn, blessed thistle, pennyroyal, red raspberry, lobelia* (very small amount). (2) *Squaw vine, black cohosh, pennyroyal, red raspberry, lobelia* (very small amount). (3) Mix equal parts: raspberry leaves, blue cohosh, false unicorn root, motherwort. These formulas will help keep the pelvic muscles elastic and relaxed.

Braxton-Hicks contractions—If this powerful tightening of the uterus and hardening of the abdomen occurs, take herbs relaxing to the uterine area, such as *cramp bark* and *wild yam*.

As pregnancy begins, be sure and carefully read the section in this Encyclopedia dealing with this subject (pp. 706-716). In order to avoid birth defects, at the very beginning of pregnancy, indeed before it occurs, it is extremely important that you are on an excellent diet of vitamins and minerals. Do not eat junk food, liquor, tobacco, or drugs.

HERBS AT CHILDBIRTH

For more information on childbirth, turn to Section 18 - **Pregnancy and Breast-Feeding** *(701-765).*

Blue cohosh— helps relax the uterine muscles, soothe the nerves, and relieve restlessness or irritability. *Black cohosh* promotes relaxation and helps regulate contractions, making them less painful and yet more productive. It helps calm pain and relax you if you get tense, overexcited, or panicky. *Raspberry leaves* relax the uterus, calm and strengthen the nerves, normalize contractions, and reduce pain. *Wild yam* is specific for those who are tense and nervous. *Cramp bark* is a general relaxant and also reduces uterine tension. *Skullcap* is an excellent relaxant; a tonic to the nervous system, it is best combined with *blue cohosh*.

Weak, irregular contractions—Any of the following herbs would be helpful: *blue cohosh, black cohosh, beth root, feverfew, raspberry leaves, wormwood, sage, calendula, goldenseal*.

Overstrong, painful contractions—Any of the following herbs: *blue cohosh, black cohosh, wild yam, cramp bark, raspberry leaves*.

Aids relaxation and relieves pain—*Skullcap, motherwort, partridge berry, lavender, chamomile, linden blossom*.

Relaxes a rigid cervix and prevents tearing—*Partridge berry, blue cohosh, motherwort, black cohosh, skullcap, passionflower.* After the birth: *lavender, ginger, raspberry leaves, false unicorn root*.

Expel afterbirth—In order to help the uterus continue to contract, so the afterbirth will be expelled: a tea of *raspberry leaves* and *beth root*. Another formula is **black haw, beth root, partridge berry, black cohosh,** and **raspberry leaves**. (Breast-feeding is a natural trigger to postpartum contractions, to expel the afterbirth.)

Heal perineum—Tinctures of **calendula, arnica, distilled witch hazel**.

Tonic after delivery—To help restore energy after the birth: A tea of **dong quai (dang gui)** has been used for centuries in China, and tastes good. Drink a tea of false unicorn three times a day.

Pain after delivery—Here are sedative and anodyne (pain-relieving) herbs; drink a tea from one or several throughout the day: **black cohosh, pulsatilla, lavender, wild yam**.

Postpartum hemorrhage—Use any of the following: **goldenseal, false unicorn root, black haw, beth root, wild yam**. In China, **Huang qi** and **dong quai (dang gui)** are used for postpartum hemorrhage or any after weakness. They also promote healing of the pelvic tissues.

Postpartum uterine infections—Drink **echinacea** tea every 2 hours. Other astringent and antiseptic herbs are **goldenseal** and **cramp bark**.

Postnatal depression—Drink teas of one or more of the following, to help your nervous system and lift depression: **rosemary, lemon balm, vervain, borage, skullcap, pulsatilla**.

HERBS FOR NURSING MOTHERS

For more information on childbirth, turn to Section 18 - **Pregnancy and Breast-Feeding** *(701-765)*.

Nursing—**Brewer's yeast** taken daily with increased milk is extremely helpful in producing enough mother's milk. **Red raspberry** and **marshmallow** are also good. **Alfalfa** provides extra nourishment. **Fennel seed** boiled in **barley water** increases mother's milk. **Blessed thistle** also increases mother's milk.

Cracked nipples—Apply a quality **vegetable oil** (almond, wheat germ, flaxseed). Thin **honey** can also be applied.

Drying up milk—**Sage** and **parsley** will dry up mother's milk.

HERBS FOR INFANT CARE

For more information on infant care, turn to Section 19 - **Infancy and Childhood** *(722)*.

Colic—**Catnip tea** is an old standby. It is outstanding. **Fennel** and **peppermint** tea are also good for babies. A tiny amount of **lobelia** is very relaxing.

Constipation—Something gentle is needed. A small amount of **mullein** added to warm water or weak **licorice** tea.

Cradle cap—Rub **vitamin E** or a quality **vegetable oil** onto the scalp.

Diaper rash—Make a paste of ground **comfrey**,

goldenseal, and **aloe vera juice**. **Vitamins E and A** are helpful.

Diarrhea—Every few hours, give one of the following: **barley water, carob flour** in clean water, carob in boiled milk. Useful herb teas include: **slippery elm, red raspberry, ginger, yarrow, oak bark tea, strawberry**.

Dry skin—A quality **vegetable oil, vitamins A** and **E, aloe vera**.

Ear infection—Place **garlic oil**, echinacea, or plantain tea in the ear. To relieve pain, bake a large **onion** until soft, cut into halves and apply over the ear and wrap it tightly.

Fever—**Catnip** tea or **red raspberry** tea. Enemas help bring the fever down; also sponging with slightly cool water bring fevers down.

Pinworms—**Chamomile** and **mint** tea. Small piece of **garlic** placed in child's rectum helps discard worms. **Raisins** soaked in **senna tea** for older children.

Teething—More **calcium** and **vitamin D** (but not too much) is needed by restless, crying babies who are teething. A weak, warm tea of **catnip**, **chamomile, peppermint,** or **fennel**. If the infant chews on **licorice root**, it will dull any irritation and pain.

Sore gums—Mix thick **honey** and a tiny pinch of **salt**, rub it on the gums. Also helpful to rub on gums: **honey** with **chamomile oil** or **peppermint oil**.

Cannot urinate—Crush **watermelon seeds** and make into a tea; frequently give small amounts.

CAUTIONS REGARDING HERBS
This is not a complete listing.

Aloe Vera *(Aloe vera, var, officinalis)*
Warning: It is an emmenagogue and should not be used during pregnancy.

Angelica *(Angelica archangelica)*
Warning: it is a strong emmenagogue and should not be used during pregnancy. Diabetics should avoid it, because it can induce weakness.

Black Cohosh *(Cimicifuga racemosa)*
An overdose will produce nausea and vomiting.

Blessed Thistle *(Cerbenia benedicta)*
Warning: Do not take alone or in large amounts during pregnancy.

Buckthorn *(Rhamnus frangula)*
Warning: It should not be used during pregnancy.

Wild Celery *(Apium graveolens)*
Use only in moderate amounts during pregnancy.

Ephedra *(Ephedra vulgaris)*
It should not be used by those with high blood pressure or who are weak or debilitated.

Goldenseal *(Hydrastis canadensis)*
Do not use large amounts during pregnancy. Used over prolonged periods of time, it will reduce B vitamin absorption and destroy intestinal bacteria. Two to three #00 capsules daily is usually adequate for most conditions.

Juniper *(Juniperis communis)*

Juniper should not be used alone, in large doses, or with prolonged use during urinary tract or inflammatory problems.

Licorice *(Glycyrrhiza glabra)*

Large does are to be avoided by those with high blood pressure or hyper-adrenal function. When it is taken daily over an extended period of time, the dosage should not exceed three grams per day. It contains a substance similar to adrenal cortical hormones that may cause edema.

Mandrake *(Polophyllum peltatum)*

Do not use during pregnancy or in large doses. Only moderate doses of this herb should be used. In large doses, it produces nausea, vomiting, and even inflammation of the intestines and membranes of the stomach. Discontinue its use if any uncomfortable symptoms are noticed.

American Mistletoe *(Viscum flavescens)*

It is known to be toxic and should be used with caution.

European Mistletoe *(Viscum album)*

Do not eat the berries! They are poisonous.

Myrrh *(Commiphora nayrrha)*

Do not take myrrh gum in large amounts or over a long period of time.

Parsley *(Petroselinum sp.)*

It should not be used if kidney inflammation exists.

Peach *(Amygdalus persica)*

The bark and leaves are used as herb medications. Avoid large doses of either for pregnant women, as they can cause a purging of the bowels.

American Pennyroyal *(Mentha pulegium)*

Do not use when there is excessive menstrual flow. Do not use during pregnancy; for the tea has been used to induce abortions.

Poke *(Phytolacca americana)*

Poke contains toxic substances; it should not be used in excess of one gram a day. Toxic effects have been noticed while using it either internally and externally.

Rhubarb *(Rheum palmatum)*

Do not use it over prolonged periods; it tends to aggravate any tendency toward chronic constipation. Do not use it during pregnancy.

Rosemary *(Rosmarinus offinalis)*

Do not drink rosemary tea in excessive amounts. Three cups daily appears to be the limit in most cases.

Sassafras *(Sassafras officinale)*

The oil is toxic and should not be taken internally. Those who are anemic or have thin blood should not use this herb.

Senna *(Cassia acutifolia)*

It should not be used when there is inflammation anywhere in the intestinal tract, piles, prolapsed intestines, or rectum. It should not be used during pregnancy.

Uva Ursi *(Arctostaphylos uva ursi)*

It should not be used in large quantities during pregnancy, because it is a vasoconstrictor to the uterus (reducing blood circulation to it).

WOMAN'S HERBAL TONIC

Dr. Daniel B. Mowrey, in his book, *The Scientific Validation of Herbal Medicine,* presents an outstanding herbal tonic for women. Here it is:

Mix equal amounts of the following powdered herbs, and place them in capsules:

Black Cohosh Root, Licorice Root, Raspberry Leaves, Passion Flower, Fenugreek, Black Haw Bark, Saw Palmetoo Berries, Squaw Vine, Wild Yam Root, and Kelp.

Dr. Mowrey recommends using the mixture, when needed, as teas to drink, in capsules to swallow, and in douches.

Use this tonic during pregnancy, delivery, menstruation, and menopause. Also use it for pain, cramping, and atony that is related to pregnancy and childbirth.

For any of the above-named problems, you will also want to take additional herbs, which are especially suited for alleviating pain, reducing bleeding, and calming the nerves.

For more information, see:

Section 14 - **Reproductive Disorders** *(672-700)*
Section 15 - **Pregnancy and Breast-Feeding** *(701-721)*.

W
H
E
R
B

"Cast thy burden upon the Lord, and He shall sustain thee: He shall not suffer the righteous to be moved." —Psalm 55:22

"Thou art my God, and I will praise Thee: Thou art my God, I will exalt Thee." —Psalm 118:28

What is the difference between a medicinal drug and an herb? Herbs contain a variety of chemical compounds placed there by God "for the healing of the nations" *(Revelation 22:2; also Ezekiel 47:12)*. Over the centuries, many have been found to be extremely useful for physical problems. Medicinal drugs are different. In order to patent them (for exclusive sales and profits), medicinal drugs cannot have the exact formulas found in herbs. Instead, they contain various man-made combinations of chemicals. Because of this, to one extent or another, they are always poisonous. Their *"contraindications"* verify the fact. The liver, kidneys, and other organs frequently suffer from them.

SPECIAL SECTIONS FOR WOMEN - 5

The **Natural Remedies Encyclopedia**

- Disease Section 18 -
Herbs for Pregnancy

PREG HERB

WHICH HERBS TO AVOID DURING PREGNANCY

During pregnancy, the following herbs must not be used. *For a much longer list, see the section on Women's Herbs (754-759).*

As a rule, use great caution when taking any herbs during the pregnancy, especially in the first 12 weeks.

• **Oxytocic plants.** Because they have a chemical similar to oxytocin (a hormone which contracts the uterus), these herbs produce contractions in the uterus. Do not take them during pregnancy! **aloe vera, birchwort, rue, Scotch broom, shepherd's purse**. But they can be taken at the time of delivery, to lessen labor.

• **Emmenagogue plants**. These herbs produce or ease menstruation. As a rule, they have a balancing and normalizing effect on the menstrual cycle. But do not use them during pregnancy, because they increase the risk of abortion: **aloe vera, basil, birchwort, buck bean, butterbur, calendula, clary sage, European pennyroyal, German chamomile, groundsil, heliotrope, jalop, juniper, laurel, lavender cotton, madder, milfoil, motherwort, mugwort, parsley, Roman chamomile, rowan, rue, saffron, sage, tansy, tarragon, Venus' hair, wood betony, wormwood, wild balm**.

• Other herbs to avoid during pregnancy: **arnica, barberry, black cohosh, bloodroot, cat's claw, celandine, cottonwood bark, dong quai, ephedra, feverfew, ginseng, goldenseal, lobelia, myrrh, Oregon grape, pennyroyal, saw palmetto, turmeric**.

THE SINGLE BEST PREGNANCY HERB

RED RASPBERRY

Either wild *(Rubus strigosus)* or cultivated *(Rubus*

idaeus) can be used.

Red raspberry helps from before pregnancy begins to after it ends. This is the most all-round good herb for the needs of pregnancy, from start to finish. It is the most widely used and safest of all pregnancy and uterine tonics. It is high in vitamins A, C, D, E, and B complex. It increases fertility, eases morning sickness, assists labor and reduces pain, promotes easier childbirth, relaxes smooth muscles and reduces tears, improves milk production.

It can be used as a tea or taken as capsules. Safe and effective, it strengthens the uterus for easier delivery; and there is less bleeding. It is also high in natural iron and helps reduce after pains. It tends to shorten labor. Drink the tea as often as you wish.

Caution: It is claimed by some that *Rubus idaeus* (the cultivated form) should not be used and may lead to miscarriages. But most women use it with no problem. You may want to avoid it if you have had a previous miscarriage.

DURING PREGNANCY
MORNING SICKNESS

GINGER
Relieves morning sickness (nausea). Ginger helps relieve nausea, reduces vomiting, and calms the stomach.

Sip 1 Tbsp. of the tea (but not more than that) whenever nausea occurs. Or take 6 capsules of the powdered herb daily. It combines well with wild yam, which also reduces morning sickness.

Caution: Do NOT take during the last trimester (last 3 months). This is because ginger increases circulation to the uterus, and could increase risk of post-partum (after delivery) infection.

PEPPERMINT TEA
Relieves morning sickness, prevents vomiting.

Peppermint is an old standby for relieving nausea and upset stomach, and preventing vomiting.

Sip the tea whenever needed.

Other dietetic aids to reduce morning sickness: catnip or spearmint tea, digestive enzymes, green drink, alfalfa. Take plenty of B_6, and B complex. Take 2 ginger capsules before each meal.

Avoid irritating food, hot spicy foods, condiments. Baking soda, fatty, fried, oily foods, caffeine, sugar. Do not lie down right after eating.

Maintain regularity in sleep, eating, and outdoor exercise.

DANDELION
Put 4-6 Tbsp. dried dandelion root in 1 quart boiling water and steep for 4 hours. Strain, cool, drink slowly throughout the day (up to 2 cups). Or

take 30 drops of undiluted tincture 3-4 times a day until nausea is gone. It calms and strengthens the stomach, and improves appetite.

ANEMIA

YELLOW DOCK
Yellow dock is almost 50% iron. Pregnant women need extra iron; yet iron tablets can be extremely dangerous! It can cause miscarriage. Obtain iron from natural sources only! Blackstrap molasses is the richest natural source of iron. Red beets are helpful. Vitamin C (500 mg) helps absorption of iron in the diet. Vitamin E (600 IU) strengthens blood cells.

INCREASE CALCIUM ABSORPTION

KALE
Calcium builds strong bones in both mother and child. It also calms the nerves and reduces pain.

The deep green leafy vegetables are excellent sources of calcium and most vitamins and minerals.

INDIGESTION OR HEARTBURN

MEADOWSWEET
Take 15-45 drops of tincture diluted in a bit of water 1-4 times a day. Find the amount which works best for you. Or put a heaping tablespoon in a cup, pour 1 cup boiling water over it, steep for 20 minutes, strain, cool, and drink 3-4 cups daily. Sip this slowly. It is a good digestive aid.

CONSTIPATION

SLIPPERY ELM BARK
This invaluable herb reduces constipation, soothes the digestive system and irritated bowels, and is an antacid. It is a safe herb to take during pregnancy for constipation.

Take 1 teaspoon of the powder with hot water and honey. Or swallow 6 capsules daily, as needed.

Eat raw vegetables and fruits daily. Also helpful is brewer's yeast and psyllium seed. If bran is taken, it should be accompanied by a large glass of water—or the bran will cause further constipation.

SWELLING

PEPPERMINT
Drink peppermint or spearmint tea with the juice of a fresh lemon.

EDEMA

CORN SILK
Make a tea of this outstanding diuretic herb and drink it as needed.

VARICOSE VEINS

WITCH HAZEL
Varicose veins are caused by increased pressure

P
R
E
G

H
E
R
B

in the abdomen, and will normally disappear after the baby is delivered.

Witch hazel (or white oak bark) tea, applied externally, will help tighten the tissue and reduce varicose veins. Saturate a cloth in the tea and wipe it on varicosities, which may be in the legs, vulva, and/or near the rectum. Also drink a quart of nettle leaf tea each day.

Other helps include eating lots of green leafy vegetables, garlic, and onions. Keep the bowels moving regularly. Avoid crossing your legs. If necessary, wear elastic stockings. In some cases, taking 1 tablet of stone root, 3 times daily, helps. Discontinue if there is no improvement within 2 weeks.

BILBERRY

This is the European blueberry. It contains flavonoid compounds, known as *anthocyanosides*, which greatly improves circulation in the smaller blood vessels. Research studies (using an extract standardized for 25% *anthocyanidin* content at dosage of 160-480 mg daily) show that they prevent and treat varicose veins during pregnancy.

HORSE CHESTNUT

In addition to daily exercise, take 5-15 drops of tincture diluted in ¼ cup water 2-3 times a day. Do this during the first trimester, to reduce varicose veins.

BLADDER INFECTION

UVA URSI

Take uva ursi tablets for 1 week at the most (if taken longer, uterine contractions could be stimulated). Drink cranberry juice. Avoid sweets, coffee, black tea, cola drinks, and panties not made of cotton. Echinacea, taken for no more than a week at a time, may also help reduce infection.

HYPERTENSION

HAWTHORN BERRY

This herb reduces hypertension during pregnancy by dilating the blood vessels and strengthening the heart. Take 8 drops of the tincture, 2 or 3 times daily. Do not take hawthorn berries if you have low blood pressure.

TOXEMIA

HERB MIX

Alfafa tea (mixed with red raspberry and comfrey) is cleansing and nourishing. Both to avoid and eliminate toxemia during pregnancy, you need fresh vegetables. Kelp, dandelion, and alfalfa is another good combination. Avoid meat, white flour and white sugar products. Add more vitamins A and C to your diet.

AVOID MIS CARRIAGE

BLACK HAW

Black haw root bark (also called cramp bark) is an astringent which increases the tone and firmness of the uterine tissues. Women, who in the past have had repeated miscarriages, would do well to take black haw when miscarriage threatens. It will help prevent premature labor. This herb was listed in 19th century pharmacy reference books as a treatment for painful menstrual cramps and threatened miscarriage. It reduces the discomforts of pregnancy and soothes the uterus. Drink 1-2 cups of tea daily and then, after symptoms cease, drink the tea for an additional 2 weeks.

Because it decreases excessive menstrual flow, black haw is also good for PMS. When needed, drink 3 or 4 cups of the tea daily. It will stop contractions.

FALSE UNICORN

This herb is a specific for threatened abortion. It increases the muscle tone of the uterus and related organs. Take 3-4 drops of the tincture 4-5 times daily during the first trimester.

FORMULAS

Here is a suggested formula to prevent miscarriage: Mix tinctures: 20 drops black haw, and 10 drops each of wild yam and false unicorn root. Add water or juice, and drink 2-4 times a day. If spotting occurs, take it every 2 hours until spotting stops.

Another formula to prevent miscarriage: Mix 2 Tbsp. lemon balm (melissa) and partridge berry leaves, and 1 Tbsp. each oatstraw, red raspberry leaves, and stinging nettle leaves. Steep in a quart of boiling water. Drink 1-3 cups a day.

LAST SIX WEEKS

LAST SIX WEEKS

HERB MIX

During the last six weeks before delivery, this formula will make labor easier and help the delivery: Drink a tea of squaw vine, black cohosh, pennyroyal, red raspberry, and a pinch of lobelia. Or take false unicorn, squaw vine, pennyroyal, black cohosh, red raspberry, and blessed thistle.

K FACTOR (ANEMIA)

NETTLE LEAF

This useful herb, taken as a tea, improves the K factor in your blood during last month. It is a blood coagulant. This means that if bleeding starts, it is more likely to stop right away. Nettle leaf tea strengthens the entire body (including the kidneys). Taken during the last month before delivery, this will increase vitamin K in both the mother and child.

PREMATURE LABOR

WILD YAM ROOT

Wild yam has antispasmodic qualities. It relaxes muscles, reduces spasms, convulsions, and cramps. It also helps the liver. It stops premature labor (miscarriage), and is also good for morning sickness because it balances female hormones. For threatened miscarriage, take 8-10 drops of the tincture every hour as long as needed. Sip the tea to reduce morning sickness.

DURING LABOR

ASSIST LABOR

BLACK COHOSH WITH BLUE COHOSH

Taken together, these two herbs assist labor from the time the baby has dropped. They should be taken together; for blue cohosh gets the contractions going and black cohosh makes the contractions rhythmic. This makes labor easier; and the contractions become consistent and regular. But it is important to take both herbs together for the best effect. They help relieve pain and soothe irritation of the uterus and cervix. Take 8-10 drops of the tincture. Either take sublingually (place under the tongue and let it dissolve) or drink with water. In order to stimulate labor contractions, start with 5 drops of black cohosh under the tongue; then alternate with 5 drops of blue cohosh. After alternating them four times, stop. These two herbs help initiate labor by stimulating contractions. They also help the afterbirth come out. Begin with 5 drops of the two herbs combined; this can be increased to 8-10. Repeat every 20-30 minutes, but stop after you have taken the drops 4 times.

Caution: Do NOT stimulate contractions UNTIL the baby's head is engaged (has dropped into the pelvic cavity). Using these two herbs to start labor increases the possibility of ruptured membranes which, in turn, increases the possibility of a prolapsed cord.

PARTRIDGE BERRY

Indian squaws living in western New York would drink it for 2-3 weeks before and during delivery, because it made the delivery so much easier.

FORMULAS

A formula to make delivery easier: Mix equal parts of black haw, red raspberry, partridge berry, blessed thistle, and licorice or sarsaparilla. Make a tea and drink it just before delivery.

A formula at time of delivery: Add 2 parts each of lemon balm, lavender, and holy basil, and 1 part each pansy flowers and borage. Alternate drinking this tea, with a tea of red raspberry leaf.

AVOID PERINEAL TEARS

ARNICA

While in labor, gently rub arnica oil over the lip of the cervix. This will help protect it from tearing. Do not take internally.

EVENING PRIMROSE OIL

Place on the cervix to help soften it. Slowly rub it into the rigid part. This is especially helpful for mothers bearing their first child (primiparas). But do NOT place it on a loose cervix; for you do not want the child to come out too rapidly.

AFTERWARD

EXPEL AFTERBIRTH

ANGELICA

Angelica root is a powerful uterine stimulant. It helps expel the retained placenta; also if a miscarriage accidentally occurs during the pregnancy, taking angelica will help complete it. It is a good uterine stimulant and helps bring on menstrual cycles. Take 8-10 drops of the tincture. Hold them under the tongue (sublingually) and let them absorb. Start with the lowest dosage and repeat if necessary.

Caution: Some are sensitive to this herb. Do not take large doses. It can affect blood pressure and the heart.

STOP POST-PARTUM BLEEDING

SHEPHERD'S PURSE

This herb reduces post-partum bleeding from the womb. It is a blood coagulant. Begin with only 8-10 drops of the tincture. Place it under the tongue. This will stop post-partum hemorrhage. If needed, take more.

Caution: Do not take shepherd's purse during pregnancy. Only use it after the baby is born. Do not take too much; for it can cause huge clots which are difficult to expel.

Caution: Some recommend taking cayenne to stop bleeding. Normally, it is good for that purpose, but not in this case. Although it may reduce bleeding, cayenne does not contract the uterus. Taken with shepherd's purse, the cayenne will stimulate circulation, causing still larger blood clots.

HEALING OF PERINEUM

COMFREY

This herb aids in more rapid healing of either a tear or episiotomy in the perineum. Put it in a sitz bath and let the mother sit in the water. Comfrey will help prevent infection and relieve pain. Comfrey tea can also be applied to the breast, for breast infections.

For a sitz bath, put 4 oz. dried leaves in ½ gallon of boiling water, steep 8 hours, strain. Then pour in tub and let mother sit in it 15 minutes twice a day.

As a compress, place a handful of dried leaves in a folded clean cloth, simmer 12-15 minutes. Apply the compress several times each day, for not over 5 minutes at a time.

ST. JOHN'S WORT OIL

Rub this blood-red oil on the perineum (the area between the vulva and anus) at the time of delivery. This will help avoid tearing this area, which tends to tear. Applying it after delivery speeds healing of perineal tears. It has a soothing action; and it reduces burning and swelling of the tissues. Like all essential oils, it must only be applied externally.

P
R
E
G

H
E
R
B

FORMULA

This formula will help repair perineal tears: Take herbal **sitz baths**, with **yarrow flowers, comfrey leaves, and calendula** added to the water.

AFTER PAINS

CHAMOMILE

Taken internally by the mother, this beneficial herb relaxes and reduces pains. It may be applied to the perineum during delivery and to help clean the infant's eyes shortly after birth. As a tea, use 1 tsp. to 1 cup of water. For the infant's eyes, do this: Place 1 oz. in 1 quart of boiling water and let it steep 1-2 hours. Very carefully, apply lukewarm with sterile cotton.

Caution: Do not drink chamomile throughout pregnancy! Doing so may calm the uterus or bring on a menstrual cycle, resulting in a miscarriage.

AFTER CESAREAN SECTION

FORMULA

A formula to use after cesarean sections: Mix a tincture of 3 parts **bupleurum**: 2 parts **dandelion root**; and 1 part each **blessed thistle, wild yam, and astragalus**. Drink it and apply it to area.

MASTITIS

ECHINACEA

This excellent antibiotic herb will reduce or eliminate mastitis. Echinacea purifies the blood, destroys viruses, and prevents the growth of bacteria. It helps build the immune system. It fights infection, both bacterial or viral (something antibiotic drugs cannot do). It can also be used for infections in the newborn infant.

Add 1 oz. echinacea to 1 pint of boiling water, and let steep 4-8 hours. Drink 2 cups daily or ½ dropper of tincture 3-6 times daily. For infants: Every 3 hours, give 1 drop of echninacea tincture per five pounds of the child's body weight. (Example: a 10-pound infant would receive 2 drops every 3 hours.) Do not give it to infants for more than 10 days.

INCREASE BREAST MILK

HOPS

This helpful herb relieves after pains, increases breast milk, and helps the mother go to sleep.

Add 1 tsp. to a cup of boiling water, steep for 20 minutes, and take a little (only as much as needed) each night.

"Happy are the parents whose lives are a true reflection of the divine, so that the promises and commands of God awaken in the child gratitude and reverence; the parents whose tenderness and justice and long-suffering interpret to the child the love and justice and long-suffering of God; and who, by teaching the child to love and trust and obey them, are teaching him to love and trust and obey his Father in heaven. Parents who impart to a child such a gift have endowed him with a treasure more precious than the wealth of all the ages—a treasure as enduring as eternity.

"In the children committed to her care, every mother has a sacred charge from God. 'Take this son, this daughter,' He says; 'train it for Me; give it a character polished after the similitude of a palace, that it may shine in the courts of the Lord forever.'

"The mother's work often seems to her an unimportant service. It is a work that is rarely appreciated. Others know little of her many cares and burdens. Her days are occupied with a round of little duties, all calling for patient effort, for self-control, for tact, wisdom, and self-sacrificing love; yet she cannot boast of what she has done as any great achievement. She has only kept things in the home running smoothly; often weary and perplexed, she has tried to speak kindly to the children, to keep them busy and happy, and to guide the little feet in the right path. She feels that she has accomplished nothing. But it is not so. Heavenly angels watch the care-worn mother, noting the burdens she carries day by day. Her name may not have been heard in the world, but it is written in the Lamb's book of life.

"There is a God above, and the light and glory from His throne rests upon the faithful mother as she tries to educate her children to resist the influence of evil. No other work can equal hers in importance. She has not, like the artist, to paint a form of beauty upon canvas, nor, like the sculptor, to chisel it from marble. She has not, like the author, to embody a noble thought in words of power, nor, like the musician, to express a beautiful sentiment in melody. It is hers, with the help of God, to develop in a human soul the likeness of the divine.

"The mother who appreciates this will regard her opportunities as priceless. Earnestly will she seek, in her own character and by her methods of training, to present before her children the highest ideal. Earnestly, patiently, courageously, she will endeavor to improve her own abilities, that she may use aright the highest powers of the mind in the training of her children. Earnestly will she inquire at every step, 'What hath God spoken?' Diligently she will study His Word. She will keep her eyes fixed upon Christ, that her own daily experience, in the lowly round of care and duty, may be a true reflection of the one true Life."—*Ministry of Healing, 375-378.*

Every day Samuel was the subject of his mother's (Hannah's) prayers "that he might be pure, noble, and true. She did not ask for her son worldly greatness, but she earnestly pleaded that he might attain that greatness which Heaven values—that he might honor God and bless his fellow men.

"What a reward was Hannah's! and what an encouragement to faithfulness is her example! There are opportunities of inestimable worth, interests infinitely precious, committed to every mother. The humble round of duties which women have come to regard as a wearisome task should be looked upon as a grand and noble work. It is the mother's privilege to bless the world by her influence, and in doing this she will bring joy to her own heart. She may make straight paths for the feet of her children, through sunshine and shadow, to the glorious heights above. But it is only when she seeks, in her own life, to follow the teachings of Christ that the mother can hope to form the character of her children after the divine pattern. The world teems with corrupting influences. Fashion and custom exert a strong power over the young. If the mother fails in her duty to instruct, guide, and restrain, her children will naturally accept the evil, and turn from the good. Let every mother go often to her Saviour with the prayer, 'Teach us, how shall we order the child, and what shall we do unto him?' Let her heed the instruction which God has given in His Word, and wisdom will be given her as she shall have need."
—*Patriarchs and Prophets, 572-573*

SPECIAL SECTIONS FOR WOMEN - 6

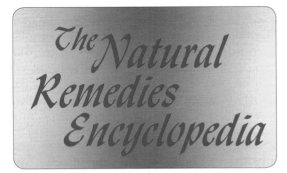

The Natural Remedies Encyclopedia

- Section 19 -
How to Deliver a Baby

INTRODUCTION

Most women today do not deliver babies; but you never know what might happen. Perhaps you live in a cabin in an isolated part of the Yukon. Or perhaps someday, because your husband is working a late shift, you might need to catch a cab, in the middle of the night, to take you to the hospital. If so, take this *Encyclopedia* with you. Who knows; if the cab driver does not make it to the hospital before the baby arrives, you might need to read this chapter to him!

However, every prospective mother will learn much helpful information from reading this brief chapter.

The woman should eat plenty of nutritious food (no sugar or junk food) during the nine months; so she will have strength, during childbirth, to avoid complications and lessen the likelihood of excessive bleeding, etc.

Reading this chapter can teach a woman the basics of midwifery! There is excellent information here.

BASIC THINGS TO HAVE READY

By the seventh month, you should have the following things ready at hand:

Soap and a clean scrub brush (for cleaning hands and fingernails). A lot of very clean cloths, alcohol for rubbing hands after washing them, and clean cotton. A new unwrapped razor blade (to cut the umbilical cord) or a pair of clean, rust-free scissors. (Boil for 15 minutes. It will be used to cut the cord.)

Sterile gauze or patches of thoroughly clean cloth for covering the navel. Two ribbons or strips of clean cloth (to tie the cord). Both should be wrapped and sealed in paper packets and then baked in an oven or ironed.

ADDITIONAL THINGS IT WOULD BE GOOD TO HAVE

Flashlight, suction bulb (for sucking mucus out of baby's nose and mouth). Two bowls: 1 for washing hands and 1 for catching and examining the afterbirth. Blunt-tipped scissors for cutting the cord

D
E
L
I
V
E
R
Y

**THIS INFORMATION IS FOR THE EMERGENCY DELIVERY OF A CHILD.
YOU USE THIS INFORMATION AT YOUR OWN RISK.**

before the baby is all the way born (to be used in an extreme emergency if the cord is wrapped around the baby's head). Rubber or plastic gloves (which can be sterilized by boiling) to wear when examining the woman while the baby is coming out, when sewing tears in the birth opening, and for catching and examining the afterbirth. Sterile needle and gut thread for sewing tears in the birth opening.

DEFINITIONS

The *fetus* is the *baby*. The *uterus* is the *womb*. The *placenta* is the sack attached to the wall of the uterus and to the *umbilical cord* (also called the *cord*) through which the baby receives food and oxygen and gives off waste. The *amniotic fluid* is the *waters* in the placenta surrounding the baby. After the baby is born, the placenta soon comes out; then it is called the *afterbirth*. The placenta contains the fluid, not only the baby. When the placenta breaks (before birth), it is said that the *bag of waters has broken*.

Commonplace terms will generally be used in this chapter: *baby, womb, waters, cord, bag of waters,* and *afterbirth*. The cervix is the birth opening which is tightly closed until the time of birth, when contractions gradually widen it; so the baby can pass down through the *vagina* and the round opening in the *pelvic bone (birth canal)* to the outside world. The baby and its position can be gauged by feeling the *abdomen*, the soft frontal area of the mother that is above the *pubic bone* and below the *ribs*. The area of the mother's skin, sometimes torn during birth, is the *perineum*. The woman helping the mother throughout the time is the *helper* or *midwife*.

GETTING CLOSER TO LABOR

You will want to see the mother more often as birth approaches. If she has already given birth to other children, ask how long labor lasted and if she had any problems. Talk with her about ways to make the birth easier and less painful. Explain the importance of adequate rest, moderate exercise, cheerful surroundings, and a good diet with very little salt intake.

Have her practice deep, slow breathing; so she can later do this during the labor contractions. Explain to her that, when labor begins, relaxing during contractions and resting between them will help her save strength, reduce pain, and speed labor. Also mention that it is best that she not do heavy work or lifting. The baby can prematurely drop and lose the

skin on top of its head. Also explain that too active exercise or putting her arms above her head too much might wrap the cord about the baby's neck.

It is helpful to keep records. Here is a summary of what you will want to write down: Date of visit, general health, minor problems, and whether there is anemia (if so, how severe?). Danger signs, swelling (where and how much?), pulse, temperature, weight, blood pressure, protein in urine, sugar in urine, position of the baby in womb, size of womb (how many fingers above or below the navel?). Much of this will be explained below.

RISK AND DANGER SIGNS

• **Severe anemia:** Signs include if the woman is weak, tired, and has pale or transparent skin. The diet needs to be improved. *See Anemia (537-540, 713).* If not treated, she might die from blood loss during labor at the time of childbirth.

• **Toxemia:** Signs include swelling of the hands, feet, and face with headache, dizziness, and sometimes blurred vision. Other indications include sudden weight gain, high blood pressure, and excessive protein in the urine. She should stay quiet in bed and eat foods rich in protein, but with only a little salt. Salty foods should not be eaten. (But a tiny amount of salt is needed.) If she does not get better quickly, swells more in the face, has trouble seeing, or has convulsions, take her to a hospital immediately.

• **AIDS:** If the woman has HIV, she can pass it on to her child while it is in the womb or at the time of birth. A medicine, called nevirapine, can help prevent the baby from getting HIV. Take 200 mg by mouth when labor begins. Give the baby 6 mg liquid nevirapine (2 mg per body weight) as soon as possible during the first 7 days after birth.

HOW TO CHECK THE GROWTH AND HEIGHT OF THE BABY IN THE WOMB

Each month write down how many finger-widths, above or below the navel, is the top of the womb (the top of the felt bulge of the womb).

Teach the mother to horizontally lay the second and third fingers of her hand by the top of the womb, and use this to measure with. Measure from her navel. Normally, the womb will be 2 fingers higher each month. At 4½ months, it is usually at the level of her navel. So measure two finger-widths down from the navel, till it reaches the navel; then start

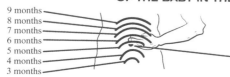

DETERMINING THE GROWTH AND POSITION OF THE BABY IN THE WOMB

9 months
8 months
7 months
6 months
5 months
4 months
3 months

The womb is usually 2 fingers higher each month. At 4 1/2 months, it is usually at the level of the navel.

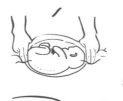

HOW TO CHECK THE HEIGHT OF THE WOMB

1 - Have the mother breathe out all the way.
2 - With the thumb and 2 fingers, push in just above the pelvic bone.
3 - With the other, feel the top of the womb below the breasts.

CHECKING IF THE BABY'S HEAD IS UP OR DOWN

The baby's *butt* is larger and wider. If it is at the top, it will feel larger and high up.

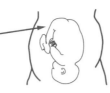

If the *butt* is down, it will feel larger and be low down.

The baby's *head* is hard and round.

measuring up from the navel. *(See illustrations on page 766.)*

If the womb seems too big, or is growing too fast, it may mean the woman is going to have twins. But, instead, the cause may be that the womb has more water (amniotic fluid) in it—which will make it more difficult to feel the abdomen and locate the position of the baby inside. Too much water in the womb means there is a greater risk of severe bleeding during childbirth and may mean the baby is deformed. Make sure the mother is on a good diet, so she is not anemic.

HOW TO CHECK THE BABY'S HEARTBEAT

Start listening for the baby's heartbeat (fetal heartbeat) after the first five months; also begin checking for movement. You may be able to hear it by putting your ear against the abdomen, but a stethoscope works better.

A baby's heart beats twice as fast as an adult's. Using a watch with a second hand, count the baby's heartbeats. Anywhere from 120 to 160 beats per minute is normal. If they are less than 120, something is wrong. However, it is possible you heard the mother's heartbeat instead. Check her pulse and see what her heart rate is. The baby's heartbeat is often difficult to hear. It takes practice.

If the baby's heartbeat is heard loudest below the navel in the last month, the baby's head is down and will probably be born head first. This is normal and best.

If the heartbeat is heard loudest above the navel, his head is probably up and it may be a breech birth (with buttocks coming out first).

HOW TO CHECK IF THE BABY'S HEAD IS UP OR DOWN

You want to make sure the baby's head is down,

which is the normal and ideal position for birth. Have the mother lay down, with the pelvic area unclothed.

In order to locate where the head is while you are standing beside her, have her breathe out all the way. Then, with thumb and 2 fingers, push in just above her pelvic bone. With the other hand, feel farther up at the top of the womb. *(See illustration on the top of this page.)*

The baby's butt is larger and wider and the head is hard and round. If the butt is up, that part will feel larger high up. If the butt is down, it will feel larger low down. *(See illustration on the top of this page.)*

Next, push gently from side to side, first with one hand and then the other. If the baby's butt is pushed gently sideways, its whole body will move also. But if the head is pushed gently sideways, it will bend at the neck and the back will not move.

HOW TO CHECK IF THE BABY HAS DROPPED YET

Has the baby dropped yet? (dropped lower into the pelvis, ready for birth). If the head is downward and the baby is still high in the womb, you can move the head a little. But if it has already engaged (dropped lower, getting ready for birth), you cannot move it. *(See illustration on the bottom of this page.)*

A woman's first baby sometimes engages 2 weeks before labor begins. Later babies may not engage until labor starts.

If the baby's head is down, his birth is likely to go well. If the head is up, it will be a breech birth and more difficult. It is safer for the mother to give birth in, or near, a hospital. If the baby is sideways, the mother should have her baby in a hospital. She and the baby are in danger.

—Important: see Signs of Pregnancy Risk (706).

CHECKING IF THE BABY'S HAS DROPPED YET

Push gently from side to side, first with one hand, and then the other.

But if the baby's *butt* is pressed gently sideways, the baby's whole body will also move.

But if the baby's *head* is pressed gently sideways, it will bend at the neck and the back will not move.

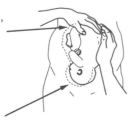

If the baby is still high in the womb, you can move the head a little. But if it has already dropped lower ("engaged") and getting ready for birth, you cannot move it.

A woman's first baby often engages 2 weeks before labor begins. Later babies may not engage until labor starts.

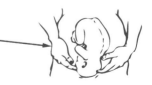

D
E
L
I
V
E
R
Y

A few days before labor begins, the baby moves lower. This lets the mother breathe easier; but urination must be more frequent (because of pressure on the bladder).

Some thick mucus may come out a short time before labor or 2-3 days earlier. It may be tinged with blood. This is normal.

Once again, explain to her that as contractions begin, relaxing during contractions and resting between them will help her save strength, reduce pain, and speed labor.

CONTRACTIONS

Labor pains are caused by contractions, tightening of the womb. Between contractions, the womb is relaxed. During each contraction, the womb tightens and lifts upward. Each contraction pushes the baby farther down the birth canal. This causes the cervix (door of the womb) to open a little more each time. *(See the illustration on the bottom of this page.)*

Contractions may begin up to several days before childbirth. At first, several minutes or hours pass between them. When they become stronger, regular, and more frequent, labor is beginning.

Some women have a few practice contractions weeks earlier. This is normal. Rarely, she may have false labor, which is this: The contractions begin coming strong and close; but then they stop for several hours or days before actual labor begins. Sometimes walking, a warm bath, or resting will help calm the contractions if they are false—or bring on childbirth if they are real.

This is what is meant by "breaking of the bag of waters": The fluid surrounding the baby in the womb usually breaks with a flood of liquid sometime after labor has begun. If the waters break before the contractions start, this usually means the beginning of labor. After they break, the mother should keep very clean: no sexual contact, no sitting in a bath of water, and no douching! Walking back and forth may help bring on labor more quickly. If labor does not begin within 12 hours after the waters break, seek medical help.

THREE STAGES OF LABOR

There are three stages of labor. *First stage:* From the beginning of the strong contractions until the baby drops into the birth canal. *Second stage:* From the dropping into the birth canal until it is born. *Third stage:* From the birth of the baby until the placenta (afterbirth) comes out.

THE FIRST STAGE

This stage usually lasts 10-20 hours or longer, when it is the mother's first birth (primaparia), and from 7-10 hours in later births (multiparia). This can vary quite a bit. During the first stage, the mother should not try to hurry the birth. It is natural for this to go slowly, as the openings gradually expand. Reassure the mother; for she may not think the process is going fast enough. Tell her most women have the same concern.

She should not try to push, or bear down, until the baby is beginning to move down into the birth canal and she feels she has to push.

During this stage, it is important that the mother keep her bladder and bowels empty. If they are full, they get in the way when the baby is being born. She should urinate often. If she has not had a bowel movement in several hours, an enema given to her will make labor easier. As the baby keeps moving downward, it fills a lot of space while pushing other things in the pelvis back.

During labor, she should drink water or other liquids often. Too little liquid in the body can slow or stop the labor. If the labor is long, she should also eat lightly. If she is vomiting, she should sip a little water, herb tea, or fruit juice between each contraction.

During labor, she should often change positions or get up and walk about every so often. She should not lie flat on her back for a long time.

During this first stage of labor, the birth attendant (nurse, midwife, or other helper) should do these three things:

• Wash the mother's belly, genitals, buttocks, and legs well with soap and warm water. The bed should be in a clean place with enough light to clearly see.

• Clean sheets or towels should be spread on the bed and changed whenever they get wet or dirty.

BETWEEN AND DURING CONTRACTIONS
Labor pains are caused by contractions (tightening of the womb), as the baby is pushed lower.

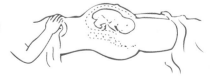

Between contractions, the womb is relaxed and appears like this.

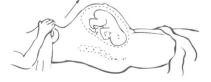

During each contraction, the womb tightens and lifts up like this.

Each contraction pushes the baby farther down. This causes the cervix (the bottom door of the womb) to gradually open, more and more.

• As mentioned earlier, have a new, unopened razor blade ready for cutting the cord or boiled pair of scissors. Keep the scissors in the boiled water in a covered pan until needed.

The helper should NOT massage or push on the belly. She should NOT ask the mother to push or bear down at this time.

If the mother is frightened or in pain, have her take deep, slow, regular breaths during each contraction and then breathe normally between them. This will help control the pain and calm her. Reassure her that the strong pains are normal and that they help to push the baby out.

THE SECOND STAGE

It is during this stage that the child is born. Sometimes this begins when the bag of waters breaks. This stage is often easier than the first stage, and usually does not last longer than 2 hours. During the contractions, the mother bears down (pushes with her inner muscles) with all her strength. Between contractions, she may seem very tired and half asleep. This is normal.

This is how to bear down: The mother takes a deep breath and then pushes hard with her "stomach" muscles as if she were having a bowel movement. If the child comes slowly after the bag of waters breaks, she can double her knees as she squats on her feet, sitting propped up as she leans against a wall with pillows under and behind her as she holds her knees toward her chest or kneels on the bed or floor, with her legs folded back under her, or lying down as she holds her legs just below the knees.

When the outside birth opening of the mother stretches—and the baby's head begins to show—the helper should have everything ready for the actual birth.

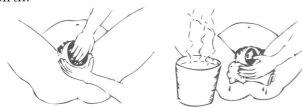

As soon as the baby's head begins to be seen, the mother should NOT try to push! Instead, she should pant and let the head come out slowly, so the birth opening is not torn.

About tearing: It is more likely to happen if this is the mother's first baby. Tearing can be prevented in this way: As soon as the baby's head begins to show, she should not bear down (that is, she should stop pushing), but instead pant (take many short, rapid breaths). This gives the birth opening time to stretch—open up wider. When the birth opening is stretching, the midwife can support it with one hand and with the other hand gently keep the head from coming too fast *(as shown in the illustration on the lower left)*. Placing warm compresses against the skin below the birth opening is also helpful *(illustration below)*. Start doing this as soon as the stretching begins. You can also massage the skin with oil. (If a tear does occur, it should be sewed closed, after the placenta comes out, by someone who knows how to carefully sew it shut with gut thread.)

In a normal childbirth, the helper should NEVER put her hand or finger inside the mother. This is the most common cause of infection to the mother after birth!

The helper should have scrubbed her hands and nails thoroughly beforehand; and, it is preferable that she wear gloves previously sterilized. This protects the mother, the baby, and the helper. *(See illustration on the bottom of this page.)*

THE THIRD STAGE OF LABOR

This stage begins as soon as the baby has been born and continues until the afterbirth (placenta) comes out. Normally, the afterbirth comes out 5 minutes to an hour after the baby is born.

While waiting for the afterbirth, do this:
• Put the baby's head down, so the mucus comes out of his mouth and throat. Do not change this position until he begins breathing.
• Keep the baby below the level of the mother until the cord is tied. This will help extra blood to flow into the baby.

If the baby does not begin breathing right away:
• Rub his back with a towel or cloth. If he still does not breathe, clean the mucus out of his nose and mouth with a suction bulb or clean cloth wrapped around your finger.

THE MOTHER AND THE HELPER UNITE IN HELPING THE BABY TO BE BORN

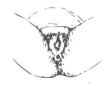
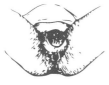
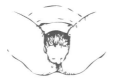
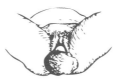
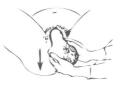
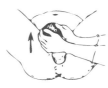

1 - Now the mother should push hard

2 - Now she should not push hard. Instead, she should take many short breaths. This will help prevent tearing of the birth opening.

3 - The head usually comes out face down. Its body then turns to one side, so the shoulders come out.

4 - The helper takes the baby's head and very gently lowers it, and a shoulder comes out.

5 - Then the head is raised so the other shoulder can come out. The helper never pulls on the baby, or twists or bends its neck.

• If the baby does not breathe within one minute after birth, start mouth-to-mouth breathing at once! *(See page 992-994, in the chapter on Emergencies, for directions.)* With babies and small children, cover the nose and mouth with your mouth and breathe *very gently* about once every 3 seconds.

• It is important that you not let the baby get chilled, especially if he is premature. Wrap him in a clean cloth.

How to cut the cord:

As soon as the infant is born, the cord will be fat and blue, and pulsing as blood flows through it from the mother to the child. WAIT. You want as much blood as possible to flow into the child. Very soon, the cord becomes thin, white, and stops pulsing. Then it will be time to cut it.

You have ready two pieces of ribbon or narrow cloth strips, recently ironed or heated in an oven. Now tie one ribbon or cloth strip close to the body of the newborn child. (Leave about ¾ inch [2 cm.] of the cord attached to the baby.) Then tie the other a short distance away. Next, wash your hands very well, unwrap the unused (clean) razor blade, and cut the cord. (Or use a freshly boiled pair of scissors.) These precautions protect the baby from tetanus.

You will want to tie the cord as soon as the pulsing has stopped, so that the baby can be brought up and placed on the mother's breast as soon as possible.

Keeping the cord clean: Keep the cord exposed to the air, so it can dry out. If the home is quite clean, with no flying insects, leave it uncovered. If dust and flies are present, cover the cord lightly with sterile gauze or a previously boiled (or recently ironed) cloth. The sooner the cord dries out, the quicker it will fall off.

As shown in the illustration just below, cut the gauze on a corner halfway to the center of one-half of the gauze. Then place it over the cut cord. Gently flip the top half over it; and then gently place a thin and loose cloth around it.

To avoid getting urine on it, the baby's diapers must not cover the navel.

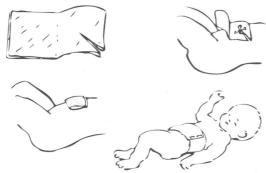

AFTERWARD

CLEANING THE NEWBORN

Use a clean, warm, soft, damp cloth and gently clean away any blood or fluid from the baby.

Do not bathe the baby until after the cord drops off (usually 5-8 days). Then bathe him daily in warm water, using a mild soap.

PUTTING THE BABY TO THE BREAST

As soon as the cord is tied (which should be as soon as the pulsing in the cord has ceased), put the baby on the mother's breast. If the baby nurses, this will help the afterbirth come out sooner and prevent or control heavy bleeding.

THE AFTERBIRTH

The placenta usually comes out 5 minutes to an hour after the baby is born. But sometimes it is delayed for many hours.

Checking the afterbirth: It is extremely important, as soon as the placenta comes out, that you pick it up and carefully examine it to see if it is complete. If it is torn or any piece seems to be missing, get medical help. At the hospital, they will scrape the womb; this is because, if any piece of the placenta is still inside the womb, it can cause continued bleeding or infection.

Wear gloves or plastic bags on your hands as you handle the placenta. Afterward, wash your hands very well.

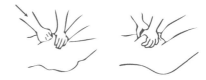

If the placenta is delayed in coming out: If the mother is not losing much blood, do nothing; just patiently wait. While waiting, do NOT pull on the cord! This could cause heavy bleeding from the uterus. Sometimes the placenta comes out if the mother squats and pushes (bears down) a little.

If the mother is losing blood, feel the womb. If it is soft, massage it carefully until it gets hard *(illustration below)*. This should make it contract and push out the placenta.

If the placenta does not come out soon and bleeding continues, push downward on the top of the womb very carefully *(illustration below, right)* while supporting the bottom of the womb.

HEAVY BLEEDING AND SHOCK

Warning: The mother may be bleeding heavily inside, with little blood coming out. Feel her abdomen from time to time. If it seems to be getting bigger, it may be filling with blood. Check her pulse often and watch for signs of shock, which include these: Weak, rapid pulse over 100 per minute. Cold sweat and pale, cold, damp skin. Blood pressure drops dangerously low. Mental confusion, weakness, or loss of consciousness.

In order to prevent or treat shock:

At the first sign of shock or if there is risk of shock: Have the woman lie down with her feet a little higher than her head. Stop any bleeding. If she feels cold, cover her with a blanket. Give her sips of water or other drinks. Keep her calm and reassure her.

If heavy bleeding continues and the placenta still does not come out, call for medical help and do this:

To help prevent or control heavy bleeding: Let the baby suck the mother's breast. If the baby will not suck and the husband is present, have him gently pull and massage the mother's nipples. This will cause her to produce pituitrin, a hormone that helps control uterine bleeding.

Even a slow, steady trickle of blood coming out can cause serious trouble. Make sure medical help is on the way. Have her drink a lot of liquid (water, fruit juices, herb tea, or soup). Put her legs up and head down. This brings blood from the legs into the trunk and head.

Massage the abdomen until you can feel the womb getting hard. If the bleeding stops, check every 5 minutes to make sure the womb is remaining hard. If not, massage it again. As soon as the womb gets hard and bleeding stops, do not massage it. But check every 5 minutes or so and begin massaging if it gets soft again.

If the bleeding still continues: This time, using all your weight, press down with both hands (one hand over the other) on the abdomen, just below the navel. You should continue this press a long time after the bleeding stops.

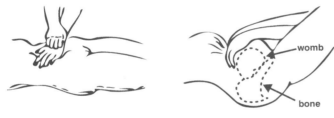

womb

bone

If bleeding still continues, do this: Press both hands into the abdomen *above* the womb. Scoop up the womb (uterus) and fold it forward (toward the legs), so the womb is pressed hard against the pubic bone. Press as hard as you can, using the weight of your leaning body if your muscles are not strong enough. Keep pressing for several minutes after the bleeding has stopped or until you can get medical help.

DIFFICULT BIRTHS

If the birth is difficult, it is important that you get medical help as soon as possible during the labor.

There are several possible causes of why **labor stops, slows down, or lasts a long time** after earlier being strong or after the waters break.

• **The mother may be frightened or upset**. This can slow or even stop the contractions. Reassure her, so she can relax. Explain that the birth is slow and there are no serious problems. Encourage her to change her body position often and to drink juices, eat some food, and urinate. Stimulating the nipples (either with a massaging or milking motion) can help speed labor.

• **The mother may be dehydrated** if she has been vomiting or has not been drinking liquids. This can slow or stop the contractions. Have her sip fruit juice after each contraction.

• **The mother's pelvis may be too small**. The baby's head may be too large to fit through the mother's pelvis (the birth canal). This is more likely if the woman is short, but unlikely in a woman who has given birth before. By feeling the pelvis, you may notice that the baby does not move down. If you suspect that this may be the problem, get her to a hospital; for she may need a cesarean section. Women who have very narrow hips, or are exceptionally short, should especially have their first child born in, or near, a hospital.

• **The shoulders may get stuck after the head comes out first**. The helper can take the baby's head in her hands and lower it very carefully, so one shoulder can come out. Then she can raise the head a little, so the other shoulder comes out.

• **The baby may not be in the best position**. As mentioned earlier, you can feel the mother's abdomen and know whether the baby is in the best position (head downward), breech (buttocks downward, legs up, and head at the top), or sideways. Sometimes the helper can carefully turn the baby with very gentle handling of the woman's abdomen. Between contractions (not during contractions!), try to work the baby around, little by little, until the head is downward. Do not use force; for this could tear the womb. If the baby cannot be turned, get the mother to the hospital as soon as possible.

[1] **If the baby's head is downward**, the head is probably facing the rear of her body. This is normal.

[2] **If the baby's head is downward, but with the head facing forward**, you may be able to feel the lumpy arms and legs rather than the rounded back. This is usually not a serious problem; but labor may be longer because the mother has more back pain. She should change positions often; for this may help turn the baby. Have her get on her hands and knees. This may help turn him.

D E L I V E R Y

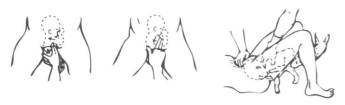

[3] **If the baby is sideways** and you cannot turn it, rush the mother to the hospital.

[4] **If the baby's buttocks is downward** and you cannot turn the baby, the buttocks will come out first. This is called a *breech* birth. The helper may be able to tell if the baby is in the breech position by feeling the mother's abdomen and listening to its heartbeat. A beech birth may be easier if the mother will get down on her hands and knees (with her hands, knees, and lower legs resting on the bed).

[5] **If the baby's legs come out first, but not the arms**. Wash your hands very well; rub them with alcohol (or wear sterile gloves). And then do this:

Slip your fingers inside and push the baby's shoulders toward the back *(illustration, above)*, pressing his arms against his body.

If the baby gets stuck, have the mother lie face up. Put your finger into the baby's mouth and push his head toward his chest. At the same time have someone push the baby's head down by pressing on the mother's abdomen. Have the mother push hard. But you must not—never—pull on the body of the baby.

[6] **A hand or arm comes out first** ("presentation of a hand or arm"). If this happens, get medical help immediately. A cesarean section may be needed.

[7] **The cord may be wrapped about the head of the baby** so tightly he cannot come out all the way. If this is the case, the birth process has stopped and he is locked in there until the afterbirth comes out. But you cannot wait for that to happen, because he might suffocate. Try to slip the loop of cord from around the baby's neck. If you cannot do this, you may have to clamp, tie, and cut the cord. If you have to do that, you must use boiled blunt-tipped scissors. (At a childbirth, which the principle author attended when he was much younger, this happened. The baby girl's head had come out, stopped, and was turning blue. He knelt and earnestly prayed—and immediately the baby came out and the afterbirth with her! Normally, the afterbirth would not have come out immediately.)

• **The mother may have twins**. Another cause of a difficult birth is if the mother is carrying twins. This is more difficult and dangerous to both mother and infants. It is best if she delivers them in a hospital. Labor often begins early with twins; so a mother expecting twins should be staying close to the hospital after the seventh month of pregnancy. She should rest a lot and be careful to avoid hard work. Doing so will help the twins not be born early. (Twins are often born small and need special care.)

Here are four signs that she may have *twins*:

• The womb grows faster and becomes larger than usual, especially in the last months.

• She is gaining weight faster than normal or the common pregnancy problems are worse than usual: morning sickness, backache, varicose veins, piles, swelling, and difficult breathing.

• If you can feel 3 or more large objects (heads and buttocks) in an extra-large womb.

• If you can hear 2 different heartbeats (other than the mother's); however, hearing both infants' heartbeats may be difficult.

PROBLEMS AT THE TIME OF BIRTH

• **Meconium may be in the waters**. When the waters break, you may see there is a dark green, almost black liquid in them. This is probably the baby's first stools (meconium). This means the baby may be in danger. If he breathes any of it into his lungs, he may die. Therefore, as soon as his head is born, tell the mother not to push, but only take short, rapid breaths. Before the baby starts breathing, you must immediately suck the feces out of his nose and mouth with a suction bulb. Even if he starts breathing right away, you must continue sucking until you get all the feces out.

• **The perineum may have torn**. The birth opening stretches a lot during delivery. Sometimes it tears; this is more likely during the first delivery. How to prevent it was mentioned earlier. If a tear does occur, someone who knows how to do it should carefully sew it shut, after the placenta comes out.

• **The cord may have been pulled too hard**. Some midwives or physicians (more often a physician than a midwife) pull on the cord, so the afterbirth will come out quicker. The cord should not be pulled at all! The afterbirth will come out when it is ready to be expelled. If pulled, it may tear loose from the wall of the uterus, leaving pieces of afterbirth inside. This can cause the mother much bleeding and suffering later on. The only reason for pulling on the cord is so the doctor can go home quicker; that is not a good enough reason.

How to check the afterbirth for tears and missing parts was explained earlier.

CARING FOR THE NEWBORN

• The care of the cord immediately after childbirth was explained earlier.

• To protect the eyes of a newborn baby from conjunctivitis, it is recommended that a drop of 1% silver nitrate be placed in each eye as soon as he is born. If either parent has ever had gonorrhea or chlamydia, this is especially important.

• Keep the baby warm, but not too warm. In

D
E
L
I
V
E
R
Y

cold weather, wrap him well. But leave him naked in hot weather or if he has a fever. Keeping the baby close to his mother's body helps keep him warm. This is especially good to do if the baby was born early or is very small.

ALTERNATIVE

IF YOU CHOOSE A HOSPITAL DELIVERY

Perhaps you would prefer to have your baby in the hospital and not try to have it at home. Here are a few things to check on:

Select an understanding physician. Do you want to try to have the baby by natural methods as much as possible? (no drugs, etc.) What is his attitude about this?

What will the hospital or other facility permit you to do while there?

Here are several more questions:

During labor, will they let you walk around or take a shower, or do they just want you to remain in bed the whole time?

How many people will be allowed to stay with you? Can your husband be with you during the childbirth? Do you want an intravenous (IV) line inserted during labor? Although it often is not necessary, in many hospitals it is routinely done.

Do you want to be given drugs (usually oxytocin [Pitocin]) to speed up labor? Often given through an IV, it can make the labor more painful. But it will mean less time spent by the physician and staff.

Do you want any pain medication? If you decide against it, will it still be available later if you change your mind during the labor?

Will it be safe to breast-feed your baby immediately after receiving pain medication?

What methods will be used to monitor the baby during labor?

Will they have you placed in the "lithotomy" position (flat on your back on a padded table, with your feet in stirrups)? Laying in this one position for hours does not give you opportunity to change positions, squat, and do other things mentioned earlier to help the baby come more easily.

Do you want an episiotomy? This is an incision made in the perineum, to enlarge the vaginal opening. This is done so forceps can be used to hasten delivery or to prevent possible tearing in this area (which might not otherwise happen). Tearing takes longer to heal than an incision.

Are you willing to have a cesarean section? Under what emergency conditions will they perform it? Although over 24% of American women who give birth in hospitals have cesareans, the World Health Organization estimates that, anywhere in the world, it is only needed 10%-15% of the time. They cost over twice as much as a vaginal birth and the mother has to remain in the hospital for about two more days. *Four reasons are given for a cesarean:* The umbilical cord is seen before the baby, the baby is in a breech or sideways position, the baby's head is too big to fit through the pelvis (a very uncommon event), or the mother has earlier had a cesarean. But many problems can be solved without resorting to a major operation, which is what a cesarean section is.

SPECIAL RESEARCH STUDY

A scientific research study disclosed the following findings. The study compared the risks of a home delivery by a competent helper vs. delivery of a baby in an average hospital in America. In each instance, hospital deliveries involved a greater risk! Part of the problem may be that some physicians and hospital staff may be anxious to hurry up the procedure. Frankly, competent and caring midwives are a great blessing. *(Source: Lewis Mehl, et al., "Outcome of Elective Home Birth: A Series of 1,147 Cases," Journal of Reproductive Medicine, Vol. 19, No. 5, November 1977, pp. 288-289)*

PROCEDURE — IN THE HOSPITAL

Cesarean operation - Three times greater.

Forceps - 20 times more used.

Oxytocin (a drug to accelerate or induce labor) - Twice as much used.

Analgesia and anesthesia - Nine times more used.

Episiotomy - Nine times greater incidence; at the same time they had more severe tears in need of major repair.

Infant distress in labor - Six times more often.

Maternal high blood pressure - Five times more cases.

Postpartum hemorrhage - Three times greater.

Infection of newborn baby - Four times more infection among the newborn.

Babies needing help to breathe - Three times more babies needed help to begin to breathe.

Birth injuries - There were 30 cases of birth injuries; these included skull fractures, facial nerve palsies, brachial nerve injuries, and severe cephalhematomas. There were no such injuries at home.

Low birth rate (2,501 grams) - 1.3% for home births and 6.4% for hospital births.

Infant death rate - Infant death rate was low in both cases and essentially the same (4.3/1000 for home births and 10.2/1000 for hospital births).

Maternal death rate - There were no maternal deaths for either home or hospital.

D
E
L
I
V
E
R
Y

"Who are those with thee? . . The children which God hath graciously given thy servant."—*Genesis 33:5.* / "Children are an heritage of the Lord, and the fruit of the womb is His reward."—*Psalm 127:3.* / "Behold, I and the children whom the Lord hath given me."—*Isaiah 8:18.* / "Thy children shall be taught of the Lord."—*Isaiah 54:13.*

SPECIAL SECTIONS FOR WOMEN - 7

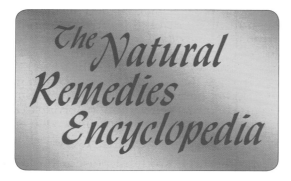

- Section 20 -
The First
Nine Months

PRENATAL GROWTH

Just a wonderful little human being! Though small, that is what he is. By **eighteen days** his little heart is already beating. **Before six weeks** (at 40 days), his electrical brain waves (electroencephalograph) has been recorded (*H. Hamilin, Life or Death by E.E.G., JAMA, October 1964*). **Prior to six weeks** his yolk sac was making his own blood cells; but, **by the sixth week,** his liver begins doing this important work. (Later it will be done within his bones.) He has been moving for quite some time. All twenty milk teeth buds are present at **six-and-a-half weeks**. He is really priceless.

And he is already sensitive to things about him. "In the sixth to seventh weeks . . If the area of the lips is gently stroked, the child responds by bending the upper body to one side and making a quick backward motion with his arms. This is called a 'total pattern response' because it involves most of the body, rather than a local part."—*Leslie B. Arey, "Developmental Anatomy," 6th Edition.*

At **seven weeks** ultrasound scanners can pick up the heart action of the infant (*T. Schawker, "Ultrasound Pictures first-trimester Fetus," Medical World News, February 1978);* and ultrasonic stethoscopes, now common in obstetricians' offices, allow the mother to hear her baby's heart beat as early as **eight weeks**. He is really doing well.

Your child is now just **two months old**—eight weeks! And the brain is completely present. At **eight weeks**, if we tickle the baby's nose, he will flex his head backward away from the stimulus. By **eight weeks** an unborn will grasp something placed in his small hand and hold onto it. Now, that's pretty nice, isn't it?

His stomach is now secreting gastric juice. And experts say that all of his body systems are present.

The nose is short and snub, and the eyes peer out from above it. But later, at the beginning of the third month (twelfth week), the eyelids will grow together,

closing the eyes. They will open again during the seventh month.

Weeks ago, the bones began to form and mature. That maturing will continue on for years. The top of the skull does not close until a year-and-a-half after birth. Yet the body skeleton will not itself be fully developed until the age of twenty-five. (That is why people before that age can so wonderfully heal when they injure their bones.)

Well, let's look at his tiny ear: The ear consists of three different parts and originates in three different regions. In the fourth week a bubble is turned inward from the skin on both sides of the rear part of the brain. This will later become the inner ear, with its delicate auditory and balance organs. In the **fifth week** the outer ear, with the auditory canal and the outer side of the eardrum, is developed at the upper end of the first of three grooves; the rest will close. The inner ear will be formed from tissue that comes from down in the pharynx. Only the God of heaven knows how to make little babies.

And yet at twelve weeks he does not weigh much. But don't let someone tell you that his life isn't important, simply because he is so small. Although tiny, he is a growing human being, just as a twelve-year-old boy is a growing human being. The only difference is that one is larger than the other. Both come from God and are fully human. Both of their lives are very important to God and to those who care for them.

From his very earliest days, this little fellow was a human being. We now have ultrasound to let us see an unborn child moving. We have electronic monitoring of an unborn baby's heart. We can identify the baby's sleep cycles. There are now techniques to sample the baby's urine, blood, and skin—and even identify sophisticated chemical reactions between the baby and the mother.

These new scientific methods clearly show that the separate individuality of the unborn child is a

9
MONTHS

scientific fact. He is not part of his mother. He is a separate human being. She nourishes his body; but, in the sight of God, she does not own it. It was given to her to protect.

When he was still very young—long **before the end of the first trimester**, the little infant could feel pain (he pulls back quickly from pinpricks). And soon noise will bother him, also.

At twelve weeks (three months) this little person weighs one ounce; at sixteen weeks, six ounces; and, at twenty weeks (four months), approximately one pound. A physician describes him:

"We know that he moves with a delightful easy grace in his buoyant world, that foetal (British variant for fetal) comfort determines foetal position. He is responsive to pain and touch and cold and sound and light. He drinks his amniotic fluid, more if it is artificially sweetened, less if it is given an unpleasant taste. He gets hiccups and sucks his thumb. He wakes and sleeps. He gets bored with repetitive signals but can be taught to be alerted by a first signal for a second different one."—*A. William Liley.*

It is now **two months** since pregnancy began, and for the first time you are certain that you are with child. It is at this time that most mothers will go to a doctor for prenatal care. Your physician will tell you that you should not be smoking, for it may damage your unborn child.

The small human being that God has given you to nourish is already remarkably developed. At **nine to ten weeks** he squints, swallows, moves his tongue; and, if you stroke his palm, he will make a tight fist. By **eleven to twelve weeks** he is also breathing fluid steadily and will do so until birth when he will breathe air.

He does not drown by breathing fluid; for he obtains his oxygen through his umbilical cord. But if he had air to breathe, he would breathe air. Certain experiments with unborn babies still in the womb have involved replacing some of the fluid with air in order to outline the baby's movements and position on X-ray film. But some of the baby's positions were such that when the mother laid on her back, the little nose and mouth extended into the air bubble. The baby breathed out the fluid in his lungs and breathed in the air. This, of course, made it possible for their vocal cords to make sound, so some of the babies cried loudly enough day and night to keep their mothers awake. The crying was loud enough to be heard by the others in the room. When the mother would roll on her side, she would submerge the nose and mouth under water again; the infant would breathe out the air, breathe in fluid and the crying would stop. This did not harm the infant; for, in the womb, he was able to breathe both ways *(A.W. Liley, Medical Professor, University of Auckland, New Zealand).*

"Maternal cigarette smoking during pregnancy decreases the frequency of fetal breathing by 20%. The 'well-documented' higher incidence of premature, stillbirth, and slower development of reading skill may be related to this decrease."—*F. Manning, Meeting of the Royal College of Physicians and Surgeons, Canada, Family Practice News, March 15, 1976.*

By eight weeks all of the body systems of your baby are present; by eleven weeks they are all working. He is a little human being; his brain is functioning, his nerves are working, he is moving about. By eleven weeks he is sucking his thumb vigorously *(A. Hellegers, Fetal Development).*

His little fingernails are present by the **eleventh week;** his eyelashes will be there by the **sixteenth week**. The muscles have already been working under the skin for some time, and their movements continue to become more coordinated. The lips open and close, the forehead wrinkles, the brow area raises and the head turns—**all this by the end of the first trimester (the first three months)** of your baby's life.

And now, with the twelfth week, the mother enters her fourth month. **The fourth through sixth months are known as the second trimester.** The little one is already assuming full-term proportions. The head is now about one-third of its entire body length with legs outstretched. The ribs are clearly visible.

Here is what this small human being—your child—looks like at only eight weeks of age. This is one of the most stunning descriptions of early human life ever recorded anywhere:

"Eleven years ago, while giving an anesthetic for a ruptured tubal pregnancy (at two months, or eight weeks), I was handed what I believed to be the smallest human being ever seen. The embryo sac was intact and transparent. Within the sac was a tiny (one-third inch) human male swimming extremely vigorously in the amniotic fluid, while attached to the wall by the umbilical cord. This tiny human was perfectly developed with long, tapering fingers, feet, and toes. It was almost transparent as regards to the skin, and the delicate arteries and veins were prominent to the ends of the fingers.

"The baby was extremely alive and swam about the sac approximately one time per second with a natural swimmer's stroke. This tiny human did not look at all like the photos and drawings of 'embryos' which I have seen, nor did it look like the few embryos I have been able to observe since then, obviously because this one was alive.

"When the tiny sac was opened, the tiny human immediately lost its life and took on the appearance of what is accepted as the appearance of an embryo at this stage (blunt extremities, etc.)."—*Paul E. Rockwell, M.D., Director of Anesthesiology, Leonard Hospital; Troy, New York (document presented to U.S. Supreme Court, Markle vs. Abele, 72-56, 72-*

9
M
O
N
T
H
S

730, p. 11).

Children can be born with quite a low birth weight and still survive. An unusual example of this is the case of Marion Chapman who was born in South Shields (County Durham), England on June 5, 1938—only 10 ounces! She was born unattended and was nursed by Dr. D.A. Shearer, who fed her hourly through a fountain pen filler. By her first birthday she had attained a weight of 13 pounds. Her weight on her twenty-first birthday was 106 pounds.

How very thankful we can be that God gives us these little babies—to hold, to love, and to raise for Him.

SPECIAL COMPLICATIONS

Unfortunately, there are instances in which a decision is made to suddenly end the growth of this child. People blame one another for what has happened. But, amid our grief, let us turn our attention to factors that are generally given little attention: **the effect of this on the mother and her later children.** This is very important, and you will want to read it. We are here discussing the long-term effects, following a medical termination of pregnancy.

First, there is the problem of immediate injuries to the mother:

American sources will not report deaths or injuries due to abortions. The Ohio State Department of Health, for example, reported in May 1977 that "there is no information available as to complications on the abortion procedure . . The reporting on this statistic has been very minimal."

But in Czechoslovakia a very careful study was made and documented. Here it is:

Charles University, in Prague, did thirteen years of research on records of carefully reported abortions. All were performed under the best-possible conditions (generally better than in America) in the gynecology department of a hospital. The limit was set at very "safe" levels: no abortions past the twelfth week (3 months) of pregnancy. The "safest method" was used: vacuum curettage [cutting the baby apart and then sucking out the pieces]. The patient stayed an average of 3 to 5 days in the hospital; and, then, another full week at home (receiving insurance benefits for lost wages). This is what they discovered:

"**Acute inflammatory conditions occur in 5%** of the [abortion] cases, whereas **permanent complications** such as chronic inflammatory conditions of the female organs, sterility, and ectopic [tubal] pregnancies are registered in **20%-30% of all women** [who received abortions] . . these are definitely higher in primagravidas [initial abortions] . . Especially striking is **an increased incidence in later ectopic pregnancies**. A high incidence of cervical incompetence resultant from abortion has raised the incidence of **later spontaneous abortions [miscarriage] to 30%-**

40%. We rather often observe complications such as rigidity of the cervical os, placenta adherens, placenta accreta, and atony of the uterus."—*A. Kodasek, "Artificial Termination of Pregnancy in Czechoslovakia," in International Journal of Gynecology and Obstetrics, 1971, Vol. 9, No. 3.*

Young girls are especially liable to physical damage as a result of abortion operations. One medical expert says that **girls of school age have extra risks** from abortion due to the fact that they have small tightly closed cervixes which are especially liable to damage of dilatation. He says: *"Evidence has accumulated steadily over the past 10 years of increased risks for these young mothers."*—*G.P. Russel, England, Statement made January 10, 1974.*

"Adolescent abortion candidates differ from their sexually mature counterparts, and these differences contribute to higher morbidity [death of the mother]."—*C. Cowell, University of Toronto, Ortho Panel 14.*

"The younger the patient and the further along she is in her pregnancy, the greater the complication rate."—*M. Bulfin, "Deaths and Near Deaths with Legal Abortions," Meeting of the American College of Obstetricians and Gynecologists, Florida, 1975.*

Less well-known, but suspected by the public, is the fact that deaths of mothers from abortion increase with the length of gestation. Abortion in the first eight weeks is the safest; but, **between the ninth and tenth week of pregnancy and onward, the number of deaths to mothers climbs. After 21 weeks, it is even greater.** Using aggregated mortality data, researchers for the Center for Disease Control noted that the abortion death rate increases 40 to 60 percent per week for each week of delay after the eighth week. Abortions performed at 9-10 weeks are nearly three times more dangerous, in terms of deaths, than earlier ones; the small number of abortions performed after 20 weeks' gestation are about 45 times riskier *(CDC, "Morbidity and Mortality Weekly Report," for July 6, 1979).* The main risks result from delay; **the most common complications are bleeding, infection, and injury to the cervix or uterus.** *(See W. Cates, et al., "The Effect of Delay and Method Choice on the Risk of Abortion Morbidity.")*

Another problem is perforation of the uterus:

Horan, et al., in an *Amicus Curiae Brief,* submitted to the Supreme Court in 1971, detailed a list of other damages that could occur to the mother as a result of an abortion. These included **perforation of the uterus; this could result in peritonitis and occasionally death, but more frequently in emergency removal of the uterus.**

Rupture (breaking) of the uterus takes place in 6 percent of all women who become pregnant after hysterectomy abortions. Substantial risk of rupture was obvious in 26% of such women. The babies born to such women tended to be smaller.

In addition, there are a number of problems which may occur in later years. First, there is the problem of premature births:

A woman who has had an abortion is more likely to have premature births thereafter. This is due to the fact that the cervix was cut and weakened by the abortion; so, thereafter, she is not as able to bear up under the weight of a growing child. It will tend to open prematurely instead of trying to bear up under the weight. This results in a number of problems, as we shall see below.

Women who have had abortions **have twice the likelihood of a premature baby later** (*G. Papaevangelou of the University Hospital, Athens, Greece, in British Commonwealth Journal of Obstetrics and Gynecology, 1973*). After just one legal abortion, **the increase of later premature births is 14% more likely**. After two, it is 18%; and, after three, it is 24% (*Klinger, "Demographic Consequences of the Legalization of Abortion in Eastern Europe," International Journal of Gynecology and Obstetrics, September, 1971*).

As mentioned earlier, Czechoslovakia is one of the few countries that has openly investigated the situation and reported all of its findings. Premature births, the aftereffects of previous abortions, are so frequent that if a pregnant woman is known to have had an earlier abortion, she now receives very special care. This is what is done: If the physicians can see scar tissue on the cervix, they will sew the cervix closed [!] in the 12th or 13th week of pregnancy. The patient will then have to stay in bed in the hospital as long as necessary, which in some cases can mean months.

The problem is that **the cervical muscle, the ring muscle between the vagina and the womb, forms the base upon which the placenta, fluid, and growing fetus must rest.** It is the cervix that bears up this continually increasing weight. When an abortion is done, the cervical muscle must be stretched open to allow the surgeon to enter the uterus. But it is "green" (as the doctors call it)—strong, tight and difficult to open. Undoubtedly, in the process, some muscle fibers will be torn and cuts in the muscle wall will be made. In some of these abrasions, the cervix is permanently weakened. In many instances this results in an "incompetent cervix" which will open prematurely in later pregnancies. It is no longer strong enough to hold the heavier weight of a baby in later stages of growth.

Here is a statement from one of the very best hospitals in America:

"In our hospital amongst nulliparous (first pregnancy) patients undergoing suction curettage for therapeutic abortions, **about one in eight required suture [stitches] of the cervix because of laceration** occurring during the process of dilatation."—*R.C. Goodlin, M.D. of Stanford University Hospital, in "Collected Letters of the International Correspondence Society of Obstetricians and Gynecologists," June 15, 1971.*

"Dilatation" occurs when the ring muscle of the cervix is opened up—in abortions, forcibly. Ironically, God has arranged it that in the course of natural events there is no problem. When there is a natural, or spontaneous, miscarriage, the cervix is automatically softened by certain body hormones triggered for this purpose. Also, when a woman who is not pregnant has a D & C for excessive menstruation, the cervix will be soft and easy to work with. The problem is people decide they want to do an abortion when nature says it is not necessary. Then the cervix is hard (because it is the "floor" of the womb and its growing contents); to open it can cause it great damage.

Another problem is later miscarriages:

Spontaneous miscarriages are more common after abortion, and are due to abortion-linked damage of the cervix and uterus.

"If that cervix is injured and this young woman who has undergone a therapeutic abortion has no problems at that time, **there may be problems encountered in future childbearing. She may have repeated spontaneous abortions** due to incompetent cervical Os . . Again, we don't even know yet whether we are causing in these women a situation which might exist for them to have repeated spontaneous miscarriages."—*Kenneth L. Wright, former abortion doctor, testimony before California State Health Department hearing, March 25, 1980.*

"There was a tenfold increase in the number of second trimester miscarriages in pregnancies which followed a vaginal abortion."—*Wright, et al., "Second Trimester Abortion after Vaginal Termination of Pregnancy," in The Lancet, June 70, 1972. (The Lancet is a British medical Journal.)*

Another problem is that of later tubal pregnancies:

Nearly every abortion involves scraping the womb, and many involve cutting up the baby into pieces; in the process, the womb receives cuts also. **A later fertilized egg cannot always locate properly in the walls of such a scarred, damaged womb**; so it fastens to the wall of the mother's tube instead. A few weeks later this will cause an acute abdominal condition because the growing child does not have room to expand. Internal hemorrhaging begins and an emergency operation takes place,—and the tube is removed. (*For more on this, see Amicus Curiae Brief, U.S. Supreme Court, 1971, Horan et al.*)

Still another problem is later sterility:

A large number of the women today who are having abortions are young women who later, after

9 MONTHS

marriage, want to have children and raise a family. **Normally, only about 10% of all marriages will be childless due to sterility. But the situation is greatly changed if an earlier abortion has taken place.** Hilgers and Shearin report that **if a woman has had one legal abortion, the likelihood of permanent sterility thereafter will be increased 10%** *(Hilgers and Shearin, "Induced Abortion, A Documented Report," 1971, p. 30).* Similar reports from Poland, Holland, Russia, Norway, and Japan produce similar statistics.

But, again, the most open and frank confessions come from Czechoslovakia. In 1974, Dr. Bohumil Stipal, Deputy Minister of Health for the nation, said this: **"Roughly 25% of the women who interrupt their first pregnancy have remained permanently childless."** And remember that it is in Czechoslovakia where women receive excellent abortion care in fully staffed, well-equipped hospitals, not in an abortionist's office.

Every mother who is going to receive an abortion should be tested for Rh sensitivity. But much of the time this is not done. A very expensive substance, called *Rhogam*, could be given. But this costs extra money; abortion clinics are notorious for ignoring this matter. The problem here is that **induced abortion, even in the early weeks, can sensitize a mother; so that, in later pregnancies, her babies will have Rh problems**, need transfusions, and occasionally be born dead or die after birth.

Another problem is that of the higher incidence of birth injuries that can result from these premature births:

Czechs have found that the increased number of abortions is resulting in, first, an increased number of premature births. But this is producing a higher percentage of brain injuries at birth. Experts in the field suspect that the outcome of all this is that in countries willing to legalize "abortion-on-demand,"—the number of babies killed by abortion will be offset by **large numbers of defective babies caused by later premature births**, resulting from those earlier abortions.

Another problem is that of brain damage to children who are born later:

"A growing number of children [are] requiring special education because of **mental deficits related to prematurity**."—*"Czechs tighten reins on abortion," in Medical World News, 1973.*

"A growing number of children who are born prematurely must attend special schools because they are not as intelligent as their full term peers."—*Vedra and Zidovsky, in Medical World News, October 12, 1973.*

Still another problem associated with abortion is infant deaths during or concluding later pregnancies:

"Prematurity was a direct or contributory cause in over 50% of deaths during the first month of life. **The death rate of the premature baby ran about thirty times higher** than among full-term infants. If premature infants survive, **they face a higher frequency of the tragic aftermath of mental retardation, neurologic diseases and blindness**."—*Dennis Cavanaugh, M.D., "The Challenge of Prematurity," in Medical World News, February, 1971.*

McDonald and Auro, two researchers in the field, tell us that **the incidence of fetal death during pregnancy and labor is twice the normal amount,** if the mother has had a previous abortion.

Another problem is perforation of the uterus:

Horan, et al., in an *Amicus Curiae Brief,* submitted to the Supreme Court in 1971, detailed a list of other damages that could occur to the mother as a result of an abortion. These included **perforation of the uterus, which could result in peritonitis and occasionally death, but more frequently in emergency removal of the uterus.**

Rupture (breaking) of the uterus takes place in 6 percent of all women who become pregnant after abortions. Substantial risk of rupture was obvious in 26% of such women. The babies born to such women tended to be smaller.

Here are conclusions of other large studies:

A wealth of facts is available—but abortion lobbies and their supporting physicians, hospitals, and clinics would have us believe that an abortion operation is far safer than bringing a child through to birth. But quite the opposite is true. It is political today to be in favor of abortion; but the common decency of telling the truth about what abortion will do to the mother cries to be heard. This statement was published in a medical journal:

"There has been almost a conspiracy of silence in declaring its [abortion's] risks. Unfortunately, because of emotional reactions to legal abortion, well-documented evidence from countries with a vast experience of it receives little attention in either the medical or lay press. This is medically indefensible when patients suffer as a result. For these reasons, we summarize the facts of our experience in this division of Obstetrics and Gynecology. We are proud neither of the number of pregnancies which have been terminated nor the complications described."—*J.A. Stallworthy, et al., "Legal Abortion, A Critical Assessment of Its Risks," in The Lancet, December 4, 1971.*

The above was a report by a British teaching hospital. The statistics of complications to the mothers requesting and receiving abortions was as follows:

• **27% complication rate is due to infection.**

• **9.5% requires blood transfusions in order to survive.**

• **5% of the suction and D & C abortions results in a tearing of the cervical muscle.**

• **1.7% have major perforation.**

"It is significant that some of the more serious complications occurred with the most senior and experienced operators."—*Ibid*. The report concluded with this comment: "[Such complications] are seldom mentioned by those who claim that abortion is safe."—*Ibid*.

Another thorough source of data on this problem comes from the 1969 Survey of the Office of the Prime Minister of Japan. After the abortions were done, the immediate complications were somehow cared for; and the patients went home—this is what happened within the next several years:

• **20% to 30% suffered abdominal pain, dizziness, headaches, and similar problems.**

• **A 400% increase in tubal pregnancies (resulting in death to the fetus and partial sterility to the mother) occurred.**

• **14% had a subsequent pattern of habitual spontaneous miscarriage.**

• **9% were rendered totally sterile.**

• **17% suffered menstrual difficulties and irregularities that they had not had before the abortion took place.**

Next to Czechoslovakia, probably one of the most careful and thorough studies into this problem of abortion-related difficulties was made in England. The *Wynn Report* constitutes one of the most important collections of scientific papers detailing the kind of damage a woman can expect if she elects to have an abortion. Interestingly enough, this exhaustive report of physical and mental complications of induced abortion (in Great Britain and elsewhere) was produced by a group of pro-abortionist doctors. For further details of this study, we refer you to *"Some Consequences of Induced Abortion to Children Born Subsequently [to the abortion],"* by Margaret and Arthur Wynn, Foundation of Education and Research in Child Bearing, in London, 1972.

Lastly, another problem is the effect that this procedure has on the mind:

"The incidence of serious permanent psychiatric aftermath [from abortion] is variously reported as being from **between 9% and 59%**."—*Report of the Council of the Royal College of Obstetricians and Gynecologists, England, 1966.*

Dr. Paul Gebhart was a foremost authority on the subject, due to his extensive research in the field of sexuality and abnormalities related to it. Testifying before the New Jersey legislature in 1968, he said there was evidence of **prolonged psychiatric trauma (mental and emotional damage) in 9%** of a sample of American women who had undergone abortion operations. That is **nearly one woman out of every ten**.

This is due to the fact that **people sense that killing other humans is wrong, whether born or unborn.** Japan is not a Christian nation; yet, in spite of abortion-on-demand for over a third of a century, a majority of women polled knew that it was wrong. A 1963 Aichi survey reported that **73.1% of women who had undergone an abortion procedure felt "anguish" afterward about what they had done.** A very large survey made in 1969 by the Prime Minister's Office reported that 88% of all women in the Japanese nation considered it to be bad. Guilt is a powerful agency keeping happiness from people who otherwise could have it.

We dislike the pain we cause an animal when we kill it, but think of what it must be when abortion doctors cause pain to a small human. During the first three months, they suck him to pieces with a vacuum cleaner; during the second three months, they cut him to pieces with a curved knife; and, during the third three months, they burn him to death with salt!

But, in this section, we have given our attention to the terrible toll on the poor mothers who have accepted the false report of their physicians who told them that what was eliminated is nothing important and doing so is perfectly safe for the mother.

What the mother is not told is the immense profits that physicians, willing to do such a procedure, make each year. They care neither for the baby nor the mother; they only want to rush through as many patients as possible each day, regardless of how many they damage in the process.

9 MONTHS

"Who are those with thee? . . The children which God hath graciously given thy servant."—*Genesis 33:5.*

"Children are an heritage of the Lord: and the fruit of the womb is His reward."—*Psalm 127:3.*

"The babe leaped in my womb for joy."—*Luke 1:44.*

"Behold, I and the children whom the Lord hath given me."—*Isaiah 8:18.*

"Thus saith the Lord, thy redeemer, and He that formed thee from the womb, I am the Lord that maketh all things."—*Isaiah 44:24.*

"Suffer little children, and forbid them not, to come unto Me."—*Matthew 19:14.*

"Thou knowest not what is the way of the spirit, nor how the bones do grow in the womb of her that is with child: even so thou knowest not the works of God who maketh all."—*Ecclesiastes 11:5.*

"Can a woman forget her sucking child, that she should not have compassion on the son of her womb? yea, they may forget, yet will I not forget thee."—*Isaiah 49:15.*

"Teach us what we shall do unto the child that shall be born."—*Judges 13:8.*

"Thy children shall be taught of the Lord."—*Isa 54:13.*

The Natural Remedies Encyclopedia

- Section 21 -
Tumors and Cancer

SPECIAL REPORT: How to Live Longer - page 797

IF YOU SUSPECT CANCER, CONSULT YOUR PHYSICIAN.

Special Note: This section was originally larger; but, after completing it, the author wrote a separate 198 page book on the subject, titled Alternate Cancer Remedies, which is now available. Also see his book, The Gerson Therapy, for additional information.

Although those two books were written for cancer researchers, students of the history of alternative therapy and those wishing to prevent cancer will find that a remarkable number of alternative cancer remedies are available to us.   Also see page 799 of this book for a Special Report.

As with everything else in this series of books, this information on cancer should not be substituted for the advice and treatment of a physician or other licensed health care professional.

FOR MORE NATURAL REMEDIES:
HERBS: Herb Contents (pp. 129-130) will help you locate the 126 most important herbs and the diseases each one can treat. How to prepare herbs (132). How to use them (141-189)
HYDROTHERAPY: Therapy Contents (pp. 206-207) and its Disease Index (263-265) will lead you to over 100 water therapies and many more remedies. DIS. INDEX: 1211- / GEN. INDEX: 1221-

VITAMINS AND MINERALS: Contents (100-101). Using 101-124. Dosages (124). Others (117-)
CARING FOR THE SICK: Home care for a sick person (28-36). The healing crisis (36-39)
WOMEN'S SECTIONS: Female Organs (672) Pregnancy (701). Childbirth (765). Infancy, Childhood (722). Women's Herbs (754, 760)
EMERGENCIES: (973-). FIRST AID: (990-)

C
A
N
C
E
R

Section 21 - TUMORS AND CANCER

TUMORS AND CANCER - 1 - TUMORS

CYSTS AND POLYPS

SYMPTOMS—*In the nose:* chronic difficulty in breathing through the nose.

In the colon: Bleeding or a mucous drainage from the rectum are common symptoms.

In the bladder: Blood in the urine.

In the cervix: A heavy watery, bloody, discharge from the vagina. Bleeding may occur after intercourse, between periods, and after menopause.

CAUSES—Polyps *(polyposis)* are growths of various sizes, and are especially found in certain portions of the mucous membranes: the nose, large intestine (colon), bladder, and cervix. They are especially common in the rectum and the portion of the colon just above that (the sigmoid). They often arise from a diet of **too much unsaturated fatty acids**.

These growths are often benign (not cancerous) and, growing on stalk-like structures, look something like narrow mushrooms. They tend to be hereditary.

Nasal polyps: Generally when the nose is clogged, the cause is a heavy cold or possibly chronic catarrh. But it can be nasal polyps. This is a special kind of tumor which usually forms as a result of a chronic infection in a sinus of a person having allergies. Surgical removal is done to remove them.

Colon and rectal polyps: These growths in the outlet end of the colon can become cancerous. *Familial polyposis* is a hereditary disease in which one hundred or more polyps develop in the colon, generally producing mucous drainage and rectal bleeding. They grow back as soon as they are removed. If they are not removed, colon cancer can result. A colectomy is the surgical removal of these polyps; but it is generally done (not by cutting out the polyps) by removing part of the colon! Sometimes the rectum is left in place and the small intestine is connected to it. But, whether or not this drastic operation is performed, the polyps generally return. Bleeding from the colon can be a sign of polyps or of cancer.

Bladder polyps: The medical route is removal of the bladder. It is important that these polyps be removed, whether by natural means or the standard medical way; because bladder cancer may result if they are not removed.

Cervical polyps: These polyps line the inside of the cervix of the uterus and are more common in women who have not had children. They rarely return after being removed.

Vocal cord polyps: These are caused by screaming or improper singing.

NATURAL REMEDIES

• Cysts are unwanted material in the body that can be dissolved and cleared with the proper use of herbs. Cysts are often caused by a rundown condition of the body where the malfunction is so intense in a specific area that the cell structure gets out of hand and grows additional unneeded lumps or polyps.

• In breaking up a cyst, the use of **walnut herbs (leaves, bark, or the green hull or dried pulp** around the shell of the nut) are excellent. The use of **chaparral** may be used internally or externally.

• A Wisconsin research team discovered that the polyps in most of their patients either lessened or disappeared entirely, when they were placed on a high **vitamin C** diet. The body is attempting to get rid of various waste products; it needs help doing the job. Vitamin C, more **water** drinking, **nutritious food**, and a **high-fiber diet** is needed. Also **eliminate foods that are processed, fried, and junk**. Take some type of supplemental fiber daily. Be sure to increase your water intake at the same time you increase your fiber intake.

• **Stop eating meat** products. They load the body with impurities which must be eliminated. Only eat wholesome food. Stop using **caffeine, tobacco, and alcohol**.

• Those who eat heavily of **saturated fats** are twice as likely to develop polyps. Use **flaxseed oil** instead.

• Spray **bayberry** powder on the growth, leave it on for 6-8 hours; wash away and repeat.

• The following herbs will help cleanse the body of toxins: **garlic, burdock, goldenseal, red clover**.

• Apply these directly to the cysts and polyps: **aloe vera, pau d' arco,** and **pycnogenol gel**.

• **Scrub your skin** with a loofah or dry skin brush regularly, to keep the sebaceous (oil) glands unblocked.

—*Read the sections on Cancer (781-796).*

ENCOURAGEMENT—Throughout the trials of life we have a never-failing Friend. God can do for you what you could never do for yourself. Ask Him for help. How very thankful we can be for peace, perfect peace, even though we are still in this dark world of sin. In the strength of Christ's enabling grace, we can have power to resist all the temptations of the evil one and come off more than conqueror.

C
A
N
C
E
R

TUMORS
(Including Fibroids)

SYMPTOMS—Tumors, swellings, or growths in the body. They seem to contain solid or semifluid material and be abnormal in their growth. This is an abnormal formation of parasitic, non-inflammatory cells or tissue arising from the cells of the host; yet their growth is progressive and independent. Tumors can be malignant or nonmalignant; they can be fast-growing or slow-growing; and they can be in many parts of the body— such as the lymphatic glands or nodes, the urinary and genital areas, or the abdominal structure.

CAUSES—When something has no apparent reason to be growing, it is growing abnormally. These structures are called tumors. They can be either benign or malignant (cancerous). Malignant tumors spread to other parts of the body; whereas benign ones generally do not spread.

Fibroids are tumors which most often occur in the uterus. Hysterectomies are done to remove them. But the effect of a hysterectomy (removal of the uterus) on a woman's hormonal system can be devastating. Avoid it, if at all possible.

Poor diet and environmental factors are special causes of tumors. Changing both can reverse the process and even eliminate these strange growths. It is best to eliminate them, whenever possible. Even the benign ones, although small, may later become cancerous.

NATURAL REMEDIES
See your physician.

• The body uses tumors as containers in which to store toxic waste collected throughout the body, when the system's natural ways of elimination are overloaded: the lungs, bowels, kidneys, liver, and skin. When these channels of elimination become clogged or inadequate to care for the excess refuse, then the body starts manufacturing garbage cans (the tumors) and placing the waste products in them.

• A physician can cut, burn, chemical, or radiate away the garbage can and its contents. But soon the body will manufacture more of them!

• The solution is to change your way of life. A **complete change of diet** is needed, along with **eating smaller amounts** and **improving ways of eliminating waste** from the body.

• Go on a short **liquid diet** to cleanse the system. Follow with a healthful diet of **fruits, vegetables, whole grains, nuts, and legumes. Avoid refined foods, fried foods, and meat**.

• Take **vitamin C** to bowel tolerance.

• Put **slippery elm poultices** or **sage poultices** on external tumors. Drink one or more of the following herb teas: **bayberry, chickweed, sage, slippery elm, or wild yam**.

• Other useful herbs include bayberry, burdock root, celandine, chickweed, coltsfoot, elder flowers, flaxseed, hops, Irish moss, mullein, mugwort, sage, sanicle, tansy, skunk cabbage, slippery elm, walnut leaves and husks (green), wild yam, witch hazel, wood sage, yellow dock.

• Use the same treatment for cancer. *Read the sections on Cancer (below); also Special Reports (815).*

ENCOURAGEMENT—How thankful we can be that we can go to God for help. He who sent His Son to die, so we could have eternal life, can help you.

TUMORS AND CANCER - 2 - CANCER
Also: Chemotherapy and Radiation Poisoning (876)

CANCER

SYMPTOMS—*The most common symptoms of cancer:* any sore that does not heal on the skin, mouth, tongue, or lips. Any irregular or unusual bleeding or discharge from any body opening. A persistent change from normal in the action of the bowels or bladder. Any persistent lump or thickening in breast or anywhere on the body. Hoarseness or nagging cough. Difficulty in swallowing. Persistent indigestion or loss of appetite, especially if accompanied by loss of weight. Sudden or rapid changes in the form, appearance, or rate of growth of a mole or wart, or if it bleeds. Persistent fatigue. Nagging cough or hoarseness.

To the basic eight cancer signs, listed above, can be added three others which are also important: any condition which does not respond to treatment, inflammation from blood clotting (thrombophlebitis), and putrid intestinal gas.

Four basic types of cancer: There are more than one hundred different varieties of cancer. They have different causes, produce different symptoms, and vary in the speed at which they spread. However, most types of cancer fall into one of four broad categories:

Carcinomas—cancers that affect the skin, mucous membranes, glands, and internal organs

Leukemias—cancers of blood-forming tissues

Sarcomas—cancers that affect muscles, connective tissue, and bones

Lymphomas—cancers that affect the lymphatic system

Fifteen most frequent types of cancer:

Skin cancer: A lump under the skin, moles which change color or size and have raised edges, an ulcer which does not heal, flat sores, lesions which look like moles. *See Skin Cancer (787).*

Mouth or throat: Chronic ulcer of the mouth, tongue, or throat which does not heal.

Larynx: Persistent cough and hoarse throat.

Lung: Persistent cough, bloody sputum, and chest pain.

Breast: Lump which is hard, does not go away, and does not move; inflammation or thickening of the skin. *See Breast Cancer (788) for more signs.*

Leukemia: Whiteness of skin, weight loss, fatigue, repeated infections, easy bruising, nosebleeds.

Stomach: Indigestion and pain after eating.

Bladder and Kidney: Blood in urine and increased urination frequency. Bloody urine is generally not a cancer symptom, but it can be.

Ovaries: Usually there are no obvious symptoms until later stages.

Endometrium: Bleeding between menstrual periods, unusual discharge, painful periods, heavy periods.

Cervical and Uterine: Bleeding between periods, unusual discharge, painful periods, heavy periods.

Prostate: Weak or interrupted urine flow. Continuous pain in lower back, pelvis, and/or upper thighs.

Testicles: Enlargement of a testicle, lumps, thickening of the scrotum, sudden excess of fluid in the scrotum, and mild ache in the lower abdomen or groin.

Colon: Blood in stools, rectal bleeding, changes in bowel habits (diarrhea and/or constipation).

Lymphoid Tissue: Enlarged, rubbery, lymph nodes. Also itching, night sweats, unexplained fever, and/or weight loss.

CAUSES—Cancer is now the second most common killer in the United States and steadily increasing. One in every three people will die from some form of it. Over 1,400 Americans die each day with it.

Cancer cells are wild, irregular, and different from other body cells. They grow rapidly and gradually invade and fill surrounding areas. They rob neighboring cells of nutrition, resulting in a gradual wasting away of the patient. They can migrate to new locations and multiply. Wherever they go, there are abnormal growths and tumors.

Cancer cells are classified by the organs they initially invade (liver, breast, colon, lung, lip, etc.). There are more than 100 different varieties of cancer. Each varies in its symptoms and how fast it spreads.

There are four main types of cancer: *Carcinomas* affect the skin, mucous membranes, glands, and other organs. *Leukemias* are blood cancers. *Sarcomas* affect muscles, connective tissue, and bones. *Lymphomas* affect the lymphatic system.

Early detection and treatment is vital. One person dies every 3 minutes from cancer.

Dr. Otto Warburg, Nobel Prize winner, stated: "More is known about the cause and prevention of cancer than most any other disease."

Dr. Ronald Raven, Chairman of the Royal College of Surgeons in London, made this comment: "Seventy-five percent of all cancer can be prevented if we utilize the facts we now possess."

At the Eighth International Cancer Congress, Dr. Kavetsky said: "It is essential in the treatment of tumorous disease, not only to act on the tumor, but to endeavor to strengthen the compensatory and defensive reaction . . of the entire system."

When a cancer becomes noticed, it is already far advanced. By the time a person has reached that stage, it is important that he place himself under the care of a competent physician who understands and uses nutritional therapy. However, he needs to understand, for himself, what is required and what he must do. There are situations in which a cancer victim has no one to help him, and he must carry out such a program entirely on His own.

But, whether helped by others or going it alone, unless the individual fully cooperates with right principles, he cannot successfully be helped. He must cease his violations of the natural laws, given by God to mankind, and live fully in accordance with them.

The type of food we eat, the way we live, and environmental factors gradually build up or weaken the body. If the organs of elimination cannot cope with the amount of toxic waste we are producing, in desperation the body eventually turns to the formation of tumors and cancers. Soft cancers are cells gone wild because of the excess waste in the system. Hard tumors are garbage cans prepared to hold the toxic waste.

Cancer generally has a lengthy incubation period of years. Nourishing the body, building up the immune system, and avoiding excess and debilitating substances enables the body to resist cancer.

Because of intemperate living, eating, sleeping, combined with stress, the body is gradually weakened over a period of many years. This produces a chronic autointoxication. Poisons have accumulated in the body. Vital organs, whose job it is to purify and eliminate wastes (primarily the skin, lungs, liver, kidneys, and bowels), become less active and efficient. The system becomes poisoned. These poisons accumulate around the weakest organs or where the body has been injured by a bruise, fall, or blow. The accumulated poisons from years of tea, coffee, tobacco, cola, meat, liquor, fried food, etc., are sent over to the weakened area. Then the body tries to build garbage cans (tumors), to hold the waste products, or the cells in that area go wild from the irritation and begin multiplying. Either way, eventually the cancer cells spill out and spread. It is well-known that irritation, such as always picking at a certain spot, can induce cancer.

Unfortunately, there are also toxic substances in the air, water, and soil. Chemicals, food additives, pesticides, air pollution, etc., make it all the more crucial that we live as carefully as we can.

Prevention of cancer requires effort; yet many people give more attention to caring for their prize dogs or their new cars. It is far more important, for your future, that you give your body the most careful attention.

Drs. Hans Nieper and Dean Burk stated that, by the time the tumor is present, a patient's malignancy is already far advanced. As noted earlier, a tumor is something of a strange parasite which has as little as 2% of normal blood circulation. Its cells are living on sugar fermentation instead of oxygen as normal cells do. It is more like a plant or fungus.

Here are two interesting facts: (1) The U.S. Government declares that the five-year survival rate from

C
A
N
C
E
R

taking the officially authorized cancer remedies (chemotherapy, surgery, or radiation) has not changed over the past 20 years. (2) Statistics reveal that patients who do not take officially authorized therapy will, as a group, survive longer than those who do. (3) There is only one form of cancer which the medical community is effectively treating, and that is skin cancer. In all other forms, the death rate is extremely high; that is, within five years after authorized treatment, most of the patients die.

A problem with the cut, burn, and poison routes is their deadly nature. Chemotherapy, for example, produces hair loss, extreme nausea, vomiting, fatigue, weakness, sterility. It also damages the liver, kidneys, and heart. Both chemotherapy and radiation treatments are designed to kill cancer cells a little faster than they are killing or weakening other cells. The effect of this greatly debilitates the entire person and his immune system. Reputable natural remedies cancer specialists, such as those at the Gerson Institute, tell us that it is far more difficult to recover a person from cancer who has previously undergone chemotherapy or radiation treatments.

What should you do? That is your decision. Fortunately, you have a right to decide for yourself. However, you should know that the government and the medical association advises that you should never treat yourself for cancer. Their counsel is that you consult a medical doctor (M.D.) and follow his advice. Not to do so, they say, could result in your death.

Cancer has been reported to be badly underdiagnosed. In one autopsy review of those found with malignancies, over half of the deaths were caused by undiagnosed cancer.

Cancer is a systemic disease, affecting the entire body and caused by conditions in the entire person. So it cannot be treated by specifics. An entire change in one's way of life is required.

NATURAL REMEDIES

PREVENTION AND TREATMENT
• It is easier to prevent cancer than to treat it. Many things which prevent it (and *many* are discussed in this article) help safeguard all of us. But, once contracted, some treatments help one person more than another. So prevention is the best way to deal with cancer. Eat right and live temperately.

"About 80% of cancer cases appear to be linked to the way people live their lives. For example, whether or not you smoke, the foods you eat, and certain industrial pollutants all affect your likelihood of getting cancer. The role of diet in the cause and prevention of cancer is particularly important. About 35% of cancer deaths may be associated with dietary influences."—*National Cancer Institute, press bureau, October 1990.*
• The NCI press bureau goes on to list seven things you must do to avoid contracting cancer:
"1. *Avoid obesity:* If you are 40% or more overweight, you increase your risk of colon, breast, prostate, gallbladder, ovary, and uterine cancer.
"2. *Cut down on total fat intake.* High-fat intake may be a factor in the development of certain cancers (particularly breast, colon, and prostate). By avoiding

fatty foods, you are better able to control body weight.
"3. *Eat more high-fiber foods.* These include whole-grain breads and cereals, fruits, vegetables, and legumes (such as dry peas and beans). These foods may help to reduce the risk of colon cancer. Furthermore, high-fiber foods are a wholesome substitution for fatty foods.
"4. *Include foods rich in vitamins A and C.* Favorable foods are dark-green and deep-yellow fresh vegetables and fruits, such as carrots, yams, peaches, and apricots for beta-carotene, the precursor of vitamin A. Also use oranges, grapefruits, strawberries, and green and red peppers for vitamin C. These foods may help lower risk for cancers of the larynx, esophagus, and the lungs.
"5. *Daily intake of cruciferous vegetables.* These are cabbage, broccoli, brussels sprouts, kohlrabi, cauliflower, and others. They have ingredients that build resistance to certain cancers.
"6. *Avoid salt-cured, smoked, or nitrite-cured foods.* Among those who eat these foods frequently, there is more incidence of cancer of the esophagus and stomach.
"7. *Keep alcohol consumption moderate if you must drink.* Heavy use of alcohol, especially when accompanied by cigarette smoking or smokeless tobacco, increases risk of cancers of the mouth, larynx, throat, esophagus, lung, and liver."—*National Cancer Institute, press bureau, October 1990.*

NUTRITION
• The person must return to a good diet and the avoidance of various pollutants and drugs which caused the problem. Anger and hate must be replaced by cheerfulness and happiness.
• Eat a high-fiber, plant-based diet. Take 16-24 oz. of fresh vegetables juice daily. And get regular exercise.
• The best cancer-fighting foods include:
Carotene-rich foods: carrots, yams, green vegetables, tomatoes. This includes all fruits that are red, orange, and yellow.
Antioxidant-rich foods: garlic, onions, broccoli, wheat germ, sea vegetables, and leafy vegetables.
Steamed cruciferous vegetables: broccoli, cabbage, cauliflower, kale.
Protease inhibitors: beans (especially soy), rice, potatoes, corn.
High-fiber foods: whole grains (especially brown rice), fruits, and vegetables.
Lignan foods: Flaxseed oil, walnuts.
• **Broccoli and dark leafy greens** are outstanding foods. They contain *lutein*, which is an anticancer agent. **Broccoli, brussels sprouts, and cauliflower** contain *D-glucaric acid* which reduces various cancers. Research shows that eating high levels of antioxidant foods provides a strong protection against cancer.
• Other very good foods include **apples, berries, Brazil nuts, cherries, legumes** (including **lentils**), **oranges, plums**.
• Daily drink juice from raw **carrots, beets, cabbages,** and a lesser amount of **asparagus**. Raw **garlic** is powerful. Blend in tomato (or V-8) juice and drink. Let

crushed garlic set out (in the air at room temperature) for 10 minutes, before putting it in the juice. This seems to increase its potency. Only drink **distilled water**.

• Eat raw **apricot kernels** daily. If you cannot obtain it, substitute with **almonds, apple seeds, or peach kernals**. They all contain *laetrile*, a cancer-fighting agent.

• Eat a little seaweed daily. Eat **tomatoes**; they contain lycopene, an antioxidant, which protects against cancer.

• **Cherries** (especially tart ones) contain anthocyanins which, by their antioxidant action, prevent cancer and heart disease.

• The only added sweetening should be a little **honey** or **blackstrap molasses**.

• **Soybeans** contain *genistein* and *diadzein*, two isoflavones which are antioxidants and protect against most forms of cancer.

FOODS TO AVOID
• Do not eat any kind of **meat**.
• Do not eat **dairy products, salt, sugar, peanuts, or white flour. No processed, refined, junk, or fried foods**. The chloride in salt is the problem. **Milk** contains saturated fat. **Milk sugar** *(lactose and galactose)* can cause ovarian cancer.
• Do not use **aluminum cooking utensils**; instead use stainless steel (or glass in the oven).

NUTRIENTS
• Nutritional supplements would include:
• **Vitamin C:** 3,000-12,000 mg daily, in divided dosages.
• **Vitamin E:** 400-800 IU daily.
• **Flaxseed oil:** 2 tsp. 3 times daily, because of its lignan and high omega-3 content.
• **Carotene complex:** 50,000-100,000 IU daily.
• **Coenzyme Q_{10}:** 150-300 mg daily.
• **Vitamins C and E** decrease the oxidation of body fats. **Vitamin B_6** (inositol) helps prevent and shrink tumors. **Niacin** has a similar effect. **Calcium** is a preventive factor against cancer. **Selenium** (not over 200 mcg daily) is also helpful.
• Do not take supplemental **iron**. It encourages the growth of cancer cells.

HERBS
• *Cancer-fighting herbs* include **pau d'arco** tea (4 cups daily), garlic (6-10 cloves, daily), **ginseng, licorice root. Comfrey** is good; but it should only be applied externally.
• **Essiac tea** has been used for decades, in Canada and more recently the U.S. and Europe, to eliminate cancer.
• **Citrus pectin** inhibits growth of cancer cells; it is especially useful against skin and prostate cancers.
• **Ojibwa herbal tea** is used to reduce cancer. This American Indian combination includes **burdock root, slippery elm bark, sheep sorrel, and turkey rhubarb root.**
• *Herbs which increase immune function* and have antitumor factors are **olive leaf extract and ginkgo biloba**. Also included in this list is **cat's claw** (but not to be used during pregnancy).

• *Antioxidant herbs* include **turmeric**. It contains *curcuma*, which helps protect against cancer and inhibit growth of cancer cells.

• *Herbs which reduce the effects of chemotherapy and radiation:* Alternate the following: **Astragus, echinaciea / goldenseal root capsules, burdock root, chaparral, dandelion, milk thistle, red clover, birch, suma**,

AVOID
• Avoid **synthetic hormones**, particularly **estrogen, X-rays, alcohol**, and **caffeine. And avoid tobacco** in all forms.
• Avoid dangerous chemicals, such as are found in **insecticides** (an important cause of cancer), **fresh paints, cleaning compounds, hair sprays, waxes, cosmetics**. And beware of **ingredients in auto products, art and craft supplies, pet supplies, foods and beverages**.
• **Medicinal drugs and street drugs** are additional sources of trouble. Regular exposure to **secondhand smoke** can increase a nonsmoker's chance of getting cancer by 30%.
• Keep your weight down. **Obesity** in men can contribute to colon and rectal cancer; in women, it has been linked to gallbladder, breast, cervical, and uterine cancer. Fat disrupts the level of sex hormones in the body. The greater the amount of a woman's body fat, the higher will be her levels of stored estrogen. Estrogen stimulates breast and reproductive cells to divide.
• **Tap water** contains chlorine, fluorine, and may contain radium. **Fluoride**, a risk factor for cancer, is in toothpaste, tap water, and every product made with tap water. Therefore, as mentioned earlier, only drink distilled water.
• Check the **radon** level in your home. Test kits for this radioactive gas can be purchased. If found, seal lower cracks, and increase upper ventilation to the outside.
• Do not sit close to **TV screens**, and do not use **microwave ovens**. Both produce radiation. If you sit at a **computer**, install a quality radiation screen.
• Avoid living or working near a high-voltage power line; it may induce cancer.

OTHER HELPS
• Especially for cancer of the internal organs, get some **sunlight** on the body every day possible. It reduces the risk of breast, colon, and prostate cancers.
• **Exercise** regularly outdoors. No healing program will succeed without some exercise.
• If you are able to do so, move to a **rural home** where the air is fresh and not polluted with auto and factory pollutants.
• **Breast-fed children** have a lower rate of leukemia.

SAMPLE RESEARCH STUDIES

Research studies have found many factors which lead to the formation of cancer. Here are a couple samples:

• A 12-year research study of more than 5,000 vegetarians and over 6,000 meat eaters found that **vegetarian diets** reduce risk of death from all causes, including cancer. People who ate no meat had a 40% lower risk of dying from cancer and a 20% lower risk than meat eaters dying from any cause. (Margaret Thorogood, Ph.D., coauthored the study.)

• A Harvard follow-up study of nearly 48,000 men, aged 40-75, found that **fat** helps tumors grow more quickly. A diet as low as possible in saturated fat was recommended. The leading sources of saturated fats are **beef, pork, processed meats, whole milk, dairy products, and fats and oils (such as butter, margarine, and mayonnaise)**.

• It has repeatedly been found that eating meat fat is a cause of cancer. But a Harvard study found that even eating **red meat** (with much less fat content) was also dangerous. A 6-year study of almost 90,000 women found that those who ate red meat as a main dish each day were 2½ times more likely to have colon cancer than those who seldom, or never, ate meat. Other studies revealed that frequent consumption of meat is also associated with an increased risk of breast cancer, according to Harvard School of Public Health.

It is remarkable how many natural remedies there are! Here are but a few samples, from among many which could be cited, which either prevent or eliminate various forms of cancer:

• A recent study of a group of Seventh-day Adventists found that men who ate at least five **tomatoes** a week had a 40% lower risk of developing prostate cancer. It is believed that a pigment (lycopene) found in tomatoes is the key factor. It is chemically similar to beta-carotene in carrots, which is also a cancer fighter *(Edward L. Giovannucci, M.D., Harvard Medical School)*.

• Forty-four cats were given a feline leukemia virus so lethal that, once cats develop clinical symptoms, 70% are dead within 8 weeks and the rest soon after. **Acemannan**, found in **aloe vera** and a potent immunostimulant, was then injected into the cats for 6 weeks and then reexamined 6 weeks later. By that time, 71% of the cats were alive and in good health *(Molecular Biotherapy, 3(1):41-5, 1991)*.

• **Berberine**, found in **goldenseal, oregon grape root, goldthread, and barberry root bark**, has been used in China, since 1972, in the treatment of cancer. Several research studies have found that berberine shows potent antitumor activity against brain, and other, tumors. Three studies could be cited. *(One is from Chinese Medical Journal, 103(3):658-65, 1990.)*

• **Bromelain** (the proteolytic enzyme in pineapple), when added to the diet, decreased metastases in lung cancers. Six studies could be cited. *(One is Cancer Investigation 6(2):241-2, 1988.)*

• **Chaparral** (creosote bush) is an evergreen desert shrub. Its primary anticancer chemical is a potent antioxidant. Research studies reveal that, when used with care, this plant reduces tumors. Attention to chaparral for this purpose began in 1969, when a man with a known malignant melanoma of the right cheek (with large metastasis) treated himself for a year with chaparral tea *(Cancer Chemotherapy Report, 53:147-51, 1969)*.

• **Chlorella**, a green algae that grows in freshwater, was added to the diet of 21 patients treated for malignant brain tumors. Two years after treatment, 7 patients were alive and showing no reappearance of their tumors *(Phytotherapy Reports 4(6):220-31, 1991)*.

• **Coumarin** is a component of several anticancer herbs (including dong quai, sweet clover, and red clover). Eight studies could be cited, which demonstrate its ability to shrink and eliminate cancers *(one study is Molecular Biotherapy, 3:170-8, 1991)*. (Note: Coumarin should not be confused with coumadin, also known as warfarin; this is rat poison, used to thin the blood).

• An extract of **echinacea** was given to patients, who were actively receiving massive doses of medical cancer drugs. Patients generally lived longer than they otherwise would have; some did not die. Four studies could be cited. *(One is Cancer Investigation 10(5):343-8.)*

• Remarkable rates of death to cancer cells were experienced by patients receiving **garlic**. Seventeen studies could be cited *(one is Journal National Cancer Institute, 81(2):162-4, 1989)*. Garlic appears to exert its effects by "direct action on tumor cell metabolism, inhibition of the initiation and promotion phase of cancer, and modulation of the host immune response" *(Nutritional Reports, 10-937-48, 1990)*.

• LaPacho, a tree in Brazil, also known as **pau d' arco** or tahebo, has a long history of use by Brazilians in the treatment of cancer. The major active component is *lapachol*. Four studies could be cited (one is Revista do Instituto de Antibioticos, 20:61-8, 1980/81, in which all 9 patients experienced a shrinkage of tumors.) Note: Two Canadian studies revealed that many commercially sold pau d'arco products contained no *Iapachol* (Canadian Health Protection Branch: Information Letter, 726, August 13, 1987).

• **Mistletoe** has been widely used in Europe for cancer therapy. They are injected because they are not absorbed if taken orally. Seven reports could be cited. *(One is Journal Ethnopharmacol, 29:35-41, 1990.)*

• Chinese or Korean **ginseng** is another inhibitor of cancer development. Nine studies could be cited. *(One is Biotherapy, 4(2):117-28, 1992.)*

• An extract of a **seaweed** (Undaria pinnantifida) stimulates immunological processes, including macrophage activity and antitumor effectiveness *(Cancer Letter, 50:71-8, 1990)*.

• **Shiitake mushrooms** are an important part of Japanese diets; they are well-known for their protection against cancer. One of its components, lentinan, is used in cancer treatment in that nation. But it must be injected. Four studies could be cited. *(One is Cancer Detection Previews [supplement], 1:333-49, 1987.)*

• **Turmeric** and its major active component, *curcumin*, exerts powerful antioxidant effects; it is helpful in the treatment of cancer, according to three studies. *(One is Cancer Letter, 29:197-2002, 1985.)*

See your physician.

ENCOURAGEMENT—Life is difficult and we cannot always see what the future will hold; but, if our trust is in God, we can have the assurance that He will care for us, regardless of what may happen. "He that hath the Son, hath life." 1 John 5:12. "The meek shall inherit the earth; and shall delight themselves in the abundance of peace." Psalm 37:11.

SKIN CANCER
(Melanoma)

SYMPTOMS—Identification is especially important in dealing with skin cancer. *Here are official warning signs of skin cancer:*

1. An open sore that bleeds, crusts over, and will not heal properly.

2. A reddish, irritated, spot that is usually on the chest, shoulder, arm, or leg. It may itch, hurt, or cause no discomfort at all.

3. A smooth growth with an elevated border and a center indentation. As it becomes bigger, tiny blood vessels develop on the surface.

4. A shiny scar-like area that may be white, yellow, or waxy. It has a shiny, taut appearance.

5. An enlarging, irregular, "angry" appearing lesion on the face, lips, or ears.

Here is a description of one of the more common types of skin cancer: large flat, tan, or brown spots, with darker black or brown areas dotted on its surface. The edges may, or may not, be clearly defined. The spot may appear mottled.

Moles should also be watched—especially those that change in size or color, are irregularly shaped, have ridges around the edges, widen, bleed, itch, or seem to be continually irritated by clothing.

Here are still more identifiers of skin cancer—the so-called "A-B-C-D checklist":

Asymmetry: Both sides of the mole should be shaped similarly. If the overall shape is irregular, then it might be skin cancer.

Border: The edges of moles should be smooth, not blurred or ragged.

Color: It should be tan, brown, or dark brown if it is normal. If it is not, it is red, white, blue, or black.

Diameter: Any mole that is larger than 1/4 inch, in diameter, or its diameter seems to be increasing, should be treated with suspicion.

CAUSES—Skin cancer is called melanoma, or *lentigo-maligna melanoma;* it appears on body surfaces which are most frequently exposed to the sunlight: the face, neck, arms, and trunk. It can also occur on the lips and even eyelids.

The best thing about skin cancer is that it is often slow in spreading and invading the deeper layers of the skin. As long as the cancer is only on the surface,

it can easily be removed.

There are three types of skin cancer: The first two are the most common; the third is the most dangerous. Yet all three types can be eliminated if treated early. The medical route or natural methods can be used to eliminate each of these. But, either way, be sure it is gone. As long as it is treated early, you can easily see if it is gone.

Basal cell carcinoma: This is the most common type, the slowest growing. It does not spread until it has been present for a number of years. It is an ulcer-like growth which spreads very slowly. The first sign is a large pearly lump, generally on the face, nose, or area around the eyes. About six weeks later, it becomes an ulcer with a moist center and a hard border which may bleed. Scabs continually form; then they drop off. But there is no healing of the ulcer. Another form is flat sores which slowly widen. Treatment is the same as for squamous cell cancer.

Squamous cell carcinoma: Due to damage to lower-skin surface, a lump forms on the skin. Looking like a wart or a nonhealing ulcer, physicians cut it off, freeze it off, chemical it off, or irradiate it off. A skin graft may be applied afterward.

Melanoma: This is the most dangerous of the three; and it can run in families. It often begins as what appears to be a mole. Most people have moles; but be especially beware of those which appear after the age of 40. Any mole that is unusual or that changes in size or color should be eliminated. If in doubt, see a physician!

A melanoma mole arises out of the deeper pigment layer of the skin. For this reason, it spreads more quickly. Melanomas most frequently occur on the upper back and legs. But they may also occur on mucous membranes or under the nails.

A fourth type of skin cancer is ***actinic*** (solar) ***keratoses***. These appear to be age spots on the neck, head, or back of the hands. But eventually 25% of them become cancerous. *See Actinic Keratoses (355).*

A fifth type is the rare ***mycosis fungoides***. For years there will be itching skin lesions. Eventually they become firm and begin ulcerating. Later they involve the lymph nodes and produce cancer of the lymph (lymphoma).

Over 600,000 Americans develop skin cancer each year; and 10,000 die of it. More than 90% of skin cancers can easily be eliminated, if done early.

NATURAL REMEDIES
See your physician.
• Wear **protective clothing** when out in the sun. Exposure to the sun is vital to good health. Unfortunately, the ultraviolet rays also cause wrinkles and 90% of all types of skin cancer. (It can cause cataracts too.) Yes, continue to get out in the sunlight; but try not to overdo it. Keep in mind that, in the early stages, it is not difficult to remove skin cancers; but you have to have a certain amount of sunlight for general physical health.

Be especially careful between 10 a.m. and 2 p.m., when sunlight is strongest. Those with a family history of skin cancer should obtain their sunlight more sparingly. In the summer, wear light-colored clothing which has a tight weave. Consider using a sunscreen of at least 15. As the **ozone layer** is gradually destroyed over the north and south poles, those living in the temperate zones throughout the world become more susceptible to skin cancer—without even being in the sun.

• **Tanning salons** and **sunlamps** are more dangerous than sunlight, because people tend to overdo them.

• Every month or so check over your body carefully and look for signs of skin cancer. Then do something about it.

Suggestions for eliminating skin cancer:

You can **go to your physician**; and he will excise it with a knife or an ointment which will burn it off. If you delay, surgery will cut more deeply; and, as with all cancer surgery, there is the very real danger that not all the cancer will be removed.

• Or you can use natural remedies. Fortunately, with skin cancer, as long as it is treated in the early stages, you can tell if it is gone!

• **Garlic** is a faithful standby. Cut a thin slice of garlic and carefully tape it over, what you consider might be, a skin cancer. Try to avoid contact of the garlic on good skin. (If you can't avoid it, the skin will redden and burn somewhat.) Russian research, from back in the 1950s, revealed that garlic is more powerful than antibiotics in destroying bacteria. It also causes moles and skin cancers to fall off. In the morning, put on the garlic patches; take them off in the evening, before bedtime, and carefully wash the area. Put on a new application. Remove it in the morning; and repeat the process. Do this for about 3 days. The mole or ulcer will dissolve and slough off. Let the area heal. If part of it remains, repeat the process at a later time. If you continue applying the garlic for more than 4 days, it will begin burning deeper into the skin (you will know, because the area will become very painful.) Such deep burning is not necessary to slough off the cancer; it could be harmful.

• The herb, **chaparral**, works well for skin cancer. Take it as a tea or in tablet form. Also good is **burdock root and red clover** tea.

• According to a 1988 medical article (*British Journal of Surgery*), eating an adequate amount of essential **fatty acids** helps protect the body against skin cancers. It even helps eliminate them, once they form.

• Get enough **rest**. Temperate living helps your body resist and throw off cancerous lesions.

• Eat a **nourishing diet,** including **leafy greens**. Green, orange, and yellow vegetables are important. The diet should be **high in antioxidants** (such as **broccoli, brussels sprouts, kale, cabbage, carrots**). It is important that you **reduce your fat intake**. Instead, take 2 tablespoons flaxseed oil daily.

• **Stop eating meat and foods that are processed, fried, sugary, and junk.** Stop smoking and drinking, including the drinking of caffeine or eating caffeine products.

• Take **vitamin C** to bowel tolerance; also take **vitamin A** and **selenium**. Eat a few **apricot kernals** daily.

• Apply a **goldenseal / myrrh** solution to the affected areas.

• **Carcelim** is a cream which you can purchase; with this, it requires 30 days to remove the melanoma. Apply **tea tree** oil cream to the area.

—*Read the sections on Cancer (782-796).*

ENCOURAGEMENT—Take your problems to God; for He can help you know what to do. He can lead you to solutions which are the best. Psalm 34:18.

BREAST CANCER

SYMPTOMS—*The most common type:* Lumps are firm, do not go away, and are generally pain free. Lumps which do not move around may be malignant or may not be. *In another type:* There is itching, redness, and soreness of the nipple. *In yet a third type:* The breast becomes extremely tender and appears infected with something.

All three are explained in more detail below.

CAUSES—Breast cancer is a leading cause of malignant death among women in the United States. Women over forty are more likely to develop breast cancer than younger women. Lung cancer kills about 56,000 women in America each year; breast cancer is responsible for the death of about 46,000.

It is vital that early detection be made. Discussions of how to carry out breast self-examination are readily available elsewhere and need not be repeated here. As you conduct it, watch for subtle changes in the breast. You are looking for special types of lumps in the breast. These lumps are firm, do not go away, and are generally pain free. Lumps which do not move around may be malignant or may be caused by normal fibrocystic changes during the menstrual cycle. The experts say a biopsy will detect what kind of lump it is.

But you should know that biopsies can be dangerous. A *biopsy* is a slice of the tissue which is then sent to a lab for microscopic examination. The problem is that slicing any suspected tissue—immediately releases its cancer (if any is present) into the body, where it can more rapidly spread. Whether or not you choose to have a biopsy made someday, you should be aware of this fact.

There are several different types of breast cancer. Most of them are similar, producing lumps described above. But a few are different:

Paget's disease of the nipple affects the nipple; it cannot be detected by a self-examination. Cancer cells have migrated to the nipple. The symptoms are itching, redness, and soreness of the nipple. This form of cancer only occurs when a different form of cancer is present elsewhere in the breast tissue.

Inflammatory carcinoma is a different type. The skin thickens and turns red. The breast becomes extremely tender and appears infected with something. The lymphatic system and blood vessels have become clogged because of a tumor. This type of cancer spreads very rapidly. Professionals recommend a biopsy; but, if you choose not to do so, you must be planning to go on an intense natural remedies cleansing, to eliminate the problem. Whatever you do, you had better set to work and do it.

It is well to keep in mind that many people have undergone the orthodox cancer routine of surgery, chemotherapy, or radiation; some have survived while others have died. There are many who have taken the natural remedies route, with the same end results; some have lived and others have died. No one can, or ought to, decide what you should do; the decision is yours.

NATURAL REMEDIES
See your physician.

IMPORTANT FACTS
• In the late 1980s, researchers discovered that women develop breast cancer far more frequently in certain localities than in others. Analyzing those locations, it was discovered that they are those areas where there tends to be **less sunlight** throughout the year. For example, northwestern California, the western slopes of Oregon and Washington, and the Northeast had a far greater number of breast cancer cases than did Florida, Texas, Arizona, and southern California. The solution: **Take sunbaths** from time to time, throughout the year; sunlight is important for maintaining good health, purifying the body, and resisting infection.

• Breast cancer more often occurs in women who previously **started menstruation early** in their youth, had a **late menopause**, **gave birth later in life**, had a **family history** of breast cancer, developed **obesity after menopause**, and had a history of **alcoholism** and eating a **high-fat diet**.

• Research indicates that those who take **oral contraceptives** are 3 times more likely to develop breast cancer. **Silicone** (used in breast implants) causes cancer in test animals. Those who develop breast cancer, and other cancers, have **less vitamin A** in their bodies.

WHAT TO DO
• Eat a **nutritious diet** centered around **fresh fruits and vegetables, whole grains, and nuts**. Eat **garlic and onions**. Drink **distilled water** and **fresh fruit and vegetable juices**.

• Get **extra fiber** in your diet. Studies have shown that breast disease is associated with poor intestinal health, constipation, and low-fiber diets. Fiber also dramatically reduces estrogen levels in a woman's body; and estrogen is a significant causative factor in this disease.

• Take **coenzyme Q_{10}**, as well as full **vitamin-mineral supplementation**. Take 40 IU of vitamin E daily. Low levels of B12 are linked to an increased risk.

• Cancer thrives in an oxygen-poor environment. Gradually build up until you are **walking** 2 miles, 4 times a week. Women who exercise outdoors have a lower incidence of this disease.

• Do not eat too much **soy or peanut products**. Do not eat **meat or dairy products. No alcohol, caffeine, or nicotine. No processed, fried, white-flour, and junk foods**. Do not eat **sugary foods**. Do not take supplements containing **iron**. There is a clear link

between drinking **alcohol** and breast cancer. Cut total **fat consumption** to 20% of total calorie intake. **Birth control pills, X-rays,** and **permanent dark hair dyes** increase the likelihood of later breast cancer.

• Herbs useful in cleansing the blood and liver include **red clover, milk thistle, and burdock root**. **Silymarin**, an antioxidant extract of milk thistle, is being used to reduce breast cancer.

• **Wearing a bra** for more than 12 hours a day increases the likelihood of breast cancer. That discovery resulted from interviews with over 4,000 women. A woman who never wears a bra is 21 times less likely to get breast cancer than a woman in the general population. Avoid bras with stiffening wires; they are the worst.

• You should **examine your breasts regularly**. Procedures for doing this, and what to watch for, are discussed in many books. You will be able to detect initial changes better than anyone else.
—*Read the sections on Cancer (782-796).*

ENCOURAGEMENT—Take all your problems to God in prayer. He can wonderfully change the most hopeless outlook. And whatever happens will be for the best, if we are trusting in Him. Psalm 147:3.

PROSTATE CANCER

SYMPTOMS—Possible pain or burning sensation during urination, frequent urination, a decrease in the size and force of urine flow, inability to urinate, blood in the urine, and continuing lower-back or pelvic discomfort just above the pubic area. But there may be no symptoms until an advanced stage or until the cancer spreads out beyond the prostate.

Many, many, times the above symptoms point to a benign enlargement of the prostate and not cancer in that organ.

CAUSES—The prostate is a walnut-sized gland at the base of the bladder and encircles the urethra, the tube through which the bladder voids urine. The prostate makes prostatic fluid which nourishes the sperm.

Prostate cancer is the second leading cause of cancer deaths in American men. **Poor diet, exposure to environmental toxins and cancer-causing chemicals, and overactivity of the sexual organs** are possible causes. There is a link between a **high-fat diet** and prostate cancer. It is believed, by some, that a **vasectomy** may increase the likelihood that this problem will later develop.

Men over 65 have 80% of the cases of prostate cancer; and 80% of 80-year-old men have it. The incidence is higher among married men and African-Americans. It is lowest among Asian-Americans.

The younger a man is, when he is diagnosed with prostrate cancer, the worse the outlook. Those with recurring prostate infections are at greater risk. Men whose ancestors had prostate cancer are more likely to develop it.

A careful, but relatively simple, rectal examination

C
A
N
C
E
R

can reveal if cancer is developing in this organ. There are also other screening methods; and PSA (prostate-specific antigen) appears to be the best. The PSA test should be taken twice if there is an indication of cancer.

The prostate glands of many men in their 70s are gradually enlarging. Having an operation can damage the ability to urinate and cause incontinence (25% of the time), resulting in much difficulty later. Fortunately, prostate cancer is slow growing. "Watchful waiting" is the method used in Europe. However, invasive prostate cancer is rapidly increasing worldwide. This deadly form rapidly engulfs the organ and spreads throughout the body; it is noticeably increasing among men in their 40s and 50s in all industrialized countries. Western diet, chemicals, and living is a major problem. There are natural remedies which can help.

An enlarged prostate can become cancerous; but, fortunately, it always proceeds very, very slowly. So slowly, in fact, that an operation to remove the prostate, because of cancer, is generally not needed. This is because, before the man is likely to die of prostate cancer, he is quite aged and dies of something else first. But, of course, you will want to consult your medical specialist.

—*Also see Cancer (782), Enlarged Prostate (668), and Prostatitis (670); also Special Report (815).*

NATURAL REMEDIES
Contact your physician.
• Go on a program with a **nourishing diet, vitamin and mineral supplementation, and outdoor exercise**.
• Make the diet rich in **vegetables**. Drink **fresh fruit and vegetable juices** daily. **Carrot, beet, cabbage juices** are especially good; they are used in cancer clinics worldwide. Only drink distilled water.
• **Do not eat meat**. There is a definite correlation between red meat consumption and prostate cancer. **Avoid processed and junk foods, saturated fats, dairy products, coffee, tea, alcohol, tobacco, tobacco smoke, food additives**.
• **Vitamins C and E, zinc, selenium, flaxseed oil** are important in avoiding and reducing this disease.
• Researchers gave 15 patients with advanced prostate cancer 600 mg, daily, of oil-based **coenzyme Q$_{10}$**; a year later, cancer had been reversed in 10 patients and stopped in 4 others.
• In one study of hundreds of men, a daily intake of 200 mg **selenium** reduced prostrate cancer incidence by 60%.
• **Saw palmetto** herb shrinks prostate tissue. Take 80 mg 2 times daily, plus 25 mg daily of **pygeum africanum**. Both inhibit the DHT form of testosterone. Another herb that may reduce prostate swelling is **pipsissewa** tincture (25 drips, 3 times daily).
• Other helpful herbs include **turmeric, echinacea, goldenseal, pau d'arco, and buchu**.
• **Exercise** is a must for men dealing with this disease, plus early morning **sunlight**
• The risk of prostate cancer is three times greater for men who have had **vasectomies**.
—*Read the sections on Cancer (782-796) for additional information. Also see Enlarged Prostate (668) and Prostatitis (670); also Special Reports (815).*

ENCOURAGEMENT—No friend can help us as wonderfully as God can. Go to Him in prayer and ask for His help. Trust your life to Him and believe that He will work everything out for the best.

LUNG CANCER

SYMPTOMS—A persistent cough, chest pain, shortness of breath, wheezing, sputum with blood, hoarseness, fatigue, recurring bronchitis or pneumonia, weight loss, swelling of face and neck.

CAUSES—This is the most common form of cancer that kills both men and women. The average age at diagnosis is 60. Nearly 200,000 people die of lung cancer yearly. Because early symptoms are not noticed, most cancers are advanced before they are discovered; so only 12% of cases recover. The rest die.

There are two types: small-cell (oat cell) and large-cell lung cancer. The small-cell type, commonly found in smokers, grows rapidly and quickly spreads to other parts of the body. About 75% of lung cancers are of the large-cell type.

Smoking is the leading cause of both types of lung cancer. But some contract the disease through **smoking marijuana and breathing secondary smoke. Lung cancer is also caused by exposure to nickel, asbestos, chromates, arsenic compounds, radon, pesticides, pollution, or radioactive substances**. Other factors include **drinking alcohol, tuberculosis, chronic bronchitis, lung scarring from pneumonia, exposure to talcum powder, and deficiency or excess of vitamin A**.

NATURAL REMEDIES
Contact your physician.
• Immediately **eliminate tobacco and alcohol** from your house and workplace.
• Eat a diet rich in **fresh fruits, vegetables, whole grains, nuts, and legumes**.
• Take **vitamins C, E, B complex, and beta-carotene**, as well as **selenium, lutein, lycopene, genistein**, and glutathione. Genistein is found in soybeans, lentinan in shiitake mushrooms.
—*Also read the sections on Cancer (782-796).*
ENCOURAGEMENT—The blessings of God are more than the hairs of our head, more than the sands of the seashore. Meditate upon His love and care for us; and may it inspire you with love that trials cannot interrupt nor afflictions quench.

BLADDER CANCER

SYMPTOMS—Early symptoms do not usually appear. The first indication is generally blood in the urine. Other symptoms may be increased urination, pain and burning during urination, or difficulty in urinating.

CAUSES—**Smoking** is the leading cause. **Breathing or ingesting chemicals** is another. Such chemicals include **aniline dyes, benzidines, saccharin, sucaryl,**

insecticides, medicinal drugs, street drugs, radiation exposure, and urinary tract infections. It is also caused by **working in the rubber, chemical, leather, or dye industries.** Previously sick with **schistosomiasis**, a tropical disease, will also cause this.

NATURAL REMEDIES
Contact your physician.
• Drink a lot of **liquids** (including fresh **carrot, cabbage, beet, and fruit juices**). Such a program continually cleans out the bladder, so it can recover from the illness.
• Research studies have found that eating **broccoli, brussels sprouts, cabbage, kale, and cauliflower** help lower the risk of this disease. Eating **fruits of various kinds** also reduces it. The same diet should also be eaten during the disease.
• Take vitamins C, A, a B-complex supplement, plus beta-carotene. DMSO also helps reduce the cancer.
• Do not eat **meat, junk, fried, or processed foods.**
—*Also read the sections on Cancer (782-796).*
ENCOURAGEMENT—If you have given yourself to God, to do His work, you have no need to be anxious for tomorrow. He, whose servant you are, knows the end from the beginning. The events of tomorrow, which are hidden from your view, are open to the eyes of Him who is omnipotent.

When we take into our hands the management of things with which we have to do, and depend upon our own wisdom for success, we are taking a burden which God has not given us and are trying to bear it without His aid. We are taking upon ourselves the responsibility that belongs to God, and thus are really putting ourselves in His place. We may well have anxiety and anticipate danger and loss; for it is certain to befall us. But when we really believe that God loves us and means to do us good, we shall cease to worry about the future. We shall trust God as a child trusts a loving parent. Then our troubles and torments will disappear; for our will is swallowed up in the will of God.

Christ has given us no promise of help in bearing today the burdens of tomorrow. He has said, "My grace is sufficient for thee"; but, like the manna given in the wilderness, His grace is bestowed daily, for the day's need. Like the hosts of Israel in their pilgrim life, we may find morning by morning the bread of heaven for the day's supply.

One day alone is ours; and, during this day, we are to live for God. For this one day we are to place in the hand of Christ, in solemn service, all our purposes and plans, casting all our care upon Him, for He careth for us. "I know the thoughts that I think toward you, saith the Lord, thoughts of peace and not of evil."

SYMPTOMS—Rectal bleeding, blood in the stool, gas pains, constipation, persistent bloating, abdominal tenderness or pain. Changes in bowel habits, anemia, significant weight loss, ulcerative colitis, unusual fatigue, or paleness.

CAUSES—This is the second most common form of cancer that kills both men and women; it primarily occurs in people over 50 (about 20% of all cancer deaths in the U.S.). The large intestine contains the colon (the upper 5-6 feet) and the rectum (the last 6-8 inches).

This cancer develops over a period of 10-15 years; it produces no symptoms until it is advanced.

It is far more prevalent in the Western world, where people eat lots of **meat** and **dairy products**; it is much lower among people groups which primarily eat grains, vegetables, and fruits. A diet rich in meat and **fat**, and **low in vegetables and fiber,** helps this cancer develop. Other factors include **obesity, alcohol, tobacco, and cancer elsewhere in the body.** A **lack of exercise** is also a factor. You are more likely to contract it if you have had **inflammatory bowel disease**.

A diet of meat and fat also encourages the growth of colon polyps, which can become cancerous.

If the disease is detected early enough and the tumor has not metastasized (spread), the survival rate is high.

NATURAL REMEDIES
Contact your physician.
• Eat a **high-fiber diet of fruits and vegetables, citrus fruits, soybeans, whole-grains** (especially **brown rice**). Broccoli, cabbage, dark leafy greens, and raw **garlic** are excellent.
• Take **vitamins C, E, folic acid** (800 mcg daily), **beta-carotene, calcium, and the B complex. Quercetin**, one of the **bioflavonoids**, has been found to also have anticancer properties.
• **Do not eat meat or even unsaturated fats.** Avoid **charbroiled, burned, wood-smoked, or fried foods.** Do not drink **coffee** or **chlorinated water.** Avoid **vitamin D** and **iron** supplements.
• Obtain adequate outdoor **exercise.**
—*Also read the sections on Cancer (780-797).*
ENCOURAGEMENT—We are living in altogether too solemn a period of the world's history to be careless and negligent. You must pray, believe, and obey. In your own strength you can do nothing; but in the grace of Jesus Christ, you can employ your powers in such a way as to bring the greatest good to your own soul and the greatest blessing to the souls of others. Lay hold of Jesus and you will diligently work the works of Christ and finally receive the eternal reward.

COLON CANCER
(Colorectal Cancer)

CERVICAL CANCER
(Uterine, Endometrial Cancer)

SYMPTOMS—No symptoms until the disease has progressed quite a bit. Bleeding between menstrual periods, bleeding after intercourse or douching. Unusual discharge. Painful or heavy periods.

CAUSES—A primary cause is HPV (**human papilloma virus**) infection, which can be transmitted sexually. Other factors include **unprotected sex, sexually transmitted infections** (including **HIV, HPV, and genital herpes**), **multiple sex partners, first intercourse before 18, early childbearing, more than five complete pregnancies, infertility, smoking, nutritional deficiencies,** and **susceptible tendencies toward it because of low socioeconomic status**.

If not treated, cervical cancer usually spreads to underlying connective tissue, nearby lymph glands, the uterus, and the genito-urinary tract.

Serious vaginal infections, such as **trichomonas** and **exposure to carcinogenic substances** (such as **heavy metals, asbestos, herbicides and nicotine**), should be warning signs. Beware of the drug, called **tamoxifen**.

The American Cancer Society now says that annual pap smears should only be obtained in case of high-risk factors.

NATURAL REMEDIES
Contact your physician.
• Eat a diet high in **fruits and vegetables, soy products, whole grains, and vitamin supplementation** (especially **vitamins C, E, A, bioflavonoids, and B complex**). **Folic acid** (800 mcg daily) can reverse precancerous changes in the cells within the cervix. Drink **green drinks** daily.
• **Do not eat meat** of any kind. Do not eat **unsaturated fatty acids,** including **eggs and butter.** Avoid **white bread, cheeses, and processed or fried foods**.
• **Smoking** secretes toxins into cervical mucus and increases risk of cervical cancer.
—*Also read the sections on Cancer (782-796).*

ENCOURAGEMENT—Blessed is the soul who can say, "I am guilty before God; but Jesus is my Advocate. I have transgressed His law. I cannot save myself; but I make the precious blood that was shed on Calvary all my plea. I am lost in Adam, but restored in Christ. God, who so loved the world as to give His only begotten Son to die, will not leave me to perish while repentant and in contrition of soul. He will not look upon me; for I am all unworthy. But He will look upon the face of His Anointed, He will look upon my Substitute and Surety; He will listen to the plea of my Advocate who died for my sin, that I might be made the righteousness of God in Him. By beholding Him I shall be changed into His image. I cannot change my own character, save by partaking of the grace of Him who is all goodness, righteousness, mercy, and truth. But, by beholding Him, I shall catch His spirit and be transformed into His likeness."

OVARIAN CANCER

SYMPTOMS—Symptoms are often absent until the disease is advanced. Abdominal enlargement, constipa-tion or diarrhea, frequent urination, or vaginal bleeding (rarely). Especially watch for any enlargement of the abdomen or persistent digestive disturbances that cannot be explained.

CAUSES—This is the leading reproductive-organ cancer killer among women. If diagnosed and treated early, the survival rate is high. But there are generally no symptoms till it is quite advanced. The risk of this disease increases after the age of 40.

Risk factors include **high dietary fat intake, the use of talcum powder in the genital area, human papilloma virus, obesity, a diet high in saturated animal fat and low in fiber. There is also previous history of breast, uterine, or colon cancer. Other risks include not having gone through pregnancy and childbirth, exposure to radiation or asbestos, early onset and/or late cessation of menstruation,**

NATURAL REMEDIES
Contact your physician.
• **Stop eating meat, grease, and all saturated fatty acids.** Do not use **tobacco, alcohol, or eat junk food**.
• Eat a high-fiber **fruit and vegetable diet,** as discussed in other articles under Cancer (782-796).

ENCOURAGEMENT—The heart that is filled with the grace of Christ will be made manifest by its peace and joy; and where Christ abides, the character will become purified, elevated, ennobled, and glorified.

TESTICULAR CANCER

SYMPTOMS—One or more lumps in the testicle. Enlargement of a testicle. Thickening of the scrotum. Sudden quantity of fluid in the scrotum. Discomfort or pain in the scrotum or a testicle. Mild ache in the back, lower abdomen, or groin. Enlarged or tender breasts. Bloody semen.

CAUSES—White men between the ages of 20 and 35 are most likely to contract this disease. Because it can enlarge and spread very rapidly, it must be detected and treated early.

Cryptorchism (undescended testicles) increases the risk, even if earlier corrected by surgery. Other factors are **inguinal hernia,** during childhood, and earlier **mumps orchitis**. The other causes are not known.

NATURAL REMEDIES
Contact your physician.
• A **low-fat diet of fruits, vegetables, and whole grains. Tomatoes** contain *lycopene,* which may protect against testicular cancer.
• Take a full vitamin-mineral supplement, high in **vitamin E**. Drink **carrot juice** for carotenes instead of taking added **vitamin A**, which may cause problems.
• **Do not eat meat, unsaturated fat foods, or junk foods**. Do not use **tobacco** or **alcohol**.
—*Also read the sections on Cancer (782-796).*
ENCOURAGEMENT—There is nothing that can

make the soul so strong to resist the temptations of Satan (in the great conflict of life) as to seek God in humility, laying before Him your soul in all its helplessness, expecting that He will be your helper and your defender.

With the trusting faith of a little child, we are to come to our heavenly Father and tell Him of all our needs. He is always ready to pardon and help. The supply of divine wisdom is inexhaustible; and the Lord encourages us to draw largely from it.

MOUTH CANCER
(Oral Cancer)

SYMPTOMS—Sometimes early symptoms appear; at other times none till the disease is advanced. Symptoms include a persistent sore on the tongue, in the mouth, or throat which does not heal. Discolored patches in the mouth or throat. Loss of feeling on the tongue or mouth. Difficulty swallowing or a feeling something is stuck in the throat. A mass in the cheek or neck. Swelling of the jaw or difficulty moving jaw or neck. Changes in the voice. Unexplained toothache. Weight loss.

CAUSES—This is another totally unnecessary disease; yet 10,000 people die from it in America each year. Nearly all (90%) of those who contract this disease either **chew smokeless tobacco or smoke cigarettes / pipes**. Other factors are ongoing use of a **mouthwash containing alcohol, ultraviolet light exposure to the lips, human papilloma virus, and immuno-depressant drugs**. When cancer occurs in the mouth, it frequently develops in other parts of the body as well.

Oral leukoplakia is a precancerous condition of the mouth, which smokers and drinkers are most likely to develop.

NATURAL REMEDIES
Contact your physician.
• Immediately **stop the use of tobacco and alcohol**.
• Eat a fiber-rich diet of **fresh fruits, vegetables, flaxseed oil,** and **vitamin-mineral supplementation. Broccoli, brussels sprouts, green leafy vegetables, soybeans, and garlic** are important.
—*Also read the sections on Cancer (782-796).*
ENCOURAGEMENT—Oh that we might have a consuming desire to know God by an experimental knowledge, to come into the audience chamber of the Most High, reaching up the hand of faith, and casting our helpless souls upon the One mighty to save. His loving kindness is better than life. He desires to bestow on the children of men the riches of an eternal inheritance. His kingdom is an everlasting kingdom.

LARYNGEAL CANCER

SYMPTOMS—Persistent cough, hoarse throat, difficulty swallowing, chronic sore throat. A pain from swallowing that radiates to the ear, continual ear pain. Blood in sputum or saliva. Difficult breathing, weight loss.

CAUSES—The larynx ("voice box") is the section of the respiratory tract between the pharynx and trachea, where the vocal chords are located. This disease especially occurs in men over the age of 50; it is primarily caused by the prolonged use of **tobacco** or **alcohol**. But repeated inhalation of **poisonous fumes, frequent straining of the vocal chords or laryngitis** can be involved. The cells lining the larynx become cancerous.

NATURAL REMEDIES
Contact your physician.
• Immediately **stop the use of tobacco and alcohol**. Eat a **nourishing diet of fruits and vegetables, whole grains, and vitamin-mineral supplementation**.
• **Vitamins A, B complex, C, E, flavonoids, and retinoids** are important.
—*Also read the sections on Cancer (782-796).*
ENCOURAGEMENT—If we would give more expression to our faith, rejoice more in the blessings that we know we have,—the great mercy and love of God,—we should have more faith and greater joy. No tongue can express, no finite mind can conceive, the blessing that results from appreciating the goodness and love of God. Even on earth we may have joy as a wellspring, never failing, because we are fed by the streams that flow from the throne of God.

ESOPHAGEAL CANCER

SYMPTOMS—No symptoms until the cancer is advanced. An increasing difficulty in swallowing (dysphagyia), often with a feeling that something is stuck in the throat or chest. Vomiting, often of blood. Spitting out excess mucus. Weight loss, pernicious anemia, chronic indigestion, stomach pain after eating.

CAUSES—Esophageal cancers occur more frequently in men and in African-Americans. Primary causes are **using tobacco and/or drinking alcohol**. Other factors include a **high-fat diet, eating wood-smoked foods, frequent heartburn or reflux** (stomach fluids going up into esophagus).

NATURAL REMEDIES
Contact your physician.
• Eat plenty of **fruits and vegetables**, especially **broccoli and cabbage**. Also **green peppers, soybeans, whole wheat, wheat bran, garlic**. Add glutathione-rich foods like **avocados, asparagus, grapefruit, oranges, and tomatoes. Spirulina** (a freshwater algae) also inhibits the growth of the tumor.
• Take **vitamins A, C, riboflavin, and selenium**.
• **Stop eating all meat, fats, salt. No processed, sugary, or fried foods**. Do not eat **moldy or pickled foods**. Do not eat **very hot or very cold foods**.
—*Also read the sections on Cancer (782-796).*

ENCOURAGEMENT—Satan has represented God as selfish and oppressive, as claiming all, and giving nothing, as requiring the service of His creatures for His own glory, and making no sacrifice for their good. But the gift of Christ reveals the Father's heart . . It declares that while God's hatred of sin is as strong as death, His love for the sinner is stronger than death. Having undertaken our redemption, He will spare nothing, however dear, which is necessary to the completion of His work. No truth essential to our salvation is withheld, no miracle of mercy is neglected, no divine agency is left unemployed. Favor is heaped upon favor, gift upon gift. The whole treasury of heaven is open to those He seeks to save. Having collected the riches of the universe, and laid open the resources of infinite power, He gives them all into the hands of Christ and says, All these are for man. Use these gifts to convince him that there is no love greater than Mine in earth or heaven. His greatest happiness will be found in loving Me.

The Father appreciates every soul whom His Son has purchased by the gift of His life. Every provision has been made for us to receive divine power, which will enable us to overcome temptations. Through obedience to all God's requirements the soul is preserved unto eternal life.

God has a heaven full of blessings that He wants to bestow on those who are earnestly seeking for that help which the Lord alone can give.

STOMACH CANCER

SYMPTOMS—Often no symptoms until the condition is advanced. Pain, indigestion, bloating after eating, stomach pain that cannot be eliminated (even by antacids), vomiting after eating, bloody vomit, black stools, fatigue, anemia, and weight loss.

CAUSES—Stomach cancer occurs twice as often in men, especially among those with a lower income. The risk increases after the age of 40.

Risk factors include **lack of dietary fiber, a high-fat diet. Too much smoked, salted, or picked foods. Foods high in starch and low in fiber. Tobacco and/or alcohol.** Other factors include **pernicious anemia, previous stomach surgery, chronic gastritis, stomach polyps, or having type A blood.**

A **high-fat, low-fiber diet** is always present in stomach polyps and stomach cancer. **Smoking** is another high-risk factor. This cancer takes as long as 15 years to develop.

NATURAL REMEDIES
Contact your physician.
• **Stop eating meat products and white-flour. No fried, processed, sugared, and junk foods**.
• Eat **fruits, vegetables, whole grains** (especially **brown rice), soybeans, and lentils, broccoli, brussels sprouts, green leafy vegetables, plus vitamin-mineral supplements. Vitamins C, E, bioflavonoids, and selenium** are important. **Garlic and pineapple** are very helpful.

—Also read the sections on Cancer (782-796).
ENCOURAGEMENT—The transforming power of grace can make you a partaker of the divine nature. The glory of God has shone on Christ; and by looking upon Christ, contemplating His self-sacrifice, remembering that in Him dwells all the fullness of the Godhead bodily, the believer is drawn closer and closer to the Source of power.

The sinner may become a child of God, an heir of heaven. He may rise from the dust and stand forth arrayed in garments of light . . At every step of advance, he sees new beauties in Christ and becomes more like Him in character.

The love that was manifested toward him, in the death of Christ, awakens a response of thankful love; and, in answer to sincere prayer, the believer is brought from grace to grace, from glory to glory, until (by beholding Christ) he is changed into the same image.

HODGKIN'S LYMPHOMA

(Hodgkin's Disease)
SYMPTOMS—Fatigue, itching, fever, general sickish feeling, night sweats, weakness, weight loss, enlargement of lymph nodes and spleen (which is generally not painful).

CAUSES—There are two types of cancer of the lymph system: Hodgkin's disease and non-Hodgkin's disease. Both are lymphomas. Hodgkin's disease is cancer of the lymph glands, which includes the lymph nodes and the spleen. It most frequently occurs in young adults. There are hundreds of lymph nodes in your body; and, together with their connecting network of tubes, they are really immense in size and scope.

The lymphatic system helps protect the body against toxins of various types. Carried off through the lymphatic vessels, those foreign substances are then temporarily stored in lymphatic organs (the spleen, nodes, tonsils, and appendix). If these are removed or become clogged because too much waste matter is being channeled through them, then trouble occurs.

NATURAL REMEDIES
Contact your physician.
• Go on a **vegetable juice fast** for 2-3 days; then eat **nourishing food** and **fast again** every few days. It is vital that you clean out the system, so it can restore itself.
• Stop eating all **refined and junk foods**. Stop **smoking and drinking** liquor. You must live right if you are to recover.
• **Exercise** is vital. Muscles move the lymphatic waste.
• **Steam baths, salt glows, and hot and cold water treatments** will invigorate the body.
• Keep the **bowels** open. **Do not strain** at the stool; for this could injure a temporarily enlarged spleen.
• Helpful herbs include **echinacea, burdock, pau d'arco, and red clover**. Other herbs include **white oak bark, plantain, vervain, and yarrow**.

—For further information, see Cancer (782-796). Also see Non-Hodgkin's Lymphoma (next).

ENCOURAGEMENT—Decide, with all your heart, that you will walk in the truth found in the Bible, and you will be safe. Cling to Jesus as your only help and stay close to Him amid the crises of life. Habakkuk 3:18.

NON-HODGKIN'S LYMPHOMA
(Non-Hodgkin's Disease)

SYMPTOMS—*If cancer is in abdomen:* vomiting, nausea, abdominal pain, or abdominal enlargement. *If in the chest:* shortness of breath and coughing. *If in the brain:* vision changes, headaches, seizures. *If in the bone marrow:* anemia. *If in the thymus:* shortness of breath or feeling of suffocation, plus coughing.

CAUSES—There are two types of cancer of the lymph system: Hodgkin's lymphoma (HL) and non-Hodgkin's lymphoma (NHL). NHL is the fifth most common cancer in the U.S.; and it is rapidly increasing. In this disease, the body's ability to resist infection is greatly reduced because fewer than normal white blood cells are being produced. In addition, the cancer is able to spread more rapidly.

Causes include **exposure to herbicides, pesticides, black hair dye, benzene, meat eating, AIDS, immune-depressant drugs, or previous organ transplantation**,

NATURAL REMEDIES

Contact your physician.

• Immediately **stop eating meat. Stop using tobacco and alcohol. Do not eat processed, fatty, and junk foods**.

• Eat a nourishing diet of **fruits and vegetables. And drink fresh juices of carrot, cabbage, and beet**.

—Read the sections on Cancer (782-796) and see Hodgkin's Disease (above).

ENCOURAGEMENT—Only those who read the Bible as the voice of God speaking to them are the true learners. They tremble at the Word of God; for, to them, it is a living reality. They study; they search for the hidden treasure. They open their understanding and heart to receive; and they pray for heavenly grace, that they may obtain a preparation for the future, immortal life. Through the study of the Bible, man sees his own frailty, his infirmity, his hopelessness in looking to himself for righteousness. He sees that in himself there is nothing to recommend him to God. He prays for the Holy Spirit, the representative of Christ, to be his constant guide, to lead him into all truth. With all his heart, he claims the precious promises of Scripture and, by faith in the empowering grace of Christ, he obeys all ten of the commandments (Exodus 20:3-17).

LEUKEMIA

SYMPTOMS—Weakness, easy fatigue, a remarkable whiteness of the skin, difficulty in breathing, spells of fever, palpitation, rapid heart, excessive sweating, loss of weight, easy bruising, soreness or ulceration of the throat and gums, swollen lymph nodes, slow-healing cuts, bone and joint pain, an enlarged spleen or liver, or a tendency to hemorrhage or nosebleeds.

CAUSES—This is called cancer of the blood; but it is actually cancer of one of the organs where the white blood cells are made (bone marrow, lymph system, or spleen).

Leukemia (which means "white blood") produces a defect in the production of white blood cells (WBCs or leukocytes), resulting in large numbers of immature WBCs in the bloodstream. WBCs are vital to physical health; and, without them, the body deteriorates. But the bone marrow is now producing an excess of them; and large numbers of those dumped into the bloodstream are essentially useless.

A blood test reveals anemia (not enough red blood cells), low platelet count, increased lymphoblasts (an excess of immature WBCs), and an elevated total WBC count.

Chronic cases run an up-and-down course for several years. Acute cases generally end fatally in a few weeks. As a rule, leukemia ends in death. A person can choose to go the medical route or try natural remedies. There will, of course, be a risk and the very real possibility of death, whatever his decision.

It occurs among both children and adults; and it is slightly more among Caucasians than among African-Americans. Causes include **exposure to radiation, radon, benzene, or certain toxic chemicals.** Other causative factors include **chronic viral infections, genetics, Down Syndrome, having a sibling with leukemia, HIV infection, commercial hair dyes, certain cancer therapies, and poor living habits**.

TREATMENT—

• Treatment may include **laetrile, germanium, selenium, vitamin A, and vitamin C** to bowel tolerance. **DMSO IV** helps mature the immature white blood cells in circulation. A moderate amount of **selenium** should be taken; for leukemia victims tend to have a low amount.

• **Quercetin**, a bioflavonoid found in citrus pulp and certain other vegetable sources has been found to have definite anti-leukemia properties. **Genistein** is another bioflavonoid which destroys leukemia cells. Bioflavonoids are essential for the absorption of vitamin C; and the two bioflavonoids should be taken together. Sources of bioflavonoids include **peppers, buckwheat, black currants,** and **the white material just beneath the peel of citrus fruits.** Other sources include **citrus pulp, cherries, apricots, blackberries,**

C
A
N
C
E
R

plums, prunes, and rose hips.

—*Also read the sections on Cancer (782-796).*

ENCOURAGEMENT—In Christ we find our hope; in Him we find our salvation. Cry to Him for help and trust that He will work everything for the best for all concerned. You can safely lean on Him. He will not fail you, no matter what the outcome.

LEPROSY

It is an intriguing fact that people get leprosy in tropical climates and cancer in cooler areas. So leprosy is listed in this chapter.

SYMPTOMS—Any unnatural patch on the surface of the skin. If void of sensibility to temperature, pain, or touch, it should be a warning of the possible onset of this disease. Other early symptoms include headache, nosebleed, and fevers. Certain areas may become insensitive, because the disease follows along nerve trunks and especially affects areas on, or close to, the skin. Eventually, even the bones decay; and fingers and toes drop off.

CAUSES—Leprosy is a strange infectious disease, caused by a bacteria which, under a microscope, looks like tuberculosis. It is mildly contagious.

There may be 2-3 years, and sometimes much longer, after exposure before symptoms appear. Once it appears, it develops very slowly.

The disease is almost unknown among vegetarians; but is prevalent among **meat eaters**, especially in hot tropical climates. People who eat heavily of meat, especially pork, are the ones most likely to contract leprosy. The worst things to take into your body are **pork, crocodile meat, lard, blood, greasy meats, coffee, alcohol, or tobacco**.

NATURAL REMEDIES

• A careful, **nourishing vegetarian diet** and **clean, hygienic living** is important. Eat plenty of **fruits, vegetables, whole grains, nuts, and legumes.** Fresh air is important.

• In tropical countries, **chaulmoogra oil** is taken. Begin by swallowing 10 drops a day, gradually increasing to 30 if the person can tolerate it.

• **Sunbathing helps.**

• Helpful herbs include **red clover blossoms, burdock seeds, myrrh, dandelion, yellow dock root, lobelia, redroot, poke root, goldenseal, myrrh, bittersweet, sassafras, poplar bark, black cherry bark, and comfrey.**

• Mix a heaping tsp. of **goldenseal** and ½ tsp. **myrrh**; steep in a pint of boiling water. Drink 1 cup ½ hour before each meal and before retiring.

• Dr. Christopher recommends making an apple cider vinegar tincture of freshly bruised **pennyroyal** and applying it externally as a fomentation. Also drink pennyroyal internally.

—*Leprosy closely resembles syphilis (804) and tuberculosis (505); so you may also wish to read those articles also.*

ENCOURAGEMENT—Find in God the help that you so much need. He can help you, day by day. Giving your life to Him is the best thing you can do. Whatever the outcome, He has your life in Hands. And that is the best way to have it. Ephesians 1:7.

By His humanity, Christ touched humanity. By His divinity, He lays hold upon the throne of God. As the Son of man, He gave us an example of obedience. As the Son of God, He gives us power to obey. The meek and lowly Saviour is God "manifest in the flesh" (1 Tim. 3:16). "God with us" is the surety of our deliverance from sin, the assurance of our power to obey the law of heaven.

In taking our nature, the Saviour has bound Himself to humanity by a tie that is never to be broken. Through the eternal ages He is linked with us. "Unto us a child is born, unto us a son is given" (Isa. 9:6). God has adopted human nature in the person of His Son, and has carried the same into the highest heaven. It is the "Son of man" who shares the throne of the universe. In Christ the family of earth and the family of heaven are bound together. Christ glorified is our brother. Heaven is enshrined in humanity, and humanity is enfolded in the bosom of Infinite Love.

"Behold, God is my salvation; I will trust, and not be afraid: for the Lord Jehovah is my strength and my song; He also is become my salvation."   —Isaiah 12:2

"I, even I, will sing unto the Lord; I will sing praise to the Lord God of Israel."
   —Judges 5:3

"Let the people praise Thee, O God; let all the people praise Thee."   —Psalm 67:3

"And when He [Christ] was come nigh . . the whole multitude of the disciples began to rejoice and praise God with a loud voice for all the mighty works that they had seen."
   —Luke 19:37

"Ye that fear the Lord, praise Him; all ye the seed of Jacob, glorify Him."
   —Psalm 22:23

"O give thanks unto the Lord; for He is good: for His mercy endureth forever."
   —Psalm 118:29

"My heart is fixed, O God, my heart is fixed: I will sing and give praise."
   —Psalm 57:7

"Thou art my God, and I will praise Thee: Thou art my God, I will exalt Thee."
   —Psalm 118:28

HOW TO LIVE LONGER

A researcher in Germany discovered that how you deal with problems can affect how long you will live and, to some extent, how you may die!

In this life, each individual is continually confronted by problems—difficulties in relation to persons, situations, and goals. Some of these problems can be quite large. Yet the attitude the person takes toward his problems can, literally, finish him off.

What you are about to read can affect your entire life, so you will want to consider it carefully. Recognize it as good advice; not only start doing it, but also share it with your friends and loved ones.

Ronald Grossarth-Maticek, a Yugoslavian oncologist, and his students were given access to mortality data in Heidelberg, Germany. They carefully studied thousands of deaths, read through autopsy reports, and interviewed relatives of the deceased. He discovered that a person's attitude greatly affects his life span—and in special ways.

There are four methods of dealing with problems. The European researcher dealt with the first three. Other research studies reveal there is also a fourth. Here they are:

Type 1 - The first way of dealing with a problem is to let it get you down. The key words are **"hopeless / helpless."** This person is unable to solve problems relating to others, situations, or goals. If relationships are sour, circumstances unfavorable, and goals seemingly unachievable, he sinks into a depression, characterized by feelings of helplessness and hopelessness. This person seems unable to change his negative view of life. He consistently holds on to depression as a habit to run into and hide. The coroner reports revealed the fact that **the person choosing this type of behavior is highly prone to cancer.**

Type 2 - The second way of dealing with a problem is to blow up. The key words are **"frustrated / angry."** This person also seems unable to deal with problems in a positive way. Instead, he becomes disgusted or loses his temper. **The person choosing this type of behavior is highly prone to heart disease.**

Type 3 - The third way of dealing with a problem is to remain positive and turn one's attention to finding a new way—a different way—to tackle the problem and resolve it. The key words are **"cheerful / positive."** The significant factor, of course, is the continued positive outlook.

The individual selecting this type of response to problems—tends not to get sick! That is what the interviews and coronary reports revealed. These people have the lowest incidence of disease. In fact, they have the lowest incidence of death due to all causes, including accidents.

Here we have two major killers and many smaller ones. The solution to forestalling many of them is a change in outlook and thinking, a change in behavior.

Type 4 - There is also a fourth way of dealing with problems, which other studies have repeatedly shown to be highly beneficial to both mind and body. **This method increases the positive outlook of Type 3 living, intensifies the healthful results, and makes it easier to switch from Type 1 and Type 2 to Type 3 behavior.**

The fourth manner of dealing with a problem is to take it to God in prayer. Here we find a person who has chosen to accept Christ as his Saviour. He has dedicated his life to Him and, by enabling grace, seeks to obey His Written Word each day.

Then when a problem arises, he takes it to God in prayer. Those who do this have found that it produces wonderful results. In some cases, a beautiful solution appears all by itself. At other times, the person will arise from prayer, greatly encouraged to press forward in a Type 3 approach: With a positive outlook, he will try a new way to solve the problem. However, there are difficulties which, unfortunately, cannot easily be solved. They would try to hang as a dead weight around the neck, year after year. Only Type 4 living can deal effectively with such problems.

A Christian can face problems more positively than others. He can cheerfully live with problems which would crush others.

Yet there is something else about Type 4 living which is special: The person who puts God first in his life—will spend much of his thought and energy trying to make the lives of others happier. The person who is busy helping others will always seem to have fewer problems. He is too busy being a blessing to others to give his personal problems much attention.

What have we learned from these four types?

When you have a problem, do this: (1) Take the problem to God in prayer. Make sure you are obeying the Ten Commandments and all that He commands in His Inspired Writings. (2) Keep positive and cheerful. If you have a personal relationship with God, you will especially be able to do this. Trust everything to Him; and believe He will work it all out for the best. (3) Change your behavior in such a way that conditions are changed for the better. Obedience to God's laws will greatly encourage you.

Amid the problems of life, when you walk up to a wall of difficulty, you can go through it, go around it, or go over it. Sometimes, with God's help, the wall just disappears as you walk toward it.

Here are several additional pointers:

Just what is the problem? What new, alternative activities would produce more positive results? Think it through; and then, prayerfully, try making the changes. Always stay on the positive. Failure should not be regarded as a reason for not trying out new types of behavior and activity. Discouragement or anger accomplish nothing. Take it to the Lord in prayer and arise ready to move forward positively again.

Some problems cannot be solved. Sometimes you live with them. This is when Type 4 living—walking hand-in-hand with God—can provide wonderful solutions, even if unfortunately circumstances do not seem to change as quickly as they might. It can also help you live in environments which would crush others.

Choose the sunshine side of life; and problems about you will evaporate. The Christian has heaven coming; he can afford to wait patiently through the days that are dark. For him, the future is bright.

Remember to use your longer life to help and bless others. That is why you were born into this world. Spend your time making others happy.

—*vf*

CANCER

The Natural Remedies Encyclopedia

Cancer Lesions on the Skin

Here you will find 16 color pictures of 5 of the cancers which produce lesions on the skin: Although most carcinomas are internal, some show evidence of their presence by lesions on the skin.

Melanoma (6) 798-799 / Basal Cell Carcinoma (3) 799 / Squamous Cell Carcinoma (2) 799-800 / Skin Cancer (1) 800 / Kaposi's Sarcoma (4) 800

CANCER

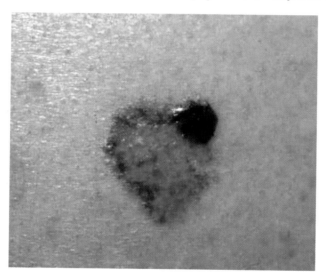

Melanoma

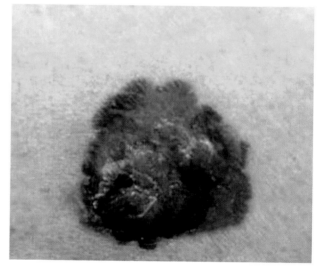

Melanoma

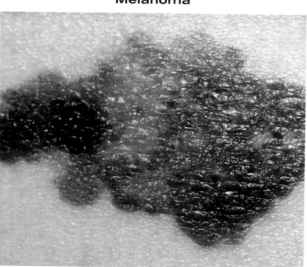

Melanoma

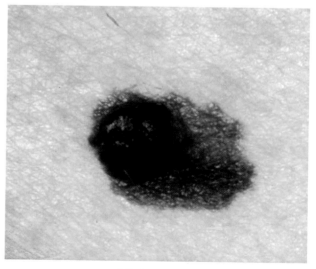

Melanoma

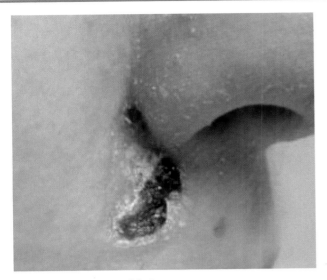

Melanoma

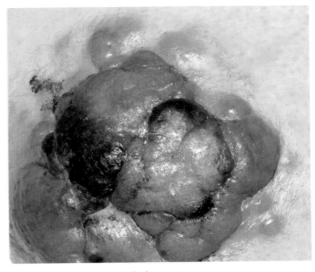

Melanoma

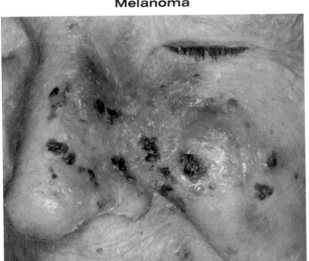

Basal cell Carcinoma

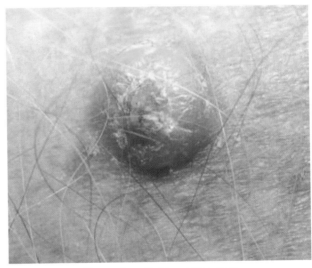

Basal cell Carcinoma

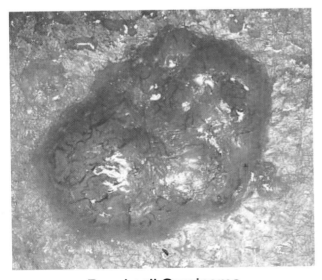

Basal cell Carcinoma

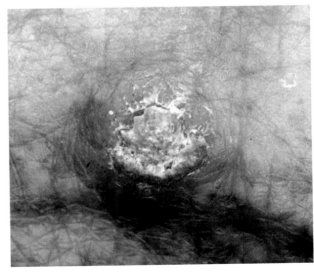

Squamous cell Carcinoma

CANCER

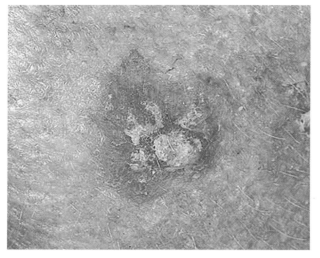

Skin Cancer

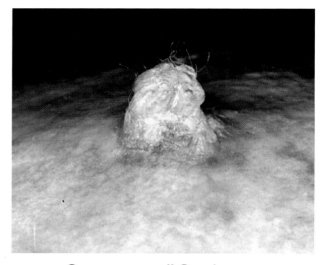

Squamous cell Carcinoma

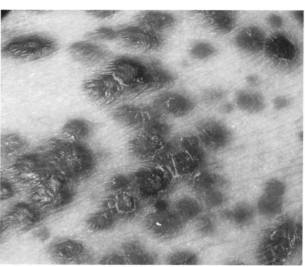

Kaposi's Sarcoma

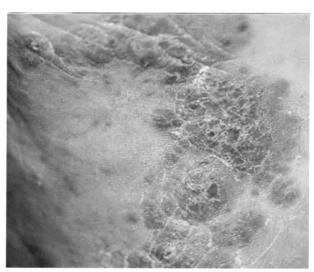

Kaposi's Sarcoma

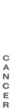

C
A
N
C
E
R

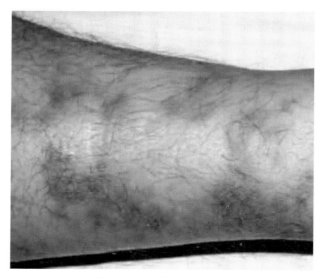

Kaposi's Sarcoma

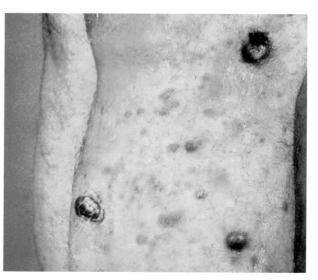

Kaposi's Sarcoma

The Natural Remedies Encyclopedia

- Section 22 -
Sexually Transmitted Diseases

"Eye hath not seen, nor ear heard, neither have entered into the heart of man, the things which God hath prepared for them that love Him."
— *1 Corinthians 2:9.*

"He hath sent Me to bind up the brokenhearted."—*Isaiah 1:1.*

"Keeping mercy for thousands, forgiving iniquity and transgression and sin."
—*Exodus 34:7.*

"Great peace have they which love Thy law: and nothing shall offend them."
—*Psalm 119:165.*

"Come out from among them, and be ye separate, saith the Lord, and touch not the unclean thing; and I will receive you."
—*2 Corinthians 6:17.*

"Who forgiveth all thine iniquities; who healeth all thy diseases."
—*Psalm 103:3.*

S
T
D

FOR MORE NATURAL REMEDIES:
HERBS: Herb Contents (pp. 129-130) will help you locate the 126 most important herbs and the diseases each one can treat. How to prepare herbs (132). How to use them (141-189)
HYDROTHERAPY: Therapy Contents (pp. 206-207) and its Disease Index (263-265) will lead you to over 100 water therapies and many more remedies. DIS. INDEX: 1211- / GEN.

INDEX: 1221-
VITAMINS AND MINERALS: Contents (100-101). Using 101-124. Dosages (124). Others (117-)
CARING FOR THE SICK: Home care for a sick person (28-36). The healing crisis (36-39)
WOMEN'S SECTIONS: Female Organs (672) Pregnancy (701). Childbirth (765). Infancy, Childhood (722). Women's Herbs (754, 760)
EMERGENCIES: (973-). FIRST AID: (990-)

Section 22 - Sexually Transmitted Diseases

STD - 1 - VENEREAL DISEASES

WHICH ONE IS IT?

Here are key symptoms of the nine leading kinds of sexually transmitted diseases:

AIDS (acquired immunodeficiency syndrome)—Headache, night sweats, unexplained weight loss, fatigue, swollen lymph glands, persistent fever, oral thrush (a heavy, whitish coating on the tongue and the insides of the mouth),recurrent vaginal yeast infections, persistent diarrhea, lung infections.

Chlamydia—*For women:* a white vaginal discharge that resembles cottage cheese, a burning sensation when urinating, itching, painful intercourse. *For men:* a clear, watery urethral discharge. Often, however, there are no symptoms at all.

Candidiasis: *Both sexes* have itching in genital area and pain when urinating. *Women:* Thick, odorless vaginal discharge.

Genital herpes: Itching, burning in the genital area, discomfort during urination. A watery vaginal or urethral discharge. Weeping, fluid-filled eruptions on penis or in vagina.

Genital warts—Soft, cauliflower-like growths appearing either singly or in clusters in and around the vagina, anus, penis, groin, and/or scrotal area.

Pelvic inflammatory disease, *Women:* Pus-filled vaginal discharge, plus fever and pain in lower abdomen.

Trichomoniasis, *Women:* Itching and pain in vagina. Foamy, greenish or yellowish, smelly discharge. *Men:* Clear urethral discharge.

Gonorrhea, *Women:* Vaginal itching, frequent and painful urination, and a cloudy vaginal discharge. Inflammation of the pelvic area, rectal discharge, abnormal uterine bleeding. *Men:* Yellowish, pus-filled urethral discharge. *Both sexes:* Very often (especially in women) there are no symptoms.

Syphilis: A sore on the genitals, sores in the mouth or anus. A rash, patches of flaking tissue, sore throat, fever.

ENCOURAGEMENT—It is only as we feel our need of a Saviour that we can receive the help that we so much need. Those who receive Christ by faith receive power to become the sons of God. Trusting in Jesus, and pleading for divine help, they will receive empowering grace to resist temptation and overcome sin. How thankful we can be that, in Christ's strength, we can live lives which are pleasing to God and have a home someday with Him, in heaven.

VENEREAL DISEASES
(STD, Sexually Transmitted Diseases)

SYMPTOMS—Blisters around the vagina, burning when urinating, anal pain, itching, pelvic inflammation, penile discharge, sore throat, flu-like symptoms, and more. *Here is a brief comparative analysis of the symptoms of nine of these STDs:*

Chlamydia: In women, there is a burning sensation when urinating. A white vaginal discharge resembling cottage cheese. Itching, painful intercourse. In men, a clear, watery, urethral discharge. This disease, which often shows no symptoms at all, can cause urinary tract infections and adhesions, resulting in sterility.

Genital Herpes: Itching and burning in the genital area. Discomfort when urinating. A watery vaginal or urethral discharge. Fluid-filled, weeping, eruptions in the vagina or on the penis.

Genital Warts: Single or clustered, soft, cauliflower-like growths in and around the vagina, anus, penis, groin, and/or scrotal area.

Pelvic Inflammatory Disease (PID): Fever and lower abdominal pain. A pus-filled vaginal discharge.

Trichomoniasis: In women, there is a foamy, greenish or yellowish, foul-smelling vaginal discharge, vaginal itching, and pain. In men, there is a clear urethral discharge.

Syphilis: A sore on the genitals is accompanied by rash, fever, patches of flaking tissue, sore throat, and sores in the mouth or anus.

Gonorrhea: In women, there is a cloudy vaginal discharge, frequent and painful urination, vaginal itching. Inflammation of the pelvic area, rectal discharge, and abnormal uterine bleeding. In men, there is a pus-filled, yellowish discharge. Often there are no symptoms for months. In women, there may never be symptoms; yet, all the while, they are infecting men.

AIDS (Acquired Immune Deficiency Syndrome): Aids has many symptoms; see AIDS (806).

Candidiasis: Itching in the genital area, pain

when urinating, a thick odorless vaginal discharge. *This is not a "venereal disease"; but it is a yeast infection which can be transmitted by sexual activity, as well as in other ways (Candidiasis, 281).*

CAUSES—Venereal diseases are transmitted by **intimate contact**, when at least one has had more than one partner. STDs can cause urinary tract problems, sterility in women, and prostatic inflammation in men.

At the present time, one teenage girl in four has a STD. Some of these diseases can kill newborn babies.

People who **smoke or chew tobacco** are three times as likely to contract an STD.

Oral contraceptives also increase the STD risk. They do this by decreasing levels of key nutrients within the body. Because of their imbalancing estrogen content, they also increase the likelihood of precancerous lesions.

We are living in an STD health crisis; it is rapidly increasing every year.

Condoms do not guarantee protection against any STD. A University of Texas research study showed that 30% of the time they do not even protect against AIDS, one of the worst killers of all.

Many STDs are increasing, due to the fact that the AIDS epidemic weakens the immune system and reduces resistance to many diseases.

Strong doses of antibiotics are the usual medical treatment; but an increasing amount of drug resistance is occurring among patients.

NATURAL REMEDIES
• The only genuine protection is **abstinence**. Marry a person who never has, and never will have, sex with another during your lifetime. Afterward, both of you remain faithful to one another to the end.
• Follow a very cleansing **liquid diet** for 3-7 days. During acute stages, take one each of the following juices daily: **potassium broth, fresh carrot juice, vegetable drink**, and **apple / parsley juice** to alkalize.
• Follow the liquid diet with a cleansing **fresh foods** diet. **Avoid refined, starchy, fried, and saturated fat foods. No meat, dairy products, caffeine, tobacco, and liquor.**
• Take **vitamin C** (3,000-8,000 mg daily), **vitamin E** (200-400 IU daily), and **flaxseed oil** (1 Tbsp. daily).
• **Fever therapy** is powerful; but you need to do it under the supervision of someone who knows how to watch the temperature closely and reduce it as needed. This is excellent for controlling virus replication. Even slight increases in body temperature can lead to considerable reduction of infection.
• If you have one of these diseases, see your physician. The directions for Cancer *(792-796)* in this book will help alleviate some of these afflictions.

ENCOURAGEMENT—When all seems dark and unexplainable, we are to trust in God's love. You need His help. In His strength, you can stand for the right and come off more than conqueror in the battle against temptation.

GONORRHEA

SYMPTOMS—In women, no symptoms may ever appear. When they do, there may be vaginal discharge, frequent and painful urination, abnormal menstrual bleeding, acute inflammation in the pelvic area, and rectal itching. Symptoms generally appear 7-14 days after sexual contact.

In men, symptoms are generally present (including difficult and painful urination, a yellow discharge of pus, and mucus from the penis). Symptoms appear 2-14 days after contact. The discharge continues 6-8 weeks.

LATER SYMPTOMS—As with syphilis *(804)*, the effects of gonorrhea keep getting worse. The secondary stage is difficult to detect; so it is often misdiagnosed as arthritis. The gonorrhea is entering the bones, joints, tendons, and other tissues. This causes mild fever, aches, inflamed joints, and sometimes skin lesions. In men, the outcome can be sterility.

As long as 10 years later, the urethra may narrow or stricture; this makes urination difficult and at times impossible, producing serious inflammation of the bladder. This occurs more often in men than in women.

Women, who unknowingly contract gonorrhea from their husbands, generally do not realize that they have the disease until it is far advanced. The infection can travel up the uterus, into the Fallopian tubes, and out into the abdominal cavity. This causes peritonitis and possibly death. If that does not occur, the tubes may eventually seal off. This is due to pus pockets of infection and pain, causing sterility.

CAUSES—Gonorrhea is caused by a microoganism, called *Neisseria gonorrhoeae*. These bacteria are commonly known as gonococci.

NATURAL REMEDIES
See your physician.
• Go on a **cleansing program**. Drink lots of **lemon juice**. An entire changeover to **a good diet and way of life** is required. Follow the program under Cancer *(613)*.
• Go to bed as soon as you know you have this disease. Have the room well-ventilated. Go on a **cleansing program of fruit juices**. Take 2 high **enemas** daily. Eat nothing that is irritating to the stomach.
• Take **beta-carotene** (150,000 IU daily) and ½ tsp. **vitamin C** powder, every hour to bowel tolerance, during the acute phase. Later reduce it to 5,000 mg daily, for a month.
• When you begin solid food, only eat simple, nourishing **fruits and vegetables.** Later include **whole grains, nuts, and legumes**.
• **Avoid refined, starchy, fried, and saturated fat foods. No meat, dairy products, caffeine, tobacco, or liquor**.
• Here is a tea with which you can wash the sores: **myrrh, goldenseal root, witch hazel, chickweed, and sorrel**.

S
T
D

• Drink 3 cups of the following tea daily: **skullcap, hops, white oak bark, uva ursi, sage, poplar, redroot, and juniper**. Take 2 high **enemas** each day.

• A tea of **red raspberry leaves and witch hazel leaves** can be used as a douche for women, including after each urination.

• A tea of one part **aloes** and two parts each of **goldenseal and myrrh** can be used as a wash on the sores and ulcers. Drink at least one quart of slippery elm tea daily. It can be mixed with fruit juice.

• A warm **sitz bath,** 2-3 times daily, will give relief from the pain. If there are pains in the legs or elsewhere, apply hot **fomentations**.

• For acute gonorrhea, mix **black willow, skullcap, and saw palmetto berries**. Steep a heaping tsp. of the mixture in a cup of boiling water for ½ hour. Take 2 Tbsp. 6 times daily. In addition, use **herbs** listed under syphilis (bellow).

• Keep in mind that all this work will be a waste of time if certain other lifestyle changes are not made.

ENCOURAGEMENT—There is hope for everyone who will seek God's face. He alone can provide for our needs; He alone can give us the solutions we need. He alone can provide the strength to resist temptation and overcome all tendencies to wrongdoing.

"Ye shall walk in all the ways which the Lord your God hath commanded you, that ye may live, and that it may be well with you, and that ye may prolong your days in the land which ye shall possess."—Deuteronomy 5:33.

SYPHILIS

SYMPTOMS—A chancre appears on the skin, either on the mouth, in the mouth, or on the genitals. It is also called a hard chancre or Hunterian sore. This is a red, painless, raised ulcer with hard, well-defined edges. It appears 10 days to 3 weeks after exposure and lasts from a few days to several weeks. In women, it sometimes develops on the cervix; so it is not recognized.

Later, a rash and patches of flaking tissue appear in the mouth or genital area. This skin eruption consists of either a few red, pimply blemishes or a profuse crop of various types of blotches. By this time, the disease is well-established throughout the system.

Later stages occur, as the disease worsens. Paralysis, insanity, and death are the final outcome.

CAUSES—Syphilis is caused by the germ, *treponema pallidum,* which is corkscrew in shape and much larger than most bacteria. The germs must remain wet; for drying quickly kills them. They generally enter the body through a living source—another person (acquired syphilis) or through the placenta to the unborn child (congenital syphilis). But,

in some instances, the disease has been transmitted to the dentist during dental work.

NATURAL REMEDIES

See your physician. Go on the treatment outlined under Cancer (792-796) in this book.

• Go on a simple diet of **fruits and vegetables**. Eat **whole grains, nuts, and legumes**. Do not eat **oysters, shell fish, or any other meat**.

• Do not eat **condiments, stimulating foods, and drinks**. No **tobacco**.

• Mix together 2 Tbsp. each of the following herbs: **buckthorn bark, uva ursi, burdock root, red clover blossoms, Oregon grape, blue flag root, prickly ash berries**, plus 1 tsp. **bloodroot**. Steep 1 heaping tsp. in a cup of boiling water ½ hour. Drink at least 4 cups daily, one an hour before each meal and one upon retiring. Take these herbs at least 1 year.

Put 1 tsp. each of **goldenseal and myrrh** into a pint of boiling water. When the eruptions appear, bathe them thoroughly with this tea.

• Heavy **sweating applications and salt glows** will help eliminate the poisons from the system. Take high **enemas** daily, using the tea of **echinacea, yellow dock root, burdock root, or bayberry bark**.

Start the above treatment as soon as the first symptoms appear, in order to not suffer too much from the disease. But a **careful diet** and **adequate rest** must be adhered to.

• Other helpful herbs include **goldenseal, pau d'arco, echinacea, sassafras, and suma**.

• **Hops tea** helps relieve pain and tension.

ENCOURAGEMENT—Determine that you will study God's Word every day and obey everything you read. Let every day begin a new page in your life. Pray earnestly and take every step in the Lord.

CHLAMYDIA

SYMPTOMS—Vaginal or urethral discharge, genital inflammation, difficulty in urinating, itching around the inflamed area, and painful intercourse.

CAUSES—According to the CDC, more people in America contract Chlamydia than any other sexually transmitted disease. Over 4 million new cases are diagnosed yearly. Nearly 20% of teenagers in the United States are known to have contracted it. But these figures do not include the large number that are not reported. Nearly 10% of men and 70% of women who have chlamydia—have no symptoms. So one can expect that the total number having, and sharing, this highly contagious disease is vast indeed.

But, whether recognized or not, the effects of chlamydia are serious. About 30% of the women become sterile; and pelvic inflammatory disease and other reproductive problems can, and do, result. In young women, the disease can also produce a form of arthritis.

In men, prostate infection and seminal vesicle inflammation may later occur. (Symptoms of prostatitis include pain when urinating and a watery mucous urethral discharge.)

The disease is transmitted through the discharge produced by both men and women. If one spouse is treated for this, the other one must be also.

To delay treatment is to intensify the effects of the disease.

NATURAL REMEDIES

• This is a complicated disease; see your physician.

• If you wish to supplement such care with natural remedies, you will need to undergo a thorough natural healing program, such as is detailed in the articles on "Cancer" (792-796).

• Mix an equal amount of powdered **goldenseal, barberry**, and **Oregon grape root** with **vitamin A oil**. Soak an all-cotton tampon and place directly in the cervix.

• Bathe sores several times daily in a **goldenseal / myrrh** solution.

• Use a vaginal suppository of **tea tree oil** nightly.

ENCOURAGEMENT—How can we solve the problems we have? Only in Christ can they be resolved. He can do for you those things you could never do for yourself.

TRICHOMONIASIS

SYMPTOMS—Some women have no symptoms. If they occur, they may include profuse, yellow, frothy, and offensive-smelling discharge from the vagina. Also there is painful inflammation. Itching and soreness of the vulva (skin around the vagina). Burning sensation when urinating. Discomfort during intercourse.

Men may also not have symptoms. If present, they may include discomfort, when urinating, and discharge from the penis.

CAUSES—This is an infection caused by Trichomonas vaginalis, a protozoan. In women, it can cause vulvovaginitis. There is also inflammation in and around the vulva, which may lead to cystitis (495). In men, it causes a mild infection of the urethra (the tube from the bladder to the outside of the body). **Unprotected sex** is the primary cause; but an infected woman who is pregnant may transmit the infection to the baby during **childbirth**.

NATURAL REMEDIES

• Practice **safe sex**; and the only effective way to do that is for a virgin man and a virgin woman to only marry once, only having sex with one another.

• If you are infected, you should not have sex until confirmation has been given that the disease has been eradicated.

• See Venereal Diseases (802), Gonorrhea (803), and Syphilis (804) for additional information on natural remedies.

—Also see Congenital Infections (724).

ENCOURAGEMENT—Christ is our example in all things if we imitate His example in earnest, importunate prayer to God that we may have strength in His name (who never yielded to the temptations of Satan, but ever resisted the devices of the wily foe), we shall not be overcome by him. Amid the perils of these last days, our only safety lies in ever-increasing watchfulness and prayer.

VENERAL WARTS

SYMPTOMS—Chronic yeast infection with heavy, pus-filled discharge. Painful intercourse. Painful, infected sores in the genital area. High fever during infection.

CAUSE—Next to genital herpes (805), this is the most common STD. It infects ovaries, fallopian tubes, cervix, and uterus. Primary causes include early age of first intercourse, multiple sexual partners, lower socio-economic level (with its traditionally nutrient-poor diet), plus smoking and oral contraceptives.

NATURAL REMEDIES

• Drink 2 cups of **pau d'arco and echinacea** tea daily.

• Take a daily **calcium** supplement to prevent lesions from becoming cancerous. Take 10 drops **grape-seed extract** daily.

• Bathe sores several times daily in a **goldenseal / myrrh** solution.

• Use a vaginal suppository of **tea tree oil**, nightly, or use **goldenseal / chaparral vaginal suppositories**, mixed with **vitamin A oil**. This has helped many women.

• Alternating **hot and cold baths, fomentations, or sitz baths** will increase immune activity in the pelvic area. Sitz baths are easiest for many to use.

• Follow the remedies outlined above under Venereal Diseases (802) and Gonorrhea (803).

ENCOURAGEMENT—There is a mighty power in prayer. Our great adversary is constantly seeking to keep the troubled soul away from God. An appeal to Heaven by the humblest child of God is more to be dreaded by Satan than the decrees of cabinets or the mandates of kings.

GENITAL HERPES (TYPE II)
(Herpes Genitalis, Venereal Herpes)

INITIAL SYMPTOMS—Recurrent fluid-filled blisters on the genitals that rupture; this leaves red, inflamed, painful lesions. These are preceded by a

S
T
D

slightly irritating tingling. When the lesion appears, it is accompanied by a sharp pain.

LATER SYMPTOMS—This viral infection can range from a symptomless infection in the nerves to a major inflammation of the liver, accompanied by fever. In women, it can lead to cervical cancer. There seems to be a link between having Type II and later developing atherosclerosis.

CAUSES—Of the 90 varieties of animal herpes, only four affect humans. Herpes is a virus that causes recurrent blisters and ulcers. Type 1 is cold sores *(322)*, also called fever blisters; these affect the lips. Type II affects the genitals; this can produce blisters either on the genitals or on, or around, the mouth. Type III is herpes zoster *(350)*, which causes chicken pox *(742)* and, as a secondary infection, shingles *(350)*.

We will here deal only with Type II, which is also called *herpes genitalis*, venereal herpes, and genital herpes. It is the most prevalent sexually transmitted disease in the United States. One-sixth of all Americans (about 30 million) have the disease, although about half never develop serious symptoms. A half million new cases are reported yearly; and 80% are 20 to 39 years of age. Herpes is a virus which enters the body through the skin and travels into nerve groups at the base of the spine. The first attack generally occurs about 4-8 days after initial **exposure to a sexual partner**. Each occurrence is quite painful and lasts up to three weeks; but, once a person is infected, the disease can be transmitted at any time. Symptoms reoccur every few weeks to once a year or less. Scarring does not usually occur, but can. Outbreaks rarely occur after the age of 50.

It remains with you the rest of your lifetime; it can be dormant for years and then appear again when the immune system is lowered by **poor diet, stress, illness, too much sunlight, or harmful chemicals**. It tends to recur especially when **sexual intercourse** takes place, as a result of irritation to the skin. It is not a newly invading infection, but one which was received from a sexual partner at an earlier time.

As a baby passes through **an infected birth canal**, it can get Type II and possibly have brain damage, blindness, or death as a result. If an attack occurs late in the pregnancy, the baby should be delivered by cesarean section. If no lesions are present, the baby is far less likely to become infected as it passes through the birth canal.

NATURAL REMEDIES

• The diet should be alkaline in reaction. Eat only **nutritious food** (especially **brown rice, vegetables, potassium** [thick white potato peeling] **broth**, and some **lentils**). Drink only **distilled water** and get plenty of **rest**. Drink plenty of fruit juices and carrot / beet / cucumber juice.

Foods to avoid are sweets, alcohol, immune-

suppressing drugs, and (for some people) **citrus.** No chocolate, peanuts, nuts, seeds. Also no **refined o processed foods.** The virus lives in red meat and fat you do well to stop eating **meat products**. There are substances in meat which encourage the growth o Type II.

• **DMSO** (Dimethyl sulfoxide), a by-product of wood processing, is a liquid which can be placed on the af fected area to relieve pain and promote healing. Only use the type sold in health-food stores.

• Some physicians prescribe BHT (butylated hy droxytoluene) for this disease; but it is known to cause perforated stomachs.

• Both internally and externally, apply to the area of the problem: **black walnut or goldenseal** extrac and /or **cayenne and red clover**.

• Other helpful herbs include **goldenseal, echin acea, myrrh, aloe vera, and burdock**.

• Lightly dab **tea tree oil** on the affected area sev eral times a day, either full strength or slightly diluted It is a powerful antiseptic. Do not get it near your eyes

• Here is a formula which one herbalist has used effectively: Mix the following powdered herbs: 25% each of echinacea and chaparral, 12% each of **sarsaparilla and Oregon grape root**, 10% of **Poria cocos**, and 8% each of **licorice root and ginger**. Put them in #00 capsules; and take 2 capsules, 3-4 times daily, for a least 3 months, along with an extremely careful diet.

• To relieve pain and inflammation, apply ice packs to lesions. Get some early morning sunlight on lesions

• Take hot baths frequently as a fever therapy remedy.

• Wear only cotton underwear.

• **Do not share drinking glasses, scratch the blisters, touch genital sores, or have sex**. Doing any of these things can spread the disease.

ENCOURAGEMENT—Jesus draws near to every one who is hurting, who needs His help. He can for give and fulfill our deepest needs. In Him we can find strength, and peace, and power to overcome.

AIDS (HIV)
(Acquired Immune Deficiency Syndrome)

SYMPTOMS—Loss of appetite, weight loss, can dida, fatigue, various infections, intestinal problems. skin diseases, immune system disorders, fevers, brain and neurological disorders, and many other symptoms.

CAUSES—AIDS (Acquired Immune Deficiency Syndrome) is a disease that does not need to happen. If people controlled themselves, it would never have got ten started and would eventually die out. But, instead. it is an exploding epidemic.

HIV (Human Immunodeficiency Virus) invades special immune cells in the body, which are called T lymphocytes, and then slowly multiplies over a long

DISEASES - List: 10-26 / Index: 1211-1224 / HERBS - Contents: 129- / Preparing: 132 / Using: 141-189 (dose:
often 1 tsp. mixed herbs in 1 cup boiled water) / VITAMINS-MINERALS - Index: 100- / Dosages: 124 / HYDRO-
THERAPY - Therapy index: 206- / Disease index: 263- / CARE OF SICK - 28-39 / EMERGENCIES - 973-, 990-

period of time. As it does so, the body's immune system gradually crumbles. All this time, the disease appears to lay dormant; only an HIV test will reveal that a person even has the disease. But, after three to ten years, enough of the body's defenses are broken down and full-blown AIDS develops. Suddenly, very pronounced symptoms appear, which are called "AIDS-related diseases." These include pneumocystis carinii pneumonia (PCP, found in 60% of those with AIDS), Karposi's sarcoma (a rare type of skin cancer), Epstein-Barr virus (EBV, *214*), cytomegalovirus (CMV), toxoplasmosis, and tuberculosis *(505)*.

The less deadly AIDS-related diseases are often the first to appear. The first sign is often the tongue coated with white bumps. This is oral thrush, a type of candida (candidiasis, *281*). Intestinal parasites *(861)* and herpes simplex virus (herpes type I, *250*) are two other relatively simple infections which can occur. All indicate that the body's immune system is damaged. Yet, it is true that candida, parasites, herpes simplex, Epstein-Barr virus, and tuberculosis can occur in individuals who do not have AIDS.

Most of those who are HIV-positive eventually develop full-blown AIDS. Once that occurs, they generally live only a few years. The median survival time, after full-blown AIDS appears, is 26 months.

Researchers are searching for an "AIDS cure"; but the HIV virus changes form so fast, it is unlikely a cure will ever be found.

Some say the origin of AIDS is unknown; the earliest documented case of it appeared in 1981 in San Francisco. However, there may have been undocumented cases of it in the 1970s.

Others say that there is a different origin of AIDS. Dr. Eva Snead feels that the virus was created in the laboratories. She insists that, if you have been vaccinated, you have the virus.

Then there is Dr. William Campbell Douglass, M.D., who, in his book, *AIDS the End of Civilization*, maintains that the vaccines were made from the kidney of the green African monkeys; and that the disease was purposely invented to eliminate certain people.

The disease is transmitted by **oral, vaginal, and anal sex.** This disease is also transmitted through **common needles for IV drugs, contaminated hospital and dental equipment, commercially prepared blood products, and immunotoxic lubricants**. In other words, HIV is transmitted by **sex, street drug IVs, blood transfusions, and getting someone else's blood into your eyes or into cuts on your skin**. It is not possible to contract HIV by giving blood.

NATURAL REMEDIES

PREVENTION

• There are definite indications that some people who test positive for HIV, yet who **take good care of their immune systems**, are less likely to develop full-blown AIDS. Those most often in this category are individuals who contracted HIV by accident (such as hemophiliacs) and normally lived **healthful, clean**

lives. Many of them never develop AIDS.

• Conduct yourself properly, so you are not likely to contract HIV in the first place. Maintain an excellent immune system through **proper diet, rest, exercise**, etc.

• **Total abstinence**, on the part of both you and your spouse prior to and after marriage, is a wonderful way to live and an excellent way to avoid a lot of misery and disease.

• **Never share a toothbrush, razor**, or anything that might have another person's blood on it.

TREATMENT
See your physician.

• But if you contract HIV, you need to think through what you need to change in your life and then set to work to rebuild your immune system.

• Eat lots of **broccoli, brussels sprouts, and cabbage. Raw foods**, such as fruits and vegetables (especially those high in **vitamins A, B complex, C, bioflavonoids, and E**) are very important. Take **vitamin C** to bowel tolerance. **Selenium, zinc, potassium, calcium**, and **magnesium** are also important.

• **Garlic, cabbage, kelp, and lots of fresh and cooked greens** are important. Eat **whole-grain products**. Also eat **beans and nuts**. Limit your intake of **soy products**, without fully dropping them.

• Drink fresh **carrot juice** (3 glasses) daily.

• It is important that you take 4,000-6,000 mg of **flaxseed oil** daily.

• Here are herbs which will help rebuild the immune system: **burdock, garlic, goldenseal, pau d'arco, psyllium, suma, and ginkgo. Garlic** contains *allicin*, which can help kill viruses.

• Also important is **black radish, dandelion root, and silymarin** (milk thistle extract), to strengthen the liver. **Aloe vera** inhibits the growth and spread of HIV. **St. John's wort** tends to inhibit retroviral infections.

• In a research study, 13 patients with HIV were given injections of **bloodroot** and **celandine**; they were found to have improved after 20 days. In another research study, an aged **garlic** preparation significantly helped AIDS patients. In yet another study, **licorice root** was found to help the patients.

• Drink concentrated **aloe vera** juice (2-4 Tbsp.) daily. It contains *carrisyn*, which appears to inhibit the growth of HIV. Although echinacea is a powerful drug, avoid it because it can increase levels of the tumor-necrosis-factor (TNF), thus stimulating replication of HIV.

AVOID
• Stop eating **meat, processed foods, and junk foods.** Banish **tobacco, alcohol, and coffee**. Avoid those who **smoke**.

Certain activities tend to tear down the immune system faster than anything else. Everyone should be aware of what those activities are:

• Using any form of **nicotine**.
• Drinking **alcohol**.
• Using **street drugs**.
• Taking **medicinal drugs**.
• Eating primarily **junk foods**.

S
T
D

• **Sexual excess**, especially non-monogamous sex.

• **Overeating** and getting **little exercise**.

• Eating lots of **pork, shellfish, and animal fat**. Follow the instructions for Cancer *(792-796)* in this book.

Jon Kaiser, M.D., in San Francisco, has stopped the progression of HIV in more than 1,000 patients by putting them on a program of whole foods, nutritional supplements, herbs, exercise, and stress reduction. Once again, natural remedies can accomplish a lot.

RISK FACTORS FOR AIDS—

Since the beginning of the epidemic in the 1980s, a number of health conditions and lifestyle factors have been identified that increase an individual's risk of contracting HIV and developing AIDS. The more of the following factors are present, the greater the risk:

• Overuse of certain drugs, especially **antibiotics and steroids**

• **High-risk sexual activity**

• Substance abuse, including the use of **alcohol, cigarettes, cocaine, amyl nitrate, marijuana, and other recreational drugs**, especially **intravenous drug use**

• Preexisting **herpes infection, hepatitis**, and/or **mononucleosis**

• Preexisting **sexually transmitted disease**, especially **syphilis**

• A diet high in **processed foods, refined sugars, and fat**

• Infection with yeast (**Candida** albicans) and/or **parasites**

ENCOURAGEMENT—You have a bright future, if you will give your earthly life to Jesus, just now. He can forgive your past and empower you, by His grace, to obey His Ten Commandment law. Everyone in the world needs Him. You can be one of those who find Him.

More Encouragement

"God never leads His children otherwise than they would choose to be led, if they could see the end from the beginning, and discern the glory of the purpose which they are fulfilling as coworkers with Him. Not Enoch, who was translated to heaven, not Elijah, who ascended in a chariot of fire, was greater or more honored than John the Baptist, who perished alone in the dungeon. 'Unto you it is given in the behalf of Christ, not only to believe on Him, but also to suffer for His sake.' Philippians 1:29. And of all the gifts that Heaven can bestow upon men, fellowship with Christ in His sufferings is the most weighty trust and the highest honor."

—Desire of Ages, 224-225

"The first thing to be learned by all who would become workers together with God is the lesson of self-distrust; then they are prepared to have imparted to them the character of Christ. This is not to be gained through education in the most scientific schools. It is the fruit of wisdom that is obtained from the divine Teacher alone."

—Desire of Ages, 250

"God takes men as they are, and educates them for His service, if they will yield themselves to Him. The Spirit of God, received into the soul, will quicken all its faculties."

— Desire of Ages, 251

Two editions of Desire of Ages, the classic (and best) book on the life of Christ are available from us.

The *Natural* *Remedies* *Encyclopedia*

STD Skin Lesions

Here you will find 10 color pictures of skin lesions produced by 6 sexually-transmitted diseases:

Syphilis (3) 809 / Gonorrhea Infant (1) 809 / Oral Herpes (2) 810 / Genital Warts (1) 810 / Genital Herpes (1) 810 / AIDS (2) 810

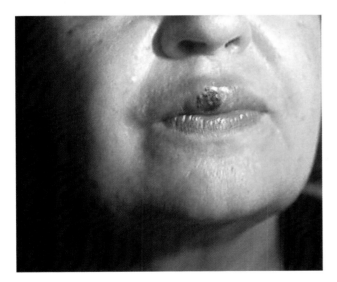
Syphilis

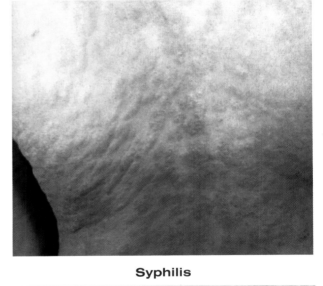
Syphilis

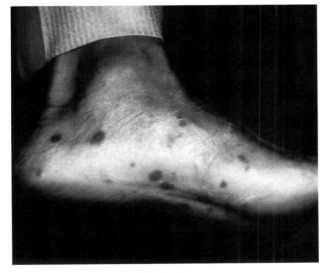
Syphilis

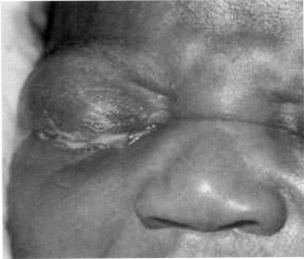
Gonorrhea infant

S
T
D

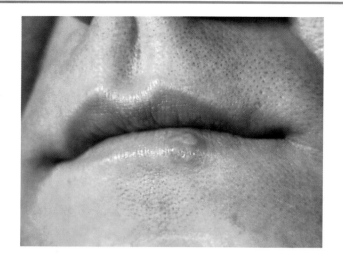

Oral Herpes

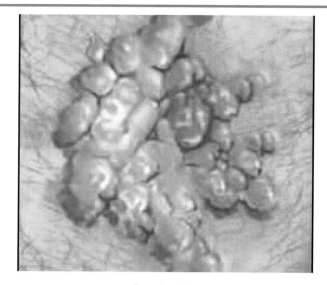

Genital Warts

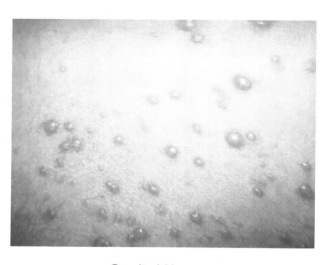

Genital Herpes

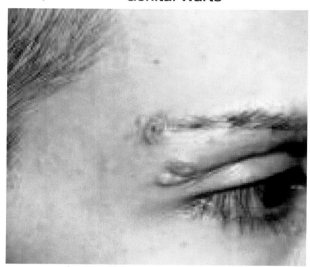

AIDS

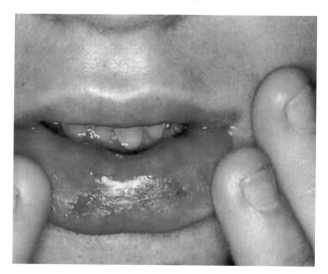

Oral Herpes

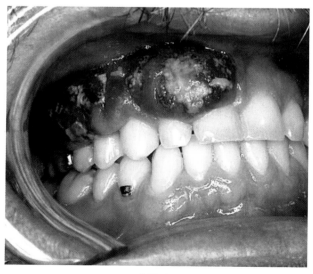

AIDS

Natural Remedies Encyclopedia

- Section 23 - Terrorist and New Diseases

Also Terrorist Attacks, How to Prepare for an Emergency 973-989

"His mercy is on them that fear Him from generation to generation."
　　　　　　　　　　　　—Luke 1:50

"And let him that is athirst come. And whosoever will, let him take of the water of life freely."
　　　　　　　　　　　　—Revelation 22:17

"There is no want to them that fear Him . . They that seek the Lord shall not want any good thing."
　　　　　　　　　　　　—Psalm 34:9-10

"God shall wipe away all tears from their eyes; and there shall be no more death, neither sorrow, nor crying, neither shall there be any more pain: for the former things are passed away."
　　　　　　　　　　　　—Revelation 21:4

N
E
W

TERRORISM ALERT DANGERS - AND OTHER NEW LISTINGS

TERRORIST AND NEW DISEASES -
1 - TERRORIST DISEASES

RADIATION POISONING

— TERRORISM ALERT —
— *The threat of "Dirty bombs" are becoming an increasing danger. Turn to page 974 for ways to protect yourself and your family.*

SMALLPOX (VARIOLA)

— TERRORISM ALERT —
— *Smallpox is far more dangerous than anthrax, because it is so easily communicated. See pages 974 for information on this important subject.*

ANTHRAX (BACILLUS ANTHRACIS)

— TERRORISM ALERT —
SYMPTOMS—Because terrorists distribute a fine, white powder to be breathed, *Pulmonary Anthrax* is the likely result. Early symptoms include low-grade fever, nonproductive cough, malaise, fatigue, myalgia, profound sweats, chest discomfort. Upper respiratory tract symptoms are rare.

One to 5 days after the onset of initial symptoms (but may be preceded by 1-3 days of improvement), there is an abrupt beginning of high fever and severe respiratory distress (dyspnea, stridor, cyanosis). Within 24-36 hours, shock and death occurs.

If the powder gets on the skin, but is not breathed, it can cause *Cutaneous Anthrax*, producing a pustule on the skin that breaks, discharging a heavy serum. In about 36 hours, that area becomes a bluish-black mass of dead tissue. This form is less dangerous if treated early. High fever, vomiting, profuse sweating, and extreme prostration result. Fatal if not treated.

CAUSES—The only cause in the Western World would be a terrorist attack. Fortunately, unlike small-pox, anthrax is not contagious. You have to breath the particles.

TREATMENT—Contact a physician immediately. If not treated early, death will follow.

EBOLA VIRUS (Ebola Hemorrhagic Fever)

— TERRORISM ALERT —
SYMPTOMS—The incubation period ranges from 2 to 21 days. Onset of illness is abrupt and characterized by fever, headache, joint and muscle aches, sore throat, and weakness, followed by diarrhea, vomiting, and stomach pain. A rash, red eyes, hiccups, and internal and external bleeding may occur.

CAUSES—This disease, named after a river in the Congo (formerly Zaire), is a severe, often fatal disease in humans and primates (monkeys and apes) that first appeared in 1976. It is mentioned here because terrorists may try to use it. There are three subgroups, but the symptoms are identical.

The primary cause is eating diseased animal meat. After the first person is infected, others can catch it from direct contact with his blood and/or secretions, while caring for him, or needle contact.

TREATMENT—Caregivers must use masks, gowns, and gloves. Contact a physician immediately.

BUBONIC PLAGUE

(Pneumonic Plague)
— TERRORISM ALERT —
— *Bubonic Plague is dealt with in detail on pp. 843. If not treated within 24-48 hours, it is generally 100% fatal. Knowing what causes it will help you avoid it.*

FOOT AND MOUTH DISEASE

(Hoof and Mouth Disease)
— TERRORISM ALERT —
This is NOT a disease which humans can contract, and does not affect food safety; but, because terrorists can use it to infect livestock and thus cripple the economy, it is mentioned here.

SYMPTOMS—It infects pigs, sheep, goats, deer, and other cloven-footed animals, and is one of the most dreaded diseases by ranchers.

CAUSES—Although rarely fatal (except among young animals), it is highly contagious and cannot be stopped till it runs its course (2 weeks to 6 months) and heavily reduces the milk and meat supply.

TREATMENT—The virus can be killed by heat, low humidity, or some disinfectants. Although they themselves cannot contract it, people can spread the virus to animals. In England, large numbers of livestock have been slaughtered in order to stop the spread of the disease.

TERRORIST AND NEW DISEASES - 2 - NEW DISEASES

WEST NILE VIRUS
(West Nile Encephalitis)

SYMPTOMS—*Mild case:* Light illness (fever, headaches, body aches). *Serious:* The virus begins with a low-grade fever and diarrhea. About a week later, it develops into encephalitis (brain infection). Permanent brain damage or death can result if people in your area are contracting the disease. Dead birds, especially crows, are another indication. It is in the elderly that the disease spreads to the nervous system and bloodstream.

CAUSES—This is an inflammation of the brain which is commonly found in Africa, West Asia, and the Middle East. It is caused by viruses transmitted by mosquitoes. The Middle East strain of the disease entered the U.S. through New York in 1999. Of those with severe illnesses, about 3% to 15% die. Fatalities generally occur from 55 years of age, onward.

Stay indoors at dawn, dusk, and early evening. When outside, wear long-sleeved shirts and long pants. Because mosquitoes can bite through thin clothing, spray clothing with repellents containing permethrin or DEET. (An insecticide with 35% DEET is best; higher than that provides no additional protection.) Insecticides are dangerous! Do not put them on the hands of children; for they may put them in their mouths or touch their eyes. Install window and door screens.

TREATMENT—Contact a physician.
—*See Viral Infections (296).*

LYME DISEASE

— *For a larger discussion of this very dangerous new disease, turn to pp. 840.*

CREUTZFELDT-JACOB DISEASE
(Mad Cow Disease, Kuru)

— *Mad Cow Disease has become a serious menace. Experts warn that it will become the most endemic plague of the 21st century, surpassing that of even AIDS. For more on this relatively new menace, turn to p. 806.*

HUNTA VIRUS

SYMPTOMS—The first signs are fever and muscle aches, which appear 1-5 weeks after infection. Then comes shortness of breath and coughing. Once this phase begins, the disease progresses rapidly. It is potentially deadly.

CAUSES—This is a lung infection which results from exposure to rodent (especially deer mouse, but also rat) droppings in warm, dry climates. New Mexico and Arizona have the most cases of this recently introduced disease. The chances that a person will become infected are rare. Poorly maintained cabins in the Southwest are usual sources of infection. It is not contagious. Rats and mice shed the viruses through their urine which, when it dries, goes into the air and is inhaled.

TREATMENT—Residents in that area are acquainted with the symptoms; and they recognize that the disease is serious enough that the patient must be rushed to the hospital.

LA CROSSE ENCEPHALITIS

SYMPTOMS—Symptoms similar to West Nile Virus (WNV): headaches, fever, neck stiffness, and confusion.

CAUSES—This disease is similar to WNV, but less common. Unlike WNV which occurs primarily in older people, La Crosse occurs in children under 16. The disease is usually mild, but long-term effects can include learning disabilities, seizures, and permanent brain damage. La Crosse was first discovered in the U.S. in 1974. The disease is transmitted by infected mosquitoes and small animals, such as squirrels and chipmunks in oak forest areas.

TREATMENT—Contact a physician.
—*See Viral Infections (296).*

FIRE ANTS
(Solenopsis Invicte)

SYMPTOMS—You will find mounds of loose dirt above ground. Worker ants are dark, small, highly variable in size, aggressive, and sting relentlessly. Be aware of your surroundings.

CAUSES—If you must work near fire ants, wear rubber boots and gloves with talcum powder. You will find mounds of loose dirt above ground. Phorid flies (which do not injure people) lay their eggs on fire ants and greatly damage their underground hives.

TREATMENT—If they crawl onto your skin, they first bite with their mandibles in order to anchor for the thrust of the sting. As soon as you feel this pinching action, quickly sweep the ants off before they actually sting and you can avoid most of the damage.
—*See Ant Bite (833) and Fire Ant Bite (833).*

NEW

KILLER BEES

SYMPTOMS—Many repeated bites from extremely ferocious bees.

CAUSES—In 1956, some colonies of African Honey Bees were imported into Brazil. When they escaped, they gradually spread northward. In 1990, they entered southern Texas and Arizona; and they entered California in 1995. They react to disturbances faster than honey bees, attack in great numbers, and chase people for a quarter mile. They have killed about a thousand people since 1956. They endanger the U.S. honey bee industry.

TREATMENT—Be aware of your surroundings, wear proper clothing, take cover as soon as possible.

SHARK ATTACK

SYMPTOMS—A deep bite. Tiger sharks are the only ones which eat people; the great white shark and bull shark only take a bite.

CAUSES—There is an increasing number of shark attacks on our coasts. It is thought that ocean warming may be causing the dangerous shark species to move farther northward. About 100 people are attacked yearly; about 35 die.

WHAT TO DO—

When you are in the water, do not carry dead fish. Do not swim alone, at night, early in the morning, or late in the evening. Stay out of murky water. Do not wear contrasting colors or flashing objects. Purchase an underwater attack gun.

When in shark waters, but no shark is in sight, watch for fins. If you see one fin cutting the surface, it is probably a porpoise. Two fins, one behind the other, is likely to be a shark.

If you spot a shark, stay calm, swim calmly and rhythmically back to land or boat. Keep the shark in sight, especially if you are underwater. In most shark attacks, the victim did not see the shark.

Sharks seem to shy away from people who look directly at them. If he comes at you, hit him on the nose. It is a very sensitive area, and he is likely to retreat.

The most dangerous sharks are the great white, tiger, and bull. Bull sharks are in the Mississippi River as far as Ohio.

FORMOSAN TERMITE

SYMPTOMS—This new pest does not injure people, but eats their homes. The most severe infestation is in New Orleans, where entire city blocks and live oaks are under attack. They eat wood faster than any other termite because they have larger colonies, produce more young, and are more aggressive. They have been known to eat through lead, asphalt, plaster, mortar, rubber and plastic—in order to get to wood.

They eat houses and living trees. They live in nests made of chewed wood, saliva, and excrement. The nests may be located above ground. Each colony forages an area of several hundred feet.

CAUSES—The Formosan Termite first entered the U.S. a number of years ago. It is now in Louisiana, Hawaii, Mississippi, Texas, Alabama, Florida, Georgia, South Carolina, southern California, North Carolina, and Tennessee.

TREATMENT—They swarm at dusk in the spring and fall, and are attracted to light. Mud tunnels show their presence; also hollow-sounding walls and floors. Nests in walls may cause them to bulge outward. Check in crawl spaces under structures. Spray for termites.

SEVERE ACUTE RESPIRATORY SYNDROME (SARS)

SYMPTOMS—In the first phase, patients get a fever of 100.4° F. or more—with chills, headaches, and muscle aches. The SARS virus incubates in the body for 2-7 days before symptoms emerge. Within a week, most develop a dry cough and difficulty in breathing. About 10%-20% require a ventilator. There are muscle aches, loss of appetite, and diarrhea which is possibly severe. Chest X-rays are suggestive of pneumonia.

CAUSES—The cause of SARS is a previously unknown virus in the coronavirus family. Those viruses often infect animals; and, until now, they caused only mild illness in people. It is believed that the virus was in poultry and jumped to humans.

SARS is spread by direct person-to-person contact. Unlike influenza *(294)* or tuberculosis *(505)*, SARS is transmitted by droplets spread when an infected person coughs or sneezes, not merely through the air. It is not yet known how long an infected person remains contagious.

TREATMENT—Officially, there is no cure, other than bed rest and the care you would give for fevers and virus infections.

But a team of doctors (Leonard Horowitz and Joseph Puleo) have developed a natural remedy for coronaviruses; this includes (1) Lomatium dissectum root extract (which was used for centuries by American Indians to treat tuberculosis and other lung infections), (2) Devil's club (oplopanax horridus; which boosts the immune function), (3) Rosaceae plants (Amelanchier ainifolia, Rosa nutkana, or Saskatoons), and edible fruits used by the Indians for stomach problems. In 1995, they were shown to fight coronaviruses. For the tincture, contact 888-508-4787.

PREVENTION—Doctors and nurses caring for SARS patients should take proper safety precautions and wear masks, gloves, and gowns. Washing hands regularly is important. A mask should be worn in areas where there are many cases. Coronaviruses can survive for 24 hours on surfaces; so carefully remove and dispose of your mask after using it.

N
E
W

AVIAN FLU (BIRD FLU)

SYMPTOMS—Eye inflammation; possibly respiratory infections, especially pneumonia.

CAUSES—This is a virus infection which jumps from chickens to humans on chicken farms; and it is then transmitted by sneezed droplets to other people.

TREATMENT—If caught early, give treatment for flu (294). But if a severe case, treat as for pneumonia (503).

GUANARITO VIRUS

SYMPTOMS—Fever, shock, and hemorrhaging.

CAUSES—This is a deadly new virus that emerged when farmers in Venezuela began clearing millions of acres of forest lands in order to grow crops. The farms drew hoards of rats and mice which, through their droppings, brought a new virus. So far, a major outbreak in America has not occurred.

TREATMENT—Treat this viral infection as for fever and pneumonia (503). Also see viral infections (296).

NIPAH VIRUS

SYMPTOMS—Fever, leading to a severe brain infection and death.

CAUSES—Another new disease (1999), Nipah virus, first appeared in Malaysia. The droppings of fruit bats, living in the rafters of pig farms, fell into hog drinking troughs. The virus soon spread from pigs to their keepers. The immediate outbreak ended when over a million pigs were slaughtered. There is reason to believe that the epidemic could reoccur and be carried to Western nations.

TREATMENT—Treat this viral infection as for fever and pneumonia (503). Also see viral infections (296).

TERRORIST AND NEW DISEASES -
3 - SPECIAL REPORTS

SPECIAL REPORT:
GULF WAR SYNDROME

Veterans of the 1990-1991 Gulf War have experienced a number of puzzling, and often severe, symptoms. This special report will provide you with additional information on this problem.

Physicians at a number of research centers have studied intensively into the problem. For example, in 1999, physicians at the University of Texas Southwestern Medical Center in Dallas presented the results of brain scans performed on victims of the syndrome, which showed depleted brain cells in three areas of the brain.

The scans performed on 12 veterans with severe cases of the syndrome found brain cell losses of between 10%-25% in three regions deep inside the brain: (1) the basal ganglia of the left hemisphere, (2) the basal ganglia of the right hemisphere, and (3) the brain stem.

Scans performed on healthy veterans of the 1990-1991 Gulf War were normal.

Astoundingly, it was found that the amount of brain cell loss in the Gulf War Veterans was comparable to that of patients with brain diseases like Amyotrophic Lateral Sclerosis (ALS or Lou Gehrig's Disease, 577), Multiple Sclerosis (580), Dementia Praecox, and other degenerative neurological disorders, even though the brain areas affected were different.

Examining this more closely, it was found that veterans with damage to the right basal ganglia appeared to share symptoms such as impaired sense of direction, memory lapses, and depression.

Brain cell losses on the left side appeared to cause more general confusion (including difficulty in understanding instructions, reading, solving problems, and making decisions). Left side damage also appeared to correlate with elevated levels of dopamine, a neurotransmitter involved in movement and emotion.

Damage to the brain stem appeared to account, at least in part, for loss of balance and dizzy spells.

These discoveries helped explain why veterans with Gulf War Syndrome show several different types of symptoms. The key appears to be which part of the brain was damaged by chemicals in the war.

There can be damage to one of the three areas, to two of them, or all three.

Earlier research disclosed three primary Gulf War Syndromes. Efforts were made to link sets of symptoms with different combinations of chemicals which were toxic to brain cells.

Syndrome 1 was commonly found in veterans who wore pesticide-containing flea collars. Apparently, the fumes from the flea collars were breathed into the lungs and produced impairment of cognition. Those veterans could not perceive or retain information as well as they could prior to going to Saudia Arabia.

Syndrome 2, called *confusion ataxia*, is the most severe and debilitating. It occurred among veterans who said they were both exposed to low-level nerve gas and had experienced side-effects from swallowing anti-nerve gas PB (*pyridostigmine*) tablets.

Researchers at the University of Texas concluded that it was the combination of low-level nerve gas exposure and the anti-gas tablets that caused the severe brain damage.

Syndrome 3 was characterized by central pain, and was found among veterans who wore both the insect collars containing high levels of DEET, an insect repellent, and had taken the anti-nerve gas tablets.

Tests were also done to verify whether the physical problems could have been caused by combat stress and post-traumatic stress. But no correlation was found to exist. The problem was the chemicals, not the war.

One out of every seven Gulf War veterans suffered later symptoms from exposure to chemicals (100,000 out of 700,000 U.S. soldiers).

Meanwhile, other investigators found additional factors which were involved:

It was discovered that 15 separate chemical agents had been mixed together and put into artillery shells. These shells had earlier been given to Saddam Hussein who, at the time was thought to be our ally. Caches of those shells, when found by our military in southern Iraq during the Gulf War, were exploded in order to eliminate them. But they forgot to watch the wind, which was blowing south at the time (there is lots of wind in the desert)—and many of our soldiers were gassed by those nerve agents. Alarm systems, previously installed to give warning of the approach of chemical agents, did not function properly.

Another problem was *mycoplasma*, also released by those explosions. Some shells contained several strains of *mycoplasma* bacteria, which had been "engineered" by the U.S. military to be more deadly against an enemy.

Another difficulty was the anthrax vaccines which were given to our soldiers. There were contaminating factors in the vaccines which later caused many soldiers serious problems. It is feared that current supplies of Anthrax vaccine in the U.S. are also contaminated.

Another aspect was the oil smoke, from oil wells set on fire at Saddam's command, which many breathed.

Lastly, there were the excitotoxins. Aspartame is marketed as *NutraSweet, Equal, Spoonful*, and *Equal Measure*. It is also found in MSG (monosodium glutamate). When the temperature of a product containing aspartame (so-called "diet foods") exceeds 86° F., the wood alcohol in aspartame converts to formaldehyde and then to formic acid. This produces methanol toxicity which mimics the symptoms of multiple sclerosis. Civilians are having problems with this and our Gulf War veterans did also. Diet drinks were the primary fluid intake for most of them, stored at temperatures approaching 120° F. It is extremely dangerous for pregnant women to drink aspartame. But it is not good for the rest of us either. Even sugar manufacturers are now adding aspartame to their sugar, because it is cheaper than the sugar. It is believed that every major food company now adds aspartame or MSG to its products, to make them more delicious. Read the labels on the food you purchase. For more on this, see the book by Russell Blaylock, M.D., *Excitotoxins: The Taste that Kills*. Also see *Defense Against Alzheimer's Disease*, by H.J. Roberts, M.D. Also available is the lengthy discussion of excitotoxins in this *Encyclopedia*.

Summarizing the problem: Pesticide collars and sprays, nerve-gas inhalation, swallowing anti-nerve gas (PB) tablets, *Mycoplasma* infection from the nerve gas, anthrax vaccines, breathing smoke from burning oil wells, and drinking "diet" ("sugarless") soft drinks heated above 86° F.

SPECIAL REPORT:
MAD COW DISEASE

The following information is adapted from the author's very popular 176-page book, *International Meat Crisis*.

It is now known that all the diseases, listed below, are caused by people or animals eating diseased animals.

1 - ***Kuru*** was once epidemic in a certain tribe in New Guinea, because people had a tradition of eating their dead relatives. Gradually, they developed CJD (described below), which they called "Kuru." Researchers from Britain and America, in the early 1950s, brought it to their laboratories. When they could not figure out what it was (because, incredibly, it is misfolded proteins—called **prions**—instead of bacteria or viruses), their samples were tossed out. The disease gradually spread to animals. (*Also see pp. 585, 813.*)

2 - ***Bovine spongiform encephalopathy*** (BSE). This is better known as **mad cow disease**. It is an infectious and incurable disease which affects the entire body while slowly attacking the brain and nervous system of cattle. Spongiform encephalopathy is Latin for "sponge brains." Cattle, which should normally eat only grass, get it from eating feed pellets which primarily consist of dead and often diseased cows, sheep, pigs, and horses. Like the Kuru people, they have been turned into cannibals. Livestock is fed this diet to hasten growth and increase profits for the meat industry.

3 - ***Scrapie*** is the form of BSE which is found in sheep. When the dead animals are fed to cattle, BSE is transmitted. Infected sheep scrape their sides and heads on trees, fence posts, or even barbed wire. The sheep got this disease because they were fed, not just grass, but pellets made from dead, diseased cows and sheep. So they were also forced to become cannibals, eating other sheep.

4 - ***Spongiform encephalopathies*** is the name given to this type of disease in various animals and in man. We get it from eating meat from farm animals which have contracted BSE by being fed diseased animals.

5 - Drs. Creutzfeldt and Jakob were researchers in Berlin who, in the early 1920s, gave their names to a strange disease, which was an extreme rarity, until the researchers brought Kuru samples to the Western World.

6 - By late 1994, a handful of people in Britain had died from the same disease, which by that time had been named ***Creutzfeldt-Jakob disease*** (CJD). This is the name, in people, for **mad cow disease**. (It is pronounced "*Crewtzfelt-Yahkob*.") Although the disease existed as a rarity prior to the New Guinea research, it did not explode on the world until after Kuru was investigated.

7 - ***Alzheimer's disease*** is a non-spongiform disease, and is not at all related to BSE, CJD, or mad cow disease. But it figures strongly into the present discussion because there is clear evidence that many people, dying in America and elsewhere from *Creutzfeldt-Jakob disease* are being misdiagnosed as the victims of Alzheimer's. This is due to the fact that the symptoms of both diseases are practically identical prior to death.

Whether it be Kuru or CJD, patients first show

symptoms of mental changes (such as problems with coordination, recent memory loss, and slurred speech). Sometimes obvious twitching of muscles can be seen, the facial expression becomes fixed, and the person may stumble and fall over. Over the next few weeks, the person becomes confused and unaware, unable to read or recognize even close relatives. **The disease is very similar to Alzheimer's; yet the cause is very different.**

Physicians at the Veterans Administration Medical Center in Pittsburgh autopsied 54 patients who died of dementia. It was found that three had actually died of CJD (mad cow disease)! That is a shockingly high ratio; it means that large numbers of people in America are now dying each year from mad cow disease, misdiagnosed as Alzheimer's.

Since the 1970s, CJD has been able to hide behind Alzheimer's, which in recent decades has had an incredible rapid increase of cases. The truth is that many cases are mad cow disease—caused by eating cattle, sheep, and pigs; all of which are routinely fed feed containing diseased animal blood and (contrary to directives) diseased animal parts.

Alzheimer's is a genetic disease; and genetic diseases do not double and triple their rates. Yet Alzheimer's is doing just that. All the while you are being told that there is no "mad cow disease in America."

Especially in the Western world, which is able to afford commercially raised meat, BSE will, even more than AIDS, eventually become the most prevalent, virulent disease to hit this planet since the bubonic plague of the Middle Ages. You can only avoid it by refusing to eat anything which contains meat. BSE is a long-term disease; people generally die 7 to 35 years after contracting it.

Rendering (turning dead animals into animal feed) is only legal in America. In all other countries, the "cash for corpses" practice is illegal. In the U.S., until 1997, it was fully legal. This firmly established BSE and scrapie in U.S. farm animals. Since 1997, it is still legal to put blood in the animal feed; yet it is known that mad cow disease affects every part of the animal, even though symptoms most heavily affect the brain. Since that year, news reports have disclosed that many meat producers are ignoring the ban and continuing to feed animal parts to U.S. cows, sheep, pigs, chickens, and pond-raised fish. Only old or sickly animals are sold to the animal feed processors, to be rendered into animal feed.

As you may know, news reports tell of wild animals (especially elk and deer) which now have a variant of mad cow disease, called wasting disease. Hunters are known to have died from eating them.

It is, indeed, unfortunate that these problems exist. We deeply wish it were not so. But since the crisis is real, and gradually worsening, it is urgent that solutions be found. *(Also see pp. 585, 813.)*

Unlike the American public which keeps eating animals that are fed diseased blood and animal parts, people in Europe are frightened. Anxious to keep eating meat they are stealing elk, reindeer, ostriches, crocodiles, and other exotic meats from the zoos *(AP, Berlin, January 28, 2001).* For more on this, and how meat eating increases the chances of other diseases, see the author's book, *International Meat Crisis.*

SPECIAL REPORT:
EXCITOTOXIN SYNDROME

Excitotoxins is the name that has been applied to a group of chemicals which is widely used as food additives, to enhance food flavors and substitute for sugar.

One of these is monosodium glutamate (MSG). Another is aspartame, which is marketed under the name, NutraSweet. *Also see Gulf War Syndrome (815).*

Eating foods containing excitotoxins can affect your child's nervous system, so that in later years he may have learning or emotional difficulties. They can cause brain tumors to develop. They can aggravate or even precipitate many of today's neurodegenerative brain diseases, such as Parkinson's disease *(582),* Alzheimer's disease *(587),* or the very rare Huntington's disease. People who eat foods containing excitotoxins are especially at risk if they have diabetes, or have ever had a stroke, brain injury, brain tumor, seizure, or have suffered from hypertension, meningitis, or viral encephalitis.

Both MSG and aspartame can cause the same brain damage. Many of the brain lesions caused by these products are irreversible and, in sufficient concentration, can result from a single exposure to these products.

MSG and aspartame are added to foods in order to increase the flavor and substitute for real sweetening. This sells more food and saves the food industry millions of dollars—since MSG and aspartame cost the manufacturers a lot less than real food. Unfortunately, the food industry frequently disguises these excitotoxin food additives (MSG and aspartame) under different names on food labels.

Here are food additives which always contain MSG: monosodium glutamate, hydrolyzed vegetable protein, hydrolyzed protein, hydrolyzed plant protein, plant protein extract, sodium caseinate, calcium caseinate, yeast extract, textured protein (including TVP), autolyzed yeast, hydrolyzed oat flour, corn oil.

Here are food additives which frequently contain MSG: malt extract, malt flavoring, bouillon, broth, stock, flavoring, natural flavors, natural flavoring, seasoning, spices.

Here are food additives which may contain MSG or excitotoxins: carrageenan, enzymes, soy protein concentrate, soy protein isolate, and whey protein concentrate.

In addition, protease enzymes of various sources can release excitotoxin amino acids from food proteins.

Next, we turn our attention to aspartame, which is an intense source of excitotoxins. Aspartame is a sweetener made up of three chemicals: Aspartic acid, phenylalanine, and methanolphenylalanine. It should be avoided at all costs! Do not eat or drink anything containing aspartame!

Aspartame is the technical name for the brand names

N
E
W

of *NutraSweet, Equal, Spoonful,* and *Equal-Measure.* Aspartame was discovered by accident in 1965, when James Schlatter, a chemist of G.D. Searle Company, was testing an anti-ulcer drug. Aspartame was approved for dry goods in 1981 and for carbonated beverages in 1983. It was originally approved for dry goods on July 26, 1974; but objections filed by neuroscience researcher Dr. John W. Olney and Consumer attorney James Turner (in August 1974), as well as investigations of G.D. Searle's research practices, caused the U.S. Food and Drug Administration (FDA) to put approval of aspartame on hold (December 5, 1974). In 1985, Monsanto purchased G.D. Searle and made Searle Pharmaceuticals and The NutraSweet Company separate subsidiaries.

Aspartame is, by far, the most dangerous substance on the market that is added to foods. Aspartame accounts for over 75 percent of the adverse reactions to food additives reported to the U.S. Food and Drug Administration (FDA). Many of these reactions are very serious (including seizures and death), as recently disclosed in a February 1994 Department of Health and Human Services report.

A few of the 90 different documented symptoms listed in the report as being caused by aspartame include: headaches / migraines, dizziness, seizures, nausea, numbness, muscle spasms, weight gain, rashes, depression, fatigue, irritability, tachycardia, insomnia, vision problems, hearing loss, heart palpitations, breathing difficulties, anxiety attacks, slurred speech, loss of taste, tinnitus, vertigo, memory loss, and joint pain.

According to researchers and physicians studying the adverse effects of aspartame, the following chronic illnesses can be triggered or worsened by ingesting aspartame: brain tumors, multiple sclerosis, epilepsy, chronic fatigue syndrome, Parkinson's disease, Alzheimer's, mental retardation, lymphoma, birth defects, fibromyalgia, and diabetes. *Also see Gulf War Syndrome (815).*

Dr. Russell L. Blaylock, a professor of Neurosurgery at the Medical University of Mississippi, recently published a book *(Excitotoxins: The Taste that Kills)* thoroughly detailing the damage that is caused by the ingestion of excessive aspartic acid from aspartame. Fully 99% of monosodium glutamate is glutamic acid. The damage it causes is also documented in Blaylock's book. Blaylock makes use of almost 500 scientific references, to show how excess free excitatory amino acids (such as aspartic acid and glutamic acid) in our food supply are causing serious chronic neurological disorders and a myriad of other acute symptoms.

The risk to infants, children, pregnant women, the elderly, and persons with certain chronic health problems from excitotoxins are great. Even the Federation of American Societies for Experimental Biology (FASEB), which usually understates problems and sides with the FDA, recently stated in a review that "it is prudent to avoid the use of dietary supplements of L-glutamic acid by pregnant women, infants, and children. The existence of evidence of potential endocrine responses *(i.e.,* elevated cortisol and prolactin) and differential responses between males and females would also suggest a neuroendocrine link and that supplemental L-glutamic acid should be avoided by

women of childbearing age and individuals with affective disorders." Aspartic acid from aspartame has the same deleterious effects on the body as glutamic acid.

The exact mechanism is currently being debated. As reported to the FDA, acute reactions to excess free glutamate and aspartate include headaches / migraines, nausea, abdominal pains, fatigue (blocks sufficient glucose entry into brain), sleep problems, vision problems, anxiety attacks, depression, and asthma / chest tightness.

One common complaint of persons suffering from the effect of aspartame is memory loss. Ironically, in 1987, G.D. Searle, the manufacturer of aspartame, undertook a search for a drug to combat memory loss caused by excitatory amino acid damage. Blaylock is one of many scientists and physicians who are concerned about excitatory amino acid damage caused by ingestion of aspartame and MSG. A few of the many experts who have spoken out against the damage being caused by aspartate and glutamate include Adrienne Samuels, Ph.D., an experimental psychologist specializing in research design. Another is Olney, a professor in the department of psychiatry, School of Medicine, Washington University, a neuroscientist and researcher, and one of the world's foremost authorities on excitotoxins. (He informed Searle, in 1971, that aspartic acid caused holes in the brains of mice.) Also included is Francis J. Waickman, M.D., a recipient of the Rinkel and Forman Awards, and Board certified in Pediatrics, Allergy, and Immunology.

As mentioned earlier, aspartame is the technical name for the brand names, *NutraSweet, Equal, Spoonful,* and *Equal-Measure.* Here are some of the food products in which you will find this substance, which is 200 times as sweet as sugar: diet foods, soft drinks, cereals, instant breakfasts, sugar-free chewing gum, cocoa mixes, coffee beverages, juice beverages, frozen desserts, gelatin desserts, milk drinks, breath mints, laxatives, shake mixes, tea beverages, instant teas and coffees, topping mixes, nonprescription pharmaceuticals, tabletop sweeteners, wine coolers, yogurt, some multivitamin supplements. Aspartame is also found in sugar-free gums, sugar-free Kool Aid, Crystal Light, children's medications, and any product claiming to be "low calorie," "diet," or "sugar free."

Aspartame breaks down within 20 minutes at room temperature into several primary toxic ingredients: (1) DKP (diketopiperazine). When ingested, it converts to a near duplicate of a powerful brain tumor-causing agent. (2) Formic acid. This is the venom which ants inject when they sting you. (3) Formaldehyde. This is embalming fluid. (4) Methanol. This substance can cause blindness.

Here is additional information on methanol: It is poisonous, even when consumed in small amounts. It can cause inflammation of the pancreas and heart muscle, swelling of the brain, and/or blindness.

What should you do in order to not eat or drink anything containing aspartame or glutamic acid? The only effective solution is to avoid using all foods containing additives. Primarily eat fresh fruits and vegetables, whole grains, legumes, and nuts. These are the foods consistently recommended throughout this *Encyclopedia.*

N
E
W

The Natural Remedies Encyclopedia

How to Quit Smoking and Drinking

The information in each of these two sections is helpful for both those who want to quit smoking and those who want to quit drinking alcoholic beverages. The principles are similar. If you want to quit one of them, it would be well to read both sections.

The information below was taken from two books by the author: *You Can Quit Smoking* and *You Can Quit Alcohol.*

HOW TO QUIT TOBACCO

The best way to quit smoking is to stop all at once—none of this tapering-off business. It is better to have a few rough days and be through with it than to drag it out for weeks and months. Slow torture is no fun.

Decide to quit—and do it with a positive enthusiasm. Do not be negative, thinking how much you miss it. Be thankful you are getting rid of the habit.

After quitting, the hardest part comes in the first three days; but, by the end of five days, the majority of individuals find the craving definitely less or gone. Continue for ten days, and you make it.

Say to yourself: "I choose not to smoke." The power of the will is important. It is the key to victory. Keep repeating your decision throughout the day from morning till night. The more you say it, the more you mean it.

You know the issues that are involved; the future—for yourself and your loved ones. You know what a miserable life it is to smoke and have it constantly getting in your eyes, costing you money, and craving it in places where smoking is not permitted. And you know it is going to shorten your life.

The facts are out there; you hear them all the time: cancer of the throat, lung cancer, emphysema, hardening of the arteries, slowing of mental activity and reflex responses, cholesterol buildup, reduced heart action and physical endurance, blood pressure problems.

Just one statistic: Dr. Harold F. Dorn studied 200,000 military veterans; and he found that the death rate among all types of cigarette smokers was 58 percent higher than among non-smokers.

There are over 2,000 known harmful chemicals in tobacco; and 400 of them are known to be carcinogenic. These are the facts.

Make a decision to quit. Make a list of reasons why you are quitting. Read over the list while you are quitting.

Learn to depend on prayer. Only God can give you the help you need. There are no atheists in foxholes; and you had better not be one now. This is a crisis in your life; and you need God's help.

If you can, find someone who will pray with and for you, someone who is a real friend and not just a critic. Call your friend on the phone and talk to him when things get rough.

Carry with you some Bible promises:

"I can do all things through Christ which strengtheneth me."—*Philippians 4:13.*

"But thanks be to God, which giveth us the victory through our Lord Jesus Christ."—*1 Corinthians 15:57.*

"Fear thou not; for I am with thee: be not dismayed; for I am thy God: I will strengthen thee; yea, I will help thee."—*Isaiah 41:10.*

Believe that these promises were written just for you and your need, just now. Repeat them often.

Get rid of all your tobacco products, including ash trays and all the rest.

Stay away from other smokers as much as possible for the next few weeks.

Two or even three times a day, take a warm bath for 15 or 20 minutes at a time. Relax and enjoy it. This will help soak the poisons out quicker.

Since you will be tense at this time, the baths will help relax you. (Frankly, while you were smoking, you

Tobacco 880, 936 / CHART 1055

D
R
U
G
S

were tense all the time!)

If you are able to take it and have no cardiac problems—hot showers, hot baths, or steam baths (best of all) will get the nicotine out quicker.

It is a known fact that the quicker the yellow nicotine leaves your body, the quicker the addiction goes with it.

When you go off tobacco, you are likely to find that your sweat at night will yellow the sheets. That is good; you want the nicotine out of your body.

After the bath or shower, take a "cold mitten friction." This water therapy is described in this *Encyclopedia*, on pp. 187-188.

Each time you crave a smoke or drink, begin slow deep breathing. Slowly take in as much air as you can; then exhale it slowly. Repeat your resolve: "I choose not to smoke; I choose not to drink."

As often as you can, go outside in the open air and breathe deeply. There is energy in fresh air; and it is helping to clean you out.

Drink at least 6-8 glasses of water daily. Do this between meals. If necessary, keep a record of how much water you are drinking. This helps flush out poisons.

Take no alcoholic beverages, none at all. They will cloud your mind, weaken your will power, and you will go back to smoking.

Eat lots of fresh fruit and vegetables. Fresh fruit is especially important now. There was a man who hitched a ride across country. He slipped into a re-frigerator car and got locked in. It was full of oranges.

By the time he got out—about six days later—he found he had no craving for cigarettes. For six days, he had nothing to eat but oranges. Eating them took away the craving. The vitamin C in the oranges also helps destroy the poisons in your body, lessening the craving.

You may find that you may gain some weight. But getting rid of tobacco is far more important than the few pounds gained!

You are increasing your will power; and you will later be able to use it to lessen the amount of food you eat, so you can get your weight back down.

Walk outdoors for 15-30 minutes after each meal, breathing deeply as you go. Don't just sit after a meal; for this is the time of day that you will especially want to smoke. Instead, get outside.

Open up the curtains, raise the windows, and let in the purifying sunlight and air. There is tobacco odor all over your house. Get it out. This is important.

Avoid mustard, spices, pepper, vinegar, ketchup, hot sauce, chili, and horseradish. These foods tend to arouse cravings.

Skip all sweets, pastries, cake, ice cream, and chocolate during the first 10 days at least. Avoid rich, sugar-heavy desserts.

Heavy smokers often like highly spiced foods; they frequently eat a heavy meat diet, plus gravies, fried foods, and other rich foods. Avoid them if you want success in kicking the habit.

If you are starting to get squeamish, ask yourself: How serious am I about this?

Do not use fish, fowl, meat, tea, coffee, or cola beverages. The uric acid, ammonia, purines, and other wastes in meat is what gives it that special flavor. It also stimulates your nerves and increases your craving for nicotine and alcohol. The caffeine in tea, coffee, and cola drinks can so trigger your nerves that, in a matter of minutes, you will have an uncontrollable desire to light up.

A lot of sugar in the diet makes you more jumpy and irritable. This is because it steals B vitamins and minerals, especially calcium. Calcium helps strengthen and calm your nerves.

Do not try to solve any major problems just now. Make life as pleasant as possible; keep on the posi-tive side.

Be thankful for your blessings and name them. Thank God for help and ongoing victory. Your prayers will be a sham if you stop praying, after you have gotten the victory over tobacco.

Avoid all sedatives and stimulants.

Tobacco raises blood sugar for 2½ to 3 minutes; and this is part of its addictive power. So, if neces-sary, carry a few pieces of honey-drop candy in the pocket you formerly kept your cigarette pack in. If the going gets rough, chew on one.

Do not go where people are drinking liquor. Avoid old friends who like to drink.

Gentian root is an herb that can be chewed. It removes the taste for tobacco. Chamomile is another helpful herb. You can chew the blossoms between meals when you want a smoke.

The most important part of this program is the earnest prayer to God. Commit your life to Him, and your future will be much happier than your past. Place your will on the side of God. Determine that, with His help, you will succeed.

A sweat bath once a week will help eliminate the nicotine from your system. Keep in the open air as much as possible.

Keep your mind occupied. When tempted, repeat, "Through the power of Christ, I choose not to smoke." When you need to, phone your prayer partner.

Carrot sticks or raw celery at the close of a meal will lessen the craving. Chewing raisins helps some-what. Carry a small package of raisins in your pocket.

You will notice that each time the craving comes, it will keep weakening more quickly in a few minutes.

When friends tell you that you can't do it, do not become angry; but pleasantly tell them to wait and see. (They only tell you that because they don't think they could do it.) Take the initiative: Tell them they need to give it up too.

If you know you are going to be in a situation where people are smoking, prepare for it. Meet it in a positive manner. Settle it, that you are not a timid rabbit. Your days of slavery to the tobacco leaf are over with.

Vitamin C is a great help for cutting the smoking habit. Take vitamin C tablets with water or juice.

Vitamin B complex is also important. Take a B complex supplement at each meal.

Hot water with lemon juice is helpful. Go on a fast for a day or two at a time, drinking only hot water and lemon juice. That will clean the poisons out the fastest. Remember that the quicker they are eliminated, the quicker the craving will go.

Keep positive. Keep busy doing something. Keep praying. Keep thanking Him. Keep thinking of the brighter future for you and your loved ones.

Now that you have kicked the habit, live for others. Find ways to bring more happiness into the lives of those around you. Regularly attend church. Live for God. Encourage others to find the better way of life you have discovered.

There are principles in *How to Quit Alcohol*, below, that will also help you quit smoking. Be sure and read them. *Also see pp. 937*

HOW TO QUIT ALCOHOL

First read over the preceding section on how to quit tobacco. Many of the same principles apply. We will not repeat many of them here. *Also see p. 608, 25.*

First, accept the fact that you have an alcohol problem. Many people refuse to accept this fact, so they continue on with the problem.

You know the situation already: Drinking alcohol shortens the life span drastically. The death records of 2 million policy holders in 43 American life insurance companies, for a 20 year period, were summarized:

People drinking 2 glasses of beer or 1 glass of whisky per day—were 18% more likely to die than the average American. Among those using over 2 glasses of beer or 1 glass of whisky daily—death was 86% higher.

Alcohol produces cirrhosis of the liver. It is progressive and leads to death. It lowers resistance to disease, especially pneumonia. Chronic alcoholism leads to mental disease. A study of 56,000 patients in Massachusetts revealed that one-fifth of all admissions were alcoholics.

Alcohol is not a food and can neither nourish nor strengthen the body. It seems to warm you; but that is only because blood is being drawn from the internal organs to the surface. Alcohol drys out brain

cells; and, over a period of time, more cells keep being destroyed. How well do you want your mind to work when you are older?

Alcoholics tend to need friends. Find a friend or several of them. Talk to them regularly on the phone. Visit them. Especially find someone that you can help recover from alcoholism. Frequently encouraging him will help you.

In a 1967 experiment by U.D. Register, M.D. (Loma Linda University in California), he found that rats fed junk food wanted to drink diluted alcohol instead of water. When he added coffee to their diet, their alcohol intake greatly increased. When they were switched over to an exclusively nutritious diet, nearly all the rats quit the alcohol entirely and returned to drinking water.

Nearly a century ago, Horace Fletcher, a researcher into the careful chewing of food, paid some drunks to go on an experiment. They could have all the liquor they wanted, free, if they did two things: eat nutritious meals—and slowly chew every mouthful of liquor before swallowing it. Those that did this lost their interest in alcohol—even though they could have all they wanted, free of charge.

Drinking alcohol causes a deficiency of the B complex vitamins. So, as you begin quitting liquor, take B complex supplements every day.

Niacin (B_3) is considered by many researchers to be the most important single vitamin in overcoming the alcohol habit. "B_3 far surpasses other therapeutic agents commonly used in the treatment of alcoholics."—*Dr. Russell F. Smith, University of Michigan.* A dose of 12 grams of niacin each day, and onward for several years thereafter, has been suggested. (Be aware that niacin tends to cause the face to flush red for a few minutes when you swallow it. This is natural and in no way harmful.)

Vitamin B_6 (pyridoxine) is also very important.

Other important vitamins include vitamins C, B_1, B_{12}, and E. The entire B complex works together; increased amounts of all the B vitamins should be supplied.

It should be mentioned that increased B_3 dosage depletes the amount of vitamin C in the body; so more vitamin C is needed (An average dose of 1000 mg. of vitamin C daily is frequently used.)

Be sure to remain on a nutritious diet and take these vitamins after you have victory over liquor.

Magnesium is an important mineral. It is significant that the symptoms of magnesium deficiency are identical to the symptoms of *delirium tremens*. Dr. Edmund G. Flink, at West Virginia University Medical School, discovered that magnesium (a trace mineral) greatly reduces the withdrawal symptoms called *delirium tremens* (the D.T.s).

Studies reveal that poor food (such as hot dogs,

Alcohol withdrawal 881

DRUGS

spaghetti meat balls, sweet rolls, and soft drinks) and/ or narcotics (coffee, tea, cigarettes, hard drugs) and/or irritating foods (spices, condiments, sauces, ketchups, gravies)—all increase the craving for alcohol.

Physicians recommend an "aversion therapy." A measured amount of an alcoholic beverage is given. But into it a certain amount of a nausea-producing agent has been mixed. Two such agents are apomorphine and emetine. This tends to develop a loathing for alcohol. Because of the severe physical reactions, this treatment should be accompanied by close medical supervision.

But such treatments are often only temporary. Far better is a nutritious dietary program, deep trust in God, continual study of the Bible, earnest prayer, resolute decision, a friend to talk to, and trying to help others break from the alcohol habit.

What about Alcoholics Anonymous? Unfortunately, it does not urge people to find the help they need in Christ. Only in His strength can we be enabled to resist temptation and addictions, and come off more than conqueror. It says to look to a "higher power," but some of the AA meetings lead people toward occult practices. You do not want that kind of "higher power" in your life. There are lords many and gods many, but there is only one Jesus Christ. He alone can deliver us from sin! He alone can strengthen a person, moment by moment. He alone can take away the thirst for liquor.

Here is a seven-point program of basic Christian principles that, for centuries, have helped many:

Step 1: We admitted that we were powerless over alcohol; our lives had become unmanageable.

Step 2: We came to believe that a Power greater than ourselves could restore us to sanity,— and that Jesus Christ was the only Power that could help us and change our lives.

Step 3: We made a decision to turn our will and our lives over to Jesus Christ, and dedicate ourselves to Him.

Step 4: We honestly searched our lives and determined, in His strength, to make many needed changes. We admitted these wrongs to Christ, and asked Him for forgiveness.

Step 5: We made a list of all persons we had harmed; and we became willing to make amends to them all.

Step 6: We made direct amends to such people whenever possible, except when to do so would injure them or others.

Step 7: Ever seeking to deepen our personal experience with Jesus, we have prayed a for knowledge of His will for us and the power to carry it out, and have tried to to carry this message to alcoholics and to practice these principles in

all our affairs.

Recently a new group therapy approach has been started. It is called the *4-DK Plan* (Four-Dimensional Key to the Cause of Alcoholism). The four dimensions are physical, mental, social, and spiritual.

The plan is educational, can be started in any community, is positive, and emphasizes good health and wholesome living. For more information, contact the International Commission for the Prevention of Alcoholism: 12501 Old Columbia Pike, Silver Spring, MD 20904-6600.

Alcohol is a problem that can be overcome. Others have done it and you can do it also. Carefully read the following information and do exactly what it says. This can mean the beginning of a new way of life for you.

First: You must accept the fact that you have a problem. You must be convinced that you have to quit, for your own sake and for the sake of your loved ones.

Second: You must accept the fact that you cannot do it by yourself. Only in the strength of Christ can it be done. You can only receive that strength through earnest prayer for help. Go on your knees alone—all by yourself—and cry to God over the whole thing. Tell Him what you've done wrong and ask Him to forgive you. And mean it. Tell Him that you are going to dedicate the rest of your life to Him. And mean it. Tell Him you are willing to sacrifice anything that such a dedication requires. And mean it. Then ask Him for strength to break from this terrible habit. Ask Him to help you to either do it by yourself or provide you with one or more friends that will provide encouragement.

Third: Accept the fact that you are not going to stay close to God unless you read His written Word—the Bible—every day; and every day send up your prayers for forgiveness and for help. Each day is a new one, and you must start it with God. There are no shortcuts; for they only lead to detours. You must start every day with Jesus Christ and then walk with Him all day long.

Fourth: Accept the fact that continued prayer for help must be mixed with continued praise. Thankfulness is powerful. Believe in Christ. Believe that He is there; believe that He will help. Believe it all day long, and at night too. Talk to Him often. —You will have the help when you need it, if you will sincerely stay with Him. Believe that He will forgive and accept you, even when you fall. Believe that He loves you deeply, more deeply than you have ever thought possible. He has tried to help you for years, but your stubborn ways have hindered Him. Let Him give you the help now that He wants to give you. Thank Him continually for it. Thank Him even when things look dark and you seem to have no one on your side.

Fifth: You must make some changes in your life. You will have to get more exercise in the open air and more rest at night. You will have to put away the things that tend to separate you from God. If television and radio and the music and magazines you are used to are pulling you away for God, then throw them out. You may find that you have to make some new friends and avoid some old ones. They don't care for your new way of life and want your company in doing things you are no longer interested in doing. The best solution is to find new friends. Go to church regularly. That's where you are more likely to find better ones.

Sixth: It will greatly help if you will go on an initial cleansing program. This will help expel the alcohol from your system more quickly. As with nicotine, the more quickly alcohol is out of your body, the more quickly the old cravings will subside. Such a program will also help you over the initial tremors.

As you know, one must stop these dangerous practices all at once; they cannot be put away simply by gradually cutting down. You want to get rid of the craving as quickly as possible.

Here is a four-day program:

In order to carry out this program, you may need someone to help you. The baths mentioned below will help expel impurities more quickly. Continue them, to a lesser extent, later on. This is a four-day program; and, in order to do it, you will need to stay home during those four days. You will be expelling impurities, getting better nutrition, and obtaining a lot of rest.

Prepare an herbal tea from the following powdered herbs: equal parts of skullcap, catnip, and blue vervain with no sweetening. Combine them in a pot and place 2 tablespoons in a quart of water that has been brought to a boil; then turn off and let it sit for 20 minutes, with the lid on. (This is called "steeping.") Two quarts should last a day and a half, and can be kept refrigerated until it is used up. An eight-ounce glass of tea should be taken every two hours, except when sleeping at night. (The skullcap and catnip will help you relax and sleep; the blue vervain will help you sweat.)

First day—At 7 a.m., drink a glass of water. At 8 a.m., drink 8 oz. of tea. This is a relaxant tea and will help you sleep. The idea here is the more sleep during withdrawal from alcohol, the less problem with the withdrawal symptoms (delirium tremens, hallucinations, etc.). And it works. Stay in bed and rest. Sleep all you can. Every two hours another glass of tea should be brought to you. At 6 p.m. each evening, take a hot and cold shower.

Second day—Same as the first day; but that evening you can have a glass of tomato juice with a ½ teaspoon of cayenne in it. The stomach is used to the bite of alcohol and the red pepper helps take its place just now. Do not use black pepper.

Third day—Same as preceding days. But now you can add a meal, in the evening, of sliced tomato; or, if you prefer, stay with the tomato juice and cayenne.

Fourth day—The usual pattern, except as follows: In the morning, a small meal of fresh fruit or soaked dried fruit; at noon a medium-sized salad, but not too much.

Fifth day—Eat normally, but of nutritious food. Be done with junk food. The program is over.

The above program was developed by an herbalist who died in the 1970s. She successfully used it with many people, and saw it work repeatedly for both those coming off alcohol and those trying to quit tobacco.

During the initial withdrawal and immediately after, sleep is essential. One method of obtaining this is by the use of prolonged baths (with the water temperature maintained at around 92° to 94° F.). Quiet surroundings during this time are absolutely essential. The diet should not include coffee, spices, and condiments; they should be permanently stopped. It is now known that these only whet the appetite to return to alcohol. Fruit, vegetables, and grains are needed, along with water in order to replace body losses.

Dr. Theron G. Randolph discovered that people who regularly drink alcohol become overly sensitive to the things that the alcoholic beverage was derived from. "Sensitivity to corn, malt, wheat, rye, grape, and potato were encountered [in alcoholics] in that order of frequency. It is well-known that alcoholic beverages consumed in this country are derived from foods in approximately the same order."

But more important, than all else, is a personal surrender to Jesus Christ and a strict obedience, by faith in Him, to all Ten of the Commandments (Exodus 20:3-17). God will help you.

**FOR MORE INFORMATION
ON QUITTING TOBACCO, ALCOHOL, COFFEE, AND DRUGS
CHECK THROUGH THE DISEASE AND GENERAL INDEXES**

Anodyne herbs lessen the excitability of the nerves and nerve centers. Most can be used externally as fomentations or internally as teas, tinctures, or powders. *Here is a list of them:* chamomile, cloves, echinacea, ginger, hops, juniper berries, kava kava, lady's slipper, mullein, pulsatilla, skullcap, valerian, vervain, white willow, wild lettuce, wild yam, wood betony. Chamomile and skullcap are among the best.

DRUGS

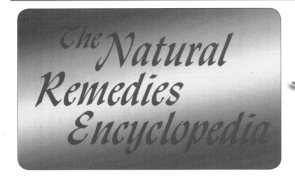

Hard Drugs Warning Signals

This chapter is excerpted from the author's book, Hard Drugs Can Ruin You.

SIXTEEN WARNING SIGNALS: A MESSAGE TO PARENTS

All of the following warning signs have been suggested by professionals in the field of detecting and caring for drug abusers and addicts. One sign alone may mean nothing; several together can be very significant.

1 - SCHOOL GRADES SUDDENLY GO DOWN—This is an important sign. The teenager may offer many different reasons and excuses; but there may be another reason—drugs. A closely related sign is the absence of report cards: They are no longer being shown to you. Check into it; you may find that your A and B student may suddenly have become a C, with occasional F, student.

2 - SUDDENLY DIFFERENT FRIENDS—Young people feel that they have a right to select their own friends; and so they may not appreciate your interest in who their friends are. Notice a strange narrowing of the circle of friends that your adolescent is chumming around with. Keep track of who their friends are. If they suddenly change, or narrow to only a few friends, or seem to drop off entirely, ask about this some evening and see what the reaction is. The kind of friends we have reveals our values and interests. Friends reveal behavior. When our values and actions change, our friendships will change also.

3 - SUDDENLY OLDER FRIENDS—If their friends suddenly change from their own age to four or five years older, this is significant. Why the new acquaintances? The older person has something that the younger wants; and the younger has something the older one wants.

4 - A MAJOR CHANGE IN ATTITUDES AND FEELINGS—Temper tantrums, extreme irritability, or no feelings at all. How did all this start? What has made the change? What caused the switch from an upbeat, energetic attitude to an apathetic, indifferent shrug which seems to be uninterested or not involved in anything worthwhile?

5 - SUDDENLY MONEY COMING IN—Does your son or daughter act as if he or she has inherited wealth? Clothes, food, drink, recreational equipment, electronics.

6 - SUDDENLY MONEY GOING OUT—This is the opposite of the previous possibility: Does your son or daughter suddenly have no money, when he used to have enough for his simple needs?

7 - PHONE CALLS AT ODD HOURS—When the phone rings at 11:30 p.m. on a school night and your son yells "I'll get it." Phone calls late at night after your known bedtime are a cause for concern. Listen in and confront him if what you have heard is the awful truth you have suspected.

8 - THE BEDROOM—What does his or her bedroom look like? Has it recently changed from neatness to sloppiness? Does it look like a cave or a horror movie? Are there blankets on the windows to shut out all light? Is there a total disregard to health and proper environment? Is there unusual equipment in the bedroom (such as hypodermic needles, smoking gadgets, spoons, saucers, white or brown powders, pills, tablets, or ampoules)?

9 - LIVING IN AN UNREAL WORLD—Does your teenager live in a totally different world than most of his or her companions? Does he dream of a great occupation as an astronaut, yet gives no attention to school studies? Does she dream of romance with a rock star, yet shuts herself away from boys her own age? Living in a fantasy world can be an early step into the drug

Drug withdrawal 883 / Opium symptoms 1055 / Street Drugs 953-963

DRUGS

culture. Becoming conditioned to not want to cope with real life can prepare one for the unreal dead-end street of drug entertainment.

10 - CONCERNED NEIGHBORS AND FRIENDS—People tend to keep to themselves and not speak up, even when they should. But if some of your friends and neighbors begin warning you about the behavior of your teenager, then you had better sit up and listen. If someone comes to you about your youngster, it may be serious. Pay attention and do something about it.

First try to solve the problem in your home; and, if that does not work, there are resources outside the home. Be a loving, helpful parent. But also be watchful. And if warning signs arise, bring it out into the open. If necessary tell them, "If you're buying dope, I want to know about it. I'm not going to throw you out. I love you, but I want to know about it."

11-16 - SIX MORE SIGNS—(1) The youngster becomes sleepy, apathetic, secretive, cranky, and unreliable. (2) He loses interest in his schoolwork, his hobbies, and in physical exertion. (3) He locks himself in the bathroom for long periods. (4) He takes money or articles of value from the home. (5) He wants to quit school and usually does. (6) His arms may be covered with the marks of a hypodermic needle.

THIRTY-FOUR WARNING SIGNS OF DRUG USE

Here are additional warning signs. The list comes from helpforteens.net. If you wish to phone for counseling, here is the number: 800-637-0701.

Neglected appearance / hygiene. Poor self-image. Grades dropping. Violent outbursts at home. Frequent use of eye wash. Unexplained weight drop. Drug paraphernalia. Slurred speech. Curfew violations. Running away. Skin abrasions. Hostility toward family members. Chemical breath. Glassy eyes. Red eyes. Valuables missing. Possessing unexplained valuables. Stealing / borrowing money. Change in friends. Depression. Withdrawal. Apathy. Reckless behavior. No concern about future. Defies family values. Disrespect to parents. Lying and deception. Sneaky behavior. Disregards consequences. Loss of interest in healthy activities. Verbally abusive. Manipulative / self-centered. Lack of motivation. Truancy.

FIFTEEN INHALANT WARNING SIGNS

Here are twelve warning signs of inhalant drug use:

Chemical smell on child or child's clothing. Correction fluid in nose, on fingers or clothing. Markers in pockets. Red eyes. Nonsensical talk. Irritability. "Drunk" appearance. Slurred speech. Unusual breath odor. Decreased appetite. Frequent headaches. Sores around mouth. Lack of concentration. Low grades. School absences.

WHY YOUNG PEOPLE DO IT: THE HELP THAT IS NEEDED

1 - TO ESCAPE FROM REALITY—The adult life is just ahead of them; but teenagers often are quite uncertain whether they will be able to successfully handle it when it arrives. They can imagine that their fears, anxieties, and sense of inadequacy can be momentarily forgotten by taking street drugs.

Before they reach the teen years, teach them to value the worthwhile real things of life: the benefits of hard work and the importance of a genuine Christian experience. Be yourself what you want your children to be, and their future will be bright.

2 - SEARCH FOR A CHEAP THRILL—They want a quick and inexpensive "kick." What they haven't learned is that the cheap thrills in life are always disappointing, always damaging in the long run.

Before they reach the teen years, teach them to value the success and self-respect that comes from bearing responsibility and carrying necessary duties in the home. Teach them how to work and appreciate what they do.

3 - LACK OF INFORMATION—Teach them the dangers in the street drugs. Give them information; they need it and want it. If you do not give them this information, they will obtain it from the drug pusher at school.

Hand them a copy of this book and let them read it from cover to cover. Read it yourself; and discuss it with them, when they have completed it. Many teenagers, having been forewarned of the dangers, choose never to indulge in the drug culture that is pervading our time in history.

4 - PROLONGING ADOLESCENCE—Many parents, having had to work hard to succeed in life, feel that their present duty is to "protect" their children from hard work and decision making. But this only prepares them to escape to the unreal world of drug fantasy, so that they can forget about the adult world that they have not been trained to meet.

From their childhood, teach them how to bear responsibility and be in charge of routine duties about the home. Take up gardening and let it be something your whole family can enjoy together. Life is real and not make-believe. The only people who succeed in it are the people who enjoy working for its own sake.

D
R
U
G
S

5 - DO NOT USE DRUGS YOURSELF—This is the downfall of many young people: Their parents do it already. Cigarettes, alcohol, chewing tobacco, cigars, a weekly drunk night, and all the rest.

Do not give this as a heritage to your children. Get off of the bad things yourself, and it will be far easier for your sons and daughters to follow your example.

6 - HAVE STANDARDS IN YOUR HOME— Far too many parents seem to care little what their children do. We live in an age of permissiveness. Do as you please. Explore and try new things. If you get burned a little, then you are finding out what life is like. But young people of all ages need parental guidance that is based on solid, worthwhile standards.

The Bible has the best standards in the world. Christianity is the only thing in the world that can change the heart, the motives, and the life for the better. Go to God and give Him your life. Win your children and loved ones. Begin attending church again. Have morning and evening family worship each day. Pray together. And when alone, pray for one another. Life is real; and it takes a personal, daily relationship with God to make it succeed.

With your family, find ways to help others. Help old folks. Paint their homes, clean outside and in. Visit nursing homes. Find people who need help. Do things that are worthwhile.

Write to the publisher of this book for a list of very helpful books that can enable you to come back to God. Peace with God: This is what many of us want and need. And peace with God is something you can have. There is no greater happiness than a conscious awareness of His forgiveness and His presence. There is no greater satisfaction than working with Him to minister to the needs of others around you.

WHERE TO OBTAIN HELP

Toll free Parent Hotline — 800-637-0701 A consultant is on standby at all times, to help you locate resources which can help you.

Free Resource Catalog — 888-200-5061 Lists residential centers, treatment programs, or specialty schools.

Free Resource Video — 800-637-0701 Parents telling of resources that they have found effective in dealing with their troubled son or daughter.

THE LEGAL PENALTIES

Federal penalties for the illegal possession or usage of narcotics were first established under the Harrison Act of 1914, which provides that illegal possession of narcotics is punishable by fines and/or imprisonment.

Prison sentences can range from 2 to 10 years for the first offense, 5 to 20 years for the second, and 10 to 20 years for further offenses.

Illegal sale of narcotics can mean a fine of $20,000 and a sentence of 5 to 20 years, for the first offense, and 10 to 40 years for further offenses. A person who sells narcotics to someone under 18 is refused parole and probation, even for the first offense. If the drug is heroin, the sentences are very stiff.

Take a good, hard look at the information given in this book and the legal penalties in this chapter; and determine that you will have nothing to do with those terrible habits. All they will do is get you in trouble. And they always will. It may take a few weeks or months; but trouble will be headed your way.

This is because once you start, you will tend to keep coming back to it. And on it goes until you are damaged physically, worn-out mentally, unable to obtain decent employment, and perhaps imprisoned.

Now it is a much easier decision to stay out of it. But if you choose to get into it, later it will be much more difficult for you to get out.

Who wants to spend their life as a slave to dope, prostitution, theft, and crime? But that is what the street drugs can bring into your life. And remember that the little things lead to bigger things. Stay away from the "innocent" drugs and narcotics, and you will never be tempted with the bigger ones. Avoid coffee, tea, cola drinks. Never take up smoking or drinking beer, wine, or any other liquor.

If someone offers you any of these things, just tell him, "I have enough problems now; I don't need anymore." He will probably just stare at you and walk away, knowing that he wishes he could get away from the problem he is trying to get you started on.

Live and act from principle. Enjoy doing right because it is right. Find the deep peace and happiness that comes from accepting Christ as your Saviour from sin. He alone can enable you, by His grace, to resist temptation and sin. He alone can empower you to obey the Ten Commandments of Exodus 20:3-17.

And this is what you really want: a better, happier life. But such a life cannot be found in swallowing, sniffing, smoking, or mainlining drugs.

The key to victory is self-control; and the key to self-control is surrender to God. He can give you the help that you can obtain nowhere else. He is your heavenly Father, the one who created you; and He loves you deeply as no other one can. In His strength, you can overcome hereditary and cultivated desires that are injuring your body and your life.

Write to me, the author of this book, at the publisher's address given on the second page of this book; and I will send you printed materials that can help you find this better life.

More Encouragement

"It is the love of self that brings unrest. When we are born from above, the same mind will be in us that was in Jesus, the mind that led Him to humble Himself that we might be saved. Then we shall not be seeking the highest place. We shall desire to sit at the feet of Jesus, and learn of Him. We shall understand that the value of our work does not consist in making a show and noise in the world, and in being active and zealous in our own strength. The value of our work is in proportion to the impartation of the Holy Spirit. Trust in God brings holier qualities of mind, so that in patience we may possess our souls."

—Desire of Ages, 330-331

"Those who take Christ at His word, and surrender their souls to His keeping, their lives to His ordering, will find peace and quietude. Nothing of the world can make them sad when Jesus makes them glad by His presence. In perfect acquiescence there is perfect rest. The Lord says, 'Thou wilt keep him in perfect peace, whose mind is stayed on Thee: because he trusteth in Thee.' Isaiah 26:3. Our lives may seem a tangle; but as we commit ourselves to the wise Master Worker, He will bring out the pattern of life and character that will be to His own glory. And that character which expresses the glory—character—of Christ will be received into the Paradise of God. A renovated race shall walk with Him in white, for they are worthy.

"As through Jesus we enter into rest, heaven begins here. We respond to His invitation, Come, learn of Me, and in thus coming we begin the life eternal. Heaven is a ceaseless approaching to God through Christ. The longer we are in the heaven of bliss, the more and still more of glory will be opened to us; and the more we know of God, the more intense will be our happiness. As we walk with Jesus in this life, we may be filled with His love, satisfied with His presence. All that human nature can bear, we may receive here. But what is this compared with the hereafter? There 'are they before the throne of God, and serve Him day and night in His temple: and He that sitteth on the throne shall dwell among them. They shall hunger no more, neither thirst any more; neither shall the sun light on them, nor any heat. For the Lamb which is in the midst of the throne shall feed them, and shall lead them unto living fountains of waters: and God shall wipe away all tears from their eyes.' Revelation 7:15-17."

—Desire of Ages, 331-332

D
R
U
G
S

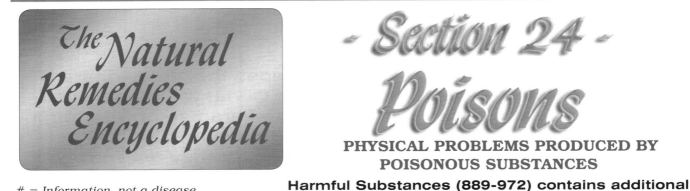

The Natural Remedies Encyclopedia

- Section 24 -

Poisons

PHYSICAL PROBLEMS PRODUCED BY POISONOUS SUBSTANCES

Harmful Substances (889-972) contains additional valuable information

"Ye shall serve the Lord your God, and he shall bless thy bread, and thy water [without poisonous substances]; and I will take sickness away from the midst of thee." *—Exodus 23:25*

Section 24 - Poisons

POISON CONTROL CENTERS

EMERGENCY - IF SOMEONE SWALLOWS A POISON OR GETS IT IN THEIR EYE OR SKIN - PHONE YOUR STATE POISON CONTROL CENTER. You may want to write yours on a sheet and place it by your phone.

UNITED STATES
Alabama - 800-462-0800
  800-292-6678 *Children*
Alaska - 800-478-3193
Arizona
  800-362-0101 *statewide*
  602-253-3334 *Phoenix area*
  602-626-6016 *Tucson area*
Arkansas - 800-376-4766
California
  800-876-4766 *CA only;*
   Sacramento, Madera
  800-876-4766 *San Diega*
  800-876-4766 *San Francisco*
   / Bay area
Colorado
  800-332-3073 *outside*
   metro Denver
  303-739-1123 *Denver*
   metro area
Connecticut - 800-343-2722
Delaware - 800-722-7112
District of Columbia - 202-625-3333
Florida
  813-253-4444 *Jacksonville area*
  800-282-3171 *Miami area*
  800-282-3171 *Tampa area*
Georgia - 800-282-5846
Hawaii - 808-941-4411
Idaho - 800-860-0620
Ilinois - 800-942-5969
Indiana - 800-382-9097
Iowa - 800-272-6477
Kansas - 800-332-6633
Kentucky - 502-589-8222
Louisiana - 800-256-9822
Maine - 800-442-6305
Maryland

  800-492-2414 *statewide*
  202-625-3333 *DC suburbs*
Massachusetts - 800-682-9211
Michigan - 800-764-7661
Minnesota - 800-POISON1
Mississippi - 601-354-7660
Missouri - 800-366-8888
Montana - 800-525-5042
Nebraska - 800-955-9119
Nevada - 800-466-6179
New Hampshire - 800-562-8236
New Jersey - 800-POISON1
New Mexico - 800-432-6866
New York
  800-252-5655 *Cen NY area (NYC to Canada)*
  800-336-6997 *Eastern New York area*
  800-333-0542 *Finger Lakes region*
  516-542-2323 *Long Island*
  212-340-4494 *New York City*
  800-888-7655 *Western New York area*
North Carolina - 800-848-6946
North Dakota - 800-732-2200
Ohio
  800-682-7625 *Statewide*
  800-762-0727 *Dayton*
  800-872-5111 *Cincinnati area*
Oklahoma - 800-764-7661
Oregon - 800-452-7165
Pennsylvania
  800-521-6110 *Hershey / Central PA*
  412-681-6669 *Western PA*
  800-722-7112 *SE PA / Lehigh Valley*
Puerto Rico - 787-726-5674
Rhode Island - 401-444-5727

South Carolina - 803-922-1117
South Dakota - 800-POISON1
Tennessee - 800-288-9999
Texas
  800-764-7661 N, S, SE,
   Panhandle, W TX
  800-POISON1 *Central TX*
Utah - 800-456-7707
Vermont - 877-658-3456
Virginia
  800-451-1428 *Central, Western VA*
  202-625-3333 *DC Suburbs*
  800-552-6337 *Eastern, Central VA*
Washington - 800-732-6985
West Virginia - 800-642-3625
Wisconsin - 800-815-8855
Wyoming - 800-955-9119
CANADA
Alberta - 800-332-1414
British Columbia - 800-567-8911
Wisconsin - 800-567-8911
Manitoba - 204-787-2591
New Brunswick
  506-857-5555 *Fredericton*
  506-648-6222 *St. John*
New Foundland - 709-722-1110
Nova Scotia
  902-428-8161 *local*
  800-565-8161 *toll free from P. E. Island*
Ontario - 800-267-1373
Prince Edward Island - 800-565-8161
Quebec - 800-463-5060
Saskatchewan
  800-667-4545 *Provincewide*
  800-363-7474 *Saskatoon*
Yukon Territory - 403-667-8726

FOR MORE NATURAL REMEDIES:

HERBS: Herb Contents (pp. 129-130) will help you locate the 126 most important herbs and the diseases each one can treat. How to prepare herbs (132). How to use them (141-189)

HYDROTHERAPY: Therapy Contents (pp. 206-207) and its Disease Index (263-265) will lead you to over 100 water therapies and many more remedies. DIS. INDEX: 1211- / GEN. INDEX: 1221-

VITAMINS AND MINERALS: Contents (100-101). Using 101-124. Dosages (124). Others (117-)

CARING FOR THE SICK: Home care for a sick person (28-36). The healing crisis (36-39)

WOMEN'S SECTIONS: Female Organs (672) Pregnancy (701). Childbirth (765). Infancy, Childhood (722). Women's Herbs (754, 760)

EMERGENCIES: (973-). **FIRST AID:** (990-)

POISONS - 1 - BITES AND STINGS

FOUR POWERFUL ANTIDOTES

NATURAL ANTIDOTES

This chapter is filled with various types of poisons which we can get—from plant stings, insect or animal bites, infestations, and poisoning. When you need it, you may not have immediate access to the recommended antidote; you may need something in a hurry. When nothing better is available, here are the best universal antidotes: The first is for poisoning and the others for infestations and disease. It is good to keep them on hand. If you go hiking, carry them with you.

CHARCOAL

There are 80 different harmful substances which charcoal can neutralize. It can stop cold 29 of the 30 leading poisons. It can handle many infections. Chew up 10 activated charcoal tablets and swallow them with water. If the problem is on or beneath the skin, also apply charcoal poultices. The sooner the charcoal is applied, the more effective it is. Activated charcoal is better than regular charcoal, because it has more surfaces to adsorb the toxic substance. (Keep in mind that some poisons are powerful acids or alkalines, and need antidotes of the opposite pH to neutralize them; however charcoal can handle many of them also.)

GARLIC

There are 45 different diseases that raw garlic can effectively deal with. It is powerful against bacterial, viral, and fungal infections. The active ingredient is germanium; and garlic has a far higher content of germanium than any other plant or food. Mice exposed to cancer cells, that had been treated with garlic, did not die of cancer. Russian scientists said it was a better antibiotic than any other substance. But the garlic must be raw.

VITAMIN C

This amazing substance helps your white blood cells powerfully fight all kinds of toxic (bacterial, viral, and fungal) substances. The Linus Pauling Institute of Science and Medicine in Palo Alto, California has been researching the benefits of this vitamin for decades. It is used in the treatment cardiovascular disease, cancer, HIV, infections, fevers, cataracts, skin problems, and hundreds of other things. It destroys free radicals and is an antihistamine. It also functions as a "cell cement" to hold your body together!

PLANTAIN

This herb is found in many areas, and is effective in many, if not most, insect bites. Chew the leaves and then apply the pulp to the affected skin area.

ENCOURAGEMENT—Of all things that are sought, cherished, and cultivated, there is nothing so valuable in the sight of God as a pure heart, a disposition imbued with thankfulness and peace. If the love of God is in our hearts, it will shine forth in words and actions.

NETTLE RASH
(Urticaria)

SYMPTOMS—Small, pale swellings on the skin, with severe itching and burning which come and go, to be replaced by others. Each lesion lasts a few hours and is succeeded by new ones in other places. They look like raised, red, inflamed areas; sometimes this is with white lumps.

CAUSES—Also known as urticaria, nettle rash is an intensely itchy rash that may affect the whole body or just a small area of skin. Although it usually lasts only a few hours, chronic urticaria can last for sever months. Both acute and chronic forms can recur.

The other forms of urticaria are dealt with under Hives (346). This present article is only concerned with the rash caused by touching stinging nettles.

Contact with the nettle plant pricks a poison into the skin.

NATURAL REMEDIES

• Sponge with very **hot water**. Also one can sponge with **hot salt or alkaline water**. Give a prolonged **neutral temperature bath**.

• Pour 4 Tbsp. powdered **calcium** into a cup of **water**. Gently cover the itchy area with it. This will help neutralize and eliminate itching.

• Use a poultice of crushed **plantain** over the area.

ENCOURAGEMENT—Pray earnestly for help in all the little things of life, and you will be ready when great crises come. Psalm 119:9.

INSECT REPELLENTS

NATURAL REPELLENTS

All of the following are to be applied only externally (to skin or clothing), unless otherwise stated:

• Mosquitoes and flies: Apply **citronella**.
• Most flying insects: Apply **eucalyptus**.
• Fleas: Apply **pennyroyal** (but not if you are pregnant).
• Fleas and ticks: Apply **cedarwood**.
• Fleas and flies: Apply **thyme, geranium, lavender, rosemary, or peppermint**.
• Insects: In India and Africa, natives rub **basil** on their skin.
• Insects: Pennyroyal (also called **fleabane, tickweed, and mosquito plant**) has been used for thousands of years as an insect repellent. Pliny (first century A.D.) said it was the best flea repellent.
• Insects: **Mountain mint** is said to be even more effective than pennyroyal.
• Insects: **Citronella** smells like a lemon and has been used for years to drive off insects. It is also the active ingredient in several non-DEET products which you can apply. Pure citronella oil can be irritating to the skin

(and should never be swallowed). Dilute the pure oil by adding some vegetable oil to it.

• Insects: **Citrus essential oils**. Any type of citrus, or other plant which smells like citrus, repels insects. Crushed **lemon thyme** has 62% of DEET's repellency. Crush **citrus leaves** and apply. Dilute citrus essential oils before applying to the skin.

• Insects: **Lemon grass** is an herb with a citrus-like odor, which is a good insect repellent.

• Insects: A combination which is powerful in driving off insects: Mix **lavender, citronella, and pennyroyal** in a **vegetable oil** base; then apply it. Never swallow essential oils. Do not use pennyroyal if pregnant.

• **Oil of cedarwood** is effective against moths, flies, and mosquitoes. A box made of soft wood, then painted with cedarwood oil, will repel moths as effectively as a cedarwood chest.

• Sprigs of **mint** leaves will repel flies and fleas. Hang springs of mint about doorways and put them anywhere flies gather.

• Make a strong tea of **chamomile** flowers and let it stand until cold. Then strain off the herb and sponge the solution over the exposed areas of your body, allowing the liquid to dry on. No insects will touch you. Fortunately, chamomile has a very pleasant odor.

• **Pyrethrum** is a herbaceous perennial chrysanthemum that is non-poisonous to man and higher animals. It has been used for thousands of years as an insecticide in China, Persia, and elsewhere. It destroys many forms of biting and sucking insects such as fleas, flies, mosquitoes, gnats, ants, roaches, moths, aphids, leafhoppers, etc. It may be used as a powder or in a water solution. As a powder, it can be puffed around the room, especially in cracks. As a concentrated liquid, it is sprayed. It can also be mixed with other insecticide herbs.

• **Quassia** is amazingly bitter; yet it is harmless to man and animals. Pour ½ pint of boiling water over ¼ oz. of quassia chips and sweeten with molasses or sugar. When cool, pour the mixture in saucers and place in rooms where flies are most numerous.

• A strong solution of **sassafras**, sprinkled or sprayed around the house, keeps flies away. Chips of sassafras, placed in bowls of fresh fruit, will eliminate gnats and fruit flies.

• As a flea repellent, fill a pad or pillow of **winter savory** and place it in the sleeping quarters of the family pet.

• This repellent formula is used in South American jungles with good success: 1 oz. each of rosemary oil, basil oil, rue oil, and wormwood oil. Put in small bottles and carry with you. Do not drink it. Label it as poisonous.

• To fumigate a room (to eliminate all insects), place a Tbsp. of **cayenne** on a bottle lid. Place over a Sterno, or candle-type food warmer, lighting the underneath candle to heat the lid. Allow the pepper to fume (smoke). Close the room. Repeat when necessary.

• Rodent repellent: Rats hate **peppermint**. Close all but one exit in a house, cellar, or barn. Place peppermint oil on clothes, and the rats will rush out. Rat catchers would use this with great success, except that they would place a large bag at the only exit, and the rats would run into it and be caught in it.

ENCOURAGEMENT—You are safe only as, in perfect submission and obedience, you connect yourselves with Christ. The yoke is easy; for Christ carries the weight. As you lift the burden of the cross, it will become light; and that cross is to you a pledge of eternal life.

INSECT BITE

SYMPTOMS—Redness, slight swelling, and possibly some itching.

Reaction to the sting can sometimes be more pronounced: hoarseness, labored breathing, confusion, difficult swallowing, and severe swelling.

Sometimes the reaction can be severe: possible closing of the airway and perhaps shock (cyanosis and a drop in blood pressure).

CAUSES—Certain stinging insects in North America can cause reactions (honeybees, bumble bees, African bees, hornets, scorpions, fire ants, yellow jackets, wasps, spiders, centipedes, and ants). Of these, the honeybee, yellow jacket, and African bee are the most dangerous.

Bee venom contains formaldehyde.

Note: Each year, bee stings cause more deaths in America than snake bites.

Anaphylactic Shock may occur! *(846)*.

NATURAL REMEDIES

• **Pull out the stinger**, if any remains. (Honeybees leave their stinger in the wound. It must be pulled out immediately; for it keeps pulsating venom into the skin.) Avoid removing the stinger with your fingers; use a knife blade to scrape it out, to avoid squeezing in more poison.

• **Do not scratch** the area. Although it provides some relief, it can lead to a secondary infection. Instead, quickly apply a natural remedy to reduce the itch.

PUT ON THE AREA

• On the area, apply a paste of **baking soda and water** or a compress that is wet with diluted **ammonia** water (which is more useful for scorpion stings).

• Wet a little **calcium gluconate** and put it on the area.

• Crush a **charcoal** tablet, place on the area, and cover with cloth. This will reduce pain and swelling. Put some wet powdered charcoal in a cloth and tie it on for 3-4 hours. Charcoal has an amazing adsorptive (not absorptive) ability to pull into itself toxins and poisons, thus neutralizing them. This is due to its large chemical surface and the fact that charcoal is pure carbon. The carbon molecules are eager to unite with other substances.

• **Clay or mud** can also be used, especially if you are out in the woods. As soon as possible, wet some dirt and put it on. Leave it on for a half hour. Try to select mud from a clean place—not from a mud hole, where animals may have polluted it. If pain persists, apply charcoal.

• **Plantain** is one of the best herbs for bug bites, and first with most herbalists for this problem. Because it is a common weed, it is frequently available. It grows where the ground is damp, heavy, and shaded. Rub the freshly picked herb on the area. Or add ¼ cup dried plantain leaves to a quart of boiled water, cover and steep for 20-30 minutes. Soak the bitten limb in cooled tea for 10-15 minutes, 3-4 times a day.

• After pulling out the sting, put a little **honey** on it. Or put on some grated **onion,** to draw out swelling and reduce pain.

• **Chamomile** and **St. John's wort** are two other useful herbs for insect stings and bites.

• Other helpful substances to apply include **goldenseal** (to stop the infection) and **bentonite clay** (to remove toxins).

• Apply powdered **comfrey,** mixed with **aloe vera** juice, to reduce the swelling.

• Put a piece of fresh **onion or garlic** on it.

• An enzyme-based **meat tenderizer** breaks down the proteins that make up insect venom; but you have to place it on the area right away for it to be effective.

• Also helpful are **calcium chloride, hydrochloric acid, or ammonium chloride** on the area.

• Apply a poultice of **white oak bark and leaves, comfrey, and slippery elm**.

• Other herbs you can place on the wound include **agrimony, yerba santa,** and **lobelia**. Make a tea and apply to the area.

• **Parsley** alleviates insect bites. Mash the plant and use as a poultice. **Lavender** is an antiseptic, a wound healer; and, in compresses, it reduces inflammation from the bite.

• Here are more things you can place on the area: **aloe vera gel, ammonia, Epsom salts dissolved in warm water, eucalyptus oil**.

• Applying **lemon juice and vinegar** removes the toxic pain.

• **Pain gels, DMSO, or Caladryl** lotions can be applied. **Calamine** lotion often reduces the itching.

OTHER HELPS

• Drink as much **yellow dock** tea as you can or take **echinacea** (tea or in capsule form).

• Ironically, either **hot or cold**, will lessen the pain, when placed on the area. Heat eases distress because it neutralizes a chemical which causes inflammation. Cold also reduces inflammation.

• A lengthy **hot tub bath** will help relieve abdominal pain that often develops after a bite.

• A **cold pack or ice pack** on the area will help relieve pain.

• To strengthen the bodies defenses, after being bitten, take **B₆** (50 mg) and **pantothenic acid** (100 mg) immediately after the bite, to help detoxify poisons and prevent allergic reactions. Thereafter, take one high-potency **B complex** tablet daily. Take **vitamin C** (1,000-2,000 mg) immediately; during the rest of that first day, take 4,000-10,000 mg in divided doses. Each day thereafter, take 3,000 mg. Adding **bioflavonoids** to the C dosage increases the protection. **Calcium** (up to 1,500 mg daily)

reduces pain and lessens stomach irritation from the acidity of vitamin C.

• Eat **citrus fruits** and **green and yellow vegetables** to boost immunity.

PREVENTIVES

• If you are sensitive to stings, **avoid situations** in which you might get stung. If you have to be in such localities, carry **adrenalin** (epinephrine) with you, so you can inject it. Be accompanied by a friend who can go for help. Reactions can occur within minutes or hours. Contact a physician. Death can result if treatment is not sought. *See Anaphylactic Shock (846).*

• If you have a known allergy to a certain venom, you can have a physician prescribe an **emergency treatment kit** which you can keep with you.

• Purchase a small **venom extractor** and keep it with you.

• Take **vitamin B₁** (thiamine, 50 mg daily). It creates a natural insect repellent in human skin.

• Squashing a yellow jacket releases a chemical that causes other yellow jackets to attack. When one stings, that also causes the others to become excited. **If stung, run**. Go indoors or jump into water. Insects have a hard time following a person through a thicket of woods.

• Always wear shoes outside. Bees love clover and yellow jackets live in the ground.

• Stinging insects prefer dark colors or brightly flowered clothes. So **wear white or light-colored clothing**.

• Insects are attracted to people who are **deficient in zinc**. Take at least 30 mg a day.

• Insects are repelled by the odor of **turpentine**.

• **Brewer's yeast or garlic** rubbed on the skin (or eating it daily) sometimes deters insects.

• **Do not use perfumes**, colognes, scented soaps, or hair sprays. These odors attract insects.

• Drinking **alcohol** or eating an excess of **sugar** attracts insect biting.

• **Avoid bright jewelry** and other metal objects.

• **Meeting an insect:** If you come in contact with a stinging insect, move away slowly. But if there is only one insect and you see him heading directly toward you, face him and wave your hands up and down in front of you. That will confuse him. But if you are outside and he may have buddies, run away fast.

• Do not touch **insect nests**. Keep **garbage cans** covered. Be especially alert **after rain**, because pollen is scarce then and insects are searching everywhere for it.

• *See Spider Bite (836),* which includes that of black widows. *Also see "Snake Bite (837).* Treatment for a black widow bite is the same as that for a snake bite.

ENCOURAGEMENT—Praise God for all His blessings, and you will have more to praise Him for. How many are the dangers He has protected you from!

CHART 1056: Malaria (306) / Mosquito Bite (832)

MOSQUITO BITE

SYMPTOMS—The itchy, red bite of a mosquito, with its attendant itching.

CAUSES—The culex, aedes, and anopheles mosquitoes are in North America. Malaria *(306)* can sometimes occur. The treatment below is for non-malarial bites.

NATURAL REMEDIES
• To relieve itching: Rub with raw **garlic** or fresh **lemon juice**; repeat as often as possible. Rub with damp **salt** or **vitamin C** powder.
• Cover the bite with **Epsom salts** dissolved in warm water, **eucalyptus oil, aloe vera gel, lemon juice, or vinegar**.
• Apply a poultice of crushed **plantain leaves**.

PREVENTION
To prevent mosquito or biting fly bites:
• Eat lots of raw **garlic**. Include vitamin **B complex** and/or **brewer's yeast** in the diet.
• Take 100 mg B_1 (niacin) immediately before exposure and every 4 hours during the problem.
• Take 30 mg **zinc** every day for a month.
• Avoid **sugar** and **white flour** in all forms.
• Wear body-covering **garments**.
• Add 4 Tbsp. **bleach** to a tub bath; and soak in it for 15 minutes. No mosquitoes will bite you for a day or two.
—*Also see Malaria (306), West Nile Virus (813), and Dengue (309).*

ENCOURAGEMENT—We strive for happiness, but rarely find it. Only in God can we find genuine, lasting peace of heart. Psalm 66:8-9.

BEE AND WASP STINGS

SYMPTOMS—You have just been painfully bitten by a bee or wasp.

CAUSES—There are hundreds of bees; but only one makes honey. Unfortunately, all of them can give us painful stings. But we still value our little honey bee. To make a pound of honey, bees have to travel 13,000 miles, or about 4 times the distance across America.
Wasps help man by eating many harmful insects. They do more good than harm. Hornets and yellow jackets are among the several kinds of wasps.

NATURAL REMEDIES
• As long as the stinger remains in the skin, it keeps pulsating and injecting more venom. So, first, gently **remove the stinger**. Try not to squeeze it as you do this.
• Next, **wash** the sting area. This will remove some of the venom. After this, apply **damp charcoal** to pull out more venom. A paste of **baking soda and water** will help neutralize the toxins. **Cold compresses** or **ice** cubes will help reduce pain still more.
• Six hours later, apply **heat**.
• If the person shows dizziness, difficulty in breathing, severe swelling, or hives, *contact a physician*
Also see Insect Bite (831), Anaphylactic Shock (846), and Hives (346-347).

ENCOURAGEMENT—If we would travel heavenward, we must take the Word of God, the Bible, as our lesson-book. In the words of inspiration we must read our lessons day by day.

ANT BITE

SYMPTOMS—A biting pain, and the ant is still there biting.

CAUSES—Most ants are no problem, but some bite ferociously. Ant venom, although very small, is quite similar to honey bee venom. What should you do?

NATURAL REMEDIES
• Apply a poultice of crushed **plantain** leaves.
• To reduce itching and swelling, apply **baking soda** to the area. Only add enough water to make a paste.
An **ice pack or cool compress** will also help.
If the person bitten manifests symptoms of shock (difficulty breathing, severe swelling, hives, or dizziness), contact a physician.
—*Also see Insect bite (831), Fire Ant Bite (below), Anaphylactic Shock (846), and Hives (346-347).*

ENCOURAGEMENT—The meekness and humility that characterized the life of Christ will be made manifest in the life and character of those who "walk even as He walked." As we humbly, prayerfully read in the Bible, our lives are ennobled; and, trusting in Jesus, we are prepared to encourage and bless those around us. This is the will of God for our lives: to be kindly, sympathetic helpers.

FIRE ANT BITE

SYMPTOMS—One or more severely burning bites from a large ant. A pustule develops within 24 hours, and then subsides over the next several day.

CAUSES—You probably stepped on a fire ant's nest. It is a low mound of loose dirt, 1-3 feet across. As soon as you stepped on it, hundreds of ants started toward your legs.
Fire ants, imported from Africa to Brazil in the 1960s, finally reached America near the end of the century. They have venom similar to that of bees, wasps, hornets, and yellow jackets. And they are still primarily in the Southern States.

NATURAL REMEDIES
• If the bitten part is an extremity, put it in **very hot water** for 30 minutes. This will neutralize the venom.
• To reduce pain, next put **baking soda, ice, vinegar and lemon juice**, or astringent herb tea (**white oak bark, witch hazel, plantain**, etc.) over the area.
• If the person shows any signs of hives, difficult breathing, dizziness, or excessive swelling, contact a physician.
—*Also see Insect Bite (831), Ant Bite (833), Anaphylactic Shock (846), and Hives (346-347).*

ENCOURAGEMENT—To be a real man or woman in the sight of God is to be like Jesus—meek and lowly of heart, always anxious to guard the interests of others more sacredly than you would your own.

CATERPILLAR STING

SYMPTOMS—Stinging sensation after touching a caterpillar.

CAUSES—A caterpillar is a worm-like creature which is the second (larval) stage in the life cycle of butterfies and moths. Many caterpillars can be handled; but some cause problems. When in doubt, avoid them all.

NATURAL REMEDIES
• The stings come from the hairs on the caterpillar, which become slightly embedded in the skin. Gently place a **sticky tape**, such as Scotch tape, over the injured area; then carefully lift it up. This will extract the hairs. Then apply crushed **plantain** leaves to the area.
—*See Insect Bite (831) for many suggestions about what to do next.*

ENCOURAGEMENT—True happiness is to be found, not in self-indulgence and self-pleasing but, in learning of Christ. Those who trust to their own wisdom and follow their own way go complaining at every step, because the burden which selfishness binds upon them is so heavy

CENTIPEDE BITE

SYMPTOMS—A painful bite caused by touching or handling a centipede, which causes swelling of the lymph glands. Symptoms generally subside within 48 hours.

CAUSES—Centipedes look like caterpillars; but they have very long legs (varying from 15 to 170 pairs). The first pair of legs are used for fighting, not walking. They are called *poison claws*, because a gland in the centipede's head fills these claws with poison. Fortunately, they travel about at night and are primarily found in the tropics.

NATURAL REMEDIES
• Immediately apply a **charcoal compress** to help draw out the poison.
• A **cool compress** or **ice cube** can be applied for pain relief.
• If the person shows dizziness, difficulty in breathing, severe swelling, or hives, contact a physician.
—*Also see Insect Bite (831), Anaphylactic Shock (846), and Hives (346-347).*

ENCOURAGEMENT—The meekness of Christ, manifested in the home, will make the inmates happy; it provokes no quarrel, gives back no angry answer; but it soothes the irritated temper and diffuses a gentleness that is felt by all within its charmed circle. Wherever cherished, it makes the families of earth a part of the one great family above.

CHIGGERS

SYMPTOMS—A red spot that itches intensely for about 3 days.

CAUSES—Chiggers, also called red bugs, are extremely tiny insects (about 1/20-inch) in the class, called *arthropoda* (eight-legged creatures). Arthropoda includes scorpions, spiders, and mites. They prefer grassy, weedy, fields; but they are also found in wooded areas and are active from May to September, especially during June and July.

Chiggers attach to humans with claws. They feed for about 3 days by secreting enzymes which liquefy skin cells; then they drop off.

Moving slowly, a chigger crawls along until he finds a tight spot in a body crease or where the clothing is tight. Then, about 2 hours after hitching a ride, he digs in by injecting fluid which dissolves tissue and produces a welt. About 3-6 hours later, the itching begins and continues for about 3 days.

NATURAL REMEDIES
• **Remove the chigger** by scratching off with a fingernail; or you can do this by applying castor oil or Vaseline.
• Another method is to apply clear **nail polish** to the spot; this smothers the creature.
• Or **lather** with soap, scrub with a brush, then rinse thoroughly.
• A **charcoal** or **plantain** poultice can be a help.
• An ice pack helps control swelling.
• **Banana** soothes chigger bites.
• **Hot baths** or a **baking powder** paste helps control the itching. If you have too many chigger bites, get into a bathtub with **cornstarch** sprinkled into it.
• Use the remedies suggested for mosquito bites *(560)*.

ENCOURAGEMENT—Find in the Lord the strength you need every day. The Lord is a great God, a great King above all gods. Oh come; let us worship and bow down, and kneel before our Maker.

ITCH MITE

SYMPTOMS—Itching occurs; but it seems to travel from place to place on the skin.
CAUSES—Beware of bird nests close to your house! Many birds are infested with mites; and these can enter your home and get on you.

NATURAL REMEDIES
• **Wash** the affected part with tar soap. **Wash clothing** in boiling water or press them with a hot iron.
• Steep 1 Tbsp. each of **burdock root, yarrow, and yellow dock root** in a pint of boiling water for half an hour. Strain, add a pound of **cocoa fat**, and keep boiling and stirring until it is a salve. Use this for an itch of any kind.

• The principle author of this *Encyclopedia* got mites while preparing the Fourth Edition. A bird raised three babies on his front porch; and, as soon as they left the nest, he took it down and could see mites crawling (at a rate of 2 inches every four seconds) up his wrist. Some managed to settle into their new home. Desirous of a simple and non-toxic solution, after praying, a highly successful plan came to mind: It was obvious that ticks hide in the clothes, bite the skin when it's very warm, then retreat to the clothes. If ticks bit during the day, he took off his clothes that evening (or the next morning if they bit at night), and pressed them down in a bucket of clear tap water till, all bubbles gone, they remained underwater. Then he showered off in clear water. After a minimum of two hours, he put the clothes in the washer on spin dry for a few minutes; then hung them up to dry. It worked. The ticks drowned.

ENCOURAGEMENT—Oh how good the Lord is to all of us; and how safely we may trust Him every-day. He calls us His little children. So obey Him in all things, and your happiness can only deepen.

LICE
(Pediculosis)

SYMPTOMS—Itching of the skin, often on the head, trunk, or pubic area. Lice eggs can be seen on one's hair. The person will feel like he is overheated or has a slight fever.

CAUSES—There are three types of lice which infect people: the head louse *(pediculosis capitis)*, the body louse *(p. corporis)*, and the crab louse *(p. pubis)*. Crab lice (also called crabs) are spread by sexual contact.

Lice can be spread by hanging coats, scarves, and caps together or using someone else's comb, brush, etc. They live on the clothing (especially in the seams), travel to the skin once a day for a meal, then back onto the clothing.

Lice live about 30 days; and the female lays about ten eggs a day. The tiny eggs (nits) are laid at the base of a hair shaft. As the hair grows, the nits are carried upward and can be seen. They look like tiny black or rust-colored spots at, or near, the base of the hair. They can even be found on the chest, beard, and eyelashes.

NATURAL REMEDIES

No drugs are needed to eradicate lice. Instead use one or more of the following methods:

• Heat **combs and brushes** to 151° F. for 5-10 minutes, soak for an hour in 2% Lysol solution, or freeze them for 30 minutes.

• Launder **clothing and bedding** in hot water. Non-washable items should be sealed in a plastic sack for 10 days.

• **Soak** the place on the body for 30 minutes in very warm, soapy, water.

• Crumble 3 Tbsp. **rue** into 1 pint **white vinegar**. Steep as long as possible (2 weeks is best). Apply to the head or other body area. It is good for body lice, skin parasites, or as a ringworm lotion.

• The **hair** can be doused in kerosene and then wrapped in a towel. Garlic compresses can be placed on the scalp for 2 hours. Hot vinegar (or a 50-50 vinegar / water mixture) applied to the scalp will loosen eggs, so they can be vigorously combed out of the hair with a fine-toothed comb. A 50-50 mixture of kerosene and olive oil can be put on the scalp, to get rid of the nits. Another hair wash: labrador tea or field larkspur. In extreme cases, the hair can be cut off.

• Be careful what you place on the **eyebrows**; you do not want to damage the eyes. Petroleum jelly has been recommended to suffocate the lice.

• Vacuuming **carpets** is as effective as spraying them. Do it frequently.

• Scrub **toilet seats** regularly.

• Whatever method you use, keep in mind that there is a 14-day cycle; you must work intensely for a little over 2 weeks on your body, clothing, and home if you are to have success.

ENCOURAGEMENT—In everything you do, put God and His standards first. You will never be disappointed if you do this. Matthew 1:21.

BEDBUGS

SYMPTOMS—Bites on your skin, which occur at night, often while you are in bed. The bites often appear in groups or lines.

CAUSES—Bedbugs are very small, flat, crawling insects that hide inside mattresses, bedding, furniture, and walls. They usually bite at night. These are especially common in the tropics.

NATURAL REMEDIES

• *To get rid of bedbugs*, **wash** bedding and pour boiling water on bed frames. Sprinkle sulfur on mattresses, cloth furniture, and rugs; and do not use them for 3 weeks. Then wash or shake out the sulfur. Clean it off well before using again.

• *To prevent bedbugs*, often spread bedding in the **sun**.

ENCOURAGEMENT—Cultivate tenderness, affection, and love that have expression in little courtesies, in speech, in thoughtful attentions. It is the kind word, the thoughtful consideration for others that God values.

TICK BITES

SYMPTOMS—You have found a tick on your body.

POISONS

CAUSES—Although the bite of most ticks are usually harmless, while drawing blood they can inject disease-causing bacteria. The mouth of a tick has a sharp probe with backward pointing barbs.

After initially digging in, it injects bacteria as it feeds on blood. So the sooner it is removed, the less infection you will receive from it.

Ticks live in marshy places, woods and forests, bushes, shrubs, and long grass. Stay on trails and avoid brushing against vegetation.

Ticks cannot jump or fly; but they wait on low vegetation for a host to pass by, with their little "arms" held upward. As soon as something does, they grab hold and start climbing in search of a place to attach and feed.

NATURAL REMEDIES

• **Avoid walking** in areas frequented by ticks: woods and open fields in the summer. They are generally not on roads or lawns.

• **To remove a tick** that is firmly attached, take care that its head does not remain in the skin, since this can cause an infection. Never pull on the body of a tick! With tweezers, grasp the tick as close as possible to its mouth—the part sticking into the skin. Try not to squeeze its swollen belly. Pull very gently on the tick. This may take as much as 30 seconds, but be patient and gently pull. He will then withdraw and come out. Do not touch the removed tick. Burn it or put some alcohol on it. Then apply crushed plantain leaves.

• If you have to go into fields or forests, you may want to dust some **sulfur** powder on your ankles, wrists, and underarms. But get that powder off later! If you ingest any of it, boils or skin rashes can result.

• *For symptoms, see Rocky Mountain Spotted Fever (840) and Lyme Disease (813, 840). For detailed information on removal of ticks, see Lyme Disease.*

ENCOURAGEMENT—Strength of character consists of two things—power of the will and power of self-control. Many youth mistake strong, uncontrolled passion for strength of character; but the truth is that he who is mastered by his passions is a weak man. The real greatness and nobility of the man is measured by his powers to subdue his feelings, not by the power of his feelings to subdue him.

BLACK WIDOW SPIDER BITE

SYMPTOMS—Within a short time the victim feels agonizing pain throughout the body, especially in the abdomen, which may be rigid as a board. Abdominal pain similar to that of appendicitis. Cold sweats, difficulty in breathing, nausea, spastic muscle contractions, vomiting, localized tissue death, and sometimes delirium and convulsions occur.

CAUSES—There are more than 29,000 known types of spiders. They are excellent at insect control; but two in the U.S. are extremely dangerous. The tarantula is the world's largest spider; it lives as far north as the southwestern U.S. But its bite is no more dangerous to a human than the sting of a bee or wasp.

Black widow venom is more potent, drop for drop, than the poison of a pit viper (rattlesnake, copperhead, or cotton mouth); yet each spider bite injects only an extremely small amount of venom. Four out of every 100 people bitten by a black widow have anaphylactic shock and death. It is possible to develop tetanus (593) from a spider bite.

DESCRIPTION—The black widow is the most dangerous spider in the U.S.; it has a shiny black body and a red (or yellow) hourglass patch on the underside of the main body segment. Only the female is dangerous to man. It weaves shapeless webs in dark corners. It may be found in the corners of barns, sheds, and other buildings near homes. It hides in its web when frightened; but it may bite if caught in clothing. Most common in the South, the black widow is in nearly every state and in Canada. There is a brown widow and red widow in Florida, which are also poisonous. Deaths usually result from complications, not from the bite.

NATURAL REMEDIES
Contact a physician.

• The bite of a black widow should be treated like a snake bite (837), except that it is not necessary to give antivenin.

• If there is swelling or pain after a spider bite, keep calm and **apply a constricting band 2-4 inches above** (above, not below) the bite. Loosen the band for 15 seconds every 10 minutes. Do not let the extremity turn blue! Do not move the affected area; and keep it below the heart level, if possible. The victim should lie down. Pack **ice** around the wound.

• Chew up and swallow 10 **charcoal** tablets with water. Crush more tablets, make a paste, and place on the bite as a compress. Charcoal will powerfully draw out the poison if applied extremely fast.

The objective, throughout the above paragraph, is to slow the blood and reduce spread of the poison.

• Drink as much **yellow dock** tea as possible or take 2 capsules of this every hour till symptoms recede. Swallow **echinacea**. Apply **white oak bark** poultices. **Slippery elm, plantain, or comfrey** are also good.

• Massive doses of **vitamin C** (a first dose of 4,000 mg; followed by 1,000-2,000 mg *each hour*). Reduce the dosage if diarrhea develops. **Calcium** gluconate (500 mg every 6 hours), to relieve pain and abdominal cramping from the venom, and prevent stomach upset from massive amounts of vitamin C. Accompany each dose of calcium with **magnesium** (1,000 mg). **Pantothenic acid** (500 mg each 8 hours for 2 days), to augment vitamin C's detoxifying effects.

—*Rattlesnake and black widow venom is similar, and so is the treatment. See Snake Bite (837) and Insect Bite (831) for much more information. Also see Brown Recluse Spider Bite (below).*

ENCOURAGEMENT—Trust Him with all your heart. He will carry you and your burdens. Find in Him the answers you need. Job 5:20.

BROWN RECLUSE SPIDER BITE

SYMPTOMS—A "bull's eye" appearance of a blister encircled by red and white rings. A few hours after being bitten, the skin around the bite becomes red and swollen. Eventually, most of this tissue dies, leaving a deep sore that may take months to heal.

CAUSES—There are more than 29,000 known types of spiders. They are excellent at insect control, but two in the U.S. are extremely dangerous. The tarantula is the world's largest spider; it lives as far north as the southwestern U.S. But its bite is no more dangerous to a human than the sting of a bee or wasp.

The bite can cause the flesh to decay; it can require extensive treatment over weeks or months. But death from a brown recluse is extremely rare. It is possible to develop tetanus (866) from a spider bite.

DESCRIPTION—The brown recluse is a brownish, poisonous spider, about 3/8-inch long, with a dark, violin-shaped mark on its upper back near the head. It prefers to hide in dark places in the house, like closets and drawers. It spins a sticky, irregular web, with threads running in all directions. It can lives for days without food or water. And it is found all over the U.S.

NATURAL REMEDIES
Contact a physician.
• Chew up and swallow 10 **charcoal** tablets with water. Crush more tablets, make a paste, and place on the bite as a compress. Charcoal will powerfully draw out the poison if applied extremely fast.
• If there is swelling or pain after a spider bite, keep calm and **apply a constricting band 2-4 inches above** (above, not below) the bite. Loosen the band for 15 seconds every 10 minutes. Do not let the extremity turn blue! Do not move the affected area; keep it below the heart level, if possible. The victim should lie down. Pack **ice** around the wound. The objective is to slow the blood and reduce spread of the poison.
• Drink as much **yellow dock** tea as possible or take 2 capsules of this every hour till symptoms recede. Swallow **echinacea**. Apply **white oak bark** poultices. **Slippery elm, plantain, or comfrey** are also good.
• Massive doses of **vitamin C** (a first dose of 4,000 mg; followed by 1,000-2,000 mg *each hour*). Reduce the dosage if diarrhea develops. **Calcium** gluconate (500 mg, every 6 hours), to relieve pain and abdominal cramping from the venom and prevent stomach upset from massive amounts of vitamin C. Accompany each dose of calcium with **magnesium** (1,000 mg). **Pantothenic acid** (500 mg each 8 hours, for 2 days), to augment vitamin C's detoxifying effects.
—*Rattlesnake and recluse venom is similar, and so is the treatment. See Snake Bite (below) and Insect Bite (831) for much more information. Also see Black*

Widow Spider Bite (836).

ENCOURAGEMENT—Trust Him with all your heart. He will carry you and your burdens. Find in Him the answers you need. The highest evidence of nobility in a Christian is self-control. Purity of heart and loveliness of spirit are more precious than gold, both for time and for eternity. Psalm 34:8.

SNAKE BITE

SYMPTOMS—One or two tiny bite holes which cause intense pain; frequently there is nausea, vomiting, and unconsciousness.

CAUSES—There are two types of poisonous serpents in North America:

The *pit viper* (which includes **rattlesnakes, copperheads, and cotton mouths** [also called **water moccasins**]) has a deep, heat-sensitive, pit on each side of the head. Pit vipers lunge forward, bite, and immediately pull back. Their venom contains a blood poison.

The **coral snake** does not jump; and, when it catches hold of the flesh, it must hold on and chew awhile for the poison to sink in. Its venom is a nerve poison.

The danger from snake bite occurs when the poison reaches the heart and, secondarily, the effect of that poison in the blood and nervous system.

The action of the venom is rapid, regardless of the type of poisonous snake. There is rapid swelling and inflammation. The greatest danger is if it is a young child or an old person, the bite is close to the heart, a large quantity of venom is injected, or immediate treatment is not given to suck out or neutralize the poison.

If treatment is not immediately given, the poison may cause death. If not death after the initial effects of pain and shock begin to wear off, extensive tissue damage begins. There is suppuration, gangrene, sloughing, and hemorrhage. If this happens, recovery time is greatly slowed.

Most cases of snakebite occur between sunrise and sunset. Non-poisonous snakebites are treated with antibiotic herbs or drugs, in order to prevent infection. If you are not sure of the identity of the snake, and you killed him, you might bring it back for identification at the emergency room.

DESCRIPTIONS—*Coral snakes:* They are found only in the southernmost areas of the United States, as well as south of the border, and have brightly colored rings. There is a non-poisonous snake which looks similar; but the colored rings are arranged differently. Remember it this way: *"Red by black, friend of Jack; but black by yellow, kill a fellow."*

NATURAL REMEDIES
CLAY POULTICE
• This is the currently recommended procedure: Keep

calm. Apply a thick, wet clay poultice (or better, ground-up activated charcoal powder mixed with the wet clay). Immediately lay down for two hours. The poultice will absorb the venom at the wound site.

HOW TO SUCTION

• An alternate remedy recommended by others: Keep on hand a small **hand-suction extractor** for immediately pulling the poison out of the wound. Continue this for half an hour. (This suction is less useful for coral snake venom; but use it on all snake bites anyway!)

• Suction can also be done with a **pop bottle** which is heated and applied. As it cools a vacuum is formed.

• Another alternative is to cut off the end of a plastic **injection syringe** at the bottom of the large end, apply to the bitten area, and pull back on the plunger.

• If there is no other way to extract the poison, another person should **suck it out**, continually spitting out the blood, for half an hour. The person doing the sucking should not have any sores in his mouth.

• The former instruction was to cut across between the two bite holes, so you could suck out more blood and poison. The current theory is that no cuts should be made, but only sucking. It might be the best to **suck and spit** for a couple minutes; this will clean the surface as well. Then **cut across**, so you can **suck** even better. But, when you are in the crisis, do what seems best.

Here is more detailed information on this:

• Cutting a snakebite to suck or suction out the venom should be done only when medical care is several hours away and when the bite is on an arm or leg. Then it should be done as soon as a tourniquet is in place.

• Sterilize a sharp knife or razor blade in a flame or alcohol. Make cuts 1/8 of an inch deep. Each cut should run the length of the limb, not across it. So, if necessary, two cuts will be made instead of one.

• For 30-60 minutes, suck out the poison and spit it out. Then rinse out the mouth (snake venom is not poison in the stomach; it is poisonous only when it gets directly into the bloodstream). Wash the wound and bandage it.

THE TOURNIQUET METHOD

• If medical help is more than 30 minutes away and if the bite is on an arm or leg, the medically recommended procedure is to apply a tourniquet between the wound and the heart during the first 5 minutes after the bite: Have the patient **lie down**, keep him **calm and warm**, apply a **tourniquet** above the limb where the wound is. (*But the clay poultice method, mentioned earlier, is far superior.*) This constricting band should be 2-4 inches above the bite and tight enough to shut off the venous blood (but not so tight that it stops the arterial circulation. It should be loose enough that a finger can be inserted between it and the skin, and a pulse can be felt below the bite site.) Loosen the band 15 seconds every 10 minutes. If the swelling reaches the tourniquet, it should be left in place and a second constricting band should be applied a few inches higher.

OTHER HELPS

• Specific **antivenin serums** are in stock for various species of snakes. Learn to identify the various snakes in your locality. (Coral snakes are primarily found only in the southeastern states.)

• Massive doses of **vitamin C** (a first dose of 4,000 mg; followed by 1,000-2,000 mg *each hour*). Reduce the dosage if diarrhea develops. **Calcium** gluconate (500 mg, every 6 hours), to relieve pain and abdominal cramping from the venom, and prevent stomach upset from massive amounts of vitamin C. Accompany each dose of calcium with **magnesium** (1,000 mg). **Pantothenic acid** (500 mg each 8 hours, for 2 days), to augment vitamin C's detoxifying effects.

• The person bitten should **keep calm** and work carefully. Excitement speeds up the blood flow to the heart.

• In most cases, the person does not die. But pray and get yourself prepared for whatever may happen.

• Do not give **liquor** to the person, thinking that this will help him. It does not!

• Take **charcoal** from the campfire, mix it with water and drink it, as follows: a half glassful of water with 1 tsp. of charcoal, and drink another one every 15 minutes until the danger is past.

• If able to do so, a couple hours later, take a **steam bath** or something similar, to sweat out the poison.

• Throughout all this time, you should **eat no food**.

• Do not apply **ice or a cold pack** to the bitten area; for this will drive the poison toward the heart.

• If, after several hours, the bite area is still swollen and painful, put **kerosene** on a cloth and apply it, keeping it wet for several hours. This will help neutralize the poison. An alternative is to grind up raw **onions** and apply to the area. Leave them there until an offensive odor, not of onions, is noticed. Remove. Bathe the area. And apply more raw, crushed onions until the pain is gone. The onion is drawing out the poison.

• **Rue** can expel poison. Drink the tea and apply it to the wound.

• Pouring **alcohol** on a bite is useless and may speed up the venom.

• Chew up and swallow 10 **charcoal** tablets with water. Crush more tablets, make a paste, and place on the bite as a compress. Charcoal will help draw out the poison if applied extremely fast.

PREVENTION

• When you go hiking or camping, include a **suction kit, charcoal, a bottle of powdered vitamin C, and a cell phone** in your pack sack. Stay on the **trails**. If you are in heavy snake country, wear **canvas protectors** on your lower legs. They can be purchased at surplus stores.

ENCOURAGEMENT—When trials and tribulations come to you, know that everything will work out well if, through dedication and prayer, you will keep close to God. Psalm 60:12.

JELLYFISH STING

SYMPTOMS—A strong stinging feeling on the legs or arms while swimming at an ocean beach. This may afterward be followed by headache, muscle cramps, coughing, shortness of breath, nausea, and vomiting.

CAUSES—Jellyfish and Portuguese men-of-war are found in warmer marine waters. The eastern beaches of Florida are one example.

Their long tentacles contain stinging cells which, touching you, pierce the skin and release poison. Even severed tentacles can poison just as intensively.

NATURAL REMEDIES

• Immediately **rinse the wound** with saltwater. Do not use freshwater, because it activates any stinging cells which have not already burst. For the same reason, **do not rub** the skin.

• Neutralize the area as soon as possible by splashing on one of the following; and do it again as needed: Use rubbing or ethyl (liquor) **alcohol, vinegar, ammonia, or meat tenderizer**. Travel tip: Take a bottle of vinegar with you to the ocean beach.

• **If any tentacles remain** on your skin, apply a paste of sand and seawater; then wrap your hand in a towel and wipe them off or scrape them off with a knife or credit card.

• Apply generous amounts of **aloe vera gel and plantain tincture** to the affected area.

ENCOURAGEMENT—God is preparing the hearts of those who dedicate their lives to Him. Soon, at His coming, they will go to heaven to ever be with Him. This is something each one of us can have.

CORAL, STINGRAY, AND SEA URCHIN BITES

SYMPTOMS—Painful abrasions and wounds while swimming, scuba diving, or snorkeling.

CAUSES—Coral polyps have the same toxic cells as jellyfish. The hard coral can cause painful abrasions; and the polyps can discharge small, poisonous barbs.

Stingrays have barbed, toxic spines at the base of their long tails. Sea urchins have spines which can inject poison. All of them can cause pain and infection.

NATURAL REMEDIES

• Do not rub; but **flush the wound** with saltwater.
• Then, to neutralize more of the poison, splash the wound with **alcohol, vinegar, ammonia, alum, or meat tenderizer** dissolved in saltwater.
• With tweezers or fingers covered with cloth, carefully **remove** coral **fragments** or small spines.
• Then, to neutralize more of the toxin, immerse the wounded area in **hot water** for 30 minutes or more.
• If medical assistance is not likely within half an hour, apply a **tourniquet** between the wound and the heart. *See Snake Bite (837) for directions on how to apply a tourniquet properly.*

ENCOURAGEMENT—There is a science of Christianity to be mastered,—a science as much deeper, broader, higher than any human science as the heavens are higher than the earth. The mind is to be disciplined, educated, trained; for we are to do service for God in ways that are not in harmony with inborn inclination. Hereditary and cultivated tendencies to evil must be overcome. Often the education and training of a lifetime must be discarded, that one may become a learner in the school of Christ. Our hearts must be educated to become steadfast in God. We are to form habits of thought that will enable us to resist temptation. We must learn to look upward. The principles of the Word of God,—principles that are as high as heaven, and that compass eternity,— we are to understand in their bearing upon our daily life. Every act, every word, every thought, is to be in accord with these principles. All must be brought into harmony with, and subject to, Christ.

POISONS -
2 - TRANSMITTED DISEASES

TYPHUS

SYMPTOMS—Sudden onset of chills, high fever, prostration, and general pains. The patient is excited, mentally alert, and has a flushed face and bloodshot eyes.

Delirium frequently occurs early. Small pink spots on neck, chest, abdomen, and limbs appear about the fifth day. They change from pink to red, then to purple, and finally turn brownish.

Heavy bronchitis, with cough and sputum. Pulse is rapid; but blood pressure is low.

In its early stages, typhus is like Rocky Mountain Spotted Fever; but the home treatment for both is essentially the same.

CAUSES—There are three main types of typhus fevers (louse fever, flea and tick fever, and mite fever); but they are all treated about the same and are caused by similar bacteria carried by **lice, fleas, ticks, or mites**.

Typhus, caused by rickettsia, occurs where people are crowded together under unsanitary conditions.

But Rocky Mountain Spotted Fever and Lyme Disease are more easily acquired by anyone who goes out into the woods. —*See Rocky Mountain Spotted Fever (840) and Lyme Disease (813, 840) for related information.*

NATURAL REMEDIES

• Typhus is a tropical disease; it rarely occurs in the northern climates. Call a physician. If none is available, give the treatment for Fevers (222, 302) or Bubonic Plague (843).
• Typhus responds to **colloidal silver, echinacea, goldenseal, garlic,** and **water** which is extensively used inside and outside of the body. Eat no food for a few days.

POISONS

It is best to call a physician if one is available.

ENCOURAGEMENT—The end of all things is at hand. Oh that we could see, as we should, the necessity of seeking the Lord with all the heart! Then we would find Him. May God teach each one of us how to pray more fervently. Matthew 11:29.

"It is a good thing to give thanks unto the Lord, and to sing praises unto Thy name, O Most High; to show forth Thy lovingkindness in the morning, and Thy faithfulness every night." Psalm 92:1-2.

"And it shall come to pass, that in the place where it was said unto them, Ye are not My people; there shall they be called the children of the living God." Romans 9:26.

What encouraging promises are these!

You must learn in the school of Christ precious lessons of patience. Do not become discouraged; but keep at the work in all humility. It will drive you to Jesus; it will lead you to study the Pattern. You want to work as Jesus worked.

ROCKY MOUNTAIN SPOTTED FEVER
(Tick Fever)

SYMPTOMS—Symptoms begin 7-12 days after being bitten: headaches, chills, weakness, fever, muscle pain, and dry cough. There is a skin rash on the wrists, ankles, palms, soles of the feet, and forearms. This then spreads to the neck, face, axilla, buttocks, and trunk.

Next comes liver enlargement and pneumonitis. If untreated, circulatory failure brings death.

CAUSES—When symptoms first appear, do not wait for a positive blood test identification before instituting treatment. Death may occur as soon as 4-10 days after appearance of symptoms. Contact a physician.

Rocky Mountain Spotted Fever is caused by a similar bacteria *(rickettsia)* that causes typhus *(839);* but it is transmitted solely by a tick. Of the reported cases, 90% occur along the eastern seaboard and 10% in the Rocky Mountains. But it can be contracted anywhere in between those regions.

May through October is when people, who are out in the woods, are especially bitten. You can also get it from your dog, which has been roaming the woods and picking up ticks as though he were a vacuum cleaner.

NATURAL REMEDIES

• Call a physician. Auxiliary home treatment is for fevers *(222, 302)* and Bubonic Plague *(843).* For preventive measures, see Lyme Disease *(840).*

• **Colloidal silver, echinacea, goldenseal,** and **garlic** are used to aid in recovery.

• If a tick is biting you, pull it off slowly, so as not to leave part behind; then rub on a little alcohol, vinegar, or lemon.

PREVENTION—Before going on a walk in the woods or fields, mix 50-50 powdered **sulphur and talcum powder**, dusting it on your legs and around your waist. An old-timer suggests putting a little turpentine around your ankles and one drop on your tongue, to discourage them.

Avoid **sleeping** where cattle graze or near your dog.

• *For detailed information on ticks, see Lyme Disease (568, 744).*

ENCOURAGEMENT—We can safely trust in God, to help us through the trials and disappointments of life. Go to Him and find in Him the help you so much need. He will give that which is best.

LYME DISEASE

SYMPTOMS—Between 2 and 32 days after the bite, symptoms appear: fatigue, flu-like symptoms, stiff neck, backache, headache, nausea, and vomiting.

Ultimately, enlargement of the lymph nodes and spleen may occur, along with irregular heart rhythm, arthritis, and brain damage.

Some of these symptoms slowly pass away over 2-3 years. But sometimes symptoms recur later without having been bitten again.

Because this disease is now so prominent, and because it can occur so mysteriously, here are more detailed symptoms on its usual 3 stages (which not everyone experiences):

1 - Small raised bumps, and/or a rash, appear on the entire body for 1-2 days or several weeks and then fades. Fever, chills, nausea, and vomiting may also occur.

2 - Weeks or months later, facial paralysis may occur. Frequently, enlargement of the spleen and lymph glands occurs and/or severe headaches, enlargement of the heart muscle, and abnormal heart rhythm.

3 - This can develop into backache, stiff neck, joint pains in the knees, swelling and pain in other joints, and even degenerative muscle and joint disease. About 70% of those who remain untreated later develop problems in the joints and central nervous system.

Physicians especially look for the following symptoms, before treating with antibiotics: a small red bump at the site of the tick bite, a bull's-eye rash surrounding that tick bite, and flu-like symptoms (such as fatigue, chills, and joint pain). If treatment is postponed until more advanced symptoms develop (heart, brain, or joint problems), drug medications do not work as well.

That **"bull's-eye" spot**, caused by the tick bite, is the best single early warning that you have been infected with Lyme Disease. Within a day it usually enlarges to a rash around tick bite that is about 3 inches in diameter. But in about 10% of the cases, no rash appears.

To complicate the situation, the tick may not only have transmitted the bacterium, *Borrelia burgdorferi* (the cause of Lyme Disease), to you, but at the same time, it may have infected you with Ehrlichiosis *(842).*

CAUSES—Lyme Disease is the most common tick-borne illness in America. It was first discovered in Old Lyme, Connecticut in 1975; it most frequently occurs where the white-tailed deer is most abundant, which is the northeastern states. But the disease has spread. Eight states report 90% of the cases: Connecticut, Massachusetts, California, Minnesota, New York, Rhode Island, Wisconsin, and New Jersey. Yet it has occurred in every state except Alaska, Arizona, Hawaii, Montana, and Nebraska. Lyme Disease is actually a very dangerous disease! Therefore, special attention is given to it here.

The bite of a tiny tick *(Ixodes dammini)* is primarily carried by deer. But it is also carried, in the eastern states, by white-footed field mice and, in the west, by lizards and jackrabbits. In California, it is also transmitted by the black-legged tick, carried by wood rats. Unfortunately, deer ticks also infest dogs and get on cats. For centuries, foxes and bobcats killed the mice carrying Lyme Disease; but now the country is overrun with the mice and the ticks they carry, which are now on deer and other animals. Researchers found that, because there are less predators, the ticks are 7 times as prevalent on 1-2 acre lots than on 10-15-acre lots.

Both deer ticks and black-legged ticks are very tiny. An adult is less than 1/10th of an inch and the nymph is a pinhead in size. They are much smaller than a dog tick.

Dogs and cats can collect these special ticks out in the woods and bring them into your home.

Tick bites are generally painless and unnoticed; so the symptoms may not at first, or later, be correctly diagnosed. Yet in advanced stages, when correct diagnosis finally occurs, the situation may have become critical.

The symptoms are similar to those of multiple sclerosis *(580)*, gout *(627)*, Epstein-Barr virus *(280)*, and Chronic Fatigue Syndrome *(279-281)*.

A test now exists which can detect the bacteria *(Borrelia burgdorferi)* which causes Lyme Disease. Antibodies are present from 3 days to 3 weeks after infection.

The majority of cases occur in the summer and fall. After a tick bites, it waits several hours before it begins to feed on the host's blood; and, once it does, it feasts for 3-4 days. The longer the tick remains attached, the greater the risk of Lyme Disease. If you remove the tick within 30 minutes after he starts biting, you are usually safe. —But can you be sure when the 30 minutes begins?

Lyme Disease is treatable and almost always curable if correctly diagnosed in the early stages. But, because the bites are usually painless, the incubation period so long, and the symptoms so varied, the problem may go unrecognized for weeks or months.

If you develop a bull's-eye type of rash anywhere on your body, see your health-care provider right away.

Significantly, many people have been bitten by the deer tick and have not gotten sick. In some Lyme-endemic parts of the U.S., 10% of the people have antibodies to the disease, showing they were earlier bitten but did not become ill. In other parts of America, about 1%-2% have already been bitten and not gotten sick. A 1995 AMA survey revealed that only about half of those diagnosed with Lyme Disease actually had it. The rest had arthritic or other physical problems from other causes.

If you walk in fields or woods at all, purchase two pairs of flat-edged tweezers, one for home and one to carry with you.

NATURAL REMEDIES

HOW TO REMOVE THE TICK

• The longer the tick is on you, the greater the risk of infection. Here is the safe way to remove it.

• A **drop of oil or alcohol** may be applied to partially immobilize the tick; but *do not use the wrong methods* to get him out. Put a **hot match** close to him to get him to back out or suffocate it with **petroleum jelly** or **nail polish**. Any of these will cause more bacteria to enter your body. Instead quickly, remove him.

• **Remove the tick** with tweezers. Keep fine-pointed tweezers in the home and in your backpack when you camp or hike.

If you find a tick embedded in the skin, carefully place the tweezers straight down over the flat side of the tick (so the tweezers are over its top and bottom). The tweezer points should close on the tick's head, right next to the skin where it is embedded. With a slight rocking motion, slowly and steadily pull the tick out of the skin. Notice that you closed the tweezers on its head, not its rear body! Do not twist. You want the entire tick out, without leaving part of it in the skin or injecting bacteria from its broken body into the skin. You may pour rubbing alcohol on the tick before pulling him out. Do not touch the tick with your hands. Do not apply kerosene, turpentine, or petroleum jelly. (If you do not have tweezers, use your fingers covered with tissue; then thoroughly wash them.) Any of its fluids could cause an infection. If you squeeze or twist the tick, its insides will get on you.

• It is important to **remove the whole tick**. If mouth parts remain in your skin, disinfect them with alcohol and consult your physician.

AFTER REMOVING THE TICK

• Wash your hands and the bite area with **soap and water**. Apply rubbing **alcohol or hydrogen peroxide** to the bite area. Then apply a small bandage, if needed.

• Two or 3 times a day, disinfect the bite area with **tea tree oil, calendula** extract, **St. John's wort** extract, or **echinacea / goldenseal** extract.

• Save the **tick in a jar**, labeled with the date, location, and where the tick bit you on your body. Place a damp towel in the jar; that will keep him fresh for up to 6 weeks.

• **Call a physician,** so you can have it tested immediately. **Watch for symptoms** over the next 3 weeks. Especially look to see if the bull's eye red rash appears within a day! Does stiffening in one or more joints—most often the knee or ankle—occur later?

• *Comparative symptoms: **Rocky Mountain Spotted Fever** (840)* will produce a fever within a week, a rash of reddish black spots on wrists and ankles. ***Lyme Disease*** starts with a red rash around the bite (70% of the time). From 3 days to 3 months, other symptoms develop: fever, joint and muscle pains, dizziness, swollen glands.

• Put suspicious **clothing in the dryer** for 30 minutes, to kill ticks by dehydration. Washing clothes, even in hot water and bleach, does not necessarily kill ticks.

• Heat relieves pain. **Hot baths** are helpful. *See Fevers (302).*

• Jim Duke recommends **garlic** capsules (equivalent to 1,200 mg of fresh garlic every day), 6 **echinacea** capsules daily (each containing 450 mg). He also recommends drinking fresh **juice from carrots, tomatoes, and fresh garlic**, along with the drug, doxiycycline.

IF YOU HAVE CHRONIC LYME DISEASE

• Eat a nourishing diet of **fruits, vegetables, whole grains, nuts, and legumes**. Omit **processed and junk foods, meat, saturated fat**. Identify **food allergies** and eliminate them. Do not use **caffeine, sugar, or alcohol**. Get regular **exercise**—in a safe place outside. Drink at least 48 oz. of **water** daily.

• Take high-potency **B complex, vitamin C** (500-1,000 mg, 3 times a day), **vitamin E** (400-800 IU), **flaxseed oil** (2 Tbsp. daily), **calcium, and seaweed** for trace minerals.

PREVENTION

During the summer and fall months:

• Keep **lawns cut short** and shrubbery to a minimum, where children play. Cut the grass or, otherwise, **clear paths** you walk on in the woods near your home.

• The best solution to this problem is prevention. **Avoid going in the woods** in the summer months when ticks are the most active (especially June to August). Stay on the **center of the trails**. **Check yourself** and your children carefully afterward.

• Wear **long pants** and tuck them into your socks. Wear a **long-sleeved shirt** with a high neck or scarf, plus hat and gloves. If the clothing is light-colored, you can see the ticks better.

• Do a careful **body inspection** every day, if you have been in the woods or live in an infested area. **Look for dark spots** on your skin, behind knees, in the scalp, crevices, and armpits. Check children before they go to bed.

• You may choose to use an **insect repellent** containing DEET (diethyl toluamide). It lasts longer than others; and it is said to be safe on the outside. But it is fatal if taken into your body. It dissolves plastics, synthetics (nylons and polyesters), and some paints; and it causes adverse reactions in children. Wash it off as soon as you go indoors!

• Avoid having a **dog or cat**; they vacuum up the ticks and bring them to the house, where they fall off and you get them. You may miss the pets; but they will be replaced with lots of songbirds and some happy chipmunks. If you still want to have a pet that roams about the countryside, give it a good bath every week. Unfortunately, deer ticks also infest dogs. They also get on cats.

• **Pregnant women** should do what is needed to keep from being bitten. The infection can be transferred to the developing fetus and causes miscarriage (but rarely).

• Not everyone bitten acquires the disease. A **high sugar and fat diet** attracts insects! The skin eliminates toxins, which attract bugs when the diet is unnatural.

• When the blood is pure and the body clean, there is far less likelihood of tick bites and lice infestation.

A diet high in fiber and natural food will help keep the body clean and protect against infections. Sugar attracts insects.

• Herbs useful in preventing infections include **echinacea, goldenseal, garlic, and burdock**. Rubbing with **lemon juice** will disinfect that part of the body you place it on. Applying **aloe vera** aids in healing.

• **Vitamins A and C** protect against infections. **B complex** vitamins help keep the blood clean. **Eat lots of greens**.

A Lyme test is now available; but false positives occur sometimes. So, if you are being treated for Lyme Disease and are not getting better, consider having a second test made. One study of nearly 800 people, diagnosed with Lyme Disease, revealed that half of them did not have it! Physicians blame false-positive tests for this.

—*Also see Rocky Mountain Spotted Fever (840).*

PET SYMPTOMS

If your cat or dog shows any of the following symptoms, it may have Lyme Disease: One or more swollen, hot joints. Poor appetite. Hot, dry nose. Fever of 103°-106°F. Wants to sit or lie in one place for long periods of time. Lameness that sometimes disappears.

ENCOURAGEMENT—If, through surrender and prayer, you are in Christ, as the trials come, the power of God will come with them. You will receive exactly that which is best at this time. Isaiah 63:9.

EHRLICHIOSIS

SYMPTOMS—Symptoms usually appear 7-10 days after the tick bites. Symptoms include severe headache, chills, fever, and joint pains. Sometimes there is nausea and vomiting; occasionally a spotted rash appears.

Rarely, serious complications develop, causing anemia and damage to the liver, kidneys, lungs, and nervous system.

CAUSES—This is another disease (caused by ehrlichia bacteria) which can be caused by a tick bite. A single tick can transmit two or more different disease bacteria; so you can come down with two or more tick-borne diseases at the same time.

So far, most cases are occurring in southern, central, and Atlantic coast states of the U.S. Walking or camping in wooded areas during the summer and early fall should be avoided.

The disease can be difficult to diagnose from the symptoms, especially if you have Lyme Disease at the same time.

NATURAL REMEDIES

• Prompt treatment can relieve the symptoms within 24-48 hours. See a physician.

• Helpful information will be found in Fevers *(302)* and Antibiotic Herbs *(297)*. Lyme Disease *(840)* is full of information on how to avoid ticks.

ENCOURAGEMENT—Have faith in Jesus as your helper. Remember that you are not to choose your own work or follow your own ways; but look to Jesus as your guide and pattern. Keep His example before you; and constantly ask what will be pleasing in His sight. Learn from Him lessons of self-denial and self-sacrifice.

LEISHMANIASIS

SYMPTOMS—Bite of a small sand fly, which can be difficult to recognize in an internal infection which has developed.

If only the skin is infected, 2-8 weeks after being bitten, a swelling appears where the fly bit. The swelling becomes an open sore, usually with pus. Sores can heal by themselves; but they may take several weeks to 2 years. Meanwhile, the sores can easily become infected by bacteria.

CAUSES—This is a disease which travelers to the Near East, India, and Asia can contract. It is occasionally found in southern Mexico, Central America, and South America.

The infection is carried from person to person by a small sand fly which infects a person when it bites.

Some forms of the disease cause internal infection, called *visceral leishmaniasis*, kala azar, or dumdum fever. These infections are very difficult to recognize and the usual medical treatment is complicated.

Other forms of the disease primarily affect the skin. These are known as *cutaneous leishmaniasis*, tropical sore, Delhi boil, espundia, forest yaws, uta, or chiclero ulcer. These skin sores are easier to treat.

NATURAL REMEDIES

• Clean the skin sore with cool water which has been boiled. Apply a hot, moist cloth to the sore for 10-15 minutes. The cloth should not be so hot that it burns the skin.

• Repeat this 2 times daily for 10 days. This treatment often brings a complete elimination of the skin disease.

• If the sore becomes red and painful, it is becoming infected. Apply goldenseal, echinacea, or another antibiotic herb *(287)*.

ENCOURAGEMENT—Had Peter walked humbly with God (hiding self in Christ), had he earnestly looked for divine help, had he been less self-confident, had he received the Lord's instruction and practiced it, he would have been watching unto prayer. Had he closely examined himself, the Lord would have given him divine help and there would have been no need of Satan's sifting. There is no power in the whole satanic force that can disable the soul that trusts, in simple confidence, in the wisdom that comes from God.

GUINEA WORM

SYMPTOMS—A painful swelling develops in the ankle, leg, testicles, or elsewhere on the body. A week later, a blister forms; and it soon bursts open, forming a sore. This often happens when standing in water or bathing. The end of a white, thread-like Guinera worm can be seen poking out of the sore.

If the sore becomes dirty and infected, the pain and swelling spreads. Eventually walking becomes impossible. Sometimes tetanus *(866)* occurs.

CAUSES—This is another disease which overseas travelers can contract. The disease is spread by drinking **infected water**. It can also be spread by **walking or bathing in pools**. An infected person with an open sore wades into a water hole. The worm extends its head and lays thousands of eggs into the water. Tiny water-fleas pick up the worm eggs. Another person drinks some of water, and fleas and worm eggs are swallowed. Some of the worms develop into worms under the skin; but the person feels nothing. About a year later, a sore forms when an adult worm breaks through the surface of the skin, to lay its eggs.

NATURAL REMEDIES

• Keep the sore clean. Soak it in cold water until the worm's head pokes out. Attach a thread to the worm and pull gently, a little more each day. This may take a week. Do not break it! The worm may be more than 3 feet in length! If broken, severe infection can result. At the same time (or if sores become infected), take antibiotic herbs *(297)*.

• To prevent infection while traveling overseas, boil all drinking water. Stay out of pools. If you must drink out of a pool, put the water into a special pot for drinking, which has a clean cloth tied over the top. The cloth will filter out the water-fleas.

• If nobody wades or bathes in water used for drinking, the infection cannot be passed on; it will eventually disappear from the area.

ENCOURAGEMENT—The answer to our prayers may not come as quickly as we desire; and it may not be just what we have asked. But He who knows what is for the highest good of His children will bestow a much greater good than we have asked, if we do not become faithless and discouraged.

BUBONIC PLAGUE
(Pneumonic Plague)

SYMPTOMS—Following an incubation period of 2-10 days, the disease begins suddenly with a high fever, severe headache, great weakness, and pains in the back and limbs. There may be vomiting and diarrhea.

The fever may go up to 104° F. the first day, accompanied by intense thirst.

Buboes (swollen places) begin to appear the second day in the groin, under the arms, and in the neck.

The disease causes great weakness; and death often occurs sometime between the third and sixth day.

The key symptoms of the *bubonic* form are swollen

lymph notes in the groin and armpits. The key symptoms of the *pneumonic* form is the severe cough and shortness of breath.

CAUSES—In the bubonic form of the plague, the lymph glands swell. When swollen, they are called "buboes."

This is a disease carried by the Norway rat. The bacteria are in its droppings, which it leaves in the food stuffs it has broken into and partly eaten.

There is also a pneumonic form of the plague, which is far less common. The symptoms are about the same as pneumonia; but it is transmitted through the air, extremely contagious, and is lethal.

In earlier centuries, several outbreaks of the plague occurred; during one, one-sixth of the people of Europe died. In the 14th century, 25 million people in Europe died from this plague.

Today, small outbreaks occur in Asia, Africa, and South America. There are only 10-12 cases a year in the U.S. So the plague essentially never occurs in the Western world today. We mention it here, so you will be aware of the symptoms. There is danger that terrorists will eventually use it against Western civilization. It is known that stored cultures of the bacterium *(Yersinia pestis)* which causes it are in Russia.

NATURAL REMEDIES

• Call a physician. Living cleanly and eating right is the best prevention. Healthy, rested, people can resist infection better than others.

• This is a serious disease; a physician will use tetracycline, if it is available. Otherwise, use **coloidal silver, echinacea, goldenseal,** and **garlic**. Drink and bathe in much water; rest and fast for a few days.

• Very helpful information will be found in Fevers *(302-308)* and Antibiotic Herbs *(297).*

ENCOURAGEMENT—All our sufferings and sorrows, all our temptations and trials, all our sadness and griefs—in short, all things work together for good to them that love God and are called according to His purpose. Romans 8:28.

DOG OR ANIMAL BITE

SYMPTOMS—You are bitten by an animal.

CAUSES—A bite from an animal carries with it a high risk of transmitted infection. Even a superficial bite should be checked by a physician. There is a special risk of infection of rabies *(844)* or tetanus *(866)*.

The first question is: "Has the skin been broken?" If the tissues have been merely squeezed, then the matter is of little importance. There may be soreness and a black-and-blue appearance; but it will soon disappear.

But, if there has been penetration (an actual wound) then action must be taken. The animal may be perfectly healthy; but you cannot be certain of that.

The animal's teeth may cause the spores of tetanus germs to enter the body or the animal may be rabid. Such bites, if not promptly treated, can result in death.

NATURAL REMEDIES

• Remove the victim from danger, if it is safe to do so.

• **Wash the area** thoroughly, to remove the animal's saliva from the wound. Use warm water and then soap and water. Clean it for 5 minutes. Splash it with hydrogen peroxide or other antiseptic. Rinse with plain water. Pat it dry. Apply a sterile dressing. An ice pack may be placed over the bandage, to relieve pain.

• If the wound is serious, treat it as for severe bleeding.

• Either catch the dog and confine it or try to learn who the owner is. Notify health authorities, so they can observe the animal.

• Ideally, the wound is superficial, the animal is a healthy pet, and the one bitten has had a tetanus shot within the past 5 years. But if there are deep gashes, the possibility of rabies, subsequent swelling, redness, or drainage, contact a physician.

—*See Rabies (below) for detailed information about this danger and what should be done. Also see **Tetanus** (866). Tetanus is less likely; yet it is still a possibility.*

ENCOURAGEMENT—All experiences and circumstances are God's workmen, whereby good is brought to us. Let us look at the light behind the cloud. Proverbs 3:6.

RABIES
(Hydrophobia)

SYMPTOMS—Symptoms begin appearing within 1-4 months after the bite, but sometimes longer. They include numbness, soreness, and tingling where the bite occurred.

These sensations spread. And it becomes difficult to swallow, breathe, and talk.

Then more extensive muscle spasms begin; and the victim gradually becomes maniacal. The final stages are depression and exhaustion. Sometimes there is paralysis, coma, and death.

If the symptoms of rabies have already begun to appear, the person will probably die.

See end of this article for symptoms in a rabid dog. Rabies can also be transmitted by the bite of infected bats, foxes, skunks, and other animals.

CAUSES—Rabies is an infectious disease which destroys the nerve cells of part of the brain and causes death. Humans and all warm-blooded animals can get rabies. Because one of the symptoms is inability to swallow water, the disease is also called hydrophobia ("fear of water"). The disease is transmitted by a bite or by getting some of the saliva in a wound. Some animals contract rabies from breathing the air in caves where millions of bats are sleeping during the day. **Dogs** and **wild animals** are the most common sources of rabies for humans.

When the virus enters the body, it travels along the nerves to the spine and brain, producing inflammation. Once symptoms appear, death is inevitable.

MEDICINAL TREATMENT
This is the standard treatment for rabies:
• Nearly all human rabies cases result from dog bites.

The animal can transmit disease before it shows symptoms of rabies; but, except in rare instances, the symptoms will appear within 10 days if it is rabid. The disease is always fatal, unless it is halted by a series of Pasteur treatments, which are started before symptoms first appear.

• If at all possible, it is crucial to confine the animal which inflicted the bite, so it can be observed. The course of the disease runs so fast that the animal should show symptoms of rabies before they begin to appear in the person. If the animal is rabid, it will show clear signs within 2 weeks; then the person bitten should begin the Pasteur series of rabies shots (unless circumstances are clear that the animal was not rabid).

• If the animal got away and cannot be found, then the person should immediately take the rabies vaccine series.

• If the series has already been started, and the animal is then found not to have rabies, the Pasteur treatments can be stopped.

• About 10%-12% of persons bitten by a known rabid animal, and not treated, will contract rabies and die. If the Pasteur series is started within 2 weeks or less after the bite, about one-third of 1% of those bitten will die.

• It is not widely known that rabies is sometimes transmitted accidentally in hospitals. Rabies in humans is sometimes misdiagnosed as a stroke. After death, some of that rabid tissue may be transplanted to another person.

• If your child's pet hamster bites him, do not think the child needs to start rabies shots. Know that, if you have had that hamster for 3 weeks or more and it shows no symptoms of rabies, the hamster does not have rabies.

• Rabies shots last 10 days and are so difficult to take that the person often goes to the hospital for respiratory support while they are in progress. Yet they will save your life, if you contract the disease.

UNUSUAL ALTERNATIVES

• A backwoodsman, who is also a nature doctor, has treated all kinds of things with remarkable success. He says to do this: Wash the wound with **water** right away; then mix half and half **vinegar and warm water**, and wash the wound with it. When dry, apply 1-2 drops of **muriatic acid** (hydrochloric acid) to each wound. Do this even if (what appears to be) a rabid dog only licks a previous wound on your body. For extra precaution, you may apply a **tourniquet** and a rubber vacuum cup as for a snake bite (837). If Muriatic acid is not available and you are far from civilization, you may **burn the wound** with a magnifying glass in the sunlight or use a red-hot iron. Then treat as for a regular burn until it is healed. This treatment usually prevents further worry. So says one backwoodsman.

• Jethro Kloss has a lengthy article on rabies in his book, *Back to Eden* (pp. 490-495). He also says to put **hydrochloric acid** on the wound, to neutralize the rabies poison in the saliva. Then, after discussing a number of herbal remedies to also use, he quotes a scientific paper by an M. Buisson, read to the French Academy of Arts and Sciences. M. Buisson had accidentally contracted rabies from a women suffering with it. By the time he discovered

he had it, the disease was advanced and he knew he was soon to die. *Kloss quotes a London newspaper which reported on the scientific paper:*

"Concluding from these various symptoms that he was suffering with hydrophobia, he [Buisson] resolved to make an end of himself by suffocating himself in a vapor [**steam**] **bath**. With this view, he raised the heat very, very, hot, but was delighted, no less than surprised, to find that all his pains disappeared. He went out of the bath completely cured, ate a hearty dinner, and drank more freely than was usual with him. He adds that he has treated more than fourscore persons who have been bitten by mad dogs in a similar manner, and they all recovered, with the exception of a child seven years old, who died in a vapour bath he was administering."—*Jethro Kloss, Back to Eden, p. 493.*

• Water therapists normally work with a **steam bath** temperature of 115°-120° F. Those with diabetes, valvular heart disease, extreme arteriosclerosis, or emaciation should not take a steam bath.

• *Kloss also quotes a German newspaper which discussed an incident which happened in Saxony:*

"A Saxon forester named Gastell, at the age of 82, unwilling to take to the grave with him a secret of so much importance, has made public in the *Leipsic Journal* the method which he used for fifty years, and he affirms he has rescued many human beings and cattle from the fearful death of hydrophobia. Wash the wound immediately with **warm water and vinegar**; let it dry, and then pour upon the wound a few drops of **hydrochloric acid**, and that will neutralize and destroy the poison of the saliva."—*Kloss, p. 494.*

• Dr. Christopher suggests the following for rabies: Steep 1 tsp. lobelia in 1 pint boiling water and drink as much as possible to induce vomiting and cleansing of the stomach. Follow this with a high enema of lobelia and catnip. Christopher's remedy is based on the theory that, by cleansing the stomach and intestinal tract, the rabies can be eliminated.

• In his book, *Hydropathic* Encyclopedia, Robert Trall, M.D., recommended the following treatment for rabies: Apply **wet sheet packs or dry sheet packs** to promote perspiration; or give a **rubbing sheet pack, followed by a wet sheet pack**. *(See the hydrotherapy indexes for more information on such treatments: pp. 206-207, 273-275.)*

Trall's method is similar to the steam bath method; both of these methods cause the body to heat up in order to burn out the rabies virus.

• Taking **garlic** and other **antibiotic herbs** are also very helpful in treating serious infections. See Fevers (302-308) and Antibiotic Herbs (297).

RABIES SYMPTOMS IN THE DOG—Was the dog who bit the person rabid? Here are symptoms of rabies in a dog:

• Initially, there is a marked change in its disposition. He will become very friendly or very snappy; the bark becomes hoarse.

• Paralysis may soon develop—first the lower jaw, then the hind legs, and gradually the rest of the body.

• But, instead, the dog wants to run away. It may run for miles, snapping at any creature which comes near it. But some dogs never show this excitative phase.

• Finally, the dog becomes exhausted and paralysis sets in. Paralysis of the jaw usually occurs.

If a dog shows signs of rabies, it must be chained (not roped) and observed for 2 weeks. If it shows signs of rabies, the person must begin a series of injections.

—*Also see Dog or Animal Bite (846) and Antispasmodic Tincture (312, 576).*

ENCOURAGEMENT—Jesus encourages you to persevere in prayer. In Him you can find the help you need for the crisis you face. How thankful we can be for the sacrifice of Christ on our behalf, that we might be saved!

TULAREMIA
(Rabbit Fever, Deer Fly Disease)

SYMPTOMS—The symptoms are similar to those of undulant fever and the plague. The first indication is a local ulceration at the infection site. About 1-7 days after infection occurs, chills, headache, prostration, and general pains suddenly begin. The disease is characterized by high fever and recurring chills with drenching sweat. A shallow, but ongoing, ulcer develops at the site of the original wound or bite. Lymph glands draining that area become swollen and painful; but they should not be lanced!

If not treated, the fever usually lasts 3-4 weeks; and it is, generally, not fatal. But convalescence is slow. Physical and mental depression can last for months.

CAUSES—Tularemia is a disease caused by *Francisella tularensis*; and it is transmitted to man from rodents, through the bite of a deer fly, and other blood-sucking insects. It can also be acquired through the bite of an animal, generally a **rabbit**. A more frequent cause today (87%) is cutting oneself while skinning and dressing infected rabbits or **ground squirrels**. The infected rabbits are often wild, not tame ones.

If you notice the appearance of symptoms (and you have been working with rabbits, especially wild ones), then have the condition immediately diagnosed. Sputum samples are highly contagious; so the lab should be warned about your suspicions.

TREATMENT—Go to a physician.
— *Helpful information will be found in Fevers (302-309) and Antibiotic Herbs (297).*

ENCOURAGEMENT—We yearn for a deeper, broader sense of God's presence. As we seek for it, we find the strength, peace, and encouragement we need. God will help you. 1 Timothy 1:15.

CAT COCCIDIA
(Toxoplasmosis)

SYMPTOMS—Symptoms can mimic the flu and cause headache, high fever, rash, swollen lymph nodes, meningitis, hepatitis, pneumonitis, myocarditis, blindness, and diarrhea.

If a pregnant woman contracts this disease, it will cause birth defects in the fetus (brain defects, blindness, and/or mental retardation).

CAUSES—Those who keep cats should be aware of this danger. Cat coccidia is caused by a tiny protozoa (*Isospora bigemina*) which lives in the intestines of cats. Apparently, it is in many cats!

This disease is acquired by inhaling or swallowing dust from contaminated **kitty litter boxes,** outdoor **sand, or dirt piles**. But it can also come from eating **rare beef**. While that protozoa is in an intermediate stage, it is outside the cat's intestines—and can enter the human body.

TREATMENT—See a physician. Diagnosis is made from a positive blood test or skin test.

PREVENTION—Women should **avoid cats** just prior to, and during, pregnancy. They should only eat **well-cooked meat**. Better yet, stop eating it entirely; since many diseases are transmitted through eating meat (including poultry, fish, and shellfish.)

Other diseases which you can get from cats, include Lyme Disease (813), Poison Ivy and Oak (854), Pinworms (863), and Toxoplasmosis (846, 864). shellfish).

ENCOURAGEMENT—You can trust God to do for you that which you cannot do for yourself. In Him is our strength and help. In Him we find the answers we need to life's problems. Deuteronomy 33:12.

POISONS - 3 - ALLERGIES

ANAPHYLACTIC SHOCK
(Anaphylaxis)

SYMPTOMS—Sudden feeling of extreme anxiety. Swollen face, lips, and tongue. Possibly an itchy, red rash and flushing of skin (hives, 346-347). There may be puffiness around the eyes. Wheezing and difficult breathing. If severe, he may lose consciousness.

CAUSES—If you have an extreme sensitivity to a substance, you may experience some or all of the above symptoms as soon as you are exposed to it.

We live in a chemical age, in which we seem to be overwhelmed with drug medications, polluted air, water, soil, chemicaled crops, and chemicals used in our cars and homes. When an insect bite or antibiotic drug is added to all this, serious trouble can develop.

Anaphylaxis, also called anaphylactic shock, is a rare and severe type of allergic reaction to a specific substance (allergen). It can develop within seconds or a few minutes.

The reaction spreads throughout the body, causing a sudden drop in blood pressure and narrowing of the airways. It can be fatal unless immediate treatment is received.

It is most commonly triggered by **insect stings or certain drugs,** such as the antibiotic **penicillin. Certain foods** (nuts, strawberries, etc.) may also trigger it.

EMERGENCY TREATMENT

• An immediate **injection of epinephrine**. He also needs oxygen right away.

• You may have been provided with syringes of injectable epinephrine (keep one at home, one at work, or with you as you travel). If anaphylaxis occurs, **inject the epinephrine into a muscle in your thigh**. Then call for an ambulance.

Epinephrine acts to reverse the swelling of the throat, narrowing of the airways, and drop in blood pressure that occurs in anaphylaxis. The drug is given by injection and doses are repeated until the condition improves.

• **Call an ambulance**. If conscious, **help him sit** in a position that makes breathing easiest. If he has a syringe of epinephrine, help him **inject it**.

• Give him **cayenne** (2 capsules or ¼ tsp.) in warm water, as a shock preventive, to strengthen the heart.

• If he loses consciousness, **open the airway, check breathing and pulse**, and be prepared to carry out resuscitation if necessary. Monitor pulse and breathing until medical help arrives. *See chapter on First Aid (990) for how to Give CPR and Rescue Breathing (991-995).*

PREVENTION

• Avoid any substance to which you are sensitive, especially if you have had a previous anaphylactic reaction. You may be given epinephrine to self-inject. You will also be advised to carry an emergency card or bracelet, to alert others to your extreme allergy.

ENCOURAGEMENT—To all who are reaching out to feel the guiding hand of God, the moment of greatest discouragement is the time when divine help is nearest. From every temptation and every trial He will bring them forth with firmer faith and a richer experience.

PULSE TEST, HOW TO DO

WHAT IT IS—The Pulse Test is occasionally mentioned in this *Encyclopedia*. It was devised by Arthur Coca, M.D., and is discussed in detail in his book, *The Pulse Test*. It is a simple home method, to determine which foods you are allergic to.

HOW TO DO THE PULSE TEST

Identifying specific food allergens can improve your health. Each test is simple enough; but, to make them more effective, they must be continued over a period of time.

Your *pulse* is the rhythmic dilation (enlargement) of an artery, produced by the increased volume of blood as it surges into the vessel by the contraction of the heart. Normal pulse is between 52 and 70 beats per minute.

How to take your pulse. Place your finger on an artery, somewhere on your body that you can easily feel.

Nurses check the pulse at the inside of the wrist. But, immediately after exercise, athletes check their pulse at the carotid artery in the neck. This is also the best way to check it when giving first aid. The carotid artery is also the easiest place for you to check it.

Place your right hand up to the right side of your neck, slightly toward the front. You will quickly find a place where a strong beat (pulse) is occurring. You are pressing the hollow between the trachea (windpipe) and the large neck muscle in the front side of your neck with two fingers on the large carotid artery which is carrying blood to your head.

Have a stopwatch in your left hand and time the beats for one full minute. (Athletes check their heart rate, immediately after strong exercise, for 15 seconds, and multiply by four. But, for accuracy in the Coca pulse test, you should take it for a full 60 seconds.)

To perform Arthur Coca's pulse test, you **first take your pulse before you eat anything.** This is called your *basal pulse* or *base pulse rate*.

Then eat a single food and check your pulse rate 15 minutes afterward, 30 minutes afterward, and 60 minutes afterward.

An elevation in pulse rate of more than ten beats (that is, **if it beats more than 10 beats faster per minute than your base pulse**) means that you are allergic to that food.

A problem is that you may wish to eat more than one food at a time. You can take your base pulse, then sit down and **eat your entire meal and keep checking your pulse** 15, 30, and 60 minutes after you finished that entire meal. In this way you will obtain an inkling that everything was all right at that meal or that something was wrong. Gradually, **over a period of time, you can narrow it down** and then **work on specific foods**. You do that by eating only one food at a time and checking your pulse afterward.

OTHER TESTS

Here are several other tests:

The Elimination Diet: **Eliminate certain foods from your meal for several days**; and see how it affects your pulse. This is a good pattern to use in connection with the Pulse Test.

Food Rotation Diets: This is said to be a good method. Grains, proteins, and other suspected foods are arranged in the diet so that **the consumption of certain types of foods are not repeated more frequently than every 4-5 days.** This helps you figure things out a little more quickly with your pulse test.

Common Allergenic Food Test: For a month or two, **remove all foods from your diet which most frequently cause allergies** or asthma. Then begin adding foods back, one at a time every 3 days, until allergic symptoms reappear.

Here would be the ones to start with: **eggs, milk, chocolate, soy, legumes, corn, citrus, and tomatoes.**

Other problem foods include **all dairy foods, grains**

(especially **wheat, rye, barley, oats, white rice, and corn**), **strawberries, bananas, peanuts, meat products, caffeine, oysters, salmon, processed and refined foods, white sugar foods, fried foods, salt, tobacco.**

The Fast Test: **Fast for five days; then add individual foods and test each one** with your pulse. This is far more accurate; but who wants to eat like a mouse all that time? The theory behind this method is that many reactions take 5 days to settle down and another 3-5 days to begin again. But following that theory, you will not be eating much for a good long time.

The Diet Diary: This method helps when offending foods afterward seem to emotionally bother you, give you headaches, etc. **Keep an ongoing meal diary, in which you note what you eat; afterward write down how it affected you.** Within minutes or hours after eating an offending food, there may be indications of problems.

Skin Patch Test: This is something you can buy at your drugstore. Perhaps it will tell you something.

The RAST Test: This test costs about $15 per food item; and you may want to use it, after narrowing the range with the other tests. The *Radioallergicabsorbent Test* (RAST Test) identifies specific antibodies in the blood to certain foods or other substances. The most common allergenic foods (such as **wheat, milk, eggs, yeast, and citrus**) are tested. But any food can be a problem. Most good laboratories do RAST tests. However, because it is extremely selective (only showing up positive Ige-mediated allergies), many false-negative reactions occur.

The Cytotoxic Allergy Test: This test exposes some of your white blood cells to a fraction of the suspected food or substance. A battery of 38 to 40 tests of common foods are routinely tested for only $80 to $90; so it is less expensive and more convenient than RAST. Even inhalants, food dyes, or other chemicals can be tested, which is a decided advantage. But the test is only done at large medical centers; and, again, many false-positives occur. Some experts question the reliability of this test, since human interpretation is required to analyze the results.

Unfortunately, results of RAST and the cytotoxic tests rarely agree. (It is said that each test locates different "systems" of allergies.) Frankly, it seems that you would do best just checking your pulse at home and saving the money.

Once you have identified specific allergenic foods, you then eliminate them from your diet.

—*See "Testing Food," under Allergies (below). Also see Hay Fever (850).*

ENCOURAGEMENT—What must it be like to be close to God? It is a little heaven on earth, to go to heaven in. Yet, by daily surrender and prayer, we can each have this experience. Through the enabling strength of Christ, obey His Ten Commandment law, and you will fulfill His plan for your earthly life.

ALLERGIES

SYMPTOMS—*Digestive (after eating) symptoms:* Dry mouth, food intolerance, stomach ulcers, canker sores, excessive tiredness, palpitations, swelled stomach,

CHART 1056: Is it a Cold (288-293), Flu (294), or Allergy (848-860) ?

sweating, mental fuzziness, stinging tongue, metallic taste, heartburn, indigestion, vomiting, nausea, diarrhea, constipation, food cravings, pains, intestinal gas, gallbladder trouble.

Muscular and skeletal symptoms: Arthritis. Aches in neck, back, or shoulders. Fatigue; spasms; joint pain.

Respiratory and throat symptoms: Cough, asthma, frequent colds, postnasal drip, wheezing, hay fever, nosebleeds, chest tightness, hoarseness, shortness of breath, dry or sore throat.

Nervous symptoms: Tachycardia (fast heart rate), palpitations, depression, anger, anxiety, confusion, irritability, hyperactivity, restlessness, learning and memory problems. After repeated contact with the allergen, a laryngeal (throat) spasm may occur and emergency intubation (a tube) is required to save the life. If the condition gets that bad, epinephrine may be necessary.

Skin symptoms: Blotches, acne, flushing, hives, dark circles under eyes, itching, eczema, psoriasis. The skin rash is the special identifying symptom.

CAUSES—An allergy is a sensitivity to some particular substance, known as an *allergen*. It may be harmless to some while causing problems for others. The allergen will not be a virus or bacteria; but it may be a food, inhalant, or chemical. It may be **smoke, molds, pollen, perfume, formalin, hair spray, fumes from gas stoves, paint fumes, or tobacco smoke**, etc. Hay fever *(850)*, one of the most common allergies, is triggered by **pollens from flowers**. A common cause is **chocolate, milk, pork, and other meat products**.

Causes vary widely: There can be urticaria (skin rash with itching) from **fish** or **strawberries**, paranoia from **sugar**, headaches from **perfume**, or asthma-like symptoms from **sulfite** (a preservative in sulphured raisins and apricots). The list goes on and on.

Mold is a special problem to many. It can be in the house, in the food, in the drugs (that is what the penicillin-type drugs are: mold!). Avoid dampness in, or around, your home.

About 25-30 million Americans suffer from hay fever *(578)* every year. Another 12 million are allergic to things other than pollen (**bee stings, certain foods, drugs**, etc.)

Unfortunately, we live in the chemical age. The body cannot handle all the problem substances entering it; and it rebels. Allergies generally are not life-threatening. But some are; and we call that anaphylaxis *(846)*.

NATURAL REMEDIES

• Begin with a short **3-day cleansing fast** on fruit and vegetable juices. This will eliminate excess mucus buildup, release allergens from your body, and pave the way for improved diet changes. If you are not thin, repeat this 3-day fast every month.

• Here is a good **liver flush** to take during the fast: 1 tsp. of olive oil, one-half tsp. of fresh ginger, 1 tsp. of fenugreek, 1 tsp. of ground dandelion, the juice of 1 fresh lemon, and a pinch of cayenne. Mix it in juice and drink every morning during the fast.

• Take **vitamin C** to bowel tolerance (the amount you can take before diarrhea results from the acidity in the C). Take 1,000 mg, with bioflavonoids, 3 times a day.

• Take **vitamin A** and **zinc**; and be sure and get enough **essential fatty acids** and vitamin **B complex**.

• Take **pantothenic acid** (50-100 mg, 3 times daily) for a few days, to stimulate the production of your own allergy-fighting cortisone. **B complex** and **B₁₂** may also help. **Pantothenic acid** (200-500 mg daily) boosts adrenal function. **Vitamin E** (400-600 IU) has allergenic properties, when taken for several days before exposure to allergens.

• Eat a balanced, moderate, **nutritious diet.** Drink more **water**, making sure it is pure; and you will find that many things in your life will improve.

• **Avoid** canned, refined, preserved, sugary, fatty foods. Avoid meat, caffeine, dairy, and alcoholic products.

• Try eating 1-2 tsp. **bee pollen** granules each day. This helps solve allergic reactions for some people. Two **acidophilus** capsules daily help others.

• Building up the body and avoiding the offensive substances is what you want. But how can you learn what you should avoid? The simplest solution is to **do a pulse test** *(847)*. Include one test item in each meal, take your pulse after each meal and see if that item raised your pulse a little. Some people are disturbed each time they ride in a car. Perhaps it is something where you work. Keep searching for causes.

• **If you suspect a certain food** to be the problem, avoid it for a week or two; then try it again and see if the symptoms reappear. **If no particular food** is suspected, test favorite foods first. This is because some allergic foods give a "lift" before giving you a letdown allergic reaction, so you tend to crave them. Sometimes a **certain combination** of foods at a meal is the problem. Write down what you are learning in a "food diary," so you will not forget. Always use a high-quality sample of the food you are testing, so you will be certain whether or not it is that food itself which is bothering you. *See Pulse Test (847) for more information on food testing.*

• **Suspect foods** most likely to cause problems: **dairy foods, eggs, grains (especially wheat, rye, barley, oats, white rice, and corn), soybeans in any form (tofu, soy milk), citrus, strawberries, tomatoes, bananas, peanuts, chocolate, meat products, caffeine, oysters, salmon, processed and refined foods, white sugar foods, fried foods, salt, tobacco.**

HERBS

• **Garlic** contains *quercetin*, which slows inflammatory reactions. Quercetin is a bioflavonoid. **Bromelain** (in pineapple) makes quercetin more effective.

• **Stinging nettle** roots and leaves have been used for centuries to treat allergic nasal and respiratory symptoms (runny nose, coughs, chest congestion, asthma, etc.).

• In Europe, **chamomile** is used to treat skin allergies and hives.

• **Wild yam** stimulates the production of hormones which reduce inflammation caused by allergies.

• **Nettles** (stinging nettles) are widely used for their antihistamine and anti-inflammatory effects. Take ½ tsp. tincture or 1-2 capsules (preferably freeze-dried) every 2-4 hours.

• **Ginkgo** contains *ginkgolides*, which reduce allergies, asthma, and inflammation. Do not use more than 60-240 mg of the standardized extract per day.

• **Horseradish** clears the sinuses, **Feverfew** treats migraines and is useful for allergies. Pregnant or nursing mothers should not take feverfew.

• The following herbs have antihistamine properties: **dandelion, eyebright, burdock, comfrey, goldenseal** (unless you are allergic to ragweed or pregnant), **fenugreek, and lobelia.**

• For excess mucus, sip **eyebright** tea.

• For irritated mucous membranes, drink 1 cup of any of these herb teas: **thyme, hyssop, marjoram, or lavender**.

• For itching eyes, apply cold compresses of **witch hazel** diluted in 4 parts boiled water.

• **Echinacea** (½-1 tsp. tincture, 3-4 times daily for 1 week) will help stimulate the immune system.

• For eye redness, drink hot **mullein** flower tea.

• The adrenal gland is weaker during the hay fever season; so drink **licorice** root tea, but not if you have high blood pressure and tend to retain water).

• Hot fluids open nasal passages. Drink hot **red clover** or **nettles** tea.

• In contrast, cold applications to the forehead and face greatly help ease very severe hay fever. Wring the **compress out of ice water** and replace them when they begin warming up. You will begin feeling better in an hour; but keep it up for 3-4 hours and see how much help it brings you.

OTHER HELPS

• **Vacuum** the house and car more often. **Air-condition** the house and car. Install an **air cleaner** in your bedroom or get one which connects to your central air conditioner. Buy a **dehumidifier**.

• Make sure the **bedroom** is as dust free as possible. Wrap your **mattress in plastic**. Use a **synthetic pillow** (polyester fiberfill) or none at all (not feather and kapok pillows). **Wash mattress pads** more often. Avoid fuzzy **blankets**. Wash **bed clothing** frequently. Wipe bed **frames** with a damp cloth. Use **cotton sheets** and **blankets** of synthetic fibers. Avoid **comforters** and **quilts**. Keep **pets** out of the bedroom.

• Get rid of the old **carpets** and clean the **floors**. You may need to install new carpets or stop using carpets; use throw rugs instead. Eliminate "dust catcher" areas.

• Clean **damp areas** in your home, such as under the sink and around the bathtub. Wear a **mask** when you clean your house. Use **dust-removing polish**. When done, **go outside** for 30 minutes so the dust can settle.

• Use a mold-proof paint on the house.

• If you have **animals in the house**, keep them clean, well-groomed, and healthy. Frequently change cages or

P
O
I
S
O
N
S

wash their bedding. Animals are not involved in allergy as frequently as people think. But if you have unmistakable evidence that a pet is the source of an allergy, try bathing it and keeping it well-groomed. If this fails, be sure to find a good home for the pet. It is a living thing also and its needs should be respected.

• Set aside **one room** which you keep air-filtered.

• **Avoid** mold, fresh paint, insect sprays, tobacco smoke, and fresh tar.

• Avoid **outdoor activities too early** in the day when pollen and mold counts are very high. Late afternoon or early evening are better.

• Remain indoors if it is **windy and dry** outside.

• Allergic dust collects in your nose. **Rinse your nose** with saltwater (¼ tsp. in 1 cup warm water).

• **Eat lightly** and maintain a regular **exercise** program. (But do not exercise next to busy, air-polluting roads and freeways.) Exercise improves air flow through the nasal passages. Three minutes of vigorous exercise has been shown to reverse nasal congestion.

• A **hot footbath** is often effective in relieving nasal congestion.

• **Do not smoke** and avoid secondhand smoke. Do not live or work near smoke-producing factories.

• **Avoid** pesticides, fungicides, phosphorus fertilizers, fluorescent lights, aluminum cookware, mercury tooth fillings, deodorants, microwave ovens, and non-filtered computer screens.

• Do not swim in a lake heavily infested with **algae**, or in pools which are heavily **chlorinated**.

• In extreme situations of severe symptoms and high pollen counts, **shower** when you come indoors or do it that night. Avoid contact with **pets** which have been outside. Do not permit them in the house.

• Here is *Gaonkar's maneuver:* Take a large swallow of salty water into your mouth. Tip your head back as if to swallow it; then try to gargle it up through your nose. While doing this, have your fingers in your ears to close them (to protect the eustachian tubes); the mouth is also closed. Then, as you bring your face downward, try to cough. This forces water into the nasal passageway, and nicely cleans out the nose and nasal cavities. Do this 3-4 times a day.

• Make sure an effective **pollen filter** is installed in your car.

MORE FACTS

• Some allergy-provoking substances, such as dust and pollen, have a positive electrical charge. **Negative ions** appear to counteract the allergenic effects of these positively charged ions on respiratory tissues. Purchasing a negative ion generator (often included in air filter machines) often helps reduce allergenic problems.

• There really are **dust mites**! They are microscopic creatures with eight legs, called house-dust mites. It eats flakes of dead skin and excretes tiny pellets which cause you to sneeze when you breathe them. They live in every type of natural or synthetic fiber in your home. They multiply fastest when temperatures are above 70°F. and the relative humidity is above 50%. They die when the humidity drops below 40%-50%. So purchase a de-

humidifier—especially for your bedroom. Before every dust mite dies about 4 months after birth, it leaves 200 times its own weight in waste matter behind—for you to inhale and sneeze over.

—Also see Hay Fever (bellow) and How to Do the Pulse Test (847). It explains how to identify food allergies.

ENCOURAGEMENT—How sweet it is to trust in God! How encouraging it is to find in Him the guidance we need for daily life. As you seek Him in prayer, He will bring you the deep peace your heart so craves. How thankful we can be every day of our lives that, through the enabling strength of Christ, we can overcome all the temptations of the devil and live clean, honest, good lives and live to help those around us. This is what Jesus wants for us.

HAY FEVER
(Allergic Rhinitis)

SYMPTOMS—Itching in the nose, throat, and eyes. Runny or stuffy nose, headaches, pain in the head and sinuses, blurred vision, red and itchy eyes, postnasal drip. A clear, watery discharge from the nose and eyes occurs. There is sneezing and nervous irritability.

CAUSES—Hay fever is most frequently caused by breathing in mold or plant pollens. **Ragweed and grass pollen** are the worst offenders. Ragweed pollen accounts for about 75% of hay fever cases in the U.S. The problem tends to be seasonal (spring or fall), according to plant cycles.

But some may have to suffer with allergies all year long if they are sensitive to **dust, feathers, or animal danders**. Such people are said to have perennial allergic rhinitis. See *Allergies (848),* which contains a lot of useful information.

Hay fever is a reaction of the mucous membranes of the eyes, nose, and air passages to such seasonal pollens, as well as to dust, feathers, animal hair, and other irritants.

Days that are dry and windy, riding in an open car, and working in the garden sometimes increase symptoms. **Morning hours (5 to 10 a.m) are the worst; mid-day is usually best**. The best days are those which are rainy, cloudy, or windless.

Stressful situations and **alcoholic beverages** can trigger an attack.

Anger, resentment, or negative thoughts can increase the symptoms.

Hay fever sufferers frequently have **asthma and dermatitis**.

The body is trying to clean out toxins and dust. If the **diet is not nutritious** or if the person is **eating too much** (perhaps eating foods, such as **milk products, ice cream, sugar, and white-flour products**), the overloaded system cannot deal properly with the additional task of resisting the effects of airborne pollens.

In the Midwest alone, in August and September a quarter of a million tons of pollen blow through those states.

NATURAL REMEDIES

• The most effective treatment is to **avoid the irritant**. Try to find what it is. *See Allergies (848) and Pulse Test (847). Also see Rhinitis (850).*

DIET

• Eating **brewer's yeast** tablets for 2 months before hay fever season has helped some.

• **Vitamin C,** in large doses of 200 mg or more daily, greatly helps many with this problem.

• **Vitamin A** is essential for proper functioning of the respiratory system. The **B complex** (especially **B$_6$** and **B$_{12}$**) help the body produce interferon, to protect the body against allergens.

• **Calcium, magnesium, potassium, selenium, and zinc** are also important.

• Be sure and eat **green leafy vegetables**. Stay on a **high-fiber diet**. Eat **whole grains, nuts, and legumes**. If you are allergic to ragweed, do not eat **cantaloupe**; it contains some of the same proteins.

• A diet with too many fats and concentrated carbohydrates can be a causal factor; adhering to a **low-fat, sugar-free diet** helps relieve hay fever in many.

• Try eating unprocessed, **raw honey**. It is rich in pollen. For several weeks before hay fever attacks are expected to begin, eat **comb honey** for 3 days, stop for 3 days, and then do it again for 3 days, etc. Try to use honey made in your area.

• Alternating 1 day of **regular meals** with 1 day of only **fresh fruits and vegetables** has helped many.

• Drink at least 1-2 glasses of **raw vegetable juices** daily (beet, carrot, cabbage, celery, parsley, spinach, and tomato).

• Include **tyrosine** (an amino acid) in your diet, to help prevent hay fever from grass pollen.

• **Grape-seed extract** contains PCO, a powerful bioflavonoid which has a strong antiallergic action. It strengthens cell membranes of basophils and mast cells, which contain the allergic chemicals, thus preventing overreaction to pollens.

• If you are allergic to **bananas**, German researchers have found that eating 3 of them will provide you with enough magnesium to stop a hay fever attack.

• Each morning and evening, take 1 tsp. grated **lemon or orange peel**, sweetened with honey.

• Eating a small **garlic** clove every 6 hours has been known to relieve congestion caused by hay fever.

• Eating **horseradish** is good for congestion and a runny nose.

• For vitamin-mineral supplementation, *see under Allergies (848).*

• **Alcoholic beverages** increase the severity of allergic reaction in some people. Do not eat **watermelons and mangos during pollen season**; for they are in the same plant family as ragweed.

• Do not consume **soft drinks, coffee, tobacco, chocolate, cake, diary products. No processed, white-flour, sugary, fatty, or junk foods**.

HERBS

• **Eyebright** tea reduces hay fever symptoms, such as runny nose and watery eyes in children.

• **Boswellia** is an Indian herb which reduces inflammatory and allergic symptoms.

• Add 1 tsp. powdered **ginseng** to herb drinks during the hay fever time.

• **Yerba mate** (2-3 tsp. in 16 oz. hot water) helps relieve allergic symptoms. Drink it between meals.

• Soak **eucalyptus** and/or **thyme** (1 oz. in 1 cup boiling water) and inhale the steam in order to reduce nasal congestion.

• **Fenugreek** helps eliminate hard mucus from the body. **Garlic** kills bacteria. **Goldenseal** helps clear out toxins from the digestive tract.

• Each day, during hay fever season, daily drink 1-2 glasses of **red clover** or **fenugreek.** Or take 2 capsules of freeze-dried **nettle**. This has helped many.

• Dr. Christopher recommends the following formula: Mix 1 handful each of **blessed thistle tansy and buckbean**; also add 5 tsp. each of **gentian root and bitter orange peel**. Simmer for 10 minutes in 1 quart water, cool, strain, and bottle. Take 1 Tbsp. with a glass of water after your noon and evening meals.

• **Mullein** leaf provides mucilaginous protection to mucous surfaces, thus inhibiting the absorption of allergens through those membranes.

• **Horehound** directly affects the respiration by dilating vessels and acting as a serotonin antagonist. In this way, it helps alleviate any respiratory distress that occurs.

OTHER HELPS

• **Water** helps flush out the system. Be sure you are drinking enough. A significant amount of water can be lost through sneezing and nasal discharge. Drink at least 2 quarts of quality water (or fruit and vegetable juices for part of it) each day.

• Because it firms up blood vessels throughout the body, **exercise** decreases nasal stuffiness.

• A **hot footbath** helps relieve nasal congestion.

• Consider these possibilities: **Cold cloths** wrung from ice water applied to the forehead greatly help. Change as soon as they warm up. Relief comes in about 45 minutes; but continue it for 3 hours. Then intermittently for 6 hours. In some, this treatment has stopped attacks for the season.

• **Build up the immune system**, and clean the blood and colon. Healthy sinuses have moist mucous membranes similar to the skin in the mouth. They are able to wash pollen and other irritants out of the nasal cavities and down the throat into the stomach, where they are neutralized.

• **Guard against chilling**. It constricts blood vessels in the skin and drives the blood elsewhere, including the nasal cavities. This causes a swelling in the sinuses, which makes the symptoms worse.

• **Cover mattress and pillows** with plastic. Avoid **wool** bedding or furniture stuffed with horsehair.

• If you have **animals** in the house, keep them clean, well-groomed, and healthy. Frequently change cages or wash their bedding.

• **Do not mow** the lawn during grass-pollen season; and avoid freshly cut grass.

• **Do not hang sheets** out to dry; they collect pollen.

• Become a pollen expert. Learn when and where pollens are the most prevalent. When the pollen count is high, stay indoors in an air-filtered room. The *American Academy of Allergy and Immunology* offers this advice:

Springtime: The East and Midwest has tree pollen (oak, sycamore, and birch). The South, South Central States, and the West have tree pollen.

Summer: The East and Midwest has grass pollen (bluegrass and redtop). The South, South Central, and West have tree pollen.

Fall: The East and Midwest has ragweed pollen. The South and South Central States have grass and ragweed pollen. The West has tumbleweed and sage pollen.

Winter: The South and South Central States have tree and grass pollen. The West has tumbleweed and sage pollen.

Throughout much of the year: The Eastern States have mold spores on soil and vegetation from April through November; frost does not kill them. The ragweed season runs from June to November in Central Florida. Much of the West, especially the higher elevations, has less ragweed pollen; and mold spores are less in higher and dryer areas.

Before you take antihistamines for hay fever, read the long list of side effects. Another primary drug medication is steroids; and if they are not safe for athletes, they are not safe for the rest of us.

—*Also see Allergies (848), Asthma (714, 852), and Pulse Test (847).*

ENCOURAGEMENT—Amid the problems to which all are exposed, we need help from God. As we come to Him, believing, we can receive all the help we need. Trust Him ever; He will never forsake you, except by your choice. Psalm 68:35.

ASTHMA

SPECIAL NOTE: Asthma is a serious respiratory disorder. But, since 80% of asthma problems are caused by allergies, the large section dealing with it is located here instead of in the chapter on Respiratory Diseases.

SYMPTOMS—Difficult breathing, coughing, wheezing, tight chest. Attacks of multiple symptoms can occur suddenly or gradually. Sometimes there is coughing with thick, persistent sputum that may be clear or yellow. There is a feeling of suffocation. Children often have coughing and vomiting episodes.

CAUSES—Asthma is a lung disease that results in blockage of the airways. During an asthma attack, the muscles around the bronchi (the small passageways of the lungs) tighten and narrow, making it difficult for air to leave the lungs.

The chronic inflammation and excessive sensitivity of the bronchi produce those constricting spasms. The bronchial tubes swell and become plugged with mucus. An attack, often occurring at night, usually begins as a nonproductive cough and wheezing; this is often followed by difficult breathing and a tight chest. After a few hours, it subsides.

But what causes an attack to come on? Only certain people have asthma; those that do may have an attack triggered by an **allergen** or **other irritant** (such as **chemicals, drugs, dust mites, feathers, food additives, pollutants, fumes, mold, animal dander, tobacco smoke**, etc.). But other things can also do it: **anxiety, fear, laughing, stress, low blood sugar, adrenal disorders, temperature changes, extremes of dryness or humidity, or respiratory infections**.

About 80% have an allergic disorder; but others do not. The experts warn that ever-increasing amounts of pollutants will cause the number of asthmatics to increase. Many workers must continually live with such things as **sulfites, urethane, polyurethane, epoxy resins, dry cleaning chemicals**, and many other chemicals common to industry. In the last decade alone, the number of asthmatics in America has increased by one third! Children under 16 and adults over 65 suffer the most from it.

Asthmatics are frequently very sensitive to **foods containing sulfite additives: potassium metabisulfite, sulfur dioxide, potassium bisulfite, sodium bisulfite**, etc. Restaurants use them, to prevent discoloration in salads and other foods. Sulfites are also added to many other foods by the food industry.

Nitrogen dioxide, sulfur dioxide, ozone, carbon monoxide, hydrocarbons, nitrogen oxide, and cigarette smoke are also known to precipitate asthma attacks.

Fumes and strong odors (such as **turpentine, paints, gasoline, perfumes**, etc.) disturb many asthmatics.

There are two types of asthma: intrinsic and extrinsic. *Extrinsic asthma* (inherited) usually begins in childhood, is seasonal, and is usually caused by a definite number of substances which can more easily be identified. Asthma is the leading cause of disease and disability in the 2-17 age group.

Intrinsic asthma is the more severe; it generally begins after 30 years of age. Attacks can occur at any time; and the causes are much more difficult to identify.

About half of asthmatics are diagnosed between 2 and 17; another third are diagnosed after age 30. The other one-sixth does not fit either the intrinsic or extrinsic category. For example, some may initiate the problem in their 20s and others may, after their 30s, develop reactions to only one or two seasonal allergens.

But asthma can be difficult to diagnose; for its symptoms are similar to those of bronchitis *(500-502)*, emphysema *(507)*, and lung infections *(502-510)*. But, if the symptoms recur every year at a certain time and your family has a history of allergies, treat as for asthma.

In order to test whether food allergies could be the cause of their problem, 322 children with bronchial asthma or rhinitis were placed on an elimination diet. As is often the case, previous food tests had proved negative. However, 91% showed significant improvement, 61% had almost complete clearing, 30% showed some improvement, and 9% no improvement. In this study, **eggs, milk, chocolate, soy, legumes, and corn** were found to be the allergen foods. (Other studies have also found **citrus and tomatoes** to be problem foods.)

About 20% of infants allergic to cow's milk are also allergic to soy products.

Over a period of time, the attacks can become more frequent; so it is best for the person with asthma to learn every possible way to lessen the problem. Here are several suggestions. *Also p. 35. More will be found in Allergies (848), Hay Fever (850), and Pulse Test (847).*

NATURAL REMEDIES

TREATMENT DURING THE ATTACK —

WATER THERAPY

• Hot **fomentations** to the back of the neck, thorax, and front of the chest are helpful, along with a hot **foot-bath**. Keep the head cool by **sponging** with cool water or use a fan.

• Pouring **cold water** on the back of the neck is useful. As the person bends over, the water is poured on the back of the neck from a container holding about a gallon of water. From about 24 inches above the neck, pour it for about 30-90 seconds. Do this 3 times a day during the critical phase.

• A **neutral bath** (94°-98° F.) is quieting to the nerves and helps relax them.

• A **vaporizer** which blows cold, moist air is helpful during an attack. **Menthol or eucalyptus oil** may be added to the water.

HERBS

• Some take 1 cup of **hot water, catnip tea, or mullein tea** each hour.

• After blending a clove of **garlic** in a cup of water, drink it. This may be vomited back out, loosening the phlegm. If vomited, give another cup. The garlic really helps.

• **Lobelia** is an herb that, when sipped slowly, relaxes the nerves and tends to stop the spasm. (If one drinks it more rapidly or in larger amounts, it has a different effect and induces vomiting.)

• **Mullein oil** is a worthwhile remedy for bronchial congestion. The oil stops coughs because it unclogs bronchial tubes. When taken with water or fruit juice, the effect is even more rapid.

• Other useful herb teas include **juniper berries, echinacea**, and (of course that old standby) **slippery elm** bark.

• Pour 1 cup cold water over 1-2 tsp. shredded **ele-campane** root. Let stand 8-10 hours. Reheat and take very hot, in small sips. You can sweeten with honey. Drink 1 cup daily.

• Three times a day, add 20-40 drops of **licorice** tinc-ture to a cup of hot water, let it cool to room temperature, and drink it.

• **Cayenne** desensitizes the respiratory system to irritants; and it is helpful in stopping an asthma attack.

• Asthma is caused by malnutrition. Only by diligent and consistent effort to change embedded habits will one get permanent relief. The cough is a result of nature's effort to expectorate mucus from the lungs, after which breathing becomes easier. Often the cause of asthma is basically a nervous condition because the nerves are irritated.

• When a person is in a convulsion there are certain herbs that will give very fast relief. One of these is tincture of **lobelia**, and a **valerian** decoction with a little **cayenne** added to relieve spasms. If such an attack comes after a meal one should use an emetic, such as a large dose of **lobelia**.

• Drink several cups of warm water, then place the middle finger deep down the throat and press the tongue until regurgitation starts. **Mustard** is also good to clean the stomach and lungs. Prior to the emetic a **peppermint** or **spearmint** tea should be used to soothe the area and alleviate the discomfort of continual vomiting. Hot fomentation of **castor oil, comfrey, lobelia, mullein**, etc., may be placed over the stomach, liver, spleen and lung areas. Frequent hydrotherapy **baths** or lengthy **sweat baths** are beneficial, followed by a **cold shower or sponging**. Another helpful method is to take a **vapor bath** twice a week, inhaling steam from a decoction of **cudweed ragwort, wormwood**, or a decoction of the following herbs, taken warm, (equal parts) will prove very beneficial: **elecampane root, horehounds, hyssop, skunk cabbage root, vervain, wild cherry bark** (and to this preparation add tincture of **lobelia** or **antispasmodic tincture**). Clear the bowels with an injection of **catnip or barberry bark**. This affliction also calls for plenty of outdoor exercise, deep breathing, and good ventilation while sleeping. The whole body system should be built up with tonic herbs such as **chickweed, comfrey, marshmallow, mullein**, etc. Diet should be mostly **fruits and vegetables**, avoiding all processed devitalized foods.

OTHER THINGS

• During *asthmatic asphexia:* Tincture of **lobelia**, or an antispasmodic tincture taken internally is excellent. One can also massage the outside of the body rubbing the tincture thoroughly between the shoulder blades, across the upper rib-cage area, through the chest and bronchial areas.

• At the first sign of an asthmatic attack, **sit up straight** in a chair for the first 10 minutes. **Inhale** through your nose and **exhale** through pursed lips. This helps press open the bronchial tubes. Slumping reduces the amount of available air.

• Then **lie on your stomach**, with your head and chest over the edge of the bed. **Cough gently** for 2-3 minutes, to bring up the sputum. (But, during an attack, some cannot tolerate this position; instead, they lie face down on the bed with 2-3 pillows under their hips and a towel under their face.)

TREATMENT THE REST OF THE TIME —

DIET

• Eat a **nourishing diet**. Include **garlic** and **onions**. **Eat lightly**. Research has revealed that a **fat-free diet** can help reduce asthma attacks. Strictly adhere to a simple diet, and not much eaten. Your only oil should be 1 spoonful of **flaxseed oil** taken raw twice a day. It is rich in *omega-3*, which reduces tissue damage from asthma.

• **Avoid bananas and melons**, especially if you are also sensitive to ragweed. Avoid **processed and junk foods**. Do not use **nicotine, alcohol, or caffeine**, **chocolate, fish, eggs**, and other common allergenic foods. Avoid foods containing **additives**. Do not use **milk products**. You may be allergic to **wheat** products. Do not eat **ice cream** or other **cold liquids**. Cold can shock the bronchial tubes into a spasm.

• Be sure and drink enough **water**. This vital fluid is greatly needed to keep your lungs and bronchi free of thickened phlegm.

• Daily nutrients in divided doses: vitamin **A** (in the form of **beta carotene**, 35,000 IU), **B complex** (a complete supplement), **vitamin C** (500-5,000 mg), bioflavonoids (500 mg), **vitamin D** (400 IU), **vitamin E** (400 IU), **calcium** (1,500 mg), **magnesium** (500 mg). Taking 1-2 calcium tablets during an attack will often reduce its severity. Calcium relaxes the muscles.

OTHER THINGS

• Go on a **juice fast**, 3 days each month, of distilled water and lemon juice, to help clean out the body of toxins and mucus.

• Reduce **stress**. Avoid worry and fear.

• Be alert to **changing weather conditions** (temperature, humidity, barometric pressure, and strong winds). All can bring on an asthma attack.

• Avoid **food additives, chemical environments, smokers**, etc. Avoid riding in **automobiles**.

BREATHING

• You need to **breathe deeply**. Learn to play a wind instrument, harmonica, or sing. Practice deep breathing when you are outdoors. Have regular physical **exercise**. Hiking, swimming, etc. are good. You need to **build up your lung capacity** and utilization. This will strengthen your entire respiratory tract. A person at rest uses only 10% of his lung capacity; hard work increases it to about 50%.

• **Exhale forcefully** through a small drinking straw into a large bottle of water. This forces the bronchial tubes to expand somewhat and become larger.

• Some asthmatics have problems when they breathe too deeply. One way to minimize exercise-induced asthma is to wear a **mask** that retains heat and moisture and limits the effects of cold, dry air.

• Spend a few minutes each day practicing **standing tall**, expanding your chest, and breathing deeply. Devise simple exercises (on the floor, against walls, etc.) which help you do this. Practice breathing through your nose rather than your mouth.

• Practice "**sleep breathing**." This is done by breathing slower and deeper than normal, with a three second pause at the top of the inspiration and at the end of the expiration.

• Move out to the **country**, where the air is purer.

DUST

• Get a good vacuum cleaner and **get rid of the dust** and dust mites in your bed, cushions, rugs, and floor. Avoid **goose feathers** (pillows and down coats). **Dead cockroaches** are also known to produce a dust which can bring on an attack. **House plants** may contain **mold spores**. Keep the bathroom clean of mold, also under the sinks.

• Eliminate things from the house which harbor dust: **carpets, venetian blinds, draperies**, etc. Washable cotton curtains are all right. Avoid the use of electric **fans**; they stir up dust.

• **No dogs, cats**, or other furry animals in your home—and no **birds**.

Cover mattresses in plastic casings. **Wash sheets** in hot water weekly.

—*Important: Also see Hay Fever (850) and Allergies (848).*

HYDRO—Neutral Bath at bedtime, **Hot Abdominal Pack, copious water drinking, Enema before retiring, graduated Cold Baths, Renal Douche. Cold Colonic** daily in cases of toxemia with dilated colon. Correct any existing stomach disturbance. If skin is inactive, give **sweating process**, followed by a **cold bath** of an appropriate form.

• Use a cold-mist **humidifier** in the room, especially during the winter when the heater dries out the air.

J.H. KELLOGG, M.D., PRESCRIPTIONS FOR ASTHMA AND ITS COMPLICATIONS (*how to give these water therapies: pp. 206-275 / list of treatments: pp. 206-207 / Hydrotherapy Disease Index: pp. 273-275*)

GENERAL TREATMENT—Neutral Bath at bedtime, Hot Abdominal Pack, copious water drinking, Enema before retiring, graduated Cold Baths, Renal Douche. Cold Colonic daily, in cases of toxemia with dilated colon. Correct any existing stomach disturbance.

INACTIVE SKIN—Sweating process, followed by a cold bath of an appropriate form.

Also see Allergies (848), Hay Fever (850), and Pulse Test (847).

ENCOURAGEMENT—All who have been born into the heavenly family are, in a special sense, the brethren of our Lord. The love of Christ binds together the members of His family; and wherever that love is manifested, souls are encouraged and helped.

POISON IVY
(Poison Oak, Poison Sumac)

SYMPTOMS—*In those only slightly sensitive to it:* One or more small round bumps with a slight pus area showing in the center. Each one is extremely itchy. It is slightly itchy until touched by something (clothing, a hand, etc.), when it suddenly becomes intensely itchy. Scratching brings momentary relief. But it causes redness, rash, and much more itching.

In those very sensitive to it: Extreme redness, rash, and large swelling of the affected area. The itch is continuous. Many large blisters develop. As the poison is spread over other parts of the body, both fever and secondary infection may develop.

Symptoms appear within a few hours to 7 days after contact with the plant.

CAUSES—These three poisonous North American plants (poison oak, poison ivy, and sumac) contain an oily, slightly sticky, sap in the flowers, fruit, stem, bark, and roots which, when touched, produces a contact papular dermatitis on the skin. The plant has the greatest amount of this sap in the spring and early summer. The poison is *urushiol,* which has both a plant resin and a volatile oil. Even dead roots and stems contain urushiol.

Scratching can transmit the toxic substance to still other parts of the body.

Contact with the poison can be made by touching an animal's fur, contaminated clothing, shoes, etc. Touching the plant is not the only way to contract the poison. Smoke from burning plants can, through droplets, transmit it to the skin, nose, throat, or lungs. In some cases, children have eaten the leaves or grayish berries and developed severe inflammation in the mouth.

Sensitivity to the plant varies from person to person and at different times in a person's life. Lightweight fabrics do not adequately protect against poison ivy or oak.

Dogs and cats are not affected by urushiol; but they can give it to you when you touch them. Wash them thoroughly while wearing rubber gloves.

NATURAL REMEDIES

• *Those slightly sensitive* to the plant can simply **avoid touching or scratching** the pimples, and the itching will be only slightly noticed. If they wish, they can **briefly apply compresses** of hot, plain, water to the area.

• Those strongly sensitive may wish to consult a physician. *Also see chapter on Poisonous Plants (200).*

WATER THERAPY

• If the possibility exists that you may have touched the plant, **wash your hands** as soon as possible. Carefully wash downward, so the water drips down off your hands rather than up your arms. Wash with soap and water, rinse in running water, wash again with soap and water, rinse. Do this several times in order to get the toxic oils off your skin. Then dry and see what happens.

• As soon as you touch the plant, **try to wash** the skin with water, even if no soap is available. Water tends to carry off the oil. If nothing else is available, in an emergency apply paint thinner, ammonia, or acetone to carry off the oils.

• **Yellow laundry soap** is best for this purpose. You want a strong cleansing soap which cuts oil and carries it away. An **alkaline laundry soap or detergent** is the best.

• In washing the skin, **never use a washcloth**; it only

moves the toxic oil around.

• Wet dressings and soaks are helpful. A **physiological saline solution** (2 level tsp. of salt to a quart of water) is useful.

• Run **hot water** (as hot as can be tolerated) over the area. This seems to wash off some of the oils. Itching may stop for several hours. Repeat when needed.

• Also very effective (even though opposite from above) is to **shower in cool water** immediately after you are exposed to the plant. The sooner and longer you shower, the better.

• Removing urushiol from the skin within 15 minutes after contact greatly reduces or eliminates the rash. Splashing with plain water will do. But 3 soapy latherings and rinses are ideal. Remove clothing and launder it as soon as possible.

• **Wash clothing and gear** in soapy water. Decontaminate everything that might have touched the plant. Use ammonia or paint thinner on most gear. Add 1 cup hydrogen peroxide to 5 gallons of water and wash shoes, tents, or dogs. Add bleach to clothes washing water.

• If you are next to the **ocean**, bathe in it. This will help neutralize the poison.

TO REDUCE ITCHING

Keep in mind that, for most people, the treatment for urushiol is to **reduce the itching until the poison eventually leaves the system**. At the point in time when the poison leaves, the rash completely clears up.

What should you put on the affected area to reduce the itching? Here are several suggestions:

• **Jewelweed** always ranks at the top of every list. This is a small plant with dark green leaves and red berries, which may be found in your locality. If you are sure it is jewelweed (and if you can find it), crush the leaves and rub them lightly on the affected area. Another method is to ball up the whole plant and wipe it over the area. Jewelweed contains *lawsone*, which chemically binds to the same areas as the plant poison, in effect locking it out. The red knobs near the roots of the plant have the most lawsone. Jewelweed grows in shady wetlands from Canada to Georgia and west to Oklahoma and Missouri. From its tall, translucent stems hang trumpet-shaped yellow or orange flowers. You can buy the seeds and grow jewelweed near your home!

• Another **jewelweed** formula is to make **ice cubes** of the tea and apply them directly to the affected area. It feels wonderful and rapidly reduces the infection.

• Other herbs include **bloodroot, echinacea, goldenseal, lobelia, myrrh, plantain, or Solomon's seal**.

• Another method is to apply a tea made of 50-50 **white oak bark** and **lime water**. Place it on a cloth, cover the area, and reapply as often as needed.

• Most poisons have a pH that is either strongly acid or alkaline. *Here are several **alkaline antidotes** to the itching:* Place some form of **powdered calcium**, mixed with water, to hold it in place, on the area. Calcium gluconate is one of the most alkaline of the dietary calcium supplements and nicely reduces the itching. A combination of **calamus and cloves oil** used topically (on the skin) eliminates the itching.

• An alternate alkaline method is to blend **oatmeal** into a fine powder and add a small amount of water, to make a paste. Add a cup of **oatmeal** (or **cornstarch**) to a bathtub with about 4 inches of lukewarm water. Splash it about for a soothing effect.

Goldenseal, a very alkaline substance, can also be used. **Banana** peels, rubbed directly on the area, bring relief for as long as 4 hours. Another way is to place **calamine** lotion on it (but beware of the antihistamine additives in some brands of it; they can produce their own allergic rash). **White shoe polish** (which contains calcium and pipe clay) has also been used; but it may contain additives you do not want.

• Dr. Christopher recommends drinking **sassafras** tea and applying it externally.

• In addition to healing skin burns, **aloe vera** soothes and heals the rash that is caused by contact with the poison.

• Combine 2 parts each of **yellow dock** and **echinacea** with 1 part **chaparral**. Put the mixed powders in capsules and take 2 capsules every 2 hours. This is a blood purifying formula which will help the body eliminate the poison quicker.

• The *New England Journal of Medicine* reported that **plaintain** poultices can help control the itching of poison ivy. Crush the leaves and place on the skin.

• To reduce itching, mix the following antispasmodic herbs: 1 part each of **valerian** and **black cohosh**, and ½ part **lobelia**. Put the powdered mixture into capsules and take 2 capsules, 3 times a day.

• Apply a poultice of equal parts **comfrey root, slippery elm, witch hazel, aloe vera, and comfrey root**.

• *There is also an **acid approach** to the problem!* Several acid substances have also been used with success, to reduce itching: Wash **lemon juice** over the area, then pat dry. Repeat as needed. **Vinegar** can be used.

• Apple cider **vinegar** washes and baths will reduce the itching.

• The fatty acids in **evening primrose oil** retard the inflammatory process and increase healing of the skin.

• Apply **tea tree oil** to disinfect and heal the skin.

NUTRIENTS

• To reduce the swelling, take **vitamin C** (up to 3,000 mg) and **pantothenic acid** (500 mg) tablets. If taken immediately, the vitamin C can greatly reduce the rash.

• Make a **paste of vitamin C,** spread it over the rash, and leave it on for 1 hour; then rise it off with cool water and pat dry. Do this 3 times a day.

• Also take **beta carotene** (25,000 IU) and **zinc** (30 mg). Swabbing the blisters with crushed zinc tablets often relieves itching. Apply **vitamin E** oil (squeezed from capsules), to reduce pain and increase healing.

OTHER HELPS

• When you are finished working on the affected area, you might wish to wash **rubbing alcohol** over the skin exposed to that area. This washes oils off your skin. (But this would appear to be a poor solution; since the

oiless skin would be likely to have a higher affinity to the urushiol than oiled skin.)

• Avoid forest fires, other outdoor **wood fires, or leaf fires**, if one of the three toxic plants may be burning.

IDENTIFYING THE PLANT

• **Poison ivy** is a small plant in the Eastern States which creeps along or grows up an nearby bush or tree. It has three leaves with a notch on the outside of the two outer ones. The central leaf is at the end of the stalk.

• **Poison oak** is a bush which, although generally smaller, can grow taller than a man. Growing in the Western states, it has the same three leaf and notch pattern; but the leaves are curly and appear thicker—more like a live oak.

• **Poison sumac** is also a bush; and, with its compound leaves, it looks very much like other sumacs. It does not have the three-leaf pattern. You are less likely to encounter poison sumac.

ENCOURAGEMENT—Amid all the perils of life, we need help from God. The shield of His grace can preserve us from yielding to temptation to sin. But we must submit our lives to God if we would have this help. Numbers 23:21.

DRUG ALLERGY

SYMPTOMS—Wheezing. Swelling anywhere on the body, but typically affecting the face and throat. Nausea and diarrhea. An itchy rash consisting of red, raised areas and, occasionally, white lumps.

CAUSES—These symptoms may be due to a prescription or over-the-counter drug. Both kinds can cause various difficulties. The underlying problem is that, unlike natural remedies, drug medications consist of artificially separated chemicals (which is done so the drug can be patented and sold for large profits). Because of this, it is unlikely you will ever find a drug which is not poisonous. They all have "side effects," many of which can be very serious.

Although called "drug allergies," drug manuals admit that most symptoms are not allergies at all, but side effects that can injure many of those taking them. A true "drug allergy" occurs when the taking of a drug produces an abnormal reaction. Some can be life-threatening (*see Anaphylaxis, 846*). But even the non-allergenic reactions can be very serious. For example, many people lose normal kidney functions because of drugs.

An allergic reaction to a drug can occur the first time it is used or after taking it for some time. Allergic reactions may occur with any drug; but it occurs most frequently with antibiotics. See your physician.

If you develop any of the above symptoms, immediately stop taking that drug and contact your physician. The problem may be that you are taking several at the same time, and are uncertain which one is causing the most immediate damage. Once it begins, an allergy to a certain drug is life-long. If it is severe, you will be advised to carry a card or bracelet at all times, in case you need emergency treatment.

One other possibility: Switch to natural remedies.
—*Also see Urticaria (346-347, 830), Anaphylaxis (846), and Allergies (848).*

ENCOURAGEMENT—There are many who are not satisfied with the work that God has given them. They are not satisfied to serve Him pleasantly in the place that He has marked out for them, or to do uncomplainingly the work that He has placed in their hands. It is right for us to be dissatisfied with the way in which we perform duty, but we are not to be dissatisfied with the duty itself.

CHEMICAL ALLERGIES

SYMPTOMS—Skin rashes and eruptions, stuffy nose, nausea, watery eyes, upset stomach, ringing in the ears, depression, headache, diarrhea, fatigue, asthma, intestinal disorders, arthritis, bronchitis, eczema. The symptom(s) may occur immediately or a day later.

CAUSES—Ours is the chemical age. We are surrounded by chemicals and doused in them. They are in the air we breathe, water we drink, and food we eat.

When the body is exposed to foreign chemicals, it may respond by producing antibodies to defend itself. We are all different; and some of us are bothered more by one substance than by another. Here is a sampling of some of the chemicals which cause such allergic reactions: **insecticides, smog, fumes of gasoline, coal, oil, disinfectants, chlorine, phenol, paint, hair sprays, formaldehyde, carbolic acid, household cleaning products.** Other chemicals causing allergies are metals that include **nickel, mercury, chrome, beryllium.** The metal may be in **watchbands, earrings, or rings.** Amalgam **dental fillings** contain **mercury.**

NATURAL REMEDIES

• Consider the **above pollutants** and try to avoid them.

• Avoid **sprayed food** or food with **artificial colors.** Avoid protective waxes and ripening agents. When possible, grow your own vegetables or buy locally raised food, grown organically. Read food product labels.

• Try to **identify** which chemicals are bothering you. What caused the problem? Where have you been? What has changed in your environment? What can you do differently?

• Take **vitamin A** (10,000 IU), **B complex** supplement, **carotene** (in carrot juice, and red and yellow vegetables), **grape-seed extract, zinc** (30 mg), **copper** (3 mg).

• At the time of a chemical allergic attack, load up on **vitamin C** (1,000-5,000 mg daily, in divided doses).

• Only eat fresh **fruits and vegetables,** plus **whole grains, legumes, and nuts. Garlic** is important.
—*Also see Chemical Poisoning (868) and Heavy Metal Poisoning (868).*

ENCOURAGEMENT—Give to God the most precious offering that it is possible for you to make; give Him your heart. He speaks to you saying, "My son, My daughter, give Me thine heart. Though your sins be as scarlet, I will make them white as snow; for I will cleanse you with My own blood. I will make you members of My family—children of the heavenly King. Take My forgiveness, My peace which I freely give you. I will clothe you with My own righteousness,—the wedding garment,—and make you fit for the marriage supper of the Lamb. When clothed in My righteousness, through prayer, through watchfulness, through diligent study of My Word, you will be able to reach a high standard. You will understand the truth; and your character will be molded by a divine influence."

AUTOIMMUNE DISEASES

SYMPTOMS—Varied, depending on the type of autoimmune disease involved.

CAUSES—Autoimmune diseases occur when the body becomes allergic to part of itself! This results from inadequate nutrition, junk foods, pollutants in the environment and workplace, mercury fillings, vaccinations, etc.

Here are several remedies which have helped some with certain autoimmune diseases:

NATURAL REMEDIES

• Only eat good, **nutritious food.** Take a full **vitamin-mineral** supplement. Avoid **meat, saturated fat, caffeine, alcohol, and tobacco.**

• Roy Swank, M.D., spent 20 years studying the problem and found that a **high-saturated fat diet** makes the problem worse. It is important you only maintain a low-fat, unsaturated fat diet (2 Tbsp. daily of raw **flaxseed oil,** and no other oil).

• Take **magnesium** (375 mg daily). **Purslane** is the herb richest in magnesium (2% on dry weight basis), followed by **poppy seeds** and **cowpeas.** Steam purslane or eat it raw in salads.

• **Black currant oil** contains *gamma-linolenic acid* GLA), useful in treating multiple sclerosis (MS). GLA is good for all autoimmune disorders. GLA is also in **borage** and **evening primrose oil.** Evening primrose oil is very good for MS.

• **Blueberries** contain *oligomeric procyanidins* (OPCs), which help prevent autoimmune destruction. They also relieve anti-inflammatory activity in it.

• **Pineapple** contains *pancreatin* and *bromelain*, two enzymes which break up protein molecules in the stomach so they can be digested better. These enzymes also reduce *circulating immune complexes* (CICs) which occur in several autoimmune diseases. The CICs activate the immune system to attack the body.

• **Ginkgo biloba** contains several unique terpene molecules *(ginkgolides)* which reduce inflammatory and allergic processes in autoimmune diseases.

• **Coenzyme Q$_{10}$** (90 mg daily) improves circulation and tissue oxygenation, and strengthens the immune system. Coenzyme A (as directed on label) works with CoQ_{10} in detoxifying many dangerous substances.

• **Methylsulfonylmethane** (MSM) helps keep cell walls permeable. It allows water and nutrients to flow freely into cells. And it helps wastes to exit. Mthylsulfonylmethane is used with vitamin C, to build new cells.

• **Chelation therapy** *(869)* helps certain autoimmune diseases.

• **Hyperbaric oxygen therapy** has been used successfully in some other countries (outside the U.S.).

• Here is folk medicine which has helped many people with certain autoimmune problems: They find **stinging nettle** plants and, handling them with gloves, slap it against exposed skin. This places the tiny, hairlike stingers into the skin and gives microinjections of several beneficial chemicals, including histamine (the chemical that often induces allergies such as hay fever). Another method is to get stung by **honey bees**. Both include similar helpful chemicals which can help the condition but will not cure it. The nettles keep regenerating new leaves.

• Other helpful herbs include **ginkgo, suma, gotu kola, kelp, hops, chamomile, skullcap, and valerian**.

ENCOURAGEMENT—The heart in which Jesus makes His abode will be quickened, purified, guided, and ruled by the Holy Spirit; and the human agent will make strenuous efforts to bring his character into harmony with God. He will avoid everything that is contrary to the revealed will and mind of God. 1 Timothy 6:12.

FOOD POISONING

SYMPTOMS—Pain, vomiting, cramping, weakness, diarrhea, dizziness.

Symptoms occur within 1-4 hours after eating the contaminated substance. They can last for a few hours or a few days.

Salmonella symptoms: pain, vomiting, and diarrhea can require several days to appear.

Staphylococcus aureus symptoms: diarrhea, nausea, and vomiting 2-6 hours after the meal. It is good to induce vomiting, to help rid the system of toxins.

Botulism symptoms: 12-48 hours after ingestion, symptoms appear. Extreme weakness, double vision, swallowing difficulty. Paralysis and death can follow.

Giardia symptoms: constipation, diarrhea, abdominal pain, loss of appetite, nausea, flatulence, and vomiting. Symptoms occur within 1-3 weeks after infection.

Campylobacter jejuni symptoms: abdominal cramps, diarrhea, fever, possibly blood in the stool. It takes 3 days for the symptoms to appear.

Scombroid poisoning (histamine poisoning) symptoms: Within a few minutes, nausea, vomiting, hives, abdominal pain, and facial flushing can occur. Symptoms usually subside in 24 hours.

CAUSES—Eating food containing harmful bacteria causes food poisoning. Each year more than 2 million Americans report food poisoning. Of course, the actual number is far higher. Unfortunately, we live in a poisoned age. Of those Americans who report food poisoning each year, 9,000 people die. A number of those who think they

have the flu really have food poisoning.

A full 90% of botulism cases in the United States are caused by **improper home canning**. The safest method is to cook the jarred food in a pressure cooker rather than in a tub on top of the stove.

Two-thirds of all food poisoning cases are related to the use of **poorly cooked eggs**.

The types of bacteria in food which cause disease (pathogenic) or produce toxins (toxigenic) cannot be seen, tasted, or smelled in the food.

Here are the most common of these food poisoning organisms:

Salmonella (Salmonellosis): This is the most common cause of food poisoning. It has especially increased since antibiotics began being placed in animal feeds, to prevent disease in crowded, unsanitary conditions. Anibiotics help animals grow faster. (More than 50% of cattle, poultry, and swine are now given antibiotics.) But, doing this, promoted the growth of antibiotic-resistant bacteria in animal intestines. A third of all chickens in America have salmonella.

Salmonella is easily transmitted on **hands, food supplies, knives, table tops, cracked eggs, partly raw food**, etc. Mechanical methods of evisceration in slaughterhouses spread salmonella to all the other birds being slaughtered. Cooks that handle **raw meat or eggs**, and then handle other food—especially **raw food**, such as **salads**—endanger many people. Vegetarians should wash their hands with soap, immediately after handling **raw egg shells**. Cook eggs well. (Beware of **mayonnaise**; it contains raw eggs.) **Milk** and **ice cream** can also be contaminated with salmonella. In 1985, 17,000 people in the northeast became ill from contaminated milk.

Outbreaks of salmonella poisoning primarily occur in the warmer months. Symptoms range from mild abdominal pain to severe diarrhea and even typhoid-like fever. This disease can so weaken the immune system that the kidneys, heart, and blood vessels are damaged. Arthritis can result.

Eating **raw or poorly cooked eggs, chicken, beef, and pork products** is the main way salmonella is eaten. But it can also be found in **clams** and **oysters**.

Of 35 food poisoning outbreaks reported between 1985 to 1987, 24 were caused by contaminated eggs or foods containing them. Boil eggs at least 25 minutes.

Here are some other sources of food-borne illness:

Staphylococcus aureus: This is said to be the second-largest source of food poisoning (25%). This can be transmitted by coughing and sneezing on food.

Clostridium botulinum: This is old-fashioned botulism. Many restaurants and roadhouses leave **food setting out at room temperature** for hours. This can also be found in **old mustard, and other sauce, jars**. It is also in **oxygen-deprived foods,** like foil-wrapped baked potatoes left out overnight. Botulin toxin likes **home-canned vegetables** with a low acidity level (such as green beans, asparagus, beets, and corn). Although easily destroyed by cold or heat, botulism is the most deadly of all the food-borne diseases. It produces toxins which block nerve impulses to the muscles.

Although it does not kill the botulin spores, heating food to 176° F. for 20 minutes or 194° F. for 10 minutes destroys the lethal toxins. **Home-canned food**, not properly cooked, can be dangerous. Never use the **contents of a bulging can or a rusty can**!

Staphylococcus and botulism toxins are found in **canned vegetables, meats, fish, soups, tuna, potato and macaroni salads, cream-filled pastries, and mushrooms.**

Giardia (giardiasis): This is found in **drinking water from lakes and streams**. It is not destroyed by water treatment, including chlorination. It can also be found in **raw food,** grown in contaminated water. Giardia grows best where it is cool and damp.

Staphylococcus: This is carried on human skin and in airborne droplets from coughs or sneezes.

Campylobacter jejuni: This is in fish, fowl, meat, and raw milk. Fortunately, heat destroys this organism which is in the intestines of many apparently healthy animals or birds before they were slaughtered for food.

Clostridium perfringens: This grows rapidly in large portions of food (meat or poultry dishes) allowed to cool slowly. Therefore, it is rather common in cafeterias, even when the food is then reheated (because the toxins are not destroyed by heating).

Escherichia coli (E. coli): A bacteria normally found in human and animal colons. Not always harmful; but when it is, it can be deadly. Sloppy slaughterhouse and packinghouse methods cause this bacteria to infect many people each year.

Ciguatera: This is in large reef fish.

Vibrio (vibrio bacteria): This is in raw or improperly cooked fish and shellfish.

Scombroid poisoning (histamine poisoning): After tuna, mackerel, mahimahi, sardines, bluefish, and abolone are caught, bacteria begin forming and histamine is produced.

Molds: Visible molds, growing on food, can produce mycotoxins or poisons—even when refrigerated. The USDA says that small spots of mold can be removed from surfaces of jams, jellies, hard cheeses, firm vegetables, hard salami, and smoked turkey. But other moldy food must be discarded. This includes grains, nuts, dried legumes, soft vegetables, dairy products, bacon, canned ham. Better yet: Discard all food with mold anywhere on it.

Solanine: Do not eat **potato sprouts** or **potatoes which have begun to sprout.** The sprouts have concentrated *solanine* which can cause hallucinations even after recovery. The green sprouts put salanine all through that potato, which cannot be destroyed by cooking.

Each of the above primarily comes from eating **meat** and, sometimes, **dairy products.** Bacterial contaminants are odorless, tasteless, and invisible. Large colonies may develop without obvious food spoilage.

Before concluding, keep in mind *trichine (trichinella),* which is found in **pork**. Also beware of **mold** found on food; it can produce poisonous toxins. When **cream-filled pastries**, potato salad, or cooked high-protein foods are contaminated through unsanitary handling,

the bacteria multiply at room temperature and produce poisonous toxins.

The very young, the very old, and those with chronic illnesses are at the highest risk of severe injury. Contact the local health department if the source was a restaurant, roadhouse, or commercially canned food. If the condition continues, contact a physician.

NATURAL REMEDIES

• As soon as you believe you have food poisoning, take a eyedropperful of alcohol-free **goldenseal** extract every 4 hours for 24 hours. This natural antibiotic will destroy bacteria in the intestinal tract. (But never take goldenseal for more than a week at a time, during pregnancy, or if you are allergic to ragweed.)

• Take 6 **charcoal** tablets immediately and again in 6 hours. They will help neutralize poisons in your bloodstream. Drink lots of good **water** (distilled is best).

• Also take 2 **garlic** capsules, 3 times a day. Research at the University of Wolverhamptom, in Britain, disclosed that all types of disease-producing intestinal bacteria died when **garlic** was present.

• Drink a tea of **wormwood, wormwood seed, and cloves** powder 3 times daily to stop symptoms and eliminate the toxin. But **charcoal** is better and cheaper.

• Drinking (or sipping) fluids (**water or fruit juices**) will help the body fight the toxins and recover. **Burdock** root tea is also helpful.

• Telephone your regional Poison Control Center. There is a different phone number for each state. Dial the operator (0) or emergency (911) and ask for that number in your state.

• Use **enemas** to clean out the colon.

• Someone should **help the one vomiting**, so he does not choke. If he does not stop vomiting within 24 hours, collect samples for analysis, to identify the poison.

• Sometimes it is best to **induce vomiting**. Lobelia will help induce vomiting. Also drinking water and putting a **finger** down the throat does this too.

• A severe headache and vomiting soon after a meal may be caused by food allergies *(848)*. Charcoal tablets will help solve that problem.

The body should be permitted to cast off the toxins by diarrhea, without being given **antidiarrhea drugs**.

Antacid or **baking soda with water** should not be given. Either of these can weaken the body's defenses against the toxins. Goldenseal, charcoal, garlic, and lots of water or fruit juices are sufficient.

PREVENTION—It is best to **stop eating meat and dairy products**. If you do, be sure they are most thoroughly cooked. **Check home-canned jars** carefully before opening them. **Beware of restaurants, roadhouses, and salad bars**. When eating out, you eat at your own risk. To help protect you, eat two **garlic** tablets before you eat anything else. Better yet, pack bag lunches and learn to buy what you need at a grocery store. You will save a lot of time and a lot of money.

Refrigerate food you buy as soon as you can. Keep

perishables refrigerated. **Keep food hot or cold**; food left at room temperature encourages bacterial growth. Keep the refrigerator set at 40° F., or below, and the freezer set at 0° F. or below. Below 40° F., most bacteria hibernate. Between 45° and 150° F., they become active and multiply. Above 165° F., they die. Two exceptions: Botulism in home-canned foods takes 20 minutes of boiling to kill; staphylococcus bacteria are not destroyed by cooking.

Meat, poultry, eggs, and seafood are especially dangerous. They must be cooked thoroughly and **hands** washed. All **utensils** touching the raw materials must be sterilized. Do not use **recipes** calling for raw eggs which will remain raw or be inadequately cooked. Do not leave mayonnaises, salad dressings, and milk products sitting out at room temperature. Be especially careful what you eat at **picnics**.

Even tasting certain raw or undercooked foods (meat, seafood, poultry, or eggs) can be risky.

Wash kitchen **towels and sponges** daily with a 1-20 bleach and water solution.

Do not handle meat or raw eggs (or eggshells) and then handle other food. Wash hands in between.

Do not use **bulging cans or products** with loose lids or cracked jars! Rusted, sticky, or bent cans should be discarded. Wash **lunch boxes** and **Thermos bottles** after each use.

Thaw all **frozen foods** slowly in the refrigerator, quickly in a microwave oven, or (completely wrapped) in hot water in the sink.

When **reheating food**, bring it to a quick boil, and cook it for a minimum of 4 minutes.

Take **acidophilus** every few days, to increase the beneficial bacteria in your intestinal tract. This encourages an ample supply of B vitamins to protect against food-borne contaminants.

Do not give **honey** to a young baby below the age of one. Fed by the honey, botulism spores will grow in the infant's intestine, producing botulism toxin. After the age of one, honey is safe for infants.

ENCOURAGEMENT—By firm adherence to the right, through the grace of Christ, each one of us can fulfill God's plan for our lives. Go to Him in prayer and find the answers you need. Isaiah 35:3-4.

POISONS - 4 - INFESTATIONS
Also: Lice (835)

HEAD LICE
(Body Lice, Crab Lice)

SYMPTOMS—The head itches intensely, but there are no other symptoms. Lice and/or small eggs (nits) may be seen. Symptoms of body and crab lice are the same; except that body lice infests the body and crab lice are on the pubic area.

CAUSES—Head lice are tiny wingless insects which live on the scalp. It is most common among children between 5 and 11; it is more frequently in girls (because of their longer hair) than boys.

These tiny, almost transparent insects are transmitted by close contact and by sharing combs, brushes, and hats, or by hanging coats together. They are also spread by scarves, carpets, upholstered furniture, bedding, coat hooks, earphones, and pets. Head lice actually prefer clean hair and skin. They live by sucking blood.

The eggs, known as nits, are visible as tiny white specks attached to the bases of the hairs. As the hair grows, the nits move higher up the hair shaft.

Here are the three types of lice which infect humans: head lice (*Pediculosis capitis*), body lice (*Pediculosis corporis*), and crab lice (*Pediculosis pubis*).

Body lice crawl onto the body for feeding; then they crawl back onto the clothing the rest of the time (often making their home in the lining). They do not get on the skin of a person with a fever or who is overheated by exercise.

Since simple remedies are available, it is best to avoid the use of toxic shampoos, containing insecticides. The EPA would like lindane (Kwell) banned because it is reported to have induced convulsions, birth defects, nerve damage, and aplastic anemia. Pyrethrins (RID [brand name]) are also toxic; they irritate the eyes, nose, and mouth. If the child is under age 2, has allergies or asthma, you will have to be careful in administering toxic drugstore shampoos. (In some instances lindane, carefully used, is effective. Avoid getting it in the eyes and mouth. But natural remedies are better.)

NATURAL REMEDIES

HEAD LICE —
• If you think your child has head lice, **check for eggs** at the root of hair. Using a fine-toothed nit comb, comb the hair over a piece of white paper to see if adult lice fall out. The nits can be seen on the hair.

• If you find any, **check the rest of the family** and notify your child's school.

• Researchers in India treated 814 people who had head lice with a combination of two herbs, **Neem** and **turmeric**. Within 3-15 days, 98% of the people were completely cured, as the paste of the two herbs was put on their bodies at the same time that they boiled all their clothes and linens. (The other 2% had not followed the program.) Neem (*Azadiracta indica*) is a large tree; its leaves and seed oil contain compounds active against a variety of insect pests. Turmeric has been used for centuries in Asia to kill vermin.

• The powdered root of **sweet flag** has lice-killing properties. Apply it as a poultice or by rubbing directly on the affected area.

• Add 2½ Tbsp. **rue** to 1 cup water; and use it in a compress to kill lice. Apply **citronella** oil to the hair. Cover with a bathing cap. Leave on for 8 hours. Shampoo, rinse, comb out remaining lice and nits. (Some are allergic to citronella. If itching or burning occurs, wash it out of the hair immediately.)

• A compress of **elecampane** root powder destroys skin parasites. **Pokeweed** destroys fungi and skin parasites; apply it as a compress.

• European **pennyroyal** repels moths and kills lice. Mix it 50-50 with rubbing alcohol and apply to the scalp. Leave it there for 10 minutes. Then shampoo, rinse, check the scalp, comb, and pick out remaining eggs and lice.

• To get rid of lice, douse the hair in **kerosene** and wrap it in a towel. To get rid of the eggs, mix equal parts **olive oil and vinegar** (or **vinegar and rubbing alcohol**) and apply to the scalp. Keep the solutions on the head for at least 2 hours; then wash the hair and inspect it. Comb out remaining lice. (Compresses of blended **garlic and water** are equally effective, but strong smelling.)

• Apply hot **vinegar** to the hair to loosen eggs; keep it there 2 hours. Then **comb out** the dead lice and eggs, using a fine-toothed comb.

• **Wash linens, combs, and towels** in very hot water. Tell the child **not to share combs or hats**.

• **Vacuuming carpets** is just as effective as spraying insecticides on them. Vacuum frequently.

Soak combs and brushes in 2% Lysol (heated to 151° F.) for 1 hour or put them in a deep **freezer** for 30 minutes.

• Items which cannot be washed or vacuumed, can be **sealed in a plastic sack** for 10 days. By that time, the lice eggs will have hatched and died.

BODY LICE —

Also read the above section on head lice (860).

• To eliminate body lice, soak for 30 minutes in a very warm bath with soap. Then launder the clothing and bedding in hot water.

ENCOURAGEMENT—Those who take the name of Christian should come to God in earnestness and humility, pleading for help. The Saviour has told us to pray without ceasing. The Christian cannot always be in the position of prayer; but his thoughts and desires can always be upward. Our self-confidence would vanish, when we talk less and pray more. 1 Thessalonians 5:17.

WORMS
(Intestinal Parasites)

SYMPTOMS—Allergies, diarrhea, constipation, gas and bloating, appetite loss, weight loss, anemia, nervousness, sleep disturbances, irritable bowels, anal itching, chronic fatigue, picking at the nose, dry cough, teeth grinding, and the appearance of worms in the toilet. Worms sometimes cause spasms or convulsions.

CAUSES—An estimated 55 million people, worldwide, are infected with intestinal parasites. Worms live in the gastrointestinal tract or burrow from that tract into the muscles. Several types of parasitic worms can live in human intestines (including tapeworms, hookworms, pinworms, whipworms, and roundworms). The degree of infestation is determined (upon examination) by the type, size, and number of worms found.

Worms tend to eat your food! In the process, they irritate your intestinal lining and reduce even more the amount of nutrients which are absorbed into your bloodstream. The worms also produce toxic waste which is harmful to your body.

Causes include eating **raw or poorly cooked meat, vegetation polluted by contaminated water**, improper disposal of **animal and human waste,** and **walking barefoot** on soil. Scratching the anus will transfer worm eggs on your fingers to anything else you touch. In some cases, the worm eggs are airborne and inhaled.

Pinworms: Very tiny white worms, which cause rectal itching at night. Contracted by eating raw or poorly cooked vegetables which have contacted contaminated water. Scratching the anal area can also transmit them on the fingers. *Also see Rectal Itching (471).*

Tapeworms: Flat worms contracted from eating poorly cooked meat (beef, pork, and fish). The most common one (beef tapeworm) can grow to 20 feet in length in the human intestine.

Hookworms: Found in southern soil and sand, they enter by boring into the feet; but they can also enter when eating with unwashed hands.

Roundworms: Most common in children, they bore through the intestinal wall and settle in other organs.

Because of the warmth of the bed, worms tend to come out of the anus. So inspect that area on children after they are asleep.

Worm infestation can lead to arthritis, colitis, fatigue, diabetes, headaches, indigestion, lupus, nausea, sinus trouble, back and neck pain, and cancer.

Metronidazole, the drug of choice, can cause severe side effects.

NATURAL REMEDIES
TO PURGE WORMS

• **Aloe vera**, taken in any form, is especially helpful in eliminating worms.

• The following herbs help expel worms: **cascara sagrada, wormwood, wormwood seed, cloves, echinacea, goldenseal, burdock, and black walnut**. Do not use wormwood during pregnancy.

• **Grapefruit-seed extract** helps destroy parasites. **Take black walnut extract and chaparral** tea or tablets. **Eat pumpkin seeds and figs**. Also can drink fig juice.

• Take **diatomaceous earth** capsules for 3 weeks, to get rid of your worms. (Do not imagine you do not have some; everyone generally does.) The worms eat this, and it causes them to disintegrate.

• Drink one cup of **wormwood** tea three times daily between meals.

• Clean the colon with **enemas and colonics**. Take 2 per week for 4 weeks.

• A hot-water **enema**, with 3 tsp. of **salt** to a quart of water, may get rid of pinworms.

• **Cinchona** bark tea (½ tsp. in 1 cup boiling water for 10 minutes) is bitter but effective.

• **Elecampane** contains 2 anti-amoebic compounds.

Add 1 tsp. to 1 cup boiling water, simmer 20 minutes, drink 1-3 cups per day.

• The Japanese use **ginger** to get rid of worms. Research has shown this to be true.

• Folk healers in India give **turmeric** for getting rid of worms, especially nematodes. It has 4 anti-parasitic compounds.

DIET

• Eat a diet high in **fiber** (primarily from **raw vegetables, whole grains, nuts, and legumes**).

• For a time, **avoid *all* sugar foods**, including fruits, with the exception of figs and pineapples.

• Eat **figs** and **pumpkin seeds**. This can be combined with **black walnuts**. Pumpkin seeds and extracts immobilize and aid in the expulsion of intestinal worms.

• Because of its high tannin content, the kernel and green hull of **black walnut** have been used to expel various worms by Asians and American Indians. External applications kill ringworm. Chinese use it to kill tapeworms.

• Eat **garlic, onions, cabbage, and carrots**. They contain natural sulphur, which helps expel worms. As you might expect, worms do not like garlic.

• **Garlic** is used for pinworms, roundworms, giardia (an amoeba), and other parasitic infections. Juice 3 cloves with 4-6 oz. carrot juice and take every 2 hours.

• Make sure you are obtaining enough **water**. Drink only pure water (distilled).

• To eliminate pinworms: Eat 1-2 **bitter melons** each day for 7-10 days. It is available in Asian markets.

• To eliminate tapeworms: Fast 3 days on raw **pineapple**. The bromelain in it destroys the worms.

• Cut up two raw **onions** and soak them 12 hours in 1 pint water; strain while squeezing out the juice. Drink a cup of this 3 times a day. Along with this, use **garlic** enemas.

• Mix **tansy, bitterroot, and wormwood.** And put in capsules. Take two capsules, 4 times a day.

• **Pomegranate** is used to expel round worms and tape worms. Grated raw **apples**, sprinkled with **anise** seed in a salad, is said to expel worms. **Yarrow** is a tonic to the bowels after worms have been expelled. Mexicans use **cayenne** to eliminate worms. Fresh **horseradish** is effective against some worms. **Tansy** seeds are used in Britain. Eat **thyme** sprigs or dried thyme mixed in food.

• Other vermifuges include: **bilberry, tarragon, European pennyroyal, quassia wood and bark, tamarind leaves, mugwort, and carline thistle**.

• For children, make **senna** tea, strain it, add enough **raisins** to soak up the tea. Give the children 1 tsp. of this 2-5 times a day. Use **garlic** enemas and put a garlic **clove** up the rectum before bedtime.

• Add ½ cup Epsom salts, per gallon of water, and take a warm bath in it. Before entering it, apply zinc oxide to the anus. Repeat this 3 days in a row.

OTHER PRECAUTIONS

• Eat a **nourishing diet**, rich in vitamins and minerals. You need all the good nourishment you can get. The worms are robbing you of so much. Make sure your children, if they have worms, are getting adequate nutrition.

• **Do not eat** sugar, partly cooked fish, beef, or pork. Do not eat raw food which might be contaminated.

• Never eat **watercress**. It grows in streams, many of which are now polluted. Watercress, which is eaten raw as a salad, can have pinworms and tapeworms.

• **Wash vegetables** thoroughly before eating them raw.

• **Keep the house clean:** Wash all underclothing, bed clothes, and sheets frequently in hot water. Clean rooms frequently, especially bedrooms. Put some ammonia on a cloth, to dampen it as a dustcloth. Sterilize toilet seats. The infected person should sleep alone.

• Have all family members **wash hands** frequently, especially after using the toilet, before meals, and bedtime. Do not bite nails.

—Also see Convulsions (573-576) and Ringworm (335).

ENCOURAGEMENT—Living day by day with God, we can pray to Him, obey Him, and walk with Him. This can bring a peace and maturity to our lives that is so much needed. The affections should center upon God. Contemplate His greatness, His mercy and excellences. Let His goodness and love and perfection of character captivate your heart. Isaiah 41:10.

ASCARIS
(Intestinal Roundworms)

SYMPTOMS—Often no symptom. In the intestines: diarrhea, abdominal pain. In the lungs: possible wheezing and coughing. Too many worms can cause appendicitis or an intestinal blockage.

CAUSES—The roundworm, *Ascaris lumbricoides*, is one of the most common parasitic infestations of humans. It is pale pink and about 8-12 inches long. About 1 in 4 people in the world have it at some time in life. It is most common in tropical and subtropical areas.

Infestation occurs by **food or water that is contaminated** with the worm eggs. **Poor sanitation, human excrement as fertilizer, poor personal hygiene** are other causes. Once swallowed, the eggs hatch into larvae in the intestine. They then travel in the blood to the lungs and later return to the intestine, where they lay eggs.

NATURAL REMEDIES
• *See Worms (861) for an abundance of remedies.*

ENCOURAGEMENT—Many stumble over this phrase, "a new heart." They do not know what it means. They look for a special change to take place in their feelings. This they term conversion. Over this error thousands have stumbled to ruin, not understanding the expression, "Ye must be born again." When Jesus speaks of the new heart, He means the mind, the life, the whole being. To have a change of heart is to withdraw the affections from the world and fasten them upon Christ. To have a new heart is to have a new mind, new purposes, new motives. What is the sign of a new heart?—a changed life. There is a daily, hourly dying to selfishness and pride.

P O I S O N S

PINWORMS

SYMPTOMS—Intense itching in the anal region at night, when the worms lay eggs. Inflammation of the anus as a result of constant scratching. Occasionally, mild abdominal pain. Tiny white pinworms can be seen wriggling in the feces after a bowel movement.

CAUSES—Pinworm infestation is caused by a very small, white roundworm, *Enterobius vermicularis*. It is the most common parasitic worm infestation affecting humans in the U.S.

It is primarily caused by eating raw vegetables, any inadequately cooked food, licking the fingers or touching them to the mouth, or inhaling house dust (especially if dogs or cats are kept in the house). Eggs can be picked up under the fingernails and then transferred to the mouth. Pinworm infestation is very common in cold areas throughout the world; it mainly affects children.

NATURAL REMEDIES
• Eating **bitter melons** is a specific for pinworms. They can be purchased in Asian markets. Eat 1 or 2 each day for 7-10 days.
• **Maintain cleanliness**: Do not scratch the anal area. Wash hands after going to the toilet. Regularly wash clothes and linens.
• *See Worms (861) for an abundance of remedies.*

ENCOURAGEMENT—To love as Christ loved means to manifest unselfishness at all times and in all places, by kind words and pleasant looks. Genuine love is a precious attribute of heavenly origin, which increases its fragrance in proportion as it is dispensed to others.

TAPEWORMS
(Taenia solium)

SYMPTOMS—Mild abdominal pain, diarrhea. You may feel segments of the worm wriggling out of your anus.

CAUSES—There are three kinds: pork tapeworm *(Taenia solium)*, beef tapeworm *(Taenia saginata)*, and fish tapeworm *(Diphyllobothrium latum)*.

Infestation is by eating raw or undercooked meat or fish. Once in the intestines, the worms mature and may reach 20-30 feet in length. Pork and beef tapeworm are the most common. Fish tapeworm occurs in areas where raw fish (such as sushi) are eaten.

Pork is an extremely dangerous food to eat. The larvae of pork tapeworm frequently burrow through the intestinal wall and travel around the body in the blood. Epilepsy *(574)* and, if they infect the eyes, blindness may result.

NATURAL REMEDIES
• Take 2 Tbsp. castor oil and then fast for 24 hours. Eat nothing but light fruits or fruit juices. Crush 2 oz. pumpkin seeds, flavor with honey, and eat it. Vomiting should be prevented if possible, at least for 30-60 minutes, by firm pressure over the stomach. At the end of 1 hour, take 2 oz. (4 Tbsp.) of castor oil. In the course of 3-4 hours, take a large enema with the hips elevated. The worm should always be examined for the head. If this is not present, the treatment must be repeated.
• *See Worms (861) for an abundance of remedies for intestinal worms (but not for pork tapeworms in the bloodstream).*

ENCOURAGEMENT—Christ's love is deep and earnest, flowing like an irrepressible stream to all who will accept it. There is no selfishness in His love. If this heaven-born love is an abiding principle in the heart, it will make itself known, not only to those we hold most dear in sacred relationship but, to all with whom we come in contact. It will lead us to bestow little acts of attention, to make concessions, to perform deeds of kindness. It leads to tender, true, encouraging words. It will lead us to sympathize with those whose hearts hunger for sympathy.

GIARDIASIS

SYMPTOMS—If symptoms develop, they usually appear within 2 weeks of infection with the parasite and may include diarrhea, excessive flatulence and belching, bloating and abdominal pain, and nausea.

CAUSES—The disease is caused by Giardia lamblia, a tiny parasite which infects the small intestine. Cysts (in dormant stages) are excreted in the feces of infected animals and people. The Giardiasis usually occurs from drinking water contaminated with cysts. But the disease can also spread from poor personal hygiene.

Infections are worse in those with reduced immunity, due to HIV *(806)* or treatment with immunosuppressant drugs.

If symptoms last longer than 1 week, the infection may cause damage to the lining of the small intestine, preventing the absorption of food and vitamins. If this happens, weight loss and (in some cases) anemia *(537-541)* may occur.

NATURAL REMEDIES
• *See Worms (861) for an abundance of remedies for intestinal worms (but not for pork tapeworms in the bloodstream).*
• Antibiotic herbs *(297)* should be taken.
See your physician.

PREVENTION
• If visiting a region where giardiasis is prevalent, **boiling drinking water** for at least 10 minutes will kill the cysts. Practice strict personal hygiene. Wash hands

after bowel movements and before preparing and eating food.

ENCOURAGEMENT—The qualities which it is essential for all to possess are those which marked the completeness of Christ's character—His love, His patience, His unselfishness, and His goodness. These attributes are gained by doing kindly actions with a kindly heart. Christians love those around them as precious souls for whom Christ has died. There is no such thing as a loveless Christian; for "God is love."

CRYPTOSPORIDIOSIS

SYMPTOMS—Sometimes no symptoms; at other times watery diarrhea, abdominal pain, fever, nausea, and vomiting may develop about a week after infection. Symptoms usually last 7-10 days. Those with reduced immunity (AIDS) may have chronic symptoms and develop severe malnutrition and dehydration, which can be fatal.

CAUSES—This is an intestinal infection which is caused by *Cryptosporidium parvium*, a protozoal parasite. It is spread through contact with infected people or animals, or by eating food or water that has been contaminated with the parasite. Poor personal hygiene helps spread the infection. The disease occurs throughout the world. In the 1990s, it became a frequent cause of diarrhea in children.

NATURAL REMEDIES
• Maintaining outstanding health is the best treatment for this disease. When that is done, you generally can easily resist it.
• If symptoms are severe, take antibiotic herbs *(297)* or contact a physician.
• if a local outbreak occurs, boil all your drinking water, to kill parasites.

ENCOURAGEMENT—The Lord will help every one of us where we need help the most in the grand work of overcoming and conquering self. Let the law of kindness be upon your lips and the oil of grace in your heart. This will produce wonderful results. You will be tender, sympathetic, courteous.

AMEBIASIS

SYMPTOMS—Most infected people do not develop symptoms; or they have mild, intermittent symptoms which may include diarrhea and mild abdominal pain. Five days or several weeks after the initial infection, amoebic dysentery may develop. Symptoms will include watery, bloody diarrhea. Severe abdominal pain. Fever. Sometimes dehydration and anemia may develop. If the disease spreads to the liver, there will be high fever, painful liver abscesses, extreme fatigue, and loss of appetite. The key symptom is bloody mucous in the stools which does *not* go away.

CAUSES—This is an intestinal infection, caused by the protozoan parasite *Entamoeba histolytica*. It is most

common outside of North America; about 500 million people, worldwide, are affected.

Infection is usually caused by water or food contaminated with the parasite, which is excreted in the feces of infected people. In severe cases, ulcers occur in the intestinal walls; it is called amoebic dysentery.

PREVENTION
• Drink only bottled or thoroughly boiled water. Avoid eating raw vegetables, salads, or fruits with skins that cannot be peeled.
• Activated **charcoal** is best. Also **wormwood**.

ENCOURAGEMENT—By beholding the character of Christ you will become changed into His likeness. The grace of Christ alone can change your heart; and then you will reflect the image of the Lord Jesus. God calls upon us to be like Him—pure, holy, and undefiled. We are to bear the divine image. 2 Corinthians 3:18.

SCHISTOSOMIASIS
(Bilharziasis)

SYMPTOMS—Fever, muscle pains, diarrhea, coughing, and vomiting. A burning sensation when urinating and an increased need to urinate. Blood in the urine, especially at the end of the stream. "Swimmer's itch" at the sight where the parasite has entered the skin, which usually occurs within a day after swimming or bathing.

CAUSES—The disease is caused by any of five species of flukes (types of flatworms) of the schistosoma group. Freshwater snails release larvae of the parasite, which penetrate the skin of bathers. Once inside, they mature into adults which lay eggs, causing inflammation. **Those who bathe in lakes, canals, or unchlorinated freshwater pools** (especially in the tropics) are at great risk.

NATURAL REMEDIES
• *See Worms (861) for an abundance of remedies for intestinal worms.*
See your physician.

ENCOURAGEMENT—The pure in heart discern the Creator in the works of His mighty hand, in the things of beauty that comprise the universe. In His written Word they read in clearer lines the revelation of His mercy, His goodness, and His grace. The truths that are hidden from the wise and prudent are revealed to babes. The beauty and preciousness of truth are constantly unfolding to those who have a trusting, childlike desire to know and to do the will of God.

TOXOPLASMOSIS

SYMPTOMS—Most people do not develop symptoms. But, in some people, mild symptoms appear 1-3 weeks after the initial infection and include fatigue, fever, and headache. There are enlarged lymph nodes, usually in the neck.

In those with reduced immunity, the heart, muscles,

skin, and eyes may become damaged. Symptoms may include fever and headache. Confusion, lethargy, partial loss of vision, paralysis of a limb or one side of the body. Seizures may occur.

If a fetus is infected, blindness may occur.

CAUSES—Contact with cats and eating raw or undercooked meat are primary risk factors. This is a protozoal infection caused by *Toxoplasma gondii*. The dormant (cysts) stage of the parasite are excreted in the feces of cats and can be passed to people by direct contact with cats or by **handling cat litter**.

People with reduced immunity, or pregnant women, can become extremely ill. If the parasites infect the fetus, abnormalities can occur. If a child pets cats frequently and then puts a finger in his own mouth, he can lose the sight in one eye.

This disease may affect the person for the remainder of his life.

Other diseases which you can get from cats, include Cat Coccidia *(846)*, Lyme Disease *(840)*, Poison Ivy and Oak *(854)*, and Pinworms *(863)*,

NATURAL REMEDIES
• Avoid contact with **cats**. Do not pet cats. Do not clean their litter boxes. If you are pregnant, do not have them in the house.
• Do not eat undercooked **meat**.
See your physician.

ENCOURAGEMENT— When we receive Christ as an abiding guest in the soul, the peace of God, which passeth all understanding, will keep our hearts and minds through Christ Jesus.

PNEUMOCYSTOSIS INFECTION

SYMPTOMS—Fatigue and not feeling well. Shortness of breath on mild exertion (later, even when resting). Dry cough, fever, pneumonia. The symptoms usually develop gradually over weeks, but sometimes quickly.

CAUSES—Pneumocystic infection is caused by **inhaling** the *Pneumocystis carinii* parasite. In those with a healthy immune system, it does not cause pneumonia. **Undernourished** children in developing countries may contract it. Less than 1 case in 10 is fatal. But, without treatment, the infection can reoccur. This is one of the diseases which HIV *(806)* can lead to.

NATURAL REMEDIES
• Use antibiotic herbs *(297)*.
See your physician.

ENCOURAGEMENT—Happiness drawn from earthly sources is as changable as varying circumstances can make it; but the peace of Christ is a constant and abiding peace. It does not depend upon any circumstances in life, on the amount of worldly goods, or the number of earthly friends. Christ is the fountain of living water; and happiness drawn from Him can never fail.

FUNGAL INFECTIONS
(Fungus Growth)

SYMPTOMS—A peculiar tiny growth on various parts of the body. It appears to be moist, red, circular patches. In the vagina, it produces a cheesy discharge.

CAUSES—This substance is fungus, which is also called yeast or mold. It can grow under the nails, causing them to become raised and misshapen *(see Ringworm, 335)*. It can grow on the feet and toes *(see Athlete's Foot, 377)*. It can grow in the throat or intestines *(see Candidiasis, 281)*, or vagina *(see Vaginitis, 695)*.

Those especially affected are those who **take antibiotics**, have a **depressed immune function, perspire heavily, live in a damp environment, or eat improperly. Also affected are those who are obese, ill, diabetic, or use oral contraceptives. Using the same bathroom, shoes, or shaver** of someone who is infected.

NATURAL REMEDIES
• Eat a **nutritious diet**, supplemented with **vitamins and minerals**. Eat plenty of fresh **fruits and vegetables**, much of them raw.
• Avoid mucous-forming foods (**milk and white- flour products**). Do not eat **meat or processed foods**. Fungi thrive on the **sugar** foods you eat. Avoid **soft drinks, caffeine, alcohol, fried and greasy foods**.
• Keep body parts **clean**; and keep them **dry**! Wear clean, dry clothing.
• Do not let an infected part of your body come in contact with healthy skin.
• Apply crushed **garlic** to the affected area on the outside of the body, alternating with honey.
• Another formula for fungal infections of any kind is **tea** (tea or tee) **tree oil**. Place some on the affected area for 2-3 weeks, and the problem will be eliminated. Tea tree oil, which smells like eucalyptus, also comes from Australia.
• The fresh husk of the **black walnut** destroys fungus better than many drugs.
• For fungus in toenails: Apply **black walnut tincture** with **plantain** and **tea tree oil** to toenails every night for 60-90 days.
• Drink 1-4 cups of tea, daily, of **lemongrass**, turmeric, or **pau d'arco**. All are good fungicides.
• Use either **chamomile** or **garlic** (or both together) internally and externally as anti-fungal remedies. Garlic, taken internally, is a powerful weapon against fungus attacks on the skin. The extract is very potent when applied externally. Studies revealed that people who took 5-6 tsp. garlic extract daily had significantly greater antifungal activity against several common fungi.
• **Licorice** contains 25 fungicidal compounds.

Goldenseal contains *berberine*, a powerful fungicide.

• *Fungus under the fingernails or toenails (paronychia):* This is a special problem which is quite difficult to solve. It may take six months of careful work before results begin to be seen. The fungus is generally under one or more toenails and causes them to warp out of shape. **Potassium permanganate** has been the remedy used on this for decades. This is a poison; yet if used externally, it seems to be one of the best solutions to the problem.

• Used externally, permanganate is a powerful fungus killer! It can be used on any fungal infection of the skin. It is deadly, do not drink it! The permanganate will stain the skin dark brown for several days. Formula: Soak the feet for half an hour in a warm 1:5,000 solution of potassium permanganate. Dry the feet thoroughly after use. This is the same formula for athlete's foot *(377)*, which is a similar fungal foot disease.

• If you need to prepare this solution at home, you dissolve a slightly rounded teaspoon of the crystals in 8 ounces of water. Keep it in a dark-colored glass bottle. One tsp. of this saturated solution in a pint of water makes a solution of about 1:1,500 strength; 1 tsp. in a quart of water makes one of about 1:3,000 strength. With this information, you will be able to prepare about any strength you might need. This is one of the few powerful poisons mentioned in this book. Do not let a child drink it!

• Another formula for under-nail fungus is soaking them in a 50-50 mixture of white distilled **vinegar** and clean water for 15-20 minutes daily.

—*See Ringworm (335), Athlete's Foot (377), Candidiasis (281), and Vaginitis (695) for much more information.*

ENCOURAGEMENT—Live to bless others, and you will find a happiness which you have not experienced before. Ezekiel 34:30.

TETANUS
(Lockjaw)

SYMPTOMS—Symptoms generally appear within 5-10 days. Possible discomfort at the site of the wound. Stiffness on opening and closing the mouth. The person becomes restless and apprehensive. Muscle stiffness and spasms increase and spread to more muscles in the body. The face becomes contorted; and the slightest noise or disturbance produces muscle spasms. Pain intensifies. High fever and exhaustion develops, followed by death.

CAUSES—Tetanus is caused by the toxin (waste product) of *clostridium tetani*, which normally lives in animal manure.

Puncture wounds from stepping on dirty nails is the most likely immediate cause. The germ only grows where there is little or no oxygen. The spores (seeds) are on that nail; and, entering the body, they begin to grow and multiply. But the spores must penetrate deep enough; they cannot grow if oxygen is present. It is the toxin which the growing tetanus produces that paralyzes voluntary muscle tissue, including the jaw muscle (the masseter).

Tetanus is not common; but, if contracted, it is extremely dangerous. See your physician.

NATURAL REMEDIES

• Squeeze the puncture wound repeatedly to **make it bleed**. Keep doing this until it bleeds freely. If necessary, **cut the area open** with a clean, sharp razor blade. You must get air to the wound and get it to bleed freely.

• Then **wash it well** with soap and water; pour in **hydrogen peroxide** and let it fizz. Get the **blood flowing again**. Then **wash** the area with pure water, pat dry with a sterile cloth, and cover with a bandage.

• Call a physician. If symptoms of tetanus begin appearing, call a physician at once! It is not too late.

Here is what nature healers in out-of-the-way places do, when there are no available physicians:

• Take **cramp bark** tea in teaspoon doses.

• Grind up some **peach leaves** and apply directly to the wound after washing it. Change this raw poultice twice a day.

• Heat some **turpentine** and apply it to the wound. Massage it over the jaw, neck, and spine when symptoms of lockjaw are suspected.

• Use 2 cups of **wood ashes** (or powdered **charcoal**), per gallon of water, and soak the limb or punctured part in it. If the wound is located where it cannot be soaked, apply the ash solution in a fomentation. Do this for an hour; repeat if danger is suspected.

• If lockjaw actually appears and the person shows stiffening, give 10 drops of **antispasmodic tincture** every 15 minutes until the stiffening is gone.

The formula for the tincture is as follows:

• Into a large-mouth, glass quart jar, put 1 ounce each of the following herbs (they should be in ground form or you should grind them first): **skullcap, skunk cabbage root or seed, gum myrrh, lobelia seed (or plant** if seed is not obtainable**), and black cohosh root**. Mix them in the jar, while dry, and add one pint of pure grain (not isopropyl or rubbing) **alcohol** of 70 to 100 proof (80 proof **Vodka** works well). Let this stand for 10-14 days, tightly covered, and shaken well once a day. Then strain it through a very fine cloth and squeeze out all the sediment you can. Keep the tincture in a tightly covered jar. Put some into a small dropper bottle. It is taken internally in 8-10 drop doses.

• In addition to the above, also give the person **lobelia and cayenne**. Prepare it by boiling a quart of water, take it off the stove, and put 1 tsp. lobelia powder and 1 tsp. ground cayenne into the water. Let it stand 20 minutes and drink ¼ cup every half hour till relieved.

ENCOURAGEMENT—Make it the law of your life, from which no temptation or side interest shall cause you to turn from honoring God. What would Jesus do if He were to make your decision? This is the question to be asked.

PARROT FEVER
(Ornithosis)

SYMPTOMS—Weakness, fever, chills, and loss of appetite. Dry coughing changes into sputum coughing.

CAUSES—The primary cause is **inhaling the contaminated dust from the feathers, cage bedding, or feces of infected birds**. These birds can include **parrots,**

parakeets, lovebirds, canaries, or pigeons. Think twice about keeping a parrot or pigeon. Yet there is danger with the other birds also.

The disease gives the appearance of an "atypical (unusual type of) pneumonia." When it first starts, it is often misdiagnosed as the flu *(294)* or confused with Legionnaires Disease *(508)* or Q fever *(509)*. Only a blood test can provide a certain diagnosis; but a history of frequent exposure to birds ought to provide an indication of the true nature of the problem.

NATURAL REMEDIES
• Call a physician. Strict bed rest while he is receiving treatment.
• If left untreated, parrot fever can be fatal.

ENCOURAGEMENT—God wants you to choose the best gifts. And only He can give them to you. Through continued prayer, study of His Written Word, and obedience to it, let Him ennoble your life. You are to be His representative, showing others what it means to be a Christian.

Make God your entire dependence. When you do otherwise, then it is time for a halt to be called. Stop right where you are and change the order of things. In sincerity, in soul hunger, cry after God. Wrestle with the heavenly agencies until you have the victory. Put your whole being into the Lord's hands—soul, body, and spirit—and resolve to be His loving, consecrated agency which is moved by His will, controlled by His mind, infused by His Spirit. Then you will see heavenly things clearly. 1 Corinthians 2:10-12.

POISONS - 5 - POISONING
Also: Toxic Shock (699)

POISONING

SYMPTOMS—Something was swallowed, smelled, or touched that caused the person to be poisoned.

CAUSES—We live in the chemical age; and it is taking us down rapidly. Sometimes the ongoing poisoning becomes especially serious.

Children are especially sensitive, because they are even less careful than the rest of us.

The cause may be **medicinal drugs, street drugs, batteries, cosmetics, paints and varnishes, pesticides, cleaning supplies, workplace chemicals, various gases, smog, etc.**

NATURAL REMEDIES
• Contact your nearest **Poison Control Center** (PCC) and describe the situation to them. Have labels of the product at hand. Every state and many large cities in America and Canada have their own PCC phone number. There is no nationwide number. Telephone the operator (0) or emergency (911), and they can direct you to your nearest Poison Control Center. Also see page 828.

• Many poisons are strong acids or strong alkalies. In such cases, the antidote will have the opposite pH. But the PCC will know what the antidote should be. The PCC will have even better data on the substance than will be found on the label of the product. Then contact a physician.

• *If the poison is on the outside* of the body, **flush with plenty of water**. If inside, follow directions on the label if no other information is available.

• Many poisons can be counteracted by taking an **emetic** to cause **vomiting**. (In the case of certain caustic poisons, vomiting is not the best.) Putting a tsp. of **salt** in 2 cups warm water, and drinking it quickly, will usually produce vomiting. Repeat a second or third time if necessary. **Tickle the throat** with a finger. After vomiting has occurred, induce more vomiting.

• *If a caustic acid has been swallowed:* First, swallow **soda, chalk, lime water, milk, or vegetable oil,** to neutralize the acid in the stomach; then induce vomiting.

• If a **strong alkali has been swallowed**, then first neutralize it by swallowing **lemon or vinegar**.

• Swallow lots of powdered **charcoal** in water.

• After swallowing the powdered charcoal, to help heal the stomach, drink a tea of **white oak bark, alfalfa, oregano, or sweet basil**.

• *If bits of glass* from a broken bottle get into the food and some is swallowed, eat lots of **soft bread**. The sticky dough will tend to wrap around the glass and may help carry it safely through the intestines.

• *To get rid of heavy metals,* eat **nutritious** food. Include lots of **fiber**, including **pectin** in apples; this helps discharge metals from the body. **Whole grains** are all high in fiber. Have a hair analysis made. It will tell you how much heavy metals you have. A urine analysis can also identify the metal excess or deficiency.

• **Vitamin A** (25,000 IU for only a few days) helps the body discharge poisons. Deficiency of vitamin A can cause lesions from radiation, antibiotics, and metal poisoning. **B complex** vitamins protect the nervous system and help the liver detoxify the blood. Deficiencies of **vitamin B_6** (200-500 mg) suppress the immune system. **Vitamin E** (400 IU) is an antioxidant and prevents free-radical damage. **Calcium** (2,000 mg) and **magnesium** (1,000 mg) are natural chelating minerals. **Selenium** (700 mcg) enhances the functions of vitamin E. **Zinc** (30 mg) is a free-radical inhibitor and helps utilize vitamin A.

• Herbs which help counteract metal poisoning include **burdock, alfalfa, chaparral, dandelion, echinacea, fennel, garlic, juniper, kelp, lobelia, and cayenne**.

• *To counteract arsenic:* Eat **onions, beans, legumes, and garlic**; all of these contain sulfur, which helps to eliminate the arsenic. But do not take inorganic sulfur into the body! It will produce boils. Only drink distilled water. Drink plenty of fruit and vegetable juices.

—*Related topics in this book include Chelation*

Therapy (869), Mineral Effects on Minerals (870), Food Poisoning (858), Chemical Allergies (857), and the poisonings listed on the next several pages: Chemical Poisoning (868), Aluminum (872), Arsenic (871), Cadmium (872), Copper (874), DDT (873), Fluoride (873), Lead (873), Mercury (874), Nickel (874), Radiation (875), Toxic Shock (699), Drug Rash (877), Tobacco (821), Toxemia (880).

ENCOURAGEMENT—There are many problems which we encounter in life; but only God can help us deal with them. Go to Him with your difficulties; He can give wisdom to know what is best to do. James 1:5.

CHEMICAL POISONING

SYMPTOMS AND EFFECTS—A remarkable variety of symptoms can occur. The following are common: stuffy nose, watery eyes, diarrhea, ringing in the ears, nausea, upset stomach, eczema, depression, headache, fatigue, bronchitis, asthma, and arthritis.

WHERE FOUND—We live in a chemical age. Chemicals are in the **air, water, earth, food, and drink**. We find them in the **materials, surfaces, and fabrics** in our lives. It is impossible to escape from them; but, with care, we can reduce the rate at which these hazards cause us harm.

Metals (such as mercury, chrome, nickel, and beryllium) produce skin rashes. Aluminum is the primary cause of Alzheimer's Disease.

• Lead causes anemia.

• Dental fillings containing mercury can poison the system.

• *Poisons:* Herbicides, pesticides, insecticides, fungicides, fumigants, and fertilizers seep into the soil, ground, water, and wells.

• These poisons are taken up by the plants which animals, birds, and humans eat. They passes on into milk, eggs, meat. The toxic substances are in the fruit and vegetables we eat.

• *Food additives:* There are food preservatives and additives. There are artificial colorings, flavorings, and odors. These come from coal tar and lead to cancer.

• Waxes are on the fruit; and added sprays are on the vegetables. There are ripening agents and defoliant chemicals.

• *Other poisons:* There are toxic fumes, dangerous chemicals, and radioactive wastes. The rivers and lakes are polluted with poisonous runoff. Smog is full of them.

• There are hair sprays, treated bedding, animal hair products, paint formulas, and exotic cleaning formulas.

• There is benzene from solvents, styrene from plastics, and formaldehyde from pressed-wood products.

• Smoke arises from cigarettes, cigars, and burning forest fires.

• We hardly have time to worry about old-fashioned dust, molds, parasites, and diseases. We now live amid an onslaught of chemicals and radiation.

—*For additional information, please see Poisoning (867), Food Poisoning (858), and the poisonings listed on the contents page of this chapter (867-884). These in-* clude Aluminum Poisoning, Arsenic Poisoning, Cadmium Poisoning, Copper Poisoning, DDT Poisoning, Fluoride Poisoning, Lead Poisoning, Mercury Poisoning, Nickel Poisoning, and Radiation Poisoning.

NATURAL REMEDIES

• Eat a **nourishing, well-balanced diet** of fresh **fruits, vegetables, whole grains, nuts, and legumes**. Obtain adequate **vitamin-mineral supplementation**. Drink lots of **water**.

• Do not overwork. Obtain **adequate rest** at night and **outdoor exercise** during the day.

• Wear **protective clothing** and gloves when handling chemicals. **Read the labels**; try to learn what type of environment you are in! Employees have died because they have been asked to work with materials which they were not aware were hazardous. If you are feeling bad effects, **consider quitting** and getting a job somewhere else.

• **Stay inside during aerial applications** of insecticides, pesticides, or defoliants. All insect poisons are dangerous.

• **If exposed** to chemicals, go to the contents page of this section *(828);* then turn to the section on the following pages which deals with that type of problem. *Also see Poisoning (867).*

• Go on a **cleansing fast** for 2-3 days every month. This will help strengthen your body.

ENCOURAGEMENT—As you try to help others, you will be helping yourself. There are those all about us who need a friend they can talk to and pray with. The more you help them, the more help you will receive for yourself.

HEAVY METAL POISONING

SYMPTOMS—Diarrhea, ringing in the ears, nausea, gastrointestinal problems, colic, rickets, extreme nervousness, headache, anemia, poor kidney and liver function, speech disturbances, memory loss, eczema, depression, headache, fatigue, bronchitis, asthma, arthritis, weak and aching muscles, and softening of bones.

CAUSES—Heavy metals, including lead, are inhaled and absorbed through the skin in the smog in cities, industry, and on the highways. They are eaten in food (especially, meat, milk, and processed food). They are in substances you place on your body. They are in your clothes, carpets, insecticides, and certain cooking utensils.

NATURAL REMEDIES

• Read labels and **use nothing containing lead, aluminum, or other dangerous metals**.

• Drink plenty of **fresh fruit and vegetable juices**. Eat **food high in fiber**, including the pectin in apples. The fiber tends to bind with metal in the colon and carry it out of the body.

• Take a full-spectrum **vitamin-mineral supplement**, to help stabilize the body's resistance to excess metal.

• The **B vitamins**, especially B_6 (200 mg), help rid the intestinal tract of excess metals.

• **Vitamin C** (5,000-20,000 mg) and **bioflavonoids** (200 mg). By taking large amounts of this detoxicant, it will combine with heavy metals and, through diarrhea, will help flush them out of the body.

• **Calcium** (1,500 mg) and **magnesium** (700 mg) bind with aluminum and some other metals, and carry them out.

• The unusually balanced mineral content in Nova Scotia **kelp** and Norwegian **dulse** helps eliminate an excess of certain metals. California kelp is not as efficient.

• **L-glutathione** is an amino acid which interrupts radiation from toxic metals and radiation.

• **Echinacea, ginkgo biloba, ginseng, and burdock root** are beneficial, when taken regularly, in blocking heavy metal and radiation absorption.

• **Acid rain** absorbs heavy metals from the soil and carries them into the groundwater, wells, and rivers which later finds its way into the city **water supplies**.

• A **hair analysis** can determine the level of heavy metals in the body.

• **Chelation therapy** is available from some health-care providers. It can remove toxic metals from the body.

—For additional information, see Chelation Therapy (bellow), Aluminum Poisoning (871), Cadmium Poisoning (872), Copper Poisoning (872), Lead Poisoning (873), Mercury Poisoning (874), Nickel Poisoning (874). Also see Poisoning (867), Chemical Allergies (857), and Chemical Poisoning (868).

ENCOURAGEMENT—If we would permit our minds to dwell more upon Christ and the heavenly world, we should find a powerful stimulus and support in fighting the battles of the Lord. Pride and love of the world will lose their power as we contemplate the glories of that better land so soon to be our home. Beside the loveliness of Christ, all earthly attractions will seem of little worth.

CHELATION THERAPY

WHAT IT IS—Chelation *(key-LAY-shun)* therapy is used to safely eliminate excess poisons, especially heavy metals, from the body.

Chelating agents are used to bind with heavy toxic metals (lead, mercury, cadmium, aluminum, etc.) and excrete them from the body.

Chelation therapy is especially useful for circulatory disorders *(523-543)*, atherosclerosis *(523)*, Alzheimer's disease *(587)*, multiple sclerosis *(580)*, Parkinson's Disease *(582)*, arthritis *(618)*, and gangrene *(367)*.

CHELATING AGENTS—There are five groups of chelating agents which can help remove toxins and heavy metals from your body. They can be purchased at a health-food store:
• **Coenzyme A**.
• **Coenzyme Q_{10}**.
• **Calcium** and **magnesium** chelate with **potassium**.
• **Alfalfa, fiber, rutin, and selenium**.
• **Copper chelate, iron, sea kelp, and zinc chelate**.

Other powerful chelating agents (which include some of the above) include:
• **Apple pectin and rutin**.
• **Calcium** (1,500 mg daily) plus **magnesium** (800 mg).
• **Selenium** (200 mcg, but not over 40 if pregnant).
• **B complex** (100 mg of each major B vitamin, 3 times daily), **B_{12}** (1,000 mcg, 3 times daily), **pantothenic acid** (50 mg, 3 times daily), **niacin** (50 mg, 3 times daily), **folic acid** (5 mg), **garlic** (fresh or Kyolic).
• **Vitamin A** (10,000 IU daily) with mixed **carotenoids**.
• **Alfalfa** liquid (2 Tbsp.).
• **Coenzyme Q_{10}** (80 mg daily).
• **L-cysteine and L-methionine** (each: 500 mg twice daily; take on an empty stomach with water or juice, not with milk; take with 50 mg **B_6** and 100 mg **vitamin C** for better absorption).
• **L-lysine and glutathione** (500 mg each daily; do not take lysine longer than 6 months at a time).
• **Vitamin C** (5,000-12,000 mg daily in divided doses).

DIET—Proper diet is important. Fresh **fruits, vegetables, whole grains, nuts, and legumes**. Eat **fiber foods** (such as **oats, wheat bran, and brown rice**). **Onions and garlic** are both good chelating agents. Include them in your diet.

• Eat foods rich in **manganese**, an important chelating agent: **whole wheat, pecans, barley, Brazil nuts, buckwheat, dried split peas**.

• **Alfalfa, kelp, and zinc** supplements also help chelate. **Iron** is helpful, only if taken in natural (not supplement) form (such as **blackstrap molasses**). If taking zinc, eat sulfur-rich foods (**garlic and onions**); because zinc will balance out the sulfur amount. Only drink distilled water.

• **Avoid processed, fried, sugar, and fast foods.** Avoid **diary products, oils, mayonnaise, meat, salt**.

INTRAVENOUS CHELATION THERAPY—In addition to home therapy, you can also receive chelation from a physician who knows how to do it (there are about 150 in America). Most serious illnesses require repeated injections of the chelating agents.

But the primary chelating agent currently used is a chemical compound that is not natural and somewhat controversial: *ethylenediaminetetraacetic acid* (EDTA). Don't try to pronounce it. A number of lab tests precede the series of injections.

A typical course includes two 3-hour treatments a week. In addition to EDTA, several supplements (including vitamin C, magnesium, and trace minerals) are also injected. This is done because the EDTA removes certain nutrients from the body, so they have to be replaced. If you wish to go this route, you would do well to take extra vitamin-mineral supplements at home.

—For additional information, see Chelation Therapy (above), Aluminum Poisoning (871), Cadmium Poi-

P
O
I
S
O
N
S

soning (872), Copper Poisoning (872), Lead Poisoning (873), Mercury Poisoning (874), Nickel Poisoning (874). Also see Poisoning (867), Chemical Allergies (857), and Chemical Poisoning (868).

ENCOURAGEMENT—Put your highest power into your effort. Call to your aid the most powerful motives. You are learning. Endeavor to go to the bottom of everything you set your hand to. Never aim lower than to become competent in the matters which occupy you. Do not allow yourself to fall into the habit of being superficial and neglectful in your duties and studies; for your habits will strengthen and you will become incapable of anything better. The mind naturally learns to be satisfied with that which requires little care and effort; it tends to be content with something cheap and inferior. Determine that you want to know God through the study of the Bible and a personal, prayerful relationship with Him each day. John 9:4.

MINERAL EFFECTS ON MINERALS

Of the 92 basic elements, 27 are especially used in the body. An excess of each one in the human body can increase or decrease the availability of certain other elements. In nutrition, they are called "minerals"; so we will call them that here.

The following information can be invaluable if you are trying to increase or reduce the amount of a certain mineral in your body. If not, the following listing is of no value to you.

Hair analysis can reveal the minerals which you have an excess of in your body. The following listing will tell you how they interact with other minerals, either helping or hindering them.

For example, an excess of molybdenum in your body will increase your body's absorption of the dangerous mineral, copper—which hair analysis may reveal that you already have too much of. This information can be very helpful, if you are determined to reduce the amount of certain dangerous elements in your body. For example, looking through the list, you will find that a slight increase in the amount of selenium and zinc taken into your body will help eliminate the dangerous lead in your body. But, of course, never take very much of the trace minerals. *You will find detailed information on dosages of major minerals and trace minerals on pp. 84-85.* You will also learn that lead in your body is interfering with your body's absorption and utilization of three very important major minerals: calcium, iron, and potassium.

Code:
[1] = increases the absorption and use of
[2] = reduces the absorption and use of
[3] = the absorption and use of is reduced by

Example:
Molybdenum (*Mo* is its chemical abbreviation) [1] increases the absorption and use of copper and sulfur. [2] Molybdenum reduces the absorption and use of phosphorus. [3] The absorption and use of molybdenum is reduced by nitrogen.

List of 27 special minerals:
Aluminum (Al) **[1]** P / **[2]** F
Arsenic (As) **[1]** Co, I / **[2]** Se
Beryllium (Be) **[2]** Mg
Cadmium (Cd) **[2]** Cu
Calcium (Ca) **[1]** Fe, Mg, P / **[2]** Cu, F, Li, Mn, Zn / **[3]** Cr, Pb, S
Chlorine (Cl) **[1]** (Interactions not documented yet)
Chromium (Cr) **[2]** Ca
Cobalt (Co) **[1]** As, F / **[2]** Fe, I
Copper (Cu) **[1]** Fe, Mo, Zn / **[2]** P / **[3]** Ag, Ca, Cd, Mn, S
Fluorine (F) **[2]** Mg / **[3]** Al, Ca
Iodine (I) **[1]** As, Co
Iron (Fe) **[1]** Ca, Cu, K, Mn, P / **[3]** Co, Mg, Pb, Zn
Lead (Pb) **[2]** Ca, Fe, K / **[3]** Se, Zn
Lithium (Li) **[2]** Na / **[3]** Ca
Magnesium (Mg) **[1]** Ca, K, P / **[2]** Fe / **[3]** Mn
Manganese (Mn) **[1]** Cu, Fe, K, P / **[2]** Mg / **[3]** Ca
Mercury (Hg) (Interactions not documented yet)
Molybdenum (Mo) **[1]** Cu, S / **[2]** P / **[3]** N
Nickel (Ni) (Interactions not documented yet)
Nitrogen (N) **[2]** Mo
Phosphorus (P) **[1]** Al, be, Ca, Fe, Mg, Mn, Zn / **[2]** Na / **[3]** Cu, Mo
Potassium (K) **[1]** Fe, Mg, Mn, Na / **[3]** Pb
Selenium (Se) **[2]** Cd, Pb / **[3]** As, S
Silver (Ag) **[2]** Cu
Sodium Na) **[1]** K / **[3]** Li, P
Sulfur (S) **[1]** Mo / **[2]** Ca, Cu, Se / **[3]** Zn
Zinc (Zn) **[1]** Cu, P / **[2]** Cd, Fe, Pb, S / **[3]** Ca

—*For additional information, see Chelation Therapy (869), Aluminum Poisoning (871), Cadmium Poisoning (872), Copper Poisoning (872), Lead Poisoning (873), Mercury Poisoning (874), Nickel Poisoning (874).*

ENCOURAGEMENT— God has given the human mind great power, power to show that the Creator has endowed man with ability to do a great work against the enemy of all righteousness, power to show what victories may be gained in the conflict against evil. To those who fulfill God's purpose for them will be spoken the words, "Well done, good and faithful servant; thou hast been faithful over a few things, I will make thee ruler over many things."

ENVIRONMENTAL TOXICITY

SYMPTOMS—Headache, stuffy nose, depression, fatigue, bronchitis, arthritic pains, and skin rashes.

CAUSES—Our world is rapidly becoming poisoned and, frankly, somewhat unsafe to live in. The petroleum, chemical, and manufacturing industries pour their pollutants into the air, water, and soil. Modern agriculture is keyed to spraying plants with poisons "to help them grow." There are pesticides, herbicides, insecticides, fungicides, fumigants, and fertilizers.

There are food additives, preservatives, artificial coloring. Toxic chemical and hazardous waste seems to be everywhere.

According to EPA findings, indoor air pollution levels in homes, offices, factories, and schools are often 2-5 times greater than outside those buildings; sometimes

100 times greater.

Pollutants include asbestos, animal hair, bedding, dust, carbon monoxide, disinfectants, formaldehyde, hair sprays, electromagnetic fields, lead, household cleaning products, radiation from TV and computer screens, paint, mold, pollen, solvents, and radon. Certain products emit poisonous fumes and vapors: carpets, certain wood products, plastics, cigarette and pipe tobacco,

NATURAL REMEDIES

• It is urgent that each of us individually maintain the highest level in our body's immune system. This can only be done as we obtain adequate **rest, fresh air, exercise, and nourishing food**.

• In addition to nutritional data in nearby sections of this *Encyclopedia*, here are several additional nutrient sources which you should be aware of. They strengthen natural immunity and help protect your body against the effects of poisonous substances of a foreign nature: **grapeseed extract, coenzyme Q$_{10}$, coenzyme A, superoxide dismutase, proteolytic enzymes, S-adenosylmethionine, and quercetin.**

ENCOURAGEMENT—We should cultivate a love for time spent alone with God, studying the Bible, praying to Him, thinking about Him and how to help others. Many seem to begrudge moments spent in meditation, the searching of the Scriptures, and prayer, as though the time thus occupied was lost. I wish you could all view these things in the light God would have you; for you would then make the kingdom of Heaven of the first importance. To keep your heart in Heaven will give vigor to all your graces and put life into all your duties. To discipline the mind to dwell upon heavenly things will put life and earnestness into all our endeavors.

ALUMINUM POISONING

SYMPTOMS AND EFFECTS—Many symptoms are similar to those of Alzheimer's Disease *(587)* and osteoporosis *(612)*.

Other symptoms include gastrointestinal problems, colic, rickets, extreme nervousness, headache, anemia, poor kidney and liver function, speech disturbances, memory loss, weak and aching muscles, and softening of bones.

It is believed, by many, that **Alzheimer's disease** *(587)* is caused by aluminum poisoning. Aluminum was little used until the 1940s, when an inexpensive method was found to extract it from bauxite, by running an electric current through that ore. Since then, Alzheimer's disease has rapidly increased. The brains of Alzheimer's patients have 10-50 times as much aluminum as those of normal people.

An excess of either aluminum or silicon in the body results in reduced absorption of calcium and other minerals. Aluminum salts in the brain produce impaired mental abilities and seizures. The autopsied brains of Alzheimer's patients had four times as much aluminum as did those of other people.

Aluminum also damages the kidneys which try to excrete it from the body.

There is so much aluminum in our daily environment, that the average person absorbs 3-10 mg of it every day. It is primarily absorbed in food and drink, but also in breathing and through the skin.

Absorbed through the skin: **Antiperspirants, deodorants, Aluminum lawn chairs, foil, and toys.**

Absorbed in food eaten: **Aluminum from pots, pans,** and other cookware that food is cooked in. Aluminum eating utensils and plates (in campware). **Bleached flour, regular table salt, tobacco smoke, processed cheese, cream of tartar, douches, canned goods, baking powder, antacids, buffered aspirin,** and **most city water. Processed cheese** is high in it; for the aluminum helps it melt when heated. Never use aluminum (or copper) cookware! Use stainless steel or glass whenever possible.

Absorbed in air inhaled: **Deodorants, aluminum dust in industry.**

NATURAL REMEDIES

• Do not use any of the **above listed products.** Read labels.

• **Use nothing containing aluminum.** Avoid aluminum sources and environments. Do not use **aluminum foil** on food. Do not take **buffered aspirin** and certain **antacids**; both are extremely high in aluminum!

• Use only **stainless steel cookwar**e. Store nothing in aluminum containers. • Do not purchase **canned juice** which is acid (pineapple juice, grapefruit juice, etc.).

• **Calcium** (1,500 mg) and **magnesium** (700 mg) bind with aluminum and some other metals, and carry them out of the body.

• **Acid rain** absorbs aluminum out of the soil, and carries it into wells and water supplies. Drink **distilled water** instead of tap water (which may contain aluminum).

A **hair analysis** can determine the level of aluminum in the body.

—For additional information and remedies, see Alzheimer's Disease (587), Heavy Metal Poisoning (868), Chelation Therapy (869), Chemical Poisoning (868), and Poisoning (867).

ENCOURAGEMENT—Do not allow the perplexities and worries of everyday life to fret your mind and come between you and God. You need Him all the more in the troubles you encounter. Do not forsake Him.

ARSENIC POISONING

SYMPTOMS AND EFFECTS—Confusion, headaches, drowsiness, convulsions, vomiting, muscle cramps, diarrhea, bloody urine, and gastrointestinal problems. Alopecia, constipation, delayed healing of skin problems, edema, burning and tingling, stomatitis. The lungs, skin,

P
O
I
S
O
N
S

and liver are primarily affected.

WHERE FOUND—**Herbicides, slug poisons, pesticides, smog, beer, water, table salt, seafood, tobacco smoke, laundry aids, smog, dolomite, bone meal. Copper smelting, mining shafts, and sheep dipping.**

Arsenic poisoning especially affects the skin, lungs, kidneys, and liver. The more the body accumulates it, the worse the symptoms. Coma and death can result.

NATURAL REMEDIES

• *EMERGENCY!* In case of accidental taking of arsenic, immediately chew up 7 **charcoal tablets** and swallow with water. Take 7 more every 15 minutes, until you reach the emergency room.

• **Avoid arsenic sources and environments**. Read labels and use nothing containing arsenic.

• **Selenium** (200 mcg daily) helps rid the body of arsenic.

• Sulphur foods help eliminate arsenic: **garlic and garlic supplements, onions, legumes, and beans**.

• Dr. Christopher has a special "iron compound" which he recommends for arsenic poisoning: 3 oz. each of cut **yellow dock** root and cut **bugle weed**. Simmer for 10 minutes in 1 pint water, strain, sweeten with honey, let cool. Take 2-3 fl. oz. every hour until you drink it all.

—*For additional information and remedies, see Heavy Metal Poisoning (868), Chelation Therapy (869), Chemical Poisoning (868), and Poisoning (867).*

ENCOURAGEMENT—Thank God there are answers! Go to Him in prayer and you will receive the help you need. He can give you guidance that you very much need.

CADMIUM POISONING

SYMPTOMS—Anemia, joint soreness, hair loss, dry and scaly skin, dulled sense of smell, high blood pressure, loss of appetite. It can lead to emphysema *(507)* and cancer *(782)*.

EFFECTS—Cadmium is a trace metal; but it is poisonous and weakens the immune system by decreasing T-cell production in the body. It is increasingly found in many substances. Cadmium stores up in the liver and kidneys, seriously weakening both organs. In the bloodstream, it produces a dangerous anemia, so body cells do not receive enough oxygen.

WHERE FOUND—**Cigarette and cigar smokers** have high cadmium levels, but you can get it from **secondhand smoke**. Cadmium is in **plastics, white paint, and nickel-cadmium batteries**. It is in **drinking water, pesticides, fungicides, fertilizers, industrial air pollution, and various foodstuffs (including rice, coffee, tea, soft drinks, and refined grains)**.

SOLUTIONS—Avoid cadmium sources and environments.

One individual lived for a year near a battery salvage plant. It permanently poisoned his body with cadmium. In order to keep his teeth from falling out, he frequently

chews on **ginger root** between meals. This has firmed up his gums and kept his teeth intact.

—*For additional information and remedies, see Heavy Metal Poisoning (868), Chelation Therapy (869), Chemical Poisoning (868), and Poisoning (867).*

ENCOURAGEMENT—As you open your door to needy ones, you are inviting angels to come in. Do what you can to be a blessing to those around you, and you will be blessed. Hebrews 13:2.

COPPER POISONING

SYMPTOMS AND EFFECTS—Excess amounts of copper can result in emotional problems, behavioral disorders, mood swings, anemia, depression, kidney damage, eczema, schizophrenia, sickle-cell anemia, and central nervous system damage.

It can produce infections, heart attack *(513)*, anemia *(537)*, cirrhosis of the liver *(450)*, mental illness *(601)*, insomnia *(547, 709)*, stuttering *(699)*, Wilson's Disease *(385)*, and niacin deficiency *(101)*.

WHERE FOUND—**Beer, copper plumbing and cookware, insecticides, permanent wave kits, pasteurized milk, oral contraceptives, tobacco, swimming pools, city water, and various foods.** Also **certain frozen foods** have copper added in order to make them greener (peas, etc.).

SOLUTIONS—Read labels and use nothing containing copper. Avoid copper sources and environments.

• **Vitamin C** (1,000 mg, 4 times daily) with rutin (60 mg daily) works as copper chelators and reduce the amount of copper in the system.

• **Zinc** (50 mg, but not over 100 mg daily) actively reduces levels of copper. (Contrariwise, if there is not enough zinc in the diet, copper levels will automatically increase.)

• **L-cysteine and L-methionine** (each: 500 mg twice daily; taken on an empty stomach with water or juice, not with milk) also reduces copper in the body. Take them with 50 mg B_6 and 100 mg **vitamin C** for better absorption.

• Hair analysis can help you determine the amount of copper poisoning in your system.

DEFICIENCY—It is also possible to not have enough copper in the body. Without a balance of copper and zinc in the body, the thyroid will not work properly. Babies fed soy milk tend to have a deficiency of copper. The result is damaged nerves, bones, and lungs. Adults lacking copper will lose protein. Excessively large doses of zinc can also produce a copper deficiency. Oral contraceptives can cause either an excess or deficiency of copper.

—*For additional information and remedies, see Heavy Metal Poisoning (868), Chelation Therapy (869), Chemical Poisoning (868), and Poisoning (867).*

ENCOURAGEMENT—Keep cheerful and sunny. This will encourage those around you to take heart. They have problems too. Kneel down and pray with them.

DDT POISONING

THE PROBLEM—We still have DDT poisoning. It was first introduced in 1939, into agriculture, to kill insects. It was banned in December 1972; however, we still have DDT. Here is why:

First, it has long-lasting effects on humans, as well as birds, fish, and animals. Second, it is still in our water and soil. Third, shipments of DDT food from overseas are not banned. Food grown in Israel is heavily laced with DDT and then shipped to America because orthodox Jews will not allow it to be sold in Israel. Fourth, it is still used on fruit trees in America!

SOLUTIONS—Avoid DDT sources and environments. Special note: Do not fast on water alone; always do it on **fruit juices**. This is because DDT is stored in your body fat. During a water fast, its sudden release can damage various organs. Drink distilled, not regular, water. Drink plenty of fruit and vegetable juices.

—*For additional information and remedies, see Heavy Metal Poisoning (868), Chelation Therapy (869), Chemical Poisoning (868), and Poisoning (867).*

ENCOURAGEMENT—Come up to the light of God's Word, where Jesus is, and you will find all the guidance you need on the pathway to heaven.

FLUORIDE POISONING

SYMPTOMS—Mottled, discolored teeth. This is a permanent change which cannot be reversed.

EFFECTS—Fluoride, a trace mineral, is added to most city water in excessively large amounts. In addition, dentists prescribe fluoride substances in order to reduce dental caries (tooth decay). A much smaller amount has that effect, but only in small children. Fluoride never helps the teeth of adults. (The true cause of dental caries is eating sugar, candies, refined carbohydrates, soda beverages, and too little of fruits and vegetables. The cause is not a lack of fluoride in the diet.)

There was an 85% increase of cancer in Manchester, England, after the introduction of fluoride in the city drinking water. Down's Syndrome increased in U.S. cities when fluoridated water supplies began. Japanese researchers found that children with mottled teeth had a higher incidence of heart disease.

Fluoride combines with calcium to make an insoluble calcium, producing bone deformities.

Because it destroys iodine, fluoride also causes thyroid problems.

SOLUTIONS—Read labels and use nothing containing fluoride. Avoid fluoride sources and environments. Only drink distilled water. Drink plenty of fruit and vegetable juices.

• Hair analysis can help you determine the amount of fluoride poisoning in your system.

—*For additional information and remedies, see Heavy Metal Poisoning (868), Chelation Therapy (869), Chemical Poisoning (868), and Poisoning (867).*

ENCOURAGEMENT—In Christ is light and peace and joy forevermore. The longer we live with Christ, the closer we draw to heaven. Let nothing separate you from His side.

LEAD POISONING

SYMPTOMS—Anxiety, confusion, chronic fatigue, diarrhea, insomnia, learning disabilities, loss of appetite, a metallic taste in the mouth, seizures, tremors, vertigo, muscle weakness, arthritis, gout, severe gastrointestinal colic. Also, gums turn blue.

EFFECTS—Lead poisoning produces hyperactivity in children, behavioral problems, and weakened minds. Chronic lead poisoning causes reproductive disorders, impotence in men, infertility in women, and anemia. Sudden infant death syndrome occurs more often in infants with high lead levels than those who die of other causes. Lead poisoning can eventually result in blindness, mental disturbances, mental retardation, paralysis of the extremities, coma, and death.

Toxic amounts damage liver, kidneys, heart, and nervous systems. Painter's colic shows severe wandering pain in the abdomen and acute muscle spasm. Sometimes you will find a lead line on the gum margin of the teeth. Lead inhibits the actions of calcium, iron, and potassium in the body. All of these are important nutrients.

WHERE FOUND—Lead is extremely toxic; it is widely found in **leaded gasoline, lead pipes, piping with solder, ceramic glazes, lead-based paints, and lead-acid batteries**. Lead arsenate is an **insecticide** used on certain plants. **Burning newspapers** throw lead into the air. Lead is in **commercial baby milk** and industrial materials (**nails, solder, plating, plaster, and putty**). **Lead pipes** put lead in **water supplies**. Copper water pipes are connected with **lead soldering**.

People also consume it when they use **tobacco**, eat **liver**, and drink domestic or imported **wines**. It can also be in **soldered cans**. Women with high lead levels give birth to infants with high levels. Such children grow more slowly and have nervous system disorders. No matter how high its lead level, your body is always ready to absorb more.

SOLUTIONS—Read labels and use nothing containing lead. Avoid lead sources and environments.

• **Vitamin E** (400-800 IU) tends to reduce the effects of lead poisoning. **Calcium** (2,000 mg daily) prevents lead from being deposited in body tissues. Take **magnesium**

(1,000 mg) with the calcium. **Garlic** binds with, and excretes, lead. **Zinc** (50 mg) reduces lead in the system. **Vitamin A** (1,000 IU) helps protect body from effects of lead.

• Drink **aloe vera** gel or liquid.

• Buy only **canned goods** which are lead-free. These cans have been welded and have no soldered side seems. Do not use imported canned goods; no regulations cover them. Only drink distilled water. Drink plenty of fruit and vegetable juices.

• Stay off main **highways** whenever possible; and do not live near them. Lead fumes and other noxious chemicals and metals are still coming out of car exhausts. Do not grow family garden crops near highways.

• Do not have lead or copper **water pipes** in your home; use PVC (plastic) pipes instead. Copper pipes are connected with lead solder. Solder leaches a significant amount of lead into the water supply, especially during the first few years after installation. Lead solder was not banned until 1986. Copper is also poisonous.

• Do not drink out of **glazed pottery**, especially if it is imported! The glaze can contain lead, which will leach into your fruit juice, etc.

Do not eat on **antique dinnerware**; they leach lead. Do not store foods or liquids in **lead crystal** glassware. Do not turn **bread bags inside out** and use them to store food. There is lead on the ink. Never use the **first water** from your tap in the morning for drinking or cooking. Let it run 3 minutes.

If safe drinking water is not available, **treat water with grapefruit-seed extract**, before using it. Add 10 drops, per gallon of water, and shake (or stir) vigorously.

Hair analysis can help you determine the amount of lead poisoning in your system.

—For additional information and remedies, see Heavy Metal Poisoning (868), Chelation Therapy (869), Chemical Poisoning (868), and Poisoning (867).

ENCOURAGEMENT—If we have Christ abiding with us, we shall be Christians at home as well as abroad. He who is a Christian will have kind words for all he associates with. As we do this, our own hearts will be warmed the more with Christ's love.

MERCURY POISONING

SYMPTOMS AND DISEASE—Allergies, anxiety, metallic taste, gastroenteritis, burning mouth pain, salivation, abdominal pain, tremors, uncontrolled crying, vertigo, nausea, and vomiting.

Mercury poisoning can lead to colitis, kidney disease, dermatitis, asthma, hair loss, gingivitis, mental and emotional disturbances, and nerve damage.

It is believed, by many, that multiple sclerosis is caused by mercury poisoning.

Arriving in the brain, it is stored there and produces dizziness, insomnia, weakness, fatigue, depression, and memory loss.

Symptoms in a child include hyperactivity, irritability, depression, and behavioral changes.

WHERE FOUND—Mercury is more toxic than lead, and can be ingested or inhaled. It is stored in the brain and in the fat.

At normal temperatures, it tends to change from a solid into a gas. This means that the mercury in the **amalgam fillings** in your mouth are always ready, when the opportunity presents itself, to pass into saliva and be swallowed. Acids in food provide that opportunity. Amalgam is over 50% mercury. Minute amounts of methyl mercury are released from the tooth filling as you chew your food. Eventually it passes into the organs and brain.

Nearly 100 chemicals are placed in mouths by dentists (including mercury, copper, nickel, beryllium, zinc, phenol, formaldehyde, disocyanate, and acetone).

Mercury is also found in streams, lakes, **fish, shellfish**, and sewage. The problem is that it is added to **insecticides, herbicides, and fungicides. Grains and seeds** are frequently treated with it, to keep out bugs. We would rather eat a stray bug than mercury. Gradually these substances have gone into the rivers and lakes, contaminating the fish.

Mercury is also included in **fabric softeners, polishes, wood preservatives, latex, solvents, plastics, ink, and some paints. It is in cosmetics, laxatives which have calomel, some hemorrhoidal suppositories, and a variety of other medications**.

SOLUTIONS—Read labels and use nothing containing mercury. Avoid mercury sources and environments.

• Remove the mercury (amalgam) fillings from your teeth.

• **Sweating** helps excrete mercury. **Selenium** (220 mcg daily) helps eliminate it.

• Hair analysis can help you determine the amount of mercury poisoning in your system.

—For additional information and remedies, see Heavy Metal Poisoning (868), Chelation Therapy (869), Chemical Poisoning (868), and Poisoning (867), Dental Amalgam (424).

ENCOURAGEMENT—Tell the one in trouble, "Let us pray." Kneel down together and unload your hearts to God. Find in Him the peace and help that both of you need.

NICKEL POISONING

SYMPTOMS AND DISEASE—Skin rashes, respiratory illness, and myocardial infarction. It also interferes with the Kreb's cycle. Later problems are pulmonary edema, and brain and liver swelling.

WHERE FOUND—Nickel is found in **hydrogenated fats and oils, baking soda, cocoa powder, refined and processed foods, and jewelry**. It is in **superphosphate fertilizers**. It is also in **automobile exhaust, cigarette smoke, and manufacturing emissions**. Absorption through the skin can come from **jewelry, hairpins, errings, tongue piercing, coins, heart valves, nickel plating, and prosthetic joints**. Some **cooking utensils**

contain nickel. Nickel carbonyl is the most toxic form.

SOLUTIONS—Read the above paragraph carefully. Avoid nickel sources and environments. Also read labels and use nothing containing nickel.

• **Do not pierce your ears** or wear **metal jewelry** containing nickel. The posts placed in pierced ears are nickel and cause nickel rash. The earrings have it also. This rash will appear everywhere on your body when you are wearing metal of any kind. Leave your ears the way God made them. Do not **pierce your tongue**.

• Avoid nickel alloys in **dental work**.

• Do not place acidic foods or liquids in **cookware** that has nickel in it.

• Do not **work** where you may breathe nickel dust or fumes. Doing so can eventually cripple or kill you. Do not work in, or live near, **nickle plating industries**.

Hair analysis can help you determine the amount of copper poisoning in your system.

—*For additional information and remedies, see Heavy Metal Poisoning (868), Chelation Therapy (869), Chemical Poisoning (868), and Poisoning (867).*

ENCOURAGEMENT—Where can we find help? Only in God! No one on earth can fill our deepest needs. Only He who created us can give what is needed, as we cry to Him in faith for help.

RADIATION POISONING
(Radiation Exposure)

SYMPTOMS AND DISEASE—Dizziness, mental fatigue, eye fatigue, severe headache, cataracts, and nausea.

WHERE FOUND—**Medical and dental X-rays, television, cellular phones, video display terminals, satellite dishes, building materials containing radon or uranium, computers, microwave ovens, satellites, high-voltage electric lines, radar devices, electronic games, smoke detectors, and tobacco**. It can also come from a **nuclear bomb,** which exploded halfway around the world, or from a terrorist's **dirty bomb** here in the U.S.

When radiation strikes a human cell, it alters, damages, or destroys it. If a cell's DNA is damaged, genetic mutations in offspring can occur. Whether a little or a lot, radiation is extremely dangerous. Living tissue is damaged when ionizing radiation strikes it. This is radiation powerful enough to shift electrons from one collection of atoms to another. Such restructuring of tissue can result in disease or cancer.

A significant percentage of women inherit a **gene** that is sensitive to X-ray exposure. In those women, even a short exposure to X-rays can lead to cancer.

Strontium-90 and **Iodine-131**, which are produced by nuclear explosions, are especially harmful because they have short half-lives and are easily absorbed by the body. In the U.S., **radon and X-rays** are the most frequent sources of radiation. You are exposed to more radiation when you climb in very high altitudes.

SOLUTIONS—**Avoid radiation sources and environments**. As a help in protecting yourself from radioactivity, you must eat enough **non-radioactive elements**. (1) If you are not obtaining enough **calcium**, your body will absorb radioactive *strontium-90* from the air. (2) Buy a bottle of **iodine** and paint a little on the top of your foot (or the inside of your thigh). If the color disappears within 24 hours, put on a little more (too much iodine can be harmful). Your body will absorb it and protect you from radioactive fallout from radioactive iodine *(iodine-131)*, which destroys the thyroid.

• The following nutrients help protect the body against radiation: **Pantothenic acid** (200 mg), **inositol** (100 mg), **lecithin granules** (1 Tsp), **B complex**, **vitamin E (400-800 IU)**, **calcium** (2,000-5,000 mg), **potassium** (5,500 mg), **magnesium** (750 mg), **zinc** (50 mg), **coenzyme Q$_{10}$** (100 mg), **dulse or kelp** (1,000 mg). **Aloe vera** has been shown to reduce radioactivity.

• During a nuclear attack, **vitamin C**, taken in large amounts (5,000-25,000 mg or more in divided doses each day), will help protect you. Be sure to get extra calcium and iodine at that time.

• Foods which protect against radiation include **fresh fruits, vegetables, whole grains, and legumes**.

• Foods which reduce one's ability to be protected against radiation include **meat, poultry, dairy products, sugar, refined food, and food with chemical additives**.

• Have your home tested for **radon**. This is a radioactive gas which seeps up from the ground. Homes which are tightly closed are especially liable to this problem.

• People who **smoke** are at special risk of injury by radon in the home.

• If you sit in front of computer monitor (screen) for long hours each day, you need to install a **radiation / glare screen filter**. If your employer will not purchase one for you, for your own protection, buy it yourself.

• Beware of unnecessary **X-rays**. Refuse them if you are pregnant.

• It is claimed that **cell phones** can irradiate your brain. Purchase an earpiece or phone guard. Use it only for short calls.

• Avoid working in an **X-ray lab**; Because, you do, you will gradually keep increasing your *rad* count.

—*For additional information and remedies, see Heavy Metal Poisoning (868), Chelation Therapy (869), Chemical Poisoning (868), and Poisoning (867), Thyroid (659-661), Cell Phones (938-944), X-rays (944), Microwave Cooking (947-948).*

ENCOURAGEMENT—Our time here is short. We can pass through this world but once. While we are here, let us do all we can to help and bless others. In Christ's strength, you can minister to many of their needs.

P
O
I
S
O
N
S

CHEMOTHERAPY AND RADIATION THERAPY POISONING

SYMPTOMS—Loss of appetite, vomiting, diarrhea, anemia, hair loss, anxiety, insomnia, pain, fatigue, mouth ulcers, yeast infections, depression.

CAUSES—The above are some of the symptoms of current medical cancer treatments, using chemotherapy and/or radiation therapy. Most cancer patients, receiving these treatments, become very ill.

Here are several things which can reduce those symptoms:

NATURAL REMEDIES

• **Maitake** is a Japanese mushroom which contains beta-glucan. It is able to heavily reduce nausea, increase appetite and energy, and strengthen the body's immune system's white blood cells. Take 2-3 drops a day of the extract.

• Take **ginger** in order to reduce the nauseous abdominal sensation that wants to make you vomit.

• **Glutamine** (5,000-15,000 mg daily) is an amino acid which helps protect the lining of your gastrointestinal tract against the damaging effects of chemotherapy and radiation.

• Physicians are taught that **antioxidant vitamins and minerals** reduce the cancer-killing power of chemo and radiation. But, in reality, by taking those vitamins and minerals, recovery is more likely to occur. *See Antioxidants (104).*

• **Siberian ginseng** (200 mg, 3-6 times, daily) helps prevent fatigue brought on by chemo and radiation. Take it with **astragalus** (1,500 mg daily). Make sure the Siberian ginseng is standardized for *eleutherosides*, the primary active ingredient.

• **Green tea** reduces the nausea. Drink several cups each day (or take 500 mg of the herb).

• **Umeboshi** is a good remedy for the nausea and vomiting from chemo and radiation. Umeboshi is a Japanese tea which contains salt plum paste, ginger, and the root of the kudzu plant.

—*For additional information, see Radiation Poisoning (875), Chemical Poisoning (868); Thyroid (659-661).*

ENCOURAGEMENT—Let every one who desires to be a partaker of the divine nature appreciate the fact that he must escape the corruption that is in the world through lust. There must be a constant, earnest struggling of the soul against the evil imaginings of the mind. There must be a steadfast resistance of temptation to sin in thought or act. The soul must be kept from every stain, through faith in Him who is able to keep you from falling. We should meditate upon the Scriptures, thinking soberly and candidly upon the things that pertain to our eternal salvation. The infinite mercy and love of Jesus, the sacrifice made in our behalf, call for most serious and solemn reflection.

CHART - 1063-1064: Information on the 9 types of vaccinations required prior to overseas travel. For more on vaccinations: 876, 928, 972

GUILLAIN-BARRÉ SYNDROME

SYMPTOMS—It begins with neurological weakness in the arms, legs, and face. As it progresses, paralysis of the motor nerves can occur. This can lead to respiratory failure. As the condition worsens, there is strong anxiety, fear, and panic, and depression. Convalescence and recovery can be slow, with the possibility of permanent nerve damage.

CAUSES—This is another disease produced by **vaccinations**. Normally, such a condition would never occur. But when fluids, drawn from animals, are injected into the human bloodstream, terrible consequences can result. *See the author's book, Vaccination Crisis, for more on dangers and ways to avoid having your children vaccinated. (See back of this book.)*

Gerald Ford's introduction of a nationwide vaccination program, in the winter of 1976-1977, was a disaster and resulted in many cases of Guillain-Barré Syndrome.

Other possible factors causing this disorder could include **surgery, viral infections** *(296),* **Hodgkin's Disease** *(794),* **Rabies** *(844),* or **Lupus** *(310).*

NATURAL REMEDIES

• There are instances in which a careful home-care recovery program has solved the problem.

• In one case, a young man was told he had a severe case of Guillain-Barré Syndrome, and that it might require 2 years to recover. Refusing cortisone shots, he used natural healing methods: heavy on **vitamins and minerals, especially B complex, plus extra pantothenic acid, and vitamin C with bioflavonoids.** In addition to other minerals, he emphasized **calcium, potassium, and additional chelated minerals.** Herbs included **blue vervain, licorice root, chamomile, echinacea, burdock, and ginkgo.** He also took **chlorophyll, green drinks, fruit and vegetable juices** (especially **carrot and beet juice**). Within a month, he was well and back to work, with no residual problems later occurring.

• Mercury poisoning is part of the vaccination problem. *See Mercury Poisoning (424, 874), Chelation Therapy (869), and Vaccination Poisoning (876).*

ENCOURAGEMENT—A lamp, however small, may be the means of lighting many other lamps. Trusting in Jesus, do what you can to encourage another, and you will be more courageous yourself.

VACCINATION POISONING

SYMPTOMS AND CAUSES—The **measles vaccine** can produce visual problems, seizures, paralysis. The **tetanus vaccine** can heavily reduce T lymphocyte blood count ratios (as occurs in HIV). The **diphtheria vaccine** can cause confused speech and a rare form of encephalitis. The **polio vaccine** can produce polio in those who handle babies receiving the live-virus (oral) vaccine. The **mumps vaccine** can cause febrile seizures, rashes, nerve deafness, and encephalitis. The **flu vaccine** can produce Guillain-Barré Syndrome or multiple sclerosis. The **rubella vaccine** can cause limb defects, mental retardation, impaired vision, damaged hearing, or heart malformation in the infant born to a mother receiving that vaccine. Those receiving them directly can experience polyneurities, arthralgia (painful joints), or arthritis. The **pertussis vaccine** can produce neurological complications, including death. It can cause fever, convulsions, blindness, and spasticity.

The **DPT vaccine** combines the diphtheria, pertussis, and tetanus vaccines (discussed above); so it is more dangerous than a vaccine for a single disease. Years later, it can result in a number degenerative diseases (including rheumatoid arthritis, leukemia, diabetes, and multiple sclerosis). Experts believe the DPT vaccine is the direct cause of sudden infant death syndrome.

The **MMR vaccine** combines the measles, mumps, and rubella vaccines; this is another source of danger. As with DPT, it can produce the terrible effects of each of the three single vaccines. The MMR vaccine is the direct cause of autism.

A significant factor is that these vaccines are given to infants and small children, when their natural immunity is not as strong as it would be later.

For an in-depth study on both adult and childhood vaccines, their dangers, and how to avoid them, obtain a copy of the author's book, *Vaccination Crisis. (See the back of this Encyclopedia for additional information.)*
—*Also see Vaccination Problems (752; also 928).*

ENCOURAGEMENT—The very first step in the path of life is to keep the mind stayed on God, to have His fear continually before the eyes. A single departure from moral integrity blunts the conscience and opens the door to the next temptation. "He that walketh uprightly walketh surely: but he that perverteth his way shall be known." It is impossible to keep a clear conscience and the approval of Heaven without divine aid and a principle to love honesty for the sake of the right.

DRUG RASH

CAUSES—It is truly surprising what a high percentage of medicinal drugs are poisonous. Yet it need not be, when their underlying *modus operandi* (method by which they work) is understood.

Medicinal drugs work by introducing a strange new poison into the body. The system immediately turns its attention from the debilitated area—and begins fighting the drug. The type of poison (the drug) introduced, and the way it operates, affects the reaction of the body. For example: The body was eliminating sulphur through a boil; but, then, a drug is introduced and the boil disappears, seemingly "healed." The body no longer lets the boil suppurate, so attention can be diverted to the radical poison which has been introduced. But the body has been weakened by the introduction of a poison; some of this may not be eliminated for years.

Natural remedies operate in a different way: They clean out the body and restore it to a healthy normalcy. Whether it be fresh air, pure water, nutritious food, simple herbs, or water treatments, the natural remedies assist the body in carrying on its work of cleansing the body. For that is what "disease" is: an effort of nature to cleanse the body of impurities and eliminate the effects of enervation.

In contrast, a drug is a foreign substance of a poisonous nature. The healing herbs are not "drugs." It is true that about five of every 100 herbs is poisonous, but natural therapy only uses the safe ones. The poisonous ones can be purchased at the drugstore or grocery counter (tobacco, coffee, black tea, chocolate, black pepper, digitalis, quinine, etc.). Such things as aspirin, Valium, phenobarbital, Dilantin, morphine, etc., are foreign chemical substances of a poisonous nature. They all produce dangerous side effects, called "contraindications."

The natural remedies were given us by the God of heaven (Genesis 1:29). We are unwise to turn from them to use poisonous substances instead. The reason the pharmaceutical firms sell poisons is because they cannot patent the natural remedies; they must invent something new. So they extract chemicals from rocks and herbs; and, in doing so, the result is a poisonous compound.

Most of the damage that drugs inflict on the body occurs beneath the skin; but *drug rashes* are effects on the skin.

Here are a few examples of drugs which produce drug rashes:

Antipyrine: Papular, erythematous rash, sometimes accompanied by edema and much irritation.

Arsenic: Papular or erythematous rash, sometimes urticarial. Prolonged use may produce pigmentation of skin.

Belladonna: Erythematous rash, usually accompanied by intense itching.

Bromides: Usually like acne vulgaris. Sometimes erythema.

Chloral: Papular erythema.

Iodides: Usually papular erythema, sometimes with acne-like pustules.

Phenolphthalein: Macular rash, sometimes purpuric.

Quinine: Very irritable erythema or urticaria.

Salicylate: Erythematous rash, possibly morbilliform.

Serum: Usually urticaria.

Sulfonal: Erythematous or urticarial rash.

Here are some other drugs which produce skin rashes: opium compounds, acetanilid, amidopyrine, barbiturates, ephedrine, novocaine, sulfanilamide, and other sulfa drugs.

Some of the drugs have been given very nice sounding names; but note the chemicals they contain: calomel (mercurous chloride), green vitriol (zinc sulfate), goulard water (lead lotion), oil of vitriol (sulfuric acid), and vermilion (mercuric sulfide). Most drugs are compounded

POISONS

from a wide range of extremely complex and very poisonous chemical mixtures, not just two.

Let it be emphasized that most drugs work their damage in a thousand other ways in the body, without always producing skin rashes. Many damage the kidneys or liver.

NATURAL REMEDIES

• **Stop using the medicinal drug**. Take **vitamin C** to bowel tolerance (all you can, before its acidity causes a slight diarrhea). Take vitamins A, B complex, and E. Be sure **selenium** and **zinc** are in your diet. Eat more **fresh fruit and vegetables**, as well as kelp or dulse.

• If the drug has an acid base, consider taking a **soda alkaline bath**. Fill a bathtub with water at 95°-98°F. Add about a cup of baking soda or sodium bicarbonate. Sitting in the tub, dip and pour it over yourself. After 30-60 minutes, stand in the tub, partially drip dry, and pat yourself dry.

—*Also see Eczema (345).*

ENCOURAGEMENT—The throne of grace is to be our continual dependence. There is strength for us in Christ. He is our Advocate before the Father.

PTOMAINE POISONING

SYMPTOMS—Intense pain in the stomach and bowels, headache, backache, shooting pains, soreness, intense vomiting, retching, diarrhea, cold and clammy sweat, weak pulse, collapse, and possible death. Inflammation of the joints, especially the knee, if ptomaine poisoning was caused by eating lobsters or shellfish.

CAUSES—Ptomaines are the waste products produced by bacteria. **Eating tainted or decomposed meat** (sausage, oysters, salmon, pork, shellfish), **cheese**, etc. Because they are not acid, home-canned **peas and beans** are especially liable to become rotten.

NATURAL REMEDIES

• Quickly **empty the stomach** with a stomach tube. Or cause **vomiting** in one of the following ways: Drink 5-6 glasses lukewarm saltwater or a glass of hot water, in which has been stirred a tablespoon of mustard. Two certain ways to induce vomiting: Reach the finger in and tickle the back of the throat or put 1 tablespoon of lobelia in a glass of warm water and immediately drink it.

• Apply **fomentations** over the stomach and bowels while keeping the feet warm; put him **to bed** and keep him **warm**. Give 2 tablespoon of **castor oil** as soon as the stomach will retain it. Allow **no food** for 24 hours; but give all the **water** the stomach will tolerate.

ENCOURAGEMENT—A character that is approved of God and man is to be preferred to wealth. The foundation should be laid broad and deep, resting on the rock Christ Jesus. There are too many who profess to work from the true foundation, whose loose dealing shows them to be building on sliding sand; but the great tempest will sweep away their foundation, and they will have no refuge.

LISTERIOSIS

SYMPTOMS—Symptoms vary. The infection is often unnoticed in healthy adults. Flu-like symptoms may develop (such as fever, sore throat, headache, and aching muscles).

CAUSES—The bacterium, *Listeria monocytogenes*, is in the soil and in most animals everywhere; this can pass to humans through **food products (especially soft cheeses, milk, meat, and prepackaged salads)**. The risk is increased by **letting food remain warm** for a time. The bacteria can multiply in the intestines and spread to the blood and other organs.

In the elderly or those with low immunity, including HIV *(806)*, listeriosis can lead to meningitis *(578)*. In pregnant women, infection can pass to the fetus, causing miscarriage or stillbirth.

NATURAL REMEDIES

• Proper food handling greatly reduces the risk.

• For mild infections, antibiotic herbs *(297)* can be given.

• Those with serious infections should be taken to the hospital.

—*Also see Fever (302-309), Inflammation (293), Flu (294).*

ENCOURAGEMENT—To dwell upon the beauty, goodness, mercy, and love of Jesus is strengthening to the mental and moral powers; and, while the mind is kept trained to do the works of Christ and to be obedient children, you will habitually inquire, Is this the way of the Lord?

MUSHROOM POISONING

SYMPTOMS—Intense stomach pains immediately after eating a mushroom.

CAUSES—There are thousands of edible mushrooms. But there are two species which are extremely poisonous, quite common, and members of the amanita group: the death angel (or death cup) and the fly amanita.

The death angel grows in the woods from June until fall. It is usually white, but sometimes somewhat colored. Its poison acts like the venom of a rattlesnake; for it separates blood corpuscles from the serum.

The fly amanita grows in the woods or along the roadside; it has a bright red, yellow, or orange cup. It paralyzes the nerves which control heart action.

IDENTIFICATION—There are three signs to look for: (1) There will be a ring about halfway up the vertical shaft. (2) The base of the mushroom in the ground will be in the form of a rounded bulb. (3) The top may have tiny flecks on it. (Other indicators are a full, wide cup on top and white spores.) It is said that no mushroom which grows on wood is poisonous.

NATURAL REMEDIES

• There is no known antidote for the death angel,

except to quickly empty the stomach. Take an **emetic** to cause **vomiting**. Put a teaspoon of **salt** in 2 cups warm water and quickly drink it. Keep repeating this. **Tickle the throat** with a finger. After vomiting has occurred, induce more vomiting.

• If the fly amanita (which is somewhat less poisonous) is eaten, the stomach must be immediately emptied and an injection of **atropine** given.

Take the person to the emergency room.

Teach your children the three identifying marks of an amanita. *Also 200-201.*

ENCOURAGEMENT—God is able to take those, who are dead in trespasses and sins, and (by the operation of the Spirit which raised Jesus from the dead) transform the human character and bring back the lost image of God to the soul. Those who believe in Jesus Christ are changed from being rebels against the law of God into obedient servants and subjects of His kingdom. They are born again, regenerated, and sanctified through the truth.

FOOD ADDITIVE POISONING

SYMPTOMS—A variety of symptoms.

CAUSES—*Here are the 10 worst food additives:* **BHA** (butylated hydroxyanisole) - food preservative - *Allergies, liver disease, cancer.* **Caffeine** - coloring, flavoring, and stimulant - *Nervousness, heart palpitations, heart defects.* **Carrageen** - thickening agent, binder - *Colitis, genetic defects.* Modified food starch - thickener, filler - *Vomiting, lung damage.* **MSG** (monosodium glutamate) - flavoring agent - *Headaches, chilling, sweating, diarrhea, chest pain, genetic damage.* **Nitrites** and **sodium nitrites** - preservative, coloring, curing - Cancer-causing. **Propylene glycol alginate** - thickener, stabilizer - *Liver damage.* Red dye 40 (Allura Red AC) - coloring - *Birth defects, cancer.* **Saccharin** - sugar substitute - *Allergic response, affects skin, heart, intestines, tumors, bladder cancer.* **Sodium erythrobate** - preservative, coloring agent - *Genetic effects.*

Here are the next 10 worst food additives: **Caramel** - *Genetic effects, possibly cancer.* **EDTA** (*calcium disodium ethylenediamine tetraacetate*) - preservative, flavoring - *Kidney disorders, cramps, skin rashes, intestinal problems.* **Gums: Arabic, cellulose, Ghatti, Karaya, Tragacanth, Xanthan** - thickener, binder, increase easy flow - *Allergic reactions, constipation, diarrhea.* **Hydroxylated lecithin** - binder - *Skin irritations.* **Lactic acid** - preservative - *Caustic.* **Maltol dextrin** - aroma and flavor enhancer - *Derived from harmful wood tars.* **Monoglycerides and diglycerides** - softeners, smoothing agents - *Genetic changes, cancer, birth defects.* **Polysorbate 60, 65, 80** - emulsifier for creaminess - *Diarrhea.* **Propyl gallate** - preservative - *Liver damage, birth defects.* **Tannin (tannic acid)** - flavoring - *Liver ailments and tumors, cancer.*

Foods containing the 20 worst food additives:

Cakes, crackers, pies, and doughnuts - contains 11 of the 20 worst additives. **Colas, soft drinks, punches, powders** - contains 9 of the 20. **Frozen pizzas** - 6 of the 20. **Gelatin and pudding desserts** - 6 of the 20. **Ice cream and ice milk** - 6 of the 20. **Beer** - 6 of the 20. **Vegetable sauces** - 5 of the 20. **Broths** - 4 of the 20.

Also avoid these food additives (which are not quite as dangerous as the 20 worst): baking soda and powder, BHT, nitrates, black pepper, sodium erythorbate, spices, and vinegar.

ENCOURAGEMENT—Reader, are you preparing to become a member of the heavenly family? Are you seeking in the home life to be fitted to become a member of the Lord's family? If so, make the home life happy by mutual self-sacrifice. If we want Jesus in our home, let kind words only be spoken there. The angels of God will not abide in a home where there is strife and contention. Let love be cherished; and peace and Christian politeness, and angels will be your guests.

MSG SENSITIVITY
(Chinese Restaurant Syndrome, Monosodium Glutamate)

SYMPTOMS—Headache, flushing, tingling, weakness, and stomachache.

CAUSES—Monosodium Glutamate is a chemical compound added to food as a flavor enhancer. It is found in some **Chinese and Japanese food** (as Aji no Moto) and is also used as a **meat tenderizer** (Accent). But MSG is being increasingly added to other processed foods (such as **textured vegetable protein, gelatin, hydrolyzed vegetable protein, yeast extracts, calcium and sodium caseinate, whey, vegetable broth, malt extract, smoke flavoring, and many other food ingredients**)—often without being mentioned on the label.

NATURAL REMEDIES

• **Avoid processed foods** in order to avoid MSG.

• It is known that a lack of **vitamin B$_6$** will increase the symptoms of MSG sensitivity. Give 50 mg for at least 12 weeks. (Pregnant and lactating women should not take more than a total of 100 mg of B$_6$.)

ENCOURAGEMENT—Through the enabling grace of Christ, each of us can be an overcomer in the battle with temptation. Let no one say, "I cannot overcome my defects of character"; for if this is your decision, then you cannot have eternal life. The impossibility is all in your will. If you will not, that constitutes the cannot.

The real difficulty is the corruption of an unsanctified heart and an unwillingness to submit to the will of God. When there is a determined purpose born in your heart to overcome, you will have a disposition to overcome. You will cultivate those traits of character that are desirable and will engage in the conflict with steady, persevering effort. You will exercise a ceaseless watchfulness over your defects of character and cultivate right practices in little things. The difficulty of overcoming will be lessened in proportion as the heart is sanctified by the grace of Christ.

TOXEMIA

HYDRO—Here are several suggestions from the *Hydrotherapy* section *(207-275)* of this *Encyclopedia* on detoxifying the body:

Adsorb toxins: Poultices made of charcoal, clay, and glycerin, etc.

Eliminate toxins: These are procedures which encourage vital resistance to disease while at the same time encouraging the destruction of toxins by stimulating the toxin-destroying cells of the thyroid, liver, spleen, lymphatics, and other tissues: Hepatic Douche, Splenic Douche, General Cold Douche. (The word, "douche," in hydrotherapy, means "spray.") Other procedures include Steam Bath *(262)* and Hot Fomentations (234).

Remove waste products: Contrast Baths to the arm, hand, leg, or foot.

Combat local toxemia, resulting degenerations, and localized inflammations: Hot blanket Pack, followed by Sweating Wet Sheet Pack. Repeat every 3-4 hours if necessary. Fomentation to throat every 2-3 hours for 15 minutes. Ice Compress to throat during intervals. If inflammation becomes intense and sloughing is threatened, the Heating Compress at 60° F., changing every hour. Warm Vapor Inhalation.

Combat toxemia: Sweating procedures, Radiant Hot Bath, Sweating Wet Sheet Pack, Steam Bath, prolonged Neutral Bath. Follow hot baths by short cold applications (such as a Wet Sheet Rub, Cold Towel Rub, Cold Shower, Spray Douche, copious water drinking). Enema daily for a week or two, at 70° F.

ENCOURAGEMENT—Give to God the most precious offering you can give. Give Him your heart. He will take it and, with your cooperation, make it pure and clean.

POISONS - 6 - ADDICTIONS
Also: Dangers of Marijuana (293)

TOBACCO WITHDRAWAL

SYMPTOMS—A continual craving for tobacco in some form.

If the person smokes, there is irritation and inflammation of throat and lungs, chronic cough, chronic bronchitis, and premature aging of the skin. This eventually leads to lung cancer, high blood pressure, osteoporosis, emphysema, respiratory ailments, heart disease, stroke, and/or many other diseased conditions and cancers. Women will have intensified problems with menstruation and menopause; and men will have greater prostate trouble. Women who smoke age twice as fast as other women. Their skin rapidly ages; and the result is a dull, lifeless, gray, deteriorating complexion and wrinkles.

If he chews tobacco, there is irritation and inflammation of the lips, mouth, teeth, throat, and esophagus. This eventually leads to cancer of the lip, mouth, tongue, larynx, esophagus, pharynx, and other diseases.

CAUSES—Nicotine is remarkable for the vast number of harmful chemicals it naturally contains, plus those which are added to it during growth or processing of the leaves. Nicotine is also remarkable for its addictive qualities. It ranks with heroin; and some who have been hooked on both declare it to be harder to quit than heroin. Like heroin, cocaine, and alcohol, tobacco gives a sense of relaxation while making the heart pump harder (12-25 beats per minute faster), causing palpitations and a generalized feeling of anxiety. For the smoker who takes the last puff before bedtime, the circulatory system is only normal 2 hours out of every 24.

Each cigarette destroys 25 mg of vitamin C; a full pack in one day eliminates more of this vitamin than is in the diet.

Nearly 500,000 die each year in the U.S. In America alone, tobacco causes 35% of all cancer deaths, 78% of all fatal heart attacks, 18% of deaths of all kinds, 85% of lung cancer, and 85% of obstructive pulmonary disease. More Americans die each year from smoking than from alcohol, illegal drugs, traffic accidents, murder, or suicide. Cigarettes, pipes, etc., are coffin nails which shorten lifespan by at least 15-20 years. Here are some of the blessings you get from the nicotine: lead, carcinogens, cadmium, hydrogen cyanide, carbon monoxide, and over 5,000 other irritating chemicals in tobacco. Tobacco not only injures you, but it also damages those around you: your spouse, your children, your unborn, and fellow workmen. Did you know that the breath of a smoker contains slightly more nicotine than the side smoke from his cigarette? Men and women who smoke are constantly exhaling air into the room for their children to breathe.

NATURAL REMEDIES

Withdrawal symptoms include cough, depression, anxiety, headaches, stomach cramps, irritability, hunger, and cravings for tobacco. This continues for about 2 weeks. If supplementary treatment is given, the crisis can be weathered easier, with less likelihood of a return to smoking.

• The craving for a smoke only lasts 3-5 minutes; then it returns later for another 3-5 minutes. As time passes, it gets easier to resist the urge.

• In order to quit, it is best to accompany a firm decision with a **cleansing program**. This helps speed up the elimination of stored-up nicotine and other poisons. The quicker this happens, the faster the cravings cease.

• A **nutritious diet** must be adhered to. **Carrot juice** and **citrus juices** are very helpful. **Vitamin C** (5,000-25,000 mg in divided doses daily) is important.

• Take the tobacco pack, or can, and throw it away. In its place put a **candy bar**. Blood sugar level is a factor in the addiction. When the cravings are successfully gone, throw away the candies.

• Take extra **calcium** and **chamomile** 3-6 times a day. Both will help to relax during the withdrawal period. Vitamin **B complex** is also important for the nerves.

• **Lobelia** contains *lobeline*, which is similar to nicotine. It is non-addictive, but helps a person quit tobacco. Here is how to use it in aversion therapy:

• Only smoke one hour each day; at which time 15 drops of lobelia, diluted in water, are swallowed every half an hour and then 15 minutes before lighting the first cigarette. With each 15-minute period, an additional 15 drops are added to the water, to drink while the cigarettes are smoked. The result will be nausea, which the mind will associate with the cigarettes. This kills the desire for the cigarettes.

• If the lobelia method is not used, the alternative must be a definite quit-all-at-once approach. *See the author's book. How to Quit Tobacco (see back of this book).*

• Keep a stick of **licorice** in your pocket; and suck on it when you want a smoke. Or munch on a raw carrot.

• Do **deep breathing** exercises, whenever you feel an urge to smoke.

• The following herbs help get you off tobacco: **ginger, catnip, skullcap, hops, burdock root, red clover, slippery elm, and cayenne**. Take whichever ones you want, together or alone. Eat **garlic. Stop eating junk food and meat**.

—*Also 208. Also see How to Quit Tobacco (819-821).. Also Dangers of Marijuana (953, and 953-963).*

HYDRO—Here are suggestions from the hydrotherapy section of this *Encyclopedia (207-275)*:

• **Heating and Sweating Packs** can be used for the elimination of nicotine from the body, thus lessening the physical craving for more tobacco .

• Taking **steam baths** during the withdrawal are also useful in tobacco addictions.

J.H. KELLOGG, M.D., PRESCRIPTIONS FOR ELIMINATING DRUG HABITS AND THEIR COMPLICATIONS (*how to give these water therapies: pp. 206-275 / Hydrotherapy Disease Index: pp. 273-275*)

TOBACCO HABIT—

GENERAL—Drop the drug at once. Put him to **bed**. **Sweating procedures** (such as Radiant Heat Bath, Steam Bath, sweating Wet Sheet Pack) twice daily. Follow with **short cold application** (as Shallow Cold Bath, Wet Sheet Rub, or Cold Douche). **Alternate hot and cold Compress** to spine, 3 times a day. **Hot Abdominal Pack** day and night, renewing 3 times daily. Copious **water** drinking and large **Colonic** daily.

ENCOURAGEMENT—God can give you the help you need. Go to Him and tell Him you need His help. Surrender your life to Him. In His strength, you can overcome the tobacco habit.

DELIRIUM TREMENS

SYMPTOMS—Visual and auditory hallucinations, convulsions, acute anxiety, wild expression on face, pulse feeble and rapid, profuse perspiration, possibly fever.

CAUSES—Severe symptoms immediately following very heavy drinking of alcoholic beverages.

The following article explains how to recover from alcoholism; this one is about the immediate crisis.

NATURAL REMEDIES

• Place him in a **neutral bath** and keep him there as long as possible, 2 or 3 hours or more. Keep the **head cool** with towels wrung out of cold water. Put these around the neck and on the head.

• While he is still in the bath, have him drink **hot, soothing, quieting herbs** (such as **catnip, skullcap, peppermint, spearmint, valerian, gentian, sweet balm, and/or calamus root**). Do not make the tea too strong. Use a small teaspoon of herbs in 1 cup of water.

• Several times, while he is in the bathtub, give him a **short, cold shower** or sponge bath.

• Just before finishing, give him a brisk **salt glow**.

• Put him back in the **warm water**, so he can become thoroughly warm. Then give a final **cold shower** or rub. Dry thoroughly.

• Put him to **bed** in a warm, well-ventilated room.

• Give 2 high **enemas** each day. Herbs kill poisons better than water; so use tea of **bayberry bark or red raspberry leaves**. Use **laxative herbs** to keep the bowels open.

• Give **bayberry bark and lobelia** as an emetic to clean out the stomach. Repeat the vomiting until the stomach and throat are entirely clean.

ENCOURAGEMENT—How thankful you can be every day of your life that, through the enabling grace of Jesus Christ, you can obey all that God asks of you in the Bible.

ALCOHOL WITHDRAWAL

SYMPTOMS—Dependence on, and addiction to, alcoholic beverages. Depression, blackouts, hangovers, arrests, ulcers, emotional problems, flushing of the face, forgetfulness, heart palpitation, indigestion, insomnia, urinary problems, hepatitis, hypertension, divorce, hard drugs, and numbness in the extremities.

CAUSES—Alcohol is absorbed directly through the walls of the stomach, without digestion. It then travels in the bloodstream to every cell in the body, where it extracts water. This weakens or kills cells. The effect on the liver, brain, and vital organs is especially damaging. Most alcoholics are either hypoglycemic or borderline diabetics.

In addition, alcohol produces severe nutritional deficiencies. The body thinks it is well-fed (alcohol contains 70 calories per ounce) while it is being slowly starved.

The liver slowly breaks the alcohol down to sugar. Eventually the difficult task weakens this vital organ, and fatty liver degeneration begins. Scar tissue develops; the experts call it cirrhosis *of the liver (450).* Binge drinking (drinking heavily for several days) can lead to cardiac arrhythmia.

Alcohol is deceptive: It makes a person feel happy, when he is miserable, and strong when he is weak. It ruins his liver, destroys his marriage, hurts his children, eliminates his employment, and makes a bum out of him. The liquor industry should be closed down.

NATURAL REMEDIES

• **Stop drinking** alcohol entirely. Begin eating very **nutritious food. Vitamins A** (5,000 IU), **B complex, C** (1,000 mg), **D** (1,000 mg), **and K** (140 mcg) are needed in addition to **zinc, iron, potassium, calcium, essential fatty acids, bioflavonoids, and adequate protein**. Sea **kelp** is important, to help the thyroid.

• **Avoid certain foods** which increase the craving for alcohol in those who indulge in it. These include **milk, wheat, corn products, chocolate, and sugar.**

• After going off alcohol, do not substitute large amounts of **sugar** products and strong **coffee**. Sugar only increases the hypoglycemic problem. Nourish the system with good food; do not sugarize it.

• The alcoholic craves **potassium**. One teaspoon of **honey**, to take the place of a beer, supplies some of the potassium which has been depleted by the alcohol. Also high in potassium is **potato peel soup**. The peelings should be about a half inch thick; discard the rest of the potatoes. Cover with water, cook well, then blend and add a little salt. He should eat it often with his meals.

• 1 teaspoon of 50-50 powdered **charcoal and honey** will help sober up a drunk person.

• People who regularly eat good nourishing food are less likely to crave stimulants or addictive substances. Especially eat **raw fruits, vegetables, and nuts**. These are nourishing and have lots of fiber.

• Meat eating will bring back the craving for alcohol; so **quit meat**. Get regular outdoors **exercise**.

• An excellent combination to help a person get off alcohol is take the amino acids, **tyrosine** and **tryptophan**, along with **vitamin B$_6$, niacin, hops, valerian,** and **passionflower**.

• **Slippery elm** is good to drink while going off alcohol.

• **Quassia chips** help destroy the taste for liquor. Put 1 teaspoon in 1 cup of boiled water and steep a half hour while covered. Take a swallow every 2 hours. Stay with someone, so you will not be tempted to go out and buy more of the cursed stuff.

• Blend up some **orange peel** with **water** and a little **cayenne**. It will help wean away from liquor.

• Drinking **angelica** tea helps produce a disgust for liquor. **Chamomile** tea helps during the withdrawal.

• **Hops tea** is good during delirium tremens.

HYDRO—Here are suggestions from the Hydrotherapy section of this *Encyclopedia (206-275):*

• The **neutral wet-sheet pack** is excellent for alcoholic delirium. A neutral bath will accomplish the same purpose as a neutral pack; it will probably do it better. Heating and sweating packs are also used for alcoholism.

• Withdraw alcohol at once. Nutritive **enemas**, copious **water** drinking. Neutral **colonic** daily, for a week.

• The **Steam Bath** is also useful in chronic alcoholism. A lot of toxins come out in the sweat.

J.H. KELLOGG, M.D., PRESCRIPTIONS FOR ELIMINATING DRUG HABITS AND THEIR COMPLICATIONS *(how to give these water therapies: pp. 206-275 / list of treatments: pp. 206-207 / Hydrotherapy Disease Index: pp. 273-275)*

ALCOHOLISM—

GENERAL—Aseptic dietary, especially fruits. Meats and flesh foods must be strictly prohibited. This includes meat juices, broths, and all preparations of flesh. **Fomentation** over the stomach twice a day with Hot **Abdominal Pack** between applications, short **sweating baths** (Radiant Heat Bath, sweating Wet Sheet Pack), followed by **Wet Sheet Rub. Graduated Cold Baths** twice a day.

INSOMNIA—Neutral Bath at bed time, 94°-96° F., 20-60 minutes. Hot **Abdominal Pack** at night. *See Insomnia (547).*

VOMITING—Ice pills swallowed, **ice bag** over stomach, **hot and cold compress** over stomach.

DELIRIUM TREMENS—Rest in bed. **Hot Full Bath** for 5 minutes. **Hot Blanket Pack**, followed by sweating **Wet Sheet Pack**, **Neutral Bath** for 1-2 hours or longer, twice a day. **Ice Cap**. Hot **Fomentations** over stomach and abdomen every 3 hours, for 15 minutes. During interval between, **Heating Compress**, changing every 30-60 minutes. Copious water drinking and large **Enema** daily. Exclusive **fruit diet** for 2-3 days.

COUNTERACT NARCOTIC EFFECTS OF ALCOHOL—Cold Shower, **water** drinking or **Enema**, followed by short **Cold Douche** to spine and lower sternum. Repeat every hour or two if necessary, until the toxic effects disappear.

NEPHRITIS—Usually present in acute alcoholism; treat as for kidney disease.

GENERAL METHOD—He must be placed in a proper environment; isolation and confinement may be required. Suitable mental and moral influences must be brought to bear.*Also p. 25.*

—*Also see Wernicke-Korsakoff Syndrome (554).*

ENCOURAGEMENT—Only in Christ's strength can you be strong to resist the temptations which assail you. Plead with God for forgiveness. Accept Christ as your Saviour and ask Him to make you a new person. If you are determined to stand true, and cry to Him moment by moment as His little child, He can help you overcome.

COFFEE WITHDRAWAL ALSO 915

PROBLEMS—Coffee and black tea are both addictive and damaging to the system. If you think you are not addicted to your coffee, try to immediately terminate its use.

When it is regularly used, the body enters into a very special chemical dependency on coffee. Immediate withdrawal can cause heart problems. Therefore, gradually go off coffee, taking less and less of it, over a seven-day period. During that time, and afterward if necessary, give the following therapy: — *Also 915.*

NATURAL REMEDIES

WATER THERAPY

The following suggestions for withdrawing from the coffee and black tea addictions are from the hydrotherapy chapter in this *Encyclopedia (206-275):*

• Discontinue the use of the drug at once. If necessary, employ some harmless cereal substitute. **Neutral Bath** at bedtime, **Fomentation** over abdomen, **alternate sponging** of the spine, **cold mitten friction or cold towel rub** before rising in the morning. **Hot abdominal pack** night and day (changing morning, noon, and night), short **sweating wet sheet pack or steam bath** 2-3 times a week. Followed by a **cold** application.

J.H. KELLOGG, M.D., PRESCRIPTIONS FOR ELIMINATING DRUG HABITS AND THEIR COMPLICATIONS *(how to give these water therapies: pp. 206-275 / Hydrotherapy Disease Index: pp. 273-275)*

TEA AND COFFEE HABIT—

WARNING—The long-term effects of caffeine are not so pleasant. Dr. Han Me and colleagues from Pusan National University in Korea reported in a 2005 study published in "Biochemical Biophysical Research Communication Journal" that long-term consumption of low doses of caffeine slowed the functions of hippocampus. This area in the brain is responsible for long-term memory and learning. The authors concluded that although caffeine might improve person's alertness for a short period of time, it actually slows down the learning and memory via decreasing the function of hippocampus.

ENCOURAGEMENT—God can help you, just where you are. He can reach down and lift you up; He can help you overcome the coffee habit.

DRUG WITHDRAWAL

SYMPTOMS—Decreased desire to work, inattentiveness, extreme drowsiness, frequent mood swings, loss of appetite, and restlessness.

Prolonged use may result in damage to cells, chromosomes, liver, kidney, and respiratory organs. There is a real danger of cancer and male sterility.

Withdrawal symptoms include insomnia, headache, diarrhea, sensitivity to light and noise, hot and cold flashes, sweating, deep depression, irritability, disorientation, and irrational thinking.

CAUSES—There are legal drugs (medicinal drugs), which you can obtain at a pharmacy. There are also illegal ones, called hard drugs or street drugs. These include narcotics, stimulants, barbiturates, and hallucinogens. In nearly every instance, drugs are toxic and dangerous. Exceptions are the natural products which the FDA erroneously classifies as "drugs." Included here are such things as charcoal tablets and peppermint tea.

People often start taking drugs (such as nicotine, alcohol, and coffee) because they think these are harmless, enjoyable, or beneficial. But they are none of these. Frequently the dose is increased, to obtain the same pleasant effect; but the body is increasingly injured.

NATURAL REMEDIES

• **Withdrawal** from the drug must be done. When a person is highly dependent on a drug, it is best that the dose gradually be reduced over a four-week period. Regarding the hard drugs, it is best that withdrawal be done under professional guidance.

• **Nutritious food** should be eaten along with heavy **vitamin / mineral** supplementation. **Vitamins C** and **B complex** are especially important. Drink lots of water and get extra **rest**. Take **sweat baths**, to help excrete poisons.

• **Valerian** root has a calming effect. Use it with **Siberian ginseng** and the amino acid, **tyrosine**.

• **St. John's wort** minimizes depression during withdrawal.

HYDROTHERAPY

The following water therapies are used for opium, cocaine, and related addictive habits:

General: **Rest** in bed. Give **sweating baths** (such as a **Steam Bath**) twice a day, for 3 days before withdrawing the drug. Follow bath by vigorous cold applications. While withdrawing the drug, the symptoms may be successfully combated with the following water therapies.

Nervousness, restlessness, "indescribable sensations": Prolonged **Neutral Bath** at 92°-94° F., for 10 minutes.

Cardiac weakness: **Cold Compress or Ice Bag** over heart, alternate (hot and then cold) applications to the spine, **Cold Mitten Friction**, **Cold Towel Rub**. Repeating treatment hourly if necessary.

Vomiting: **Hot and Cold Truck Pack**, **Ice Bag** over stomach and spine, **Hot Leg Pack**.

Diarrhea: **Hot Enema** after each movement. **Cold Compress** over abdomen, changed every 30 minutes.

Local pain: Revulsive **Compresses** or a compress that alternates hot and cold.

Insomnia after withdrawal: **Wet sheet pack**. Prolonged **Neutral Bath**, 20-60 minutes. Heating **Leg Pack**, Hot **Abdominal Pack**, cold **Ice Cap**.

—Also see Alcohol Withdrawal (881), Tobacco Withdrawal (880), Drug Rash (877), Hard Drug Warning Signals (824-827). Also Dangers of Marijuana (953).

ENCOURAGEMENT—Every wrong habit can be resisted and overcome in the strength of Christ. He died to forgive your sins and strengthen you to resist the temptations of the devil. Trust in Him, live for Him, and determine that you will do what is right.

Since Jesus came to dwell with us, we know that God is acquainted with our trials and sympathizes with our griefs. Every son and daughter of Adam may understand that our Creator is the friend of sinners. In every promise of joy, every deed of love, every divine attraction presented in the Saviour's life on earth, we see "God with us" (Matt. 1:23). Jesus cares for each one of us as though there were not another individual on the face of the earth. As Deity, He exerts mighty power in our behalf while, as our Elder Brother, He feels for all our woes. The Majesty of heaven held not Himself aloof from degraded, sinful humanity. We have not a high priest who is so high, so lifted up, that He cannot notice us or sympathize with us, but one who was in all points tempted like as we are, yet without sin.

More Encouragement

"The Elder Brother of our race is by the eternal throne. He looks upon every soul who is turning his face toward Him as the Saviour. He knows by experience what are the weaknesses of humanity, what are our wants, and where lies the strength of our temptations; for He was in all points tempted like as we are, yet without sin. He is watching over you, trembling child of God. Are you tempted? He will deliver. Are you weak? He will strengthen. Are you ignorant? He will enlighten. Are you wounded? He will heal. The Lord 'telleth the number of the stars;' and yet 'He healeth the broken in heart, and bindeth up their wounds.' Psalm 147:4, 3. 'Come unto Me,' is His invitation. Whatever your anxieties and trials, spread out your case before the Lord. Your spirit will be braced for endurance. The way will be opened for you to disentangle yourself from embarrassment and difficulty. The weaker and more helpless you know yourself to be, the stronger will you become in His strength. The heavier your burdens, the more blessed the rest in casting them upon the Burden Bearer. The rest that Christ offers depends upon conditions, but these conditions are plainly specified. They are those with which all can comply. He tells us just how His rest is to be found.

" 'Take My yoke upon you,' Jesus says. The yoke is an instrument of service. Cattle are yoked for labor, and the yoke is essential that they may labor effectually. By this illustration Christ teaches us that we are called to service as long as life shall last. We are to take upon us His yoke, that we may be coworkers with Him.

"The yoke that binds to service is the law of God. The great law of love revealed in Eden, proclaimed upon Sinai, and in the new covenant written in the heart, is that which binds the human worker to the will of God. If we were left to follow our own inclinations, to go just where our will would lead us, we should fall into Satan's ranks and become possessors of his attributes. Therefore God confines us to His will, which is high, and noble, and elevating."

—Desire of Ages, 329

The Natural Remedies Encyclopedia

Poisonous Creatures

Sixteen color pictures of the most poisonous creatures in the U.S.: This is a rather complete color picture identification guide to poisonous reptiles and insects, plus the general appearance of their bites and stings. Many of these are described in the preceding chapter. Rattlesnake 885 / American Copperhead 885 / Eastern Diamondback Rattlesnake 885 / Coral Snake 885 / Cottonmouth 886 / Brown Recluse 886 / Female Black Widow 886 / Black Widow Bites 886 / Male Black Widow 886 / Brown Recluse Bites 886 / Mosquito Bite 887 / Lice 887 / Tick Bite 887 / Lice Bite 887 / Chigger Bites 887 / Mite Bite 887

— Plus 17 more pictures on 888

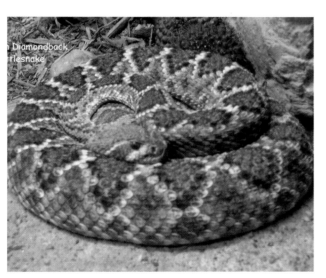

Rattlesnake

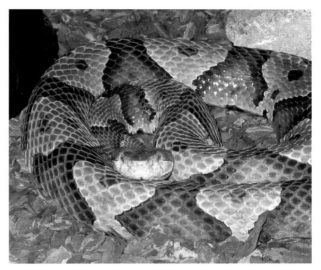

American Copperhead

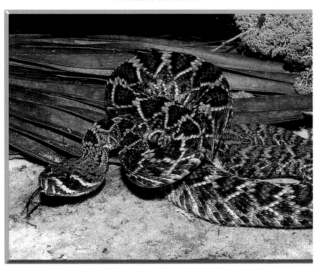

Eastern Diamondback Rattlesnake

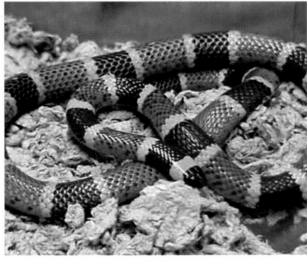

Coral Snake

CREATURES

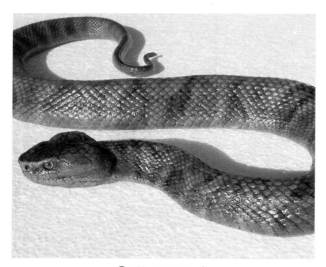

Cottonmouth

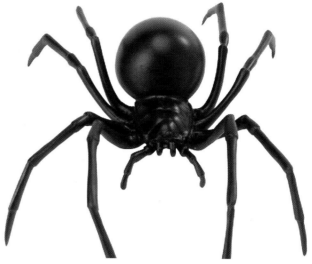

Female Black Widow

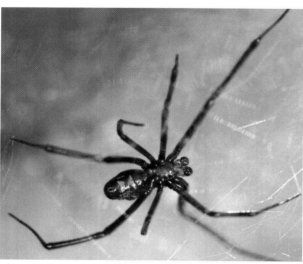

Male Black Widow

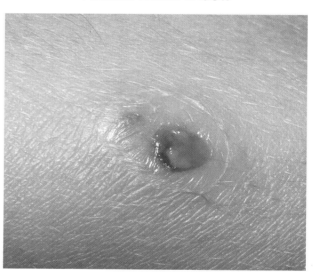

Black Widow Bites

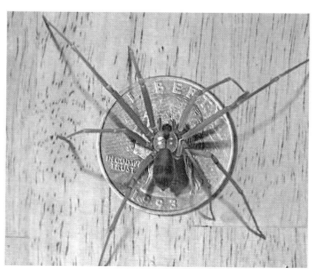

Brown Recluse

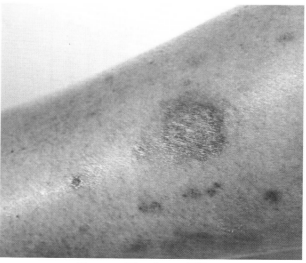

Brown Recluse Bites

CREATURES

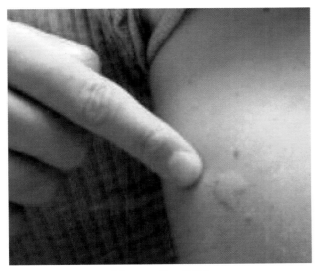

Mosquito Bite

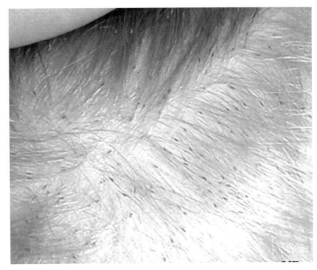

Lice

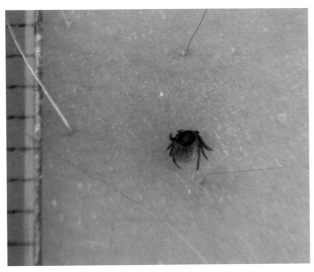

Tick Bite

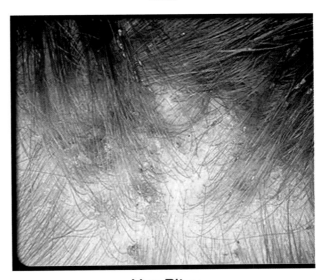

Lice Bites

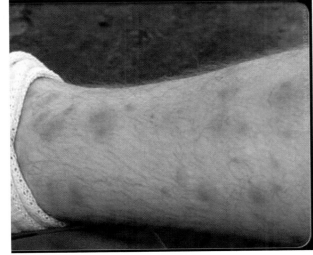

Chigger bite

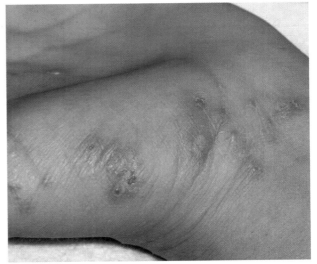

Mite Bites

CREATURES

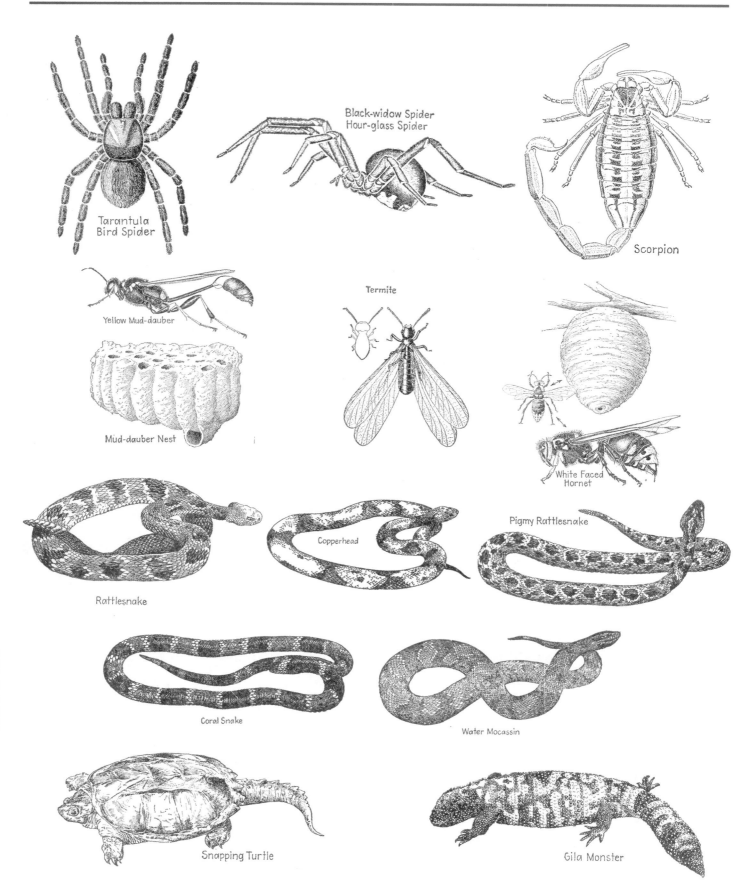

Tarantula
Bird Spider

Black-widow Spider
Hour-glass Spider

Scorpion

Yellow Mud-dauber

Mud-dauber Nest

Termite

White Faced
Hornet

Rattlesnake

Copperhead

Pigmy Rattlesnake

Coral Snake

Water Mocassin

Snapping Turtle

Gila Monster

CREATURES

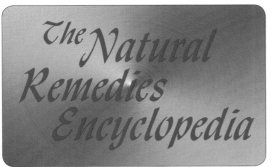

The Natural Remedies Encyclopedia

Harmful Substances

GUIDE TO OVER 200 HARMFUL STUBSTANCES IN AND AROUND YOU HOME

Poisons (828-884) contains additional valuable information

1 - HARMFUL SUBSTANCES GUIDE

OVER 200 DANGEROUS SUBSTANCES

Table of Contents

In the back of this book will be found A SPE-CIAL INDEX to these HARMFUL SUBSTANCES (1084-1086) found in this chapter.

HARMFUL

I – Processed Foods

The processed food industry loads fat, sugar, and salt into their products because they are cheap. They use chemicals to change these cheap, raw materials into brightly colored, tasty products with a long shelf life. Food producers buy the cheapest raw materials, manufacture the product as quickly as possible, then sell it for the highest price. Good business sense, but what is lost in the manufacturing is quality.

Aluminum compounds are added to baking powder, aspirin, antacids, beer, table salt, and antiperspirants. It also leaches into our food and water through cookware, soft drink cans, and aluminum foil. It has been discovered, in high concentrations, in the brains of Alzheimer's patients and is suspected in contributing to this most hideous disease.

A child consuming a soup containing **MSG (monosodium glutamate)** plus a drink with **NutraSweet** will have a blood level of excitotoxins six times the blood level that destroys hypothalamus neurons in baby mice. The younger the child, the greater the danger to the brain. Baby mice fed MSG grow up to be short and grossly obese, despite dietary intake in normal amounts for mice.

Ice cream producers use **propylene glycol**, the same substance in antifreeze and paint remover. **Carboxymethylcellulose** is a stabilizer that is used in ice cream, salad dressing, cheese spreads, and chocolate milk. It has produced tumors in 80% of rats injected.

Sodium levels in most manufactured foods need

to be lower, according to the *World Action on Salt and Health* (WASH), representing 194 medical experts in 48 countries. They pressured food companies to lower the salt content of prepared foods, but without success.

Synthetic color adds nothing to nutritional value. Numerous colors have been banned after twenty years on the market, because they were carcinogenic. All **certified food colors** in use today are of a class of chemicals called *polycyclic aromatic hydrocarbons* (derived from coal tar) that are carcinogenic.

Fast foods are relatively inexpensive foods that are prepared and served quickly. The fast-food industry had its beginnings around the mid-twentieth century; and it has grown tremendously since then.

The most common type of U.S. **fast-food restaurants** specializes in a meal consisting of a hamburger, French fries, and a beverage. Many fast foods are fried; are high in fat and sodium; and low in fiber, vitamins, and some minerals. The "added value" option, whereby customers can order larger sizes for a minimal additional charge, adds to the total calorie and fat intake.

The fetus cannot deal with foreign chemicals. Whatever toxic substances the mother eats flow largely unimpeded into the unborn child. Unlike an adult, the fetus lacks protective, detoxifying systems. *Teratogens* are toxins which harm fetal development. Certain food additives are considered teratogenic.

Toxicology testing cannot accurately predict the long-term combined effect of **3,000 additives** and environmental toxins on children, the elderly, newborn, the fetus, and people with cancer. The combined effect of these toxins on humans is unknown.

How to live longer—Do not eat commercially processed foods such as **cookies, cakes, crackers, TV dinners, soft drinks, packaged sauce mixes**, etc.

• Avoid all **refined sweeteners** such as **sugar, dextrose, glucose and high-fructose corn syrup**.

• Avoid white flour, **white flour products,** and **white rice**. Avoid **fried foods**.

• Avoid all **hydrogenated or partially hydrogenated fats and oils**. Avoid **most grocery store vegetable oils** made from soy, corn, safflower, canola, or cottonseed. They are highly processed for longer shelf life.

• Do not use polyunsaturated oils for cooking, sauteing, or baking. Keep them refrigerated and use them raw at the table.

• Avoid products containing **protein powders**.

• Avoid **processed meat** and **pasteurized milk**. Do not consume lowfat milk, skim milk, powdered milk or imitation milk products.

• Avoid **rancid and improperly prepared seeds, nuts, and grains** found in granolas, quick-rise breads, and extruded breakfast cereals; since they block mineral absorption and cause intestinal distress.

• Avoid **canned, sprayed, waxed, bioengineered, or irradiated fruits and vegetables**.

• Avoid **artificial food additives** (especially **MSG, hydrolyzed vegetable protein, and aspartame**) which are neurotoxins. Most soups, sauce and broth mixes, and commercial condiments contain MSG.

HARMFUL

• Avoid **caffeine-containing beverages**—such as **coffee, tea, soft drinks, and chocolate drinks**.

• Avoid **aluminum-containing foods** such as commercial **salt, baking powder, and antacids**. Do not use **aluminum** cookware or aluminum-containing deodorants.

• Do not drink **fluoridated water**. Purchase a water distiller or a good-quality water filter. They can eliminate chlorine, fluorine, iron, or other contaminants in the water.

• Avoid **synthetic vitamins** and foods with them.

• Do not use **GM (genetically modified) foods**. Genetic engineering brings about combinations of genes that would never occur naturally, and can result in the random incorporation of new genes into the DNA of the one eating them. GM foods are not safe. It will be years before we will understand all their dangers.

THE HIDDEN DANGERS IN PROCESSED FOODS

Every day, 7 percent of the U.S. population visits a McDonald's, and 20-25 percent eat fast food of some kind, says Steven Gortmaker, professor of society, human development, and health at the Harvard School of Public Health. As for children, 30 percent between the ages of 4 and 19 eat fast food on any given day.

But that's just the tip of the iceberg. Americans get processed food not only from fast-food restaurants but also from their neighborhood grocery stores. As it stands, about 90 percent of the money that Americans spend on food is used to buy processed foods.

Is your diet filled with harmful ingredients that are damaging your health? For example, saturated fats may be increasing not only your risk of a heart attack, but the severity as well. A report by the *National Institute of Medicine* concluded that there is no level of trans fats that is safe to consume. Salt has been called one of the deadliest ingredients in the food supply and some organizations believe sugary foods, like soft drinks, are so detrimental to health they should carry warning labels. What can you do about it? Read more to find out where they lurk, why you should limit them, and how to do it.

Processed, packaged foods have almost completely taken over the diet of Americans. It is an astounding fact, as mentioned above, that according to industry estimates nearly 90 percent of our household food budget is spent on processed foods.

Unfortunately, most processed foods are laden with sweeteners, salts, artificial flavors, factory-created fats, colorings, chemicals that alter texture, and preservatives. But the trouble is not just what has been added, but what has been taken away. Processed foods are often stripped of nutrients designed by nature to protect your heart, such as soluble fiber, antioxidants, and "good" fats. Combine that with additives and the lack of many basic nutrients, and you have a recipe for disaster.

Here are several very important ingredients in processed foods which you should beware of:

TRANS FATS

Trans fats are man-made or processed fats, which are made from a liquid oil. When you add hydrogen to liquid vegetable oil and then add pressure, the result is a stiffer fat, like the fat found in a can of Crisco. Trans fats are also called *hydrogenated fats.*

Trans fats are found in many processed foods. Including cookies, bakery muffins, various crackers, microwave-popcorn, snack foods, some deep-fried foods (french fries, donuts, chicken nuggets, etc.), and especially fast-food "French Fries", even the stick margarine you may rely on as a "heart-healthy" alternative to saturated-fat-laden butter likely contains it.

The restaurant industry (especially fast food places!) is the very worst for trans fat. When dining out avoid deep-fried foods or ask whether the oil used is free of these fats.

The U.S. Food and Drug Administration shed light on a potentially serious health threat recently when it announced that products containing trans fatty acids require stringent nutritional labeling starting in 2006. And one city in the U.S. has gone further. In December 2006, New York City became the first city in the nation to ban artificial trans fats at all restaurants. Restaurants in the city will be required to eliminate the artificial trans fats from all of their foods by July 2008.

Once hailed as a cheap, heart-friendly replacement for butter, lard, and coconut oil, **trans fats have, in recent times, been denounced by one Harvard nutrition expert as "the biggest food-processing disaster in U.S. history."** Why? Research now reveals trans fats are twice as dangerous for your heart as saturated fat, and cause an estimated 30,000 to 100,000 premature heart disease deaths each year.

In the *Harvard Nurses' Health Study* involving over 80,000 women, those women who consumed the most trans fats were 50% more likely to develop heart disease and almost 40% more likely to develop type 2 diabetes. According to this comprehensive health sttudy—the largest investigation of women and chronic disease—trans fats double the risk of heart disease in women.

In the *Seven Countries Study* involving over 11,000 men, a diet high in saturated fat was identified as one of the most important risk factors causing death from heart disease.

Trans fats are especially bad for your heart than saturated fats because they boost your levels of "bad" LDL cholesterol in the blood, and decrease "good" HDL cholesterol in the blood. That's double trouble for your arteries. These fats also make the arteries stiff and may increase the risk of type 2 diabetes. And unlike saturated fats, trans fats also raise your levels of artery-clogging lipoprotein and triglycerides. They may also increase the risk of type 2 diabetes, Alzheimer's disease and some cancers.

Trans fats is supposed to be listed on the "Nutrition Facts" panel on food packages. Also check the ingredient list for any of these words: "partially hydrogenated," "fractionated," or "hydrogenated" (fully hydrogenated fats are not a heart threat, but some trans fats are mislabeled as "hydrogenated"). The higher up the phrase "partially hydrogenated oil" is on the list of ingredients, the more trans fat the product contains.

Replacing trans fats with good fats could cut your heart attack risk by a surprising 53 percent.

Recommended intake is no more than 2 grams daily (ideally as close to 0 grams as possible). Check the labels, and look for products that are trans fat free.

Trans fats pose a higher risk of heart disease than saturated fats, which were once believed to be the worst kind of fats. While it is true that saturated fats—found in butter, cheese and beef, for example—raise total cholesterol levels, trans fats go a step further. Trans fats not only raise total cholesterol levels, they also deplete good cholesterol (HDL), which helps protect against heart disease.

The stiffer and harder that the regular fats are, the more they clog up your arteries. **Artificial trans fats have the same effect in your body as grease**; the same as what bacon grease does to kitchen sinks. Over time, they can "clog the pipes" that feed the heart and brain, which can lead to heart attack or stroke risk.

No human body has any need for these man-made fats. **Food manufacturers started putting them in products because they allow for a longer shelf life.** Crackers, for example, can stay on the shelf and stay crispy for years in part because of the hydrogenated fats in them.

Children are at an even greater risk. Because trans fats increase the risk for heart disease, therefore children who start at age 3 or 4 eating a steady diet of fast food, pop tarts, commercially prepared fish sticks, stick margarine, cake, candy, cookies and microwave popcorn can be expected to get heart disease earlier than kids who are eating foods without trans fats.

While a person may not get heart disease until they are in their 40s, some research at the University of Maryland has shown that kids as young as 8, 9 and 10 already have the high cholesterol and blood fats that clog arteries. By starting healthy eating habits early, parents can help their children avoid heart attacks and stroke.

What Steps Can Parents Take to help their children? Model healthy eating behaviors. Make healthy choices available. Try new fruits, vegetables, beans, chicken and other foods and recipes. Cook or prepare food more often as a family. Guard against fatigue because a tired parent can rely too heavily on fast foods or highly processed foods.

Learn how to identify high fat and trans fat foods. Because the U.S. Food and Drug Administration began requiring food labels to list trans fats in January 2006, trans fats are listed under the Fat category of the Nutrition Facts panel. Many foods are now formulated to be trans fat free. Naturally low fat foods are generally the best: fruits of all types, vegetables, beans, whole grains, breads and some cereals. These foods can be fixed in fun ways that your children will enjoy.

Learn the categories of foods that are likely to have trans fats: Fast foods - fried chicken, biscuits, fried fish sandwiches, French fries, fried apple or other pie desserts. Donuts, muffins. Crackers. Many cookies. Cake, cake icing, & pie. Microwave popped corn. Canned biscuits. International and instant latte coffee beverages parents are more likely to use.

High fat milk products (whole and 2% milk, cheese, butter, cream, ice cream) and fatty meats (ground beef, hamburgers, hot dogs, sausages, salami, bologna, ribs, chicken wings), as well as tropical oils (coconut oil, palm oil, palm kernel oil).

Be a smart shopper. Don't shop when you're hungry because you're more likely to make poor choices and buy on impulse when you shop on an empty stomach. If you take the children with you, give them a satisfying snack before you go. Stand firm in your plans about what you will and will not purchase.. Shop the perimeter of the store. Most of the processed foods, which contain a lot of trans fats, are on the inner isles of the supermarket.

When you do purchase processed foods, choose the lower fat versions of crackers, cereals and desserts. Finally, remember that you are responsible for the quality of the foods you bring into the house for your children. Children eat the foods that are available to them.

The dangers and risks of eating meat are still not understood by many, despite the evidence. Here are facts you should be aware of: Eating meat is one of the biggest health hazards today. Cows, pigs, lambs, hens, and turkeys are, among other ingredients, given a diet of reject meat mixed with fecal matter to eat. When an animal is killed for food, about half of its weight is not sold to the human food industry, but instead ground up and put as pellets into the feed of food animals. No animal is too decomposed to be omitted from the feed.

CANOLA OIL

Rapeseed oil was a monounsaturated oil that had been used extensively in many parts of the world, notably in China, Japan, and India. It contains almost 60 percent monounsaturated fatty acids (compared to about 70 percent in olive oil). Unfortunately, **about two-thirds of the monounsaturated fatty acids in rapeseed oil are erucic acid**, a 22-carbon monounsaturated fatty acid that had been associated with Keshan's disease, characterized by fibrotic lesions of the heart.

In the late 1970s, using a technique of genetic manipulation involving seed splitting (*R.K. Downey, Genetic Control of Fatty Acid Biosnythesis in Rapeseed. Journal of the American Oil Chemists' Society, 1964;41:475-478.*), Canadian plant breeders came up with a variety of rapeseed that produced a monounsaturated oil low in 22-carbon erucic acid and high in 18-carbon oleic acid.

The new oil, referred to as LEAR oil for *Low-*

Erucic-Acid Rapeseed, was slow to catch on in the U.S. In 1986, Cargill announced the sale of LEAR oil seed to U.S. farmers and provided LEAR oil processing at its Riverside, North Dakota plant; but prices dropped and farmers took a hit *(Journal of the American Oil Chemists' Society, December 1986;63(12):1510).*

Before LEAR oil could be promoted as a healthy alternative to polyunsaturated oils, it needed a new name. Neither "rape" nor "lear" could be expected to invoke a healthy image for the new "Cinderella" crop. In 1978, the industry settled on *"canola,"* for "Canadian oil," since most of the new rapeseed at that time was grown in Canada.

"Canola" also sounded like "can do" and "payola," both positive phrases in marketing lingo. However, the new name did not come into widespread use until the early 1990s.

An initial challenge for the Canola Council of Canada was the fact that rapeseed had never been given GRAS *(Generally Recognized as Safe)* status by the U.S. Food and Drug Administration. A change in regulation would be necessary before canola could be marketed in the U.S. *(Canola - a new oilseed from Canada. Journal of the American Oil Chemists' Society, September 1981:723A-9A).* Just how this was done has not been revealed, but GRAS status was granted in 1985. Why? Because the Canadian government paid the FDA the sum of $50 million to have rape registered and recognized as "safe" *(Source: John Thomas, Young Again, and others).*

Canola was primarily aimed at the growing numbers of health-conscious consumers rather than the junk food market. Therefore more subtle marketing techniques than merely television advertising were needed. The industry had managed to manipulate the science, to make a perfect match with canola oil: It claimed it to be very low in saturated fat, very rich in monounsaturates, and very safe healthwise *(Canola - a new oilseed from Canada. Journal of the American Oil Chemists' Society, September 1981:723A-9A).*

In addition, canola oil contains about 10 percent omega-3 fatty acids—the most recent discovery by establishment nutritionists. Most Americans are deficient in omega-3 fatty acids, which had been shown to be beneficial to the heart and immune system. The challenge was to market this dream-come-true fatty acid profile in a way that would appeal to educated consumers.

The canola industry's approach was immensely successful: scientific conferences, promotion to upscale consumers through books (like *The Omega Diet),* and articles in the health section of newspapers and magazines. By the late 1990s, canola use had soared, not just in the U.S.

Today China, Japan, Europe, Mexico, Bangladesh, and Pakistan all buy significant amounts.

How canola oil is processed: The oil is removed by a combination of high temperature mechanical pressing and solvent extraction. Traces of the solvent (usually *hexane)* remain in the oil, even after consider-able refining.

Like all modern vegetable oils, canola oil goes through the process of caustic refining, bleaching, and degumming—all of which involve high temperatures or chemicals of questionable safety. And because canola oil is high in omega-3 fatty acids (which easily become rancid and foul-smelling when subjected to oxygen and high temperatures), it must be deodorized. The standard deodorization process removes a large portion of the omega-3 fatty acids by turning them into trans fatty acids. Remember that fact.

The trans fatty acid content of canola oil: Although the Canadian government lists the trans fat (trans fatty acid) content of canola at a minimal 0.2 per cent, research at the University of Florida, in Gainesville, found trans fat levels as high as 4.6 per cent in commercial liquid oil *(S. O'Keefe and others, "Levels of Trans Geometrical Isomers of Essential Fatty Acids in Some Unhydrogenated U.S. Vegetable Oils," Journal of Food Lipids, 1994;1:165-176).* The consumer does not know that trans fatty acids are in canola oil because they are not listed on the label.

A large portion of canola oil used in processed food has been hardened through the hydrogenation process, which also introduces levels of trans fatty acids into the final product—as high as 40 per cent *(J.L. Sebedio and W.W. Christie, eds, Trans Fatty Acids in Human Nutrition, The Oily Press, Dundee, Scotland, 1998, pp. 49-50).* In fact, canola oil hydrogenates beautifully, better than corn oil or soybean oil, because modern hydrogenation methods hydrogenate omega-3 fatty acids preferentially; and canola oil is very high in omega-3s. Higher levels of trans fat mean longer shelf life for processed foods, a crisper texture in cookies and crackers—and more dangers of chronic disease for the consumer *(M.G. Enig, Trans Fatty Acids in the Food Supply: A Comprehensive Report Covering 60 Years of Research, 2nd Edition, Enig Associates, Inc., Silver Spring, MD, 1995).*

Look closely at the ingredients list on peanut butter labels. The peanut oil has been removed and replaced with canola oil. Notice that you can turn the jar nearly upside down. It has been hardened into a grease.

As explained earlier, **canola is a genetically engineered plant developed in Canada from the rapeseed plant.** According to *AgriAlternatives,* The Online Innovation, and Technology Magazine for Farmers, "By nature, these rapeseed oils, which have long been used to produce oils for industrial purposes, are . . toxic to humans and other animals."

Canola oil is genetically engineered rapeseed. Do you want to eat genetically engineered rapeseed?

Here is more about rapeseed: Derived from the *mustard family,* it is a toxic and poisonous weed which, when processed, becomes rancid very quickly.

Rapeseed oil is poisonous to living things and is an excellent insect repellent. You can use it (in very diluted form, following instructions) to kill the aphids on your roses and other plants. Available at your nursery, it works very well; it suffocates the aphids.

The industrial uses of rapeseed oil are well-known. It is used as an lubricant, fuel, soap, synthetic rubber base, and as an illuminate for color pages in magazines. It is an industrial oil, used to make varnish, and as an insecticide. It is not a food.

Rape oil is also the source of the infamous chemical-warfare agent, mustard gas, which was banned after blistering the lungs and skin of hundreds of thousands of soldiers and civilians during WW1. Recent French reports indicate that it was again used during the Gulf War.

Between 1950 and 1953, white mustard (rape) seed was irradiated in Sweden, to increase seed production and oil content. Irradiation is the process the experts want use to make our food "safe" to eat.

Here are health problems induced by rapeseed: Rape oil is strongly related to symptoms of emphysema, respiratory distress, anemia, constipation, irritability, and blindness in animals and humans. Rape oil was widely used in animal feeds in England and Europe between 1986 and 1991, when it was discontinued. It has been shown to cause lung cancer *(Wall Street Journal, June 7, 1995)*.

Reports on the dangers of rapeseed oil are rampant on the internet. One is an article, *"Blindness, Mad Cow Disease and Canola Oil,"* by John Thomas, which first appeared in *Perceptions* magazine, March/April 1996.

Hemagglutinins, substances that promote blood clotting and depress growth, are found in the protein portion of the seed; and traces are in rapeseed and canola oil.

The feeding of canola oil may make cattle more susceptible to several diseases *(M. Purdey. Educating Rita. Wise Traditions, Spring 2002;3(1):11-18)*.

There are reports of allergies to canola. And internet articles describe a variety of symptoms—including tremors, shaking, palsy, lack of coordination, slurred speech, memory problems, blurred vision, problems with urination, numbness and tingling in the extremities, and heart arrhythmias which cleared up on discontinuance of canola.

The canola industry is deeply disturbed about such reports; and so it arranges for the publication of articles to counteract them. In an article in the *Washington Post*, Robert L. Wolke declared that the publishers of these reports are spreading "hysterical urban legends about bizarre diseases."

When you purchase food products, check them for ingredients. If the label says, "may contain the following" and lists canola oil as a possible ingredient, you know canola oil is in it—because it is the cheapest oil and the Canadian government subsidizes it to industries involved in food processing.

Nearly all processed foods now contain canola oil. Fortunately, fresh fruits and vegetables contain none.

More problems with canola oil: Bird breeders check labels to ensure that there is no rape seed in their food. They will tell you, "The birds will eat it, but they do not live very long." One individual, who worked for only nine months as a quality control taster at an apple-chip factory where Canola oil was used exclusively for frying, developed numerous health problems.

Rape seed oil, used for stir-frying in China, was found to emit cancer-causing chemicals. "Rapeseed oil smoke causes lung cancer."—*Wall Street Journal, June 7, 1995.*

Chemically, canola breaks down at 5% saturated fat, 57% oleic acid, 23% omega–6, and 10%–15% omega–3. The reason canola is particularly unsuited for consumption is because it contains a very–long–chain fatty acid, called erucic acid, which under some circumstances is associated with fibrotic heart lesions.

A key problem is that the omega–3 fatty acids of processed canola oil (the only good part before processing) are transformed during the deodorizing process into *trans fatty acids*—something very bad. As reported in *Acres USA, March 2001* (one of the most respected agriculture journals in America), one study indicated that canola oil (which the industry calls "heart-healthy") actually creates a deficiency of vitamin E, which, as many of us know, is essential to our cardiovascular health.

Because of its high sulphur content, canola oil goes rancid easily and baked goods used with the oil develop molds rather quickly.

It has been very much in vogue in health-food circles to praise canola oil as very healthy oil, "high in poly-unsaturates," while condemning tropical oils such as coconut or palm oil as being saturated and unhealthy.

"The high praise for canola is propaganda put forth by the Canadian government because 'canola,' a hybridized rape plant, is one of that nation's chief export products."—*Acres USA, March 2001.*

What high temperatures produce: All food-grade canola, including the varieties sold in health-food stores, are deodorized from its natural, terrible odor—by the use of 300 degree F. high–temperature refining. You cannot cook a vegetable oil at that temperature and leave behind anything that is very edible. Most of the omega-3s in canola oil are transformed into trans fats during that deodorization process.

Oils high in omega-3 are not capable of taking high temperatures. Heating canola distorts the fatty acid, turning it into an unnatural form of trans fatty acid that has been shown to be harmful to health.

Udo Erasmus, Ph.D., a highly regarded international expert on fats and oils, says **the only safe oil to use to fry or bake with is water.** All oils are damaged by very high temperatures. He says no fat can stand the temperatures used in food processing without being adversely affected. (If you must use oil, olive oil is the best.)

A form of plastic: Research at the University of Florida, in Gainesville, determined that as much as 4.6% of all the fatty acids in canola are *trans isomers* (a type of plastic), due to the refining process. Contrary to popular opinion, saturated fats, especially those found in coconut oil are not harmful to health, but are important nutrition. There are no trans isomers in unrefined coconut butter, for example. Mary Enig, Ph.D., has published a number of research papers on this; she refutes all the establishment propaganda defending canola oil.

Any "food" substance that depletes vitamin E rapidly is extremely dangerous. Vitamin E is absolutely essential to human health. It is critically necessary in the body when processed fats are eaten; because tocopherols control the lipid peroxidation that results in dangerous free-radical activity, which in turn causes lesions in arteries and other problems.

A research study using piglets discovered that canola oil damages tocopherols (vitamin E), with the potential for rapidly depleting a body of the important vitamin. The researchers did not know what factors in the canola oil were responsible. They reported that other vegetable seed oils did not appear to cause the same problem in piglets.

Dangerous chemicals inside: Canola oil contains large amounts of *isothiocyanates*. These are cyanide-containing compounds. Cyanide inhibits mitochondrial production of *adenosine triphosphate* (ATP), which is the energy molecule that fuels the *mitochondria*. ATP energy powers the body and keeps us healthy and young!

Many substances can bind metabolic enzymes and block their activity in the body. In biochemistry, these substances are called inhibitors.

Toxic substances in canola and soybean oil encourage the formation of molecules with covalent bonds which are normally irreversible. They cannot be broken by the body once they have formed.

For example, consider the pesticide, *malathion*. It binds to the active site of the enzyme, *acetylcholinesterase,* and stops this enzyme from doing its job, which is to divide acetylcholine into choline and acetate.

Acetylcholine is critical to nerve-impulse transmission. When acetylcholinesterase is inhibited, as by pesticide residues, nerve fibers do not function normally and muscles do not respond. Partial paralysis gradually occurs. There has been a tremendous increase in disorders like systemic lupus, multiple sclerosis, cerebral palsy, pulmonary hypertension, and neuropathy.

Another group of chemicals in our modern, chemically modified food oils are the *organophosphates*. These are also used in insecticides, such as *malathion*.

Acetylcholinesterase inhibitors cause paralysis of the striated (skeletal) muscles and spasms of the respiratory system. That is why *malathion* is the pesticide of choice by the experts; it kills insects by paralysis—just as *rotenone* from soybeans does! It inhibits the insects' enzymes and those of humans, too!

Agents Orange and Blue, that were used in Vietnam to defoliate jungle cover, are also *organophosphorus* compounds. The Vietnam veterans and the Vietnamese people know about them firsthand. Government experts who okayed their use and chemical companies that manufactured them have finally admitted their toxic effects on people and the environment. Nonetheless, present-day experts in academia and government continue to claim that cheap junk food is relatively harmless.

Canola oil is also high in *glycosides* that cause serious problems by blocking enzyme function and depriving us of our life force. Glycosides interfere with the biochemistry of humans and animals. Their presence in rattlesnake venom inhibits muscle enzymes and cause immobilization of the victim.

OLESTRA

Olestra is a fat substitute used in some potato chips. It is not taken up by the body during digestion and is passed through the small and large intestine intact. For this reason, it is considered to have zero calories, but **it causes a whole host of gastrointestinal related symptoms such as abdominal cramps, bloating, flatulence, diarrhea and loose stools. Fluid will leak out of the anus during the day.** What we won't do to have our cake or chips and eat them too

GOOD OILS: FLAXSEED OIL AND SOME OTHERS

You want good oil that is nutritious and healthful! **Butter and tropical fats—coconut, palm, palm kernel, cocoa, and shea nut oil—are good. Better still is wheat germ oil. The best oil is flaxseed oil.**

Here is the ideal way to use it:

Order a bottle of *Barlean's Flaxseed Oil.* When it arrives, place it in the freezer. When you want some oil, defrost the bottle and pour some in a pint-sized canning, glass jar. Put the Barlean's back in the freezer and put the glass jar in the refrigerator. At mealtime, take out the jar and, during the meal, pour a little into a spoon and put it into your mouth along with some food. Soon after, put the jar back in the refrigerator.

In this way, you will be taking the very richest source of Omega-3; this is an outstanding source of fresh, polyunsaturated oil.

Evening primrose oil capsules are also good, but much more expensive and unnecessary if you have flaxseed oil.

An alternative method is to **daily grind fresh, raw flaxseed and sprinkle that on your meal**. But, of course, your intake of flaxseed oil will be greatly reduced. Combining the taking of ground flaxseed with flaxseed oil is a good choice. Important: Ground flaxseed must be fresh, or only kept in the refrigerator a few days at the most before it is used up.

Another alternative is **chia seed**, which is also rich in omega-3. It has several advantages: It stores well at room temperature. You do not have to grind it. Just sprinkle the seeds in your health drinks or on your food (after cooking). It is tasteless, and forms a gel which will also help keep you regular.

Here is some chemical data which will help you understand why omega-3 is so important:

Saturated fatty acids are chains of carbon atoms that have *hydrogen* filling every bond. In foods, they normally range in length from four to 22 carbons. Because of their straight configuration, saturated fatty acids pack together easily and tend to be solid at room temperature. **Butter, tallow, suet, palm oil, and coconut oil** are classified as saturated fats because they contain a preponderance of saturated fatty acids. Saturated fats are stable and do not become rancid when subjected to heat, as in cooking.

Monounsaturated fatty acids are chains of carbon atoms that have one double bond between two carbons *and therefore lack two hydrogens*. Normally they range from 16 to 22 carbons. They have a kink or bend at the position of the double bond; so the molecules do not pack together as easily as in saturated fatty acids. Monounsaturated oils tend to be liquid at room temperature but become solid when refrigerated. **Olive oil, peanut oil, lard, rapeseed, and canola oils** are classified as monounsaturated oils. The most common monounsaturated fatty acids are **palmitoleic** (16 carbons), **oleic** (18 carbons) and **erucic** (22 carbons). Monounsaturated oils are relatively stable and can be used for cooking.

Polyunsaturated fatty acids have two or more double bonds. As there is a bend or kink at each double bond, these fatty acids do not pack together easily and tend to be liquid, even when cold. **Polyunsaturated oils are very fragile.** They tend to develop harmful free radicals when subjected to heat and oxygen, as in cooking or processing. **Soybean oil, safflower oil, sunflower oil and flax oil** are polyunsaturated oils. **Omega-6** fatty acids have the first double bond at the sixth carbon from the end of the fatty acid chain. The most common omega-6 fatty acid is **linoleic acid**, which is called an essential fatty acid (EFA) because your body cannot make it.

Omega-3 fatty acids have the first double bond at the third carbon. The most common omega-3 fatty acid is the EFA alpha-**linolenic acid**. The consensus among lipid experts is that **the American diet is too high in omega-6 fatty acids (present in high amounts in commercial vegetable oils) and lacking in omega-3 fatty acids** (which are present in **egg yolks, organic vegetables, and flaxseed oil**). A surfeit of omega-6 fatty acids and deficiency in omega-3 fatty acids has been shown to depress immune system function, contribute to weight gain, and cause inflammation.

REFINED GRAINS

We have discussed trans fats and saturated fats. Refined grains are the next type of problem in processed foods.

Choosing refined grains such as **white bread, rolls, sugary low-fiber cereal, white rice, or white pasta over whole grains can boost your heart attack risk by up to 30 percent.** You've got to be a savvy shopper. Don't be fooled by deceptive label claims such as "made with wheat flour" or "seven grain." Or by **white-flour breads** topped with a sprinkling of oats, or colored brown with molasses. Often, they're just the same old refined stuff that raises risk for high cholesterol, high blood pressure, heart attacks, insulin resistance, diabetes, and belly fat.

At least seven major studies show that women and men who eat more whole grains (including dark bread, whole-grain breakfast cereals, popcorn, cooked oatmeal, brown rice, bran, and other grains like bulgur or kasha) have 20 to 30 percent less heart disease. In contrast, those who opt for refined grains have more heart attacks, insulin resistance, and high blood pressure.

Read the ingredient list on packaged grain products. If the product is one of those that are best for you, the first ingredients should be whole wheat or another whole grain, such as oats. The fiber content should be at least 3 grams per serving.

The grains that make up the typical American diet are highly refined. What this means is that the bran (fiber-rich outer layer) and the germ (the nutrient-rich inner part) of the grain are removed during the milling process. **Only the endosperm (middle part) remains.** Although this process makes grains easier to use in cooking,—**gone are many of B vitamins, iron, vitamin E, selenium, fiber, and other disease-fighting components**.

Examples of refined grain products include: White breads. Baked goods. Pasta. Crackers. White rice. Corn flakes cereal.

Some refined grain products are "enriched", which means that some of the nutrients such as niacin, riboflavin, thiamin, and iron, are added back. However, enrichment does not restore insoluble fiber and other nutrients that are lost during the milling process.

Why whole grains are more wholesome: Whole grains contain the **bran, the endosperm, and the germ**. Because they haven't gone through the refining process, they are good sources of **fiber, B vitamins, iron, zinc, magnesium, vitamin E, and selenium**. They also contain plant chemicals called **phytochemicals**, which are believed to have many health-promoting effects.

Whole grains can help with the following physical problems: Reducing constipation, hemorrhoids, and diverticular disease. They are also good at lowering cholesterol levels and decreasing the risk of cardiovascular disease. They reduce the risk of cancer, and type 2 diabetes.

They increase absorption of nutrients, because they take longer to digest.

Examples of whole grains include the following: Whole wheat. Barley. Brown rice. Bulgur. Corn. Whole oats. Quinoa. Rye. Amaranth. Buckwheat. Millet. Spelt.

How do you know if the product is a whole grain? Don't rely on the name or appearance of the product. Bread may be brown because it contains molasses,

H
A
R
M
F
U
L

brown sugar, or food coloring, not because it's whole wheat. Product names that conjure up images of health and "back to nature" can still be made with mainly white, refined flour.

Instead, look at the ingredients on the wrapper or package. **It should always say "whole grain" or "whole wheat."** Note that ingredients are listed in descending order by weight. If white flour is the first ingredient, that means that, by weight, there is more white flour than any other kind of flour in the product.

Do not be deceived by terminology. "Wheat flour," "unbleached wheat flour," or "stoned wheat." These are not the same as whole wheat. Beware of products that say "made with whole wheat," "made with whole grain," or "made with oatmeal." This does not tell you how much whole wheat, whole grain, or oatmeal is in the product. You may find that it is way down on the ingredient list.

There are many benefits to eating more whole grains. They are more nutritious, healthful, and filling than refined grains, and have more texture and flavor. The 2005 FDA Dietary Guidelines recommend consuming three or more ounce-equivalents of whole-grain products per day, and making sure that at least half of your total intake of grains is from whole grains. Stock you pantry with whole grain cereals, brown rice, whole grain bread, and whole wheat pasta, crackers, breads, and rolls. Experiment with some delicious new whole grains and whole grain recipes. You will be feel better because you did!

SALT

Three-quarters of the sodium in our diets isn't from the saltshaker. It's hidden in processed foods, such as **canned vegetables and soups, condiments like soy sauce and Worcestershire sauce, fast-food burgers (and fries, of course), and cured or preserved meats like bacon, ham, and deli turkey.**

Some sodium occurs naturally in unprocessed edibles, including milk, beets, celery, even some drinking water. But that is helpful, because sodium is necessary for life. It helps regulate blood pressure, maintains the body's fluid balance, transmits nerve impulses, makes muscles—including your heart—contract, and keeps your senses of taste, smell, and touch working properly. You need a little every day to replace what is lost to sweat, tears, and other excretions.

But what happens when you eat more salt than your body needs? Your body retains fluid simply to dilute the extra sodium in your bloodstream. This raises blood volume, forcing your heart to work harder; at the same time, it makes veins and arteries constrict. The combination **raises blood pressure**.

Your limit should be 1,500 milligrams of sodium per day, about the amount in three-fourths of a teaspoon of salt. (Table salt, by the way, is 40 percent sodium, 60 percent chloride.) Older people should eat even less, to counteract the natural rise in blood pressure that comes with age. People over 50 should strive for 1,300 mg; those over 70 should aim for 1,200 mg.

Only the "Nutrition Facts" panel on a food package will give you the real sodium count. Don't believe claims on the package front such as "sodium-free" (foods can still have 5 mg per serving); "reduced sodium" (it only means 25 percent less than usual); or "light in sodium" (half the amount you'd normally find).

Look for soups or frozen dinners that contain less than 500 to 600 mg per serving (this is still not low sodium, but is about as good as it gets). Choose snack foods like crackers, popcorn, or nuts that are unsalted or lower in sodium (120 mg per serving or less). Compare brands - the sodium content in the same food can vary tremendously from one brand to another.

Here are more dangers in excess sodium: Sodium (salt) can **increase blood pressure**, which increases the risk of **stroke, heart attack, heart failure and kidney disease**. It's also linked to a higher risk of **stomach cancer** and may be detrimental to **bone health**.

Food Sources of high sodium are these: soup, frozen dinners, cold cuts, bacon, sausages, pickled foods, tomato sauce, salsa, salad dressing, fast food and restaurant meals.

The DASH-Sodium trial (Dietary Approach to Stop Hypertension) looked at the effect of a high, medium and low sodium intake (3,300 mg, 2,400 mg and 1,500 mg per day) on blood pressure. Results were consistent: the greater the reduction in sodium, the greater the reduction in blood pressure.

As much as 80% of the sodium most people eat comes from either processed, packaged foods or from restaurant meals. Buy more fresh foods, like fruits and vegetables. When you do buy processed foods, learn to read food labels. At restaurants, ask that food be prepared without salt and if nutritional data is available, choose less salty options.

SUGAR

Sugar provides no nutritional value, other than calories. High intakes of sugar-rich, nutrient-poor foods, like soft drinks, are linked to an increased risk of **obesity** and **type 2 diabetes**, and can crowd more nutritious foods out of the diet.

Some foods are naturally high in sugar (fruit juices, dried fruit, honey, maple syrup, jam/jellies) and **many foods contain added sugar** (desserts, candy, ice cream, cereal, granola bars, yogurt, chocolate milk).

It is recommended that you consume no more than 12 teaspoons of "free sugars" daily. (All recommended intakes are based on a 2000 calorie diet.) This is sugar added to foods, plus sugars naturally present in honey, syrups and fruit juices. **To determine how many teaspoons of sugar a product contains, divide the grams of "sugars" listed on the food label by four.** For example, if a granola bar contains 12 grams of sugars, that translates to 3 teaspoons of sugar per bar.

In the **Nurses Health Study II** involving over 80,000 women, drinking one or more regular soft drinks daily was linked to an 83% higher risk of **type 2 diabetes** and an **increase in body weight**.

Use sugar in small amounts to make healthy foods taste better. For example, jam on whole-wheat toast or sugar on whole-grain cereal. **Choose healthy, pre-sweetened foods like whole-grain cereals, yogurt, chocolate milk and canned fruit that contain less added sugar. Eat most of your fruits and vegetables whole.** Most important, avoid sugar-only foods, such as soft drinks. Cakes, pies, cookies, and candy are also nutrient-poor, but sugar-rich.

Load your diet with health-protective foods including fruits, vegetables, whole grains, nuts, beans and healthy fats.

HIGH-FRUCTOSE CORN SYRUP

Compared to traditional sweeteners, high-fructose corn syrup costs less to make, is sweeter to the taste, and mixes more easily with other ingredients. That is why food manufacturers prefer it over any other kind of sweetener. Today, **we consume nearly 63 pounds of it per person per year** in **drinks and sweets**, as well as in other products. High-fructose corn syrup is in many **frozen foods**. It gives **bread** an inviting, brown color and soft texture, so it's also in **whole-wheat bread, hamburger buns, and English muffins**. It is in **beer, bacon, spaghetti sauce, soft drinks, and even ketchup.**

Research is beginning to suggest that **this liquid sweetener may upset the human metabolism, raising the risk for heart disease and diabetes**. Researchers say that high-fructose corn syrup's chemical structure **encourages overeating**. It also seems to force the liver to pump more heart-threatening **triglycerides** into the bloodstream. In addition, fructose may lower your body's reserves of chromium, a mineral important for healthy levels of cholesterol, insulin, and blood sugar.

To spot fructose on a food label, **look for the words "corn sweetener," "corn syrup," or "corn syrup solids" as well as "high-fructose corn syrup."**

THE THREE LEADING PROCESSED FOOD DISEASES

Obesity—**The World Health Organization (WHO) says processed foods are to blame for the sharp rise in obesity, and much of the chronic disease seen around the world.**

In one study by Ludwig and colleagues, **children who ate processed fast foods in a restaurant ate 126 more calories than on days they ate none.** Over the course of a year, this could translate into 13 pounds of weight gain just from fast food.

Ludwig says, "The food industry would love to explain obesity as a problem of personal responsibility, since it takes the onus off them for marketing fast food, soft drinks, and other high-calorie, low-quality products."

But the foods in our modern culture appeal to overeating: "When you have calories that are incredibly cheap, in a culture where 'bigger is better,' that's

a dangerous combination," says Walter Willett, M.D., D.P.H., professor of epidemiology and nutrition at the Harvard School of Public Health.

Diabetes—Researchers have found that, in the last 50 years, the extent of processing has increased so much that **prepared breakfast cereals—even without added sugar—act exactly like sugar itself.**

As far as our hormones and metabolism are concerned, there's no difference between a bowl of unsweetened corn flakes and a bowl of table sugar. Starch is 100-percent glucose (table sugar is half glucose, half fructose) and our bodies can digest it into sugar instantly.

We are not adapted to handle fast-acting carbohydrates. Glucose is the gold standard of energy metabolism. The brain is exquisitely dependent on having a continuous supply of glucose: too low a glucose level poses an immediate threat to survival. [But] too high a level causes damage to tissues, as with diabetes.

Heart Disease—**Many processed foods contain trans fatty acids (TFA), a dangerous type of fat.** According to the American Heart Association, "TFAs tend to raise LDL ("bad") cholesterol and lower HDL ("good") cholesterol. These changes may increase the risk of heart disease."

In addition, **most processed foods are extremely high in salt**, another blow to the heart. One-half cup of Campbell's Chicken Noodle Soup, for instance, has 37 percent of the daily-recommended amount of sodium.

"Probably the single, fastest way to reduce strokes in this country is to halve the amount of salt that's added to processed food," says Tim Lang, professor of food policy at the City University, London.

Cancer—A seven-year study of close to 200,000 people by the University of Hawaii found that **people who ate the most processed meats (hot dogs, sausage) had a 67 percent higher risk of pancreatic cancer** than those who ate little or no meat products.

A Canadian study of over 400 men aged 50 to 80 found similar results. Men whose eating habits fell into the **"processed" pattern (processed meats, red meat, organ meats, refined grains, vegetable oils and soft drinks)** had a significantly higher risk of prostate cancer than men in the other groups. Men who ate the most processed foods **had a 2.5-fold increased prostate cancer risk**.

Yet another study published in the journal *Cancer Epidemiology, Mile Markers, and Prevention* found that refined carbohydrates like **white flour, sugar and high fructose corn syrup was also linked to cancer**. This study of more than 1,800 women in Mexico found that **those who got 57 percent or more of their total energy intake from refined carbohydrates had a 220 percent higher risk of breast cancer** than women who ate more balanced diets.

Processed meats like hot dogs, lunch meats, bacon and other sausages have been linked to various forms of cancer.

Acrylamide, a carcinogenic substance that forms

when foods are heated at high temperatures, such as during baking or frying, is also a concern. Processed foods like **French fries and potato chips** have shown elevated levels of the substance, according to the *Center for Science in the Public Interest*.

"I estimate that acrylamide causes several thousand cancers per year in Americans," said Clark University research professor Dale Hattis.

2 – Food Additives

Most food additives have many effects which are not known. Those which we do know are generally not good.

The Food and Drug Administration (FDA) maintains a list of over 3,000 chemicals that are added to the processed food supply. These compounds do various things to food: **add color, stabilize, texturize, preserve, sweeten, thicken, add flavor, soften, emulsify and more.**

Some of these additives have never been tested for safety—and require no government approval—but instead belong to the FDA's *"Generally Recognized as Safe"* (GRAS) list. An item is "safe," as defined by Congress, if there is "reasonable certainty that no harm will result from use of an additive."

Some compounds that are known to be toxic to humans or animals are also allowed, though at the level of 1/100th of the amount that is considered harmful.

Potential side effects from the additives vary, and are controversial. **For example, just one common food additive, monosodium glutamate (MSG) has the following reported symptoms:** Numbness. Burning sensation. Tingling. Facial pressure or tightness. Chest pain. Headache. Nausea. Rapid heartbeat. Drowsiness. Weakness. Difficulty breathing for asthmatics

As is the case with most food additives, **some people show no side effects, while others may become ill.**

If the list of ingredients is long, there is probably a lot of chemical additives in the product. It's best to avoid these foods because of the unknown health effects of combinations of food additives.

If the list of ingredients is short, it may or may not have harmful additives in it. Look it up in *FOOD ADDITIVES: A Shopper's Guide To What's Safe And What's Not*, before you decide to purchase it.

Ingredients are listed on the label in order of predominance by weight: the ingredient that weighs the most is listed first, the ingredient that weighs the least is listed last. **If there's a questionable additive on the list, the closer it is to the top of the list, the more you put yourself at risk.**

Food Additive Safety Codes—**The following codes indicate the safety of the additives in the table below.** Many additives have more than one code used to describe their safety.

§ - FDA approved colorant

S - There is no known toxicity. The additive appears to be safe.

A - The additive may cause allergic reactions.

C - Caution is advised. The additive may be unsafe, poorly tested, or used in foods we eat too much of.

C1 - Caution is advised for certain groups in the population, such as pregnant women, infants, persons with high blood pressure, kidney problems, etc.

X - The additive is unsafe or very poorly tested.

EIGHTEEN FOOD ADDITIVES

Some Common Food Additives—**Here are 18 of these common food additives:**

X - Acesulfame-K - "Sunette"; may cause low blood sugar attacks; causes cancer, elevated cholesterol in lab animals.

X - Acesulfame-potassium - same as acesulfame-K.

C - Animal or vegetable shortening - associated with heart disease, hardening of the arteries, elevated cholesterol levels.

X - Artificial color FD & C, U.S certified food color - contribute to hyperactivity in children; may contribute to learning and visual disorders, nerve damage; may be carcinogenic; see FD&C Colors.

X, A - Artificial flavoring - may cause reproductive disorders, developmental problems; not adequately tested.

X - Artificial sweeteners - associated with health problems; see specific sweetener.

X - Aspartame - may cause brain damage in phenylketonurics; may cause central nervous system disturbances, menstrual difficulties; may affect brain development in unborn fetus.

X, A - *BHA* - can cause liver and kidney damage, behavioral problems, infertility, weakened immune system, birth defects, cancer; should be avoided by infants, young children, pregnant women and those sensitive to aspirin.

X, A - BHT - see BHA; banned in England.

X, A - Brominated vegetable oil - linked to major organ system damage, birth defects, growth problems; considered unsafe by the FDA, can still lawfully be used unless further action is taken by the FDA .

X - Caffeine - psychoactive, addictive drug; may cause fertility problems, birth defects, heart disease, depression, nervousness, behavioral changes, insomnia, etc.

§, X - FD&C Colors – colors considered safe by the FDA for use in food, drugs and cosmetics; most of the colors are derived from coal tar and must be certified by the FDA not to contain more than 10ppm of lead and arsenic; certification does not address any harmful effects these colors may have on the body; most coal tar colors are potential carcinogens, may contain carcinogenic contaminants, and cause allergic reactions.

X - Free glutamates - may cause brain damage, especially in children; always found in autolyzed yeast, calcium caseinate, enzymes, flavors & flavorings, gelatin, glutamate, glutamic acid, hydrolyzed protein, hydrolyzed soy protein, plant protein extract, protease, protease enzymes, sodium caseinate, textured protein, yeast extract, yeast food and yeast nutrient; may be in barley malt, boullion, broth, carrageenan, malt extract, malt flavoring, maltodextrin, natural flavors, natural chicken flavoring, natural beef flavoring, natural pork flavoring, pectin, seasonings, soy protein, soy protein concentrate, soy protein isolate, soy sauce, soy sauce extract, stock, whey protein, whey protein concentrate, whey protein isolate, anything that is enzyme modified, fermented, protein fortified or ultrapasteurized and foods that advertise NO MSG; see MSG.

X, A - Hydrogenated vegetable oil - associated with heart disease, breast and colon cancer, atherosclerosis, elevated cholesterol.

X, A - Hydrolyzed vegetable protein - may cause brain and nervous system damage in infants; high salt content; may be corn, soy, or wheat based. Contains free glutamates.

§ - MSG - may cause headaches, itching, nausea, brain, nervous system, reproductive disorders, high blood pressure; pregnant, lactating mothers, infants, small children should avoid; allergic reactions common; may be hidden in infant formula, low fat milk, candy, chewing gum, drinks, over-the-counter medications, especially children's, binders and fillers for nutritional supplements, prescription and non-prescription drugs, IV fluids given in hospitals, chicken pox vaccine; it is being sprayed on growing fruits and vegetables as a growth enhancer; it is proposed for use on organic crops.

X, A - Natural flavors - may be chemically extracted and processed and in combination with other food additives not required to be listed on the label; may contain free glutamates; see MSG.

X - Nitrates - form powerful cancer-causing agents in stomach; can cause death; considered dangerous by FDA but not banned because they prevent botulism.

X - Nitrites - may cause headaches, nausea, vomiting, dizziness; see nitrates.

These are only a few of the thousands of food additives commonly added to our food.

3 - Flavor Enhancers

Monosodium Glutamate (MSG) is a flavor enhancer. Because it makes processed food taste better, people buy and eat more of it, and the food processing companies make more money.

In the next section, we will discuss **artificial sweeteners**, which including such products as **saccharin, cyclamate, aspartame, equal measure, nutrasweet spoonful, canderal, splenda**, and **acesulfame potassium.**

Researchers tell us that, because of the harmful effects of certain substances within them on the human body, all of these products are termed "excitotoxins."

Just now, we will discuss excitotoxins, followed by monosodium glutamate. Then, in the next section, we will explain the dangers in the synthetic sweeteners.

EXCITOTOXINS

Excitotoxins are amino acids that also serve as neurotransmitters in the brain, such as glutamate, aspartate and cysteine. When brain neurons are exposed to these *excitatory neurotransmitters* in too high a dose, they can become very excited and fire their impulses very rapidly until they reach a state of exhaustion.

Sometime later, these neurons suddenly die as if they were "excited" to death. Because of this progression, neuroscientists have named this class of chemicals *"excitotoxins"*.

Becausse excitotoxins are amino acids that are also *neurotransmitters*, our brain, nervous system and entire body cannot operate without these chemical messengers. They are not destructive or toxic of themselves; it is an issue of balance.

A consistent supply of energy to the brain is required if neurons are to be protected against the damaging effects of excitotoxins in all forms. The brain uses 20% of the body's oxygen and 25% of its glucose while making up only 2% of its weight. Conditions like hypoglycemia can cause an energy shortage in the brain leading to failure of the main systems in place to regulate neurotransmitter concentration around neurons and calcium accumulation inside neurons. **Zinc and magnesium play important roles in calcium channel regulation.** Zinc causes the channel to remain closed, allowing no calcium into the cell. We can see how zinc in excess could present a problem. Magnesium also causes the calcium channel to remain closed, but if the nerve fires, the MG lock is blown and calcium allowed to enter the cell.

Neuroscientific research by Russell Blaylock, John Olney, George Schwartz and others has shown that **factors provided by nature are the best defense against the technological "advancements" which have produced excitotoxin food additives.**

Magnesium (mg), as we have seen, plays a key role. There is no doubt that the average American's diet is deficient in magnesium. Those deficient in magnesium have an increased risk of neural damage from exposure to excitotoxins. This is too important to guess about.

Serum magnesium that is below reference range on blood chemistry indicates a need for magnesium. The problem with serum magnesium (mg) blood studies is that mg is not a serum mineral but a cellular mineral. I know of several cases where the patients serum mg was within range but their red cell mg was decreased, indicating a need for magnesium. To be sure, it is worth the extra expense to use red cell magnesium to rule out or establish magnesium need for each individual.

HARMFUL

Adequate magnesium equals increased protection from the damaging effects of excitotoxin food additives, inadequate magnesium equals increased risk of neural damage from excitotoxin exposure. **With repeated exposure and accumulating neural damage the patient will begin to present symptoms of Alzheimer's disease, Parkinson's disease, Amyotrophic Lateral Sclerosis (ALS), or Huntington's disease, depending on which area of the brain was damaged.** Neurologists have found that the symptoms of these diseases do not begin to appear until 80 to 90% of the neurons in the involved nuclei have died. Prevention is of utmost importance!

Hypoglycemia and other sugar-handling problems are on the increase. Obesity is epidemic. **Hypoglycemia and obesity (if the person is following a low calorie weight loss diet) can both contribute to critically low energy in the brain and failure of the neuroprotective systems.** These are highly efficient pumping systems that remove excess glutamate, etc from the extracellular space and excess calcium from the inside of the neuron. This pumping system has been likened to a bucket brigade used in putting out a fire or to bail out a sinking boat. Enormous amounts of energy are needed to power this system. If not enough energy is available; the system fails, leaving the brain cells exposed to the effects of excitotoxins.

The *only* reason for the addition of excitotoxins, such as MSG, hydrolyzed vegetable protein, aspartame, etc to foods is to enhance the *taste* of the food thereby greatly increase sales. This is death by profit margin, because the research is clear regarding the damaging effects of these additives. **As far as the food processors are concerned, profits are more important than people!**

Still more information about excitotoxins—If you are not careful, the poisons being put into your food will get you. If you manage to avoid them, the medicinal drugs you are prescribed will do you in. In the chemical age in which we live, the rule must be: "Let the buyer beware."

Russell L. Blaylock, M.D., a neurosurgeon at the University of Mississippi Medical Center, has researched extensively into this little-known set of substances called ***excitotoxins***. What you don't know can kill you, by inches if not faster.

MSG (monosodium glutamate), Aspartame (Nutrasweet, Equal), hydrolyzed vegetable protein, and cysteine—are all examples of excitotoxin amino acids. **They are added to human foods and drinks in order to enhance the flavor. But careful research on animals reveals that they destroy brain cells.**

These flavor enhancing chemicals are found naturally in very small amounts in plants. But, anxious to get you to buy more of their products, the food companies use man-made, highly concentrated forms of those chemicals. Fearful that their competitors will sell more food than they do, **every (every) major food company**

uses them to heighten the flavor. **The presence of those chemicals in the food causes you to want to eat more of the product than you normally would.** Excitotoxins are especially added to foods that have a bland taste or little flavor.

But when the same amount of these chemicals, that you ingest in a bottle of Flavor Cola or a bowl of Nutty Crisps, is added to the rations of test animals (including mice, cats, and chimpanzees), it produces brain damage. **The excitotoxins stimulate the neuron brain cells so vigorously, that the cells die of exhaustion! This effect is especially seen in the hypothalamus and temporal lobes** which control behavior, emotions, onset of puberty, sleep cycle, hormones, immunity, and a number of other body functions. Short term memory and the ability to learn are also affected.

Several factors determine how much damage occurs at a given meal: **the amount that is eaten and how frequently such foods are eaten.** Some people eat such food every day or at certain times day after day. Some people drink no water, but derive all their fluids from soft drinks! Guess what is in those soft drinks? Hypoglycemia also makes the brain nerves very sensitive to these chemicals.

Dr. Blaylock recommends that **those with a family history of neurodegenerative diseases should make every effort to avoid foods containing excitotoxins.** These diseases include Alzheimer's disease, Parkinson's disease, Huntington's disease, and Amyotrophic Lateral Sclerosis (Lou Gehrig's disease). They markedly decrease the blood brain barrier, making a person more sensitive than normal to chronic exposure to these dangerous chemicals and consequent brain damage.

Now, let us consider some doctored foods in which these substances are found:

Beware of canned soup, fast foods, junk food, and food found in fast-food or Chinese restaurants. They will generally contain large amounts of MSG.

A meal of this so-called "food" can, in a child, raise the blood level of excitotoxins six times—which, in primates, destroys brain cells! **A child's brain is four times more sensitive to damage by excitotoxins than an adult's brain.** But the brain damage will not be evident until the child is more mature. Is tasty junk food really worth the damage it is going to bring to you?

The following food additives contain 30% to 60% MSG: monosodium glutamate, hydrolyzed vegetable protein, hydrolyzed protein, hydrolyzed plant protein, plant protein extract, sodium caseinate, calcium caseinate, yeast extract, textured protein, autolyzed yeast, hydrolyzed oat flour, Accent.

The following food additives contain 12% to 40% MSG: malt extract, malt flavoring, bouillon, broth, stock, flavoring, natural flavoring, natural beef or chicken flavoring, seasoning, spices.

The following additives may contain MSG: Carrageenan, enzymes, soy protein concentrate, soy protein isolate, whey protein concentrate, some types of soy milk.

MONOSODIUM GLUTAMATE

Monosodium Glutamate (MSG) is a strange chemical added to food, which the food industry says is placed there "to make the food taste better." But the real reason it is added is because MSG is *addictive*—so you will want to keep eating and buying that food product! *Here are important facts about MSG:*

MSG causes obesity!—John Erb was a research assistant at the University of Waterloo, and spent years working for the government. Later, he made an astounding discovery while going through scientific journals for a book he was writing, called *The Slow Poisoning of America.* **In order to study diabetes in test animals, in hundreds of studies around the world scientists feed mice and rats MSG so they will become extremely overweight!**

No strain of rat or mice is naturally obese, so the scientists somehow have to make them that way. They produce these morbidly obese creatures by injecting them with a chemical, known as MSG, when they are first born. **The MSG triples the amount of insulin the pancreas creates, causing them to become very obese!** Scientists even have a title for these fat rodents: They call them "MSG-Treated Rats."

MSG causes nerve damage in children!—MSG, added to the food you serve on your table or eat at restaurants, causes **brain damage in children**. It also affects how their nervous systems form during development; so that, in later years, they may have **learning or emotional difficulties**. Women should not eat MSG during pregnancy! Parents should not allow their children to eat it! —Frankly, the grown-ups should not eat it either!

There is scientific evidence that MSG permanently damages a critical part of the brain known to control hormones, so that **later in life a child might have endocrine problems**.

What MSG is found in—**MSG seems to be in just about every type of processed food!** Campbell's soups, Hostess Doritos, Lays flavored potato chips, Top Ramen, Betty Crocker Hamburger Helper, Heinz canned gravy, Swanson frozen prepared meals, Kraft salad dressings (especially the "healthy low fat" ones).

MSG (also called *hydrolyzed vegetable protein*) is a key ingredient in foods sold at Burger King, McDonald's, Wendy's, Kentucky Fried Chicken, and Taco Bell. Even the sit-down ones like TGIF, Chilis, Applebees, and Denny's use MSG in abundance.

Why MSG is added to foods—Manufacturers claim that MSG makes the food "taste better." But **the real reason it is added to food is the addictive effect it has on the human body.**

And we wonder why the nation is overweight? The MSG manufacturers themselves admit that it addicts people to their products. It urges people to choose their product over others, and makes people eat more of it than they would if MSG was not added.

So not only has MSG been scientifically proven to cause obesity,—it is an addictive substance!

Since its first introduction into the American food supply over fifty years ago, MSG has been added in even larger doses to the prepackaged meals, soups, snacks, and fast foods we are tempted to eat everyday.

Ignoring the research studies—The FDA has set no limits on how much of it can be added to food. They claim it is safe to eat in any amount, in spite of the fact that **there are hundreds of scientific studies with titles like these:**

• The monosodium glutamate [MSG] obese rat as a model for the study of exercise in obesity. *Gobatto CA, Mello MA, Souza CT, Ribeiro IA. Res Commun Mol Pathol Pharmacol. 2002*

• Adrenalectomy abolishes the food-induced hypothalamic serotonin release in both normal and monosodium glutamate-obese rats. *Guimaraes RB, Telles MM, Coelho VB, Mori RC, Nascimento CM, Ribeiro Brain Res Bull. 2002 Aug*

• Obesity induced by neonatal monosodium glutamate treatment in spontaneously hypertensive rats: an animal model of multiple risk factors. *Iwase M, Yamamoto M, Iino K, Ichikawa K, Shinohara N, Yoshinari Fujishima. Hypertens Res. 1998 Mar*

• Hypothalamic lesion induced by injection of monosodium glutamate in suckling period and subsequent development of obesity. *Tanaka K, Shimada M, Nakao K, Kusunoki Exp Neurol. 1978 Oct*

Yes, that last study is not a typo, *it was written in 1978*. Both the medical research community and food "manufacturers" have known MSG's side effects for decades!

Leads to dangerous diseases—MSG is linked to **diabetes, migraines, headaches, autism, ADHD, and Alzheimer's.** A drug that blocks the effects of MSG is being used to treat Alzheimer's disease! Yet the unsuspecting continue to eat MSG daily in their food.

Researchers have found a relationship between MSG and some of the dreaded **neurodegenerative diseases** such as **ALS, Parkinsonism, Huntington's disease, and Alzheimer's disease**, which all affect the elderly. Scientists used to think that in adults, brain cells were protected from invasion of MSG. Now, however, researchers realize that there are at least five areas in the brain that are not well-protected.

Hidden Sources of MSG—MSG manufacturers and the processed food industries are continually devising new "disguise names" for the MSG added to food. **Here is a partial list of the most common names for disguised MSG:**

• *Food additives that always contain MSG:* Monosodium Glutamate, Hydrolyzed Vegetable Protein, Hydrolyzed Protein, Hydrolyzed Plant Protein, Plant Protein Extract, Sodium Caseinate, Calcium Caseinate, Yeast Extract, Textured Protein (Including TVP), Autolyzed Yeast, Hydrolyzed Oat Flour, and Corn Oil.

• *Food additives that frequently contain MSG:* Malt Extract, Malt Flavoring, Bouillon, Broth, Stock, Flavoring, Natural Flavors/Flavoring, Natural Beef or Chicken Flavoring, Seasoning, Spices.

H
A
R
M
F
U
L

The tricky part for consumers is that, because current labeling requirements permit it, **free glutamate can be hidden under more than 40 different names.** Some common names are natural flavoring, natural chicken flavoring, natural turkey flavoring, etc., or basically any new name a manufacturer chooses. **If MSG is not harmful, it would not be hidden in the labeling.**

Additional information—When any product contains at least 79% *free glutamic acid*, it must be called MSG. Quantities of less than this amount do not fall under MSG labeling restrictions, and can be called any number of innocent sounding names, such as "natural flavoring." In larger quantities, **free glutamate is toxic to everyone**; but, for those who cannot metabolize it effectively, even very small doses can act like a poison. MSG stimulates or damages glutamate receptors, making them more sensitive to subsequent ingestion of MSG. Science suggests that **free glutamates may act as a "slow neurotoxin" with damage, such as dementia, only becoming apparent years later.**

Brain lesions have been produced again and again experimentally using hydrolyzed vegetable protein (MSG). Also, it has been determined that **when these substances are combined together, as can be found in the lengthy ingredient list of many prepared foods, they become much more toxic** than when used individually. Commercial soups, sauces, and gravies that are in liquid form are even more toxic than solid form, because **liquids are rapidly absorbed and attain high concentrations in the blood.**

The **glutamic acid in vaccines** are often described as "stabilizers," *i.e.*, ingredients to keep the virus alive. In reality, they are a hidden source of processed free glutamic acid (MSG). **This, along with mercury (a brain poison which is in all vaccines to kill viruses and bacteria in it), are two of the causes of autism in infants and small children.**

Although most vaccines are included, here are two examples which have MSG:

The Chicken pox Vaccine by VariVax (Merck & Co., Inc.). This vaccine includes "L-monosodium glutamate" and "hydrolyzed gelatin."

Another example would be Merck's M-M-R vaccine. The product insert states that the growth medium for measles and mumps includes "amino acids" and "glutamate." It also states that the medium for rubella includes "amino acids" and "hydrolyzed gelatin." Finally, it states that the "reconstituted vaccine" for subcutaneous administration includes hydrolyzed gelatin.

It is common knowledge, among chemists, that the amino acids—"glutamic acid," "aspartic acid," and "L-cysteine" are neurotoxic. It is also known that **any hydrolyzed protein, such as the hydrolyzed gelatin, will contain some processed free glutamic acid** (MSG), some aspartic acid, and some L-cysteine, all considered to be neurotoxic by neuroscientists. Even without hydrolyzing gelatin, **gelatin contains over 11% processed free glutamic acid (MSG) and some**

aspartic acid and L-cysteine. It is present as a result of the manufacturing process that results in gelatin.

One of the things that makes immediate diagnosis of MSG as the cause of a sudden physical problem is the different reaction times experienced by different people. **Some people eat MSG and react immediately with headaches, etc.** Some react as late as 48 hours after ingesting MSG. A second consideration is the fact that some react to a small dose of MSG in a meal, while others are distressed by a larger amount. But a given person will always react in the same way to MSG.

In research studies, H. Schaumburg found that approximately **30% of our population suffered immediate, adverse reactions when fed MSG in an ordinary diet** at levels readily available on a given day. Other independent researchers confirmed his observations.

MSG is always in the following:

Autolyzed yeast. Calcium caseinate. Gelatin. Glutamate. Glutamic acid. Hydrolyzed protein. Monopotassium glutamate. Monosodium glutamate. Sodium caseinate. Textured protein. Yeast extract. Yeast food. Yeast Nutrient

MSG is often in each of these:

Barley Malt. Bouillon. Broth. Carrageenan. Enzyme-modified substances. Flavoring. Flavors. Malt Extract. Malt flavoring. Maltodextrin. Natural flavor/flavorings. Natural pork/beef/chicken flavoring. Pectin. Protein-fortified substances. Seasonings. Soy protein. Soy protein isolate or concentrate. Soy sauce. Soy sauce extract. Stock. Vegetable gum. Whey protein. Whey protein isolate or concentrate

The Food and Drug Administration (FDA) has given a name to the cluster of physical problems which MSG can produce in your body. It is called the *MSG Symptom Complex*. That does not sound too bad, does it? **Here are the eleven different things that can happen to your body when you eat or drink something with MSG:**

Numbness. Burning sensation. Tingling Facial pressure or tightness. Chest pain. Headache. Nausea. Rapid heartbeat. Drowsiness. Weakness. Difficulty breathing for asthmatics.

In terms of labeling requirements, the FDA says that **"monosodium glutamate" must only be listed on the label only if MSG is added to a food. But it need not be mentioned if it is added to a food additive!** Therefore, manufacturer will list "No MSG," or "No Added MSG" on foods if sources of free monosodium glutamate is mingled with other additives, such as hydrolyzed protein. In addition, items listed as "flavors," "natural flavors," or "flavorings" may actually include MSG, hydrolyzed proteins or autolyzed yeast. You can thank highly-paid lobbyists in Washington D.C. for such deceptive rules.

Dr. Russell Blaylock, an author and neurosurgeon, recently explained **a link between sudden cardiac death, particularly in athletes, and excitotoxic damage** caused by food additives like MSG and artificial sweeteners. According to Dr. Blaylock, **excitotoxins are "a group of excitatory amino acids that can cause sensitive neurons to die."** He explains this further:

"When an excess of food-borne excitotoxins, such as MSG, hydrolyzed protein soy protein isolate and concentrate, natural flavoring, sodium caseinate and aspartate from aspartame, are consumed, these **glutamate receptors are over-stimulated, producing cardiac arrhythmias. When magnesium stores are low, as we see in athletes, the glutamate receptors are so sensitive that even low levels of these excitotoxins can result in cardiac arrhythmias and death.**"

Many consumers have personally experienced the ill effects of MSG, which leave them with a headache, nausea or vomiting after eating MSG-containing foods.

Said Cathy Evans Wisner in her article *"The MSG Myth,"* "I know from personal experience that the chemical is not as harmless as vinegar or salt. When I ingest a fair amount of MSG, I immediately have **nausea, stomach cramps, "spaciness," heart palpitations and a "pins-and-needles" headache**, followed the next day by **lethargy and overall weakness.**"

Headaches are one of the most commonly reported side effects of MSG, which may occur because it can increase blood flow to the brain. According to Ann Turner, director of the *Migraine Action Association*, "Food additives can be triggers [for headaches]. MSG, although still not fully understood, may be a culprit."

If you wish to keep eating some of the processed foods, you should **be diligent in reading processed food labels**. Hopefully, you may be able to determine whether a product is contaminated with MSG.

In general, **the more highly processed a food is (or the more ingredients listed on its label), the more likely it is to contain MSG**. Meanwhile, try to limit the number of processed foods you eat overall and you'll inevitably reduce your chances of eating MSG, too.

4 – Artificial Sweeteners

These are heavily found in so-called "diet products" and "sugar-free" processed foods and drinks. Keep in mind that all of these contain excitotoxins, which, over a period of time, severely damage the body.

These **artificial sweeteners**, include such products as **saccharin, cyclamate, aspartame, equal measure, nutrasweet spoonful, canderal, splenda**, and **acesulfame potassium.**

SACCHARIN

The first noncaloric artificial sweetener, saccharin was discovered in 1879, when it was accidentally produced by a student at Johns Hopkins University. Constantin Fahlberg was working on coal-tar deriva-

tives, and noticed a substance on his hands and arms that tasted sweet. No one knows why Fahlberg decided to lick it to see what it tasted like, but unfortunately he did.

Despite an early attempt, in 1911, to ban the substance (because skeptical scientists said it was an "adulterant" that changed the makeup of food), saccharin grew in popularity, and was used to sweeten foods during sugar rationings in World Wars I and II. Though it is about 300 times sweeter than sugar and has zero calories, **saccharin leaves an unpleasant, metallic aftertaste. And, of course, it produces all the effects of an excitotoxin.**

Widely available as Sweet-'nLow. saccharin is still used in canned fruits and chewing gums and in unexpected places, including toothpaste. Its use has declined somewhat since the advent of newer sweeteners.

Although initially tasting 350 times sweeter than sugar, saccharin produces a bitter aftertaste. It also causes an increased risk of **bladder cancer** in humans. The strange substance became mired in controversy in 1977, when a study indicated that the substance might contribute to cancer in rats.

But the manufacturers fought back—and won: When the FDA recommended that it be banned from use; the government responded by requiring a warning label to put onto products containing saccharin. The diet industry in 1997 petitioned the World Health Organization, and the U.S. and Canadian governments to remove saccharin from their list of cancer causing chemicals. The governments buckled by removing the requirement that products containing saccharin have a warning label. This will likely increase usage. This product has been shown to cause bladder and other cancer in rats and mice. Products containing saccharin are supposed to carry a warning label regarding the cancer risk.

CYCLAMATE

In 1951, cyclamate came on the market. Food and beverage companies jumped at the chance to sweeten their products with something that tasted more natural. By 1968, Americans were consuming more than 17 million pounds of the calorie-free substance a year in snack foods, canned fruit and soft drinks like Tab and Diet Pepsi.

But in the late 1960s, studies began linking cyclamate to **cancer**. One noted that chicken embryos injected with the chemical developed **extreme deformities**, leading scientists to wonder if unborn humans could be similarly damaged by their cola-drinking mothers. Another study linked the sweetener to **malignant bladder tumors** in rats. Because a 1958 Congressional amendment required the FDA to ban any food additive shown to cause cancer in humans or animals, on Oct. 18, 1969, the government ordered cyclamate removed from all food products.

Although cyclamate, a popular sweetener in the 1950s and 1960s, was banned in the U.S. in late 1969, because it was linked to **bladder cancer, shrinking** testes, and other health risks in laboratory animals—it has continued to be added to processed foods that is sold overseas.

American manufacturers still market cyclamate to many other countries, where it is used alone, or combined with saccharin. So, if you travel overseas, read labels very carefully to avoid products that contain cyclamate and/or saccharin.

ASPARTAME

Aspartame can produce serious damage in your body. If you want a sweet way to die, here it is.

Aspartame is widely available as Equal and NutraSweet. (Also as Nutrasweet, Equal Measure, Spoonful, and Canderal.) Used in soft drinks and in countless types of diet foods. **It breaks down at high temperatures, however, and therefore cannot be used in baked or cooked foods.**

Although 150 to 200 times sweeter than sugar, early tests revealed that aspartame may have caused an increased incidence of **brain tumors** in rats.

A board of public inquiry revoked the Food and Drug Administration's (FDA) 1974 approval of aspartame on the grounds that the research did not conclusively show that aspartame does not cause brain tumors. Three of five members of an FDA panel selected to review the board's decision agreed with it. **But the FDA commissioner overturned the board's decision and reapproved aspartame anyway.**

Here are more details on how this happened: For over eight years, the Food and Drug Administration (FDA) refused to approve aspartame. **Evidence was abundant that it caused seizures, brain tumors, and sudden heart attacks in laboratory animals.**

In 1981, when Ronald Reagan (a friend of the head of G.D. Searle, Inc.) took office, he fired the FDA Commissioner, who steadfastly refused to approve aspartame, and appointed Dr. Arthur H. Hayes. But there was so much opposition to its approval that a board of inquiry was set up, which demanded that aspartame not be approved either for humans or animals. Hayes overruled his own board and approved it. Shortly afterward, he resigned and accepted a position with Searle's.

When, in 1981, the synthetic compound aspartame was approved for use, it capitalized on saccharin's bad publicity by becoming the leading additive in diet colas.

The 1998 Survey—A 1998 survey conducted by the Calorie Control Council reported that **144 million American adults routinely eat and drink low-calorie, sugar-free products** such as desserts and artificially sweetened sodas.

Products containing aspartame must carry a warning label for people with phenylketonuria (PKU), a genetic problem that afflicts one in 20,000 people. They cannot metabolize a component of aspartame.

Aspartame is a presciption for disaster. **Fully 10% of aspartame consists of methanol. Methanol is a deadly poison. It is found in wood alcohol.** Methanol

is gradually released in the small intestine when the methyl group of aspartame encounters the enzyme chymotrypsin (*Steglink 1984, p. 143*).

But methanol is more readily absorbed by the body (thus becoming even more dangerous) **when it is heated above 86° F. (30° C.) before being ingested.** This occurs when soft drinks are left out in the sun or foods containing aspartame (such as Jello) are heated. A temperature of 86° F. is hardly warm! It is believed that **Gulf War Syndrome** was partly caused by the thousands of cases of bottled Diet Cokes which stood in the broiling, 120° Saudi Arabian sun for weeks at a time. It was the only fluid our soldiers could drink through the day.

Methanol breaks down into formaldehyde and formic acid in the body. Formaldehyde is a deadly neurotoxin. According to an EPA assessment, methanol "is considered a cumulative poison, due to the low rate of excretion, once it is absorbed. In the body, it is oxidized to formaldehyde and formic acid; both of which are toxic."

Full-strength **formaldehyde is embalming fluid**, because nothing can live in its presence. In the body, part of the formaldehyde is broken down into **formic acid, which is an activator to strip epoxy and urethane coatings**. Imagine what it does to your tissues! **Formic acid has been shown to slowly accumulate** in various parts of the body. **It inhibits oxygen metabolism.** Both the brain and heart muscle need lots of oxygen.

Toxic buildup in the body greatly increases when more than 7.8 mg / day of methanol is ingested. One liter (about 1 quart of aspartame-sweetened beverage) contains about 56 mg of methanol. Heavy users consume as much as 250 mg of methanol per day, or 32 times the EPA limit.

Formaldehyde is a known carcinogen; and it causes retinal damage of the eye. It interferes with DNA replication and causes birth defects. Because we lack a couple of key enzymes, humans are many times more sensitive to the toxic effects of methanol than animals. Formaldehyde is toxic to humans in even small doses.

Although very small amounts of methanol occur in fruit juices, it is never alone in natural food products. Ethanol, which is an antidote to methanol toxicity in humans, is always present in fruit juices.

Phenylalanine and aspartic acid constitute 90% of aspartame. When taken into the body, without other foods, they are neurotoxic. "Diet drinks" are loaded with aspartame and no food. The empty stomach increases the damage. Components of aspartame go straight to the brain, causing headaches, mental confusion, faulty balance, and seizures. Lab animals die from brain tumors.

As mentioned earlier, in the early 1990s, Desert Storm troops were given large quantities of aspartame-sweetened beverages which had been heated to high temperatures in the Saudi sun. Many of them returned home with a variety of mysterious disorders, called "Gulf War Syndrome," **similar to what occurs in persons chemically poisoned by formaldehyde**. Other breakdown products of aspartame, such as DKP, may also have been a factor. (The troops were also ordered to swallow insecticides and take anti-poison gas pills.)

The 1998 FDA Decision—**In a 1993 decision, the FDA approved aspartame as an ingredient in numerous food items which require heating.** On June 27, 1996, without giving public notice, the FDA removed all restrictions from aspartame and allowed it to be used in every possible type of food, including all heated and baked goods! This is astounding!

Be careful what you buy at the store! Your only safety is to not purchase processed foods in any form.

The amount of **methanol** people are putting into their bodies (by ingesting aspartame) is unprecedented in human history. Persons who eat or drink aspartame-containing products are often dieting (eating very small amounts), and thus more likely to have nutritional deficiencies. This intensifies the harmful results. More on this later.

Because these poisons gradually accumulate in the system, the full effects, in the form of chronic diseases, may not be seen until years later.

The 2002 CDC Report—On February 15, 2002, the Centers for Disease Control in Atlanta released a stunning report on the astounding fact that **more than 60% of heart disease deaths in 1999 were sudden and nearly half occurred outside of hospitals!**

This CDC report stated that **Sudden Cardiac Death (SCD) is now the nation's Number 1 killer**; it prematurely ended the lives of 460,000 Americans in 1999. **When the heart stops abruptly without warning, the diagnosis is SCD.** It kills its victims within minutes. It is estimated that 95% of victims die before reaching the hospital. SCD often happens to outwardly healthy people, such as high school, college and professional athletes, plus thousands of children—all usually with no known heart problems. Here is the official CDC press release, dated February 15, 2002. (Because it is a press release, the CDC is spoken of in the third person.)

"Despite advances in the prevention and treatment of heart attacks and improvements in emergency transportation, **more than 60% of heart disease deaths in 1999—more than 460,000—were unexpected or 'sudden,' and nearly half of all heart deaths (46.9%) occurred outside of the hospital**, according to an analysis of state data by the centers for Disease Control and Prevention (CDC).

"Of the 728,743 heart disease deaths in 1999, 462,340 (63.4%) were defined as sudden cardiac deaths (SCD). Of those, 46.9% occurred outside of the hospital, and 16.5% occurred in the emergency room or were pronounced dead upon arrival at the hospital, **according to the latest death certificate data from the National Center for Health Statistics**. Women were more likely than men to die before reaching the hospital (51.9% compared to 41.7%) . . [A list of states

with the highest and lowest percentages is then given in the report; but all were high, varying between 58.5% and 72.9%.] . .

"Possible reasons for the high percentages, according to the CDC researchers, are the unexpected nature of SCD and the failure to recognize early warning symptoms of heart disease, particularly heart attack. Early recognition of symptoms can lead to early treatment that results in less heart damage and fewer deaths.

" 'These high numbers of sudden deaths from heart disease, and the fact that they occur outside of the hospital, are alarming,' said CDC Director Jeffrey P. Koplan, MD, MPH. 'CDC and its partners are working closely with states to educate Americans—and their health care providers—about the common and uncommon signs of heart attack and to encourage them to dial 9-1-1 immediately.'

"Uncommon **symptoms** of heart attack that the public and health care providers should watch for include **breaking out in a cold sweat, nausea, and light-headedness**. More common symptoms are **chest discomfort or pain; pain or discomfort in one or both arms or in the back, neck, jaw, or stomach; and shortness of breath**.

"Douglas Zipes, MD, president of the American College of Cardiology, concurred. 'Because **almost one of every two Americans will die of cardiovascular disease, and because about half of those deaths will be sudden**, we need to train people in **cardiopulmonary resuscitation** and in use of the **automated external defibrillator**, and make that equipment widely available,' Zipes said . . [Paragraph lauding CDC's efforts to warn the public about health dangers.] . .

"**Cardiovascular disease—principally heart attack, stroke, and high blood pressure—kill nearly a million Americans each year, making it the leading cause of death among men and women and all racial and ethnic groups.** About 62 million Americans live with cardiovascular disease, which in 2002 is expected to cost the nation an estimated $329.2 billion in health care expenditures and lost productivity. This burden continues to grow as the population ages.

"Besides being aware of the warning signs of heart disease and responding immediately when they occur, **people can reduce their chances of disease through lifestyle changes: being physically active, eating a diet low in fat and high in fruits and vegetables, and stopping or never starting smoking**."—*CDC Press Release, February 15, 2002; contact: Kathryn Harben, CDC.*

The above press release assumed that the sudden cardiac disease (SCD) deaths were the result of some kind of early, and previously unrecognized, heart disease. The true cause of many of those deaths is dramatically different.

Only in recent medical history has it ever been said that people have a habit of simply "dropping dead" from routine exertion.

Now consider this fact: **Aspartame triggers an**

irregular heart rhythm and interacts with cardiac medication. It damages the cardiac conduction system and is a direct cause of this sudden death.

Since the approval of the excitotoxin, aspartame, millions of American have fallen victim to numerous chronic and degenerative diseases—and death. The most shocking aspect is its relationship to incidents of sudden death among children and adults. **Nearly half a million Americans are simply "dropping dead" each year.**

Numerous medical journal reports and articles in magazines and newspapers have acknowledged this fatal problem; they generally do not explain its cause. The evidence points to aspartame. Just stop using all aspartame foods, and suddenly you will begin feeling better.

James Bowen, M.D., believes that the evidence is pointing to aspartame as the toxin responsible for sudden death in many of these instances. This is because the combination of aspartame consumption, along with the stresses of athletic competition, lead to activation of the shock mechanism, including arginine vasodepression in the hypothalamus. This results in cerebral edema, cardiac congestion, and pulmonary edema. **In connection with this, there is severe potassium loss**—which is a sure ticket to sudden death, especially because of the many other damages produced by aspartame.

Sudden death during seizures is almost always from cardiac standstill, due to arrhythmia (irregular heart beat). There are several ways that aspartame can cause this damage. **The methyl alcohol within it damages the myocardium (heart muscle) as well as the cardiac electrical system itself.** It also causes immense damage to the mitochondria. The result is that the myocardium and cardiac conduction system (which sends beats to the heart) never get to slow down and rest, but are constantly pumping blood.

The damaged mitochondria in the heart produce larger amounts of free radicals, resulting in increasingly irregular heartbeats (arrhythmia). This is not noticed until a bigger incidence occurs and the person drops over dead.

The problem is intensified by the fact that **many people, anxious to keep their weight down, fill up on "diet" foods and drinks while not obtaining enough vitamins, minerals, and co-enzyme factors.** This increases the likelihood of arrhythmia. Seizures put unusual demands on the cardiorespiratory system. **When anti-seizure medication is then taken, the toxicity of aspartame in the body is increased.**

Please understand that **Sudden Cardiac Death (SCD) is not only a "heart attack" or mycardial infarction caused by clogged arteries; it is an electrical problem in which the cardiac conduction system that generates the impulses regulating the heart suddenly puts out rapid or chaotic electrical impulses, or both.** The heart ceases its rhythmic contractions, the brain is starved of oxygen, and the victim

loses consciousness in seconds. He is then reported to have had a sudden, mysterious heart attack, without apparent cause.

The 1984 and 1994 Reports—In November 1984, the CDC compiled a report, reviewing 213 of 592 cases of aspartame complaints. Some of these included **cardiac arrest, seizures, disorientation, hyperactivity, extreme numbness, excitability, memory loss, loss of depth perception, liver impairment, severe mood swings, and even death**. The executive summary, prepared by Frederick L. Trowbridge, concluded that all the complaints were "generally of a mild nature." He then retired.

Monsanto consistently claims that aspartame is "safe," with the exception of a few people who are "allergic" to it.

The 1994 DHHS Report—In February 1994, the U.S. Department of Health and Human Services (DHHS) released a listing of adverse reactions reported to the FDA *(DHHS 1994)*. **Aspartame accounted for more than 75% of all adverse reactions** reported to the FDA's Adverse Reaction Monitoring System (ARMS). The FDA has admitted that fewer than 1% of consumers ever report a problem they had with a food. Therefore the 10,000 registered complaints about aspartame actually represent a million. Many of those reactions were very serious, including seizures and sudden death. Here are some of these symptoms:

Abdominal pain, anxiety attacks, arthritis, asthma, asthmatic reactions, bloating, edema (fluid retention), blood sugar control problems (hypoglycemia or hyperglycemia), breathing difficulties, burning eyes or throat, burning urination, can't think straight, chest pains, chronic cough, chronic fatigue, confusion, death, depression, diarrhea, dizziness, excessive thirst or hunger, fatigue, feel unreal, flushing of face, hair loss or thinning of hair, dizziness, hearing loss, heart palpitations, hives, hypertension (high blood pressure), impotency and sexual problems, inability to concentrate, infection susceptibility, insomnia, irritability, itching, joint pains, laryngitis, marked personality changes, memory loss, menstrual problems or changes, migraines and severe headaches, muscle spasms, nausea or vomiting, numbness or tingling of extremities, panic attacks, phobias, poor memory, rapid heartbeat, rashes, seizures and convulsions, slurring of speech, swallowing pain, tachycardia, "thinking in a fog," tremors, tinnitus, vertigo, vision loss, weight gain.

According to the CDC, 100,000 young athletes die each year from all cardiovascular disorders, including cardiomyopathy, as a result of participation in sports. **This is twice as many as die in auto accidents.** Of the 100,000 who die annually, 45,000 of them play basketball, not boxing or football.

On April 20, 1995, the DHHS issued a report listing symptoms attributed to aspartame, in complaints received from the general public about that product in food and drink.

Of the more than 100 types of problems, **here are**

the 23 that were mentioned the most, with the number of complaints for each:

Headache, 1,847 complaints / dizziness, poor equilibrium, 735 / change of mood, 656 / vomiting or nausea, 647 / abdominal pain and cramps, 483 / change in vision, 362 / diarrhea, 330 / seizures and convulsions, 290 / memory loss, 255 / fatigue, weakness 242 / other neurological, 230 / rash, 226 / sleep problems, 201 / hives, 191 / change in heart rate, 185 / itching, 175 / grand mal seizures, 174 / numbness, tingling, 172 / local swelling, 114 / change in activity level, 113 / difficulty in breathing, 112 / oral sensory changes, 106 / changes in menstrual pattern, 107.

It is obvious that aspartame does not spare any structural system in the body.

Which products are the worst—**That same 1995 DHHS report also listed the distribution of reactions to aspartame by product name. This is an extremely helpful list**, because **it lists the worst of these "sugar-free" products** and gives us a glimpse of the wide variety of aspartame products on the market.

Diet soft drinks, 3,021 complaints / **table top sweetener**, 1,716 / **puddings, gelatins**, 633 / **lemonade**, 410 / **Kool Aid**, 339 / **iced tea**, 319 / **chewing gum**, 319 / **hot chocolate**, 318 / **frozen confections**, 136 / **cereal**, 119 / **sugar substitute tablets**, 71 / **breath mints**, 62 / **punch mix**, 45 / **fruit drinks**, 24 / **non-dairy toppings**, 8 / **chewable multi-vitamins**, 8 / **dried fruit**, 1 / **other**, 346.

Filling the land with defibrillators—When a person drops from SCD (if he is not given **a defibrillator shock to his heart** to get it started beating again) within five to ten minutes, he cannot be resuscitated.

A small model which can be operated by anyone is now selling like hot cakes: Push a button, and a voice instructs you to place one paddle over the heart and the other over the other side of the chest. Push another button; and the heartbeat is automatically checked and the voice announces whether or not he needs the shock (defibrillation). If so, the voice says not to touch the patient, but to push another button. An instant later, the voice says that the shock has been given; and then it tells whether the heart is working properly or another shock is needed.

These handy gadgets are being placed in malls, airports, office buildings, and on passenger airplanes all across America. Everywhere, people are suddenly dropping dead. New York State has mandated *automatic external defibrillators* (AEDs) be provided for all schools and athletic events, on and off campus. Illinois enacted a similar law. In California, they talk of making defibrillators as common as fire extinguishers.

The Philadelphia Trial Lawyers Association donated 73 AEDs to school gyms and playing fields in the area. The Philadelphia School District estimates that **7,000-10,000 children and youth in America die annually from SCD**. Victora Vetter, M.D., Chief of cardiology at Children's Hospital, said, "I diagnose, treat and follow hundreds of children from the Philadelphia

region with cardiac issues."

The *Atlanta Journal Constitution*, for September 11, 2003, said, "**Sudden death in high school athletes is a topic that has received a lot of attention recently.**" It mentioned an article in *Science* magazine in 2002 which said that **450,000 people each year are victims of sudden death**.

A 2001 article in the *Journal of Athletic Training* reported, "**In the U.S. each year, sudden cardiac arrest kills 350,000, which is approximately 1,000 people per day . . The exact incidence of Sudden Cardiac Arrest in athletes is unknown because no universal, standard surveillance method is used.**"

Some sample cases—American Airlines co-pilot Neill was drinking a diet drink, and suddenly fell over dead. The captain landed the plane, so the body could be removed and to get a new co-pilot.

Sonny Bono, the U.S. Congressman who (while skiing down a hill in Colorado) suddenly veered, hit a tree, and died. It was reported that Bono was not drinking alcohol, but only a "Diet Coke." His heart may suddenly have stopped beating.

President Bush had a fainting spell and claimed it was due to eating a pretzel. They contain aspartame. Blackouts are common in aspartame victims; and President Bush regularly drinks diet soft drinks.

Kathy Fulford was certain she was dying, because she was having blackouts. One day she almost hit a car head-on. Ten physicians were unable to diagnose the cause. Then a friend suggested she stop using aspartame products; and her health problems disappeared.

A friend of hers, a 46-year-old beautician, drank diet drinks to keep her weight down. She too had blackouts and was recently found dead on the floor—another SCD victim.

SPLENDA

Some of the most popular artificial sweeteners on the market today are: Splenda (sucralose), Aspartame, Saccharine, and Acesulfame Potassium (aka - acesulfame K).

These artificial sweeteners are used in abundance in almost every "diet" drink, "lite" yogurts, puddings, and ice creams, most "low-carb" products, and almost all "reduced-sugar" products.

The artificial sweetener **Splenda** is quickly gaining popularity in a market that was previously dominated by aspartame-based Equal and saccharin-based Sweet 'N Low. In January 2003, Splenda even surpassed Equal in dollar-market share. **Splenda, the brand name for sugar-derivative sucralose**, is converted from cane sugar to a no-calorie sweetener. It isn't recognized as sugar by the body and therefore is not metabolized. Splenda is marketed as a "healthful" and "natural" product since it is derived from sugar. However, **its chemical structure is very different from that of sugar and sucralose is actually a chemical substance.**

The chemical sucralose, marketed as "Splenda", has replaced aspartame as the #1 artificial sweetener in foods and beverages. Aspartame has been forced out by increasing public awareness that it is both a neurotoxin and an underlying cause of chronic illness worldwide. Dr. James Bowen, researcher and biochemist, reports:

"Splenda/sucralose is simply chlorinated sugar; a chlorocarbon. **Common chlorocarbons include carbon tetrachloride, trichlorethelene and methylene chloride, all deadly.** Chlorine is nature's Doberman attack dog, a highly excitable, ferocious atomic element employed as a biocide in bleach, disinfectants, insecticide, WWI poison gas and hydrochloric acid.

"Sucralose is a molecule of sugar chemically manipulated to surrender three hydroxyl groups (hydrogen + oxygen) and replace them with three chlorine atoms. Natural sugar is a hydrocarbon built around 12 carbon atoms. **When turned into Splenda it becomes a chlorocarbon, in the family of Chlorodane, Lindane and DDT.**

"It is logical to ask why table salt, which also contains chlorine, is safe while Splenda/sucralose is toxic? Because salt isn't a chlorocarbon. When molecular chemistry binds sodium to chlorine to make salt, carbon isn't included. Sucralose and salt are as different as oil and water.

"Unlike sodium chloride, **chlorocarbons are never nutritionally compatible with our metabolic processes and are wholly incompatible with normal human metabolic functioning.** When chlorine is chemically reacted into carbon-structured organic compounds to make chlorocarbons, the carbon and chlorine atoms bind to each other by mutually sharing electrons in their outer shells. This arrangement adversely affects human metabolism because our mitochondrial and cellular enzyme systems are designed to completely utilize organic molecules containing carbon, hydrogen, oxygen, nitrogen, and other compatible nutritional elements.

"By this process chlorocarbons such as sucralose deliver chlorine directly into our cells through normal metabolization. **This makes them effective insecticides and preservatives.** By their nature, preservatives kill anything alive in order to prevent bacterial decomposition."

Doctor Bowen has spent 20 years researching artificial sweeteners after his own use of aspartame resulted in being diagnosed with Lou Gehrig's disease. Dr Bowen's intention is to warn the world of the toxicity of tabletop poisons like aspartame, Splenda and Neotame.

Dr. James Bowen believes ingested chlorocarbon damage continues with the formation of other toxins: "**Any chlorocarbons not directly excreted from the body intact can cause immense damage to the processes of human metabolism and, eventually, our internal organs.** The liver is a detoxification organ which deals with ingested poisons. **Chlorocarbons damage the hepatocytes, the liver's metabolic cells, and destroy them.**

In test animals Splenda produced swollen livers, as do all chlorocarbon poisons, **and also calcified the kidneys** of test animals in toxicity studies. The **brain and nervous system** are highly subject to metabolic toxicities and solvency damages by these chemicals. **Their high solvency attacks the human nervous system and many other body systems, including reproductive genes and the immune function. Thus, chlorocarbon poisoning can cause cancer, birth defects, and immune system destruction.** These are well known effects of Dioxin and PCBs which are known deadly chlorocarbons."

"Synthetic chemical sweeteners are generally unsafe for human consumption. **This toxin was given the chemical name "sucralose" which is a play on the technical name of natural sugar, sucrose. One is not the other.** One is food, the other is toxic; don't be deceived."

A long list of harmful effects—**Research in animals has shown that sucralose can cause many problems. Here are a few of them:**

Reduced growth rate in newborns and adults at levels above 500 mg/kg.day. **Decreased red blood cells**—sign of anemia (at levels abofe 1500 mg/kd/. **Decreased thyroxine levels**, that is, the thyroid function. Mineral losses of both magnesium and phosphorus. **Decreased urination. Enlarged colon. Enlarged liver and brain.** Shrunken ovaries. Shrunken thymus above 3 grams per day. Enlarged and calcified kidneys. Increased adrenal cortical hemorrhagic degeneration. Increased cataracts. Abnormal liver cells.

McNeil Nutritionals, the manufacturer of Spenda, announced that most of the above findings, made by independent researchers, have "no toxicological significance"! But, in reality, many of these are symptoms of serious pathology.

What about FDA-approved research? **As of 2006, only six human trials have been published on Splenda** (sucralose). Of these six trials, only two of the trials were completed and published before the FDA approved sucralose for human consumption. The two published trials had a grand total of 36 total human subjects. Thirty-six people sure doesn't sound like many, but wait, it gets worse, **only 23 total were actually given sucralose** for testing and now for this astounding fact: **The longest trial at this time had lasted only four days and looked at sucralose in relation to tooth decay, not human tolerance!**

Everyone needs to be warned about Splenda. Splenda, best known for its marketing logo, *"made from sugar so it tastes like sugar,"* has taken the sweetener industry by storm. Splenda has become the nation;s number one selling artificial sweetener in a very short period of time.

Between 2000 and 2004, the percentage of US households using Splenda products jumped from 3 to 20 percent. In a one year period, Splenda sales topped $177 million compared with $62 million spent on aspartame-based Equal and $52 million on saccharin-based Sweet 'N Low.

McNeil Nutritionals, in their marketing pitch for Splenda emphasizes that Splenda has endured "some of the most rigorous testing to date for any food additive." Enough so to convince the average consumer that it is in fact safe.

There were no long-term human toxicity studies published until after the FDA approved sucralose for human consumption. Following FDA approval a human toxicity trial was conducted, **but lasted only three months**, hardly the extended length of time most Splenda users plan to consume sucralose. No studies have ever been done on children or pregnant women.

Much of the controversy surrounding Splenda does not focus just on its safety, but rather on its false advertising claims. The competition among sweeteners is anything but sweet. **The sugar industry is currently suing McNeil Nutritionals for implying that Splenda is a natural form of sugar with no calories.**

Is It REALLY Sugar?—There is no question that sucralose starts off as a sugar molecule, it is what goes on in the factory that is concerning. **Sucralose is a synthetic chemical that was originally cooked up in a laboratory.** In the five step patented process of making sucralose, three chlorine molecules are added to a sucrose or sugar molecule. A sucrose molecule is a disaccharide that contains two single sugars bound together; glucose and fructose.

The chemical process to make sucralose alters the chemical composition of the sugar so much that it is somehow converted to a fructo-galactose molecule. **This type of sugar molecule does not occur in nature and therefore your body does not possess the ability to properly metabolize it.** It can only cause trouble in your body. As a result of this "unique" biochemical make-up, McNeil Nutritionals makes it's claim that Splenda is not digested or metabolized by the body, making it have zero calories.

It is not that Splenda is naturally "zero calories". If your body had the capacity to metabolize it then it would no longer have zero calories.

How much Splenda remains in your body after you eat it?—If you look at the research (which is primarily extrapolated from animal studies) you will see that in fact, on the average, **15% of sucralose is absorbed into your digestive system and ultimately is stored in your body.** To reach a number such as 15% means some people absorb more and some people absorb less. In one human study, one of the eight participants did not excrete any sucralose even after 3 days. Clearly his body was absorbing and storing this chemical—and perhaps doing strange things with it.

The bottom line is that we all have our own unique biochemical make-up. Some of you will absorb and react to Spenda more than others. **If you are healthy and your digestive system works well, you may be at higher risk for breaking down this product in your**

stomach and intestines. Please understand that it is impossible for the manufacturers of Splenda to make any guarantees based on their limited animal data.

If you feel that Splenda affects you adversely, it is valid. Don't let someone convince you that it is all in your head. You know your body better than anyone else.

How to Determine if Splenda is Harming You— The best way to determine if Splenda or sucralose is affecting you is to perform an elimination/challenge with it. First eliminate it and other artificial sweeteners from your diet completely for a period of one to two weeks. After this period reintroduce it in sufficient quantity.

For example, use it in your beverage in the morning, and eat at least two sucralose containing products the remainder of the day. On this day, avoid other artificial sweeteners so that you are able to differentiate which one may be causing a problem for you. Do this for a period of one to three days. Observe how your body is feeling, particularly if it feels different than when you were artificial-sweetener free.

Splenda May Still Be Harming You

If you complete the elimination/challenge trial described above and do not notice any changes then it appears that Splenda is only damaging your body more slowly. Some comfort!

Keep in mind that **Splenda has a closer chemical similarity to DDT than it does to sugar**. And remember that fat soluble substances, such as DDT, can remain in your fat for decades and devastate your health.

ACESULFAME K

Acesulfame K is widely sold under the names Sunette and Sweet-One. This artificial sweetener, also called Ace-K, is used in Coke Zero.

This is the newest substance to be approved for use as a tabletop sweetener. It has not yet been approved for any additional uses.

While it is 200 times sweeter than sugar, it has not been thoroughly tested. Long-term rat studies produced **lung, breast and other tumors**. It may slightly increase the risk of **cancer** and should not have been approved for any human use. It failed to meet FDA standards.

HONEY: A GOOD SWEETENER

Honey is an easily-assimilable carbohydrate compound. It generates heat, produces energy, and helps form certain tissues. It supplies your body with substances for the formation of enzymes and other biological ferments to promote oxidation. It has distinct germicidal properties, and in this respect greatly differs from milk which is an exceptionally good breeding-ground for bacteria. Honey is a most valuable food, which today is not sufficiently appreciated.

The first *International Symposium on Honey and Human Health* was held in Sacramento, California, in January 2008. **Many significant findings were**

HARMFUL

presented, including but not limited to these:

Buckwheat honey has been found to be a more **effective cough remedy** than dextromethorphan for children from two to eighteen years.

Compared to other substances used as sweeteners, honey is **much better tolerated by the body**, leading to **better blood sugar control and sensitivity to insulin**.

Honey **promotes immunity**, as demonstrated by findings that 32 percent of cancer patients in an immunity study reported improvement in their quality of life as a result of fewer infections.

Honey **promotes wound healing**, its most useful application in medicine and has been **proven to heal burns quicker**.

The two primary sugars that make honey (fructose and glucose) both attract water. When applied to an open wound, **honey absorbs the fluid in the wound**. Most bacteria need a moist environment to grow; honey makes the wound drier.

Honey stored in airtight containers **will keep for indeterminate periods of time**. Airtight will prevent the honey from absorbing ambient water and will keep the flavor from changing. It should be kept in a cool, dry place.

If your honey crystallizes do not heat it in the microwave, as this will alter the flavor. **Place the container in hot water for about fifteen minutes** in order to return it to a liquid state.

If you substitute honey for sugar in a recipe, use only about three-quarters of a cup for every cup of sugar. Baking temperature needs to be lowered by twenty-five degrees Fahrenheit. Food made with honey will brown easier during the baking process.

Avoid feeding honey to children under the age of two years. It is possible for honey to sometimes contain the bacteria that causes botulism food poisoning, an often fatal infection. It is best to simply avoid the risk.

The universal and natural craving for sweets of some kind proves best that there is a true need for them in the human system. Children, who expend lots of energy, have a real "passion" for sweets. Proteins will replace and build tissues, but it is the function and assignment of carbohydrates to **create and replace heat and energy**.

Honey contains two invert sugars, levulose and dextrose, has many advantages as a food substance. While cane-sugar and starches, as already intimated, must undergo during digestion a process of inversion which changes them into grape and fruit-sugars, **in honey this is already accomplished because it has been predigested by the bees, inverted and concentrated**. This saves the stomach additional labor. For a healthy human body, which is capable of digesting sugar, the actuality that honey is an already predigested sugar has less importance, but **in a case of weak digestion, especially in those who lack invertase and amylase and depend on monosaccharides, honey can be an invaluable aid to digestion and health**.

The consummation of this predigestive act is ac-

complished by the enzymes invertase, amylase and catalase, which are produced by the worker bee in such large quantities that they can be found in every part of their bodies. However, there is plenty of it left in the honey they produce.

The remarkable convertive power of these enzymes can be proven by a simple experiment. If we add one or two tablespoonful of raw honey to a pint of concentrated solution of sucrose, the mixture will soon be changed into invert sugar. The addition of boiled honey, in which the enzymes have been destroyed, will not accomplish such a change.

OTHER SAFE SWEETENERS

Here are four safe sweeteners:

Honey, Stevia, Agave, Dried Cane Juice (from Florida cane juice crystals).

STEVIA IS ALSO SAFE

Stevia Rebaudiana (pronounced stee-vee-ah re-bau-dee-ah-nah) is an herb in the chrysanthemum family which grows wild as a small shrub in different parts of the world including South America and Asia.

The glycosides in its leaves, including up to 10% *stevioside*, **account for its incredible sweetness, making it unique among the nearly 300 species of stevia plants.** There are indications that stevia (also called Ca-he-he) has been used to sweeten a native beverage called mat since Pre-Columbian times. However, natural scientist, Antonio Bertoni first recorded its usage by native tribes in 1887.

In 1970 the Japanese began extracting the pure sweet powder found in the leaf for testing and commercial use. **Stevia sweeteners have been fully approved and widely used in Japan since 1970 in food products and soft drinks and for table-top use. It is also fully approved and in use in Brazil, where it is also recommended for diabetics.**

Realizing that stevia could ruin their artificial sweetener business, the food processors got the FDA to ban the use of stevia as a food additive in processed foods.

Here is more of the story: **This totally natural product has zero calories, zero carbohydrates, and zero chance of a spike in blood sugar levels.**

Stevia is all natural and derived from an herbal plant grown primarily in Asia and South America, whereas artificial sweeteners are made with chemicals in a laboratory. **Stevia also has no known side effects, whereas other alternatives do.** Reports indicate that aspartame, a well-known artificial sweetener, actually has had the highest number of consumer complaints reported to the FDA.

Several companies are just out with new products derived from the leaves of the Latin American herb *stevia*, which contain a substance hundreds of times more potent than sugar.

Arizona-based Wisdom Natural Brands was the first to start aggressively marketing packets of its powdered

SweetLeaf earlier this summer. Agribusiness giant Cargill, working in collaboration with Coca-Cola, followed with Truvia. And PepsiCo, with Whole Earth Sweetener Co., has developed a new line of beverages sweetened with a stevia product called PureVia.

"Soon you'll see stevia in pretty much every food product you can imagine," predicts Oscar Rodes, the founder of Texas-based producer Stevita Co., who is hoping that the herb could eventually account for 20 percent of the overall sweetener market.

Industrial research in Japan has shown that **stevia and stevioside extracts are extremely heat stable in a variety of everyday cooking and baking situations.** Please note, **stevia does not caramelize nor brown as sugar does.**

Is stevia safe? **Stevia has been thoroughly tested around the world and found to be completely nontoxic.** It has also been consumed safely in massive quantities (thousands of tons annually) for the past 30 years.

Stevia has long been sold by health food stores as a dietary supplement. The Food and Drug Administration still has not approved the "safety" of the new stevia products as food additives (even though Japan and Brazil has years ago), but the companies claim they've met requirements to establish stevia as "generally recognized as safe" by scientists.

It is claimed that the herb is far more healthful than either sugar or artificial sweeteners. A packet of sugar has about 11 calories, 3 grams of carbohydrates, and an estimated "glycemic load" of 2, for example.

Dietitians recommend keeping your glycemic load, a measure of how much particular foods raise blood sugar levels, below about 100 a day. A packet of sucralose (Splenda) has 3 calories, 1 gram of carbohydrates, and a glycemic load of 1, according to NutritionData.

Indeed, some research suggests that stevia may improve health. Jan Geuns, a biologist in Belgium who has organized symposiums to explore the substance's pharmacological effects on humans, points to two Chinese studies that have found it can significantly lower blood pressure among people with mild hypertension.

Danish researchers have reported that stevia seems to reduce blood glucose levels among patients with type 2 diabetes. But Geuns adds that the effects were seen only at doses far greater than those for stevia when used as a sweetener. So the typical user would experience little effect.

But read this: Stevia has been slow in being accepted by mainstream consumers, partly because of a bitter licorice aftertaste. Makers of the new stevia sweeteners claim to have found ways around that; since the degrees of processing and purity vary significantly— some products contain added flavors, bulking agents, or fiber—consumers may want to try several brands. For the best taste, Rodes recommends using products that are at least 95 percent pure; Geuns says to look

for products rich in a substance called *rebaudioside A.*

Thus we see that, although stevia is totally derived from a natural plant, yet it still involves a fair amount of processing.

It's not just taste that has hampered consumer acceptance; the herb has been trapped in a regulatory limbo. Since the 1960s, a trickle of animal studies has suggested that stevia might cause potentially cancerous mutations or reproductive problems. Though the studies' methodologies were criticized and **stevia had a good safety record in countries where it was widely used at the time, such as Japan, yet FDA regulators imposed an import ban in 1991.** The stevia industry howled, charging that artificial-sweetener makers just wanted to clear the market of competition. Which is probably true.

In 1994, a new law that revamped the way foods are regulated led to a lift of the import ban and put stevia in the odd position of being considered safe if marketed as a dietary supplement but not if used in foods or drinks. "It's a completely absurd and confusing situation for consumers," says James Turner, a partner at Swankin & Turner, a consumer rights law firm based in Washington, D.C., who has expertise on the regulation of sweeteners. The intent, according to the FDA, is to prove stevia safe through rigorous research before people start widely consuming it in food.

I will personally continue to prefer honey, and no processed foods of any kind. However, if you want a zero sweetener, then stevia is probably what you may want.

REGULAR SUGAR

Here are 125 reasons why sugar is harmful.

In addition to throwing off the body's homeostasis, excess sugar may result in a number of other significant consequences. **The following is a listing of some of sugar's metabolic consequences from a variety of medical journals and other scientific publications.** The following data is from the book, *Lick the Sugar Habit,* by Nancy Appleton. In her book, she lists research sources for each and every item, listed below:

1. Sugar can suppress the immune system
2. Sugar upsets the mineral relationships in the body
3. Sugar can cause hyperactivity, anxiety, difficulty concentrating, and crankiness in children
4. Sugar can produce a significant rise in triglycerides
5. Sugar contributes to the reduction of defense against bacterial infection (infectious diseases)
6. Sugar causes a loss of tissue elasticity and function; the more sugar you eat the more elasticity and function you loose
7. Sugar reduces high density lipoproteins
8. Sugar leads to chromium deficiency
9. Sugar leads to cancer of the breast, ovaries, prostrate, and rectum

10. Sugar can increase fasting levels of glucose

11. Sugar causes copper deficiency

12. Sugar interferes with absorption of calcium and magnesium

13. Sugar can weaken eyesight

14. Sugar raises the level of a neurotransmitter: dopamine, serotonin, and norepinephrine

15. Sugar can cause hypoglycemia

16. Sugar can produce an acidic digestive tract

17. Sugar can cause a rapid rise of adrenaline levels in children

18. Sugar malabsorption is frequent in patients with functional bowel disease

19. Sugar can cause premature aging

20. Sugar can lead to alcoholism

21. Sugar can cause tooth decay

22. Sugar contributes to obesity

23. High intake of sugar increases the risk of Crohn's disease and ulcerative colitis

24. Sugar can cause changes frequently found in a person with gastric or duodenal ulcers

25. Sugar can cause arthritis

26. Sugar can cause asthma

27. Sugar greatly assists the uncontrolled growth of Candida Albicans (yeast infections)

28. Sugar can cause gallstones

29. Sugar can cause heart disease

30. Sugar can cause appendicitis

31. Sugar can cause multiple sclerosis

32. Sugar can cause hemorrhoids

33. Sugar can cause varicose veins

34. Sugar can elevate glucose and insulin responses in oral contraceptive users

35. Sugar can lead to periodontal disease

36. Sugar can contribute to osteoporosis

37. Sugar contributes to saliva acidity

38. Sugar can cause a decrease in insulin sensitivity

39. Sugar can lower the amount of vitamin E in the blood

40. Sugar can decrease growth hormone

41. Sugar can increase cholesterol

42. Sugar can increase the systolic blood pressure

43. Sugar can cause drowsiness and decreased activity in children

44. High sugar intake increases advanced glycation end products (AGEs)(Sugar bound non-enzymatically to protein)

45. Sugar can interfere with the absorption of protein

46. Sugar causes food allergies

47. Sugar can contribute to diabetes

48. Sugar can cause toxemia during pregnancy

49. Sugar can contribute to eczema in children

50. Sugar can cause cardiovascular disease

51. Sugar can impair the structure of DNA

52. Sugar can change the structure of protein

53. Sugar can make our skin age by changing the structure of collagen

54. Sugar can cause cataracts

55. Sugar can cause emphysema

56. Sugar can cause atherosclerosis

57. Sugar can promote an elevation of low density lipoproteins (LDL)

58. High sugar intake can impair the physiological homeostasis of many systems in the body

59. Sugar lowers the enzymes' ability to function

60. Sugar intake is higher in people with Parkinson's disease

61. Sugar can cause a permanent altering of the way the proteins act in the body

62. Sugar can increase the size of the liver, by making the liver cells divide

63. Sugar can increase the amount of liver fat

64. Sugar can increase kidney size and produce pathological changes in the kidney

65. Sugar can damage the pancreas

66. Sugar can increase the body's fluid retention

67. Sugar is enemy #1 of the bowel movement

68. Sugar can cause myopia (nearsightedness)

69. Sugar can compromise the lining of the capillaries

70. Sugar can make the tendons more brittle

71. Sugar can cause headaches, including migraine

72. Sugar plays a role in pancreatic cancer in women

73. Sugar can adversely affect school children's grades and cause learning disorders

74. Sugar can cause an increase in delta, alpha, and theta brain waves

75. Sugar can cause depression

76. Sugar increases the risk of gastric cancer

77. Sugar can cause dyspepsia (indigestion)

78. Sugar can increase your risk of getting gout

79. Sugar can increase the levels of glucose in an oral glucose tolerance test over the ingestion of complex carbohydrates

80. Sugar can increase the insulin responses in humans consuming high-sugar diets compared to low-sugar diets

81. Highly refined sugar diet reduces learning capacity

82. Sugar can cause less effective functioning of two blood proteins, albumin, and lipoproteins, which may reduce the body's ability to handle fat and cholesterol

83. Sugar can contribute to Alzheimer's disease

84. Sugar can cause platelet adhesiveness

85. Sugar can cause hormonal imbalance; some hormones become underactive and others become overactive

86. Sugar can lead to the formation of kidney stones

87. Sugar can lead the hypothalamus to become highly sensitive to a large variety of stimuli

88. Sugar can lead to dizziness

89. Diets high in sugar can cause free radicals and oxidative stress

90. High sucrose diets of subjects with peripheral

vascular disease significantly increases platelet adhesion

91. High sugar diet can lead to biliary tract cancer

92. Sugar feeds cancer

93. High sugar consumption of pregnant adolescents is associated with a twofold increased risk for delivering a small-for-gestational-age (SGA) infant

94. High sugar consumption can lead to substantial decrease in gestation duration among adolescents

95. Sugar slows food's travel time through the gastrointestinal tract

96. Sugar increases the concentration of bile acids in stools and bacterial enzymes in the colon

97. Sugar increases estradiol (the most potent form of naturally occurring estrogen) in men

98. Sugar combines and destroys phosphatase, an enzyme, which makes the process of digestion more difficult

99. Sugar can be a risk factor of gallbladder cancer

100. Sugar is an addictive substance

101. Sugar can be intoxicating, similar to alcohol

102. Sugar can exacerbate PMS

103. Sugar given to premature babies can affect the amount of carbon dioxide they produce

104. Increase in sugar intake can increase emotional instability

105. The body changes sugar into 2 to 5 times more fat in the bloodstream than it does starch

106. The rapid absorption of sugar promotes excessive food intake in obese subjects

107. Sugar can worsen the symptoms of children with attention deficit hyperactivity disorder (ADHD)

108. Sugar adversely affects urinary electrolyte composition

109. Sugar can slow down the ability of the adrenal glands to function

110. Sugar has the potential of inducing abnormal metabolic processes in a normal healthy individual and to promote chronic degenerative diseases

111. I.Vs (intravenous feedings) of sugar water can cut off oxygen to the brain

112. High sucrose intake could be an important risk factor in lung cancer

113. Sugar increases the risk of polio

114. High sugar intake can cause epileptic seizures

115. Sugar causes high blood pressure in obese people

116. In Intensive Care Units: Limiting sugar saves lives

117. Sugar may induce cell death

118. Sugar may impair the physiological homeostasis of many systems in living organisms

119. In juvenile rehabilitation camps, when children were put on a low sugar diet, there was a 44% drop in antisocial behavior

120. Sugar can cause gastric cancer

121. Sugar dehydrates newborns

122. Sugar can cause gum disease

123. Sugar increases the estradiol in young men

124. Sugar can cause low birth weight babies

5 – Beverages and Water

CAFFINATED BEVERAGES

(Coffee withdrawal: 882)

Caffeine is an alkaloid found in coffee, tea, chocolate and guarana. **Americans are hooked on caffeine. Ninety percent consume it in one form or another every single day. Over half consume more than 300 milligrams of caffeine** every day. **It is our nation's most popular drug. It is in coffee, tea, cola, chocolate, and a variety of other things.**

Caffeine is an addictive drug. It operates on the brain, using the same mechanisms as amphetamines, cocaine, and heroin to stimulate the brain. Although it is milder than the others, it is manipulating the same channels. This is one of the reasons it is addictive.

If you think that you cannot function every day with it, and must consume it every day—you are addicted to caffeine.

Caffeine is *trimethylxanthine*. Its chemical formula is $C_8H_{10}N_4O_2$. When isolated in pure form, caffeine is a white crystalline powder that tastes very bitter.

Physicians use it as a cardiac stimulant and also as a mild diuretic (increases urine production). But regular folk take it for the apparent "boost of energy" or feeling of heightened alertness it gives. It is often used to help people stay awake longer.

Obviously, what is happening is that **the body is tired and needs rest; but, instead, it is whipped into action. Beating a horse always hurts it. The body, repeatedly pushed into greater activity when it wants to stop for rest, is gradually damaged. Instead of recovering, organs gradually weaken. Eventually, the weakest ones become diseased**, and the person wonders why it happened.

Caffeine occurs naturally in many plants, including coffee beans, tea leaves, and cocoa nuts. Because of this, it is found in a wide variety of food products. In addition, caffeine is added to many other foods, including beverages.

Caffeine is a stimulant that **causes heart rate and respiration to increase**. It also has a **diuretic effect** and delays fatigue. One cup instant coffee equals 90-150mg caffeine 1 cup brewed tea equals 30-70mg caffeine Caffeine has been implicated in the development of **osteoporosis**. The *Journal of the American Medical Association* reported "significant association between caffeinated coffee and decreasing bone mineral density (in women. Except when) women reported drinking at least one glass of milk per day." Caffeine has been found to inhibit the activity of some anti-epileptic drugs. It is possible to overdose on caffeine: it is estimated that it would take 50-100 cups to result in death. This figure was arrived at by employing the LD50 test.

Here is a dangerous menu to think about:

• *Coffee:* Typical drip-brewed coffee contains 100 milligrams (mg.) per 6-ounce (oz.) cup. Whether you are buying it at Starbucks or a store, drinking it at home or at the office, out of a mug or commuter's cup, you are consuming it in one of three sizes: 12 oz. (200 mg.), 14 oz. (234 mg.), or 20 oz. (334 mg.). That is a lot of caffeine!

• *Tea:* Typical brewed tea contains 70 mg. in each 6-oz. cup.

• *Cola drinks:* Coke, Pepsi, Mountain Dew, etc., contain 50 mg. per 12-oz. can. Jolt contains 70 mg. per 12-oz. can.

• *Chocolate:* Typical milk chocolate contains 6 mg. per oz.

• *Drugs:* Anacin contains 32 mg. per tablet. No-doz contains 100 mg. per tablet. Vivarin and Dexatrim contain 200 mg. per tablet.

Sit down and calculate how much you are taking each day, and you might be surprised. **Many people consume a gram (1000 mg.) or more every single day**, without realizing it.

Just what does caffeine do when it gets into the body?—As your body becomes fatigued, adenosine is made in the brain, and binds to adenosine receptors. This causes drowsiness by slowing nerve cell activity. You want to stop and rest. You want to go to sleep. This is good, for you need the rest. In the brain, the adenosine also causes blood vessels to dilate (enlarge), so more oxygen can reach the brain during sleep.

But when caffeine is taken into the stomach, it travels quickly to the brain. Once there, it does what adenosine normally does; it binds to the adenosine nerve receptors. **But, instead of slowing cellular activity, it speeds it up.** The cell can no longer bind with adenosine, because caffeine is linked up with all its available receptors.

The cell begins accelerating its activity. Because adenosine is shut out, the brain's blood vessels began to constrict (narrow).

The increased neuron firing in the brain awakens the pituitary gland to action. Some kind of emergency must be taking place! So the pituitary signals the adrenal glands to produce adrenaline (epinephrine), the "fight or flight" hormone.

The longer-term effects of using caffeine tend to spiral down. **Once the adrenaline wears off, you face even greater fatigue—and also depression.** More caffeine is taken, and soon the body is jumping into emergency levels all day long. You become jumpy and irritable.

Because the half-life of caffeine is six hours, by the time you go to bed, you cannot get to sleep or you will not obtain the deep sleep you need. (If the last cup of coffee was taken at 3 p.m., by 9 p.m., you will still have 100 mg. in your body.) **So the next morning you feel worse—and you need caffeine to get you out of bed.**

You have started another day, beating the horse.

This is why 90% of Americans consume caffeine every day. **But if you try to stop, you will get terrible, splitting headaches** as blood vessels in the brain dilate. So you go back to caffeine.

Its addictive nature—Scientific studies show that **drinking more than two cups of coffee a day cuts your remaining amount of life, on average, by a year.** While some people are dependent on their morning cup of coffee for their 'get up and go,' experts claim this apparent need is actually just the physiological nature of the addictive properties of caffeine manifesting them in your mind. **You are trying to use caffeine to take the place of proper rest.**

Most people are aware of the ill affect of drinking coffee because it contains caffeine. Actually, coffee is a narcotic beverage. **The caffeine in the coffee belongs to the same alkaloid group of chemicals as morphine, cocaine, and strychnine.** It is no surprise then why people have such a difficult time, at first, letting go of coffee and replacing it with healthier beverages.

Adrenal exhaustion—Coffee overworks the adrenals and slows sports performance. **Coffee has an acid-based oil which is an irritant to gastric mucosa. It simulates the secretion of gastric acidity; and this results in secretion of adrenaline. The secretion of adrenaline stimulates insulin secretion with consequent secondary hypoglycemia.** The end results are tension, mild rise in blood pressure, 2-3 hours later a craving for sweets, low energy and mood levels, and overworking of the adrenal glands. All of this negatively affects health, exercise and sports performance.

Just one caffeinated drink—whether it's a soft drink, caffeinated tea or coffee—starts your body on a "caffeine roller coaster." When you consume caffeine, the drug begins its effects by initiating uncontrolled neuron firing in your brain. **This excess neuron activity triggers your pituitary gland to secrete a hormone that tells your adrenal glands to produce adrenaline.** When this adrenal high wears off later, you feel the drop in terms of fatigue, irritability, headache or confusion. After prolonged "caffeinism," your body enters a state of adrenal exhaustion. Your caffeine consumption has simply pushed your adrenal glands so much that they've burned out. **Over the years, it takes more and more coffee to get the same result.** That's severe adrenal depletion. In other words, caffeine affects your body just like any drug. You start taking it slowly; but, as your body develops a tolerance to it, you need more and more to feel the same effects. Eventually, your body reaches a point where it can't be without it; otherwise, you will start to experience withdrawal symptoms.

Liver tries to get rid of it—Caffeine combines with the stomach's hydrochloric acid and forms a potent toxin, *caffeine hydrochloride*. As this toxin is absorbed into your portal circulation and hits your liver, it releases bile in an attempt to flush the toxin from your system. This accounts for the increase in bowel "regularity," which some consider helpful. But ask yourself, "Is such a toxin-induced flush really very health promoting? Or Isn't there a healthier way for me to be regular?" The answer, of course, is "No" to the first question and "Yes" to the second.

Harmful chemicals—**Drinking decaffeinated coffee is no better than drinking regular coffee** because of the large concentration of the chemical, *Trichloroethylene*. It is used mainly as a degreasing agent in the metal industry and as a solvent and dry cleaning agent in the clothing industry. *Trichloroethylene* is related to plastic chemical *vinyl chloride*, which has been linked to certain types of liver cancer. Columbian coffee planters have regularly used deadly pesticides on their plants for over 20 years. Some include *Aldrin, Dieldrin, Chlordane, and Heptachlor.* **Some speculate that coffee beans are the most significant source of these deadly toxins in U.S. diets.**

The extreme temperatures in the roasting process of coffee beans depletes the beans of its natural oils. **Though it may enhance their aroma, high heat actually causes the oils to become rancid.** The *chlorogenic acid* found in coffee has also been linked to toxic side effects.

Injures the body—The secondary rise in *plasma epinephrine*, due to the low blood sugar, will undo whatever good medications are doing to counteract the hyperactive dopaminergic system in patients suffering from pain, obesity, hypertension, or depression. **A few minutes after drinking coffee, the stimulation of the dopaminergic system results in cold extremities with simultaneous rise in visceral temperature.** A patient with high fever is harmed by coffee, but helped by lemon juice. The decaffeinated coffee contains the same acid oil, and thus is no better than regular coffee.

Causes nutritional deficiencies—Heavy coffee drinkers create *Thiamine* (vitamin B_1) insufficiency. Symptoms of B_1 insufficiency range from fatigue, nervousness, general malaise, general aches and pains to headaches.

Regular use of coffee prevents some of the nutrients in your food from being absorbed effectively in your small intestines, which leads to further vitamin and mineral deficiencies.

Rebound fatigue—The "buzz," or stimulation, you get from coffee actually contributes to rebound fatigue when the stimulating effects wear off. **Repeated stimulation can contribute to the exhaustion of key organs like the liver, pancreas, and adrenal glands.**

Caffeine forces your glands to secrete when they don't have much left to give; and they have to keep digging deeper and deeper, making you more and more tired over time.

CARBONATED BEVERAGES

Bone loss in a can—**The carbonation in all soft drinks causes calcium loss in the bones through a three-stage process:**

The carbonation irritates the stomach.

The stomach "cures" the irritation the only way it knows how. It adds the only antacid at its disposal: calcium. It gets this from the blood.

The blood, now low on calcium, replenishes its supply from the bones. If it did not do this, muscular and brain function would be severely impaired.

But, the story doesn't end there. **Another problem with most soft drinks is they also contain phosphoric acid (not the same as the carbonation, which is carbon dioxide mixed with the water). This substance also causes a drawdown on the store of calcium.**

So, soft drinks soften your bones (actually, they make them weak and brittle) in three ways:

Carbonation reduces the calcium in the bones.

Phosphoric acid reduces the calcium in the bones.

The beverage replaces a calcium-containing alternative, such as milk or water. Milk and water are not excellent calcium sources, but they are sources.

A study of 500 high school athletes found that **drinking just one carbonated beverage a day increased the fracture rate of bones from 200% to 500%**, depending on the amount of carbonation in the bottle. Coke was said to be the worst offender. **Carbonation destroys the body's ability to absorb minerals.**

Diabetes in a can—**The picture gets worse when you add sugar to the soft drink. The sugar, dissolved in liquid, is quickly carried to the bloodstream, where its presence in overload quantities signals the pancreas to go into overdrive.** The pancreas has no way of knowing if this sugar inrush is a single dose or the front-end of a sustained dose. The assumption in the body's chemical controls is the worst-case scenario. **To prevent nerve damage from oxidation, the pancreas pumps out as much insulin as it can. Even so, it may not prevent nerve damage.**

But, this heroic effort of the pancreas has a hefty downside. **The jolt of insulin causes the body to reduce the testosterone in the bloodstream, and to depress further production of it. In both men and women, testosterone is the hormone that controls the depositing of calcium in the bones.** You can raise testosterone through weight-bearing exercise, but if you are chemically depressing it via massive sugar intake (it takes very small quantities of sugar to constitute a massive intake, because refined sugar is not something the human body is equipped to handle), then your body won't add calcium to the bones.

Add this to what we discussed above, and you can see that drinking sweetened colas is a suicidal endeavor. And now you know why bone damage formerly apparent only in the very old is now showing up in teenagers.

Stomach acid dissolves tissue—that is its purpose. The stomach lining does not extend into the esophagus, so **the lower esophagus gets damaged by acid far**

HARMFUL

more frequently in soft drink users than in non-soft drink users. This results in a radical increase in cell mutations, along with a far higher level of free radicals.

Heart damage in a can—But carbonated beverages also cause problems for the heart.

An Australian study revealed that **giving magnesium to heart attack victims immediately improved their condition 41% of the time.** Remember that; and keep some on hand. This is because magnesium is essential in the body's manufacture of enzymes that tell the heart to beat. There are 300 of these magnesium heart-related enzymes in the human heart.

The body needs both calcium and magnesium together. Calcium makes it possible for the heart to physically beat. Every muscle contraction requires calcium.

Drinking a carbonated beverage blocks the ability of the body to absorb both calcium and magnesium.

Two other important nutrients for healthy heart action are vitamin E and selenium, which are co-factors to one another. (The FDA commissioned a study of vitamin E without selenium and happily concluded that vitamin E was of little value.)

Copper is also important. A deficiency of this mineral can cause varicose veins, heart fibrillations, and brain aneurysms. **Copper works with zinc**; and both should be taken together.

Why is it that people are so determined to drink chemically colored and chemically sweetened water, when plain water is so much better?

Oh, yes, what about plain water?

THE WATER YOU DRINK

The water in our wells and rivers are becoming thoroughly contaminated. **With safe drinkable water being a problem for half of the world's population, it seems ludicrous that we should want to pollute such a precious resource.** Our water may be accidentally contaminated by **nitrates, lead or agrochemicals**; or purposely by **aluminium** (added to make the water clear), **chlorine** (to prevent algae bloom) and **fluoride** (claimed to reduce dental decay).

The toxicity of chlorine is well-known, however **the need for chloriination could be ended** by UV treatment , ozone treatment and improved filtration could be used to end the need for chlorine. **Steps could be taken to reduce water contamination** in the home by replacing lead and copper piping (both poisonous) with PVC, and filtering drinking water. Filters are targeted to remove specific chemicals, so water testing is required before fitting one.

Use cold water to fill your kettle, as the copper in hot water pipes dissolves into the warm water. Filters are targeted to remove specific chemicals, so water testing is required before fitting one.

DISTILLED WATER
- A WONDERFUL SOLUTION

Here are facts you should know about the best

drinking water you can drink and use for cooking: It is:

• It is water that has been turned into vapour so that its impurities are left behind. Upon condensing, it becomes pure water.

• It is the only type of water which meets the definition of water: hydrogen + oxygen.

• It is perfectly natural water.

• It is odorless, colourless and tasteless.

• It is free of virtually all inorganic minerals including salt.

• It is the only natural solvent that can be taken into the body without damage to the tissues.

• It acts as a solvent in the body by dissolving nutrients so they can be assimilated and taken into every cell.

• It dissolves the cell wastes so the toxins can be removed.

• It dissolves inorganic mineral substances lodged in the tissues of the body so that the substances can be eliminated in the process of purifying the body.

• It does not leach out organic body minerals but does collect and remove the toxic inorganic minerals, which have been rejected by the cells of the body and are therefore, nothing more than harmful debris obstructing he normal functions of the body.

• It is indeed the most ideal and beneficial water for all humans and also for animals.

• It leaves no residue of any kind when it enters the body.

• It is the most perfect water for the healthy functioning of those great sieves, the kidneys.

• It is the perfect liquid for the blood.

• It is the ideal liquid for efficient functioning of the lungs, stomach, liver and all other vital organs.

• It is universally accepted as the standard for bio-medical applications and for drinking water purity.

• It is so pure that all drug prescriptions are formulated with distilled water.

• It is fresh, clean and pleasing to the palate.

• It makes foods and drinks prepared with it taste noticeably better. The flavour is subtle enough not to interfere with the food it is mixed with.

• It is the only pure water left on our polluted planet!

6 - Food Colors

25 FOOD COLORS AND/OR FLAVOR ENHANCERS

Did you know that if a food additive is animal derived, the item need not be stated on the ingredient label at all, leaving vegetarians without knowing that they are consuming products that they are ethically opposed to?

Here are two naturally derived colorants which are animal derived, and thus not subject to FDA certification: carmine or cochineal extract comes from the female cochineal insect (commonly used in Campari, fruits, yogurts, processed foods and cosmetics). **Canthaxanthin**, which can be derived from ocean crustaceans, but is mostly made synthetically (in the U.S. is commonly used for chicken feed).

Though past research showed no correlation between Attention Deficit Hyperactivity Disorder and food dyes, new studies now point to **synthetic preservatives and artificial coloring agents as aggravating ADD & ADHD symptoms**, both in those affected by these disorders and in the general population. Older studies were inconclusive quite possibly due to inadequate clinical methods of measuring offending behavior. Frankly, **parental reports were more accurate indicators of the presence of additives than clinical tests.**

Several major studies show **academic performance increased and disciplinary problems decreased** in large non-ADD (attention deficit disorder) student populations when artificial ingredients, including artificial colors, were eliminated from school food programs.

Norway banned all products containing **coal tar and coal tar derivatives** in 1978. New legislation lifted this ban in 2001 after EU regulations demanded it. As such, many FD&C approved colorings have been banned.

Tartrazine (Yellow) causes **hives** in at least 0.01% of those exposed to it.

Erythrosine (Cherry Pink) is linked to **thyroid tumors** in rats.

Cochineal (Red), also known as **carmine**, is derived from insects and therefore is neither vegan nor vegetarian. It has also been known to cause **severe, even life-threatening, allergic reactions** in rare cases.

Yellow dye #6 is the most dangerous of all! Beware of yellow dyes in processed food! It can cause **SEVERE abdominal pain with vomiting & diarrhea.** Some people with Irritable Bowel syndrome benefit from removing **food items colored orange and yellow** from their diet. Yellow dye #6 will probably be eventually classified as a cancer causing agent.

A new study in Britain has found that **food coloring and preservatives can increase hyperactivity, including ADHD** in kids age 3-9, and also have adverse effects on the general population.

Food colorings are chemicals foreign to the body. Anything foreign to the body has the potential to be harmful.

Food colorings have been shown to be especially harmful to children. —Yet the processed food in your grocery store for kids is now in bright colors of all kinds! It can and does make children allergic, and even get sick.

Children tested showed significant differences in their behavior based on whether their fruit drink had added colorings and preservatives, versus those drinks that were more natural. The additive-laden drinks increased **hyperactivity**.

Here are a list of several colorants which could be harmful or not depending upon which expert you listen to:

Citrus Red #2 is **carcinogenic** and used to enhance

the color of the skin in some Florida oranges and other fruits. Since most people don't eat the skin of oranges, the FDA isn't concerned, **but for those of you who candy orange peels or use orange zest, be cautious of where your oranges come from.** We thought we were safe from additives with fresh fruit, but apparently, we were wrong.

Red dye #3 is in marishino cherries. Studies were done in 1983 that showed **thyroid tumors** in rats on high amounts of this dye. As a result of these studies, the FDA recommended that Red dye #3 be banned in the U.S., but the governmental powers that be overruled the FDA's decision and subsequently, this colorant is still used, but only as a straight color additive; not in "lake form". What does that mean? Straight color additives are water soluble and are ideal for use in foods that have a lower fat content, or a higher liquid content. Lakes are the water insoluble form of the same colorant and are used in products that have a low moisture content such as tablets, or in high fat products, such as icing.

FD&C Blue #1 is Brilliant Blue FCF, and was previously banned in many EU countries, but most have removed the ban. It is on the list of approved colorants in the U.S. The *International Agency for Research on Cancer* concluded in 1998, that this colorant causes **cancer** in rats. Studies have found this substance to be a **skin and eye irritant and allergen**.

There is a wonderful website called *Toxicology Advice and Consulting* that summarizes recent studies on over 600 different chemicals. You need only type the name of the chemical into the database and press enter. The *Material Safety Data Sheet* for Blue 2 states that it is "**hazardous in case of ingestion, of inhalation**"; although this may refer to people who use this dye in large amounts.

FD&C Green #3 has been linked to studies showing **tumors** in rats that were injected with this dye.

Tartrazine, also known as **FD&C Yellow #5 or E-102**; an ingredient that I have taught my 4 and 6 year old to recognize on a package of candy. It provides the color **yellow** and as such, can also be found **in green and blue candies**. There is currently a petition to the FDA to ban tartrazine from food. Some schools have banned products containing tartrazine and subsequently noticed a big difference in the overall behavior of their students. Tartrazine is a coal tar derivative, like most artificial colorings, and **is one of the most controversial of the azo dies** used in food. Norway has banned the substance. This chemical has been linked to **severe allergic reactions, especially in asthmatics** and is one of the food additives thought to be a cause of **hyperactivity** in children.

FD&C Yellow #6 – Sunset Yellow is **Sudan 1** that has been sulfonated. Sudan 1 often remains as an impurity in Sunset Yellow. It is banned in Norway and Finland and the Food Standards Agency in Britain has called for a voluntary removal of Sunset Yellow from food and drink by 2009. It has been linked with a small percentage of skin irritations and asthmatic reactions. In addition, it may cause **hyperactivity in children when** combined with **Sodium Benzoate** (a preservative). The *Carcinogenic Potency Project* at Berkeley has revealed no positive results for a cancer test summary. Basically this website is a summary of all of the studies done with regards to potential carcinogenic agents.

Sudan 1, also called **CI Solvent Yellow 14** has been banned in the EU. Lab tests on exposed rats revealed **bladder and liver tumor growth**. Sudan 1 is banned in the U.S. As a result of all the negative publicity for this colorant, the nation of Sudan has asked to have that name changed.

Ferrous Gluconate is a naturally derrived, mineral colorant added to **olives**. It is also a medication used for treating anemia, and **as a drug has side effects, and contraindications**.

Color and Flavor Enhancers

Aristolochic acid is **an ingredient used in "traditional medicines" or "dietary supplements"** that is known to potentially cause **irreversible and fatal kidney failure**.

Sodium nitrate and nitrite are added to **meats** to stabilize them, give them their **red color** and provide that characteristic **smoked flavor**. They mix with the acid in your stomach to form **nitrosamines**, which are **very strong cancer causing** cells. They are especially present in **fried bacon**. Recently, food companies have been adding ascorbic acid and erythorbic acid to nitrate and nitrite treated meat to slow the formation of nitrosamines in the stomach which has significantly reduced the harm that these ingredients cause, but does not eliminate it completely. **Hot dogs** are also filled with nitrites; without them, both bacon and hot dogs would be an unappetizing shade of gray.

Chloropropanols are a family of drugs commonly found in **Asian food sauces like black bean, soy, and oyster sauce**. There are two specific substances within this category that are known **carcinogens** and that are banned in Canada and the **UK:3-MCPD** and **1,3 DCP**. They are not banned in the United States, although the FDA has recommended that foreign products containing these materials be banned from entering the U.S.

Diacetyl, the chemical that imparts the **buttery flavor in microwave popcorn** has a disease named after it due to the large amount of microwave popcorn factory workers that came down with the **lung condition**. It is called *Diacetyl Induced Bronchiolitis Obliterans*; or *"Popcorn Worker's Lung"*. There is no official ban in the EU, and U.S. companies are starting to volunarily replace this ingredient in the microwave popcorn. The CDC has issued a safety alert for workers in factories that use diacetyl.

Potassium Bromate is a chemical added to **flour** to make bread rise better and give it a uniform consistency. Most of what is added to flour breaks down during the cooking process into bromide, which at this time, is shown little to no health risk, but what hasn't been broken down remains in the baked good and is a known **carcinogen**. Numerous petitions have been made to the FDA to ban this ingredient and many flour mills

have voluntarily stopped adding it to their products. It is banned in most countries except the U.S. and Japan.

Ephedra is an herb used in many supplements. This drug is illegal in the U.S. for use in supplements but does turn up in other products. It is commonly promoted for its effects on "enhancing manhood". **The list of effects on the body is about as long as my arm and include almost every system in the body**. I do want to note, that this substance has been used for years in pharmaceutical preparations as an effective **bronchodilator**, but physicians are opting for newer, as effective drugs with less side effects. Ephedra is very strictly controlled in the United States because it can be used to make Methamphetamine.

Here are several additional food colors—and where they are found:

E102 Tartrazine, used in sweets, biscuits, mushy peas. Causes **hyperactivity, asthma, and rashes**.

E124 Ponceau 4R, used in sweets, biscuits, drinks. Causes **allergy**.

E110 Sunset Yellow, used in sweets, drinks, ice cream. Causes **gastric upset, allergy**.

E122 Carmoisine, used in biscuits, jelly, sweets, and ready meals. Causes **allergy**.

E104 Quinoline Yellow, used in sweets, smoked haddock, pickles. Causes **hyperactivity, asthma, rashes**.

E129 Allura Red, used in soft drinks, cocktail sausages. Causes **hypersenstivity**.

E211 Sodium Benzoate. used in soft drinks, baked goods, candy. Causes **hyperactivity, asthma**.

7 - Preservatives

6 PRESERVATIVES

Chlorphenesin and Phenoxyethanol. The FDA has issued a consumer warning that these two substances cause **depression of the central nervous system, vomiting and diarrhea in infants**. Phenoxyethanol is used as a preservative in medications and cosmetics.

Sulfites are used as preservatives to maintain shelf life, color and inhibit bacterial growth in food products. They are also used to enhance the potency of certain medications. For most people, sulphites are not of particular concern, but people who are sensitive to them have experienced **severe allergic reactions including anaphalactic shock**. In addition, sulfites destroy thaimin (vitamin B1). People with sulfite sensitivities should avoid any product containing sulfites.

BHA is a preservative used in cereals, potato chips and chewing gum to stop them from becoming rancid. It has been shown to cause **cancer** in mice, rats and hamsters. The U.S. Department of Health and Human Services considers BHA to be a carcinogen and that it poses a reasonable risk to health. Despite this warning, the FDA still allows BHA to be used.

Methyl mercury is **found in nearly all fish and shellfish** and gets more concentrated up the fish food chain you go. Researches have concluded that most of us don't eat enough for it to be a health concern, but some larger fish such as shark, swordfish, pike and walleye can contain up to 1ppm, the highest allowable safe limit for human consumption.

Benzene is **carcinogenic** and found in some foods. It can occur as a result of **benzoate and ascorbic acid chemically combining** in some soft drinks. The soft drink industry was made aware when tests came back positive for benzene. In 2005, additional tests revealed benzene in soft drinks, but the FDA decided that the amount was too small to be of concern, but will continue to take random samples to monitor the situation.

Bisphenol A is used to package food and has been found to **mimic the effects of estrogen**, both in mice and human studies. It has been linked to **obesity**, causing the body to trigger fat cell activity and has be shown to have **carcinogenic** effects on developing fetuses, creating **breast cancer** precurser cells. World wide studies are underway to re evaluate the safety of using this product as it is still widely available although many companies including Nalgene, Mountain Equipment Coop and Patagonia are voluntarily ceasing to make products with Bisphenol A. In addition, Wal Mart (Canada) has discontinued sales of soothers, baby bottles, sippy cups, food and water containers and has made a commitment to do away with Bisphenol A in U.S. stores by 2009. How do you know if your container is made from Bisphenol A? Look on the bottom for the recycling triangle. If it has a 7 or 3, it contains Bisphenol A.

8 - Antioxidants

2 ANTIOXIDANTS

Butyl compounds—**Butylated Hydroxyanisole (BHA)and Butylated Hydroxytoluene (BHT)** are the most widely used antioxidants, found in breakfast cereals, dry beverage mixes, cake mixes, candy, gum, margarine, glazed fruit, chips, peanuts, polyethylene food wraps, adhesives and vegetable oils. Not permitted in infant foods. In the top ten of most commonly used preservatives in cosmetics. Also used in many petroleum products including jet fuels, paints, adhesives, printing products and plastics. Known to accentuated **tumor growth** and cause **liver damage** in rat tests, may trigger **hyperactivity**, and other intolerances; serious concerns over **carcinogenicity**; BHA (additive no 320) is banned in Japan; in 1958 & 1963 official committees of experts recommended that BHT (additive no 321) be banned in the UK, however due to industry pressure it was not banned; McDonald's eliminated BHT from their US products by 1986. Also responsible for **contact dermatitis** in some people. See also toxicity 'toluene'.

9 - Genetically Modified Foods

DANGERS OF GM FOODS

The term GM foods or GMOs (**genetically-modified organisms) is most commonly used to refer to crop plants created for human or animal consumption using the latest molecular biology techniques.** These plants have been modified in the laboratory to enhance desired traits such as increased resistance to herbicides or improved nutritional content.

European environmental organizations and public interest groups have been actively protesting against GM foods for years, and recent controversial studies about the effects of genetically-modified corn pollen on monarch butterfly caterpillars have brought the issue of genetic engineering to the forefront of the public consciousness in the U.S.

Environmental activists, religious organizations, public interest groups, professional associations and other scientists and government officials have all raised concerns about GM foods, and criticized agribusiness for pursuing profit without concern for potential hazards, and the government for failing to exercise adequate regulatory oversight. It seems that everyone has a strong opinion about GM foods. **Most concerns about GM foods fall into three categories: environmental hazards, human health risks, and economic concerns.**

Environmental hazards—Unintended harm to other organisms. Last year a laboratory study was published in Nature[21] showing that pollen from B.t. corn caused **high mortality rates in monarch butterfly caterpillars**. Monarch caterpillars consume milkweed plants, not corn, but the fear is that if pollen from B.t. corn is blown by the wind onto milkweed plants in neighboring fields, the caterpillars could eat the pollen and perish. Although the Nature study was not conducted under natural field conditions, the results seemed to support this viewpoint. Unfortunately, B.t. toxins **kill many species of insect larvae indiscriminately**; it is not possible to design a B.t. toxin that would only kill crop-damaging pests and remain harmless to all other insects. This study is being reexamined by the USDA, the U.S. Environmental Protection Agency (EPA) and other non-government research groups, and preliminary data from new studies suggests that the original study may have been flawed. This topic is the subject of acrimonious debate, and both sides of the argument are defending their data vigorously. Currently, there is no agreement about the results of these studies, and the potential risk of harm to non-target organisms will need to be evaluated further.

This may be what is killing our honey bees!

Reduced effectiveness of pesticides Just as some populations of mosquitoes developed resistance to the now-banned pesticide DDT, many people are concerned that insects will become resistant to B.t. or other crops that have been genetically-modified to produce their own pesticides.

Gene transfer to non-target species—**Another concern is that crop plants engineered for herbicide tolerance and weeds will cross-breed, resulting in the transfer of the herbicide resistance genes from the crops into the weeds.** These "superweeds" would then be herbicide tolerant as well. Other introduced genes may cross over into non-modified crops planted next to GM crops. The possibility of interbreeding is shown by the defense of farmers against lawsuits filed by Monsanto. The company has filed patent infringement lawsuits against farmers who may have harvested GM crops. Monsanto claims that the farmers obtained Monsanto-licensed GM seeds from an unknown source and did not pay royalties to Monsanto. **The farmers claim that their unmodified crops were cross-pollinated from someone else's GM crops planted a field or two away.**

Allergenicity—Many children in the US and Europe have developed life-threatening allergies to peanuts and other foods. There is a possibility that **introducing a gene into a plant may create a new allergen or cause an allergic reaction in susceptible individuals.** A proposal to incorporate a gene from Brazil nuts into soybeans was abandoned because of the fear of causing unexpected allergic reactions. Extensive testing of GM foods may be required to avoid the possibility of harm to consumers with food allergies. Labeling of GM foods and food products will acquire new importance, which I shall discuss later.

Unknown effects on human health There is a growing concern that **introducing foreign genes into food plants may have an unexpected and negative impact on human health.** A recent article published in Lancet examined the effects of GM potatoes on the digestive tract in rats. This study claimed that there were appreciable differences in the intestines of rats fed GM potatoes and rats fed unmodified potatoes. Yet critics say that this paper, like the monarch butterfly data, is flawed and does not hold up to scientific scrutiny[34]. Moreover, **the gene introduced into the potatoes was a snowdrop flower lectin, a substance known to be toxic to mammals**. The scientists who created this variety of potato chose to use the lectin gene simply to test the methodology, and these potatoes were never intended for human or animal consumption

Economic concerns—Bringing a GM food to market is a lengthy and costly process, and of course agri-biotech companies wish to ensure a profitable return on their investment. Many new plant genetic engineering technologies and GM plants have been patented, and patent infringement is a big concern of agribusiness.

Yet **consumer advocates are worried that patenting these new plant varieties will raise the price of seeds so high that small farmers and third world countries will not be able to afford seeds for GM crops**, thus widening the gap between the wealthy and the poor. It is hoped that in a humanitarian gesture, more companies and non-profits will follow the lead of the Rockefeller Foundation and offer their products at reduced cost to impoverished nations.

Patent enforcement may also be difficult, as the contention of the farmers that they involuntarily grew Monsanto-engineered strains when their crops were cross-pollinated shows. One way to combat possible patent infringement is to introduce a "suicide gene" into GM plants. These plants would be viable for only one growing season and would produce sterile seeds that do not germinate. Farmers would need to buy a fresh supply of seeds each year. However, this would be financially disastrous for farmers in third world countries who cannot afford to buy seed each year and traditionally set aside a portion of their harvest to plant in the next growing season. In an open letter to the public, Monsanto has pledged to abandon all research using this suicide gene technology.

How are GM foods labeled?—Labeling of GM foods and food products is also a contentious issue. On the whole, agribusiness industries believe that labeling should be voluntary and influenced by the demands of the free market. If consumers show preference for labeled foods over non-labeled foods, then industry will have the incentive to regulate itself or risk alienating the customer. But c**onsumer interest groups are demanding mandatory labeling. People have the right to know what they are eating**, argue the interest groups, and historically industry has proven itself to be unreliable at self-compliance with existing safety regulations. The FDA's current position on food labeling is governed by the Food, Drug and Cosmetic Act which is only concerned with food additives, not whole foods or food products that are considered "GRAS"—generally recognized as safe. **The FDA contends that GM foods are substantially equivalent to non-GM foods, and therefore not subject to more stringent labeling.** If all GM foods and food products are to be labeled, Congress must enact sweeping changes in the existing food labeling policy.

It would be nice to think the FDA can be trusted with these matters, but think again. **Monsanto has succeeded in ensuring that government regulatory agencies let Monsanto do as it wishes.**

To offer up one glaring example as reported on the Organic Consumers Association's Millions Against Monsanto website:

In order for the FDA to determine if Monsanto's growth hormones were safe or not, Monsanto was required to submit a scientific report on that topic.

Margaret Miller, one of Monsanto's researchers put the report together.

Shortly before the report submission, Miller left Monsanto and was hired by the FDA. Her first job for the FDA was to determine whether or not to approve the report she wrote for Monsanto. In short, Monsanto approved its own report. Assisting Miller was another former Monsanto researcher, Susan Sechen. Deciding whether or not rBGH-derived milk should be labeled fell under the jurisdiction of another FDA official, Michael Taylor, who previously worked as a lawyer for Monsanto.

10 – Pesticides and Herbicides

POISONOUS EFFECTS OF PESTICIDES

(Also on chemical poisoning: 868)

A pesticide is a substance or mixture of substances used to kill what is considered to be a pest. A pesticide may be a chemical substance, biological agent (such as a virus or bacteria), antimicrobial, disinfectant or device used against any pest. Pests include insects, plant pathogens, weeds, molluscs, birds, mammals, fish, nematodes (roundworms), microbes. **But, unfortunately, many other things are killed, include song birds and beneficial insects. Animals and humans are injured.**

Pesticides can be absorbed through the skin, swallowed, or inhaled (most toxic). During application pesticides drift and settle on ponds, laundry, toys, pools, and furniture. People and pets track pesticide residue into the house. **Only 5% of pesticides reach target weeds. The rest runs off into water or dissipates in the air.** Drift from landscaping ranges from 12 feet to 14.5 miles. More serious effects appear to be produced by direct inhalation of pesticide sprays than by absorption or ingestion of toxins

Studies show that, primarily from pesticides on the food they eat, **Americans have an average of 12 parts per million of DDT in the fatty tissues of their bodies. This is more than twice the amount allowed in fish sold commercially.** It has also been discovered that the blood of the average American contains more DDT than is permitted in meat. Chlorinated insecticides can cause chronic poisoning in people most exposed to them, and liver and kidney damage are known to be hazards. **Breast-fed babies were found to be getting from their mother's milk twice the quantity of pesticides recommended as the limit by the World Health Organization.** Swedish toxicologist Dr. Goran Lofroth noted that when such amounts are present in animals, they begin to show biochemical changes.

Traces of pesticides have been found in the tissues of stillborn and unborn babies. In some cases the concentrations of poisons were as high as existed in the mother. The pesticides were found in the babies' liver, kidney and brain, with the greatest concentration being in the fatty tissue.

Some of these poisons are skin absorbed (for example, black leaf 40) and so are some herbicides, too!

The very worst thing is that **some of these cannot be washed out of your clothes, and they then spread from you to everything you touch!** (We will learn below that some herbicides do this also.)

So if you wash your babies clothes with yours, and, if they touch them and later put their hand in their mouth—they get that poison into their little bodies also!

A recent Seattle research study found that the urine and saliva of children eating a variety of conventional foods from area groceries contained biological markers of organophosphates, the family of pesticides spawned by the production of nerve gas agents in World War II.

But when those same children ate organic fruits, vegetables and juices, signs of pesticides were not found. That is significant evidence that it is indeed true that organic produce is the best for you.

In a study carried out by the University of Granada, the researchers analyzed samples, and measured 6 different POC concentration levels in human volunteers: DDE, a principal metabolite in DDT (a pesticide used in Spain until the 1980's); hexachlorobenzene, a compound used as fungicide and currently released by industrial processes; PCB's: compounds related to industrial processes; and Hexaclorociclohexano, used as an insecticide and currently used in scabies and pediculosis treatment.

In another study, all 387 adults analyzed had at least one kind of persistent organic compound in their bodies; some many of them. All of these were substances internationally classified as potentially harmful to a persons health.

Here is still more information on this deadly collection of poisons—Pesticides are the most widespread and insidious form of poisoning on earth. Traces of pesticides were found in the bodies of wildlife in the Antarctic were none had ever been used. They are detectable in every body of water, in the soil and all that grows in it, in the air and dust of our homes. An American study reported that **82% of adults have traces of chloropyrifos (an organochlorine) in their urine.**

Organophosphates are recognized as the most dangerous risk of 'quick poisoning': **as little as a teaspoon of Parathion (used on fruit trees) spilt undiluted on the skin can cause death.** Organophosphates are frequently used by farmers for quick control of insects, fungus and weeds.

The chlorine in organochlorine pesticides causes them to persist in the environment, **effecting a 'slow' poisoning to the exposed.** They are often used where the

HARMFUL

effect is meant to be long term as for termites. Dieldrin and chlordane, now restricted to termite use, were once popular in household pest control. Today diazinon, dichlorvos and chloropyrifos are commonly used. Chlorinated hydrocarbons are known to accumulate in human fatty tissue.

We can be exposed to pesticides in many ways: **they are readily absorbed through the skin, eyeballs and scalp; breathed in during spraying; or consumed as residue on and in foods**. One study found that tinned foods contained less pesticide residue than fresh, and that **broccoli, parsley, sweet potato and squash were moderately contaminated, recommending purchasing only organically grown of these vegetables**. Rice had little contamination, cereals grains were moderate.

The legacy of acute exposure to pesticides is often lifelong chemical sensitivity thereafter. Beside this, **all pesticides have been shown to cause damage to the nervous system, immune system, genetic damage, birth defects and cancer**. The anecdotal evidence pointing to poisoning is overwhelming, however most scientific research on the safety of pesticides is carried out by the companies who make them who release their results only to government agencies under strict secrecy. Because of this, the issue of bio-accumulation, or 'slow-poisoning' is denied existence. **Governments are irresponsible in their denial of the harmful effects of pesticides**, departments will always assure us that levels in our food too low to be toxic. However, the US Environmental Protection Agency has advised pregnant women in particular to avoid exposure to any pesticides

Because escaping pesticides is an impossible task, we must boycott their use and support those using organic methods of pest control by purchasing their products.

For alternatives to pesticides in the home garden, see Gardening.

This may be what is killing our honey bees!— Just as some populations of mosquitoes developed resistance to the now-banned pesticide DDT, many people are concerned that **either crops poisoned with insecticides, and/or those that have been genetically-modified to produce their own pesticides (!) are the cause of the widespread death of our honeybees.** More and more honey bees die each year. It is fast becoming an international disaster. **Without them, over 50% of our food crops will not grow!**

There is no perfect solution, since pesticide poisons are everywhere. But here are three things, each of which, may greatly help you:

1. Grow your own food in your own garden.
2. Only purchase and use organic foods.
3. Wash your foods carefully. The *Iotus Home Cleaning System* is the best I have found. Go to tersano.com if you wish to purchase it.

Are government-approved pesticides safe?— They are not. **Many of the "safety tests" used to test these products are fundamentally inadequate**: They test for the acute (not chronic) effects of single (not multiple) chemicals on healthy (not sick, chemically

sensitive, or immuno-suppressed etc.) adult (not fetal or young) animal (not human) subjects exposed over short (not long) periods of time. Some of the companies testing pesticides have been charged and convicted of falsifying residue and environmental studies that were used to support pesticide registration in the U.S. and Canada. **Some pesticides become even more toxic as they break down.** (In the U.S. it is a violation of federal law to state that the use of pesticides is safe.)

Here is a list of several of the health risks in pesticides: Increased risk of leukemia. Cancers (lung, brain, testicular, lymphoma). Increase in spontaneous abortions. Greater genetic damage. Decreased fertility. Liver and pancreatic damage. Neuropathy. Disturbances to immune systems (asthma/allergies). Increases in stillbirths. Decreased sperm counts.

Here are several of the special risks for children: Cancer: Leukemia and brain cancer. Asthma and allergies. Polyneuritis with numbness and pain in lower limbs. Altered neurological functioning and long-lasting neuro-behavioral impairments. Birth defects. Neurotoxicity. Gangrene (tissue death) of the extremities.

Children whose homes and gardens are treated with pesticides have 6.5 times greater risk of leukemia than children living in untreated environments.

Who is most susceptible?—Children, infants and fetuses. Children have more rapid breathing and metabolic rates, greater surface to body mass ratios, thinner skins, spend more time in contact with the ground, more frequently place their fingers in their mouths, and are less likely to be able to read hazard signs. Adults—especially those with asthma, lupus erythematosus, vasculitis, dermatitis and chemical sensitivities. Animals: pets, wildlife of all kinds and their habitat.

What is their effect on wildlife?—Birds die after eating granular pesticides. Animals may develop: cancer, abnormal thyroid function, decreased fertility, decreased hatching success, demasculinization and feminization of males, and alteration of immune function.

Other known effects of pesticides—These include developmental and behavioral effects in various animal species, non-Hodgkin's lymphoma, reproductive and endocrine disruptions, cancer in dogs (canine malignant lymphoma), increased number of abnormal sperm in exposed farmers, and decreased fertility in male rats.

The chemical compound, 2, 4-D, is the most common herbicide used by lawn companies. It is present in pesticides and fertilizers found in stores (under names that sound safe like "Weed 'n Feed"). **Yet it is a component of *Agent Orange*—**that deadly poison which injured so many American soldiers in the Vietnam War. **It also contains *dioxin* contaminants.** Dioxin is one of the most dangerous of all industrial chemical wastes.

What are the "inert" ingredients in insecticides?—**These "inert" ingredients are not harmless,** as you might suppose. They can comprise up to 97% of products like weed killers. These so-called inerts are often insecticides, such as DDT, or contaminants, such as dioxin. The "inerts" may be even more toxic than the active ingredients listed on the labels. Dr. J. Irwin declares that **3700 chemicals can legally be concealed in pesticides**. Fertilizer sprays also may contain poisonous solvents. Inerts sometimes include benzene, a known human carcinogen. (If it were spilled on the highway, it would be considered a toxic chemical spill.) Applicators (those applying them) do not know the danger of their product because they do not know the identity of the "inert" ingredients. Reyes Syndrome is linked to an ingredient additive that allowed the pesticide to stick on the trees.

Additional information—Most people are unaware of pesticide dangers. (Most companies claim they are "Safe"!) Most people do not know that nontoxic lawn care is available.

Chemical fertilizers and pesticides on lawns weaken the grass and destroy the natural balance of microbes and beneficial insect predators, thus promoting weed and insect proliferation. Despite a tenfold increase in insecticide use, studies have shown a proliferation in types of pests from fewer than 10 to more than 300. Of the 25 most serious insect pests in California in 1970, 24 were secondary pests (produced because of insecticides) and 73% are resistant to one or more insecticides.

ENDURING EFFECTS OF HERBICIDES

Herbicides are poisons used to kill plants. Used in yards, farms and parks throughout the world, Roundup has long been a top-selling weed killer. But now **researchers have found that one of Roundup's inert ingredients can kill human cells**, particularly embryonic, placental and umbilical cord cells. The new findings intensify a debate about so-called "inerts"—the solvents, preservatives, surfactants and other substances that manufacturers add to pesticides. Nearly 4,000 inert ingredients are approved for use by the U.S. Environmental Protection Agency.

In addition, herbicides cause large changes in the habitat available on clear-cuts and plantations, and these might be expected to diminish the suitability of sprayed sites for the many species of song birds, mammals, and other animals that utilize those habitats. This means that **the only ground suitable for growing crops is gradually being ruined by these substances.**

Agent Orange, sprayed on jungles in Viet Nam in the late 1960s, was a super herbicide like Roundup. Later research found **it not only permanently injured our own troops as well as the Vietnamese,—but it has passed down generation to generation throughout time,—and never will go away!**

Modern, intensively managed agricultural and for-estry systems continue to rely on herbicides and various pesticides. **Unfortunately, the use of herbicides and other pesticides carries risks to humans through exposure to these potentially toxic chemicals, and to ecosystems through direct toxicity caused to non-target species, and through damages to food crops and the soil.**

Both organochlorines and organophosphates have been shown to cause cancer, birth defects and nervous system damage, acute toxicity kills. 2,4-D is the most commonly used in the US and Australia, containing both chlorine and dioxin which can been stored in the body's fatty tissues and has been found in breast milk. see also Pesticides.

II – Infected Meat

NUMEROUS EFFECTS OF INFECTED MEAT

The present author's low-cost book, International Meat Crisis, *presents the full scope of the dangers of meat-eating in detail. The book is available at remarkably low prices in boxful amounts, for easy distribution.*

Global meat consumption has increased from under 50 million tons annually to over 200 million tons in the last 50 years. The amount of animal manure produced in the U.S. is 130 times greater than the amount of human waste. This is causing more environmental and health problems than ever seen before. **Here are 15 good reasons to stop eating meat:**

Health Reasons:

Lower risk of cancer—The Physicians Committee for Responsible Medicine has reported that vegetarians are less likely to get cancer by 25 to 50 percent.

Lower risk of heart disease—Researchers Dr. Dean Ornish and Dr. Caldwell Esselstyn have a program that includes a vegetarian diet and is currently one of the few programs that has been proven to reverse heart disease. A vegetarian diet reduces cholesterol.

Lower risk of osteoporosis—Studies have shown that too much protein in our diet causes loss of bone calcium. Meat eaters generally get far more protein than they need or can use.

Lower risk of kidney and gallstones—The calcium leached from the bones by the body's efforts to neutralize the acids produce by too much protein intake can end up forming kidney stones and gallstones.

Factory farmed animals carry disease—According to the FDA poultry is the number one source of food-borne illness. Despite the heavy use of pesticides and antibiotics, up to 60% percent of chickens sold at the supermarket are infected with live salmonella bacteria. Approximately 30% of all pork products are contaminated with toxoplasmosis. We are increasingly

H
A
R
M
F
U
L

at risk from highly contagious diseases like Mad Cow Disease and Foot and Mouth disease in sheep and cattle.

Factory-farmed animals contain toxic chemicals—Meat contains accumulations of pesticides and other chemicals up to 14 times more concentrated than those in plant foods. Half of all antibiotics used in the U.S. are used in farm animals and 90% of those are not used to treat infections but are instead used as growth promoters.

Environmental Reasons:

Inefficient use of agriculture—70% of U.S. grain production is used to feed farm animals. The grains and soybeans fed to animals to produce the amount of meat consumed by the average American in one year could feed seven people for the same period.

Inefficient use of water. It takes 2640 gallons of water to produce one pound of edible beef. The water used to raise animals for food is more than half the water used in the United States.

Inefficient use of energy—4 calories of fossil fuel needed to produce 1 calorie of protein in beef: 1 calories of fossil fuel needed to produce 1 calorie of protein in soybeans.

Environmental Pollution—Raising animals for food is the biggest polluter of our water and topsoil. Factory farm animal waste pollutes the ground and groundwater horribly.

Destruction of natural habitat—It takes more land to raise animals for food than it does to produce the equivalent nutritional value by raising edible plants. Rain forests are being destroyed to make room for huge cattle ranches. Coyotes and other animals are poisoned and shot by western cattle ranchers who consider federal land to be their land for grazing.

Animal Rights Reasons:

Animals on factory farms are over-crowded—They spend their brief lives in crowded and ammonia-filled conditions, many of them so cramped that they can't even turn around or spread a wing.

Animals on factory farms are tortured—Within days of birth, for example, chickens have their beaks seared off with a hot blade. Animals are hung upside down and their throats are sliced open, often while they're fully conscious.

Animals on factory farms are treated like machines—They are pumped up with drugs, fed their own waste and forced to grow or produce as fast as possible. They are subjected to 24-hour artificial lighting while being crammed into tiny cages one on top of the other to make it easier to harvest.

We do not need to eat animals—Most of us in the U.S. don't eat animals because we must in order to survive. We eat them because we want to. We are subjecting animals to torture, damaging the environment unnecessarily and subjecting ourselves to greater risk of disease just to satisfy a desire, not a need.

You can get a totally balanced diet without eating meat. All vegetables contain protein and too much protein consumption is unhealthy. Grains, legumes and soybeans contain plenty of protein. Vegetarian foods do not have to be boring. Spice it up! For example, veggies and rice with some Teriyaki sauce is delicious and as filling as any meat dish you can think of while being far more healthy for you and easier on animals and the environment. Why not give a vegetarian diet a try and give our environment a break. Your body will thank you and so will the Earth!

FEDS HIDING MAD COW CASES: American Records Not Credible, Former Packing Plant Vet Says. *The Edmonton Journal, April 7, 2005*—Edmonton, Canada: **A former American government packing plant veterinarian says the United States government is hiding cases of mad cow disease.**

Dr. Lester Friedlander said Wednesday that colleagues with the United States Department of Agriculture have told him of cases that the USDA has chosen not to announce. Friedlander, who has been invited to speak to Parliament's agriculture committee next week on proposed changes to Canadian inspection legislation, refused to give details. He said the USDA employees are close to retirement and risk losing their pensions.

He has previously spoken out, however, about **a Texas cow that had mad cow symptoms and went untested to a rendering plant after a USDA veterinarian condemned it at a packing plant in San Angelo.**

Mad cow cases in America

There have been U.S. news reports that just three cows processed by the plant were tested for bovine spongiform encephalopathy over two years. The plant, Lone Star Beef, processes older dairy cows considered at higher risk of carrying BSE.

Friedlander said **it's not credible that the USDA has found just one BSE case and only in a cow that entered the United States from Alberta rather than being raised in the U.S.**

"You've found four cases (including a cow from Alberta discovered in Washington state with the disease) out of 12 million cattle and the United States has found none out of 120 million," Friedlander said in an interview during a speaking visit to Edmonton.

He said production practices in the two countries are similar enough that the USDA should be finding more BSE cases.

New Agency Needed

Friedlander was in charge of meat inspectors at the largest U.S. culled-cow packing plant, in Pennsylvania, until 1995. **He lost his job for, in his words, "doing too good a job."**

He has since become a public speaker on food and animal safety issues. He was in Edmonton as a guest of the Edmonton North Environmental Society.

The USDA's record looks worse than the Canadian Food Inspection Agency's, but Canada needs a new "consumer" agency to oversee packing plant inspections, he added. **He said the USDA and CFIA both suffer from having too much influence from politicians eager to please the food industry.** His proposed consumer agency would be a government body but would have more safeguards against political influence.

Marc Richard, speaking from Ottawa for the CFIA, said the agency enforces rules set by Parliament and does its job well.

He said it reports to Agriculture Minister Andrew Mitchell and a replacement government agency would have to do the same.

Friedlander also warned against intensive livestock operations, such as cattle feedlots and large hog operations. He said they are ideal breeding grounds for bacteria and disease; and authorities have tended to react slowly when there's an outbreak.

Delayed reaction to avian flu last year at a British Columbia poultry operation led to a large and costly outbreak, he said.

U.S. Hiding Mad Cow Cases:: Expert Says

Ottawa Citizen, March 7, 2005— . . . Mr. Friedlander is a former veterinarian with the U.S. Department of Agriculture. And, since he left in 1995, he is now a well-known whistle-blower. He used to supervise meat inspection at a slaughterhouse in Pennsylvania that processed 1,800 cows a day, including many "downers," or suspect animals no longer able to walk.

In April, he intends to travel to Ottawa to speak to parliamentarians reviewing our rules for food inspection. They're in for an earful.

Mr. Friedlander says, flat out, that mad cow is probably prevalent in the U.S., but has so far been kept out of the public eye. "There's no doubt in my mind."

Mr. Friedlander said he was one of the first government vets to begin looking for mad cow in the late 1980s when he used to extract cattle brains and send them to labs for testing . . .

The problem, he explained, can be traced to the way cattle are fed. Until 1997, it was common to use rendered cattle remains as a component in cattle feed. **"They're all eating from the same contaminated source."**

In the early 1990s, he said he was speaking to the USDA's chief pathologist about mad cow when the following exchange took place:

"Lester, **if you ever find mad cow disease, promise me one thing?" he was asked. "What's that?" he responded. "Don't tell anybody."**

Mr. Friedlander says he would take a lie-detector test to back up his story. "Once I heard that, then I knew this whole thing was a joke."

A FEW OF THE REASONS WHY EATING MEAT CAUSES CANCER—First of all, understand that during a cancer treatment, a person should not eat anything **that is not building the immunity system or killing cancer cells.** Meat does not contribute to curing the cancer, so meat is normally forbidden in cancer diets. There are plenty of foods that help cure cancer, so there is no need to eat meat.

For some kinds of cancer, meat eaters (especially red meat) have a higher probability of getting those kinds of cancer, such as colon cancer and prostate cancer.

Meat also uses up the two critical enzymes trypsin and chymotrypsin, which are critical to allowing the immune system to kill cancer cells, though more potent enzymes have now been found. Vegetable proteins do not use up those enzymes.

Another reason to avoid meat is the accumulation of fecal matter in the colon. The colon should be relatively clear during a cancer treatment so that the body can absorb as many nutrients as possible. **"All foods which ferment in the bowel should be avoided.** Absolutely no meat or fish!"

Then there are the hormones in meat: *Diethylstilbestrol* (Des) has been shown by the FDA to cause cancer of the uterus, breast and other reproductive organs. This is an artificial sex hormone widely used in food production. Dangerous residues of stilbestrol are in 85% of all the meat sold in the United States. This is the main reason why 15 countries around the world now refuse to import American meat; 21 nations have a total ban on the use of stilbestrol in food production or processing.

And there is more:

Nitrosamines **cause cancer of the liver, stomach, brain, bladder, kidneys and several other organs**. Dr. William Lijinski, of the University of Nebraska, says **they are "perfect carcinogens."** When chemical preservatives and color enhancers are ingested, they cause the body to produce nitrosamines. **Another source is nitrates and nitrites, which are heavily added to meat during processing.** Runoff of nitrates and nitrites from fields sprayed with chemical fertilizers get into aquifers and wells and, when the water is drunk, can lead to cancer. Avoid amines, which are in cheese and meat.

Another problem with meat is toxins: avoid meat if the digestive system is weak, **digestion of meat could produce toxins in blood.**

Avoid meat in all forms. **It is dead matter, low in minerals, and produces uric acid in excess which is a waste product. The incidence of cancer is in direct proportion to the amount of animal proteins, particularly meat, in the diet.**

However it is true that devitalized, processed, and sugared food can also cause cancer—even in vegetarians. But far more often, when cancer strikes, those eating the junk foods are also eating meat. Nations and groups which consume less meat have less cancer. **Hospital records show that Seventh-day Adventists, who eat little or no meat, suffer far less from cancer than the average meat-eating American.** Dr. Willard J. Visek, research scientist at Cornell University, stated that the high protein diet of Americans is linked to the high incidence of cancer in the U.S.

Another cancer physician, who also worked with hundreds of cancer patients, said that **anyone who does not eat meat, eats only good food, and does all he can** to protect his liver, **may never get cancer.** Cancer is less a disease than a condition existing in the whole body. **Cancer would be almost unheard of if no devitalized food or meats were eaten.** Cancer cannot exist where there is a pure bloodstream.

Meat production—It has been estimated that **the amount of grain used to fatten one cow for meat could feed up to 16 people for the same period of time.**

In the US **cattle consume 90% of the soybean crop, 80% of all corn grown** and yet 20 million people will die from starvation this year. (The US department of Agriculture and Oxfam America statistics)

Not only do **cattle consume half the worlds grain crops**, but meat farming contributes significantly to **soil erosion, desertification and deforestation** especially of rainforests, global warming through the use of fossil fuels in transport, slaughter, processing and storage; and produce 20% of the total production of methane. Meat farming contributes to **pollution of waterways with manure and pesticides in amounts greater than the amount of pollution caused by cities and industry combined**. (Cross and Byers, etal 1990)

Meat production involves much suffering and degradation of the animals at all stages. Animals are branded with hot irons, sheep undergo Mulesing (a brutal process which involves cutting away the flesh at either side of the anus), dipped or sprayed with toxic chemicals, whipped and nipped by dogs, packed tightly into trucks or ships for transport where they are often dehydrated and may die in transit. At the slaughterhouse animals may be strung up by their feet alive and unstunned, as is the practice for "Halal" slaughter, their killing may be botched, so that the animal is not yet dead when it is bled and dismembering begins. The whole process is brutal, immoral even, resulting in much avoidable torment and waste of life and resources.

12 - Vaccines

VACCINES: PROBLEMS AND CONTENTS

(Also on vaccination poisoning: 876)

The evidence suggests that vaccination is an unreliable means of preventing disease—The medical literature has a surprising number of studies documenting vaccine failure. **Measles, mumps, smallpox, polio and Hib outbreaks have all occurred in vaccinated populations.** [11, 12, 13, 14 ,15] In 1989 the CDC reported: "Among school-aged children, [measles] outbreaks have occurred in schools with vaccination levels of greater than 98 percent. [16] **[They] have occurred in all parts of the country, including areas that had not reported measles for years.**" [17] The CDC even reported a measles outbreak in a documented 100 percent vaccinated population.

CHART - 1063-1064: Information on the 9 types of vaccinations required prior to overseas travel. For more on vaccinations: 876, 928, 972

[18]

A study examining this phenomenon concluded, **"The apparent paradox is that as measles immunization rates rise to high levels in a population, measles becomes a disease of immunized persons."** [19] A more recent study found that measles vaccination "produces immune suppression which contributes to an increased susceptibility to other infections." [19a]

These studies suggest that the goal of complete immunization is actually counterproductive, a notion underscored by instances in which **epidemics followed complete immunization of entire countries**. Japan experienced yearly increases in smallpox following the introduction of compulsory vaccines in 1872. By 1892, there were 29,979 deaths, and all had been vaccinated. [20]

Early in this century, the Philippines experienced their worst smallpox epidemic ever after 8 million people received 24.5 million vaccine doses; **the death rate quadrupled as a result**. [21] In 1989, the country of Oman experienced a widespread polio outbreak six months after achieving complete vaccination. [22] In the U.S. in 1986, 90% of 1300 pertussis cases in Kansas were "adequately vaccinated." [23] 72% of pertussis cases in the 1993 Chicago outbreak were fully up to date with their vaccinations. [24]

Vaccination causes significant death and disability at an astounding personal and financial cost to families and taxpayers—The FDA's VAERS (*Vaccine Adverse Effects Reporting System*) receives about 11,000 reports of serious adverse reactions to vaccination annually, some 1% (112+) of which are deaths from vaccine reactions. [1]

The majority of these reports are made by doctors, and **the majority of deaths are attributed to the pertussis (whooping cough) vaccine**, the "P" in DPT series of shots. This figure alone is alarming, yet it is only the "tip of the iceberg." **The FDA estimates that only about 10% of adverse reactions are reported**, [2] a figure supported by two National Vaccine Information Center (NVIC) investigations. [3]

In fact, the NVIC reported that **"In New York, only one out of 40 doctor's offices [2.5%] confirmed that they report a death or injury following vaccination,"** A full 97.5% of vaccine related deaths and disabilities go unreported there. Implications about the integrity of medical professionals aside (doctors are *legally required* to report serious adverse events), these findings suggest that vaccine deaths actually occurring each year may be well over 1,000.

With pertussis, the number of vaccine-related deaths dwarfs the number of pertussis disease deaths, which have been about 10 annually for recent years according to the CDC, and only 8 in 1993, the last peak-incidence year (pertussis runs in 3-4 year cycles, though vaccination certainly doesn't). Simply put, the vaccine is 100 times more deadly than the disease.

Given the many instances in which highly vaccinated

populations have contracted disease, and the fact that **the vast majority of disease decline this century occurred before compulsory vaccinations** (pertussis deaths declined 79% prior to vaccines), this comparison is a valid one—and this enormous number of vaccine casualties can hardly be considered a necessary sacrifice for the benefit of a disease-free society.

Unfortunately, the vaccine-related-deaths story doesn't end here. **Both national and international studies have shown vaccination to be a cause of SIDS** [4,5] (SIDS is "Sudden Infant Death Syndrome," a "catch-all" diagnosis given when the specific cause of death is unknown; estimates range from 5 - 10,000 cases each year in the U.S.).

One study found the peak incidence of SIDS occurred at the ages of 2 and 4 months in the U.S., precisely when the first two routine immunizations are given, [4] while another found a clear pattern of correlation extending three weeks after immunization. **Another study found that 3,000 children die within 4 days of vaccination each year in the U.S.** (amazingly, the authors reported no SIDS/vaccine relationship), while yet another researcher's studies led to the conclusion that **half of SIDS cases—that would be 2500 to 5000 infant deaths in the U.S. each year—are caused by vaccines.** [4]

There are studies that claimed to find no SIDS-vaccine relationship. However, many of these were invalidated by yet another study which found that "confounding" had skewed their results in favor of the vaccine. [6] **Shouldn't we err on the side of caution?** Shouldn't any credible correlation between vaccines and infant deaths be just cause for meticulous, widespread monitoring of the vaccination status of all SIDS cases?

In the mid 70's Japan raised their vaccination age from 2 months to 2 years; their incidence of SIDS dropped dramatically. In spite of this, the U.S. medical community has chosen a posture of denial. Coroners refuse to check the vaccination status of SIDS victims, and unsuspecting families continue to pay the price, unaware of the dangers and denied the right to make a choice.

Low adverse event reporting also suggests that the total number of adverse reactions actually occurring each year may be more than 100,000.

Due to doctors' failure to report, no one knows how many of these are permanent disabilities, but statistics suggest that it is several times the number of deaths. This concern is reinforced by a study which revealed that 1 in 175 children who completed the full DPT series suffered "severe reactions," [7] and a Dr.'s report for attorneys which found that 1 in 300 DPT immunizations resulted in seizures. [8]

England actually saw a drop in pertussis deaths when vaccination rates dropped from 80% to 30% in the mid 70's. Swedish epidemiologist B. Trollfors' study of pertussis vaccine efficacy and toxicity around the world found that "pertussis-associated mortality is currently very low in industrialized countries and no difference can be discerned when countries with high, low, and zero immunization rates were compared." He also found that **England, Wales, and West Germany had more pertussis fatalities in 1970 when the immunization rate was high than during the last half of 1980, when rates had fallen.** [9]

Vaccinations cost us much more than just the lives and health of our children. **The U.S. Federal Government's *National Vaccine Injury Compensation Program* (NVICP) has paid out over $724.4 million to parents of vaccine injured and killed children, in taxpayer dollars.** The NVICP has received over 5000 petitions since 1988, including over 700 for vaccine-related deaths, and there are still over 2800 total death and injury cases pending that may take years to resolve. [10]

Meanwhile, pharmaceutical companies have a captive market: vaccines are legally mandated in all 50 U.S. states (though legally avoidable in most), yet yet these same companies are "immune" from accountability for the consequences of their products. Furthermore, they have been allowed to use "gag orders" as a leverage tool in vaccine damage legal settlements to prevent disclosure of information to the public about vaccination dangers. **Such arrangements are clearly unethical; they force a non-consenting American public to pay for vaccine manufacturer's liabilities, while attempting to ensure that this same public will remain ignorant of the dangers of their products.**

It is interesting to note that insurance companies refuse to cover vaccine adverse reactions. They do the best liability studies, and understand what is involved. Profits appear to dictate both the pharmaceutical and insurance companies' positions.

Vaccines are the main reason for low disease rates in the U.S. today—According to the British Association for the Advancement of Science, **childhood diseases decreased 90% between 1850 and 1940, paralleling improved sanitation and hygienic practices, well before mandatory vaccination programs.** Infectious disease deaths in the U.S. and England declined steadily by an average of about 80% during this century (measles mortality declined over 97%) prior to vaccinations. [25]

In Great Britain, the polio epidemics peaked in 1950, and had declined 82% by the time the vaccine was introduced there in 1956. Thus, at best, vaccinations can be credited with only a small percentage of the overall decline in disease related deaths this century. Yet even this small portion is questionable, as **the rate of decline remained virtually the same after vaccines were introduced.**

Furthermore, **European countries that refused immunization for smallpox and polio saw the epidemics end along with those countries that mandated it.** (In fact, **both smallpox and polio immunization campaigns were followed initially by significant disease incidence *increases*; during smallpox vaccination campaigns, other infectious diseases continued their declines in the absence of vaccines. In England and Wales, smallpox disease and vaccination rates eventually declined simultaneously over a period of several decades. [26])

A recent World Health Organization report found that the disease and mortality rates in third world countries have no direct correlation with immunization procedures or medical treatment, but are closely related to the standard of hygiene and diet. [27] Credit given to vaccinations for our current disease incidence has simply been grossly exaggerated, if not outright misplaced.

Vaccine advocates point to incidence statistics rather than mortality as proof of vaccine effectiveness. However, **statisticians tell us that mortality statistics can be a better measure of incidence than the incidence figures themselves, for the simple reason that the quality of reporting and record-keeping is much higher on fatalities.** [28]

For instance, a recent survey in New York City revealed that only 3.2% of pediatricians were actually reporting measles cases to the health department. **In 1974, the CDC determined that there were 36 cases of measles in Georgia, while the Georgia State Surveillance System reported 660 cases.** [29]

In 1982, Maryland state health officials blamed a pertussis epidemic on a television program, "D.P.T.— Vaccine Roulette," which warned of the dangers of DPT; however, when former top virologist for the U.S. Division of Biological Standards, Dr. J. Anthony Morris, analyzed the 41 cases, only 5 were confirmed, and all had been vaccinated. [30] **Such instances as these demonstrate the fallacy of incidence figures, yet vaccine advocates tend to rely on them indiscriminately.**

1 - National Technical Information Service, Springfield, VA 22161, 703-487-4650, 703-487-4600.

2 - Reported by KM Severyn,R.Ph.,Ph.D. in the Dayton Daily News, May 28, 1993. (Ohio Parents for Vaccine Safety, 251 Ridgeway Dr., Dayton, OH 45459)

3 - National Vaccine Information Center (NVIC), 512 Maple Ave. W. #206, Vienna, VA 22180, 703-938-0342; "Investigative Report on the Vaccine Adverse Event Reporting System."

4 - Viera Scheibner, Ph.D., Vaccination: 100 Years of Orthodox Research Shows that Vaccines Represent a Medical Assault on the Immune System.

5 - W.C. Torch, "Diptheria-pertussis-tetanus (DPT) immunization: A potential cause of the sudden infant death syndrome (SIDS)," (Amer. Adacemy of Neurology, 34th Annual Meeting, Apr 25 - May 1, 1982), Neurology 32(4), pt. 2.

6 - Confounding in studies of adverse reactions to vaccines [see comments]. Fine PE, Chen RT, REVIEW ARTICLE: 38 REFS. Comment in: Am J Epidemiol 1994 Jan 15;139(2):229-30. Division of Immunization, Centers for Disease Control, Atlanta, GA 30333.

7 - Nature and Rates of Adverse Reactions Associated with DTP and DT Immunizations in Infants and Children" (Pediatrics, Nov. 1981, Vol. 68, No. 5)

8 - The Fresno Bee, Community Relations, 1626 E. Street, Fresno, CA 93786, DPT Report, December 5, 1984.

9 - Trollfors B, Rabo, E. 1981. Whooping cough in adults. British Medical Journal (September 12), 696-97.

10 - National Vaccine Injury Compensation Program (NVICP), Health Resources and Services Administration, Parklawn Building, Room 7-90, 5600 Fishers Lane, Rockville, MD 20857, 800-338-2382.

11 - Measles vaccine failures: lack of sustained measles specific immunoglobulin G responses in revaccinated adolescents and young adults. Department of Pediatrics, Georgetown University Medical Center, Washington, DC 20007. Pediatric Infectious Disease Journal. 13(1):34-8, 1994 Jan.

12 - Measles outbreak in 31 schools: risk factors for vaccine failure and evaluation of a selective revaccination strategy. Department of Preventive Medicine and Biostatistics, University of Toronto, Ont. Canadian Medical Association Journal. 150(7):1093-8, 1994 Apr 1.

13 - Haemophilus b disease after vaccination with Haemophilus b polysaccharide or conjugate vaccine. Institution Division of Bacterial Products, Center for Biologics Evaluation and Research, Food and Drug Administration, Bethesda, Md 20892. American Journal of Diseases of Children. 145(12):1379-82, 1991 Dec.

14 - Sustained transmission of mumps in a highly vaccinated population: assessment of primary vaccine failure and waning vaccine-induced immunity. Division of Field Epidemiology, Centers for Disease Control and Prevention, Atlanta, Georgia. Journal of Infectious Diseases. 169(1):77-82, 1994 Jan. 1.

15 - Secondary measles vaccine failure in healthcare workers exposed to infected patients. Department of Pediatrics, Children's Hospital of Philadelphia, PA 19104. Infection Control & Hospital Epidemiology. 14(2):81-6, 1993 Feb.

16 - MMWR, 38 (8-9), 12/29/89).

17 - MMWR (Morbidity and Mortality Weekly Report) "Measles." 1989; 38:329-330.

18 - Morbidity and Mortality Weekly Report (MMWR). 33(24),6/22/84.

19 - Failure to reach the goal of measles elimination. Apparent paradox of measles infections in immunized persons. Review article: 50 REFS. Dept. of Internal Medicine, Mayo Vaccine Research Group, Mayo Clinic and Foundation, Rochester, MN. Archives of Internal Medicine. 154(16):1815-20, 1994 Aug 22.

19a-Clinical Immunology and Immunopathology, May 1996; 79(2): 163-170.

20 - Trevor Gunn, Mass Immunization, A Point in Question, p 15 (E.D. Hume, Pasteur Exposed-The False Foundations of Modern Medicine, Bookreal, Australia, 1989.)

21 - Physician William Howard Hay's address of

H
A
R
M
F
U
L

June 25, 1937; printed in the Congressional Record.

22 - Outbreak of paralytic poliomyelitis in Oman; evidence for widespread transmission among fully vaccinated children Lancet vol 338: Sept 21, 1991; 715-720.

23 - Neil Miller, Vaccines: Are They Safe and Effective? p 33.

24 - Chicago Dept. of Health.

25 - See Note 23 pp 18-40.

26 - See Note 23 pp 45,46 [NVIC News, April 92, p12].

27 - S. Curtis, A Handbook of Homeopathic Alternatives to Immunization.

28 - Darrell Huff, How to Lie With Statistics, p 84.

29 - quoted from the internet, credited to Keith Block, M.D., a family physician from Evanston, Illinois, who has spent years collecting data in the medical literature on immunizations.

30 - See Note 20, p 15.

31 - See Note 20 p 21.

32 - See Note 20, p 21 (British Medical Council Publication 272, May 1950)

33 - See Note 20, p 21; also Note 23 p 47 (Buttram, MD, Hoffman, Mothering Magazine, Winter 1985 p 30; Kalokerinos and Dettman, MDs, "The Dangers of Immunization," Biological Research Inst. [Australia], 1979, p 49).

34 - Archie Kalolerinos, MD, Every Second Child, Keats Publishing, Inc. 1981

35 - Reported by KM Severyn,R.Ph,Ph.D. in the Dayton Daily News, June 3, 1995.

36 - Vaccine Information and Awareness, "Measles and Antibody Titre Levels," from Vaccine Weekly, January 1996.

37 - NVIC Press Release, "Consumer Group Warns use of New Chicken Pox Vaccine in all Healthy Children May Cause More Serious Disease".

38 - See note 35 (quoted from The Lancet)

39 - Hearings before the Committee on Interstate and Foreign Commerce, House of Representatives, 87th Congress, Second Session on H.R. 10541, May 1962, p.94.

40 - Ullman, Discovering Homeopathy, p 42 (Thomas L. Bradford, Logic Figures, p68, 113-146; Coulter, Divided Legacy, Vol 3, p268).

41 - See Note 27.

42 - See Note 27.

43 - Golden, Isaac, Vaccination? A Review of Risks and Alternatives.

Dangerous metals, poisonous chemicals, half-dead viruses, and animal pus is what you will find in vaccines—The vaccine used in the mandated 1976 supposed swine flu "epidemic" caused the deaths of 2,000 people before it was removed; and 4,000 filed injury law suits. Before that, it was the Salk polio vaccine, also fast-tracked with $9-million of tax-payer money, to inoculate 57-million Americans before it was even proved to be safe to use. And it wasn't.

African green monkey kidney tissue was used to grow the polio virus; and it proved to have long-term and deadly effects. In 1955, the "British Medical Journal warned against the used of the Salk polio vaccine."(2) The warning, and there were others as well, was ignored. Before genetic engineering opened a Pandora's Box, **this vaccine "was an uncontrolled experiment in interspecies viral transmission."**(3) Long-term, but not known then (in the financial rush to get this vaccine produced), **the use of this monkey's tissue was to be the cause of cancers detected much later.** This cancer-causing monkey virus, known as SV40 (still debated in some medical circles) is documented in "The Virus and the Vaccine: The true story of a cancer-causing monkey virus, contaminated Polio Vaccine, and the millions of Americans Exposed."(4)

There are countless stories of vaccinations causing death, seizures, and other permanent injuries. Over many years, Robert F. Kennedy has waged a valiant campaign about the dangers of vaccines. His article about what he calls "Deadly Immunity" has been re-printed just this past week.(5) It is yet another reminder of a path continuously trodden by rapacious multi-national corporations, and always with grave consequences that the public bears. **Manufacturing vaccines has now become a multi-billion dollar investment by international pharmaceutical corporations. With this enormous investment, there is total lack of precaution.** Money trumps safety every time. Now, we are talking about millions of people getting vaccinated without any safety data or long-term studies. We are the guinea pigs.

Who benefits from all this? Follow the money trail. Novartis will receive from the US HHS [Health and Human Services] $346-million for antigen and $348.8-million for adjuvant. They also have orders from 30 other countries. Baxter has orders from five countries for 80-million doses, but has not received FDA approval. GlaxoSmithKline has received $250-million to supply the US with various "pandemic products." This is not small change; and more vaccine purchases are planned. Dr. Mae-Wan Ho and Prof. Joe Cummins, in their new article (see below), report that **the total US vaccine figure for these orders amounts to $7 billion.**

In a lengthy article posted on July 27, the distinguished British geneticist and biophysicist Dr. Mae-Wan Ho and biologist Prof. Joe Cummins have written that **"Vaccines themselves can be dangerous, especially live, attenuated viral vaccines or the new recombinant nucleic acid vaccines, they have the potential to generate virulent viruses by recombination and the recombinant nucleic acids could cause autoimmune diseases.** A further major source of toxicity in the case of the flu vaccines are the adjuvants, substances added in order to boost the immunogenicity of the vaccines. There is a large literature on the toxicities of adjuvants. **Most flu vaccines contain dangerous levels of mercury in the form of thimerosal, a deadly**

H
A
R
M
F
U
L

preservative 50 times more toxic than the mercury itself. At high enough doses, it can cause long-term immune, sensory, neurological, motor, behavioural dysfunctions. Also associated with mercury poisoning are autism, attention deficit disorder, multiple sclerosis, and speech and language deficiencies. The *Institute of Medicine* has warned that infants, children, and pregnant women should not be injected with thimerosal, yet the majority of flu shots contain 25 micrograms of it."(6)

It should be noted that Dr. Mae-Wan Ho is the Director of the prestigious London non-profit organization, the *Institute of Science in Society* [ISIS]. She has written several important books and, for more than a decade, also has been writing about the dangers of genetically engineered organismslong before anyone was writing about these issues in the US. This ISIS article is absolutely essential reading for anyone who wants additional and unbiased background information on the questionable safety of these flu vaccines.

In order to be well informed, there also are other important questions that we all must ask every public official. (1)What vaccines are actually going to be used? There are numerous websites that list ingredients for all the pharmaceutical companies involved in this multi-million dollar so-called "pandemic." **Far too many of the ingredients listed are highly toxic. Some vaccines are not recommended at all for children.** (2) How many injections are going to be forced on children (some reports say four!) and adults? If this goes forward in the Fall, using schools as medical clinics, how will parents know what is in these vaccines? **Given the governmental immunity for the pharmaceutical companies, what recourse does anyone have for serious immune damage or death from these vaccines?**

These extremely dangerous vaccines are classified as bioweapons by the US government's own definition.

NOTE: *Adjuvants* are added to all vaccines to make dispersal faster and easier in the body (but not more safely). It affects the "action of the drug's active ingredient." It also then requires less adjuvant, so the product then can be expanded to cover many more vaccinations with less vaccine. This also means a faster production of vaccines, and more money for the drug companies with less production output of vaccine. However, the trial tests this month on children will not contain a squalene adjuvant, even though it is an ingredient in all three of the vaccines listed below. According to Jane Burgermeister's July 29 report, **these three companies "will conduct their own trials under secret contract with Health and Human Services."**(1) Why are they secret, when our lives are all at such risk? Again, there is a long history of rigged trials [the outcome always favoring the company, and rarely emphasizing the serious health risks and toxicity], especially when conducted by the same company that will produce a drug.

Wendy Scholl's testimony before a Congressional committee—"My name is Wendy Scholl. I reside in

the State of Florida with my husband, Gary, and three daughters, Stacy, Holly, and Jackie. Let me stress that all three of our daughters were born healthy, normal babies. **I am here to tell of Stacy's reaction to the measles vaccine** . . where, according to the medical profession, anything within 7 to 10 days after the vaccine to do with neurological sequelae or seizures or brain damage fits a measles reaction.

"**At 16 months old, Stacy received her measles shot. She was a happy, healthy, normal baby, typical, curious, playful until the 10th day after her shot**, when I walked into her room to find her lying in her crib, flat on her stomach, her head twisted to one side. Her eyes were glassy and affixed.

"She was panting, struggling to breathe. Her small head lay in a pool of blood that hung from her mouth. It was a terrifying sight, yet at that point I didn't realize that my happy, bouncing baby was never to be the same again.

"When we arrived at the emergency room, Stacy's temperature was 107 degrees. The first 4 days of Stacy's hospital stay she battled for life. She was in a coma and had kidney failure. Her lungs filled with fluid and she had ongoing seizures.

"**Her diagnosis was 'post-vaccinal encephalitis' and her prognosis was grave.** She was paralyzed on her left side, prone to seizures, had visual problems. However, we were told by doctors we were extremely lucky. I didn't feel lucky.

"**We were horrified that this vaccine, which was given only to ensure that she would have a safer childhood, almost killed her.** I didn't know that the possibility of this type of reaction even existed. But now, it is our reality."—*Wendy Scholl, testimony given to Hearings Before the Subcommittee on Health and the Environment; 98th Congress, 2nd Session, December 19, 1984; in Vaccine Injury Compensation, p. 110.*

What is in these childhood vaccines?—**Every childhood vaccine contains viruses and mercury.** Diphtheria, pertussis, and tetanus vaccines are generally given in one dose, called the *"DPT vaccine."* **Formaldehyde, thimerosal (a form of mercury), and aluminum phosphate—all strong poisons—are used to "stabilize" the germs** in DPT, as well as the other vaccines.

For just for a moment, let us discuss this matter of "stabilized" and "attenuated" viruses: If you half-kill a plant or animal, it is in bad shape. It may become diseased, it may die, it might recover its full strength. The same applies to the half-killed ("attenuated") viruses in vaccines. **The poisonous chemicals used to "stabilize" the viruses have caused some to become diseased, some dead, and some to recover quite well. —*Then the whole mess is pumped into the arm of a small child.* And we wonder why he develops a strange sickness afterward.**

One child will develop one kind of disease, another a different kind. It all depends on which direction a majority of the weakened viruses injected into that particular child happened to go—before and after being injected. It also depended on what other viruses happened to be in the bovine or monkey pus which the viruses came from. It also depended on the child's general health and diet at the time. It also depended on how many vaccines he received at one time. It also depended on whether this was the first vaccination or the third or fourth in a series.

After being injected, **the fast-flowing bloodstream carries off the entire collection of chemicals and viruses in the vaccine to the liver—and quickly separates the viruses from the chemicals which kept them in a weakened condition.** What happens to the viruses next, now that they are back in an ideal growth environment? What do the deadly chemicals do? Very likely, the chemicals weaken the body's immune system, as the foreign viruses set to work to grow and multiply.

A 60-Minute documentary, entitled "DPT: Vaccine Roulette," produced by reporter Lea Thompson, was aired over WRC-TV, Washington, D.C., in April 1982. **It reviewed a shocking number of incidents of neurological damage to children** following DPT vaccination.

"To health professionals, of course, the dangers of DPT are nothing new . . Almost from the inception of widespread DPT immunization, severe reactions have been reported, beginning with Byers' and Moll's study of vaccine-associated encephalopathy in 1948."—*Journal of the American Medical Association, July 2, 1982.*

"We have shown that triple antigen injections (DTP) given to scorbutic children [low in vitamin C] can result in massive immunological insults which may cause death *(as reported in Medical Journal of Australia, April 7, 1973).* Obliged to investigate this phenomenon, we were surprised to find the whole subject of herd [mass] immunization is controversial and not nearly so well authenticated as we would have our recipients believe.

"It is now seriously suggested that **the slow virus may be the cause of a number of degenerative diseases including rheumatoid arthritis, leukemia, diabetes, and multiple sclerosis. It is further possible that some of the attenuated [chemically weakened] strains of vaccines that we advocate may be implicated with these diseases.** Of polio immunization . . Fred Klenner (North Carolina) has stated, 'Many here voice a silent view that **the Salk and Sabin vaccines, being made of monkey kidney tissue, have been directly responsible for the major increase of leukemia** in this country."—*Glen C. Dettman, "Immunization, Ascorbate, and Death," Australian Nurses Journal, December 1977.*

Rep. Burton demands action—On Thursday, April 26, 2001, Rep. Dan Burton (R-Ind.), chairman of the House Government Reform Committee, confronted officials from the FDA, CDC, and NIH (National Institutes of Health).

Earlier that week, an Institute of Medicine (IOM) panel issued a report, that there was no causal connection between the combination MMR vaccine and an increased risk of autism in children.

Burton angrily wanted to know why these officials had not recalled the MMR vaccine, in view of the fact that it contains *thimerosal*, **a preservative which uses the toxic element, mercury, as an active ingredient (as does most other vaccines).**

The officials replied that pulling MMR from the market would cause shortages in available vaccine and would send unjustified panic throughout the public about the safety of immunizations.

Burton told them his own grandson developed autism shortly after receiving the recommended vaccination shots. "If you at the federal health agencies think this issue is going to go away, you guys are blowing smoke," he said. "If the health agencies don't deal with this and deal with it quickly, you're going to have a big problem over here."

MMR puts measles virus in boy's brain—**A child developed severe epilepsy after receiving the MMR vaccination.** Careful investigation has revealed that measles virus from the vaccine went to his brain and caused his debilitating condition. The tragedy was reported in the *London Telegraph (January 21, 2001).*

Her son developed an allergic rash eight days after he received the MMR vaccination, when he was 15 months old. Progressively, he began to have more and more seizures until he was having 10 to 12 every month. In the summer of 1998, he descended into *status epilepticus,* which is a state of continuous convulsions.

By this time he was 9 years old; and physicians at a London hospital decided that he needed emergency brain surgery in the hope of saving his life. It was at this juncture that a brain biopsy was taken—and it was revealed that the cause of the problem was the MMR vaccine. The biopsy had been sent to a reputable laboratory for analysis, and the results revealed that some of the measles virus had entered his brain.

Medical Journal article—The following research article explains how, in the laboratory, one or several poisonous chemicals are stirred into a solution of viruses in order to kill or weaken them.

It would be difficult to later extract the toxic chemicals used to kill the dead viruses and the poisonous chemicals must remain there anyway; since they are needed to keep the "attenuated" viruses (the live viruses) in a partially weakened condition. They are injected into a small child's arm.

"Besides introducing foreign proteins, and even live viruses into the bloodstream, each vaccine has its own preservative, neutralizer, and carrying agent, none of which are indigenous to the body. For instance, triple antigen DPT (diphtheria, pertussis, and tetanus) contains the following poisons: **formaldehyde, mercury (thimersal), and aluminum phosphate** *(Physician's Desk Reference, 1980).* The packet insert accompanying the vaccine (Lederle) lists these poisons: **aluminum potassium sulfate, a mercury derivative (thimersal), and sodium phosphate.**

"The packet insert for the polio vaccine (Lederle)

lists **monkey kidney cell culture, lactalbumin hydrolysate, antibiotics, and calf serum**. The packet insert (Merck Sharp & Dohme) for the MMR (measles, mumps, and rubella) vaccine lists **chick embryo and neomycin, which is a mixture of antibiotics**. Chick embryo, monkey kidney cells, and calf serum are foreign proteins, biological substances composed of animal cells, **which, because they enter directly into the bloodstream can become part of our genetic material** (*World Medicine, September 22, 1971, pp. 69-72; New Medical Journals Limited, Clareville House, pp. 26-27, Oxendon St., London, J.W. 1X4 EL1 England. Reprinted in part in The Dangers of Immunization, published by the Humanitarian Publishing Company, Quakertown, Pennsylvania, 1979, pp. 20-31*).

"These foreign proteins as well as the other carriers and reaction products of a vaccine are potential allergens **and can produce anaphylactic shock**."—*W. James, Immunization: Reality Behind the Myth, p. 10.*

The following is an incomplete (but significant) list of vaccine ingredients:

GlaxoSmithKline Plc based in London Vaccine Ingredients:

Aluminum adjuvant: an aluminum-containing compound. It releases the antigen [an active substance that is capable of generating an enhanced immune response from the body, and then reacting with the products from that response], causing strong, enhanced antibody response -what Dr. Mercola calls a "turbo charge" to the body's immune system. It has been linked to Gulf War Syndrome that has caused tremendous permanent damage to thousands of military.(7) Aluminum is a known cause of cognitive dysfunction.

AS03: The company's proprietary squalene adjuvant. (See: squalene below)

Daronrix: Glaxo's H5N1 bird flu vaccine.

Disodium phosphate: a white powder, water-soluble salt. It is used as an anti-caking additive in powdered products. This inorganic chemical is also used as a fungicide and microbiocide.

Formaldehyde: a known carcinogen and reproductive or developmental toxicant. Interestingly, according to PANNA, in 2007, California used 30,328 pounds of this carcinogen, as a microbiocide [a drug or other agent that can kill microbes] on the top 50 crops grown in the state.

Octoxynol 10: (Also known as Triton X-100) A detergent, emulsifier, wetting and defoaming agent. [Octoxynol-9 is a spermatocide.] It can alter metabolic activity, damage membranes, and cause a rapid decline in cell function.

Polysorbate 80: Also known as Tween 80. It is used as an emulsifier in cosmetics, and is one of the ingredients in Gardasil, the cervical cancer vaccine that is being mandated/promoted for teen-age girls. This ingredient is known to cause infertility, grand mal convulsions, spontaneous abortions, and life-threatening anaphylactic shock. So far, 28 Gardasil deaths have

been reported.

Sodium Chloride: Refined table salt. Salt is a naturally occurring complex mineral that balances the water inside and outside our cells. Refined salt, sodium chloride, is chemically treated and contains many other hidden chemicals that destroy natural salt's healing abilities. The body can get most of its daily requirement by eating a well-balanced, organic diet —eliminating processed foods. A good source is untreated, natural sea salt.

Squalene: A natural oil found in sharks (mostly found in their livers) and humans. The American Journal of Pathology (2000) reported that rats injected with squalene triggered "chronic, immune-mediated joint-specific inflammation," -i.e., rheumatoid arthritis. How will this affect people who already have an immune inflammation, or will it cause untold new cases (lupus, chronic fatigue)? Squalene is being added to all new vaccines. It is linked to the thousands of military who have contracted "Gulf War Syndrome" and have suffered irreparable auto-immune damage, including lupis, multiple sclerosis, fibromyalgia, and rheumatoid arthritis.

Thimersol: (MERCURY). Put in all multiple doses of vaccines. Any amount of mercury is highly toxic. There is no safe level. This is has been repeatedly linked to the increasing rates of autism, multiple sclerosis, and ADD.

Baxter International Based in Chicago.

"Celvapan" or its common name: pandemic influenza vaccine [H5N1] NOTE: Adverse reactions include: headaches, dizziness, vertigo, nasopharyngitis, chills, fatigue, malaise, injection site pain. There is "no data on Celvapan vaccination dose and schedule for subjects under 18 years of age" and for subjects who are immuno-supressed. Vaccine Ingredients: African Green Monkey: Cultured cells are taken from this species of monkey through a process called "vero cell technology." This species of monkey (and the tissue derived from it) have been implicated in transmitting several viruses, including HIV and polio. Baxter has "applied for a patent on a process using this type of cell culture to produce quantities of infecting virus, which are harvested, inactivated with formaldehyde and ultra violet light, and then detergent. Baxter has produced H5N1 [bird flu] whole virus vaccine in a Vero cell line derived from the kidney of an African green monkey."(11) According to Dr. Mae-Wan Ho and Prof. Cummins, "details of the production of this vaccine have not yet been released to the public."

Whole virus (H5N1) influenza vaccine, vero-celled derived. (See above.)

Trometamol: Also known as Tris (or Tris buffer) or THAM. An organic compound used as a buffer. May be harmful if inhaled. Avoid contact with eyes, skin, and clothing. Long-term effects: no data. Ecological information: no data.(12)

Novartis International AG Based in Basel, Switzerland.

Called "Focetria" or its common name: **pandemic influenza vaccine. Licensed May 8, 2007.** NOTE: Adverse reactions include: headaches, sweating, joint pain, fever malaise, shivering, and pain at injection site. Vaccine Ingredients: Virus: The company is using a proprietary cell line. [Unknown is whether they are using dog or green monkey tissue.] By using this process, instead of growing the virus strain in chicken eggs, it "has cut weeks off the time required to begin vaccine production [to be done at its cell-based facility in Germany."(13) According to the European Assessment Report (May 2007), "Focetria should not be given to patients who have an anaphylactic reaction (severe reaction) to any of the components of the vaccine, or to any substances found at trace levels in the vaccine, such as egg, chicken protein, kanamycin, or neomycin sulphate (two antibiotics), formaldehyde, cetyltrimethylammonium bromide (CTAB, a disinfectant used to sterilize utensils and instruments) and Polysorbate 80." The CTAB Material Safety Data Sheet notes that its "chemical, physical, and toxicological properties have not been thoroughly investigated" but it "is irritating to mucous membranes and upper respiratory tract."(14) PANNA also lists this as an herbicide and microbiocide.

Squalene: see above.

MF59: A proprietary oil-based adjuvant that and contains (according to Dr. Mae-Wan Ho and Prof. Cummins's ISIS article, already cited) Tween 80, Span85, and squalene. The authors also note that MF59 has "substantially higher local reactogenicity and systemic toxicity than alum." This adjuvant is part of a new generation of potent vaccine enhancers. In their book, "New Generation Vaccines" authors Levine, Kaper, Rappuoli, and Good note that "The precise mechanisms of action of most adjuvants still remain only partially understood."(15) Animal rat studies using oil-based adjuvants have demonstrated severe reactions to them, including paralysis, crippling, auto-immune disorders, and severe arthritis, and immune system impact. The FDA has yet to approved this for used in any vaccine, according to Jane Burgermeister's July 29 online report (previously cited).

Span85: Patented by the now defunct Chiron (bought by Novartis). Its chemical name is Sorbitan Trioleate. It is an oily liquid used in medicine, textiles, cosmetics, and paints as an emulsifier, anti-rust agent, and thickener. [Some factories in China specialize only in manufacturing Tween 80 and Span 85.] According to the Pesticide Action Network North America [PANNA], this chemical is used as a pesticide. It is also used as an adjuvant and is "toxic to humans, including carcinogenicity, reproductive and developmental toxicity, neurotoxicity, and acute toxicity."(16)

1. A. True Ott, Ph.D., ND. "Startling New Evidence That The 'Swine Flu' Pandemic Is Man-Made." July 26, 2009: www.rense.com/general86/manmd.htm; and Jane Burgermeister's website has a complete dossier of all her reports, as well as daily updates with her ongoing investigation: www.birdflu666.wordpress.com. For Dr. Lanctôt, see: Kurt Nimmo. "Canadian Doctor: H1N1 Vaccination: A Eugenics Weapon for 'Massive & Targeted Reduction of the World Population.'" July 10, 2009.

2. Eleanor McBean. "The Poisoned Needle."

3. Interspecies viral transmission:
www.sunnewsonline.com/webpages/features/goodhealth/2009/jan/20/goodhealth-20-01-2009-002.htm

4. Azoma Chikwe. "Polio vaccine dangers revealed." See: Note above, #3; and Tam Dang-Tan et al. "Polio vaccines, Simian Virus 40, and human cancer: the epidemiological evidence for a causal association." Oncogene. (2004) Vol. 23: 6535-6540.

5. Robert F. Kennedy Jr. "Deadly Immunity." July 23, 2009.

6. Dr. Mae-Wan Ho and Prof. Joe Cummins. "Fast-tracked Swine Flu Vaccine under Fire." Institute of Science in Society. London.

7. Petrik MS, Wong MC, Tabata RC, Garry RF, Shaw CA (2007). "Aluminum adjuvant linked to gulf war illness induces motor neuron death in mice". Neuromolecular Med 9 (1): 83-100. PMID 17114826. Also, see: Gary Matsumoto. "Vaccine A: The Covert Government Experiment That's Killing Our Soldiers and Why GI's Ae only the First Victims of This Vaccine." NY: Basic Books.

11. Dr. Mae-Wan Ho, ISIS already cited, NOTE #6. Baxter filed for a "Swine flu patent in August 2008, a year before any flu outbreak. See: Lori Price. "Big Pharma: Baxter Files Swine Flu Vaccine Patent a Year Ahead of Outbreak. July 18, 2009.

12. See: bsd.leica-microsystems.com/pdfs/msds/ebv-k_msds.pdf. Interestingly, it is a prohibited substance for racing horses.

13. Novartis Hopeful of H1N1 Flu Vaccine by Autumn."

15. MF59: Myron Max Levine, James B. Kaper, Rino Rappuoli, and Michael F. Good. "New Generation Vaccines." 2004. p. 260.

16. Span85/Sorbitan Trioleate. PANNA Pesticide Data Base - Chemicals:

17. WHO changes its mind: Mark Prigg. "Vaccine from swine flu may be unsafe warns WHO." London Evening Standard. July 27, 2009

[NEW 18. Emily P. Walker. "FDA Likely to Approve H1N1 Vaccine In Advance of Data." July 23, 2009: www medpagetoday.com/PrimaryCare/Vaccines/15230; and "Evidence of Harm Has Been Linked To Various Vaccines Challenging Prevailing Public Recommendations." May 28, 2009:

19. Jim Kirwan. "Legacy of the Bush Brigades." July 31, 2009: www.rense.com/general86/legacy.htm; and also: "State of the Union." August 1, 2009: www. rense.com/general86/stateuu.htm

20. Michel Chossudovsky. "Martial Law and the Militarization of Public Health. The Worldwide H1N1 Flu Vaccination Program." July 26, 2009

21. Banks: Dennis Kucinich. "The Federal Reserve is paying banks NOT to make loans to struggling Americans."

It is said that vaccines contain "monkey pus." While it is true that some do, vaccines contain a lot more than just mare's urine or fluid from animal pustules. When you take your small child in for his "shots," this is a sampling of what will be injected into him:

• *Formaldehyde*—Also known as formalin, this is a major constituent of embalming fluid. It is a powerful killer of living cells and is poisonous to the nervous, reproductive, immune, and respiratory systems. It also damages the liver. It is a carcinogen and linked to leukemia and cancer of the brain, colon, and lymph.

• *Tri (n) butylphosphate*—A suspected nerve and kidney poison.

• *Polysorbate 80*—This absorbent is known to cause cancer in test animals.

• *Ammonium sulfate*—This poisonous salt damages the gastrointesinal tract, the liver, and nerve and respiratory systems.

• *Animal, bacterial, and viral DNA*—Taken into the human body, these substances are absorbed by the DNA, resulting in genetic mutations.

• *Mercury*—In the form of Thimerosal, it is included in vaccines to kill some of the dangerous bacteria and viruses in vaccine fluid. But thimerosal is, itself, one of the most poisonous substances known to mankind. It especially affects the brain, intestines, liver, kidneys, and bone marrow. Extremely small amounts can cause nerve damage, paralysis, and death. It is a major cause of autism in children; even in extremely small amounts, it is one of the most dangerous substances in this list.

• *Beta-propiolactone*—This preservant is known to cause cancer; it is poison to the liver, respiratory organs, skin, sense organs, and alimentary tract.

• *Latex rubber*—Minute amounts of this can cause life-threatening allergic reactions.

• *Monosodium glutamate*—Also known as MSG, glutamate, and glutamic acid, this substance is mutagenic and teratogenic; that is, it is known to cause developmental malformation and monstrosities. This is because it is a neurotoxin, producing allergic reactions ranging from mild to severe.

• *Gentamicin sulfate*—This antibiotic causes mild to life threatening allergic reactions.

• *Aluminum*—A cause of brain damage and a suspected factor in Alzheimer's disease, dementia, seizures, and comas. Allergic reactions can occur on the skin.

• *Microorganisms*—These include both live and dead viruses, bacteria, and toxins emitted by them. For example, the polio vaccine was contaminated with a monkey virus which is now being found in the bones, lung lining (mesothelioma), brain tumors, and lymphomas of humans.

• *Neomycin sulfate*—This antibiotic interferes with vitamin B$_6$ absorption. When B$_6$ is not properly absorbed, a rare form of epilepsy and mental retardation can occur.

Allergic reactions can vary from mild to life threatening.
• *Polymyxin B*—A powerful antibiotic which can produce dangerous allergic reactions.

• *Genetically modified yeast*—Absorbed by the recipient's DNA, it causes genetic mutations.

• *Glutaraldehyde*—Poisonous, if ingested. It causes birth defects in experimental animals.

• *Gelatin*—This is produced from pig's feet and skins, calf and cattle skins, and demineralized cattle bones. Allergic reactions have been reported.

• *Phenol*—Also known as phenoxyethanol (2-PE), this substance is also used as antifreeze. When animals drink antifreeze, they die a horrible death. Phenol is toxic to all cells and capable of disabling the immune system's primary response mechanism.

• *Human cells*—These are taken from aborted fetal (human baby) tissue and human albumin.

• *Animal cells*—Also included in vaccines will be found a variety of the following substances: pig blood, horse blood, and calf serum. Pieces of guinea pigs, rabbit brain, dog kidney, cow heart, monkey kidney, chick embryo, and eggs of chickens and ducks. No check is made to guarantee that these included animal parts will not be diseased. The vaccine manufacturer hopes that all the various poisonous chemicals included in the vaccine will kill the bacteria and viruses.

13 - Tobacco

According to the World Health Organization (WHO), there are 1.1 billion smokers around the world. That is about one third of the entire adult global population. **Smoking causes more deaths and disabilities than any other single disease, accounting for 7% of all deaths**, with about 13,700 people dying each day of tobacco-related illnesses.

The WHO's projection, that states that **tobacco will result in more than 10 million deaths annually by the year 2020, will at that time make it the leading cause of death and disability.** Thus it becomes more lethal than HIV, tuberculosis, car accidents, maternal mortality, suicide, and homicide combined.

There is an estimated 42% of men and 24% of women that smoke in developed countries; while, in developing countries, 48% of men and 7% of women smoke. **There are 800,000 smokers and an estimated one million people who die annually from tobacco in developing countries.**

An estimated 80% of adult smokers began smoking before the age of 18. Each day, approximately 5,000 children and youth under the age of 18 smoke their first cigarette.

In the United States, smoking is the leading cause of preventable death leading to more than 440,000 deaths annually. The health-care costs associated with tobacco-related illnesses in the U.S are more than $75 billion.

In developing countries, cigarette sales have increased by 80% since 1990. In Africa, the annual rise in the rate of smoking is estimated to be 2.5% higher than in other developing countries. It is anticipated that, **in the next 20 years, tobacco-related diseases will become the number one cause of deaths in Africa.**

Not only does smoking affect the person who chooses to smoke, exposure to secondhand smoke can and does affect nonsmokers, especially children whose bodies are still developing. **Parents who smoke around their children increase their risk of occurrence of sudden infant death syndrome (SIDS) and middle ear infections. This smoke also causes an increased incidence of respiratory diseases**: such as bronchitis, pneumonia, asthma, and lower respiratory tract infections.

In adults who are lifetime *nonsmokers*, secondhand smoke is also a cause of lung cancer and coronary heart disease. *Environmental tobacco smoke* (ETS) is listed by the National Institutes of Health as a human carcinogen. Therefore exposure to ETS is a causative factor of human cancer. Around 3,000 deaths caused by lung cancer occur each year among adult nonsmokers. Studies also show that ETS is the cause of 35,000 deaths from ischemic heart disease in the U.S each year.

Studies have shown that children can become addicted to tobacco after smoking only a few cigarettes. According to a report in the journal *Tobacco Control*, a study performed on nearly 700 schoolchildren in the U.S., with an average age of 12, showed that **a quarter of the children who smoked, initially had cravings within two weeks of beginning to smoke.** Some even had symptoms of addiction within days of starting to smoke.

Over 6.4 million children living today will die prematurely due to smoking. The global tobacco epidemic is predicted to prematurely claim the lives of some 250 million children and adolescents, a third of who are in developing countries.

Women who smoke during pregnancy place their babies at an increased risk of miscarriage, low birth weight, and intrauterine growth and brain retardation.

Smoking has become a worldwide epidemic, an unnecessary killer that everyone could avoid.

14 – Alcoholic Beverages

Alcohol enters into the blood stream and is circulated throughout the body. It acts as a depressant of the central nervous system when it reaches the control center of the brain, causing a dulling of the senses. Inhibitions, thought processes, judgment, and physical coordination are all impacted by drinking alcohol.

Liver damage—**Cirrhosis is a serious effect of** heavy, long-term drinking. With cirrhosis, the tissue of the liver suffers irreversible damage that prevents the organ from functioning properly. In instances of severe cirrhosis, the scar tissue leads to liver failure. This means that a liver transplant is necessary to stay alive.

Other Body Systems—Alcohol also interacts with the **digestive tract** to irritate the lining of the **stomach** and prevent the healthy production of metabolism regulating **hormones**. This can lead to **obesity**. Drinking alcohol in excess over a significant period of time may also contribute to **high blood pressure** and other health issues that may cause **heart attacks and strokes**.

Fetal Alcohol Syndrome—When pregnant women consume alcohol, **their unborn baby is exposed to the drug.** The brain of a fetus is rapidly developing, and **any alcohol consumed by the mother permanently damages the part of the brain that is developing at the time of consumption.** Children born with a fetal alcohol spectrum disorder have varying degrees of brain damage, depending on the amount of alcohol the mother consumed during her pregnancy and at what stages of brain development. These children typically struggle with cause and effect reasoning, retardation, social immaturity, and other physical complications related to the mother's drinking.

Legal Ramifications—Many laws regulate the sale and consumption of alcohol, and the consequences for breaking these laws can be damaging both personally and professionally. **Underage drinking typically occurs in settings where the amount of alcohol consumed is not being regulated by a responsible party**, which dramatically increases the likelihood of over consumption and recklessness. Supplying alcohol to minors is a criminal offense. **Drinking and driving is not only potentially deadly for the driver and everyone else on the road, but also a criminal offense.** A person who has received a drunken driving charge will have to pay fines, may serve jail time, and may have his license suspended or permanently revoked.

Withdrawal—When a person consistently drinks large quantities of alcohol for a significant length of time, **the central nervous system reacts to the cessation of drinking by going into a form of shock. Withdrawal is characterized by tremors, physical pain and sometimes even seizures.** If a person with a serious, long-term drinking problem is planning to detoxify, she should do so under the supervision of a medical professional to help manage the symptoms of withdrawal.

Physical and social problems—**About 2/3 of violent behaviors on campus.** Almost half of all physical injuries. About 1/3 of all emotional difficulties among students. Just under 30% of all academic problems. $15 billion in health care costs (12% of total adult).

In the short run, physical problems include **reduced physical coordination, reduced mental alertness, poor decision making**, staggering, slurred speech, double vision, mood swings, unconsciousness.

Long term chronic consumption of high levels of alcohol leads to **higher risk for heart disease for liver disease, circulatory problems, peptic ulcers, various forms of cancer, irreversible brain damage.**

Alcohol is addictive: Phase 1—Alcohol dependency **may start with social drinking and is accompanied by psychological relief. It proceeds to use of alcohol for stress management** with developing tolerance.

Alcohol is addictive: Phase 2—

As drinking increases, memory blackout periods occur. The dependency sets in - **alcohol becomes a need and consumption is heavy,** but the person may seem to function normally. Drinking before social situations is common.

Alcohol is addictive: Phase 3—

Taking a drink sets up a chain reaction—**and he cannot stop.** Although he may try to stop ("go on the wagon"), this will not continue very long. Morning drinking begins.

Alcohol is addictive: Phase 4—

Daily intoxication, all day long. Loss of job, and social problems set it. Tolerance drops. **Physical problems become obvious.**

15 – Cell Phones

How to safely use a cell phone: **(Full information on how to do this is given at the end of this report. You will want to read it.)**

Here are the facts about cell phones:

CELL PHONE CRISIS:
1993 TO TODAY

Cell phones use microwave beams (also known as fields of radiation) to connect to the nearest cell tower. Contrary to what some people think, **the cell phone makes that contact by emitting the same radiation in all directions.** It does not just carefully avoid your head and send the signal straight up into the air.

Research studies have shown that this radiation can penetrate an inch or so into an adult's skull.

However, in the case of a child's head, it penetrates even farther. It goes halfway through a 5-year-old's brain, and almost a third of the way into a 10-year-old's brain (O.P. Gandi, G. Lazzi, C.M. Furse, *"Electromagnetic Absorption in the Human Head and Neck for Mobile Telephones at 835 and 1900 mhz," in Transactions on Microwave Theory and Techniques,* 1996, 44(10): 1884-1897).

What do those microwaves do inside your head? There is the obvious factor of heat; for that is what microwaves do in a microwave oven. But research studies have shown that, long before any heat is produced,

difficulties arise.

It should be kept in mind that we have only been holding microwaves to our brain for a relatively few years. **The long-term effects will not be known for quite some time.** That is the way it was with tobacco and lead paint.

Dr. Lennart Hardell, M.D., Ph.D., of Sweden conducted a series of case-control studies, in which his group examined long-term cell phone users. **He discovered a marked increase in brain and auditory nerve cancer on the cell-phone side of the head.** His research group found the same amount of risk in his research study, of 1,617 brain tumor victims, as that of the Lonn study, just below (L. Hardell, K.H. Mild, M. Crilberg, *"Further Aspects on cellular and Cordless Telephones and Brain Tumors," International Journal of Oncology [cancer], 2003; 22(2):399-407*).

Another research study found a 3.9-fold (390%) increase in risk of auditory nerve cancer on the same side of the head where the phone was normally used by those who had used a cell phone for more than 10 years (S. Lonn, A. Ahlbom, P. Hall, M. Feychting, *"Mobile Phone Use and the Risk of Acoustic Neuroma [nerve cancer]," Epidemology 2004 15(6):653-659*).

Then there is the *Interphone Case Study,* which was carried out in five European countries. **It found an 80% increased risk of a tumor on the same side of the head where the phone was used,** in individuals who had used cell phones for more than 10 years (M.J. Schoemaker, A.J. Swerdlow, A. Ahlborn, A. Auvinen, K.G. Blaasas, E. Cardis, et al., *"Mobile Phone Use and Risk of Acoustic Neuroma. Results of the Interphone Case-Control Study in Five North European Countries," British Journal of Cancer 2005; 93(7):842-848*).

So apparently there is a connection between extensive use of cell phones, over a lengthy period of time, and brain and/or nerve tumors.

But the problem does not seem to manifest symptoms prior to about 10 or 15 years of continued use of those phones.

Then there is Dr. Jerry Phillips, Ph.D. Motorola sponsored him to do research studies which would exonerate their products. When he discovered only horror stories and negative research conclusions, Motorola told him to rewrite his report. He refused to comply, and instead published his findings in a research report (J.L. Phillips, O. Ivaschuk, T. Ishida, R.A. Jones, M. Campbell-Beachler, W. Haggren, *"DNA Damage in Molt-4-t-lymphoblastoid Cells Exposed to Cellular Telephone Radio-frequency Fields in Vitro," Biochemistry and Bioenergetics, 1998; 45:103-110*).

Phillips is today an outspoken critic of the "all is safe" public image of cell phones; nor does he trust the studies being paid for by the cell-phone industry.

Thus we have found that cell phones emit a form of radiation which has negative biological impact on the human brain. We have also discovered that

long-term use drastically increases the likelihood that a person will eventually develop a brain cancer.

It would appear best to only use them when absolutely necessary. (There are emergencies when they are needed.) The rest of the time, use a regular phone.

Also discovered: The headsets, used with cell phones, concentrate local EMF waves to your head, increasing your EMF dose by 2-3 times as much as the cell phone would! **Cordless phones also emit nearly as much radiation as a cell phone.**

A huge public health crisis is looming, both for our nation and the entire world, from one particular threat: *electromagnetic radiation* (EMR) from cellular phones. This includes both the radiation from the handsets and from the tower-based antennas carrying the signals.

EMRs are produced by electrical appliances, power lines, wiring in buildings, and many other technologies that are part of modern life. From the dishwasher and microwave oven in the kitchen and the clock radio next to your bed, EMRs are there. **But none of them are as serious as the intensity of EMRs entering your brain from a cell phone held next to your ear.**

Studies have linked EMRs to development of brain tumors, genetic damage, and other exposure-related conditions. **Yet the government and a well-funded cell phone industry media machine continue to mislead the unwary public about the dangers of a product used by billions of people.** Most recently, a Danish epidemiological study announced to great fanfare the inaccurate conclusion that cell phone use is "completely safe".

George Carlo, PhD, JD, is an epidemiologist and medical scientist who, from 1993 to 1999, headed the first telecommunications industry-backed studies into the dangers of cell phone use. That program remains the largest in the history of the issue. But he ran afoul of the very industry that hired him when his work revealed preventable health hazards associated with cell phone use.

The cellular phone industry was born in the early 1980s, when communications technology that had been developed for the Department of Defense was put into commerce by companies focusing on profits. **This group, with big ideas but limited resources, pressured government regulatory agencies—particularly the Food and Drug Administration (FDA)—to allow cell phones to be sold without pre-market testing.** The rationale, known as the "low power exclusion," distinguished cell phones from dangerous microwave ovens based on the amount of power used to push the microwaves. At that time, the only health effect seen from microwaves involved high power strong enough to heat human tissue. The pressure worked, and **cell phones were exempted from any type of regulatory oversight, an exemption that continues today.** An eager public grabbed up the cell phones.

Today more than two billion cell phone users are being exposed every day to the dangers of electromagnetic radiation (EMR). Government regulators and the cell phone industry refuse to admit that these dangers exist.

These EMR dangers include: genetic damage, brain dysfunction, brain tumors, and other conditions such as sleep disorders and headaches. The amount of time spent on the phone is irrelevant, according to Dr. Carlo, as t**he danger mechanism is triggered within seconds**. Researchers say if there is a safe level of exposure to EMR, it's so low that we can't detect it.

The cell phone industry is fully aware of the dangers. In fact, **enough scientific evidence exists that some companies' service contracts prohibit suing the cell phone manufacturer or service provider, or joining a class action lawsuit**.

Still, the public is largely ignorant of the dangers, while the media regularly trumpets new studies showing cell phones are completely safe to use. Yet, Dr. Carlo points out, "None of those studies can prove safety, no matter how well they're conducted or who's conducting them." What's going on here? While the answer in itself is simplistic, how we got to this point is complex.

The flawed Danish study—In December, 2006, an epidemiological study on cell phone dangers published in the *Journal of the National Cancer Institute* sent the media into a frenzy. **Newspaper headlines blared: "Danish Study Shows Cell Phone Use is Safe,"** while TV newscasters proclaimed, "Go ahead and talk all you want—it's safe!" The news seemed to be a holiday gift for cell phone users.

But unfortunately, **that was a flawed study, funded by the cell phone industry designed to encourage sales.**

According to Dr. George Carlo, **the Danish research study was done in such a way that it could not have identified even a very large risk.** Therefore, any claim that it proves there's no risk from cell phones is a blatant misrepresentation of the data that will give consumers a very dangerous false sense of security. "Epidemiological studies are targets for fixing the outcome because they're observational in nature instead of experimental," Dr. Carlo explains. **"It is possible to design studies with pre-determined outcomes that still fall within the range of acceptable science."**

Key problems with the Danish study—The people defined as exposed to radiation were pretty much the same as those defined as not exposed to radiation. With few differences, it's nearly impossible to find a risk. Users were defined as anyone who made at least one phone call per week for six months between 1982 and 1995.

The "exposed" people used ancient cell phone technology bearing little resemblance to cell phones used today. The results, even if reliable, have no relevance to the 2 billion cell phone users today.

From 1982 to 1995, cell phone minutes cost much more than today, so **people back then used their phones much less**. Thus there was very little radiation exposure at that time.

During those years (1982-1995), people likely to use their cell phones the most were commercial subscribers. Yet **this highest exposed group, in whom risk would most easily be identified, was specifically excluded from the study.**

Ignored were mechanisms of disease found in other studies of cell phone radiation effects, including genetic damage, blood-brain barrier leakage, and disrupted intercellular communication. **The possibility of mental or physical damage was totally ignored.** The study did not discuss any research supporting the notion that cell phones could cause problems in users.

The study itself was inconsistent with cancer statistics published worldwide addressing the Danish population. **While this cell-phone study claimed a low risk of cancer overall;—in reality, Denmark has some of the highest cancer rates in the world.** This inconsistency suggested that something in the data does not add up.

Because the cell phone industry constantly guards its financial interests, an unwitting public can be harmed in the process, says Dr. Carlo. "Industry-funded studies in many cases now produce industry-desired outcomes. By tampering with the integrity of scientists, scientific systems and public information steps over the lines of propriety that are appropriate for protecting business interests—especially when the casualty of the interference is public health and safety."

To learn more about the dangers of cell phones and to read Dr. George Carlo's full formal analysis of the Danish cell phone study, visit the Safe Wireless Initiative website at www.safewireless.org.

How the George Carlo research began—Cell **phones were originally developed for the Department of Defense, and therefore these devices were never tested for safety.** They entered the marketplace due to a regulatory loophole by the FDA.

Questions about cell phone safety arose in the early 1990s, when a Florida businessman filed a lawsuit alleging that cell phones caused his wife's death due to brain cancer. The evidence he presented was powerful, and the media reported it widely.

In order to deal with the questions surrounding cell phone safety, the cell phone industry set up a non-profit organization, *Wireless Technology Research* (WTR). **Dr. George Carlo was appointed to head WTR's research efforts.** The manufacturers made the mistake of not paying attention to what he was discovering.

Oversight of the issue was charged to the *Food and Drug Administration* (FDA), though it should have gone to the *Environmental Protection Agency* (EPA), which fought hard for jurisdiction. But the industry had enough influence in Washington to keep that from happening. It simply didn't want to tangle with EPA because, says Dr. Carlo, "The EPA is tough. Anything that's ever made a difference in terms of public health has come from the EPA." He adds, "Safety issues that are covered in corruption and questions seem to always

have a connection to the FDA, which has been manipulated by pharmaceutical companies since it was born." Unfortunately, under later pressure from the industry, it concluded that cell phones are totally harmless.

Shocking research discoveries: Under Dr. Carlo's direction, scientists found that **cell phone radiation caused DNA damage, impaired DNA repair, and interfered with cardiac pacemakers**.

It was assumed that when Dr. Carlo was handpicked by the cell phone industry to head this research project, his conclusions would only back up the industry's claim that cell phones are safe.

But when called to help with the cell phone issue, **Dr. Carlo quickly recruited a group of prominent scientists to work with him,** bulletproof experts having long lists of credentials and reputations that would negate any perception that the research was predestined to be a sham. He also created a *Peer Review Board* chaired by Harvard University School of Public Health's Dr. John Graham, something that made FDA officials more comfortable since, at the time, the agency was making negative headlines due to the breast implant controversy. In total, **more than 200 doctors and scientists were involved in the project.**

Strict Study Guidelines imposed—Dr. Carlo established a strict list of criteria for the research:

First, "the money had to be independent of the industry—they had to put the money in trust and couldn't control who got the funds," he says. "**Second,** everything had to be peer reviewed before it went public, so if we did find problems after peer review, we could use that information publicly to recommend interventions."

A **third** requirement was for the FDA to create a formal interagency working group to oversee the work and provide input. The purpose of this was to alleviate any perception that the industry was paying for a result, not for the research itself. But the **fourth** and last requirement was considered by Dr. Carlo to be highly critical: "Everything needed to be done in sunlight. The media had to have access to everything we did." —**Dr. Carlo had established four criteria which made the outcome of the study uncorruptible!**

The research begins—The program began, but Dr. Carlo soon discovered that everyone involved had underlying motives. "The industry wanted an insurance policy and to have the government come out and say everything was fine. The FDA, which looked bad because it didn't require pre-market testing, could be seen as taking steps to remedy that. By ordering the study, law makers appeared to be doing something."

Dr. Carlo and his team developed new exposure systems that could mimic head-only exposure to EMR in people, as those were the only systems that could approximate what really happened with cell phone exposure. **These studies identified the micronuclei in human blood, for example, associated with cell phone near-field radiation. They also identified DNA damage and other genetic markers.**

Says Dr. Carlo: "**We also conducted four different**

epidemiological studies on groups of people who used cell phones, and we did clinical intervention studies. For example, **studies of people with implanted cardiac pacemakers** were instrumental in our making recommendations to prevent interference between cell phones and pacemakers. **In all, we conducted more than fifty studies that were peer-reviewed and published in a number of medical and scientific journals.**"

Industry tries to discredit findings—Manipulation by the industry, in its separate announcements to the media, began almost immediately at the start of research. While Dr. Carlo and his team had never defined their research as being done to prove the safety of cell phones, the industry internally defined it as an insurance policy to prove that phones were safe. **From the outset, what was being said by the cell phone industry in public was different from what was being said by the scientists** behind closed doors.

Results showed that cell phones do indeed interfere with pacemakers, but moving the phone away from the pacemaker would correct the problem. Amazingly, the industry was extremely upset with the report, complaining that the researchers went off target. **When Dr. Carlo and his colleagues published their findings in the *New England Journal of Medicine* in 1997** (Hayes DL, Wang PJ, Reynolds DW, et al. *Interference with cardiac pacemakers by cellular telephones. N Engl J Med. 1997 May 22;336(21):1473-9.*)**, the industry promptly cut off funding for the overall program.**

It took nine months for the FDA and the industry to agree on a scaled-down version of the program to continue going forward. Dr. Carlo had volunteered to step down, since he was clearly not seeing eye-to-eye with the industry, but his contract was extended instead, as no one wanted to look bad from a public relations standpoint.

The research continued, and what it uncovered would be a dire warning to cell phone users and the industry's worst nightmare. When the findings were ready for release in 1998, the scientists were suddenly confronted with another challenge: **the industry wanted to take over public dissemination of the information, and it tried everything it could to do so.** It was faced with disaster and had a lot to lose.

Dr. Carlo publishes—Fearing the industry would selectively release research results at best, or hold them back at worst, **Dr. Carlo and his colleagues took the information public on their own**, creating a highly visible war between the scientists and the industry. An ABC News expose on the subject increased the wrath of the industry.

European research confirmed Dr. Carlo's findings. Studies suggest that cell phone radiation contributes to **brain dysfunction, tumors, and potentially to conditions such as autism, attention deficit disorder, neurodegenerative disease, and behavioral and psychological problems**.

When Dr. Carlo was fired after cell phone manufacturers learned what he had discovered, **he independently brought safety information about cell phones to the public through his book**, *Cell Phones: Invisible Hazards in the Wireless Age.*

Instead of taking a break, **Dr. Carlo began working behind the scenes, setting up an organization and a registry for the benefit of consumers.** He also started the *Safe Wireless Initiative and the Mobile Telephone Health Concerns Registry*. It was a creative solution as part of the settlement of a lawsuit brought by an Illinois citizen against the cell phone industry, WTR, and Dr. Carlo personally. The lawsuit alleged that the cell phone industry, WTR, and Dr. Carlo were conspiring to hide the dangers of cell phones. Dr. Carlo was offered a way out of the suit because his book had made it clear he wasn't on the same page as the industry. That was how his new organization was set up.

"I wanted to make sure the litigation brought at least some value to consumers. We created **the *Safe Wireless Initiative*** (www.safewireless.org) for disseminating information on the dangers and on prevention, and **the *Mobile Telephone Health Concerns Registry*** (www.health-concerns.org) to track information voluntarily provided by cell phone users, particularly those who believe they're experiencing health effects. Post-market surveillance hadn't been done before, and the registry does that. It will help direct future research of potential health effects related to cell phone use. In the end, we did the best we could to get some benefit for consumers."

The industry attack—According to Dr. Carlo, "**The industry played dirty.** It actually hired people to put negative things about me and the other scientists who found problems on the internet, while it tried to distance itself from the program. Auditors were brought in to say we misspent money, but none of that ever held up. They tried every angle possible."

This included discussions with Dr. Carlo's ex-wife to try to figure out ways to put pressure on him, he says. **Threats to his career came from all directions**, and Dr. Carlo learned from Congressional insiders that the word around Washington was that he was "unstable." But all the character assassination paled in comparison to what happened next.

Toward the end of 1998, Dr. Carlo's house mysteriously burned down. Public records show that authorities determined the cause of the blaze was arson, but the case was never solved. Dr. Carlo refuses to discuss the incident and will only confirm that it happened. By this time, enough was enough. Dr. Carlo soon went "underground," shunning the public eye and purposely making himself difficult to find.

Why Cell Phones are Dangerous—**A cellular phone is basically a radio that sends signals on waves to a base station.** The carrier signal generates two types of radiation fields: a *near-field plume* and a *far-field plume*. Living organisms, too, generate electromagnetic fields at the cellular, tissue, organ, and

H
A
R
M
F
U
L

organism level; this is called the biofield. **Both the near-field and far-field plumes from cell phones and in the environment can wreak havoc with the human biofield**, and when the biofield is compromised in any way, says Dr. Carlo, so is metabolism and physiology.

"**The near field plume is the one we're most concerned with. This plume that's generated within five or six inches of the center of a cell phone's antenna is determined by the amount of power necessary to carry the signal to the base station**," he explains. "The more power there is, the farther the plume radiates the dangerous information-carrying radio waves."

A *carrier wave* oscillates at 1900 megahertz (MHz) in most phones, which is mostly invisible to our biological tissue and doesn't do damage. **The information-carrying *secondary wave* necessary to interpret voice or data is the problem**, says Dr. Carlo. **That wave cycles in a hertz (Hz) range familiar to the body.** Your heart, for example, beats at two cycles per second, or two Hz. **Our bodies recognize the information-carrying wave as an "invader," setting in place biochemical reactions that alter physiology and cause biological problems that include intracellular free-radical buildup, leakage in the blood-brain barrier, genetic damage, disruption of intercellular communication, and an increase in the risk of tumors.** The health dangers of recognizing the signal, therefore, aren't from direct damage, but rather are due to the biochemical responses in the cell.

Here is what happens in your body—In an effort to protect themselves, cell membranes harden, keeping nutrients out and waste products in.

Waste accumulating inside the cells creates a higher concentration of free radicals, leading to both disruption of DNA repair (micronuclei) and cellular dysfunction.

Unwanted cell death occurs, releasing the micronuclei from the disrupted DNA repair into the fluid between cells (interstitial fluid), where they are free to replicate and proliferate. This, says Dr. Carlo, is the most likely mechanism that contributes to **cancer**.

Damage occurs to proteins on the cell membrane, resulting in disruption of intercellular communication. When cells can't communicate with each other, the result is impaired tissue, organ, and organism function. In the blood-brain barrier, for example, cells can't keep dangerous chemicals from reaching the brain tissue, which results in damage.

The effects from the near and far-fields are very similar. Overall, says Dr. Carlo, almost all of the acute and chronic symptoms seen in electrosensitive patients can be explained in some part by disrupted intercellular communication. **These symptoms of electrosensitivity include inability to sleep, general malaise, and headaches**. There has been, in recent years, a large increase in conditions such as **attention-deficit hyperactivity disorder (ADHD), autism, and anxiety disorder**.

Dr. Carlo says, "Here in the US, we're six years behind in getting the brain tumor database completed, and currently the best data are from 1999. By the time you see any data showing an increase, the ticking time bomb is set." **We are not going to see the complete brain tumor research findings completed and published—before it is too late** and large numbers of the population have been disastrously affected.

European funding was provided for independent research to corroborate or confirm the work of Dr. Carlo and his team. The work was completed in mid-2004 (*Diem E, Schwarz C, Adlkofer F, Jahn O, Rudiger H. Non-thermal DNA breakage by mobile-phone radiation (1800 MHz) in human fibroblasts and in transformed GFSH-R17 rat granulosa cells in vitro. Mutat Res. 2005 Jun 6;583(2):178-83).*

When it was released, it not only provided independent scientific corroboration of the work done by Dr. Carlo's group, but **it also took the work a step further and showed how the problems were occurring mechanistically. This information formed a biologically plausible hypothesis for how cell phone radiation could be related to so many diseases.**

Dr. Carlo noted, "**The industry exerted pressure** on the scientists who conducted the work, including renowned German scientist Dr. Franz Adlkofer. **It first tried to change the conclusions of the work, then to delay its public release.** Then Dr. Adlkofer, the lead scientist, was attacked in the media and threatened privately with no more research money, a ruined reputation—similar to what we experienced in the WTR. **But this situation attracted the attention of a German documentary filmmaker, who decided to do a film on the cell phone issue.**"

It was enough to bring Dr. Carlo into view again, as he was asked to participate. The film, *The Boiling Frog Principle*, by Klaus Scheidsteger, builds on information from his first film, *The Cell Phone War*, and was released in 2007. **Its intent was to integrate the latest political and scientific evidence from around the world**, and bring forth to consumers important information on cell phone dangers that was previously withheld.

A floood of lawsuits ahead—**Currently in the US, there are seven class action lawsuits moving forward against the cell phone industry**, says Dr. Carlo, and nine other cases that are personal injury cases brought by people with brain cancer. In the past two years, two workers compensation awards were given to people with brain tumors based on a link between their tumors and their cell phone use in the workplace. Both of these cases occurred in California.

"**What we have now is a major litigation burden, a vulnerability the cell phone industry has never before been under**," Dr. Carlo says. "**They're uninsured for these health risk claims and are already positioning themselves for a congressional bailout**, like the Savings and Loan crisis of the late 1980s. They'll lose a couple of these lawsuits and once they do, there'll be an onslaught of new litigation against them."

It has now been been over a decade since the WTR was funded. Despite Dr. Carlo's revealing research and the corroborating research of other scientists from around the world that continue to follow, a search of **media reports today on the subject of cell phone dangers tends to suggest one of only two conclusions: There is no risk, or no one has yet proven the risk. That's at odds with more than 300 studies in the peer-reviewed scientific literature supporting an increased risk of disease.**

"When you put all the science together, we come to the irrefutable conclusion that **there's a major health crisis coming, probably already underway**," warns Dr. Carlo. "**Not just cancer, but also learning disabilities, attention deficit disorder, autism, Alzheimer's, Parkinson's, and psychological and behavioral problems**—all mediated by the same mechanism. That's why we're so worried. Time is running out. When you put the pieces of the puzzle together, it's such a wide ranging problem. It's unlike anything we've ever seen before."

HOW TO SAFELY USE A CELL PHONE

(1) When you need to contact someone on a cell phone, make sure it is set on "speaker phone." Then listen and talk while holding it down below your chest. In this way the most intense radiation (that which is nearest the phone) is not close to your brain.

Here is more information on this:

The best protection against cell phone radiation is keeping a safe distance from the cell phone itself—Always use a headset to minimize exposure to harmful cell phone radiation. The wire will lead to the radiation transmitter.

The most effective technique for protecting yourself against the dangers of cell phone radiation is keeping the phone at a distance from the body. Simply using a hands-free headset is a big step. Headsets **keep the cell phone's antenna at a distance of six to seven inches away from the body**, thus eliminating near-field exposure. **Wired headsets** can act as an antenna to draw some ambient EMR, but not much, so using one is still preferable to holding the phone to your head. **Wireless headsets** should be avoided, as they draw much more far-field EMR.

The safest headsets have hollow air tubes, similar to those used in stethoscopes, instead of wires.**They offer protection against both near-field and far-field exposure.**

If possible, **avoid wearing the phone at your waist, which exposes the hip bones to radiation. Eighty percent of red blood cells are formed in the hip bones.** Also **do not place it in a pocket near your heart!**

There are also newer cell phones available capable of functioning in **speaker phone mode. This enables you to talk on the phone while keeping it at a safe distance from your body.** If you are able to conduct most of your conversations using a speaker phone, this could enable you to use a cell phone without encountering the intense radiation exposure that occurs when holding it to your ear.

(By the way, the **wireless mouse** at your computer also sends radiation outward. So use a wired mouse. Another source of radiation is **wireless extension phones to your regular telephone**. That wireless extension, held next to your ear is also dangerous!)

Special note—Invisible electromagnetic radiation surrounds us each day, emanating from diverse sources such as power lines, home wiring, computers, televisions, microwave ovens, photocopy machines, and cell phones.

While undetectable to the eye, scientists have proposed that **electromagnetic radiation may pose serious health effects, ranging from childhood leukemia to brain tumors.**

As scientists continue to unravel the precise health dangers of electromagnetic radiation, **it makes good sense to avoid the "hot spot" locations of these potentially dangerous frequencies as much as possible. A *gauss meter* is a useful tool you can use to measure electromagnetic radiation in your home and work environments.**

Using the gauss meter at varied locations, you can easily detect electromagnetic radiation hot spots where exposure to these ominous frequencies is the greatest. Armed with this crucial information, you can then avoid these areas, re-arranging furniture or electronic devices as needed in order to avoid unnecessary exposure to electromagnetic radiation.

For additional study, here are several technical studies which support the findings in this present report:

1. Lahkola A, Auvinen A, Raitanen J, et al. Mobile phone use and risk of glioma in 5 North European countries. Int J Cancer. 2007 Apr 15;120(8):1769-75.

2. Lonn S, Ahlbom A, Hall P, Feychting M. Mobile phone use and the risk of acoustic neuroma. Epidemiology. 2004 Nov;15(6):653-9.

3. Hardell L, Carlberg M, Hansson Mild K. Pooled analysis of two case-control studies on the use of cellular and cordless telephones and the risk of benign brain tumours diagnosed during 1997-2003. Int J Oncol. 2006 Feb;28(2):509-18.

4. Hardell L, Mild KH, Carlberg M, Hallquist A. Cellular and cordless telephone use and the association with brain tumors in different age groups. Arch Environ Health. 2004 Mar;59(3):132-7.

5. Schreier N, Huss A, Roosli M. The prevalence of symptoms attributed to electromagnetic field exposure: a cross-sectional representative survey in Switzerland. Soz Praventivmed. 2006;51(4):202-9.

6. Westerman R, Hocking B. Diseases of modern living: neurological changes associated with mobile phones and radiofrequency radiation in humans. Neurosci Lett. 2004 May 6;361(1-3):13-6.

7. Available at: http://www.ijhg.com/text.asp?2005/11/2/99/16810. Accessed May 17, 2007.

HARMFUL

8. Available at: http://www.medscape.com/view-article/408066_1. Accessed May 17, 2007.

9. Available at: http://www.starweave.com/reflex. Accessed May 17, 2007.

10. Schuz J, Jacobsen R, Olsen JH, Boice JD Jr, McLaughlin JK, Johansen C. Cellular telephone use and cancer risk: update of a nationwide Danish cohort. J Natl Cancer Inst. 2006 Dec 6;98(23):1707-13.

11. Hayes DL, Wang PJ, Reynolds DW, et al. Interference with cardiac pacemakers by cellular telephones. N Engl J Med. 1997 May 22;336(21):1473-9.

12. Diem E, Schwarz C, Adlkofer F, Jahn O, Rudiger H. Non-thermal DNA breakage by mobile-phone radiation (1800 MHz) in human fibroblasts and in transformed GFSH-R17 rat granulosa cells in vitro. Mutat Res. 2005 Jun 6;583(2):178-83.

16 - X-Rays

REGULAR X-RAYS

(Also on radiation poisoning: 602, 603)

People are routinely x-rayed (x-rays, fluoroscopes, dental x-rays, CT scans, etc.) as part of their diagnosis; and it has now become fashionable to get CT scans to check one's health. —Yet all are extremely dangerous.

X-rays *(roentgen rays)* were discovered in December 1895. They were introduced so rapidly into medicine that, until about 1906, they "were tried out [as therapy] on nearly every chronic disease" *(MacKee, 1938, pp. 15-16)*.

After World War I, fluoroscopes were introduced. They emit even higher radiation dosage than medical x-rays. From 1970 onward, the use of fluoroscopy, which delivers x-rays at a full 2 to 20 rads (the measure of radiation doses) per minute, has greatly expanded, especially during catheterizations, surgeries, and other common procedures. A leading expert in radiology, Henry D. Royal, M.D., estimates that **average per capita x-ray doses are 2 or 3 times higher now than they were in 1980**, due to expanded use of CT *(Royal, in Veterans 200, pp. 260-261)*.

One expert declares that **medical x-rays were, and remain, a necessary cofactor in over half the U.S. mortality rates, from cancer and ischemic heart disease** *(Gofman, 1999)*. The *Committee for Nuclear Responsibility* is trying to prevent some 250,000 premature deaths per year in the U.S., by cutting average per capita x-ray exposure in half.

Although x-rays have been widely used in medical practice for over 100 years, **in no decade have x-ray doses been measured.** Indeed, for about the first 40 years, the response of the skin (whether or not it got red!) was the only "measure"!

Have you ever sat or stood in front of an x-ray machine, covered with a bulky lead apron, waiting for someone who was standing behind a lead wall to press a button that would send ionizing radiation through your body?

For decades, the scientific community has known that x-rays cause a variety of mutations. There is no risk-free dose of x-rays. Exposure of the body cells and tissue to large doses of X-radiations, which have a very high ionising power, can result in **DNA abnormalities** that may further lead to cancer and birth defects. Even the weakest doses of x-rays can cause cellular damage that cannot be repaired.

X-rays are known to cause **instability in our genetic material**, which is usually the central characteristic of most aggressive **cancers**. There is strong epidemiological evidence to support the contention that x-rays can contribute to the development of every type of human cancer. There is also strong evidence to support the contention that x-rays are a significant cause of **ischemic heart disease**.

X-rays are produced in X-ray tubes by the deceleration of energetic electrons, by placing a metal target in their path or by accelerating electrons moving at relativistic velocities in circular orbits.

They are detected by their photochemical action in photographic emulsions or by their ability to ionize gas atoms. X-ray photons result in current pulses, whose rate can be measured to find their intensity. Dosage badges are used for this purpose.

X-rays can be very harmful and can quickly and easily kill living cells, if dosed in high quantities. Even though safer low-energy X-rays are today being used often in hospitals, dentists' offices and laboratories, lead shielding is still recommended to prevent prolonged exposure to these harmful radiations to the attendants.

We're all exposed to radiation sources—the sun, X-rays, mammograms, CT scans, dental exams; and to a far much less degree, the sun and even some underground rocks—and we are just now finding out whether those rays, combined, are dangerous.

So how much radiation is too much? Scientists have found worrying signs that radiation exposure is on the rise, thanks largely to the popularity of high-tech medical exams like **CT scans**. Here is information that you need to know:

The odds of developing cancer from radiation exposure are very small, but **risks increase the more you get zapped and the younger you are when you are radiated**, according to the National Academy of Sciences. This means **putting off radiating medical scans, if they're not medically necessary, is always best** because radiation can damage cell DNA—and that damage can lead to cancer years down the road. It's true that your body can repair the damage or the cell may simply die. But **the earlier you get radiated, the more opportunity there is for uncorrected errors to start cropping up in your DNA.**

If you break your ankle on vacation, an X-ray cannot be avoided. But you can ask for copies of the X-ray so that you do not need a second one when you get home. And do you really need dental X-rays every six months to look for hidden cavities? If your teeth are generally healthy and you brush and floss regularly, ask your dentist about annual or biannual bitewing X-rays instead.

Frequent flying theoretically ups your cancer risks. After all, seven miles above sea level, there's much less atmosphere to absorb radiation from the sun. The *Association of Flight Attendants* takes the risk seriously enough that it recently warned members (who fly an average 100,000 to 450,000 miles a year) that some researchers have found "a significant increased risk of **breast cancer** among female flight attendants."

We absorb radiation from a variety of sources. How much is too much? Experts say 3 mSv per year is probably OK for most of us; 20 mSv for those who *must* have medical tests.

How Much Radiation Are You Getting?—Here are the radiation sources and how much radiation each will give you:

Single airplane flight, coast-to-coast—0.01–0.03 mSv*

Dental X-ray (bitewing)—0.02 mSv

DEXA (bone-density) scan—0.01–0.05 mSv

X-ray of chest (or ankle to look for broken bones)—0.1–0.6 mSv

High-mileage frequent flying (100,000–450,000 miles per year)—1–6.7 mSv

Mammogram—1–2 mSv

Natural background radiation from living at sea level (e.g., Chicago)—3 mSv (per year)

Natural background radiation (from sunlight, radon gas, etc.) from living in high-altitude cities (e.g., Denver, Salt Lake City)—6 mSv (per year)

CT scan, chest or pelvis—4–8 mSv

CT scan, full body—10–12 mSv

*mSv=millisievert, the scientific unit of measurement for radiation dose. At high levels, radiation can mutate the structure (genetic components) of a body's dividing or reproducing cells and increase cancer risks. Sources: American College of Radiology; Radiological Society of North America; American Association of Physical Medicine; *The New England Journal of Medicine*; University of California, San Francisco, Cancer Center.

Some Practical Recommendations on Taking or Not Taking X-rays—So what does all of this mean for you the next time that your doctor recommends taking an x-ray?

If a health practitioner recommends that you have an x-ray or CT scan done, **find out exactly what the health practitioner is looking for.** More importantly, **find out what the practitioner will recommend that you do for each possible major finding.**

If you cannot see yourself following through on any of the practitioner's recommendations for each possible major finding, it seems logical not to expose yourself to unnecessary ionizing radiation to begin with. If your practitioner is unwilling to address all of your concerns, you really need to find a practitioner who will.

If you decide that taking an x-ray will help you figure out what the problem is and/or help you figure out how to get better, **ask the person who will take the x-ray exactly what the dose will be.** If he or she cannot tell you exactly what the dose will be, it is likely that you will be exposed to a higher dose than is necessary. If this is the case, you need to find another x-ray facility, one that is fully committed to using the lowest possible dose for its x-rays.

If you have x-rays taken, **know that these x-rays belong to you.** If you don't feel good about your doctor's interpretation of your x-rays, you can take your x-rays to other practitioners to ask for as many other opinions as you wish. You may be asked to sign a form in order for your doctor or x-ray facility to release your x-rays to you, but make no mistake about it - *your x-ray films belong to you.*

Babies, growing children, and pregnant women should not be exposed to x-rays unless they are faced with a life or limb-threatening situation. Fetuses, babies, and growing children have rapidly growing cells that are much more susceptible to genetic damage when exposed to ionizing radiation than the slower growing cells of adults.

FLUOROSCOPY

Fluoroscopy is an imaging technique commonly used by physicians to obtain real-time moving images of the internal structures of a patient through the use of a fluoroscope. In its simplest form, **a fluoroscope consists of an x-ray source and fluorescent screen between which a patient is placed.** However, modern fluoroscopes couple the screen to an x-ray image intensifier and CCD video camera allowing the images to be recorded and played on a monitor.

The use of x-rays, a form of ionizing radiation, requires the potential risks from a procedure to be carefully balanced with the benefits of the procedure to the patient.

While physicians always try to use low dose rates **during fluoroscopic procedures, the length of a typical procedure often results in a relatively high absorbed dose to the patient.** Recent advances include the digitization of the images captured and flat-panel detector systems which reduce the radiation dose to the patient still further.

Because fluoroscopy involves the use of x-rays, a form of ionizing radiation, **all fluoroscopic procedures pose a potential health risk to the patient. Radiation doses to the patient depend greatly on the size of the patient as well as length of the procedure**, with typical skin dose rates quoted as 20–50 mGy/min. **Exposure times vary depending on the procedure being performed, but procedure times up to 75 minutes have been documented.** Because of the long length of some procedures, in addition to standard cancer-inducing stochastic radiation effects, deterministic radiation effects have also been observed ranging from mild erythema, equivalent of a sun burn, to more serious burns.

A study has been performed by the Food and Drug Administration (FDA) entitled *Radiation-induced Skin Injuries from Fluoroscopy* with an additional publication to minimize further fluoroscopy-induced injuries, *Public Health Advisory on Avoidance of Serious X-Ray-Induced skin Injuries to Patients During Fluoroscopically-Guided Procedures*.

CT SCANS

Computed tomography (CT) is a medical imaging method employing tomography created by computer processing. **Digital geometry processing is used to generate a three-dimensional image of the inside of an object from a large series of two-dimensional X-ray images taken around a single axis of rotation.**

CT produces a volume of data which can be manipulated, through a process known as "windowing", in order to demonstrate various bodily structures based on their ability to block the X-ray/Röntgen beam.

What is the financial cost of having a CT scan?—If you don't have any insurance, the cost of a CT (with injectable contrast) is around $3,000. Without the contrast, subtract about $130.

What is the physical harm to your body? It is immense! Each CT scan irradiates you with a far greater dose than any other kind of radiation! CT scan, chest or pelvis—4–8 mSv. CT scan, full body—10–12 mSv. —**Although fluoroscopy is almost as bad.**

A recent study in *The New England Journal of Medicine* warned that **up to one-third of all CT scans may be medically unnecessary—and that 20 million Americans may be radiated unnecessarily every year.** In view of the fact that some **65 million CTs are performed annually in the United States**, study authors David Brenner, PhD, and Eric Hall, PhD, of Columbia University Medical Center in New York City suggested that **up to 2% of all future cancers may be caused by radiation from CTs**.

While your odds of cancer from one CT scan are minuscule—1 in 2,000—the study also reported that some scans may be riskier than others.

Full-body CT scans are often used in emergency rooms to check for internal injuries after car accidents. **A typical, full-body CT scan can emit 200 to 250 times as much radiation as a chest X-ray.**

The same dangerously high numbers apply to full-body scans at boutique medicine storefronts designed for healthy people wondering if they have undiscovered diseases.

There is no doubt that CTs can be incredibly useful, but some experts believe that **doctors may order full-body CTs to protect themselves from possible malpractice suits following emergencies, on the off chance that they'll miss something.**

Always ask if a CT scan is absolutely necessary, says William McBride, PhD, a radiation-oncology expert at the University of California, Los Angeles, Jonsson Cancer Center.

Even more dangerous than single x-rays are CT scans. They are the latest way to have your body flooded with radiation. Let us consider them next:

Body scans are the current "health fad." **Extensive media attention, praising CT scans as a way to increase health and lengthen life, has caused many perfectly healthy people to get their bodies scanned** for possible indications that, somewhere in the body, a disease may just be starting.

High-tech machines, known as CTs *(computed tomography)* use **high-power, wide-area body x-rays** to "photograph" internal organs, producing wafer-thin serial images that are then viewed on a computer screen. Theoretically, CT scans are supposed to reveal cancer, heart disease, osteoporosis, and other conditions at their earliest stages. **The scans are said not to injure you.** They are fast; and, for just $700 to $1300, you can take a look at your insides.

It may sound great; but the amount of radiation you will receive is immense.

According to a 2000 *Life Extension* report, for the doses needed to produce the CT scans, **one CT chest scan is equivalent to 400 chest x-rays. A scan of the abdomen is equal to 500 chest x-rays. A scan of the head is equivalent to 115 chest x-rays. Combine the x-rays of the chest, abdomen, and head in the scan and you have over 1,000 x-rays.** Imagine having 1,000 x-rays at one time! This is not healthy living.

Please understand that the above amounts are "effective doses." That is, they are the minimum amount needed to produce the CT scan. **In reality, you are likely to have received a lot more radiation than that** listed above.

Frankly, this is as bad as the radioactive baths some wealthy people were taking back in the 1920s!

Back then, you could buy radioactive bath salts. They were supposed to be a cure for insomnia. Then, when you climbed out of the tub, nicely irradiated for the evening, you could get in bed and apply your *Radium Ore Heating Pad*—a nifty device said to be good for stomach, liver, and spine.

The FDA's Dr. Thomas Shope has cautioned that multiple CT scans can expose a person to radiation approaching the lower levels of Hiroshima and Nagasaki. A controversial new report estimates that **if 600,000 children get head and abdomen CT scans, 500 will get cancer from those scans.**

You might wonder why there is such a serious danger here; but **the body does not forget radiation. It keeps count of every rad you get** and the amount you get, whether it be from x-rays, CT scans, fluoroscopes, dental x-rays, etc. **Most of the radiation you get stays with you for a lifetime.** Radiation damage to DNA can never be completely repaired.

Beware of any physician or medical institution that offers to give you a "health scan" or a "body scan."

Dr. Stanley, president of the *American Roentgen Ray Center*, is highly critical of whole body CT screening in people who have no symptoms. He says that **the damage from a body scan might not be evident for many years.**

So do not listen to some medical expert who suggests that a whole body scan would be good for you.

It may be good for his wallet; but it will not be good for you, now or later.

CT scanners were not originally intended to be used in people with no symptoms and unknown risk. There are many safer diagnostic tools.

Ask yourself: Do I really need to undergo the equivalent of 1,000 x-rays to find out that I am not exercising, eating right, or that I need to buy a better mattress for my aching back?

AIRPORT FULL-BODY SCANNERS

Now they are giving people *full-body X-Ray scans* **at many airports in Europe and America.**

Full-body scans are conducted with the use of radio waves *(Millimeter Wave Scanners)* or radiation (**B**ackscatter Scanners), depending on the type of full body scanner.

Could Radio Frequency (RF)/Millimeter Wave Scanners cause cancer? While the FDA does not have a category for Security devices using *ultra-high frequency radio waves*, which are used in Millimeter Wave Scanners, they do provide safety information for cell phones. According to the U.S. Transportation Security Agency, the radiation emitted by the full-body scanners used in airports is less than the amount emitted by a cell phone.

—Yet the U.S. government has officially stated the amount of radiation in a cell phone is relatively harmless! *(Read the section in this book on cell phones to learn how very dangerous they are! p. 938).*

Dangers of RF radiation

High levels of radio frequency radiation can be extremely harmful to the body. RF energy in high levels heats tissues, in what is known as the **thermal effect** (This is what makes microwave ovens work). While the levels of energy used in a **full-body scanner** are far less than in a microwave oven, a malfunction in the scanner could theoretically cause energy due to the thermal effect of the RF energy.

What are Backscatter Scanners?

Backscatter scanners are a type of full-body scanner that use low-level X-rays to reflect back from skin and clothing. The person being scanned is exposed to a small amount of X-rays during the procedure.

WIRELESS COMPUTER NETWORKS

Any type of wireless operation produces radiation, especially a series of computers connected wirelessly (instead of on cables) to a central station. Read this:

"Wireless Computers Linked to a Network, From The London Times, November 20, 2006—Health fears lead schools to dismantle wireless computer networks **Radiation levels blamed for illnesses Teacher became too sick to work**.—

"Parents and teachers are forcing some schools to dismantle wireless computer networks amid fears that they could damage children's health.

"**More schools are putting transmitters in classrooms to give pupils wireless access from laptops to the school computer network and the internet**.

"But many parents and some scientists fear that **low levels of microwave radiation emitted by the transmitters could be harmful, causing loss of concentration, headaches, fatigue, memory and behavioural problems and possibly cancer in the long term.** Scientific evidence is inconclusive, but some researchers think that children are vulnerable because of their thinner skulls and developing nervous systems . .

"At the Prebendal School, a prestigious preparatory in Chichester, West Sussex, a group of parents lobbied the headteacher, Tim Cannell, to remove the wireless network last month. Mr Cannell told The Times: "We listened to the parents' views and they were obviously very concerned. We also did a lot of research. The authorities say it's safe, but there have been no long-term studies to prove this.

" **"We had been having problems with the reliability of it anyway, so we decided to exchange it for a conventional cabled system."**

"Vivienne Baron, who is bringing up Sebastian, her ten-year-old grandson, said: "I did not want Sebastian exposed to a wireless computer network at school. No real evidence has been produced to prove that this new technology is safe in the long term. Until it is, I think we should take a precautionary approach and use cabled systems." . .

"Judith Davies, who has a daughter at the school, said: "Many people campaign against mobile phone masts near schools, but there is a great deal of ignorance about wireless computer networks. Yet **they are like having a phone mast in the classroom and the transmitters are placed very close to the children**."

"Stowe School, the Buckinghamshire public school, also removed part of its wireless network after a teacher became ill. Michael Bevington, a classics teacher for 28 years at the school, said that **he had such a violent reaction to the network that he was too ill to teach**.

" "I felt a steadily widening range of unpleasant effects whenever I was in the classroom," he said. "**First came a thick headache, then pains throughout the body, sudden flushes, pressure behind the eyes, sudden skin pains and burning sensations, along with bouts of nausea**. Over the weekend, away from the classroom, I felt completely normal."

"Anthony Wallersteiner, the head teacher of Stowe School, said that **he was planning to put cabled networks in all new classrooms and boarding houses**.

"Professor Sir William Stewart, chairman of the Health Protection Agency, said that **evidence of potentially harmful effects of microwave radiation had become more persuasive over the past five years**."

MICROWAVE OVENS

(Also on radiation poisoning: 875)
A microwave oven is an X-Ray generator. It is

H
A
R
M
F
U
L

a heating device in which the waves generated are tuned to the frequency that can be absorbed by the water and fat in the food, but not by the dish, which is relatively dry, and is thus not heated up. When a microwave photon strikes a water molecule, the latter, being polar, rotates to align itself with the incoming electromagnetic field. This movement increases the temperature of the substance in which that particular water molecule is present.

Microwaves ovens play an increasingly wide role in heating and cooking food quickly, and are being widely used today.

Radiation leakage can occur during cooking if the oven door is faulty. A more significant problem with microwaves is the tendency of some additives found in plastics "particularly those which make it pliable, (to) migrate [enter] into food." Soft plastic containers designed for storing frozen or refrigerated items should not be put into microwave ovens.

The heating effect of microwaves destroys living tissue when the temperature of the tissue exceeds 43° C (109° F). Accordingly, prolonged exposure to intense microwaves to body surface can be harmful. In extreme cases, it can lead to cataracts, and can have adverse effects on the electrochemical balance of the brain, if the frequency equals the brain wave frequencies.

There was a lawsuit in 1991 in Oklahoma. A woman named Norma Levitt had hip surgery, but was killed by a simple blood transfusion when a nurse "warmed the blood for the transfusion in a microwave oven!"

Logic suggests that if heating is all there is to microwave cooking, then it doesn't matter how something is heated. Blood for transfusions is routinely warmed, but not in microwave ovens. Does it not therefore follow that microwaving cooking does something quite different?

Two researchers, Blanc and Hertel, confirmed that microwave cooking *significantly* changes food nutrients. Hertel previously worked as a food scientist for several years with one of the major Swiss food companies. He was fired from his job for questioning procedures in processing food because they denatured it. He got together with Blanc of the *Swiss Federal Institute of Biochemistry* and the *University Institute for Biochemistry.*

They studied the effect that microwaved food had on eight individuals, by taking blood samples immediately after eating. They found that after eating microwaved food, hemoglobin levels decreased. "These results show anemic tendencies. The situation became even more pronounced during the second month of the study."

Who knows what results they would have found if they had studied people who ate microwaved food for a year or more?

The violent change that microwaving causes to the food molecules makes new life forms called radiolytic compounds. These are mutations that are unknown in the natural world. This causes deterioration in your blood and immune system.

In addition, they found that the number of leukocytes increases after eating microwaved food.

Also, after eating microwaved food, cholesterol levels increased. Hertel said "Common scientific belief states that cholesterol values usually alter slowly over longer periods of time. In this study, the markers increased rapidly after the consumption of the microwaved vegetables." He believes his study tends to confirm new scientific data that suggest cholesterol may rapidly increase in the blood secondary to acute stress. "Also," he added, "blood cholesterol levels are less influenced by cholesterol content of food than by stress factors. Such stress-causing factors can apparently consist of foods which contain virtually no cholesterol - the microwaved vegetables."

The Russian research report—After World War II, the Russians experimented with microwave ovens. From 1957 up to recently, their research has been carried out mainly at the Institute of Radio Technology at Klinsk, Byelorussia. According to U.S. researcher, William Kopp, who gathered much of the results of Russian and German research and was apparently prosecuted for doing so (*J. Nat. Sci, 1998; 1:42-3*)—the following effects were observed by Russian forensic teams:

1. Heating prepared meats in a microwave sufficiently for human consumption created: (1) *d-Nitrosodiethanolamine* (a well-known cancer-causing agent). (2) Destabilization of active protein biomolecular compounds. (3) Creation of a binding effect to radioactivity in the atmosphere. (4) Creation of cancer-causing agents within protein-hydrosylate compounds in milk and cereal grains.

2. Microwave emissions also caused alteration in the catabolic (breakdown) behavior of glucoside and galactoside.

3. Microwaves altered catabolic behavior of plant alkaloids when raw, cooked, or frozen vegetables were exposed for even very short periods.

4. Cancer-causing free radicals were formed within certain trace-mineral molecular formations in plant substances, especially in raw root vegetables.

5. Ingestion of microwaved foods caused a higher percentage of cancerous cells in blood.

6. Due to chemical alterations within food substances, malfunctions occurred in the lymphatic system, causing degeneration of the immune system capacity to protect itself against cancerous growth.

7. The unstable catabolism of microwaved foods altered their elemental food substances, leading to disorders in the digestive system.

8. Those ingesting microwaved foods showed a statistically higher incidence of stomach and intestinal cancers, plus a general degeneration of peripheral cellular tissues with a gradual breakdown of digestive and excretory system function.

9. Microwave exposure caused significant decreases in the nutritional value of all foods studied,

particularly: (1) A decrease in the bioavailability of **B-complex vitamins, vitamin C, vitamin E, essential minerals and lipotrophics**. (2) Destruction of the nutritional value of **nucleoproteins** in meats. (3) Lowering of the **metabolic activity** of alkaloids, glucosides, galactosides and nitrilosides (all **basic plant substances** in fruits and vegetables). (4) Marked acceleration of **structural disintegration** in all foods.

As a result, microwave ovens were banned in Russia in 1976.

Standing in front of a microwave is also highly damaging to your health. Perhaps you have already felt this intuitively? We know that cells explode in the microwave. Just fry an egg in your microwave. We are made up of trillions of cells. So work out how many are getting damaged if you or your child stands in front of your microwave for 5 minutes.

ULTRAVIOLET LIGHT

Ultra-violet rays can have wavelengths as short as 10^{-9}m. They have high frequencies, though not as much penetrating power to sufficiently enter the skin. They are invisible to human eyes, but can be seen by many insects.

Ultra-violet radiation of very short wavelengths can be very harmful to the skin, and are responsible for causing our sunburns. Tanning and natural body pigments prevent the destruction of skin cells by ultraviolet light to a certain extent. But **prolonged exposure can cause skin cancer, cataract and damage to the human immune system**.

However, we are protected from the large amounts that the Sun releases by the ozone layer in the atmosphere, which absorbs a major part of the small-wavelength rays. A small dose of UV rays is thought beneficial to the human body, and can be used to treat some skin diseases as they can kill some harmful bacteria. Scientists today, have developed a UV index to help people protect themselves from these harmful ultraviolet waves.

The layer of ozone (O_3) that protects us from the ultra-violet radiation emitted by the Sun, by absorbing the short wavelength ultraviolet rays (between 2000 and 2900 Å), and attenuates those with higher wavelengths, is produced about 10 to 50 kilometres above the Earth's surface by reaction between upward-diffusing molecular oxygen (O_2) and downward-diffusing ionized atomic oxygen (O^+).

Many scientists today believe that this life-protecting stratospheric ozone layer is being reduced by the chlorofluorocarbon gases released into the atmosphere by different sources on the earth. Many environment groups are vehemently protesting against the use of these gases, and their use in many places in the world has been banned. Pollution on the earth has already caused a hole in the ozone layer above the Antarctic.

17 – Amalgam Fillings

MERCURY TOOTH FILLINGS

(Also on mercury poisoning: 874)

Any filling in the mouth that looked silver when it was new and is gray or black now is probably 50% mercury, the rest being copper, silver, tin, and zinc.

Over the past 150 years, the amalgam filling has evolved from a commonplace cavity remedy to a hot button health issue. It is now known that the long-term safety of amalgam dental fillings are harmful to your body. They should not be in your mouth!

Known by their color rather than content, amalgam fillings are commonly called silver fillings due to their silver/gray hue. The word *amalgam* is used to denote the mixture of metals used for the material, namely silver, tin, copper, and mercury.

Mercury is the most controversial element in amalgam fillings. It has the highest percentage of any ingredient in the filling, up to 50 percent. Mercury is a known toxin to many animals and body organs.

Fish consumption during pregnancy is discouraged or limited due to increasing levels of mercury in the fish, and mercury spills are treated with extreme caution to limit exposure for those involved in the cleanup. Yet, somehow, mercury persists as a key ingredient in dental practices.

The *American Dental Association* states that the mercury used poses no threat to the rest of the body. But what does the evidence say? This type of filling began being used in teeth fillings decades before any research was done to ascertain its possible harmfulness.

It was initially thought that, as the mixture of mercury, tin, silver and other metals hardened, no mercury vapor could be released. —But this has been disproved.

Researchers are concerned that the release of higher levels of mercury burden the body and are related to chronic diseases like **heart disease** and **dementia**.

A World Health Organization study revealed that amalgam fillings were a major source of mercury exposure for many people.

The FDA recently settled a lawsuit among many consumer groups who argued that the mercury fillings were unsafe. As part of their agreement, **the FDA has agreed to alert consumers to the threat mercury fillings may pose to certain groups, including children and pregnant or breast-feeding women**. Yet mercury fillings in teeth are still permitted!

Mercury is extremely toxic to the developing structures of the brain and nervous system, such as those of children or developing fetuses. Women of childbearing age should know that some research has connected high levels of mercury in the umbilical cord with the number of mercury fillings the mother had.

Individuals with compromised immune systems may also be at risk for complications with increased mercury exposure. While these groups are at a higher risk, all populations should be aware of potential dangers.

A cause of autoimmune diseases—Many medical professionals believe that mercury toxicity from dental amalgam is an **Autoimmune Disorder.** Autoimmune disorders **include rheumatoid** arthritis, Hashimoto's thyroiditis, human adjuvant disease, multiple sclerosis, amyotrophic lateral sclerosis (Lou Gehrig's disease) and MCTD (mixed connective tissue disease).

Add to this, **Crohn's disease, Raynaud's disease, systemic candidiasis, diabetes, and even Alzheimer's disease**. Each of these are now believed to also be autoimmune disorders. When patients are afflicted with such disorders, they come into their physician's office with all, or some, of these autoimmune symptoms:

- **generalized morning stiffness**
- **skin rashes**
- **dry eyes and mouth**
- **joint pain**
- **immune dysfunction**
- **axillary lymph node swelling**
- **subcutaneous nodules (skin bumps)**
- **neurological symptoms (ringing in ears, burning and numbness sensations)**
- **chronic fatigue**
- **depression and/or environmental sensitivities.**

The clinical assessment usually shows a connective tissue disorder, the result of the immune system attacking the tissues of the body. **The immune elements of T-lymphocytes, B-cells and "PAC-man" cells, instead of attacking bacterial, viral and yeast fungal invaders, attack the cells of the thyroid (HT), joint surfaces (RA), peripheral vascular bed (Raynaud's) or the skin cells with patches across the nose and cheeks (lupus erythematosus).**

In addition to the reports from the United States, Canada and Japan, European researchers have observed many adverse reports concerning amalgams. On February 18, 1994, **mercury fillings were banned in Sweden for children and youth 19 years of age because evidence showed them to be a trigger of autoimmune disorder.**

A study in Canada has shown that **pregnant sheep with new silver amalgams have elevated levels of mercury in their fetuses within two weeks of placement of the fillings.** Further studies on monkeys showed the same findings. These studies were done by Vimy, Takahasi and Lorscheider at the University of Calgary, Faculty of Medicine.

Research that has been done and reported in scientific literature demonstrates that:

1 Mercury escapes from fillings in the form of vapor created by chewing. It then enters the bloodstream and is delivered to all parts of the body, including the brain. For example: A recent autopsy of an 82-year old woman from St. Paul with confirmed Alzheimer's disease had studies done by the Mayo Heavy Metals Lab. **Brain tissue examination showed 5.3 UGIG mercury (53 times normal levels).** The pathologist reported **"neurofibrillary tangle" in the brain sections that are common in Alzheimer's** patients. She had multiple amalgam fillings.

2 People with mercury fillings have higher levels of mercury in their urine, blood and brain than people without fillings.

The European community had significant developments in the availability and use of mercury amalgam fillings when:

1. Degussa AG, the largest producer of dental amalgams in Germany announced **it would no longer provide mercury amalgams because of pending and future lawsuits.** This was based on a German Federal Court ruling that dentists who use such amalgams face legal liability.

2. A series of studies by Dr. Catherine Kousmine of France, reported that **illnesses like multiple sclerosis (MS) and chronic polyarthritis, both autoimmune diseases, are triggered by silver amalgams.** This is outlined in her book, *La Sclerosa and Plaques Est Guerissable (Multiple Sclerosis is Curable).*

3. A study of multiple sclerosis from Great Britain reports that **the highest incidence of MS is found in Northern Ireland and the Scottish Islands of Orkeny and Shetland—which also have the highest incidence of dental cavities and dental amalgam fillings.** This provides more suspicion that mercury is a possible link to autoimmune dysfunction.

When amalgams were introduced to the US in 1833 by two French entrepreneurs, the Crawcour brothers, amalgam use was denounced by a substantial number of American dentists. So strong was the opposition to amalgams that the American Society of Dental Surgeons, formed in 1840, required its members to sign pledges promising not to use them.

It is an intriguing historical note that the common term for mercury in Germany in those years was "quick silver." The German pronunciation for "quick" is "quack." Thus, those dentists who used mercury were called "quacks." This term has now come to mean anyone who is an "ignorant pretender to medical skill" *(The Random House Dictionary of The English Language).*

What you should know about amalgam removal—Many people ask what they should do about existing amalgam fillings. Clearly this is an important topic, as many patients dealing with chronic illness have removed their mercury fillings. Some have benefited greatly from removal, while the conditions of others have worsened. **The problem is that the amalgam must be very carefully removed from the teeth!**

Exposure to mercury is highest whenever the filling is drilled. A dentist must be experienced in methods used to limit exposure. When making the decision to have the mercury fillings replaced, take current health, personal and family history, and strength of the detoxifying organs such as the kidneys and bowels into consideration. Always discuss with your dentist any precautions that need to be taken prior to, as well as after having any fillings removed.

For example, **chronic fatigue syndrome** (CFS) is another amalgam caused problem. If you have decided that you have a toxicity problem causing CFS (chronic fatigue syndrome), you can ill afford more toxin exposure from mercury amalgam fillings.

Whether you believe the fillings caused your CFS problem or only contribute to your problems, it makes no difference. **The amalgam fillings are exposing you to mercury all the time from the fillings in your mouth**.

A person with CFS has a greatly diminished ability to deal with the constant mercury flow from their mercury amalgam fillings. **The mercury releasing fillings have got to go!** Ridding yourself of further mercury exposure is imperative if you desire to become well and stay well.

Proceed carefully. **Removing mercury amalgam can give you a big one time exposure if it is not done correctly. This is because mercury is released when the dentists high speed drill is applied to the amalgam.**

Studies have shown that a person's mercury exposure increases far above the normal amount as a direct result of an unsafe amalgam removal process.

There are three ways mercury can enter your body during amalgam removal.

1. The **hot mercury vapor** created by the drill can pass directly into the tissue of the oral cavity.

2. **Particles of amalgam can fall into the throat** and pass into the GI track where the mercury amalgam experiences further dissolution by your own bodies digestion, and bacterial flora inhabiting the GI.

Both digestion and flora can release more mercury from the particles. Worse, GI organisms change the dental mercury into the even more toxic methyl mercury.

3. Mercury vapor released during drilling is **inhaled into the lungs**. The dentist suffers this exposure as well. Fully 80% of respired mercury is absorbed into the lungs. From the lungs the mercury ions travel in the blood until a binding location is found.

If you are already ill with CFS, all of these exposures are of great concern. If the smell of gasoline can make you sick, you can know that a mercury rush from dental drilling has the potential to really cause you problems.

Safe amalgam removal—**Here is how this is done:**

1. **The dentist at minimum has to use a rubber dam** to keep some of the hot vapors from entering the tissues of your mouth directly. The dam can be effective at keeping amalgam particles from tumbling down your throat.

Many dentists use rubber dams. The mercury ignorant dentist just wants to keep his work area clean and dry. You will not raise too many eyebrows with this request, though don't expect much understanding for your mercury concerns.

Sam Ziff believes **a rubber dam is less than fool proof, since experiments have shown mercury vapor to collect in the mouth under the rubber dam** during amalgam drilling.

2. **The mercury free dentists are placing respira-** tors on their patients during drilling. This is an invaluable help, for it sucks the air, fumes, etc. out of the mouth during all drilling operations—either to install amalgam or to remove it.

The special, knowledgable dentists are also employing scavenging systems to clear the operating room of any mercury vapor that escapes the suction device in your mouth. If you press for a respirator, the dentist is going to think you are bonkers. If you are one who is severely ill with CFS, you really need that respirator.

3. **There is a water cooled drill from Sweden now in use to keep mercury vaporization at a minimum. The dentists using this equipment will section the amalgam, removing it in pieces.** The unsafe dentist is going to grind away the entire filling.

Make sure it is all gone!—There is also hidden mercury. **Endodontists use amalgam to cover the root apex after doing a root canal *from the gum side*.** An endodontic root canal is an unpleasant surgery to endure. They cut open your gums, and saw away the bottom of the tooth to get at the nerve and pulp of the tooth.

The amalgam on the root apex can produce great irritation with the chin bone. Examination of the extracted tooth may reveal that all the tooth contact points with the amalgam are heavily corroded. The only portion of the amalgam not black is the surface facing out to the gums.

Dentists will use amalgam to cover a root canal, and to build a post for a crown. This is the worst possible use of amalgam. When gold and amalgam touch they produce the most effective galvanic reaction available for dental mercury release.

The result of this "battery" (for that is the effect it produces) is a rapid release of mercury and other metal ions into your body as the amalgam corrodes. Cement does not form a trustworthy insulated barrier between the amalgam and the crown.

J.P. Dewald, C.J. Arcoria and V.A. Marker of Baylor College of Dentistry published a report in 1992 titled: *"Evaluation of the interactions between amalgam, cement, and gold castings"*. They conducted a complete double blind experiment "in vitro" on 3 variables: cement A vs cement B; cement vs no cement; and thermal cycle vs no thermal cycle. (A "thermal cycle" is going from hot to cold and back again; something that regularly occurs in your mouth as you drink cold water or then or later eat hot food or fluids.)

What they found is that there is cement loss in all thermal cycled cases. They found that the amalgam corroded in all cases. **Amalgam corrosion rate went up with thermal cycles in all cases.** Thermal cycles simulate what happens when you eat hot food, and drink hot fluids. **Mercury releasing amalgam corrosion was at it's maximum when thermo-cycled and there was direct contact between a gold crown and mercury amalgam.**

H
A
R
M
F
U
L

Don't Mix Metals Any Longer Than Needed—Next worst for amalgum loss into your body, after direct contact between gold and amalgam, is **the same galvanic reaction using your saliva, tissue, bone and tooth as conductive intermediaries**. Very likely gold in some form will be used as a replacement if you have large molar fillings.

The saliva in your mouth is an excellent conductor. Ever witness a kid get a jolt by placing his tongue across a 9V battery's connectors? It was the saliva that short circuited the battery.

Dentists use a small electrical current to detect nerve sensitivity in teeth.**The galvanic effect with gold through your mouth will hasten the release of mercury from your remaining amalgams. Don't let the amalgam reside in your mouth with other metals any longer than possible.** You do not want mixed metals in your mouth. It can produce chronic illness you cannot trace to its cause.

The only good mercury amalgam is the one that never got placed!

How to find a dentist who will safely remove your mercury fillings—In your computer, type in **http://mercuryfreedentists.com** and you will find all of those in your area who can help you.

Here is an additional research report on this topic, which the present author wrote earlier:

DENTAL AMALGAM FILLINGS

When you have your tooth cavities filled, ask for filling material that is not amalgam; do this because it contains the deadly poison, mercury. Try to find a dentist who will replace all your amalgam fillings with a different substance. *We have so many excellent dentists in our nation, and many will be glad to help you in this matter.* **The following article was written by John Whitman Ray, N.D., M.D.**

"1. I have had the pleasure of testing several hundred patients and students with the *Mercury Vapor Analyzer*. I have found only two people in all my testing who have not evidenced a continual toxic exposure to mercury vapor emanating from silver amalgam dental fillings under normal chewing compression. **The amount of mercury vapor emitted under normal chewing compression exceeded in ten seconds what the maximum allowable mercury exposure would be in industry in a 40 hour work week as is indicated by both Russian and U.S.A. standards.** This amount of exposure to mercury vapor is totally unacceptable to the scientific mind.

"2. Dental Association literature frequently claims that the amalgam filling material is harmless, and does not leak into the mouth. The sad fact is that there is absolutely no scientific research in existence to support this hypothesis. To the contrary, all evidence indicates that so-called "silver" **amalgam, which contains approxi-**mately 50% mercury, is a source of extremely toxic elemental mercury adversely affecting the health of the human body.**

"3. Evidence now demonstrates that surface particles of the amalgam filling material are being chemically broken down and released into the oral cavity. **These minute particles of mercury filling are acted upon by oral and intestinal bacteria to produce** *methyl mercury*, **an even more toxic form of mercury** than elemental mercury with target areas being primarily the pituitary gland, thyroid gland, and the brain.

"4. It has been demonstrated that **dissimilar metals in the mouth can also contribute to electrical activity and corrosion** (much like a battery) and can result in unexplained pain, ulcerations, inflammation and disruption of corresponding meridians in the body. This may result in a wide range of unexplained symptoms and disease.

"5. The presence of mercury in dental amalgam fillings has been shown conclusively to **adversely affect the body's immune response**. It has been shown that, after amalgam removal, the red and white blood cell levels tend to seek normal range with a corresponding increase in the body's immune response as evidenced by T-lymphocyte count increase.

"6. Research has indicated that **mercury is the single most toxic metal that has been investigated, even more toxic than lead, cadmium, or arsenic.**

"7. The *International Conference on Bio-compatibility of Materials* was held in November 1988 in Colorado Springs, Colorado, U.S.A. Many of the world authorities on mercury and mercury toxicity met to discuss the issue of dental amalgam and other materials used in dentistry. Their official conclusion was drafted and signed which read: **Based on the known toxic potential of mercury and its documented release from dental amalgams, usage of mercury containing amalgam increases the health risk of the patients, the dentists, and the dental personnel.**

"8. Autopsy studies from Sweden and Germany show a positive [definite] **statistical correlation between the number of occlusal surfaces [tooth to tooth contact] of dental amalgam [in the mouth] and mercury levels in the brain and kidney cortex.** It would be wise to point out that both elemental mercury and organic methyl mercury were found in brain tissue upon autopsy.

"9. Dr. David Eggleston, of the University of California, found a T-lymphocyte count of 47% (ideal levels are between 79%-80%) in patients with silver amalgam fillings. After removal of the amalgams, the T-lymphocyte count rose to 73%.

"10. **Multiple Sclerosis patients have been found to have 8 times higher levels of mercury** in the cerebrospinal fluid compared to neurologically healthy controls. Inorganic mercury is capable of producing symptoms which are indistinguishable from those of multiple sclerosis.

"11. **It is the responsibility of every dentist and doctor to inform and educate** their patients to the effect that:

"(I) **Mercury is contained in most dental filling material and all silver amalgam material.**

"(2) Manifestations of the disease of mercury poisoning only starts to become apparent three to ten years after the insertion of the mercury.

"(3) **There are alternative materials that could be used** for dental filling that could have no aftereffects on the individual.

"(4) **The patient has the right to insist that an alternative material be used.** The freedom of individual choice in health care shall be inherently respected and preserved as an individual right and responsibility of free men everywhere.

"12. One must remember that **the diagnosis of mercury intoxication is extremely difficult to ascertain because of the insidious nature of the onset of symptoms** and because of most physicians' unfamiliarity or misinformation concerning proper testing techniques. Unfortunately, **mercury is so toxic to the human organism, that there can be cell death or irreversible chemical damage long before clinical observable symptoms appear** and indicate that something is wrong. Since organic mercury in some body tissues (e.g. brain) has a half- life of over 25 years (*i.e.* it takes the body 25 years to get rid of ½ of a single dose of mercury under normal circumstances), it is only a matter of time and degree of exposure until some form of symptomology appears. **With all this in mind, we dare not delay having the safe removal of silver amalgam fillings by the hands of a knowledgeable and responsible dentist.**"

18 – Street Drugs

MARIJUANA

Marijuana is the most common, illegal drug. Also called grass, pot, weed, or ganja, it is a dry, shredded mix of flowers, stems, seeds, and leaves of a crude drug made from the plant *Cannabis sativa*.

The main mind-altering (psychoactive) ingredient in marijuana is THC (delta-9-tetrahydrocannabinol), but more than 400 other chemicals are also in the plant. A marijuana "joint" (cigarette) is made from the dried particles of the plant. **The amount of THC in the marijuana determines how strong its effects will be.** The type of plant, the weather, the soil, the time of harvest, and other factors determine the strength of marijuana. The strength of today's marijuana is as much as ten times greater than the marijuana used in the early 1970s. This more potent marijuana increases physical and mental effects and the possibility of health problems for the user.

Hashish, or hash, is made by taking the resin from the leaves and flowers of the marijuana plant and press-ing it into cakes or slabs. Hash is usually stronger than crude marijuana and may contain five to ten times as much THC. Pure THC is almost never available, except for research. Substances sold as THC on the street often turn out to be something else, such as PCP.

Some of the immediate effects of smoking marijuana—Some immediate physical effects of marijuana include a **faster heartbeat and pulse rate, bloodshot eyes, and a dry mouth and throat**. No scientific evidence indicates that marijuana improves hearing, eyesight, and skin sensitivity. Studies of marijuana's mental effects show that the drug **can impair or reduce short-term memory, alter sense of time, and reduce ability to do things which require concentration, swift reactions, and coordination**, such as driving a car or operating machinery.

Are there any other adverse reactions to marijuana?—A common bad reaction to marijuana is the **"acute panic anxiety reaction."** People describe this reaction as an extreme fear of "losing control," which causes panic. The symptoms usually disappear in a few hours.

What about psychological dependence on marijuana?—Long-term regular users of marijuana may **become psychologically dependent**. They may have a hard time limiting their use, **they may need more of the drug to get the same effect**, and **they may develop problems with their jobs and personal relationships**. The drug can become the most important aspect of their lives.

What are the dangers for young people?—One major concern about marijuana is its possible effects on young people as they grow up. Research shows that **the earlier people start using drugs, the more likely they are to go on to experiment with other drugs**. In addition, when young people start using marijuana regularly, **they often lose interest and are not motivated to do their schoolwork**. The effects of marijuana can interfere with learning by **impairing thinking, reading comprehension, and verbal and mathematical skills**. Research shows that **students do not remember what they have learned** when they are "high".

How does marijuana affect driving ability?—Driving experiments show that **marijuana affects a wide range of skills needed for safe driving—thinking and reflexes are slowed, making it hard for drivers to respond to sudden, unexpected events**. Also, **a driver's ability to "track" (stay in lane) through curves, to brake quickly, and to maintain speed and the proper distance between cars** is affected. Research shows that these skills are impaired **for at least 4-6 hours after smoking** a single marijuana cigarette, long after the "high" is gone. **If a person drinks alcohol, along with using marijuana, the risk of an accident greatly increases**. Marijuana presents a definite danger on the road.

H
A
R
M
F
U
L

Does marijuana affect the human reproductive system?—Some research studies suggest that **the use of marijuana during pregnancy may result in premature babies and in low birth weights**. Studies of men and women may have a **temporary loss of fertility**. These findings suggest that **marijuana may be especially harmful during adolescence**, a period of rapid physical and sexual development.

How does marijuana affect the heart?—Marijuana use **increases the heart rate as much as 50 percent**, depending on the amount of THC. **It can cause chest pain** in people who have a poor blood supply to the heart - and **it produces these effects more rapidly than tobacco smoke** does.

How does marijuana affect the lungs?—Scientists believe that **marijuana can be especially harmful to the lungs** because users often inhale the unfiltered smoke deeply and hold it in their lungs as long as possible. Therefore, the smoke is in contact with lung tissues for long periods of time, which irritates the lungs and damages the way they work. Marijuana smoke contains some of the same ingredients in tobacco smoke that **can cause emphysema and cancer**. In addition, many marijuana users also smoke cigarettes; **the combined effects of smoking these two substances creates an increased health risk**.

Can marijuana cause cancer?—Marijuana smoke has been found to **contain more cancer-causing agents than is found in tobacco smoke**. Examination of human lung tissue that had been exposed to marijuana smoke over a long period of time in a laboratory showed **cellular changes of the lungs called metaplasia that are considered precancerous**. In laboratory test, the tars from marijuana smoke have produced tumors when applied to animal skin. These studies suggest that it is likely that marijuana may cause **cancer** if used for a number of years.

How are people usually introduced to marijuana?—Many young people are introduced to marijuana by their peers—usually acquaintances, friends, sisters, and brothers. **People often try drugs such as marijuana because they feel pressured by peers to be part of the group. Children must be taught how to say no** to peer pressure to try drugs. Parents can get involved by becoming informed about marijuana and by talking to their children about drug use.

What is marijuana "burnout"?—"Burnout" is a term first used by marijuana smokers themselves to describe the effect of prolonged use. Young people who smoke marijuana heavily over long periods of time **can become dull, slow moving, and inattentive**. These "burned-out" users are sometimes so unaware of their surroundings that **they do not respond when friends speak to them, and they do not realize they have a problem**.

How long do chemicals from marijuana stay in the body after the drug is smoked?—When marijuana is smoked, **THC, its active ingredient, is absorbed by most tissues and organs in the body; however, it is primarily found in fat tissues.** The body, in its attempt to rid itself of the foreign chemical, chemically transforms the THC into metabolites. Urine tests can detect THC metabolites for up to a week after people have smoked marijuana. Tests involving radioactively labeled THC have traced these metabolites in animals for up to a month. **Source:** *National Institute on Drug Abuse, 1984.*

In summary—Marijuana *(cannabis)* is the most commonly-used illegal drug in America and England. *Research studies reveal the following facts about this strange substance:*

The THC *(tetrahydrocannabinol)* in it passes from the lungs through the blood into the brain. Enzymes in the brain cannot break down the THC as quickly as nicotine, so some THC will linger in the body for a full week.

An average marijuana stick in the 1960s contained 10 mg THC, but today as much as 150 mg. The THC interferes with normal **brain waves**, and depresses electrical activity of the frontal cortex (the center of character and moral strength). **Recent memory** is damaged. THC **reduces motivation, cognition, learning, focused ability, and concentration**. Marijuana smokers are **less likely to finish school**.

Chronic use of marijuana reduces aggression if the environment is placid. But if problems, stress or hunger occur, **strong aggression** can occur. There is a greater tendency to **suicide**, especially in females. It is a valid risk factor for **anti-social, criminal, sexual, and other behavioral aberrations**.

There is a two-fold increase of **psychosis** in steady marijuana users. **Severe psychiatric reactions**, including **schizophrenia**, can occur.

Even small amounts of THC can **weaken mitochondria**, the source of cell energy, thus reducing body strength. THC **inhibits the immune system, especially in the brain**. There are significant amounts of **cancer**-causing chemicals in marijuana tar. In addition to damaging the brain and immune system, THC **damages the heart and blood vessels in the eye**. It causes more problems than it solves.

COCAINE AND CRACK

Cocaine and crack are toxic, addictive, psychoactive substances that have significant physiological and psychological consequences for users. Perhaps even more significant and unfortunate, however, are the negative effects that cocaine and crack users have on their families, communities, workplaces, and society.

Domestic violence and random violence are often fueled by cocaine or crack. Children are often the victims of cocaine- or crack-using parents and suffer from prenatal exposure or parental abuse.

What is Cocaine?—**Cocaine is a central nervous system stimulant, the most powerful found in nature.** Most often seen in the form of cocaine hydrochloride, a white, crystalline powder, it is extracted from the leaves of the coca plant, *Erythroxylon coca*, which is native to the highlands of the Andean mountains in South America. The Incas used coca leaves as a part of their native ceremonies thousands of years ago. Over the centuries, laborers of the Andes, who toil under harsh conditions, have either chewed coca leaves or brewed tea from them to relieve apoxia (mountain sickness that occurs at high altitudes), hunger, and fatigue and for refreshment.

This stimulant drug, cocaine, comes in the form of a white powder. Street names for the drug include snow, nose candy, coke, "C," toot, and blow. People snort cocaine through their nose or inject it into their muscles or veins.

Drug dealers mix it with other substances so they can have more of the drug to sell. **These "fillers" make the drug even more dangerous because the user does not know how much cocaine he or she is taking.** The fillers also can add harmful side effects to an already unsafe drug.

Cocaine in the United States—**Cocaine was first isolated from the coca leaf in the late 1800s.** It quickly became popular as an ingredient in patent medicines (throat lozenges, tonics, etc.) and other products (including Coca Cola, from which it was later removed). **Concern soon mounted due to instances of addiction, psychotic behavior, convulsion, and death.** A series of steps, including passage of the Pure Food and Drug Act of 1906, were taken to combat health and behavioral problems associated with the use of cocaine and other drugs. Finally, the Harrison Act of 1914 was enacted, outlawing the use of cocaine and opiates in over-the-counter products and making these drugs available only by prescription. Cocaine use soon dropped dramatically and remained at minimal levels for nearly half a century. It continued to be used as a local anesthetic in eye, nose, and throat surgery, however, and still is used today.

In the 1960s, illicit cocaine use rebounded. Although cocaine powder was expensive, selling at about $100 per gram, use of the drug had become common among middle- and upper-middle-class Americans by the late 1970s. A kind of generational forgetting had occurred. Lost were the lessons about cocaine's toxicity and the dangers of abuse that had been learned from the cocaine epidemic earlier in the century. By the mid-1980s, **there was widespread evidence of physiological and psychological problems among cocaine users, with increased emergency-room episodes and admissions to treatment.**

The primary route of administration for cocaine powder is through inhalation, commonly referred to as "snorting."

What is Crack?—**Crack is a smokable, rapidly reacting form of cocaine base,** which is processed from cocaine hydrochloride. It usually appears as off-white chips, rocks, or chunks. There are many theories about the origin of the crack form of cocaine. It is probable that cocaine traffickers, seeking a broader market for an existing glut of the drug, developed the process to expand their user base, since this method allows small amounts to be sold at very low prices.

Crack is cocaine that has been processed so that it can be smoked. Crack looks like small pieces or shavings of soap but has a hard, sharp texture. The user inhales the fumes.

When a person smokes crack, **cocaine reaches the brain more rapidly and in higher doses than when taken as a powder.** The user feels an intense "rush" followed by a "crash" that can produce a strong craving for more of the drug.

America's Crack Epidemic—**Soon after crack first appeared, in the early to mid-1980s,** crack abuse swept through the country. Three factors contributed to this: first, the drug was cheap and affordable; second, it was easy to smoke; and third, its effects were rapid and intense. Smoking crack brings users to a euphoric state twice as fast as "snorting." **Because of this rapid high, crack is more quickly addicting; it is also cheap enough to be available to poor and young users.** This has made crack an extremely marketable product.

How Do They Affect You?—**Cocaine in all its forms stimulates the central nervous system. It causes the heart to beat more rapidly and blood vessels to constrict.** This results in the demand for a greater supply of blood. But the narrowed blood vessels are unable to deliver the volume of blood demanded, which **significantly increases the risk of cardiovascular incidents or strokes.** Initially, use of these drugs reduces appetite and makes the user feel more alert, energetic, and self-confident—even more powerful.

With high doses, users can become delusional, paranoid, and even suffer acute toxic psychosis. Blood pressure increases, which can cause strokes or heart attacks. In some cases these effects have proven fatal. **As the drug's effects wear off, a depression (often called a "crash") can set in, leaving the user feeling fatigued, jumpy, fearful, and anxious.**

Crack causes the same effects as powder cocaine. Because it is smoked, however, onset is more rapid and intensity greater. Thus, the effects may be significantly exacerbated. **The depression following use is considerably deeper and more profound.** The likelihood of **cocaine psychosis** after binging on crack may be greater and notably more intense. Crack use is associated with incidents of **hyperactive violence by users** and is capable of doing significant harm to fetuses of pregnant users.

Paying the Price of Cocaine and Crack Use—A broad range of consequences include:

• **Dependence and addiction**. Cardiovascular problems, including **irregular heartbeat, heart attack, and heart failure**.

• Neurological incidents, including **strokes, seizures, fungal brain infections, and hemorrhaging** in tissue surrounding the brain.

• Pulmonary effects, such as **fluid in the lungs, aggravation of asthma and other lung disorders, and respiratory failure**.

• Psychiatric complications, including **psychosis, paranoia, depression, anxiety disorders, and delusions**.

• **Increased risk of traumatic injury from accidents and aggressive, violent, or criminal behavior.**

• Other effects include: **sleeplessness, sexual dysfunction, diminished sense of smell, perforated nasal septum, nausea, and headaches.**

• Fetal cocaine effects include **premature separation of the placenta, spontaneous abortion, premature labor, low birthweight and head circumference at birth, greater chance of visual impairment, mental retardation, genitourinary malformations, and greater chance of developmental problems.**

• For intravenous (IV) cocaine users, there is increased risk of **hepatitis, HIV infection, and endocarditis**.

• For addicts, whether they smoke, inject, or snort, **promiscuous sexual activity can increase the risk of HIV infection**.

Even after one try, a person can experience: **Brain seizures. Irregular heartbeat. Depression. Stroke. Violent actions. Paranoia.**

A **person who is addicted often loses control of his life. He will do anything to get more cocaine. He spends hundreds of thousands of dollars on his habit He loses interest in friends, family, and social activities. He has a need to take the drug just to feel "normal"**

Why do people become addicted to cocaine?—
Cocaine causes chemical changes in the brain that control happiness and trigger an intense craving for the drug. These chemical changes stay in the brain even after the person stops using cocaine. They account for the extreme pleasure the user feels, as well as the depression that occurs when the user stops taking the drug.

Though an addict may further use cocaine to relieve bouts of depression, **an even stronger withdrawal state, called anhedonia, influences addiction. Anhedonia is the inability to experience pleasure**. The user can overcome depression, but still feel as if he or she cannot enjoy life without cocaine. Anhedonia can last for years, which is one reason why cocaine addiction can be so difficult to treat.

*Here are the signs that someone is addicted to cocaine—*Periods of severe depression, alternating with euphoria. Weight loss. Decline in personal hygiene or appearance. Constant runny nose. Frequent upper respiratory infections. Changes in sleep patterns. Loss of interest in friends, family, and social activities. Loss of interest in food, sex, or other pleasures. Hearing voices when nobody has spoken, or feeling paranoid. Expressing more anger, becoming more impatient or nervous. Hallucinations. Money trouble. Stealing. Selling personal possessions

How can I help someone who is addicted?—
Most drug users deny that they have a problem and push family and friends away. You may feel helpless, frustrated, and unable to cope. **You can get help by contacting a local drug abuse treatment center.** *You should also:*

Maintain established limits and rules. Don't change your actions to suit the needs of the addict. Don't cover up for the addict when he or she fails to meet responsibilities at work, school, or home. Don't make excuses for the addict's drug use. Don't lend money for drugs. Encourage the user to seek help. Get help from Alanon or NarAnon. These organizations are for family members.

*How are cocaine and crack addiction treated?—*Recovery often begins with "detox," the body's physical withdrawal from cocaine. **Physical symptoms of withdrawal can begin within a few hours and last up to seven days.** *Withdrawal symptoms include:*

• Extreme agitation and nervousness
• Depression and suicidal thinking
• Extreme craving for more cocaine

After the body is clean of cocaine and other drugs or alcohol, the addict enters a counseling program. The goal of counseling is to help the addict understand the effects of cocaine use, confront issues that lead to drug use, and learn ways to abstain from cocaine.

HEROIN

*Effects of heroin substance abuse on the body—*Heroin depresses, or slows down, the central nervous system. This can cause the heart rate to slow, and blood pressure to drop. Respiratory functions can also be impaired. **Prolonged use of heroin can lead to heart and/or lung failure. Heroin creates conditions of bad health over all, making the body susceptible to illness. Liver disease and pneumonia** are just a couple of the problems that can result from the body's lowered immune system abilities.

Heroin is also a drug for which the body develops a tolerance. This means that **as the body becomes used to the effects of heroin, more and more is needed in order to produce the "rush."** Eventually, as increasingly high dosages are needed just to achieve the same thing that the first dose did, the body becomes dependent on the drug. This means that the body almost needs heroin to function. The heroin has negative effects of the body overall, but the body has become used to having the drug present in its system.

Indirect effects of heroin substance abuse— The culture of heroin substance abuse lends itself to certain effects that may not be directly related to the drug's effects on the body. However, these other effects can have very real and lasting effects on someone's long-term health.

1. The repeated use of needles: Many people do not think about the effects the repeated use of needles can have in terms of heroin substance abuse. However, these effects should not be discounted. Because the fastest way to experience a "rush" is to inject the heroin directly into the blood stream, **needle use is very common amongst heroin users.** *Unfortunately, the repeated use of needles can have very negative consequences:*

• **Collapsed veins.** Eventually, continually injecting heroin into the same spot can result in collapsed veins. This leads some heroin users to move on to another vein. Some heroin addicts have collapsed several veins as they move on to "usable" entrance points for needles.

• Chronic users may develop **collapsed veins, infection of the heart lining and valves, abscesses, cellulitis, and liver disease.** Pulmonary complications, including various types of **pneumonia,** may result from the poor health condition of the abuser, as well as from heroin's depressing effects on respiration.

• **Infectious diseases.** Many heroin users actually use the drug in groups, often even at the dealer's location. This often results in **shared needles. This means that it is possible to get diseases from infected users. Hepatitis and HIV/AIDS can be contracted this way.** These are two diseases that, while they are often "managed," cannot be cured.

2. Effects of additives to heroin: Sometimes heroin dealers mix the drug with other substances to stretch supply and make more money. This can be very dangerous. **Some of the additives do not dissolve as well as heroin does,** and this can result in **clogging the blood vessels that lead to the lungs, liver, kidneys, or brain. This can cause infection or even death of small patches of cells in vital organs.**

3. Heroin affects unborn children: It is important to remember that **heroin will also affect a fetus.** Heroin use can result in **spontaneous abortion** as well. **Low birth rate** among children that do survive prenatal heroin exposure is common, and this can cause **developmental problems.**

Heroin substance abuse results in very real problems. The Drug Abuse Warning Network found that **eight percent of emergency room visits that are drug related are a result of heroin use.** Another **four percent of drug related emergency room visits were the result of "unspecified" opiates - some of which could include heroin.** It is vital to recognize the danger that heroin substance abuse can expose the user to.

As higher doses are used over time, physical dependence and addiction develop. With physical dependence, the body has adapted to the presence of the drug and **withdrawal symptoms occur if use is reduced or stopped.**

Withdrawal, which in regular abusers may occur as early as a few hours after the last administration, produces **drug craving, restlessness, muscle and bone pain, insomnia, diarrhea and vomiting, cold flashes with goose bumps, kicking movements,** and other symptoms. Major withdrawal symptoms peak between 48 and 72 hours after the last does and subside after about a week. Sudden withdrawal by heavily dependent users who are in poor health can be fatal.

METHAMPHETAMINE
(Crystal Meth)

Methamphetamine, also known as "speed," "crank," "crystal," or "ice" is a powerful central nervous system stimulant. It can be snorted, smoked, injected, or ingested by mouth. The color and texture of meth can vary; most commonly it is usually white or slightly yellow in a crystal-like powder or rock-like chunks. Street names, or slang terms, for methamphetamine are speed, ice, chalk, meth, crystal, fire, or glass.

Meth is used in various age groups, lifestyles, and neighborhoods. Users range from curious teens, college students attracted by the drug's reputation for increasing energy and sexuality, truck drivers, shift workers who use the drug to keep alert for extended periods of time, and girls and women who view it as a way to lose weight.

Quickly becoming the drug of choice in the USA, **meth is a deadly drug that is highly addictive** and detrimental to the human central nervous system. Its stimulant properties can cause **serious brain damage** in passive smokers and inhalers of the drug as well.

A horrible nightmare—While evaluating an outpatient and residential treatment program in northern California, Karol Kumpfer, now director of the U.S. Center for Substance Abuse Prevention in Washington, D.C., found herself staring at young women "who looked like they had come from Auschwitz." Their faces were pale and haggard, their eyes shrunken into their sockets. Much of their hair had fallen out. She was looking at the effects of methamphetamine.

Treatment guidelines issued this year, by the *U.S. Center for Substance Abuse Treatment,* say "some of the most frightening research findings about meth suggest that its prolonged use not only modifies behaviors but **literally changes the brain** in fundamental and long-lasting ways." In layman's language, **meth rewires the brain; and, while recovery may be possible, the brain will not be the same.**

Dr. Daniel Amen, a clinical neuroscientist who specializes in nuclear brain imaging in northern California, **ranks meth's addictive qualities second only to**

HARMFUL

heroin's. But he says **it's far more dangerous to users, and the people around them, because of the paranoia and psychosis that inevitably follow**. "Our scans basically show that the use of meth has caused these people to have **defective brains**," Amen said.

In Bellingham, Washington, Dr. Greg Hipskind discovered that **meth decreases the flow of blood to the brain and causes people to live in a perpetual daze**.

For a short time, it can help people lose weight and appear more attractive. But soon the situation changes. It can cause people to **lose so much weight, that they become emaciated**. One woman of average height, dropped to 80 pounds while she was pregnant. High-intensity users can shed 50 to 100 pounds.

Addicts become **prematurely aged**. Their **skin looks horrible** and their **internal organs are in terrible shape**.

Meth use also produces **severe sleep losses**. Dr. Alex Stalcup, an addiction physician in Concord, California, regularly treats people who have gone without sleep for as long as 10 days. The record holder was a woman with 21 days of no sleep. "Politely put, she was crazier than a barn owl," he says.

For a short time, the use of meth can produce strong sexual experiences. That is why it is so popular at "raves" in nightclubs and in gay bathhouses.

But eventually the drug **inhibits sexual functioning** in both sexes. The consequences, cited in the guidelines from the *Center for Substance Abuse Treatment*, include **men developing breasts, losing interest in sex, and experiencing impotence** and **women developing menstrual problems, infertility, and difficulty achieving orgasm**.

For a short time, meth gives one extra energy and a sense of being able to accomplish a lot. But soon he begins to crash. He begins producing **behavior that is persistent, repetitive, and compulsive**. Federal treatment guidelines describe the following activities as very typical of meth use: "vacuuming the same part of the floor over and over, repeatedly popping knuckles, picking at scabs, or taking apart and reassembling mechanical devices." **A lot of mindless activity that is useless**.

Experts believe **people between ages 18 to 25 are the most likely to use meth; and women account for 45 percent of addicts** seeking treatment—more than for any other drug. That is largely because women have reported to using meth to help lose weight while maintaining high energy levels.

Instead, it has **made users' teeth and hair fall out**. Meth "is as bad, or worse, than most of those drugs for most of those people who have encountered it. **It makes them the walking dead**," John P. Walters, director of the *White House Office of National Drug Control Policy*, said.

A former meth user, in Pacific Beach, California, said, "It's like selling your soul to the devil. When I was high, I felt alive for the first time in my life. While I was using it, I thought nothing could touch me. I was beautiful and perfect in my meth world. In the real world, my body was rotting from the inside out."

How does meth work?—Meth tells the brain's pleasure center to release more dopamine and endorphins, two natural chemicals that make people feel good. They cause people to feel more confident, lose weight, work quicker at a myriad of tasks, and enjoy sex more.

For the first few days on meth, the user will feel absolutely wonderful. But **very quickly, he finds he must keep taking more and more to feel good**. (Overdosing is called "amping.")

After six months of use, 94 percent of those who smoke meth become addicted, as do 72 percent who snort it.

The person continues to chase—but can never recapture—the intensity of the initial euphoric sensation of the first day. Over three to 15 days, he will help himself to more and more meth, as **he begins feeling more and more worthless when without it**.

Dosing more and more heavily, soon the user begins experiencing "tweakings." This is **intense anger, aggression and paranoia** (a type of insanity) during this tweaking stage, which can persist 24 hours. (Afterward, the body must collapse, so the user sleeps for one to three days.)

The only thing more dangerous than a tweaker is a tweaker when around others, notably those who are weaker. Tweakers, with extreme sleep deprivation, need no provocation to lash out. **Terrible domestic violence often follows**.

In his San Diego emergency room, Dr. J.R. Sise repairs the handiwork of tweakers far too often. He has stitched together the heart of a woman who was stabbed by the meth dealer who stole her money. He removed a blood clot from the gangrenous leg of a young binger. He told a woman her daughter died of a gunshot wound, suffered during an argument with her meth-using boyfriend.

When they hear of abnormally violent acts, the first thought of police and emergency responders is meth. Two years ago an Arizona man repeatedly stabbed his 14-year-old son, then decapitated him and threw his head out the window of a van. The man, now serving a 30-year sentence, had gone into a combination of temporary insanity and rage from meth—and was convinced that the devil was inside the van.

Meth abusers die at higher rates from suicide, traffic accidents and murder, and commonly drop dead from overdoses or malnutrition.

More facts about Meth—

Magic Johnson, the retired basketball player who is conducting a national campaign against meth, says that 51% of those involved with meth are blacks. According to a study at the *Centers for Disease Control & Prevention*, **of all the gay men in America, 15%-17% of them used meth** in the three months prior to August 2005; and **up to 20% have used it in the preceding year. Illegal immigrants and migrant workers are another major category of meth users.**

Barry R. McCaffrey, Former Drug Czar, said, "Methamphetamine has "exploded" from a West Coast bikers' drug into America's heartland and could replace cocaine as the nation's primary drug threat." **At the present time, meth has become the second most-used street drug in America. It is also invading European nations.**

In the short term, meth causes **mind and mood changes such as anxiety, euphoria, and depression**. But the user tends to keep taking it—and long-term effects begin. They include **chronic fatigue, paranoid or delusional thinking, and permanent brain damage**.

Producing a false sense of energy, the drug pushes the body faster and further than it is meant to go. Methamphetamine use not only causes addiction, psychotic behavior, and brain damage,—but it also **increases a person's heart rate and blood pressure, thereby increasing the risk of stroke**. An overdose of meth can also result in **heart failure**. Its long-term physical effects—such as **liver, kidney, and lung damage**—can be fatal.

Meth use can cause **heart palpitations, nausea, damage to blood vessels in the brain, shortness of breath, mental confusion, malnutrition, anorexia, severe anxiety, and depression**. A more severe manifestation of chronic toxicity is a state of **paranoia** closely resembling paranoid schizophrenia.

Users can also exhibit **psychotic behavior—including auditory hallucinations, mood disturbances, delusions, and paranoia**—possibly resulting in homicidal or suicidal thoughts.

New research shows that those who use methamphetamine risk **long-term damage to their brain cells similar to that caused by strokes, epilepsy, or Alzheimer's disease**. Even very short-term use of meth produces damage to the brain that is detectable months after the use of it is stopped. It can produce **irreversible damage to blood vessels in the brain**.

Psychological symptoms of prolonged meth use are characterized by **paranoia, hallucinations, repetitive behavior patterns, and delusions of parasites or insects under the skin**. Users often obsessively scratch their skin, to get rid of imagined insects. Meth addicts often have scabs and scratch marks on their faces and arms, from "picking" and scratching at imaginary "bugs."

The "high" effects of methamphetamine can last 6 to 8 hours. After the initial 'rush,' however, there is typically a state of **intense agitation that can lead to violent behavior**. Users coming down from a meth high or who are trying to abstain from continued use may suffer **withdrawal symptoms that include depression, anxiety, fatigue, paranoia, aggression, and intense cravings for more meth**.

Meth users tend to quickly develop a tolerance, causing them to need to take even larger amounts to get high. This leads to longer binges. **Some users avoid sleep for 3 to 15 days** while binging.

When using methamphetamine, the user feels energetic and powerful; but a "crash" inevitably follows the "high." In order to avoid or counteract the crash, the user takes more meth. Tolerance develops rapidly, often leading to addiction in a relatively short time.

Meth injectors who share syringes and "works" (spoon, cotton, rinse water, etc.) **have an increased risk of HIV and viral Hepatitis infections**.

Meth use in combination with another drug—such as alcohol, heroin, or cocaine—can be fatal. Between 1993 and 1995, deaths due to meth rose 125 percent nationally. Between 1996 and 1997, meth-related emergency room visits doubled. Users who inject meth and share needles risk exposing themselves to the **AIDS virus** and passing it to others.

Use by 12- to 17-year-olds has increased dramatically in the past few years. Meth use has been closely linked to **teen suicide**.

Dangerous manufacturing process—In addition to the dangers of methamphetamine abuse, the manufacturing process presents its own hazards. The production of methamphetamine **requires the use of hazardous chemicals. Many of these chemicals are corrosive or flammable. The vapors that are created in the chemical reaction attack mucous membranes, skin, eyes, and the respiratory tract**. Some chemicals react dangerously with water; and **some can cause fire or explosion**.

The chemicals used to cook meth (and the toxic compounds and by-products resulting from its manufacture) produce **toxic fumes, vapors, and spills**. A child living at a meth lab may inhale or swallow toxic substances or inhale the secondhand smoke of adults who are using meth. Exposure to low levels of some meth ingredients may produce **headache, nausea, dizziness, and fatigue**. Exposure to high levels can produce **shortness of breath, coughing, chest pain, dizziness, lack of coordination, eye and tissue irritation, chemical burns (to the skin, eyes, mouth, and nose), and death**. Corrosive substances may cause **injury through inhalation or contact with the skin**.

Normal cleaning will not remove methamphetamine and some of the chemicals used to produce it. They may remain on eating and cooking utensils, floors, countertops, and absorbent materials. Toxic byproducts of meth manufacturing are often improperly disposed of outdoors. These endanger children and others who live, eat, play, or walk near the site.

Approximately 15% of meth labs are discovered as a result of a fire or explosion. Careless handling and overheating of highly volatile hazardous chemicals and waste and unsafe manufacturing methods cause solvents and other materials to burst into flames or explode. Improperly labeled and incompatible chemicals are often stored together, compounding the likelihood of fire and explosion. Highly combustible materials left on stove tops, near ignition sources, or on surfaces accessible to children can be easily ignited by a single spark or cigarette ember. Hydrogenerators, used in il-

H
A
R
M
F
U
L

legal drug production, "constitute bombs waiting to be ignited by a careless act." Safety equipment is typically nonexistent or inadequate to protect a child.

Meth dealers and "cookers" typically have guns or other weapons, including booby traps, to protect their operation. The chemical imbalances in the user's brain, and the sleep deprivation associated with chronic meth use, can result in hallucinations and extreme paranoia which may cause the user to act out in bizarre, violent ways.

Children are often found living in environments where meth is being manufactured or sold. In San Diego's North County alone, an average of seven children a month are removed from meth environments.

For each pound of finished methamphetamine, seven pounds of highly toxic waste is produced. Ingredients include substances which **can cause chemical burns or can easily ignite**. Fumes generated during the manufacturing process can **contaminate porous surfaces such as walls, carpets, and countertops**. Cleanup of labs is dangerous and very expensive. The only lab sites that get cleaned up are the ones that are found.

This waste includes **corrosive liquids, acid vapors, heavy metals, solvents, and other harmful materials** that can cause **disfigurement or death** when contact is made with skin or breathed into the lungs. Lab operators almost always dump this waste illegally, in ways that severely damage the environment. National parks and other preserved sites have been adversely affected.

(Sources of the above data: U.S. Drug Enforcement Agency, California Office of Criminal Justice, Newsletter of the Federal Courts, Drug Rehabilitation Center, and San Diego County)

The meth-HIV-VD connection—With an estimated 35 million users, methamphetamine is the second most popular illegal substance in the world. Here in the United States, the epidemic grew in the last few years, moving eastward, from Hawaii to the West Coast, through the Midwest, and is now putting down roots in Philadelphia, Washington, Atlanta, Miami, and New York *(Ana Oliveira, Executive Director of Gay Men's Health Crisis [GMHC], 2003).*

The Centers for Disease Control and Prevention (CDC), in collaboration with the San Francisco Department of Public Health, concludes that **men using crystal meth were more likely than nonusers to be infected with HIV or other STDs**. Compared to nonusers, **crystal meth users were more than twice as likely to be HIV infected, 1.7 times more likely to test positive for gonorrhea, 1.9 times more likely to test positive for chlamydia, and 4.9 times more likely to be diagnosed with syphilis**. Crystal meth users also reported an average of four sexual partners over the four-week period prior to a clinic visit, compared to two partners reported by nonusers. This study suggests that **meth use plays an important role in the transmission of HIV and STDs**.

According to an August 2005 study at the *Centers for Disease Control & Prevention*, **of all the gay men in America, 15%-17% of them used meth (methamphetamine) in the preceding three months**. Up to 20% have used it in the preceding year.

A recent study of 19,000 men in Los Angeles showed that **new HIV infections were three times higher among methamphetamine users** than among nonusers.

A substantial body of data now confirms that sexual risk behaviors among gay and bisexual men have significantly increased over the last several years, in part due to the sexual disinhibitions associated with crystal use. In New York City, **syphilis rates have doubled in the last three years, with men who have sex with men**. This accounts for virtually all of the increase in cases. Investigation by city health authorities indicate that a syphilis diagnosis is strongly associated with crystal use; HIV seropositivity; and having sex in a bathhouse, at a sex party, or via an Internet connection.

Researchers found that **methamphetamine users with advanced HIV infection had evidence of a specific type of brain damage** not usually seen in HIV-infected patients with HAD: the loss of a specific group of neurons (nerve cells) and an increase in the number of glial cells (cells that repair damaged neurons) *(Journal of Acquired Immune Deficiency Syndrome*, 2003).

Seizures of clandestine meth labs in the Midwest increased tenfold from 1995 to 1997.

Additional data collected by the Center for HIV/AIDS Education Studies and Training (CHEST) at New York University indicate that, in New York City, among gay or bisexual male party/club drug users, approximately **62% of the participants indicated significant and frequent use of crystal meth**. This is an increase from the early 1990s, when usage rates among gay and bisexual men ranged between 5% and 25%. CHEST also found that MSM who reported crystal meth use were diverse in terms of ethnicity, age, income, and HIV status; **45% of the samples were men of color. In terms of HIV status, half the men using crystal meth reported being HIV positive** *(Meth Report, National Coalition of STD Directors, November 2004).*

Warning signs that it is being used—
1. *People are using it:* Hyperactivity, wakefulness, loss of appetite, incessant talking, extreme moodiness and irritability, repetitive behaviors such as picking at skin or pulling out hair, false sense of confidence and power, aggressive or violent behavior, and loss of interest in previously enjoyed activities. As effects of the drug wane, the user may sleep for extended periods (24-48 hours or more) and exhibit prolonged sluggishness and severe depression. **The paraphernalia of meth use may be observed: syringes, razor blades, drinking straws cut down to 3"-4," small zipper-closure plastic bags, and small glass pipes.**

2 - *Dealers:* Signs of meth dealing include lots of

traffic. **People coming and going at unusual hours, especially at night. Residences with windows blacked out**. Large amounts of cash, for example renters who pay their landlords in cash.

3. *Manufacturing sites:* At a location where methamphetamine is being made, **there are signs of use, dealing, and smells of strong odors (often described as smelling like cat urine). There are also large amounts of trash, canisters of denatured alcohol, camping fuel, muriatic acid, and/or lye, multiple packages of over-the-counter medications containing pseudoephedrine** (most often cold/allergy tablets or diet aids), **coffee filters stained red** (from red phosphorus used to accelerate the manufacturing process), rock salt, plastic tubing, glass jars, flasks, and cookware. Most of these items have legitimate household uses; but the typical consumer will not possess ten cans of camping fuel or 20 packages of cold medication.

HYDROCODONE

Hydrocodone is antitussive; that is, it is sold as a cough suppressant. This is a prescription drug for mild to severe pain that has been abused for its neurotic qualities. It is one of the most popular cough suppressants and is equally **as powerful in pain neutralizering as morphine**.

Signs of Hydrocodone overdose—include **dizziness, slower respiration, cool and damp skin, diminished muscular strength, confusion, smaller pupils, physical fatigue, nausea and diaphoresis, and in a few cases, coma.** Ahydrocodone overdose can cause **death**.

Many medical experts believe dependence or addiction can happen between 1-4 weeks at higher doses of Hydrocodone, depending on an individuals tolerance to it. Reports in medical journals of high profile movie stars, TV personalities and professional athletes who are recovering from Hydrocodone addiction provide evidence of its harmful effects.

OXYCONTIN

OxyContin® is actually a prescription drug that in some countries can be found over the counter (OTC). **It is a painkiller prescribed for moderate and acute pain relief** caused by physical injuries, arthritis, back pains, and pain felt during cancer treatments.

OxyContin contains the narcotic drug oxycodone. OxyContin, manufactured by Purdue Pharma, has a time-release mechanism meant to prevent overdoses, but crushing or dissolving the pill can release the entire dose at one time and produce an overdose. Mixing OxyContin with alcohol can also result in an overdose.

Overdoses can cause death, coma, and brain damage, often brought on by respiratory failure. The symptoms can begin soon after the drug is taken.
Symptoms of OxyContin overdose include:
Slowed breathing. Unconsciousness. Dizziness. Weakness. Contracted pupils. Confusion. Clammy or cold skin. Seizure. Coma.

Oxycodone, the active ingredient of OxyContin, is a highly addictive drug, similar to morphine. It is classified as a Schedule II controlled substance by the DEA (Drug Enforcement Agency). **Addiction can occur after only 5 to 7 days of use. Symptoms of OxyContin withdrawal are the same as any withdrawal from narcotic addiction.** These symptoms can begin within hours of the last use **and last up to 1 week!**
The symptoms include:
• **Nausea and diarrhea. Intense body pain. Abdominal cramping. Tremors. Muscle cramps and spasms. Chills. Running nose and eyes. Heavy sweating. Insomnia. Anxiety. Paranoia. Depression**
Other less serious side effects of OxyContin include:
• **Altered mental states. Confusion. Light headedness. Constipation. Dry mouth**.

If you or a family member has suffered side effects from OxyContin, you may be able to recover damages from the drug firm that manufacturers it. Your first step in doing that is to have your case evaluated by a qualified attorney.

INHALANTS

This is not just any one drug but **a combination of volatile solvents, nitrates, and gases**. The inhalants are sniffed, snorted and inhaled to acquire a drunk feeling much like that of alcohol. The most popular inhalants are glue, cigarette lighter fluid, household cleaning fluids, and painting products. This is the most popular drug for minors to abuse as it is normally found around the home and access is free.

What are the most serious short-term effects of inhalants?—Deep breathing of the vapors, or using a lot over a short period of time may result in **losing touch with one's surroundings, a loss of self-control, violent behavior, unconsciousness, or death**. Using inhalants can cause **nausea and vomiting**. If a person is unconscious when vomiting occurs, death can result from aspiration.

Sniffing highly concentrated amounts of solvents or aerosol sprays can produce **heart failure and instant death**. Sniffing can cause death the first time or at any later time. High concentrations of inhalants cause **death from suffocation** by displacing the oxygen in the lungs. Inhalants **can also cause death by depressing the central nervous system so much that breathing slows down until it stops**.

Death from inhalants is usually caused by a very high concentration of inhalant fumes. Deliberately inhaling from a paper bag greatly increases the chance of suffocation. Even when using aerosol or volatile (vaporous) products for their legitimate purposes, i.e, painting, cleaning, etc., it is wise to do so in a well-ventilated room or outdoors.

What are the long-term dangers?—Long-term use can cause **weight loss, fatigue, electrolyte (salt)**

imbalance, and muscle fatigue. Repeated sniffing of concentrated vapors over a number of years can cause **permanent damage to the nervous system**, which means **greatly reduced physical and mental capabilities**. In addition, long-term sniffing of certain inhalants can damage the **liver, kidneys, blood, and bone marrow**.

Tolerance, which means the sniffer needs more and more each time to get the same effect, is likely to develop from most inhalants when they are used regularly.

What happens when inhalants are used along with other drugs?—As in all drug use, taking more than one drug at a time multiplies the risks. **Using inhalants while taking other drugs that slow down the body's functions, such as tranquilizers, sleeping pills, or alcohol, increases the risk of death** from overdose. Loss of consciousness, coma, or death can result. Source: *National Institute on Drug Abuse, 1986*

MDMA (Ecstasy)

MDMA is a terrible drug that is synthetic and psychoactive dedicated to creating a hallucinogenic fervor. Acting as a stimuli and psychedelic, Ecstasy creates an energy effect and creates distortions in reality, time and perception of the taker and ultimately creates a seemingly joyful experience.

Horrible mental effects—In addition to several other harmful ones, three dangerous reactions are these: **serotonin syndrome, stimulant psychosis, and/or hypertensive crisis**.

The symptoms can include the following:
• Psychological disorientation and/or confusion **Anxiety, paranoia, and/or panic attacks**.
• Hypervigilance or increased sensitivity to **hypomania or full-blown mania**.
• Depersonalization. **Hallucinations and/or delusions**. Thought disorder or disorganized thinking.
• **Cognitive and memory impairment** potentially to the point of retrograde or anterograde **amnesia**.
• **Acute delirium and/or insanity**.
Horrible physical effects—
• Myoclonus or **involuntary and intense muscle twitching**. Hyperreflexia or over responsive or **overreactive reflexes**. Tachypnea or **rapid breathing** and/or dyspnea or **shortness of breath**.
• **Palpitations** or abnormal awareness of the beating of the heart. Angina pectoris or **severe chest pain**, as well as **pulmonary hypertension** (PH).
• Cardiac arrhythmia or **abnormal electical activity of the heart**. Circulatory shock or cardiogenic shock
• Vasculitis or **destruction of blood vessels** Cardiotoxicity or **damage to the heart**. **Cardiac arrest**, myocardial infarction or **heart attack**, and/or **heart failure**. **Hemorrhage and/or stroke**. Severe **hyperthermia**, potentially resulting in **organ failure**.
Miscellaneous effects—
• Syncope or **fainting** or loss of consciousness. Seizures or **convulsions**. Organ failure (as mentioned

above). Severe neurotoxicity or **brain damage. Coma and/or death**.
• Potential incarceration, hospitalization, institutionalization, and/or death, on account of extreme erratic behavior which may include **acts of crime, accidental or intentional self-injury,** and/or suicide, as well as illicit drug abuse, may ensue under such circumstances.

ANABOLIC STEROIDS

These are laboratory produced variants of male hormone testosterone. They are used to promote muscle growth, however has some very damaging side effects such as **brain damage and heart attacks**.

Are Steroids Illegal?—Without a doctor's prescription for a medical condition, it is against the law to possess, sell, or distribute anabolic steroids.

Legal prosecution can be a serious side effect of illicit steroid use. Under federal law, **first-time simple possession of anabolic steroids carries a maximum penalty of one year in prison** and a $1,000 fine. For first-offense trafficking in steroids, the maximum penalty is five years in prison and a fine of $250,000. Second offenses double this penalty. In addition to federal penalties, state laws also prohibit illegal anabolic steroid use.

Anabolic steroids are powerful hormones. They affect the entire body. Some of the side effects are common to all users. Other side effects are specifically related to your sex and age.

Men who take anabolic steroids may:
• **Develop breasts. Get painful erections. Have their testicles shrink. Have decreased sperm count. Become infertile. Become impotent.**
Women who take anabolic steroids may:
• **Grow excessive face and body hair. Have their voices deepen. Experience menstrual irregularities. Have an enlarged clitoris. Have reduced breast size. Have a masculinized female fetus.**
Both men and women who take anabolic steroids may:
• **Get acne. Have an oily scalp and skin. Get yellowing of the skin (jaundice). Become bald. Have tendon rupture. Have heart attacks. Have an enlarged heart. Develop significant risk of liver disease and liver cancer. Have high levels of "bad" cholesterol. Have mood swings. Fly into rages. Suffer delusions.**
Teens who take anabolic steroids may:
• **Have short height due to arrested bone growth. Girls may suffer long-term masculinization.**

Since steroids are often taken by injections, there is also the risk of getting **HIV or hepatitis infection** from an unsterile needle or syringe.

LSD

LSD is a lysergic acid compound that is a derivative of from ergot, a poisonous fungus that sometmes develops on rye grass.

There are two long-term effects of LSD: **persistent psychosis** and **hallucinogen persisting perception disorder** (HPPD), more commonly referred to as "flashbacks," have been associated with use of LSD. The causes of these effects, which in some users occur after a single experience with the drug, are not known.

Psychosis—The effects of LSD can be described as **drug-induced psychosis-distortion or disorganization of a person's capacity to recognize reality, think rationally, or communicate with others.** Some LSD users experience **devastating psychological effects that persist after the trip has ended, producing a long-lasting psychotic-like state.** LSD-induced persistent psychosis may include **dramatic mood swings from mania to profound depression, vivid visual disturbances, and hallucinations.** These effects may last for years and can affect people who have no history or other symptoms of psychological disorder.

Hallucinogen Persisting Perception Disorder (HPPD)—Some former LSD users report experiences known colloquially as **"flashbacks"** and called "HPPD" by physicians. **These episodes are spontaneous, repeated, sometimes continuous recurrences** of some of the sensory distortions originally produced by LSD.

The experience may include **hallucinations**, but it most commonly consists of **visual disturbances** such as **seeing false motion on the edges of the field of vision, bright or colored flashes, and halos or trails attached to moving objects.** This condition is typically persistent and in some cases remains unchanged for years after individuals have stopped using the drug.

No Known Treatment—Because HPPD symptoms may be mistaken for those of other neurological disorders such as stroke or brain tumors, sufferers may consult a variety of clinicians before the disorder is accurately diagnosed. There is no established treatment for HPPD, although some antidepressant drugs may reduce the symptoms.

19 – Other Food Ingredient Sources

Aluminium—implicated in the development of **Alzheimer's disease**, higher levels than normal have been observed in the brains of sufferers. Large amounts of aluminium are known to cause **muscle and bone pain and weakness**, as well as **placental weakness**. It is believed that aluminium cookware contributes to overdose. Aluminium is used as **an anti-caking agent in white flour, salt and dried milk substitutes**. Also **in eye makeup moisturisers, face powders and anitperspirants**.

Aspirin—used as a pain killer and blood-thinner for people susceptible to blood clots, initially derived from the bark of a willow-tree, now synthetically produced from salicylic acid. It causes **bleeding from the stomach**.

Benzoic acid—used in mouthwashes and deodorants, as a food preservative and in medicines, contained in **coal tar and resins**, as benzoin. May be derived from vertebrates. Also added to soft drinks, processed juice and cordial. Sensitivity can provoke **asthma and stomach pains**.

Clothes powders—may contain phosphorus (common pollutant of waterways), ammonia, naphthalene or phenol. Sodium nitrilotriacetate (NAT) is commonly used in clothes detergents, recognized by the U.S. *National Cancer Institute* as **carcinogenic** 12, 17

Contraceptives—Responsibility for contraception has largely been left to women and it is women who must decide what is to happen to their bodies. Breast feeding has long been an effective way of spacing pregnancies, though few women continue it long enough to be effective. For couples who plan to have no more children, sterilization is an effective method, and certainly an excellent economical form of population control. Modern chemical contraceptives (the pill) have many unwanted side-effects on health including **migraine, increased risk of cancer of the cervix, liver and breast, gall-bladder disease, thrush, blood clots, strokes, diabetes, fluid retention, skin disorders, depression and heart disease.** In addition to this, **most contain animal products** and have been tested on them. **IUD's are not 100% effective and work by causing abortion and may damage a foetus through copper poisoning even six months after it has been removed.** In an age where sexually transmitted diseases like AIDS and Hepatitis can be fatal, abstinence is becoming increasing expedient. Condoms offer protection from impregnation, and often from transmission of disease.

Cortisone—hormone **from cattle**, used in medical creams.

Creams (skin)—many skin creams and sunscreens contain **animals products**. The ingredients to look out for include: *stearates* derived **from beef fat** (stearic acid and anything with the prefix stear-, although not all are derived from animals it is hard to know unless specified on the label), lanolin, beeswax, casein (derived from milk), honey, eggs or albumin, allatoin, reticulin, keratin, arachidonic acid, benzoic acid (may be derived from vertebrates, though can be found in berries), cholesterol, L-cysteine, lecithin (may be derived from eggs), myristic acid (also called Isopropyl Myristate, Myristyls, Oleyl Myristate, Myristal Ether Sulfate), oleic acid, palmitic acid, squalene (**derived from sharks**), tallow (**from pigs**), Cetyl Palmitate (**derived from whales**).

The following companies produce skin creams that are definitely VEGAN : Aquarius, Dial, Evoke, In Essence, Nature's Remedy, The Good Oil.

Deodorants—may contain **aluminium** (reputed to be in a form not readily absorbed by the body and

HARMFUL

therefore safe), **ammonia, formaldehyde (carcinogenic)**, and/or ethanol. Varieties that contain tea-tree oil (a powerful antiseptic) are available.

Dioxins—**chlorinated compounds**, known to cause **cancer, developmental and reproductive problems**. There is no safe dose, cancer being produced in laboratory animals even at very low doses. It accumulates in the body, increasing risk with longer exposure and age. "2,3,7,8-TCDD" is **one of the most toxic substances known**. Dioxins are produced as **a by product of chlorine based chemicals** in their manufacture, use and disposal. A major source of dioxin production is rubbish burning which releases dioxins into the air where they are easily ingested by people. Dioxins **may also be present in drinking water and food**. The BHP Steelworks at Port Kembla and Newcastle account for 90% of total dioxin emissions for the whole of NSW, Australia.

Estrogen—often derived **from cow ovaries**, but also found in significant amounts in soy milk. Estrogen is used in contraceptive pills and skin creams (though there is no proof of their benefits in creams), large doses can be **harmful to children**. Those estrogen sensitive may need to avoid soy products.

Ethanol—Undenatured **alcohol**. Not permitted as a food additive in Australia, however ethanol is used **in mouthwashes** as well as **hairspray** and **perfumes**. Also used in **cough elixirs**.

Fish—Industrial dumping and runoff in the many parts of the world has rendered major bays and harbours toxic with **lead, cadmium, chromium and mercury** as well as high levels of **aromatic hydrocarbons**, known **carcinogens**. With many fish harvested from these areas, little wonder there is concern for humans. **Mercury poisoning** from fish and other sea creatures in Japan in 1950s led to an epidemic know as **Minamata disease**, where **mercury accumulated in the brains of the victims** causing irreparable damage to the central nervous system.

Overfishing by wasteful industrial fishing concerns has rendered stocks low in all the oceans of the world, endangering the livelihood of small-time survival fishermen, mostly in the third world. 27 million tons (one quarter of the total catch) is thrown back, mostly already dead. The world's fishing fleet has increased twice as fast as the total catch since 1970, more than three and a half million fishing vessels. A decrease in the population of birds, turtles and sharks is the obvious corollary to irresponsible large-scale commercial fishing, who rely on fish as a principal food source, or are accidentally killed in fish nets. Greenpeace estimate that millions of dolphins have been killed by Tuna seine nets, and thousands of albatrosses are killed by Tuna longliners.

Fluorine (and Fluoride)—a **poisonous gas** that occurs only in compound with other elements. It is used in small amounts **to purify water and decrease tooth decay**. The fluoride ion, in combination with other chemicals is the basis of many **psychoactive** drugs, such as Rohypnol and Prozac. The **nerve gas Sarin**, used in the 1995 Tokyo subway poisonings, is also a fluoride mixture. The effect of these drugs is to **inhibit enzyme production in the brain**, the mildest and most common of the side effects being memory loss.

As early as 1944 the US government was aware that fluoride caused **confusion, drowsiness and listlessness**, as enlisted men were exposed to it reputedly at an atomic weapons base. In 1995, Dr Phyllis Mullenix, a toxicologist at the Children's Hospital in Boston, published a study (and there are others) that came to the conclusion that the most likely effects of long term fluoride exposure was "**motor-sensory dysfunction, IQ deficits and/or learning disabilities**." Another researcher (Issacson, 1992) found that, in combination with aluminium (sometimes added as a water clarifier), there was the added risk of an increase in the incidence of **Alzheimer's disease**. The synergistic (in combination) effects with other contaminants already in the environment and our bodies (such as lead, mercury and chlorine) have not been measured, though the prognosis is not good, as **combinations with other metals in particularly seem to increase its derogatory effects**. Other studies have shown that fluoride, administered for the treatment of osteoporosis, can actually **weaken and decrease bone mass**, though these results are controversial. It has also been implicated as a mutagen, "**producing chromosome aberrations and gene mutations** in cultured mammalian cells." (Zeiger, Shelby & Witt: 1993, National Institute of Environmental Health Sciences, Carolina)

Fluoride has been proven by the American Dental Association, no less, to be responsible for **fluoridosis** in children and has be the cause of a spate of compensation claims paid out by Colgate in the UK, one claim resulted in a payment of ú1000 to the parents of a child whose **teeth were damaged** by their product.

Food Poisoning—It has been estimated that **meat eaters have an 80% greater chance of suffering a bout of food poisoning** than their vegetarian contemporaries. This is partly the result of more people buying take-away foods, and unscrupulous vendors trying to make their products last longer. **Salmonella** is common in livestock given prolonged doses of antibiotics, especially in factory farming situations, effecting chickens and their eggs, as well as pigs. Cooking destroys salmonella, but recontamination may occur from utensils. Salmonella was responsible for the 1996 peanut butter poisoning scare, it is thought that the bacteria may have come from rat faeces. **Poisoning can also occur where heavy metals have built up in the flesh of animals, such as mercury and cadmium in fish.**

Botulism is caused by **bacteria that may grow in preserved vegetables and fruit which have not been adequately sterilized**. Alkaline foods are more acceptable to the bacteria, so adding citrus juice to preserves helps eliminate the spores. Other vegetable poisoning risks are **green potatoes**, containing **solanine** which is not destroyed by cooking, see also alkaloids and caffeine.

Formaldehyde—Used to make 'staypress' fabrics, as an adhesive used to bond particle board. The US EPA estimated in 1987 that almost 5,000 workers would contract **cancer** as a direct result of exposure to formaldehyde. Formaldehyde causes **mucus membrane irritation, headaches, depression, memory loss and dizziness, and ultimately cancer**. Fumes may leak out from the resin for years after use. Formaldehyde is contained in many household products including **shampoos, deodorants, detergents and mouthwashes**.

Fungicides—Some wood preservative fungicides contain **organochlorines, tributyltin oxide or dioxin**, all are poisonous. Wood treated with these fungicides emits **toxic gas** for years after application and are implicated in causing **leukemia and asthma**.

Hair products—Like cosmetics, many commercially available hair products contain animal products. Herbal rinses for the hair are easily prepared in the home and are both ethical and economical. See Shampoo.

Heavy Metals—including **mercury, cadmium, chromium, lead and arsenic** to name a few, all are associated with poisoning animals and humans

Hormones—**Estrogen, progesterone, testosterone**; all are of animal origin

Hydrolized animal protein—used in **cosmetics, and shampoo**. Soy and vegetable proteins can be substituted.

Lactic acid—derived **from blood, muscle, milk**, and used **in skin fresheners** and as **plasticiser** and **food preservative**.

Lanolin—(lanosterol, lanoinamide DEA, wool fat, wool wax) a **moisturising agent** derived from sheep wool, often after the animal has been slaughtered and skinned, lanolin may contain **pesticide residues** from sheep dipping, and can cause **allergic reactions**. Used in **sunscreens, moisturisers, perfumes, pharmecueticals, hair products, dish detergents, baby products**.

"LD50"—The toxicity of many products is estimated by employment of the LD50 test, where animals (usually rats) are force fed a substance until 50 percent of the test population dies, having consumed a 'lethal dose'. Used in **toothpaste**.

Lard—This is rendered **pig fat**.

Lead—Lead may enter the body **inhaled from car exhaust**, consumed from **vegetables contaminated by exhaust**, or from **lead-based paint, lead water pipes, copper pipes soldered with lead**. It is proven to cause

infertility, sperm deformity, and lower intelligence in children. Some other sources of lead may include some **Indian eye liners** and **hair blackeners**. An item in the Courier Mail in June 1997 claimed that "**certain hair dyes contain so much lead that consumers, bathrooms, hair dryers, hands and dyed hair are contaminated**".

Margarine - **vegetable oils hydrogenated** to make them solid. This process convert oils into **saturated fats**. Sometimes milk or fish oils such as **cetyl palmitate or spermaceti (derived from whales and dolphins**) may be used. During processing, the oils are also degummed, bleached, hydrogenated, deodorized and combined with salt, color preservatives, flavor, emulsifiers and vitamins.

Marine Oil—This is fish oil, also used in **margarine** and **soap**.

Mercury—Exposure to high levels of mercury is proven to cause serious **fetal abnormalities**. Mercury may be present **in canned fish**, especially tuna fish, who are contaminated by factory effluent. Some **weedkillers and fungicides** contain mercury, so take care handling seeds dusted in fungicides. In Iraq 6,000 people were hospitalized and 500 died as a consequence of **eating bread made from flour made from grain treated with a mercurial fungicide. Dental amalgam** contains mercury. **Garlic has been found to help prevent mercury been absorbed by the body**. Phenylmercuric salts are used as a preservative in some eye medications and cosmetics. See also toxicity, fish, phenylmercuric salts.

Milk—like meat production, the animals concerned are often treated as commodities, **fed hormones and doused in pesticides**. In order for a cow's milk to be taken for human consumption, its young must suffer, first being taken from their mother prematurely.

Fully 5.5 million dairy cows from the United States are said to live under factory conditions. **Cattle are forced to eat sawdust, ammonia, feathers, toxic ink, processed sewage, poultry litter, grease, and plastic hay**. The female calves born to dairy cows are bred for milk production and the male calves are immediately processed for veal. The calves raised for veal are confined to small, dark, damp cells where **they are fed only iron-deficient gruel that they will become anemic so that their flesh will become tender**. Small calves may be chained by their necks for months at a time while milking machines are wheeled to them. The life expectancy of cattle raised for milk production is usually decreased by 15 years in factory farms. These cows are always pregnant and give three or more times the milk they would natually give. **Hormones are injected into the cows** causing their udders to swell and drag on the ground getting cut, bruised, and infected.

Milk products are often mixed with additives. These include peroxide and gelatine, milk is sometimes fortified with Vitamin D derived from fish oils.

Hormones and antibiotics are often present in dairy products because of these drugs are used on most farms. **Genetically engineered Bovine-Growth Hormone**, is supposed to increase milk production when injected into dairy cows. BGH is manufactured by the Monsanto Corp., was approved by the FDA despite potential human health problems associated with consuming milk from BGH cows: "the drug was approved without one single test examining its impact on humans ingesting products from animals treated with it." (Ronnie Cummins, national director of the Pure Food Campaign, a consumer advocacy group in the US).

Milk replacements—Soy drink is an excellent milk substitute. But **coffee whitening powders** usually contain hydrogenated palm oil, corn syrup and sodium caseinate -the latter is derived from milk.

Mink oil—derived from dead minks left over from fur production, **used in shampoos, conditioners and skin creams**.

Mineral oil—often called 'baby oil', or white mineral oil and found **in many cosmetics**, mineral oil is **petroleum derived liquid paraffin**. Paraffin is not easily absorbed by the skin.

Mineral salts—increase moisture retention, modify flavors. **Mineral oil is sometimes used to polish apples and cucumbers**, and **liver abnormalities** have been attributed to ingestion of it.

Moisturizers and facial creams—Many **commercial moisturizers** are made with **animals fats**, including **stearates** derived from beef fat, and **lanolin**. The more expensive brands are often in excessive packaging .

There are simple and cheap alternatives to hand, face and body moisturizers: sorbolene is inexpensive and available at chemists and supermarkets. Health food stores often sell unperfumed bases in bulk containers.

Home remedies are also effective: Lemon juice restores the skins acid mantle. Almond oil is an excellent moisturiser and suitable for use on baby's skin. Acne scrubs can be made from colloidal oatmeal and almond meal mixed 2:1 and added to soap when cleansing. Other facial scrubs can contain alfalfa, corn meal and/or carrot juice for acne, grated apple and almond oil for rough skin, cucumber and oatmeal for oily skins, or apple cider vinegar. Raw cucumber rubbed on the face helps reduce oiliness and is astringent and is soothing on sunburnt skin. see also cosmetics, shampoo, draize test.

Musk—extracted from the **genitals of musk deer, muskrats, civet and beavers** by a cruel and painful process. Used in **perfumery**, as a **flavouring**. Musk can be replaced with plant based labdanum oil.

Musk ambrette—is a synthetic product, containing **toluene (a known carcinogen)** although it is on the USFDA's GRAS list. It is used to **simulate blackberry flavor** in foods; as a fixative **in fragrances, dentifrices and deodorants**. Musk ambrette can cause **contact dermatitis**.

Myristic acid—Isopropyl myristate. Myristyl. etc. In most animal and vegetable fats, and **in butter acids**. Used in **shampoos, creams, cosmetics, food flavorings**.

Nappy sterilizers—some contain hypochlorite, which contributes to **organochlorin pollution**. *Instead use:* vinegar, bicarbonate soda, lemon juice or eucalyptus may be added to the rinse water, or use hot water and sunlight to help destroy bacteria and make nappies white.

Nitrosamines—compound formed in the stomach in the presence of amino acids, **especially from meat**. Known **carcinogen**. The consumption of Vitamin C with amino acids halts the reaction.

Organo-chlorines—organic compounds containing **chlorine**. Commonly used as **pesticides**, eg. **DDT, Chlordane and Aldrin**. See Pesticides.

Organo-phosphates—**pesticides**, see Roundup.

Ozone depletion—Thinning of the ozone layer allows more UV rays to penetrate the Earth's atmosphere. Increased exposure to UV is **harmful to plants and animals** alike and has been linked to increased levels of **skin cancers** in Australia. Could lead to global warming The notorious 'hole' located over Antarctica gets larger each year. Concern for the state of the ozone layer is becoming an important force in the choices made by consumers. This is the result of findings that indicate **CFCs and halons, (and some other chlorine-based chemicals) all commonly used in refrigeration and propellants**, are the primary cause of the thinning of the ozone layer. Depletion, combined with continuing use of **HFCs, fossil fuels, carbon dioxide and nitrous oxide emitting industries, and methane leaks** from gas pipelines are contributing to a world-wide increase in temperatures: the Greenhouse Effect. We cannot stop ozone depletion (although it can replenish itself given time), but we can reduce the amount of ozone depleting chemicals we emit into the atmosphere. Alternatives to the chlorine based chemicals responsible and proper disposal of those currently in use is vital. see also, Energy consumption

Packaging—see active packaging, plastic contamination, dioxins

Paints—derived primarily from petrochemicals, most paints are toxic in production, use and disposal. **Pentachlorphenol (PCP) was once a fungicide used in many paints**, banned in 1984 due to its links with **cancer**. **Paint strippers** are often made from **chlorinated hydrocarbons**, which are toxic at all levels and give off fumes in use. During the 19th and early 20th centuries, **lead was added to paint** to increase its durability. Lead is **known to reduce intelligence, attention, and hearing, irreversibly**. It continues to be a problem in old buildings where children eat peeling paint, or renovators inhale the dust created by sanding it. Lack of action on the part of authorities in the light of such knowledge has been described as 'environmental racism' in the US where the majority of poisoned children are black, hispanic, and/

or poor. Lead was banned in paints in 1982.

Paints are still made today containing **acrylonitrile and chromates** (suspected **carcinogens**), **glycol ether** as a solvent (causes **anemia and infertility**), **mercury as a fungicide, and formaldelhyde (a carcinogen** that may 'outgas' for up to 5 years after application).

Citric acid has proved a good alternative in paints, thinners and cleaning products for brushes. On the internet: EZicare makes a range of artist quality products using citric acid. Bio Products in Australia also produces a range of clean-up, solvents, and paints based on wood resins, plant oils, earth pigments and citrus. Some of their paints do contain casein (milk protein).

Palmitic acid—contrary to the name, not always derived from palm oil, Palmitic acid is **often mixed with stearates**, which are the major saturated fat found in meat, Stearates are 40% of the fat in palm oil. Used in **hair products** and **shaving preparations**.

Panthenol—also called Dexpanthenol, Provitamin B-5, Vitamin B-complex factor. Panthenol can be derived from plants, animals or synthetically produced. Used in **shampoos, emollients and foods**.

Parabens—(methyl-, ethyl-, propyl-, butyl-) synthetic agent used as a **preservative to prevent mould growth**. Used **in drugs** including Narcan, Xylocaine and topical creams; most often **in cosmetics, especially those labelled "hypoallergenic"**. In foods including **alcohol, bakery goods, cheese, oils, frozen dairy, gelatine, preserves, processed fruit and vegetable products, cordials and soft drinks, sugar substitutes and sauces**.

Parrafin—**Wax** that is **petroleum based**.

PCB's—Dioxins and PCBs are environmental contaminants which find their way **in very low concentrations into many food sources**. They are particularly found **in fatty foods like meat and milk**. They are now banned worldwide, but are very persistent and will remain in the environment for many years.

In 1929 the Monsanto Corporation started selling PCBs (polychlorinated biphenyls). PCBs are oily liquids that are very stable, even when they get hot, and they don't conduct electricity but they do conduct heat. Therefore, they make good **insulators in electrical transformers and capacitors**. They have also been used as **hydraulic fluid**, and **in metal finishing**. They are found **in electrical systems and other components of automobiles**. For a time, **carbonless carbon paper** was made with PCBs.

Then scientists in the 1970s studying damage to wildlife from DDT realized that there was something else causing the same problems as DDT, and soon they identified PCBs as the culprit. It turns out that PCBs **interfere with birds' reproductive systems just the way DDT does—they cause egg shells to become thin**, so the eggs get crushed when the mother sits on them, and they never hatch.

PCBs are **estrogenic in their effect on humans and animals** (see also Estrogenic effect of chemicals)

"Other evidence about hazards from PCBs came to light and in 1976 the US Congress banned PCB production. Nevertheless, Monsanto had already sold a lot of PCBs, there are 1.2 million tons (2.4 billion pounds) of PCBs loose somewhere in the world. Sixty-five percent of them are still in use in **electrical equipment** that will be getting old and ready for replacement during the '90s, or are in landfills. Twenty percent have already reached the oceans. Eleven percent are in terrestrial soils and sediments; 4% have been incinerated or otherwise degraded.

PCBs accumulate **in fatty tissues of living things** (birds, fish, people, etc.) and they readily pass through the walls of cells. PCBs can cause **cancer**, either alone or in combination with other chemicals. PCBs also cause **birth defects** in humans and animals. PCBs **damage the human immune system** (and probably the immune systems of other creatures as well). PCBs also cause **hypertension (high blood pressure)** and they cause **strokes** in humans. Women who ate fish from the Great Lakes mildly polluted with PCBs (at or below legal limits) bore **children with small heads** and who suffer from significant **learning and behavioral defects**.

Because PCBs can become airborne when they are released into the environment, they have spread everywhere on earth. Recent studies in sparsely populated areas of Canada have revealed that rainfall now carries 17 parts per trillion (ppt) of PCBs. As a matter of law, the Ontario government allows only 1 ppt of PCBs to be discharged into the environment, but it has been difficult to get a court injunction against rainfall.

By the year 2005, the average polar bear had 50 parts per million (ppm) PCBs in their fatty tissue (adipose tissue), so they now meet the EPA (U.S. Environmental Protection Agency) criteria for being classified as a hazardous waste. Some species of cetaceans (the whale family) already far exceed polar bears in PCB concentrations. Killer whales from the deep ocean have 410 ppm PCBs in their blubber, and blue-white dolphins off the coast of Europe have 833 ppm. Thus these creatures must definitely now be classified as hazardous wastes by EPA criteria. In the food chain, the concentration of animals at the top of an oceanic food chain (like whales) will have a concentration of PCBs in their bodies 10 million times greater than the concentration in plankton at the bottom of the chain. (This is called biomagnification or bioconcentration, and it is the reason why dilution is no solution to pollution.)

The next-to-last chapter in our unfolding story is that marine mammals (seals, porpoises, whales, etc.) have a **genetic predisposition to reproductive failure** caused by PCBs. PCBs act like hormones in marine mammals, **interfering with their ability to reproduce**. Joseph Cummins, Associate Professor of Genetics at University of Western Ontario, writing in the journal, The Ecologist, says that **if even as little as 15% more of the world's stock of PCBs gets into the oceans, "the extinction of marine mammals would be inevitable."** He adds, "The consequence of failing to control PCB releases to the oceans will be the extinction of marine mammals and **the**

H
A
R
M
F
U
L

chemical fouling of the ocean fisheries, rendering them unsuitable for use by humans." Dr. Cummins is concerned that the developing world hasn't the financial resources to control the PCBs now in use in its domain. He therefore suggests that Monsanto should purchase back all its PCBs from wherever they are located in the developing world, to avoid PCB-induced calamity for all the world's oceans in the coming decades.

For its part, Monsanto makes no apology for its behavior. It continues to operate very profitably, introducing new chemicals into use at every opportunity." (Rachel Environment and Health Weekly)

See also Pesticides, Roundup, Gene Technology, Milk

Pepsin—derived from **pig's stomachs**, used in **cheese making**. see Rennet

Petrolatum—also called yellow petroleum jelly, **petroleum jelly**, vaseline officinal. Derived from steam or vacuum distillation of petroleum. May contain aromatic hydrocarbons (see separate entry) known **carcinogens**. *There are four types of petrolatum:* natural (distilled from petroleum), artificial (created from natural solid hydrocarbons, such as paraffin wax and mineral oil), gatsch (derived from the by-products of lubricating oil and mixed with mineral oil), and synthetic petrolatum (made by ethylene polymerization). It is used **in foods, cosmetics** as a **hair conditioner**, and **drugs** as a **skin protectant and ointment base**. It is flammable, and may cause **acne**.

Polution by motor vehicles—Oil consumption by cars creates pollution that harms humans and the natural environment: **Smog particles** contribute to **respiratory illness**, especially the consumption of **lead enriched fuels** which is a known mutagen and teratogen, and contributes to **retarded intellectual development** of children. Smog causes **acid rain** which can kill off plant life and consequently causes fauna deaths. **Fumes and noise** can render some areas unpleasant, indeed dangerous, for pedestrians and animals alike. Traffic congestion magnifies the pollution aspects as well as increasing stress levels of drivers which may have serious social implications: for instance the increased incidence of 'road-rage' that sometimes leads to murders. Ultimately, **exhaust fumes** from cars are contributing in a big way to global warming.

Infrastructure to accommodate cars creates a vast tracts of bitumen, soil lost to roads and carparks, while using up a sizable portion of council budgets. Paving over of soil and loss of vegetation causes stormwater runoff problems, including increased pollution of creeks. With housing expansion, fertile farming land may be lost. Expanded suburbs reduce neighbourhood interaction, and preferred car use over walking rendered neighbours virtual strangers. Suburbs increase the isolation and alienation of the car-less and youth, for whom mass transit is not easily accessible in so called 'dormitory suburbs'.

Phenol—a member of the group of compounds called '**aromatic hydrocarbons**', phenol is derived **from petroleum or coal tar. Phenol and Cresol are the primary ingredients in disinfectants and both are toxic**, and known to damage the **central nervous system**. Phenol is also used to make resins that bind plywood and chipboard, some pharmaceuticals and in some pesticides. It is also used as an antimicrobial preservative in **medications** and **cosmetics** such as **mouthwash** and **skin creams**.

Phenylmercuric salts—despite the fact that **Mercury** is toxic to humans, it continues to be used in drugs (such as **eye preparations, vaginal products and nasal drops**), and **cosmetics (eye shadow, mascara, eyeliner and makeup removers)** as a **preservative**. The FDA banned its use in vaginal drugs based on animal tests. See also Mercury.

Pigs—Pigs are usually intensively farmed indoors, spending their entire lives in pens barely big enough to turn around in. Bearing sows are often chained down in small pens so that they cannot crush their young. Pigs are **given antibiotics and hormones** to prevent disease and promote unnatural growth. Pig farming commonly **pollutes the surrounding area**, runoff **causing nitrate problems in waterways, resulting in algae bloom and fish deaths**.

Consumers are eating **hormone-treated pork** without knowing or being aware of the consequences. The hormone has only been approved in Australia and so Australian consumers are now guinea pigs for the rest of the world. Mr Copeman says what is known is that **growth hormones** can cause pigs to suffer **painful bone and joint problems** and also decreases the fat content and flavor of the pork." - Courier Mail, October 1997

Plastics—Plastics are based on **petrochemicals** and are not fully biodegradable. Many **emit toxic gases** in degradation or burning. Plastic is become widely recycled. **PVC** is the most toxic (see separate entry) *Plastic codes on the base of product will help you identify them:* 1=PET polyester E/G, 2=HDPE high density polyyethylene, 3=PVC polyvinyl chloride and vinyl, 4=LDPE low density polyethylene, 5=PP polypropylene, 6=PS polystyrene.

Plastic contamination—CSIRO: "The Australian Food Standards Code set maximum migration levels for three specific monomers (basic plastic compounds): **vinyl chloride, acrylonitrile and vinyllidene chloride**. They are singled out because of their known **potential toxicity**". **The risk of food contamination from plastics increases with heating**, so it is advised that only microwavable plastics be used. **Styrene and inks used to color plastic** have also been known to taint flavor and odor of food packaged in them.

"Toys made with **PVC** (polyvinyl chloride) contain **hazardous chemicals** which can injure the **brain**.

HARMFUL

Polyethylene Glycol—PEG, Carbowax, Macrogol. PEG 100-700 are liquids, PEG 1000-10,000 are solids. Used in **soft gelatin capsule**, **oral liquids** and **other medications** as solvents. The solid forms are used in **ointment bases, tablet binders and lubricants**. They are also found in **cosmetics** as solvents and humectants for **bath oils, fragrances and hair products, skin products and eyeliner, mascara and foundations**. Known to cause **renal failure** if used on burn patients.

Polysorbates—These are **emulsifiers** derived **from fatty acids of animal origin**. sometimes called polyethelene 20 (40, 60, 80) sorbitan, sorlate or tween. Used in foods as an **emulsifier, synthetic flavouring, surfactant, opacifier, and dough conditioner**. In **drugs and cosmetics** as an **emulsifier (shampoos, fragrance powders, skin products, eye makeup, bath products)**, the most widely used in cosmetics is **Polysorbate 20**. May become an indirect **food additive via adhesives, emulsifiers and surfactants**. The deaths of 40 infants in the early eighties resulted when they were given a vitamin E product containing polysorbates 20 and 80 in ten times the usual amount accepted as safe.

Polystyrene—commonly used **in disposable food containers and insulation, in adhesives, foams, coating and some plastics. Releases benzene and styrene** when it is burnt, the former a **carcinogen**, the latter, a **systemic toxin**. Polystyrene also degrades in sunlight, releasing **toxic gasses**.

Polyvinyl Chloride (PVC)—used in **water-based emulsion paints, plastic pipe, plastic wrap and vinyl coated fabrics**. It is **toxic when burned, emitting vinyl chloride, HCl, dioxins, phosgene and furans**, all of which have been linked to **cancer** or **systemic poisoning**. Polyethylene is a safer substitute. See alo dioxins.

Chemicals are added to PVC to make it soft and flexible. Laboratory studies show that some of these chemicals are linked to **cancer** and **kidney damage** and may interfere with the **reproductive system and development**. In addition, recent testing by the governments of Denmark and the Netherlands concludes that **children can ingest hazardous chemicals from PVC toys during normal use**—sometimes at unacceptable levels!

"Should babies be chewing on **PVC toys**? No. They are toxic chemicals. They are easily absorbed. We know they **show up in children's bloodstream**." (Dr. Michael McCally, Director of Community Medicine, Mt. Sinai, USA)

Some PVC toys have already been taken off the market. The Dutch and Danish governments are urging retailers not to sell soft PVC toys. PVC toys also have been taken off the shelves in Sweden, Spain, Italy, Argentina and Greece."

Pristane—**shark oil and whale ambergris**. Used as a **lubricant** and **anti-corrosive**, also in **cosmetics**

Propylene Glycol—**petroleum product** used as

a **humectant, plasticizer, solvent with preservative properties**. In foods such as **baked goods, sweets, soft drinks, salad dressings and cakemixes, snack foods and frozen cakes**. Its glycerin like taste has made it popular for **children's medications** and other elixirs, and it is used in many **topical creams** and **ointments**. It is also used in **cosmetics, hair products and deodorants**. Propylene Glycol has been linked with **fatal heart attacks** (when given intravenously), **central nervous system depression**, and **cosmetic or pharmacuetical contact dermatitis**.

Propyl Gallate—used as an **anti-oxidant** to **prevent rancidity in oils, margarine, butter, meat products, snack foods, baked goods, nuts, grain products, gum and sweets, frozen dairy, and beverages**. Also commonly used in **lipsticks, balms and skin lotions**. May cause **contact dermatitis**.

Quaternium 7—derived from **tallow**.

Quaternium 15 - **formaldehyde** based **preservative** used in many **shampoos, conditioners and cosmetics**. Formaldehyde is known to be **carcinogenic**. Can cause **contact dermatitis** and sensitization to formaldehyde.

Quaternium 27—derived from **tallow**. In **deodorants** and **skin care products**.

Quorn—meat substitute derived from **fungi**, **often mixed with egg white**.

Rennet—an **enzyme extracted from a calf's stomach lining**. Used in **cheese making** and **Junket**. Substitutes can be derived from a fungus (Mucor Miehei) which makes it suitable for vegetarian consumption. Rennet is more often genetically engineered: synthesized from yeast genetically altered with **calf genes**.

Reticulin—**animal protein**.

Rosin—Resin, pine resin, colophane. Gum tapped from pine trees. Used in chewing gums, and as a polishing agent for coffee beans. Used to coat some tablets, and in depilatory products, hair tonics, makeup and mascara. Also used to produce glues, solder flux, paints, furniture polish, wood preservative and wax, paper and an additive in cigarettes. **Up to 3.6% of Europe is supposed to be sensitive to Resin.**

Roundup—a popular glyphosphate **herbicide, the manufacturers refuse to release the names of other ingredients**. Roundup was proven to have caused the **death** of three species of frogs in Western Australia in 1996, when used near aquatic environments. The manufacturer, Monsanto, has reported "**severe local effects and testicular effects** in rabbits" giving wider implications for other species as well as humans. It has yet to be tested in movement and accumulation studies.

Monsanto, however, claims that "Comprehensive toxicological studies in animals have determined that glyphosate, the active ingredient in Roundup, does not cause cancer, birth defects, mutagenic effects, neuro-

H
A
R
M
F
U
L

toxic effects or reproductive problems." See also Gene technology, addresses for action.

Saccharin—sweetening agent banned in 1977, but reinstated subject to strict labelling stating "Use of this product **may be hazardous to your health**. This product contains saccharin which has been determined to cause **cancer** in laboratory animals". Smolinske writes: "It is generally recommended that saccharin be avoided in nondiabetic c**hildren, patients with sulfonamide allergy, pregnant women, and young women of childbearing age**. Excessive use should be discouraged"

Salt—Sodium is a vital though often over-consumed mineral found throughout the body, usually in the form of sodium chloride or table salt. It is **added to every processed food** and occurs naturally in many fresh fruits and vegetables. Iodine is usually added to salt, although it is only required in trace amounts. See also, Iodine.

Shampoo—Many shampoos contain **formaldehyde**, a **carcinogen**. Alkylphenyl ethoxylates, commonly used in **detergents, shampoos, and cleaners** as well as in many industrial chemicals, have been found to have **estrogenic effects** on the human body. "Exposure to **excess estrogenic compounds can cause developmental and reproductive problems in both sexes, but especially males**. Excess estrogen may possibly be linked to **breast cancer** in women." (See also estrogen). Concern is high because **exposure to these chemicals is so widespread**. They are commonly used in many **detergents**, **shampoos**, and **cleaners** as well as in many industrial chemicals.

A herbal substitute for commercial shampoos: an infusion of soapwort leaves, simmered for five minutes, to which may be added (3:1) a small amount of the infused leaves of another herb such as rosemary (for dark hair), chamomile (for blonde hair), sage (for its conditioning properties) or lavender and rose (for scent). Almond oil, rosemary and nettle can be used to strengthen the hair. Supermarkets stock a range of compassionate alternatives. See also moisturisers, cosmetics, draize test.

Shellac—a varnish made from the **wings of an insect**, sometimes used to **wax fruit**. Also used to coat **tablets** (including Sudafed), in **hair sprays, eyeliners and mascara** .

Smog—**Nitrogenous and Sulphurous emissions in the air undergo photochemical conversion to ozone, sulphuric acid and nitric acid gas**. These chemicals then contribute to a**cid rain, respiratory illnesses like asthma, and breathing difficulties, even deaths**, not to mention the filth added to the environment. **Particulate matter and gases emitted from car exhausts and industrial pollution forms a haze** in the air over cities when anti-cyclonic weather conditions occur which prevent the smog from being dispersed by wind. Solutions: reducing car emissions through a combination of pollution controls devices on vehicles and reduced numbers of vehicles. Encouraging public transport usage.

Sodium Benzoate—Additive 211. An **antimicrobial preservative**. **Orange soft drinks** contain a high amount of it, up to 25mg per 250ml. Also **in milk and meat products, relishes and condiments, and baked goods**. Used in many **oral medications** including Actifed, Phenergan, and Tylenol. Known to cause **nettle rash**, and **aggravate asthma**.

Sodium benzoate is a **commonly found preservative in such food and drink products as fruit juice, soft drinks, coffee flavoring syrups, as well as a variety of condiments**. Although the FDA has previously classified sodium benzoate as a safe preservative, this classification is now being questioned. It appears that **sodium benzoate forms a chemical known as benzene when in the presence of vitamin C**. Benzene not only causes damage to DNA, the genetic material, **it is also a known carcinogen and appears to play a role in a variety of diseases due to it's DNA damaging capabilities**.

Another reason sodium benzoate may be considered an unhealthy preservative is its effect on children. Some studies have shown that **sodium benzoate along with artificial food colorings can cause children with ADHD to be more hyperactive**. This can be a particular problem for kids who consume soft drinks on a regular basis since most carbonated beverages have sodium benzoate as a preservative. Because of increasing awareness of this problem, Coke is planning on removing this unhealthy preservative from its soft drink products this year.

Because the conversion of sodium benzoate to benzene occurs in the presence of vitamin C, **this unhealthy preservative may be particularly unsafe when used in fruit jellies, jams, and fruit juices where high vitamin C fruits are present**. It's also thought that heat plays a role in the conversion to benzene, so **heating products containing this preservative could increase the risk of negative health effects**.

Sodium Lauryl Sulfate—sometimes contains **formaldehyde** as a preservative. Used in some **medications, medicated shampoos**. The lauryl component is derived from fatty acids, sometimes found in **spermaceti in whales**, but more widely sourced from laurel oil derived from trees in the bay family. Widely used in **cosmetics, especially shampoos, bubble baths and hair dyes**. Known to cause **dermatitis**.

Sodium Stannate—salt of **tin**.

Soap—most soaps contain **animal fats** in the form of **sodium tallowate**. An inexpensive and plentiful source, sodium tallowate can also be found in some **shampoos** and **shaving creams**. Don't be fooled by glycerine soaps either, many contain sodium tallowate. Vegetable oils soaps are readily available, and more palatable than the alternative of smearing ones body with animal fat!

Squalem, squalene—**shark oil** used in **hair colours, cosmetics, perfumes**.

Stearates—**stearic acid, stearamine, stearamide**, etc. Mainly derived from **animal fats**, usually obtained from **pigs**. Found in **cosmetics, soaps, shampoos and hair products, food flavouring**.

Steroids—derived from **animal glands** or plant tissues. Used in **hormone medications, creams, conditioners and perfumes**.

Sugar Decolorizers—despite the fact that purified sugar has no nutritional value, it makes a lot of otherwise unpalatable foods edible. Sugar is detrimental nutritionally when it is used to replace complex carbohydrates available from fruit, vegetables and grains.

White sugar is decolorized by mixing liquid sugar with activated carbon. Ten years ago, this probably would have been bone char, but now they use coal or wood charcoal. A third alternative is a chemical resin, albeit more expensive. **Sugar produced from cane in the US may have been decolorized with bone char**.

Sulphur dioxide—preservative derived from **coal tar** used to control the growth of bacteria. **All sulphur drugs are toxic** and restricted in use. **Sprayed on grapes after harvesting** and frequently used in **wines. Produced by the combustion of sulphur or gypsum**. See also active packaging.

Sulphites—**along with aspartame, are the most often blamed for adverse reactions to food additives.** The Adverse Reaction Monitoring System in the US has recorded that **half these reactions can be classed as serious**. Symptoms include: "**difficulty breathing or seizures**", especially in those susceptible to **asthma**. Most of the poisonings were traced to **salad bars where a sulphite preservative had been used to keep the food looking fresh**. Sulphites are commonly used **in processed orange juice, wine, packet potato chips, sweets, jams, condiments, processed vegetables, soups, sauces, and dried fruit**. Banned in the US in 1986 for use with fresh fruits and vegetables (excepting potatoes) Also used as a preservative in **hair permanent wave products** and **some medications**.

Synthetic fabrics—Around 25 thousand barrels of oil a day are used to create synthetic fabrics! Being of **petrochemical origin**, they do not biodegrade. Burning nylon fabrics **release nitrous oxide**, a gas contributing to **ozone depletion**.

Talcum powder—usually contains **hydrated magnesium sulphate or magnesium carbonate**, the fine particles of which can **cause lung problems** if inhaled often. Also known to cause cancer. A cornstarch variety is available as a safe alternative. Talc itself is used in **capsules and tablets**, as well as **other medications**. Also in **cosmetic powders**. Inhalation is know to cause

Foods which contain Sulfites (1072) / More about Sulfites (971)

emphysema, especially in smokers. Use corn starch instead of talc to dry baby bottoms.

Tallow—hard, white fat derived **from animals**, used to make **soap** and **candles**, and in the **dressing of leather**. Also used in **wax paper, crayons, margarines, paints, rubber, lubricants, soaps, shampoos, lipsticks, shaving creams, other cosmetics**. May contain **pesticide residues**.

Tea—Black (China) tea contains the stimulant **caffeine** in smaller amounts than in coffee. Tea also contains the alkaloids **theobromine** and **theophylline** which **stimulate the heart rate** and have the added effect of relaxing smooth muscle, and dilating blood vessels. Tea **accumulates aluminium when growing**, so that prepared tea may contain 2-6mg of aluminum per liter. **Tea bags** may have been bleached with **chlorine**, causing the release of **dioxins**. See Dioxins.

Teflon—a coating applied to cooking utensils for its non-stick quality. Teflon contains **fluorine**

Titanium dioxide—pigment used in **white paint** and **toothpaste** derived from mineral rocks, pollutes many rivers and oceans.

Toothpaste—*Toothpastes usually contain* an abrasive (calcium phosphate or carbonate), a softening agent (glycerine), a foaming agent (often sodium laurel sulphate), a thickener (often sodium carboxymethyl cellulose), a flavouring (usually spearmint or peppermint oil) and water. **Calcium carbonate** is sometimes derived from **bones**; **Titanium dioxide** is often used to **whiten** the paste (a pollutant in many waterways) and **Fluoride** (a potential **systemic poison**) is added for its reputed cavity preventing properties. Many brands are tested using the LD50 process, force feeding rats and guinea pigs. Tubes are sometimes made of **aluminum** and leaching may occur (see aluminum).

Toothpaste has had a long history of animal abuse and chemical toxicity: the ancient Romans used ground bones of burnt rodent's skulls, dog's bones have also been used and some toothpastes still contain bone ash. Toothpastes once contained hexachlorophene, chloroform and/or cyclamate, all toxic in various ways. Tubes were once made of lead until it was discovered that the lead leached into the paste!

There are herbal toothpastes readily available in supermarkets and health food stores that do not test on animals or contain fluoride. A simple home-made toothpaste can be made from powdered charcoaled bread to which peppermint, cloves or rosemary oil have been added, or a simple mixture of bicarbonate of soda and salt. see also Fluoride.

Toxicity: 14 Highly-toxic chemicals—the 'dirty dozen' commonly leached from waste sites include: **trichloroethylene, lead, toluene, benzene, chromium, tetrachloroethene, trichloroethane, chloroform, arsenic, PCBs, cadmium and zinc. Petroleum/**

H
A
R
M
F
U
L

chlorine compounds are always toxic, persistent and accumulative in the bodies of plants and animals. Nine studies analysed by the Environmental Research Foundation in 1992 showed that **many forms of cancer have been linked with exposure to these chemicals**, including **leukemia, stomach, lung, and lymph system cancers, as well as links with increased incidence of diabetes, suicide and cancer of the brain**. Industries which used solvents (pathologists and printers), adhesives (rubber, plastics and synthetic chemical industries), dyes, perfumes, paints, and other inorganic substances, in oil refineries, and those who handle and transport those products were shown to have higher incidence of cancers than the general population.

Tyrosine—derived from **milk casein**, found in **skin products**.

Urea—(Carbamide) in **urine and bodily fluids**, can be synthetically produced. Used in **mouthwashes, hair colours and creams**.

Uric acid—produced by the body accompanying a high fat diet, combined with alcohol, contributes to **gout**

Vaccines—vaccines are **often prepared using the blood of animals** or people who have contracted the disease in question and built up an immunity to it.

"Health authorities credit vaccines for disease declines, and assure us of their safety and effectiveness. Yet these seemingly rock-solid assumptions are directly contradicted by government statistics, medical studies, Food and Drug Administration (FDA) and Centers for Disease Control (CDC) reports, and reputable research scientists from around the world.

Vichyssoise—*potato and leek soup usually containing chicken stock.*

More Encouragement

"In the heart of Christ, where reigned perfect harmony with God, there was perfect peace. He was never elated by applause, nor dejected by censure or disappointment. Amid the greatest opposition and the most cruel treatment, He was still of good courage. But many who profess to be His followers have an anxious, troubled heart, because they are afraid to trust themselves with God. They do not make a complete surrender to Him; for they shrink from the consequences that such a surrender may involve. Unless they do make this surrender, they cannot find peace.

"It is the love of self that brings unrest. When we are born from above, the same mind will be in us that was in Jesus, the mind that led Him to humble Himself that we might be saved. Then we shall not be seeking the highest place. We shall desire to sit at the feet of Jesus, and learn of Him. We shall understand that the value of our work does not consist in making a show and noise in the world, and in being active and zealous in our own strength. The value of our work is in proportion to the impartation of the Holy Spirit. Trust in God brings holier qualities of mind, so that in patience we may possess our souls . .

"When our will is swallowed up in the will of God, and we use His gifts to bless others, we shall find life's burden light."
—Desire of Ages, 330-331

Two editions of Desire of Ages, the classic (and best) book on the life of Christ, are available from us.

H
A
R
M
F
U
L

ALSO SEE <u>FIRST AID</u>   990-1009

The Natural Remedies Encyclopedia

Preparing for an Emergency

WHEN SUDDEN PERIL STRIKES OR A MAJOR DANGER OCCURS

Also see Terrorist
and New Diseases 811-818

1 - PREPARATION FOR EMERGENCIES AND NATURAL DISASTERS

Table of Contents

"A prudent man foreseeth the evil, and hideth himself; but the simple pass on, and are punished."

EMER

—Proverbs 22:3

"Come, My people, enter thou into thy chambers, and shut thy doors about thee. Hide thyself as it were for a little moment, until the indignation be overpast."
—Isaiah 26:20

"By faith Noah, being warned of God of things not seen as yet, moved with fear, prepared an ark to the saving of His house."
—Hebrews 11:7

"Let them which be in Judea flee into the mountains."
—Matthew 24:16

This chapter and the next chapter (990-1009) enlarges on information given in an earlier chapter in this book.

EMERGENCY SUPPLY LIST

Water—One gallon a day per person. Household liquid bleach, to purify water.

Food—Ready-to-eat canned food (including peanut butter, bread, crackers, and multi-vitamins).

Clothing and bedding—Sturdy shoes or work boots, warm socks, rain gear, hats and gloves. Extra warm clothing. Thermal underwear. Blankets or sleeping bags.

Other supplies—*Items you would need whether you remain home or evacuate:* Mess kits, paper cups, plastic utensils, can opener. Batteries and battery-operated radio. Flashlight and extra bulbs. Signal flare. Paper and pencil. Plastic sheeting. Maps. Money, utility knife, paper towels. Plastic garbage bags and ties, and cell phone. Important family documents. Do not forget your Bible.

Items you would need if you remained at home: Duct tape, wooden matches in waterproof container, aluminum foil, plastic storage containers, needles and thread, shovel and other useful tools. Fire extinguisher. Plastic bucket with tight lid.

You will also need other special items if you have a baby or an elderly person is in your group.

Disaster supplies kit—You may have to evacuate or remain at home. Either way have some essential supplies on hand in an easy-to-carry container or two, such as a duffel bag or small plastic trash can. Include "special needs" items (infant formula, items for those with disabilities), first aid supplies (including prescription medications), change of clothing for each one, a sleeping bag or bedroll for each, battery-powered radio and extra batteries, bottled water, and tools. Include some cash and

copies of important family documents (birth certificates, passports, licenses). Outside your home in a safe location (safe-deposit box or in the home of a family member or friend), keep copies of essential documents (powers of attorney, birth and marriage certificates, insurance policies, life-insurance beneficiary designations, your will).

If you are in a position to do so, consider moving to a safer location. Some parts of the nation, especially large cities and certain strategic sites, are more likely to receive terrorist attacks than others.

INDIVIDUAL EMERGENCIES

In each of the following instances, provide emergency help; and, if the situation is serious, call 911 and get him to the hospital.

BASIC PREPARATION

Two of the most valuable preparations you can make for the coming crisis are these:

1 - Surrender your life to God, and let Him guide your life. By faith in Christ, as your personal Saviour and through His enabling grace, obey the Ten Commandments and the words of Scripture. Trust Him to care for you and cooperate with Him. Do your part to prepare for what is inevitably coming.

2 - Live in the country. This is a great solver of life's problems. Many of the situations discussed in this book will be minimized if you live in a rural area and have a well, a garden plot, and some trees. Such a setting will also provide you with room around your home for emergency activity and storage.

—Get out of the cities! They will become very dangerous places in which to live, when the crisis breaks. Get a little plot of land in the country, sink a well, clear space for a garden, have trees around you for firewood. Country living is the best kind of living. Breathe fresh air for a change.

Food, water, heating fuel, electricity, and computers will be the Achilles' heel of most Americans in the coming crisis

The government may enact antihoarding laws within the next 6-12 months. So it is good to start preparing right now. Those storing up needed supplies may be blamed as "hoarders" and the cause of the panic and crisis.

You should provide basic supplies to last you for at least 6 weeks. Some people plan to stock up for 3 to 6 months. Some are preparing for a crisis which may last for a year or two.

There are several basics you should stock in your home: water, food, clothing, bedding, first aid supplies, tools, emergency supplies, and special items. You should also have a reliable nonelectric

CHART 1067: 16 types of triangular Bandages (sketches)

EMER

heat source and, of course, shelter.

Even more basic: Write down everything—in any possible way—that you use in a day. Note other items which you use, but not every day. Then stockpile those items, so you can weather storms ahead.

WATER

Without water, you will be dead in 5 days. So it is a good place to begin our preparation list.

If you live in a city or town, you have a real problem. If you live on even a little acreage in the country, where you can sink a well, you can have water!

Get out of the cities—before it is too late and you cannot get out! Government controls could restrict travel from place to place. Beware, trouble is ahead. You can know that major problems are coming to the cities.

Where will you get your water when your local electrical power station stops providing it, and your local water utility ceases operations or no longer can treat the water?

You need water to drink, bathe, wash dishes and clothes, and operate the toilet. If you live in the country, you do not need to rely on an inside toilet. Then you only need water for drinking, washing, and bathing.

If you live in the country, you want to make sure you have a well, a stream, or a spring where you can get your water.

If you live in a city or town, you will need to haul in bottled water and store up a lot of it. But, even if you have a well, it would be good to have some extra water stored up.

A normally active person needs to drink at least two quarts of water each day. Hot environments and intense physical activity can double that amount. Children, nursing mothers, and ill people will need more.

Store 1 gallon of water per person per day (2 quarts for drinking, 2 quarts for food preparation and sanitation). Keep at least a three-day supply of water in your home. Better yet, have more than that stockpiled.

Store water in thoroughly washed plastic, glass, fiberglass, or enamel-lined metal containers. Never use a container that has held toxic substances because residue can be retained in the surface pores of the container. If you are not sure if a container is clean enough, only use the water in it for sanitation purposes, such as flushing the toilet.

Gradually stock up on water. Fill a number of gallon jugs. Purchase plastic 5-gallon buckets, clean them thoroughly (!), and then gradually fill a number of them with clean water. Because they are flat on top and bottom, they stack well. Fill them and stack them along a wall.

You may have a distiller, and can put water in bottles . Another option is to gradually buy filtered or ozonated water (purchase extra bottles every week for months).

I always keep several 5-gallon buckets full of well water on hand. Where we live, storms knock out the electricity every so often. But the crisis ahead will require more than a few buckets. You should be able to purchase empty mayonnaise buckets at a local fast-food restaurant; then clean them out and store water, grains, or beans in them.

Avoid using containers that will decompose or break. Do not store plastic bottles where the sun lights on them, lest the UV rays destroy them.

One expert suggests taking a water bed and filling it with water. But you would need to add purification tablets, if you were going to later drink from it. A water bed will hold approximately 175 gallons of water.

A relatively 15-foot plastic swimming pool will hold over 5,000 gallons of water. But, because of the various chemicals used to purify them, it is best to use the water only for washing and sanitary purposes.

You can purchase used 55-gallon metal drums (about $10 each), but beware of what was originally stored in them. Check with growers; you might be able to purchase drums which formerly held apple juice ($60 a drum). Legally, they are only supposed to be used once, so are available for you to purchase afterward. Many parts of the country grow apples. You can also buy new water tanks.

Place a washed-out drum at each corner of your house, and let the water from the gutters pour down into them. This water will prove to be a great help in the middle of a dry summer, when water is scarce.

Those 55-gallon drums are difficult to move, and difficult to get the water out of—unless you have a pumping device or some kind of spigot on the side. For household use, you would do well to gather lots of 5-gallon jugs. Military containers are the best, but Walmart and other stores carry commercial containers for campers. These 5-gallon jugs are ideal for hauling water; but 1-gallon jugs are also very useful.

Consider 55-gallon plastic drums made specifically for water storage. Another more permanent solution is an underground, fiberglass storage tank. They can hold thousands of gallons of water but are relatively expensive compared to the other solutions mentioned above. A 6 x 16-foot tank will hold 3,000 gallons.

Know where you can go to get more water, in an emergency.

If you have a well, purchase a well bucket, rope, and a pulley. Then you can manually haul water out of your well when there is no electricity. (A well bucket

EMER

is a bucket narrow enough to fit down a drilled, lined well hole.)

An alternate method is to purchase a hand pump. However, many find the bucket works more efficiently. Hand and solar pumps are also available. You should have a hand pump or a solar pump on hand as a backup—just in case.

There are special catalogs where you can purchase special items like hand pumps for wells, well buckets, and solar well pumps. We will list some later. For example, on p. 112 of the latest *Lehman's Nonelectric Catalog*, solar well pump kits are listed (330-857-5757). Another source for solar pumps is Golden Genesis Company, Scottsdale, Arizona (602-948-8003).

Another alternative is to rig up gutters and downspouts, to drain water from your roof into barrels or a cistern. If you filter the roof water runoff through an old nylon stocking, cheese cloth, or other thin cloth, this water can be boiled and used. (However, nearly 40 years ago, I found that roof water generally contains asphalt or aluminum, depending on whether it comes from a house roof or the top of a mobile home.) Be careful what kind of water you drink! One source says that painting your roof with white *Cool Seal* will reduce the asphalt in the water runoff from the roof.

Because it may contain asphalt, it is best to only use roof water for washing, bathing, flushing the toilets, and watering your garden.

Then there is water purification. This can be a key to long-term survival, if you are not sure of the water in the creek or well. If you have water purification equipment, a wider range of water sources are available to you. Water filters today can literally purify swamp and sewer water, and should be obtained now while they are still available. Katadyn, Pur, and Sweetwater are a few of the best brand names. Purchase a portable filter unit for each member of your family, and get one or two counter-top drip models if possible.

If you store water, an excellent way to preserve and keep it potable [which means drinkable] is to add one tablespoon of 3% hydrogen peroxide per gallon, keep it tightly closed and in a cool place, and it will store indefinitely.

If you live in an area where it is difficult to store water, or you do not have a well, consider purchasing a large water tank you can place on a trailer or in the bed of a truck.

Military water buffalo trailers are a good solution for those who can afford them. Each one holds at least 400 gallons and some are insulated. You can use it to haul water from a water source to your home. But you must be able to pump and, if necessary, purify water without electricity.

If you live in a city, the need to flush toilets can be a problem; and you will need water for this purpose also. Without electricity, your municipal sewage system will probably shut down. Portable toilets with chemicals to neutralize waste are available. Do not ignore basic sanitation. Cholera is not something to be desired.

Here is more detailed information on purifying water:

Untreated water could be unsafe because of disease carrying microbes or because of chemical contaminants such as heavy metals, salts, or pesticides. Contaminated water may be present, even though the water smells okay. It might contain microorganisms that cause diseases such as dysentery, typhoid, and hepatitis. You should purify all water of uncertain purity before using it for drinking, food preparation, or personal hygiene.

There are four ways to purify water:

1. *Boiling:* Bring water to a rolling boil for 3-5 minutes, keeping in mind that some will evaporate. Let it cool before drinking. Boiled water will taste better if you pour it back and forth between two clean containers, to restore the oxygen content. This technique will also improve the taste of stored water. Boiling will kill microbes, but will not remove chemical contaminants.

2. *Disinfection:* Liquid bleach (Chlorox, Purex, etc.) can be used to kill microorganisms in the water. But do not use bleach which is color-safe, scented, or has added cleaners. Add 16 drops of bleach per gallon of water, stir, and let it stand for 30 minutes. If the water does not have a slight odor of bleach, add another 16 drops and let it stand another 15 minutes.

3. *Filtration:* This removes microbes, but not chemicals. There are two kinds:

a. The inexpensive kinds use paper or charcoal to do the filtering, but they need to be replaced frequently (Pur Explorer and First Need are two such brand names).

b. The expensive kinds are ceramic filters. They cost nearly $200, but can treat as much as 15,000 gallons of water before needing replacement. Both the UN and Red Cross use the Swiss Katadyn brand. It can use a 50-psi hand pump to treat up to 1.2 quarts of water per minute. It is said to be able to purify very dirty water.

4. *Distillation:* Water is boiled and the vapor is condensed and collected. This is the only method which will remove both microbes and chemicals. Tie a cup right-side-up to the central-top handle of a lid. Then put the lid upside down over a pot of water and let it boil. Water will flow down the lid into the cup, producing distilled water.

Solar still uses the heat of the sun to produce distilled water. Very little water is produced each hour, but no fuel is required.

FOOD

In the United States, at any given time there is a three-day supply of food on hand. The lettuce you buy was picked four days ago. When a disaster (such as a hurricane) occurs, there is a rush on grocery stores and the food is gone within three hours.

Increase your food supply to a minimum of 6 weeks, especially canned goods. (Some knowledgeable experts warn that you should have as much as a two-years' supply for each family member.) Make sure you have a manual can opener. Especially select foods which require no refrigeration, preparation, or cooking, and take little or no water to prepare. Such foods would include:

Ready-to-eat canned fruits and vegetables
Canned juices and soup
Staples: grains, dry beans (if you are planning to cook), salt
High-energy foods: peanut butter, granola bars, trail mix, honey, molasses
Vitamin supplements
Foods for infants, elderly persons, or persons on special diets
Possibly dried fruit, if you can afford it (Freeze-dried foods are excellent, but very expensive.)
Some recommend that you plan not to heat food; and, if so, include a few cans of Sterno.

However, if you are properly prepared, you will have a woodstove and can cook on top of that. More on heating and cooking below.

Food is becoming more expensive every day. It may be a real problem later. The problem is not the supply of grain in the field. It is the delivery system. First, as we neared the end of 1999, there was an increasing demand for rice, beans, etc. This could cause shortages. Second, computers control the shipping of food and other commodities throughout the nation. When the computers go down, the food supply could be cut off for an undisclosed period of time.

It is estimated that one adult needs 1,000 pounds of food per year. The diet should consist of about 50% grains, beans, and rice. Vegetables should be another 50%. In addition, you will need a little vegetable oil, salt, etc.

Bulk foods to stock up on would include corn, rice, wheat, pinto and navy beans, oats, salt, and honey in bulk. If you have wheat, soybeans, and corn,—you have a perfect protein!

Go to a cheap food outlet (such as Sam's Club or Costco) and buy such staples: beans, rice, and corn. Or purchase your wheat and soybeans at a local co-op. (But if you get anything at a co-op, make sure it is not treated seed! Insecticides might have been added.)

Wheat in the field is only $2.50 a bushel (60 lbs.), or 4 cents a pound. At that rate, it would only cost $1.50 to fill one of your buckets with good wheat! Wheat at the co-op costs more, but still far less than the flour at the grocery store. When you go to the co-op, make sure you get triple-cleaned wheat. Lacking the bits of sand, it is less likely to wear out your high-speed grinder as quickly.

If you do not know where to start, here is a basic suggestion: Estimate how much wheat, corn, and beans you would use in a week, if you did have any other source of carbohydrates and proteins. Then go out and purchase a year's supply of whole wheat, corn, and beans. If you buy 50 lb. sacks, this will only cost a couple hundred dollars or so. Be sure and specify that you want food-grade product; otherwise you could get seed wheat, etc., which has a poisonous coating to repel insects.

Purchase garbage cans (tinned steel or plastic) with tight-fitting lids. Store your dry staples in them.

Also useful are 5-gallon buckets, especially those with screw-on lids. *M&M Industries* makes a good one. A case of 6 (with lids), shipped, is about $40, depending on address mailed to (316 Corporate Place, Chattanooga, TN 37419 / 800-331-5305). An excellent source for 5-gallon buckets (but without the screw-on lids), are the fast-food restaurants. Buy their empty buckets for 50 cents or $1 each; take them home and wash them out well. These can be used for food or water. You can estimate that about 35 pounds of grain or beans will fill each bucket.

Have a manual grain grinder; so you can make flour when you need it from your staples.

Learn to make good bread. Grind your wheat, soybeans, and corn in your grinder (use a high-speed electric grinder before the crisis; a hand grinder during it). Mix them together in these proportions: $40% wheat, $40% corn, and 20% soybeans. Add some yeast, knead it, let it rise, then bake. You will have all the major amino acids in that bread. (However, you will have to learn to like the taste; it is a little different.)

Over a period of time, you will be stocking up on the various foodstuffs. But then, during storage, insects will want to claim their share.

As soon as you get your latest order of dry staples (wheat, beans, corn, etc.), put it in your freezer for 3 days. This will help kill a majority of the bugs that were included in the shipment. But that will not eliminate them all.

E
M
E
R

Next, the experts advise that you mix a cupful of diatomaceous earth (DE) into each bucketful of wheat. This primarily consists of calcium. Yet it is a special kind, which big bugs and post-larval bugs choke on. DE is said to be harmless to people, if the silica content is 1% or less. It kills bugs by dehydrating them. DE costs about 90 cents to a dollar per pound, plus shipping. Your co-op may sell it. (*Nitron Industries* is an organic gardening company which sells DE for about $24 for 20 lbs. P.O. Box 1447, Fayetteville, AR 72702 / 501-587-1777.)

Unfortunately, not only the bugs but the very air is hazardous to your stored foods. As you may know, it is the air in the jar (the oxygen and humidity in that air) which, along with warmth, works to destroy the food value of the contents of each jar. There is now a gadget which removes the air from the jar so you can seal it! Normally, one has to boil the jar and contents in order to create a "vacuum pack." But foods you do not want to boil can be sealed with a Pump-n-Seal.

Pump-n-Seal is used to seal both jars and good-quality zipper locking plastic freezer bags. Recommended jarred foods include soups, salads, berries, beans, cooking oils, chips, nuts, etc. It can be used on nut mixes, cooking oils, and other oil foods. It helps prevent freezer burn and preserve freshness in frozen foods. Of course, it would also be excellent, not only for food but, for storing garden seeds in jars.

Pump-n-Seal, Pioneering Concepts, Inc., P.O. Box 2346, Naperville, IL 60567 (630-553-2340; fax 630-553-2380)

For long shelf life food reserves, call International Collectors Associates (800-525-9556).

Get to know farmers who will sell or barter their produce to you. More on bartering later in this book.

FOOD FROM THE GARDEN

If you do not know much about gardening, begin practising! Plant a garden this summer! Do not wait for a crisis to begin learning how to raise your own food. Buy nonhybrid garden seed, and plant some this summer. Learn how to save some of the seed for the next year.

This fall, stock up on nonhybrid seed for the next year. Nonhybrid (reproducible seeds) are available from Pinetree Garden Seeds, Box 300, New Gloucester, ME 04260; also from R.H. Schumway: Box 1, Graniteville, SC 29829.

After the growing season, buy small packets of garden seeds (then available at lowest cost) and store them for barter or future gardens.

Keep your food storage program very private, known only to your immediate family or closest friends. You can, and should, share with whom you like; but it should not be because hungry, unprepared neighbors or marauders forcibly beat your door down and seize your reserves.

You can always grow a variety of foodstuffs in the summer months; but you also need food for winter.

Hubbard squash (a winter squash) and kale are two of the best. Grow the squash this summer and harvest it this fall. Spread it out on newspapers in a cool, dry place—and it will last through the winter and provide you with excellent starchy food. Hubbard is one of the best-keeping of the winter squashes. (If you did not know it, pumpkins very quickly spoil.)

Then there is kale. Collards do better in the heat of the summer, and for use in the summer and early fall. But, in many parts of the nation, kale can overwinter in the ground! Order a sizeable amount of kale and plant it in late summer. (Where I live, in eastern Tennessee, August 1-15 is the date to plant it.) It will provide fresh cooking greens throughout the winter and early spring! All through the winter you can go out and harvest some leaves. It will not grow during the winter, but it will not die—unless a severe freeze occurs.

You will want to have seed on hand for the next summer. Asgrow (Kalamazoo, Michigan) is a large company which sells vacuum-packed cans of seeds. Buy a few cans and you will have lots of seeds for summer and fall planting. But remember: as soon as you open the can, outside moisture will began degrading the quality of the seed.

If you only have a lawn around your home, tear up part of it—and plant a summer and fall garden. But be sure and check the pH. Do a soil test and find out if you need to add some lime to sweeten the soil. Most vegetables like a soil which is generally more alkaline than most in the eastern states. (Out West, the soil is less acid.)

If you do not have a soil test kit, you can collect a few samples from various areas of your proposed garden plot—and mail it to your state agriculture station, or to a state college. For $10 or so, they will test the soil for you and send you a report in a few weeks. Phone your local ag agent and he will explain what to do. You will find him listed in your phone book under "(County name) Extension Service."

If you have access to rotted manure, put some on your garden plot in order to help build it up. But you must begin preparing your garden now; do not wait until later. If you can only haul in fresh manure, get it this spring and let it set for six months. If you know how to compost, all the better. Crops grow far better in soil which has been properly fertilized. But do not use chemical fertilizers! They only injure your soil and kill the earthworms and microzyma.

If you garden, you will need canning jars and

related supplies; and a hand grinder for corn, wheat, and other grains. That was discussed in the preceding section on food.

HEATING FUEL

One or more heat sources are also needed, not only to warm you and cook your food, but also to keep the pipes from freezing.

You must have an alternative to electricity! Purchase a nonelectric heating source. The simplest is a stand-alone, nonvented propane heater.

If you are relying on propane, make sure your tank is full. Consider having a second tank installed for awhile.

If you have a source of firewood, install a woodstove! A good woodstove can heat 2,000 sq. ft. of living space. There are places out West where firewood is difficult to find; but there is usually plenty of it in the eastern states.

Be sure and use insulated pipe, where it runs through the wall. Make sure the chimney has a liner in it. Woodstoves can cause chimney fires; so you must take special precautions with them, which would not be necessary with propane. Wood heat can produce a lot of rather sudden heat in the chimney. In addition, wood smoke tends to build up a creosote which occasionally can start a chimney fire.

What kind of woodstove should you get? The better-made (and more expensive) are lined with firebrick, or something similar, and will last a long time. They are tighter, and will hold wood heat through the night. In this way, if you select a large log in the evening, and bank down the stove, you will not have to wake up to an alarm clock in the middle of the night to refill the stove! Make sure the stove top is flat, so you can cook on it. The stove should be large enough to heat your home.

If you cannot afford such an expensive stove, you can buy a cheap, thin-walled model at the hardware store. It can be of value, even though it will not last for many years. Such a stove generally will have to be refilled halfway through the night (unless you want to let it go out and then start a fire in a cold house the next morning.)

Used good stoves are most often available in the spring. That is the best time to buy a good one at a lower price.

If the woodstove does not have an integral blower fan—to push out the hot air,—place a fan behind or above the stove. This applies to any other kind of house-heating source. (Of course, when there is no electricity, you will not be able to use that fan.) It is possible to purchase stove fans which run from the heat and move the heated air.

If you have always wished to have a fireplace, you might want to build it this year and stock plenty of wood for it by wintertime. (However, woodstoves provide far more heat than fireplaces.) If you have a fireplace, you can increase the heating efficiency with an insert. You can go from 15% to 80%-90% efficiency by purchasing and installing one.

If you live in the city, the experts recommend that you keep the firewood in your garage, out of sight. Otherwise it might be stolen at night. (That is what happened in Watertown, New York during a three-week power blackout during an icestorm.) If you live in the country, you will need a shed or tarp to keep the wood dry.

Stoves, firewood, and a number of other things mentioned in this book should be purchased prior to the crisis. Do not forget to purchase and store 1 or 2 complete sets of interior chimney pipes (elbows, joints, etc.)

Purchase 1 or 2 good wood-splitting mauls, axes, hatchets, and some extra handles.

You might want to get a crosscut saw and Swede saw. A chain saw and supplies (oil, gas, tools, spare chains, and a sharpener) is a must if you are going to cut your own wood.

Cast-iron cooking utensils are great for a woodstove.

Those who live in apartments can get a small camper's cooking stove or a small wood or propane stove. However, camping-type stoves and heaters should only be used outdoors in a well-ventilated area. If you do purchase an alternative heating device, make sure it is approved for use indoors and is listed with the Underwriters Laboratories (UL). It is best not to heat the house with the oven or top burners of a propane cookstove. This is because of the fumes emitted. (However, in an emergency, use them anyway.)

There are numerous camping cookstoves available. Be sure to have extra fuel and matches for the stove; and only use it outdoors. A dozen or two large cans of sterno for cooking could be useful.

In case the power fails, plan to use alternative cooking devices in accordance with manufacturer's instructions. Do not use open flames or charcoal grills indoors.

You will need a reliable nonelectric way to heat your home and cook your food. Propane is very handy. (LP [liquid propane] gas is another name for propane.) You cannot store electricity, but you can store propane. Getting this propane early avoids the rush, in stores, for availability of this product during an emergency.

For those who are interested, solar heat is avail-

E
M
E
R

able—if you live in an area which has lots of cloudless days. One source of solar equipment is Kent Morgan, 8534 E. 37th Place, Suite 200, Indianapolis, IN 46226 (317-465-8496). More on solar energy in the next section.

ALTERNATE ELECTRICITY SOURCES

If you live in an area where you can legally and functionally have one, a generator can be very useful. (Another reason why you want to live in the country; they are not appreciated in urban areas because they are noisy). Frankly, none of us appreciate their noise; yet, in an emergency, they will be very much appreciated.

Generators designed for camping or recreational vehicle usage (1,000 - 5,000 watts) have insufficient capacity to handle the load requirements of even a small home. Only a few pieces of equipment can be operated at a time.

An adequately sized, high-quality generator (16,000 - 20,000 watts), on the other hand, will be quite expensive to purchase ($6,000-$8,000), and will require large amounts of fuel whenever it is running.

(One expert recommends that, if you wish to use a backup generator for an extended period, you need to install a group of deep-cycle marine or industrial batteries, an electronic controller, and a converter which converts direct current (DC) to alternating current (AC). If you choose this system, you will need to get an expert to design and install it for you.)

If you plan to use a portable generator, connect what you want to power directly to the generator. Do not connect the generator to your home's electrical system. Reason: If the power company suddenly turned the electricity on, it could burn up your generator!

We had a direct line to a generator wired into our office. Another was installed in the print shop. When the crisis comes, we turn the generators on. When not in use, the generators are on wheels and are stored in a sheltered place, such as a garage.

Select those appliances you wish to have on a special wiring circuit to the generator. Ideally, this would include the following:

Washing machine
Dryer (or omit)
Freezer
Refrigerator
Certain kitchen outlets for table-top appliances (blenders, etc.)
Certain lights, preferably those in the kitchen

Keep in mind the following principle:

Electric heating devices (dryers, water heaters, cookstoves, heaters) use a lot of power! Larger mo-

tors do also. Motors require extra power when they first start. Therefore, do not operate electric heating devices from your generator. Only operate one or two larger appliances at a time.

Depending on the size of your generator, you might (might not) be able to operate the freezer, refrigerator, radio (for the latest news), and kitchen lights at the same time. But do not start the motor items (freezer and refrigerator) at the same time! Pull the plug on one before starting the generator.

You may wish to purchase a 5,000 watt model. However, some folk have been successful buying two 1,200 watt models. They can be used in different places.

But even the 5,000 watt generators will only operate a few things at a time. Check it out in advance and find what you can do. Have the special wiring circuit installed and tested before the crisis comes. Know ahead of time what you can, and cannot do, with your generator. Then operate the generator several hours each day. During that time, the food is being chilled again and you are rushing around the kitchen while listening to the news, to find out what the government and the cities are doing.

At the end of this book is a voltage reference guide—so you can know in advance what a generator can handle. In this way, you will be able to make a wiser choice when selecting the size of a generator to purchase!

If you have a generator which can operate several hours each day to keep your home freezer cold, this will greatly help. However, you can never know what may happen. It is terrible to lose a freezer full of food! If in doubt as to what is ahead, eat all the food in your freezer by the end of the year. (The only way you can know you can make it is to install a generator, and test it on your refrigerator and freezer a few hours a day, for several days, and see if it can handle the load and keep the food cold as it should be.)

Keep the generator in a well-ventilated area (because it has gasoline in it), either outside or in a garage, keeping a door ajar. Do not put a generator in your basement or anywhere inside your home.

Plan ahead: Arrange to operate the generator so that it is not so loud when running. To lessen the noise, either have some insulation board partially around it, or place it in a hole in the ground, ensuring that surface water will not flow into it.

If possible, the generator should have a multi-fuel capacity (able to operate on either propane or diesel). Buy one between 8 Kwh to 12 Kwh, if possible.

Generators can use gasoline, diesel fuel, natural gas, or propane. Either of the last two options is recommended for safety and greater ease of fuel storage.

Honda generators are the best gasoline generators on the market. They run longer on a gallon of gasoline, are quieter, and easier to start than the cheap models with a Briggs and Straton engine. Honda engines are also easier to work on.

Then there is the matter of fuel tanks. Check with a local agriculture supply house or with local farmers and ranchers. They may have used tanks no longer in use which they will be glad to dispose of at low cost, if you will haul it off.

Diesel fuel is more stable than gasoline, stores better and longer, and is less explosive. Be sure you place any fuel storage tanks in a safe area, away from your home and any machinery that may spark or ignite the fuel. Gasoline or diesel tanks (300 or 500 gallon size), the kind you see standing on stands in farmers' and ranchers' yards in the country, can be bought from agriculture supply houses in small towns and refilled monthly.

Regarding fuel in tanks, keep in mind that there may be disruptions in delivery and the possibility of rationing, should shortages develop.

If you are going to store gasoline over 4 months, treat it all with Sta-bil. Sta-bil is a compound which keeps the gas in stabilized form for months.

If you put Stabil in the gas tank of the generator and run it for a few minutes, you can shut it off and not worry about the gas that is in the carburetor gumming up and making future starting difficult. The gas can remain in your machine for a whole year and still crank up easily.

Solar grids can also be used to produce electricity. Solar cooking and solar lanterns are available. Kits are available.

A solar energy system, though initially more expensive, is ultimately simpler, safer, easier to maintain, and requires no fuel (except sunlight). If you are considering this, consult an expert on whether you should use either a generator/battery/converter system or a solar system.

Wind generators can also be used as an alternate electrical energy source. But you need to live in the midwest or on a mountaintop, where there is a lot of wind.

For more information on energy back-up systems, send $10 to Year 2000 Survival Newsletter, P.O. Box 84910, Phoenix, AZ 85071 (800-528-0559). for the special issue on back-up energy systems.

An emergency generator, or power source of some kind, is important. Keep in mind that, without electricity, you cannot pump water out of a 300-foot well (although you can get it out with a well bucket).

Consider converting all or part of your appliances (dryers, water heater, cookstove, freezer, and/ or refrigerator) to either propane or natural gas. Buy or lease the largest gas tank and keep it topped off monthly.

Before concluding this section, before you spend money on solar power or wind generator systems, know that it will work where you live!

Solar power is great in states such as New Mexico and Arizona. But it is far less efficient in the eastern part of the country, especially east of a north-south line running through Chicago. Too cloudy.

Wind generators are outstanding if you live in very windy areas, but less so elsewhere. From Texas north to the Dakotas is windy country. Mountain ridges where the wind can blow in from the west or north are good. The first ridge next to the Pacific Ocean and the tops of mountains are also good. It has been said that if most of North Dakota were covered with wind generators, there would still be room for the same number of cattle—yet a sizeable portion of America could be electrified from it.

ALTERNATE LIGHTING

Buy several dozen candles and at least a dozen boxes of strike-anywhere matches. Butane lighters are also good.

Purchase some kerosene lamps and several gallons of kerosene. If you suspect the crisis may last for some time, you may want 5-10 gallons. Also get spare wicks.

Aladdin lamps are best, but cost up to $65 and require special Aladdin oil. Like Coleman lamps, they require special fuel and provide a white light. Such lamps burn cleaner and, in the evening, are much brighter to read by.

Kerosene lamps can be purchased at Wal-Mart or at surplus stores, generally for under $25 each.

Purchase several flashlights, a dozen or more rechargeable batteries, and a 12-volt battery charger. Or, if you will have no alternate electrical energy source to recharge batteries, purchase a quantity of alkaline batteries (they store better and outlast regular batteries). Do not forget replacement flashlight bulbs.

CLOTHING AND BEDDING

Basically, you should have extra blankets, coats, hats, and gloves to keep warm. Buy warm winter clothing, long underwear, etc., and lots of it. You want enough to last several years. When you can dress warm, you are better prepared for whatever may happen.

You need durable work clothing, shoes, and boots. A lot of our clothing is imported from China; and the shipping industry may cease functioning.

Important items to have on hand:
Warm shirts
Durable pants or dresses

EMER

Sturdy shoes or work boots
Rain gear
Blankets or sleeping bags
Pull-down thick caps or wool hats
Leather work gloves
Thermal underwear
Protective clothing (coveralls, overalls, etc.)
Sunglasses

Ladies should make sure they own some comfortable, durable walking shoes.

Bedding is also important:

You should have several warm, wool army blankets for each member of the family, and a dozen more for other friends or relatives who may arrive. Warm sleeping bags, which can withstand temperatures down to zero, are very useful.

Make sure you have several hot-water bottles, to help keep you warm in bed. You cannot be sure how the heating situation may turn out.

PREPARING THE HOUSE

In addition to other points mentioned in this book, here are a few more:

The crisis may begin in the dead of winter. Prepare your house for the possibility. Install storm windows, to help hold the heat in. Or purchase a roll of clear, plastic sheeting. Have it ready and, if you need to next winter, tack it up over leaky windows to keep the cold out.

Locate those passageway areas where you should drive nails and put up blankets to help keep the heat in certain quarters. Figure out which rooms you can close off and not heat.

If you have a fireplace, place a board plywood over it, to close it off. (Otherwise air from the living room will keep going up the fireplace chimney.) Install a good woodstove.

HOUSEHOLD ITEMS

List the items you regularly use in your home over a week's time. These are the things you need to have extra on hand!

Liquid soap
Detergent
Toilet paper
Matches and disposable butane lighters

A little thought will suggest many other household items you will need.

Sam's Club has a 50-page catalog of all its standard products. Ask the manager for a copy. From it, make a list of what you need! If you are able to do so, you can place an order and then borrow a pickup and get it.

Here are some sample prices at Sam's:
Laundry detergent: 40-lb. bucket - $10
Toilet paper: Case (60 rolls, 500 sheets, double-

ply) - $25
Disposable lighters: 50 - $10
You will need trash bags, paper towels, razors, etc.

Also keep in mind light bulbs, duct tape (several rolls), stamps, and envelopes.

If soap may become scarce, laundry disks are helpful. They can do hundreds of loads with little or no soap.

Do not forget canning equipment, jars, etc. Keep this ratio in mind: For each 100 jars, you need 100 rings and 300 lids.

Purchase a hand-powered mill for grinding flour or meal.

SANITATION

Here is a list of sanitation items you will want to keep on hand:

Toilet paper, towelettes
Soap, liquid detergent
Feminine supplies
Personal hygiene items
Plastic garbage bags, ties
Plastic bucket with lid
Disinfectant
Household chlorine bleach
Baking soda (for odors)
Agricultural lime (for sanitation purposes)

SPECIAL ITEMS

There will be family members who have special needs which should be considered.

For the infant:
Formula
Diapers
Bottles
For adults:
Heart and blood pressure medication
Insulin
Prescription drugs
Denture needs
Contact lenses and supplies
Extra eye glasses
Books
A sewing kit with polyester thread

MEDICAL SUPPLIES

Do you need a regular supply of medical products? If so, store them up gradually ahead of time; so you will have a 3-4 months' supply. This would include both prescription and nonprescription medications which you regularly use.

Begin purchasing any special medications in 90-day quantities and renew your prescriptions early.

FIRST AID KIT

Assemble a first-aid kit for your home and one

for each car. The experts advise that you include all of the following:

Sterile adhesive bandages in assorted sizes
2-inch sterile gauze pads (4-6)
4- to 9-inch sterile gauze pads (4-6)
Hypoallergenic adhesive tape
Triangular bandages (3)
2-inch sterile roller bandages (3 rolls)
3-inch sterile roller bandages (3 rolls)
Scissors
Tweezers
Needle
Moistened towelettes
Antiseptic
Thermometer
Tongue blades (2)
Tube of petroleum jelly or other lubricant
Assorted sizes of safety pins
Cleansing agent/soap
Latex gloves (2 pairs)
Sunscreen
Activated charcoal

Herbal remedies (preferably in tincture form which retain their potency the longest) should also be included in your medical chest. Have extra cayenne pepper powder on hand. It can be used to stop bleeeding, arrest a heart attack, and do many other things. Slippery elm powder is excellent for the stomach, dysentery, and as a food supplement. Also keep white willow bark, ginger, Barley Green, rice bran, and Hawthorn berry syrup on hand. Store up extra vitamins.

Echinacea, astragalus, Dr. Christopher's Anti-Plague Formula, and vitamin C are useful. Taking all four every hour helps neutralize an emerging cold or flu.

There are many herbal supply houses. One source of pure, high-strength herbs is *American Botanical Pharmacy*, P.O. Box 3027, Santa Monica, CA 90408 (310-453-1987).

Essential oils have the longest shelf life of all plants. Their antimicrobial, antiviral, antibacterial, antifungal properties are very powerful. For a personalized family health kit, call *Essential Oils for You (712-203-2045)*.

HOUSEHOLD EQUIPMENT

Buy extra batteries of all sizes for radios, clocks, and other battery operated products. Hand-pumped flashlights do not require batteries and are useful.

For reliable fire starters, obtain a large supply of long-burning candles, matches, and butane lighters.

Certain household equipment should be checked on, including your smoke alarms. If they are wired into your home's electrical system (most newer ones are), check to see if they have battery backups. Each

fall, replace all batteries in the smoke alarms as a general fire safety precaution.

Check on other equipment. Know what will still operate when the electricity goes off. Keep extra batteries on hand.

A washtub and hand wringer would be handy to have. But, if you have a generator, you can turn it on at certain hours and cool the refrigerator and freezer while you wash clothes and hear the latest news on the radio.

It was mentioned earlier that, in view of what is ahead, a gas (propane or natural gas) washer, dryer, water heater, cookstove, freezer, and refrigerator are better than the electric operated kind.

Cast-iron cookware that can be used on stoves or open fires are useful.

ALTERNATIVE COMMUNICATIONS

Purchase a shortwave band radio receiver, so you can keep up with what is happening in the world. This is vital in case of riots in the cities and subsequent government takeover because of the severity of the crisis. The radio equipment should have an optional battery pack. Or listen to an electric one at those times you operate your generator to cool the refrigerator and freezer, etc. Sony has an excellent shortwave model that can be received worldwide; yet is small enough to fit into the palm of your hand. Grundig is another good brand.

Some survival experts recommend that you also get small, hand-held two-way shortwave radios (transceivers) for each member of your family (15 years old and up). Each one will transmit 10-15 miles. However, a general-class amateur license or technician-class amateur license is required. An alternate method is small hand-held walkie-talkies, which can communicate on citizen band about half a mile. Transceivers on amateur radio frequencies can reach out to 10 miles.

A scanner can be used to tell you what is happening locally; but the local radio news may substitute. Here are some ham and radio equipment sources: *Ham Radio Outlet* (800-854-6046); *Amateur Electronic Supply* (800-558-0411); *Texas Towers* (800-272-3467); Radio Shack sells transceivers for citizens band. Radios which operate on solar or hand-crank power are also available.

You might want to buy an inexpensive used CB (civilian band) radio home station and car CB for inexpensive local emergency communications.

ELECTRONIC EQUIPMENT

Check with manufacturers of any essential computer-controlled electronic equipment in your home or business, to see if that equipment may be affected. This would include fire and security alarm

E
M
E
R

systems, programmable thermostats, appliances, consumer electronics, garage-door openers, electronic locks, and any other electronic equipment in which an embedded chip may control its operation.

Sell your computer and purchase a new one with new softwear and Windows XP. It is the best Microsoft computer available.

The following items would be very helpful during emergency conditions:

Solar battery charger ($15)
Solar powered am/fm/sw radio ($20)
Quartz battery powered clock ($10)
Battery tester ($5)

TOOLS AND SUPPLIES

Some of the following items reflect the fact that you may need to relocate:

Mess kits (paper cups, plates, and plastic utinsils)
Emergency preparedness manual
Battery operated radio and extra batteries
Flashlight and extra batteries
Cash or traveler's checks, change
Nonelectric can opener, utility knife
Fire extinguisher (small canister, ABC type)
Tube tent
Pliers
Tape
Compass
Matches in a waterproof container
Aluminum foil
Plastic storage containers
Signal flare
Paper, pencils
Needles, thread
Shutoff wrench, to turn off household gas and water
Whistle
Plastic Sheeting
Map of the area (for locating shelters)

We earlier mentioned the need for a chain saw and supplies, axes, mauls, hatchets.

Do not forget adequate garden tools.

SURVIVAL KIT

This is what the U.S. Armed Forces tells its men to include in their survival kit:

Lightweight, roll-up raincoat
A broad-brimmed, lightweight hat (in hot climates)
A knitted cap, to cover head and ears, and extra gloves or mittens (in cold climates)
A change of underwear and socks
Roll-up 4-foot seine (Poles can be fashioned from available sticks or other wood found near a stream. A seine is a fishing net, especially a long one that hangs vertically in the water and

is supported by floats on its upper edge and kept taut by weights on the bottom edge.]
Waterproof, stike-anywhere matches
Waterproof, batteryless flashlight
Candle stub (besides light, candle wax is useful for plugging, patching, and starting fires.)
Fire starter
Toilet paper
Insect repellent in plastic squeeze bottle
Sunscreen lotion or cream
Sunglasses
Signal mirror
Two smoke signals
Two flares
Compass
Appropriate topographic maps
Halazone tablets for purifying water
Two dozen assorted fishhooks
50 feet of 50-lb. monofilament line
Brass swivels and 25 feet of light wire for rigging snares
Swiss Army-type pocket knife
Needle and thread
25 feet of parachute cord or other heavy-duty nylon line
Short file or whetstone
Ax or hatchet
A strong saw (one that is easily stored, yet sturdy enough to take down trees many inches in diameter)
Plastic pack of bouillon cubes and chocolate packs to mix with water
1 square yard of aluminum foil
Antiseptic cream
Small pad and pencil

TRANSPORTATION

Many of us remember the lineup of cars waiting to be served at gas stations, when their was a shortage of gas; and the price went up. As soon as the electricity goes out, it will be impossible to pump gas at gasoline stations.

Consider contacting a fuel company and having them set a gasoline tank on your property. They will be glad to do this; since they will be selling you the gasoline. But do not wait; get the tank installed early!

Disadvantages of a tank installation are these: (1) You may pay a little more per gallon for gasoline. (2) The inside of the tank can gradually acquire water in the bottom of the tank from condensation; yet the outlet is generally a little higher than the tank bottom. In other words, gasoline in one of those home tanks can be a little dirty. The larger the tank the cleaner it is. (3) You will not have the brand of gasoline you normally prefer (if you care about such matters).

However, in a crisis, the advantages far outweigh

the disadvantages! That tank, filled, will hold from 50 to 150 gallons, and would provide you with enough gasoline to run your car for quite some time. And that could be worth a lot to you!

Acquire alternate transportation in the event that the system goes down for a long time and fuel becomes scarce or unavailable. This might include bicycles, mountain bikers, motor scooters, trail bikes, or motorcycles. Some of these use fuel, but in smaller amounts.

IMPORTANT DOCUMENTS

There will be important family documents which you should keep in a waterproof, portable container. Make sure the following includes addresses and phone numbers.

Will, insurance policies, contracts, deeds, stocks and bonds

Passports, social security cards, immunization records

Bank account numbers, credit card account numbers, and companies

Inventory of valuable household goods, important telephone numbers, family records (birth, marriage, death certificates)

PERSONAL FINANCES

There is the possibility that you may have difficulty withdrawing money from your bank at certain times because so many people will panic and withdraw their savings. Therefore, you may find it wise to withdraw enough to tide you through the crisis. Have all your cash in small denominations.

If the banking system shut down for a month, what would happen to you, to your employer, your employment, your retirement fund, and your pension?

When the banks reopen, would more bank runs shut them down again?

This is why you would do well to slowly begin removing funds from the bank. Keep the cash in a safe place. Withdraw money from your bank in small amounts. In this way, you will avoid long lines at the bank near the end. You should also be aware that computer-controlled electronic transactions involving ATM cards, credit cards, and the like cannot be processed in certain emergencies.

If you wish to remove very large amounts from your bank account, go to a bank officer and tell him what you are doing. You can mention that the Federal Reserve understands the problem and is printing an additional $50 billion to facilitate such demand. Tell him that you understand that you must fill out a form in order to arrange for such a large withdrawal. Be very courteous; but know that it is your money; and you have a legal right to withdraw the money.

You are breaking no laws by doing so. Smaller bills will be more useful in a time of crisis. A growing number of businesses today will not accept $50 and $100 bills. Several hundred dollars in rolled change could also be useful.

If you live in the country, it is rather easy to store money in jars in the ground outside your home. (Plastic lids cannot be detected by metal detectors.) If you live in the city, you may wish to purchase a safe. A safe is only safe when it contains certain substances which will turn to water if a fire occurs. That will limit the amount of heat buildup possible inside the safe. Then wait a week after the fire is past, before opening the safe. (Otherwise, the papers will burst into flame as soon as you open it.)

Tell no one except your spouse or a close family member about your stored savings.

Frankly, the welfare of the nation is better off if everyone only withdraws a small amount from the bank. But the amount you should withdraw will be an individual decision.

Pay all 30-day accounts by the latter part of the month! Do not wait until too late to pay them! If you pay in cash, get receipts. If you pay by check, you would do well to get receipts also.

Have paper records of all types of financial data.

Then there is the stock market. Get out of it! Trouble is coming. There are several reasons why we can expect a depression when the crisis hits. Experts advise that you sell all your bonds (including municipal bonds) and equity mutual funds.

Keep in mind that, if the government shuts down the stock market in a panic, you probably will not get your money back. This would also be true of every electronic promise to pay, including bank accounts. If it is a digital promise, it is a risky promise.

Here is another suggestion: End your automatic deposit of paychecks; have them given to you instead. End automatic utility payments; instead pay them by check (not cash, so you can prove your payment). Cash your checks at the grocery store or bank, and no longer at automatic teller machines. Carry $60 in rolled quarters and dimes in your car.

POSSIBILITY OF RELOCATION

Be prepared to relocate to a shelter for warmth and protection during a prolonged power outage.

Keep items you would most likely need during an evacuation in an easy-to-carry container. Be prepared to leave. Depending on the situation and the mode of transportation, this might be a large garbage can with a lid, a camping backpack, or a duffle bag.

Store this kit in a convenient place known to all family members. Or give one to each member. Keep a smaller version of this Disaster Supply Kit in the trunk of your car. Keep items in airtight plastic bags.

Be sure to take blankets, sleeping bags, etc., with you.

Plan first, second, and third choice places (homes, relatives, business) where you will go to reunite your family. Select two out-of-state relatives you will call if your family members are separated in a crisis. Have a secret hiding place at each location where you have food and supples and/or can leave a message if you must leave the location. Each family member should carry a copy of this information. Even your small children will have this, so adults can notify you if they become lost.

Give each family member a message beeper. Then have a few practice "emergencies." Teach each one how to turn off the household gas and electricity, and put out fires with salt, baking soda, water. Hold practice sessions. We put out a dangerous trailer fire by throwing wet towels over the beginning fire.

OTHER PREPARATIONS TO MAKE

Develop a sense of urgency; and pursue that strategy with a vengeance.

Make sure your computers are backed up properly! Have the information on them stored, so you can later retrieve it.

Have a battery operated radio for information about what is happening, where shelters are located. Knowing what is happening locally and in the nation during a crisis would be information you should have. Are riots taking place? Are the banks still open? Is the economy collapsing?

If possible, change your stored drinking water every 6 months, so it stays fresh. Rotate your stored food every 6 months.

Rethink your family needs at least once a year. Replace batteries, update clothes, etc. Ask your physician or pharmacist about storing prescription medications.

Contact your local emergency management of civil defense office and your local American Red Cross chapter. Find out which disasters are most likely to happen in your community. Ask how you would be warned. Find out how to prepare for each.

Meet with your family and discuss the types of disasters that could occur. Explain how to prepare and respond. Discuss what to do if advised to evacuate. Practice what you have discussed.

Plan how your family will stay in contact, if separated by disaster. Pick two meeting places: (1) a location a safe distance from your home, in case of fire, and (2) a place outside your neighborhood, in case you cannot return home. Choose an out-of-state friend as a "check-in-contact" for everyone to call.

Also do this: Post emergency telephone numbers by every phone. Show responsible family members

how and when to shut off water, gas, and electicity at the main switches. Install a smoke detector on each level of your home, especially near bedrooms. Test them monthly and change the batteries twice a year.

Meet with certain neighbors; plan how you could work together after a disaster. Know their skills (medical, technical). Consider how you could help neighbors who have special needs, such as the elderly and disabled persons. Make plans for child care in case parents cannot get home.

Remember to practice and maintain your plan.

STILL MORE THINGS TO CONSIDER

Request copies of all your medical records ahead of time.

Save canceled checks; so you can prove you made your payments.

Try to get out of debt, except for your home mortgage.

If you want to remove cash from banks, do not wait until everyone else will be doing it! If a run on the banks is made, laws could be quickly passed to shut down the banks.

If you have an unused RV or travel trailer in your driveway with a propane stove, fill up the propane tank and hang onto the camper rig.

HOME PROTECTION

In a time of local or national crisis, you will need the guardianship of angels. Plead with God for help and protection.

One expert recommends that everyone have a shotgun and rifle for personal protection and hunting wild game in time of crisis, as well as a supply of pepper spray. Another survival expert suggests purchasing 6 wasp and hornet sprays (cheaper than tear gas and as powerful). But the Lord is the best protection you can have.

Some may wish to install dead bolts on outside doors and windows.

SPECIAL CATALOGS

An outstanding catalog is Lehman's Non-Electric Catalog ($3.00). Order a copy today. P.O. Box 321, Kidron, Ohio 44636 (Phone: 330-857-5757) (Lehmans.com). —All kinds of things are in this catalog! The variety is fabulous. It includes grain mills, cast-iron cookware, canning and juicing equipment, heating and cookstoves, refrigerators (propane and diesel), solar power, toilets, washing machines, water pumps and buckets, water heaters, tools, wagons, buggies, and gardening and farming tools and equipment.

Here are more catalogs:

Natural Lifestyle: (phone: 800-752-2775; web: natural-lifestyle.com).

Campmor Catalog: P.O. Box 700-A, Saddle River,

New Jersey 07458-0700; phone: 800-226-7667. Camping gear especially.

Richters Herb Catalog: Goodwood, Ontario L0C 1A0; phone: 905-640-6677; fax 905-640-6641; web: richters.com

Heirloom Organics: address: 3388 Merlin Road, Ste 400, Grants Pass, OR. Phone number: 877-980-7333; www.heirloomorganics.com. They provide, for sale, nonhybrid, open-pollinated vegetable and fruit seeds in specialty packs (amounts for one person households, family, farms) of greens, fruit, beans, mixed, etc. at reasonable prices. Also for storing for emergency use.

BARTER ITEMS

Here is something to consider while there is still time to do it. You might wish to acquire some barter items. These are things you can later trade with the neighbors for garden food, etc.

There are five criteria which make a product useful for barter: (1) Not easily made at home. (2) High consumer demand. (3) Durable in storage. (4) Divisible in small quantities. (5) Its authenticity is easily recognizable.

You may not stock up on all of the following, but having a few would be good:

Liquid detergent, laundry detergent, rubbing alcohol, bleach, toothbrushes, razor blades, toilet paper, aluminum foil, writing paper, typing paper, pens, pencils, erasers, shoelaces, string, cord, rope, fishing line, insect repellent, water repellent, paint, varnish, matches, watches, tape, light bulbs, sewing supplies (such as needles, thread, zippers, buttons) aspirin, vitamins, seeds, grain, burn ointments, safety pins, manual can opener, knives, canning jars, lids, rings, socks, underwear, winter clothes, coats, blankets, quarts of multiviscosity motor oil, antifreeze, wire, glues, bolts, screws, and/or nails.

AND MORE THINGS TO CONSIDER

Every time you shop, purchase double or triple amounts. Stock up. You may be able to help others when the crisis comes. Remember Joseph in Egypt. He helped his family when they had their major crisis.

Find alternate methods of doing things.

Eliminate nonessentials from your life. Eliminate all those time wasters and money wasters and extra belongings you do not need. Get rid of your television set.

Simplify your lifestyle. Learn to say no to things or activities which do not make you self-sufficient.

Begin treating things as though they were not replaceable. Figure out how to do without. Buy things that will last. Obtain equipment which does not need electricity.

Always have more than one way to do something.

Organize your life. If you live in a disordered manner, it will cause you grief later on.

Eliminate distractions from your life. Be God-centered. He should be first, last, and best in all your plans and activities.

Believe that, with God's help, you can do it; then go ahead and tackle the job. Toughen up. Learn to get in and work, and carry it through to success.

Do not be spread too thin in your daily life. Take time with God and with others. Only certain things in life really matter.

Train your family to be guarded. Teach your children to not give information to a stranger. Be prepared for trouble ahead.

Get rid of things you do not use or need.

What items do you use daily that must be replaced by a third party? Could you make them in a pinch? If you could not, do you have spares?

Your first big mistake would be failure to prepare. Your second big mistake would be to rely on those preparations. Seek God for the help you need! He alone can guide and care for you through the coming crisis—and all the others.

Begin immediately. Start preparing!

Begin incrementally. Start preparing little by little. Every week add to your preparation.

Work with others. Some are better on water, others on electricity. Working together, you will accomplish more.

APPENDIX 1 - PREPARATION TIME LINE

This is a very brief sprinkling of points discussed in the preceding pages; but it will help you see the forest from the trees:

Rededicate your life to God. You only have a little time left. Death comes quickly to all of us.

If you have not moved out of the city yet, look for a place in the country to move to.

Select your garden area. Collect soil samples and send them off for testing.

Haul in manure; so it can rot and later be used on the garden.

Apply the recommended amount of lime, to make the soil a little more alkaline. Rely on the manure, leaf mold, etc., to supply the nitrogen, phosphorus, and potash.

Order some of the catalogs listed here; ask friends about other sources. We have listed only a few.

Go through this book and underline in black everything you need to stock up on; and start doing so.

Go through the book again and underline in red all the equipment you could get. Circle those items you want to order. Start doing so.

EMER

Review all your financial assets. Begin getting out of stocks and bonds. Gradually, week by week, withdraw more savings from the bank. Pay your debts.

Get rid of all your excess baggage.

Begin installation of the various equipment you are getting. Test it out.

Install the special electrical circuit for your generator backup electrical system.

Following a family preannouncement, turn off the electricity for one day that you and others in your family will be at home all day. Proceed with a variety of regular duties. Try to include washing some clothes and drying them. What could you not do? Did you need to? What other preparations yet need to be made?

If you have small ones, decide whether you will stock up on boxes of diapers or will return to the old-fashioned method. Try it for a day, and you will know what will work best for you.

Turn off the water another day. Better yet, turn it off the same day you turn off the electricity. —Because that is what is likely to happen later.

Turn off the propane on another day, and see how well you do.

Go back to the drawing board, and list other things to be done.

Set to work doing them.

By late spring plant your garden and learn from your mistakes. What went wrong? How could you have done better?

Late summer is time to plant your kale. Plant a lot of it, enough for your family and nearby friends.

Harvest the last of your crops, including the Hubbard squash. Spread it out, one layer high, on newspapers in a room which will stay dry and cool, but will not freeze. You can harvest and cook it throughout the winter as a fresh, starchy food.

By late September, you should have ordered nearly all your equipment and supplies. You might try to obtain more, but may have a much more difficult time doing so.

By this time, you have sold your stocks and bonds, and pulled all the money out of the bank which you intended to remove. Before the end of the year, serious runs on the bank could occur.

By this time, you have obtained copies of all your legal, medical, and personal records. Those papers are all organized in large envelopes in one place, preferably a box of some kind.

By this time, hopefully, you have your equipment and fuel storage facilities; and they are full of fuel. From this point onward, there are several more things to be done:

Finalize on obtaining receipts for every purchase, etc., and obtaining the latest copies of your financial records (bank statements, credit card account sta-

tus, home mortgage papers, etc.).

At some point in the last two months of the year, vaccum and clean your house thoroughly. Also thoroughly clean around your home. You may not easily be able to do so later for quite some time. If there are extra things to be washed or dry-cleaned, do it now.

Listen to the hourly news on the radio. If you have shortwave or web, you can also use it to keep in contact with what is taking place elsewhere in America and overseas.

Gas up the car frequently, keeping it full.

Pray for God's blessing on those who need it, and be aware of what is happening in the world.

Your heavenly Father will provide you with more complete wisdom as to what needs to be done, as you seek Him in prayer.

APPENDIX 2 - VOLTAGE REFERENCE GUIDE

Actual running watts may vary. Refer to your owner's manual for actual wattage. On the left, below, is listed the appliance or machine; and on the right is the *running watts*. (That is not the *starting watts!* Allow 3 times the listed watts for starting devices which have motors.)

Air Conditioner (12,000 BTU) 1700	
Battery Charger (20 amp)	500
Belt Sander (3-in.)	1000
Chain Saw	1200
Circular Saw (6½ in.)	600-1000
Coffee Maker	1000
Compressor (1 HP)	2000
Compressor (¾ HP)	1800
Compressor (½ HP)	1400
Curling Iron	700
Deep Freeze	500
Disc Sander (9 in.)	1200
Edge Trimmer	500
Electric Nail Gun	1200
Electric Range (I element)	1500
Electric Skillet	1250
Furnace Fan (1/3 UP)	1200
Hair Dryer	1200
Hand Drill (1 in.)	1100
Hedge Trimmer	450
Lawn Mower	12000
Light Bulb	100
Microwave Oven	700-1000
Milk Cooler	1100
Oil Burner on Furnace	300
Oil Fired Space Heater (140,000 BTU)	400
Oil Fired Space Heater (85,00 BTU)	225
Paint Sprayer, Airless (1/3 HP)	600
Paint Sprayer, Airless (handheld)	150
Radio	50-250

Refrigerator	600
Slow Cooker	200
Submersible Pump (1½ HP)	2800
Submersible Pump (1 HP)	2000
Saw Pump	600
Table Saw (10")	1750-2000
Television	200-500
Weed Trimmer	500

Allow 3 times the listed watts for starting these devices.

APPENDIX 1 - NATURAL DISASTERS

FLOOD—Find out if you live in a flood plain. If so, do the following: Learn the safest route to high, safe ground if you have to evacuate quickly. Have an emergency supply kit ready. It should include a portable radio, emergency cooking equipment, and flashlights.

If you live in a frequently flooded area, have shovels and sandbags. Fill the bags half full of sand immediately before or during the storm. (If done earlier, the bags will rot.) They will not completely seal out water. Keep children away from creeks, streams and storm drains. Water can rise fast.

Have check valves installed in your home's sewer traps, to prevent flood waters from backing sewage up into house. Use large corks or stoppers to plug showers, basins, etc. Move valuable things to upstairs floors. Fill bathtubs, sinks, and jugs with clean water, in case water becomes contaminated. If instructed to do so by local authorities, turn off all utilities. Be prepared to evacuate.

If outdoors, climb to high ground and stay there. If moving swiftly, even water 6 inches deep can sweep you off your feet. If in a car and you come to a flooded area, turn around and go another way. If car stalls, immediately leave it and go to higher ground. If indoors, move to the second floor or the roof. Take warm clothing, flashlight, and a portable radio with you. Do not try to swim to safety. Do not touch any electrical equipment, unless it is in a dry area and you are standing on a piece of dry wood while wearing rubber gloves and rubber-soled boots or shoes.

Afterward, throw away all food, including canned goods, that has come in contact with flood waters—for they have harmful bacteria. Until public drinking water is declared safe, boil drinking and cooking water 10 minutes before using it.

TORNADO—Keep alert to weather news. Know how likely you are to have a tornado in your area. In case of trouble, a storm cellar provides the best protection against a tornado. The next best place is a basement corner, a small interior room, or lay flat beneath a table or bed, away from windows. It is best to crouch in the southwest corner; since debris usually falls in the northeast corner. If you

are in a car, do not try to outrun a tornado. Get out and take shelter in a ditch or on low ground, but not under a tree.

HURRICANE—Read the sections, above, on floods and tornadoes. Watch news reports. Have an emergency kit, board up all windows, and go inland. The full fury of a hurricane only affects the 12 miles near the ocean; inland, the danger is from flooding.

EARTHQUAKE—In advance, know the safe spots in your house (inside walls, under sturdy tables, in stout doorways. And be sure those places are away from windows, fireplaces, tall furniture). It is not the shaking that can kill or injure; but it is the collapsing walls, flying glass, and falling objects. If inside, stay there. Take cover in a safe place—and hold on. If outdoors, move into the open—away from buildings, street lights, and utility wires. Stay there until the shaking stops. If in a car, slow down, stay in the vehicle, and move to a clear area away from buildings, trees, overpasses, or utility wires. When the shaking stops, proceed with caution; and avoid bridges or ramps that may have been damaged. Be prepared for aftershocks which might come even months later. They can be strong enough to topple more buildings and sever utility lines.

WILDFIRE—If you live near wildlands or woodland areas, be on guard. Have a portable gas-powered water pump, in case electricity fails. Install hose spigots on at least two sides of the house and near remote buildings, like garages. Install more outlets at 50 feet from the home.

Have a garden hose long enough to reach anything that is burning. It is good to have a small pond you can draw water from. Have a ladder as tall as your roof, rake, ax, handsaw or chainsaw, shovel, and buckets.

Be ready to evacuate. Tune radio to fire reports. Until then, protect your home. Wear sturdy shoes, protective clothing, gloves, and handkerchief to protect your face. Back car into garage or in open space, facing direction of escape. Leave key in ignition. Shut doors and windows, but leave unlocked. Disconnect automatic garage door openers. Shut off gas at meter, turn off pilot lights. Open fireplace damper; close fireplace screens. Move flammable furniture away from windows. Turn on a light in each room to increase visibility in heavy smoke. Turn off propane tanks. Put lawn sprinklers on roof and above ground fuel tanks. Turn them on and wet everything down. Wet or remove shrubs within 15 feet of house.

When you return after the fire, check roof and attic immediately and put out any sparks or embers. Watch for hot spots in the area that may start burning again. Recheck the house for hours afterward.

EMER

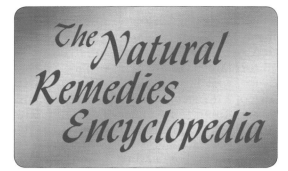

The Natural Remedies Encyclopedia

Emergency First Aid

WHEN AN EMERGENCY TREATMENT IS SUDDENLY NEEDED

F
I
R
S
T

A
I
D

POISON CONTROL CENTERS - 829
EMERGENCY PRESSURE POINTS - TO STOP BLEEDING - 2008-2009

This special section provides quick, basic information on dealing with a variety of emergency situations. Unlike the rest of the book, which deals with folk-based natural remedies, the information in this section is derived strictly from current medical advice and has been reviewed for accuracy by authorities in the field.

Relatively noncritical situations such as minor burns and insect stings that do not cause systemic reactions are dealt with elsewhere in this book, in alphabetical order. Here, we are dealing with those injuries that can potentially cause permanent or fatal damage.

This is not a complete guide to first aid. It does not cover, for instance, severe multiple injuries that might result from violent accidents. For a more complete guide to first aid, we recommend that you buy and keep on hand a first aid book published by an authoritative source such as the American Medical Association or the American Red Cross.

BREATHING CRISIS (CPR)
Breathing Crisis Procedure

Without oxygen a person can die in minutes. So, regardless of other injuries, if there is no breathing, artificial breathing becomes the first priority.

If you encounter someone who appears not to be breathing, the first step is to quickly determine if the person is conscious.

1. Gently shake the person's shoulder and ask loudly if he or she is all right. If he can answer, he can breathe. Watch for any breathing difficulties while you tend to other injuries.

If there is no response, check the breathing.

2. Clear and open the airway. This is done as follows:

A. Lay the person on his back on a hard surface, such as the floor or ground.

B. With your finger, quickly clear the mouth of any foreign matter.

C. If there appears to be no neck injury, place one hand under the neck and lift. Place the heel of the other hand on the forehead and press down. Now the victim's head will be tilted back as far as possible ("head-tilt").

D. If there is suspicion of a neck injury, either by the nature of the injury or by complaint of neck pain, do not tilt the head back. Put your forefingers and two middle fingers at the corners of the jaw by the earlobes and lift the jaw up toward you ("jaw-thrust").

Certified First Responders in the U.S.

A certified first responder is a person who has completed a course and received certification in providing pre-hospital care for medical emergencies. They have more skill than someone who is trained in basic first aid but they are not a substitute for advanced medical care rendered by emergency medical technicians (EMTs), emergency physicians, nurses, or paramedics. First responder courses cover cardiopulmonary resuscitation (CPR), automated external defibrillator usage, spinal and bone fracture immobilization, oxygen and, in some cases, emergency childbirth as well as advanced first aid. The term "certified first responder" is not to be confused with "first responder", which is a generic term referring to the first medically trained responder to arrive on scene (police, fire, EMS). Most police officers and all professional firefighters in the US and Canada, and many other countries, are certified first responders. This is the required level of training. Some police officers and firefighters take more training to become EMTs or paramedics.

First Responders in the US can either provide emergency care first on the scene (police/fire department/park rangers) or support Emergency Medical Technicians and Paramedics, provide basic first aid, CPR, Automated external defibrillator use, spinal immobilization, oxygen, and assist in emergency childbirth (in some areas they are trained in the use of suction and airway adjuncts. CFRs can also assist with providing glucose, aspirin, and epipens. They are also trained in packaging, moving and transporting patients.

First responder training differs per state or country. Lifesaving skills in the first responder course include recognizing unsafe scenarios and hazardous materials emergencies, protection from blood borne pathogens, controlling bleeding, applying splints, conducting a primary life-saving patient assessment, in-line spinal stabilization and transport, CPR, and calling for more advanced medical help. Some areas give more training in other life-saving techniques and equipment.

When a person is unconscious the tongue can drop back and block the throat or airway as it is called. The above head-tilt or jaw-thrust lifts the tongue and opens the airway.

E. On a victim with no neck injury, if the head-tilt does not open the airway, do a jaw-thrust also.

3. Put the side of your face and ear close to the person's mouth and nose, and look at the chest. Is he or she breathing now? Is the chest rising and falling, and do you feel and hear air being exhaled? Take about five seconds for this. Sometimes,

QUICK PICTURE GUIDE

IF CONCIOUS, BUT CHOKING —
Give abdominal thrusts until
the object comes out. *(755)*

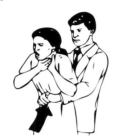

**IF UNCONSCIOUS AND NOT BREATHING,
DO RESCUE BREATHING—**
Give 1 slow breath about every 5 seconds. If you breaths are not going in, retilt head and give more breaths. *(755)*

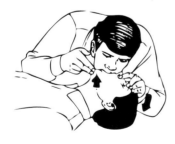

IF AIR STILL WON'T GO IN—
Give up to 5 abdominal thrusts.
(755)

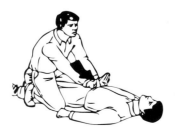

Then pause, and with a hooked fingersweep, remove any object from his mouth. Then give two slow breaths to check if throat cleared. If not, give 5 more thrusts. *(756)*

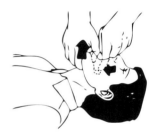

IF NOT BREATHING, AND THERE IS NO PULSE — GIVE CPR
Count aloud, "one and two and three, etc." as you do the compressions. Maintain a smooth, steady rhythm. When you give breaths, be sure to open the victim's airway with a head tilt and a chin lift. *(753)*

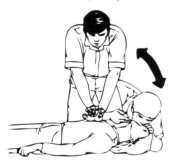

Do cycles of 15 chest compressions and 2 slow breaths. After 4 continuous cycles, check for a pulse. If there is no pulse, continue CPR. Begin with chest compressions and recheck for a pulse every few minutes. If you do find a pulse, check for breathing. If the victim has a pulse but is not breathing, go to rescue breathing.

F
I
R
S
T

A
I
D

simply by opening the airway, a person begins breathing on his own.

If there is no breathing: (**How to do RESCUE BREATHING**)

4. Keep the person's airway open with a head-tilt and/ or jaw-thrust.

5. While the heel of your one hand remains on the victim's forehead, use the thumb and forefinger of that hand to pinch closed the victim's nose. When trying to inflate the victim's lungs through the mouth, air must not come out the nose when it should be going to the lungs. Another way of doing the same thing is to press your cheek against the person's nose while blowing into the mouth.

6. Inflate the victim's lungs with four full quick breaths. Here's how:

A. Open your mouth wide and take a deep breath.

B. Cover the victim's mouth with your mouth and form a seal.

C. Quickly blow four full breaths allowing very little air to escape from the victim's lungs in between the breaths. Before you begin rhythmic breathing, the lungs need to be inflated as much as possible. Also, the victim may begin breathing. This is why the initial four strong breaths are necessary.

7. Again, put the side of your face and ear close to the person's mouth and nose, and look at the chest while maintaining the head-tilt and/or jaw-thrust. Is the victim breathing now? Also, check for a pulse. Take at least five seconds to check for a pulse, but no more than ten seconds.

8. Check for a pulse in the neck. Find the Adam's apple and move in either direction to one of the grooves in the neck. Feel with the tips of your forefinger and two middle fingers. The carotid artery is in those grooves.

If there is no pulse:

9. If you have had cardiopulmonary resuscitation (CPR) training, begin that technique.

10. Call (or preferably have someone else call) an ambulance or paramedics. If necessary, have someone drive you and the victim to a hospital while you perform artificial breathing or CPR en route.

If there is a pulse, but no breathing, or if you do not know CPR, try to restore breathing.

11. Blow into the person's mouth once every five seconds (12 times per minute) as described below:

A. Each time take a deep breath, form a seal, and blow until the victim's chest rises and expands. Moderate resistance is expected. But if the chest won't rise, add a jaw-thrust to the head-tilt.

B. Then raise your mouth and turn your head to the side to watch the victim's chest fall, and to feel and hear the air leaving the lungs.

C. After each breath count five seconds with, "one- one thousand, two-one thousand, three-one thousand, . . ." and so on.

12. Continue the mouth-to-mouth resuscitation until the person begins to breathe well on his own, until medical help comes, or until a doctor tells you to stop. If necessary, have someone drive you and the victim to a hospital while you perform artificial breathing en route.

Babies and Small Children

With infants and small children the procedure for restoring breathing is basically the same except that you should not tilt the head back as far as you would an adult's or large child's head. Instead:

1. Tilt' the baby's head by putting one of your hands under the baby's back and shoulders and lifting slightly. That will allow the head to drop back.

2. Put your mouth over the infant's mouth and nose. You do not pinch a baby's nose closed.

3. Use only small puffs of air until you see the chest rise and expand. Babies require much less air to inflate their lungs than adults.

4. Inflate the chest every three seconds (20 times per minute).

5. In infants check for the heartbeat below the left nipple.

No Air Exchange

If for some reason air is being obstructed from going in and out of the victim's lungs:

1. Repeat the steps for tilting the head and/ or thrusting the jaw. That may open the airway for breathing.

If there is still no air being exchanged, then there must be an obstruction which needs to be cleared out. Here is what to do:

2. Turn the person on his side facing you. Rest the person's chest against your knees.

3. Deliver four sharp hits between the shoulder blades, as rapidly as possible.

If the obstruction is not cleared out:

4. Roll the victim on his back and deliver four forceful, rapid upward abdominal thrusts. Perform the thrusts in the manner described below:

A. Straddle the victim at his hips or one thigh.

B. Put one hand on top of the other and place the heel of the lower hand slightly above the victim's navel but below the ribs. Keep your arms straight—elbows locked.

C. Push quickly and forcefully with forward and downward thrusts, four times directly toward the person's head. Do not push to the right or left or you may damage the liver or spleen.

If there are still no results, perform a finger sweep.

5. With one hand, grab the victim's lower jaw and tongue and lift away from the back of the throat.

6. Put the index finger of your other hand on the inside of one of the victim's cheeks. Go down the cheek into the throat by the base of the tongue.

7. Using your finger like a hook, attempt to dislodge the obstruction and bring it up and out of the person's mouth. Be careful not to push the object further into the throat. Never use any instrument (such as forceps) to remove a foreign object.

8. Do not stop until the obstruction is dislodged or until medical help comes. You may be able to at least partially dislodge the obstruction so that breathing or artificial breathing can be done enough to keep the person alive.

9. When the object has been dislodged and breathing is restored, seek medical assistance. Even if you get the victim breathing, there may be damage to the respiratory tract or some other injury which could lead to other problems.

Obstructed Breathing in Babies and Small Children

Because of the smaller size, there are differences when dislodging an object from the throat of a baby or small child. The procedure is basically the same as for adults except for the following:

1. Put a baby or small child face down across your forearm or lap. The head should be lower than the rest of the body.

2. Deliver four quick blows with the heel of your hand between the shoulder blades. The blows are less forceful than those needed for an adult.

If hitting the back is unsuccessful, give four thrusts as described below:

3. Put the infant face up across your forearm or lap. The head should be lower than the rest of the body.

4. Place two or three fingertips on the breastbone between the infant's nipples on the sternum and press into the chest with four quick inward thrusts. For a child you could use the heel of one hand. Thrusting is done gently with a baby or small child. It can be done at the abdomen, but there is the possibility of injury.

5. With one of your smaller fingers, do a finger sweep. Because their mouths are so small compared with your fingers, there is the risk of pushing the obstruction further down the infant's throat. If you believe that even your smallest finger is too large, then do not do any finger sweeps.

6. Repeat the steps until the obstruction is dislodged.

A. Attempt an air exchange.
B. Four blows to the back.
C. Four chest thrusts.
D. Finger sweep, if your fingers are small enough.

Choking in Fat or Pregnant People

The abdominal thrust is different than that for other adults. The rest of the procedure is the same.

1. For the abdominal thrusts, put a fist, with your other hand over it, on the middle of the breastbone between the breasts. (Don't get off to either side onto the ribs.)

Deliver four quick, forceful thrusts.

Drowning

A drowning victim's stomach may be bloated with swallowed water. You may still perform artificial breathing, but be aware that the person may regurgitate the water.

You could quickly attempt to empty the stomach as follows:

1. Turn the person on his stomach.
2. Put both hands under the stomach and lift. If no water comes out after about ten seconds, turn the person back over.
3. Turn the person on his back and resume artificial breathing.

BURNS

Third-Degree Burns

The most severe burns are called third degree. All the layers of skin tissue are destroyed.

While first- and second-degree burns are red in appearance, third-degree burns look white or charred. Oddly enough you may also notice the lack of severe pain. That is because third-degree burns are so extensive that the nerve endings are also destroyed.

Part of the immediate treatment for a victim of third- degree burns is not to do certain things.

1. Do not remove any clothing that is stuck to the burn. That should be done only by a doctor.
2. Do not use ice or ice water on the burn. That will make the shock reaction work.
3. Do not put any ointments, sprays, antiseptics or home preparations on the burn. No matter what is written on the label or said in the ads.

Do take the following steps:

4. Check the person's breathing. Frequently a burn victim will develop problems with breathing. You must maintain an open airway and look for any difficulties with breathing. (See Breathing Crises this section.)
5. Put a cold cloth or cool water (not iced) on burns of the face, feet or hands. For burns on the face, feet or hands, this can be soothing. These areas are particularly sensitive.
6. Cover the burn with a thick sterile dressing or with a clean linen. Sterile dressings can be purchased at drugstores. If you don't have any dressings, you can use a clean pillowcase or sheet, or even a baby's disposable diaper.
7. Call an ambulance. The victim must be transported to a hospital promptly. You should always consult a doctor even with what appears to be a small third-degree burn.

Once you have done all of the above, continue to care for the person in the following ways until help arrives:

8. Keep burned hands and arms higher than the level of the person's heart. Pillows. or blankets are good for elevating limbs. Remove rings or bracelets.
9. Keep burned legs and feet higher than the level of the person's heart. Use pillows or blankets.
10. For burns of the face or neck, have the person sit up or prop him up with pillows. Check his breathing frequently. A person burned about the face will develop difficulty breathing within minutes.
11. Treat for shock reaction. As long as the person does riot have face or neck injuries (in which case he would be propped up), treat for shock as follows:
    A. Keep the person lying down.
    B. Elevate the person's feet about 12 inches. If the person complains of pain, lower the feet. Do not raise the feet if there are injuries of the neck, spine, head, chest, lower face or jaw.
    C. Keep the person comfortably warm, but not hot. IF the person is outside on the ground, try to place a blanket underneath him.
12. Keep the person calm and reassure him that he will be all right. This is very important, especially for shock reaction.

If the burn victim is unconscious or facial damage is extensive, put the person on his side. This is to allow fluids (saliva, blood, vomit) to drain out of the mouth. Otherwise the person could choke. If the person is having trouble breathing, slightly elevate the head and shoulders, but keep him on his side.

Immediate medical attention is needed for any burn (not just third degree) that covers over 15 percent of the adult body or 10 percent of a child's body. How can you tell area size? One of the hands {front and back) and its fingers is about 1 percent of total body area. An adult hand is about 3 to 4 percent of a baby's body.

You will also want to be watchful of a person who has inhaled smoke or the fumes of any burning substance, or who has facial burns. Lung damage could develop, and as a result, breathing problems. Get him to a doctor as soon as possible.

If it appears that medical help is over two hours away, give the person the following mixture in the appropriate amount:

Take one quart of cool water. Mix in 1 level teaspoon of salt and 2 level teaspoon of baking soda. Give an adult (over 12 years old) 1/2 cup (four ounces); give a child (1 to 12 years old) 1/4 cup (two ounces); give an infant (less than 1 year old) one ounce. Have the adult, child or infant sip the appropriate amount slowly over a 15-minute period. Clear fruit juices (like apple juice) may also be given.

Never give fluids to a person who is unconscious, having convulsions, vomiting, or who is likely to need surgery because of serious injuries.

Chemical Burns

Treatment for chemical burns is immediate irrigation of the area. Use plenty of water. The longer the chemical is in contact with the body, the more extensive the injury.

1. Flush the burn area with running water for at least five minutes. Think about heading for the nearest garden hose, shower or tub. Or even buckets of water if that's closer. Try not to use too powerful a stream of water. Use whatever normally feels comfortable to you in the shower.
2. Remove any clothing from the burned area while you wash the area. The chemical substance will be on the clothing too. You want to get it off the person to avoid further contact with the chemical.
3. After flushing the burn with water, read the label of the chemical container and follow any first aid instructions offered.
4. Cover the burn with a clean bandage or cloth. A clean towel might be the handiest, or use a pillowcase or sheet.
5. Get medical attention.

As with third-degree burns there are certain things you must never do.

6. Do not apply antiseptics, ointments, sprays or home preparations. This could complicate or increase the severity of the burn.

Chemical Burns of the Eye

Again, the important thing is to act fast because damage may occur in one to five minutes. You will need water to flush the chemical out of the eye, or you can use milk if water isn't available.

1. Have the person lie down or lean over something. Leaning over a sink or a drinking fountain would be best. But don't waste time looking for a sink if there is a closer source of running water.
2. Turn the person's head to the side with the burned eye closest to the floor.
3. Hold the upper and lower lid apart with your thumb and forefinger and pour water all over the eye, from the inner corner (by the nose) of the eye outward. This procedure is important because it avoids washing the chemical into the unaffected eye. If both eyes are affected, pour water over both of them. Separate the eyelids and reach all parts of the eyes with the water.
4. Flood the eye for at least ten minutes.
5. Close the eye and cover it with a piece of sterile dressing. (Do not use cotton balls. Cotton fibers will come out and stick to the wound and eyelashes.) Sterile gauze pads are available in drugstores. A clean folded handkerchief would also work.
6. Tell the person not to touch his eyes. Rubbing the eyes could increase the damage.
7. Get medical assistance. If possible, call an eye specialist or go to the nearest hospital emergency room.

CHOKING

The signs of choking are:
- Noisy breathing and gasping (crowing sounds) as the choking victim tries to inhale.
- Victim usually grasps his throat.
- Inability to speak.
- Victim may cease breathing.
- Skin turns pale, blue or gray.
- Alarmed expression and behavior. Panic.
- Finally, unconsciousness.

Victim is Conscious

1. As long as the person can speak, breathe or cough, do not interfere. Coughing is the body's natural mechanism for expelling an obstruction from the larynx. Be calm and reassuring.
2. Do not give the victim anything to eat or drink to "wash the object down."
3. If the person is standing or sitting, perform four abdominal thrusts:
   A. Stand behind the victim and put your arms around his waist.
   B. Make a fist and place it (thumb side toward you) the person's navel, but below the ribs and breastbone. Hold that fist with your other hand.
   C. Perform four fast, strong upward thrusts. You are pushing on the abdomen which in turn pushes the diaphragm and forces air (and hopefully the obstruction) out of the victim's mouth.
   D. Do not squeeze with your arms. Use your fists only.
4. If the person is lying down, deliver four abdominal thrusts:
   A. Roll the victim onto his back. Kneel beside him, or straddle his hips or one thigh.
   B. Put one of your hands on top of the other with the heel of the lower hand placed slightly above the victim's navel, but below his ribs and breastbone.
   C. Perform four fast, strong upward thrusts directly toward the victim's head. Do not push off to either side. Keep your elbows locked and thrust with your upper body.
5. If the object is not yet dislodged, repeat the four abdominal thrusts until the object is coughed up or the person loses consciousness. (See following page for unconscious victim.)
6. Keep checking the person's mouth and top of his throat to see if the object appears. If it does, pull it out with your fingers.

Victim is Unconscious

1. Put the person on his back on a hard surface.
2. Try to open the airway with a head-tilt or jaw-thrust. Attempt an air exchange. (See Breathing Crises this section.)
3. If there is still an obstruction and no air exchange, roll the victim onto his back and deliver four strong abdominal thrusts. (See step 4 above, Conscious Victim.)
4. If still unsuccessful, perform a finger sweep:
   A. Grasp the person's lower jaw and tongue and lift up. That lifts the tongue from the back of the throat and maybe away from the obstruction.
   B. Put your forefinger inside one of the victim's cheeks. Slide it down the inside of the cheek into the throat to the base of the tongue. Sweep your finger across the back of the throat.
   C. Using your finger like a hook, try to dislodge the object and bring it out along the inside of the other cheek.
   D. Be careful. Do not push the object farther down the throat.
   E. Never try to remove an obstruction with any kind of instrument. Use only your finger.
5. Repeat the steps of attempting an air exchange—four abdominal thrusts and a finger sweep until the obstruction is dislodged and the person is breathing or until medical help comes. Do not give up.
6. Even if the object is dislodged, get medical help for all choking victims. Damage may have occurred to the respiratory tract.

Choking in Infants and Small Children

The procedure is basically the same as for adults except for the following:

1. Put a baby or small child face up across your forearm or lap. The head should be lower than the rest of the body.
2. Place two or three fingertips between the child's nipples and press into the chest with four quick inward thrusts. Thrusting is done gently with a baby or small child. It can be done at the abdomen, but there is the possibility of injury.
3. With one of your smaller fingers, do a finger sweep. Because their mouths are so small compared with your fingers, there is the risk of pushing the obstruction further down the infant's throat. If you believe that even your smallest finger is too large, then do not do any finger sweeps.

4. Repeat the steps until the obstruction is dislodged.

Choking in Fat or Pregnant People

The abdominal thrust is different than that for other adults. The rest of the procedure is the same.

1. For the abdominal thrusts, put a fist, with your other hand over it, on the middle of the breastbone between the breasts. (Don't get off to either side onto the ribs.)
2. Deliver four quick, forceful thrusts. Do not squeeze with your arms. Just use your fists.

DIABETIC EMERGENCIES

Diabetic Coma

A diabetic coma is the result of too little insulin in the victim's body. The person may have forgotten his insulin injection, eaten the wrong food or may have an infection.

The symptoms of a diabetic coma which are the opposite of those of insulin shock (see below for Insulin Shock) are:

- Symptoms begin gradually.
- Person is very thirsty, but not hungry.
- Hot, dry skin. May be flushed.
- Drowsiness.
- Fruity odor to breath. Breathing is deep and rapid. Dry mouth and tongue.
- Nausea and vomiting.
- Frequent urination.

Your only job is to obtain medical help immediately. If possible, go to the nearest hospital emergency room.

Insulin Shock

Insulin shock is the result of too little blood sugar in the victim's body. The person may have injected too much insulin, not eaten enough or exercised too much.

The symptoms of insulin shock which are the opposite of those of diabetic coma are:

- Symptoms begin abruptly.
- Person may be hungry, not thirsty.
- Perspiration, pale skin.
- Nervous behavior or belligerent.
- Breath does not smell fruity. Shallow to normal breathing. Moist mouth and tongue.
- No vomiting.

If the person is conscious, give him or her food containing sugar, such as honey, fruit juice or just sugar in water. Then obtain medical help.

If the person is unconscious, quickly get medical help. If possible, go to the nearest hospital emergency room.

DROWNING

It is possible to save a drowning person even if you can't swim, but be careful not to risk your own life. Don't overestimate your strength or ability. A drowning victim may panic and pull you under the water with him.

1. If the person is near the edge of a swimming pool, a dock, a pier, etc., don't get in the water. Extend your hand or foot to him, or a life preserver, board, pole, deck chair, stick, towel, rope, etc., and pull the person in.
2. If the person is too far away, either wade into waist- deep water and extend an object or, if necessary, row a boat to the victim and extend the oar or some object to him and pull him to the boat. The victim should hold onto the back of the boat while you row in. If he can't hold on, carefully try to get the victim into the boat.
3. If the person has lost consciousness or if you suspect a neck or back injury (as might happen in a surfing accident), put a board (like a surfboard) beneath the victim's head and back while he is still in the water. Remove the person from the water on the board. That procedure prohibits movement and might prevent paralysis.

If the Victim is Not Breathing

Begin artificial breathing as soon as the victim's body can be supported (see Breathing Crises this section), in a boat, for instance. Once you have the person out of the water, lay him down on a hard surface and continue mouth-to-mouth breathing.

People drown from lack of air, not because there is water in the lungs or stomach. So do not waste time trying to empty the lungs or stomach, but be aware that the victim may regurgitate water.

Get medical help. Call an ambulance or paramedics and tell them of the drowning. If necessary, have someone take you to the nearest hospital emergency room while you perform artificial breathing en route.

Treat for shock.

If the Victim is Breathing

1. Remain for a while to be sure that the person is breathing well on his own.
2. Turn the person on his side. Extend the head backward to allow fluids to drain from the mouth.
3. Victim should be comfortably warm. Use blankets, clothes or towels. If he is on a cold wet surface, attempt to put a blanket beneath him.
4. Never give the victim water or food.
5. Be kind, cairn and reassuring.
6. Get immediate medical attention.

Cold Water Drowning

There have been people totally submerged in cold water (below 70°F) for as long as 38 minutes who have survived. Young children, especially, are able to survive long immersion, often without brain damage. The body reacts to the cold water by slowing the heartbeat and reserving the oxygen present in the blood for the brain and heart.

Artificial breathing or cardiopulmonary resuscitation (if you have had CPR training) must be started as soon as possible. (See Breathing Crises this section.) Victims of cold water drowning may not respond to mouth-to-mouth breathing for three or more hours. Until they do respond, they may appear dead. Do not give up!

ELECTRIC SHOCK

Do not touch a person directly if he or she is still in contact with a "live electric current. Wait until the electricity is turned off or until the victim is no longer in contact with the electric current. Otherwise, you also will receive an electric shock.

A person who has been struck by lightning may he touched immediately.

Remember, chances of survival are better the sooner the person has broken contact with the electric current.

1. Try to turn off the electric current. You can do this by removing the fuse or by pulling the main electrical switch.

You can also call the electric company and ask them to cut off the electricity.

If the current can't be turned off or you just don't know how, the following steps may be taken:

2. It may be necessary to remove the victim from a live wire or electrical source. Be very careful not to touch the victim directly.
3. Make sure you are standing on something. You can use a piece of wood, a newspaper, a piece of clothing, a rubber mat or a blanket.
4. If available, wear dry gloves.
5. Move the victim off the wire using something dry. Do not touch the victim directly. You can use a dry piece of wood or a broom handle. Or try to loop a rope around an arm or leg, and pull.
6. Never use anything that is wet, damp or has any metal on it.
7. If you cannot pull or push the person from the live wire (maybe because the person is too heavy), very carefully push or pull the electrical source away from the person.
   A. Never touch the wire directly.
   B. Stand on something dry. If possible something made of rubber or a dry board.
   C. If possible wear dry gloves, or even insulated gloves.
   D. Push or pull the wire with something dry like a broom handle. If available, use an instrument made of rubber or plastic.

After you have the person away from the electrical current:

8. Check his breathing. If necessary, begin artificial breathing. (If artificial breathing is needed, see Breathing Crises this section.) You may have to do this a long time so don't get discouraged. Even if the person is breathing, he should be examined by a doctor.
9. Obtain medical help. If that is not possible, get someone else to drive you and the victim to a hospital emergency room while you give artificial breathing en route.
10. Even small electrical burns may cause severe damage. Seek medical attention for any electrical burn.

EYE INJURIES

For chemical burns in the eyes, see Burns this section. Any sudden pain, blurring or loss of vision requires immediate medical help.

F
I
R
S
T

A
I
D

Foreign Particles in the Eye

Foreign particles such as eyelashes, cinders or small bugs may be blown or rubbed into the eye. Such particles are irritating to the eyeball and there is always the danger that the particle could scratch the eyeball or might even become embedded.

If you suspect that something is actually sticking into someone's eyeball, take the following steps:

1. Do not let the person rub his eye.
2. Before examining the eye, wash your hands thoroughly with soap and water.
3. If there is something sticking into the eyeball, do not attempt to remove it.
4. Cover both eyes with sterile compresses or clean cloths. Loosely bandage the compresses in place. (Covering both eyes lessens the possibility that the victim will move his affected eye.) If you don't have a bandage, use a scarf, a tie or anything long enough to tic around the victim's head.
5. Get medical help immediately, an eye specialist if possible. If you take the person to a hospital emergency room, keep the victim lying down.

If the particle is just floating on the eyeball or inside the eyelid, do the following:

1. Do not let the person rub his eye.
2. Before examining the eye, wash your hands thoroughly with soap and water.
3. Gently pull the upper eyelid down over the lower eyelid. Hold for a moment. This will cause tearing and may flush out the particle.
4. If the tears do not wash the particle out, get a medicine dropper. Fill it with warm water and squeeze it over the eyeball to flush out the particle.
5. If the flushing is unsuccessful, then pull down the lower lid and see if the particle is there. If it is on the inside of the lower lid, carefully lift the particle with the moistened corner of a clean handkerchief, cloth or paper tissue. Do not use dry cotton balls because loose fibers can become stuck to the eye.
6. If the particle is not on the inside of the lower lid, look at the upper lid. Have the person look down through this entire procedure. Pull the eyelashes of the upper eyelid downward. While holding the eyelid

down, place a matchstick or cotton swab across the outside of the lid. Then fold the eyelid back over the matchstick by gently pulling upward on the eyelashes. While the victim holds the matchstick, carefully remove the particle with a moistened corner of a clean handkerchief, cloth or paper tissue. Gently replace the eyelid.

7. If the particle is still in the eye, cover both eyes with sterile compresses and get medical assistance promptly.

Cuts of the Eye

Cuts to the eye or eyelid can be very serious. There is the danger of blindness if treatment is not immediate.

1. Put a sterile gauze pad over both eyes (to stop movement). Bandage the pad in place, but apply no pressure.
2. Get medical help immediately, preferably an eye specialist. If necessary, take the person to a hospital in a lying position.

Blunt Injuries

A blunt injury usually results in a black eye. Even though the injury may not appear to be serious, there is the possibility of internal bleeding. So treat the victim as follows:

I. Put cold compresses on the injured eye.
2. Try to keep the victim lying down with his eyes closed.
3. Get medical help. If it's necessary to take the victim to a hospital, transport the person lying down.

Contact Lenses

When there is an eye injury to a person wearing contact lenses, the lenses should be removed as soon as possible but only by a physician, preferably an ophthalmologist.

FROSTBITE AND COLD EXPOSURE

Frostbite

Frostbite is the freezing of fluids in the skin and the underlying soft tissues. It usually happens to small areas on cheeks, the toes, fingers, nose and ears when they've been exposed for a long period of time to extreme cold. Wind and humidity can speed the freezing. Thawing and refreezing a frostbitten part can worsen the injury.
The signs of frostbite are:

- At first the affected skin is red and painful.
- The skin becomes white or grayish yellow and looks pale and glossy. It feels waxy and firm, and the pain disappears, replaced by cold and numbness.
- Typically the victim does not know he has frostbite. Someone else usually observes the symptoms first.

Immediate first aid has three objectives. First, to protect the affected part from further injury. Second, to quickly warm the area. And third, to monitor the victim's breathing.

1. Cover the frozen part. If you're still outside, use extra clothing. If the hands are affected, put them under the armpits to make use of body heat. Get the person inside as quickly as possible and cover with blankets.
2. Warm the frostbitten part quickly by putting it in warm (never hot) water. The water should be 100°F to 104°F. Use a thermometer or test the water on the inside of your arm.
3. If there isn't any warm water, gently wrap the area with a blanket or sheet.
4. Stop warming the frostbitten area as soon as the skin turns pink and/or feeling returns.
5. Get medical help.

You must never do the following. These actions can increase the severity of the injury.

1. Do not rub the part with your hand or anything else. That may cause gangrene (tissue death).
2. Do not use heat lamps, hot water bottles or heating pads.
3. Do not break the blisters.
4. Do not let the person hold the frostbitten part near a hot stove or radiator. The affected area could burn before feeling returns.
5. Do not give the person alcoholic beverages.
6. Do not let the victim walk if the feet or toes are involved.
7. Do not apply dressings or bandages unless you have to transport the victim to a medical facility.

Until medical help comes, you can continue to care for the victim in the following manner:

I. Give the person something warm to drink like tea or soup.
2. Tell the person to exercise toes and fingers after they are warmed.
3. Use dry, sterile gauze to separate frostbitten fingers or toes.
4. Make certain thawed areas do not refreeze.
5. If possible, elevate frostbitten part. Use pillows or blankets.
6. If you must transport the victim, keep the affected parts elevated and covered with clean cloth.

Cold Exposure

Cold exposure or hypothermia is the chilling or freezing of the entire body. The victim could have any one or all of these symptoms:

- Shivering.
- Numbness.
- Drowsiness or sleepiness.
- A low body temperature.
- Muscular weakness.
- If severely chilled or frozen, the victim may lose consciousness.

If the person is unconscious, you must proceed as follows:

1. Monitor person's breathing. (See Breathing Crises this section.)
2. Quickly get the person into a warm room.
3. Remove any wet, frozen or constricting clothing.
4. Warm the person by wrapping in warm blankets, sheets or towels.
5. Get immediate medical help.

Until medical help comes you may:

6. Give a conscious victim something warm to drink. Do not give alcoholic beverages.
7. See the above treatment for frostbite.

HEART ATTACK

IMMEDIATELY TURN TO PAGE 513!!

A heart attack results from the lack of blood and oxygen getting to a portion of the heart muscle. The deprived portion of the heart muscle may die if it is without blood and oxygen for a long period of time.

A heart attack is complex. The person may have a history of heart disease or an attack could come with no warning at all. The victim may or may not lose consciousness. And the degree of pain the victim is having is not a good indicator of the seriousness of the attack.

FIRST AID

Any one or all of the following could be a symptom of a heart attack:

- A persistent central chest pain, usually under the breastbone. The pain is not sharp, but the victim feels as though something is hugging the chest and crushing it. The pain usually spreads to the shoulders and arms, especially the left arm, or to the neck or jaw, mid-back or the upper abdomen.
- Shortness of breath. Gasping, perhaps.
- Victim is very weak.
- Pale skin, or the lips, skin and fingernail beds may look blue.
- Heavy sweating.
- The person is anxious and afraid.
- The victim may be nauseated or vomiting.
- A good sign of heart disease is swollen ankles.
- Frequently the pain and discomfort is mistaken for indigestion.

If the Victim is Conscious

1. Gently put the victim in what he feels is a comfortable position. This is usually sitting up because breathing is easier. Use pillows to make him as comfortable as possible.
2. Loosen any tight clothing, especially around the neck.
3. Close off any drafts or coldness. Keep the victim comfortably warm.
4. Be calm and reassuring.
5. Call an ambulance or paramedics. Tell them the problem and that oxygen is needed. If that is not possible, take the victim to a doctor or hospital immediately.
6. The person could have a history of heart disease and be under medical care. Help him with his medication. (The victim may be wearing an emergency medical identification. Look for a necklace or bracelet.)

If the Victim is Unconscious and Not Breathing

See Breathing Crises this section.
Initiate cardiopulmonary resuscitation (CPR) if you are trained in it.

You Are Alone and Having a Heart Attack

1. Call an ambulance or paramedics. Tell them the problem and that you need oxygen.
2. Get comfortable. That usually means sitting

up or in a semi-sitting position. Pillows will help make you feel more comfortable.

3. Loosen any tight clothing, especially around the neck.
- Painful stomach cramps and possible cramping elsewhere in the body.
- Breathing and speaking difficulties or tightness in the chest.

You need to slow down the absorption and spread of the spider's venom. The immediate treatment is as follows:

BROWN RECLUSE SPIDER BITE

The brown recluse spider is also very dangerous, especially to young children. Its distinctive marking is a dark brown violin-shaped marking located on the top front portion of its body. (It's also called a fiddler spider.)

After being bitten by a brown recluse spider, any one or all of the signs below may appear:

- At the time of the bite there is stinging.
- At first redness, then a blister.
- Pain increases severely over the next 8 hours.
- Within the next 48 hours, the victim may develop chills, fever, nausea, vomiting, pains in the joints and a rash.
- There is destruction of red blood cells and other changes in the blood.

The first aid for a bite from the brown recluse spider is the same as for the black widow described previously.

If the Victim is Conscious

1. Monitor the person's breathing. (See Breathing Crises this section.)
2. The bite area should be kept lower than the level of the victim's heart.
3. Apply cold compresses or ice wrapped in cloth to the bite area.
4. Quickly obtain medical help. Go to the nearest hospital emergency room and take the dead spider with you, if possible.

Until medical help is obtained, continue to care for the person:

5. Keep the person quiet.
6. If necessary, treat for shock.

POISONING
Swallowed Poisons

Common poisonous substances found in

and around the house are cosmetics, hair preparations, petroleum products (like gasoline and kerosene), paints and turpentine, detergents and other cleaning products, bleach, lye, glue, ammonia, acids, poisonous plants and non-edible mushrooms. Although the symptoms from swallowing a poison may vary, look for the following:

• Information from the victim or from observers.
• A container of the poisonous material. Save the label and/or container.
• Victim is suddenly ill or has a sudden pain.
• Burns around the mouth.
• Strange odor on the breath.

The objectives of emergency treatment arc: to dilute the poison as soon as possible; to call a poison center (or a doctor, paramedics or hospital emergency room) for instructions; to monitor breathing, blood circulation, and vital functions; and to get medical help.

1. Quickly dilute the poison by giving at least one eight- ounce glass of water, unless the victim is unconscious or having convulsions. Never give milk, fruit juice, vinegar, olive oil, etc. Only water.

2. Call a poison center, a doctor, paramedics or a hospital emergency room to get further instructions. Be sure to have the following information when you call:
   A. Person's age.
   B. Poison's name.
   C. How much poison was swallowed.
   D. When the poison was swallowed.
   E. If the person has vomited.
   F. How long it will take to get to the nearest medical facility.

3. Only on medical advice (preferably from a poison center) do you induce vomiting. Never induce vomiting if you do not know what was swallowed or if the victim swallowed a strong acid (like rust remover) or a strong alkali (like dishwasher detergent). If vomited, strong acids and alkalines can cause additional damage to the throat and esophagus. Petroleum products might be inhaled into the lungs and cause a chemical pneumonia.

4. Always follow the instructions of a poison center. A center may give instructions to induce vomiting for some petroleum products due to other, more harmful effects to the body.

5. If the person vomits, position him face down with the head lower than the rest of the body. Position a child face down across your lap. Such positions prevent choking.

6. Get immediate medical help. Take the poison container and any vomited material with the victim to the hospital where it will be inspected.

7. Do not give activated charcoal ("universal antidote"), except if told to do so by a doctor or poison center. It must be in powdered form, and the dose must be adequate (25 grams for children, 50 grams for adults). Activated charcoal is given only after Syrup of Ipecac.

Be careful about the antidotes or instructions on the labels of poisonous substances. The antidotes are not always correct and may be out of date. Always consult a poison center.

Remember, induce vomiting only if a poison center or other medical personnel instructs you to do so. However, if no medical help can be contacted, induce vomiting only if the swallowed substance was not an acid, alkali or petroleum product. To induce vomiting:

1. Give an adult (over 12 years old) two tablespoons of Syrup of Ipecac (available in drugstores); give a child one tablespoon (of Syrup of Ipecac); and give an infant (less than one year old) two teaspoons. Then give one or two glasses of water (8 to 16 ounces). If after 15 to 20 minutes there has been no vomiting, repeat dose of Syrup of Ipecac and water only once more. Never give any other substance to induce vomiting.

2. If there is no Syrup of Ipecac, tickle the back of the person's throat with your finger.

3. If the victim vomits, position the head face down, lower than the rest of the body to avoid choking. Put a small child across your lap with his face down.

4. Continue to seek medical help. Be sure to take the poison container and any vomited material with the victim to the hospital.

SEIZURE

A seizure is brought on by a disturbance in the brain's electrical activity. Most will last only a few minutes, and even though they appear serious, they usually do not cause serious problems in themselves. Injuries may conic about if the person falls or knocks into surrounding objects while the seizure is in progress.

A person experiencing a seizure may show any number of the following signs:

- For a few seconds the body's muscles are rigid. That is followed by jerking and twitching movements. When the muscles are rigid, the person may stop breathing, possibly lose bladder and bowel control or bite the tongue.
- Face and lips look bluish.
* Foaming (may be bloody) or drooling at the mouth.
- Person may give a short cry or scream.
- Eyes could roll upward.
- After the seizure, victim will be sleepy and confused.
- During the seizure, the person is unre-sponsive.

The main objective for a first-aider is to pre-vent the person from injuring himself.

1. If the person begins to fall, try to catch him and lay him down gently. If the person is too large, it is most important that you protect the head—grab his shoulders and at least break the fall.
2. Clear a space around the victim. Push away items such as chairs, tables, doors, etc., so the person won't knock against them.
3. During the seizure don't let the victim bang his head on a hard floor. Try to slip a pillow, a coat or something soft under the head.

- An overall weakness.
- A fast (over 100) but weak pulse. You may feel no pulse at the wrist.
- An increased rate of breathing. It may be shallow and irregular, or it may be like sighing.
- Restlessness or anxiety.
- Severe thirst.
- Vomiting.

The following signs will appear later:

- Unresponsiveness.
- A dull, sunken look to the eyes. The pupils will look larger than usual.
- The skin looks blotchy or streaked. That is an indication that the person's blood pres-

sure is very low.

In a severe case of shock, or if left untreated, a person will . .

- Lose consciousness.

Your main objectives will be to help the blood circulate better, to provide an adequate supply of oxygen, to maintain a normal body temperature and get medical aid.

Take the following steps:

1. Check for any difficulties in breathing. (See Breathing Crises, this section.)
2. If possible, treat the injury which is the cause of the shock.
3. Keep the person lying down. That is the best position for good circulation. But some injuries may not permit this. In that case, put the person in whatever position feels most comfortable.
4. Keep the person comfortably warm, but not hot. This is to prevent the loss of body heat. If the victim is outside or on a damp surface, try to put a blanket beneath them.

For continued care until help comes:

5. Do not move a person with the possibility of head, neck or back injuries unless they are in danger of being injured again.
6. Elevate the feet 8 to 12 inches. Elevating the feet improves circulation. A pillow or blanket works well. If the person experi-ences chest pain, a red face or has diffi-culty breathing, lower the feet.
7. If there is unconsciousness or severe facial injuries, turn the victim on his side to al-low fluids (blood, saliva, vomit) to drain out the mouth. Otherwise the person could choke.
8. Always reassure the person and be gentle.

In the rare instance when medical attention is more than two hours away, the following solution may be given in the manner speci-fied:

Take one quart of cool water. Mix in 1 level teaspoon of salt and 1/2 level teaspoon of baking soda. Give an adult (over 12 years old) 1/2 cup (four ounces); give a child (1 to 12 years old) 1/4 cup (two ounces); and give an infant (less than 1 year old) one ounce. Have the adult, child or infant sip the appropriate amount slowly over a 15-minute period. Clear fruit juices (like apple juice) may also be given.

Never give fluids to a person who is unconscious, having convulsions, vomiting, or who is likely to need surgery because of serious injuries.

SNAKEBITE

Any snakebite causes fear and anxiety. But it is important for the rescuer to know whether or not the snake is poisonous. If possible, the snake should be killed and taken to a medical facility with the victim. If the snake gets away, try to remember what it looked like.

The poisonous snakes found in the United States are the rattlesnake, the cottonmouth (or water moccasin), the copperhead and coral snake. The severity of reaction from their bites depends upon several things: how much venom is injected and how fast the victim's bloodstream absorbs it; the size of the person; what protective clothing is worn, like boots, gloves or long pants; how quickly the person obtains antivenom therapy; and what part of the body is bitten.

Bites by a Rattlesnake, Cottonmouth, or Copperhead (Not Coral)

If a person is bitten by a rattlesnake, cottonmouth or copperhead, he or she may have any or all of the following symptoms:

- Extreme pain; fast swelling.
- Puncture wounds left by the snake's fangs and discoloration of the skin around the bite.
- General weakness; nausea and vomiting.
- Shortness of breath; blurred or dim vision.
- Shock reaction.
- Convulsions.

You need to slow the blood circulation through the bitten area to delay the spread of the venom. The victim's respiration should be monitored and the wounded area aggravated as little as possible.

1. Check the person's breathing. (See Breathing Crises this section.)
2. Do not let the victim move around.
3. Immobilize the bitten area and keep it lower than the level of the heart.
4. If the bite is on the arm or leg, put a light constricting band, 3/4 to 1 1/2 inches wide (like a belt or watchband), 2 to 4 inches above the wound. Do not make it so tight as to cut off the circulation. The band should be loose enough for a finger to be slipped underneath. Discharge should come out the wound.

5. If swelling reaches the band, move the band up another 2 to 4 inches.
6. Do not remove the band until medical help is reached.
7. Thoroughly wash the bite area with soap and water.
8. If you are more than one hour from medical help, make an incision and provide suction immediately after the person has been bitten. Use a snakebite kit, if that is available, which provides a blade and suction cup. Or use a sharp, sterilized knife and your mouth.
   A. Carefully make a cut. 1/8 to 1/4 inch deep (no deeper) and no more than 1/2 inch long, through each fang mark. Cut down the length of the arm or leg, not across it. Do not cut snakebites on the head, neck or trunk.
   B. Suction should be done for at least 30 minutes. Use the suction cup in the snakebite kit. Or use your mouth if it is free of cuts and sores. Spit the venom out. Rinse your mouth when finished.
9. Do not put cold or ice compresses on the bites. That could cause tissue damage.
10. Get medical help. If you transport the person to a hospital, try to phone ahead and tell them what has happened. The antivenom serum will need to be prepared. If the snake has been killed, bring it to the hospital.

Until help comes, continue to care for the person:

11. Put a clean, sterile bandage over the wound.
12. Be calm and reassuring. Keep the victim quiet.
13. If necessary, treat for shock.
14. If the victim absolutely must walk, then move slowly.
15. Only small sips of water may be given if the victim can swallow without difficulty. Don't give water if there is nausea, vomiting, convulsions or unconsciousness. Never give alcoholic beverages.

Bites by a Coral Snake

The coral snake is a member of the cobra

FIRST AID

family and is smaller than pit vipers (such as rattlesnakes, cottonmouths and copperheads). Like nonpoisonous snakes, the coral snake has rounded eyes, but it has long fangs. Its venom is highly toxic and affects the nervous system. The coral snake "chews" and does not make the usual two puncture wounds.

The coral snake has bright yellow, red and black bands of color, with narrow yellow rings always separating the wide red bands from the black. Its nose is always black.

It is found along the coastal plains from the middle of North Carolina through Florida and the other Gulf states; west into Texas; and up the Mississippi Valley to Arkansas.

The symptoms from a coral snakebite may not appear immediately. *For a coral snakebite, do the following:*

1. Immediately wash the wound area.
2. Immobilize the area and keep the person still.
3. Quickly get medical assistance. Preferably, go to the nearest hospital. Try to have someone phone ahead and tell the hospital what has happened so that antivenom serum may be prepared.

Nonpoisonous Snakebite

If a person has been bitten by a snake believed not to be poisonous, then do these four things:

1. Keep the wounded area below the level of the victim's heart.
2. Wash the area thoroughly with soap and water.
3. Place a sterile bandage or clean cloth over the snakebite.
4. Seek medical assistance. Medication or a tetanus shot may be required. If the snake has been killed, bring it to the hospital.

STROKE

A stroke is usually the result of an interruption in the blood circulating to a part of or all of the brain. That may be caused by a blood clot in an artery going to the brain; by a blood vessel becoming narrow; or by the rupture of an artery within the brain.

Major Stroke

The signs of a major stroke are given below. Any or all may be present.

- The victim may lose consciousness or be mentally confused.
- His speech may be slurred or lost.
- There may be a weakness, numbness or paralysis on one side of the body, particularly in the face, arm or leg. One side of the mouth may drop.
- A sudden headache.
- The person could have difficulty in talking, chewing or swallowing.
- Breathing may be difficult.
- The person may lose control of the bowels and bladder.
- Sudden falls.
- The pupils of the eyes will be unequal in size.
- The pulse will be slow and strong.

The following things should be done immediately:

1. Get medical assistance.
2. Keep the victim's airway open. (See Breathing Crises this section.) Begin artificial breathing if needed.

Until medical help arrives, you can continue to care for the person.

3. Keep the person comfortably warm.
4. Turn him on his side so that secretions can drain from the mouth. Clean out the mouth and hold it open to prevent choking.
5. Keep the victim quiet.
6. Put cold cloths on the person's head.
7. Be calm and reassuring.
8. Never give fluids or anything to drink. That could cause vomiting or choking.

Minor Stroke

Only small blood vessels are involved in a minor stroke and the victim usually remains conscious. The signs depend where in the brain the rupture and bleeding take place and how much brain damage there is. The stroke could occur while the victim is asleep.

The signs are:

- A headache.
- Mental confusion.
- Minor dizziness. Perhaps ringing in the ears.
- Slight difficulties with speech.
- Muscle weakness.

There are two things to do:

1. Get medical help.

F
I
R
S
T

A
I
D

2. Prevent any further injury or physical exertion.

If you begin to feel the symptoms of a minor stroke yourself, proceed as follows:

1. Call for medical help.
2. Lie down on your side. This will allow any secretions to drain out of your mouth and avoid choking.
3. Stay quiet until help comes.
4. Stay comfortably warm. Not hot.
5. Never eat or drink anything.

WOUNDS

With a severe open wound, there are four primary objectives:

1. Stop the bleeding.
2. Prevent contamination and infection.
3. Treat for shock.
4. Get medical assistance.

In addition, monitor the person's breathing. (See Breathing Crises this section.)

Stopping the Bleeding

A person can bleed to death in a very short time so you must quickly stop any rapid, large loss of blood and then treat for shock.

Never clean a large, severe wound or put any medication or home remedy on it.

1. Place a thick, clean compress over the entire wound and press firmly with the palm of your hand. Sterile compresses are available in drugstores. You could also use a handkerchief, towel, pillowcase, undershirt or any clean, soft cloth.

If no cloth is available, use your bare hand a id fingers (they should be clean).

2. Apply direct steady pressure. In most instances this will stop the bleeding and will not interfere with the person's normal circulation.
3. Do not remove the compress. The thick cloth will absorb blood and help it to clot. If the cloth is moved, the blood clots will be disturbed allowing more bleeding. If blood soaks through the first cloth, apply additional cloths on top of it and press more firmly.
4. If a limb or the neck is involved, elevate it above the level of the victim's heart and continue direct pressure. Do not elevate the limb or neck if it appears to be fractured. Elevation uses gravity to reduce the blood pressure in the limb.

5. If the bleeding stops or slows down, you may use a pressure bandage to hold the compress in place. (Maintain elevation.) Place the center of a gauze strip directly over the compress. Wrap the ends around the wound, pulling steadily to maintain pressure. Tie a knot directly over the wound.

Preventing Contamination and Infection

The procedure for controlling contamination and infection in an open wound depends upon the amount of bleeding.

If there is severe bleeding, do not remove the original compress (see Stopping the Bleeding above). No attempt should be made to clean the wound. The important steps are to halt the loss of blood, get medical help, give treatment for shock, immobilize the injured area and elevate the wounded area.

If the bleeding is not severe, clean the skin as thoroughly as possible before a dressing and bandage are applied, especially if medical help is not immediately available.

Do not remove any foreign objects in deep tissues or muscles. Only a physician should do that.

For open wounds with no severe bleeding, treat as follows:

1. First, wash your hands thoroughly to prevent further contamination.
2. If necessary, apply direct pressure with a clean cloth to stop any bleeding.
3. Carefully wash in and around the wound with soap and water. Gentle scrubbing may be necessary to remove all dirt and prevent infection. Rinse.
4. Particles, such as wood splinters and glass fragments, embedded in the skin's surface, may be removed. (But do not remove anything stuck in deep tissues or muscles. This should be done only by a physician.) Use tweezers that have been sterilized over a flame or in boiling water, or use the tip of a needle that has been sterilized over a flame.
5. With a sterile gauze pad or clean cloth, pat the wound dry. Sterile gauze pads are available in drugstores.
6. Do not use any antiseptic sprays or home preparations until a physician instructs

F
I
R
S
T

A
I
D

you to do so.

7. Put a sterile dressing over the wound and secure it in place.

8. Get medical assistance if the injury is severe; if the bleeding will not stop; if the wound was caused by a dirty object; if a foreign object is stuck in the wound; if there is a question about tetanus immunization; or if there appears to be an infection.

9. Infection, caused by the invasion and growth of bacteria, may develop in hours or days after the injury. Get to a doctor if it develops. The symptoms are: swelling around the wound, redness or a feeling of heat around the wound, tenderness, evidence of pus, red streaks leading from the wound to the body or fever.

Puncture Wounds

A puncture wound is caused by an object (such as a bullet, nail or ice pick) piercing the skin and underlying tissues. It resembles a hole. The wound is deep and narrow, and there is little external bleeding. Since bleeding helps to wash out germs, a puncture wound is more susceptible to infection. Therefore, tetanus is a danger. Also, there may be damage to internal organs and internal bleeding.

Treat a puncture wound as follows:

1. Wash your hands with soap and water before you touch the wound.

2. Do not touch or attempt to remove any object which has broken "off or become lodged in the wound. That should be done only by a doctor.

3. With a minor puncture wound, such as a wood splinter, you may remove objects stuck only into the skin's surface. Use tweezers which have been sterilized over a flame or in boiling water.

4. Do not poke into the wound. Do not apply any type of ointment.

5. Encourage bleeding by gently pressing around the wound edges. Do not cause further injury by doing this.

6. Wash a minor puncture wound with soap and water. Rinse with running water. Do not wash a large, deep puncture wound.

7. Put a clean dressing over the wound and bandage it in place.

8. Treat for a shock reaction if necessary.

9. Get medical attention.

EMERGENCY PRESSURE POINTS - TO STOP BLEEDING

PRESSURE POINTS

Fingers usually can be applied without worsening a victim's condition to control bleeding at a pressure point. There are a half-dozen pressure points where bleeding from an artery can be stopped or reduced by pressing the artery against a bone located next to it. See page 1067 for bandages

PRESSURE POINTS FOR NECK, MOUTH, OR THROAT

To stop bleeding from the neck, mouth, or throat area, apply pressure at a point on the neck where an artery passes alongside the trachea, or windpipe. Place the thumb of the hand against the neck and the fingers on the neck just below the larynx, or Adam's apple. Then push the fingers against the artery.

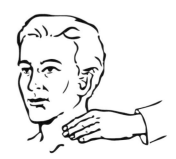

STOP BLEEDING FROM TWO-THIRDS OF ARM

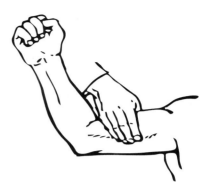

An artery supplying the lower arm passes close to the bone of the upper arm about halfway along the length of the upper arm. By applying pressure at that point, pressing the artery against the arm bone, bleeding from nearly any point beyond can be stopped.

PRESSURE POINTS IN UPPER ARM

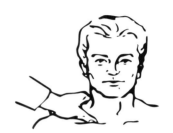

A pressure point for controlling the loss of blood in the upper arm, shoulder, or armpit should be found where an artery passes over the outer surface of the top rib. Place the thumb in the position shown (the top rib is indicated in the drawing) and the fingers over the shoulder so they press against the area behind the collarbone. Apply pressure to the artery crossing the top rib.

BLEEDING BELOW THE EYE AND ABOVE THE JAWBONE

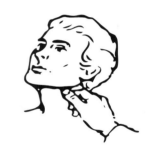

Bleeding from an artery supplying the area of the face below the level of the eye usually can be controlled by finding the pressure point that is located along the edge of the jawbone.

BLEEDING FROM THE HEAD ABOVE THE EYE LEVEL

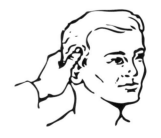

For bleeding above the level of the eye, the rescuer should be able to find a pressure point where an artery passes over one of the skull bones front of the upper portion of the ear, as shown in the drawing.

PRESSURE POINT FOR THE LEG

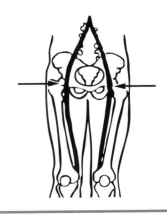

To stop bleeding from a leg or foot, apply pressure at a point in the area of the groin where the femoral artery passes over one of the bones of the pelvis, as shown in the drawing. If the blood flow slackens or stops you can be sure you have found the pressure point.

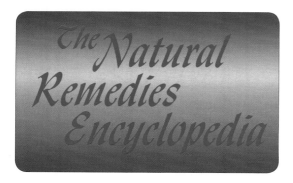

Basic Physiology

INTRODUCTION

Anatomy is the study of the structure of the human body; and **physiology** is the study of how it functions. But, since the word physiology is frequently used to summarize both, it will be so used in this chapter.

This is a very important study. We need to better understand the house we live in, so that we can give it better care.

As you read this section, be aware of the fact that you are reading an astounding, ongoing miracle. Two tiny cells come together—and grow into all this utter complexity of a human being!

It is a basic theory of evolution that everything in our world was produced by purposeless, random effects. Sloshing seawater mixed with sand, one day, and produced the first organisms. These creatures kept changing into ever larger ones, till we have our present world of living plants and animals. That is the theory.

Yet, in the study of the human body, as in every other aspect of the natural world, you will find that each tiny detail reveals super-human planning. Only God, the Creator of heaven and earth, could make the human body! Read and believe.

BODY SYSTEMS

Tissues—Cells of the same kind are joined together to form **tissues**. There are as many tissues as there are kinds of cells. Every tissue has a special function.

• **Epithelial** - Covers surfaces and lines cavities (skin, hair, nails, lining of parts of the body, including gastro-intestinal tract, urinary tract, etc.).

• **Connective** - Anchors and holds other tissues together (ligaments, tendons, cartilage, bone).

• **Muscular** - Contracts (muscle tissue).

• **Nerve** - Sends and receives sensations (brain, spinal cord, nerves).

• **Blood** - Carries food and oxygen to the cells, and carries wastes away. Through a network of blood vessels, it fights infections and poisons.

Organs—Different kinds of **tissues** are grouped together to form **organs**. The heart, for example, is a combination of muscle, nerve, blood, and epithelial tissues. Every organ has one or more special functions. Each organ works with the other organs. They are so marvelous that only God could have made them.

Systems—This is a still larger category, and includes organs which work together.

1. Skeletal - The bones are the body's framework.

2. Muscular - The muscles; these are attached to the bones, and make body movements possible.

3. Circulatory - The heart, blood, blood vessels, lymph, and lymph vessels. They carry food, water, oxygen, and wastes in the body.

4. *Digestive* - The mouth, salivary glands, pharynx, esophagus, stomach, intestines, liver, and pancreas. They liquefy and absorb food.

5. *Respiratory* - The nose, pharynx, larynx, trachea, bronchi, and lungs. They bring in the body's supply of oxygen and eliminate carbon dioxide waste.

6. *Urinary* - The kidneys, ureters, urinary bladder, and urethra. They eliminate waste products from the body. Sometimes this is included, with the respiratory and digestive systems and skin, as part of the excretory system.

7. *Reproductive* - The ovaries, fallopian tubes, uterus, vagina, and mammary glands in the woman. The testes, accessory glands, and penis in the man. They perpetuate the human race.

8. *Endocrine* - The endocrine or ductless glands. They secrete hormones that regulate various body organs.

9. *Nervous* - The brain, spinal cord, and nerves. They control and coordinate the activities of the body.

10. *Sense organs* - The eyes, ears, tongue, and certain nerves. These are the means by which we make contact with the world.

1 - THE SKIN

Function—The **skin** protects the body, excretes fluids, regulates body temperature, and produces vitamin D upon exposure to the sun.

Layers—The **epidermis** is the outside layer of the skin and contains **pigment** which colors the skin. The cells on top die and drop off continually. Below it is the **dermis** (*corium*), the inner layer or true skin. It has live cells in a network of lymph vessels, capillaries and nerves projecting out to form ridges. The nerves regulate the size of the capillaries, and produce blushing and paling (blanching) of the skin.

Hairs—Except in a few areas (such as the palms of the hands and the soles of the feet), the skin is covered with tiny hairs. The part of the hair above the skin is the **shaft**; the part below is the **root**. The bottom of the roots are in tiny sacs, the hair **follicles**. Organs of touch lie close to the hairs, which is why you sense when those hairs are touched. As long as the hair follicle is alive, a new hair will continue to grow. Brushing the hair or massaging the scalp will help increase hair growth.

Glands—There are two kinds of glands in the skin: the **sebaceous glands**, or *oil glands*. These lie close to the hair follicles and discharge oily **sebum** into them. This keeps the hair soft and pliable. There are also **sweat glands** (*sudoriferic glands*), which remove waste from the body in **perspiration**. They extract water and salt wastes from the blood and discharge them through tiny outlets on the skin surface, the **pores**. Perspiration also helps control body temperature.

Nails—These are tightly packed cells of the epidermis, and are made of cartilage. The roots are alive and the outer ends are dead. Fingernails grow 1/10th of a millimeter per day; toenails grow at half that rate.

2 - THE SKELETAL SYSTEM

Number—There are 206 bones in the human body. Six of them are the **ossicles** in the ear. Infants have about 350 bones; but many of these eventually connect, forming the 206 bones in the adult.

Function—The bones provide a solid framework, supporting and shaping the body. They protect delicate or soft parts and anchor the muscles.

Substance—**Bones** are *osseous cells* hardened by calcium and phosphorus from the food we eat. **Periosteum** is a membrane that covers every bone. It is filled with blood vessels that carry bone-building materials and minerals to the bone cells, to keep them alive and harden the bone by filling in the spaces between the cells. The bones of a baby are partly cartilage, which is bone cells not fully hardened. Bones are not completely hardened until a person is about 20 years old. This is why adults can break their bones easier than children. Bone cells multiply rapidly during the growing years, but slowly thereafter as bones needs to be repaired. With age, bones become harder and more brittle.

Long bones—The **shaft**, or *diaphysis*, is the lengthy section, and is hard and compact. The **end**, or *epiphysis*, is sponge-like and covered by a shell of harder bone. The shaft and end do not fuse until full growth is achieved.

Joints—These are the places where the bones are attached to one other. They enable you to move your arms and legs. Strong, fibrous bands, called **ligaments**, hold them together. The moving joints are lined with a membrane that secretes a fluid, called **synovial fluid**. This keeps the joints "oiled" and working smoothly. *Cartilage plates* on the ends of bones make a slick surface for rotation.

Types of joints—Finger joints move like a door on hinges, and are called **hinge joints**. Shoulder and hip joints are **ball-and-socket joints**, and allow rotating movement. The rounded end of one bone fits into the hollowed-out end of the other.

Joint problems—*Arthritis* and *rheumatoid arthritis* occurs in the joints. Other types include *tubercular (TB) arthritis, gonerrheal arthritis,* and *gout. Synovitis* is inflammation of the lining of the joint. (Rheumatism is an inflammation in the muscles.)

Vertebral column—Your **spine** supports your head, stiffens the mid-portion of your body, and anchors your ribs and pelvic bones. It also protects the **spinal cord**, which passes from the brain down through its bony rings. The spine also carries the

P
H
Y
S

body weight, and consists of 26 irregularly shaped bony rings called **vertebrae** (**Vertebra** is singular). On the inner side of each of the vertebra is a bony structure, called the **arch**, which forms an opening or **spinal foramen** through which the spinal cord passes. Jutting from the arch are several finger-like extensions or **processes** on which ligaments and tendons are anchored. The **discs** are plates of cartilage between these rings, which are shock absorbers when you walk, sit, or fall. They make the joints flexible, so you can bend and turn.

Spinal curves—The spine has four normal curves. Disease, injury, or poor posture distort these curves, producing **kyphosis** (hunchback), **lordosis** (swayback), or **scoliosis** (lateral curvature).

The seven top vertebra (in your neck) are the **cervicals**. The next 12 in your upper back are the **thoracics**. The next five, below that, are the **lumbar** in your lower back. Then come five **sacral** vertebra and, lastly, four **coccygeal** in your, so-called, "tail bone." Without that section, you could not sit properly.

Ribs—Your **rib cage** is formed by 12 ribs on each side of a central divide. The **sternum** is the **breast bone**, a flat bone in the upper center of your chest. The upper seven pairs of ribs are attached to the sternum in front. The next three pairs are attached to each other and indirectly to the sternum. The last two are free in front and are called **floating ribs**. They help your chest expand as you inhale.

Pelvic bones—Your **pelvic girdle** is formed from several bones. In women, the central opening is called the **birth canal**. If it was not larger than in men, babies could not be born.

Leg bones—The **femur** is the upper bone of the leg and is the longest and strongest bone in your body. Its upper end is attached to the pelvic bone in a ball-and-socket joint. Try to avoid falls, which could break that joint, called "breaking the hip." There are two bones in the lower leg: the **tibia,** or **shin bone** in front, and the **fibula** in back. The **knee cap (patella)** covers the knee joint, so you can kneel.

Ankle and foot bones—There are seven **tarsal bones** in the ankle, with the largest in the heel. They join the five **metatarsals** (instep bones), to form two **arches**—one lengthwise across the foot (the longitudinal arch) and the other from side to side (the metatarsal arch). Weak muscles reduces the "spring"; and flat feet can result. The 14 bones of the toes, the **phalanges**, are attached to the metatarsal bones. The great toe has two phalanges; each of the others has three.

Shoulder bones—In front are two long, thin bones—the **clavicles** or **collarbones**. In back, there are the two scapula (**scapulars**), or **shoulder blades**. Because all these bones are only attached

to the sternum, you can freely move your shoulders and arms up, down, forward, and back.

Arm bones—The **humerus** (no, it's not the "funny bone") is the single long bone in the upper arm. The upper end is attached to the scapula; the lower end connects with the ulna to form the elbow joint (and that is what people call your "funny bone"). There are two bones in the forearm. The larger is the **ulna** and the other is the **radius**. Because God gave you two bones in your forearm, instead of one, you can rotate your hand in a semicircle. As you extend your hand with the thumb up, the radius is on top and is the one that rotates.

Hand bones—There are eight **carpal**, or **wrist, bones**. Next come five **metacarpal bones,** forming the palm of your hand; then come the **phalanges** (finger bones). There are three phalanges in each finger and two in the thumb. You have 29 (!) joints in each wrist and hand; so you can produce fine movements.

3 - THE MUSCULAR SYSTEM

Muscles—Without muscles, you could not move an inch. Muscles are connected to bones by **tendons,** which enable muscles to move the bones. Muscle cells are tiny elastic threads of protein, wrapped together in bundles; several bundles make a muscle. Each muscle is covered by a sheath of connective tissue called fascia, the ends of which lengthen into tough cords, called **tendons**, which are attached to bones.

Bursas—The tendons have sheaths lined with **synovial membrane** that allows a smooth, gliding movement. **Bursas** (Bursae) are small sacs lined with synovial membrane found wherever pressure is exerted over moving parts. When bursae become inflamed, bursitis is the result. Often this occurs in the knee joint, and is commonly called "housemaid's knee."

Muscles work in pairs. Nerves in the muscle bundles direct movements, and blood vessels carry food materials. An overstretched or damaged muscle hurts.

Flexion and extension—When you bend your arm, your arm muscle becomes shorter and thicker; that is **flexion**. When you straighten it out, the muscles lengthen and narrow; that is **extension**. A muscle is most powerful when contracted. By keeping your arm muscles close to your body, and your back straight when you move something, you are less likely to overstrain. Pick things up with your muscles, not your spine.

Power—Muscles use oxygen and a type of sugar to provide the power to do things. The result is energy and heat. In fact, most of the heat in the body is produced by muscles (with the liver in second place as a heat source). Using muscles build them up. Otherwise they become flabby.

Waste products—Two waste products are produced when a muscle works. **Carbon dioxide** is carried to the lungs while **lactic acid** is removed through the kidneys and sweat glands. If you work too hard, so much lactic acid remains in the muscles that they ache and feel sore afterward.

Rehabilitation—An injured or inactive muscle can be retrained to do its work. This must be done slowly and carefully. The person you are helping must be encouraged to persevere.

Control—There are two types of muscles: You consciously control the **voluntary (skeletal) muscles**. The **involuntary (smooth) muscles** work automatically. These latter muscles include the stomach, heart, kidneys, etc.

Breathing muscles—Of the 325 muscles in the body, some are especially important for breathing. The **diaphragm** is between the abdominal and chest cavities, and helps you breathe. Muscles between the ribs, the **intercostals**, also help enlarge the chest cavity.

Abdominal muscles—These are mentioned because they are the ones most likely to produce hernias. They are arranged to give support by overlapping in layers from various angles. There are also special places where **rupture (hernia)** with **protrusion** of part of the intestine may occur. These weak places are areas where blood vessels, nerves, ligaments, and cords pass through the muscles. The **inguinal rings,** the **femoral rings,** and the **umbilicus** are common sites for hernias.

Shoulders and buttocks—These muscles are important in for moving the arms and legs. In addition, the shoulder muscles sometimes become chilled and aches develop in them.

Leg muscles—The **Achilles tendon** is the name for the large tendon which attaches the calf muscle to the heel bone. Sometimes it becomes strained or injured.

4 - THE CIRCULATORY SYSTEM

Blood—Blood is composed of liquid, red and white cells, and various other elements; all of them are extremely important. An adult usually has 1 to 1½ gallons of blood.

Blood plasma—This is the carrying agent for blood cells, carbon dioxide, and other dissolved wastes. It also brings hormones and antibodies to the tissues. It is composed of water, dissolved food materials, and a substance (**fibrinogen**) that helps blood clotting. About 55% of the blood is plasma.

Red blood cells—These are tiny pink disks, with the outer part bulged, which are called **erythrocytes** or **RBCs**. These are mature cells in the body which have no nucleus. They are very tiny; approximately

3,000 of them could lie side by side in a distance of one inch. A person who has a decreased amount of RBCs has *iron deficiency anemia.*

Hemoglobin—This is a substance which contains *iron* and gives the red blood cells their color. As the blood passes through the lungs, the hemoglobin picks up oxygen which it carries to the body cells. When hemoglobin is saturated with oxygen, it is bright red. Body waste makes it a darker red. It takes trillions of red cells to carry the body's oxygen supply. In a blood count, the average number of RBCs is 4½ to 5 million per cubic millimeter (in an amount of blood smaller than a tiny drop). They wear out in less than a month, and are then destroyed in the spleen and liver. Red blood cells are made in the red marrow of the bones. Leukemia is a cancer of the bone marrow, which results in RBCs not being made. Decreased RBCs and increased WBCs are the sign of this.

White blood cells—These are also called **leukocytes** or **WBCs**. They are colorless cells that protect the body against disease organisms or irritants. There are two main types: *granular* and *nongranular* leukocytes.

Since the number of WBCs in the blood varies with certain diseases, a common aid to diagnosis is a **white cell count**. A tiny drop of blood is viewed under a microscope, and the number of WBCs is estimated. Normally, they would average from 7,000 to 9,000 per cubic millimeter. This number may be increased from 15,000 to 25,000 when infection is present. For example, an increased number of WBCs indicates infection, allergies, hookworm, etc. A decreased number is a sign of typhoid fever, toxins, influenza, or tuberculosis.

At the first sign of danger, the white cells multiply and rush to the spot where the threatening organisms are at work; they gobble them up, destroy their poisons, and dissolve the damaged tissues.

Differential count—In some diseases, the relative proportion of the two kinds of WBCs may vary. Therefore a *differential count* is made, in which the number of granular and nongranular WBCs are compared.

Platelets—These are also called **thrombocytes**. Like the red and white cells, they are formed elements in the blood. Platelets help in the clotting of blood. A blood count of 250,000 to 500,000 could be considered normal.

Blood clotting—When a blood vessel is cut, **fibrinogen** and **platelets (clotting factors)** in the escaping plasma go into action. The fibrinogen suddenly changes into a tangled mass of threads which traps the blood cells and makes a **clot**, which stops the blood flow and tends to draw the cut edges together. If a clot forms inside a blood vessel and remains there, it is called a *thrombus*. A deficiency of *vitamin K* lowers the amount of clotting substance in

P
H
Y
S

the blood. Green leafy vegetables contain this vitamin (frozen foods lack it). *Hemophilia* (bleeder's disease) is caused by an improper function of the platelets.

Hemorrhage—The word means the escape of blood from blood vessels, but we generally use it to refer to the loss of a considerable amount of blood. If too much blood is flowing or there is a lack of clotting factors, clotting does not occur adequately.

Blood transfusion—Severe hemorrhage is serious because of the loss of fluid, food materials, and oxygen-carrying red blood cells. A blood transfusion from one person to another will replace the volume of fluid and the blood cells. Tests must first be made to match blood types of donor's and recipient's blood.

Blood types—All bloods fall into one of 4 groups: *AB, A, B, and O*. Blood from a person in your group would match yours safely. *Type O* can be given to any other blood group and is called the **universal donor**. *Type AB* can receive blood of any other group and is called the **universal recipient**. If the blood is incompatible, it will form dangerous blood clots in the recipient's blood vessels. Plasma transfusion is always safe and quicker than a transfusion of whole blood, but blood plasma does not contain red and white blood cells.

Blood pressure—Blood in the *arteries (arterial blood)* always exerts some pressure against their walls. When the heart muscle is contracting, the pressure is higher than when it is relaxed. The higher pressure is more important because it shows the condition of the arteries—their resistance to the blood flow. When a physician says that a blood pressure is 140 over 100, he means these two pressures. When the heart muscle is contracted, this is the **systolic** (higher) pressure. When it is relaxed, this is the **diastolic** (lower) pressure. Throughout a typical day, blood pressure can vary—depending on activity, emotion, and strain. But this is normal and only temporary.

Blood pressure and age—Children generally have lower blood pressures than adults. From the ages of 20 to 50, most people show little change. However, women often develop high blood pressure in their forties; it occurs more frequently after 50 in men.

Blood pressure and elasticity—If the walls of the *arteries* become hardened and less elastic *(arteriosclerosis)*, the heart has to pump harder to force the blood through them. When the pressure in the arteries remains high *(hypertension;* generally a systolic over 160), the heart muscles become thicker, and the heart enlarges. The arteries lose some of their elasticity with age; but diet, emotional strain, or overweight can cause it to occur in younger people.

Low blood pressure—Some people have lower than average blood pressure. Unless this is caused by disease, their prospects for a long life are good.

Rh factor—The Rh factor is an inherited blood type characteristic. About 85% of white Americans have this Rh factor (they are **Rh positive**). The others (15%) are **Rh negative**. The percentage of Rh negative people is lower in other races. For example, only 7% of blacks and 1% of Chinese are Rh negative.

Rh factor marriages—If an Rh-positive man and an Rh-negative woman marry (only about 13% of marriages), and only if a baby inherits the father's Rh-positive blood,—then the mother's body may produce antibodies that destroy the baby's red blood cells. This may not cause trouble with the first baby; but it may affect later pregnancies. Usually such a baby is born successfully, but its life is threatened by the destruction of its red blood cells. This condition is called *erythroblastosis fetalis*. Physicians can test the parents before birth and be ready to give the baby an Rh-negative blood transfusion, if necessary, to replace its Rh-positive blood.

Heart—Your heart is a powerful pump that may drive 5 to 6 quarts of blood per minute through thousands of feet of tubes in your body. Every stroke of the pump is a heart beat. A healthy man can increase his cardiac output from 5 quarts per minute during rest to as much as 20 quarts during active exercise.

Heart muscle—Your heart, about the size of your doubled-up fist, lies in the left lower part of your chest cavity. It has four **chambers**. The two upper ones, the **atria,** or **auricles**, receive blood, and the two lower ones, the **ventricles**, pour it out. The heart is divided into a left and right half by a complete wall, the **septum**.

(Clarification: We are here speaking of the person's own "right" and "left." This is standard medical nomenclature. Therefore, if you are working with someone else, his "right" side will appear on your left as you look at him. Example: When looking at a person in front of you, think of four quarters to his heart; his top right is the right atria, top left is the left atria; bottom left is the left ventricle, bottom right is the right ventricle.)

Blood circulation—Blood, having delivered its oxygen, flows into the heart through **the right auricle**, goes down into the **right ventricle**, and is pumped to the lungs to pick up a fresh load of oxygen. This trip to the lungs is called **pulmonary circulation**. It returns, brighter red, because it has exchanged its carbon dioxide waste for oxygen. Entering the **left auricle**, it goes down into the **left ventricle** and is pumped out again, through the *aorta*, and then to the **arteries** on another trip to carry oxygen to the body. At one point, it arrives at the liver and picks up a load of food; at another, it enters the kidneys and is cleaned. Finally, it returns through the veins to the heart.

The heart nodes—These special bundles of unique tissue are simply astounding. The first is embedded in the wall of the right atrium, and is called the **sinoatrial node (S.A. node)** and is the **"pace-maker"** of the heart. (Artificial pacemakers derive their name from it.) The other bundle is in the lower part of the septum, and is the **atrioventricular node (A.V. node)**. The **bundle of His** is also in this area, and is called the **coordinator**.

Heartbeat—The heartbeat originates in the S.A. node, and immediately the entire auricle contracts. Then the A.V. node picks up the message and relays the signal to the muscle fibers of the ventricle, which contracts. *Heart block* is a condition which occurs when disease of the bundle of His interrupts communication between the auricle and the ventricles. A proper balance of calcium, sodium, and potassium is needed for the heart to function properly. If you eat only good food, you should have the proper nutritional balance.

Heart rate—The heart rate is controlled by the *medulla* in the brain and *sensory nerve impulses* to the heart. It is speeded up by emotional reaction, fever, or physical exertion. It is decreased by increased blood pressure, a lack of oxygen, or excess carbon dioxide.

Heart valves—The openings into the aorta and the pulmonary artery are fitted with flaps, called valves. There are similar valves at the openings between the auricles and ventricles. The valve between the right auricle and right ventricle is called the **tricuspid valve**. The valve between the left auricle and left ventricle is called the **mitral,** or **bicuspid valve**. After the blood is squeezed into the ventricles, these valves close, and those over the artery outlets open. This keeps the blood from flowing back when the heart relaxes.

Blood vessels—These are the tubes which carry blood throughout the body. Those that carry blood away from the heart are the **arteries**; those that take it to the heart are the **veins**. (One oddity in following this rule is the pulmonary circulation, which sends blood to the lungs and back to the heart. Arteries carry deoxygenated blood away from the heart and veins carry fresh, oxygenated blood to the heart. Elsewhere in the body, only arteries carry the fresh blood.)

Coronary arteries—These are especially important arteries because they are the ones supplying food and oxygen to the heart muscle itself. If these arteries become narrowed, or if a blood clot blocks part of them, the heart is not supplied with blood and serious trouble may occur. We call this **coronary heart disease**; it is the cause of most of the deaths from heart trouble after middle age.

Brain arteries—If a blockage occurs in a brain artery, a **stroke** can occur.

Capillaries—Blood travels out from the heart through the **aorta**, and thence through smaller **arteries**, and finally through very small arteries **(arterioles)** into the **capillaries** (the smallest blood vessels). From there, the blood travels into the smallest veins **(venules),** then into **veins,** and finally to **superior**

and **inferior venae cava** and back into the heart.

Special systems—We have already mentioned the pulmonary circulation, which takes blood from the heart to the lungs and back again—so the blood can pick up oxygen. Another important one is the **portal system**. All the veins from the stomach, intestines, spleen, and pancreas empty into the portal vein, which leads to the liver—so the blood can pick up food. Blood leaves the liver through the **hepatic vein** and goes to the heart.

Lymphatic system—Your body is filled with lymphatic vessels. They do not carry blood; they carry excess fluids and waste and empty into the **thoracic duct** and **right lymphatic duct**, from whence it goes into veins at the back of the neck. Body muscles keep the lymph flowing; valves in the vessels keep it from flowing backward.

Lymph nodes—There are lymph nodes at several places in your body; these filter out harmful substances such as bacteria and cancer cells. They also manufacture *lymphocytes* (one type of white blood cell). There are six places where these **nodes** are found: under the arms, on the right and left side of the groin, and the right and left side of the neck. If they become infected, the disease is called *adenitis*.

Spleen—The spleen lies directly below the diaphragm, above the left kidney, and behind the stomach. It destroys old red blood cells, makes one type of white blood cell, and filters toxins from the blood. It also produces antibodies, which give us immunity to certain diseases. It stores iron, bile pigments, and antibodies. It becomes enlarged in anemia, malaria, and leukemia.

Tonsils—The three tonsils in the pharyngeal wall at the back of your throat strain out toxins and make *lymphocytes*. It is significant that the tonsils guard the entrance to the gastro-intestinal tract and the appendix guards the outlet of the small intestine.

5 - THE DIGESTIVE SYSTEM

The G.I. tract—This system starts when food enters your body and ends when the waste leaves it. The process is called **digestion** and it takes place in the *digestive tube*, also called the **alimentary canal**, the **gastro-intestinal system**, or the **G.I. tract**. The entire length is from 30 to 40 feet long. The tract is lined with a protective tissue, called **mucous membrane**. It is always moist and smooth, has many nerves, and helps the food to slide along.

Organs in the system—The **mouth, pharynx, esophagus, stomach, small intestine,** and **large intestine** are the **alimentary canal organs**. Other organs in the system which help in digestion include the **teeth, tongue, salivary glands, pancreas,** and **liver**.

Absorption—After food is processed, it passes through the walls of the digestive tube, into the circulation, and is taken by the bloodstream to the cells or to storage places in the body. This is known as absorption.

Types of foods—The purpose of digestion is to extract the basic food materials from the food that is taken in and convert them into a form the body can absorb. There are three main food materials: *carbohydrates, proteins,* and *fats.* The chemicals that most of these digestive processes use are called *enzymes.* Each type of enzyme acts only on a specific substance. Some act on protein, others on fat, etc.

Mouth—Digestion begins in the mouth, which has *lips, cheeks, the tongue, a hard palate* on top, and *a soft palate* on the bottom. Food is cut up by the teeth, rolled around by the tongue, and moistened by *saliva* from the *salivary glands*; then it is rolled into a ball (the *bolus*) and swallowed.

Teeth—Everyone develops 2 sets of teeth. There are 20 in the first set of *deciduous,* or *baby teeth.* These first begin to come when the baby is 6 to 8 months old, and he has them all when he is about 2½ years old. When he is about six, the *permanent teeth* begin to appear. There are 32 in the permanent set. The front and side teeth are biters (*incisors*) and cutters (*canines*); the back teeth are grinders (*molars*). The last upper and lower teeth, at the far back, are the *wisdom teeth*, and sometimes do not appear before the 25th year.

Parts of the tooth—A tooth has 3 parts: the exposed part (the crown), the narrowed *neck* at the gum line, and the root in the bony socket. A root may have from 1 to 4 branches. Most of a tooth is hard dentin. The dentin in the crown is covered by enamel, which is harder than bone. Cement covers the dentin on the root of the tooth. A cavity inside the root opens into a canal that connects the tooth with the covering of the bony socket. Blood vessels go into the cavity through this canal.

Tongue—The rough upper surface is sprinkled with small bumps *(papillae)*; some of these are *taste buds*. They distinguish between sweet (on the top), sour (sides), salty (tip and sides), and bitter (at the back). The tongue mixes food with saliva from several salivary glands.

Salivary glands—Three pairs of glands from the mouth, cheek, and jaw pour *saliva* into the mouth. The saliva moistens the food and begins the process of digestion by changing starches into sugars. Proper chewing in the mouth is important for good digestion.

Pharynx—The tongue lifts the food and passes it into a muscular tube behind the mouth, the pharynx. This tube contracts, pushing the food down into the esophagus. The pharynx connects with the ear through the *eustachian tube*. The *tonsils* are in back of the pharynx. The pharynx is also the top part of the airway into the lungs.

Esophagus—This is another muscular tube, about 10 inches long. It extends from the pharynx down through the neck and chest and into the stomach. It takes about 6 seconds for semisolids to pass from the top of esophagus into the stomach. They are pushed along by contraction waves, called *peristalsis*. Liquids just drop down, without any contraction.

Stomach—This is a collapsible pouch-like sac which is capable of great *distension* (enlargement). It is located in the upper left portion of the *abdominal cavity*. Food enters the stomach through *the cardiac orifice* (also called the *esophageal opening*), and leaves at the bottom through the *pyloric orifice*. Both are guarded by round *sphincter muscles* which can tightly close.

(*Note:* At various points in the G.I. tract, there are sphincter muscles which act as closure valves on tubes. A sphincter muscle works like the drawstring on a sack.)

Stomach digestion—The rounded top portion of the stomach is the *fundus*. Some food can remain here, being partly digested by saliva from the mouth, while the food below it is washed by *stomach (gastric) juices*. Digestion continues in the stomach, where the gastric juices mix with the food; the mass is churned and moved about by the *contraction* (*peristalsis*) of the muscular stomach walls. When the bottom part of the food is digested well enough, the pyloric valve relaxes, and food begins traveling into the small intestine.

Vomiting—The contraction waves are usually downward; but, if the stomach is too full or contains an irritating substance, the waves may reverse. This forces the material back up into the lower part of the esophagus. Stomach and esophagus contractions force the food up during vomiting.

Gastric juices—Gastric juices are secreted by glands in the stomach wall. Two of these digestive juices are especially important. *Pepsin* (*gastric protease*) digests protein. *Renin*, a milk casein, breaks up milk by curdling it. *Hydrochloric acid (HCl)* makes everything so acid that the enzymes in the other gastric juices can work. HCl also destroys organisms and helps regulate the pyloric valve at the stomach outlet. The digestion of protein is the primary work done in the stomach.

Digestion time in stomach—It usually takes 5 or 6 hours for an ordinary meal to move on out of the stomach. (A very large meal will take longer, because it is difficult for the stomach to digest it.) For this reason, nutritionists will tell you not to eat more than three meals a day; and, if you digest food well, only two. If you are overweight, try it. Unpleasant emotions at mealtime slow digestion because they prevent digestive juices from flowing freely.

Stomach ulcers—Continual negative attitudes or problems can overstimulate the gastric nerve, causing an ongoing excess of HCl into the stomach. Since its objective is to digest protein, the stomach wall, blanched of blood because of nervous tension, begins being eaten by the hydrochloric acid. We call that a *gastric ulcer*.

Small intestine—The food (now called *chyme*) is thin and watery as it passes from the stomach, a little at a time, into the intestine. The small intestine is 1½ inches wide and 23 feet long.

Duodenum—The top 10 to 12 inches of the small intestine is the duodenum, a "C"-shaped area. Digestive juices from the pancreas and liver pour into this area. One objective is to alkalinize the food. Another is to aid in digestion. **Pancreatic juice** comes in from the pancreas and other juices from the walls of the duodenum (**intestinal juice glands**). These break down proteins, sugars, and starches into materials the body can use. (More digestive juice will also flow in from the lower small intestine.) Greenish **bile**, made by the liver, pours in from the **liver ducts** through the **gallbladder**. It breaks down fats.

Rest of the small intestine—As the food travels on, it first passes through 7½ feet of small intestine, called the **jejunum**. Then it goes into the **ileum**, the remaining 15 or so feet.

Food absorption—Throughout the whole length of small intestine are tiny, fingerlike projections, called **villi**. In the center of each is a **lymph channel (lacteal)**, with surrounding blood capillaries. The intestinal juice glands are located in the areas between the villi. The digested food passes into the villi, then is taken into the *bloodstream* and carried throughout the body, to nourish the *cells*. That part of the fat that is not absorbed by the villi is absorbed directly into the lacteals and is mixed with lymph. This mixture eventually reaches the bloodstream through the thoracic duct. Most of the food has been absorbed by the time the large intestine is reached.

Large intestine—This is a large tube, also called the **colon**, which is 2½ inches wide and about 5 feet in length. Its entrance, called the **cecum**, has the **appendix** attached to it. Another sphincter muscle (**ileocecal valve**) guards it, so nothing from the colon can travel back into the small intestine.

The colon then proceeds upward on your right side **(ascending colon)**, goes horizontally **(transverse colon)** across the upper part of the abdomen, and then descends **(descending colon)** down the left side. The bottom of it is "S"-shaped, called the **sigmoid flexure**. Then comes the **rectum**, about 5 inches long, which ends at the **anal canal**, about 1 to 1½ inches long. The opening, the **anus**, is guarded by an internal and external sphincter muscle.

Activity in the colon—As the contents move along, most of the water passes through the intestinal walls into the circulation, to keep up the body's water supply. The woody fibers, left from food, mass together as the water leaves and passes on to the rectum. This solid waste, the **feces**, contains bacteria and normally a small amount of water.

Constipation and diarrhea—The contents presses against the sphincter muscles of the anus, signaling the need for a bowel movement. If this signal is not obeyed, the impulse dies. If the contents remain in the rectum too long, they continue to lose water and become drier and harder. Dry, hard feces are difficult to expel. This is *constipation*. Irritants in the intestine will stimulate contraction waves that rapidly rush the contents through, water and all; this is *diarrhea*.

Liver—Although not in the digestive tract, the **liver, gallbladder,** and **pancreas** are part of the digestive system. The liver is the largest and heaviest gland in the body. Located just below the diaphragm, it fits in front of and over the right kidney, part of the colon, and most of the stomach. The liver weighs from 3 to 3½ pounds and is divided into 4 lobes.

Functions of the liver—The liver has over 2,000 functions; about 400 of these are primary ones! (1) It is a filtration plant; for it removes products from the bloodstream. (2) It is a manufacturing plant and chemical laboratory; for it produces bile, *glycogen* (a form of stored sugar), and substances which aid in blood clotting (*prothrombin* and *fibrinogen*) and prevent clotting (*heparin*). (3) It is a warehouse; for it stores iron, vitamins, copper, glycogen, *amino acids* (the absorbable form of proteins), and fats. (4) It is a heating plant; for it produces large amounts of heat, second only to the amount produced by the muscles. (5) It is a waste disposal plant, because it prepares substances for excretion and tries to remove harmful substances from various poisons (including medicinal drugs), so they can be excreted.

Gallbladder—Bile produced in the liver is carried by two bile ducts into the gallbladder for storage, until it is needed to digest (*emulsify*) fats. Sometimes **gallstones** form. If bile cannot pass out of the intestines normally, it will be absorbed into the blood, causing the skin to become yellow or **jaundiced**. The *stool* is then *clay-colored*, due to the absence of bile and poor fat absorption.

Pancreas—This is a long fish-shaped gland behind the stomach, and is made of two different tissues. The ducted cells in one of them secretes *pancreatic juice* for food digestion. The ductless cells in the other tissue, called the **islands (islets) of Langerhans**, secrete **insulin**, a hormone which body cells must have. Without it, they cannot use sugar. *Diabetes* is caused by lack of insulin.

Metabolism—The food materials, which have been

absorbed into the bloodstream, travel to the cells. The cells burn some foods, to supply the body with heat and energy. They build and repair tissues with others. Certain materials help the cells do their work more efficiently. Normally, the process continues evenly, with some food used up and other food stored. The amount of food burned up and the amount of heat produced can be measured, and is called the metabolic rate. If an inactive person overeats, the cells are provided with too much food; so the excess is stored, and he becomes overweight.

6 - THE RESPIRATORY SYSTEM

Introduction—Your cells must have oxygen to burn food, and air is about 20% oxygen. You breathe it in through your respiratory system. In the food-burning process, carbon dioxide is formed; your blood carries it to the air passages, where you breathe it out. *Inspiration* is breathing in and *expiration* is breathing out.

Nose—Air enters your body through your nose (which has two compartments, divided by a **septum**) and passes into the **nasal cavities**. Nerve endings in the septum and nasal passages provide you with the **sense of smell**. Two **eustachian tubes** go from the **nasal cavity** to your ears. They are needed because your middle ear has to have air in it, and the eustachian tubes equalize air pressure. As you know, they can become infected. The nasal cavities are lined with hair-like (*ciliated*) mucous membranes that are richly supplied with blood, which aid in warming and moistening the air before it reaches the lungs. The mucous secretion is sticky and catches impurities in the incoming air. Small hairs in the nose help stop some larger items.

Pharynx—Air passes from the nose into the tube, called the pharynx, a passageway for both air and food. It lies behind the nose and mouth. The part behind the mouth is called the *throat*. The *tonsils* are at the back of the throat. A leaf-shaped cartilage, the **epiglottis**, covers the air passage that leads out of the pharynx so that, when you swallow, food does not enter the lungs and choke you.

Larynx—The air passes from the pharynx into the larynx, a box-like area made of tough cartilages that are held together by ligaments and located in front of the neck. The cartilages move when you talk. Inside are two triangular folds of mucous membrane and the **vocal cords** which extend from back to front. They vibrate as air passes over them.

Trachea and bronchi—Air passes into the trachea, a tube made of membranes inside horseshoe-shaped bars of cartilage. At the lower end, it divides into two smaller tubes (the **bronchi**), one **bronchus** going to each lung. Within the lung, they divide into many smaller branches, the **bronchioles**. These keep thinning out (quite similar to branches of a tree) and end in sac-like air spaces, called **atria**. Each atria has many irregular projections, called **alveoli** or air cells. It resembles a bunch of grapes. The lungs have over 400 million alveoli, along with blood and lymph vessels, nerves, and connective tissue.

Lungs—The lungs are two cone-shaped organs which fill the chest cavity. They are separated by the heart. The top of each cone is called the *apex*; the *base* is the lower, wider portion above the diaphragm. This is where the blood exchanges *carbon dioxide* for *oxygen*. The lungs have **lobes**; infection in only one lobe is called *lobar pneumonia*.

Pleura—The chest cavity is lined with a membrane, the pleura, that folds back against the lungs. The surface is moist, so the lungs can move smoothly without friction when you breathe. Infection of the pleura is *pleurisy*.

Breathing—There are two kinds of breathing: breathing which occurs within body cells and lung breathing. The lungs hold about 3½ quarts of air. You normally take in and let out about a pint with every breath. The **diaphragm**, that dome-shaped muscle between your breathing and digestive apparatus, helps push in and let out the air.

7 - THE URINARY SYSTEM

Why it is needed—Activity in the human body produces wastes of various kinds. Carbon dioxide is removed through the respiratory system, but there are other wastes which result when body cells burn food. Many of these wastes are in the circulating blood. Some of them are removed in the blood filtration and removal plant, which is the **urinary system**.

Location and appearance of the kidneys—These are two reddish-brown, bean-shaped organs, located in the small of the back at the lower edge of the ribs, on either side of the spine. Because their appearance is so similar, "kidney beans" are named after them. Each kidney is embedded in fatty tissue; and, in turn, all this is surrounded by a fibrous covering, called the **renal fascia**. This attaches to muscles of the lower pelvis and helps hold the kidneys in place.

Inside the kidneys—The kidneys receive a rich supply of blood. Each kidney has two distinct portions: the outside (**cortex**) and the inner portion (**medulla**). In addition to blood and lymph vessels and nerve fibers, most of the kidney consists of over a million tiny units, called **nephrons**.

Nephrons—Each nephron is a capillary cluster with a coiled tube (known as a **convoluted tubule**) attached to it. As the blood passes through the capillary cluster, water and waste products filter through the capillary walls and into the tubule. Much of this water is reabsorbed back into the body. But the wastes remain behind in a concentrated solution. It is very important that you drink enough water, so you will not wear out your kidneys!

Ureters—This concentrated mixture of waste products and water is *urine*. A tube (the *ureter*) leads from each kidney to the bladder. Each tube is 10 to 12 inches long and the size of a goose quill (1/5-inch in diameter). The upper end of the ureter extends into the hollowed-out area of the kidney (remember the shape of that kidney bean). That hollowed-out area is called the *renal pelvis*. Infection in that area is called *pyelitis*.

Bladder—Both tubes lead down into the bladder. It is a muscular sac that lies in front in the lowest part of the *abdominal cavity*. The bladder is the reservoir where the urine collects. It has 3 layers of muscle and is lined with mucous membrane (as is the entire urinary system). The bladder can greatly enlarge, so much so that it can rise to the height of the *umbilicus (belly button)*. Although capacity varies, the desire to void is generally present when it fills to about 200 cc. A total of 1 pint can be retained before voiding.

Sphincters—The *external* and *internal* *sphincter muscles* are valves keeping the bladder outlet closed. When enough urine has collected to stretch the bladder walls, nerve signals relax the inner sphincter and more signals reach the brain. The decision is made to *void*, and this causes other nerve signals to tell the outer sphincter to relax. Urine flows and the bladder is emptied.

Urethra—Urine leaves the bladder through the urethra. In the male, it extends the length of the *penis*, and has a total length of about 7 inches. In the female, it is about 1½ inches long.

Urine—Normal urine contains water (about 95%), salt, and protein wastes filtered out of the blood by the kidneys. It is a yellowish, clear fluid with an ammonia-like odor. Its color, odor, composition and amount are influenced by diet, amount of liquid drunk, perspiration, hemorrhage, diarrhea, vomiting, fever, emotional disturbances, drugs, as well as diseases affecting the pancreas, kidneys, bladder, heart, and blood vessels. *Albumin* in the urine is a sign of *kidney damage*. *Sugar* in varying amounts indicates *diabetes*.

Water intake—A healthy person usually eliminates a quart or more of urine each day. It is of extreme importance that you drink enough water! People who obtain their fluid intake only from coffee or soft drinks are not only taking harmful substances into their bodies, but they generally are not getting enough water. Learn to drink plain water, and enough of it! Water is not only needed for thousands of body functions, but it also helps reduce heat. On a hot day, you lose heat through perspiration.

8 - THE NERVOUS SYSTEM

Autonomic nervous system—Many functions are done automatically, without any thinking on your part. This is called the autonomic nervous system. This includes such things as the digestion of food and circulation of blood, activity within the cells, and control of the muscles in the glands and blood vessels.

Central nervous system—The central nervous system includes the *brain* and *spinal cord* (which are also used by the autonomic nervous system). The brain and spinal cord are the switchboard, and the *nerves* are the wires that carry incoming and outgoing messages.

Brain—The human brain is the center for thinking. It weighs about 3 pounds and is in the *skull*, which protects its delicate structure. It has several sections.

Cerebrum—The cerebrum is divided into two halves, one on either side, called *hemispheres*. The outside portion *(cerebral cortex)* is soft grayish, wrinkled matter that is mostly nerve cells. Underneath is the *white matter*, containing nerve fibers, that help store and move data around. Some centers in the cerebrum record and store data; others are connected with hearing, seeing, moving, and speaking.

Hemispheres—The cerebrum has a right and left side, with duplicate motor control centers in each side. The right side controls muscles on the left side of the body and vice-versa. Thus an injury to the left side would affect the right side of the body.

Thalamus—Directly beneath the cerebral hemispheres are the thalamus and hypothalamus. The thalamus is a relay station. It receives impulses from every part of the body and relays them to appropriate parts of the cortex. The thalamus also tells you whether sensations are pleasant or unpleasant.

Hypothalamus—This structure regulates the action of various body organs, so normal conditions can be maintained. It helps maintain body temperature by causing us to shiver when we are cold. It sends messages to the *pituitary*, which, in turn, sends messages to the *thyroid,* to send out more *thyroxin* to the cells to increase energy levels. The hypothalamus also regulates the expression of certain emotions.

Cerebellum—The cerebellum helps you keep your balance. It coordinates groups of muscles, so they can work together. You could not handwrite or typewrite without the help of your cerebellum. It keeps you walking straight and makes your movements graceful.

Midbrain—At the top of the brain stem is a small bit of tissue, called the midbrain. It is an important reflex center. A *reflex* is an action that takes place automatically in response to some stimulus. As an example, if you look in a mirror and shake your head from side to side, you will see your eyes continue to look straight forward. That is a reflex effect, controlled by the midbrain.

Pons—The word means "bridge"; the pons bridge between the cerebral cortex and the cerebellum, carrying messages back and forth.

Medulla—Lying just below the pons, the medulla rests on the *floor of the skull*. It connects the spinal cord with the brain. It also directly controls such things as changing breathing rate, in response to carbon dioxide rate, and changing the rate of heartbeat and muscles in the smallest arteries.

Spinal cord—The spinal cord is inside the column of vertebral rings; it is a long mass of nerve cells and fibers, extending from the medulla down the backbone. It conducts impulses from various nerves to the brain and vice-versa. It is also a reflex center. If you touch something hot, the message goes from your hand to the spine, which immediately sends back the message to remove your hand. The truth is that part of your brain is in your spine!

Nerves—The nerves connect the body, brain, and spinal cord. A complete nerve cell consists of a cell body with thread-like fibers. The whole thing is called a **neuron**. Each one can be rather long, and transmits impulses in only one direction. **Axons,** on one end, conduct impulses away from the cell body. **Dendrites**, on the other end, conduct impulses to the cell.

Cranial nerves—There are 12 pairs of cranial nerves and 31 pairs of spinal nerves. The cranial nerves attach directly to the brain; and most of them carry impulses to and from the brain and various structures about the head (sensory organs, swallowing, speech, jaw muscles, etc.). Other cranial nerves act on the organs of the thorax (upper chest and back area) and abdomen.

Spinal nerves—Spinal nerves are attached to the spinal cord and carry sensory messages (pain, pleasure, etc.) from the skin to the central nervous system. They also send motor impulses to the skeletal muscles.

Sensory and motor nerves—Sensory neurons receive messages from all parts of the body and transmit them to the central nervous system. Motor neurons transmit messages from the central nervous system to points throughout the body. The message may be to alter muscle activity or to cause glands to secrete.

Nerve covering—A sheath, called a **myelin sheath,** covers the outside of the brain and spinal cord. It is like the insulation on electric wires, and has the same purpose. An outer covering over this sheath is the **Neurilemma**. Its function is to grow new nerve tissue. This is slow growth, so paralysis or numbness may persist for months. Sometimes nerve tissue does not repair itself at all.

Message routes—Nerve messages can be routed in many different paths; yet they always follow the shortest, quickest one.

9 - THE ENDOCRINE SYSTEM

Endocrines—This is another amazing part of your body. Without your glandular secretions, you could not survive; yet, as with most of the rest of the human body, they are a bewildering complexity which could not be originated by chance. There are eight main types of endocrine glands: ***pineal, pituitary, parathyroids, thyroid, thymus, adrenals, islets of Langerhans, gonads (testes and ovaries)***. Located in different parts of the body, they pour their secretions directly into the bloodstream; so they are called **ductless glands**. A *duct* is a tubular structure that a fluid passes through. Examples of *ducted glands* would be gastric and duodenal glands, which secrete digestive juices through ducts.

Hormones—The endocrine glands produce substances, called hormones, which speed up or slow down activities of various body organs. They also affect each other's actions. Too much or too little of one hormone not only affects one organ, but also interferes with the work of other hormones.

Thyroid—Located in the front of the neck, the thyroid covers the sides and lower front of the *larynx* (your voice box). It looks something like a butterfly with wings 2 to 3 inches wide. The thyroid secretes the hormone, ***thyroxine***. (T_3 is the most active subtype of thyroxine.)'

Thyroxin—This substance regulates the rate at which the cells burn food. If not enough hormone is secreted, the cells burn food too slowly; and this interferes with the development of the body and slows its activities. If too much is secreted, the body burns food so rapidly that it uses up its daily supply and draws on the stored reserves of food. All activities are speeded up.

Iodine—Over half of what is in thyroxin is iodine. The thyroid gland gets iodine from the blood. If not enough is available in the diet, the thyroid grows larger in its effort to make enough thyroxin. This enlarged condition is *goiter*. A *basal metabolism* test can help indicate how close the person's body is to the *normal metabolic rate* (the normal rate of burning food in the cells).

Parathyroids—These are four small glands, each about the size of a pea. Two are on each side behind the thyroid. If removed, the person immediately dies. They secrete a hormone **(parathyroid hormone)** that regulates the amount of *calcium in the blood*, thus affecting the amount of nerve and muscle irritability. Too little calcium produces muscle spasms and convulsions and lead to death within hours. If too much hormone is secreted, the diet cannot supply enough calcium and calcium salts are drawn from the bones, making them soft and unable to support weight (*osteitis fibrosa cystica*).

P
H
Y
S

Adrenals—The two adrenal glands are located at the upper end of the kidneys. Each one is curved and the size of the last joint in the little finger. Each adrenal gland is actually two separate glands in one.

Adrenal medulla—The central part of each one is the medulla, secreting *epinephrine (adrenaline)*. This brings many body processes into action quickly. It makes the heart beat faster, raises blood pressure, increases muscle power, raises blood sugar level, and makes blood clot more rapidly. It is the "fight or flight" hormone, needed for sudden emergencies. Emotions of fright, anger, pain, love, or grief trigger it to action.

Adrenal cortex—The outer part of the adrenals, the cortex, secretes several hormones. One is *Cortin*, which regulates the behavior of salt and water content in the body. If part of the gland is destroyed, Addison's disease develops. This is a condition of extreme muscle weakness, highly pigmented (bronzed) skin, and decreased kidney activity. Both male and female sex hormones are also secreted by the adrenal cortex. Disorders of the cortex can produce tumors, hasten sex development in boys, or cause male characteristics in girls (facial hair, absence of menses).

Pancreas—There are small bunches of tissue scattered through the pancreas, called the *islets (islands) of Langerhans*. They secrete *insulin*, which regulates the amount of sugar in the blood. If they secrete too little insulin, sugar accumulates, and the kidneys try to get rid of it in the urine. This condition is called *diabetes mellitus*, and is controlled by injections of insulin.

Pituitary—This is one of the most protected glands in your body. Located at the base of the brain and behind your eyes, it is almost in the center of your skull. About the size of a pea, it probably secretes more potent hormones than any other gland, and has been called the "master gland." It is made up of two parts: the anterior lobe and the posterior lobe.

Pituitary posterior lobe—This rear lobe secretes two hormones that affect the smooth muscles, raise blood pressure, and stimulate the reabsorption of water in the kidney tubules, thus affecting water balance.

Pituitary anterior lobe—This frontal lobe secretes several hormones. One *(ACTH)* controls the adrenal cortex. Others regulate the thyroid, stimulate the activity of sex and mammary glands, and regulate growth of bone and fibrous tissue. Too little of this hormone in youth results in *dwarfism*. Too much of the growth hormone in youth causes *gigantism*; in adults, it makes the hands and feet and head abnormally large, a condition called *acromegaly*.

Gonads—The testes and ovaries are the glands of reproduction and sexual characteristics.

Testes—These secrete the male sex hormones, *androgens*. One of these, *testosterone*, controls the development of sex characteristics—such as male body form, hair distribution, and voice.

Ovaries—These produce two hormones: *Estrogen* helps maintain normal menstrual cycle and controls and maintains sex growth. *Progesterone* is necessary for implantation of the fertilized ovum and continuation of pregnancy. Both hormones prepare the endometrium for pregnancy and are necessary for a woman's normal emotional life.

Thymus—This gland lies behind the sternum (breast bone). It has two main lobes and aids in attaining sexual maturity. It atrophies (ceases to function) following puberty.

Pineal gland—This gland, located in the brain behind the pituitary, affects body growth.

Other hormones—There are other hormones which are not often discussed. The stomach wall secretes a hormone, *gastrin*, that affects the blood vessels and secretions of the stomach digestive juice glands. The lining of the upper part of the small intestine (duodenum) secretes *secretin*, which stimulates the pancreas to send pancreatic juice to help digest food. The duodenal lining also secretes another hormone that tells the gallbladder to open and send gall to emulsify fat. The *placenta* acts as a temporary endocrine gland, helping in the maintenance of pregnancy.

10 - THE REPRODUCTIVE SYSTEM

Introduction—Asexual reproduction is done by mitosis, as in protozoa. Human beings reproduce by sexual methods. Each female and male possesses sex glands *(gonads)* which produce special sex cells *(gametes)*. When the male gamete is brought into contact with the female gamete, they unite and form a new single-celled individual (a *zygote*). The zygote undergoes repeated divisions, resulting in another individual, a composite of its parents and other ancestors.

MEN

Testes—These are two oval-shaped glands which produce large numbers of *sperm cells*. They are suspended in a sac, called the *scrotum*. The sperm cells are in a fluid called *semen*; most of this is produced by the testes. Hormones which aid in the development of changes occurring at puberty are also produced by the testes. The *sperm* is a microscopic cell with a whip-like tail, and it swims rather rapidly in the semen. Millions of sperm are in 1 drop of *seminal fluid* (semen).

Epididymis—This is a 20 foot tube, which is coiled along the top and side of the testes; it is so narrow it can barely be seen by the naked eye. The sperm swims through this tube.

Seminal duct—This duct is also called the *vas*

PHYS

deferens or **ductus deferens**. It is a tube which goes from the epididymis tube, through the **inguinal canal**, all the way up and around the bladder and into the prostate gland. (An *inguinal hernia* can occur at the inguinal canal opening into the abdomen.)

Seminal vesicles—These are pouches which secrete additional fluid for the semen. They also store sperm which has traveled that far. Ducts (tubes) leading from them join with the seminal ducts at the entrance to the prostate gland.

Prostate gland—This is a doughnut-shaped gland located just below the bladder. It contains 30 to 50 *alveola glands*, and encircles the seminal duct and the urethra (the tube that carries urine to its final outlet). The prostate adds an alkaline fluid to the seminal fluid which greatly increases how fast the sperm, which pass beyond it, are able to swim.

Urethra—As the seminal duct is about to exit the prostate, it joins with the urethra (normally used as a urine tube). It is well-known that, in older men the prostate sometimes enlarges, reducing the flow of urine through the urethra. Less well-known is the reason why the prostate gland surrounds the urethra: A little before sexual intercourse, a signal is sent to the prostate, to clamp down and close off the urine tube so it is empty. The inflowing semen purifies it, prior to ejaculation. Just beyond the prostate, two **cowper's glands** each the size of a pea, add a mucous-like lubricating fluid into the semen in the urethra. The urethra continues on down to its outlet, at the tip of the penis.

Penis—This is a cylinder-shaped organ located externally. It has cavern-like spaces in it which can greatly engorge with blood. At the end of this organ is a fold of loose skin which forms the hood-like **foreskin (prepuce)**. *Circumcision* is the cutting off of this foreskin.

WOMEN

Ovaries—The **ovum** is the female cell of reproduction. The **ova**, or eggs (**ovum** is singular), are produced by the ovaries, which are two glands about the size of an unshelled almond, located within the abdominal cavity just below the top of the pelvis; one is on each side. Imbedded in the ovaries are thousands of microscopic structures called **graafian follicles**. The ova are encased inside these follicles. A female infant has 400,000 follicles; an adult has 200,000, of which about 400 mature into ova and are discharged. The ovaries also secrete hormones that help regulate reproduction.

Menstruation—Upon reaching menstrual age, the ova begin maturing in the follicles. Once each month one follicle ripens, pushes its way to the surface of the ovary, breaks open, and discharges the egg (ova) into the pelvic cavity. This is **ovulation**.

Fallopian tubes—There are two fallopian tubes (*uterine tubes*), one on each side. Each of these tubes is about 4-5 inches in length. The mature ovum bursts from the ovary into the **peritoneal cavity**. Just beneath it is the open end of a fallopian tube. Finger-like projections (called **processes**) on that open end wave the ovum into one of the tubes, where it travels on down into the uterus.

Uterus—The fallopian tubes are attached to the uterus (**womb**), which is a hollow, very muscular, pear-shaped organ in the center of the pelvic cavity. It is about three inches long and has two parts, the body and the neck (**cervix**). The body rounds into a bulging surface, about the level where the tubes enter it. This area is called the **fundus**. The cervix, below it, is narrow and thicker. Its lower portion is called the **cervical canal**. The opening of the cervix is the **external os**. ("Os" means a mouth or opening.) The inside is lined with a tissue filled with blood vessels. This tissue is a mucous membrane layer called **endometrium**. Strong ligaments keep it in position. The uterus is capable of great expansion, since it is the organ in which the baby grows.

Vagina—The neck of the uterus opens into a muscular canal, the vagina, which opens into the **vulva**, which has the external genital organs (the **labia**, two sets of lip-like folds on each side of the vaginal opening, and the **clitoris**). The vagina is the female organ of intercourse and is part of the **birth canal**. (The birth canal is the route taken by the baby in the process of being born into the world.) The **urinary meatus**, the urinary outlet, is between the clitoris and vaginal opening (orifice). Initially, the **hymen** partially closes the external opening of the vagina.

Perineum—This is the space between the lower end of the vagina and the rectum. During childbirth, it is sometimes torn or deliberately cut. If either occurs, it requires special care after birth.

Breasts—These are the **mammary glands**. They are stimulated by endocrines to secrete **milk**, after a child is born. Each breast, composed of glandular tissues and fat, is divided into 16 to 20 separate *lobes* that secrete milk. Each lobe has a main duct; these ducts converge toward the **nipple (areola)**, like the spokes of a wheel. They terminate in tiny openings on the surface of the nipple. The breasts enlarge during pregnancy, and the skin around the nipples become pigmented (darker in color).

Fertilization—An ovum leaves the ovary about halfway between menstrual cycles; it enters the fallopian tube and travels down toward the uterus. During intercourse, millions of sperm cells (200 million to 400 million) are discharged by **ejaculation** into the vagina. They enter the uterus and move into the fallopian tubes. These sperm, earlier nourished by the semen, only live about 24 hours (since they swim upward, away from the semen). If one of the sperm cells meets an ovum, the two cells join. The new cell (a **zygote**) then proceeds down the tube and attaches itself to the wall of the uterus, and **pregnancy** is established. It rarely attaches to the wall of the fallopian tube, which results in **tubal pregnancy** and is a serious problem.

Menstruation—About every 28 days a rhythmical series of changes occurs, called the **menstrual cycle (period)**. The various changes that occur are the result from several hormones.

During 7 to 10 days after the flow has ceased, a graafian follicle and an ovum are maturing (caused by a hormone from the pituitary). As the follicle matures, it produces a hormone called **estrogen**, which, in turn, causes the lining (endometrium) of the uterus to greatly thicken in preparation for a possible pregnancy.

At the end of this time (about the 7th to 10th day following cessation of the flow), ovulation occurs. As soon as the ovum is released, the follicle it used to be in now becomes a yellow body with a new name: **corpus luteum**. This secretes a second female hormone, **progesterone**, which continues the work begun by estrogen in further preparing the uterus for pregnancy.

Nonfertilization—The ovum can only be fertilized for a day or two following its release. If that does not occur, the ovum soon perishes and the corpus luteum stops producing progesterone. Without that hormone, the blood supply to the endometrium is affected and it begins to disintegrate. Soon the endometrium is sloughed off, and a discharge (the **menstrual flow**) from the uterus occurs. This lasts one to five days, during which time a new follicle starts to ripen and another cycle begins.

Fertilization—If fertilization (the uniting of the sperm with the ovum) occurs, it usually takes place while the ovum is in the fallopian tube. The fertilized ovum (now a zygote) moves to the uterus and implants itself in the uterine wall. This immediately causes the corpus luteum to increase its production of progesterone. Because there is now a use for the endometrium, menstruation ceases.

Menopause—As long as ovarian hormones act on the uterine lining, menstruation continues. The ovaries gradually become less active as forties approach. In women between 45 and 55 (usually beginning 45-50), mature egg cells and the hormones that act on the uterine line cease being produced. Then menstruation ceases. This span of time is called menopause. It should be a gradual change that the body can adjust to with little difficulty. But sometimes there are problems, such as hot flashes (sudden warm flushes over the skin, induced by the thyroid, that are temporary disturbances of the circulation). When menopause is excessive or prolonged, head-

aches, sweating, dizzy spells, worry, fear, irritability, and/or persistent depression may occur.

11 - THE SPECIAL SENSES

External ear—This is the only visible part. It is mostly cartilage, shaped to receive sounds, with the small end opening into a tube, the **auditory canal (meatus)**. This canal ends at a thin wall, called the **ear drum (typanic membrane)**. The lining of the auditory canal is covered with tiny hairs and secretes a waxy substance, called **cerumen**. This aids the transmission of sound and the taste of it causes entering insects to hurriedly exit.

Middle ear—This is a small cavity, behind the ear drum, in the temporal bone of the skull. It has two openings: one into the **mastoid cells** behind it and the other into the **eustachian tube** that goes down to the back of the nose (nasopharynx). If the eustachian tube was not there, your ear drum would be destroyed as soon as you climbed or descended a few thousand feet. Because it is there, the ear drum can vibrate freely, transmitting sound. The tube only opens during swallowing. Infection can travel from the throat to the middle ear through that tube.

Three small bones **(the ossicles)** hang between the ear drum and the cavity side wall, which are named for their strange shapes: the **hammer (malleus),** the **anvil (incus),** and the **stirrup (stapes)**. Sound waves start vibrations of the ear drum that set these bones in motion, and they carry the sound across the middle ear.

Inner ear—The internal ear has two parts: the **cochlea** and the semicircular canals. The cochlea looks like a snail shell. Its coils are filled with fluid that carries the sound waves that enter from the middle ear. The base of the stirrup bone fits into the opening between the middle ear and the inner ear. When the stirrup sets the fluid in the cochlea in motion, the tiny receptive nerve endings pass the vibrations on to the **auditory nerve**, which carries them to the **brain**. The brain interprets these vibrations as **sounds**.

Semicircular canals—The three semicircular canals in each ear, shaped like horseshoes, lie beside the cochlea. They are partly filled with fluid that is set in motion by head or body movements. Because this fluid also has communication with the brain, we are able to sense and maintain proper balance.

Eye—As with everything else in the human body, the human eye is astounding. Instead of being a camera, the eye registers every new image, one immediately after the other (about 20 per second). In addition, because there are two eyes, **in-depth (binocular) vision** is accomplished. Because the eyeballs can move separately, and the lens can change thickness, you can see things both closer and at a distance. The eye lies in a circular cavity within several bones which, before birth, fused together. Each eye has optical equipment, muscles, conjunctiva, tear apparatus, and eyelids. Here is a very simplified description of the many wonders in the eye:

Eyeball—As you look at the eye, the white of the eye is the *sclera*. Inside that is the colored part, or *iris*. Inside that is the black spot, the *pupil*. Light passes into the eyeball through the pupil, which can enlarge (dilate) or shrink (contract) in size. (A camera has a similar mechanism, which is called the diaphragm or "stop").

Behind the pupil, the light travels through the *lens*, double convex in shape. Behind that is a clear fluid throughout the middle of the eyeball *(vitreous humor)*. At the back of the eyeball, the light strikes the *retina*, which contains nerve fibers of the *optic nerve* and the *nerve cells* sensitive to light. Two types of cells are there: rods and cones. There are 100 million *rods* in each retina, which can see things as light and dark ("black and white"), even in very dim light. There are less *cones*; they see color, but only in brighter light. This is why, at night, you only see objects as dark and light, without any color to them.

The lens bends thicker or thinner in order to focus the light into a sharp image. This focusing is called *accommodation*. The light image is then carried to the cells and nerves in the retina and is sent through the optic nerve, to the sight center in the brain.

Eye muscles—Smooth muscles in the eye control the size of the pupil and focusing action of the lens. Three pair of eye muscles outside the eyeball move the eyeball. Another muscle holds the *eyelid* open (or relaxes and lets it shut).

Tear glands—The *lacrimal (tear) glands* are above the eyeball. They secrete tears which keep the eyeball moist. They drain into the *conjunctival sacs* and then drain into the inner corners of the eyelids. From there, they drain through small ducts into the nose. When they flow rapidly, tears run down the cheeks.

Eye problems—When a lens becomes cloudy, the condition is called *cataract*. If the eyeball is too short, the light rays focus behind the retina instead of on it. This causes *far-sightedness (hyperopia)*. Corrective convex lenses are needed. In *near-sightedness (myopia)*, the eyeball is too long or the lens too strong, and the light rays are focused in front of the retina. Corrective concave lenses are needed. *Presbyopia* is lack of lens elasticity, which tends to occur in old age. If the eye has a defective shape, the rays do not exactly focus on a point on the retina. This is *astigmatism*. Corrective lenses must be slightly cylindrical. *Cross eyes* converge excessively. *Wall eyes* diverge too much.

Smell—The sense of smell is obtained through the *olfactory cells*, which are nerve receptors in the walls of the nasal cavity. Tiny particles of odorous substances in the air, in these cells, are dissolved in a special secretion. A message is then sent to the brain, where they are interpreted as a particular odor.

Taste—The taste receptor nerves are called taste buds. Buds on the sides sense *sour* (which is acid). Those on top sense *sweet* (organic products, especially carbohydrates). Those on the tip and sides sense *salty* (chlorides). Those at the back of the tongue sense *bitter* (alkaloids and bile).

Touch—You have sensory organs in your skin, so you know when you touch or are touched. You can sense pressure, heat, cold, and pain. These receptors vary from 16,000 for heat to 4 million for pain.

Kinesthetic—This is the sense of position *(proprioceptive sense)*. You are able to sense your position, erect posture, muscle tonus, weight, pressure, and coordinated body movements. You have sense organs in certain skeletal muscles *(interfusal fibers and neuromuscular spindles)*. You also have sense organs in your tendons *(neurotendinous spindles)*. *And, of course, you have the semicircular canals in your ears which, by locating the pull of gravity, help you maintain balance.*

IMPORTANT MUSCLES

The human body has over 600 muscles. *Smooth muscles* include the heart and liver, and are involuntary. *Skeletal muscles* are under your control. Here are the most prominent of them:

Shoulder muscle - Deltoid
Back shoulder-to-neck muscle - Trapezius
Top upper arm muscle - Biceps
Lower upper arm muscle - Triceps
Chest muscle - Pectorals
Abdominal muscle - Rectus abdominis
Rump muscle - Gluteus maximus
Front upper leg muscle - Quadriceps femoris
Rear lower leg muscle - Gastrocnemius
Also: ankle tendon - Achilles tendon

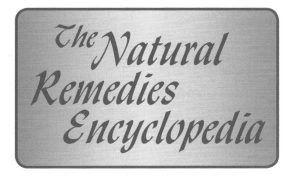

The *Natural* *Remedies* *Encyclopedia*

Basic Anatomy

Here are 50 color pictures of the 50 primary parts of your body:
Integumentary System 1025 / Skelatal System Front 1026 / Skelatal System Back 1026 / Skull Front 1027 / Skull Side 1027 / Ribs Side 1027 / Ribs Front 1027 / Foot 1027 / Spinal Column 1028 / Lumbar Vertebrae 1028 / Tooth 1028 / Adult Teeth 1028 / Muscular System Front 1029 / Muscular System Back 1030 / Muscular System Front Detailed 1031 / Muscular System Back Detailed 1032 / Main Arteries of the Body 1033 / Main Veins of the Body 1033 / Circulatory System 1033 / Views of the Heart 1034 / Coronary Arteries 1034 / Brain 1035 / Spinal Nerves 1036 / Nerve Cell 1036 / Sensory System 1036 / The Ear 1037 / Views of the Eye 1037 / Liver 1038 / Pancreas 1038 / Digestive System 1038 / Stomach 1038 / Respiratory System 1039 / Urinary System 1040 / Male Reproductive System 1040 / Female Reproductive System 1040

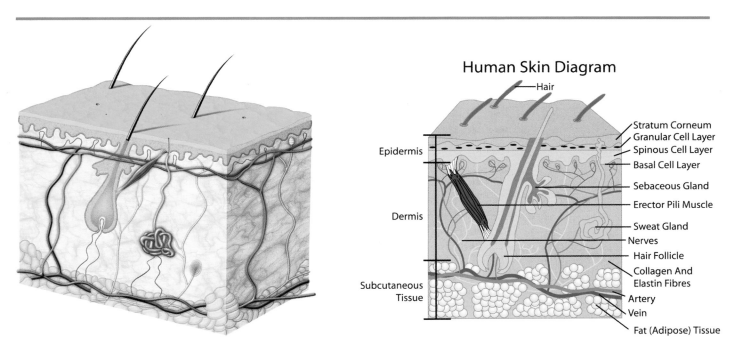

Human Skin Diagram

INTEGUMENTARY SYSTEM (Skin & Body Surfaces)

"Wash you, make you clean." Isaiah 1:16

ANATOMY

SKELETAL ANATOMY (ANTERIOR VIEW)

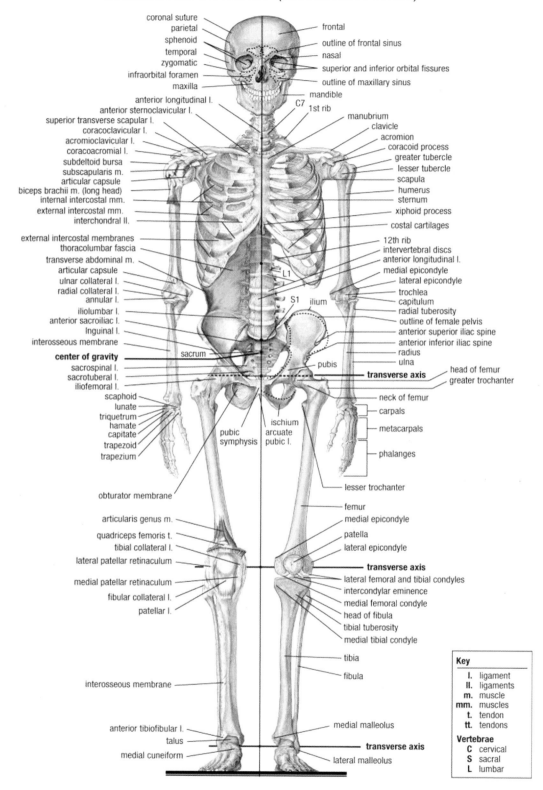

coronal suture
parietal
sphenoid
temporal
zygomatic
infraorbital foramen
maxilla
anterior longitudinal l.
anterior sternoclavicular l.
superior transverse scapular l.
coracoclavicular l.
acromioclavicular l.
coracoacromial l.
subdeltoid bursa
subscapularis m.
articular capsule
biceps brachii m. (long head)
internal intercostal mm.
external intercostal mm.
interchondral ll.
external intercostal membranes
thoracolumbar fascia
transverse abdominal m.
articular capsule
ulnar collateral l.
radial collateral l.
annular l.
iliolumbar l.
anterior sacroiliac l.
Inguinal l.
interosseous membrane
center of gravity
sacrospinal l.
sacrotuberal l.
iliofemoral l.
scaphoid
lunate
triquetrum
hamate
capitate
trapezoid
trapezium
obturator membrane
articularis genus m.
quadriceps femoris t.
tibial collateral l.
lateral patellar retinaculum
medial patellar retinaculum
fibular collateral l.
patellar l.
interosseous membrane
anterior tibiofibular l.
talus
medial cuneiform

frontal
outline of frontal sinus
nasal
superior and inferior orbital fissures
outline of maxillary sinus
mandible
C7
1st rib
manubrium
clavicle
acromion
coracoid process
greater tubercle
lesser tubercle
scapula
humerus
sternum
xiphoid process
costal cartilages
12th rib
intervertebral discs
anterior longitudinal l.
medial epicondyle
lateral epicondyle
trochlea
capitulum
radial tuberosity
outline of female pelvis
anterior superior iliac spine
anterior inferior iliac spine
radius
ulna
transverse axis
head of femur
greater trochanter
neck of femur
carpals
metacarpals
phalanges
lesser trochanter
femur
medial epicondyle
patella
lateral epicondyle
transverse axis
lateral femoral and tibial condyles
intercondylar eminence
medial femoral condyle
head of fibula
tibial tuberosity
medial tibial condyle
tibia
fibula
medial malleolus
transverse axis
lateral malleolus

L1
S1
ilium
sacrum
pubis
ischium
arcuate
pubic l.
pubic
symphysis

Key
l.   ligament
ll.   ligaments
m.   muscle
mm.   muscles
t.   tendon
tt.   tendons

Vertebrae
C   cervical
S   sacral
L   lumbar

"Thou hast clothed me with skin and flesh, and hast fenced me with bones and sinews." Job 10:11

SKELETAL ANATOMY (POSTERIOR VIEW)

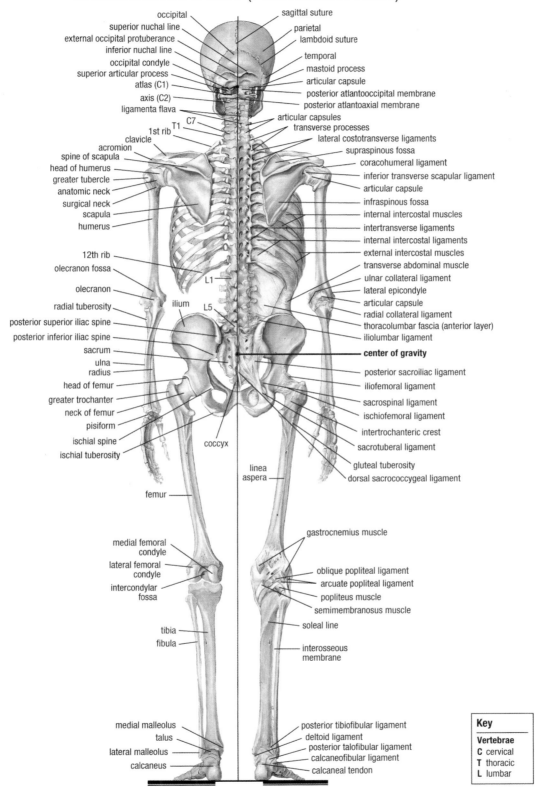

occipital
superior nuchal line
external occipital protuberance
inferior nuchal line
occipital condyle
superior articular process
atlas (C1)
axis (C2)
ligamenta flava
C7
T1
1st rib
clavicle
acromion
spine of scapula
head of humerus
greater tubercle
anatomic neck
surgical neck
scapula
humerus
12th rib
olecranon fossa
olecranon
radial tuberosity
posterior superior iliac spine
posterior inferior iliac spine
sacrum
ulna
radius
head of femur
greater trochanter
neck of femur
pisiform
ischial spine
ischial tuberosity

sagittal suture
parietal
lambdoid suture
temporal
mastoid process
articular capsule
posterior atlantooccipital membrane
posterior atlantoaxial membrane
articular capsules
transverse processes
lateral costotransverse ligaments
supraspinous fossa
coracohumeral ligament
inferior transverse scapular ligament
articular capsule
infraspinous fossa
internal intercostal muscles
intertransverse ligaments
internal intercostal ligaments
external intercostal muscles
transverse abdominal muscle
ulnar collateral ligament
lateral epicondyle
articular capsule
radial collateral ligament
thoracolumbar fascia (anterior layer)
iliolumbar ligament
center of gravity
posterior sacroiliac ligament
iliofemoral ligament
sacrospinal ligament
ischiofemoral ligament
intertrochanteric crest
sacrotuberal ligament
gluteal tuberosity
dorsal sacrococcygeal ligament

ilium
L1
L5
coccyx

linea
aspera

femur

medial femoral
condyle
lateral femoral
condyle
intercondylar
fossa

gastrocnemius muscle

oblique popliteal ligament
arcuate popliteal ligament
popliteus muscle
semimembranosus muscle
soleal line
interosseous
membrane

tibia
fibula

medial malleolus
talus
lateral malleolus
calcaneus

posterior tibiofibular ligament
deltoid ligament
posterior talofibular ligament
calcaneofibular ligament
calcaneal tendon

Key	
Vertebrae	
C	cervical
T	thoracic
L	lumbar

A
N
A
T
O
M
Y

"Pleasant words are as an honeycomb, sweet to the soul, and health to the bones."
Proverbs 16:24

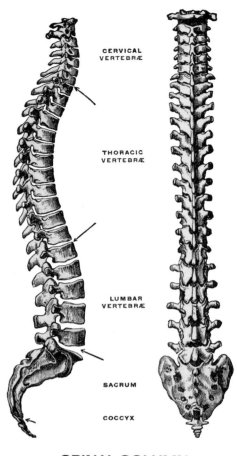

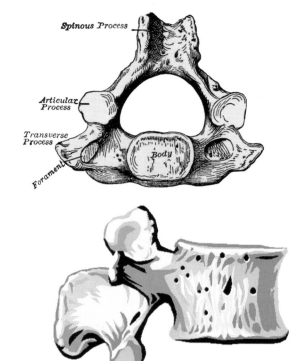

SPINAL COLUMN

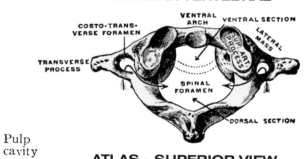

LUMBAR VERTEBRAE

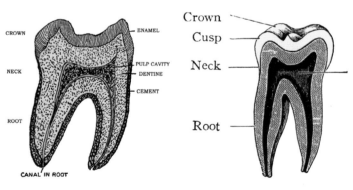

TEETH

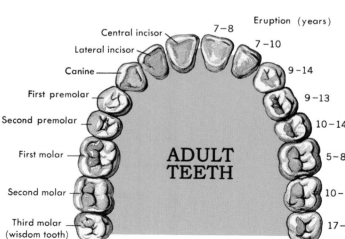

ATLAS - SUPERIOR VIEW

*"And the LORD shall guide thee
continually, and satisfy thy soul in
drought, and make fat thy bones."*
Isaiah 58:11

Muscles of the Body (Front)

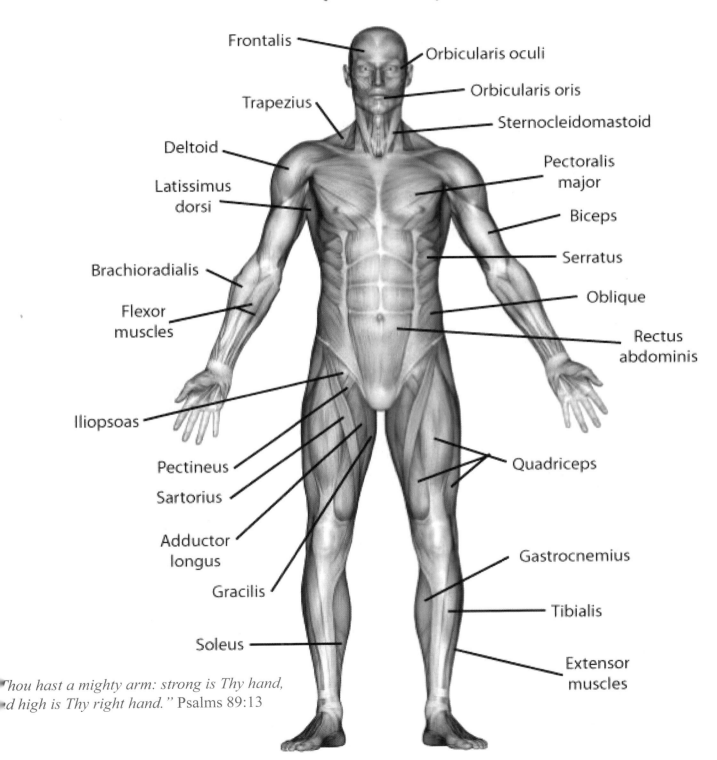

Frontalis
Orbicularis oculi
Orbicularis oris
Trapezius
Sternocleidomastoid
Deltoid
Pectoralis major
Latissimus dorsi
Biceps
Serratus
Brachioradialis
Oblique
Flexor muscles
Rectus abdominis
Iliopsoas
Pectineus
Quadriceps
Sartorius
Adductor longus
Gastrocnemius
Gracilis
Tibialis
Soleus
Extensor muscles

*"Thou hast a mighty arm: strong is Thy hand,
and high is Thy right hand."* Psalms 89:13

ANATOMY

Muscles of the Body (Back)

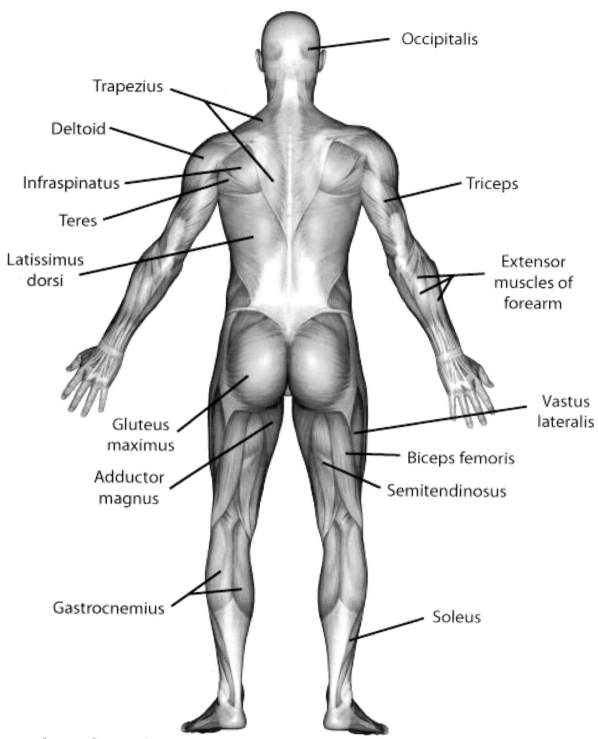

Occipitalis

Trapezius

Deltoid

Infraspinatus

Teres

Latissimus dorsi

Triceps

Extensor muscles of forearm

Gluteus maximus

Adductor magnus

Vastus lateralis

Biceps femoris

Semitendinosus

Gastrocnemius

Soleus

"God is our refuge and strength, a very present help in trouble." Psalms 46:1

MUSCULAR SYSTEM (ANTERIOR VIEW)

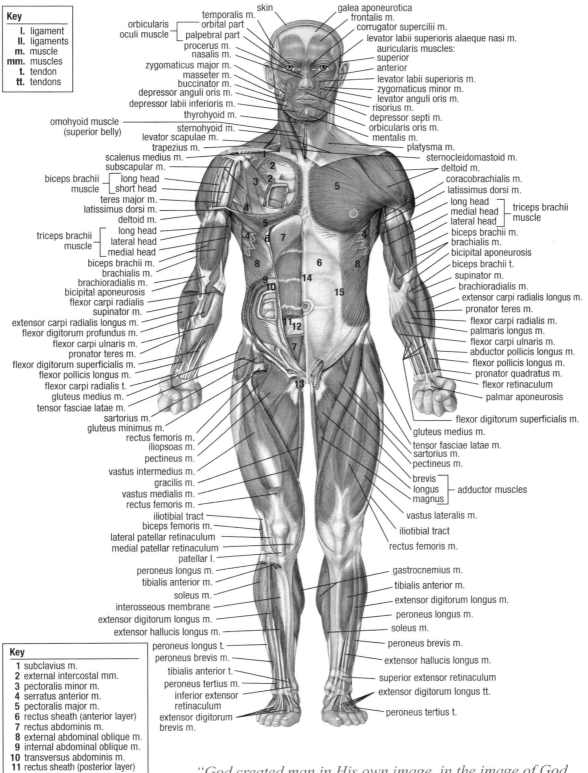

Key
l.	ligament
ll.	ligaments
m.	muscle
mm.	muscles
t.	tendon
tt.	tendons

skin
temporalis m.
orbicularis
oculi muscle
  orbital part
  palpebral part
procerus m.
nasalis m.
zygomaticus major m.
masseter m.
buccinator m.
depressor anguli oris m.
depressor labii inferioris m.
thyrohyoid m.
omohyoid muscle (superior belly)
sternohyoid m.
levator scapulae m.
trapezius m.
scalenus medius m.
subscapular m.
biceps brachii muscle
  long head
  short head
teres major m.
latissimus dorsi m.
deltoid m.
triceps brachii muscle
  long head
  lateral head
  medial head
biceps brachii m.
brachialis m.
brachioradialis m.
bicipital aponeurosis
flexor carpi radialis
supinator m.
extensor carpi radialis longus m.
flexor digitorum profundus m.
flexor carpi ulnaris m.
pronator teres m.
flexor digitorum superficialis m.
flexor pollicis longus m.
flexor carpi radialis t.
gluteus medius m.
tensor fasciae latae m.
sartorius m.
gluteus minimus m.
rectus femoris m.
iliopsoas m.
pectineus m.
vastus intermedius m.
gracilis m.
vastus medialis m.
rectus femoris m.
iliotibial tract
biceps femoris m.
lateral patellar retinaculum
medial patellar retinaculum
patellar l.
peroneus longus m.
tibialis anterior m.
soleus m.
interosseous membrane
extensor digitorum longus m.
extensor hallucis longus m.
peroneus longus t.
peroneus brevis m.
tibialis anterior t.
peroneus tertius m.
inferior extensor retinaculum
extensor digitorum brevis m.

galea aponeurotica
frontalis m.
corrugator supercilii m.
levator labii superioris alaeque nasi m.
auricularis muscles:
  superior
  anterior
levator labii superioris m.
zygomaticus minor m.
levator anguli oris m.
risorius m.
depressor septi m.
orbicularis oris m.
mentalis m.
platysma m.
sternocleidomastoid m.
deltoid m.
coracobrachialis m.
latissimus dorsi m.
triceps brachii muscle
  long head
  medial head
  lateral head
biceps brachii m.
brachialis m.
bicipital aponeurosis
biceps brachii t.
supinator m.
brachioradialis m.
extensor carpi radialis longus m.
pronator teres m.
flexor carpi radialis m.
palmaris longus m.
flexor carpi ulnaris m.
abductor pollicis longus m.
flexor pollicis longus m.
pronator quadratus m.
flexor retinaculum
palmar aponeurosis
flexor digitorum superficialis m.
gluteus medius m.
tensor fasciae latae m.
sartorius m.
pectineus m.
adductor muscles
  brevis
  longus
  magnus
vastus lateralis m.
iliotibial tract
rectus femoris m.
gastrocnemius m.
tibialis anterior m.
extensor digitorum longus m.
peroneus longus m.
soleus m.
peroneus brevis m.
extensor hallucis longus m.
superior extensor retinaculum
extensor digitorum longus tt.
peroneus tertius t.

Key
1 subclavius m.
2 external intercostal mm.
3 pectoralis minor m.
4 serratus anterior m.
5 pectoralis major m.
6 rectus sheath (anterior layer)
7 rectus abdominis m.
8 external abdominal oblique m.
9 internal abdominal oblique m.
10 transversus abdominis m.
11 rectus sheath (posterior layer)
12 arcuate line
13 cremaster m.
14 linea alba
15 aponeurosis of external abdominal oblique m.

"God created man in His own image, in the image of God created He him; male and female created He them."
Genesis 1:27

ANATOMY

MUSCULAR SYSTEM (POSTERIOR VIEW)

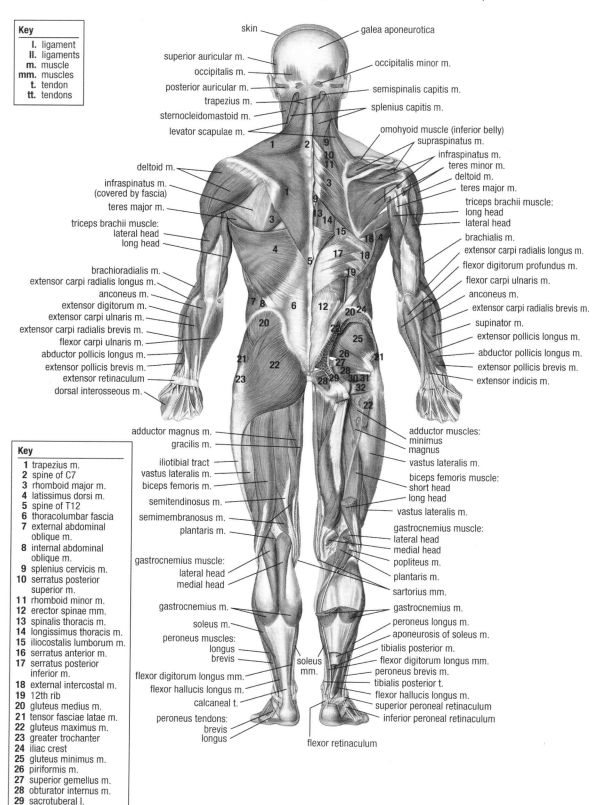

Key

I. ligament
II. ligaments
m. muscle
mm. muscles
t. tendon
tt. tendons

skin
galea aponeurotica
superior auricular m.
occipitalis minor m.
occipitalis m.
semispinalis capitis m.
posterior auricular m.
splenius capitis m.
trapezius m.
omohyoid muscle (inferior belly)
sternocleidomastoid m.
supraspinatus m.
levator scapulae m.
infraspinatus m.
teres minor m.
deltoid m.
deltoid m.
infraspinatus m.
(covered by fascia)
teres major m.
teres major m.
triceps brachii muscle:
long head
lateral head
triceps brachii muscle:
lateral head
long head
brachialis m.
extensor carpi radialis longus m.
flexor digitorum profundus m.
brachioradialis m.
flexor carpi ulnaris m.
extensor carpi radialis longus m.
anconeus m.
anconeus m.
extensor carpi radialis brevis m.
extensor digitorum m.
supinator m.
extensor carpi ulnaris m.
extensor pollicis longus m.
extensor carpi radialis brevis m.
abductor pollicis longus m.
flexor carpi ulnaris m.
extensor pollicis brevis m.
abductor pollicis longus m.
extensor indicis m.
extensor pollicis brevis m.
extensor retinaculum
dorsal interosseous m.

adductor magnus m.
adductor muscles:
gracilis m.
minimus
magnus
iliotibial tract
vastus lateralis m.
vastus lateralis m.
biceps femoris muscle:
biceps femoris m.
short head
long head
semitendinosus m.
vastus lateralis m.
semimembranosus m.
gastrocnemius muscle:
plantaris m.
lateral head
medial head
popliteus m.
gastrocnemius muscle:
plantaris m.
lateral head
sartorius mm.
medial head
gastrocnemius m.
gastrocnemius m.
peroneus longus m.
soleus m.
aponeurosis of soleus m.
peroneus muscles:
tibialis posterior m.
longus
flexor digitorum longus mm.
brevis
peroneus brevis m.
soleus
tibialis posterior t.
flexor digitorum longus mm.
mm.
flexor hallucis longus m.
flexor hallucis longus m.
calcaneal t.
superior peroneal retinaculum
inferior peroneal retinaculum
peroneus tendons:
brevis
longus
flexor retinaculum

Key

1 trapezius m.
2 spine of C7
3 rhomboid major m.
4 latissimus dorsi m.
5 spine of T12
6 thoracolumbar fascia
7 external abdominal
  oblique m.
8 internal abdominal
  oblique m.
9 splenius cervicis m.
10 serratus posterior
   superior m.
11 rhomboid minor m.
12 erector spinae mm.
13 spinalis thoracis m.
14 longissimus thoracis m.
15 iliocostalis lumborum m.
16 serratus anterior m.
17 serratus posterior
   inferior m.
18 external intercostal m.
19 12th rib
20 gluteus medius m.
21 tensor fasciae latae m.
22 gluteus maximus m.
23 greater trochanter
24 iliac crest
25 gluteus minimus m.
26 piriformis m.
27 superior gemellus m.
28 obturator internus m.
29 sacrotuberal l.
30 inferior gemellus m.
31 obturator externus m.
32 quadratus femoris m.

MAIN ARTERIES OF THE BODY

External jugular v.
Internal jugular v.
Superior vena cava
Hepatic v.
Inferior vena cava
Renal v.
Brachial vv.
Gonadal vv.
Radial vv.
Ulnar vv.
Venous palmar arches
Deep femoral v.
Femoral v.
Popliteal v.
Anterior tibial vv.
Small saphenous v.
Great saphenous v.
Dorsal venous arch

Brachiocephalic v.
Subclavian v.
Axillary v.
Diaphragm
Kidney
Cephalic v.
Basilic v.
Common iliac v.
Internal iliac v.
External iliac v.
Median antebrachial v.
Dorsal venous network
Femoral v.
Posterior tibial vv.
Fibular vv.
Plantar venous arch

MAIN VEINS OF THE BODY

Superior sagittal sinus
Inferior sagittal sinus
Straight sinus
Right transverse sinus
Sigmoid sinus
Right internal jugular
Right external jugular
Right subclavian
Right brachiocephalic
Superior vena cava
Right axillary
Right cephalic
Right hepatic
Right brachial
Right median cubital
Right basilic
Right radial
Right ulnar
Right palmar venous plexus

Pulmonary trunk
Coronary sinus
Great cardiac
Hepatic portal
Splenic
Superior mesenteric
Left renal
Inferior mesenter
Inferior vena cava
Left common iliac
Left internal iliac
Left externa iliac
Left femoral
Left great saphenous
Left popliteal
Left small saphenous
Left anterior tibial
Left posterior tibial
Left dorsal venous arch

Pulmonary artery
Superior cava or vein from head and neck
Right auricle
Inferior vena cava
Right ventricle
Portal circulation
Second renal circulation

Pulmonary capillaries.
Pulmonary veins
Aorta
Arteries to head and neck
Left auricle
Left ventricle
Gastric and intestinal vessels
First renal circulation
Systemic capillaries

"I will praise Thee; for I am fearfully and wonderfully made." Psalms 139:14

ANATOMY

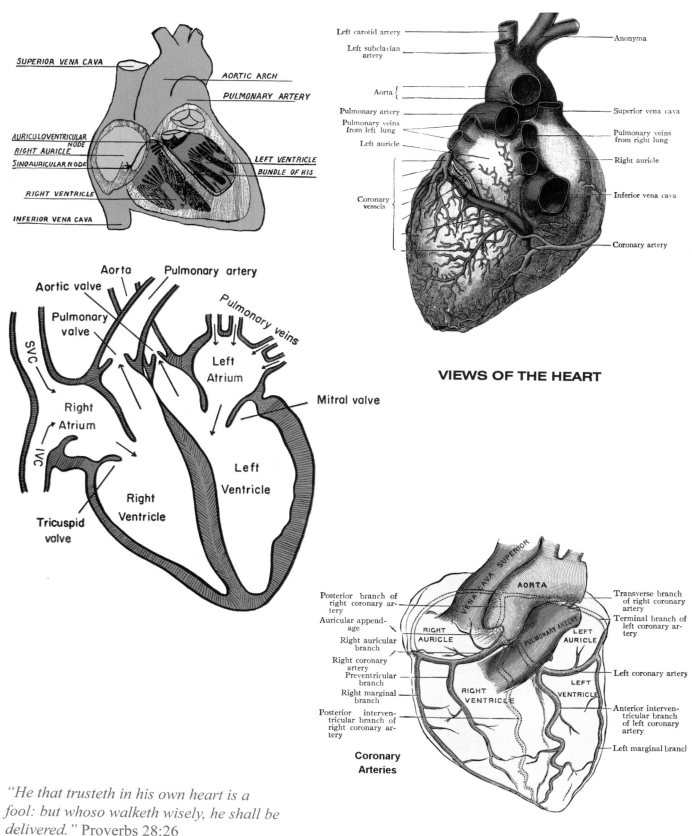

SUPERIOR VENA CAVA

AORTIC ARCH

PULMONARY ARTERY

AURICULOVENTRICULAR
NODE
RIGHT AURICLE
SINOAURICULAR NODE

LEFT VENTRICLE
BUNDLE OF HIS

RIGHT VENTRICLE

INFERIOR VENA CAVA

Aorta   Pulmonary artery

Aortic valve

Pulmonary
valve

Pulmonary veins

SVC

Left
Atrium

Right
Atrium

Mitral valve

IVC

Left
Ventricle

Right
Ventricle

Tricuspid
valve

Left carotid artery

Left subclavian
artery

Anonyma

Aorta

Pulmonary artery

Superior vena cava

Pulmonary veins
from left lung

Left auricle

Pulmonary veins
from right lung

Right auricle

Coronary
vessels

Inferior vena cava

Coronary artery

VIEWS OF THE HEART

Posterior branch of
right coronary ar-
tery

Auricular append-
age

Right auricular
branch

Right coronary
artery
Preventricular
branch

Right marginal
branch

Posterior interven-
tricular branch of
right coronary ar-
tery

VENA CAVA SUPERIOR

AORTA

RIGHT
AURICLE

PULMONARY ARTERY

LEFT
AURICLE

RIGHT
VENTRICLE

LEFT
VENTRICLE

Transverse branch
of right coronary
artery

Terminal branch of
left coronary ar-
tery

Left coronary artery

Anterior interven-
tricular branch
of left coronary
artery

Left marginal branch

**Coronary
Arteries**

A
N
A
T
O
M
Y

*"He that trusteth in his own heart is a
fool: but whoso walketh wisely, he shall be
delivered."* Proverbs 28:26

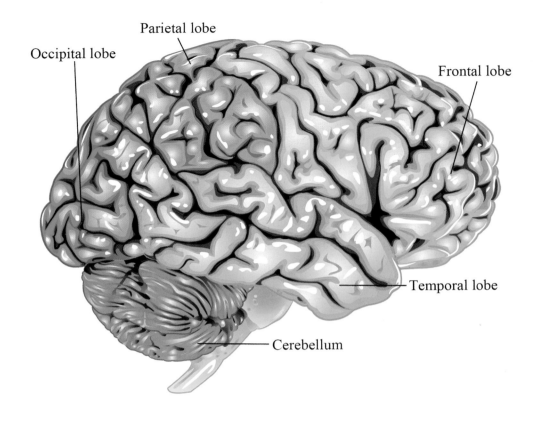

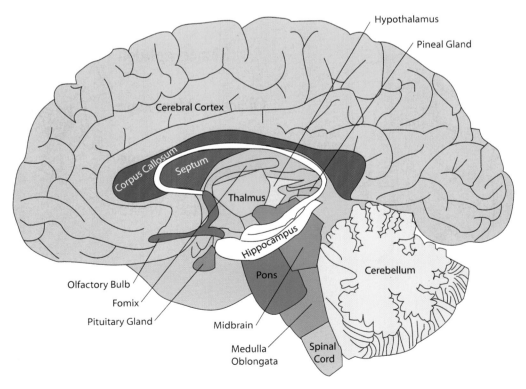

"Keep thy heart with all diligence; for out of it are the issues of life." Proverbs 4:23

ANATOMY

PONS   Spinal accessory nerve

CERVICAL
PLEXUS

I

II

III

IV

CERVICAL
NERVES

V

VI

VII

VIII

BRACHIAL
PLEXUS

SUPERIOR CERVICAL
GANGLION OF
SYMPATHETIC

MIDDLE CERVI-
CAL GANGLION

INFERIOR CERVI-
CAL GANGLION

I

II

III

IV

V

VI

VII

VIII

IX

X

XI

XII

T H O R A C I C   N E R V E S

T H O R A C I C   G A N G L I A

I

II

III

IV

V

LUMBAR
PLEXUS

LUMBAR
NERVES

LUMBAR
GANGLIA

SACRAL
GANGLIA

I

II

III

IV

V

CO.

SACRAL
NERVES

SACRAL
PLEXUS

COCCYGEAL
PLEXUS

SPINAL NERVES

NERVE CELL

Olfactory Bulb

Brunn's Membrane

Rhinencephalon

Olfactory Membrane

Tongue

Olfactory Nerve

SENSORY SYSTEM

"Thou wilt keep him in perfect peace, whose mind is stayed on Thee: because he trusteth in Thee."
Isaiah 26:3

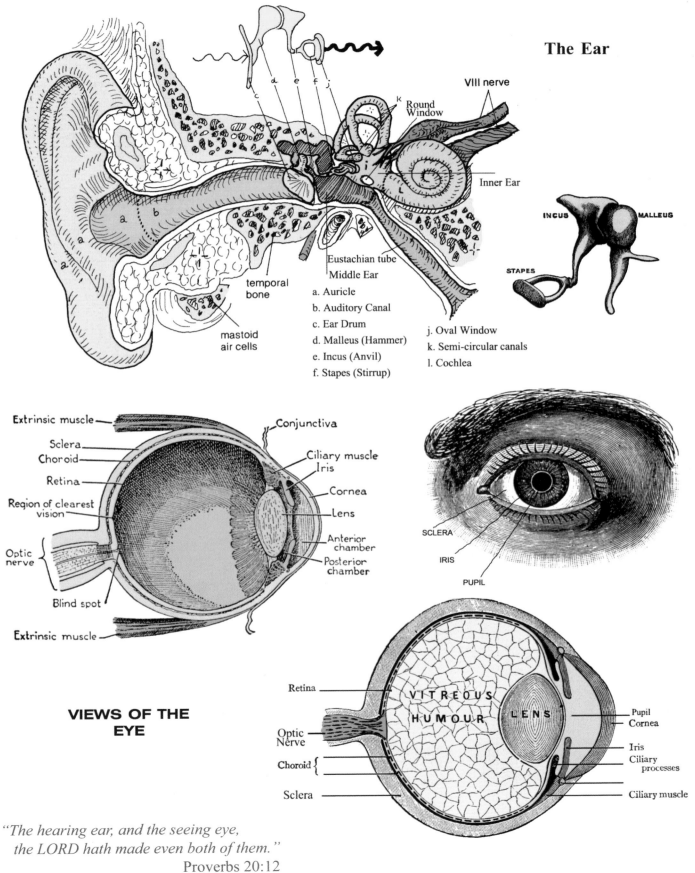

The Ear

VIII nerve

k Round Window

Inner Ear

INCUS   MALLEUS

STAPES

Eustachian tube
Middle Ear
a. Auricle
b. Auditory Canal
c. Ear Drum
d. Malleus (Hammer)
e. Incus (Anvil)
f. Stapes (Stirrup)

j. Oval Window
k. Semi-circular canals
l. Cochlea

temporal bone

mastoid air cells

Extrinsic muscle
Sclera
Choroid
Retina
Region of clearest vision
Optic nerve
Blind spot
Extrinsic muscle

Conjunctiva
Ciliary muscle
Iris
Cornea
Lens
Anterior chamber
Posterior chamber

SCLERA

IRIS

PUPIL

VIEWS OF THE EYE

Retina
Optic Nerve
Choroid {
Sclera

VITREOUS HUMOUR
LENS

Pupil
Cornea
Iris
Ciliary processes
Ciliary muscle

ANATOMY

"The hearing ear, and the seeing eye,
the LORD hath made even both of them."
Proverbs 20:12

LIVER

RIGHT LOBE

LEFT LOBE

GALL BLADDER

PANCREAS

- body of pancrease
- bile duct
- accessroy pancrease duct
- head of pancrease
- duodenum

DIGESTIVE SYSTEM

- Mouth cavity proper
- Sublingual gland and duct
- Submaxillary gland and duct
- Parotid salivary gland and duct
- Pharynx
- Esophagus
- Gall bladder
- Liver
- Hepatic duct
- Cystic duct
- Common bile duct
- Duodenum
- Stomach
- Pylorus
- Pancreas with duct
- Transverse colon
- Descending colon
- Ascending colon
- Vermiform appendix
- Rectum

STOMACH

- Gall bladder
- Hepatic duct
- Cystic duct
- Stomach
- Common bile duct
- Artery to duodenum
- Head of pancreas

Aorta
Celiac artery
Gastric artery

LIVER
PANCREAS
STOMACH
SPLEEN
GREAT OMENTUM

B — X-ray view when empty
C — X-ray showing peristalsis

Esophagus
Cardiac area
Fundus
A
Lesser curvature
Duodenum
Body
Pyloric area
Greater curvature
Full

"Hearken diligently unto Me, and eat ye that which is good." Isaiah 55:2

ANATOMY

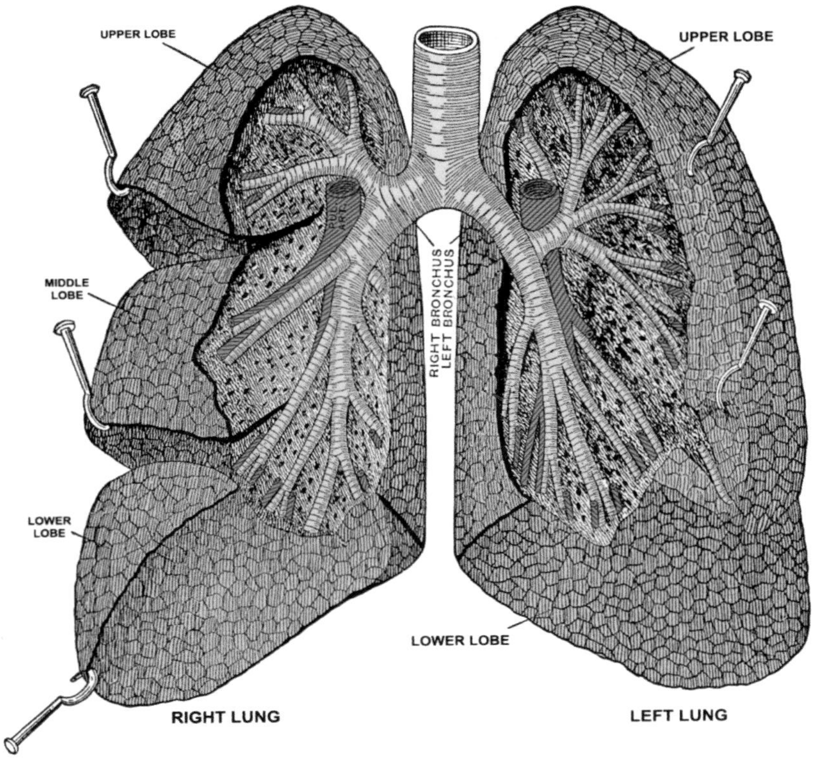

UPPER LOBE

UPPER LOBE

MIDDLE LOBE

RIGHT BRONCHUS
LEFT BRONCHUS

LOWER LOBE

LOWER LOBE

RIGHT LUNG

LEFT LUNG

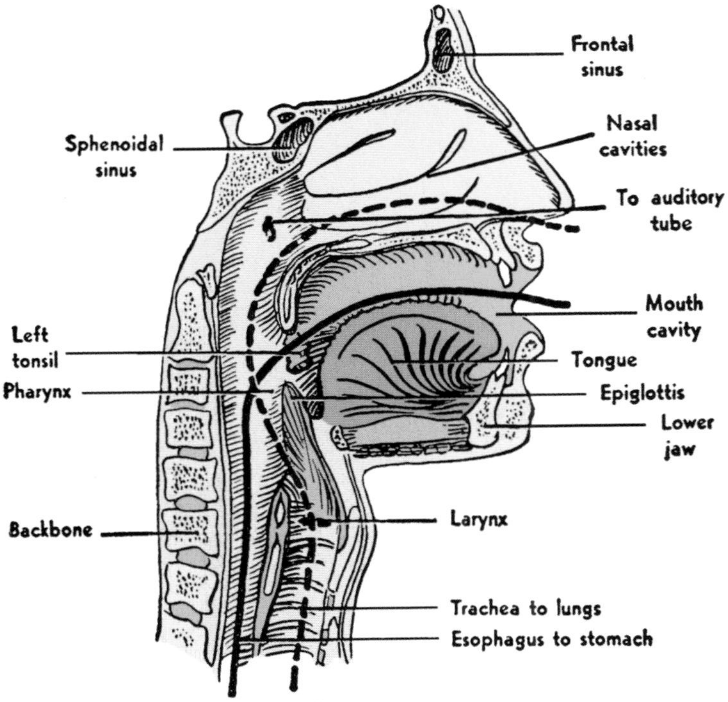

Frontal sinus

Sphenoidal sinus

Nasal cavities

To auditory tube

Mouth cavity

Left tonsil

Tongue

Pharynx

Epiglottis

Lower jaw

Backbone

Larynx

Trachea to lungs

Esophagus to stomach

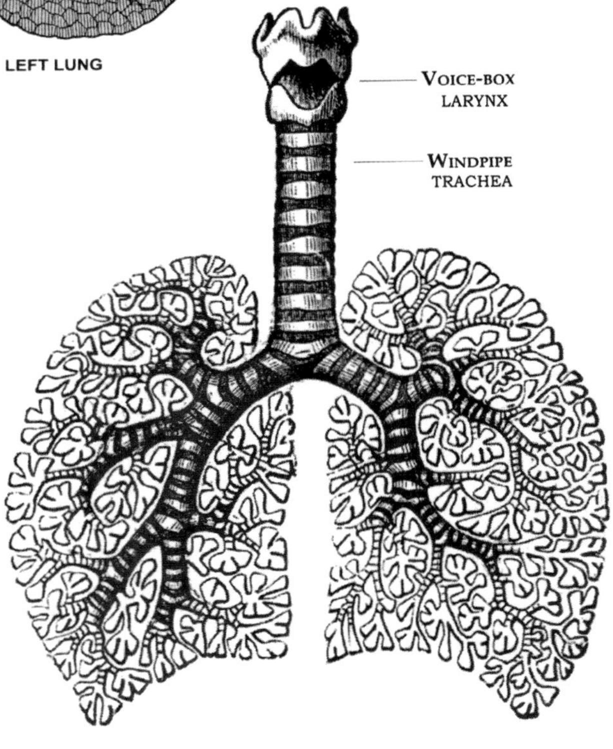

Voice-box
Larynx

Windpipe
Trachea

RESPIRATORY SYSTEM

"Beloved, I wish above all things that thou mayest prosper and be in health, even as thy soul prospereth." 3 John 1:2

ANATOMY

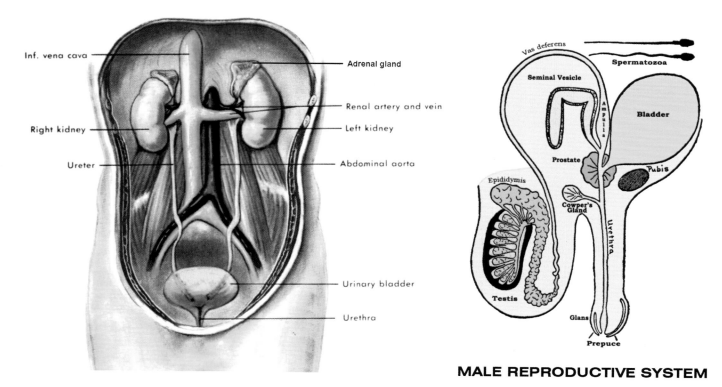

URINARY SYSTEM

MALE REPRODUCTIVE SYSTEM

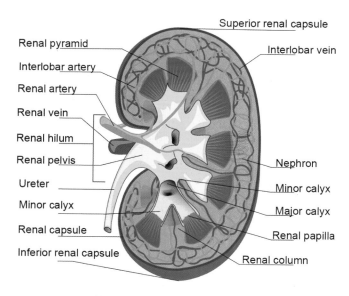

KIDNEY STRUCTURES

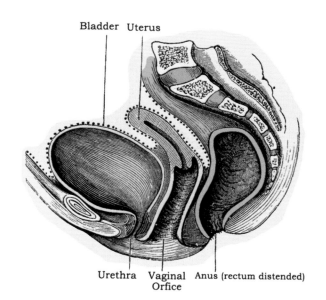

FEMALE REPRODUCTIVE SYSTEM

A
N
A
T
O
M
Y

"Fear thou not; for I am with thee: be not dismayed; for I am thy God: I will strengthen thee." Isaiah 41:10

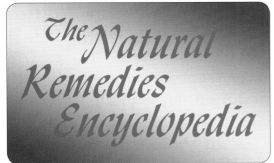

The Natural Remedies Encyclopedia

Disease Comparison Charts

HELPING YOU TO BETTER HELP OTHERS

It is helpful to be able to compare symptoms and physical indicators which are able to differentiate between different diseases, show their progress, or provide other useful information.

There are 40 very helpful Disease Comparison (and other) Charts in this chapter. In the coming years, you will find many of these charts to be extremely helpful as you minister to the needs of your sick family and friends. **ALL HAVE BEEN CROSS REFERENCED**

CHARTS

SOME QUOTATIONS TO THINK ABOUT

More quotations on pages 062 and 1064

"My dear Kepler, what do you say of the leading philosophers here, to whom I have offered a thousand times of my own accord to show my studies, but who, with the lazy obstinacy of a serpent who has eaten his fill, have never consented to look at the planets or moon, or telescope? Verily, just as serpents close their ears, so do men close their eyes to the light of truth."—*Galileo in a letter to Johannes Kepler, c. 1630; both men pioneered in teaching the truth that the earth circles the sun, and not vice versa. They were opposed by all the 'great men' of their time.*

"Let thy food be thy medicine and thy medicine be thy food."—*Hippocrates (460-377 B.C.) is considered by medical doctors to be the Father of Medicine.*

"I believe that you can, by taking some simple and inexpensive measures, extend your life and years of well-being. My most important recommendation is that you take vitamins every day in optimum amounts, to supplement the vitamins you receive in your food."—*Linus Pauling, Ph.D.; Two-time Nobel Prize Winner.*

"The ultimate cause of human disease is the consequence of our transgression of the universal laws of life."—*Paracelsus; 1493-1541, a leading Middle Ages physician and the first systematic botanist.*

"Medicine is a collection of uncertain prescriptions, the results of which, taken collectively, are more fatal than useful to mankind. Water, air, and cleanliness are the chief articles in my pharmacopeia."—*Napoleon Bonaparte.*

"It has always been one of the most difficult practical problems in the world: how to present new truths so as not to offend old errors; for persons are very apt to regard arguments directed against their opinions as attacks upon their persons. And many there are who mistake their own ingrained prejudices for established principles."—*R.T. Trall, M.D.; leading 19th century authority on healing with water therapy treatments and natural foods.*

"It is more important to know what sort of person has a disease than to know what sort of disease a person has."—*Hippocrates (460-377 B.C.).*

"To gain health once it has been lost we need to begin to reverse some, and ideally all, of those processes which may be negatively impacting us, and over which we have some degree of control."—*Leon Chaitow, N.D., D.O.*

"Medicine is for the patient. Medicine is for the people. It is not for the profits."—*George Merck. (George W.E. Merck was the president of Merck & Co. from 1925 to 1950.)*

"Unless we put medical freedom into the Constitution, the time will come when medicine will organize into an undercover dictatorship . . To restrict the art of healing to one class of men and deny equal privileges to others will constitute the Bastille of medical science. All such laws are un-American and despotic and have no place in a republic . . The Constitution of this republic should make special privilege for medical freedom as well as religious freedom."—*Benjamin Rush, M.D., Signer of the Declaration of Independence and leading American physician in the late 18th century (from the autobiography of Benjamin Rush).*

"Most over-the-counter and almost all prescribed drug treatments merely mask symptoms or control health problems. Or in some way they alter the way organs or systems, such as the circulatory system, work. Drugs almost never deal with the reasons why these problems exist, while they frequently create new health problems as side effects of their activities."—*John R. Lee, M.D.*

"Even if conventional medicine tells you that your condition is incurable or that your only option is to live a life dependent on drugs with troublesome side effects, there is hope for improving or reversing your condition."—*Leon Chaitow, N.D., D.O.*

"As long as providers make their income and fame largely by delivering 'rescue' medicine, they will have less economic interest in prevention."—*Paul Mencel, from his book, Medical Costs and Moral Choices.*

MAIN CATEGORIES OF DISEASES AND DISORDERS - 1

Group	Subgroup	Examples
BLOOD Diseases of the blood and blood forming organs and disorders involving the immune mechanism	nutritional anemias	iron deficiency anemia, vitamin B12 deficiency anemia
	hemolytic anemias	thalassemia, sickle-cell disorder
	aplastic and other anemias	acquired pure red cell aplasia, acute posthemorrhagic anemia
	coagulation defects, purpura, and other hemorrhagic conditions	hereditary factor VIII deficiency, hereditary factor IX deficiency
	other diseases of the blood and blood forming organs	agranulocytosis, diseases of spleen, methaemoglobinemia
ENDOCRINE Endocrine and metabolic diseases	disorders involving the immune mechanism	immunodeficiencies, sarcoidosis
	disorders of thyroid glad	iodine-deficiency syndrome, hypothyroidism, thyroditis
	disorders of glucose regulation and pancreatic internal secretion	non-diabetic hypoglycemic coma
	disorders of other endocrine glands	hyper-or hypofunction of pituitary gland, Cushing's syndrome, diseases of thymus, polyglandular dysfunction
	metabolic disorders	lactose intolerance, cystic fibrosis, amyloidosis
NERVES Diseases of the nervous system	inflammatory diseases of the central nervous system	Meningitis, encephinitis, myeiitis, encephalomyelitis
	systemic atrophies primarily affecting the central nervous system	Huntington's disease, hereditary ataxia
	extrapyramidal movement disorders	Parkinson's disease, dystonia
	other degenerative metabolic disorders of the nervous system	Alzheimer's disease
	demyelinating diseases of the central nervous system	multiple sclerosis
	episodic and paroxysmal disorders	epilepsy, migraine, other headache syndromes, sleep disorders
	nerve, nerve root, and plexus disorders	trigeminal nerve, facial, cranial nerve, mononeuropathies
	polyneuropathies and other disorders of the perypheral nervous system	hereditary, idiopathic, inflammatory
	diseases of the myoneural junction and muscle	myashtenia gravis
	cerebral palsy and other paralytic syndromes	infantile cerebral palsy, hemiplegia, paraplegia, tetraplegia
	other disorders of the nervous system	hydrocephalus, toxic encephalopathy
EYE Diseases of the eye and adnexa	disorders of the eyelid. lacrimal system, and orbit	hordeolum and chalazion
	disorders of conjunctiva	conjunctivitis
	disorders of sclera, cornea, iris, and ciliary body	keratitis, iridocyclitis
	disorders of tens	cataract
	disorders of choroid and retina	retina detachments and breaks
	glaucoma	glaucoma
	disorders of vitreous body and globe	various
	disorders of optic nerve and visual pathways	optic neuritis
	disorders of ocular muscles, binocular movement, accommodation, and refraction	strabismus
	visual disturbances and blindness	low vision
	other disorders of the eye and adnexa	nystagmus
EAR Diseases of the ear and mastoid process	diseases of external ear	otitis externa and perichondritis
	diseases of middle ear and mastoid	Bezold's abscess, Cholesteatoma, Gradenigo's syndrome, Otitis media, Perforated eardrum, Tympanic membrane retraction, Tympanosclerosis, and Tympanostomy tube

Ear: 407-415 / Eye 387-404 / Nerves 546-605 / Endocrine 652-662 / Cardiovascular: 512-545

CHARTS

MAIN CATEGORIES OF DISEASES AND DISORDERS - 2

Group	Subgroup	Examples
URINARY Diseases of the genito-urinary system	glomerular diseases	nephritis syndrome
	renal tubulo-interstitial diseases	nephritis
	renal failure	acute, chronic
	urolithiasis	calculus of kidney, ureter, lower urinary tract
	other disorders of the kidney and ureter	unspecified contracted kidney, small kidney of unknown cause
	other disorders of the urinary system	Cystis, urethritis
	diseases of male genital organs	disorders of prostate, male infertility, disorders of penis
	disorders of breast	benign mammary dysplasia, hypertrophy of breast
	inflammatory diseases of female pelvic organs	uterus, cervix uteri, vagina, vulva
	non-inflammatory disorders of female genital tract	endometriosis, conditions related to menstruation and menstrual cycle, female infertility
	other disorders of the genito-urinary system	postprocedural disorders, not elsewhere classified
REPRODUC-TIVE Congenital malformations, deformations, and chromosomal abnormalities	congenital malformations of eye, ear, face, and neck	anophthalmos, micro-and macrophthalmos
	congenital malformations of the circulatory system	of cardiac chamber, connections, septa; of great arteries; of great veins
	congenital malformations of the respiratory system	of nose, larynx, trachea, bronchus, lung
	cleft lip and cleft palate	either or both
	other congenital malformations of the digestive system	of tongue, mouth, esophagus, intestines
	congenital malformations of genital organs	of ovaries, fallopian tubes, uterus, cervix, female genitalia; undescended testicle, hypospadias, malformations of male genitalia; indeterminate sex and pseudohermaphroditism
	congenital malformations of the urinary system	renal agensis, cystic kidney disease
	congenital malformations and deformations of the musculoskeletal system	polydactyly, syndactyly, osteochondrodysplasias
	other congenital malformations	congenital ichthyosis, epidermolysis bullosa
	chromosomal abnormalities, not elsewhere classified	Down's syndrome, Edward's syndrome, Patau's syndrome, Turner's syndrome
MISCELLA-NEOUS Symptoms, signs, and abnormal clinical and laboratory findings, not elsewhere classified	symptoms and signs involving the circulatory and respiratory systems	gangrene, not elsewhere classified; cardiac murmurs; cough; pain in throat and chest
	symptoms and signs involving the digestive system and abdomen	abdominal and pelvic pain, nausea and vomiting, hertburn, dysphagia, fecal incontinence
	symptoms and signs involving the skin and subcutaneous tissue	rash, localized swelling; distrubances of skin sensation
	symptoms and signs involving the nervous and musculoskeletal system	abnormal involuntary movements, lack of coordination
	symptoms and signs involving the urinary system	unspecified urinary incontinence, retention of urine
	symptoms and signs involving the congnition, perception, emotional state, and behavior	somnolence, stupor, and coma; dizziness and giddiness; disturbances of smell and taste: symptoms and signs involving appearance
	symptoms and signs involving speech and voice	dyslexia, speech disturbances [not elsewhere classified]
	general symptoms and signs	fever, headache, malaise and fatigue, senility, syncope and collapse, enlarged lymph nodes, lack of expected physiological development, other general symptoms and signs, unknown and unspecified causes of morbidity

Miscelaneous Systems / Birth Defects: 724-727 / Reproductive: M - 667-671 / W - 672-700

MAIN CATEGORIES OF DISEASES AND DISORDERS - 3

Group	Subgroup	Examples
RESPIRATORY Diseases of the respiratory system	acute upper respiratory infections	acute nasopharyngitis (common cold), acute sinusitis, acute laryngitis, acute obstructive laryngitis (croup)
	influenza and pneumonia	influenza, pneumonia
	other acute lower respiratory infections	acute bronchitis
	other diseases of upper respiratory tract	chronic rhinitis, chronic sinusitis, nasal polyp, chronic laryngitis
	chronic lower respiratory diseases	bronchitis (non-acute and non-chronic), emphysema, asthma
	lung diseases due to external agents	coalworker's pneumoconiosis; pneumoconiosis due to asbestos, other mineral fibers, dust containing silica; conditions due to inhalation of chemical gases, fumes, and vapors
	other respiratory diseases primarily affecting the interstitium	pulmonary edema
	suppurative necrotic conditions of lower respiratory tract	abscess of lung and mediastinum, pyothorax
	other diseases of pleura	pleural effusion, pleural plaque
	other diseases of the respiratory system	respiratory failure, not elsewhere classified
DIGESTIVE Diseases of the digestive system	diseases of oral cavity, salivary glands, and jaws	dental caries, gingivitis and periodontal diseases, stomatitis
	diseases of esophagus, stomach, and duodenum	esophagitis, gastric ulcer, duodenal ulcer, peptic ulcer, dyspepsia
	diseases of appendix	acute appendicitis
	hernia	inguinal, femoral, umbilical, ventral, diaphragmatic hernia
	non infective enteritis and colitis	Crohn's disease
	other diseases of the intestines	irritable bowel syndrome
	diseases of peritoneum	peritonitis
	diseases of liver	alcoholic liver disease, toxic liver disease, fibrosis and cirrhosis of the liver
	disorders of gallbladder, hiliary tract, and pancreas	choletithiasis, cholccystitis, pancreatitis
	other diseases of the digestive system	intestinal malabsorption
SKIN Diseases of the skin and subcutaneous tissue	infections of skin and subcutaneous tissue	impetigo, cutaneous abscess, furuncle, carbuncle, cellulitis
	bullous disorders	pemphigus
	dermatitis and eczema	dermatitis, eczema, pruritus
	papulosquamous disorders	psoriasis, pityriasis rosea, lichen planus
	urticaria and erythema	urticaria, erythema
	radiation-related disorders of the skin and subcutaneous tissue	sunburn, radiothermatitis
	disorders of skin appendages	nail disorders, hair disorders, acne, rosacea, sweat disorders
	other disorders of skin and subcutaneous tissue	vitiligo, sebothric keratosis, corns and callouses, lupus erythematosus
MUSCLES, BONES, JOINTS, CONNECTIVE Diseases of the musculoskeletal system and connective tissue	arthropathies	infectious arthropathies, inflammatory polyarthropathics, arthrosis
	systemic connective tissue disorders	polyarteritis nodasa, dermatopolymyositis
	dorsophathitis	deforming dorsopathies, spondylopathies
	soft tissue disorders	of muscles, of synovium and tendon
	osteopathics arid chondropathies	disorders of bone density and structure (including osteoporosis); osteomyelitis, osteonecrosis
	other disorders of the musculoskeletal system and connective tissue	other acquired deformities, postprocedural disorders, not elsewhere classified

Skeletal-Muscular: 606-651 / Skin: 314-355 / Digestive: 419-484 / Respiratory: 497-511

CHARTS

POSSIBLE CAUSES OF VARIOUS PHYSICAL PROBLEMS

Abdominal pain, cramping across the abdomen: Bladder or kidney disorder, pelvic inflammatory disease, premenstrual syndrome, uterine prolapse. **Around the navel:** Appendicitis; constipation, gas. **Lower left side:** Colitis; Crohn's disease, diarrhea, diverticulitis, lactose intolerance, ovarian cyst, regional enteritis, uterine fibroids, or polyps. **Lower right side:** Acute appendicitis, colitis, Crohn's disease, uterine fibroids, or polyps. **Upper left side:** Food allergies, heartburn, hiatal hernia, irritable bowel syndrome, peptic ulcer. **Upper right side of rib cage:** Liver or gallbladder problems. **Any location:** Endometriosis, food poisoning, internal injury, indigestion, miscarriage, stress.

Anal bleeding, itching, pain, swelling: Abscess, allergies, anal fissure, bruising, cancer, candidiasis; Crohn's disease, cysts, diverticulitis, food poisoning; genital warts, hemorrhoids, infection, muscle spasms, pinworms, polyps, sexually transmitted diseases, tumor, ulcers, ulcerative colitis.

Back pain: Aortic aneurysm, arthritis, awkward sleeping/sitting position, cancer, disc disease, endometriosis, gallbladder disorders, heart attack, improper lifting, injury, kidney disease, lack of exercise, menstrual cramps, muscle spasms, obesity, osteoporosis, Paget's disease of the bone, pelvic inflammatory disease, peptic ulcer, pneumonia, poor posture, pregnancy, scoliosis, spinal tumor, sprain, strained muscle and/or ligament, urinary tract infection, uterine fibroids.

Bad breath: Abscessed tooth, bulimia, constipation, diabetes, dry mouth, gum disease, indigestion, infection (especially sinus and lung infection), liver disease, lung disease, mouth ulcers, breathing through the mouth, periodontal disease, poor oral hygiene, kidney failure, liver malfunction, disorders of the metabolism, sinusitis, tooth decay.

Bleeding, menstrual, heavy, or irregular: Blood-clotting disorders, cancer, endometriosis, endocrine disorders, hormonal imbalance, menopause, miscarriage, obesity, overzealous dieting or exercise, urinary tract infection, use of improper oral contraceptives, thyroid disorder, uterine polyps or fibroids, vaginal infection,

weight loss or gain.

Blinking, frequent: Anxiety, dry eyes, foreign body in the eye, injury, mimic spasm or tic (may occur in Tourette's syndrome), Parkinson's disease, stroke, or use of contact lenses.

Bloating: Allergies, appendicitis, bowel or kidney obstruction, adrenal disorders, diverticulitis, edema, gallbladder disorders, heart failure, irritable bowel syndrome, kidney disease, lactose intolerance, menstruation, overeating, peptic ulcer, tumor.

Blood in sputum, vomit, urine, stools, or from vagina or penis: Blood clots and swelling of lung tissue, cancer of colon, bladder, hemorrhoids, infection, peptic ulcer, polyps, prostatitis, prostate cancer, ruptured blood vessel, sexually transmitted disease, tumor.

Body aches: Arthritis, infection, influenza, lupus, Lyme disease, overexertion.

Body odor: Constipation, diabetes, excess toxins, gastrointestinal abnormalities, indigestion, infection, liver dysfunction, poor hygiene.

Breast lumps: Boils, cancer, cysts, fibrocystic disease, injury, infected milk duct, infected sweat gland or lymph node, premenstrual syndrome.

Breast tenderness: Blood clots in veins of breast, breast-feeding related problems, cancer, estrogen therapy, excessive consumption of fat, salt, caffeine, fibrocystic breast disease, hormonal imbalance, menopause, pregnancy, premenstrual syndrome, stress.

Bruising, easy: AIDS, anemia, cancer, Cushing's syndrome, drug reaction, hemophilia, liver or kidney disorder, vitamin C deficiency, vitamin K deficiency, weakened immune system.

Breath, shortness of: Asthma, cardiovascular disease (especially in women), chronic bronchitis, cystic fibrosis, emphysema, obesity, panic attacks, pneumonia.

Chest pain: Angina, anxiety, bruised or broken rib, carditis (inflammation of the muscles of the heart), coronary artery disease, gas, heart attack, heartburn, hiatal hernia, hyperventilation, pleurisy, pneumonia, strained muscle, stress.

Chills: Acute infection, anemia, exposure to cold, fever, hypothermia, shock.

Cold sweats: AIDS, cancer, diabetes, food

poi-soning, influenza, menopause, mononucleo-sis, severe heart or circulatory disease, shock, tuberculosis.

Cough, persistent: Allergies, asthma, cancer, chronic bronchitis, emphysema, pneumonia, postnasal drip, tuberculosis.

Delirium: Alcohol abuse, appendicitis, diabetes.

Drug overdose: Drug reaction, epilepsy, high fever, manic episode, stroke.

Disorientation: Alcohol abuse, Alzheimer's disease, anemia, acute anxiety (panic attack), drug reaction or overdose, hypoglycemia, poor circulation, schizophrenia, seizure, stroke, transient ischemic attack (TIA, temporary interference with blood flow to the brain).

Dizziness, light-headedness: Acute anxiety (panic attack), allergies, anemia, brain tumor, inhaling chemical products, diabetes, drug reaction, heart disease, high blood pressure, hypoglycemia, infection, low blood pressure, Mbnibre's disease, motion sickness, stress; stroke or impending stroke, vertigo.

Double vision: Cataracts, concussion, excessive alcohol consumption, eye disorders, hyperthyroidism.

Drooling: Drug withdrawal, ill-fitting dentures, Parkinson's disease, pregnancy related problems, salivary gland disorders, seizure; stroke.

Drowsiness: Acute kidney failure, allergies, caffeine withdrawal, drug reaction or overdose, encephalitis, narcolepsy, skull fracture, sleep disorders.

Dry mouth: Aging, breathing through the mouth, diabetes, dehydration, drug reactions, Sjögren's syndrome.

Ear discharge: Clogged eustachian tube, earwax buildup, immune system dysfunction, infection, middle-ear infection, ruptured eardrum, severe head injury, tumor.

Eye, bulging: Aneurysm, blood clot or hemorrhage, glaucoma, hyperthyroidism, infection.

Eyelid, drooping: Botulism, diabetes, head or eyelid injury, hypothyroidism, muscle weakness, stroke.

Fever, persistent: AIDS, autoimmune diseases, cancer (especially leukemia, kidney cancer, lymphoma), chronic bronchitis, chronic infection, diabetes, hepatitis, influenza, mono-

nucleosis, rheumatic disorders.

Flushing: Alcohol consumption, anxiety, dehydration, diabetes, heart disease, high blood pressure, hyperthyroidism, menopause, pregnancy, rosacea, use of high doses of niacin or of cholesterol-lowering medications.

Gas, frequent burping: Allergies, candidiasis, digestive problems, gallbladder disorders, intestinal obstruction, intestinal parasites, irritable bowel syndrome, lactose intolerance, stomach acid deficiency, swallowing air.

Hands and/or feet, cold: Circulatory problems; exposure to cold, Raynaud's phenomenon, stress.

Headaches, persistent: Allergies, asthma, brain tumor, cluster headaches, drug reaction, eyestrain, glaucoma, high blood pressure, migraine, sinusitis, stress, vitamin deficiency.

Heartbeat, irregular or rapid: Anemia, anxiety, arteriosclerosis, asthma, caffeine, alcohol, tobacco consumption, calcium, magnesium, and/or potassium deficiency, cancer, cardiovascular disease, drug reaction, fever, heart attack, high blood pressure, hormonal imbalance, low blood pressure, obesity, overeating, overzealous exercising.

Hot sweats, then chills: Acute infection, excessive alcohol or sugar consumption, fever, hypoglycemia, thyroid disorders, tuberculosis (mainly night sweats).

Incontinence: Advanced neurological disease, Alzheimer's disease, atrophic vaginitis, bladder infection, diabetes, excessive liquid consumption, loss of muscle tone, multiple sclerosis, prostatitis, psychological problems, restricted mobility, spinal cord trauma, stroke, urinary tract infection.

Intercourse, painful: Endometriosis, inflammation or infection of the vulva, muscle spasms, unaccustomed position during sex, urinary tract infection; vaginal dryness.

Irritability, mood swings: Alcohol or drug abuse, Alzheimer's disease, anxiety, brain tumor, depression, diabetes, drug reactions, excessive sugar intake, food allergies, hormonal imbalance, hyperthyroidism, hypoglycemia, hypothyroidism, menopause, nutritional deficiencies, premenstrual syndrome, schizophrenia, stress, stroke, virtually any chronic or disabling illness.

See the Disease Index for additional information on these 37 physical difficulties

CHARTS

Identifying Eleven Eruptive, Infective, and Contagious Diseases

Name	Period of Incubation	Time of Eruption	Duration of Eruption	Period of Quarantine
1 Scarlet Fever	2 to 5 days	12-24 hr. after onset	4 to 5 days	21 days
2 Smallpox	8 to 12 days	3rd day of fever	14 to 21 days	21 days
3 Measles	10 days	4th day of fever	5 to 10 days	14 days
4 Roetheln	5 to 21 days	2nd day of fever	3 days	5 days
5 Mumps	14-21 days			Until all swellings have subsided
6 Wooping Cough	7 to 27 days			28 days
7 Chickenpox	4-27 days	2nd day of fever	7 days	7 days
8 Diphtheria	5 days			7 days , until 2 successive nose and throat cultures, 24 hours apart, are negative
9 Typhus Fever	12 days	5th or 6th day of fever	14 days	14 days
10 Typhoid Fever			20 days	Release after 2 sucessful active cultures of urine and feces not less than 24 hours apart
11 Erysipelas	3 to 7 days	2nd day of fever	4 days	

Left margin: Scarlet Fever 745 / Smallpox: 304 / Measles: 743 / Mumps: 743 / Whooping Cough: / Chickenpox: 742 / Diphtheria: 747 / Typhus: 839 / Typhoid Fever: 307 / Erysipelus: 353

Differential Symptoms of Heatstroke vs. Heat Exhaustion

Heatstroke vs. Heat Exhaustion

Left margin: Heatstroke and Heat Exhaustion: 286

Heat or Sunstroke Definition: A condition or derangement of heat-control centers due to exposure to the rays of the sun or very high temperatures.
  History: Exposure to sun's rays
  Differential Symptoms:
  Face: Red, dry, and hot
  Skin: Hot, dry, and no diaphoresis
  Temperature: High, 108° to 110° F.
  Pulse: Full strong bounding
  Respirations: Dyspneic and sonorous
  Muscles: Tense and possible convulsions
  Eyes: Pupils are dilated but equal
Treatment: Absolute rest with the head elevated. Use cold packs to prolong radiation of body heat.
Drugs: Allow no stimulants; give infusion of normal saline (to force fluids)

Heat Exhaustion Definition: A state of very definite weakness produced by the loss of normal fluids and sodium chloride of the body.
  History: Exposure to heat, usually indoors
  Differential Symptoms:
  Face: Pale, cool, and moist
  Skin: Cool, clammy, with profuse diaphoresis
  Temperature: Slight elevation to subnormal
  Pulse: Weak, thready, and rapid
  Respirations: Shallow and quiet
  Muscles: Tense and contracted
  Eyes: Pupils and normal
Treatment: Keep patient quiet; head should be lowered. Keep body warm to prevent shock symptoms.
Drugs: Aromatic spirits of ammonia. Salt tablets and fruit juices in abundant amounts.

Method of Transfer in Eleven Common Communicable Diseases

Cholera 306 / Tuberculosis: 506 / Syphilis: 804 / Smallpox: 304 / Influenza: 294 / Pneumonia: 503 (512) / Scarlet Fever 745 / Diphtheria: 747 / Typhoid Fever: 307

Disease	How the Bacteria Leave the Bodies of the Sick	How They May Be Transferred	How They May enter the Bodies of the Well
Typhoid	Feces and urine	Direct contact. Hands of nurse or attendant. Linen and all articles used by and about patient. Hands of "carriers" soiled by their own feces. Water polluted by excreta. Food grown in or washed with such water. Milk diluted or milk cans washed with such water. Flies.	Through mouth in infected food or water and thence to intestinal tract.
Diphtheria	Sputum and discharges from nose and throat.	Direct contact. "Droplet infection" from coughing. Hands of nurse. Articles used by and about patient.	Through mouth to throat or nose to throat.
Scarlet fever	Discharges from nose and throat.	Direct contact. "Droplet infection" from patient coughing. Hands of nurse. Articles used by and about patient.	Through mouth and nose.
Pneumonia	Sputum and discharges from nose and throat.	Direct contact. Hands of nurse. Articles used by and about patient.	Through mouth and nose to lungs.
Influenza	as Pneumonia	as Pneumonia	as Pneumonia
Smallpox	Discharges from nose and throat. Skin lesions.	Direct contact. Hands of nurse. Articles used by and about patient.	Thought to be through mucous membrane of respiratory tract.
Syphilis	Infected tissues. Lesions.	Direct contact. May be by kissing or by sexual intercourse. Dishes, food, toilets, towels, bathtubs, drinking cups, etc.	Directly into blood and tissues through breaks in skin or membrane.
Tetanus	Excreta from infected herbivorous animals and man.	Soil, especially that with manure or feces in it. Dust, ect. Articles used about stables.	Directly into blood stream through wounds. (Its anaerobe and prefers deep incised wound.)
Tuberculosis Human	Sputum Lesions Feces	Direct contact, such as kissing. "Droplet Infection" From person caughing with mouth uncovered. Sputum from mouth to fingers, thence to food and other things. Soiled dressings.	Same as Tuberculosis Human.
Tuberculosis Bovine		Milk	Same as Tuberculosis Human.
Cholera	Exreta from intestinal tract.	As in Typhoid, through feces	As in Typhoid, through mouth to intestinal tract.

CHARTS

Comparison of the Four Major Types of Joint Diseases

	Acute Rheumatism	Rheumatoid Arthritis	Osteoarthritis	Gout
Age	Children and young adults	25 and over	Middle and old age	Middle and old age
Sex	Either	Mainly women	Either	Mainly men
Cause	Unknown ? allergic reaction to streptococci	Often focal sepsis (streptococci)	Trauma, old age, degenerative changes	Uric acid in blood, clue to disordered purine metabolism
Joints	Usually large joints, subsiding in one and commencing in another	Multiple, including small joints of hands and feet	Usually on large joint, e.g., hip, knee, shoulder	Several, e.g., great toe, knee, elbow, hands.
Pyrexia	At onset	In acute stages	Nil	During acute attack
Permanent Deformity	Nil	Spindle-shaped joints. Often gross deformity	Often slight.	Deformity mainly from "chalky" deposits.
Heart	Often affected	Not affected	Not affected	Often arteriosclerosis

Five Temperatures at Seven Ages

Temperature	Abnormal	Pulse	Abnormal	Respiratory	Abnormal	Age
Rectal....99.6°	99°	140-130	90	44	20	at birth
Rectal....99.6°	100°	130-115	100	35	22	at 1st year
Rectal....99.6°	101°	115-100	110	25	24	at 2nd year
Mouth....98.6°	102°	85-80	120	20	26	at 15th year
Mouth....98.6°	103°	85-75	130	18	28	at 25 years
Mouth....91.2°	104°	75-70	140	16	30	at 50 years
Mouth.......93°	105°	65-50	150	14-16	36	at 70 years

Respiration, Pulse, and Temperature Ratios

Respiration	Pulsations	Temperature
18	80	99° F.
19 (plus)	88	100° F.
21	96	101° F.
23	104	102° F.
25 (minus)	112	103° F.
27	120	104° F.
28	128	105° F.
30	136	106° F.

Eight Diseases in Which Sputum Occurs

Variety of Sputum	Character of Sputum	Diseases in Which the Various Types Occur
Mucoid	Clear, thin, may be somewhat viscid	Early stages of Bronchitis
Mucopurulent	Thick, viscid, greenish color, inoffensive, frothy, may have sweetish odor.	Later stages of Bronchitis, Phthisis, Pneumonia.
Purulent	Thick, viscid yellow, often offensive.	Abscess of lung, empyema, advanced phthisis
Nummular	Mucopurulent, with small round, semisolid masses which sink in water.	Advanced phthisis
Rusty	Mucopurulent, very viscid and gelatinous, rusty tinge.	Pneumonia.
Prune juice	Dark brown, offensive, often semisolid.	Later stages of Pneumonia, gangrene of the lung, new growth of lung.
Red current jelly	Blood clots resembling current jelly.	New growth of lung
Blood (hemoptysis)	Bright red, frothy, with air bubbles; blood may be in streaks or mixed with sputum, fluid, or clotted, or sputum may consist of pure blood.	Phthisis (ulceration of a vessel in a cavity); other diseases of the lung (pneumonia, new growth, gangrene, abscess, bronchiectasis); mitral stenosis; aneurysm rupturing into bronchial tubes.

Bronchial and Lung Problems: 500-507

Comparing Eight Symptoms of Coronary Thrombosis vs. Angina Pectoris

Symptoms	Coronary Thrombosis	Angina Pectoris
Onset	At rest	With effort
Character of pain	Continuous	Paroxysmal
Duration of attack	Hours or days	Seconds or minutes
Patient Blood pressure	Often restless	Remains still
Pulse	Falls	Rises Regular
Vomiting	Sometimes irregular	Uncommon
Treatment	Common	Amyl nitrite
	Morphia	Morphia
	Amyl nitrite has no effect	

**Coronary Thrombosis 521
Angina Pictoris 530**

CHARTS

"The Lord is my strength and song." —Exodus 15:2

Significant Causes of Acid, High Acidity, and Alkalinity Characteristics of Urine

Normal	Abnormal	Significance
Acid (slight)		Diet of acid-forming foods (meats, eggs, prunes, wheat, etc.) overbalacing the base-forming foods (vegetables fruits).
	High acidity	Acidosis, diabetes mellitus, many pathological disorders (fevers, starvation).
	Alkaline	Putrefying bacteria change urea into ammonium carbonate. Infection or ingestion of alkaline compounds.

Characteristics of Urine in Nine Different Diseases

Examination of Urine

Table Giving the More Important Characters of the Urine in Some of the Commoner Diseases.

	Names of Diseases	Condition of Urine
I.	Gastric Catarrh	Quantity normal; high colored; sp. gr. often raised; acid. Urates, oxalates, or phosphates may be deposited.
II.	Jaundice	Urine greenish-brown in color, frothy; acid reaction; contains bile. Quantity and sp. gr. usually normal.
III.	Heart and Lung Disease	Urine often diminished, dark in color, acid; high sp. gr. Urates deposited; albumin often present.
IV.	Fevers, General and Special	Quantity nearly always diminished, high colored, usually acid; high sp. gr.; turbid; urates. May be albumin, blood and tube casts. Urea usually increased.
V.	Diabetes Mellitus	Quantity increased, pale, usually acid, sweet odor; high sp. gr. Sugar in greater of less quantity. Sometimes diacetic acid and (or) acetone amount of urea usually increased.
VI.	Acute Nephritis	Quantity diminished. Urine may be suppressed. Sp. gr. at first raised, then lowered. Albumin; sometimes blood, tube casts; sometimes urates, urea diminished.
VII.	Chronic Nephritis	Urine increased in quantity, pale; sp. gr. low. Albumin in small amount, or absent; no blood; a few tube casts.
VIII.	Chronic Cystitis	Quantity not usually altered, turbid, often alkaline and offensive. Mucus and pus (muco-pus) often present.
IX.	Acute Gout	Quantity usually diminished, high colored; sp. gr. rashed. Abundant deposit of urates.

"The fear of the Lord is the instruction of wisdom; and before honour is humility." —Proverbs 15:33

Urine analysis: Various diseases refer to chapter on urine for this informatnion 485-496

C
H
A
R
T
S

Significance in Changes in Amount, Color, Transparency, and Odor of Urine in Different Diseases

Urine analysis: Various diseases refer to chapter on urine for this information 485-496

Significance of Changes in amount of Urine

Normal	Abnormal	Significance
1000-1500 cc. (96% H_2O)		Depends upon water and fluid foods consumed, exercise, temperature, kidney function, etc.
	High (polyuria)	Diabetes millitus, diabetes insipidus, nervous diseases, certain types of chronic nephritis (kidney disorder), diuretics (drugs such as caffeine, calomel, digitalis, causing increased urinary excretion).
	Low (oliguria)	Acute nephritis, heart disease, fevers, eclampsia, diarrhea, vomiting.
	None (anuria)	Uremia (urinary substances in blood), acute nephritis, metal poisoning, e.g., due to bichloride of mercury.

Color

Normal	Abnormal	Significance
Yellow to amber		Depends upon concentration of pigment (urochrome).
	Pale	Diabetes insipidus, granular kidney, due to a very diluted urine.
	Milky	Fat globules, pus corpuscles in genitourinary infections.
	Reddish	Blood pigments, drugs, or food pigments.
	Greenish	Bile pigment, associated with jaundice.
	Brown-black	Poisoning (mercury, lead, phenol), hemorrhages.

Transparency

Normal	Abnormal	Significance
Clear		No significance.
Cloudy on standing		Precipitation of mucin from urinary tract. Not pathological.
Turbid		Precipitation of calcium phosphate. Not pathological.
	Milky	Presence of fat globules. Pathological.
	Turbid	Presence of pus as result of inflammation of urinary tract. Pathological.

Odor

Normal	Abnormal	Significance
Faintly aromatic		No significance.
	Pleasant (sweet)	Acetone, associated with diabetes mellitus.
	Unpleasant	Decomposition or ingestion of certain drugs or foods.

Detailed Comparisons of Different Types of Ulcers

CHART 1054: Comparing different kinds of ulcers - Stomach 442-443 / Skin 321

Detailed Comparisons of Different Types of Ulcers

Type of Ulcer	Healing	Weak	Callous	Irritable	Inflamed	Syphilitic	Tubercular
SURFACE	Smoothing and healing	Raised and flabby granulations.	Granulations absent or pale and ill-formed.	Congested, no granulations.	Sloughing irregular, no granulations.	Circular or irregular.	Pale, unhealthy granulations.
EDGES	Smoothing and regular	Smooth and healthy	Raised, firm, hard, dense, white	Dark red, irregular.	Sharp and turned outwards, irregular and undermined.	Steep and sharp cut, dull red, undermined.	Pale, bluish, thin, undermined.
SURROUNDINGS	Healthy	Usually healthy	Pigmented, indurated, eczematous	Normal, Tender spots	Dusky, swollen and inflamed, skin brawny.	Smoothing, slistening, pigmented, old cicatrices.	Enlarged glands; purplish, old cicatrices.
DISCHARGE	Sweet pus or serum	Watery, copious.	Scanty, thin, serous.	Scanty, thin, serous.	Serous, bloody, putrid.	Breaking down debris.	Thin yellowish-green scanty debris.
PAIN	Absent	Absent	Intense	Intense	Severe constitutional fever.	None	None
CICATRIZATION	All round	None	None	None	None	Often in center	None
TREATMENT	Rest and clean lines skin grafting	Removal of cause elevation, stimulating lotions or caustics	Rest, elevation, antiseptics, ointments astraping, excision of the whole ulcer followed by skin grafting of the raw surface, Amputation.	Improved general health, opiates, caustics locally, operation to divide nerve.	Rest, elevation, soothing applications; constitutional.	Iodide of potash and mercury internally, poultices, followed by black wash. Intravenous injection of salvarsen.	Pare edges, scrape base, Use Iodine type antiseptic.

Common Causes of Unconsciousness in Nine Diseases or Disorders

CHART - 1055: Alcoholism (821-823, 937) Apoplexy [Stroke] (529) Cerebral Compression (573) Brain Concussion (573) Diabetes and Insulin (656) Epilepsy (574) Opium (953-963) Uremia (486)

Causes	Onset	General Condition	Pupils	Pulse	Respiration	Muscles	Temperature	Special Points
Acute alcoholism	Gradual	Can be roused.	Dilated.	Full.	Deep, slightly stertorous.	Twitching	Below normal	Odor in breath, face is flushed
Apoplexy	Sudden	Cannot be roused.	Unequally dilated and fixed.	Slow, full, and tense.	Slow, stertorous.	One side paralyzed	Below normal	Face dusky
Compression	Gradual	Cannot be roused.	Pin point at first, then dialated, fixed and unequal.	Slow and full.	Slow, irregular, and stertorous	Paralysis of certain groups	First below normal, later above.	
Concussion	Sudden	Can be roused.	Equal and react to light.	Slow and weak.	Slow, irregular, and shallow.	Relaxed and flacid	Below normal	
Diabetes	Gradual	Cannot be roused.	Normal.	Slow.	Slow, deep, and sighing	Relaxed	Below normal	Dry skin, odor of acetone in breath, sugar and acetone in urine.
Insulin	Fairly sudden	Gradually deepening coma, preceded by exitement.	Normal.	Weak and rapid.		Relaxed, twitching in advanced stages.		Sweating
Epilepsy	Preceded by fits	Cannot be roused.	Variable.	Becoming less rapid.	Noisy or stertorous.	Relaxed	Raised	
Opium	Gradual	Cannot be roused.	Pin point.	Slow	Labored, irregular, stertorous, and slow.	Relaxed		Face pallid, skin sweating.
Urimia	Sudden or Gradual	Cannot be roused.	Usually contracted.	Hard.		Frequent convulsions.	Below normal	

Is it a Cold (288-293), Flu (294), or Allergy (848-860) ?

COLD, FLU, OR ALLERGY?

Chest infection or cough
COLD - Common. Mild to moderate
FLU - Common. Can become severe
ALLERGY - Rare

Fever
COLD - Rare (except in young children)
FLU - Pneumonia is a common complication
ALLERGY - Not present

General aches and pains
COLD - Mild
FLU - Usually high fever (102°-104°F). May last for 3-4 days
ALLERGY - Rare

Headache
COLD - Rare
FLU - Usual. Can be severe
ALLERGY - Rare

Sneezing/red, watery, itchy eyes
COLD - Usual, but more prevalent in allergies
FLU - Common
ALLERGY - Usual, especially sneezing. These symptoms come on quickly, without the warning signs of a cold, and can last longer.

Sore throat
COLD - Usual
FLU - Rare
ALLERGY - Occasional

Stuffy nose
COLD - Usual
FLU - Occasional
ALLERGY - Occasional

Tiredness
COLD - Mild
FLU - Severe
ALLERGY - Rare

Primary season
COLD - Late August through April
FLU - Winter
ALLERGY - March through September

Duration
COLD - 7-10 days
FLU - Up to a month
ALLERGY - As long as the allergen is present

TABLE COMPARING DISEASES OF JOINTS

Diseases of the Joints 615-633

	Acute Rheumatism	Rheumatoid Arthritis	Osteoarthritis	Gout
Age	Children and young adults	25 and over	Middle and old age	Middle and old age
Sex	Either	Mainly Women	Either	Mainly Men
Cause	Unknown? alergic reaction to strepto-cocci.	Often focal sepsis (stretococci).	Trauma, old age, de-generative changes.	Uric acid in blood, due to disordered purin metabolism.
Joints	Usually large joints, subsideing in one and commencing in another.	Multiple, including small joints of the hands and feet.	Usually one large joint, e.g., hip, knee, shoulder.	Several, e.g., great toe, knee, elbow, hands.
Pyrexia	At onset	In acute stages	Nil	During acute attack
Permanent Deformity	Nil	Spindle-shaped joints. Often gross deformity	Often slight	Deformity mainly from "chalky" deposits
Heart	Often affected	Not affected	Not affected	Often arteriosclerosis

Termination of Fever: Crisis and Lysis

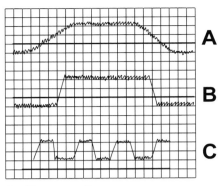

A= Fever continues
B= Fever continues to abrupt
   onset and remission
C= Fever remittent

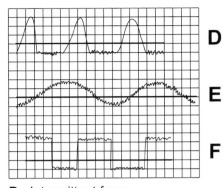

D= Intermittent fever
E= Undulant fever
F= Relapsing fever

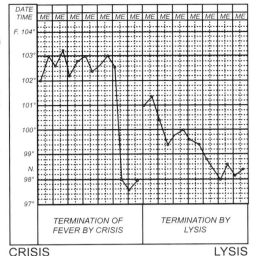

TERMINATION OF FEVER BY CRISIS

TERMINATION BY LYSIS

CRISIS   LYSIS

Termination of Fever Crisis and Lysis - Fevers 302-309

Chart 1 (above, left)—
This chart explains the temperature patterns of six types of fevers: (A) Continuous (as in scarlet fever, typhus, and pneumonia), in which there is a slight daytime variation. (B) Fevers that continues to abrupt onset and remission. (C) Remittent (as in typhoid fever, septice fever, and remittent fever), in which it partially leaves during the day and then returns at night. (D) Intermittentant (malaria, Malta fever), with minimum normal and subnormal temmperature, and with marked daytime variation. (E) Undulant fever - Brucellosis, also called Bang's disease, Crimean fever, Gibralter fever, Malta fever, Malta fever, Maltese fever, Mediterranean fever, or rock fever. (F) Relapsing fever, synonym: typhinia, is an infection caused by certain bacteria in the venus Borrelia. It is a vector-borne disease that is transmitted through the bites of lice or soft-bodied ticks.

Charts 2 (above, right)—
A normal fever generally has two distinct stages; first the crisis and then, after a sudden drop in temperature, the concluding phase, or lysis. The crisis is the turning point of a disease, and is a very critical period often marked by a long sleep and profuse perspiration. It may also be marked by a sudden descent of a high temperature to normal or below, generally within 24 hours (as shown on the chart, below left).

Diagnosis of Diabetic and Hypoglycemic Coma
[Diabetic (656) and Hypoglycemic (653) Coma]

	Diabetic Coma	Hypoglycemic Coma
Onset	Gradual	Often sudden
History	Often of acute infection in a diabetic or no previous history of diabetes	Recent insulin injection, or inadequate meal or excessive exercise after insulin
Skin	Flushed, dry	Pale, sweating
Tongue	Dry	Moist
Breath	Smell of acetone	No acetone
Respiration	Deep (air hunger)	Shallow
Pulse	Rapid, feeble	Normal or bounding
Eyeball Tension	Low	Normal or raised
Urine	Sugar and acetone	None, unless bladder has not been emptied for some hours
Blood Sugar	Raised (over 200)	Subnormal (40 -70)
Blood Pressure	Low	Normal
Abdominal Pain	Common and often acute	Sometimes sense of constriction

CHARTS

Locations, Functions, and Diseases
of the Seven Principle Endocrine Glands

Name	Position	Function	Disease Connected With It
The Thyroid Gland	Two lobes in the neck joined by a narrow band called the isthmus	Influences growth and nutrition through its hormone thyroxin.	1. Goiter - an enlargement of the gland 2. Cretinism 3. Myxedema 4. Exophthalmic goiter
The Parathyroid Glands	Four tiny glands, 2 on each side. In the neighborhood of the thyroid.	Influence nutrition of muscle tissue	Tetany, a disease in which the painful spasms of the hands and feet occur. Mainly seen in the muscles of children.

The Surarenal (or adrenal) Capsules	One lies above each kidney. Each has an outer layer, the cortex (bark), and an inner layer, the medulla (pith).	Hormone of cortex influences growth and sexual development. Hormone of medulla is called adrenaline, affects blood pressure, keeps up muscle tone, has some effect on the coloring matter in the skin.	Addison's disease:
			  Symptoms:
			    Muscular weakness
			    Low blood pressure
			    A darkening of the skin
			    Vomiting

The Pituitary Gland	About the size of a pea, lying in the floor of the skull. It is in 2 lobes, an anterior and posterior.	Anterior lobe influences growth, especially of the bones. Posterior, has an action somewhat like that of adrenaline.	Acromegaly, a disease in which there is enlargement of the bones of the hands, feet, and head.
The Thymus Gland	Found just beneath the sternum. Weighs about half an ounce at birth, develops up to puberty, after which it atrophies.		
The Pineal Gland	About the size of a small cherry stone, connected with the upper surface of the brain.		
The Testicles and Ovaries		Cause the development of the secondary sexual characters such as the growth of hair and deepening of the voice in the male.	Dementia precox

Important Results of Diseases of Four Endocrine Glands

Gland	Name of Hormone	Hypersection		Hyposecretion	
		In Children	In Adults	In Children	In Adults
Thyroid	Thyroxin	Hyperthyroidism (exophthalmic goiter)		Cretinism	Myxedema
Parathyroid	Parathormone	Generalized osterits fibrosa, with high blood calcium.		Tetany, with low blood calcium.	
Suprarenal (cortex) (mendula)	Cortin or Eucortione	Sexual precocity	Obesity, increased hairiness.	Addison's disease	
	Adrenaline	--	--	--	
Pituitary (anterior lobe) (posterior lobe)	--	Giganitsm	Acromegally	Infantilism	?
	Pituitrin	? Disorder of carbohydrate metabolism		Diabetes insipidus	

HORMONES AND THEIR FUNCTIONS

Gland	Hormone	Function
Posterior pituitary gland	Antidiuretic hormone (ADH)	Water reabsorption from kidney tubules.
	Oxytocin	Contraction of the uterus during birth.
Anterior pituitary gland	Growth hormone (GH)	Growth
	Prolactin	Milk production and secretion.
	Follicle-stimulating hormone (FSH)	In females, maturation of the Graafian follicle; in males, sperm production.
	Luteinizing hormone (LH)	In females, ovulation, forming corpus luteum; in males, testosterone synthesis.
	Thyroid stimulating hormone (TSH)	Stimulates the thyroid to release thyroid hormones.
	Adrenocorticotrophic hormone (ACTH)	Stimulates the adrenal cortex to produce corticosteroid hormones.
Ovary	Estrogen	Female secondary sexual characteristics.
Ovary placenta	Progesterone	Prepares uterus for pregnancy; maintains it during pregnancy.
Testes	Testosterone	Male secondary sexual characteristics.
Adrenal gland (cortext)	Adrenaline	"Fight or flight": increases heart activity, rate and depth or breathing, blood flow to muscles; inhibits digestion and excretion.
Thyroid	Thyroxine	Regulates metabolism and growth.
	Calcitogen	Regulates blood calcium levels by reducing release of calcium from bones.
Parathyroid	Parathormone	Regulates blood calcium levels by stimulating release of calcium from the bones.
Pancreas (islets of Langerhans)	Insulin	Regulates blood glucose levels by stimulating conversion of glucose to glycogen.
	Glucagon	Regulates blood glucose levels by stimulating conversion of glycogen to glucose.

CHARTS 1068-1061: Endocrine System 652-662

Malaria
life cycle of teh malaria parasite,
split between mosquito and human

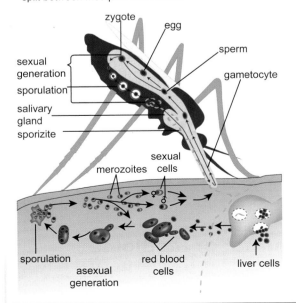

LIFE CYCLE OF THE MALARIA PARASITE

The life cycle of the malaria parasite is split between mosquito and human hosts. The parasites are injected into the human bloodstream by an infected Anopheles mosquito and carried to the liver. Here they attack red blood cells, and multiply asexually. The infected blood cells burst, producing spores, or merozoites, which reinfect the bloodstream. After several generations, the parasite develops into a sexual form. If the human host is bitten at this stage, the sexual form of the parasite is sucked into the mosquito's stomach. Here fertilization takes place, the zygotes formed reproduce asexually and migrate to the salivary glands ready to be injected into another human host, completing the cycle.

—Malaria (306) Mosquito Bite (832)—

C H A R T S

CHARTS 1068-1061: Endocrine System 652-662

ESTROGEN'S BENEFITS

Relief from the classic symptoms of menopause: hot flashes, mood swings, vaginal dryness, thinning skin

Proven reduced bone loss (osteoporosis) associated with menopause, including a probable reduction in hip fractures

Probable reduced risk of heart disease by improving cholesterol levels and the flexibility of blood vessels

Possible improved memory and better mental functioning of women with mild to moderate Alzheimer's disease

Possible lowered risk of colon cancer

ESTROGEN'S RISKS

An increased risk of endometrial cancer which may be partially countered by adding progesterone to a regimen of estrogen

Symptoms similar to premenstrual ones (swelling, bloating, breast tenderness, mood swings, headches)

A menstrual discharge (when progesterone is taken with estrogen)

Increased risk of breast cancer

Stimulation of the growth of uterine fibroids and endometriosis

Probable increased risk of gallstones and blood clots

Possible weight gain

— New England Journal of Medicine

THE GLYCEMIC INDEX

Glycemic index (GI) has become a popular term; it is more meaningful than the label, "simple carbohydrate." <u>GI refers to the rise in your blood sugar after you ingest a specific food</u>. This numerical value is compared to the GI of glucose at a value of 100. It is recommended that people with obesity, diabetes, and insulin resistance eat foods that have lower glycemic values. For example, a Coca-Cola soft drink has a glycemic index of 63; whereas a serving of kidney beans has a value of 23.

<u>A GI of 70 or more is considered high</u>. A GI of 56 to 69 is considered medium. A GI of less than 55 is considered low.

THE GLYCEMIC LOAD

Recently, doctors and researchers have placed more value on the glycemic load (GL) value of foods. <u>The glycemic load takes into account the amount of carbohydrates in one serving of a particular food</u>. The glycemic index tells us how quickly a carbohydrate turns into blood sugar; but it neglects to take into account the amount of carbohydrates in a serving, which is important. The higher the glycemic load value, the higher the blood-sugar level and the resulting stress on insulin levels. <u>This value is derived by multiplying the amount of carbohydrates contained in a specified serving size of the food by the glycemic index value of that food, and then dividing by 100</u>. For example, an apple has a GI of 40, compared to that of glucose, which is the baseline at 100, but the amount of carbohydrates available in a typical apple is 16 grams. The GL is calculated by multiplying the 16 grams of available carbohydrates times 40 and then dividing by 100, to arrive at a decimal number of approximately 6. Compare this to a serving of Rice Krispies which has a GI of 82, 26 available carbohydrates, and a glycemic load of 21. A serving of macaroni and cheese has a glycemic load of 32.

<u>A GL of 20 or more is considered high. A GL of 11 to 19 is considered medium. A GL of 10 or less is considered low</u>.

Complex carbohydrates should be the dominant type of carbohydrates in the diet. They provide a longer-lasting energy source; help us to feel full; maintain our blood-sugar balance; contain fiber that helps us with elimination; and contain more vitamins, minerals, and phytonutrients than carbohydrates do. <u>Examples of complex carbohydrates include whole grains (such as whole wheat pasta, whole grain breads and cereals, and oatmeal), beans, brown rice, peas, and most root vegetables</u>.

<u>Consuming carbohydrates along with protein, fiber, and fat (good fats) helps to smooth out their effect on blood-sugar levels</u>. This is another reason why a balance of all the nutrients is so important.

C
H
A
R
T
S

THE MOST POWERFUL, NATURAL BACTERIA AND VIRUS KILLERS

Bacteria vs. virus— What is the difference between a bacterial infection and a viral infection?

Bacterial infections are caused by bacteria and viral infections are caused by viruses. **Infections caused by bacteria include strep throat, tuberculosis and urinary tract infections. Diseases that result from viruses include chicken pox, AIDS and the common cold.**

Bacteria are single-celled microorganisms that thrive in many different types of environments. Some varieties live in extremes of cold or heat, while others make their home in people's intestines, where they help digest food. Most bacteria cause no harm to people.

Viruses are even smaller than bacteria and require living hosts (people, plants or animals) to multiply. Otherwise, they cannot survive. When a virus enters your body, it invades some of your cells and takes over the cell machinery, redirecting it to produce the virus.

Perhaps the most important distinction between bacteria and viruses is that **antibiotic drugs usually kill bacteria, but they are not effective against viruses.** In some cases, it may be difficult to determine whether a bacteria or a virus is causing the symptoms. Many ailments (such as pneumonia, meningitis and diarrhea) can be caused by either type of microbe.

Antibiotic drugs can be dangerous, while herbal antibiotics are generally safe. In addition, inappropriate use of antibiotics has helped create strains of bacterial disease that are resistant to treatment with different types of antibiotic medications.

Here is a list of the most powerful antibiotic natural remedies:

Vitamin C—**This is a remarkably powerful destroyer of bacteria and viruses.** Lack of it causes scurvy, loose teeth, superficial bleeding, fragile blood vessels, poor healing, compromised immunity, and anemia.

It has many functions in the body, a primary one being to produce collagen in the connective tissue. Vitamin C literally helps hold your body together! It is also important in the transfer of energy to the cell mitochondria. It is a strong antioxidant.

Vitamin C, taken with one or more antibiotic herbs, will help provide for powerful germ and virus fighting. If too much is taken, it will cause diarrhea.

The tissues with the greatest percentage of vitamin C—over 100 times the level in blood plasma—are the adrenal glands, pituitary, thymus, corpus luteum, and retina.

The brain, spleen, lung, testicle, lymph nodes, liver, thyroid, small intestinal mucosa, leukocytes, pancreas, kidney, and salivary glands usually have 10 to 50 times the concentration present in blood plasma.

Garlic—**This is one of the most powerful antiseptic substances ever discovered.** It is also one of the most readily available and easily used medicinal substances.

In the 1950s, Soviet scientists found it to be equal to penicillin, yet without the harmful effects of that powerful drug.

Internally, garlic detoxifies the entire body and protects against infection by enhancing immune function. **It is good for virtually every infection and disease.** Its beneficial effect on blood circulation and heart action can bring relief for many common body complaints. It is used for **all lung and respiratory ailments, colds, tuberculosis, fevers, and blood diseases;** and it can be used as a tea or added to syrups for coughs.

It is used for **arteriosclerosis, cancer, contagious disease, coughs, cramps, diverticulitis, emphysema, gas, heart problems, high blood pressure, indigestion, liver congestion, rheumatism, sinus congestion, and ulcers. It aids in the treatment of arthritis, asthma, circulatory problems, cold and flu, digestive problems, heart disorders, insomnia, liver diseases, sinusitis, ulcers, and yeast infections.**

Garlic is helpful in all intestinal infections, including dysentery, typhoid, cholera, and paratyphoid fever. It lowers blood lipid levels. **It works to eliminate putrefactive intestinal bacteria.**

Echinacea—**Internally, echinacea is used for bladder infections, blood poisoning, as a blood purifier, fevers, inflammation of mammary glands, intestinal antiseptic, leukopenia (reduction in blood leukocytes), lymphatic congestion, uremic poisoning, venereal disease, and all chronic and acute bacterial and viral infections. It has been used for years for syphilis, gonorrhea, and in douches for all vaginal infections. Combine it with myrrh, to rid the body of pus, abscess formations, and for typhoid fever.** The rootstock helps dispel flatulence. Echinacea aids digestion and is a digestive tonic.

Echinacea is an excellent antibiotic, and ranks with goldenseal and red clover. For acute ailments, it must be taken every hour or two, as a tincture (one tsp.) or a powder in two #00 capsules.

Echinacea fights viruses in two ways. It contains three compounds with specific antiviral activity—*caffeic acid, chicoric acid, and echinacin.* Root extracts of echinacea have also been shown to act like interferon, the body's own antiviral compound. In addition, echinacea is an immune stimulant that helps the body defend itself against viral infection more effectively.

Although echinacea as an excellent **immune booster,** scientists still do not fully understand how it stimulates the immune system. Some suggest that it increases the body's levels of a compound, known as properdin, which activates the specific part of the immune system, called the complementary pathway, that is responsible for sending disease-fighting white blood cells into infected areas to battle viruses and bacteria.

Other researchers maintain that other compounds in the herb, *lipophilic amides* and *polar caffeic acid derivatives,* are at the root of its immunostimulant activity. One compound, chicoric acid, inhibits integrase, an enzyme that is important in viral reproduction

Goldenseal—This is another powerful antiseptic (germ killer). Like echinacea, **it is good for nearly every disease.** Taken with any herb, it increases the tonic effects on the specific organs being treated. Add it when giving eyebright for the eyes, squaw vine for the female genito-urinary system, gotu kola for the brain, and cascara sagrada for the lower bowel. Add it to salves for the skin, douches for vaginal infections, and reducing hemorrhoids. It especially acts on mucous membranes and can be used for all catarrhal conditions, including those in the intestines. **Used at the first sign of possible symptoms, it can stop a cold, flu, or sore throat.**

Goldenseal contains berberine and hydrastine, and is a broad-spectrum herlbal antibiotic. Berberine, is an immune stimulant. (Berberine is also in barberry root bark and Oregon grape root, two other antibiotics.

Goldenseal is a powerful alkaloid and should not be overused. Two or three #00 capsules per day are safe and adequate for most conditions. Normally, do not use it more than a week at a time, then switch to echinacea or another antibiotic herb (myrrh, chaparral, pau d'arco). Excessive use diminishes vitamin B absorption, by killing certain intestinal bacteria.

Chaparral—Internally, chaparral is **one of the best herbal antibiotics. It is useful against bacteria, viruses, and parasites, both internally and externally.** It fights free radicals and chelates heavy metals. **It has anti-HIV activity. It protects against harmful effects of radiation. It may be taken internally for colds and flus, inflammations of the respiratory and intestinal tracts, diarrhea, and urinary tract infections.**

Chaparral protects against the formation of tumors, cancer cells, and over-exposure to sunlight. It contains a substance, called NDGA (nordihydroguararetic acid), which is a powerul antioxidant, useful in preserving fats and oils and a powerful antitumor agent. American Indians used it to treat cancer. It relieves pain and is good for skin disorders. It is excellent as an addition to an herbal formula in the treatment of kidney and bladder infections.

Chaparral is very bitter and is usually mixed with other herbs or taken in tincture form. Pau d'arco (Tabebuia heptaphylla), also called lapacho or taheebo, has similar antibiotic and anticancer properties, but is less harsh than chaparral.

Pau d'arco—Aiso called Lapacho or Taheebo, pau d'arco is a South American herb which, **internally, fights bacterial and viral infections;** cleanses the blood; and is useful for **AIDS, cancer, tumors,** ulcers, candidiasis, smoker's cough, allergies, cardiovascular problems, inflammatory bowel disease, rheumatism, and **all types of infections.** Only the inner bark is used. It has similar antibiotic and anticancer properties to chaparral, but is less harsh.

Red Clover—internally, red clover is considered **among the very best anticancer herbs.** It is a powerful blood purifier, either used alone or in combination with yellow dock, dandelion root, sassafras, or other blood purifiers. **It fights infection,** suppresses appetite, relaxes the system, stops spasms, and induces expectoration. It is soothing to the nerves and is good for whooping cough, psoriasis, rheumatism, and stomach problems. It is used for **coughs, bronchitis, inflamed lungs, kidney problems, liver disease, weakened immune system, bacterial infections, HIV, and AIDS. Externally, it can be applied as a poultice or fomentation on cancerous growths.**

Olive Leaf—This remarkable herbal supplement is **effective against nearly all the viruses and bacteria.** It helps protect against infection by **influenza, herpes, and other viruses.** It is used to deal with **sore throat, rashes, skin diseases, shingles,** sinusitis, pneumonia, and chronic infections. It is good for **bacterial infections, and even stubborn fungal infections.**

Here are several other excellent antibacterial, antiviral herbs:

Juniper Berries—These contain deoxypodophyllotoxin, which inhibits a number of different viruses.

Licorice—This has eight active antiviral compounds, including glycyrrhizin, which keeps viruses from replicating. Licorice has the most bactericidal compounds (up to 33% antibacterial compounds on a dry-weight basis). It also has saponins, which increase the availability of other antibiotic compounds.

Ginger—This contains 10 antiviral compounds, called sesquiterpenes.

Shitake—This is a tasty Asian mushroom which contains lentinan, an antiviral, immune-stimulating and anti-tumor compound.

HOW INFECTIOUS DISEASES ARE SPREAD

Infectious Diseases (293-302) / Also see in Disease Index (1211-1221) for each of the 21 types of infectious diseases

Disease	Agent	Transmission
AIDS (acquired immune deficiency syndrome)	Virus	Contract of the body fluid (semen, blood, vaginal secretions) with that of an infected person. Sexual contact and sharing of unclean paraphernalia for intravenous drugs are the most common means of transmission.
Blatomycosis	Fungus	Inhaling contaminated dust
Botulism	Bacteria	Consuming contaminated food
Chicken Pox	Virus	Direct or indirect contact with the infected person
Common Cold	Virus	Direct or indirect contact with the infected person
Diptheria	Bacteria	Direct contact with the infected person
Encephalitis	Virus	Mosquito bite
Gonorrhea	Bacteria	Sexual contact
Hepatitis	Virus	Direct or indirect contact with the infected person
Herpes simplex	Virus	Direct contact with the infected person
Histoplasmosis	Fungus	Inhaling contaminated dust
Hookworm	Nematode	Contact with contaminated soil
Infectious mononucleosis	Virus	Direct or indirect contact with the infected person
Influenza	Virus	Direct or indirect contact with the infected person
Lyme disease	Bacteria	deer tick bite
Malaria	Protozoa	Mosquito bite
Measles	Virus	Direct or indirect contact with the infected person
Mumps	Virus	Direct or indirect contact with the infected person
Pertussis (whooping Caugh)	Virus	Direct or indirect contact with the infected person
Poliomyelitis	Bacteria	Direct contact with the infected person
Rubella (German Measles)	Virus	Direct or indirect contact with the infected person

MORE QUOTATIONS TO THINK ABOUT

More quotations on pages 1042

"A search of the Medlars' Data Base at the National Library of Medicine shows that, since 1966, there have been 12,869 studies on vitamin C, of which 5,546 deal with humans, and 7,043 studies on vitamin E, of which 3,205 deal with humans. In total, there probably have been more than 75,000 studies on nutrients now being consumed as dietary supplements. Many of these studies provide the kind of evidence that would persuade anyone—except, of course, the FEDA—of the health benefits of dietary supplements."—*Saul Kent, President, The Life Extension Foundation.*

"We don't need to have more restrictions on supplements and herbs. This will only act to benefit the pharmaceutical companies and doctors who are already making enorous profits in this field and make it more expensive for people to take care of themselves."—*Konrad Kail, N.D., past President, American Association of Naturopathic Physicians.*

"It's supposed to be a professional secret, but I'll tell you anyway. We doctors do nothing. We only help and encourage the doctor within."—*Albert Schwizer, M.D. (1875-1965), a Franco-German physician who founded an important hospital in Lambaréné, now in Gabon, west central Africa; Nobel Prize Winner.*

WHAT PEOPLE ARE REQUIRED TO TAKE BEFORE TRAVELING OVERSEAS !

Disease	Immunization	Timing	Reaction	Protection	Duration of precautions	Other precautions	Notes
Cholera	2 injections not less than a week apart	1 week to 1 month before departure	soreness where injected, fever, headache, fatigue	50-60%	6 months	avoid food or water that may be dirty	low risk in reasonable tourist accommodation; infants under 6 months should not be vaccinated
Hepatitis A	(a) injection of immunoglobulin or (b) a vaccine consisting of 2 injections 1 month apart, then a 3rd injection 6 - 12 months later	(a) just before travel (b) 2 months before	(a) immunoglobulin - some may experience soreness and swelling at the injection site and, in some cases, hives (b) vaccine - soreness where injected, sometime headache and fatigue	(a) prevents illness (b) lessens it's severity	(a) 3 months (b) 10 years	as typhoid	
Hepatitis B	2 injections of vaccine 1 month apart, then booster 4 months later	last injection 1 month before travel	soreness where injected	80-90%	perhaps 5 years		given to those at high risk, such as health workers, and is now also part of the recommended childhood vaccination series
Malaria	none; take preventative tablets from 1 week before to 4 weeks after leaving malaria area	order tablets 2 weeks before travel	side effects are rare	90%	only while tablets are taken	use antimosquito sprays, mosquito nets; keep arms and legs covered after sunset	some antimalarial drugs are not recommended for pregnant mothers or children under 1 years
Polio	(a) oral vaccine - 3 - 4 doses (b) injections -3 -4 shots, the best way to be protected is to get 4 doses of polio vaccine; immunized adults; 1 booster dose	for travelers who are not up-to-date with their vaccination it may be necessary to allow as much as 7 months for the full recommended vaccination schedule, depending upon other vaccines that may be necessary for the trip	very rare cases develop polio	95+%	10 years		(a) should not be given to pregnant mothers (b) (injections) recommended only for people 18 years and older who have not yet been vaccinated, and for people who cannot take the oral vaccines because of health reason; should not be given to a person who has had an allergy problem with the antibiotics neomycin or streptomycin. The overall risk to travelers is too low
Rabies	3- doses series of injections, usually given on days 0,7, and 21, or 28	5 weeks before travel	swelling and itching where injected, headache, abdominal pain, muscles aches, nausea	opinion divided as to whether vaccine prevents or promotes a faster response to treatment	3 months	avoid bites, scratches, or licks from any animal; wash any bites or scratch with antiseptic or soap as quickly as possible and get immediate medical attention	The overall risk to travelers is too low

CHART - 1063-1064: Information on the 9 types of vaccinations required prior to overseas travel. For more on vaccinations: 876, 928, 972

CHARTS

CONCLUDED ON NEXT PAGE

Much more on Vitamin C (108-109)

Disease	Immunization	Timing	Reaction	Protection	Duration of precautions	Other precautions	Notes
Tetanus	normally given in childhood with booster every 10 years; unimmunized adults; 2 injections 1 month apart then 3rd injection 6 months later	not critical	headache, lethargy in rare cases	>90%	about 10 years	wash any wounds with antiseptic	recommended for those visiting countries with poor food and water sanitation
typhoid	3 types of vaccine: (a) 1 - 2 injections 4 - 6 weeks apart (b) single injection (c) 4 oral doses, every-other-day series on days 1,2,4 and 6	5-7 weeks before departure	soreness where injected, nausea, headache (worst in those over 35 and on repeat immunizations) may last 36 hours	50 - 70%	(a) 1 -3 years (b) 3 years (c) 1 year	avoid food, milk or water that may be contaminated by sweage or by flies	may only be available from special centers
Yellow Fever	1 injection	at least 10 days before departure, but not more than 10 years before (arrival)	possible slight headache and low fever muscle ache	almost 100 %	10 years	against mosquitoes, as for malaria	

VITAMIN C CONTENT OF DIFFERENT FOODS
(In milligrams per 3½-ox (300-g per serving)

More quotations on pages 1042 and1062

Acerola	1300	Cabbage, red	61	Okra	31
Peppers, red chili	369	Strawberries	59	Tangerines	31
Guavas	242	Papayas	56	New Zealand spinach	30
Peppers, red sweet	190	Spinach	51	Black-eyed peas	29
Kale leaves	186	Oranges & juice	50	Soybeans	29
Parsley	172	Cabbage	47	Lima beans, young	28
Collard leaves	152	Lemon juice	46	Green peas	27
Turnip greens	139	Grapefruit & juice	38	Radishes	26
Peppers, green sweet	128	Elderberries	36	Raspberries	25
Broccoli	113	Turnips	36	Chinese cabbage	25
Brussels sprouts	102	Mangoes	35	Yellow summer squash	25
Mustard greens	97	Asparagus	33	Loganberries	24
Watercress	79	Cantaloupe	33	Honeydew melons	23
Cauliflower	78	Swiss chard	32	Tomatoes	23
Persimmons	66	Green onions	32		

STILL MORE QUOTATIONS TO THINK ABOUT

"I don't feel comforable using a substance [mercury, the major constituent in the dental filling, amalgam] designated by the Environmental Protection Agency to be a waste disposal hazard. I can't throw it in the trash, bury it in the ground, or put it in a landfill; but they say it's okay to put it in people's mouths. That doesn't make sense."—*Richard D. Fischer, D.D.S.*

"Although it is not clear whether denal amalgams and other metals used in dental work are the primary or secondary cause of many health problems, both doctors and dentists have to be concerned with evaluating the clinical implications of using toxic metals in the human body."—*Theron Randolph, M.D.*

"Mercury vapors from tooth fillings damage both brain and body."—*Kendrick J. Wellington, D.D.S.*

C
H
A
R
T
S

Eight Types of Bandages

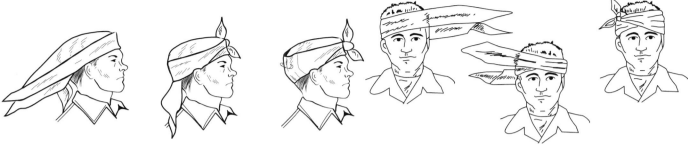

Applying a triangular bandage to the head

Applying a cravat bandage to the head

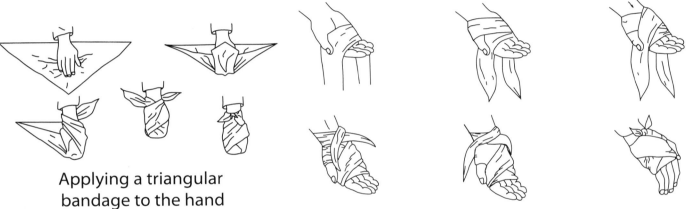

Applying a triangular
bandage to the hand

Applying a cravat bandage to the hand

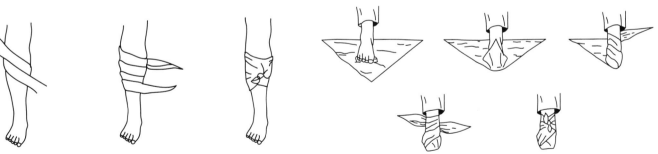

Applying a cravat bandage to the leg

Applying a triangular bandage to the foot

Method 1

Method 2

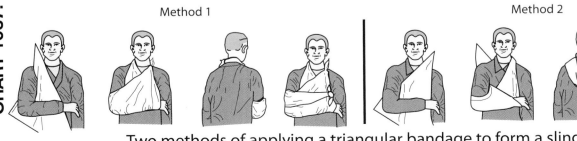

Two methods of applying a triangular bandage to form a sling

CHART 1067: Also see First Aid Handbook (990-1009) / Preparing for Emergencies (973-989)

CHARTS

Recommended Weight Tables, by ages for men and women / Also see Obesity (480, 899)

RECOMMENDED WEIGHT TABLES

Height		Small frame weight		Medium frame weight		Large frame weight	
m	ft/in	kg	lbs	kg	lbs	kg	lbs
Men Aged 25 and Over							
1.55	5'1"	48-51	105-113	50-55	11-122	54-61	119-134
1.57	5'2"	49-53	108-116	52-57	114-126	55-62	122-137
1.60	5'3"	50-54	111-119	53-59	117-129	57-64	125-141
1.63	5'4"	52-55	114-122	54-60	120-132	58-66	128-145
1.65	5'5"	53-57	117-126	56-62	123-136	59-68	131-149
1.68	5'6"	55-59	121-130	58-64	127-140	61-70	135-154
1.70	5'7"	57-61	125-134	59-66	131-145	64-72	140-159
1.73	5'8"	59-68	129-149	61-68	135-149	65-74	144-163
1.75	5'9"	60-65	133-143	63-69	139-153	67-76	148-167
1.78	5'10"	62-67	137-147	65-72	143-158	69-78	152-172
1.80	5'11"	64-69	141-151	67-74	147-163	71-80	157-177
1.83	6'0"	66-70	145-155	69-76	151-168	73-83	161-182
1.85	6'1"	68-73	149-160	70-79	155-173	76-85	168-187
1.88	6'2"	69-74	153-164	73-81	160-178	78-87	171-192
1.91	6'3"	71-76	157-168	75-83	165-183	79-89	175-197
Women Aged 25 and Over							
1.45	4'9"	41-44	90-97	43-48	94-106	46-54	102-118
1.47	4'10"	42-45	92-100	44-49	97-109	48-55	106-121
1.5	4'11"	43-47	95-103	45-51	100-112	49-56	108-124
1.52	5'0"	45-48	98-106	47-53	103-116	50-58	111-127
1.55	5'1"	46-49	101-109	48-54	106-118	52-59	114-130
1.57	5'2"	47-51	104-112	49-51	109-112	53-61	117-134
1.60	5'3"	49-52	107-115	51-57	112-126	55-63	121-138
1.63	5'4"	50-54	110-119	53-59	116-131	57-64	125-142
1.65	5'5"	52-56	114-123	54-62	120-136	59-66	129-146
1.68	5'6"	54-58	118-127	56-63	124-139	60-68	133-150
1.70	5'7"	55-59	122-131	58-65	128-143	62-70	137-154
1.73	5'8"	57-62	126-136	60-67	132-147	64-72	141-159
1.75	5'9"	59-64	130-140	62-69	136-151	66-74	145-164
1.78	5'10"	61-65	134-144	64-70	140-155	68-77	149-169

LIFE EXPECTANCY TABLES - 1

Age (years)	Expectation of life in years					Expected deaths per 1000 alive at specified age				
		White		Black			White		Black	
	Total	Male	Female	Male	Female	Total	Male	Female	Male	Female
At birth	74.6	71.7	78.7	65.4	73.6	11.15	10.79	8.6	21.05	17.23
1	74.5	71.5	78.4	65.9	73.9	0.75	0.80	0.59	1.22	0.92
2	73.5	70.5	77.4	64.9	72.9	0.59	0.60	0.47	1.00	0.76
3	72.6	69.6	76.4	64.0	72.0	0.47	0.47	0.37	0.81	0.62
4	71.6	68.6	75.5	63.0	71.0	0.39	0.39	0.31	0.66	0.51
5	70.8	67.6	74.5	62.1	70.1	0.33	0.35	0.26	0.54	0.42
6	69.7	66.6	73.5	61.1	69.1	0.30	0.33	0.23	0.45	0.34
7	68.7	65.7	72.5	60.1	68.1	0.26	0.30	0.20	0.38	0.29
8	67.7	64.7	71.5	59.2	67.2	0.23	0.27	0.18	0.33	0.25
9	66.7	63.7	70.6	58.2	66.2	0.20	0.22	0.16	0.30	0.23
10	65.7	62.7	69.6	57.2	65.2	0.18	0.19	0.14	0.30	0.22
11	64.7	61.7	68.6	56.2	64.2	0.18	0.18	0.14	0.32	0.23
12	63.7	60.7	67.6	55.2	63.2	0.22	0.25	0.17	0.38	0.25
13	62.8	59.8	66.6	54.3	62.2	0.31	0.39	0.21	0.48	0.27
14	61.8	58.8	65.8	53.3	61.2	0.44	0.60	0.28	0.61	0.31
15	60.8	57.8	64.6	52.3	60.3	0.59	0.83	0.36	0.75	0.36
16	59.8	56.9	63.7	51.4	59.3	0.73	1.04	0.43	0.91	0.41
17	58.9	55.9	62.7	50.4	58.3	0.84	1.22	0.49	1.10	0.47
18	57.9	55.0	61.7	49.5	57.3	0.92	1.34	0.51	1.32	0.54
19	57.0	54.1	60.7	48.5	56.4	0.97	1.41	0.51	1.55	0.61
20	56.0	53.1	59.8	47.6	55.4	1.02	1.47	0.50	1.81	0.69
21	55.1	52.2	58.8	46.7	54.4	1.07	1.53	0.50	2.06	0.77
22	54.2	51.3	57.8	45.8	53.5	1.10	1.57	0.50	2.27	0.84
23	53.2	50.4	56.9	44.9	52.5	1.12	1.58	0.51	2.42	0.90
24	52.3	49.4	55.9	44.0	51.6	1.13	1.57	0.52	2.53	0.94
25	51.3	48.5	54.9	43.1	50.6	1.13	1.55	0.53	2.62	0.98
26	50.4	47.6	54.0	42.2	49.7	1.14	1.52	.54	2.74	1.04
27	49.4	46.7	53.0	41.3	48.7	1.14	1.51	0.55	2.88	1.09
28	48.5	45.7	52.0	40.4	47.8	1.16	1.50	0.56	3.05	1.16
29	47.6	44.8	51.0	39.6	46.6	1.18	1.51	0.57	3.26	1.24
30	46.6	43.9	50.1	38.7	45.9	1.21	1.52	0.59	3.49	1.33
31	45.7	42.9	49.1	37.8	45.0	1.24	1.54	0.61	3.72	1.43
32	44.7	42.0	48.1	37.0	44.0	1.28	1.57	0.65	3.93	1.53
33	43.8	41.1	47.2	36.1	43.1	1.33	1.61	0.69	4.12	1.65
34	42.8	40.1	46.2	35.3	42.2	1.38	1.66	0.74	4.30	1.77
35	41.9	39.2	45.2	34.4	41.2	1.46	1.73	0.81	4.50	1.91
36	41.1	38.3	44.3	33.6	40.3	1.54	1.82	0.80	4.73	2.07
37	40.0	37.3	43.3	32.7	39.4	1.64	1.92	0.96	4.99	2.24
38	39.1	36.4	42.3	31.9	38.5	1.76	2.04	1.05	5.26	2.42
39	38.2	35.5	41.4	31.0	37.6	1.89	2.18	1.15	5.57	2.61

CHART 1069: Life Expectancy Tables - by Race, Gender, Age
How to estimate how long you will live 127

CHARTS

What to do if you have a heart attack (513) / How to tell if he is about to have a stroke (529) / Your heart attack risk (127)

Distilled water (918)

C
H
A
R
T
S

LIFE EXPECTANCY TABLES - 2

| Age (years) | Expectation of life in years | | | | | Expected deaths per 1000 alive at specified age | | | | |
| | Total | White | | Black | | Total | White | | Black | |
		Male	Female	Male	Female		Male	Female	Male	Female
40	37.2	34.6	40.4	30.2	36.7	2.05	2.35	1.27	5.89	2.81
41	36.3	33.6	39.5	29.4	35.8	2.23	2.55	1.40	6.26	3.05
42	35.4	32.7	38.5	28.6	34.9	2.44	2.78	1.55	6.75	3.33
43	34.5	31.8	37.6	27.8	34.0	2.69	3.06	1.71	7.40	3.67
44	33.6	30.9	36.7	27.0	33.1	2.97	3.39	1.90	8.16	4.05
45	32.7	30.0	35.7	26.2	32.2	3.29	3.76	2.10	9.02	4.47
46	31.8	29.1	34.8	25.4	31.4	3.64	4.17	2.33	9.90	4.92
47	30.9	28.2	33.9	24.7	30.5	4.02	4.64	2.58	10.74	5.39
48	30.0	27.4	33.0	23.9	29.7	4.45	5.17	2.88	11.51	5.89
49	29.1	26.5	32.1	23.2	28.9	4.91	5.77	3.20	12.23	6.41
50	28.3	25.7	31.2	22.5	28.1	5.42	6.42	3.56	12.97	6.98
51	27.4	24.8	30.3	21.8	27.3	5.97	7.12	3.94	13.81	7.58
52	26.6	24.0	29.4	21.1	26.5	6.56	7.90	4.34	14.81	8.24
53	25.8	23.2	28.5	20.4	25.7	7.20	8.76	4.76	16.02	8.97
54	24.9	22.4	27.7	19.7	24.9	7.89	9.70	5.19	17.40	9.75
55	24.1	21.6	26.0	19.1	24.1	8.63	10.72	5.64	18.85	10.56
56	23.3	20.8	25.9	18.4	23.4	9.42	11.80	6.15	20.35	11.41
57	22.6	20.1	25.1	17.8	22.7	10.28	12.59	6.72	22.03	12.36
58	21.8	19.3	24.3	17.2	21.9	11.22	14.14	7.37	23.94	13.46
59	21.0	18.6	23.4	16.6	21.2	12.23	15.41	8.10	26.02	14.66
60	20.3	17.9	22.6	16.0	20.5	13.33	16.76	8.89	28.35	16.01
61	19.6	17.2	21.8	15.5	19.9	14.49	18.22	9.74	30.74	17.37
62	18.8	16.5	21.0	14.9	19.2	15.71	19.83	10.61	32.81	18.55
63	18.1	15.8	20.3	14.4	18.6	16.98	21.63	11.51	34.37	19.44
64	17.4	15.2	19.5	13.9	17.9	18.31	23.62	12.45	35.54	20.13
65	16.7	14.5	18.7	13.4	17.3	19.72	25.74	13.45	36.43	20.69
70	13.5	11.5	15.1	10.9	14.1	29.70	39.52	20.78	51.45	30.79
75	10.7	9.0	11.8	9.0	11.5	44.31	60.15	32.76	68.22	42.55
80	8.1	6.9	8.8	7.1	9.0	66.98	90.04	53.49	93.33	62.99
85 and over	6.1	5.2	6.5	6.0	7.4	1,000.00	1,000.00	1,000.00	1,000.00	1,000.00

HOME WATER TREATMENT METHODS

Activated Carbon: (Faucet Mounted Under Sink or Counter) - Water is filtered through a carbon trap that absorbs the contaminants.

Carbon Filtration: (Countertop Freestanding Whole House) - Water is passed through charcoal granules or a solid block of charcoal that captures contaminants. When carbon is used up or plugged, cartridge is replaced.

Distillation: (Countertop Undersink Whole House) - Raises water temperature to boiling, leaving contaminants behind. Pure condensate is collected. *This is the best method. "Water Wise" has an outstanding countertop water distiller.*

Reverse Osmosis: (Countertop Undersink Whole House) - Forces pressurized water through a semipermeable membrane and sends improved water to a holding tank.

Water Softener: (Whole House) - Replaces calcium and magnesium with sodium to "soften" the water. This much sodium is not good for you!

CHEMICAL CONSTITUENTS OF THE BODY

Proteins

Elements	Symbol	Percent	End Products
1. Carbon	C	.53 %	
2. Hydrogen	H	.07 %	Urea, uric acid, H_2SO_4, CO_2, H_2O
3. Oxygen	O	.22 %	Salts set free.
4. Nitrogen	N	.16 %	Proteins are tissue, muscle, nerve and brain builders and also furnish heat and energy.
5. Sulfur	S	.015 %	
6. Phosphorus	P	.005 %	
7. Other Minerals			
		1.00 %	

Simple Plant Proteins

Globulins	Glutelins (Gluten)
Legumes	Wheat
Nuts	Several Grains

Conjugated/Derived Proteins (Animal Based)

Casein (phospho-protein) / Whey	Flesh/Meat Based
Milk	Poultry
Cheese	Fish
	Other (Beef, pork, etc.)

Carbohydrates (Cx(H_2O)y)

Elements	Symbol	Percent	End Products
1. Carbon	C	76 %	
2. Hydrogen	H	12 %	Salts set free.
3. Oxygen	O	12 %	CO_2 and H_2O
		100 %	

Classification of Carbohydrates

Glucose	Cane Sugar	Cellulese
$C_4H_{12}O_6$	$C_{12}H_{23}O_{11}$	$C_6H_{10}O_5$

Carbohydrates as well as fats are heat and energy producers, but neither can take the place of proteins, as they contain no nitrogen. They consist principally of the sugars, starch, cellulose and fibers.

Fats

Elements	Symbol	Percent	End Products
1. Carbon	C	76 %	CO_2 and H_2O
2. Hydrogen	H	12 %	Fats are heat and energy producers and not tissue or cell builders.
3. Oxygen	O	12 %	
		100 %	

Classification of Fats

Fats	Oils	Nuts	Olives
Butter			

Food Accessories
Water, mineral, Vitamins

TEMPERATURE BEST SUITED FOR STORAGE OF FOODS

Fruits

	Degrees F.		Degrees F.
Apples	31 - 32	Lemon	36
Bananas	34 - 36	Oranges	36
Berries	34 - 36	Watermelons	32
Cantaloupe	32		
Cranberries	33 - 34	**Vegetables**	
Dried Fruits	35 - 40		
Fresh Fruits	33 - 40	Fresh Vegetables	33 - 35

CHARTS

FOODS WHICH CONTAIN SULFITES

Sulfites are a frequent cause of "unknown" allergies. They are common food additives used as sanitary agents and preservatives to prevent discoloration of foods. They are usually used in restaurant salad bars and are also present in many supermarket foods, including frozen foods, dried fruits, and certain fresh fruits and vegetables. Many people are allergic to sulfites. The types and severity of reactions to sulfites in sensitive individuals vary, and may include breathing difficulties, anaphylactic shock, severe headaches, abdominal pain, stuffy and/or runny nose, flushing of the face and a "hot flash" feeling, diarrhea, irritability, and/or feelings of anger. These symptoms tend to occur quickly, usually within twenty to thirty minutes after consuming sulfites. Sulfites pose a greater danger to some people than to others. People with asthma; a history of allergies; or a deficiency of the liver enzyme, sulfite oxidase, can suffer great harm. Sulfites have been implicated in at least thirteen deaths in the United States. It is not always easy to determine if a food product contains sulfites. Sulfiting agents appear in food ingredient lists in a variety of ways, including *sodium sulfite, sodium bisulfite, sodium metabisulfite, potassium bisulfite, potassium metabisulfite, and sulfur dioxide.* Any ingredient ending in *sulfite* should be assumed to be a sulfiting agent. If you have ever suffered a reaction after ingesting a food you believe contained

sulfites, you should beware of the foods and beverages listed in the table below, which often contain these substances. Sulfite-free forms of some of these foods may be found in health-food stores.

Foods that often contain sulfites:

Beware of the following foods! Avocado dip (guacamole), prepared cut fruit or vegetable salads, cole slaw, mushrooms, fish, canned seafood, commercial soups, dried fish, oysters, clams, shellfish, scallops, crabs, shrimp, lobster, prepared/processed foods, cornstarch, horseradish, sauerkraut, breading mixes, dietetic processed foods, jams and jellies, shredded coconut, commercial breakfast cereals, dried or canned soups, maraschino cherries, trail mixes, brown sugar, dry salad dressing mixes, noodle and rice mixes, wine vinegar, canned fruit pie fillings, olives (frozen, canned, or dried), canned mushrooms, onion relish, caramels, frozen french fries, pickles, glazed fruits, potato chips, pancake syrups, hard candies, sauces and gravies, apple cider (bottled, canned, or frozen), cordials, gelatin, commercial baked goods, commercial vegetable juices, cornmeal, instant tea mixes, beer, cocktail mixes, frozen doughs, wines, fruit juices (bottled, canned, or frozen), colas, and commercial fruit drinks.

SOURCES OF 20 VALUABLE PHYTOCHEMICALS

In recent years, laboratory researchers have discovered the existence of phytochemicals. These are substances which protect the human body against a variety of diseases, including cancer. Twenty are currently known to exist; and they are only found in fruits and vegetables. Here are the names of these substances, plus the foods you would need to eat in order to absorb them into your body:

Allyl sulfides - garlic, onions, leeks, chives
Carotenoids - yellow-orange vegetables and fruits; green, leafy vegetables; red fruits
Coumarins - celery, parsnips, figs, parsley
Curcumins - turmeric, ginger
Dithiolthiones - cruciferous vegetables (cabbage, broccoli, cauliflower, brussels sprouts, kale, collards)
Ellagic acid - grapes, strawberries, raspberries, nuts
Flavonoids - most fruits and vegetables
Indoles / isothiocyanates - broccoli, cabbage, cauliflower, brussels sprouts, radish
Isoflavones - soybeans, tofu
Glucarates - citrus fruits, grains, tomatoes, bell peppers
Lignans - flaxseed, flaxseed oil, soybeans
Liminoids - citrus fruits

Phthalides / polyacetylenes - celery, caraway, cumin, dill, fennel, parsley, carrots, coriander
Phenolic acids - berries, grapes, whole grains, nuts
Phytates - grains, legumes
Phytosterols - seeds, legumes
Protease inhibitors - grains, seeds, nuts, legumes
Saponins - beans, herbs
Terpenes - cherries, citrus fruits, herbs
Tocotrienols - seeds, nuts

Phytochemicals not only provide color, texture, and flavor to plant foods; they also protect the plants against microorganisms and insects. When eaten, these substances protect us against disease! A high intake of fruit and vegetables protects the human body against various cancers, coronary heart disease, and stroke. A Harvard study found that the risk of stroke, alone, was reduced by 31%. A Finnish study found that phytochemicals reduce the likelihood of death by 35%.

For example, there are over 600 types of carotenoids in plants. Rich in antioxidants, they reduce or eliminate cancers in research animals, stimulate the immune system, and protect against age-related macular degeneration. Another example is the glucarates (found in the white portion under the peel of citrus) which protect against breast cancer.

Much more on important nutrients 99-128

FACTS AND FIGURES ABOUT YOUR ASTONISHING BODY

• Doubling a child's height on the second birthday gives a close estimate of his or her final adult height. A boy of 2 has usually grown to 49.5 percent of his adult height; a girl of 2 is 52.8 percent of her adult height.

• Each fingernail and toenail takes about 6 months to grown from its base to the tip.

• During pregnancy a woman's blood volume can increase by 25 percent. Most of the increase is due to the growing fetus and the needs associated with its development in the womb. The augemted blood volume can also aid the mother in case of excessive hemorrhaging during delivery.

• The brain accounts for about 2 percent of the body weight. But it uses 20 percent of all the oxygen we breathe, 20 percent of the calories in the food we eat, and about 15 percent of the body's blood supply. It has more than 100 billion (10^{11}) neurons, or nerve cells, and over 100 trillion (10^{14}) synapses, or nerve connections, so that the interconnections in the brain are virtually limitless.

• The adult human body contains approximately 650 muscles, more than 100 joints, and 50,000 miles of blood vessels and capillaries. An adult has 206 bones, nearly half of them in the hands and feet. A baby has 300 bones at birth, but 94 fuse together during childhood.

• For supporting weight, human bone is stronger than granite. A block of bone the size of a matchbox can support 10 tons, or four times more than concrete can.

• A man's testicles manufacture several hundred million new sperm cells a day, enough to double the population of the United States and Canada combined.

• The heart beats more than 2.8 billion times during the average human life span, and in that time will pump around 60 million gallons of blood. Even during sleep, the fist-sized heart of an adult pumps almost 80 gallons per hour —enough to fill an average small car's gas tank every 9 to 10 minutes. It generates enough muscle to power every day to lift a small car about 50 feet.

• The average pulse rate is 72 beats per minute at rest for adult males and 75 for adult females. The rate can increase to as much as 200 beats per minute during extremely active exercise. Resting pulse rates for athletes can be much slower than 72 to 75 range.

• The lungs contain about 300 million little air sacs called alveoli. If the alveoli were flattened out, they would cover an area of about 1,000 square feet.

• The body of the average adult contains 79 pints of water, about 65 percent of a person's weight.

• Each kidney contains some 1 million individual filters, and between them the two kidneys filter an average of about 8 quarts of blood every hour. The waste products are expelled as urine at the rate of about 3 pints a day.

• In general, the larger you are, the greater your blood volume. A 155 pound person has about 11 pints of blood. The body's entire blood supply washes through the lungs about once a minute. Human red blood corpuscles are created by bone marrow at the rate of about 2 million corpuscles per second. Each lives for 120 to 130 days. In a lifetime, bone marrow creates about half a ton of red corpuscles.

• The body's largest organ is the skin. In an adult man it covers about 20 square feet; a woman has about 17 square feet. The skin is constantly flaking away and being completely replaced by new tissue about once every 4 weeks. On average, each person sheds about 105 pounds of skin and grows about 1,000 completely new outer skins during a lifetime.

• The smallest human muscle is in the ear; it is a little over 0.04 inch long. The ear also contains one of the few parts of the body that has no blood vessels. Cells in part of the inner ear, where sound vibrations are converted to nerve impulses, are fed by constant bath of fluid instead of blood. Otherwise the sensitive nerves would be defeated by the sound of the body's own pulse.

• You grow almost 0.3 inch every night when you are asleep but shrink to your former height the following day. During the day cartilage discs in the spine are squeezed like sponges by gravity while you stand or sit. But at night when you lie down to sleep, the pressure is relieved and the discs swell again. For the same reason, astronauts can temporarily be 2 inches taller after a long space flight.

• Digestion is a precarious balancing act between actions of strong acids and powerful bases. The stomach's acids are strong enough to dissolve zinc, but they are prevented from quickly destroying the stomach lining by bases in the stomach. Nonetheless, 500,000 cells of the lining die and must be replaced every minute, and the entire lining is renewed every 3 days.

• The retina at the back of the eye, which covers only about 1 square inch (650 sq mm), contains approximately 130 million light sensitive cells: about 125 million rod cells for black-and-white vision and 7 million cone cells for color vision.

• In a lifetime the average U.S. resident eats more than 50 tons of food and drinks more than 13,000 gallons of liquid.

C
H
A
R
T
S

THE HIPPOCRATIC OATH
(WHICH MOST PHYSICIANS AGREE TO AT THE TIME OF GRADUATION)

Medical ethics around the world are often measured against the Hippocratic oath, thought to have been written by the Greek physician Hippocrates (c. 460-370 s.c.). In some medical schools and universities, graduating doctors are still obliged to swear to a form of the oath. Here is a translation of the original oath:

I swear by Apollo the healer, invoking all the gods and goddesses to be my witnesses, that I will fulfill this oath and this written covenant to the best of my ability and judgement.

I will look upon him who shall have taught me this art even as one of my own parents. I will share my substance with him, and I will supply his necessities if he be in need. I will regard his offspring even as my own brethren, and I will teach them this art, if they would learn it, without fee or covenant. I will impart this art by precept, by lecture, and by every mode of teaching, not only to my own sons but to the sons of him who has taught me and to disciples bound by covenant and oath, according to the law of medicine.

The regimen I adopt shall be for the benefit of the patients according to my ability and judgement, and not for their hurt or for any wrong. I will give no deadly drug to any, though it be asked of me, nor will I counsel such, and especially I will not aid a woman to procure abortion. Whatsoever house I enter, there will I go for the benefit of the sick, refraining from all wrongdoing or corruption, and especially from any act of seduction, of male or female, of bond or free. Whatsoever things I see or hear concerning the life of men, in my attendance on the sick or even apart therefrom, which ought not to be noised abroad, I will keep silence thereon, counting such things to be as sacred secrets. Pure and holy will I keep my life and my art.

CHARTS

The Natural Remedies Encyclopedia

Resources

HERBS - PLANTS - CATALOGS - ORGANIZATIONS
JOURNALS - LIFESTYLE CENTERS- COOKBOOKS

HERB SUPPLY SOURCES

This chapter will provide you with sources of herbal powders and extracts, plus live herbal seeds and plants!

DRIED HERBS AND EXTRACTS

Albi Importa Limited, P.O. Box 35151, Station E, Vancouver, B.C., Canada.

Kwan Yin Chinese Herb Co., P.O. Box 18617, Spokane, WA 99208 —Special Chinese herbs.

Bio-Botanica Inc., 2 Willow Park Center, Farmingdale, NY 11735 —Herbal extracts, done with a cold (not heat) process. Such extractions keep well (but, because they are extracts, they are in alcohol).

Capriland's Herb Farm, Silver St., Coventry, CT 06238 — Live herb plants and seeds.

Geological Botany Co., 622 W. 67th St., Kansas City, MO 64113.

Golden Gate Herbs, Inc., 140 Market St., San Rafael, CA 94901.

Herb Research, Box 77212, San Francisco, CA 94107.

Herbs of Mexico, 3859 Whittier Blvd., Los Angeles, CA 90023 —Herbs from all over the world.

Indiana Botanic Gardens, Inc., P.O. Box 5, Hammond, IN 46325 —Herbs, gums, oils, resins.

Kiehl Pharmacy, 109 Third Ave., NY, NY 10003.

Larsen's Country Herb Shop, Box 253, Orem, UT 84057

—herbs, extracts, tinctures, ointments, capsules, live aloe vera plants.

Magus, P.O. Box 254, Cedar Grove, NJ 07009 —Claims that many of their herbs are organic and picked wild.

Meadowbrook Herb Farm, Route 138, Wyoming, RI 02898 —Dried herbs, spices.

Kudus, 8513 S Cottage Grove Ave., Chicago, IL 60619.

D. Napier & Sons, 17 Bristo Place, Edinburgh, EHI, Scotland   —Started in 1860, many special products.

Nature's Herb Company, 281 Ellis Street, San Francisco, CA 94102 —Herbs for medical use, essential oils.

Paprikas Weiss, Importers, 1546 Second Ave. NY, NY 10028 —Herbs, spices, misc.

S.B. Penick & Co., 100 Church Street, NY, NY 1007 —Bulk imported botanicals at lower cost.

The Redwood City Seed Co., P.O. Box 361, Redwood City, CA 94064 —Rare nuts, berries, herbs.

Otto Richter & Sons, Ltd., Locust Hill, Ontario, Canada —Rare herbs.

Rocky Hollow Herb Farm, Lake Wallkill Road, Sussex, NJ 47461 —Dried herbs in packages.

A. Shamrock, P.O. Box 40900, San Francisco, CA 94110 —Herb brokers, mail order herbs.

San Francisco Herb Co., 47444 Kato Rd. Fremont, CA 94538 —Wholesale herbs at low prices. Minimum orders $50.00.

Star Herb Co., 352 Miller Ave.,

Mill Valley, CA 94941 —Importers and distributors of botanicals and ginseng.

Wide World of Herbs, Ltd., 11 Saint Catherine St., East Montreal, 129, Canada —Fairly inexpensive source.

Wunderlich-Dietz Corp., State Highway 17, Hasbrouck Heights, NJ 07604 —Many European herbs.

LIVE HERB PLANTS AND SEEDS

Capriland's Herb Farm, Silver St., Coventry, CT 06238 —Live herb plants and seeds.

Carroll Gardens, P.O. Box 310, East Main St., Westminster, MD 21157 —Live herbs and medicinal shrubs.

Clearwater Farms, Des Arc, MO 63636 —Live ginseng seed.

Country Herbs, 3 Maple Street, Stockbridge, MA 01262 —130 varieties of organically grown medicinal, culinary, aromatic, and dye plants.

Ferndale Nursery & Greenhouse, P.O. Box 218, Askov, MN 55704 —Wild ginger, blue cohosh.

Gilberties Herb Garden, Sylvan Avenue, Westport, CT 06860 —200 varieties of herb plants and shrubs.

M. Girvan, Stanhope, IA 50246   —Jewelweed seed (Jewelweed juice is the best antidote for poison ivy on your skin).

Green Herb Gardens, Greene, RI 02827 —Herb seeds.

Halcyon Gardens, Gibsonia, PA 15044 —100 varieties of medical, culinary, and fragrant herbs.

J.H. Hudson, Seedsman, P.O. Box 1058, Redwood City, CA 94064 —Big source of medicinal and other herb seeds.

Johnny's Selected Seeds, Foss Hill Road, RR 1, Box 2580, Albion, ME 04910 —Organic seeds for luffa sponge, white clover, burdock.

Leslie's Wildflower Nursery, 30 Summer St., Methuen, MA 01844 —Wildflowers, ferns, wild ginger, vervain, boneset, arnica, cinquefoil.

Midwest Wildflowers, Box 64, Rockton, IL 61072— Many medicinal wild flowers, plus other herbs.

Nichols Garden Nursery, 1190 North Pacific Highway, Albany, OR 97321 —Hard-to-get herbs, plants. Also peppermint oil.

Ohio Comfrey Growers, Rt. 1, Box 289A, Millersport, OH 43046 — Comfrey roots.

Plant Oddities, Box 127, Basking Ridge, NJ 07926 —Unusual nursery stock.

Otto Richter & Sons, Ltd., Box 26A, Goodwood, Ontario, Canada LOCIAO —300 varieties of herb seeds.

Clyde Robin, P.O. Box 2091, Castro Valley, CA 94546 — Rare wildflower plants and seeds.

Taylor's Herb Gardens, Inc., 1535 Lone Oak Road, Vista, CA 92083 —200 live medicinal, culinary, and aromatic herb plants. Good source.

Three Laurels, Rt. 3m, Marshall, NC 28753 —Wildflower and garden plants, witch hazel, goldenseal, berries.

Tillotson's Roses, 802 Brown's Valley Road, Watsonville, CA 95076 —Rose hips, other rose products.

Woodstream Nursery, Box 510, Jackson, NJ 08527 —Good wildflower and medicinal herb source.

Yankee Peddler Herb Farm, Rt. 4, Box 76, Hwy. 36N, Brenham, TX 77933 —chia, arnica, fenugreek, jewelweed, mullein, shepherd's purse, marshmallow, borage, etc.

LARGEST GARDENING CATALOGS

Burgess Seed and Plant Co., Galesberg, MI 49053.

W. Atlee Burpee Co., 6350 Rutland, Riverside, CA 92502.

Ferry-Morse Seed Co., Box 200, Fulton, KY 42041.

Henry Field Seed & Nursery Co., Shenandoah, IA 51602.

Gurney Seed & Nursery Co., Yankton, SD 57078.

J.H. Hudson, Seedsman, P.O. Box 1058, Redwood City, CA 94064.

Miller Nurseries, Inc., Canandaigua, NY 14424

R.H. Shumway, Seedsman, P.O. Box 777, Rockford, IL 61101.

HEALTH ORGANIZATIONS AND JOURNALS

National Food Association, P.O. Box 210, Atlanta, TX 75551 — A large organization concerned with organic farming and food resources.

National Health Federation, 212 Foothill Blvd., Monrovia, CA 91016 —Defends natural remedies, health foods, and proper nutrition.

Prevention, Emmaus, PA 18048 —The largest and oldest journal dealing with the prevention of disease.

Organic Gardening and Farming, Emmaus, PA 18048 — The other Rodale publication; this one is concerned with promoting the best in natural gardening, and avoidance of chemicals and insecticides.

VEGETARIAN COOKBOOKS

Country Kitchen Collection
Subtitle: Fantastically Delicious and Nutritious Vegetarian Meals
Phil and Eileen Brewer

Family Health Publications
8777 E Musgrove Hwy
Sunfield, MI 48890

Country Life Vegetarian Cookbook
Subtitle: Cholesterol Free
Diana J. Fleming, editor
Family Health Publications
8777 E Musgrove Hwy
Sunfield, MI 48890

Of These Ye May Freely Eat
Subtitle: A Vegetarian Cookbook
JoAnn Rachor
Family Health Publications
8777 E Musgrove Hwy
Sunfield, MI 48890
Taste and See
Subtitle: Allergy Relief Cookbook
No meat, dairy products, vinegar, sugar, wheat, baking powder or eggs and little or no salt or fat
Penny King
Family Health Publications
8777 E Musgrove Hwy
Sunfield, MI 48890

The Seventh-day Diet
Subtitle: How the "Healthiest People in America" Live Better, Longer, Slimmer—and How You Can Too!
Random House, New York

Ten Talents
Subtitle: Natural Foods, Vegetarian Food-Combining Cookbook and Health Manual
Frank J. Hurd, D.C., M.D. and Rosalie Hurd, B.S.
Hurd Publications
P.O. Box 5209
Grants Pass, OR 97527

Newstart Lifestyle Cookbook
Subtitle: More than 260 Heart-Healthy Recipes Featuring Whole Plant Foods
Weimar Institute
800-525-9192

100% Vegetarian
Subtitle: Eating Naturally from Your Grocery Store
Julianne Pickle
Pickle Publishing Company
Route 1, Box 441

Seale, AL 36875

Tastefully Vegan
Creative Vegetarian Cooking
Kathryn J. McLane
Lifestyle Center of America
Route 1, Box 4001
Sulfur, OK 73086
Phone: 800-596-5480

LIFESTYLE CENTERS

SEVERAL SPECIAL CENTERS

1 - U.S. LIFESTYLE CENTERS

For more information, please contact the institutions directly, by using the contact info listed.

Desert Spring Therapy Center
66705 East Sixth Street
Desert Hot Springs, CA 92240
Phone: 760-329-5066
Fax: 760-251-6206
E-mail: dsrtspgt@gte.net

Types of programs offered:
Smoking cessation, weight reduction, addiction recovery, muscular and skeletal disorders. Live-in and walk-in sessions.

Duke University Health and Fitness Center
804 West Trinity Ave.
Durham, NC 27201
1-800-677-2177
(919) 684-6331

Eden Valley Lifestyle Center
6263 N County Road #29
Loveland, CO 80538
Phone: 970-669-7730
Fax: 970-663-7072
Lifestyle Center: 970-669-7730

Emerald Valley Wellness Clinic
600 Dale Kuni Road
Creswell, Oregon 97426
Phone # (541) 895-5300
FAX # (541) 895-5319

Types of programs offered:
Website: **emeraldwellness.com**
Medical Director, Dr. Richard Hansen, MD. Emerald Valley provides treatment that leans less towards the prescription pad and more toward natural remedies. Other services include Outpatient Clinic, Health education classes/seminars, books and more. See web site.

Hartland Wellness Center
P.O. Box 1
Rapidan, VA 22733
Phone: 800-763-9355

Lifestyle Center of America
Route 1, Box 4001
Sulfur, OK 73086
Phone: 800-596-5480
Fax: 405-993-3902

Poland Spring Health Institute
226 Schellinger Road
Poland, ME 04274-6134
207-998-2795
207-998-2894
Lifestyle Center
207-998-2164 lax

Pritikin Longevity Center
1910 Ocean Front Walk
Santa Monica, CA 90405
1-800-206-5813
(310) 450-5433

Uchee Pines Lifestyle Center
30 Uchee Pines Road
Seale, AL 36875-5702
Phone: 334-855-4764
E-mail: center@ucheepines.org
Web site: ucheepines.org

Types of programs offered:
Treatment of lifestyle related disorders by board-certified physicians, including obesity, diabetes, heart disease, hypertension, stress, substance abuse, and chronic diseases. Lifestyle modification includes an emphasis in hydrotherapy, herbs, and faith in God. Live-in and walk-in sessions.

Tennessee Institute of Lifestyle Education
Thirty minutes north of Crossville, TN
Phone: 931-863-3553

Types of programs offered:
Daily massage and water treatments, exercise facility, organic cuisine, country setting.

Weimar Lifestyle Center
P.O. Box 486
Weimar, CA 95736
Phone: 916-637-4111

Types of programs offered:
NEWSTART® lifestyle education (individualized nutrition, exercise, and hydrotherapy under medical supervision), reversing diabetes, cooking schools, medical examinations and screening. Live-in and walk-in sessions. Contact for Newstart: Trevor Louw, Guest Services Director

Wildwood Lifestyle Center
P.O. Box 129
Wildwood, GA 30757
Phone: 706-820-1493

2 - FOREIGN LIFESTYLE CENTERS

Bella Vista Hospital
Carretera 349 km 2.9
Box 1750
Mayaguez, PR 00681
Phone: 787-834-2350, Ext. 6216
Fax: 787-831-6315

Types of programs offered:
Smoking cessation, alcohol and drug education, diabetes control, prenatal and parenting classes, nutrition, natural remedies, sexually transmitted diseases. Walk-in sessions.

Cedarvale Health Centre
2999 Moss Vale Road
Fitzroy Falls, NSW 2577
Australia
Phone / fax:+61-44-651-362

Delhuntie Park Youth Care & Lifestyle Centre, Inc.
RMB 5540
Trafalgar East, Vic 3824
Australia
Phone: +61-356-331688
Fax: +61-356-331683

Health & Preventive Medicine Center (Centrul de Sanatate &

Medicina Preventiva-Romania)
   Str. A. Fannon rer 16
   Tim Mures, Jud. Mures
   4300 ROMANIA
   Phone and fax +40-65-165-353

Fredheim Health Center
   Bergmannsveien 600
   3600 Kongsberg
   Norway
   Phone: +47-32-76-6050
   Fax: +47-32-76-7150

Silver Hills Guest House
   RR2, Site 10, Comp 18
   Lumby, BC V0E2G0
   Canada
   Phone: 604-547-9433
   Fax: 604-547-9488

LARGER U.S. LIFESTYLE CENTER LIST BY STATES

ALABAMA

Uchee Pines Lifestyle Center
   30 Uchee Pines Road #75
   Seale, AL 36875-5702
   Phone: 334-855-4764
   Fax: 334-855-9014
   E-mail:lifestylecenter
       @ucheepines.org
   Web site: ucheepines.org

Types of programs offered:
Treatment of lifestyle related disorders by board-certified physicians, including obesity, diabetes, heart disease, hypertension, stress, substance abuse, and chronic diseases. Lifestyle modification includes an emphasis in hydrotherapy, herbs, and faith in God. Live-in and walk-in sessions.

CALIFORNIA

Desert Spring Therapy Center
   66705 East Sixth Street
   Desert Hot Springs, CA 92240
   Phone: 760-329-5066
   Fax: 760-251-6206
   E-mail: dsrtspgt@gte.net

Types of programs offered:
Smoking cessation, weight reduction, addiction recovery, muscular and skeletal disorders. Live-in and walk-in sessions.

Pacific Health Education Center
   5300 California Avenue, Suite 200
   Bakersfield, CA 93309
   Phone: 661-633-5300
   Fax: 661-633-5302

Types of programs offered:
Smoking cessation, weight reduction, stress management, parenting classes, vegetarian cooking classes, health education training seminars, training courses in how to give health seminars; Heartbeat, a national outreach program for churches. Live-in and walk-in sessions.

Paradise Valley Hospital
   Center for Health Promotion
   2400 East Fourth Street
   National City, CA 91950
   Phone: 619-470-4784
   Fax: 619-470-4281

Types of programs offered:
Classes on cholesterol/nutrition/ hypertension, individual nutrition, weight management, diabetes management, juvenile diabetes support group, smoking cessation, asthma, osteoporosis, stress management, breast health. Walk-in sessions.

St. Helena Hospital
and Health Center
   650 Sanitarium Road
   Post Office Box 250
   Deer Park, CA 94576
   Phone: 1-800-358-9195
   Fax: 707-967-5618
Web: sthelenacenterforhealth.org

Types of programs offered:
Smoking and alcohol programs (seven days), McDougall program to prevent and care for lifestyle diseases (10 days), the Brain and Innate Giftedness Program (two days). Live-in and walk-in sessions.

Weimar Institute
   20601 West Paoli Lane
   Post Office Box 486
   Weimar, CA 95736
   Phone: 916-637-4111;
     or (800) 525-9192 Toll Free
   Web sites: newstart.com
    and weimar.org

Types of programs offered:
NEWSTART® lifestyle education (individualized nutrition, exercise, and hydrotherapy under medical supervision), reversing diabetes, cooking schools, medical examinations and screening. Live-in and walk-in sessions. Contact for Newstart: Trevor Louw, Guest Services Director

COLORADO

Eden Valley Lifestyle Center
   6263 North County Road 29
   Loveland, CO 80538
   Phone: 800-637-9355
   Fax: 970-667-1742
   E-mail: edenvalley@juno.com
   Website: eden-valley.org

Types of programs offered:
18-day lifestyle program designed for smoking cessation, stress management, and weight loss; treatment of heart disease, hypertension, diabetes, arthritis, allergies, cancer, and other degenerative diseases; physician-guided use of diet, exercise, herbal remedies, hydrotherapy, and message therapy. Live-in sessions.

FLORIDA

East Pasco Medical Center
   Wellness Center
   7050 Gall Boulevard
   Zephyrhills, FL 33541
   Phone: 813-788-0411
   Fax: 813-715-6607

Types of programs offered:
Wellness Challenge, a 21-day, total vegetarian, exercise and behavioral modification lifestyle change program (not live-in), support groups (cancers, Parkinson's disease, bereavement, etc.) Cocaine Anonymous, Alcoholics Anonymous, Overeaters Anonymous, seminars (depression, healthy cooking, smoking cessation, etc.), prayer groups, message and water therapy, and a fitness center. Walk-in sessions

GEORGIA

Wildwood Lifestyle Center and Hospital
435 Lifestyle Lane
P. O. Box 129
Wildwood, GA 30757
Phone: 706-820-1493/1-800-634-9355
Fax:706-820-1474
Website: tagnet.org/wildwood

Types of programs offered:
17- or 10-day lifestyle program using natural healing. Includes medical clinic and 13-bed hospital; also offers a 6-month lifestyle educators' course. Live-in sessions.

MAINE

Parkview Hospital
Health Education Department
329 Maine Street
Brunswick, ME 04011
Phone: 207-373-2000
Fax: 207-373-2161

Types of programs offered:
CPR, babysitting, sign language, smoking cessation, grief recovery, lifestyle choices, prenatal and parenting classes, vegetarian cooking, weight control, diabetes control, asthma control, blood pressure and cholesterol control, men's health, executive health, stress reduction, breast cancer reduction, lecture series. Walk-in sessions.

Poland Spring Health Institute
226 Schellinger Road
Poland, ME 04274
Phone: 207-998-2894
Fax: 207-998-2164
E-mail: PSH1226@aol.com
Website: PSHI.org

Types of programs offered:
7-day, 14-day, and 21-day coronary heart reconditioning and general health programs.

MICHIGAN

Lifestyle Plus, Inc.
Wellness and Lifestyle Treatment Center
4686 South Street
Gagetown, Michigan 48735
Phone: (989) 665-0076

Website: lifestyleplus.org
Bill Pineo, Chief Operating Officer

Types of programs offered:
Offers a ten day treatment program for hypertension, heart disease, cancer, diabetes, obesity and others. Offers advantage of modern medical resources, blended with an emphasis on natural, proven methods of treatment.

NORTH CAROLINA

Duke University Health and Fitness Center
804 West Trinity Ave.
Durham, NC 27201
1-800-677-2177
(919) 684-6331

OKLAHOMA

Lifestyle Center of America
Route One, Box 4001
Sulphur, OK 73086
Phone: 800-213-8955
Fax: 405-993-3902
E-mail: life@brightok.net
Web site: lifestylecenter.org

Types of programs offered:
One-day, three-day, seven-day, 10-day, 12-day, 19-day residential, physician-supervised, lifestyle education specializing in the prevention/reversal of heart disease, diabetes, hypertension, weight reduction, smoking cessation, stress-related illnesses, corporate physicals, group wellness retreats. Live-in and walk-in sessions.

OREGON

Emerald Valley Wellness Clinic
600 Dale Kuni Road
Creswell, Oregon 97426
Phone # (541) 895-5300
FAX # (541) 895-5319

Types of programs offered:
Website: emeraldwellness.com
Medical Director, Dr. Richard Hansen, MD. Emerald Valley provides treatment that leans less towards the prescription pad and more toward natural remedies.

Other services include Outpatient Clinic, Health education classes/seminars, books and more. See website.

SOUTH DAKOTA

Black Hills Health and Education Center
Post Office Box 19
Hermosa, SD 57744
Phone: 800-658-5433
Fax: 605-255-4687
Web site: BHHEC.org

Types of programs offered:
Wellness program provides 13- or 20-day live-in assistance for diabetes, heart and vascular diseases, obesity, smoking, depression, allergies, arthritis, fatigue, and general health. Live-in sessions.

TENNESSEE

MEET Ministry and Our Home Health Center
480 Neely Lane
Huntington, TN 38344
Phone: 731-986-3518
Fax: 731-986-0582

Types of programs offered:
19-day lifestyle program for weight management, smoking cessation, stress management, arthritis, diabetes, high blood pressure, cancer prevention, etc. Medical Missionary training programs and workshops. Live-in sessions.

Takoma Adventist Hospital
401 Takoma Avenue
Greenville, TN 37743
Phone: 423-639-3151
Fax: 423-636-2374

Types of programs offered:
Diabetes management, prenatal health education, fibromyalgia. Walk-in sessions

VIRGINIA

Hartland Wellness Center
P.O. Box 1
Rapidan, VA 22733
Phone: 800-763-9355

Introduction

Starting on the Path

HERE IS A MAN who was born in an obscure village, the child of a peasant woman. At His birth, those trying to protect Him had to flee with Him, lest He be slain. He worked in a small village carpenter shop until He was thirty, and then for three years He was an itinerant preacher. He never owned a home. He never wrote a book. He never held an office. He never had a family. He never went to college. He never put His foot inside a big city. He never traveled two hundred miles from the place where He was born. He never did one of the things that usually accompany greatness. He had no credentials but Himself.

While still a young man, the tide of popular opinion turned against Him. His friends ran away. One of them denied Him. He was turned over to His enemies. He went through the mockery of an illegal trial. He was nailed to a cross of rough wood, between two thieves. While He was dying His executors gambled for the only piece of property He had on earth—his coat. When He was dead, He was taken down and laid in a borrowed grave through the pity of someone who barely knew Him.

Twenty long centuries have come and gone, and today He is the centerpiece of the human race and the inspiration of human progress in all things worthwhile. I am far within the mark when I say that all the armies that ever marched, and all the kings that ever reigned, put together, have not affected the life of man upon this earth as powerfully as has that one solitary life.

Who was this Man? His birth terrorized the reigning monarch. In childhood His questions baffled the most highly educated men of the nation. In manhood He ruled the course of nature, walked upon billows of water as if on pavement, and hushed the sea to sleep. He healed multitudes with a kindly look and touch, and never charged for what He did. He condemned sin, but freely forgave and accepted every sinner who came to Him for the healing of his soul.

He never wrote a book, and yet all the libraries of the country could not hold the books that have been written about Him. He never wrote a song, and yet His life has furnished the theme for more songs than have all the songwriters combined. He never founded a college, but all the schools put together cannot boast of having as many devoted students.

The names of the proud emperors of Greece and Rome have crumbled into dust. The names of the great generals and philosophers of all ages have vanished into nothingness. But the name of this Man abounds more and more. Though twenty centuries have passed since the scenes of His crucifixion, yet He still lives. The people of His time could not destroy Him, and the grave could not hold Him.

He stands forth upon the highest pinnacle of human greatness and heavenly glory, proclaimed of God, acknowledged by angels, adored by His closest followers, and feared by devils,—as the living, personal Christ, our Lord and Saviour.

(Adapted from Phillips Brooks)

"I am far within the mark when I say that all the armies that have ever marched, and all the navies that were ever built, and all the parliaments that ever sat, and all the kings that ever reigned, put together, have not affected the life of man upon this earth so powerfully as has that one solitary life."—*Quoted in Albert Henry Newman, A Manual of Church History, Vol. 1, p. 80.*

IN THIS BOOK, I want to tell you how to come to Jesus Christ and make Him you own. I want to tell you how to live in such a way that you can live with Him in heaven later on.

This is an *extremely readable* book and it is full of guidance from that best of all books, the holy Bible. The most important teachings of Scripture are given here. These are truths we all need to know. And each quotation will be from that most accurate translation: the King James Bible, loved and trusted by generations of Christians for nearly 400 years.

This is a book which can change your life.

WE NEED GOD more than we need anything else. We need His help to find a way out of our sins, and into a close, loving relationship with our Creator. We have tried and tried, and we cannot fix our own lives. Our best efforts are a bunch of patchwork. Everything keeps unraveling. Our best resolutions fall to pieces.

The night that Aaron Burr flung open the shutters of his window at Princeton University and shouted, "Good-bye, God," he closed the windows of his soul.

But he who today will open wide the shutters of his soul to God will find the light of God's presence shining in.

"Still, still with Thee, when purple morning breaketh! When the bird waketh, and the shadows flee;

"Fairer than morning, lovelier than the daylight, Dawns the sweet consciousness, I am with Thee!

"When sinks the soul, subdued by toil, to slumber, Its closing eye looks up to Thee in prayer.

"Sweet the repose beneath Thy wings o'ershading, But sweeter still, to wake and find Thee there.

"So shall it be at last, in that bright morning, When the soul waketh, and life's shadows flee;

"Oh, in that glad hour, fairer than day dawning,

Shall rise the glorious thought, I am with Thee!"

— PART ONE —

THE BIBLE AND CHRIST

Chapter One

How to Understand the Bible

Provided by a God of Love and Power

A voice crackled over the shortwave radio. "Turn your ship 23° to starboard."

An irritated voice replied, "Turn *your* ship starboard 23°!"

Back came the response, "Turn your ship 23° to larboard—*to the left!*"

Now, thoroughly aroused, in an authoritative voice came the reply, "*You turn to the right! 23°!*"

The unknown voice ahead of them responded, "Turn your ship 23° to the left."

In his most commanding voice, the captain replied, "*I am the commander* of a U.S. Naval vessel, and we are part of the Sixth Fleet. We have two destroyers and a fuel ship accompanying us. *I command you: Turn your ship 23° to the right! Do it now!*"

Back came that totally self-assured, calm voice: Turn your ship 23° to the left. I am the lighthouse."

—This was an actual shortwave communication which occurred at night a number of years ago, before radar and satellite communications, during a heavy coastal fog in the Northeast.

The captain instantly issued orders to swerve his entire fleet to the left—out to sea,—narrowly missing collision with the rocky coast of Maine. He had yielded to a higher authority, and his obedience saved many lives.

The Bible is the only solidly grounded source we can turn to for guidance in these difficult times. We dare not rely on our own ideas, or the suggestions of friends. Only in the Word of God can we find the help we need if we are to steer a safe course through the narrow channel of life, and miss the rocks on either side.

The Word of God sends the light we need to guide us in every emergency.

Someone has said that "light travels at remarkable speed, until it meets the human mind."

"Thy Word is a lamp unto my feet, and a light unto my path." *Psalm 119:105.* When this light strikes

natural human minds, it is not appreciated because "the god of this world hath blinded the minds of them" (*2 Corinthians 4:4*).

THE BOOK FROM GOD

The Bible comes to us from God.

"For the prophecy came not in old time by the will of man: but holy men of God spake as they were moved by the Holy Ghost."—*2 Peter 1:21 (also Acts 1:16; Hebrews 1:1-2).*

The Scriptures were given so we can learn special truths God wants us to learn.

"All Scripture is given by inspiration of God, and is profitable for doctrine, for reproof, for correction, for instruction in righteousness: that the man of God may be perfect, thoroughly furnished unto all good works."—*2 Timothy 3:16-17. (Also see Romans 15:4 and Psalm 119:105.)*

Only in the Bible is there absolute truth.

"Sanctify them through Thy truth: Thy Word is truth."—*John 17:17.*

"To the law and to the testimony: if they speak not according to this Word, it is because there is no light in them."—*Isaiah 8:20.*

How then can our confused minds understand and receive the heavenly light of God's divine Book?

Here are five simple steps which will prove a help to you:

1 - PRAY FOR DIVINE GUIDANCE

We need help in understanding God's Word, and only its Author can give us that help. We must ask Him for that guidance! Amid the terrible crises of life, we need help which only He can give!

We must pray for divine guidance when we open and study God's Word, and we must ask for the guidance of the Holy Spirit in order to understand the Bible.

"Open Thou mine eyes, that I may behold wondrous things out of Thy law."—*Psalm 119:18 (also Ephesians 1:17; Proverbs 2:3-5).*

"But God hath revealed them unto us by His Spirit: for the Spirit searcheth all things, yea, the deep things of God. For what man knoweth the things of a man, save the spirit of man which is in him? even so the things of God knoweth no man, but the Spirit of God."—*1 Corinthians 2:10-11 (also John 14:26; 1 Corinthians 2:14).*

The writing of God's book, the Holy Bible, was inspired by His Holy Spirit; yet "the natural man receiveth not the things of the Spirit of God" (*1 Corinthians 2:14*). Therefore we need His Spirit to guide us. The Apostle Paul confirmed that this was the only way it could be done: "Now we have received . . the spirit which is of God; that we might know the things that are freely given to us of God." *Verse 12.* And the promise is given:

"If ye then, being evil, know how to give good gifts unto your children: how much more shall your heavenly Father give the Holy Spirit to them that ask Him?"—*Luke 11:13.*

Alexander McLeod tells of two young men who crept at night into a factory to discover the secret of a new machine that a clever man had invented, so they could make secret drawings of it and enrich themselves.

But while still in their hotel room, before heading across town to the factory, one of them saw a Bible on the table. Picking it up, it seemed to open in his hands to Exodus 20; and he read the Ten Commandments.

When he came to the eighth one, he could go no farther. Its words seemed to flash like fire, and smote his conscience. *"Thou shalt not steal."*

Those men went home without the secret of the machine, but with the secret of personal power.

"Wherewithal shall a young man cleanse his way? by taking heed thereto according to Thy Word."—*Psalm 119:9.*

We need special guidance so we can see aright. God has warned us that, if we walk in the light of our own fire and the sparks of our own kindling, we shall lie down in sorrow *(Isaiah 50:11).* But if, trusting in Him, our blind eyes are opened, we shall with the psalmist "behold wondrous things out of Thy law" *(Psalm 119:18).* And we shall receive the help we need!

"The God of our Lord Jesus Christ, the Father of glory, may give unto you the spirit of wisdom and revelation in the knowledge of Him."—*Ephesians 1:17.*

"Holy Spirit, light divine, Shine upon this heart of mine. Chase the shades of night away, Turn my darkness into day."—*Andrew Reed.*

2 - STUDY THE SCRIPTURES

A curious-minded boy prowling about the house picked up a dust-covered Bible. Addressing his mother, he said, "Mamma, is this God's book?" "Why, yes, of course," was her quick response. "Well, then," said the boy, "I think we might as well send it back to Him. We never use it."

Many will not permit any other article to be placed on top of a Bible, yet never lift a finger to open the Book that would get down to the very bottom of the greatest questions and problems of their own personal lives.

We want to start digging into this holy Book. We want to search it in order to understand its deep truths. Here is guidance telling us how to begin our search:

Jesus said: "Search the Scriptures; for in them ye think ye have eternal life: and they are they which testify of Me."—*John 5:39.*

"Man shall not live by bread alone, but by every word that proceedeth out of the mouth of God." —*Matthew 4:4*

Paul said: "Study to show thyself approved unto God, a workman that needeth not to be ashamed, rightly dividing the Word of truth."—*2 Timothy 2:15.*

"Take heed unto thyself, and unto the doctrine."—*1 Timothy 4:16.*

"Consider what I say; and the Lord give thee understanding in all things."—*2 Timothy 2:7.*

Isaiah said: "Seek ye out of the book of the Lord, and read."—*Isaiah 34:16.*

Jeremiah said: "Thy words were found, and I did eat them; and Thy Word was unto me the joy and rejoicing of mine heart."—*Jeremiah 15:16.*

The truths in the Bible are to be read over and over again, shared with others, and repeated to our children.

And, yes, don't forget your children! Be sure to teach them God's Word also! The mother and grandmother of Timothy did *(2 Timothy 1:5)*—and as a result he grew up to become an hard-working missionary and pastor.

"From a child thou hast known the holy Scriptures, which are able to make thee wise unto salvation through faith which is in Christ Jesus."—*2 Timothy 3:15.*

A visitor found a young mother with her babe in her lap and her Bible in her hand. "Are you reading to your baby?" was the humorous query. "Yes," the young mother replied. "But, do you think he understands?"

"I am sure he does not understand now, but I want his earliest memories to be that of hearing God's Word."

It is impossible to overestimate the importance of learning God's Word all through life—beginning with our earliest years.

We should compare one passage of Scripture with another as we study, and ask God to send His Holy Spirit to guide us.

"For precept must be upon precept, precept upon precept; line upon line, line upon line; here a little, and there a little."—*Isaiah 28:10.*

In this way, we avoid drawing a wrong conclusion from the study of one text or some limited portion of the Bible.

The more we value God's Word, the more it can help us!

"Sing them over again to me, Wonderful words of life; Let me more of their beauty see, Wonderful words of life."—*P.P. Bliss.*

3 - BE WILLING TO LEARN

The story is told of a young man who came to the famous Greek scholar Socrates, asking, "What shall I do to become a learned man?" Whereupon Socrates led him into a pool of water, plunged his head under, and held it there awhile. When the youth came up and got his breath, Socrates said, "When your head was under the water, what did you most wish?"

"Air," gasped the young man.

"Very well," answered the sage; "when you want knowledge as much as you wanted air, you will find ways to get it."

Tragically, many do not want knowledge when it is revealed in the Word of God. A closed mind is like a jug, corked and sealed;—you cannot get anything into it. "A man convinced against his will is of the same opinion still."

Someone has said, "If an angel brought a message of great wisdom that people did not want, few would be impressed. But they will readily accept a great speech by a man that tells them what they wish to hear and already know."

One who would learn from the Bible must follow a different path. Here is counsel from a humble man who was willing to learn:

"As newborn babes, desire the sincere milk of the Word, that ye may grow thereby."—1 Peter 2:2.

Of those in one town, Berea, in which he first opened the Word of God, Paul later said:

"These were more noble than those in Thessalonica, in that they received the Word with all readiness of mind, and searched the Scriptures daily, whether those things were so."—Acts 17:11.

The Bereans did not just listen; they began studying God's Book for themselves!

Let a man pray, "Lord, save me I plead, deliver me from the sin of prejudice. Keep my soul filled with the love and the grace and the power of God, and my eyes open to light."

Study it through. —Never begin a day without mastering a verse from its pages. *Make it your own.* —Never lay aside your Bible until the verse or passage you have been studying becomes a part of your being. *Work it out.* —Live the truth you obtained that morning throughout each hour of the day.

Dr. George Washington Carver, the great black scientist of Tuskegee Institute, spent his life helping others. For years he urged farmers in the Southeast to plant crops besides cotton, for if that crop failed all was lost. He finally persuaded them to plant peanuts. However, they raised more peanuts than they knew what to do with.

So Dr. Carver prayed for wisdom whereby the peanut might be put to new uses. His prayers were answered; and he discovered how to make oils, varnishes, colorings, medicines, and a hundred other things from peanuts.

When invited to testify before a Senate Committee in Washington, D.C., he was asked, "Dr. Carver, how did you learn all these things?" He replied, "From an old Book." The chairman asked, "What book?" Carver answered, "the Bible."

Puzzled, a committeeman then inquired, "Does the Bible tell about peanuts?" To this Carver answered, "No, Mr. Senator, but it tells about the God who made the peanut. I asked Him to show me what to do with the peanut, and He did."

4 - ALSO BE WILLING TO UNLEARN

To be willing to give up an idea which we have long held, even though we now see it is contrary to Scripture, can be very difficult. It is like getting a horse to back a heavy load up a hill.

We have many lessons to learn, and many to unlearn. Our fathers believed the world was flat and tomatoes were poisonous. It took them a long time to change their minds. Some never did.

Galileo turned a telescope, invented only a few years before in the Netherlands, upon the skies. It made objects seem thirty-three times nearer,—and helped him prove that the earth moves. But such news was a standing rebuke to the highly educated of his day. They said the world was flat, motionless, and the center of everything. Finally, he was summoned to Rome where, after four months in prison, he was set free when he agreed that the earth does not move. But under his breath he whispered, "But it does move."

Only the Bible has the right answers. "What is the chaff to the wheat? saith the Lord." *Jeremiah 23:28.*

"To the law and to the testimony: if they speak not according to this Word, it is because there is no light in them."—*Isaiah 8:20.*

But some still choose the chaff. Jesus uttered these significant words:

"Laying aside the commandment of God, ye hold the tradition of men . . Full well ye reject the commandment of God, that ye may keep your own tradition."—*Mark 7:8-9.*

Old Edwin Rushworth had been a skeptic all his life, but he resolved to read for an hour a day the book that he had so long derided. "Wife," he said, as he looked up from his first perusal, "If this is right, we are all wrong!"

He continued his readings for several more days. "Wife," he exclaimed, "If this book is right, we are lost!"

He went on reading, more earnestly than ever.

"Wife!" he said suddenly a few nights later. "If this book is right, we may be saved!"

And they were! Both of them.

5 - BE WILLING TO OBEY

The fifth and final rung in the ladder to Bible learning is *willingness to obey* what we learn in the Scriptures. God can give us the guidance we need—if we will pray for guidance; study diligently; be willing to learn, to unlearn, and to obey. Christ said this:

"If any man will do His will, he shall know of the doctrine, whether it be of God, or whether I speak of Myself."—*John 7:17.*

"But He said, Yea rather, blessed are they that hear the Word of God, and keep it."—*Luke 11:28.*

How simple, how fair! **God is telling us, "If you will choose to follow Me, I will show you the way.** If, more than anything else, you want to do My will, I will make clear to you whether a doctrine is true or false." Nothing in all this wide world can take the place of absolute honesty with God.

This fifth step of willingness to obey is the climax. It proves our sincerity in taking the four preceding steps. When Jesus called Matthew as he sat in the taxgather's booth, He said, "Follow Me." What did Matthew do when he heard those words? "He arose, and followed Him" *(Matthew 9:9).*

This is what it takes. Nothing less, nothing else. **Christ is calling to you and me today:**

"If any man will come after Me, let him deny himself, and take up his cross, and follow Me."— *Matthew 16:24.*

Christ had His cross. We have ours. **The way of obedience to God's Written Word is the way of learning the will of God.**

"I have more understanding than all my teachers: for Thy testimonies are my meditation. I understand more than the ancients, because I keep Thy precepts."—*Psalm 119:99-100.*

The Word of God, accepted into the heart and obeyed, will change our lives.

"Being born again, not of corruptible seed, but of incorruptible, by the Word of God, which liveth and abideth forever."—*1 Peter 1:23.*

"Wherewithal shall a young man cleanse his way? by taking heed thereto according to Thy Word. With my whole heart have I sought Thee: O let me not wander from Thy commandments. Thy Word have I hid in mine heart, that I might not sin against Thee."—*Psalm 119:9-11.*

"Whereby are given unto us exceeding great and precious promises: that by these ye might be partakers of the divine nature, having escaped the corruption that is in the world through lust."—*2 Peter 1:4.*

"Let the Word of Christ dwell in you richly in all wisdom."—*Colossians 3:16 (also 1 Thessalonians 2:13; Psalm 107:20; Hebrews 4:12; Deuteronomy 8:3; John 6:57-58).*

There is so much help and power and glory in the Bible that we never see unless we carefully, thoughtfully read it. As an old Scottish shepherd

was tending his flock in the springtime pastures, he came upon a man examining wild flowers in the grass through a magnifying glass.

The old man's new friend plucked a tiny flower, placed it under the glass, and invited the shepherd to take a look. He did. He kept on looking. His lips quivered. A tear stole down his weather-beaten face.

"Why are you troubled?" inquired his friend.

"I was just thinking," was the old man's wistful reply, "as I looked at the gorgeous beauty of that little flower, how many thousands of them I have trampled under my heavy shepherd boots, and never paid any heed to them."

"O Word of God Incarnate, O wisdom from on high, O Truth unchanged, unchanging, O Light of our dark sky. We praise Thee for Thy radiance, That from the hallowed page, A lantern to our footsteps, Shines on from age to age.

"It is the golden casket, Where gems of truth are stored; It is the heaven-drawn picture Of Christ, the living Word. O teach Thy wandering pilgrims By this their path to trace, Till, clouds and darkness ended, They see Thee face to face."
— *W.W. Howe*

A POWERFUL, INDESTRUCTIBLE BOOK

For centuries, men have tried to destroy the Bible, but it stands solid.

Voltaire said the Bible was an exploded book. His theory is what exploded; for he has been dead over 230 years, and the Book is still here, read and loved by more people than ever.

Voltaire said that in 100 years, the Bible would be an outmoded and forgotten book, to be found only in museums. When the 100 years were up, Voltaire's house was owned and used by the Geneva Bible Society as a Bible storehouse. Recently, 92 volumes of Voltaire's writings (a part of the Earl of Derby's library) were sold for two dollars.

Ingersoll, another skeptic, declared that the Bible would not be read in ten years. It has been long years since he died, yet the Bible today outsells any one hundred other books put together.

Like a cube of granite, the Bible is right side up no matter how many times you overturn it, and it leaves its imprint everywhere it goes.

This divinely inspired volume has been translated into more languages and dialects than any other book. Completed nearly two thousand years ago the Bible or portions of it may be read today in more than one thousand tongues, and it is the most up-to-date book in the world.

"Within this precious volume lies the mystery of mysteries. Happiest they of the human race, who have received God's grace to read, to fear, to hope, to pray; to lift the latch and force the way. —And better had they ne'er been born, who read to doubt, or read to scorn."—*Sir Walter Scott.*

Someone has written:

"The empire of Caesar is gone; the legions of Rome are mouldering in the dust; the avalanches Napoleon hurled upon Europe have melted away; the pride of the Pharaohs is fallen; the pyramids they raised to be their tombs are sinking every day in the desert sands; Tyre is a rock for fishermen's nets; Sidon has scarcely a rock left behind;—but the Word of God survives.

"All things that threaten to extinguish it have aided it, and it proves every day how transient is the noblest monument that man can build, how enduring the least word God has spoken. Tradition has dug a grave for it; intolerance has lit for it many a fagot; many a Judas has betrayed it with a kiss; many a Peter has denied it with an oath; many a Demas has forsaken it; but the Word of God still endures."

"Last eve I passed beside a blacksmith's door,
     And heard the anvil ring the vesper chime;
Then looking in, I saw upon the floor
     Old hammers, worn with beating years of time.
" 'How many anvils have you had,' said I,
'To wear and batter all these hammers so?'
'Just one,' said he and, then, with twinkling eye,
'The anvil wears the hammers out, you know.'
"And so, thought I, the anvil of God's Word,
for ages skeptic blows have beat upon;
yet, though the noise of falling blows was heard,
The anvil is unharmed—the hammers gone."
                              — *Author unknown*

"Hammer away, ye hostile hands; Your hammers break; God's anvil stands."—*Samuel Zwemer.*

The Bible is a never-failing fountain from which God's people, down through the ages, have dipped up eternal life.

"We've traveled together, my Bible and I, When life had grown weary, and death even was nigh, But all through the darkness, while avoiding wrong, I found there a solace, a prayer, and a song."

Other leaders before our time have found this treasure book of the ages, and dug deeply into its riches. Here is what some of them have said:

George Washington: "It is impossible to rightly govern any nation in the world without God and the Bible."

Daniel Webster: "If we abide by the principles taught in the Bible, our country will go on prospering and to prosper, but if we and our posterity neglect its instruction and authority, no man can tell how sudden a catastrophe may overwhelm us and bury our glory in profound obscurity."

John Wesley: "I want to know one thing—the way to heaven: how to land safe on that happy shore. God Himself has condescended to teach the way. He hath written it down in a Book! Oh, give me that Book! At any price, give me that Book of God!"

Dwight L. Moody: "I never saw a useful Christian who was not a student of the Bible. If a man neglects his Bible, he may pray and ask God to use him in His work, but God will not be able to make much use of him."

Patrick Henry: "The man who once exclaimed, "Give me liberty or give me death!" wrote "There is a Book worth all others which were ever printed—the Bible."

Abraham Lincoln: "In addition to Christ, the Bible is the best gift God ever gave to man."

David Livingstone: "All that I am I owe to Jesus Christ, revealed to me in His divine Book."

Dyson Hague: "The depth of the Bible is infinite. Millions of readers and writers, age after age, have dug in this unfathomable mine and its depths are still unexhausted. You cannot gild gold. You cannot brighten diamonds, and no artist can touch with final touch this finished Word of God. The great accomplishments of this century can add nothing to it. It stands as the sun in the sky. It has the glory of God shining on its pages."

H.L. Hastings has provided an able defense of God's book:

"This wonderful volume is in reality a library, filled with history, law, ethics, prophecy, poetry, medicine, and perfect rules for the conduct of personal and social life. It contains all kinds of writing, but what a jumble it would be if 66 books were written in this way by ordinary men. Suppose, for instance, that we get 66 medical books written by 35 or 40 different doctors, bind them all together and attempt to doctor a man according to the book. Or suppose you get 35 ministers to write a book on theology and then see if you can find leather strong enough to hold the books together."

—*H.L. Hastings, Will the Old Book Stand?*

Regarding the accuracy of Bible prophecy, Hastings wrote:

"So long as Babylon is in heaps; so long as Nineveh lies empty, void, and waste; so long as Tyre is a place for the spreading of nets in the midst of the sea; so long as the great empires of the world march on in their predicted courses,—so long we have proof that one Omniscient Mind produced the predictions of that book, and that 'prophecy came not in old time by the will of man.' "—*Ibid.*

A minister went far into a backwoods settlement to hold a meeting; and its was necessary that he return late in the very dark night. A woodsman provided him with a torch of pitch-pine wood.

The minister, never having seen anything of the kind, said, "It will soon burn out." "It will light you home," answered the other.

"The wind may blow it out," said the preacher. "It will light you home," was the response.

"But what if it should rain?" "It will light you home."

And contrary to the minister's fears, the torch did last him all the way home. The Word of God is a torch placed into the hands of each one of us. But what if it rains? What if the wind blows? What if the fires of persecution come? If you will hold the torch high it will light you all the way home.

> "We search the world for truth; we cull
> The good, the pure, the beautiful,
> From graven stone and written scroll,
> From all old flower fields of the soul;
> And, weary seekers of the best,
> We come back laden from our quest,
> To find that all the sages said
> Is in the Book our mothers read."
> —*John G. Whittier*

COMING NEXT—How to begin a new life in Christ, or, if you are already a Christian, how to deepen your experience with Him.

Chapter Two

Taking God's Hand

How to Begin a Changed Life

A number of prominent writers were assembled in a literary club in London one evening in 1825. The conversation veered to a discussion of some of the illustrious figures of the past, and one of the company suddenly asked: "Gentlemen, what would we do if Milton were to enter this room?"

"Ah," jubilantly replied one in the circle, "We would give him such an ovation as might compensate for the tardy recognition accorded him for his *Paradise Lost* by the men of his own day."

"And if Shakespeare entered?" asked another.

"We would arise and crown him master of song," was the triumphant answer.

"And if Jesus Christ were to enter?" asked yet another.

An intense silence followed for fully a minute. And then Charles Lamb spoke softly, "We would all fall on our faces."

It is when we come into the presence of Christ that our lives are changed. We are told:

"In that day there shall be a fountain opened ... for sin and for uncleanness."—*Zechariah 13:1.*

That fountain is the precious blood of Jesus. **The sacrifice of Christ, made for sinners by His death on the cross, is the central fact of the gospel.** It is the blazing sun, around which all other truths revolve. Indeed, it is the very essence of the gospel; for, if it be taken away, nothing of the gospel remains. It forms the ground of faith, the very basis of the sinner's hope.

"There is a fountain filled with blood, Drawn from Immanuel's veins; And sinners plunged beneath that flood, Lose all their guilty stains.

"E'er since by faith I saw the stream Thy flowing wounds supply, Redeeming love has been my theme, and shall be till I die."—*William Cowper.*

The teachers of modernism have been trying to shut off the stream of Christ's precious, healing blood, which was shed for sinful men. By their skeptical theories, they seek to rob Christ of His divinity, His perfect humanity, and His power to save men. Yet if this fountain be successfully sealed, then is the doom of the world also sealed; and man will never be admitted to the Paradise of God. For "without shedding of blood is no remission of sin" *(Hebrews 9:22).*

But there are those who ignore the jibes of the worldlings about them, and press through to Christ.

I have a question to ask you, which I cannot answer. You cannot answer it. If an angel from heaven were here, he could not answer it. If the devil were here, he could not answer it. **The question is this:**

"How shall we escape, if we neglect so great salvation?" Hebrews 2:3.

Both angels and demons know that if we neglect the salvation offered us—*we shall not escape!*

We want to learn, just now, how we can neglect no more to take hold of such a great salvation!

UNDERSTANDING GENUINE CONVERSION

To the degree that a man is willing to enter this experience and continue in it, a complete transformation takes place in that person's life as he is born again. This is genuine conversion. The new birth is as actual as the natural birth he had as an infant. The change is recognized both by the individual and by those who know him. The new birth affects the heart (that is, the mind), and it affects the daily life. It is produced by the Spirit of God as the newly converted person cooperates with Him.

"A new heart also will I give you, and a new spirit will I put within you: and I will take away the stony heart out of your flesh, and I will give you an heart of flesh. And I will put My spirit within you, and cause you to walk in My statutes, and ye shall keep My judgments, and do them."—*Ezekiel 36:26-27.*

God did not originate sin, but He did originate a remedy for sin. "Sin is the transgression of the law." *1 John 3:4.* But law is not the remedy for sin.

It is true, as the Apostle Paul proclaims, "The law is holy, and the commandment holy, and just, and good" *(Romans 7:12).* But the difficulty lies in the fact that man is not holy and just and good. The man cries out, "We know that the law is spiritual: but I am carnal, sold under sin. For that which I do I allow not: for what I would, that do I not; but what I hate, that do I" *(Romans 7:14-15).*

Jesus wants to bring us into harmony with the rules of His moral government. It is true that God's law is eternal, and no man or men can change or abolish it. "All His commandments are sure. They stand fast forever and ever, and are done in truth and uprightness" *(Psalm 111:7-8).* The problem is that the law is eternal, but we are temporary. "The grass withereth, the flower fadeth: because the spirit of the Lord bloweth upon it: surely the people is grass. The grass withereth, the flower fadeth: but the word of our God shall stand forever" *(Isaiah 40:8).* "For what is your life? It is even a vapour, that appeareth for a little time, and then vanisheth away" *(James 4:14).*

David declared, "The law of the Lord is perfect" *(Psalm 19:7).* The evangelist, D.L. Moody, agreed with this when he said, "Now men may cavil as much as they like about other parts of the Bible, but I have never met an honest man that found fault with the Ten Commandments" *(D.L. Moody, Weighed and Wanting, p. 11).*

The trouble is not that none can find one jot or tittle of fault with any of the Ten Commandments,— the real problem is that this moral code finds so many serious faults with us.

What, then, is the remedy? It is always and ever the same. It was announced in Eden in these words: "I will put enmity between thee and the woman, and between thy seed and her seed; it shall bruise thy head, and Thou shalt bruise His heel" *(Genesis 3:15).* Jesus told it to us in these words:

"For God so loved the world, that He gave His only begotten Son, that whosoever believeth in Him should not perish, but have everlasting life."—*John 3:16.*

God gave us His Son! Only Christ could solve the problem. There is no other solution to the sin problem that we can find anywhere. There is no other way that we can become cleansed and live godly lives. Only Jesus can provide all the answers.

The law is holy, and Christ is holy, "Who did no sin" *(1 Peter 2:22).*

The law is eternal, and Christ is eternal. "Whose goings forth have been from of old, from everlasting" *(Micah 5:2).*

The law is perfect, and Christ kept that perfect law. "I have kept My Father's commandments." *John 15:10.* Said Pilate, "Behold, . . I find no fault in Him" *(John 19:4).*

God gave this holy, perfect, eternal Christ, of whose character the law was a written transcript, and whose life was a living revelation of that same law—to save you and enable you by His grace to keep that law!

"Since the divine law is as sacred as God Himself, only one equal with God could make atonement for its transgression."—*Patriarchs and Prophets, p. 63.*

"Just now, your doubtings give o'er. Just now, reject Him no more; Just now, throw open the door; Let Jesus come into your heart!"—*Mrs. C.H. Morris.*

THREE THINGS ACCOMPLISHED BY CALVARY

There are three things which were glorified by Calvary:

First, Christ's death on the cross glorified the law of God. God's holy law had to be safeguarded, and men had to be shown the importance of that moral law of Ten Commandments.

This law was "ordained to life" *(Romans 7:10).* Obedience brought happiness. Sin brought death. **Had it been possible for God to abolish His law, the problem of sin could have been solved without Christ's death. But since the law was a very transcript—written copy—of God's character, He could not change its principles without changing His own character.** This He would not do and will not do. Stealing, murder, etc., will always be wrong and evil in God's sight.

When someone jumps out a window, God will not protect him from the effects of the law of gravity. Likewise, **when we break His moral law, the Lord cannot change that law so we will not experience the consequences of wrongdoing. To do so would mean the destruction of His government, of which the law is the foundation!**

"Justice and judgment are the habitation [Hebrew: "foundation"] of Thy throne."—*Psalm 89:14.*

The law could not save men because "all have sinned" *(Romans 3:23).* Men could not save themselves. Angels were powerless to provide the needed help. **Since the divine law is as sacred as God Himself, only One equal with God could make atonement for its transgression.**

Second, the cross glorified the love which God has for mankind, and for all His creatures. God is love, and has always been love. But not until Calvary was the depth of that love so fully revealed. Satan had rebelled in heaven, and then, by causing our first parents to sin, had spread it down here.

Far back in eternity, the Son had offered to lay down His life, if man sinned, to redeem those who would accept Him as their Saviour and obediently cooperate with Him in their restoration. The Father had accepted this pledge.

"Forasmuch as ye know that ye were not redeemed with corruptible things, as silver and gold, from your vain conversation received by tradition from your fathers; but with the precious blood of Christ, as of a lamb without blemish and without spot: Who verily was foreordained before the foundation of the world, but was manifest in these last times for you."—*1 Peter 1:18-20.*

Thank God every day for this love! He loves you! He loves me!

"O Love that wilt not let me go, I rest my weary soul in Thee; I give Thee back the life I owe, That in Thine ocean depths its flow May richer, fuller be."—*George Matheson.*

Third, the cross glorified the value of each human soul. When Napoleon was planning one of his military campaigns, Metternich, Austrian minister at the French court, remarked, "This campaign will cost a million men." To this Napoleon replied, "What are a million men to me!"

Oh, how different is God than the evil, self-centered hearts of men! While on earth, Christ repeatedly demonstrated that God loves mankind and wants to save them.

Every one who will let Him save him will be worth more to Him throughout eternity than all the treasures of the universe. Those of us who accept this great truth, and submit our lives to God's guidance and control, will experience the truth of that surrender throughout eternity.

But, tragically, there are those who will still choose to be lost. Outside the gates of heaven, they will say, "The treasures of earth were but glittering sand, compared with what I have lost. Salvation in heaven would have been worth more than anything the world had to offer."

Christ came to our planet to give His life a ransom for man, and He would have paid that price for just one soul. He spoke of His concern for the *one* lost sheep, the *one* lost coin, the *one* lost prodigal. The cross of Jesus glorified the law of God, the love of God, and the value of a human soul saved in eternity. Have you been down to Calvary?

"In the cross of Christ I glory, Towering o'er the wrecks of time; All the light of sacred story. Gathers round its head sublime."—*Sir John Bowring.*

There is the remarkable story, from over two centuries ago, of a Britisher who one day visited the slave market in Cairo, Egypt. He there saw a strong, intelligent young man about to be sold as a slave.

Scarcely realizing it, he found himself bidding against the other buyers. Up and up went the price, but finally the Britisher had purchased the young man.

His new slave eyed him with suspicion and anger,

saying to himself, "Why should this man be free, and I a slave? If I get a chance, I will kill him and run away."

The owner then led him away a short distance and said to him, "I bought you to set you free." Hearing this astounding news, the young man wept and falling down, cried, *"Oh, let me serve you forever!"*

"All to Jesus I surrender, All to Him I freely give; I will ever love and trust Him, In His presence daily live."

How thankful we can be that Christ, the divine Son of God, came down to our world to save us! He is "Christ . . who is over all, God blessed forever. Amen" *(Romans 9:5).* Adam Clarke, in his *Commentary,* wrote "This verse contains such a powerful proof of the deity of Christ; no wonder that the opposers of His divinity should strive with their utmost skill and cunning to destroy its force." And they have. But we accept the Bible, and rejoice in the blessings it brings to us!

There was a little girl who, although a child, had learned how to keep close to Jesus. When asked how she did it, she replied, "It's just this way: Jesus is my Friend. He lives in my heart, and when Satan knocks at the door, I say, 'Jesus, please answer.' When Satan sees Jesus at the door of my heart, he says, 'Oh, excuse me, I came to the wrong door; and he goes away.' "

BEHOLD CHRIST AT CALVARY

Behold Christ! He lived for you *(Matthew 20:28).* He died for you *(1 Peter 2:24).* He offers pardon to you *(Isaiah 55:7).* He offers grace and power to you *(Hebrews 4:16).* He offers heaven to you *(Matthew 7:21; 5:3, 10).*

Do you hesitate and say, "I do not understand how these things can be?"

God did not say, "Whosoever understandeth the science and philosophy of the atonement of My Son on Calvary shall have everlasting life." He said, "Whosoever believeth in Him."

"Believe on the Lord Jesus Christ, and thou shalt be saved." *Acts 16:31.*

The dying thief looked, believed, and received assurance of Paradise *(Luke 23:42-43).*

The living centurion, watching the dying Christ, said, "Truly this was the Son of God" *(Matthew 27:54).*

The sinful, conscience-smitten publican cried out, "God be merciful to me a sinner" *(Luke 18:13).*

David, who had sinned a great sin, pleaded, "Cleanse me from my sin." "Create in me a clean heart." —And God heard his prayer *(Psalm 51:2, 10).*

I tell you today: If you will believe, you shall receive! Do not trust to feeling. **Take your sins to the cross. Exchange them for forgiveness. Ask God to give you a new heart, and write His holy law upon it, that you may love it and keep it.** Believe that, as you have prayed in the name of Jesus, God does this. Surrender your all to Him. Make no reservation. Give all. Receive all that God offers you.

"These blessings we by faith receive; By simple, childlike trust; In Christ 'tis God's delight to give; He promised, and He must."

There is the old story of the man who wandered all over the world seeking true repentance. But to no avail. **At last he came to Calvary. There he found what he had been longing for.** There he heard a Voice saying, "You will always find Me here, and the way of the cross leads home."

Have you been down to Calvary and found out why Christ was bleeding there? This is the first place you should always come to.

"O, never till my latest breath Can I forget that look; It seemed to charge me with His death, Though not a word He spoke."—*Isaac Watts.*

"Let not the wise man glory in his wisdom" (Jeremiah 9:23). Let not the scientist glory in his science, the philosopher in his philosophy, or the inventor in his genius. These cannot save us.

Let the world go down to Calvary, find there repentance and regeneration. When will the whole world go? Never. It will only be as individuals that any of us will go there. Salvation is not by masses but by individuals. From beginning to end, it is a personal matter between you and God. It involves individual surrender, individual obedience.

"Down at the cross where my Saviour died, Down where for cleansing from sin I cried, There to my heart was the blood applied. Glory to His name."—*E.A. Hoffman.*

ENTERING INTO THE EXPERIENCE

The greatest question facing every human being is this: "What must I do to be saved?" This question comes to every individual; for "all have sinned and come short of the glory of God" *(Romans 3:23).* Man by nature is lost. No man has the slightest claim upon immortality.

When the jailer at Phillipi pled with the Apostle Paul, "What must I do to be saved?" Paul replied without the slightest hesitation, "Believe on the Lord Jesus Christ, and thou shalt be saved" *(Acts 16:30-31).*

Later this same apostle wrote to the believers in Rome. He declared:

"But what saith it? The word is nigh thee, even in thy mouth, and in thy heart: that is, the word of faith, which we preach; That if thou shalt confess with thy mouth the Lord Jesus, and shalt believe in thine heart that God hath raised Him from the dead, thou shalt be saved.

"For with the heart man believeth unto righteousness; and with the mouth confession is made unto salvation. For the Scripture saith, Whosoever believeth on Him shall not be ashamed."—*Romans 10:8-11.*

An equally important question is this: What then must we believe about Jesus?

We must believe that Jesus is the Son of God, and that He is able and willing to save from sin—and to bestow upon His followers the priceless gift of eternal life. We must believe in Him as *our personal Saviour.* We must believe that He died for us *individually,* and that His death on the cross was the penalty for *our sin,* which He paid in *our* behalf.

We must also believe that He is able to empower us to resist temptation; put away our darling sins; and live clean, godly lives.

Believing this, the next step is to bow before Him in utter repentance for those sins; confess them to Him, and then believe with all the heart that He forgives and cleanses.

"If we confess our sins, He is faithful and just to forgive us our sins, and to cleanse us from all unrighteousness."—*1 John 1:9.*

Jesus is calling to us today:

"Return, thou backsliding Israel, saith the Lord; and I will not cause Mine anger to fall upon you: for I am merciful, saith the Lord, and I will not keep anger forever. Only acknowledge thine iniquity, that thou hast transgressed against the Lord thy God."—*Jeremiah 3:12-13.*

Having accepted the pardon so freely offered through Jesus Christ, the believer must be ready and willing to follow Him by obeying all His commands and serving Him in the day-to-day life. That is a description of a genuine Christian life. Jesus said, "Without Me ye can do nothing" *(John 15:5).* We cannot repent and put away our sins without His help; nor can we obey His holy, Ten Commandment law without His help.

We must accept the fact that we can do nothing to save ourselves. Christ will change us from our previous sinful state to a new life of godly living—but only as we cling to Him daily and plead for His enabling strength.

"Consecration" is signing your name at the bottom of a blank sheet of paper and letting God fill in the space as He wills. It is total dedication.

"I felt His love, the strongest love, That mortal ever felt; Oh, how it drew my soul above, And made my hard heart melt!

"My burden at His feet I laid, And knew the joy of heaven. As in my willing ear He said, The blessed word, 'forgiven.' "

We already looked at one unanswerable question in the Bible. But did you know that there are yet two others? Jesus asked them, and here they are:

"For what is a man profited, if he shall gain the whole world, and lose his own soul? or what shall a man give in exchange for his soul?"—*Mat-*

thew 16:26.

The only safe response we can give to those questions is to fall down before God; repent of our sins; hand them over to Him to get rid of; and henceforth give Him our lives in humble, obedient service.

"Neither is there salvation in any other: for there is none other name under heaven given among men, whereby we must be saved."—*Acts 4:12.*

Just now, we may come to Him for cleansing and the beginning of a new life with Him.

"And the Spirit and the bride say, Come. And let him that heareth say, Come. And let him that is athirst come. And whosoever will, let him take the water of life freely."—*Revelation 22:17.*

"In looking thro' my tears one day, I saw Mount Calvary, Beneath the cross there flowed a stream of grace enough for me.

"While standing there, my trembling heart, Once full of agony; Could scarce believe the sight I saw Of grace enough for me.

"When I behold my ev'ry sin Nailed to the cruel tree, I felt a flood go thro' my soul Of grace enough for me.

"When I am safe within the veil, My portion there will be To sing thro' all the years to come Of grace enough for me.

"Grace is flowing from Calvary, Grace as fathomless as the sea, Grace for time and eternity, Grace enough for me."—*E.O. Excell.*

BIBLE SUMMARY

Whether or not we cooperate with Christ in making the needed changes will affect our eternal destiny. Here is why:

Sin is transgression of God's moral law.

"Whosoever committeth sin transgresseth also the law: for sin is the transgression of the law."—*1 John 3:4.*

"By the law is the knowledge of sin."—*Romans 3:20.*

All have sinned.

"All have sinned, and come short of the glory of God."—*Romans 3:23.*

The right kind of sorrow for sin leads to repentance.

"For godly sorrow worketh repentance to salvation not to be repented of: but the sorrow of the world worketh death."—*2 Corinthians 7:10.*

"For I will declare mine iniquity; I will be sorry for my sin."—*Psalm 38:18.*

We must confess our sins to God, and forsake them.

"All things are naked and opened unto the eyes of Him with whom we have to do."—*Hebrews 4:13.*

"When a man or woman shall commit any sin that men commit, to do a trespass against the Lord, and that person be guilty; then they shall confess their sin which they have done."—*Numbers 5:6-7.*

"But if ye will not do so, behold, ye have sinned against the Lord: and be sure your sin will find you out."—*Numbers 32:23.*

If we truly repent and confess our sins to God, He will forgive.

"He that covereth his sins shall not prosper: but whoso confesseth and forsaketh them shall have mercy."—*Proverbs 28:13.*

"If we confess our sins, He is faithful and just to forgive us our sins, and to cleanse us from all unrighteousness. If we say that we have not sinned, we make Him a liar, and His Word is not in us."—*1 John 1:9-10.*

"I acknowledged my sin unto Thee, and mine iniquity have I not hid. I said, I will confess my transgressions unto the Lord; and Thou forgavest the iniquity of my sin."—*Psalm 32:5.*

"Let the wicked forsake his way, and the unrighteous man his thoughts: and let him return unto the Lord, and He will have mercy upon him; and to our God, for He will abundantly pardon."—*Isaiah 55:7.*

"There is joy in the presence of the angels of God over one sinner that repenteth."—*Luke 15:10.*

After being forgiven, we should not return to those sins.

"Bring forth therefore fruits meet for repentance."—*Matthew 3:8.*

"For if ye forgive men their trespasses, your heavenly Father will also forgive you."—*Matthew 6:14.*

"Be ye kind one to another, tenderhearted, forgiving one another, even as God for Christ's sake hath forgiven you."—*Ephesians 4:32.*

"We know that we have passed from death unto life, because we love the brethren. He that loveth not his brother abideth in death."—*1 John 3:14.*

"Conversion" means to become changed. It is also called the "new birth."

"Verily I say unto you, Except ye be converted, and become as little children, ye shall not enter into the kingdom of heaven."—*Matthew 18:3.*

"Jesus answered and said unto him, Verily, verily, I say unto thee, Except a man be born again, he cannot see the kingdom of God."—*John 3:3.*

"Therefore if any man be in Christ, he is a new creature: old things are passed away; behold, all things are become new."—*2 Corinthians 5:17.*

The converted man lives a new life in Christ.

"Whosoever is born of God doth not commit sin; for his seed remaineth in him: and he cannot sin, because he is born of God."—*1 John 3:9.*

"There is therefore now no condemnation to them which are in Christ Jesus, who walk not after the flesh, but after the Spirit."—*Romans 8:1.*

COMING NEXT—How to maintain a close walk with Christ, day after day. Heaven is worth it! Jesus wants you to have it!

Chapter Three

Living by Faith

How to Continue That Changed Life

Two infidels once sat in a train, headed to Chicago, discussing Christ's amazing life. One of them said, "I think an interesting book could be written about Him." The other replied, "And you are just the man to write it. But set forth the correct view of His life and character. Tear down the prevailing sentiment as to His divineness and paint Him as He was—just another man among men."

The suggestion was acted upon and the book was written. The man who made the suggestion was Colonel Robert G. Ingersoll, the well-known agnostic attorney; the author of the book was General Lew Wallace, governor of the New Mexico Territory; and the book was *Ben Hur: A Tale of the Christ,* published in 1880.

In the process of constructing it, he found himself facing the unaccountable Man. The more he studied His life and character the more profoundly he was convinced that Christ was more than a man among men; until, at length, like the centurion under the cross, he was constrained to cry, *"Verily, this was the Son of God!"*

A CHANGED LIFE AT CONVERSION

At conversion, the entire life is regenerated and changed. The old carnal desires, the tendency to sin, and the love of the world become subdued. These are replaced by a desire to serve God and do right. Through the new birth men and women become "new creatures."

We are born again into the family of God.

"Verily I say unto you, Except ye be converted, and become as little children, ye shall not enter into the kingdom of heaven."—*Matthew 18:3 (John 3:3).*

"If any man be in Christ, he is a new creature: old things are passed away; behold, all things are become new."—*2 Corinthians 5:17*

"Being born again, not of corruptible seed, but of incorruptible, by the Word of God, which liveth and abideth forever."—*1 Peter 1:23.*

"Even when we were dead in sins, hath quickened [made us alive] us together with Christ."—*Ephesians 2:5.*

The promise of God is that if we "walk in the Spirit," we *"shall not* fulfill the lust of the flesh" *(Galatians 5:16).*

Here is a passage from a Christian writer of many years ago, which clearly shows the remarkable transformation which occurs when this miracle of the new birth occurs:

"A person may not be able to tell the exact time or place, or to trace all the circumstances in the process of conversion; but this does not prove him to be unconverted. By an agency as unseen as the wind, Christ is constantly working upon the heart. Little by little, perhaps unconsciously to the receiver, impressions are made that tend to draw the soul to Christ. These may be received through meditating upon Him, through reading the Scriptures, or through hearing the Word from the living preacher. **Suddenly, as the Spirit comes with more direct appeal, the soul gladly surrenders itself to Jesus.** By many this is called sudden conversion; but it is the result of long wooing by the Spirit of God,—a patient, protracted process.

"While the wind is itself invisible, it produces effects that are seen and felt. So **the work of the Spirit upon the soul will reveal itself in every act of him who has felt its saving power. When the Spirit of God takes possession of the heart, it transforms the life.** Sinful thoughts are put away, evil deeds are renounced; love, humility, and peace take the place of anger, envy, and strife. Joy takes the place of sadness, and the countenance reflects the light of heaven. No one sees the hand that lifts the burden, or beholds the light descend from the courts above. **The blessing comes when by faith the soul surrenders itself to God. Then that power which no human eye can see creates a new being in the image of God.**"—*Desire of Ages, 172-173.*

Changing a sinner into a Christian is a miracle of God's grace. The entire life is altered. He is "a new man." —But this only happens because the man continually remains close to Christ, prays to Him, reads the Bible, and continually looks to Him for guidance in everything he does.

"He that overcometh, the same shall be clothed in white raiment; and I will not blot out his name out of the book of life, but I will confess his name before My Father, and before His angels."—*Revelation 3:5.*

Whereas before the sinner delighted in the practice of sinful habits and indulgences, the Holy Spirit is now impressing him with better thought patterns. **Abhoring his former evil thoughts and actions, he now happily serves God and tries to help those around him.**

"He lives, He lives, Christ Jesus lives today! He walks with me and talks with me Along life's narrow way.

"He lives, He lives, salvation to impart! You ask me how I know He lives? He lives within my heart!"
—*A.H. Ackley*

When the surrendered heart is cleansed and renewed by divine power, Christ sets up His throne within. **Thus the converted sinner becomes a son or daughter of God. He becomes a member of God's family and now knows God as His loving Father.** He now lives to help and bless others around him.

A doctor once found a little dog with a broken leg by the roadside. Taking the little fellow with him, he put the leg in splints and kept him until he was well.

But as soon as the dog was able to run about the house, he disappeared. "That's gratitude," thought the doctor. "As soon as he didn't need me anymore, he ran away."

The next day, there was a scratching at the back door, and there was the little dog. But another little dog was with him. And that other little dog was lame! The secret cannot be kept. It has to be shared!

BEGINNING THE NEW LIFE

What shall the new believer now do with his life? He has been given a clean page. What shall he write upon it? **If he would retain the ground he has gained through faith in Christ, what kind of life must he now live?** Shall it be one of sin—which will return him to the chains of Satan's control? Or will it be willing, cheerful obedience to God's Ten Commandments?

Here is the answer. The Apostle Paul explains it to us:

"What shall we say then? Shall we continue in sin, that grace may abound? God forbid. **How shall we, that are dead to sin, live any longer therein?** Know ye not, that so many of us as were baptized into Jesus Christ were baptized into His death?

"Therefore we are buried with Him by baptism into death: that like as Christ was raised up from the dead by the glory of the Father, **even so we also should walk in newness of life.**

"For if we have been planted together in the likeness of His death, we shall be also in the likeness of His resurrection:

"Knowing this, that **our old man is crucified with him, that the body of sin might be destroyed, that henceforth we should not serve sin.** For he that is dead is freed from sin.

"Now if we be dead with Christ, we believe that we shall also live with Him: Knowing that Christ being raised from the dead dieth no more, death hath no more dominion over him. For in that He died, He died unto sin once: but in that He liveth, He liveth unto God.

"**Likewise reckon ye also yourselves to be dead indeed unto sin, but alive unto God through Jesus Christ our Lord. Let not sin therefore reign in your mortal body, that ye should obey it in the lusts thereof.**"—*Romans 6:1-12.*

Converted men and women are not free to break the law of God. True, they are free from its condemnation for sins of the past, which they were powerless to undo, but which God has now freely pardoned. But **permission has not been given them to presume upon God's goodness by continuing in transgression.** To do that is to have the responsibility for one's past sins rolled back on him.

A man who never before kept the law can be forgiven and justified before God, but he cannot remain in this new, justified state without keeping it. **Unless, in the enabling strength of Christ he obeys God's moral law, the Ten Commandments, he will not continue as a genuine Christian**; for Christians do not return to their evil, vile ways of the past.

"Know ye not that the unrighteous shall not inherit the kingdom of God? Be not deceived: neither fornicators, nor idolaters, nor adulterers, nor effeminate, nor abusers of themselves with mankind, Nor thieves, nor covetous, nor drunkards, nor revilers, nor extortioners, shall inherit the kingdom of God. And such were some of you: but ye are washed, but ye are sanctified, but ye are justified in the name of the Lord Jesus, and by the Spirit of our God."—*1 Corinthians 6:9-11.*

"But be ye doers of the Word, and not hearers only, deceiving your own selves. For if any be a hearer of the Word, and not a doer, he is like unto a man beholding his natural face in a glass: For he beholdeth himself, and goeth his way, and straightway forgetteth what manner of man he was.

"But whoso looketh into the perfect law of liberty, and continueth therein, he being not a forgetful hearer, but a doer of the work, this man shall be blessed in his deed."—*James 1:22-25.*

The Bible is full of passages commanding God's people to obey His laws. Here is what Jesus said:

"Not every one that saith unto Me, Lord, Lord, shall enter into the kingdom of heaven; **but he that doeth the will of My Father** which is in heaven.

"Many will say to Me in that day, Lord, Lord, have we not prophesied in Thy name? and in

Thy name have cast out devils? and in Thy name done many wonderful works? And then will I profess unto them, I never knew you: depart from Me, ye that work iniquity.

"Therefore whosoever heareth these sayings of Mine, and doeth them, I will liken him unto a wise man, which built his house upon a rock: And the rain descended, and the floods came, and the winds blew, and beat upon that house; and it fell not: for it was founded upon a rock.

"And every one that heareth these sayings of Mine, and doeth them not, shall be likened unto a foolish man, which built his house upon the sand: And the rain descended, and the floods came, and the winds blew, and beat upon that house; and it fell: and great was the fall of it."—*Matthew 7:21-27.*

Christ warned men not to think that He had come to destroy God's holy moral law.

"Think not that I am come to destroy the law, or the prophets: I am not come to destroy, but to fulfill. For verily I say unto you, **Till heaven and earth pass, one jot or one tittle shall in no wise pass from the law**, till all be fulfilled. Whosoever therefore shall break one of these least commandments, and shall teach men so, he shall be called the least in the kingdom of heaven: **but whosoever shall do and teach them, the same shall be called great in the kingdom of heaven**."—*Matthew 5:17-19.*

Never forget that the power to live a godly life comes only through a day by day, moment by moment, reliance upon Jesus Christ for help! Of ourselves, we can do no good thing. Here is the formula for successful living in Christ:

"I am crucified with Christ: nevertheless I live; yet not I, but Christ liveth in me: and the life which I now live in the flesh I live by the faith of the Son of God, who loved me, and gave Himself for me."—*Galatians 2:20.*

A LIFE WHICH OVERCOMES SIN

Strengthened by the enabling grace of Christ, we live clean, godly lives.

"Ye know that every one that doeth righteousness is born of Him."—*1 John 2:29.*

"Now the just shall live by faith."—*Hebrews 10:38.*

"I can do all things through Christ which strengtheneth me."—*Philippians 4:13.*

"That ye might walk worthy of the Lord unto all pleasing, being fruitful in every good work, and increasing in the knowledge of God; strengthened with all might, according to His glorious power, unto all patience and longsuffering."—*Colossians 1:10-11.*

"**Now the God of peace . . make you perfect in every good work to do His will**, working in you that which is well pleasing in His sight, through Jesus Christ; to whom be glory forever and ever."—*Hebrews 13;20-21.*

A life in Christ overcomes sin.

"To him that overcometh will I give to eat of the tree of life, which is in the midst of the paradise of God."—*Revelation 2:7.*

"He that overcometh shall not be hurt of the second death."—*Revelation 2:11.*

"To him that overcometh will I give to eat of the hidden manna, and will give him a white stone, and in the stone a new name written, which no man knoweth saving he that receiveth it."—*Revelation 2:17.*

"He that overcometh, and keepeth My works unto the end, to him will I give power over the nations."—*Revelation 2:26.*

"He that overcometh, the same shall be clothed in white raiment; and I will not blot out his name out of the book of life, but I will confess his name before My Father, and before His angels."—*Revelation 3:5.*

"Him that overcometh will I make a pillar in the temple of My God, and he shall go no more out: and I will write upon him the name of My God, and the name of the city of My God, which is new Jerusalem, which cometh down out of heaven from My God: and I will write upon him My new name."—*Revelation 3:12.*

"To him that overcometh will I grant to sit with Me in My throne, even as I also overcame, and am set down with My Father in His throne."—*Revelation 3:21.*

"He that overcometh shall inherit all things; and I will be his God, and he shall be My son."—*Revelation 21:7.*

—What a glorious collection of promises!

A life in Christ is a victorious life.

"Now unto Him **that is able to keep you from falling**, and to present you faultless before the presence of His glory with exceeding joy, To the only wise God our Saviour, be glory and majesty, dominion and power, both now and forever. Amen."—*Jude 24-25.*

"For this cause I bow my knees unto the Father of our Lord Jesus Christ, of whom the whole family in heaven and earth is named, that He would grant you, according to the riches of His glory, to be strengthened with might by His Spirit in the inner man; that Christ may dwell in your hearts by faith; that ye, being rooted and grounded in love, may be able to comprehend with all saints what is the breadth, and length, and depth, and height; and to know the love of

W
A
Y

Christ, which passeth knowledge, that ye might be filled with all the fullness of God.

"Now unto Him **that is able to do exceeding abundantly above all that we ask or think,** according to the power that worketh in us, unto Him be glory in the church by Christ Jesus throughout all ages, world without end. Amen."—*Ephesians 3:14-21.*

Christ enters the citadel of your heart, made vacant by the departure of sin and the demons which previously harassed you. Jesus takes control of your life. Having done this, He is "abundantly" able to provide you with all the help you need in resisting temptation and fighting the battle of faith to keep praying, reading the Bible, and obeying His will. And then, as a victorious overcomer, you can declare:

"I can do all things through Christ which strengtheneth me."—*Philippines 4:13.*

To us the promise is given:

"Wherefore He is able also to save them to the uttermost that come unto God by Him, seeing He ever liveth to make intercession for them."—*Hebrews 7:25.*

At the end of his epistle to the Hebrews, Paul says it even more strongly:

"Now the God of peace, that brought again from the dead our Lord Jesus, that great shepherd of the sheep, through the blood of the everlasting covenant, **make you perfect in every good work to do His will**, working in you that which is well pleasing in His sight, through Jesus Christ; to whom be glory forever and ever. Amen."—*Hebrews 13:20-21.*

Those who have the sweet, abiding presence of Jesus in their hearts will declare with David:

"O how love I Thy law! it is my meditation all the day."—*Psalm 119:97.*

"Was it for crimes that I have done, He groaned upon the tree? Amazing pity! grace unknown! And love beyond degree!

"Well might the sun in darkness hide, And shut His glories in, When Christ the mighty Maker died For man, the creature's sin.

"Thus might I hide my blushing face, While His dear cross appears, Dissolve my heart in thankfulness, And melt mine eyes to tears.

"But drops of grief can ne'er repay The debt of love I owe; Here, Lord, I give myself away; 'Tis all that I can do."—*Isaac Watts.*

CONTINUAL JUSTIFICATION AND SANCTIFICATION

What is the difference between justification and sanctification, and when does each occur? Many are confused about this, but the answer is simple:

Justification occurs when we come to God, ask for and receive forgiveness, and begin life anew with Him. This is a daily experience in the new birth, and is renewed every day. Paul said, "I die daily" *(1 Corinthians 15:31).* This also is to be our experience each day.

We begin life anew each day through earnest prayer; and, as we pass through each day in Christ's strength resisting temptation and doing what we know to be right, we continue growing spiritually. Each day we become more mature Christians: patient, kindly, helpful. **This daily growth in Christ is sanctification.** Thus we are covered by Christ's righteousness. By justification, we are forgiven and accounted righteous. By sanctification, we are becoming more and more like Him whom we so much love.

If we are betrayed into wrongdoing by the devil, we run back quickly to Jesus and plead for forgiveness, and continue on the path which will one day lead us to heaven.

Both justification and sanctification come from God and prepare us for heaven.

"That being justified by His grace, we should be made heirs according to the hope of eternal life."—*Titus 3:7.*

"Much more then, being now justified by His blood, we shall be saved from wrath through Him."—*Romans 5:9.*

"For therein is the righteousness of God revealed from faith to faith: as it is written, The just shall live by faith. For the wrath of God is revealed from heaven against all ungodliness and unrighteousness of men, who hold the truth in unrighteousness."—*Romans 1:17-18.*

"That as sin hath reigned unto death, even so might grace reign through righteousness unto eternal life by Jesus Christ our Lord."—*Romans 5:21.*

"All Thy commandments are righteousness. Let Thine hand help me; for I have chosen Thy precepts."—*Psalm 119:172-173.*

"I know that His commandment is life everlasting."—*John 12:50.*

"And the very God of peace sanctify you wholly; and I pray God your whole spirit and soul and body be preserved blameless unto the coming of our Lord Jesus Christ."—*1 Thessalonians 5:23.*

"For this is the will of God, even your sanctification."—*1 Thessalonians 4:3.*

"Be not conformed to this world: but be ye transformed by the renewing of your mind, that ye may prove what is that good, and acceptable, and perfect, will of God."—*Romans 12:2.*

"But grow in grace, and in the knowledge of our Lord and Saviour Jesus Christ. To Him be glory both now and forever."—*2 Peter 3:18.*

"I beseech you therefore, brethren, by the mercies of God, that ye present your bodies a living sacrifice, holy, acceptable unto God, which is your reasonable service. And be not conformed to this world: but be ye transformed by the renewing of your mind, that ye may prove what is that good, and acceptable, and perfect, will of God."—*Romans 12:1-2.*

COMING NEXT—What prayer can do in our lives—to make us strong, vibrant followers of Christ!

Chapter Four

Prayer and Thankfulness

Two Powerful Helps in Your Life

How much does a prayer weigh? The only man I ever knew who tried to weigh one still does not know.

Once upon a time he thought he did. That was when he owned a little grocery store over on the west side. It was the week before Christmas, just after World War I. A tired looking woman came into the store and asked him for enough food to make up a Christmas dinner for her children. He asked her how much she could afford to spend.

She answered, "My husband was killed in the war and I have nothing to offer but a little prayer."

This man confesses that he was not very sentimental in those days. A grocery store could not be run like a bread line. **So he said, "Write it on a paper," and returned to his business.**

To his surprise, the woman plucked a piece of paper out of her bosom and handed it to him over the counter and said, "I did that during the night watching over my sick baby."

The grocer took the paper before he could recover from his surprise, and then regretted having done so! For what would he do with it, what could he say?

Then an idea suddenly came to him. He placed the paper, without even reading the prayer, on the weight side of his old-fashioned scales. **He said, "We shall see how much food this is worth."**

To his astonishment the scale would not go down when he put a loaf of bread on the other side. To his confusion and embarrassment, it would not go down though he kept on adding food, anything he could lay his hands on quickly, because people were watching him.

He tried to be gruff and he was making a bad job of it. His face got red and he was unsure what to do

next. So finally, he said, "Well, that's all the scales will hold anyway. Here's a bag, You'll have to put it in yourself. I'm busy."

With what sounded like a gasp or a little sob, she took the bag and started packing in the food, wiping her eyes on her sleeves every time her arm was free to do so. He tried not to look, but he could not help seeing that he had given her a pretty big bag and that it was not quite full. So he filled another sack with beans and potatoes, and tossed it down the counter, but he did not say anything; nor did he see the timid smile of grateful appreciation which glistened in her moist eyes.

When the woman had gone, he went to look at the scales, scratching his head and shaking it in puzzlement. Then he found the solution. The scales had broken.

The grocer is an old man now. His hair is white. But he still scratches it in the same place and shakes it slowly back and forth with the same puzzled expression. He never saw the woman again. And, come to think if it, he had never seen her before either. Yet for the rest of his life he remembered her better than any other woman in the world and thought of her more often.

He knew it had not been just his imagination, for he still had the slip of paper upon which the woman's prayer had been written: "Please, Lord, give us this day our daily bread."

PRAYERLESS LIVES MISS SO MUCH

Oh, my friend, how much we need prayer in our lives! We need it every day. We need it hourly. The only footprints on the sands of time that will really last are the ones made after knee-prints!

Some go a whole week without prayer, yet seven days without prayer makes one weak. Many only pray when they are in an emergency. Such people seem to look upon prayer as a spare tire, something only to be gotten out and used when they are in trouble. Yet the truth is that there is immense strength in frequent prayer to God. The humblest saint can see further on his knees than the most learned philosopher can see from the world's highest eminence.

How little we realize what a mighty force is the simple act of talking with God. There is nothing which lies outside the reach of the hand extended up to heaven in prayer, except that which lies outside the will of God. Those who pray often and earnestly know well the depth of comfort and help they can receive from those precious moments with their Maker.

It is the name at the foot of the check which gives it value when handed to the cashier in the bank. Prayer becomes priceless through the name in which it is presented, regardless of how impoverished may be the one sending it up to heaven.

"More things are wrought by prayer than this world dreams of."—*Alfred Lord Tennyson.*

W
A
Y

In the previous two chapters, we viewed the wondrous power of God at the moment of conversion, and as the soul begins a new life in Him.

But there is a tendency with some to expect that all conflict will end at conversion. They assume that the happiness and peace they experienced in that initial coming to Christ will continue on, uninterrupted, month after month. For a time, there is a new power within, new strength to overcome weakness, and a sense of forgiveness that makes the person radiantly happy in his newfound faith.

But in the experience of many, this deep peace gradually fades away. Old temptations, old feelings, old thoughts, may clamor again for recognition. A man may yield momentarily to these old impulses. He may find himself suddenly irritable and bad-tempered. —Yet he thought he would never be that way again!

What happened? What went wrong? Let me tell you this, and let it sink deep into your thinking: *It was not God's fault.* We are quick to blame God for whatever happens. But that is the worst thing we can do, for doing so only deepens our separation from Him. *Fact one:* **God never errs or does anything wrong.** *Fact two:* **All our problems originate either with ourselves, our environment, or the devil.** God is always good. He permits trials to come, but He never does anything evil.

But now, back to our question: What went wrong? When you stop to think about it, the answer is quite simple. **How did you first find God? By humbling your heart before Him, pleading with Him for His help, and surrendering your life to Him.**

Why did you later lose Him? You stopped walking with Him! The prayer, praise, and thankfulness that you had when you first found Him had ended. Without realizing it, you had severed your connection with Heaven, and the devil quietly began moving back in and tantalizing your mind, and drawing you back to you old ways and former miseries.

"If My people, which are called by My name, shall humble themselves, and pray, and seek My face, and turn from their wicked ways; then will I hear from heaven, and will forgive their sin, and will heal their land. Now Mine eyes shall be open, and Mine ears attent unto the prayer that is made in this place."—*2 Chronicles 7:14-15.*

Christianity is living with Jesus. It is not something you do once in a while. It has to be an ongoing experience, day after day, or it is not real.

Face the fact: **Do you really want to be with Jesus, or do you just want to live your own life and manage yourself?**

In special gardens in Japan, you will find trees which should be forest giants, yet are only 12 inches high. Each tree is a dwarf of what it could be. Its growth has been stunted—so much so that it is now smaller than a common bush.

The puzzle is solved when the gardener explains that the taproots of these trees have been carefully cut back for decades, so they cannot grow normally. They are only supplied by nourishment from tiny roots which lie close to the surface.

Many people live anxious, complaining lives because, for years, they have kept their taproots cut off. They go through life, never realizing what they are missing. For it is the roots that feed the tree, and theirs are stunted. Such people live on their surface roots (their connections with those around them), while the taproots, which would go down deep into the soil, have been chopped off.

When the great ocean liner, *Titanic*, was filling with water on that fateful night of April 14, 1912, the orchestra switched from the dance music it had been playing for days—to a hymn of prayer: "Nearer, my God, to Thee . . daylight all gone, darkness be over me . . Nearer, my God, to Thee, nearer to Thee!"

Why is it that people wait till they are confronted by a terrible emergency before they think of praying?

WHAT PRAYER IS

"Prayer is the opening of the heart to God as to a friend. Not that it is necessary in order to make known to God what we are, but in order to enable us to receive Him. Prayer does not bring God down to us, but brings us up to Him . .

"Our heavenly Father waits to bestow upon us the fullness of His blessing. It is our privilege to drink largely at the fountain of boundless love. What a wonder it is that we pray so little! God is ready and willing to hear the sincere prayer of the humblest of His children, and yet there is much manifest reluctance on our part to make known our wants to God. What can the angels of heaven think of poor helpless human beings, who are subject to temptation, when God's heart of infinite love yearns toward them, ready to give them more than they can ask or think, and yet they pray so little and have so little faith?"— *Steps to Christ, p. 94.*

The taproots of the soul, which connect you to God, are prayer, study of God's Word, thankfulness, and living to help those around you.

"Lord, what a change within us one short hour Spent in Thy Presence will prevail to make! What heavy burdens from our bosoms take! What parched grounds refresh as with a shower! We kneel and all around us seems to lower, We rise, and all, the distant and the near, Stands for us in sunny outline, bright and clear, We kneel how weak, we rise how full of power!"—*William Trench.*

It is only by clinging to Christ that we are safe for a day or even a moment. It is the decision to make Him first, last, and best in everything that brings that peace and deep joy into your life. But, unfortunately, many only experienced that for a few hours or days when they first found Christ. Later on, by their neglect, they went back on out into the world.

During World War I, two men were crawling together through the darkness toward an advanced position in the frontline trenches. One whispered to the other, that they were approaching an outpost. But his comrade was unable to distinguish it in the darkness. Back came the reply, "Lieutenant, the best way to see in the dark is to get close to the ground and look up against the sky." Good advice for the dark days of life: **Get close to the ground—and look up in prayer.**

Prayer is talking to God. That is simple enough. There is nothing complicated about it. Prayer is something that a fervent Christian engages in quite frequently, when he is reading God's Word, is about his daily work, walking the streets, and driving down the road. **When alone, he generally prays out loud; but when others are around, he sends up silent prayers.** He prays for protection and for guidance. He sends up expressions of thankfulness and praise to God for all the blessings of life. He asks for help in knowing what to do next, how to find others he can help, and how he can help them in the best way. I can tell you that living this way results in very happy living.

He is putting God first in his life. He is fulfilling the words of Joel: "Turn ye even to Me with all your heart." *Joel 2:12.*

"I have been driven many times to my knees by the overwhelming conviction that I had nowhere else to go."—*Abraham Lincoln.*

When the first Atlantic cable was laid in 1850, great celebrations broke out on both sides of the Atlantic. Two great continents, which had been separated through the ages, were now united.

When the deluge of sin first separated heaven and earth, a mighty cable of prayer was laid in the love of God, and never from that day to this has it been broken. The tempted and tried of earth can communicate with the God of heaven! They can pray for help and they can receive help.

Prayer puts man in touch with God. It forms the connecting link between human weakness and God's omnipotent strength. "Out of weakness" a man is "made strong" (*Hebrews 11:34*).

Conversion brings you into God's family, and you now have the rights of sonship. Before you is a standing invitation to bring all your petitions and present them before your heavenly Father in full expectation that they will receive attention. The ear of God is bent to hear the faintest cry of His children. His greatest joy is helping them, and He always knows when it is the best time to do this.

One writer has said, "Prayer is the key in the hand of faith to unlock heaven's storehouse, where are treasured the boundless resources of Omnipotence"

(Steps to Christ, pp. 94-95).

Prayer brings definite results. It was when Daniel prayed that God sent the angel to shut the mouths of the hungry lions. It was when Paul and Silas prayed that the doors of the prison were opened and they were set free. It was when Elijah prayed that God shut up the heavens, so that there was no rain.

"Prayer is not the overcoming of God's reluctance; it is the taking hold of God's willingness."—*Phillips Brooks.*

Concerning the power of prayer, the Apostle James declared, "The effectual fervent prayer of a righteous man availeth much" (*James 5:16*).

Christ told us that men must ask if they would receive, seek if they would find, and knock if they would have the door opened (*Matthew 7:7*).

"This is the confidence that we have in Him, that, if we ask anything according to His will, He heareth us. And if we know that He hear us, whatsoever we ask, we know that we have the petitions that we desired of Him."—*1 John 5:14-15.*

But we must ask according to His will. He knows that it would not be best to give us some of the things we ask for.

Every prayer that is made in simple faith is answered, but the answer is given according to God's understanding of the needs, and not according to the asking. His wisdom is infinite, and His love is boundless. He loves His earthly children far too well to give them things that would be injurious to them. Therefore, **in His great love He sometimes says "Yes"; at other times He says "No"; and at other times He says "Wait."** The answer may be delayed, but it will be fulfilled in the best way and at the right time to work most for our eternal interest.

"God knows; He cares; He loves. Nothing this truth can dim. He does the very best for those Who leave their choice with Him."

In the 1960s, Billy Graham's wife, Ruth, told an audience of Minneapolis women, "God has not always answered my prayers. If He had, I would have married the wrong man—several times."

Henry Wadsworth Longfellow said, "What discord we would bring into the universe if our confused prayers were all answered! Then we would govern the world, and not God. And do you think we would govern it better?"

A child may see a beautiful, gleaming knife and plead his parent for it. His desire and request are intense, but the parent knows that the bestowal of such a gift would bring danger and harm to him. So the request is refused.

"As parents may in deepest love Refuse their child's request, Our loving Father may say no; He, too, knows what is best."

Although most prayers are not answered immediately, the prayer for forgiveness always is. If you will let Him, He is determined to provide you with help to resist and overcome sin.

Prayer is the Christian's greatest and highest privilege. Through this means he is able to hold constant communion with the King of the universe. He is in touch with God. To him heaven's store of eternal riches is open. And to him the promise is given:

"My God shall supply all your need according to His riches in glory by Christ Jesus."—*Philippians 4:19.*

The reason many so-called prayers receive no answer is the fact that they are made all too casually. They are *said*, perhaps *repeated*, but not prayed. Prayer to be real must become the breathing forth of the inner spiritual longings of the soul into the ear of One who is recognized as the heavenly Father.

It cannot just be a selfish asking for more things for ourselves, and it cannot just be a form to be repeated over and over.

Andrew Carnegie, one of the wealthiest men at the beginning of the 20th century, remarked, "What is the use of praying? I already have everything I want. What more could I ask for?"

A small boy, when asked if he ever prayed, answered, "Sometimes I pray, but sometimes I just *say* my prayers."

Another little boy said to his mother, "Mommie, I don't have to say my prayers anymore. *I know them now.*"

"If we keep the Lord ever before us, allowing our hearts to go out in thanksgiving and praise to Him, we shall have a continual freshness in our religious life. Our prayers will take the form of a conversation with God as we would talk with a friend. He will speak His mysteries to us personally.

"Often there will come to us a sweet joyful sense of the presence of Jesus. Often our hearts will burn within us as He draws nigh to commune with us as He did with Enoch.

"When this is in truth the experience of the Christian, there is seen in his life a simplicity, a humility, meekness, and lowliness of heart, that show to all with whom he associates that he has been with Jesus and learned of Him."—*Christ's Object Lessons, 129-130.*

CONDITIONS OF ANSWERED PRAYER

They had nearly reached the summit of the mountain high in the Alps. Then, suddenly, they were there! Exultantly, the young man leaped up, but his guide immediately pulled him down, *"Get down! You're only safe here on your knees!"* In this life, we are only safe when we are frequently on our knees.

God promises to hear our prayers.

"O Thou that hearest prayer, unto Thee shall all flesh come."—*Psalm 65:2.*

God answers prayer.

"If ye then, being evil, know how to give good gifts unto your children, how much more shall your Father which is in heaven give good things to them that ask Him?"—*Matthew 7:11.*

"He that spared not His own Son, but delivered Him up for us all, how shall He not with Him also freely give us all things?"—*Romans 8:32.*

Here is how to pray so your prayers will be answered in such a way, and at such a time, as God sees best.

In order to receive answers, prayer must be made in absolute faith.

"Without faith it is impossible to please Him: for He that cometh to God must believe that He is, and that He is a rewarder of them that diligently seek Him."—*Hebrews 11:6.*

"If any of you lack wisdom, let him ask of God, that giveth to all men liberally, and upbraideth not; and it shall be given him. But let him ask in faith, nothing wavering. For he that wavereth is like a wave of the sea driven with the wind and tossed. For let not that man think that he shall receive any thing of the Lord."—*James 1:5-7.*

Another condition of answered prayer is implicit obedience to God's Word. Unless we are willing to follow His instruction and live in conformity to His will, we have no claim whatsoever upon the least of His mercies.

"Beloved, if our heart condemn us not, then have we confidence toward God. And **whatsoever we ask, we receive of Him, because we keep His commandments, and do those things that are pleasing in His sight**."—*1 John 3:21-22.*

"**If I regard iniquity in my heart, the Lord will not hear me**."—*Psalm 66:18.*

"No good thing will He withhold from them that walk uprightly."—*Psalm 84:11.*

Solomon said it in even stronger words:

"He that turneth away his ear from hearing the law, even his prayer shall be abomination."—*Proverbs 28:9.*

But this, of course, is only reasonable. If men will not ally themselves with God by following Jesus' example of obedience to God's requirements, they are actually enemies of His and not disciples. "He that is not with Me," said Jesus, "is against Me" *(Matthew 12:30).* This is the test. If we are with Him, He is also with us to bless and keep.

"**He that hath My commandments, and keepeth them, he it is that loveth Me**: and he that loveth Me shall be loved of My Father, and I will love him, and will manifest myself to him."—*John 14:21.*

When we recognize the true character of God, as a God of deepest love, our deepest thanks pours out in words and songs of praise for His constant revelations of love and mercy to us,

"In everything by prayer and supplication with thanksgiving let your requests be made known unto God. And the peace of God, which passeth all understanding, shall keep your hearts and minds through Christ Jesus."—*Philippians 4:6-7.*

True prayer must be accompanied with the spirit of forgiveness. Jesus explained how serious a matter this is:

"But if ye do not forgive, neither will your Father which is in heaven forgive your trespasses."—*Mark 11:26.*

"When ye stand praying, forgive, if ye have ought against any: that your Father also which is in heaven may forgive you your trespasses."—*Mark 11:25.*

The more we praise God, the greater strength we will have for our daily duties.

"For the joy of the Lord is your strength."—*Nehemiah 8:10.*

"When we bless God for mercies we prolong them, and when we bless Him for miseries we usually end them. Praise is the honey of life, which a devout heart drinks from every bloom of providence and grace. As well be dead as be without praise; it is the crown of life." —*Charles H. Spurgeon*

As the armies of Napoleon were sweeping across Europe, one of his generals decided to attack the little town of Feldkirch on the Austrian border. A council of citizens quickly gathered. They knew that to defend themselves was hopeless. So, after praying, they decided to rejoice in God that He would somehow care for them. So they rang the bells of the church and sang praises to the Lord. The enemy, hearing the sudden peal, concluded that the Austrian army had arrived during the night. Quickly, they broke camp and fled; and, before the bells had ceased ringing, the danger had been lifted.

Our prayers should often be sent up to God.

"**Praying always** with all prayer and supplication in the Spirit."—*Ephesians 6:18.*

"Rejoice evermore. **Pray without ceasing.** In everything give thanks: for this is the will of God in Christ Jesus concerning you."—*1 Thessalonians 5:16-18.*

"**Evening, and morning, and at noon**, will I pray, and cry aloud: and He shall hear My voice."—*Psalm 55:17.*

"And when He had sent the multitudes away,

He went up into a mountain apart to pray: and when the evening was come, He was there alone."—*Matthew 14:23.*

"**Watch and pray**, that ye enter not into temptation."—*Matthew 26:41.*

"**Watch ye therefore, and pray always**, that ye may be accounted worthy to escape all these things that shall come to pass, and to stand before the Son of man."—*Luke 21:36.*

Every day should open and close with prayer. In the morning our prayer should be one of dedication, giving ourselves anew to God for the day's work and service, and asking His care and protection. In the evening, our prayer should confess our sins of the day, thank God for His mercies, and commit ourselves in childlike faith into His hands for the coming hours of darkness and sleep.

"The morning is the gate of day; But ere you enter there, See that you set to guard it well, The sentinel of prayer. So shall God's grace your steps attend; but nothing else pass through. But what can give the countersign, The Father's will for you.

"When you have reached the end of the day, Where night and sleep await, Set there the sentinel again To bar the evening's gate. So shall no fear disturb your rest, No danger and no care; For only peace and pardon pass The watchful guard of prayer."

Even the lowly camel can teach us important lessons:

"The camel at the close of day, Kneels down upon the sandy plain, To have his burden lifted off, And rest to gain.

"My soul, thou too shouldst to thy knees, When daylight draweth to a close, And let thy Master lift Thy load, And grant repose.

"The camel kneels at break of day, To have his guide replace his load; Then rises up anew to take The desert road.

"So thou shouldst kneel at morning dawn, That God may give thee daily care; Assured that He no load too great, Will make thee bear."

We should often pray for others. Oh, there are so many, both near and far, who need help!

"All his thoughts of people gradually turned to prayers" was the remark made concerning the missionary John Forman. How is it with you and me? Are we as faithful in offering up our pleas for God's help for others in need?

I wish there was space in this book to quote ten or fifteen astounding stories of how God has answered prayer, but here is one:

Dr. Harry A. Ironside, a powerful preacher in the early 20th century, told the story of an unsaved man who had gone to sea. One night his mother awoke with a deep sense of need. A burden for her unsaved boy rested heavily upon her heart. She earnestly prayed for his salvation. After a time, peace came to her, and she went back to sleep.

Weeks passed. Then, one day, there was a knock at her door and there stood her son! "Mother, I've found Jesus!" he exclaimed joyfully. Then he told her what had happened:

"A few weeks ago, our ship was caught in a fearful storm. The waves seemed mountain high. Hope of our outriding the storm vanished. Suddenly the ship gave a lurch and I was swept overboard. As I began to sink, the awful thought came to me: **'I'm lost forever!** Where will I spend eternity?' In agony of heart I cried out, **'O God, I look, I look to Jesus!'** Then I lost consciousness. After the storm had abated, the sailors came up from below deck,—and they found me lying, unconscious, against a bulwark!"

How fully will our kind Father provide for us?

"Now unto Him that is able to do exceeding abundantly above all that we ask or think."—*Ephesians 3:20.*

"**But my God shall supply all your need** according to His riches in glory by Christ Jesus."—*Philippians 4:19.*

FAMILIES NEED PRAYER ALSO

Not only is personal prayer important,—but family prayer is also. If at all possible, you want to have family prayer and reading of God's Word every morning and evening. Set aside definite times for this, and you will be blessed—and everything will go better all day long.

In the life of so many, prayer is often crowded out. No longer do many children in Christian homes hear their parents praying for them, as at the family prayer circle each one is presented before God. Thus a mighty Christian influence is lost. Far too often, the children grow up and wander out into the world.

Prayer involves thanksgiving. Recognizing this great truth can make your prayers more powerful.

Husbands and wives, prayer can change your marriage! Robert Newton, a well-known nineteenth-century pastor, and his bride, began their married life by each going alone twice each day and praying for one another. When an old man, Pastor Newton said, "My wife and I have just passed our fiftieth wedding anniversary, and I knew not, during the past fifty years of our union, an unkind look or unkind word has ever passed between us."

PREACHERS MADE POWERFUL BY PRAYER

Before closing, we should not forget the preachers. They should pray earnestly, both before and after their sermons. It is because so many do not do this that what they present to the people is so devoid of life and strength.

A pastor, while watching a marble cutter at work, exclaimed, "I wish I could deal such clanging blows on stony hearts!" The workman replied, "Maybe you could if you worked like me, *on your knees.*"

Martin Luther once said, "I am so busy now that I find if I did not spend two or three hours each day in prayer, I could not get through the day. If I should neglect prayer but a single day, I should lose the fire of my faith."

It is known that **John Wesley** regularly spent at least two hours each day in prayer. And **D.L. Moody** declared, "Every great movement of God can be traced to a kneeling figure!" Such are the kind of men who, in the past, accomplished things for God!

George Whitefield, the eighteenth-century evangelist, always took with him on his preaching missions a little crippled man who utterly believed in prayer. Very rarely did the crippled man attend the meetings. Often he did not leave his hotel room. It was his prayers, even more than Whitefield's preaching, which were the cause of the wonderful results which followed.

John Hyde graduated from McCormick Seminary in 1892 and then went to India as a missionary. **He had always sought the Lord earnestly in prayer for others. But, in India he saw such great needs that he spent even more time in prayer.** As a result, both his and his fellow missionaries who were working with him, were able to make many more conversions. Soon he became known as "Praying Hyde."

Dr. Wilbur Chapman wrote to a friend: "At one of our missions in England, the audience was exceedingly small; but then I received a note saying that an American missionary was on furlough from India and was going to pray for God's blessing on our work. He was known as Praying Hyde. Almost instantly the tide turned. The hall became packed, and at my first invitation fifty men accepted Christ as their Saviour. (Nearly all of these afterward proved to be genuine conversions.)

"As we were leaving the hall that night, I said, 'Mr. Hyde, I want you to pray for me.'

"He came to my room, turned the key in the door, and dropped on his knees, and five minutes passed without a single syllable coming from his lips. I could hear my own heart thumping, and his beating. I felt hot tears running down my face. I knew I was with God. Then, with upturned face, while the tears were streaming, he said, 'O God.' Then for five minutes at least he was still again; and then, when he knew that he was talking with God, there came from the depths of his heart such petitions for me as I had never heard before. **I rose from my knees to know what real prayer was.** We believe that prayer is mighty and we now believe it as we never did before."

It has been said that prayer is the greatest unused power in the world, and faith is the greatest

undiscovered resource. Oh, my friends, how much we need the strength and closeness to God which an ongoing prayer experience can bring into our lives!

The next two chapters are summarized from the best
single book that the present author has ever found on how to come to Christ and stay with Him. Reading them will provide you with an even deeper understanding of how to remain solid
in your daily walk with Christ.

Chapter Five

Summarizing the First Steps

How to Come to Christ

Abridgement of the book, Steps to Christ, in the author's own words - in this and the next chapter.

Nature and revelation alike testify of God's love. It is transgression of God's law—the law of love—that has brought woe and death. **Yet even amid the suffering that results from sin, God's love is revealed.** "God is love" is written upon every opening bud, upon every spire of springing grass.

Jesus came to live among men to reveal the infinite love of God. Love, mercy, and compassion were revealed in every act of His life; His heart went out in tender sympathy to the children of men. He took man's nature, that He might reach man's wants. **The poorest and humblest were not afraid to approach Him. Such is the character of Christ as revealed in His life. This is the character of God.**

It was to redeem us that Jesus lived and suffered and died. He became a "Man of Sorrows," that we might be made partakers of everlasting joy. But this great sacrifice was not made in order to create in the Father's heart a love for man, not make Him willing to save. No, no! "God so loved the world, that He gave His only begotten Son." *John 3:16.* The Father loves us, not because of the great propitiation, but He provided the propitiation because He loves us. None but the Son of God could accomplish our redemption.

What a value this places upon man! Through transgression the sons of man become subjects of Satan. Through faith in the atoning sacrifice of Christ the sons of Adam may become the sons of God. The matchless love of God for a world that did not love Him! The thought has a subduing power upon the soul and brings the mind into captivity to the will of God.

Man was originally endowed with noble powers and a well-balanced mind. He was perfect in his being, and in harmony with God. His thoughts were pure, his aims holy. But through disobedience, his powers were perverted, and selfishness took the place of love. His nature became so weakened through transgression that it was impossible for him, in his own strength, to resist the power of evil.

It is impossible for us, of ourselves, to escape from the pit of sin in which we are sunken. Our hearts are evil, and we cannot change them. There must be a power working from within, a new life from above, before men can be changed from sin to holiness. That power is Christ. His grace alone can quicken the lifeless faculties of the soul, and attract it to God, to holiness. To all, there is but one answer, "Behold the Lamb of God, which taketh away the sin of the world." *John 1:29.* Let us avail ourselves of the means provided for us that we may be transformed into His likeness, and be restored to fellowship with the ministering angels, to harmony and communion with the Father and the Son.

How shall a man be just with God? How shall the sinner be made righteous? It is only through Christ that we can be brought into harmony with God, with holiness; but how are we to come to Christ?

Repentance includes sorrow for sin and a turning away from it. We shall not renounce sin unless we see its sinfulness; until we turn away from it in heart, there will be no real change in the life.

But **when the heart yields to the influence of the Spirit of God, the conscience will be quickened**, and the sinner will discern something of the depth and sacredness of God's holy law, the foundation of His government in heaven and on earth. Conviction takes hold upon the mind and heart.

The prayer of David, after his fall, illustrates the nature of true sorrow for sin. His repentance was sincere and deep. There was no effort to palliate his guilt; no desire to escape the judgment threatened inspired his prayer. David saw the enormity of his transgression; he saw the defilement of his soul; he loathed his sin. It was not for pardon only that he prayed, but for purity of heart. He longed for the joy of holiness, to be restored to harmony and communion with God. A repentance such as this is beyond the reach of our own power to accomplish; it is obtained only from Christ.

Christ is ready to set us free from sin, but He does not force the will. If we refuse, what more can He do? Study God's Word prayerfully. **As you see the enormity of sin, as you see yourself as you really are, do not give up in despair. It was sinners that Christ came to save.** When Satan comes to tell you that you are a great sinner, look to your Redeemer and talk of His merits. Acknowledge your sin, but tell the enemy that "Christ came into the world to save sinners" and that you may be saved *(1 Timothy 1:15).*

"He that covereth his sins shall not prosper: but whoso confesseth and forsaketh them shall have mercy." *Proverbs 28:13.* **The conditions of obtaining the mercy of God are simple and just and reasonable.** Confess your sins to God, who only can forgive them, and your faults to one another. Those who have not humbled their souls before God, in acknowledging their guilt, have not yet fulfilled the first step of acceptance. We must be willing to humble our hearts and comply with the conditions of the Word of truth. **The confession that is the outpouring of the inmost soul finds its way to the God of infinite pity.** True confession is always of a specific character, and acknowledges particular sins. All confession should be definite and to the point. It is written, "If we confess our sins, He is faithful and just to forgive us our sins, and to cleanse us from all unrighteousness" *(1 John 1:9).*

God's promise is, **"Ye shall seek Me, and find Me, when ye shall search for Me with all your heart."** *Jeremiah 29:13.* The whole heart must be yielded, or the change can never be wrought in us by which we are to be restored to His likeness.

The warfare against self is the greatest battle that was ever fought. **The yielding of self, surrendering all to the will of God, requires a struggle; but the soul must submit to God before it can be renewed in holiness.**

In giving ourselves to God, we must necessarily give up all that would separate us from Him. There are those who profess to serve God while they rely upon their own efforts to obey His law, to form a right character and secure salvation. Their hearts are not moved by any deep sense of the love of Christ, but they seek to perform the duties of the Christian life as that which God requires of them in order to gain heaven. Such religion is worthless.

When Christ dwells in the heart, the soul will be so filled with His love, with the joy of communion with Him, that it will cleave to Him; and in the contemplation of Him, self will be forgotten. Love to Christ will be the spring of action. Such do not ask for the lowest standard, but aim at perfect conformity to the will of their Redeemer.

Do you feel that it is too great a sacrifice to yield all to Christ? Ask yourself the question, "What has Christ given for me?" The Son of God gave all - life and love and suffering - for our redemption. And can it be that we, the unworthy objects of so great love, will withhold our hearts from Him? **What do we give up, when we give all?** A sin-polluted heart, for Jesus to purify, to cleanse by His own blood, and to save by His matchless love. And yet men think it hard to give up all! God does not require us to give up anything that it is for our best interest to retain. In all that He does, He has the well-being of His children in view.

Many are inquiring, "*How* am I to make the surrender of myself to God?" You desire to give yourself to Him, but you are weak in moral power, in slavery to doubt, and controlled by the habits of your life of sin.

Your promises and resolutions are like ropes of sand. You cannot control your thoughts, your impulses, your affections. The knowledge of your broken promises and forfeited pledges weakens your confidence in your own sincerity, and causes you to feel that God cannot accept you; but you need not despair.

What you need to understand is the true force of the will. This is the governing power in the nature of man, the power of decision, or of choice. Everything depends on the right action of the will. The power of choice God has given to men; it is theirs to exercise. **You cannot change your heart, you cannot of yourself give to God its affections; but you can *choose* to serve Him.** You can give Him your will; He will then work in you to will and to do according to His good pleasure. Thus your whole nature will be brought under the control of the Spirit of Christ; your affections will be centered upon Him, your thoughts will be in harmony with Him.

Desires for goodness and holiness are right as far as they go; but if you stop here, they will avail nothing. Many will be lost while hoping and desiring to be Christians. They do not come to the point of yielding the will to God. They do not *now choose* to be Christians.

Through the right exercise of the will, an entire change may be made in your life. You will have strength from above to hold you steadfast, and thus through constant surrender to God you will be enabled to live the new life, even the life of faith.

As your conscience has been quickened by the Holy Spirit, you have seen something of the evil of sin, of its power, its guilt, its woe; and you look upon it with abhorrence. It is peace that you need. **You have confessed your sins, and in heart put them away. You have resolved to give yourself to God. Now go to Him, and ask that He will wash away your sins and give you a new heart.**

Then believe that He does this *because He has promised.* The gift which God promises us, we must believe we do receive, and it is ours. You are a sinner. You cannot atone for your past sins; you cannot change your heart and make yourself holy. But God promises to do all this for you through Christ. **You *believe* that promise. You confess your sins and give yourself to God. You will to serve Him. Just as surely as you do this, God will fulfill His word to you.** If you believe the promise, God supplies the fact. Do not wait to *feel* that you are made whole, but say, "I believe it; it is so, not because I feel it, but because God promised."

Chapter Six

Summarizing the Later Steps

How to Remain Close to Christ

Jesus says, **"What things soever ye desire, when ye pray, believe that ye receive them, and ye shall have them"** *(Mark 11:24)*. There is a condition to this promise, that we pray according to the will of God. But it is the will of God to cleanse us from sin, to make us His children, and to enable us to live a holy life. So we may ask for these blessings, and believe that we receive them, and thank God that we *have* received them.

Henceforth you are not your own; you are bought with a price. Through this simple act of believing God, the Holy Spirit has begotten a new life in your heart. You are a child born into the family of God, and He loves you as He loves His Son.

Now that you have given yourself to Jesus, do not draw back, do not take yourself away from Him, but day by day say, "I am Christ's; I have given myself to Him," and ask Him to give you His Spirit and keep you by His grace. **As it is by giving yourself to God, and believing Him, that you become His child, so you are to live in Him.**

Here is where thousands fail; they do not believe that Jesus pardons them personally, individually. They do not take God at His Word. It is the privilege of all who comply with the conditions to know for themselves that pardon is freely extended for every sin. **Put away the suspicion that God's promises are not meant for you. They are for every repentant transgressor.**

Look up, you that are doubting and trembling; for Jesus lives to make intercession for us. Thank God for the gift of His dear Son.

"If any man be in Christ, he is a new creature: old things are passed away; behold, all things are become new." *2 Corinthians 5:17.*

A person may not be able to tell the exact time or place, or trace all the chain of circumstances in this process of conversion; but this does not prove him to be unconverted. **A change will be seen in the character, the habits, the pursuits. The contrast will be clear and decided between what they have been and what they have become. Who has the heart? With whom are our thoughts?** Of whom do we love to converse? Who has our warmest affections and our best energies? If we are Christ's, our thoughts are with Him. **There is no evidence of genuine repentance unless it works reformation.** The loveliness of the character of Christ will be seen in His followers. It was His delight to do the will of God.

There are two errors against which the children of God especially need to guard: The first is that of looking to their own works, trusting to anything they can do, to bring themselves into harmony with God. All that man can do without Christ is polluted with selfishness and sin. It is the grace of Christ alone, through faith, which can make us holy.

The opposite and no less dangerous error is that belief in Christ releases men from keeping the law of God; that since by faith alone we become partakers of the grace of Christ, our works have nothing to do with our redemption.

Obedience is the fruit of faith. Righteousness is defined by the standard of God's holy law, as expressed in the ten commandments *(Exodus 20:3-20)*. That so-called faith in Christ which professes to release men from the obligation of obedience to God, is not faith, but presumption. **The condition of eternal life is now just what it always has been - just what it was in paradise before the fall of our first parents - perfect obedience to the law of God, perfect righteousness.** If eternal life were granted on any condition short of this, then the happiness of the whole universe would be imperiled. The way would be open for sin, with all its train of woe and misery, to be immortalized.

Christ changes the heart. He abides in your heart by faith. **You are to maintain this connection with Christ by faith and the continual surrender of your will to Him; and so long as you do this, He will work in you to will and to do according to His good pleasure.**

The closer you come to Jesus, the more faulty you will appear in your own eyes; for your vision will be clearer. This is evidence that Satan's delusions are losing their power. **No deep-seated love for Jesus can dwell in the heart that does not realize its own sinfulness. The soul that is transformed by the grace of Christ will admire His character. A view of our sinfulness drives us to Him who can pardon**; and when the soul, realizing its helplessness, reaches out after Christ, He will reveal Himself in power. The more our sense of need drives us to Him and to the Word of God, the more exalted views we shall have of His character, and the more fully we shall reflect His image.

The change of heart by which we become children of God is in the Bible spoken of as birth. Again it is compared to the germination of the good seed sown by the husbandman. It is God who brings the bud to bloom and the flower to fruit. It is by His power that the seed develops.

As the flower turns to the sun, that the bright beams may aid in perfecting its beauty and symmetry, so should we turn to the Sun of Righteousness, that heaven's light may shine upon us, that our character may be developed into the likeness of Christ.

Do you ask, "How am I to abide in Christ?" In the same way as you received Him at first. "As ye have therefore received Christ Jesus the Lord, so walk in Him." *Colossians 2:6.* By faith you became Christ's, and by faith you are to grow up in Him - by giving and taking. **You are to give all**, - your heart, your will, your service - give yourself to Him to obey all His requirements; **and you must take all** - Christ,

W
A
Y

the fullness of all blessing, to abide in your heart, to be your strength, your righteousness, your everlasting helper - to give you power to obey.

Consecrate yourself to God in the morning; make this your very first work. Let your prayer be, "Take me, O Lord, as wholly Thine. I lay all my plans at Thy feet. Use me today in Thy service. Abide with me, and let all my work be wrought in Thee." This is a daily matter. **Each morning consecrate yourself to God for that day. Surrender all your plans to Him**, to be carried out or given up as His providence shall indicate. Thus day by day you may be giving your life into the hands of God, and thus your life will be molded more and more after the life of Christ.

A life in Christ is a life of restfulness. There may be no ecstasy of feeling, but there should be an abiding, peaceful trust. When the mind dwells upon self, it is turned away from Christ, the source of strength and life. Hence, it is Satan's constant effort to keep the attention diverted from the Saviour and thus prevent the union and communion of the soul with Christ.

When Christ took human nature upon Him, He bound humanity to Himself by a tie of love that can never be broken by any power, save the choice of man himself. Satan will constantly present allurements to induce us to break this tie - to choose to separate ourselves from Christ. But **let us keep our eyes fixed upon Christ, and He will preserve us. Looking unto Jesus, we are safe.** Nothing can pluck us out of His hand. All that Christ was to the disciples, He desires to be to His children today.

Jesus prayed for us, and He asked that we might be one with Him, even as He is one with the Father. What a union is this! **Thus, loving Him and abiding in Him, we shall "grow up into Him in all things, which is the head, even Christ"** (Ephesians 4:15).

God is the source of life and light and joy to the universe. **Wherever the life of God is in the hearts of men, it will flow out to others in love and blessing.** Our Saviour's joy was in the uplifting and redemption of fallen men. For this He counted not His life dear to Himself, but endured the cross, despising the shame. When the love of Christ is enshrined in the heart, like sweet fragrance it cannot be hidden. **Love to Jesus will be manifested in a desire to work as He worked for the blessing and uplifting of humanity.** It will lead to love, tenderness, and sympathy toward all the creatures of our heavenly Father's care.

Those who are the partakers of the grace of Christ will be ready to make any sacrifice, that others for whom He died may share the heavenly gift. They will do all they can to make the world better for their stay in it. This spirit is the sure outgrowth of a soul truly converted. No sooner does one come to Christ than there is born in his heart a desire to make known to others what a precious friend he has found in Jesus. **If we have tasted and seen that the Lord is good, we shall have something to tell.** We shall seek to present to others the attractions of Christ and the unseen realities of the world to come. There will be an intensity of desire to follow in the path that Jesus trod.

And the effort to bless others will react in blessings upon ourselves. Those who thus become participants in labors of love are brought nearest to their Creator. **The spirit of unselfish labor for others gives depth, stability, and Christlike loveliness to the character, and brings peace and happiness to its possessor.** Strength comes by exercise. We need not go to heathen lands, or even leave the narrow circle of the home, if it is there that our duty lies, in order to work for Christ. **With a loving spirit we may perform life's humblest duties "unto the Lord."** *Colossians 3:23*. If the love of God is in the heart, it will be manifested in the life. You are not to wait for great occasions or to expect extraordinary abilities before you go to work for God. The humblest and poorest of the disciples of Jesus can be a blessing to others.

Many are the ways in which God is seeking to make Himself known to us and bring us into communion with Him. If we will but listen, Nature speaks to our senses without ceasing. God's created works will teach us precious lessons of obedience and trust.

No tears are shed that God does not notice. There is no smile that He does not mark. If we would but fully believe this, all undue anxieties would be dismissed. Our lives would not be so filled with disappointment as now; for everything, whether great or small, would be left in the hands of God.

God speaks to us through His providential works and through the influence of His Spirit upon the heart. **God speaks to us in His Word. Here we have in clearer lines the revelation of His character, of His dealings with men, and the great work of redemption. Fill the whole heart with the words of God.** They are the living water, quenching your burning thirst. They are the living bread from heaven.

The theme of redemption is one that the angels desire to look into; it will be the science and the song of the redeemed throughout the ceaseless ages of eternity. Is it not worthy of careful thought and study now? **As we meditate upon the Saviour, there will be a hungering and thirsting of soul to become like Him whom we adore.**

The Bible was written for the common people. The great truths necessary for salvation are made as clear as noonday. There is nothing more calculated to strengthen the intellect than the study of the Scriptures. But there is little benefit derived from a hasty reading of the Bible. One passage studied until its significance is clear to the mind and its relation to the plan of salvation is evident, is of more value than the perusal of many chapters with no definite purpose in view and no positive instruction gained.

Keep your Bible with you. As you have oppor-

tunity, read it; fix the texts in your memory.

We cannot obtain wisdom without earnest attention and prayerful study. Never should the Bible be studied without prayer. Before opening its pages, we should ask for the enlightenment of the Holy Spirit, and it will be given. **Angels from the world of light will be with those who in humility of heart seek for divine guidance.** How must God esteem the human race, since He gave His Son to die for them and appoints His Holy Spirit to be man's teacher and continual guide!

Through nature and revelation, through His providence, and by the influence of His Spirit, God speaks to us. But these are not enough; **we need also to pour out our hearts to Him.** In order to commune with God, we must have something to say to Him concerning our actual life.

Prayer is the opening of the heart to God as to a friend. Not that it is necessary in order to make known to God what we are, but in order to enable us to receive Him. Prayer does not bring God down to us, but brings us up to Him.

Our heavenly Father waits to bestow upon us the fullness of His blessing. What a wonder it is that we pray so little! God is ready and willing to hear the sincere prayer of the humblest of His children. What can the angels of heaven think of poor helpless human beings, who are subject to temptation, when God's heart of infinite love yearns toward them, ready to give them more than they can ask or think, and yet they pray so little and have so little faith?

The darkness of the evil one encloses those who neglect to pray. The whispered temptations of the enemy entice them to sin; and it is all because they do not make use of prayer. Yet **prayer is the key in the hand of faith to unlock heaven's storehouse, where are treasured the boundless resources of Omnipotence.**

There are certain conditions upon which we may expect that God will hear and answer our prayers:

One is that we feel our need of help from Him. If we regard iniquity in our hearts, if we cling to any known sin, the Lord will not hear us; but the prayer of the penitent, contrite soul is always accepted. When all known wrongs are righted, we may believe that God will answer our petitions.

Another element of prevailing prayer is faith. When our prayers seem not to be answered, we are to cling to the promise; for the time of answering will surely come, and we shall receive the blessing we need most. But to claim that prayer will always be answered in the very way and for the particular thing that we desire is presumption.

When we come to God in prayer, **we should have a spirit of love and forgiveness in our own hearts.**

Perseverance in prayer has been made a condition of receiving. We must pray always if we would grow in faith and experience.

We should pray in the family circle, and above all we must not neglect secret prayer, for this is the life of the soul. Family or public prayer alone is not sufficient. Secret prayer is to be heard only by the prayer-hearing God.

There is no time or place in which it is inappropriate to offer up a petition to God. In the crowds of the street, in the midst of a business engagement, we may send up a petition to God and plead for divine guidance.

Let the soul be drawn out and upward, that God may grant us a breath of the heavenly atmosphere. **We may keep so near to God that in every unexpected trial our thoughts will turn to Him** as naturally as the flower turns to the sun. Keep your wants, your joys, your sorrows, your cares, and your fears before God. You cannot burden Him; you cannot weary Him. He is not indifferent to the wants of His children.

We sustain a loss when we neglect the privilege of associating together to strengthen and encourage one another in the service of God. If Christians would associate together, speaking to each other of the love of God and the precious truths of redemption, their own hearts would be refreshed and they would refresh one another.

We must gather about the cross. **Christ and Him crucified should be the theme of contemplation, of conversation, and of our most joyful emotion.** We should keep in our thoughts every blessing we receive from God, and when we realize His great love we should be willing to trust everything to the hand that was nailed to the cross for us.

The soul may ascend nearer heaven on the wings of praise. As we express our gratitude, we are approximating to the worship of the heavenly hosts.

Many are at times troubled with the suggestions of skepticism. God never asks us to believe, without giving sufficient evidence upon which to base our faith. Disguise it as they may, the real cause of doubt and skepticism, in most cases, is the love of sin. We must have a sincere desire to know the truth and a willingness of heart to obey it.

This ends this abridgment of the book, Steps to Christ, in the author's own words.

COMING NEXT—The amazing prophecy which predicted over a thousand years of world history! It is another evidence of the inspiration of God's holy Bible.

—PART TWO—

CHRIST'S SECOND ADVENT

Chapter Seven

The Prophecy of Daniel Two

Modern Nations in Bible Prophecy

He was said to be the master man of destiny— an Italian by blood, a Corsican by birth, a Frenchman by nationality—Napoleon Bonaparte!

Born in 1769, he grew to a stature of only five feet, two inches. Although thin-faced and round shouldered, he had one of the most rapid, clear-thinking, tireless brains ever to function, and a body that only required four hours of rest out of every twenty-four.

After winning battle after battle for the French, in 1799 he overturned the government and seized control of France. For the next 16 years, he won nearly every battle.

He established the Napoleonic order in Europe, placing his relatives in leadership and arranging marriages to cement the nations together. **But, without realizing it, Napoleon was smashing his fist against the prophecy of Daniel 2**, so he was bound to fail.

On the morning of Sunday, June 18, 1815, two immense armies faced each other across a shallow three-mile wide valley in Belgium close to the French northeastern border. Nearby was a little town no one had ever heard of before. It was called Waterloo.

On the eastern side of the valley was a large army, primarily composed of British soldiers under the command of the Duke of Wellington. On the western side was a far larger army under Napoleon. He had won every skirmish and battle in the preceding days. Wellington had sent a message for Blücher, with his Austrian army, to come as quickly as possible. But, slow to respond, he still had not arrived. The situation looked hopeless for those trying to resist the French forces.

But, because God had spoken nearly 2,300 years earlier in Scripture, Napoleon would not be able to become master of Europe.

It had rained heavily overnight on the 17th, so Napoleon delayed starting the battle until noon on the 18th, to allow the ground to dry out. Because the ground was still too saturated, he could not move up to the front. His cavalry (armed horsemen) were still not useable. So repeatedly, for the rest of that day, he sent wave after wave of foot soldiers across the valley. Although many were wounded and dying on both sides, the British were narrowly able to repulse them and hold their position.

Then, late in the afternoon, Wellington gave the signal: Riding on his horse along the eastern ridge, he repeatedly waved his hat. This was the signal for

the counterattack. The entire British army (many of whom had been hidden from the French behind the ridge) headed through the valley toward the French lines.

Meanwhile, unbeknown to both, Blücher suddenly arrived with his army from the south just at that moment. —And his forces broke through Napoleon's right flank, adding their weight to the attack. Losses were heavy on all sides.

As they began to be driven back, a strange panic seized the French. It was in vain that Napoleon tried to stop their flight. His army was in total rout.

Leaving the battlefield in total disarray, the French fled to their homes, wherever they might be in France. Napoleon rode a horse back to Paris, but was unable to prevent Coalition forces from entering France and restoring King Louis XVIII to the French throne. Exiled to Saint Helena, Napoleon died six years later in 1821.

When, in his earlier years, someone told Napoleon that divine Providence would not permit him to rule all Europe, he replied, "Providence is on the side with the heaviest artillery." He had the heaviest artillery, and the largest army. But God's warm June rains came, and the heaviest artillery could not move. His fine cavalry (horsemen) could only slog slowly through the soaked roads. And then Blücher arrived at exactly the right moment to help throw Napoleon's forces into disarray.

God had said that, before the arrival of the Stone Kingdom, "the kingdom shall be divided" *(Daniel 2:41).* When God speaks, His Word stands.

THE REMARKABLE DREAM

This chapter contains God's preview of the nations, extending down to our own time—2,500 years of world history in a few brief sentences. It was written over five centuries before Christ was born, at a time when, because of its apostasy, Jerusalem had been captured by the Babylonians and many of leading Hebrews had been carried captive to Babylon. One of them was a young man named Daniel.

Because he and his three friends were faithful and obedient to God in the midst of corruption and idolatry, God chose to reveal through him the future to Nebuchadnezzar, the king who ruled over most of the then-known world.

One night, Nebuchadnezzar had a dream that greatly disturbed him. But the next morning he could neither remember it nor understand what it meant. So he ordered all his pagan astrologers and soothsayers to tell him the dream and its meaning. But, of course, they could not do this.

No one, of course, could tell the king what it was that he had dreamed. Enraged, Nebuchadnezzar ordered many people in the palace to be slain, including Daniel and his three Hebrew friends.

Upon learning about the crisis, they asked for time to pray about it. **That night, in vision, Daniel**

was shown both the king's dream and its meaning.

The next morning, the four young men knelt and thanked God for revealing the matter to Daniel. In his prayer of thanks, Daniel said:

"Blessed be the name of God forever and ever: for wisdom and might are His: And He changeth the times and the seasons: He removeth kings, and setteth up kings: He giveth wisdom unto the wise, and knowledge to them that know understanding."—*Daniel 2:20-21.*

He then went to the king and told him the dream and the interpretation. Recognizing immediately that it was that exact dream, Nebuchadnezzar knew the interpretation was correct.

As a result of this incident, Daniel was given one of the highest positions in the empire, and his three friends were also placed in leading offices.

You will want to read the whole story in Daniel 2. *We shall now begin with verse 28.*

Daniel, God's prophet, told the king that it was only through the direct power of God, that the dream and its meaning could be told to him.

"But there is a God in heaven that revealeth secrets, and maketh known to the king Nebuchadnezzar what shall be in the latter days. Thy dream, and the visions of thy head upon thy bed, are these."—*Daniel 2:28.*

Daniel was about to explain to the king about four great world powers, beginning with Babylon itself.

The vision which had been given to the king was simple. It portrayed a gigantic statue of a man, most of which was composed of various metals.

"Thou, O king, sawest, and behold a great image. This great image, whose brightness was excellent, stood before thee; and the form thereof was terrible. This image's head was of fine gold, his breast and his arms of silver, his belly and his thighs of brass, his legs of iron, his feet part of iron and part of clay."—*Daniel 2:31-33.*

But then, in his dream, the king had seen something *very unusual* happen to that giant metal image!

"Thou sawest till that a stone was cut out without hands, which smote the image upon his feet that were of iron and clay, and brake them to pieces. Then was the iron, the clay, the brass, the silver, and the gold, broken to pieces together, and became like the chaff of the summer threshingfloors; and the wind carried them away, that no place was found for them: and the stone that smote the image became a great mountain, and filled the whole earth."—*Daniel 2:34-35.*

As he heard all this, the dream immediately came back to the king's memory. He had been thinking about the future, and planning for his kingdom. Babylon was, at that time, the greatest nation on earth. Nebuchadnezzar had renewed and rebuilt the city into its present state, and he was quite proud of what he had done.

In verses 37 to 43, Daniel explained that **this dream revealed future events, which would extend down even to our own time**. One nation would arise after another.

But finally, according to the dream and its interpretation, the God of heaven would step in and eliminate all the kingdoms of the world! He would set up an incorruptible kingdom which would last forever! What a promise is that for us today who live at the end-time of this master Bible prophecy!

"And in the days of these kings shall the God of heaven set up a kingdom, which shall never be destroyed: and the kingdom shall not be left to other people, but **it shall break in pieces and consume all these kingdoms, and it shall stand forever.**

"Forasmuch as thou sawest that the stone was cut out of the mountain without hands, and that it brake in pieces the iron, the brass, the clay, the silver, and the gold; the great God hath made known to the king what shall come to pass hereafter: and the dream is certain, and the interpretation thereof sure."—*Daniel 2:45.*

King Nebuchadnezzar was astounded by this revelation of future events.

"The king answered unto Daniel, and said, Of a truth it is, that your God is a God of gods, and a Lord of kings, and a revealer of secrets, seeing thou couldest reveal this secret.

"Then the king made Daniel a great man, and gave him many great gifts, and made him ruler over the whole province of Babylon, and chief of the governors over all the wise men of Babylon.

"Then Daniel requested of the king, and he set Shadrach, Meshach, and Abednego, over the affairs of the province of Babylon: but Daniel sat in the gate of the king."—*Daniel 2:2:47-49.*

Daniel had told the king, "Thou art this head of gold" *(Daniel 2:38)*, and that other kingdoms would arise after his monarchy *(verses 39-40)*.

Well, that was nice to hear. But the prophet had also told the king, "After thee shall arise another kingdom inferior to thee" *(Daniel 2:39)*. That shattered Nebuchadnezzar's hope of having an endless kingdom. God had different plans for the future.

THE FOUR GREAT EMPIRES

Let us briefly consider these kingdoms:

BABYLON

Babylon was the first of what history knows as the four great monarchies. Its glorious capital was laid out in a perfect square, 15 miles on each side; a total of sixty miles around its walls—which are said to have been over 300 feet high and wide enough on top for five chariots to race abreast.

Gleaming in the sun, its lofty palaces and temple towers stabbed the sky above the towering walls and massive fortifications. Through the city flowed the river Euphrates, flanked by great inner walls and giant brass gates. The streets of the city were broad and straight, crossing at right angles. The famous Hanging Gardens were here, rising terrace upon terrace, one of the seven wonders of the ancient world.

But God through Daniel said that Babylon, the "head of gold," was to pass away. The prophet Isaiah had also predicted it.

"Babylon, the glory of kingdoms, the beauty of the Chaldees' excellency, shall be as when God overthrew Sodom and Gomorrah. **It shall never be inhabited**, neither shall it be dwelt in from generation to generation: neither shall the Arabian pitch tent there; neither shall the shepherds make their fold there. But wild beasts of the desert shall lie there; and their houses shall be full of doleful creatures; and owls shall dwell there."—*Isaiah 13:19-21.*

"And Babylon shall become heaps, . . **without an inhabitant**."—*Jeremiah 51:37.*

"Therefore the wild beasts of the desert with the wild beasts of the islands shall dwell there, and the owls shall dwell therein: and **it shall be no more inhabited forever**; neither shall it be dwelt in from generation to generation."—*Jeremiah 50:39.*

In 1845, and again in 1850, the famous archaeologist Layard explored the site where Babylon had once been. This is how he described what he saw:

"Shapeless heaps of rubbish cover the face of the land . . On all sides, fragments of glass, marble, pottery, and inscribed brick are mingled with the pitrous and blanched soil, which destroys vegetation, and renders the site of Babylon a naked and hideous waste. Owls start from the scanty thickets, and the foul jackal skulks through the furrows."—*Austen H. Layard, Discoveries in the Ruins of Nineveh and Babylon (1853), p. 484.*

If you go to Iraq today, you will find a town called "Babylon." **But it is located several miles from the ancient city.** This is because an Arab superstition forbids any of them from staying in the rubble-strewn remains of the ancient city overnight. The Babylonian Empire, pride of the nations, had gone down into oblivion; never again to be inhabited or rebuilt.

MEDO-PERSIA

Through the prophet Isaiah, God had predicted exactly how the city of Babylon would be captured, and the name of the man who would conquer it— nearly 200 years before it happened!

About the year 712 B.C., God declared in Isaiah 45:1-3 that the "gates of brass" in the river, which passed through the middle of the city, would be left open for the armies of a man named *"Cyrus"* to enter and take the city. It was also predicted that he would permit the Israelites to return to their home in Palestine. —*And that is exactly what happened!*

Daniel later showed Cyrus the prophecy and he decided to fulfill the prediction that he would let the Hebrews return to Jerusalem. His decree is found in the book of Ezra, chapter one.

Cyrus' general, Darius the Mede, conquered the city in 538 B.C. while Nebuchadnezzar's grandson, Belshazzar was having a riotous feast. The story of the conquest is told in the fifth chapter of Daniel. This occurred about 65 years after the dream of Daniel 2.

The new empire was called Medo-Persia, because young Cyrus had grown up in the Median province of Persia, then conquered the entire kingdom—and led his forces to subjugate the other nations of the Near East, including the Babylonian Empire.

In a different prophecy, nearly 200 years earlier, about the year 712 B.C., God through Isaiah also predicted that *"Media"* would be the nation which would conquer Babylon *(Isaiah 13:17-19).*

The "head of gold" *(Daniel 2:32, 37-38)* had been replaced by the second kingdom, represented by the "breast and arms of silver" *(Daniel 2:32, 39).* This silver kingdom of Medo-Persia (which became known as the "Persian Empire") maintained supremacy for 207 years (538-331 B.C.)

GREECE

In 331 B.C., Persia was conquered by Alexander the Great at the Battle of Arbela. After conquering Greece, Alexander had headed eastward and rather quickly became ruler of the entire Near East. His army did not stop until it had subjugated most of India. **Known as the Grecian Empire, this was the "kingdom of brass, which shall bear rule over all the earth"** *(Daniel 2:39, also 32).*

The rapidity with which Alexander, with his trained Greek phalanxes, made conquest after conquest was amazing. After only eight years (334-330 B.C.) he annexed an area a little less than 2 million square miles, containing a population of more than 20 million persons.

Returning from India, Alexander stopped in the ruins of Babylon and planned to rebuild the city (which God had predicted would never be rebuilt). But then he suddenly died. During a drunken orgy which lasted several days, Alexander contracted a violent fever and died eleven days later from this, on June 13, 323 B.C., at the age of 33. Immediately, his generals began fighting among themselves for control of the empire. Within 22 years (by 301 B.C.), his empire was divided among four of the generals.

ROME

But gradually, a nation in the west, called Rome, kept enlarging its territory. After the Battle of Pydna in Macedonia in 168 B.C., no power in the world was strong enough to withstand the Roman legions. That is considered to be the date when Rome became the next great empire. It was **"the legs of iron"** *(Daniel 2:33)*, and was known as the "iron kingdom."

"The fourth kingdom shall be strong as iron: forasmuch as iron breaketh in pieces and subdueth all things: and as iron that breaketh all these, shall it break in pieces and bruise."— *Daniel 2:40*.

In describing the ongoing Roman conquests, the eighteenth-century historian, J.W. Edward Gibbon, uses the very imagery that we find in the vision of Daniel 2:

"The arms of the republic, sometimes vanquished in battle, always victorious in war, advanced with rapid steps to the Euphrates, the Danube, the Rhine, and the ocean; and the images of *gold* or *silver*, or *brass*, that might serve to represent the nations and their kings, were successfully broken by the *iron* monarchy of Rome."—*Gibbon, The History of the Decline and Fall of the Roman Empire, Chap. 38, par. 1. Italics ours.*

The empire of the Caesars reached from the Rhine and the Danube on the north to the burning sands of the Sahara on the south. It was an immense empire, bound together by its excellent system of roads and laws. Over these roads, the first Apostles carried the good news of Christ. Greek was the common language of the empire.

Rome, known as the "iron monarchy," ruled for nearly 600 years. Jesus was born in this era and was crucified under Rome's authority.

THE TEN DIVISIONS

But Daniel had predicted that this fourth empire would be split into ten divisions—the toes, partly of iron and partly of clay.

"And whereas thou sawest the feet and toes, part of potters' clay, and part of iron, **the kingdom shall be divided**; but there shall be in it of the strength of the iron, forasmuch as thou sawest the iron mixed with miry clay."—*Daniel 2:41*.

This division (also predicted in Daniel 7; more on that later in this book), occurred in the century preceding A.D. 476, as tribes from central Europe kept invading it. The Roman empire was broken into fragments by the barbarian invasions of the fourth and fifth centuries.

The ten main divisions, corresponding to the ten toes, are given as the *Alamanni* (Germans), the *Franks* (French), the *Burgundians* (Swiss), the *Suevi*

(Portuguese), the *Saxons* (English), the *Visigoths* (Spanish), the *Lombards* (Italians), the *Huruli*, the *Vandals*, and the *Ostrogoths*. (Later in our study of Daniel 7, we will learn that God predicted that these last three tribes would be uprooted and destroyed.)

Gradually, these tribes began having victories against Roman forces as early as A.D. 351. History gives A.D. 476 as the date of Rome's fall, when Emperor Augustulus (Little Augustus) was deposed.

The modern nations of Europe developed from these barbarian tribes of the old Roman Empire. As predicted, some were to be strong and some weak. Thus it has been and continues to be.

"And as the toes of the feet were part of iron, and part of clay, so the kingdom shall be partly strong, and partly broken."—*Daniel 2:42*.

We have learned that the Bible declares with the utmost simplicity and clarity that the European nations of our time cannot be permanently united by warfare, or in any other way.

Repeated efforts have been made to unite the nations of Europe by royal marriages. But, as predicted, they have all failed.

"And whereas thou sawest iron mixed with miry clay, they shall mingle themselves with the seed of men: but **they shall not cleave one to another**, even as iron is not mixed with clay."—*Daniel 2:43*.

Before World War I, practically all the kings and rulers of Europe were related. Yet family ties failed to prevent the outbreak of that terrible conflict.

SIX WHO TRIED TO BREAK THE PROPHECY

Of the many men who, down through the centuries, tried to reunite Europe into one mammoth kingdom, *six especially stand out*:

Charlemagne tried to restore the original empire by welding its fragments together into, what he called, a "holy Roman empire." But it miserably failed. Voltaire, a witty infidel later said it was neither holy nor Roman nor an empire. Weary from nearly half a century of fighting all over Europe, Charlemagne could not make the clay and iron fuse together.

Charles V also tried it without success, and wore out his life battling Protestantism. He ended up in a monastery, trying to make a number of clocks run together.

Louis XIV of France tried it and deluged Europe in blood.

Napoleon the Great tried it, but his glory vanished at Waterloo.

Then **Kaiser Wilhelm II** said he was determined to restore all Europe into the one empire. World War I was the disastrous result.

Adolf Hitler followed, declaring that his new

W
A
Y

Third Reich would last "a thousand years."

Europe has repeatedly been drenched in blood in efforts to unite the nations, but it remains divided.

In addition to the six, more recently, the **League of Nations**, and then the **United Nations**, have tried to bring these nations together. Men may wonder whether there will be success, but God's Word says, **"They shall not cleave one to another." Those seven words form a barrier to every dream of world conquest.** No plan to rule the world will succeed.

The **European Union** is the latest attempt—but God's decree will not be broken. The nations of Europe will not be able to stick together!

"In the annals of human history, the growth of nations, the rise and fall of empires, appear as if dependent on the will and prowess of man; the shaping of events seems, to a great degree, to be determined by his power, ambition, or caprice. But in the Word of God the curtain is drawn aside, and we behold, above, behind, and through all the play and counterplay of human interest and power and passions, the agencies of the All-merciful One, silently, patiently working out the counsels of His own will."—*Prophets and Kings, 499-500.*

A KINGDOM AS DURABLE AS ROCK

Four-fifths of the prophecy of Daniel 2 has been fulfilled; the last fifth will also be fulfilled—the setting up of Christ's kingdom. For it is written:

"And in the days of these kings [that is, in the days of the kingdoms of Western Europe: Britain, France, Germany, Italy, Spain, Portugal, Switzerland, Belgium, etc.] shall the God of heaven set up a kingdom, which shall never be destroyed: and the kingdom shall not be left to other people, but it shall break in pieces and consume all these kingdoms, and it shall stand forever."—*Daniel 2:44.*

Think of it! In the days of these broken fragments of mighty Rome, called the nations of Western Europe—in their day, while they are still nations, God will actually set up His kingdom! "It shall break in pieces and consume all these kingdoms, and it shall stand forever." *Daniel 2:44.*

This is a tremendous prophecy!

CERTAINTY OF THE PREDICTION

In this basic prophecy of the Bible, six facts stand out: (1) There is a God in heaven. (2) He has servants on earth. (3) His hand is in earthly affairs. (4) He predicted the history of the world from Babylon—580 years before Christ—on down to our own time. (5) He forecast man's failure, in every instance, to truly unite the nations of the world. (6) God's glorious and eternal kingdom is to be set up—in the process of destroying all the kingdoms of mankind. **—*Today we live in the feet and toes of history!***

We are now awaiting the Kingdom of Stone.

"The kingdoms of this world are become the kingdoms of our Lord, and of His Christ; and He shall reign forever and ever."—*Revelation 11:15.*

It will smite the image and fill the whole earth *(Daniel 2:35).* We are told that it is cut out of a mountain "without hands"—that is, without human intervention. It is of divine origin. It smites the image on the feet. Notice that it will fill the whole earth.

Someone may ask, "Is this really likely to happen?" In answer, we read verse 45: "The dream is certain, and the interpretation thereof sure."

The kingdom of God will be set up by no human agencies or powers. **Christ will appear the second time, as He has promised, and the history of earthly empires will end.** The destruction of sin and a world where there is no death, no sorrow, no battles, no disease, will in God's own time be a reality. This dream of the ages will be the kingdom of eternal peace.

We must remember that this remarkable prophetic dream of Daniel 2 is part of the Holy Scriptures. In briefest form, but with great clearness, it outlines the successive world empires from the time of Nebuchadnezzar, down to the setting up of Christ's everlasting kingdom.

How can we be sure of that statement? because of verse 44, which are the words of the prophet as he continued speaking to the king:

"And in the days of these kings shall the God of heaven set up a kingdom, which shall never be destroyed: and the kingdom shall not be left to other people, but it shall break in pieces and consume all these kingdoms, and it shall stand forever."—*Daniel 2:44.*

Christ gave us more information about this Stone,—which is Himself. This is what Christ said about it:

"The stone which the builders rejected, the same is become the head of the corner. Whosoever shall fall upon that stone shall be broken; but on whomsoever it shall fall, it will grind him to powder."—*Luke 20:17-18.*

Are you willing to fall in submission upon that Stone, the foundation of the God's eternal church? Are you willing to be broken upon Jesus Christ? We must know Him now in order to meet Him in peace. **Jesus, the King of the ages, wants to be the King of your heart.** Then you can truly pray: "Thy kingdom come. Thy will be done in earth, as it is in heaven." *Matthew 6:10.*

As we near the end of this chapter, here is another story about Waterloo:

For long, dreary years, England had fought against Napoleon. Then came that final battle in that valley near Waterloo. Everything was at stake. Because there was no telegraph, telephone, or radio, news could only be sent by a living messenger or, if the weather was clear, by semaphore. These were hand-waved flags which gradually spelled out words.

The news of the battle reached England by a sailing vessel which, landing on the far south coast, was carried overland by semaphore to the top of Winchester Cathedral, and on to London.

Suddenly, the flags could be seen and **slowly the words were spelled out: "W-e-l-l-i-n-g-t-o-n-d-e-f-e-a-t-e-d."**

Then the fog closed in. *"Wellington defeated!"* Hope changed to despair as the darkness of night closed in. Orders were given to fortify the roads and the bridges, and plans were made for entrenchments along the coast.

But near noon the next day, the fog lifted again, and once again the semaphore was seen: *"Wellington defeated Napoleon at Waterloo!"* Fear changed to joy, defeat to victory! The tyrant had been overthrown, a new age had dawned for Europe.

It was dark at Calvary, and apparently Satan had gained a great victory over the world, for he had slain the Redeemer who had come to save mankind.

Although crucified in weakness, Christ arose in strength, with the message, "All power is given unto Me in heaven and in earth. Go ye therefore, and teach all nations" *(Matthew 28:18-19).*

The message, "Christ defeated," had been changed to "Christ defeated Satan at Calvary!" It is now victory for all who will accept Him! It is victory for the entire universe!

That recalls to mind Queen Victoria, who was about to visit the castle of Lord Leicester in the midlands of the British Isles. As she stepped across the threshold, in her honor the great timepiece of the castle was stopped, never again to be started, forever marking the moment of her arrival.

The King of the universe is about to step across the threshold of time, when He arrives. Every clock, every watch, every timepiece the world around, will be forever stopped, never to be started again. Time will turn on its hinge and become eternity!

Will you place yourself on God's side? This is the moment to decide. Eternity has no clock. The decision that will determine your destiny belongs to time. Time is now; and, it is soon to end for each of us personally either by Christ's coming or at death.

COMING NEXT—The glorious truth that Jesus is coming back soon! Oh, how we long for that day when we will be with Him forever!

Chapter Eight

The Second Coming of Christ

He is Coming Soon!

A great prairie fire, driven by a strong wind, swept relentlessly toward a farmer's homestead. The man quickly hitched his horses to the plow and made several furrows in the form of a large circle around his home. Then he set fire to the dry grass within the circle and totally burned it.

The roaring, terrifying demons of the prairie, with giant tongues of leaping flames, charged down upon that home. But when it struck the furrows and the ground already burned over, it swirled around both sides of the circle. For a brief time, there was thick smoke everywhere.

Then the air cleared; and the fire, now downwind, could be seen receding in the distance as it went on its way. The farmer and his family, his house and barns, his machinery and stock, had all been saved.

The fire cannot come where the fire has already been! **The fires of God's wrath against sin burned over Calvary.** All of us who are willing to gather about the cross, and there obediently give our lives to Jesus and henceforth serve Him, will be safe from the fires of final destruction.

CHRIST IS SOON TO RETURN

We must prepare for what is ahead. **Christ is going to return for His faithful ones soon. It will be His Second Coming.** Only those who are trusting in Him at that time will be secure when this final crisis of the ages occurs.

In 1860, the French scientist Pierre Berchelt spoke these words, "Within a hundred years of physical and chemical science, man will know what the atom is. It is my belief that not long after science reaches that point, God will come down to earth with His big ring of keys and will say to humanity, *'Gentlemen, it is closing time.'* "

Pitirim Sorokin wrote in his *Crisis of Our Age:*

"The history of human progress is a history of incurable stupidity. In the course of human history, several thousand revolutions have been launched with a view to establishing paradise on earth. None of them has ever achieved its purpose."

Today, we daily see more immense catastrophes,—and on a global scale that is greater than ever before. Everything about us—in international events, deepening calamities, and natural disasters—proclaims in trumpet tones that the coming of Christ is near!

"A little while, and He shall come, The hour draws on apace, The blessed hour, the glorious morn, When we shall see His face; How light our trials then will seem! How short our pilgrim way! Our life on earth, a fitful dream, Dispelled by dawning day!"

W A Y

THE FIRST ADVENT PREDICTED

All through the Old Testament Scriptures, we find promises that Christ would come. We find it in the very first prophecy, which is also the first promise in the Bible. When Adam and Eve, our first parents, sinned, God promised that one of their descendants would eventually come and destroy the power of Satan:

"I will put enmity between thee and the woman, and between thy seed and her seed; it shall bruise thy head, and thou shalt bruise His heel."—*Genesis 3:15.*

"There shall come a Star out of Jacob, and a Sceptre shall rise out of Israel."—*Numbers 24:17.*

The entire 53rd chapter of Isaiah told about the coming Messiah. The promise was that "Shiloh would come" *(Genesis 49:10).* He would be "the Prince of Peace" *(Isaiah 9:6).*

He came the first time as a "Lamb" (John 1:29). Isaiah 53:7-8 predicts this:

"He was oppressed, and He was afflicted, yet He opened not His mouth: He is brought as a lamb to the slaughter, and as a sheep before her shearers is dumb, so He openeth not His mouth. He was taken from prison and from judgment: and who shall declare His generation? for He was cut off out of the land of the living: for the transgression of My people was He stricken."—*Isaiah 53:7-8.*

The purpose of this first coming was to offer pardon to the guilty sinner.

"Let the wicked forsake his way, and the unrighteous man his thoughts: and let him return unto the Lord, and He will have mercy upon him; and to our God, for He will abundantly pardon."—*Isaiah 55:7.*

We are told that this was made possible by Christ's life and death.

"Behold the Lamb of God, which taketh away the sin of the world."—*John 1:29.*

"She shall bring forth a son, and thou shalt call His name Jesus: for He shall save His people from their sins."—*Matthew 1:21.*

But we are also told about another coming of Christ, which would complete the work of saving man from sin:

"So Christ was once offered to bear the sins of many; and unto them that look for Him shall He appear the second time without sin unto salvation."—*Hebrews 9:28.*

Did the Old Testament prophets also see beyond the first coming of Christ—*to the second?*

"Repent ye therefore, and be converted, that your sins may be blotted out, when the times of refreshing shall come from the presence of the Lord; and He shall send Jesus Christ, which before was preached unto you: Whom the heaven must receive until the times of restitution of all things, which God hath spoken by the mouth of all His holy prophets since the world began."—*Acts 3:19-21.*

Here we are assured that *all* the prophets of old understood that there was to be a glorious coming of the Messiah which would restore God's original plan for mankind.

Dwight L. Moody estimated that the second coming of Christ is referred to 2,500 times in the Bible. For every prophecy predicting the first coming of Christ, there are eight which promise His second advent.

The psalmist, David, wrote:

"Our God shall come, and shall not keep silence: a fire shall devour before Him, and it shall be very tempestuous round about Him. He shall call to the heavens from above, and to the earth, that He may judge His people. Gather My saints together unto Me; those that have made a covenant with Me by sacrifice."—*Psalm 50:3-5.*

Jude, next to the last book of the New Testament, names one of the first Old Testament prophets who preached the Second Advent of Christ.

"And Enoch also, the seventh from Adam, prophesied of these, saying, Behold, the Lord cometh with ten thousands of His saints, to execute judgment upon all, and to convince all that are ungodly among them of all their ungodly deeds which they have ungodly committed, and of all their hard speeches which ungodly sinners have spoken against Him."—*Jude 14-15.*

Enoch was only the seventh generation from Adam. Living long before the Flood, Enoch, as quoted above, painted a word picture of Christ's coming which fairly matches that which John wrote in the Revelation.

The message of the Old Testament rings forth: "He is coming!" Coming in humility and suffering, then later coming in power and glory. But always without a wavering note. *He is coming!*

A TRIUMPHANT MESSAGE

The first great message of the New Testament is that *He has come!*

"For unto you is born this day in the city of David a Saviour, which is Christ the Lord."—*Luke 2:11.*

He came as a babe born of a virgin, as a man clothed in the garb of a carpenter, as the Messiah baptized of John in the Jordan River, and anointed with the Holy Spirit. He came as the overcomer, tempted in all points as we are, yet without sin. He came as the master teacher, the divine healer, the great comforter. He died on Calvary for the sins of men. He rose from the tomb with the keys of hell and death snatched from the sealed and stony sepulchre, and ascended into heaven as the Son of man. All this *He has done*. Yes, He *has* come. That was the *first advent*.

But there is more! The second wonderful message of the New Testament is, *"He is coming again!"*

Here is what Jesus said, when questioned by His disciples:

"And then shall appear the sign of the Son of man in heaven: and then shall all the tribes of the earth mourn, and they shall see the Son of man coming in the clouds of heaven with power and great glory."—*Matthew 24:30*.

On trial before the high priest a few hours before Calvary, **Jesus was put under oath to answer the question as to whether He was the Son of God.** Standing there, bound with ropes before the arrogant Caiaphas, Christ unhesitatingly declared:

"Hereafter shall ye see the Son of man sitting on the right hand of power, and coming in the clouds of heaven."—*Matthew 26:64*.

These words affirmed in open testimony before the highest Jewish court in the land that which He had privately said to His disciples only a few hours earlier:

"Let not your heart be troubled: ye believe in God, believe also in Me. In My Father's house are many mansions: if it were not so, I would have told you. I go to prepare a place for you. And if I go and prepare a place for you, I will come again, and receive you unto Myself; that where I am, there ye may be also."—*John 14:1-3*.

Then, only 43 days later at Christ's ascension, we find the testimony of the angels:

"Ye men of Galilee, why stand ye gazing up into heaven? this same Jesus, which is taken up from you into heaven, shall so come in like manner as ye have seen Him go into heaven."—*Acts 1:11*.

The Apostle Paul, ready for execution by Nero's decree, exclaimed in triumph:

"I have fought a good fight, I have finished my course, I have kept the faith: Henceforth there is laid up for me a crown of righteousness, which the Lord, the righteous judge, shall give me at that day: and not to me only, but unto all them also that love His appearing."—*2 Timothy 4:7-8*.

Did you know that Christian believers who lived back during those ancient persecutions said to one another, *"Maranatha!"* when passing on the streets of Rome. This meant "The Lord is coming!" **Down through the centuries, God's faithful have waited, watched, and prayed for the coming of the Lord Jesus Christ** in the clouds of heaven.

The Apostle Peter solemnly declared to the believers the importance of preparing their lives for that great event.

"But the day of the Lord will come as a thief in the night; in the which the heavens shall pass away with a great noise, and the elements shall melt with fervent heat, the earth also and the works that are therein shall be burned up.

"Seeing then that all these things shall be dissolved, what manner of persons ought ye to be in all holy conversation and godliness, looking for and hasting unto the coming of the day of God, wherein the heavens being on fire shall be dissolved, and the elements shall melt with fervent heat?"—*2 Peter 3:10-12*.

In Revelation, Christ also warns us to prepare for His coming:

"Behold, I come quickly; and My reward is with Me, to give every man according as His work shall be."—*Revelation 22:12*.

We earlier read the first promise in the Bible. Now we come to the last promise in the Bible;

"He which testifieth these things saith, Surely I come quickly."—*Revelation 22:20*.

March 11, 1942, was a dark day for the freedom-loving peoples of the world. General Douglas MacArthur was ordered by his superior to leave the Philippines. The overwhelming forces of the enemy were sweeping in. In that black and bitter night, as he prepared to step into a departing ship, he uttered the promise, *"I shall return!"*

MacArthur later fulfilled that promise, when on October 20, 1944, he stepped on shore, and his forces began the triumphant liberation of the Philippines.

The Captain of our salvation is soon to return also, for He has repeatedly declared, *"I will return!"*

HOW WILL CHRIST RETURN?

Yes, this is the question we want answered. **For it is only as we learn from Scripture how Christ will actually return for His faithful ones—that we can recognize the false christs which He predicted would try to deceive us.**

"And Jesus answered and said unto them, Take heed that no man deceive you. For many shall come in My name, saying, I am Christ; and shall deceive many."—*Matthew 24:4-5*.

Here are four facts about the Second Advent of Christ which neither men nor devils can imitate:

***First*, Christ will return with ten thousand of thousands of shining angels!**

"The Son of man shall come in His glory, and all the holy angels with Him."—*Matthew 25:31*.

"They shall see the Son of man coming in the clouds of heaven with power and great glory. And He shall send His angels with a great sound of a trumpet, and they shall gather together His elect from the four winds, from one end of heaven to the other."—*Matthew 24:30-31.*

Second, **the righteous dead will be resurrected.**

"For the Lord Himself shall descend from heaven with a shout, with the voice of the archangel, and with the trump of God: and the dead in Christ shall rise first."—*1 Thessalonians 4:16.*

Third, **the righteous living will be taken up.**

"Then we which are alive and remain shall be caught up together with them in the clouds, to meet the Lord in the air: and so shall we ever be with the Lord."—*1 Thessalonians 4:17.*

Fourth, **the bodies of the righteous dead will be changed**.

"In a moment, in the twinkling of an eye, at the last trump: for the trumpet shall sound, and the dead shall be raised incorruptible, and we shall be changed. For this corruptible must put on incorruption, and **this mortal must put on immortality**."—*1 Corinthians 15:52-53.*

"For our conversation is in heaven; from whence also we look for the Saviour, the Lord Jesus Christ: who shall change our vile body **that it may be fashioned like unto His glorious body**, according to the working whereby He is able even to subdue all things unto Himself."—*Philippians 3:20-21.*

"So also is the resurrection of the dead. It is sown in corruption; it is raised in incorruption."—*1 Corinthians 15:42.*

Those of God's faithful ones who died of wasting disease, or were killed in accidents, will come forth in eternal vigor and health.

"He will gather the wheat in His garner,
But the chaff will He scatter away;
Then how shall we stand in the judgment
Of the great resurrection day?"

The answer to those words is always the same. **We may wear the crown of everlasting life** *in that great day*, **if** *now* **we will surrender our lives to Christ and live clean, godly lives in obedience, by enabling faith in Christ, to His Written Word, the Bible.**

"Oft me thinks I hear His footsteps, Stealing down the paths of time, And the future dark with shadows, Brightens with this hope sublime; Sound the soul-inspiring anthem, Angel hosts, your harps attune; Earth's long night is almost over, Christ is coming."

SIGNS THAT HIS COMING IS NEAR

We see all about us, on a massive scale, the wars and fear, the famines and disasters which the Bible predicted would occur in these last days.

"For nation shall rise against nation, and kingdom against kingdom: and there shall be famines, and pestilences, and earthquakes, in divers places."—*Matthew 24:7. (Also see Luke 21:11, 25-26; Daniel 12:1; Joel 3:9-14; Revelation 11:18.)*

We see false christs arising, false prophets, and deceivers of all kinds.

"For there shall arise false Christs, and false prophets, and shall show great signs and wonders; insomuch that, if it were possible, they shall deceive the very elect."—*Matthew 24:24 (also 1 Timothy 4:1; 2 Timothy 4:3-4; Matthew 15:9).*

We see intense evil, as in Noah's day.

"And God saw that the wickedness of man was great in the earth, and that every imagination of the thoughts of his heart was only evil continually . . The earth also was corrupt before God, and the earth was filled with violence."—*Genesis 6:5, 11.*

Oh, how few are preparing for that great event, when Christ shall return for His own!

A man visiting a certain school told the pupils that he would give a prize to the one whose desk he found in the best order when he returned. "But when will you return?" some of them asked.

"That I cannot tell," was the answer.

One little girl, who had been noted for her disorderly habits, announced that she meant to win the prize. "You!" her classmates jeered. "Why, your desk is always out of order."

"Oh, but I mean to clean it the first of every week." "But suppose he should come at the end of the week?" Someone asked. "Then I will clean it every morning."

"But he may come at the end of the day." For a moment the little girl was silent. **"I know what I'll do,"** she said decidedly; *"I'll just keep it clean."*

We cannot know the exact hour when Jesus will come; but, **trusting in Him for courage and strength to press on, we must make sure that we are ready when that great day comes!**

"Down the minster aisles of splendor, from betwixt the cherubim, Through the wondering throng, with motion strong and fleet, Sounds His victor tread approaching, with a music far and dim—*the music of the coming of His feet.*

"Sandaled not with sheen of silver, girded not with woven gold, Weighted not with shimmering gems and odors sweet, But white-winged and shod with glory in the Tabor light of old—*The glory of the coming of His feet.*

"He is coming, O my friend, with His everlasting peace, With His blessedness immortal and complete; He is coming, O my friend, and His coming brings release—*I listen for the coming of His feet.*"

BIBLE SUMMARY

Here is a brief summary of part of what we are learning in this chapter. These are truths to be read over and over again, repeated to our children, and shared with others:

Christ promises that He will return for us.

"In My Father's house are many mansions: if it were not so, I would have told you. I go to prepare a place for you. And if I go and prepare a place for you, I will come again, and receive you unto Myself; that where I am, there ye may be also."—*John 14:2-3.*

Jesus explained why many will not be prepared for His coming.

"But and if that evil servant shall say in his heart, My lord delayeth his coming; and shall begin to smite his fellow-servants, and to eat and drink with the drunken; the lord of that servant shall come in a day when he looketh not for him, and in an hour that he is not aware of."—*Matthew 24:48-50.*

"And as it was in the days of Noe, so shall it be also in the days of the Son of man. They did eat, they drank, they married wives, they were given in marriage, until the day that Noe entered into the ark, and the flood came, and destroyed them all. Likewise also as it was in the days of Lot; they did eat, they drank, they bought, they sold, they planted, they builded; but the same day that Lot went out of Sodom it rained fire and brimstone from heaven, and destroyed them all. Even thus shall it be in the day when the Son of man is revealed."—*Luke 17:26-30.*

Descriptions of those who are preparing for His Second Advent:

"Beloved, now are we the sons of God, and it doth not yet appear what we shall be: but we know that, when He shall appear, we shall be like Him; for we shall see Him as He is. And every man that hath this hope in him purifieth himself, even as He is pure."—*1 John 3:2-3.*

"I have fought a good fight, I have finished my course, I have kept the faith: Henceforth there is laid up for me a crown of righteousness, which the Lord, the righteous judge, shall give me at that day: and not to me only, but unto all them also that love His appearing."—*2 Timothy 4:7-8.*

"And it shall be said in that day, Lo, this is our God; we have waited for Him, and He will save us: this is the Lord; we have waited for Him, we will be glad and rejoice in His salvation."—*Isaiah 25:9.*

"For the Son of man shall come in the glory of His Father with His angels; and then He shall reward every man according to his works."—*Matthew 16:27.*

His coming will be a time of judgment of the wicked.

"For He cometh to judge the earth: He shall judge the world with righteousness, and the people with His truth."—*Psalm 96:13.*

"Behold, the Lord cometh with ten thousands of His saints, to execute judgment upon all."—*Jude 14-15.*

"The Lord Jesus Christ, who shall judge the quick and the dead at His appearing and His kingdom."—*2 Timothy 4:1.*

"If Jesus should come at this moment To catch up with Him in the air, All those who love His appearing, Forever to be with Him there, How would He find you, I wander—Watching, waiting, faithful, true? Dearly beloved, consider—How would it be with you?"

COMING NEXT—Why is there sin? Is there a devil, and where did He come from? Here are important facts everyone needs to know.

— PART THREE —

ETERNAL LIFE IN CHRIST

Chapter Nine

The Truth about Satan and Sin

God Did Not Create Evil

When the great Italian artist, Leonardo da Vinci, was asked to paint a mural of Christ and His disciples at the Last Supper for the wall of the convent in Milan, he began work on the project in the year 1494. He wanted to portray that moment, in John 13:21, when Jesus announces that one of His twelve disciples would betray Him.

As the painting *(L'Ultima Cena* is its Italian name) was nearing completion, **only the figures of Christ and Judas needed to added**. But, so far, he had been unable to find a model for either one: a face sublime and godly for Christ, and one grim with sin-etched lines on it for Judas Iscariot.

The months passed, and then one day entering a small church—he saw the young choir leader. It was the man he wanted for the portrayal of Christ. His name was Pietro Bandinelli.

After many days seated before da Vinci, that part of the painting was completed. When it was finished, the young man gazed at it wistfully and said, "Oh, that I could be more like Him!" The artist replied, "You can be, if you will follow His example."

Months turned into years, and the painting remained unfinished. That other face Leonardo searched for—fallen, bitter, cruel and depraved—

W
A
Y

could not be found.

Then four years later, on a cool, crisp evening in 1498, he met a beggar. Clothed in rags, the man had deep-set eyes which were clouded by remorse and sin.

Greatly excited, Da Vinci hired him as a model and began painting Judas. The tramp's features were painted into the face of the betrayer.

One day, as he was finishing on the face, the beggar began to weep. Then he confessed, *"You see, I am Pietro, the one who sat for your Christ!"* He had been the young choir director which Leonardo had painted from only four years earlier.

WHY IS OUR WORLD LIKE THIS?

The age-old question of the skeptic has always been, "Why would God create an evil world like this and let it continue?"

First, God did not create an evil world. Inspiration tells us that, in the beginning —

"God saw every thing that He had made, and, behold, it was very good."—*Genesis 1:31.*

God is love. His law is love. All His dealings with all His creatures, when properly understood, are a demonstration of unchanging love. God did not create an evil world.

Second, it is the people down here that have made it evil.

"Wherefore, as by one man sin entered into the world, and death by sin; and so death passed upon all men, for that all have sinned."—*Romans 5:12.*

Sin begins one way and ends in a thousand ways. And all lead to one place, marked "death"!

Third, God will not violate the free will of sinners who want to sin. But He has provided a solution for all willing to accept it. He gave us His Son who died for our sins, and offers to save us if we will humbly confess and forsake our sins, and yield our lives to His control.

"As Moses lifted up the serpent in the wilderness, even so must the Son of man be lifted up: That whosoever believeth in Him should not perish, but have eternal life.

"For God so loved the world, that He gave His only begotten Son, that whosoever believeth in Him should not perish, but have everlasting life.

"For God sent not His Son into the world to condemn the world; but that the world through Him might be saved.

"He that believeth on Him is not condemned: but he that believeth not is condemned already, because he hath not believed in the name of the only begotten Son of God."—*John 3:14-18.*

WHAT IS SIN?

Dr. Harry Emerson Fosdick, a well-known liberal preacher of half a century ago, wrote:

"Today we and our hopes and all our efforts after goodness are up against a powerful antagonism, something demonic, tragic, terrific in human nature, that turns our loveliest qualities to evil and our finest endeavors into failure. *Our fathers called it sin, but we no longer do.*"

Another writer said this:

"Man calls sin an accident; God calls it an abomination. Man calls it a chance; God calls it a choice. Man calls it an error; God calls it enmity. Man calls it fascination; God calls it fatality. Man calls sin a luxury; God calls it lawlessness. Man calls sin a trifle; God calls it a tragedy. Man calls sin a mistake; God calls it madness."

What is sin? According to the Bible, sin has *only one* comprehensive definition.

"**Whosoever committeth sin transgresseth also the law: for sin is the transgression of the law.**"—*1 John 3:4.*

That is what the Bible says. Sin is breaking God's moral law of Ten Commandments. And so we see that it is disobedience to God's will that has brought all the sorrow and wretchedness into our world.

WHY DOES GOD NOT STOP THE SIN?

Why does God not stop all this sin and misery right now? He could have done so long ago, but then you and I would not have had a chance to be saved! **God decided that every person born into this world must have an opportunity to make a decision.** Each person would be given opportunity, through the enabling strength of God, to choose to live a clean, godly life, or instead resist the movings of the Holy Spirit speaking through his conscience,—and cling to his selfish, evil ways.

How long will all this continue? God has promised that, when the wickedness throughout the world reaches a certain point, He is going to step in and put an end to it. *Sin will not continue forever.* More about this in later chapters.

WHO GOT SIN STARTED?

How did all this evil begin? Who got it started? God, who made all things, did not create evil in the beginning. There was a time when there was no sin.

But there can be no sin without a sinner! It is not something that a person catches, like a disease. He becomes a sinner because of personal choices that he makes. Sin is connected with the seat of conscience—the will.

Somebody, somewhere willed to sin. Evidence of this is everywhere. Who was it? The answer is in the Bible:

"He that committeth sin is of the devil; for the devil sinneth from the beginning."—*1 John 3:8.*

Here we have the name of the original—*the*

first—**sinner.** His name is "the devil." In Revelation 12:9, he is there described as "the great dragon . . that old serpent, called the Devil, and Satan." Isaiah refers to him as "Lucifer, son of the morning" *(Isaiah 14:12).* We are told that he first sinned "in the beginning."

Lucifer was a created being. Ezekiel, presenting Satan under the symbol of the king of Tyrus, says of him, "the day that thou wast created" *(Ezekiel 28:13).*

It is well to recall here that God "created all things by Jesus Christ" *(Ephesians 3:9).* This includes all things in heaven as well as on earth.

"For by Him were all things created, that are in heaven, and that are in earth, visible and invisible, whether they be thrones, or dominions, or principalities, or powers: all things were created by Him, and for Him."—*Colossians 1:16.*

The next verse says that Christ existed "before all things" *(verse 17).* Thus Christ, working with the Father, created Lucifer.

LUCIFER DECIDES TO SIN

"Why did God make the devil?" is a question often asked. The answer is that God made everything; so He made the being who, by his own choice, became a devil.

Like every other one of God's creatures, Lucifer was originally a perfect being, kind and loving, in full harmony with the principles of heaven.

"Thou sealest up the sum, full of wisdom, and perfect in beauty. Thou hast been in Eden the garden of God . . Thou art the anointed cherub that covereth; and I have set thee so: thou wast upon the holy mountain of God."—*Ezekiel 28:12-14.*

It seems certain that Lucifer was the wisest of all the angelic host. He was not only "full of wisdom," he was "perfect in beauty." In addition, he was also "the anointed cherub." This means he stood very close to the throne of God.

In the Old Testament sanctuary, which was patterned after the heavenly sanctuary *(Hebrews 8:5),* we read, "And the cherubims shall stretch forth their wings on high, covering the mercy seat with their wings" *(Exodus 25:20).* Because their wings were arched above the mercy seat—which represented the throne of God,—they stood in the immediate presence of God. Prior to his fall, Lucifer had been one of those anointed cherubs.

How did Lucifer begin to be sinful? He transgressed God's law. We have already learned that this is the definition of sin:

"Whosoever committeth sin transgresseth also the law: **for sin is the transgression of the law.**"—*1 John 3:4.*

God's holy law tells what He is like. Sin is not living in accordance with the character of God.

Any transgression against the law of God is

sin; and sin always brings dissension, confusion, and sadness to many. Breaking God's law is disloyalty, and an act of treason against Him.

Before Lucifer sinned, wickedness had never existed. God's loving ways had never before been called into question. **By disobeying God's law, Lucifer actually rebelled against God's government**—for His law governs the universe and is the foundation of His throne.

Everyone that violates it brings misery to themselves. Soon they are trying to make life miserable for those around them.

When Lucifer decided to rebel against God and His government, he could only use deception to win many others to his side. Gradually, he began to talk other angels into joining him in imagining that God was unjust.

WHY GOD PERMITTED SIN TO BEGIN

Why did the Lord let Lucifer sin?

There are only two ways in which God could have created the higher orders of His creatures. He could make them with the power of choice or without that power.

If He had made them without the power of making decisions on their own, the power of choice, they would have been mere machines, automatons. As a train follows along the track, they would have automatically done whatever they were told. Their obedience would be mechanical, slavish. But God made us all—both angels and men—to be free, moral agents. That could only be done by giving us the power of choice, the power to obey or disobey.

Worship, prayer, praise, obedience—and most everything else that makes our higher levels of intelligent thinking and acting possible—come from the fact that **God has given us this power so we can decide for ourselves, the power of the will, the power of choice.** We can think and choose. We can decide whether we will serve God or our own selfish interests.

Because God made all of us this way, those who choose to serve God—do so because they love Him and know His laws are just, and ought to be obeyed.

Because we are creatures with the power of choice, **genuine Bible religion is based on persuasion and decision-making, not on force.** Only Satan tries to force people to do something.

Willpower, the kingly power of reason is the key. Do you and I want to be on God's side in the worldwide struggle of good against evil? This is the decision placed before all men.

"If it seem evil unto you to serve the Lord, choose you this day whom ye will serve; whether the gods which your fathers served that were on the other side of the flood, or the gods of the Amorites, in whose land ye dwell: but as for me and my house, we will serve the Lord."—*Joshua 24:15.*

If we will choose God's side,—He will give us enabling strength to resist tempation and obey His law.

Each person shall decide for himself whether he wants to be saved or lost; and those who are redeemed will, through the grace of Christ, have carried that decision to success.

"Let him that heareth say, Come. And let him that is athirst come. And whosoever will, let him take the water of life freely."—*Revelation 22:17.*

Was the entrance of sin inevitable? No, but the power of choice makes possible the choosing of either good or evil. **The angels in heaven had the power to choose evil, the same power we have down here.**

Because of this, the rise of sin and rebellion was always a possibility lurking in the background. Unfortunately, one day, evil thoughts began in Lucifer's mind.

"Thou wast perfect in thy ways from the day that thou wast created, till iniquity was found in thee."—*Ezekiel 28:15.*

Solomon truly said, "Pride goeth before destruction, and an haughty spirit before a fall" *(Proverbs 16:18).* **Strangely, in the loving, unselfish atmosphere of heaven, Lucifer began thinking he should be first. He became proud.**

"Thine heart was lifted up because of thy beauty, thou hast corrupted thy wisdom by reason of thy brightness."—*Ezekiel 28:17.*

Lucifer decided that he was so great,—that he should be considered a god.

"For thou hast said in thine heart, I will ascend into heaven, I will exalt my throne above the stars of God: I will sit also upon the mount of the congregation, in the sides of the north: I will ascend above the heights of the clouds; I will be like the Most High. Yet thou shalt be brought down to hell, to the sides of the pit."—*Isaiah 14:13-15.*

Because God did not recognize the imagination of this proud angel as correct, Lucifer became jealous, and began falsely complaining to the other angels that he was being mistreated.

Both God and Christ, and the good angels, tried to reason with Lucifer, and also with the angels who began allying with him. But these rebels were determined to gain new rights. **Lucifer said that God's law was unjust and that everyone could make better decisions by not obeying it.**

Why did God not instantly destroy Lucifer as soon as he began sinning? If God had done this, everyone would thereafter have served God from fear, rather than love. The loving Creator had to let each make his own decision. God never uses compulsion

to keep anyone by His side.

Lucifer had said, "I will exalt my throne. I will have a government of my own. I will rebel against God." But in doing this, he ignored the great truth that "whosoever exalteth himself shall be abased" *(Luke 14:11).* He began filling his mind with hatred against God's leadership and government.

Later, when Christ came to earth, He said that Satan was the originator of all lies and murders, because "whosoever hateth his brother is a murderer" *(1 John 3:15).* Christ told some evil men:

"Ye are of your father the devil, and the lusts of your father ye will do. He was a murderer from the beginning, and abode not in the truth, because there is no truth in him. When he speaketh a lie, he speaketh of his own: for he is a liar, and the father of it."—*John 8:44.*

Cloaking himself under a guise of great interest for the well-being of the angels, Lucifer told one lie after another, until he had won many angels to his side. Satan could do what God could not do; he could say that which was not true, and use evil methods, deceptive practices, and lying words.

So it was that Lucifer "the light bearer" became Satan "the adversary."

When every angel in heaven had taken a definite stand either for or against God and His government,—the time had come for Satan and his followers to be cast out of heaven.

"There was war in heaven: Michael and His angels fought against the dragon; and the dragon fought and his angels, and prevailed not; neither was their place found anymore in heaven. And the great dragon was cast out, that old serpent, called the Devil, and Satan, which deceiveth the whole world: he was cast out into the earth, and his angels were cast out with him."—*Revelation 12:7-9.*

The Bible tells us that "Michael" is Christ *(Jude 9; 1 Thessalonians 4:16; John 4:25-29).*

SATAN ENTERS THE GARDEN

Arriving down here, about the time of the Creation of our world, Satan decided to tempt our first parents *(Genesis 1-3).*

Life is full of tests. We need them in order to show on whose side we stand. Adam and Eve had one also. **God specified that they were not to eat the fruit of just one of the multitude of fruit trees in the Garden of Eden. That was the lightest test which could possibly be given**—whether or not they would eat some fruit.

By this simple device man's faith, love, loyalty, and obedience were to be tested. If they disobeyed God's command, they would show that they distrusted His love, disbelieved His Word, and disobeyed His laws. It was as simple as that. *No sin is ever small!* **The** very lightness of the prohibition would make the sin great. It could not be said to have resulted from their inability to do something, for no action was required. Just don't eat that one fruit.

And, God added: If you do eat of it, *you will die.* Why? Because by so doing they would agree with Satan that it was all right to disobey what God said! They would have joined Satan's side.

"And the Lord God took the man, and put him into the garden of Eden to dress it and to keep it. And the Lord God commanded the man, saying, Of every tree of the garden thou mayest freely eat: But of the tree of the knowledge of good and evil, thou shalt not eat of it: for in the day that thou eatest thereof thou shalt surely die."—*Genesis 2:15-17.*

But Adam and Eve failed the simple test. Satan took the form of a snake and was waiting at the forbidden tree. When Eve dared to walk over close to that tree, Satan was ready with deceptive words. Here is what happened:

"Now the serpent was more subtle than any beast of the field which the Lord God had made. And he said unto the woman, Yea, hath God said, Ye shall not eat of every tree of the garden? And the woman said unto the serpent, We may eat of the fruit of the trees of the garden: But of the fruit of the tree which is in the midst of the garden, God hath said, Ye shall not eat of it, neither shall ye touch it, lest ye die.

"And the serpent said unto the woman, **Ye shall not surely die.** For God doth know that in the day ye eat thereof, then your eyes shall be opened, and ye shall be as gods, knowing good and evil.

"And when the woman saw that the tree was good for food, and that it was pleasant to the eyes, and a tree to be desired to make one wise, she took of the fruit thereof, and did eat, and gave also unto her husband with her; and he did eat."—*Genesis 3:1-6.*

Notice that Satan told Eve four specific lies: (1) God is not telling you the truth. (2) You will not die if you eat it. Instead, (3) you yourself will become god, (4) and be filled with far greater wisdom.

Adam and Eve gained nothing by committing that sin. Instead, their minds became confused and filled with worry. Sin always separates us from God, and that is what had happened to them.

"Behold, the Lord's hand is not shortened, that it cannot save; neither His ear heavy, that it cannot hear: But your iniquities have separated between you and your God, and your sins have hid His face from you."—*Isaiah 59:1-2.*

When God came to see them that evening, for the first time in their lives—they were filled with fear. When He asked them what had happened, they began blaming one another and the snake. They were really blaming God and trying to make excuses why their sin was not so bad, for it was not their fault.

THE PROMISE OF A REDEEMER

God had earlier said that the day they ate of the forbidden tree, they would be doomed to finally die an eternal death. But, in the first promise recorded in the Bible, *He now told them that a Redeemer would come later through whom they might be saved!* It was because of the promised Redeemer that they did not die that day. Instead, Speaking to Satan, God said:

"I will put enmity between thee and the woman, and between thy seed and her seed; it shall bruise thy head, and Thou shalt bruise His heel."—*Genesis 3:15.*

What a glorious promise! If we will repent; surrender our lives to God's control; and, through the enabling grace of Christ be obedient to Him,— eventually heaven will be ours, there to live with Christ and holy angels throughout eternity!

As a result of their sin, Adam and Eve had to leave the garden; so they would not continue eating of the Tree of Life, which could keep them from ultimately dying *(Genesis 3:22-24).* Later, their first son killed his younger brother! *(Genesis 4:1, 8).* How quickly one little sin began leading to many more terrible ones!

SATAN CLAIMS DOMINION OVER THE WORLD

Because our first parents and their descendants sinned, Satan was able to try to gain control of our planet. Mankind had, by their sinning, chosen the devil as their leader.

"While they promise them liberty, they themselves are the servants of corruption: for of whom a man is overcome, of the same is he brought in bondage."—*2 Peter 2:19.*

When God created our world, He gave the dominion—the control of it—to our first parents *(Genesis 1:28).* But Satan usurped that dominion.

"The god of this world hath blinded the minds of them which believe not, lest the light of the glorious gospel of Christ, who is the image of God, should shine unto them."—*2 Corinthians 4:4.*

Satan claimed this dominion to be his, when he tempted Christ:

"The devil said unto Him, All this power will I give Thee, and the glory of them: for that is delivered unto me; and to whomsoever I will I give it. If Thou therefore wilt worship me, all shall be Thine."—*Luke 4:6-7.*

When the devil tempts you and me,—he uses the same kind of lying reasoning!

W
A
Y

Christ, by His life of obedience and His death on the cross, recovered the lost dominion. He made possible the restoration of man and all that man had lost.

"For the Son of man is come to seek and to save that which was lost."—*Luke 19:10*.

HOW SATAN WORKS

There was no reason for sin. To give a reason would be to justify the deed. To offer an excuse would be inexcusable. At first in heaven, Lucifer had everything that God could give him, except being part of the Godhead. But he believed his own lies which he imagined out of nothing. Later, down here on earth, man, who had every possible blessing, also chose to believe the devil's lies.

Jesus called Satan "the prince of this world" *(John 12:31; 14:30)*. Paul said he was "the prince of the power of the air" *(Ephesians 2:2)*. The Pharisees called Him "the prince of devils" *(Matthew 12:24)*.

Satan is the "accuser of our brethren" *(Revelation 12:10)*; "your adversary" *(1 Peter 5:8)*; and "the spirit that now worketh in the children of disobedience" *(Ephesians 2:2)*.

In the Bible, the work of Satan is compared with a hunter setting out snares *(Psalm 91:3)*, to a wolf ravaging the flock *(John 10:12)*, and to a lion seeking to catch and devour his prey *(1 Peter 5:8)*.

Satan has special methods of getting people to follow him to destruction. The following true story illustrates one way this is done:

Over a hundred years ago, a preacher named Rowland Hill was walking on a country street when **he saw a drove of pigs following a man**. Intrigued, he followed the procession—and found that the man led the pigs to the slaughterhouse! Astonished, Hill asked the man how this was done, and was told this: "Oh, you did not notice. I was carrying a sack of beans, and I dropped a few as I went along—and the pigs kept following me. It works every time."

There is a parallel story, which not only contrasts the methods of Christ and Satan, but also reveals another method of Satan:

There was a party of tourists in Palestine. The guide who was with them was explaining the interesting customs of the Near East. He said, "In the West, the shepherd and his dog drive the sheep, but over here the opposite occurs. The shepherd always leads his sheep, going on before them. They know his voice and they follow him, as we read in Scripture: "My sheep hear My voice, and I know them, and they follow Me" *(John 10:27)*.

Just then, they saw a man driving a flock of sheep down the road. Startled, the guide asked him what he was doing. The reply was, "You are right, shepherds over here lead their sheep. **But I am not a**

shepherd. **I am the butcher**, and I am driving them to market."

Satan has two methods. He keeps offering little trinkets and apparent pleasures to keep people in his ranks. He then affects their minds and tries to drive them relentlessly into resentments, depression, violence, and worse.

But regardless whether he has been captured by beans or a storm of sinful emotions, a person can, if he chooses to do so, immediately flee to God in prayer—and Satan will be forced to flee.

FIVE FACTS ABOUT SIN

Here are five crucial facts about sin:

First, as mentioned earlier, it is the transgression of God's law.

"Whosoever committeth sin transgresseth also the law: for sin is the transgression of the law."—*1 John 3:4*.

The second fact is that, unless repented of and forsaken, it always leads to an eternal death.

"For the wages of sin is death; but the gift of God is eternal life through Jesus Christ our Lord."—*Romans 6:23*.

"Every man is tempted, when he is drawn away of his own lust, and enticed. Then when lust hath conceived, it bringeth forth sin: and sin, when it is finished, bringeth forth death."—*James 1:14-15*.

The third fact is that Christ died to help us stop sinning.

"He was manifested to take away our sins; and in Him is no sin. Whosoever abideth in Him sinneth not: whosoever sinneth hath not seen Him, neither known Him. Little children, let no man deceive you: he that doeth righteousness is righteous, even as He is righteous. He that committeth sin is of the devil; for the devil sinneth from the beginning. For this purpose the Son of God was manifested, that He might destroy the works of the devil. Whosoever is born of God doth not commit sin."—*1 John 3:5-9*.

The fourth fact is that, in mercy, God keeps giving us time to repent and return to Him. —And to those willing to come, God gives them the strength to do so!

"The Lord is not slack concerning His promise, as some men count slackness; but is longsuffering to us-ward, not willing that any should perish, but that all should come to repentance."—*2 Peter 3:9*.

"For I have no pleasure in the death of him that dieth, saith the Lord God: wherefore turn yourselves, and live ye."—*Ezekiel 18:32*.

"And the Spirit and the bride say, Come. And let him that heareth say, Come. And let him that is athirst come. And whosoever will, let him take the water of life freely."—*Revelation 22:17*.

The fifth fact is that God is going to step in before long—and put a stop to sin and unrepentant sinners. Sin will never arise again after that.

We dare not wait! It is now that we must make our decision to remain God's faithful, obedient children to the end!

"But the day of the Lord will come as a thief in the night; in the which the heavens shall pass away with a great noise, and the elements shall melt with fervent heat, the earth also and the works that are therein shall be burned up.

"Seeing then that all these things shall be dissolved, what manner of persons ought ye to be in all holy conversation and godliness, looking for and hasting unto the coming of the day of God, wherein the heavens being on fire shall be dissolved, and the elements shall melt with fervent heat? Nevertheless we, according to His promise, look for new heavens and a new earth, wherein dwelleth righteousness.

"Wherefore, beloved, seeing that ye look for such things, be diligent that ye may be found of Him in peace, without spot, and blameless."—*2 Peter 3:10-14*.

"What do ye imagine against the Lord? He will make an utter end: affliction shall not rise up the second time."—*Nahum 1:9*.

"And God shall wipe away all tears from their eyes; and there shall be no more death, neither sorrow, nor crying, neither shall there be anymore pain: for the former things are passed away."—*Revelation 21:4*.

IT IS TIME TO MAKE YOUR OWN DECISION

Keep in mind that it was impossible for Eve in Eden to believe what the devil said—*without first doubting* the words of God.

"In the Judgment, men will not be condemned because they conscientiously believed a lie, but because they did not believe the truth, because they neglected the opportunity of learning what is truth."—*Patriarchs and Prophets, 55*.

Our safety lies in loving and obeying the truths of God's Word, and remaining loyal to God.

"The working of Satan with all power and signs and lying wonders, and with all deceivableness of unrighteousness in them that perish; because they received not the love of the truth, that they might be saved."—*2 Thessalonians 2:9-10*.

Eve distrusted God's love, doubted His Word, and transgressed His law. She disobeyed His express words. She sinned.

"O could we know the love that bendeth o'er us, O could we understand the Father's heart,

Hear how the angels chant their loving chorus.

"But when down our cheeks the bitter teardrops start, See how all Heaven is moved to consolation, And all the mysteries of Calvary mark.

"We should not doubt the coming of salvation, Not think all hope is lost when it is dark."
—*Fanny Bolton*

To His faithful children in every age, Jesus says, "in the world ye shall have tribulation: but be of good cheer; I have overcome the world" *(John 16:33)*. It was Richard Baxter who said, "The way may seem strange to me, but not to Christ."

"Then trust in God through all thy days; Fear not, for He doth hold thy hand; Though dark thy way, still sing and praise, Sometime, sometime, we'll understand."

Man is not foredoomed to evil or predestined to good. There are two ways, two principles, two powers. There is the upward way, and there is the downward way. There is the good principle, and there is the evil principle. There is the power of Christ, and there is the power of Satan.

"Once to every man and nation comes the moment to decide, In the strife of Truth with Falsehood, for the good or evil side."
—*James Russell Lowell*

Which way shall we take? Which principle shall reign within us? Who shall be our master, Christ or Satan? The choice is ours. A delicate balance scale, that will determine our destiny, has been entrusted to each one of us. God will not tip it. Christ will not force it. Angels may not touch it. Satan cannot move it. **Only man, by casting in the weight of his own personal choice**, may decide which way the horizontal beam on the scale moves—down or up,—and what power shall be dominant in his life.

Back in the time of Rome, there were great open-air theaters that even today remain scattered over the Greco-Roman world.

This earth is a mighty stage and a great drama is going on. The controversy between good and evil is being played to its very end—as every person in the world chooses whom he will serve. On this gigantic stage, the principles of both the kingdom of God and the kingdom of Satan are being worked out, side by side.

We are nearing the end. When it comes, the whole universe will see that love is stronger than sin and that God has been good and just in all that He did and still does. When the curtain falls on evil down here, there will be no more sin or sorrow, nothing wrong with the universe, only eternal harmony and happiness.

William E. Henley concluded his atheist work, *Invictus*, with these words: "I am the master of my fate; I am the captain of my soul." Although strangely proud of the fact that he was going to die separated from God and eternal life, yet that sentence by Henley is true. **Each of us does decide the master we will serve!** It is within our power to determine whether we will accept Christ or live in captivity to the devil and die in the misery of our sins.

HOW TO OVERCOME THE DEVIL

There are three things which, in the strength of Christ, we can do to overcome Satan:

First, we can individually go to Calvary and, kneeling there, cry to God every day for help. "They overcame him by the blood of the Lamb" *(Revelation 12:11).* Although Satan sought to make Golgotha the final hour of defeat, Jesus made it the glorious, triumphant hour of victory.

"That through death, He might destroy him that had the power of death, that is, the devil."— *Hebrews 2:14.*

Begin your journey to heaven at the cross of Calvary. Keep close to Christ all along the pathway of enabled obedience—all the way to heaven.

The second thing we can do to resist Satan is to use the powerful "sword of the Spirit, which is the Word of God" *(Ephesians 6:17).*

Christ overcame Satan in the wilderness of temptation through "It is written." Three times that day Christ used the Bible to withstand the devil's attacks *(Matthew 4:1-10).*

The third thing is to "resist the devil and he will flee from you" *(James 4:7).* Down through the ages, the faithful "overcame him . . by the word of their testimony" *(Revelation 12:11).*

We must "contend for the faith which was once delivered to the saints" *(Jude 3).* We must speak up and bear our testimony for God, for Christ, and for the truths of His Word. We must stand up and be counted for God; and, taking the shield of faith and the sword of the Spirit,—go forth to "fight the good fight of faith," thus laying "hold on eternal life" *(1 Timothy 6:12).*

A young man attending college was noted for his Christian character. One morning the president of the college called him to his office for a personal interview. Questioning the youth about his spiritual experience, his heart was warmed with the young man's answers. "**I would give all I have in this world to have what you possess**," said the president.

"**Then you may have it, sir**," was the student's reply. "**That is exactly what it takes**. That is what it cost me."

———

COMING NEXT—The Bible truth about what happens when a man dies. This is a very important subject which you will want to understand.

W
A
Y

Chapter Ten

Eternal Life Only through Christ
What the Bible Says about Death

"I'll give a million dollars for each year you can add to my life," a wealthy American said to his medical advisers when he was eighty years old.

"Millions of money for an inch of time!" cried Queen Elizabeth I, the queen of England in 1603, upon her dying bed. Unhappy woman, reclining upon a couch, with ten thousand dresses in her wardrobe, a kingdom on which the sun never sets, at her feet—all now valueless. She had lived 70 years and ruled 45 years, yet never had time to come to Christ.

In contrast, Queen Victoria on her deathbed, called for her beloved hymn to be sung: "Rock of Ages, cleft for me. Let me hide myself in Thee." "It is enough," she said, "I am still with Him and will see Him at the resurrection!" She had lived 82 years and ruled 63 years, yet amid all her activities, she made Christ her personal Saviour.

The two most important queens in British history—yet how differently did each of their lives end!

Some time ago, a businessman was seated at his dinner table reading aloud a letter he had just received from a friend. "And so his illness grew suddenly worse until the doctors admitted that they could do nothing for him. A few weeks later he died. Then—

"Daddy, what does 'die' mean?" asked his little girl, looking up from her plate. Everyone said nothing. They could think of nothing to say. Yet few subjects are more clearly explained in the Bible.

The ancient Christians of Rome, so heavily persecuted for their faith, would gather about their loved ones in the Catacombs as they were dying, and sing, "Good night, beloved, sleep and take your rest. Lay down your head upon the Saviour's breast."

When death comes, some are ready, and some are not. This chapter will give you information you need to know. It will help you get ready.

WHAT IS MORTAL AND IMMORTAL?

Men wish they could live forever, but they are mortal. The word means "subject to death, destined to die." In contrast, the word, "immortal," means "not mortal; exempt from liability to die; imperishable; everlasting" *(Webster's New International Dictionary).*

Did God plan that sinless man, created in the image of God, should die? All will agree that He did not. God made man to live.

But our Creator did not purpose that man should live if he sinned. This is how it was explained to Adam:

"Of the tree of the knowledge of good and evil, thou shalt not eat of it: for in the day that thou eatest thereof **thou shalt surely die**."—*Genesis 2:17.*

The Hebrew original reads "dying thou shalt die." This means **the day you eat it you will begin to die; and, after a time, you will be entirely dead.** The sentence of death would be pronounced the day that man sinned, and the process of dying would immediately begin.

Denying this definite statement of God's, Satan told Eve, "Ye shall not surely die" (*Genesis 3:4*). But Christ said the devil was a liar *(John 8:44).*

Eve believed the words of Satan because they seemed more pleasant than the words of God. Men and women are still doing that.

The evening of the day that our first parents chose to sin, God told them, "Dust thou art, and unto dust shalt thou return" *(Genesis 3:19).*

However, there was another tree in the garden, the fruit of which would extend life, if one continued to eat of it. This was the Tree of Life. But Adam and Eve were told that they would have to leave the Garden of Eden, for they could no longer be permitted to eat of the life-sustaining tree.

WHO HAS IMMORTALITY?

Mark this in your mind: **The Bible teaches that God did not intend that sinners should live forever.** Even though it may be taught from a thousand pulpits, and printed in an equal number of books, the Bible says sinners will not live forever.

So, from what we have learned already, man was created with the *possibility* of immortality, on condition that he meet the test of obedience. **But he was not created with *inherent* immortality.** He was "subject to death" if he sinned, and was therefore "mortal." **There are no immortal sinners** and never will be, regardless of what anyone tells you.

About man, the Bible says, "Shall mortal man be more just than God?" *(Job 4:17).*

About God, the good Book says, "Who only hath immortality" *(1 Timothy 6:16).*

In other words, God is immortal and man is mortal. In fact, the word *"immortal"* is found but once in the Bible and is applied to God:

"Now unto the King eternal, immortal, invisible, the only wise God, be honour and glory forever and ever."—*1 Timothy 1:17.*

Man does not have innate (inherent) immortality. The theory of the natural immortality of the soul originated in paganism, and was adopted into the Christian church by the apostate church in the Dark Ages. Martin Luther said it was one of the "monstrous fables that form part of the Roman dunghill of decretals" (quoted in E. Petavel, The Problem of Immortality, p. 255). Commenting on the words of Solomon in Ecclesiastes 9:5-6, that the dead know not anything, the Reformer wrote:

"[This is] another place proving that the dead have no . . feeling. There is, saith he, no duty, no science, no knowledge, no wisdom there. Solomon judgeth that the dead are asleep, and feel nothing at all. For the dead lie there, accounting neither days nor years, but when they are awaked, they shall seem to have slept scarce one minute."—*Martin Luther, Exposition of Solomon's Book Called Ecclesiastes, p. 152.*

There is a profound lesson in the following story:
One evening, King Charles II stopped in at a meeting of the Royal Society of England, which was attended by the leading scientists of the nation.

The king said something like this: "Suppose I take a pail of water and it tips the beam of the scale at 10 pounds. Then I drop into the water 5 pounds of live fish. Why is it that, instead of now being 15 pounds, the scale still stands at 10 pounds?"

Various wise men arose and, in profound and complex words, suggested that air-filled fish sacs, theoretical vacuum, or nongravitating gravity might be the cause.

Then the king spoke. "You are all wrong, because when you add 5 pounds of fish to 10 pounds of water, you get a total weight of 15 pounds,—*as you learned gentlemen should all well know.*"

These men had been misled by trusting too much to a prominent man. Men and women today are still doing that.

Let us turn to the Bible, which will always lead us aright. Here are four facts it presents us with:
Man only is mortal.
"Shall mortal man be more just than God?"—*Job 4:17.*
God is immortal.
"Now unto the King eternal, immortal, invisible."—*1 Timothy 1:17.*
Only God has immortality.
"Who only hath immortality."—*1 Timothy 6:16.*
Man must seek for immortality.
"To them who by patient continuance in well doing seek for glory and honour and immortality, eternal life."—*Romans 2:7.*

WHO ONLY WILL RECEIVE IMMORTALITY?

The possibility of receiving immortality is only possible through the gospel; that is, through Christ.

"Our Saviour Jesus Christ, who hath abolished death, and hath brought life and immortality to light through the gospel."—*2 Timothy 1:10.*

It will not be given until the Second Advent, and only to God's faithful followers.

"Behold, I show you a mystery. We shall not all

sleep, but we shall all be changed, in a moment, in the twinkling of an eye, at the last trump: for the trumpet shall sound, and the dead shall be raised incorruptible, and we shall be changed. For this corruptible must put on incorruption, and this mortal must put on immortality. So when this corruptible shall have put on incorruption, and this mortal shall have put on immortality, then shall be brought to pass the saying that is written, Death is swallowed up in victory. O death, where is thy sting? O grave, where is thy victory?"—*1 Corinthians 15:51-55.*

In view of these Bible facts, it is strange that some still imagine that man has something immortal about him which not even God can destroy. This is stranger than the king's scientists who were talked into believing that 10 + 5 = 10.

SOUL NOT SEPARATE FROM THE BODY

Man does not have a separate "living soul." However, someone will say, "But man is a living soul, and therefore cannot die." Well, *what does the Bible say about this?* Here is the record:

"The Lord God formed man of the dust of the ground, and breathed into his nostrils the breath of life; and man **became** a living soul."—*Genesis 2:7.*

First, God made Adam's body from the dust of the ground. Any scientist will tell you that we consist of minerals to be found in the ground and in the air.

Second, God breathed into Adam's nostrils *the breath of life.* **Here is no indication of any "immortal soul" being put into Adam.** No such "spirit Adam" ever existed. None was here created. God simply breathed into his nostrils the breath of life.

As a result, "man *became a living soul.*"

Body + breath of life = a living soul! Note carefully: God did not breathe into Adam a living soul, but only the breath of life. **As a result, the man *became* a living soul.**

By itself an electric light bulb gives no light. But, when electricity is sent into its inner wiring, light is produced.

Adam's body, lying on the ground was useless, until God switched on the current of life—and Adam became a living, active, functioning living soul.

Only while the switch is on does man have life and a soul.

SOUL AND SPIRIT

The Hebrew and Greek words from which we translate our English words, *soul* and *spirit,* are found about 1,700 times in the Bible. Actually, the word *soul* as used in the Bible does not always have exactly the same meaning. The same holds true of the word *spirit.*

But in not one of the 1,700 places is either soul or spirit said to be immortal, never dying, imperishable, indestructible, everlasting, eternal, or having immortality.

Nor are the dead said to have a conscious existence apart from the body.

Did you know that, in the Bible, animals also have "the breath of life" *(Genesis 7:15)*? This is because they are also living beings. In Genesis 7:22, margin, they are said to have "the breath of the spirit of life."

(Actually, the words, "breath" and "spirit," which come from the same Hebrew word, are interchangeable in many passages. For example, James 2:26 has "the body without the spirit is dead." In the margin, we find "breath" instead: "The body without the breath is dead." It is the breath which keeps the body alive. In Job 27:3, we read "All the while my breath is in me, and the spirit of God is in my nostrils." The margin says it may be translated "breath.")

Just like us, an animal may have a perfect body, but it may be perfectly dead. *It also must have the current of life switched on, in order to be alive.*

We are told that animals also have life *(Genesis 1:30).* The margin of that passage reads "a living soul" instead of "life."

WE NEED ETERNAL LIFE!

When God breathed life into Adam, He was putting life into the masterpiece of earthly creation. Our bodies and minds are amazing! The psalmist said:

"I will praise Thee; for I am fearfully and wonderfully made: marvelous are Thy works."—*Psalm 139:14.*

Indeed, we are even told that we are not far below the angels!

"What is man, that Thou art mindful of him? and the son of man, that Thou visitest him? For Thou hast made him a little lower than the angels, and hast crowned him with glory and honour."—*Psalm 8:4-5.*

Yet man is nothing without life. What he needs is eternal life!

We can only have life—life that lasts forever—through a connection with Jesus Christ! Here is what the Bible teaches about this:

"He that believeth on the Son of God hath the witness in himself: he that believeth not God hath made Him a liar; because he believeth not the record that God gave of His Son.

"And this is the record, that God hath given to us eternal life, and this life is in His Son. He that hath the Son hath life; and he that hath not the Son of God hath not life."—*1 John 5:10-12.*

"For God so loved the world, that He gave His only begotten Son, that whosoever believeth in Him should not perish, but have everlasting life."—*John 3:16.*

Only Jesus "hath brought life and immortality to light through the gospel" *(2 Timothy 1:10).*

We can conclude that **man does not by nature possess an immortal soul**. It takes the body and the spirit (or breath) of life together to make a living soul. Christ came to save all there is of man. For this to be done we must let Him sanctify all there is of us.

In order to possess immortality, man must acquire it; and, since immortality is an attribute of God, it can be obtained by man only as a gift from the One who possesses it. This is why Paul declared that the gift of God is eternal life through Jesus Christ our Lord.

"Who will render to every man according to his deeds: to them who by patient continuance in well doing seek for glory and honour and immortality, eternal life."—*Romans 2:6-7.*

It is the way of the cross which leads to immortality. Christ gave us the promise:

"Be thou faithful unto death, and I will give thee a crown of life."—*Revelation 2:10.*

He also said:

"For whosoever will save his life shall lose it: and whosoever will lose his life for My sake shall find it."—*Matthew 16:25.*

That is a sentence worth thinking about a long time. **Christ is telling us, "You cannot have life, unless you come to Me."** "Please come," He says, "I am waiting!" Submission and willing obedience to God's will is the only road to holiness, heaven, and immortality.

A person who weighs 140 pounds contains enough fat for seven cakes of soap, carbon for 9,000 lead pencils, phosphorus for 2,000 match heads, magnesium for one dose of Epsom salts, iron enough to make one medium-sized nail, sufficient lime to whitewash a chicken coop, enough suphur to rid one dog of fleas, and water enough to fill a ten-gallon can.

—Yet if that person accepts Christ as his Saviour, and lives all his days in cheerful obedience to his Lord and Master—*he can inherit eternal life!*

THE JOURNEY TO DEATH

What happens when a man dies? We want to find out. Only the Bible can tell us the truth of the matter.

Dr. Alexander Bogomoletz was a Russian scientist who believed he could devise a serum which would retard the aging of the body's connective tissues. This scientist was determined to extend human life to 150 years.

He called his chemical solution ACS, or *"antireticular cytotoxic serum."* But the doctor died at the age of 64, or 86 years short of the mark. His heart gave out when he took his own serum.

—However, whether a man lives to be 70 or 170,

he is still short of what God originally planned for him: *a life that measures with the life of God, a life that continues on forever!*

And this is still in God's plan! But it is only for those who accept Jesus Christ as their Saviour, and humbly, obediently, live their lives as truehearted followers of the Lamb of God.

Yet, because of sin, "it is appointed unto men once to die" *(Hebrews 9:27).* That death is the death we all experience. Most men will die twice; Christians, but once.

The unsaved of earth will die twice. The first death, which is the common lot of all men, is temporary. **The *second death*, which will be experienced only by the wicked, will be eternal.** The gospel of Christ does not save men from the first death; but it promises emphatically that the righteous "shall not be hurt of the second death," for over them it shall have "no power." See *Revelation 2:11; 20:6.* More on that second death in the next chapter.

According to a 2008 U.S. Census Bureau Report, 55.5 million people die every year; 6,300 die every month; and 105 every minute.

"There is no man that hath power over the spirit to retain the spirit; neither hath he power in the day of death."—*Ecclesiastes 8:8.*

One man has described the journey of life:

"Ten thousand human beings set forth together on their journey. After ten years, at least a third have disappeared. At the midpoint of the usual measure of life, but half are still on the road.

"Faster and faster the ranks grow thinner. Nearly all that remained until now grow weary and lie down to rise no more.

"At ninety these have been reduced to a handful of trembling patriarchs . . One lingers, perhaps, a lonely marvel till the century is over. We look again and the work of death is finished."—*Burgess*

"One dieth in his full strength, being wholly at ease and quiet . . Another dieth in the bitterness of his soul" *(Job 21:23-25).* Death's sharpest impact comes to those with plenty, yet who are unprepared.

"How shocking must thy summons be, O Death, To him that is at ease in his possessions; Who counting on long years of pleasure here, Is quite unfurnished for that world to come!"

—*Robert Blair, "The Grave"*

WHAT HAPPENS AT DEATH?

In the beginning—

"The Lord God formed man of the dust of the ground, and breathed into his nostrils the breath of life; and man became a living soul."—*Genesis 2:7.*

When man was created, his body was **first formed of dust**. **Then God breathed** the breath of life into him and man *became* "a living soul." It is the combination of the two (dust and the breath of life) that makes man a "living soul." **He does not have a soul that is separate from his body!** Only while the breath of life is in him, does man have life and a living soul.

When the breath of life is removed at his death, he ceases to be a living soul. He ceases to be alive. Man does not have a separate "spirit," nor does he have immortality.

While he is alive:

Body + breath of life = a living soul

When a man dies:

Body – (minus) breath of life = a dead body

God did not breathe into Adam a living soul, but only the breath of life. As a result, the man *became* a living soul. At death, the breath of life departed; and there was nothing left but a dead person, who is then buried.

So we see that, **at death, the opposite of the creative process occurs**. First "his breath goes forth" (*Psalm 146:4*). This is because, as Job explained, "The breath of the Almighty hath given me life" (*Job 33:4*). And again, "The spirit of God is in my nostrils" *Job 27:3).* This is the "spirit of life" which God gives to all men; which, at death, is removed from him. "The spirit shall return unto God who gave it" (*Ecclesiastes 12:7*).

"His breath goeth forth, he returneth to his earth; in that very day his thoughts perish."— *Psalm 146:4.*

(The Hebrew word for "breath" and "spirit" is the same.)

Here is the complete equation in the Bible:

When man is given life, and while he has it:

"The Lord God formed man of the dust of the ground, and breathed into his nostrils the breath of life; and man became a living soul."— *Genesis 2:7.*

Body + breath of life = a living soul

When a man dies, and no longer has life:

"Then shall the dust return to the earth as it was: and the spirit shall return unto God who gave it."—*Ecclesiastes 12:7.*

Body – (minus) breath of life = a dead body

Here is an illustration which will help explain this:

A boy takes six wooden boards, and nails them together. The result is a box.

Boards + nails = box

Then he removes the nails from the wood, and there is no more box.

Boards – (minus) nails = no box

The box came from the combination of the boards and the nails. **When separated, there is no more box. It did not go anywhere; it just ceased to be a box.**

Now for a second illustration:

Here is a candle. It stands ready to give light, but it has no light of its own. We strike a match and light the wick. Then we have a lighted candle. Blow on the flame of the candle and it goes out. Where did it go? Out—that is all. And with the passing of the flame, the light also goes out.

Man is like that candle. **It takes divine energy to light him—to impart life to him. God strikes the match and man is a living soul.** Intelligence shines out of that human being. But **when the life is snuffed out of that man, the light goes out. The living soul dies.** Intelligence can no more be a part of that dead man than can the extinguished flame be a part of the candle. Like the flame, the soul, or life, has gone out. The human organization disintegrates in death.

Death is an enemy. It robs us of life. But death will not reign in this old world forever. Someday its power will be broken, and it too will be destroyed, never again to haunt the footsteps of a people redeemed from the grave and living with Christ forever.

In God's blessed tomorrow we shall be reunited with loved ones "whom we have loved . . and lost awhile." We are looking forward to that!

WHERE DOES A MAN GO AT DEATH?

At death, a man goes to the grave and remains there.

"What man is he that liveth, and shall not see death? shall he deliver his soul from the hand of the grave?"—*Psalm 89:48.*

"For I know that Thou wilt bring me to death, and to the house appointed for all living."—*Job 30:23.*

"All go unto one place; all are of the dust, and all turn to dust again."—*Ecclesiastes 3:20.*

HOW MUCH DOES HE KNOW AFTER DEATH?

A lawyer once told a judge that he had eight reasons why his client was not present in court. Then, starting to enumerate them all, he said the first was that his client was dead. Immediately, the judge interrupted him and said he did not need to mention the others, as his first reason was sufficient.

At death, a man's thoughts cease.

"Put not your trust in princes, nor in the son of man, in whom there is no help. His breath goeth forth, he returneth to his earth; in that very day his thoughts perish."—*Psalm 146:3-4.*

"For the living know that they shall die: but the dead know not any thing."—*Ecclesiastes 9:5.*

"For in death there is no remembrance of Thee."—*Psalm 6:5.*

"His sons come to honour, and he knoweth it not; and they are brought low, but he perceiveth it not of them."—*Job 14:21.*

"If I wait, the grave is mine house: I have made my bed in the darkness."—*Job 17:13.*

"Whatsoever thy hand findeth to do, do it with thy might; for there is no work, nor device, nor knowledge, nor wisdom, in the grave, whither thou goest."—*Ecclesiastes 9:10.*

What of the feelings and emotions? Do they also cease at death? —***All a person's thought processes end at death!***

"Also their love, and their hatred, and their envy, is now perished."—*Ecclesiastes 9:6.*

The Scripture is plain. **When death comes, all thinking and feeling end.** —If they do not, then the Bible is false and unreliable. **Thinking and feeling did not exist before God breathed life into man, and they stop entirely when the man dies.** When the electric current is turned off, the bulb is there, but the light is gone.

There is no probationary opportunity to accept Christ after the grave, for all thought and action has ceased. **If we are to be saved, it must be done during these present probationary hours.** None of us can know how soon we might have an accident and sudden death.

WHERE THE ERROR CAME FROM

Who started the theory of natural immortality? Who started this peculiar error that man has an immortal soul and lives forever? **It began in ancient Egypt, and spread throughout the world.** The Egyptians believed that man lives forever after death. The Hindus in India added to that yet another error—that man has lived forever *both before and after* he lives here on earth. That is the theory of reincarnation.

But the belief in natural or innate immortality actually started with Satan in the Garden of Eden. **God had said, "Thou shalt surely die"** *(Genesis 2:17).* **The devil said, *"Ye shall not surely die"*** *(Genesis 3:4).*

Countless millions live in fear and religious tyranny because of the devil's lie that there is continuing life—and even endless suffering—after death. (More on this in the next chapter.)

But the Bible teaches that, after man sinned, God removed him from the tree of life, lest he live forever *(Genesis 3:22-23).* God did not purpose to have everlasting sinners.

WHAT IS DEATH LIKE?

It is like a sound sleep. There is no consciousness, for the brain is totally gone. When David is resurrected it will seem but the next instant after he died: "the twinkling of the eye," as it were.

In the Bible, it is significant that death is called "sleep" 54 times. Paul said this about death:

"But I would not have you to be ignorant, brethren, concerning them which are asleep, that ye sorrow not, even as others which have no hope."—*1 Thessalonians 4:13 (also 1 Corinthians 15:18-20).*

The Bible is very certain about this matter: "The dead know not any thing" *(Ecclesiastes 9:5).*

The prophet Daniel wrote: "Many of them that sleep in the dust of the earth shall awake, some to everlasting life, and some to shame and everlasting contempt." *Daniel 12:2.*

Jesus described death in very clear words:

"Our friend Lazarus sleepeth; but I go, that I may awake him out of sleep. Then said His disciples, Lord, if he sleep, he shall do well. Howbeit Jesus spake of his death: but they thought that He had spoken of taking of rest in sleep. Then said Jesus unto them plainly, Lazarus is dead."—*John 11:11-14.*

Thomas Gray, in his well-known poem *"Elegy Written in a Country Churchyard,"* wrote this:

"The boast of heraldry, the pomp of power, And all that beauty, all that wealth e'er gave, Await alike the inevitable hour: **The paths of glory lead but to the grave.**

"Can storied urn or animated bust, Back to its mansion call the fleeting breath? Can Honor's voice provoke the silent dust, Or Flattery soothe the dull cold ear of Death?"

THERE IS HOPE BEYOND THE GRAVE

Is there hope beyond the grave? Yes, there is! for the faithful who, during this life loved God and served Him!

The promise is given us in the Old Testament:

"I will ransom them from the power of the grave; I will redeem them from death: O death, I will be thy plagues; O grave, I will be thy destruction."—*Hosea 13:14.*

Two prominent men were avowed skeptics. One was the eminent Gilbert West; the other was Lord Lyttelton, the famous English statesman. The two men agreed that Christianity should be destroyed. But they decided that, in order to do it, they must disprove His resurrection. If Christ was not raised from the dead, they said, He could not later raise anyone else from the grave.

The two men divided the task between them. At a much later time, they once again met to compare notes. Both had been confronted with the indisputable facts about the resurrection. Each one confessed that a remarkable change had occurred in his own life as a result of having, through his study, met the risen Christ—and each had become a confirmed Christian!

THE TRUTH OF THE RESURRECTION

The error, that the righteous dead go to heaven when they die, undermines—and destroys—the great truth of the resurrection!

W
A
Y

But the clear teaching of the Bible is that there will be a resurrection. It is as certain as the fact that Christ has already risen from the dead.

"If Christ be not raised, your faith is vain; ye are yet in your sins. Then they also which are fallen asleep in Christ are perished. If in this life only we have hope in Christ, we are of all men most miserable.

"But now is Christ risen from the dead, and become the firstfruits of them that slept.

"For since by man came death, by man came also the resurrection of the dead. For as in Adam all die, even so in Christ shall all be made alive.

"But every man in his own order: Christ the firstfruits; afterward they that are Christ's at His coming."—*1 Corinthians 15:17-23.*

Christ is the source of life. If we have Christ, we have the promise of life! There may be an interruption for a time in the silence of the grave, but afterward, the joyful reunion with Him forever.

Because Christ was raised from the dead, just so surely His faithful ones will one day soon, at Christ's Second Advent, come forth to an eternal, glorious life. Paul said that "Christ" was "the firstfruits of them that slept" *(1 Corinthians 15:20).* Elsewhere he said, "Afterward they that are Christ's at His coming" *(verse 23).*

"For the Lord Himself shall descend from heaven with a shout, with the voice of the archangel, and with the trump of God: and the dead in Christ shall rise first.

"Then we which are alive and remain shall be caught up together with them in the clouds, to meet the Lord in the air: and so shall we ever be with the Lord.

"Wherefore comfort one another with these words."—*1 Thessalonians 4:16-18.*

This is why the resurrection from the dead is the real hope of those who "sorrow not, even as others" *(verse 13).*

But, in addition, the Apostle Paul made it clear that **Christians who live to see the Second Coming of Christ will go to heaven "together with" the resurrected righteous.** They will "not prevent [Old English for "go before"] them which are asleep" *(verse 15).*

Those who have already died will not reach heaven before those who live to see Christ return for His faithful ones.

"God having provided some better thing for us, that they without us should not be made perfect."—*Hebrews 11:40.*

Paul said he would receive his reward at Christ's Second Advent, and not before.

"Henceforth there is laid up for me a crown of righteousness, which the Lord, the righteous judge, shall give me at that day: and not to me only, but unto all them also that love His appearing."—*2 Timothy 4:8.*

Peter declared that a thousand years after David's death, he still was not yet in heaven *(Acts 2:29, 34).*

Paul goes so far as to say that if the dead do not rise, then those who have died believing in Christ are perished; and that is the end of it all *(1 Corinthians 15:16-18).* **How thankful we can be that, for God's faithful ones, death will not be the end of it all!**

THE TIME TO RECEIVE IMMORTALITY

Christ paid the ransom price, by His death on the cross, so His faithful followers could be redeemed from the grave.

"I will ransom them from the power of the grave; I will redeem them from death: O death, I will be thy plagues; O grave, I will be thy destruction."—*Hosea 13:14.*

At Christ's return, all His redeemed ones will, for the first time, receive *immortality*, and will forever keep it!

"Behold, I show you a mystery. We shall not all sleep, but we shall all be changed, in a moment, in the twinkling of an eye, at the last trump: for the trumpet shall sound, and the dead shall be raised incorruptible, and we shall be changed. For this corruptible must put on incorruption, and this mortal must put on immortality. So when this corruptible shall have put on incorruption, and this mortal shall have put on immortality, then shall be brought to pass the saying that is written, Death is swallowed up in victory."—*1 Corinthians 15:51-54.*

"Blessed rest for the weary righteous! Time, be it long or short, is but a moment to them. They sleep; they are awakened by the trump of God to a glorious immortality."—*Great Controversy, 550.*

What will God's faithful ones look like when, at Christ's coming, they will become immortal?

Speaking of Christ and His Second Coming, Paul finishes with these words:

"For our conversation is in heaven; from whence also we look for the Saviour, the Lord Jesus Christ: Who shall change our vile body, that it may be fashioned like unto His glorious body, according to the working whereby He is able even to subdue all things unto Himself."—*Philippians 3:20-21.*

"Whosoever believeth" on Christ will have "everlasting life" *(John 3:16).* Everlasting life is a gift of God to believers. "I am the way, the truth, and the life," said Jesus *(John 14:6).* It is those who follow Him who shall live eternally

"My sheep hear My voice, and I know them, and they follow Me. And I give unto them eternal life; and they shall never perish, neither shall any man pluck them out of My hand."—*John 10:27-28.*

HOW SHOULD WE PREPARE?

What must we do now in order to receive this eternal life?

We must humbly, obediently, follow the Lamb. We must partake of Christ, as we study His Word and put it into our lives. Through His enabling grace, we must daily become more and more like Him.

"Verily, verily, I say unto you, Except ye eat the flesh of the Son of man, and drink His blood, ye have no life in you. Whoso eateth My flesh, and drinketh My blood, hath eternal life; and I will raise him up at the last day."—*John 6:53-54.*

"And this is the record, that God hath given to us eternal life, and this life is in His Son. He that hath the Son hath life; and he that hath not the Son of God hath not life. These things have I written unto you that believe on the name of the Son of God; that ye may know that ye have eternal life, and that ye may believe on the name of the Son of God."—*1 John 5:11-13.*

"He that heareth My Word, and believeth on Him that sent Me, hath everlasting life, and shall not come into condemnation; but is passed from death unto life."—*John 5:24.*

An inscription on a crypt in Allegheny Observatory, University of Pittsburgh, reads:

"We have loved the stars too fondly to be fearful of the night."

If we have seen Jesus, the Light of the world, the Bright and Morning Star, we need never be fearful of the night of death which is ahead of so many of us.

One day, when Michael Faraday, the great scientist, entered his laboratory, he found that one of his workmen had accidently dropped a little, highly valued silver cup into a strong acid bath. Within a short time it had totally dissolved.

Faraday cast in another acid—and soon all of the silver precipitated in the form of a shapeless mass. In a few days it came back from the silversmith a more beautiful cup than before.

So it is at death. The bodies of Christ's faithful ones molder into dust and nothing more can be found of them. But when He shall return,—He will restore to each one a more beautiful body—one which is immortal.

The voice of Jesus, sounding as clear as a trumpet, will, at His Second Coming, open the tomb of every saint; and with the righteous living they will be rewarded together with eternal life with Christ.

"At the sounding of the trumpet, when the saints are gathered home, We will greet each other by the crystal sea; When the Lord Himself from heaven to His glory bids them come, What

a gathering of the faithful that will be!"

What a gathering of the faithful that will be! It will be greater than any church service you have ever attended! Oh, my friend, we must be faithful now, so we can be there at that time!

"Let us sing a song that will cheer us by the way, In a little while we're going home; For the night will end in the everlasting day, In a little while we're going home."

COMING NEXT—What will finally happen to those who have never accepted Christ. Are any of them suffering now? Here are important facts you will want to know.

Chapter Eleven

The Final Death of the Wicked

What the Bible Says about Hell

In a publication of "religious instruction" for children, published a number of years ago, is found the following word picture of hell and its tortures.

"Look into this prison. In the middle of it there is a boy, a young man. He is silent; despair is on him. He stands straight up. His eyes are burning like two burning coals. Two long flames come out of his ears. His breathing is difficult. Sometimes he opens his mouth and a breath of blazing fire rolls out of it.

"But listen! There is a sound just like that of a kettle boiling. Is it really a kettle which is boiling? No; then what is it? Here is what it is:

"The blood is boiling in the scalded veins of that boy. The brain is boiling and bubbling in his head. The marrow is boiling in his bones! Ask him, put the question to him: why is he thus tormented? His answer is, that when he was alive, his blood boiled to do very wicked things, and he did them, and it was for that he went to dancing-houses, public-houses, and theaters.

"Ask him, does he think the punishment greater than he deserves? 'No,' he says, 'my punishment is not greater than I deserve; it is just.' I knew it not so while on earth, but I know now that it is just. There is a just and a terrible God. He is terrible to sinners in hell—but He is just!"—*J. Furniss, "The Sight of Hell," in Tracts for Spiritual Reading, Sec. 27, p. 20.*

At the front of the above booklet, an important churchman wrote that this was good reading for children!

"I have carefully read over this Little Volume for Children and have found nothing whatever in it contrary to the doctrines of Holy Faith; but, on the contrary, a great deal to charm, instruct and edify our youthful classes, for whose benefit it has been written."—*William Meagher, Vicar General, Dublin, Ireland, December 14, 1855.*

It is tragic that such information is given to children to read, *when it is just not true!* It portrays God as an evil beast that everyone should want to run away from. When, in fact, He is our kind, loving heavenly Father. **Yes, there will be hellfire someday,—but it will only be for** *an extremely short period of time*—**and then those who are lost will mercifully no longer exist—forever.** In this chapter we are going to prove this to you from God's Inspired book, the Bible.

There is a time coming when God will do "His work, His strange work; and bring to pass His act, His strange act" *(Isaiah 28:21)*. It will indeed be a *strange act* for the One who died to save all of mankind. It will be a *strange act* for One who prayed while they crucified Him, "Father, forgive them; for they know not what they do" *(Luke 23:34).*

It is a tragedy that millions of people have become unbelievers and skeptics, *because they accepted the error that God will burn people forever!* Many have been driven to insanity by the harrowing thought of unsaved loved ones in the never-ending torments of a burning hell. Yes, it is indeed tragic! Men and women are simply not able to reconcile the false teaching of eternal torment with the wonderful truth of God's deep love for mankind.

The brilliant attorney Robert Ingersoll is an example of one who would not have become a leading infidel—had it not been for a misunderstanding of the truth about the final punishment of the wicked.

When he was a child, Robert's father told him that there were infants in hell not longer than a span in length, who were destined to burn throughout eternity.

Young Robert thought, "If that is what God does, I want nothing to do with Him!" His logical mind correctly recognized that eternal punishment for the sins of a brief lifetime on earth would not be just.

THE TRUTH ABOUT
THE THREE WORDS FOR "HELL"

In the Bible, our English word, "hell," has three meanings:

1 - Our English word, "hell," is sometimes translated from the Hebrew word for the "grave." The Hebrew word frequently used for "grave" is *sheol*. One example would be Psalm 16:10, where *sheol* ("grave") has been translated as "hell."

"For Thou wilt not leave My soul in hell; neither wilt Thou suffer Thine Holy One to see corruption."—*Psalm 16:10.*

The above text is quoted by Peter in Acts 2:27, where the Greek word for "grave" *(hades)* is used. But,

unfortunately, it is incorrectly translated as "hell."

Then, in verse 31, Peter explains that Psalm 16:10 was a prophecy about Christ!

"He seeing this before spake of the resurrection of Christ, that His soul was not left in hell, neither His flesh did see corruption. This Jesus hath God raised up, whereof we all are witnesses."—*Acts 2:31-32.*

Of course, we know that Christ was not burning in hell! In reality, Christ went into the grave at His death after His crucifixion. But He was not left in the grave, but was raised from the dead early on the third day.

The word, *hades*, is used eleven times in the New Testament. In 1 Corinthians 15:55 it is translated "grave." But elsewhere it is translated "hell," signifying the grave or "state in the grave."

2 - Hell correctly signifies a "place of burning." In the New Testament the word is *gehenna, or the "Valley of Hinnom."* This was a deep, narrow glen south of Jerusalem, which was used as a garbage dump, where the bodies of dead animals and city refuse were cast.

What the fire did not destroy, the worms consumed. It was thus a type of *complete* annihilation. *Gehenna*, the place of burning, is used twelve times, and is always translated "hell."

3 - In one place the Greek word for "a place of darkness" is translated as "hell."

"God spared not the angels that sinned, but cast them down to hell, and delivered them into chains of darkness, to be reserved unto judgment."—*2 Peter 2:4.*

The Greek word here is *tartaroo* (derived from *tartarus*), not *gehenna* or *hades*. The above text pictures it as a place of darkness, which describes the darkness surrounding Satan and his angels when they were separated from God and heaven. Wherever Satan and his followers are, a dark cloud of evil and misery surrounds them.

WHERE DO ALL MEN GO AT DEATH?

All men go to the grave at death, that is, to *hades* or *sheol.* Job said,

"For I know that Thou wilt bring me to death, and to the house appointed for all living."—*Job 30:23.*

This house of death is the grave. "If I wait, the grave is mine house" *(Job 17:13).*

The grave is an impartial one, for everyone goes there at death. "There is one event to the righteous, and to the wicked" *(Ecclesiastes 9:2).*

"What man is he that liveth, and shall not see death? shall he deliver his soul from the hand of the grave?"—*Psalm 89:48.*

The rich and the poor, the high and the low, the righteous and the wicked; all go to that place, the grave.

"All go unto one place; all are of the dust, and all turn to dust again."—*Ecclesiastes 3:20.*

Yes, death is an enemy *(1 Corinthians 15:26),* and the grave is not a comforting thought,—but we can thank God that there is hope beyond the grave!

"Blessed are the dead which die in the Lord from henceforth: Yea, saith the Spirit, that they may rest from their labours; and their works do follow them."—*Revelation 14:13.*

And we can also rejoice that **the wicked (and everyone else) slumbers in silence in the grave, rather than screaming in torture and agony. There is no pain in the grave.**

WHEN WILL THE RIGHTEOUS DEAD COME OUT OF THE GRAVE?

God's faithful ones will come out of their graves at the Second Coming of Christ: at the sound of the "last trump: for the trumpet shall sound, and the dead shall be raised incorruptible" *(1 Corinthians 15:52).*

"For the Lord Himself shall descend from heaven with a shout, with the voice of the archangel, and with the trump of God: and the dead in Christ shall rise first:

"Then we which are alive and remain shall be caught up together with them in the clouds, to meet the Lord in the air: and so shall we ever be with the Lord.

"Wherefore comfort one another with these words."—*1 Thessalonians 4:16-18.*

Christ promised His faithful ones that He would one day return for them.

"Let not your heart be troubled: ye believe in God, believe also in Me. In My Father's house are many mansions: if it were not so, I would have told you. I go to prepare a place for you.

"And if I go and prepare a place for you, I will come again, and receive you unto Myself; that where I am, there ye may be also."—*John 14:1-3.*

This promise will soon be fulfilled! At the sound of the "trump of God," the saints who have slept in silence, unconscious of the passing of time, will suddenly be awakened. Some have slumbered for thousands of years; others only for a brief rest in the grave. But, to all, the time will seem the same—as in a moment, or "the twinkling of an eye." They will come forth with faces glowing with joy, health, and immortality,—and will go with Christ to heaven.

WHEN WILL THE WICKED COME OUT OF THE GRAVE?

Paul tells us that **there will be "a resurrection of the dead, both of the just and the unjust"** *(Acts 24:15).* Other passages of Scripture confirm this:

"Many of them that sleep in the dust of the earth shall awake, some to everlasting life, and some to shame and everlasting contempt."—*Daniel 12:2.*

"Marvel not at this: for the hour is coming, in the which all that are in the graves shall hear His voice,

"And shall come forth; they that have done good, unto the resurrection of life; and they that have done evil, unto the resurrection of damnation."—*John 5:28-29.*

The righteous are raised at the Second Advent of Christ. But the wicked are not raised until one thousand years later.

"The rest of the dead lived not again until the thousand years were finished."—*Revelation 20:5.*

This thousand years, or "millennium" as it is called, will be discussed in much greater detail later in this book.

WHAT WILL HAPPEN TO THE WICKED?

Soon after the wicked are resurrected, they together with the devil, his evil angels, death, and the grave, will be cast into the lake of fire *(Revelation 20: 10-15).* **This is the gehenna, the actual burning hell.**

The Apostle Peter declared:

"The Lord knoweth how to deliver the godly out of temptations, and to reserve the unjust unto the day of judgment to be punished."—*2 Peter 2:9.*

He also said that the earth itself is "reserved unto fire against the day of judgment" *(2 Peter 3:7),* and that "the elements shall melt with fervent heat" *(verse 10).*

John explains that **fire will come down from God out of heaven and devour the wicked**, along with the devil, death, and the grave, in a "lake of fire." This is called the "second death" *(Revelation 20:9-14).*

WHERE WILL THIS FIRE OCCUR?

It is important that we understand that **this fire occurs *on the surface of the earth,* not somewhere beneath it!**

"As therefore the tares are gathered and burned in the fire; so shall it be in the end of this world."—*Matthew 13:40.*

"Whose fan is in His hand, and He will thoroughly purge His floor, and gather His wheat into the garner; but He will burn up the chaff with unquenchable fire."—*Matthew 3:12.*

"These both were cast alive into a lake of fire burning with brimstone."—*Revelation 19:20.*

"And death and hell were cast into the lake of fire. This is the second death. And whosoever was not found written in the book of life was cast into the lake of fire."—*Revelation 20:14-15.*

"Fire came down from God out of heaven, and

devoured them."—*Revelation 20:9.*

God has promised that He will bring Satan to ashes upon the earth *(Ezekiel 28:18)*—not underground somewhere.

This fire on the surface of the earth will end in death, not eternal life.

"But the fearful, and unbelieving, and the abominable, and murderers, and whoremongers, and sorcerers, and idolaters, and all liars, shall have their part in the lake which burneth with fire and brimstone: which is the second death."—*Revelation 21:8.*

"He that overcometh shall not be hurt of the second death."—*Revelation 2:11.*

This fact, **that hell will burn on the surface of the earth, provides yet another proof that there could be no burning hell now. It must be yet future—for it is not now burning anywhere in our world.**

Since the wicked perish in this burning gehenna, and the earth itself becomes a molten lake of fire, we can understand more clearly the Bible statement that the wicked will be "recompensed" here on the earth *(Proverbs 11:31),* and that they shall be "brought forth" from the grave to this "day of wrath" *(Job 32:30).*

Jesus Himself said that "the tares are the children of the wicked one," and "as therefore the tares are gathered and burned in the fire; so shall it be in the end of the world" *(Matthew 13:38, 40).*

All of these passages provide ample evidence that the fiery end to the wicked, this fiery hell, is yet future. At the present time, not one person is burning in hell.

Second, this fact also shows **that the burning hell cannot last very long—because the promise has been given to God's faithful ones that** *they* **will inherit the earth!** But they will never be able to inherit it—if the stifling smoke and fire of hell were to continue here forever.

"Blessed are the meek: for they shall inherit the earth."—*Matthew 5:5. (See also Psalm 37:11, 29; Isaiah 65:17-25.)*

"Then shall the righteous shine forth as the sun in the kingdom of their Father."—*Matthew 13:43.*

"But the saints of the Most High shall take the kingdom, and possess the kingdom forever, even forever and ever . .*

"And the kingdom and dominion, and the greatness of the kingdom under the whole heaven, shall be given to the people of the saints of the Most High, whose kingdom is an everlasting kingdom."—*Daniel 7:18, 27.*

The fire will be on the surface of the earth, although not for very long. Then it will end.

ADDITIONAL EVIDENCE THAT THIS FIRE IS YET FUTURE

In a later chapter, we will discuss the future millennium, at the end of which the wicked will be raised from their graves and be burned up. Here are two other passages which show that this hellfire is yet future:

"The harvest is the end of the world; and the reapers are the angels. As therefore the tares are gathered and burned in the fire; so shall it be in the end of this world."—*Matthew 13:39-40.*

"So shall it be at the end of the world: the angels shall come forth, and sever the wicked from among the just, and shall cast them into the furnace of fire."—*Matthew 13:49-50.*

HOW MUCH OF MAN WILL BE CAST INTO THIS FIRE?

The error is taught that only part of people will go into hell. But the Bible teaches that the entire bodies of the wicked will be consumed in it.

Jesus warned us nine times about the "burning" hell, the *gehenna* fire. Here are two of them. They make it clear that **the whole man, soul, and body is cast into hellfire.**

"Fear not them which kill the body, but are not able to kill the soul: but rather fear him which is able to destroy both soul and body in hell."—*Matthew 10:28.*

"If thy hand or thy foot offend thee, cut them off, and cast them from thee: it is better for thee to enter into life halt or maimed, rather than having two hands or two feet to be cast into everlasting fire. And if thine eye offend thee, pluck it out, and cast it from thee: it is better for thee to enter into life with one eye, rather than having two eyes to be cast into hell fire."—*Matthew 18:8-9.*

We have earlier learned that, at death, the entire person goes into the grave,—*and there is no fire in the grave!* All this adds to the evidence that the burning hell is yet future.

WHO IS THE FIRE FOR?

This fire was not intended for people, but for the devil and his angels. However, those who choose Satan as their leader will also be destroyed with him in that fire.

"Then shall He say also unto them on the left hand, Depart from Me, ye cursed, into everlasting fire, prepared for the devil and his angels."—*Matthew 25:41.*

Satan is the root, his followers are the branches. All will alike perish.

"For, behold, the day cometh, that shall burn as an oven; and all the proud, yea, and all that do wickedly, shall be stubble: and the day that cometh shall burn them up, saith the Lord of hosts, that it shall leave them neither root nor branch."—*Malachi 4:1.*

HOW LONG DOES THIS FIRE LAST?

The meaning of everlasting and eternal—**This fire of the future is called "everlasting" or eternal.** "These shall go away into everlasting punishment" *(Matthew 25:46).* **It is a punishment which will end when the fire goes out, but the consequences are everlasting. The wicked receive a punishment which is "everlasting" in its effects.**

The question may be asked: If whatever is cast into this fire is completely consumed, why would the fire always be kept burning? The answer is that it will not.

Sodom and Gomorrah are examples of how this kind of fire works. The Bible says they were totally "destroyed" long ago *(Genesis 19:29; Luke 17:29).* But Jude says they were burned up by "eternal fire."

"Even as Sodom and Gomorrha, and the cities about them in like manner, giving themselves over to fornication, and going after strange flesh, are set forth for an example, suffering the vengeance of eternal fire."—*Jude 7.*

We know where those two cities were located; and, although they were burned with "eternal fire," **they are not burning today.** They received fire *with eternal effects.* Peter explains how the fire affected those two cities:

"And turning the cities of Sodom and Gomorrha into ashes condemned them with an overthrow, making them an ensample unto those that after should live ungodly."—*2 Peter 2:6.*

So those two cities received "eternal fire" which, after it ended, left only "ashes." Elsewhere, we are told that they were quickly destroyed ("overthrown as in a moment"; *Lamentations 4:6).*

The meaning of unquenchable—**This is fire which devours so thoroughly, that it cannot be put out until it has completed its work. For this reason, it is called *"unquenchable"*;** that is, it cannot be quenched or put out until it is finished. But when the wicked—including Satan—are totally destroyed, then the fire will go out.

"He will . . gather His wheat into the garner; but He will burn up the chaff with unquenchable fire."—*Matthew 3:12.*

Here is a Bible example which shows that "unquenchable fire" does not last forever:
Because of continued Sabbath desecration by the Jews, **God threatened the destruction of Jerusalem by a fire that "shall not be quenched"** *(Jeremiah 17:27).* That fire later occurred *(Jeremiah 52:12-13; 2 Chronicles 36:19).*

Jerusalem is not still burning today. "Unquenchable" fire is fire that cannot be put out until it has

consumed everything. **Unquenchable fire burns everything up and then burns out.** In the same way the wicked will be destroyed.

"Where their worm dieth not, and the fire is not quenched."—*Mark 9:44.*

A city-wide conflagration once enveloped Chicago. It was an unstoppable fire which could not be quenched. But that does not mean that Chicago is still burning.

The meaning of "their worm that dieth not"—The "worm that dieth not" is a figure taken from the refuse dump in the Valley of Hinnom, on the south side of ancient Jerusalem. The fact that garbage was constantly thrown into this dump, which kept the fires always burning there, was the surest proof that whatever was cast into it would be entirely consumed. —But when nothing more was thrown in, the fire eventually ended, after having done a thorough job of destruction.

Speaking of the enemies of the Lord, Isaiah said, "The worm shall eat them like wool" *(Isaiah 51:8).* This is a picture of being put out of existence.

What the fire did not destroy the worms devoured. It is a symbol of complete and final destruction—total annihilation of sinners.

The Bible also speaks of "eternal redemption" *(Hebrews 9:12)* and "eternal judgment" *(Hebrews 6:2).* But this does not mean redemption going on through all eternity, or an unending work of judgment. No, both are eventually finished, but with results which will last forever.

The meaning of forever and ever—**Why is this fire said to be "forever and ever"?** *(Revelation 14:11 and 20:10).* In order to understand it, we must see how this phrase is used elsewhere in the Bible. When we do, we discover that **the Bible usage means "as long as it lasts," which should frequently be translated, "as long as he lives."**

For instance, in 1 Samuel 1:22 we find that **Hannah lent Samuel to the Lord "forever." It means, "as long as he lives." Verse 28 translates it in that manner: "As long as he liveth he shall be lent to the Lord."** (Similar passages are 1 Samuel 27:12; Job 41:4.) In Exodus 21:6, a man can volunteer to be a slave "forever"; but, if it really meant *forever,* there would be slavery in heaven! Christ is called "a priest forever" *(Hebrews 5:6);* yet, after sin is blotted out and the Second Advent occurs, Christ's work as a priest will end.

Jonah was said to be in the belly of the great fish forever *(Jonah 2:6),* yet it only lasted three days and nights *(Jonah 1:17).* Leprosy was said to cleave to Gehazi and his offspring forever *(2 Kings 5:27),* and Philemon was counseled to receive Onesimus forever *(Philemon 15).* The Passover was to be kept "forever" *(Exodus 12:24),* but it ended at the cross *(see Hebrews 9:24-26).* Aaron and his sons were to offer incense "forever" (1 Chronicles 23:13), and have an "everlasting priesthood" (Exodus 40:15), Yet this priesthood, with its offerings of incense, ended at Calvary (see Hebrews 7:11-14).

Liddell and Scott's Greek Lexicon, the most exhaustive research work of its kind, gives the following definition of the Greek word, translated "forever," in the KJV:

"A space or period of time, especially a lifetime, life . . Also one's time of life, age: the age of man . . 2. A long space of time, eternity . . 3. Later, a space of time clearly defined and marked out, an era, age, . . this present life, this world."

As long as the wicked live, as long as consciousness lasts, they will be in the flames. For some this will only be a few moments. For Satan it will be longest of all. Yet we are told that even he will eventually cease to exist. "Nevermore shalt thou be" (Ezekiel 28:19) will be what God says of Satan, who is destroyed in that fire. And the verse before it says:

"And I will bring thee to ashes upon the earth."—Ezekiel 28:18.

It is clear that these words, "forever" and "forever and ever," must be compared with other passages of Scripture in order to properly understand them. In this chapter we have found abundant evidence that the wicked do not burn without end. "They shall be destroyed forever" (Psalm 92:7) means that *the results* of that destruction will last forever. The wicked "shall not see life" (John 3:36). "No murder hath eternal life abiding in him" (1 John 3:15).

This fire will be so thorough in destroying the wicked, that when it is done, not a hot coal or any fire will remain:

"Behold, they shall be as stubble; the fire shall burn them; they shall not deliver themselves from the power of the flame: there shall not be a coal to warm at, nor fire to sit before it."—Isaiah 47:14.

While it is taught in many pulpits that all the wicked will burn forever, the Bible, in stark contrast, clearly teaches that **some will suffer only a short time, while other more wicked people will suffer a little longer.**

"And that servant, which knew his lord's will, and prepared not himself, neither did according to his will, shall be beaten with many stripes. But he that knew not, and did commit things worthy of stripes, shall be beaten with few stripes."— Luke 12:47-48.

God does not delight in punishment. *It is His strange act.*

"He shall be wroth . . that He may do His work, His strange work; and bring to pass His act, His strange act."—Isaiah 28:21.

But sin must be eradicated. In fairness to the

universe there is no other way to deal with it. The rebellion has to be brought to an end. This planet, if one sinner were left on it, would be a deadly virus forever threatening the universe.

A QUICK, TOTAL DESTRUCTION

The Bible is quite clear about this. **The *gehenna* hell will burn until "both soul and body" are destroyed.** "Fear Him which is able to destroy both soul and body" (Matthew 10:28).

This hell will burn until the wicked are devoured (Revelation 20:9). That will be the "second death." **It will be a total everlasting *death*—oblivion,—not an everlasting, burning *life* (verse 14).**

"The Lord preserveth all them that love Him: but all the wicked will He destroy."—Psalm 145:20.

Some of the strongest words are used by the Scripture writers, in the original Hebrew and Greek in which the Bible was written, to emphasize the total destruction of the wicked. They will not only "burn" (katio; Revelation 19:20; 21:8), but they shall be "burned up" (katakaio; 2 Peter 3:10; Matthew 3:12). They shall not only be "destroyed" (apollumi; Matthew 21:41; Mark 1:24), but be "utterly destroyed" (exolothreuo; Acts 3:23, R.V.). They shall not only be "consumed" (tamam; Psalm 104:35), and "consume away," (kalah; Psalm 37:20), but be "utterly consumed" (apollumi in the Septuagint; Psalm 73:19).

It is obvious that the wicked will be completely blotted out of existence by this fire. That is why it is called "the second death." At the first death, the wicked go into the grave, as does everyone else. But only the wicked experience this second death, which marks the end of the sinner, the end of death, and the end of the grave.

The fact that the wicked "will be cut off" is frequently mentioned in the Old Testament. The word, "cut off," is *karath* and means "totally destroy" (as it is used in Ezekiel 28:16). "All the wicked will He destroy" (Psalm 145:20).

"Mark the perfect man, and behold the upright: for the end of that man is peace. But the transgressors shall be destroyed together: the end of the wicked shall be cut off."—Psalm 37:37-38.

Notice in the two following statements that, as soon as the wicked are destroyed, the redeemed will inherit the earth:

"For evildoers shall be cut off: but those that wait upon the Lord, they shall inherit the earth. For yet a little while, and the wicked shall not be: yea, thou shalt diligently consider his place, and it shall not be. But the meek shall inherit the earth; and shall delight themselves in the abundance of peace."—Psalm 37:9-11.

"Wait on the Lord, and keep His way, and He shall exalt thee to inherit the land: when the wicked are cut off, thou shalt see it."—*Psalm 37:34.*

THE WICKED ARE LIKENED TO VERY PERISHABLE MATERIALS

During that brief period of time in which they finally perish forever, **the wicked are compared to fragile substances which are burned up quickly.**

Nothing burns as quickly as hay and stubble! After a fire goes out, only the "ashes" remain, and soon they are gone also. The following passage compares those burned as being like "stubble," and the rather quick result to "ashes."

"For, behold, the day cometh, that shall burn as an oven; and all the proud, yea, and all that do wickedly, shall be stubble: and the day that cometh shall burn them up, saith the Lord of hosts, that it shall leave them neither root nor branch.

"But unto you that fear My name shall the Sun of righteousness arise with healing in His wings; and ye shall go forth, and grow up as calves of the stall.

"And ye shall tread down the wicked; for they shall be ashes under the soles of your feet in the day that I shall do this, saith the Lord of hosts."—*Malachi 4:1-3.*

The wicked are said to be like "the chaff which the wind driveth away" *(Psalm 1:4).* Isaiah says that "the whirlwind shall take them away as stubble" *(Isaiah 40:24).*

The wicked are to be utterly destroyed—consumed away as quickly as animal "fat," changed into "smoke," and brought to "ashes."

"But the wicked shall perish, and the enemies of the Lord shall be as the fat of lambs: they shall consume; into smoke shall they consume away."—*Psalm 37:20.*

GOD'S MERCIFUL PLAN

Sin and sinners will be forever gone from the universe. The righteous could not be happy throughout eternity if they knew that loved ones were forever suffering in flames! No, no. God has something wonderful planned for all. The righteous will live in continual happiness forever. **The wicked, who could not be happy in the peace of heaven, will no longer exist. It will be merciful of God to put them out of their selfish misery.**

The destruction of the wicked will be quick and complete, leaving only stubble burned into ashes *(Malachi 4:1-3).* And it will be final.

"They shall be as though they had not been."—*Obadiah 16.*

It will not take long for the wicked to be con-sumed.

"As the whirlwind passeth, so is the wicked no more."—*Proverbs 10:25.*

"For yet a little while, and the wicked shall not be: yea, thou shalt diligently consider his place, and it shall not be.

"But the meek shall inherit the earth; and shall delight themselves in the abundance of peace."—*Psalm 37:10-11.*

Through sin they have forfeited the right to life and an immortal existence. Instead, they have chosen the way of death and destruction. Because of the way in which they used their probationary time while living in this world, they squandered their final opportunities to return to God.

Their destruction will, in fact, be an act of love and mercy on the part of God; for to perpetuate their lives would only be to perpetuate sin, sorrow, suffering, and misery.

We are told that God takes "no pleasure in the death of the wicked" *(Ezekiel 33:11).* He would have saved every one of them if He could. But they would not come to Him that they might be saved.

"Cast away from you all your transgressions, whereby ye have transgressed; and make you a new heart and a new spirit: for why will ye die, O house of Israel? For I have no pleasure in the death of him that dieth, saith the Lord God: wherefore turn yourselves, and live ye."—*Ezekiel 18:31-32.*

The power and authority of the divine government shall be employed to put down rebellion; yet **all the manifestations of retributive justice will be perfectly consistent with the character of God as a merciful, long-suffering, benevolent being.**

"For the wages of sin is death; but the gift of God is eternal life through Jesus Christ our Lord."—*Romans 6:23.*

"See, I have set before thee this day life and good, and death and evil; in that I command thee this day to love the Lord thy God, to walk in His ways, and to keep His commandments and His statutes and his judgments, that thou mayest live."—*Deuteronomy 30:15-16.*

However, there must come a time when they perish, and He has reserved them unto the day of judgment. In view of that fact, why should anyone wish to rush them off to hell as soon as they die?

The wicked will burn in fire on the surface of the earth, yet God's promise is that the righteous will inherit the earth and make it their home forever.

Here are three Bible passages which tell us that **the wicked will be blotted out before the redeemed inherit the earth:**

"Wait on the Lord, and keep His way, and **He shall exalt thee to inherit the land**: when the

W
A
Y

wicked are cut off."—*Psalm 37:34.*

"For evildoers shall be cut off: but **those that wait upon the Lord, they shall inherit the earth**. For yet a little while, and **the wicked shall not be**: yea, thou shalt diligently consider his place, and it shall not be. **But the meek shall inherit the earth**; and shall delight themselves in the abundance of peace."—*Psalm 37:9-11.*

"For, behold, **the day cometh, that shall burn as an oven**; and all the proud, yea, and all that do wickedly, shall be stubble: **and the day that cometh shall burn them up**, saith the Lord of hosts, **that it shall leave them neither root nor branch.**

"But unto you that fear My name shall the Sun of righteousness arise with healing in His wings; **and ye shall go forth**, and grow up as calves of the stall. And **ye shall tread down the wicked; for they shall be ashes** under the soles of your feet in the day that I shall do this, saith the Lord of hosts."—*Malachi 4:1-3.*

Then, when the fire ends, the experience of sin will be forever over, and God's original plan of peopling the earth with a race of holy, happy beings will be carried out.

"Nevertheless we, according to His promise, look for new heavens and a new earth, wherein dwelleth righteousness. Wherefore, beloved, seeing that ye look for such things, be diligent that ye may be found of Him in peace, without spot, and blameless."—*2 Peter 3:13-14.*

"God Himself was crucified with Christ; for Christ was one with the Father. **Few give thought to the suffering that sin has caused our Creator.** All heaven suffered in Christ's agony; but that suffering did not begin or end with His manifestation in humanity. The cross is a revelation to our dull senses of the pain that, from its very inception, sin has brought to the heart of God. **Every departure from the right, every deed of cruelty, every failure of humanity to reach His ideal, brings grief to Him.** When there came upon Israel the calamities that were the sure result of separation from God—subjugation by their enemies, cruelty, and death—it is said that 'His soul was grieved for the misery of Israel.' 'In all their affliction He was afflicted: . . and He bare them, and carried them all the days of old' *(Judges 10:16; Isa. 63:9).*"—*Amazing Grace, 189.*

"His Spirit 'maketh intercession for us with groanings which cannot be uttered.' As **the 'whole creation groaneth and travaileth in pain'** *(Romans 8:26, 22),* **the heart of the infinite Father is pained in sympathy.** Our world is a vast lazar house, a scene of misery that we dare not allow our thoughts to dwell upon. Did we realize it as it is, the burden would be too terrible. **Yet God feels it all**."—*Education, 263-264.*

"Not a sigh is breathed, not a pain felt, not a grief pierces the soul, but the throb vibrates to the Father's heart."—*Desire of Ages, 356.*

"He who knows the depths of the world's misery and despair, knows by what means to bring relief . . Although human beings have abused their mercies, wasted their talents, and lost the dignity of godlike manhood, the Creator is to be glorified in their redemption."—*Education, p. 270.*

SUMMARY

One of the most beloved verses in the Bible—John 3:16—clearly states that the unrepentant ones will not live forever, but will "perish." The entire passage also explains that they will perish because they refused to accept Christ as their Saviour.

"Whosoever believeth in Him *should not perish*, but have eternal life.

"For God so loved the world, that He gave His only begotten Son, that whosoever believeth in Him *should not perish*, but have everlasting life.

"For God sent not His Son into the world to condemn the world; but that the world through Him might be saved.

"He that believeth on Him is not condemned: but he that believeth not is condemned already, because he hath not believed in the name of the only begotten Son of God."—*John 3:15-18.*

The righteous will be "recompensed [rewarded] at the resurrection of the just" *(Luke 14:14). Oh, what a glorious day that will be!*

"As for me, I will behold Thy face in righteousness: I shall be satisfied, when I awake, with Thy likeness."—*Psalm 17:15.*

The bodies of the redeemed will come forth from the grave without any traces of age, sickness, or flaws *(1 Corinthians 15:42-44; Philippians 3:20-21; 1 Corinthians 15:54-55; Luke 20:36).*

But a thousand years later, the wicked will be raised—and then forever perish. It will be a death, and total destruction which lasts forever.

"What shall the end be of them that obey not the gospel of God?"—*1 Peter 4:17.*

"For the wages of sin is death."—*Romans 6:23.*

"The soul that sinneth, it shall die."—*Ezekiel 18:4.*

"Who shall be punished with everlasting destruction."—*2 Thessalonians 1:9.*

"But the wicked shall perish, and the enemies of the Lord shall be as the fat of lambs: they shall consume; into smoke shall they consume away."—*Psalm 37:20.*

"And fire came down from God out of heaven, and devoured them."—*Revelation 20:9.*

"But the fearful, and unbelieving, and the abominable, and murderers, and whoremongers, and sorcerers, and idolaters, and all liars, shall have their part in the lake which burneth with fire and brimstone: which is the second death."—*Revelation 21:8.*

"The last enemy that shall be destroyed is death."—*1 Corinthians 15:26.*

"Then shall the righteous shine forth as the sun in the kingdom of their Father."—*Matthew 13:43.*

"Wherefore," the Apostle Paul tells us, "comfort one another with these words" *(1 Thessalonians 4:18).*

―――――――

COMING NEXT—Answers to several important questions which people ask about the other side of death. This will help fill in many important details.

Chapter Twelve

Questions and Answers about Death

Additional Important Bible Facts

Clarence Darrow, the famous criminal lawyer, once held a debate with a rabbi, a priest, and a minister on the subject of immortality. All three clergymen used symbols, similes, and allegories to defend their position that the soul of man is indestructible and not subject to the power of death.

When Darrow arose, he said, "These gentlemen never once used the Bible to prove their assertions, much less did they quote from its pages."

However, there are some difficult passages in the Bible which are "hard to be understood" *(2 Peter 3:15-16).* When there is apparent contradiction or seeming difference of meaning, two things should be kept in mind.

First, difficult texts should be studied in the light of the general teaching of the Bible on that particular subject. **Second, all lines of Bible doctrine should run parallel.** For instance, the Bible teaches that the judgment occurs down at the end of time. So we would be out of harmony with Scripture if we believed God took good people to heaven at death and put bad people into flames at death, when as yet they had not yet been judged in the final judgment.

QUESTIONS ANSWERED

So here are six answers to difficult passages concerning death:

1 - The thief on the cross—Jesus told the repentant thief, "Verily I say unto thee, Today shalt thou be with Me in paradise" *(Luke 23:43). Did Jesus take the thief to heaven that day?*

First, **Jesus did not Himself go to paradise that day.** Paradise is where the tree of life is *(Revelation 2:7).* That is in heaven at the throne of God *(Revelation 22:1-2).* Jesus did not ascend to heaven until the day of His resurrection. To Mary, He said at that time, "Touch Me not; for I am not yet ascended to My Father" *(John 20:17).*

Second, **although Jesus died that day, the thief did not** *(John 19:30-33).* He was taken down from the cross just before sunset, while still alive, so he could be put back onto a cross after the hours of the Sabbath. Although the thief was taken down from the cross over the Sabbath, historians tell us that he would have been put back on it on the day after the Sabbath. This is because death by crucifixion usually took several days.

Third, **there is no punctuation in the original.** When Luke wrote those words, punctuation marks had not yet been invented.

So, in order to make the verse agree with the above Bible facts, **the comma should be moved from before "today" to after "today": "Verily I say unto *thee today, thou shalt be* with Me in paradise."** It was on that day—the day of Christ's worst humiliation—that He could give the glorious promise that the thief would be saved and later be with Christ in heaven! What a promise is that for the rest of us!

Notice that **the thief did not ask to be taken to paradise then.** He asked, "Lord remember me when Thou comest into Thy kingdom." That is exactly when he will be remembered and taken into that kingdom.

2 - Shall never die—What did Christ mean when He told Mary that those who believed in Him would never die? The entire passage explains it:

"Jesus said unto her, I am the resurrection, and the life: he that believeth in Me, though he were dead, yet shall he live: And whosoever liveth and believeth in Me shall never die."—*John 11:25-26.*

Both the righteous and wicked will be resurrected, but only those believing in Christ will live forever. The rest will die the second death *(Revelation 20:13-15).*

God is looking to the future when He says that the wicked are dead even while they live *(1 Timothy 5:6).* They go down into Christless graves, rise in the resurrection to receive judgment, and go down in the "second death" *(Revelation 21:8).* And God is looking to the future when He says that the righteous have eternal life.

W
A
Y

This also explains why Christ said to the unbelieving Jews, "Ye will not come to Me that ye might have life" *(John 5:40).*

But the Christian, who has accepted Christ, has life in his heart. He has everlasting life abiding in him—as long as he remains faithful to Christ. This also explains why Paul said that Christ "abolished death" *(2 Timothy 1:10);* whereas, he elsewhere said that God's faithful ones do not conquer death until the resurrection, when "death is swallowed up in victory" *(1 Corinthians 15:54).* Thank God that the time is coming when "death and hell" are "cast into the lake of fire" *(Revelation 20:14).* Then, and not till then, will death truly be abolished.

3 - The spirits in prison—Some believe that during the time between His crucifixion and His resurrection, Christ went and preached to the spirits in prison. Here is the unusual passage:

"For Christ also hath once suffered for sins, the just for the unjust, that He might bring us to God, being put to death in the flesh, but quickened by the Spirit: by which also He went and preached unto the spirits in prison; which sometime were disobedient, when once the longsuffering of God waited in the days of Noah, while the ark was a preparing, wherein few, that is, eight souls were saved by water."—*1 Peter 3:18-20.*

First, notice that **Christ preached to them by "the Spirit,"** and that word is capitalized. So whatever preaching was done was accomplished through the Holy Spirit.

Second, **this preaching was done while Noah was building the Ark**, not long before the Flood covered the earth *(Genesis 6).*

"And the Lord said, My Spirit shall not always strive with man."—*Genesis 6:3.*

In other words, God's Spirit pleaded with men through the preaching of Noah.

Third, **the preaching was done to "spirits which are in prison."** The words, "spirit" and "soul" are often used when talking about people. David prayed, "Bring my soul out of prison" *(Psalm 142:7),* Paul spoke of being into captivity to sin *(Romans 7).*

It was the work of Christ to open "the prison to them that are bound" *(Isaiah 42:7).*

In summary, Christ preached by the Holy Spirit, while Noah was building the Ark, and He did it to the "spirits in prison," that is, to those individuals whose sinful lives were bound in the prison house of sin.

4 - Under punishment until the judgment—In the *Revised Standard Version* of 2 Peter 2:9, we read:

"The Lord knows how to rescue the godly from trial, and to keep the unrighteous under punishment until the day of judgment."—*2 Peter 2:9, RSV.*

This suggests that, after death, the wicked suffer punishment prior to the day of judgment.

First, this concept contradicts the whole teaching of Scripture.

Second, "to punish" may be translated to show immediate activity, or eventual purpose.

The RSV translates it to show immediate activity:

". . to keep the unrighteous under punishment until the day of judgment."—*2 Peter 2:9, RSV.*

The *King James Version* translates it to show eventual purpose:

". . **and to reserve the unjust unto the day of judgment to be punished.**"—*2 Peter 2:9, KJV.*

There is a great difference between the two translations! **The KJV agrees with the rest of Scripture, and the RSV does not.**

Elsewhere in this same epistle, the RSV correctly translates the word: "kept until the judgment" *(2 Peter 2:4, RSV),* indicating that the fallen angels are not at present suffering punishment, but later will in the time of the judgment.

5 - The rich man and Lazarus—In the parable of Luke 16:19-31, the rich man died and went to hell. "Being in torments," he called to the beggar Lazarus, who had also died and was in Abraham's bosom.

What is the meaning of this?

First, God sometimes speaks of the future as present.

"God, who quickeneth the dead, and calleth those things which be not as though they were."—*Romans 4:17.*

However, **the story of the rich man and Lazarus is a parable, and cannot be regarded as literal. It comes in the midst of a long series of parables.** Parables often teach some main lesson, but should not be held to every detail. (See Judges 9:6-20, for example.)

As He prepared to give this parable, Jesus was rebuking the covetous Pharisees *(Luke 16:14),* by showing that the rich may fare well here, but not hereafter. **He used one of their own traditions to drive this point home.**

First, let us consider Lazarus, and then the rich man.

Lazarus is represented as being carried by the angels to "Abraham's bosom." However, **it is at the Second Coming of Christ, not at death, that the angels gather the elect** *(Matthew 24:31).*

In addition, **Abraham would find it difficult to hold all the redeemed next to his chest.** So this cannot possibly be literal.

There was another Lazarus, a literal one, who died *(John 11:14-44).* He was the brother of Mary and Martha. After four days dead in the grave, when Jesus called him to life, He said, "Lazarus, come forth." He did not say, "Come from Abraham's bosom."

After being restored to life, this literal Lazarus

had nothing to say about Abraham's bosom, or anything else that had happened during those four days; for "the dead know not anything" *(Ecclesiastes 9:5).* When a real person dies, "his thoughts perish" *(Psalm 146:4).* So the Lazarus of the parable cannot be taken literally.

Then there is the rich man in the parable. In the symbolism of this story, he was in hell with a body. He had eyes, tongue, etc. *(Luke 16:23-24).* **How did his body get into hell fire instead of into the grave?**

Of this rich man we read, "And in hell he lifted up his eyes, being in torments, and seeth Abraham afar off, and Lazarus in his bosom. And he cried and said, Father Abraham, have mercy on me, and send Lazarus, that he may dip the tip of his finger in water, and cool my tongue; for I am tormented in this flame" *(Luke 16:23-24).* **The word "hell" used here is *hades,* which means "the grave." But there is no fire in the grave,** so we here have still further evidence that this parable cannot be taken literally.

The request of Lazarus, to dip the tip of his finger in water and come through the flames to cool the rich man's tongue, is obviously not literal. **How much moisture would remain on the finger and how much relief would it give?**

The climactic point of the entire parable is found in verse 31:

"If they hear not Moses and the prophets, neither will they be persuaded, though one rose from the dead."—*Luke 16:31.*

Astoundingly, not long afterward—a literal Lazarus was raised from the dead *(John 11:43)*—and the Jews that Jesus was speaking to would not believe that either!

The real lesson of the parable is that prosperity in this life does not guarantee prosperity hereafter,—but that it is now that we must prepare for eternity!

"For the grave cannot praise Thee, death cannot celebrate Thee: they that go down into the pit cannot hope for Thy truth."—*Isaiah 38:18.*

There is no second chance!

"Behold, now is the accepted time; behold, now is the day of salvation."—*2 Corinthians 6:2.*

Now is the time to speak words of kindness, and do deeds of love. Now is the time to accept Christ as our Saviour and faithfully obey all that He tells us in Scripture.

Someone has said, "The more of earth we want, the less of heaven we'll get."

Early in World War II, Colonel Warren J. Clear was ordered by his superior officer to leave Corregidor just before it fell. He was to board a submarine at midnight. In his orders were these words, *"Be ready to go aboard. No personal baggage."*

When we say good-bye to this world and breathe our last breath, we will only take our character with us. If we died holding tightly to Christ, we will be raised in the resurrection to live with Him forever.

***6 - Departing and being with Christ*—**Here is the Bible passage:

"For I am in a strait betwixt two, having a desire to depart, and to be with Christ; which is far better."—*Philippians 1:23.*

Paul did not say in this text that he would go to be with Christ when he died. He undoubtedly was using the word "depart" in reference to his death. But the Bible clearly reveals that **Paul did not believe his "departure" would mean immediate entrance into heaven.** Here is the proof:

"For I am now ready to be offered, and the time of My departure is at hand. I have fought a good fight, I have finished My course, I have kept the faith. Henceforth there is laid up for me a crown of righteousness, which **the Lord, the righteous judge, shall give me at that day: and not to me only, but unto all them also that love His appearing**."—*2 Timothy 4:6-8.*

Since he obviously did not expect to get his eternal crown at his departure in death, **when did Paul anticipate actually being with Christ?** Here is the answer:

"For the Lord Himself shall descend from heaven with a shout, with the voice of the archangel, and with the trump of God: and the dead in Christ shall rise first. Then we which are alive and remain shall be caught up together with them in the clouds, to meet the Lord in the air: and so shall we ever be with the Lord. Wherefore comfort one another with these words."—*1 Thessalonians 4:16-18.*

COMING NEXT—What is the millennium? When does it begin? How long is it? What happens when it ends? This is a very important subject.

Chapter Thirteen

The Millennium
What Happens During the Millennium

How long can a man live? Most are fortunate to make it to 70 or 80. Dr. Edward L. Bortz, president of the American Medical Association in the late 1940s, declared that the human body should be able to survive to the age of 150. Other researchers agree with him.

But the time is coming when people will live a thousand years—and continue living on after that.

Let us turn to a passage which describes that time. First, we will quote the entire passage, then,

W
A
Y

comparing Scripture with Scripture, we will discover its meaning:

"And I saw an angel come down from heaven, having the key of the bottomless pit and a great chain in his hand. And he laid hold on the dragon, that old serpent, which is the Devil, and Satan, and bound him a thousand years, and cast him into the bottomless pit, and shut him up, and set a seal upon him, that he should deceive the nations no more, till the thousand years should be fulfilled: and after that he must be loosed a little season.

"And I saw thrones, and they sat upon them, and judgment was given unto them: and I saw the souls of them that were beheaded for the witness of Jesus, and for the Word of God, and which had not worshiped the beast, neither his image, neither had received his mark upon their foreheads, or in their hands; and they lived and reigned with Christ a thousand years.

"But the rest of the dead lived not again until the thousand years were finished. This is the first resurrection.

"Blessed and holy is he that hath part in the first resurrection: on such the second death hath no power, but they shall be priests of God and of Christ, and shall reign with Him a thousand years.

"And when the thousand years are expired, Satan shall be loosed out of his prison, and shall go out to deceive the nations which are in the four quarters of the earth, Gog and Magog, to gather them together to battle: the number of whom is as the sand of the sea.

"And they went up on the breadth of the earth, and compassed the camp of the saints about, and the beloved city: and fire came down from God out of heaven, and devoured them."—*Revelation 20:1-9.*

This is the only place in the Bible where the thousand-year period is specifically named, and it is here mentioned six times. The word *millennium* is not found in the Bible. It comes from two Latin words, *mille*, meaning "a thousand," and *annum*, meaning "a year." Thus we have *millennium*, a thousand years.

Twice in the foregoing brief Bible record of the millennium **we are told that Satan is a deceiver. During the millennium he cannot deceive the nations. At its close, for a short time, he will again deceive men.**

He works today with great diligence, knowing that his time is limited before Christ returns for His people, and the millennium begins.

"Woe to the inhabiters of the earth and of the sea! for the devil is come down unto you, having great wrath, because he knoweth that he hath but a short time."—*Revelation 12:12.*

The Apostle Paul declares that **"there shall be a resurrection of the dead, both of the just and the unjust"** *(Acts 24:15).*

One of these resurrections will take place at the beginning of the one thousand years; the other, at the end. These two resurrections will be one thousand years apart.

EVENTS AT THE BEGINNING OF THE MILLENNIUM

At the beginning of the millennium comes the resurrection of the righteous, which is called the *first* resurrection.

"Blessed and holy is he that hath part in the *first* resurrection: on such the second death hath no power, but they shall be priests of God and of Christ, and shall reign with Him a thousand years."—*Revelation 20:6.*

What then happens to the wicked dead, those who went into Christless graves, at that time? The answer is brief and plain:

"But the rest of the dead lived not again until the thousand years were finished."—*Revelation 20:5.*

So the wicked dead (the "rest of the dead") will not live again until the end of the thousand years.

Now that we know that the righteous dead are raised to life at the beginning of the one thousand years, *if we can learn what other events occur when God's faithful ones are raised from the dead,—we know that these also will be at the beginning of the millennium.*

The primary event that marks the beginning of the millennium is the Second Coming of Christ. We know that from the following passage:

"For the Lord Himself shall descend from heaven with a shout, with the voice of the archangel, and with the trump of God: and the dead in Christ shall rise first."—*1 Thessalonians 4:16.*

What else happens at that time? The next verse tells us.

"Then we which are alive and remain shall be caught up together with them in the clouds, to meet the Lord in the air: and so shall we ever be with the Lord."—*1 Thessalonians 4:17.*

But there is more that happens then.

"For our conversation is in heaven; from whence also we look for the Saviour, the Lord Jesus Christ: Who shall change our vile body, that it may be fashioned like unto His glorious body, according to the working whereby He is able even to subdue all things unto Himself."—*Philippians 3:20-21.*

What a glorious promise! **So the bodies of both the righteous living and the righteous dead will be changed, glorified, and made immortal when**

W
A
Y

Jesus returns the second time!

"Behold, I show you a mystery. We shall not all sleep, but we shall all be changed, in a moment, in the twinkling of an eye, at the last trump: for the trumpet shall sound, and the dead shall be raised incorruptible, and we shall be changed. For this corruptible must put on incorruption, and this mortal must put on immortality.

"So when this corruptible shall have put on incorruption, and this mortal shall have put on immortality, then shall be brought to pass the saying that is written, Death is swallowed up in victory."—*1 Corinthians 15:51-54.*

This all occurs at the Second Advent, which is at the beginning of the millennium.

What happens next? Both the living righteous and those just raised from the dead "are caught up together . . in the clouds, to meet the Lord in the air: and so shall we ever be with the Lord" *(1 Thessalonians 4:17).*

Notice that the feet of Jesus does not touch the earth at His Second Advent. *This fact is important,* for it helps us now be able to identify "false christs" who claim to be Christ, returned to the earth.

The above verse says that, after meeting Christ in the air, we will "ever be with the Lord." Another wonderful promise! Those who have learned to love Jesus deeply while on earth will rejoice that, when He returns for them, they can be with Him forever.

But what does this verse mean?

"For this we say unto you by the word of the Lord, that we which are alive and remain unto the coming of the Lord *shall not prevent* them which are asleep."—*1 Thessalonians 4:15.*

When the King James Version was translated, the word *"prevent"* meant *"not go before."* In other words, the living righteous will not go to heaven ahead of, prior to, God's faithful ones who have died and are in the grave.

Contrariwise, we are told that the righteous dead will not go to heaven before those who are alive when Christ returns.

"And these all, having obtained a good report through faith, received not the promise: God having provided some better thing for us, that they without us should not be made perfect."—*Hebrews 11:39-40.*

So *all of God's faithful ones* will go to heaven at the same time! Yet another good promise! Jesus has wonderful things planned for those who, here on earth, have proved loyal to Him in spite of the difficulties and opposition they have encountered.

"Let not your heart be troubled: ye believe in God, believe also in Me. In My Father's house are many mansions: if it were not so, I would have told you. I go to prepare a place for you. And if I go and prepare a place for you, I will come again,

and receive you unto Myself; that where I am, there ye may be also."—*John 14:1-3.*

But there is more that happens when Christ returns the second time. **We are told that the wicked who are still alive will die "with the brightness of His coming"** *(2 Thessalonians 2:8).*

"And as it was in the days of Noe, . . the flood came, and destroyed them all. Likewise also as it was in the days of Lot, . . it rained fire and brimstone from heaven, and destroyed them all. Even thus shall it be in the day when the Son of man is revealed."—*Luke 17:26-30.*

The unrepentant wicked who are alive when Christ comes in the clouds of heaven will be consumed by the very glory of His coming. "The Lord thy God is a consuming fire" *(Deuteronomy 4:24).*

There is another important event which occurs at Christ's return, at the beginning of the millennium. Satan is bound "that he should deceive the nations no more, till the thousand years should be fulfilled: and after that he must be loosed a little season" *(Revelation 20:3).*

This is done in a very simple, effective way: The wicked will all be dead. The righteous will all be gone to heaven. There will be no human being on earth to deceive and tantalize. **Satan is bound by this chain of events at the beginning of the millennium.** Until some kind of change later occurs on earth, he cannot work at his trade of controlling human minds.

EVENTS DURING THE MILLENNIUM

There are four things to keep in mind about this lengthy, thousand-year period:

First, the earth is desolate. It is likened to a "bottomless pit" *(Revelation 20:3).* The original Greek for this phrase means "abyss." In the Septuagint Greek Version of the Old Testament, this Greek word is translated "without form and void" *(Jeremiah 4:23).* The rest of the passage is also describing the millennium.

"I beheld the earth, and, lo, it was without form, and void; and the heavens, and they had no light. I beheld the mountains, and, lo, they trembled, and all the hills moved lightly. I beheld, and, lo, there was no man, and all the birds of the heavens were fled. I beheld, and, lo, the fruitful place was a wilderness, and all the cities thereof were broken down at the presence of the Lord, and by His fierce anger."—*Jeremiah 4:23-26.*

Second, the wicked are dead. In the verses just quoted, Jeremiah says "there was no man."

Third, Satan is bound in this bottomless pit. On this desolated earth there is no one to deceive. Without having anyone to tempt, he will have a thousand years to think about all the havoc, grief, suffering, and death he has caused.

Having earlier read Revelation 20, Satan will know what is to happen at the close of the thousand

W
A
Y

years—so he will have time to plan what he will do then: a final assault against God and His faithful ones, in a last, desperate attempt to destroy them.

Fourth, the righteous are engaged in a work of judgment in heaven. John describes it:

"And I saw thrones, and they sat upon them, and judgment was given unto them."—*Revelation 20:4.*

Paul provides us with still more information:

"Do ye not know that the saints shall judge the world? and if the world shall be judged by you, are ye unworthy to judge the smallest matters? Know ye not that we shall judge angels?"—*1 Corinthians 6:2-3.*

During this period, the redeemed have an opportunity to see how difficult it was for God to try and save those who, choosing to remain in their sins, refused to be saved. When sin and sinners are totally gone, we will say, "True and righteous are Thy judgments." Because there will then be no room for doubts as to why some will not saved, "God shall wipe away all tears from their eyes."

EVENTS AT THE END OF THE MILLENNIUM

There are seven events which occur at the close of the millennium.

1 - The wicked dead are resurrected. The mighty host of all those who have ever lived on our planet, who were not saved, are raised from the dead and stand upon the earth once more.

"But the rest of the dead lived not again until the thousand years were finished."—*Revelation 20:5.*

2 - Satan is "loosed out of his prison" *(verse 7).* The raising of the wicked dead from their graves gives him opportunity to deceive once more.

3 - Satan "shall go out to deceive the nations" *(verse 8).* How can he deceive them when they are already lost? As usual, the devil has a scheme in mind.

4 - The Holy City, New Jerusalem, descends from heaven *(Revelation 21:2).* That this takes place in close connection with the loosing of Satan is obvious from what follows.

5 - Satan marshals the vast host of the wicked, and they surround the holy city. At that time occurs the final judgment.

"And shall go out to deceive the nations . . to gather them together to battle: the number of whom is as the sand of the sea. And they went up on the breadth of the earth, and compassed the camp of the saints about, and the beloved city."—*Revelation 20:8-9.*

Rejoicing that the wicked are once again alive, Satan goes among them, and convinces them that they are well able to conquer the city and gain control of its riches. We would expect that extensive prepara-

tions are made at that time for the oncoming attack.

And all the while the righteous inside the Holy City see that all those outside the city—including their former loved ones—*are devising ways to kill God's faithful ones in the Holy City!*

When the wicked, under Satan's generalship, surround the holy city, then the final judgment against them is executed. This is referred to, in a dramatic way, in Revelation 20:11-13:

"And I saw a great white throne, and Him that sat on it, from whose face the earth and the heaven fled away; and there was found no place for them.

"And I saw the dead, small and great, stand before God; and the books were opened: and another book was opened, which is the book of life: and the dead were judged out of those things which were written in the books, according to their works. And the sea gave up the dead which were in it; and death and hell delivered up the dead which were in them: and they were judged every man according to their works."—*Revelation 20:11-13.*

6 - "Fire came down from God out of heaven, and devoured them" *(verse 9).* Fire will descend from heaven and devour unnumbered billions of rebellious, unrepentant sinners. "Who shall be punished with everlasting destruction from the presence of the Lord" *(2 Thessalonians 1:9);* that is, *with a destruction which lasts forever.* The wicked come to a total end.

"For as ye have drunk upon My holy mountain, so shall all the heathen drink continually, yea, they shall drink, and they shall swallow down, and they shall be as though they had not been."—*Obadiah 16.*

"For yet a little while, and the wicked shall not be: yea, thou shalt diligently consider his place, and it shall not be. But the meek shall inherit the earth; and shall delight themselves in the abundance of peace."—*Psalm 37:10-11.*

"For, behold, the day cometh, that shall burn as an oven; and all the proud, yea, and all that do wickedly, shall be stubble: and the day that cometh shall burn them up, saith the Lord of hosts, that it shall leave them neither root nor branch

"But unto you that fear My name shall the Sun of righteousness arise with healing in His wings; and ye shall go forth, and grow up as calves of the stall."—*Malachi 4:1-2.*

Nothing shall remain of the wicked, but, as it were, a few "ashes" on the ground, which quickly disappear.

"And ye shall tread down the wicked; for they shall be ashes under the soles of your feet in the day that I shall do this, saith the Lord of hosts."—*Malachi 4:3.*

As for the devil and his angels, they will also die in that fire. Sin and sinners will then be totally gone—forever!

"And the devil that deceived them was cast into the lake of fire . . and death and hell delivered up the dead which were in them . . And death and hell were cast into the lake of fire. This is the second death. And whosoever was not found written in the book of life was cast into the lake of fire."—*Revelation 20:10, 13-15.*

7 - Then the righteous will inherit the new earth.

Sin and sinners will then be totally gone—forever! The entire universe will be pure, clean, and good for all eternity. "There shall be no more curse" *(Revelation 22:3).*

"He God will make an utter end: affliction shall not rise up the second time."—*Nahum 1:9.*

"And God shall wipe away all tears from their eyes; and there shall be no more death, neither sorrow, nor crying, neither shall there be any more pain: for the former things are passed away."—*Revelation 21:4.*

You and I have no idea of the glories that await us in the earth made new! Oh, my friend, we must cling to Jesus, obey His Word, and be faithful to the end! He has a wonderful future in store for us. *You and I must be there!*

"Eye hath not seen, nor ear heard, neither have entered into the heart of man, the things which God hath prepared for them that love Him."—*1 Corinthians 2:9.*

"Blessed are the meek: for they shall inherit the earth."—*Matthew 5:5.*

"Wait on the Lord, and keep His way, and He shall exalt thee to inherit the land: when the wicked are cut off, thou shalt see it."—*Psalm 37:34.*

"And there shall be no more curse: but the throne of God and of the Lamb shall be in it; and His servants shall serve Him: And they shall see His face; and His name shall be in their foreheads. And there shall be no night there; and they need no candle, neither light of the sun; for the Lord God giveth them light: and they shall reign forever and ever."—*Revelation 22:3-5.*

"And the kingdom and dominion, and the greatness of the kingdom under the whole heaven, shall be given to the people of the saints of the Most High, whose kingdom is an everlasting kingdom, and all dominions shall serve and obey Him."—*Daniel 7:27.*

The sin problem has been a difficult one. The entire universe has watched to see how it would work out. But, as we have learned in this chapter, God is going to end it in such a satisfactory way that there will be no more questions, so sin will never arise a second time.

COMING NEXT—One of the most sinister dangers of our time! And one that is rapidly increasing! For your own protection, this is a topic you need to understand.

Chapter Fourteen

The Danger of Spiritualism
The Deceptive Lure of the Spirit World

Spiritualism, also called spiritism, is a belief in communication with departed spirits of loved ones. We have already learned that belief in the immortality of the soul began with the Egyptians. Spiritualism also began there. **If it is believed that people live on after death, then it is logical to imagine that we can talk to them.**

"Ancestor-worship, in most cases is simply the Spiritualism of the East, and survives today through a belief in human immortality."—*Dr. James H. Hyslop, Contact with the Other World, p. 14.*

Humans do not go to another world, but to the silence of the grave at death. Therefore, **those who think they are in contact with "departed spirits" are really receiving messages that are not from men and women but from demons**—Satan's fallen angels.

MEN WHO HAVE TALKED WITH DEMONS

Some of the most evil men in history have been in communication with demons. Here are four of the more recent ones: Each one greatly affected modern history for the worse:

Charles Darwin (1809-1882) was the first of the four. During his nearly five-year expedition on the ship, *HMS Beagle* (December 27, 1831-October 2, 1836), he spent most of his time exploring on land (mostly in South America) with native guides and camping with them;—three years and three months on land, compared with only 18 months at sea. Very curious about everything around him, young Darwin wanted to learn about everything he saw. **During this time, he was initiated by natives into witchcraft ceremonies.**

One Argentine trip with native Argentinians across the pampas began on August 13, 1833; another (a 400-mile trip) inland near the Uruguay River, was made after that. On April 19, 1834, he set out in boats up the river Rio Santa Cruz, also in Argentina.

At Valparaiso, Chile, Darwin bought horses and set off into the high country for an extensive trip.

Back in Valparaiso, he set out on another trek up toward the Andes, and reached the continental divide on March 21.

Darwin's theories, turning men and women from belief in God and the Bible, have destroyed the faith of millions.

Kaiser Wilhelm (1797-1888) of Germany, a prime-mover in starting World War I, **consulted the famous German medium Augusta Schoen as well as others**. The spirits told him to start the war which, although it would cost the lives of millions, would enable him to conquer all of Europe.

Josef Stalin (1878-1953) **is believed to have also been in contact with spiritualist mediums**, which told him how to govern the Russian people. Satan delights in bringing misery to people and causing their death. In the 1930s, Stalin initiated a purge of the Communist Party of the Soviet Union, which has become known as the *Great Purge*, an unprecedented campaign of political repression, persecution and executions that reached its peak in 1937. Confiscations of grain and other food by the Soviet authorities under his orders contributed to a famine between 1932 and 1934, especially in the key agricultural regions of the Soviet Union, Ukraine, Kazakhstan and North Caucasus that resulted in millions of deaths.

Adolf Hitler (1889-1945) **consulted a spirit which would visit him alone each evening in his bedroom**, which was separate from the room in which Eva Braun stayed. Taking visible form, it would tell him that if he would militarize Germany and begin invading other nations, he would soon be in possession, not only of Europe but also Britain, Russia, and North Africa. Millions died because Hitler listened to demons.

Many **rock stars** have, by their own statements, made contact with demons. They have found that this enables them to have more control over their audiences and make them wild.

Jesus said, "By their fruits ye shall know them *(Matthew 7:20)*. Demon control by the spirits of spiritualism is the fruit of the error that men do not die when they die.

THE BIBLE CONDEMNS SPIRITUALISM

The Bible condemns spiritualism for three reasons:

First, because it is not true that we can communicate with those who have died. Men and women who die go to the grave; they do not live on in another afterlife.

"For the living know that they shall die: but the dead know not any thing, neither have they any more a reward; for the memory of them is forgotten. Also their love, and their hatred, and their envy, is now perished."—*Ecclesiastes 9:5-6*.

"His breath goeth forth, he returneth to his earth; in that very day his thoughts perish."—*Psalm 146:4*.

There is a total cessation of thought at death. Sight, hearing, mental activity, and speaking all end at the grave.

"As the cloud is consumed and vanisheth away: so he that goeth down to the grave shall come up no more. He shall return no more to his house, neither shall his place know him anymore."—*Job 7:9-10*.

Although a sincere Christian who has died "will no more return to his house" in this present world, yet when Christ returns and calls him from the grave, he will be with Jesus forevermore *(1 Thessalonians 4:15-18)*. What a glorious promise!

But, contradicting the clear statements of Scripture, spiritualism claims that we who are alive can communicate with those who have died, and learn wonderful truths from them.

The second reason why the Bible is against spiritualism is that Satan, the archenemy of God, claims that death is not real. To Eve, mother of all, he spoke the first lie—and it laid the foundation for spiritualism.

"And the serpent said unto the woman, Ye shall not surely die: For God doth know that in the day ye eat thereof, then your eyes shall be opened, and ye shall be as gods, knowing good and evil."—*Genesis 3:4-5*.

Satan's message is all there! (1) You will not die if you disobey God, but be immortal and live forever. (2) You will obtain marvelous knowledge if you will sin against God.

Satan's lie about death led the human race into sin and misery. God is against Satan, who is "a liar, and the father of it" *(John 8:44)*.

The third reason why the Bible opposes spiritualism is because it turns people from the Bible, from God, and destroys their lives.

The spirits tell people that everyone will be saved, and the most wicked people are in a higher state of heavenly existence than the most godly Christians who have died. **Everything that comes from this satanic source is designed to produce atheism, misery, and death.**

Dr. L.S. Forbes Winslow, an expert on mental illness, wrote:

"I could quote many instances where **men of the highest ability have followed the doctrines of spiritualism, only to end their day ruined.**"—*Spiritualistic Madness, p. 29*.

J. Godfrey Raupert, another expert on spiritualism, stated:

"They drive men and women to destruction

and to the madhouse. **They undermine religious faith and confidence** and, in a thousand instances, bring about an utter weariness and detestation of the duties of the present life . . I have, during the last ten years, spent much of my time in answering the inquiries of persons whose lives have been shipwrecked by spiritistic practices, and it is upon painful facts and incontrovertible evidence that I base my conclusions."

WHAT THE BIBLE TEACHES ABOUT SPIRITUALISM

God commanded His people in Bible times to have nothing to do with witchcraft and spiritistic mediums.

"When thou art come into the land which the Lord thy God giveth thee, **thou shalt not learn to do after the abominations of those nations.** There shall not be found among you any one that maketh his son or his daughter to pass through the fire, or that useth divination, or an observer of times, or an enchanter, or a witch, Or a charmer, or a consulter with familiar spirits, or a wizard, or a necromancer. **For all that do these things are an abomination unto the Lord**: and because of these abominations the Lord thy God doth drive them out from before thee. Thou shalt be perfect with the Lord thy God."—*Deuteronomy 18:9-13.*

The most sweeping condemnation is given in the above passage to astrology, fortune-telling, charms, spiritist mediums ("consulters of familiar spirits"), and other methods of making contact with supernatural beings.

This warning is also given in the New Testament:

"Now the Spirit speaketh expressly, that in the latter times some shall depart from the faith, giving heed to seducing spirits, and doctrines of devils; speaking lies in hypocrisy; having their conscience seared with a hot iron."—*1 Timothy 4:1-2.*

These are urgent words of warning, and tell us that **spiritist manifestations will increase as we approach the end of time, just before Christ returns.**

Repeatedly, the Bible has warned us to have nothing to do with all forms of spiritualism!

"Regard not them that have familiar spirits, neither seek after wizards, to be defiled by them: I am the Lord your God."—*Leviticus 19:31.*

"And I will come near to you to judgment; and I will be a swift witness against the sorcerers, and against the adulterers."—*Malachi 3:5.*

"Therefore hearken not ye to your prophets, nor to your diviners, nor to your dreamers, nor to your enchanters . . **For they prophesy a lie unto you**, to remove you far from your land;

and that I should drive you out, and ye should perish."—*Jeremiah 27:9-10.*

In Old Testament times, God commanded that witches and wizards should be killed. "Thou shalt not suffer a witch to live" *(Exodus 22:18).*

"A man also or woman that hath a familiar spirit, or that is a wizard, shall surely be put to death."—*Leviticus 20:27.*

SOMETHING TO BE AVOIDED

Because the dead are unconscious, they cannot make intelligent contact with anyone. **The purported communications from the dead are fakery. They are the fakery of the medium or fakery performed by the "spirits of devils"** masquerading as people who have died.

"I frankly admit that there is not only triviality and contradiction but fraud and trickery in the psychic field."—*Sherwood Eddy, You Will Survive After Death.*

Please do not be confused! **God's message for this critical hour in history is simply not found in the trivial disclosures of sometimes truthful and sometimes lying spirits.** Saving truth is found in the Bible,—not in the "profound" information that two sisters had a ring, or in the materialization of an ash tray, or the medium being able to see a table fork when someone in the audience thinks about one.

Satan and his "seducing spirits" who were "cast out into the earth" possess information known only to the dead loved ones and their relatives or friends. When men and women dare to consult mediums, or spiritistic devices such as ouija boards, they are lured on and on to their ruin. **Evil angels even appear in the form of a deceased loved one.**

An intelligent lady was studying the Bible on this subject. She had been very much interested in communication with the dead. But when she came to this particular point in her study, she exclaimed, *"Then who is writing on my slate?"*

Yes, who is it that gives the messages in the darkened room? Who is masquerading in the disguise of those loved ones who died? What are the powers that are unquestionably operating in the psychic world? It is Satan and his evil angels.

"**For they are the spirits of devils, working miracles**."—*Revelation 16:14.*

With their superior intelligence, **Satan and his angels can appear to work miracles**, which will deceive all who are not grounded in a knowledge of the Bible.

"For such are false apostles, deceitful workers, transforming themselves into the apostles of Christ. And no marvel; for Satan himself is transformed into an angel of light."—*2 Corinthians 11:13-14.*

One of the newest forms of ancient paganism which has entered the West in recent decades is

W
A
Y

Yoga. Both Hinduism and Buddhism use it to make contact with "master spirits." **Beware of the Eastern religions!**

We have come to a time when we cannot always trust our eyes, ears, and feelings. We must found all our beliefs on the written Word of God. We must study and obey what the Bible says.

Remember that "the dead know not anything." Our only safety is to flee from such things—and plead with Christ for help! Thank God, He is more powerful than the devil and all his demons!

It is easy to be deceived, or to deceive ourselves. "Take heed that no man deceive you (Matthew 24:4). "Let no man deceive himself" (1 Corinthians 3:18). "Satan, which deceiveth the whole world" (Revelation 12:9), wants everyone to believe that it is all right to ignore the Bible, disobey God's Ten Commandments, and refuse to accept Christ as one's Saviour.

Although there is trickery and showmanship by the mediums, witches, and psychics,—there is also satanic involvement. Have nothing to do with such things, not even horoscopes and astrology.

"Wherefore if they shall say unto you, Behold, he is in the desert; go not forth: **behold, he is in the secret chambers; believe it not**."—Matthew 24:26.

Millions of dollars are spent each year on fortune-tellers of one kind or another. "Wherefore do ye spend money for that which is not bread?" Isaiah 55:2).

We should not read witchcraft novels, such as the Harry Potter books! Their author has filled them with instruction from her large collection of spiritist books written for witches. Here are several quotations from the present author's book, The Demons of Witchcraft:

"**She [J.K. Rowling] has an extremely well-developed and sophisticated knowledge of the occult world**, its legends, history and nuances."—Richard Abanes, Harry Potter and the Bible, p. 24.

"**There is a general nastiness underneath the mantle of cuteness.** The kids lie, they steal, they take revenge. This is a disturbing moral world, and it conflicts with what I am trying to teach my children."—Ken McCormick, quoted in Baptist Press, July 13, 2000.

"The ordinary person is typified as being bad because they have no [magic] powers, and heroes are the people who are using the occult. **This is an inversion of morality**."—Robert Frisken of Christian Community Schools in Australia, quoted in Sydney Morning Herald, March 27, 2001.

"Out of the shadows, a hooded figure came crawling across the ground like some stalking beast . . The cloaked figure reached the unicorn, lowered its head over the wound in the animal's

side, and began to drink its blood."—Sorcerer's Stone, p. 256.

"Where there should have been a back to Quirrell's head, there was a face, the most terrible face Harry had ever seen. It was chalk white with glaring eyes and slits for nostrils, like a snake . . 'See what I have become?' the face said. 'Mere shadow and vapor . . Once I have the elixir of Life, I will be able to create a body of my own.' "—Sorcerer's Stone, pp. 293-294.

"**Harry Potter gives children an appetite for the occult**."—Robert Knight, Family Research Council, in Tulsa World, June 20, 2000.

Here is an outstanding passage of Scripture which is a safe guide for any willing to follow it:

"And when they shall say unto you, Seek unto them that have familiar spirits, and unto wizards that peep, and that mutter: **should not a people seek unto their God?** [instead of] for the living to the dead?

"**To the law and to the testimony: if they speak not according to this Word, it is because there is no light in them**."—Isaiah 8:20.

One day a small boy, from a non-Christian home, was curious to learn what it was like inside a church. So he began going to one. His mother had a morbid fear of death. After listening to the story of the resurrection of Christ, the child ran home with a shining face and exclaimed, "Oh, Mother! you need not be afraid to die anymore, for Jesus went through the grave and, when He came out, He left a light behind! —For He has risen from the dead!"

Yes, one of the comforting truths in all of God's Book is that **a person rests quietly, undisturbed by memories of a troubled life or by concern for his loved ones, until the promised resurrection day.**

Notice how consistent God's plan is. **Why would we need a resurrection at the end of time if men go to their reward immediately at death?** Why would Jesus need to return to this earth a second time, as He has promised, to gather His people,—if they are already with Him now in Paradise? Why do the Scriptures teach a judgment in the last days if men are already judged at death?

The dead do not return to their house. Their power to think ceases. **They know nothing until Jesus calls them forth at the resurrection.**

SAUL AND THE WITCH OF ENDOR

It is altogether possible for a fallen angel to masquerade as another being, to actually appear to be the form of a loved one. This helps explain what happened when **King Saul dared to visit a witch in a cave in the region of Endor.** The story of what happened is told in 1 Samuel 28. Notice verses 6 and 7:

"And when Saul inquired of the Lord, the Lord

answered him not, neither by dreams, nor by Urim, nor by prophets. Then said Saul unto his servants, Seek me a woman that hath a familiar spirit, that I may go to her, and inquire of her. And his servants said to him, Behold, there is a woman that hath a familiar spirit at Endor."—*1 Samuel 28:6-7.*

Although Saul knew that witches were representatives of Satan, he went to visit one—so he could receive counsel from Samuel who had died.

"And Saul disguised himself, and put on other raiment, and he went, and two men with him, and they came to the woman by night: and he said, I pray thee, divine unto me by the familiar spirit, and bring me him up, whom I shall name unto thee . . Then said the woman, Whom shall I bring up unto thee? And he said, Bring me up Samuel."—*1 Samuel 28:8, 11.*

Why did the witch say, "Whom shall I bring up?" **If Samuel went to heaven when he died, why would not the medium call him down from heaven**—instead of up from down below, as she did?

This medium said she saw several beings arriving: **"I saw gods ascending out of the earth."** *Verse 13.* She saw evil spirits entering the cave. First she said she saw several, and then said she only saw one. When Saul asked, "What form is he of?" she said, "An old man cometh up; and he is covered with a mantle" *(verse 14).* Saul accepted that as Samuel.

But how could Saul speak to Samuel, when "the dead know not anything"? Samuel was in the grave. However, **because Saul dared to visit a witch's den, Satan had direct access to the king and could affect his mind with what he thought he was seeing!**

It was only an evil demon playing the part of Samuel in psychic drama forbidden by God!

Satan is able to predict some things correctly. He knew that the king, who would get almost no sleep that night, would be so distraught with a message that he would die the next day in battle—that it would be a self-fulfilling prophecy. —Especially so, since the Lord had now fully left him!

And so the prediction came true. **Because Saul dared to do this, he died the next day.** We are told that **part of the reason he died was because he consulted a spirit medium.**

"So Saul died for his transgression which he committed against the Lord, even against the word of the Lord, which he kept not, and also for asking counsel of one that had a familiar spirit, to inquire of it."—*1 Chronicles 10:13.*

Some who read this incident in the Bible imagine that Samuel actually spoke to Saul. But, *first,* "the dead know not anything." And *second,* **if Samuel were actually in heaven—would God permit him to go at the call of a witch to talk to Saul?**

God writes over the seance, over every attempt to contact the dead, "Evil and deadly!" The same satanic powers that operated back then are working today.

A well-known spiritualist medium wrote this:

"The phenomenal aspect of modern spiritualism reproduces all of the essential principles of the magic witchcraft and sorcery of the past. The same powers are involved, the same intelligences operating."—*F.F. Morse, Practical occultism, p. 85.*

"The road to Endor is the oldest road
And the craziest road of all;
Straight it runs to the witch's abode
As it did in the days of Saul.
And nothing has changed of the sorrow in store
For those that go down on the road to Endor."
        — *Rudyard Kipling*

Commenting on that poem, Jane T. Stoddard, in her book, *The Case against Spiritualism,* wrote, **"That old road has never been more crowded than it is today."**

SPIRITUALISM IN THE LAST DAYS

Scripture declares that there will be a dramatic increase in the popularity of witchcraft as we near the end of the world.

As of January 2008, 180 million copies of **the Harry Potter books**, alone, have been printed. You will find them in over 45 languages, in 135 countries. The worldwide gross dollars for the Harry Potter films is $3.8 billion. Over 1.5 million audio versions have been sold. The author, J.K. Rowling, is now the richest woman in Britain, and the first billionaire in history who obtained it by writing books.

Yet such books portray hate, violence, murder, and crimes of the most grotesque and sordid type.

Satan is planning for a "satanic spectacular" in these last days.

"Now the Spirit speaketh expressly, that in the latter times some shall depart from the faith, giving heed to seducing spirits, and doctrines of devils."—*1 Timothy 4:1.*

He will do wonders, even appearing as "an angel of light."

"And no marvel; for Satan himself is transformed into an angel of light."—*2 Corinthians 11:14.*

His agents will pretend to be very righteous and holy.

"Therefore it is no great thing if his ministers also be transformed as the ministers of righteousness."—*2 Corinthians 11:15.*

Satan and his agents will even attempt to counterfeit the coming of Christ, and work signs and wonders to confirm their boastful claims.

"Then if any man shall say unto you, Lo, here is Christ, or there; believe it not. For there shall arise false Christs, and false prophets, and shall show great signs and wonders; insomuch that, if it were possible, they shall deceive the very elect."—*Matthew 24:23-24.*

Satan will make it appear that fire is coming down from heaven.

"And he doeth great wonders, so that he maketh fire come down from heaven on the earth in the sight of men, and deceiveth them that dwell on the earth by the means of those miracles which he had power to do."—*Revelation 13:13-14.*

Satan will work with special power and deceptive wonders just prior to Christ's Second Coming.

"Whose coming is after the working of Satan with all power and signs and lying wonders."—*2 Thessalonians 2:9.*

Even though many will be deceived by these wonders, and accept the false christs that appear, **Christ's faithful ones know the Bible teaching that Christ will not touch the earth when He comes to take His redeemed to heaven.**

"For the Lord Himself shall descend from heaven with a shout, with the voice of the archangel, and with the trump of God: and the dead in Christ shall rise first: Then we which are alive and remain shall be caught up together with them in the clouds, to meet the Lord in the air: and so shall we ever be with the Lord."—*1 Thessalonians 4:16-17.*

We must cling to Jesus, study His Word, and by His enabling grace obey what we read.

"Be sober, be vigilant; because your adversary the devil, as a roaring lion, walketh about, seeking whom he may devour."—*1 Peter 5:8.*

ONLY WITH JESUS ARE WE SAFE

The spiritualists hate the Bible, Christ, God, and the plan of salvation. Sir Arthur Conan Doyle, who spent his life writing mystery novels to preoccupy minds with crime, also went deeply into spiritualism. He wrote, "Spiritualism will sweep the world and make it a better place in which to live. When it rules the world, it will banish the blood of Christ."

But those in the world who do not have Christ are desolate and lonely. **There is no help or comfort to be found in worldly entertainment, reading Harry Potter books, or attending seances.** Only in Jesus can we find the peace of heart for which we so much long.

A little cottage in the West caught fire. In a few seconds the thatched roof and wooden timbers were ablaze. The villagers stood around helpless.

Suddenly, a young man who had recently arrived in the area, ran up—and into the burning house. **Soon he emerged through the smoke, bearing under each arm a little child.** They were unhurt, for Andy had hidden them under his coat. But he was terribly burned.

Scarcely had he got out before the roof of the cottage fell in with a sickening crash. The parents were never seen alive again.

A kind old woman took Andy into her home and nursed him carefully. Meanwhile, there was much discussion in the village as to what was to become of the two rescued children. **A council meeting was called, and two claimed the little ones.** One was the squire of the village. He had money, position, and a home to offer the children.

The other was Andy! **When asked what right he had to the little ones, he said "I was willing to die for them," and held up his hands**—burned and scarred on their account. Everyone agreed that Andy should have the children.

The Lord Jesus Christ, our divine Intercessor, holds up His hands before the Father—and claims you and me as His own. Will we accept Him? He is waiting.

"I know not how Calvary's cross, A world from sin could free. I only know its matchless love, Has brought God's love to me."

———

COMING NEXT—It is a solemn fact that God has a moral law which has never been abolished, and never will be. It has been in force all through the Bible, and continues to be the moral code for all mankind today.

———

— PART FOUR —
CHRIST'S MORAL LAW

———

Chapter Fifteen

Heaven's Law for Mankind
Obedience by Faith in Christ

IN THE OLD TESTAMENT

A woman married a man whom she did not love. He made her get up every morning at five o'clock, cook his breakfast, and serve it at six sharp. He made her wait on him, was exacting in his demands on her time. Her life was made miserable trying to satisfy him.

After a few years, he died and she married again. This time she married a man whom she really loved. One day while clearing out some old papers, she came across the strict set of rules her former husband had written out for her to obey. Looking down through them, *she discovered that she was* *actually doing all of them now!* Then she realized that she was doing them all because of her deep love for the one to whom she was married.

It is not difficult to serve God and obey His laws when we really love Him.

According to the Bible, God is a king—the "king of nations" *(Jeremiah 10:10)*. With His throne in the heavens, He is also the king of the universe "and His kingdom ruleth over all" *(Psalm 103:19)*. "He removeth kings, and setteth up kings" *(Daniel 2:21)*.

God shares this rulership with Christ. We are told about Christ, that "the government shall be upon His shoulder" *(Isaiah 9:6)*. The last book in the Bible pictures Him coming as "King of kings, and Lord of lords" *(Revelation 19:16)*.

At that time He shall "set up a kingdom, which shall never be destroyed: and the kingdom shall not be left to other people, but it shall break in pieces and consume all these kingdoms, and it shall stand forever" *(Daniel 2:44)*.

GOD'S GOVERNMENT HAS LAWS

God, who "ruleth over all," has a kingdom based on law. Without laws, everything would soon become chaotic, with each person a law unto himself.

Not even earthly governments can exist without laws. It is one of the greatest tragedies of our time, that so many teach that Christ died to abolish the moral law of Ten Commandments. The truth is that **Christ died (1) to vindicate God's just and holy law, and (2) to enable us by His grace to obey it.**

Belief in the importance of good laws, and obedience to them, is the very foundation of human society. Without this no people can be truly peaceful and happy.

We can be thankful that in Heaven's government, there are laws!

"The Lord is our judge, **the Lord is our lawgiver**, the Lord is our king."—*Isaiah 33:22*.

"**There is one lawgiver**, who is able to save and to destroy."—*James 4:12*.

God's law tells what He is like. It describes His character, showing that He is pure and holy.

"**Wherefore the law is holy, and the commandment holy, and just, and good**."—*Romans 7:12*.

His law is as stable and enduring as His character. "For I am the Lord, I change not." *Malachi 3:6*.

"**All His commandments are sure. They stand fast forever and ever**, and are done in truth and uprightness."—*Psalm 111:7-8*.

The perfection of God's law is the proof of its divine origin.

"**The law of the Lord is perfect**, converting the soul: the testimony of the Lord is sure, making wise the simple. The statutes of the Lord are right, rejoicing the heart: **the commandment of the Lord is pure, enlightening the eyes**."—*Psalm 19:7-8*.

"And knowest His will, and approvest the things that are more excellent, being instructed out of the law."—*Romans 2:18*.

"Friends and foes alike acknowledge that the Ten Commandments are the basis of our civilization."—*James D. Rankin*.

Here is a statement from a Lutheran publication about the perfection of God's law:

" 'The law of the Lord is perfect, converting the soul.' Psalm 19:7. Is there such a thing as a perfect law? Everything that comes from God is perfect . . **In a very real sense the law of God is the manifestation of the nature of the Lord. It could no more be imperfect than He is**."—*Augsburg Sunday School Teacher, August 1937, p. 483*.

GOD'S LAW IS THE STANDARD IN THE JUDGMENT

It is urgent that, through the enabling strength which Christ offers us, that we live clean, godly lives in accordance with God's holy Ten Commandment law. *For it will be the law book in the Judgment.*

"**Let us hear the conclusion of the whole matter: Fear God, and keep His commandments: for this is the whole duty of man. For God shall bring every work into judgment**, with every secret thing, whether it be good, or whether it be evil."—*Ecclesiastes 12:13-14*.

"**For whosoever shall keep the whole law, and yet offend in one point, he is guilty of all.** For he that said, Do not commit adultery, said also, Do not kill. Now if thou commit no adultery, yet if thou kill, thou art become a transgressor of the law. **So speak ye, and so do, as they that shall be judged by the law of liberty**."—*James 2:10-12*.

NO SIN WHERE THERE IS NO LAW

If it were possible for God's law to be abolished, there would be no definition of what is sinful. Any horrible thing could be done with impunity.

Where there is no law there is no sin, for **"sin is the transgression of the law"** *(1 John 3:4)*. It tells us what is sinful. **"For by the law is the knowledge of sin."** *Romans 3:20*. Therefore, in the strength which Christ offers us, He wants us to live clean, godly lives.

"Every man that hath this hope in him purifieth himself, even as He is pure. **Whosoever committeth sin transgresseth also the law: for sin is the transgression of the law**."—*1 John 3:3-4*.

THE LAW FROM ADAM TO ABRAHAM

W
A
Y

Adam knew the principles of God's law, otherwise his disobedience could not be considered sinful. This is because "where no law is, there is no transgression [sin]" (Romans 4:15).

"For until the law [was written on stone on Mount Sinai] sin was in the world: but sin is not imputed when there is no law."—Romans 5:13.

The fact that, before the law was given at Sinai, God recognized men's disobedience to be sinful—is conclusive proof that the law existed before it was spoken on that mountain. So, since Adam sinned, he transgressed the law of God.

"Wherefore, **as by one man sin entered into the world, and death by sin; and so death passed upon all men, for that all have sinned**."—Romans 5:12.

"For as by one man's disobedience many were made sinners."—Romans 5:19.

The Bible teaches that men are not held accountable for sin when no law exists, and also that everyone born into this world is under God's law.

"**Sin is not imputed when there is no law.**" Romans 5:13. But Adam was counted as a sinner, because "the wages of sin is death" (Romans 6:23), and "death reigned from Adam to Moses" (Romans 5:14). Paul sums it up when he says, "**So death passed upon all men, for that all have sinned**" (Romans 5:12).

The expression in Romans 5:13, "Until the law sin was in the world," means "prior to the giving of the *written* law on Mount Sinai, sin was in our world."

God said that Adam's son, Cain, had sinned (Genesis 4:6-7). That which Cain did was evil (1 John 3:12). Noah and Lot lived among lawbreaking men who were punished for their sins (2 Peter 2:4-8). "The men of Sodom were wicked and sinners before the Lord exceedingly." Genesis 13:13. They did "unlawful deeds" (2 Peter 2:7-8). **So there was a standard which defined right and wrong back then. God's law was in existence, and governed every human being.**

John Wesley was faithful to always teach the importance of obedience to God's moral law.

"**As he a Methodist loves God, so he keeps His commandments**; not only some, or most of them, but all, from the least to the greatest. He is not content to 'keep the whole law, and offend in one point;' but has, in all points, 'a conscience void of offense towards God and towards man.' "—*John Wesley, The Character of a Methodist, in Works, Vol. 8, p. 344.*

THE LAW FROM ABRAHAM TO EGYPT

God called Abraham out to represent Him and give an example of obedience to His laws. Abraham could do this because He knew God's laws.

"Because that **Abraham obeyed My voice, and kept My charge, My commandments, My**

statutes, and My laws."—*Genesis 26:5.*

Abraham was selected because he obeyed whatever God asked him to do.

"By faith Abraham, when he was called to go out into a place which he should after receive for an inheritance, obeyed; and he went out, not knowing whither he went."—*Hebrews 11:8.*

The promise was made to Abraham that, **through his example of obedience, everyone on earth could be helped**—and he would be the ancestor of the coming Messiah. Whoever wished to, could also become an obedient child of God.

"Abraham shall surely become a great and mighty nation, and all the nations of the earth shall be blessed in him . . **For I know him, that he will command his children and his household after him, and they shall keep the way of the Lord**, to do justice and judgment; that the Lord may bring upon Abraham that which he hath spoken of him."—*Genesis 18:18-19.*

"Now the Lord had said unto Abram, Get thee out of thy country, and from thy kindred, and from thy father's house, unto a land that I will show thee:

"And I will make of thee a great nation, and I will bless thee, and make thy name great; and thou shalt be a blessing: And I will bless them that bless thee, and curse him that curseth thee: and in thee shall all families of the earth be blessed."—*Genesis 12:1-3.*

The promises to Abraham were not made to the Jews alone, but to all who would submit humbly to the rule of the true God and obey His requirements.

"If ye be Christ's, then are ye Abraham's seed, and heirs according to the promise."—*Galatians 3:29.*

God blessed Joseph in Egypt because, determining to remain obedient to God, he refused to sin. When tempted, he said, "How then can I do this great wickedness, and sin against God?" (Genesis 39:9).

While in bondage to the Egyptians, the Israelites were punished for trying to keep the fourth of the Ten Commandments, which was God's command that they keep the seventh-day Sabbath holy.

"And the king of Egypt said unto them, Wherefore do ye, Moses and Aaron, let the people from their works? get you unto your burdens. And Pharaoh said, Behold, the people of the land now are many, and ye make them rest from their burdens."—*Exodus 5:4-5.*

Angered by this, Pharaoh ordered that their taskmasters make their work even harder, so they would not be able to get it all done in six days each week (verses 6-9).

O.C.S. Wallace, in his book, What Baptists Believe

(p. 80), wrote this:

"In the moral government of the universe God acts in harmony with a rule . . We cannot conceive of an age when the moral government of the universe shall be changed, because **we cannot conceive of God becoming different morally from what He is now and ever has been . . This Law of God is holy as He Himself is holy . . It is a universal law** . . The Law of God is full of the love of God."

THE LAW FROM EGYPT TO SINAI

The Bible specifically tells us that God brought the Israelites out of Egypt so they could faithfully, without hindrance, keep His laws.

"He brought forth His people with joy, and His chosen with gladness: And gave them the lands of the heathen: and they inherited the labour of the people; **that they might observe His statutes, and keep His laws.**"—*Psalm 105:43-45.*

When Moses led the Israelites out of Egypt, they already knew God's law. In Exodus 16, four chapters before Mount Sinai, they were tested on whether they would obey the Sabbath commandment, which they already knew.

"And he said unto them, This is that which the Lord hath said, **Tomorrow is the rest of the holy Sabbath unto the Lord**: bake that which ye will bake today, and seethe that ye will seethe; and that which remaineth over lay up for you to be kept until the morning.

"And they laid it up till the morning, as Moses bade: and it did not stink, neither was there any worm therein. And Moses said, Eat that today; for **today is a Sabbath unto the Lord**: today ye shall not find it in the field. Six days ye shall gather it; but on the seventh day, which is the Sabbath, in it there shall be none."—*Exodus 16:23-26.*

When some went out to gather manna on the Sabbath, God said this:

"**How long refuse ye to keep My commandments and My laws**?"—*Exodus 16:28.*

Even before receiving the law, spoken and written on tablets, at Mount Sinai (*Exodus 20:1-17; 24:12; 31:18*), **Moses was already explaining God's law to the people.**

"The people come unto me to inquire of God: When they have a matter, they come unto me; and I judge between one and another, and **I do make them know the statutes of God, and His laws.**"—*Exodus 18:15-16.*

Dwight Moody wrote in his book, *Weighed and Wanting, p. 16:*

"The people must be made to understand that **the ten commandments are still binding, and**

that there is a penalty attached to their violation.** The Sermon on the Mount did not blot out the ten commandments."

THE LAW AT MOUNT SINAI

At Mount Sinai, the Israelites entered into a solemn covenant that, in order to be God's special people, they would obey His laws.

"Ye have seen what I did unto the Egyptians, and how I bare you on eagles' wings, and brought you unto Myself.

"Now therefore, **if ye will obey My voice indeed, and keep My covenant, then ye shall be a peculiar treasure unto Me** above all people: for all the earth is Mine: And ye shall be unto Me a kingdom of priests, and an holy nation. These are the words which thou shalt speak unto the children of Israel.

"And Moses came and called for the elders of the people, and laid before their faces all these words which the Lord commanded him. And all the people answered together, and said, **All that the Lord hath spoken we will do**."—*Exodus 19:4-8.*

God was deeply grateful that the people, that day, agreed to obey His moral law! He knew that if they did not do so, they would perish in their sins.

"And the Lord heard the voice of your words, when ye spake unto me; and the Lord said unto me, I have heard the voice of the words of this people, which they have spoken unto thee: they have well said all that they have spoken.

"**O that there were such an heart in them, that they would fear Me, and keep all My commandments always, that it might be well with them, and with their children forever!**"—*Deuteronomy 5:28-29.*

Prior to this time, the facts of Creation and the Fall, and the knowledge of God and His law had been handed down from father to son until this time, but not in written form.

After the Ten Commandments were proclaimed by God from the top of Mount Sinai with His own voice (*Exodus 20:1-17; Deuteronomy 5:4, 22-26*) to the assembled people below, in a very impressive ceremony (*Exodus 20*), **God wrote the law with His own finger on solid rock.**

"And He gave unto Moses, when He had made an end of communing with him upon mount Sinai, two tables of testimony, tables of stone, written with the finger of God."—*Exodus 31:18.*

These stone tablets were broken by Moses when the Israelites sinned by worshiping a graven image (*Exodus 32:19*). Later God wrote them again (*Deuteronomy 10:4*).

Of the 31,072 verses of Scripture that are in the

W
A
Y

Bible, only fifteen verses were written by God. All the rest of the Bible, except these fifteen verses were written by men under the inspiration and guidance of the Holy Spirit.

"For the prophecy came not in old time by the will of man: but holy men of God spake as they were moved by the Holy Ghost."—*2 Peter 1:21.*

This small portion of Scripture is so important that God Himself came down to this earth, spoke these words in tones of thunder, and then with His own divine finger wrote them on tables of stone. These fifteen verses are the Ten Commandments.

Here are the TEN COMMANDMENTS, as God gave them to us on Mount Sinai:

"And God spake all these words, saying,

"I am the Lord thy God, which have brought thee out of the land of Egypt, out of the house of bondage.

[1] "Thou shalt have no other gods before Me. [2] Thou shalt not make unto thee any graven image, or any likeness of any thing that is in heaven above, or that is in the earth beneath, or that is in the water under the earth: Thou shalt not bow down thyself to them, nor serve them: for I the Lord thy God am a jealous God, visiting the iniquity of the fathers upon the children unto the third and fourth generation of them that hate Me; and showing mercy unto thousands of them that love Me, and keep My commandments.

[3] "Thou shalt not take the name of the Lord thy God in vain; for the Lord will not hold him guiltless that taketh His name in vain.

[4] "Remember the Sabbath day, to keep it holy. Six days shalt thou labour, and do all thy work: But **the seventh day is the Sabbath of the Lord thy God: in it thou shalt not do any work,** thou, nor thy son, nor thy daughter, thy manservant, nor thy maidservant, nor thy cattle, nor thy stranger that is within thy gates: For in six days the Lord made heaven and earth, the sea, and all that in them is, and rested the seventh day: wherefore the Lord blessed the Sabbath day, and hallowed it.

[5] "Honour thy father and thy mother: that thy days may be long upon the land which the Lord thy God giveth thee.

[6] "Thou shalt not kill.

[7] "Thou shalt not commit adultery.

[8] "Thou shalt not steal.

[9] "Thou shalt not bear false witness against thy neighbour.

[10] "Thou shalt not covet thy neighbour's house, thou shalt not covet thy neighbour's wife, nor his manservant, nor his maidservant, nor

his ox, nor his ass, nor any thing that is thy neighbour's."—*Exodus 20:1-17.*

After the Ten Commandments were written down at Mount Sinai, the tables of stone were placed inside the ark of the covenant *(Deuteronomy 10:2),* also called the ark of the testament or testimony *(Exodus 25:22; Revelation 11:19).* The ark was given these names because the law was God's "testimony" to the people *(Exodus 31:18).* It was also God's "covenant" with them *(Deuteronomy 5:1-21).*

It is of the highest significance that this Ten Commandment law, which was the basis of God's covenant with mankind, was placed in the ark of the covenant in the most holy place (the second apartment) of the sanctuary. Above the ark, in which rested this law, the presence of God was manifested in the glory of the Shekinah. **The ark represented the foundation of God's throne. That is why the Moral Law was placed inside it.** —*In this way, God taught the people the sacredness of these moral principles, and that they are the foundation of His government.*

It is also very significant that it was on the mercy seat of the ark, above the law, that the high priest sprinkled the blood of atonement once in the year.

"The wages of sin is death" *(Romans 6:23),* and "without shedding of blood is no remission" of sin *(Hebrews 9:22).* **The blood of the victim represented the blood of Christ, which was shed on Calvary—not to destroy God's moral law—but to satisfy its demands so that by Christ's grace, God's humble, repentant, believing children could come to Him, be forgiven of their sins and strengthened to obey that law.**

There were also other statutes, the ceremonial laws governing sacrifices which prefigured Christ's death, which God also gave to Moses. But they were only temporary, and ended at the death of Christ. These were only placed on the side of the ark—not within it with the eternal moral law *(Deuteronomy 31:24-26).*

Here is a nice summary statement by W.C. Proctor, a Bible scholar at the Moody Bible Institute:

"We should not suppose that the Ten Commandments were new enactments when they were proclaimed from Sinai; for, the Hebrew word *torah* [law] is used in such previous passages of the Old Testament as Genesis 26:5; Exodus 12:49; Genesis 35:2; Exodus 13:9; 16:28; 18:16, 20. [Genesis 2:3 and Exodus 16:22-30 for the fourth; Genesis 9:6, for the sixth; and Genesis 2:24 for the seventh.]

"The decalogue, given to us in Exodus 20:3-17, may therefore be regarded as the full and solemn declaration of duties which had been revealed previously, and this public enunciation took place under absolutely unique circumstances. We are told that 'the ten words' were spoken by God's own voice (*Exodus 20:1; Deuteronomy 5:4, 22-26*), and twice afterward 'written on tables of stone with the finger of God' (*Exodus 24:12; 31:18; 32:16; 34:1, 28; Deuteronomy 4:13; 5:22, 9-10; 10:1-4*), thus appealing alike to the ear and eye, **and emphasizing both their supreme importance and permanent obligation**."—*William C. Proctor, Moody Bible Institute Monthly, October 1933, p. 49.*

Someone set the Ten Commandments to verse:
"Thou shalt have no more gods but Me,
Before no idol bow the knee,
Take not the name of God in vain,
Nor dare the Sabbath to profane.
Give both thy parents honor due,
Take heed that thou no murder do.
Abstain from words and deeds unclean;
Nor steal, though thou be poor and mean;
Nor make a willful lie, nor love it,
What is thy neighbor's dare not covet."

Several years before becoming president, Abraham Lincoln addressed a group of young people in a church in Springfield, Illinois. Lincoln had earlier made a study of some of the different religions of the world, searching for a foundation which could guide men aright. He presented to this group of young people what he found to be the outstanding law of each religion, while pointing out flaws in each one. Then in summary, he said this:

"It seems to me that **nothing short of infinite wisdom could by any possibility have been devised and given to man this one excellent and perfect moral code: the Ten Commandments.** It is suited to men in all conditions of life, and summarizes all the duties they owe to their Creator, to themselves, and to their fellow men."

William Jennings Bryan said it this way:

"Sinai is inseparably connected with the Ten Commandments given by the Almighty for the guidance of humanity. **It is now the foundation of law for the entire civilized world.** Like the Lord's Prayer, in a few words it covers all the important relations of life."

THE LAW FROM MOSES TO CHRIST

After God's people entered Canaan and settled there, they repeatedly rebelled against God's authority, and refused to obey His moral law. But there were faithful ones who, in their lives, drew close to God and carefully obeyed the Ten Commandments, so they could be more like Him. *Here are some of their divinely inspired statements:*

"Blessed are the undefiled in the way, who walk in the law of the Lord."—*Psalm 119:1.*

"**The law of the Lord is perfect, converting the soul**: the testimony of the Lord is sure, mak-

ing wise the simple. The statutes of the Lord are right, rejoicing the heart: the commandment of the Lord is pure, enlightening the eyes . . **More to be desired are they than gold, yea, than much fine gold: sweeter also than honey** and the honeycomb. **Moreover by them is Thy servant warned: and in keeping of them there is great reward**."—*Psalm 19:7-8, 10-11.*

"**Great peace have they which love Thy law: and nothing shall offend them.** Lord, I have hoped for Thy salvation, and done Thy commandments. My soul hath kept Thy testimonies; and I love them exceedingly."—*Psalm 119:165-167.*

"**The fear of the Lord is the beginning of wisdom: a good understanding have all they that do His commandments**: His praise endureth forever."—*Psalm 111:10.*

But, tragically, those who refuse to obey God's holy law will eventually come to a miserable end.

"**Depart from evil, and do good; and dwell for evermore.** For the Lord loveth judgment, and forsaketh not His saints; they are preserved forever: but the seed of the wicked shall be cut off. The righteous shall inherit the land, and dwell therein forever. The mouth of the righteous speaketh wisdom, and his tongue talketh of judgment. **The law of his God is in his heart; none of his steps shall slide**."—*Psalm 37:27-31.*

"Blessed is the man that walketh not in the counsel of the ungodly, nor standeth in the way of sinners, nor sitteth in the seat of the scornful. **But his delight is in the law of the Lord; and in His law doth he meditate day and night.** And he shall be like a tree planted by the rivers of water, that bringeth forth his fruit in his season; his leaf also shall not wither; and whatsoever he doeth shall prosper.

"**The ungodly are not so: but are like the chaff which the wind driveth away.** Therefore the ungodly shall not stand in the judgment, nor sinners in the congregation of the righteous. **For the Lord knoweth the way of the righteous: but the way of the ungodly shall perish.**"—*Psalm 1:1-6.*

"**O that thou hadst hearkened to My commandments! then had thy peace been as a river**, and thy righteousness as the waves of the sea."—*Isaiah 48:18.*

"**If ye be willing and obedient, ye shall eat the good of the land**: But if ye refuse and rebel, ye shall be devoured with the sword: for the mouth of the Lord hath spoken it."—*Isaiah 1:19-20.*

"**He that turneth away his ear from hearing the law, even his prayer shall be abomina-**

tion."—*Proverbs 28:9.*

"**I have written to him the great things of My law, but they were counted as a strange thing**."—*Hosea 8:12.*

Isaiah declared God's law to be the divine test of all teaching.

"**To the law and to the testimony: if they speak not according to this Word, it is because there is no light in them**."—*Isaiah 8:20.*

The entire 119th psalm—the longest chapter in the Bible—is entirely about the law of God and what a blessing and help it is to us!

In the Baptist Church Manual, Article 12, p. 54, we read:

"**We believe that the law of God is the eternal and unchangeable rule of His moral government**; that it is holy, just, and good; and that the inability which the Scriptures ascribe to fallen man to fulfill its precepts arise entirely from their love of sin."

IN THE NEW TESTAMENT JESUS CHRIST AND THE LAW

What did Jesus have to say about God's law while He was here on earth? Did He obey it Himself? *These are very important questions!*

It was predicted that, when Christ came to earth, He would not only carefully obey God's moral law, but would emphasize its importance.

"The Lord is well pleased for His righteousness' sake; **He will magnify the law**, and make it honourable."—*Isaiah 42:21.*

It was predicted that God's law would be in Christ's heart; in other words that He would carefully obey it.

"Then said I, Lo, I come: in the volume of the book it is written of Me, I delight to do Thy will, O My God: yea, **Thy law is within My heart**."—*Isaiah 40:7-8.*

The Apostle Paul said it even more forcefully.

"Then said I, Lo, I come (in the volume of the book it is written of Me) **to do Thy will**, O God."—*Hebrews 10:7.*

It should be mentioned here that this is the *true meaning* of the Bible promise that **God will write the law on the heart of His faithful ones. That is, He will enable them by the grace of Christ to obey it.**

"I will put My law in their inward parts, **and write it in their hearts**; and will be their God, and they shall be My people."—*Jeremiah 31:33.*

"**I will put My laws into their mind**, and write them in their hearts: and I will be to them a God, and they shall be to Me a people."—*Hebrews 8:10.*

In the sermon on the mount, Christ declared that He had not come to abolish the law, but to give a perfect example of obeying it.

Christ had spoken less than two minutes of His wonderful sermon on the mount, when He declared before the multitude:

"**Think not that I am come to destroy the law**, or the prophets: **I am not come to destroy, but to fulfill.**

"For verily I say unto you, Till heaven and earth pass, **one jot or one tittle shall in no wise pass from the law**, till all be fulfilled."—*Matthew 5:17-18.*

What did Christ mean when He said, *"fulfill"?* Some people say that it meant that Christ came to earth to destroy God's moral law. *But that is not true!* **Christ did not come down here to abolish the moral principles we should live by! Instead, He came to give us, in His life, a perfect example of obedience to God's Ten Commandment law and enabling grace to obey it ourselves.**

The word, *"fulfill,"* when used in relation to prophecy, means *"to bring to pass,"* as in: "That it might be fulfilled which was spoken by Isaias the prophet" *(Matthew 4:14).* In order to fulfill prophecy, Christ had to do what the prophets predicted. This He did, when He said in Nazareth, "This day is this Scripture fulfilled in your ears" *(Luke 4:21).*

But **when used in relation to God's law, "fulfill" means "to obey it, perform it, act in accordance with it,"** *as in these passages:*

"Bear ye one another's burdens, and so **fulfill** the law of Christ."—*Galatians 6:2.*

"If ye **fulfill** the royal law according to the Scripture, thou shalt love thy neighbour as thyself, ye do well. But if ye have respect to persons, ye commit sin, and are convinced of the law as transgressors."—*James 2:8-9.*

To fulfill God's moral law, Jesus had to obey its requirements. This He did; for as He approached the hour of Gethsemane, He declared, **"I have kept My Father's commandments and abide in His love"** *(John 15:10).* **God could not love Christ if He was immoral!** But Christ obeyed the Ten Commandments. We know that He kept them with His whole heart, for God Himself testified of Christ: "Thou hast loved righteousness, and hated iniquity." *Hebrews 1:9.*

In order to fulfill, *that is to fill up,* a full example of godly living, Christ told John the Baptist to baptize Him as an example for us to follow.

"I have need to be baptized of Thee, and comest Thou to me? And Jesus answering said unto him, Suffer it to be so now: for thus **it becometh us to fulfill all righteousness**. Then he suffered Him. And Jesus, when He was baptized, went up straightway out of the water."—*Matthew 3:14-16.*

In His teaching, **Christ magnified the law, making it apply not only to outward deeds but to** inward thoughts *(Matthew 5:21-22, 27-28)*. In His life He fulfilled the law. Indeed, He was the living law. Speaking to His enemies, He asked, "Which of you convinceth Me of sin?" *(John 8:46)*. Peter later said of Christ, that He "did no sin" *(1 Peter 2:22)*.

Let us get it clear in our minds, *Christ died, not because He sinned, but because we sinned. He died not to abolish the law, but to vindicate it and give us enabling strength to obey the law!*

In Matthew 5:17-18, quoted earlier, Jesus *did not say*, "I am not come to destroy the law, but to destroy it." The word for "destroy" in the Greek is *katalusai* ("to utterly destroy," as in Matthew 26:61). That Greek word is not used in Matthew 5:17-18.

Instead, Jesus said, **"I not come to destroy the law, but to fill up (provide you with) a perfect example of obeying it."** The Greek word in verses 17 and 18 is *pleroo*. **That same word is used in "that your joy may be full,"** that is, may be made richer, more abundant, in 1 John 1:4: "These things write we unto you, **that your joy may be full."** Here are other passages which also have *pleroo*, "to make more deep, intense, perfect":

"These things have I spoken unto you, that My joy might remain in you, and **that your joy might be full.**"—*John 15:11. (Other examples are in John 16:24; John 17:13; 2 John 12.)*

"**Fulfill ye My joy**, that ye be likeminded, having the same love, being of one accord, of one mind."—*Philippians 2:2.*

Pleroo is also used in regard to preaching more fully *(Colossians 1:25)*, **and obeying more fully** *(2 Corinthians 10:6)*. It does not mean to stop preaching or stop obeying!

In the sermon on the mount, Christ also declared that whoever does not obey this law will not be saved! Here is the rest of that passage:

"Think not that I am come to destroy the law, or the prophets: I am not come to destroy, but to fulfill. For verily I say unto you, Till heaven and earth pass, one jot or one tittle shall in no wise pass from the law, till all be fulfilled.

"**Whosoever therefore shall break one of these least commandments, and shall teach men so, he shall be called the least** in the kingdom of heaven: **but whosoever shall do and teach them, the same shall be called great** in the kingdom of heaven."—*Matthew 5:17-19.*

Jesus is here saying that the entire universe would have to be destroyed before the *smallest part* of God's moral law could be done away with!

In His words, quoted above, **Christ gave a solemn warning to anyone who might tell others that they did not have to obey the Ten Commandments!** The phrase, "kingdom of heaven," as used in the book of Matthew, refers to all those who on earth accept Christ as their Saviour. But **God will consider those who**

disobey His law, and teach others to transgress it, to be the ones who will be on the bottom of the list—*and ultimately discarded*, and not later taken to Christ's heavenly kingdom.

Christ reproved the Pharisees for requiring obedience to their man-made rules, as a way to avoid obeying God's laws. On one occasion, He told how the Pharisees taught the people how to avoid keeping the sixth commandment, in a way that would enrich the Pharisees! *(Matthew 15:3-6)*. Christ then said this.

"**But in vain they do worship Me, teaching for doctrines the commandments of men.**"—*Matthew 15:9.*

Christ unsparingly condemned those who claimed to be children of God, while refusing to obey God's commandments.

"**Every tree that bringeth not forth good fruit is hewn down**, and cast into the fire. Wherefore **by their fruits ye shall know them.**

"Not every one that saith unto Me, Lord, Lord, shall enter into the kingdom of heaven; **but he that doeth the will of My Father** which is in heaven.

"Many will say to Me in that day, Lord, Lord, have we not prophesied in Thy name? and in Thy name have cast out devils? and in Thy name done many wonderful works? And then will I profess unto them, I never knew you: **depart from Me, ye that work iniquity.**"—*Matthew 7:19-23.*

When someone asked Christ what he must do to inherit eternal life, Christ replied,

"**If thou wilt enter into life, keep the commandments.**"—*Matthew 19:17.*

But, along with this, **Christ was very clear about the fact that we must be united to Him by faith in order to do *any* good thing!** Apart from Christ, it is impossible to please God by our actions.

"**Abide in Me, and I in you.** As the branch cannot bear fruit of itself, except it abide in the vine; no more can ye, except ye abide in Me. I am the vine, ye are the branches: He that abideth in Me, and I in him, the same bringeth forth much fruit: for **without Me ye can do nothing.**

"**If a man abide not in Me, he is cast forth as a branch, and is withered**; and men gather them, and cast them into the fire, and they are burned."—*John 15:4-6.*

No more soul-destroying doctrine could ever be inspired by Satan than that Christ, during His earthly life, set aside His Father's law and left man at liberty to violate it.

Christ came to earth "to save His people from their sins" *(Matthew 1:21)*,—not in their sins. Christ is "the power of God" *(1 Corinthians 1:24)*, enabling us to live godly lives. It was His mission to take "away the sin of the world" *(John 1:29)*. He will do it today for anyone who will come and submit to His authority.

John Wesley (1703-1791) **was a genuine Christian who combined both law and grace in his life**. Because of this, he gave the most powerful Christian witness of the 18th century. The founder of the Methodist Church, he wrote these words:

"The moral law, contained in the Ten Commandments, and enforced by the Prophets, He [Christ] did not take away. It was not the design of His coming to revoke any part of this . . **Every part of this law must remain in force upon all mankind, and in all ages**; as not depending either on time or place, or any other circumstances liable to change, but on the nature of God, and the nature of man, and their unchangeable relation to each other."—*John Wesley, "Upon Our Lord's Sermon on the Mount," Discourse 5, in Works, Vol. 5, pp. 311-312.*

THE APOSTLES AND GOD'S LAW

What Paul wrote—**The Apostle Paul upheld God's moral law. He declared that the law was holy, just, good, and spiritual** *(Romans 7:7, 12-14)*. In strong language, he asserted that through faith "we establish the law" *(Romans 3:27-31)*. Finally he testified in a Roman court at his own trial, "so worship I the God of my fathers, believing all things which are written in the law and in the prophets" *(Acts 24:14)*.

It is a device of the devil to quote the apostles of Christ as being against the law of God. Had Paul turned against the law of God, he himself would thereby have become a leader of apostasy, paving the way for the man of sin who was to "think to change times and laws" *(Daniel 7:25; see also 2 Thessalonians 2:3-4)*.

Paul declared that it is those who are evil who refuse to obey God's laws.

"For to be carnally minded is death; but to be spiritually minded is life and peace. Because **the carnal mind is enmity against God: for it is not subject to the law of God**, neither indeed can be."—*Romans 8:6-7.*

Paul was called by God to proclaim the truth about Jesus Christ to the Gentiles; that is, those who were not of the Jewish race.

"He is a chosen vessel unto Me, to bear My name before the Gentiles."—*Acts 9:15.*

"I have set thee to be a light of the Gentiles, that thou shouldest be for salvation unto the ends of the earth."—*Acts 13:47.*

Paul considered it his special work to bring Gentiles to faith in God and obedience to Him, "to make the Gentiles obedient, by word and deed" *(Romans 15:18)*, so they could live clean, godly lives.

Although he opposed the keeping of the ceremonial laws (since the death of Christ had abolished

their significance), **Paul was very careful to teach his converts not to be lawless, as were the heathen. Godly living, good works, was what Paul urged on the believers.**

"Let us draw near with a true heart in full assurance of faith, having our hearts sprinkled from an evil conscience, and our bodies washed with pure water. Let us hold fast the profession of our faith without wavering; for He is faithful that promised. **And let us consider one another to provoke unto love and to good works.**"—*Hebrews 10:22-24.*

To those who suggested, as many do today, that it would be all right to keep sinning and still be saved, Paul said that to do so, would mean they were still dead outside of Christ!

"What shall we say then? **Shall we continue in sin, that grace may abound?** God forbid. How shall we, that are dead to sin, live any longer therein?

"Know ye not, that so many of us as were baptized into Jesus Christ were baptized into His death? Therefore we are buried with Him by baptism into death: that like as Christ was raised up from the dead by the glory of the Father, **even so we also should walk in newness of life**."—*Romans 6:1-4.*

What John wrote—**If someone wants to abide in Christ, he should walk in obedience to God's moral law, just as Jesus did. Here is how the Apostle** John described the way we should live:

"And hereby we do know that we know Him, if we keep His commandments. **He that saith, I know Him, and keepeth not His commandments, is a liar, and the truth is not in him.** But whoso keepeth His Word, in him verily is the love of God perfected: hereby know we that we are in Him. **He that saith he abideth in Him ought himself also so to walk, even as He walked.**"—*1 John 2:3-6.*

It is clear from the above statement, that **one cannot really know God, if he does not keep His commandments.**

John also said this:

"And every man that hath this hope in Him purifieth himself, even as He is pure. **Whosoever committeth sin transgresseth also the law: for sin is the transgression of the law.**

"And ye know that He was manifested to take away our sins; and in Him is no sin. **Whosoever abideth in Him sinneth not**: whosoever sinneth hath not seen Him, neither known Him. Little children, let no man deceive you: he that doeth righteousness is righteous, even as He is righteous."—*1 John 3:3-7.*

The above text says that sin *is* (not *was*) the

transgression of the law, thus showing that the law is still in force in the gospel dispensation.

And that word, "whosoever," shows the universality of its binding claims. Everyone who commits sin transgresses the law.

John said that those who love God, always love to obey His commandments.

"By this we know that we love the children of God, **when we love God, and keep His commandments. For this is the love of God, that we keep His commandments**: and His commandments are not grievous. For whatsoever is born of God overcometh the world."—*1 John 5:2-4.*

What James wrote—**The Apostle James, years after the Christian Era began, clearly emphasized the obligation of the Christian to keep the law of Ten Commandments,**—not merely one precept, but all. **He declared this law to be the standard by which men will be judged in the great day of God.**

As Christians, we are required to keep this law as much as were God's people in ancient times. **The only basic standard of human morality that God gave to us is the Ten Commandments.**

James was very clear in his defense of God's moral law:

"**For whosoever shall keep the whole law, and yet offend in one point, he is guilty of all**. For he that said, Do not commit adultery, said also, Do not kill. Now if thou commit no adultery, yet if thou kill, thou art become a transgressor of the law. **So speak ye, and so do, as they that shall be judged by the law of liberty**."—*James 2:10-12.*

James also spoke against those who say they are Christians, but who are not obedient to the commands of God.

"Wherefore lay apart all filthiness and superfluity of naughtiness, and receive with meekness the engrafted Word, which is able to save your souls. But **be ye doers of the Word, and not hearers only, deceiving your own selves.**

"For if any be a hearer of the Word, and not a doer, he is like unto a man beholding his natural face in a glass: For he beholdeth himself, and goeth his way, and straightway forgetteth what manner of man he was.

"But whoso looketh into the perfect law of liberty, and continueth therein, **he being not a forgetful hearer, but a doer of the work, this man shall be blessed in his deed.**"—*James 1:21-25.*

Here is part of the official creed of the Church of England:

"I. **God gave to Adam a law by which He bound him and all his posterity to personal,** entire, exact, and perpetual obedience; promised life upon the fulfilling, and threatened death upon the breach of it; and endued him with power and ability to keep it.

"II. **This law after his fall, continued to be a perfect rule of righteousness**; and, as such, was delivered by God upon Mount Sinai in ten commandments, and written in two tables; the first four commandments containing our duty towards God, and the other six our duty to man."—*The Westminster Confession of Faith, Chapter 19, quoted in Philip Schaff, The Creeds of Christendom, Vol. 3, p. 640.*

If someone tells you that we don't need to keep the law anymore, ask him which of the Ten Commandments he thinks we don't need to keep anymore. He will generally have no answer to that.

"Now men may cavil as much as they like about other parts of the Bible, but **I have never met an honest man that found fault with the Ten Commandments**."—*Dwight L. Moody, Weighed and Wanting, p. 11.*

THE WAGES OF SIN IS DEATH

The Bible teaches that sin is the transgression of God's moral law, and everyone has broken it. "Whosoever committeth sin transgresseth also the law: for sin is the transgression of the law." *1 John 3:4.* And "all have sinned and come short of the glory of God" *(Romans 3:23).* "Both Jews and Gentiles . . are all under sin." *Verse 9.* "All have sinned." *Romans 5:12.*

If we continue in our sins, we will perish. "The wages of sin are death." *Romans 6:23.* "In the day that thou eatest thereof thou shalt surely die." *Genesis 2:17.* The soul that sinneth, it shall die." *Ezekiel 18:4.*

"Because sentence against an evil work is not executed speedily, therefore the heart of the sons of men is fully set in them to do evil."—*Ecclesiastes 8:11.*

"Say ye to the righteous, that it shall be well with him: for they shall eat the fruit of their doings. Woe unto the wicked! it shall be ill with him: for the reward of his hands shall be given him."—*Isaiah 3:10-11.*

Martin Luther wrote this:

"God threatens to punish all who transgress these commandments. We should, therefore, fear His anger, and do nothing against such commandments. But **He promises grace and every blessing to all who keep them. We should, therefore, love and trust in Him, and gladly obey His commandments.**"—*Martin Luther, Luther's Small Catechism, quoted in Philip Schaff, The Creeds of Chistendom, Vol. 3, p. 77.*

Jonathan Edwards, a leading Protestant revivalist of the eighteenth century in the American Colonies, wrote that **the law of God became even more important because Christ died**, so that, through Him, we could become obedient to it and be saved. The alternative would have been for Christ not to die on Calvary—and, without hope, everyone die in their sins.

"**Through the atonement of Christ more honor is done to the law, and consequently the law is more fully established**, than if the law had been literally executed, and all mankind had been condemned."—*Jonathan Edwards, Works (1842 ed.), Vol. 2, p. 369.*

It is a serious thing to trample upon God's law.

"Against every evildoer, God's law utters condemnation. He may disregard that voice, he may seek to drown its warning, but in vain. It follows him. It makes itself heard. It destroys his peace. If unheeded, it pursues him."—*Education, 144-145.*

GOD'S GIFT IS ETERNAL LIFE

But, thank God, *there is hope!* **Those who surrender their lives to God's dear Son, Jesus Christ, and humbly "follow the Lamb whithersoever He goeth"** (Revelation 14:4) **will be able to be saved—and live forever with Him in heaven!** Oh, my friend, we must obtain this glorious prize! God offers it; we can have it.

"And as Moses lifted up the serpent in the wilderness, even so must the Son of man be lifted up: That whosoever believeth in Him should not perish, but have eternal life. For God so loved the world, that **He gave His only begotten Son, that whosoever believeth in Him should not perish**, but have everlasting life."—*John 3:14-16.*

"When ye were the servants of sin, ye were free from righteousness. **What fruit had ye then in those things whereof ye are now ashamed? for the end of those things is death.**

"But now being made free from sin, and become servants to God, ye have your fruit unto holiness, and the end everlasting life.

"**For the wages of sin is death; but the gift of God is eternal life** through Jesus Christ our Lord."—*Romans 6:20-23.*

How thankful we can be that, **through the power of Christ's sacrifice on Calvary, He can empower us to live godly lives.**

"**But as many as received Him, to them gave He power to become the sons of God**, even to them that believe on His name."—*John 1:12.*

John Calvin wrote this:

"**We must not imagine that the coming of Christ has freed us from the authority of the law**; for it is the eternal rule of a devout and holy life, and must, therefore, be as unchangeable as the justice of God."—*John Calvin, Commentary on a Harmony of the Gospels, Vol. 1, p. 277.*

FAITH, LOVE, AND THE LAW

Some say that all we need is "faith." But **does faith in God make void His moral law; that is, set aside the need to obey it?**

"**Do we then make void the law through faith? God forbid: yea, we establish the law.**"—*Romans 3:31.*

The truth is that **genuine faith in Christ—provides enabling strength to keep God's law. But those who profess to accept Christ, yet refuse obedience to the will of God—do not have faith, but presumption.** They imagine that their words and expressions of faith will save them. Yet, because they are not connected with Christ, they are in terrible danger! For they think their profession of faith and their church attendance will save them—while they are actually separated from Christ and living in an unsaved state.

More than all else, **the fact that "Christ died for our sins"** (1 Corinthians 15:3) **makes it certain that the law could not have been abolished!**

If the moral law could have been abolished when mankind sinned, then Christ need not have died. But this wonderful gift of Christ proves the unchangeableness of God's law. Christ had to come and die on the cross, to satisfy the demands of the law,—or the world must perish. The law could not give way.

Although His great sacrifice was sufficient to save everyone on earth, the great tragedy is that most people will reject it. They would rather remain in their sins.

The fact that the law is to be the standard in the judgment is another proof of its enduring nature. If the law was destroyed at Calvary, how could it be standard in the judgment later on?

"Let us hear the conclusion of the whole matter: **Fear God, and keep His commandments: for this is the whole duty of man.**

"**For God shall bring every work into judgment**, with every secret thing, whether it be good, or whether it be evil."—*Ecclesiastes 12:13-14.*

By His grace, Christ can enable us to fully keep the law of God. In doing so, we are liberated—freed—from slavery to sinful habits. But those who refuse to be freed will be judged and condemned by that law.

"Whosoever shall keep the whole law, and yet offend in one point, he is guilty of all. For He that said, Do not commit adultery, said also, Do not kill. Now if thou commit no adultery, yet if thou kill, thou art become a transgressor of the law. **So speak ye, and so do as they that shall be judged by the law** of liberty."—*James 2:10-12.*

Actual obedience is required of the Christian, not just talk.

"For not the hearers of the law are just before God, **but the doers of the law shall be justified**."—*Romans 2:13 (also Matthew 21:28-31).*

"But whoso looketh into the perfect law of liberty, and continueth therein, he being not a forgetful hearer, **but a doer** of the work, this man shall be blessed in his deed."—*James 1:25.*

How can we know that we have passed from death to life?

"We know that we have passed from death unto life, because we love the brethren."—*1 John 3:14.*

How can we know that we genuinely love the brethren?

"By this **we know that we love the children of God, when we love God, and keep His commandments**."—*1 John 5:2.*

What does it mean to really love God?

"For this is the love of God, that we keep His commandments**: and His commandments are not grievous."—*1 John 5:3.*

Martin Luther said this:

"He who destroys the doctrine of the law, destroys at the same time political and social order . . as to the law in itself, I never rejected it."—*Martin Luther, quoted in M. Michelet's Life of Luther, p. 315.*

IN THE LAST DAYS

Now as always before, **Christ does not save men in sin,** but He saves them *from their sins.* Since sin is the transgression of God's law, Christ must save His people from lawbreaking, or He can never qualify them for heaven.

In the final crisis, just before Christ returns for His faithful ones, the world will become so wicked—that men will be required to disobey God's law. But the remnant, those of God's children who live down at the end of time, will be true to Him.

This final remnant will be distinguished by the fact that they keep all ten of God's commandments! —And they do it by the enabling grace of Christ!

"And the dragon was wroth with the woman, and went to make war with **the remnant of her seed, which keep the commandments of God,** and have the testimony of Jesus Christ."—*Revelation 12:17.*

"Here is the patience of the saints: **here are they that keep the commandments of God,** and the faith of Jesus."—*Revelation 14:12.*

The promise is rich and abundant. Those who faithfully obey God—will inherit eternal life!

"Blessed are they that do His commandments, that they may have right to the tree of life, and may enter in through the gates into the city."—*Revelation 22:14.*

The next verse lists many people who will not be permitted to enter those gates. Yet **only a few verses later, God pleads with each of us, while there is still time, to come—so we too can receive the glorious future He has in store for the redeemed!**

"The Spirit and the bride say, Come. And let him that heareth say, Come. And let him that is athirst come. **And whosoever will, let him take the water of life freely**."—*Revelation 22:17.*

We are told that the devils also believe in Christ, and tremble because they will eventually perish.

"**Even so faith, if it hath not works, is dead, being alone.** Yea, a man may say, Thou hast faith, and I have works: show me thy faith without thy works, and I will show thee my faith by my works.

"Thou believest that there is one God; thou doest well: **the devils also believe, and tremble.**

"But wilt thou know, O vain man, that **faith without works is dead**?"—*James 2:17-20.*

IN CONCLUSION

In this chapter, **we have learned that believing in Christ includes obeying Christ and becoming like Him.** That makes that most famous of all verses—all the more precious to us.

"**For God so loved the world, that He gave His only begotten Son, that whosoever believeth in Him should not perish, but have everlasting life**."—*John 3:16.*

There are two striking things in the above text: **When God loves, He loves a world. When He gives, He gives His Son.** Such is the boundless love of the eternal Father and Son for mankind.

How deep is that love?

"Thou hast in love to my soul delivered it from the pit of corruption."—*Isaiah 38:17.*

"He brought me up also out of an horrible pit."—*Psalm 40:2.*

How high is it?

"And hath raised us up together, and made us sit together in heavenly places in Christ Jesus."—*Ephesians 2:6.*

What is its length and breadth?

"That in the ages to come He might show the exceeding riches of His grace in His kindness toward us through Christ Jesus."—*Ephesians 2:7.*

As we have learned in this chapter, **God has rules for our lives, so that, by obeying them through the enabling grace of Christ, we will be prepared to live through eternity in the happiness of heaven.**

While there is yet time to do it, each of us have a choice to make. On God's side is Calvary's sacrifice, the commandments made more sure by it, and eternal life. On Satan's side is sin, and self, and death; nothing pleasant, nothing worth having.

To every one of us, God sends this urgent, personal, appeal:

"I call heaven and earth to record this day against you, that **I have set before you life and death, blessing and cursing: therefore choose life, that both thou and thy seed may live: that thou mayest love the Lord thy God, and that thou mayest obey His voice**."—*Deuteronomy 30:19-20.*

Earlier in this chapter, the words of John Wesley who loved the law of God were quoted. Here is a poem by another child of God who also loved that law: Isaac Watts, one of the greatest Christian songwriters of history.

"O that the Lord would guide my ways, To keep His statutes still! O that my God would grant me grace To know and do His will!

"O send Thy Spirit down to write Thy law upon my heart; Nor let my tongue indulge deceit, Nor act the liar's part.

"From vanity turn off my eyes, Let no corrupt design Nor covetous desires arise Within this soul of mine.

"Make me to walk in Thy commands, 'Tis a delightful road; Nor let my head, nor heart, nor hands, Offend against my God."—*Isaac Watts.*

———————

COMING NEXT—A very important chapter, which carefully explains how Christ enables us to obey His moral law of Ten Commandments. This is information that each of us needs to know.

Chapter Sixteen

Saved by Grace
What Christ Does in Our Lives

In a certain Midwest village, there was a dishonest man who sold firewood to his neighbors—but always cut it a little short of the required four feet.

One day people heard that he had been converted, but that seemed impossible; for everyone knew what he had been like earlier. So no one believed the report. But one man slipped quietly out of the grocery store where they were discussing this,—and soon came back running. **"It's so! He has been converted!"** They all asked, "How do you know?"

"Why," he said, "I went over and measured the wood that he cut yesterday. It is all a good four feet in length."

The person who accepts Christ as His Saviour becomes a new man, obedient to the Ten Commandments.

The moral law of God is closely connected with

Jesus Christ. Apart from the conviction of sin which the law brings, none will come to Him. And apart from His forgiving, enabling grace the Ten Commandments can do nothing to change our hearts and lives.

In this chapter we want to discover how wonderfully the two are connected. In doing so, we discover that Christ did not make the supreme sacrifice of dying on Calvary—just so a bunch of sinners, reveling in their delicious sins, could be taken to heaven.

No, no. **His sufferings and death were designed to bring us into total harmony with, and obedience to, God's moral law—so we could be transformed** into godly people who, in thought, word, and conduct, become like Jesus.

But, of course, all this could not happen if Christ destroyed the Ten Commandments when He died!

In the early days of America, a band of explorers gave an Indian chief a sundial. He was so happy to have it that he built a shelter over it, to protect it from sun and rain. But, because it was hidden from the sunlight, it could no longer indicate the time of day—and thus became a useless piece of brass, unable to be used according to its original purpose.

Perfect as is the holy Ten Commandment law, there are some things it cannot do.

We want to learn (1) what the law can do for the sinner, (2) what it cannot do for him, (3) what the grace of Christ can do for him, and (4) what the law can do for the person receiving the grace of Christ.

WHAT THE LAW DOES FOR THE SINNER

First, the law gives a knowledge of sin.

"For **by the law is the knowledge of sin**."—*Romans 3:20.*

"What shall we say then? is the law sin? God forbid. Nay, **I had not known sin, but by the law**: for I had not known lust, except the law had said, Thou shalt not covet."—*Romans 7:7.*

The law that does this is the Ten Commandment law, of which "thou shalt not covet" is the tenth commandment.

Second, the law brings a sense of guilt.

"Now we know that what things soever the law saith, it saith to them who are under the law: that every mouth may be stopped, and all the world may become guilty before God."—*Romans 3:19.*

A man drives fast through a stop sign, and then hears a police siren behind him, and suddenly he is gripped with fear. Disobedience has placed him "under the law;" that is, under its condemnation. The presence of the law intensifies guilt and fear in the heart of the violator. Before God's law, all the world must plead guilty, for "all have sinned" *(Romans 3:23).*

(It is true that some refuse to admit guilt, pleading

the excuse for their ongoing sins by saying that Christ destroyed the law at Calvary—so they are going to be saved anyway, merely by saying they are Christians. But such folk are living in fools' paradise, and they will one day have to answer in the Judgment for their conduct, and the way their flimsy excuses influenced others to continue their rebellion against God.)

The third function of the law is to act as a spiritual mirror. By looking at it, we see the flaws in ourselves which need correcting.

"For if any be a hearer of the Word, and not a doer, he is like unto a man beholding his natural face in a glass: For he beholdeth himself, and goeth his way, and straightway forgetteth what manner of man he was.

"But whoso looketh into the perfect law of liberty, and continueth therein, he being not a forgetful hearer, but a doer of the word, this man shall be blessed in his deed."—*James 1:23-25.*

Shortly afterward, James explains that this "law of liberty" is the Ten Commandments *(James 2:9-12).* He says that we are to be "judged by the perfect law of liberty," and identifies it as the one which says, "Do not commit adultery," and "Do not kill."

It was Abraham Lincoln who said, "It seems to me that nothing short of infinite wisdom could by any possibility have devised and given to man this excellent and perfect moral code." Thank God that we have those ten rules to govern our lives, and that we have Christ to write them on our hearts (that is, our minds), so we can be pure and clean like Him!

John Brown, an evangelist of the nineteenth century, said, **"The human heart cannot receive the healing thread of the Gospel—unless it is first pierced by the needle of the law."**

WHAT THE LAW CANNOT DO FOR THE SINNER

The sinner desperately needs two things which the law cannot provide.

First, he needs forgiveness, or justification. He needs to be forgiven of his past sins so he can become God's child. The publican cried for forgiveness, and went down to his house "justified" *(Luke 18:13-14).* But "by the deeds of the law there shall no flesh be justified" *(Romans 3:20).*

Perfect as it is, the law of God cannot forgive sin. It can only tell us that we are sinners and under its condemnation. That is what it means to be "under the law." **Only the *Lawgiver* can forgive; and He died on Calvary and rose afterward, so He can forgive the truly repentant and enable them to be genuine overcomers.** The needle of the law cannot ever sew up the wounds that sin has made.

The second thing the sinner needs is power to resist sin, or sanctification. But God's holy law can-

not provide this either. The sinner must be changed, and the law cannot do this.

"Is the law then against the promises of God? God forbid: for if there had been a law given which could have given life, verily righteousness should have been by the law."—*Galatians 3:21.*

Those who want to remain in their sins will accept any theory which seems to eliminate God's law. Indeed, the error that it is all right to continue in sin is taught in most pulpits of every major religion both in Christianity and the other world religions. Why? Because men want such a religion.

"The carnal mind is enmity against God: for it is not subject to the law of God, neither indeed can be."—*Romans 8:7.*

A mirror may reveal a dirty face, but it cannot cleanse it or make it clean.

WHAT THE GRACE OF CHRIST CAN DO FOR HIM

An acquaintance of a certain minister committed a crime for which he was sentenced to years in the penitentiary. After he had served a year or two, the minister went to the governor of the state and persuaded him that it would be to the best interest of society to grant this young man a pardon. "And," said the governor, "I will make you the bearer of his pardon."

With the pardon in his pocket, the minister went to the penitentiary. Before handing him the paper which would make him a free man, the minister asked him, "John, if you should receive a pardon from the governor, what would you do?"

"Mr. Johnson, if I ever get out of this place, the first thing I will do is buy a gun and kill old Lawton who testified against me at the trial."

Sorrowfully, the minister left, taking the pardon with him. **This was a case where a man had violated the law, and grace could not help him.**

The forgiveness which the law cannot provide, Christ will give to the one who genuinely wants to separate from his sins.

"For God sent not His Son into the world to condemn the world; but that the world through Him might be saved."—*John 3:17.*

Those who refuse to come to Him are "condemned already" *(verse 18).* They are still under the law's condemnation.

It is the grace of Christ which makes this forgiveness and transformation possible. His grace is unmerited favor. This marvelous love awakens love in the repentant, believing, forgiven sinner. By not resisting this love, the newly converted soul becomes determined to serve and obey God.

Forgiveness of sin and power to resist sin comes through the exercise of faith in God's promises, given in the Bible, and a full surrender of the heart to Jesus

W
A
Y

Christ.

"For by grace are ye saved through faith."—*Ephesians 2:8.*

"For what the law could not do, in that it was weak through the flesh, God sending His own Son in the likeness of sinful flesh, and for sin, condemned sin in the flesh. That the righteousness of the law might be fulfilled in us, who walk not after the flesh, but after the Spirit."—*Romans 8:3-4.*

The sinner comes to Christ and cries:

"Create in me a clean heart, O God; and renew a right spirit within me. Cast me not away from Thy presence."—*Psalm 51:10-11.*

And Christ gives him "righteousness and sanctification" *(1 Corinthians 1:30).*

"Herein is love, not that we loved God, but that He loved us, and sent His Son to be the propitiation for our sins."—*1 John 4:10.*

Choking with feeling at such a great sacrifice for us individually, we exclaim—

"We love Him, because He first loved us!"—*1 John 4:19.*

"Plunged in a gulf of dark despair, We wretched sinners lay, Without one cheering gleam of hope, Or spark of glimmering day.

"With pitying eyes the Prince of peace Beheld our helpless grief. He saw—and oh, Amazing love! He came to our relief!"

WHAT THE LAW CAN DO FOR THE PERSON RECEIVING THE GRACE OF CHRIST

First, it can show that he is a new creature in Christ. After someone has come to Christ and received forgiveness and acceptance (justification) in His sight, what can the law now do for this individual?

"Now the righteousness of God without the law is manifested, being witnessed by the law and the prophets."—*Romans 3:21.*

—What a most wonderful promise! **The law can now point to this man as someone living in accordance with it!** God's moral law testifies that, depending moment by moment on Jesus Christ for empowering grace, he continues to put away his sins and live a decent, honest, kindly life.

Fleeing to the fountain at Calvary, we plunge beneath the flood—and are forgiven and cleansed. Looking now into the mirror of the law, we see that, indeed, we are clean.

Second, he must continue to live in accordance with that law. Because we have accepted Christ as our Saviour, **we must not think we can now smash the mirror of God's law, thinking that we no longer need it. Instead, we must live in continued obedience to it!**

We must remain submissive, humble, and obedient to Christ—or we will erelong drift back into our sins! Satan will see to that. He will be there to tempt us to do the things we once did, associate with the evil friends we once liked to be with, indulge in the evils we once loved.

"What then? shall we sin, because we are not under the law, but under grace? God forbid. Know ye not, that to whom ye yield yourselves servants to obey, his servants ye are to whom ye obey; whether of sin unto death, or of obedience unto righteousness?"—*Romans 6:15-16.*

Wholehearted obedience to the law of God is the supreme responsibility and privilege of each one who has come to Christ.

"Where sin abounded, grace did much more abound . . **What shall we say then? Shall we continue in sin, that grace may abound? God forbid.** How shall we, that are dead to sin, live any longer therein? . . **Let not sin therefore reign in your mortal body,** that ye should obey it in the lusts thereof."—*Romans 5:20, 6:1-2, 12.*

Godliness is a battle and a march! Christianity is clinging constantly to Christ. Victory over temptation is something won anew all through the day. There is no let up. There is no time out.

But, oh, how happy the experience of living in Christ! It is worth all the seeming "sacrifices" that we make in order to have it.

"Through the gates to the city, in a robe of spotless white, He will lead me where no tears shall ever fall; In the glad song of ages I shall mingle with delight; But I long to meet my Saviour first of all.

"I shall know Him I shall know Him, As redeemed by His side I shall stand. I shall know Him, I shall know Him, By the print of the nails in His hands."—*Fanny Crosby.*

Yet, in this battle, let us not become like the foolish man or the vain man:

***The foolish man* tries to be saved by his own efforts to keep the law.** Recognizing that the mirror shows him to be a sinner, he does not go to Christ but decides that his own good deeds are sufficient. He is trying to use the mirror to wash himself! "Works of penance" is not the solution.

"O **foolish** Galatians, who hath bewitched you, that ye should not obey the truth, before whose eyes Jesus Christ hath been evidently set forth, crucified among you? This only would I learn of you, Received ye the Spirit by the works of the law, or by the hearing of faith?"—*Galatians 3:1-2.*

The vain man thinks he can be saved "by faith alone," apart from obedience to God's law. Finding that the mirror condemns his sins, he takes a hammer and tries to break the mirror. He excuses his actions, and continued sins, by repeating the error that Christ did away with the law, so we could be saved in our sins—as long as we call ourselves Christians and attend church once in a while.

"But wilt thou know, O **vain man**, that faith without works is dead?"—*James 2:20.*

The blessed man also looks into this perfect mirror,—but then **runs to Christ in repentance, pleading for forgiveness for past sins, and strength to resist sin and live right in the future.** Receiving forgiveness by grace through faith, he exclaims:

"**Blessed** is he whose transgression is forgiven, whose sin is covered. **Blessed** is the man unto whom the Lord imputeth not iniquity, and in whose spirit there is no guile."—*Psalm 32:1-2.*

"**Blessed** is the man that walketh not in the counsel of the ungodly, nor standeth in the way of sinners, nor sitteth in the seat of the scornful. But his delight is in the law of the Lord; and in His law doth he meditate day and night. And he shall be like a tree planted by the rivers of water, that bringeth forth his fruit in his season; his leaf also shall not wither; and whatsoever he doeth shall prosper."—*Psalm 1:1-3.*

It was H.M.S. Richards who once said,

"A few years ago, almost everyone could repeat the Ten Commandments. Fewer can today, but all should be able to do so. There would be far less juvenile and adult delinquency in the world if both old and young not only memorized, but obeyed, the Ten Commandments. It would change our world!"

Grace is like a governor's pardon to a prisoner. It forgives him the past, but it is not a license to once again violate any of the laws on the statute books.

Faith is like a man's hand. It reaches out and accepts the pardon. —But at the same time, it reaches up and takes hold of Christ's hand for continued strength to keep obeying in the future.

Love "is the fulfilling of the law" *(Romans 13:10).*

"This is the love of God, that we keep His commandments."—*1 John 5:3.*

"But God be thanked, that ye were the servants of sin, but ye have obeyed from the heart . . Being then made free from sin, ye became the servants of righteousness."—*Romans 6:17-18.*

This holy, perfect, eternal Christ, of whose character the law was a written transcript, and whose life was a living revelation of that same law;—this Christ, God gave to save you. No one else in God's universe could meet the demands of the holy, unchangeable law of the Eternal God, and make that obedience available to you.

He lives for you *(Matthew 20:28)*. He died for you

(1 Peter 2:24). He offers pardon to you *(Isaiah 55:7; 1 John 1:9)*. He offers grace and power to you *(Hebrews 4:16)*. He offers heaven to you *(Matthew 19:27-29)*.

Do not hesitate. "Believe on the Lord Jesus Christ, and thou shalt be saved." *Acts 16:31.* He will strengthen you to live like Him—a clean, godly life.

If you will believe, you shall receive. Do not trust to feeling. Take your sins to the cross. Exchange them for forgiveness. Ask God to give you a new heart, and write His holy law upon it, that you may love it and keep it. Believe that, as you have prayed in the name of Jesus, God does this. Surrender your all to Him. Make no reservation. Give all. Receive all that God wants to give you.

"I felt His love, the strongest love,
That mortal ever felt."

———————————

SPECIAL SUPPLEMENT

There are two peculiar errors which some use to excuse the fact that they would rather keep sinning than obey God's Moral Law. One is an error about the *human nature of Christ.* The second is an error about *the nature of sin.*

THE NATURE OF CHRIST

In an attempt to evade God's requirement that we must overcome sin and obey His holy law, **some say that Christ did not really take a human nature like ours,—for if He had, while on earth He could not have resisted sin and would have fallen.** Frankly, that is blasphemous and very evil, for it downgrades both the character of Christ and the enabling power of grace.

This strange error teaches that **Christ inherited the nature of Adam before he fell into sin, and that Christ had the same type of Catholic "immaculateness" that it is claimed that the Virgin Mary had: *an inability to sin!*** It is said that Christ could not sin if He had wanted to. The theory goes on and says that, if He had inherited the same fallen nature which we inherit (a nature which can be tempted and can fall into sin), Christ could not have resisted temptation and would have become a sinner. Why? Because, **according to the theory, it is impossible for anyone living on earth—including Christ while He was here—to either keep from sinning or stop doing it!**

This strange teaching that, during His life on earth, Christ was unable to sin, originates with Catholic error about a supposed "immaculate nature" which the Virgin Mary is supposed to have had, which Catholicism teaches that her Son Jesus also shared.

"We define that the Blessed Virgin Mary in the first moment of her conception . . **was preserved free from every taint of original sin. The soul**

W
A
Y

of Mary was never subject to sin."—*Cardinal Gibbons, Faith of Our Fathers, pp. 203-204.*

There is an abundance of evidence from the Bible which totally disproves this error.

The Bible teaches that **Christ took our *exact nature*—the one you and I have—which is able to sin. Then, in our nature, He never once yielded to sin** in any way. He was totally sinless. He relied on His Father for help, as we now may rely on Christ. **Therefore, Christ is able to be our perfect Example, and provide us with forgiving and enabling grace to resist sin as He did.** He provides all willing to humbly, obediently accept it, with a perfect atonement.

Unfallen Adam was able to—and did—fall into sin *(Genesis 3)*, so how could it be that unfallen Christ could not? The angels in heaven also had unfallen natures, yet a third of them fell *(2 Peter 2:4; Revelation 12:4, 7-9)*!

Abraham lived 4,000 years after Adam, and **Christ took the nature of Abraham's descendants.**

"Forasmuch then as the children are partakers of flesh and blood, **He also Himself likewise took part of the same**; that through death He might destroy him that had the power of death, that is, the devil; and deliver them who through fear of death were all their lifetime subject to bondage. For verily **He took not on Him the nature of angels; but He took on Him the seed of Abraham. Wherefore in all things it behoved Him to be made like unto His brethren**, that He might be a merciful and faithful high priest in things pertaining to God, to make reconciliation for the sins of the people. For in that **He Himself hath suffered being tempted**, He is able to succour them that are tempted."—*Hebrews 2:14-18.*

Although Christ was tempted in all points like us, yet He never once sinned.

"For we have not an high priest which cannot be touched with the feeling of our infirmities; **but was in all points tempted like as we are, yet without sin.** Let us therefore come boldly unto the throne of grace, that we may obtain mercy, and find grace to help in time of need."—*Hebrews 4:15-16.*

Christ was not only a descendant of Abraham, He was a descendant of David, who lived 3,000 years after Adam.

"The book of the generation of Jesus Christ, the son of David, the son of Abraham."—*Matthew 1:1.*

"If ye be Christ's, then are ye Abraham's seed, and heirs according to the promise."—*Galatians 3:29.*

Christ fully took our nature so He could fully bear our sins in the atonement.

"For **He hath made Him to be sin for us**,

who knew no sin; that we might be made the righteousness of God in Him."—*2 Corinthians 5:21 (also Philippians 2:6-8).*

Christ can keep us from sinning. That is why He came to earth.

"And she shall bring forth a son, and thou shalt call His name Jesus: **for He shall save His people from their sins.**"—*Matthew 1:21.*

He was made the way we are made, so He could redeem us and enable us to obey the law.

"When the fullness of the time was come, God sent forth His Son, **made of a woman, made under the law, to redeem them that were under the law**, that we might receive the adoption of sons."—*Galatians 4:4-5.*

Because He was made in the likeness of sinful flesh, He is able to *condemn sin in the flesh*. If He could not do that, He could not provide the atonement.

"For what the law could not do, in that it was weak through the flesh, God sending His own Son **in the likeness of sinful flesh, and for sin, condemned sin in the flesh**: that the righteousness of the law might be fulfilled in us, who walk not after the flesh, but after the Spirit."—*Romans 8:3-4.*

Christ really came in the flesh. Here is a strong warning not to accept this error about the human nature of Christ which denies that, here on earth, He was really in our flesh.

"And every spirit that confesseth not that Jesus Christ is come in the flesh is not of God."—*1 John 4:3.*

It is because Christ fully took our nature, that He is able to provide us with a perfect example of obedience—and the Bible teaches that we are to follow His example.

"**He that saith he abideth in Him ought himself also so to walk, even as He walked.**"—*1 John 2:6.*

"For even hereunto were ye called: because **Christ also suffered for us, leaving us an example, that ye should follow His steps: Who did no sin**, neither was guile found in His mouth."—*1 Peter 2:21-22.*

ORIGINAL SIN

This strange error was also invented as an attempt to excuse those who want to keep enjoying their sins. Augustine (A.D. 354-430), a Catholic monk who could not control his lusts (and admitted the fact in his writings), theorized that God did not want people to stop sinning, that they could not escape from it in this life, and that they were born in sin; that is, *born sinners* ("original sin"). Therefore, we are not individually responsible for our sins. (Augustine was later "sainted" for also teaching that, outside of the Catholic Church there is no salvation.)

The Bible truth is that we are born with a fallen nature (which we inherit from Adam),—but we were not born sinful; we were not born sinners. We do not inherit sin, and we do not inherit guilt.

Through Christ's sacrifice on the cross and His mediation in the Sanctuary in heaven, He provides enabling grace to those who surrender their lives to Him, so they can resist temptation and overcome sin.

Here are several Bible verses which show that we are individually responsible for our own sins:

Ezekiel 18:14-25 is very important, but too long to quote here. It teaches that **we are individually responsible for our own sins and that we do not inherit them from our fathers.**

"The fathers shall not be put to death for the children, neither shall the children be put to death for the fathers: **every man shall be put to death for his own sin**."—*Deuteronomy 24:16.*

"**Every one shall die for his own iniquity**."—*Jeremiah 31:30 (Proverbs 9:12; Romans 2:6; Galatians 6:5, 7).*

Here are additional passages: *Isaiah 3:10-11; Psalms 128:1-2; 1:3-5; 11:4-6; Ecclesiastes 8:12-13; Galatians 6:7-9; Romans 2:6-9; 2 Corinthians 5:10;* and *Hebrews 6:12.*

The closest that this error can come to proving original sin is found in two Bible verses:

Here is the first of the two verses:

"Wherefore, as **by one man sin entered into the world**, and death by sin; and so death passed upon all men, **for that all have sinned**."—*Romans 5:12.*

The first phrase, which they rely on, is a statement of fact, with no explanation offered. The explanation comes in the last part of the verse: "for that all have sinned." **The verse does not say because all have inherited guilt from Adam, but *because all have personally sinned.*** They have guilt of their own, and do not have to borrow any from Adam.

Here is what the Bible teaches:

"**For the wages of sin is death**."—*Romans 6:23.*

"**The soul that sinneth, it shall die. The son shall not bear the iniquity of the father**, neither shall the father bear the iniquity of the son: the righteousness of the righteous shall be upon him, and **the wickedness of the wicked shall be upon him**."—*Ezekiel 18:20.*

The next verse after that says that **the person is not locked into his sin, as original sin teaches, but can turn from it:**

"But **if the wicked will turn from all his sins** that he hath committed, and keep all My statutes, **and do that which is lawful and right, he shall surely live**, he shall not die."—*Ezekiel 18:21.*

Here is the second of the two verses:

"Behold, I was shapen in iniquity, and in sin did my mother conceive me."—*Psalm 51:5.*

Augustine's theory was that the very act of procreating a child is sinful. How horrible! But that error is disproved by this verse:

"**Marriage is honorable** in all, and the bed undefiled."—*Hebrews 13:4.*

"For Thou art my hope, O Lord God: Thou art my trust from my youth. **By Thee have I been holden up from the womb**: Thou art He that took me out of my mother's bowels: my praise shall be continually of Thee."—*Psalm 71:5-6. (Another example is Psalm 22:9-10.)*

In accordance with Romans 3:23, David was simply saying, in poetic language, that he was a sinner and his mother was a sinner too.

COMING NEXT—Many are confused about the word "law" in the New Testament. We are going to discover that there were two laws; one which was abolished at the cross, and the other which was placed on an even more solid foundation by Christ's death.

Chapter Seventeen

Who Nailed What to the Cross

The Two Laws

Martin Luther, a Roman Catholic monk, was a leading professor at the Catholic University of Wittenberg, Germany. On October 31, 1517, he tacked on the Castle Church door a paper containing ninety-five points, or principles, of protest which he had written against what he believed to be unholy practices of the Catholic Church.

Luther's bold act was a world-shaking event. Because small printing presses had by that time been invented, his paper was quickly copied, printed, and circulated throughout Europe. **It led men and women everywhere to want to return to the Bible as the basis of Christianity**, rather than the dogmas and rituals of the official church.

Nearly 2,000 years ago, Roman soldiers nailed, not a holy protest to a church door, but a holy Man to a tree. These men did not realize who the Man was or what they were really doing. And the Man prayed, "Father, forgive them; for they know not what they do" *(Luke 23:34).*

The crucifixion of Jesus Christ was a universe-shaking event, opening a new era of world history and making certain a future time when sin and sinners will be no more and all the intelligent creation will worship the true God and obey the precepts of His holy law.

SOMETHING NAILED TO THE CROSS

The dying Son of God Himself is said to have nailed something to that cross. The Apostle Paul speaks of it in these words:

"Blotting out the handwriting of ordinances that was against us . . **and took it out of the way, nailing it to His cross**."—*Colossians 2:14.*

This does not mean that Jesus actually took a hammer and nailed a roll of ordinances to His cross. **But it does signify that some law or set of laws ended at His death.** What could this be?

Later, in another passage, Paul speaks of this again:

"Having abolished in His flesh the enmity, even the law of commandments contained in ordinances."—*Ephesians 2:15.*

It is quite obvious that there must be more than one type, or kind, of law in the Bible. We know that the moral law of God—the Ten Commandments—did not end at Calvary. Hundreds of passages in the Bible tell us that. It is just as wrong today for one to steal, kill, commit adultery, or break any other of the Ten Commandments as it ever was.

Christ did not come to destroy the moral law, but He came to fulfill it; that is, give us a perfect example of how to live in accordance with it. In addition, He gave us the enabling strength, as we remain by His side, to fully obey it.

Indeed, if God had wanted to abolish the law which is the standard of all morality, Christ would not have died to meet its holy demands. God's moral law is as enduring as His own character!

THREE TYPES OF BIBLE LAWS

There are several types of laws in the Bible.
First, there is the great moral law of Ten Commandments. This law was written by the finger of God Himself on solid rock *(Exodus 31:18).* This is the law, of which Christ Himself said:

"Think not that **I am come to destroy the law**, or the prophets: I am not come to destroy, but to fulfill. For verily I say unto you, **Till heaven and earth pass, one jot or one tittle shall in no wise pass from the law**."—*Matthew 5:17-18.*

Second, there are the ceremonial, sacrificial sanctuary laws, which governed the animal sacrifices which foreshadowed the death of Christ.

Third, there are the civil laws of the Jewish nation, which regulated a multitude of matters pertaining to crime, court procedures, disease control, and so forth.

When the Jewish nation, as God's chosen instrument, came to an end, the civil laws naturally lapsed. For example, by the law of Exodus 22:1, if

someone stole an ox, when caught he had to repay the owner five oxen. Although this law was a good one, it would not necessarily be followed in a nation today. **However, the underlying principles are still applicable.** For instance, it is just as obligatory upon a Christian to abide by the principles of healthful living, which the Hebrews were to obey.

WHEN THEY WERE ABOLISHED

So what was it that was nailed to the cross? It was the ceremonial laws, the rules and regulations governing animal sacrifices—all of which foreshadowed the death of Christ. Those rules had been given to remind the people, down through the centuries, that their sins could only be forgiven by the Messiah who would someday come.

It was the ceremonial laws which were nailed to the cross, "the law of commandments **contained in ordinances**" *(Ephesians 2:15)*, "the **handwriting of ordinances** that was against us" *(Colossians 2:14)*.

The Ten Commandments were not "ordinances," and they were not "handwriting" produced by any human hand. God wrote them with His own finger on rock.

So it was that at the moment that Christ died on the cross,—gone were the blood offerings, the meat and drink offerings, the special yearly holy days, such as Passover, Pentecost, etc.

All these typical services and yearly holy days pointed forward to Christ and His death on Mount Calvary.

It is of the highest significance that, **at the exact moment of Christ's death, the great inner veil of the Jewish Temple in Jerusalem—the veil dividing the first apartment from the second apartment—was torn from top to bottom**—ripped into two pieces! *(Matthew 27:51).* This clearly signified that the ceremonial system of laws and regulations—had come to an end, as far as God was concerned.

In order to express this in a dramatic way, Paul said that Christ nailed those ordinances to the cross.

THE YEARLY SABBATHS

Included in these ordinances which were abolished at Calvary—were the shadow sabbaths. *These were yearly (not weekly) gatherings.* **All of them came to an end, as far as God was concerned, at the death of Christ.**

For example, **an important one was the Passover service**, which was also held in the spring of the year. It is explained in detail in Exodus 12:21-49.

On that night, as He had warned Pharaoh, the angel of God was about to slay all the firstborn in the land of Egypt. But all who gathered in the homes of the Israelites would be safe. This was because **God's people were instructed to place blood from a slain lamb on the door posts (sides) and lintels (top) of the entrance door to each of their homes.**

"Draw out and take you a lamb according to your families, and kill the Passover."—*Exodus 12:21.*

"Ye shall say, It is the sacrifice of the Lord's Passover, who passed over the houses of the children of Israel in Egypt, when He smote the Egyptians, and delivered our houses."—*Exodus 12:27.*

This symbol obviously pointed to Christ's death on the cross to redeem all those who would accept Him as their Saviour.

TWO KINDS OF SABBATHS

Now it is very important that we clearly recognize that there are two kinds of sabbaths!

First, there is the weekly Sabbath. This is always written in the singular, "Sabbath" (never "sabbaths"). God's people are commanded to rest on the seventh day of every week, week after week. **This weekly Sabbath is commanded in the Fourth Commandment:**

"**Remember the Sabbath day, to keep it holy. Six days shalt thou labour, and do all thy work.**

"**But the seventh day is the Sabbath** of the Lord thy God: in it thou shalt not do any work, thou, nor thy son, nor thy daughter, thy manservant, nor thy maidservant, nor thy cattle, nor thy stranger that is within thy gates.

"For in six days the Lord made heaven and earth, the sea, and all that in them is, and rested the seventh day: **wherefore the Lord blessed the Sabbath day, and hallowed it.**"—*The Fourth Commandment, Exodus 20:8-11.*

This is not a "shadow law" to be done away at the death of Christ! This is part of the moral law of Ten Commandments.

Indeed, not only will it be kept all the way down to just before Christ returns for His people,—but also after that in the earth made new!

"And the dragon was wroth with the woman, and went to make war with **the remnant of her seed, which keep the commandments of God**, and have the testimony of Jesus Christ."—*Revelation 12:17.*

"Here is the patience of the saints: **here are they that keep the commandments of God**, and the faith of Jesus."—*Revelation 14:12.*

"For as the new heavens and the new earth, which I will make, shall remain before Me, saith the Lord, so shall your seed and your name remain. And it shall come to pass, that . . **from one Sabbath to another, shall all flesh come to worship before Me**, saith the Lord."—*Isaiah 66:22-23.*

Notice that **while the ceremonial sabbaths (plural) prefigured (looked forward to)** the death

of Christ, when they would end, **the Bible Sabbath (singular) was kept as a memorial (looking back)** to the great facts of the seven-day Creation of our world.

This is because God specifically set the seventh day aside as a special weekly rest day,—and He did this on the seventh day of Creation Week *(Genesis 2:1-3).*

"Thus the heavens and the earth were finished, and all the host of them.

"And **on the seventh day, God ended His work which He had made; and He rested on the seventh day** from all His work which He had made.

"**And God blessed the seventh day, and sanctified it**: because that in it He had rested from all His work which God created and made."—*Genesis 2:1-3.*

So that there should be no uncertainty about whether mankind was to keep this weekly Sabbath, God wrote it with His own finger into the Ten Commandments *(Exodus 20:8-11).* He placed it in the very heart of the moral law.

In contrast, the ceremonial laws ended at the cross, and are referred to as "shadow sabbaths," for they foreshadowed Christ's death. They are also called "feast days."

Here is one passage in the New Testament, where Paul mentioned these yearly, ceremonial sabbaths:

"Let no man therefore judge you in meat, or in drink, or in respect of an holyday, or of the new moon, **or of the sabbath days: which are a shadow of things to come**; but the body is of Christ."—*Colossians 2:16-17.*

COMPARING THE TWO LAWS

Let us now compare the two laws: the moral law (the Ten Commandments), and the ceremonial laws (commandments contained in ordinances):

1 - The moral law is a perfect law.

"The law of the Lord is perfect, converting the soul."—*Psalm 19:7.*

"All Thy commandments are righteousness."—*Psalm 119:172.*

"Thy righteousness is an everlasting righteousness, and Thy law is the truth."—*Psalm 119:142.*

The ceremonial law is an imperfect law.

"For there is verily a disannulling of the commandment going before for the weakness and unprofitableness thereof. **For the law made nothing perfect, but the bringing in of a better hope did**; by the which we draw nigh unto God."—*Hebrews 7:18-19.*

"**For the law having a shadow of good things**

to come, and not the very image of the things, **can never with those sacrifices which they offered year by year continually make the comers thereunto perfect**. For then would they not have ceased to be offered?"—*Hebrews 10:1-2*.

2 - The moral law is in itself spiritual.

"We know that the law is spiritual."—*Romans 7:14*.

The ceremonial law is not in itself spiritual.

"**Which was a figure for the time then present, in which were offered both gifts and sacrifices, that could not make him that did the service perfect**, as pertaining to the conscience; which stood only **in meats and drinks, and divers washings, and carnal ordinances, imposed on them until the time of reformation**."—*Hebrews 9:9-10*.

3 - The moral law gives a knowledge of sin.

"By the law is the knowledge of sin."—*Romans 3:20*.

"**What shall we say then? is the law sin? God forbid.** Nay, I had not known sin, but by the law: for I had not known lust, except the law had said, Thou shalt not covet."—*Romans 7:7*.

The ceremonial law was instituted in consequence of sin *(see Leviticus 3 to 7)*.

4 - The moral law was spoken by God Himself.

"And the Lord spake unto you out of the midst of the fire: ye heard the voice of the words, but saw no similitude; only ye heard a voice. And **He declared unto you His covenant, which He commanded you to perform, even ten commandments**."—*Deuteronomy 4:12-13 (Exodus 20:1-17)*.

"And He added no more."—*Deuteronomy 5:22*.

The ceremonial law was spoken by Moses.

"**And the Lord called unto Moses, and spake unto him** out of the tabernacle of the congregation, saying, **Speak unto the children of Israel, and say unto them**, If any man of you bring an offering unto the Lord, ye shall bring your offering of the cattle, even of the herd, and of the flock."—*Leviticus 1:1-2*.

"[Moses said:] **This is the law of the burnt offering, of the meat offering, and of the sin offering**, and of the trespass offering, and of the consecrations, and of the sacrifice of the peace offerings."—*Leviticus 7:37. (Also see Leviticus 8:13-17.)*

5 - The moral law was written by the Lord, with His own finger, upon two tables of stone.

"**These words the Lord spake unto all your assembly** in the mount out of the midst of the fire, of the cloud, and of the thick darkness, with a great voice: and He added no more. And He wrote them in two tables of stone**, and delivered them unto me."—*Deuteronomy 5:22 (Exodus 31:18; 24:12)*.

The ceremonial law were written by Moses in a book.

"Thou shalt not offer the blood of My sacrifice with leaven . . **And the Lord said unto Moses, Write thou these words**."—*Exodus 34:25, 27*.

"**And Moses wrote this law**, and delivered it unto the priests the sons of Levi, which bare the ark of the covenant of the Lord, and unto all the elders of Israel."—*Deuteronomy 31:9 (Nehemiah 8:1; 2 Kings 22:8-16)*.

6 - The moral law was placed in the ark of the covenant.

"**And he [Moses] took and put the testimony into the ark**, and set the staves on the ark, and put the mercy seat above upon the ark."—*Exodus 40:20 (1 Kings 8:9; Hebrews 9:4)*.

The ceremonial law was placed outside the ark, by its side.

"And it came to pass, **when Moses had made an end of writing the words of this law in a book**, until they were finished, that Moses commanded the Levites, which bare the ark of the covenant of the Lord, saying, **Take this book of the law, and put it in the side of the ark** of the covenant of the Lord your God, that it may be there for a witness against thee."—*Deuteronomy 31:24-26*.

7 - The moral law is eternal, and therefore requires obedience from all.

"Do we then make void the law through faith? God forbid: yea, **we establish the law**."—*Romans 3:31*.

"**Think not that I am come to destroy the law**, or the prophets: I am not come to destroy, but to fulfill."—*Matthew 5:17*.

"It is easier for heaven and earth to pass, than one tittle of the law to fail."—*Luke 16:17*.

"**If thou wilt enter into life, keep the commandments**."—*Matthew 19:17*.

"Circumcision is nothing, and uncircumcision is nothing, **but the keeping of the commandments of God**."—*1 Corinthians 7:19*.

"**Blessed are they that do His commandments, that they** may have right to the tree of life, and **may enter in through the gates into the city**."—*Revelation 22:14*.

The ceremonial law has been abolished, and obedience to it is no longer required.

"**Having abolished in His flesh the enmity, even the law of commandments contained in ordinances**; for to make in Himself of twain one new man, so making peace."—*Ephesians 2:15.*

"Blotting out the handwriting of ordinances that was against us, which was contrary to us, and took it out of the way, nailing it to His cross; and having spoiled principalities and powers, He made a show of them openly, triumphing over them in it. **Let no man therefore judge you** in meat, or in drink, or in respect of an holyday, or of the new moon, or **of the sabbath days: which are a shadow of things to come**; but the body is of Christ."—*Colossians 2:14-17.*

"Forasmuch as we have heard, that **certain which went out from us have troubled you with words, subverting your souls, saying, Ye must be circumcised, and keep the law: to whom we gave no such commandment.**"—*Acts 15:24.*

OTHERS AGREE

"Although the law given from God by Moses as touching ceremonies and rites, doth not bind Christians; yet, notwithstanding, **no Christian whatsoever is free from the obedience of the commandments which are called moral.**"—*Methodist Episcopal Church Doctrines and Discipline, p. 23.*

"Ques.—**Are we under obligation to keep the ceremonial law?**

"Ans.—**No**, the ordinances which it enjoined were only types and shadows of Christ; and when **they were fulfilled by His death**, and the distinction between Jew and Gentile was removed, the ceremonial law was abolished, because it was no longer necessary.

"Ques.—**Are we under obligation to keep the moral law?**

"Ans.—**Yes, because that is founded on the nature of God and cannot be changed**; it is of universal application, which was impossible with respect to the ceremonial and civil laws. Christ demands obedience to His law."—*The Lutheran Catechism.*

The ceremonial laws are like the scaffolding of a building, to be removed when the building is finished. The moral law is like the foundation of the building.

Throwing away the Ten Commandments, when the ceremonial law is discarded, is like tearing down the building when removing the scaffolding!

BUILT ON A ROCK

Many years ago, a bridge was to be built across the Conemaugh River in Pennsylvania. It would in time come to be known as the "Stone Bridge." The contract for the job was assigned to a contractor, who then set to work.

On each side of the river he dug down, farther

and still farther, until he reached bedrock. Others told him it was too expensive to do this, but he was determined to build solidly. Finally, his arched, stone bridge was finished, and the extra cost was forgotten.

In the late spring of 1889 melting snows in the mountains, plus heavy rains, brought more and more water down the streams. The South Fork Reservoir, built 36 years earlier, was gradually filled to the very top. Its walls were weak, and finally gave way, permitting an avalanche of water to sweep down the valley. Trees, houses, buildings—everything was swept before the **gigantic liquid wall.**

What would happen when all this water and wreckage would strike the bridge, 14 miles below the dam, which had been built many years before? With awful impact it struck. The bridge stood solid!

The flood swept on, spreading death and desolation in one of America's greatest disasters—the Johnstown Flood of May 31, 1889. More than 20 million tons of water poured downstream, killing over 2,200 people.

But that bridge, built on the solid rock, stood like a lone and mighty stronghold in the midst of ruin and desolation. **It had stood the test of storms and floods—because it was fastened to the rock.** Holding back a massive amount of debris, it prevented many deaths downstream.

Let us build upon the rock, Christ Jesus, and upon the foundation of His unchangeable, everlasting law.

"**Think not that I am come to destroy the law**, or the prophets: I am not come to destroy, but to fulfill. For verily I say unto you, Till heaven and earth pass, one jot or one tittle shall in no wise pass from the law . .

"**Therefore whosoever heareth these sayings of Mine, and doeth them, I will liken him unto a wise man, which built his house upon a rock.** And the rain descended, and the floods came, and the winds blew, and beat upon that house; and it fell not: for it was founded upon a rock."—*Matthew 5:17-18, 7:24-25.*

COMING NEXT—We are about to study a very important topic which our present world has almost entirely lost sight of. The truths revealed in this chapter will bring great comfort to your heart, as you accept it into your life.

— PART FIVE —

CHRIST'S SPECIAL DAY

Chapter Eighteen

The Sign and Seal of God

Proof That God Created Our World

Someone has said that "craftsmen are men who cannot help doing whatever is given them to do better than others think worthwhile."

God is the great architect and supercraftsman of the universe.

"To whom then will ye liken Me, or shall I be equal? saith the Holy One. Lift up your eyes on high, and **behold who hath created these things**, **that bringeth out their host by number: He calleth them all by names** by the greatness of His might, for that He is strong in power; not one faileth."—*Isaiah 40:25-26.*

ACCURACY IN TIMEKEEPING

The starry wheels of God's huge and intricate clock never fail. At the U.S. Naval Observatory in Washington, D.C., men have checked the stars of God to ascertain the correct time for men. From their observations they have set the nation's standard clock. In England, the Royal Observatory at Greenwich has maintained a similar service. (More recently, another of God's time-measuring wonders, *cesium*, an atom which is the basis of the NIST-F1 clock in Colorado is being used.)

The source of such accuracy in timekeeping comes from God, the Master Mechanic of the universe and the atom.

"Hast thou not known? hast thou not heard, that the everlasting God, the Lord, the Creator of the ends of the earth, fainteth not, neither is weary? **there is no searching of His understanding**."—*Isaiah 40:28.*

God's clocks never run down, because He keeps them running, and always on time.

Everyone honors a man who puts skill and effort and conscience into the creation of superior products. Let all men honor the Craftsman of all craftsmen, the Creator of the vast, intricate, mysterious universe.

A PERFECT CREATOR

What does the Bible teach about how our world, and all its forms of life, were first created?

In the first verse of the Bible we read: "In the beginning God created the heaven and the earth." *Genesis 1:1.* Immediately after that, is the story of how God created one thing after another:

The first day, light. The second day, atmosphere. The third day, dry land and vegetation. The fourth day, the light of the sun, moon, and heavenly bodies. The fifth day, fish and fowl. The sixth day, animals and man.

It boggles our minds to grasp how God did all

this. But the problem is not solved by the fool who simply says, "There is no God" *(Psalm 14:1).* Nor is it solved by simply forgetting the whole matter. **We need to have certainty about this, for "without faith it is impossible to please Him** [God], for he that cometh to God must believe that He is [that He exists]" *(Hebrews 11:6).*

The order, system, and intelligence that we clearly observe all about us makes the truth of God's existence the most rational explanation of all. The foolish theories of evolution, the vague talk of atheists—all ring hollow in comparison with the great facts of the Created Universe.

Without God, men have never yet been able to solve the riddle of which came first—the hen or the egg.

"**Through faith we understand that the worlds were framed by the Word of God**, so that things which are seen were not made of things which do appear."—*Hebrews 11:3.*

"For He spake, and it was done; He commanded, and it stood fast."—*Psalm 33:9.*

Everywhere we turn, in the vast Creation, we see the evidences of His footsteps.

"The heavens declare the glory of God."—*Psalm 19:1.*

"**For the invisible things of Him from the creation of the world are clearly seen, being understood by the things that are made, even His eternal power and Godhead; so that they are without excuse.**"—*Romans 1:20.*

Long before the modern scientist declared that the earth has no visible means of support, Job said, "He . . hangeth the earth upon nothing" *(Job 26:7).* Having made the world from nothing, He hung it upon nothing tangible.

This world and all worlds are upheld "by the Word of His power" *(Hebrews 1:3).*

AN ETERNAL REMINDER OF HIS CREATORSHIP

This is the God who declared something we should never forget:

"Thus shall ye say unto them, The gods that have not made the heavens and the earth, even they shall perish from the earth, and from under these heavens."—*Jeremiah 10:11.*

For, you see, **God makes the act of Creation as the proof which distinguishes Him from all false gods.** Write that principle deep in your thinking, for it will explain a lot that we are going to now discover.

So that we would have no doubt about the matter, He gave us a special gift—that through all time to come, we would know that He is the Creator God—our God.

For this is what He did on the seventh and last

day of Creation Week:

"And God saw every thing that He had made, and, behold, it was very good. And the evening and the morning were the sixth day.

"Thus the heavens and the earth were finished, and all the host of them."—*Genesis 1:31-2:1.*

MADE FOR MANKIND
AT THE CREATION OF OUR WORLD

"**And on the seventh day God ended His work which He had made; and He rested on the seventh day from all His work which He had made.**

"**And God blessed the seventh day, and sanctified it**: because that in it He had rested from all His work which God created and made."—*Genesis 2:2-3.*

What a beautiful truth: **God gave the seventh-day Sabbath to mankind at the very creation of our world!** On the seventh day of Creation Week, **It was to always remain the special sign, or mark, of His Creatorship.**

This is the plain, unmistakable record given us in the Bible.

By three distinct acts, then, was the Sabbath made: God *rested* **on it; He** *blessed* **it; He** *sanctified* **it.** *Sanctify* means "to make sacred or holy; . . to set apart to a sacred office or to religious use."—*Webster's New International Dictionary.*

Only God could make one day holy. Only He could command that we keep it also. Only He could explain the great truth that **we are to keep it because it identifies us as the only people on earth who recognize Him as the Creator God.**

It shows that we are His people! We gladly acknowledge Him as our Lord; the One who made us.

That is why He placed this special command in the very heart of the Ten Commandments:

"**Remember the Sabbath day, to keep it holy. Six days shalt thou labour, and do all thy work.**

"**But the seventh day is the Sabbath** of the Lord thy God: in it thou shalt not do any work, thou, nor thy son, nor thy daughter, thy manservant, nor thy maidservant, nor thy cattle, nor thy stranger that is within thy gates.

"**For in six days the Lord made heaven and earth**, the sea, and all that in them is, and rested the seventh day: wherefore the Lord blessed the Sabbath day, and hallowed it."—*Exodus 20:8-11.*

How good our God is to give us the Bible Sabbath. **There is a blessing in keeping it that we could receive in no other way, for we are obeying His express command.** When we do not obey Him, we always get into trouble.

Here is what one writer said about this:

"In Eden, God set up the memorial of His work of creation, in placing His blessing upon the seventh day. The Sabbath was committed to Adam, the father and representative of the whole human family. **Its observance was to be an act of grateful acknowledgment, on the part of all who should dwell upon the earth, that God was their Creator and their rightful Sovereign; that they were the work of His hands and the subjects of His authority.** Thus the institution was wholly commemorative, and given to all mankind. There was nothing in it shadowy or of restricted application to any people.

"**God saw that a Sabbath was essential for man**, even in Paradise. He needed to lay aside his own interests and pursuits for one day of the seven, that he might more fully contemplate the works of God and meditate upon His power and goodness. **He needed a Sabbath to remind him more vividly of God and to awaken gratitude** because all that he enjoyed and possessed came from the beneficent hand of the Creator."—*Patriarchs and Prophets, 48.*

God gave the Bible Sabbath to our first parents before they had sinned. **The Sabbath and marriage are two holy institutions that came from Eden to bless the world.**

The seventh-day Sabbath is for us to keep. **In the Fourth of the Ten Commandments, God commanded us to keep it.** Let us read it again:

"Remember the Sabbath day, to keep it holy. **Six days shalt thou labour, and do all thy work. But the seventh day is the Sabbath** of the Lord thy God: in it thou shalt not do any work."—*Exodus 20:8-10.*

Then He explains the reason why we must do this:

"**For in six days the Lord made heaven and earth**, the sea, and all that in them is, and rested the seventh day: wherefore the Lord blessed the Sabbath day, and hallowed it."—*Exodus 20:11.*

THE SIGN OF HIS CREATORSHIP
AND HIS RIGHT TO RULE

Elsewhere we read:

"**It is a sign** between Me and the children of Israel forever: **for in six days the Lord made heaven and earth, and on the seventh day He rested**, and was refreshed."—*Exodus 31:17.*

The Sabbath is thus the sign of God's creatorship; our acknowledgement that He made us!

But notice that it is not the sign because Jews are Jews, but because God is God and He is the Creator.

He created the world in six days and rested on the seventh day—2,500 years before the Jewish nation came into existence!

The Bible Sabbath is not merely a day for physical rest, although we need that. By keeping it, we acknowledge that the Creator God is our God! For we are obeying His express command to keep that day holy! **We cannot select some other day; we must keep the exact day which He gave us—the seventh day of each weekly cycle.** (Later we shall discover absolute evidence that the weekly cycle has not changed, going all the way back to Moses and before. So our "seventh day" of the week—is the same seventh day that Moses kept and Jesus kept.)

On God's part, **the Sabbath is a sign of His creatorship. It is the sign of His right to rule over us**, the symbol of His gracious and timeless sovereignty.

On our part, it is the sign that we gratefully acknowledge Him as our Creator—and accept His rulership.

"My Maker and My King, to Thee my all I owe; Thy sovereign bounty is the spring whence all my blessings flow. The creatures of Thy hand, on Thee alone I live; My God, Thy benefits demand more praise than I can give.

"Lord, what can I impart when all is Thine before? Thy love demands a thankful heart; the gift, alas! how poor. O let Thy grace inspire my soul with strength divine; Let every Word and each desire and all my days be Thine."

God tells us in Scripture that the Bible Sabbath is the seventh-day Sabbath, for there is no other weekly sabbath in the Bible.

IT IS THE SEAL OF THE LAW

He also tells us it is "the seal" of His holy Ten Commandment law. *What is meant by this?*

The seal of a law gives the name of the lawgiver, his official title, and the extent of his dominion. For example, "Elizabeth II [name], Queen [title], of England [extent of dominion]."

Carefully examining all ten of the commandments, we find that the fourth, or Sabbath, commandment is the only one that qualifies as a seal.

Read it again carefully (Exodus 20:8-11), and you will find in it God's seal:

The Lord thy God [name], Creator [title], of heaven and earth [dominion].

Thus when God wrote His law upon tables of stone, He engraved His seal in the law itself.

The Bible Sabbath is the Creator's sign of His right to rule. It therefore becomes the seal of His law.

So far we have learned that the Sabbath is (1) **the sign of God's creative power and His right to rule**; and (2) **it is the seal of His holy law**.

IT IS THE MEMORIAL OF CREATION

The Sabbath is also the memorial of Creation. The Sabbath "commemorated" the Creation of our world. **It was given to the Hebrews to be shared** with the entire world, so others could also become His special people.

"**It is a sign** between Me and the children of Israel forever: **for in six days the Lord made heaven and earth**, and on the seventh day He rested, and was refreshed."—*Exodus 31:17.*

"Remember the Sabbath day, to keep it holy . . **For in six days the Lord made heaven and earth**, the sea, and all that in them is, and rested the seventh day: wherefore the Lord blessed the Sabbath day, and hallowed it."—*Exodus 20:8, 11.*

"**He hath made His wonderful works to be remembered.**"—*Psalm 111:4.*

Since the purpose of the Sabbath was to remember God as the Creator, if it had always been faithfully kept, there would be no atheists or idolaters today.

Another example of something done to commemorate a great event occurred when Joshua had men carry stones from the center of the Jordan river in flood stage, after the people had miraculously crossed over it—as a perpetual memorial.

"And these stones shall be for **a memorial** unto the children of Israel forever."—*Joshua 4:7.*

"And he spake unto the children of Israel, saying, When your children shall ask their fathers in time to come, saying, **What mean these stones?** Then ye shall let your children know, saying, Israel came over this Jordan on dry land."—*Joshua 4:21-22.*

THE SIGN OF HIS REDEEMING POWER

The Bible also tells us that the Sabbath is not only the sign of His creatorship and rulership,—**but also the sign of His redeeming power to save those who submit to His rule.**

"Verily My Sabbaths ye shall keep: for it is a sign between Me and you throughout your generations; **that ye may know that I am the Lord that doth sanctify you**."—*Exodus 31:13.*

What a glorious promise is this! **God wants to use the seventh-day Sabbath as part of His plan to save us from sin!**

"Moreover also I gave them My Sabbaths, to be a sign between Me and them, **that they might know that I am the Lord that sanctify them**."—*Ezekiel 20:12.*

Like the work of creation itself, sanctification also requires creative power. For, with their cooperation, God changes sinful men into humble, obedient children whom He can take to heaven. But if they pull back and rebel against His authority, He cannot work these changes in their lives.

"**Create in me a clean heart, O God**; and renew a right spirit within me."—*Psalm 51:10.*

"Jesus answered and said unto him, Verily,

verily, I say unto thee, Except a man be born again, he cannot see the kingdom of God."— *John 3:3*.

"**For we are His workmanship, created in Christ Jesus unto good works.**"—*Ephesians 2:10*.

As God rested from His creative works on the seventh day, so the believer rests from his activities and, on the Sabbath, enters into the rest of God. **The Sabbath is the sign of this rest which we enter into.** Paul mentions this in Hebrews 4:4-10.

The Sabbath, which is the memorial of God's creative power, will never cease to exist.

When this sinful world will end, and life in God's sinless world shall begin—God's faithful ones will continue keeping the Sabbath.

"For as the new heavens and the new earth, which I will make, shall remain before Me, saith the Lord, so shall your seed and your name remain. And it shall come to pass, that from one new moon to another, and **from one Sabbath to another, shall all flesh come to worship before Me**, saith the Lord."—*Isaiah 66:22-23*.

So the holy Sabbath is the sign of creatorship, rulership, and fellowship,—and also the sign of God's plan to redeem His faithful ones so they can live with Him forever.

He who would dare to attempt to abolish the Bible Sabbath—is directly challenging God the Creator and Redeemer, who gave the Sabbath to mankind.

D.L. Moody wrote this:

"**The Sabbath was binding in Eden, and it has been in force ever since.** This fourth commandment begins with the word 'remember,' showing that the Sabbath already existed when God wrote this law on the tables of stone at Sinai. **How can men claim that this one commandment has been done away with when they will admit that the other nine are still binding?**"—*D.L. Moody, Weighed and Wanting, pp. 46-47*.

THE FORTY-YEAR TEST OF OBEDIENCE

A special test came to God's people *before they arrived at Mount Sinai*, where the Ten Commandments were written on stone tablets.

All of the commandments, including the Sabbath commandment, had been known ever since Eden. So God tested the Israelites. He said He would give them "bread from heaven" (called manna), and the people should go out and gather it daily,—but they should not go out and gather any on the Sabbath.

"Then said the Lord unto Moses, Behold, I will rain bread from heaven for you; and the people shall go out and gather a certain rate every day,

that I may prove them, whether they will walk in My law, or no.

"And it shall come to pass, that on the sixth day they shall prepare that which they bring in; **and it shall be twice as much** as they gather daily."—*Exodus 16:4-5*.

"And it came to pass, that on the sixth day they gathered twice as much bread, two omers for one man: and all the rulers of the congregation came and told Moses. And he said unto them, This is that which the Lord hath said, **Tomorrow is the rest of the holy Sabbath** unto the Lord: bake that which ye will bake today, and seethe that ye will seethe; and that which remaineth over lay up for you to be kept until the morning."—*Exodus 16:22-23*.

But some of the people went out on the Sabbath to collect more manna, thus violating God's command.

"And it came to pass, that there went out some of the people on the seventh day for to gather, and they found none.

"**And the Lord said unto Moses, How long refuse ye to keep My commandments and My laws?**

"See, for that the Lord hath given you the Sabbath, therefore He giveth you on the sixth day the bread of two days; abide ye every man in his place, let no man go out of his place on the seventh day."—*Exodus 16:27-29*.

Commenting on Exodus 16:4-30, *Martin Luther wrote this:*

"Hence you can see that **the Sabbath was before the law of Moses came, and has existed from the beginning of the world.** Especially have the devout, who have preserved the true faith, met together and called upon God on this day."—*Martin Luther, translated from Auslegung des Alten Testaments (Commentary on the Old Testament), in Sammtiliche Schriften (Collected Writings), ed. by J.G. Walch, Vol. 3, Col. 950*.

A striking example of how important God considered it to be that the people keep the Sabbath—*is the miracle of the manna*. For forty years, or 2,080 weeks, God worked a number of miracles every week, thereby pointing out the true Sabbath 2,080 times.

God sent manna for each of the first five days of each week. That was a miracle. Then on the sixth day, He sent twice as much. Another miracle. And then on the seventh day, He sent none. It is very obvious that God wanted His people to keep the Bible Sabbath. When, after all this evidence, some went out and broke the Sabbath, He clearly showed His will in the matter.

CENTURIES OF DISOBEDIENCE

It is a tragic fact that, repeatedly, God's people

W
A
Y

in Old Testament times refused to keep His moral law. In fact, this is the great lesson we discover, over and over again, all through the Old Testament! As a result, they suffered great affliction.

In the time of Jeremiah, God promised to greatly bless the Israelites if they would remain loyal to Him.

"And it shall come to pass, **if ye diligently hearken unto Me, saith the Lord, to bring in no burden through the gates of this city on the Sabbath day, but hallow the Sabbath day, to do no work therein,** then shall there enter into the gates of this city kings and princes sitting upon the throne of David, riding in chariots and on horses, they, and their princes, the men of Judah, and the inhabitants of Jerusalem: **and this city shall remain forever**."—*Jeremiah 17:24-25.*

What a glorious promise that was! **But then followed a prediction of what would happen if they refused to keep the Bible Sabbath:**

"But if ye will not hearken unto Me to hallow the Sabbath day, and not to bear a burden, even entering in at the gates of Jerusalem on the Sabbath day; **then will I kindle a fire in the gates thereof, and it shall devour the palaces of Jerusalem, and it shall not be quenched.**"—*Jeremiah 17:27.*

This prediction was exactly fulfilled! Nebuchadnezzar, king of Babylon, came and destroyed Jerusalem—and **the Word of God said it was because the inhabitants refused to keep the Sabbath!**

"And all the vessels of the house of God, great and small, and the treasures of the house of the Lord, and the treasures of the king, and of his princes; all these he brought to Babylon. And they burnt the house of God, and brake down the wall of Jerusalem, and burnt all the palaces thereof with fire, and destroyed all the goodly vessels thereof. And them that had escaped from the sword carried he away to Babylon; where they were servants to him and his sons until the reign of the kingdom of Persia:

"**To fulfill the word of the Lord by the mouth of Jeremiah, until the land had enjoyed her Sabbaths: for as long as she lay desolate she kept Sabbath,** to fulfill threescore and ten years."—*2 Chronicles 36:18-21.*

Years later, after returning from Babylon, Nehemiah warned the people to not again forsake the Sabbath,—lest the city be destroyed again!

"Then I contended with the nobles of Judah, and said unto them, What evil thing is this that ye do, and profane the Sabbath day? **Did not your fathers thus, and did not our God bring all this evil upon us, and upon this city? yet ye bring more wrath upon Israel by profaning the Sabbath.**"—*Nehemiah 13:17-18.*

HE LOVED US TO THE DEATH

The cross of Calvary upheld, between heaven and earth, the Upholder of the universe. **Bound to its rough wood were the hands that had made the worlds and set the stars in limitless space, hands that had made the very wood in the cross on which He hung.**

"He had a way with wood, He touched the cross's ugly span, Barren and bloodstained where it stood, And built a bridge from God to man."

He touched that cross and stayed there for you and me. **If we love Him, we will obey Him! We will not, as others do, study our convenience or what others will think of us.**

As the poem says:

" 'Twas not the nails, but His wondrous love for me, kept My Lord on the cross of Calvary. Oh, what power could hold Him there—All my sin and shame to bear? Not the nails, *but His wondrous love—for me!*"

COMING NEXT—We next want to learn what Jesus, while here on earth, thought about the Bible Sabbath. Did He obey it Himself? Did He tell His disciples to obey it? Did He want them to obey it after His death on Calvary? These are important truths.

Chapter Nineteen

The Sabbath of Jesus

Learning about the Lord's Day

A man who did not believe in Christ, and His intercession for sinners, felt miserable one evening while his wife was at prayer meeting. Locking himself in his room, he tried to get away from his past, but he could not do so. It all rose up like a mountain on his soul.

Finally, he knelt down and, because he did not believe in Jesus Christ, asked God to forgive His sins; but there was no response.

Afterward, telling what happened, he said, "I did not say "for Jesus' sake," for I was a Unitarian and did believe that He had died for me."

Then in utter desperation, he cried, "Please God, I accept Jesus as my Saviour. For His sake, please—forgive my sins!" Immediately, a peace of heart flowed into his soul. In the days and months to come, he still had much to learn and he faithfully began searching God's Word, and obeying the truths he found, in the strength of Christ, until he discovered the Bible Sabbath. **The more he searched God's**

Word, the more he discovered, and the deeper became his peace and his connection to Jesus Christ.

We can be thankful that the Word of God, if carefully studied, will clearly direct men on the pathway to heaven.

CHRIST'S SPECIAL DAY

The Bible definitely states that Christ has a special day. We want to learn what it is. First, let us read Revelation 1:10.

"I was in the Spirit on the Lord's day."—*Revelation 1:10.*

There is nothing in Revelation 1:10 that tells us what day that is. Some think it is Sunday, the first day of the week. *But only the Bible can tell us.* And it gives us the answer over and over again!

The Fourth Commandment clearly explains it.

"But **the seventh day is the Sabbath of the Lord** thy God."—*Exodus 20:10.*

But there are many other passages which say the same thing.

The seventh day is the Sabbath of the Lord **is mentioned six times in the Bible!** Here they are: Exodus 16:26; 23:12; 31:15; 35:2; Leviticus 23:3; and Deuteronomy 5:14.

The only day which the Bible has ever mentioned as being the Lord's day is the seventh day of the week. The expression found in Isaiah 58:13 is a good example of this:

"If thou turn away thy foot from the Sabbath, from doing thy pleasure on *My holy day* . . then shalt thou delight thyself in the Lord."—*Isaiah 58:13-14.*

God is here describing the seventh-day Sabbath.

What day is the "Lord's day" in the Scriptures? The Bible tells us that **the Sabbath is *the day unto the Lord*** (Exodus 16:23, 25; 31:15; 35:2). **It is *the day of the Lord*** (Exodus 20:10; Leviticus 23:3; Deuteronomy 5:14), **and *His own day—His holy day*** (Isaiah 58:13).

Jesus called Himself the Lord of the Sabbath.

"The Son of man is Lord also of the Sabbath."—*Mark 2:28.*

The Apostle John speaks of it as "the Lord's day" (Revelation 1:10).

"I was in the Spirit on the Lord's day."—*Revelation 1:10.*

John well knew which day was the Lord's day. This day is the memorial day of the Creator *(Genesis 2:1-3; Exodus 31:17),* and the memorial day of the Redeemer *(Ezekiel 20:12, 20).*

It is the Lord's Day! God's own day. A day He wants to share with you.

Don't refuse Him. He wants to give you better things than you could ever give yourself. **Do not try to make a sabbath out of something man-made that others offer you. Choose instead the best—*the***

only Sabbath God ever gave to mankind—*the seventh-day Sabbath.*

CHRIST MADE THE SABBATH

How did Christ become Lord of the Sabbath?

The reason Jesus claims the Sabbath as belonging to Him is because, **in the beginning, God and Christ worked together in the Creation of the world. *Jesus made the Sabbath and gave it to us!***

"God . . hath in these last days spoken unto us by His Son . . by whom also He made the worlds."—*Hebrews 1:1-2.*

"To make all men see what is the fellowship of the mystery, which from the beginning of the world hath been hid in God, who created all things by Jesus Christ."—*Ephesians 3:9.*

In other words, the same Christ who came to this earth to redeem man worked closely with God the Father in creating all things in the beginning. This truth is taught again and again.

"In the beginning was the Word, and the Word was with God, and the Word was God. The same was in the beginning with God. **All things were made by Him; and without Him was not anything made that was made**, . . He was in the world, and the world was made by Him."—*John 1:1-3, 10.*

"**God, who created all things by Jesus Christ**."—*Ephesians 3:9.*

"Who is the image of the invisible God, the firstborn of every creature. **For by Him were all things created, that are in heaven, and that are in earth**, visible and invisible, whether they be thrones, or dominions, or principalities, or powers: all things were created by Him, and for Him. And He is before all things, and by Him all things consist."—*Colossians 1:15-17.*

Christ was the active agent in creation. The Creator rested on the seventh day from the work of creation. **Therefore, Christ must have rested on the seventh day with the Father. So it is His rest day as well as the Father's.**

How thankful we can be that Jesus shares His Sabbath with us! Since God's children are members of His family *(Ephesians 3:14-15),* we would expect that they would have special fellowship with Him on His rest day. So **it is not only the Sabbath of God, but also of man.**

"The Sabbath was made for man."—*Mark 2:27.*

Christ, who was born into the human race, is the Son of man who died that we might inherit eternal life. He is also Lord of the Sabbath.

"The Son of man is Lord also of the Sabbath."—*Mark 2:28.*

IS OUR SEVENTH DAY

W
A
Y

THE SAME AS CHRIST'S SEVENTH DAY?

But now we come to a very important question: Is the seventh day of the week in Christ's time, the same as it is in our time?

The little town of Nazareth is located on the most southerly of the mountain ranges of southern Galilee. Quietly it lies nestled on the side of a shallow ridge that runs in the shape of a horseshoe. Here, among the dwellings and groves of this small town, is where Jesus grew to manhood.

But, just now, come back with me in imagination to that village, where so many years ago, the Master walked among men. Another day is quietly dawning, as the early rising sun chases away the bright mists that hang over the slope of Nazareth. From the home of the carpenter, Jesus steps forth and walks to the little church in the center of town. It is Sabbath in Nazareth on this morning!

Oh, how much you and I would like to go to church with Jesus! And, perhaps more important— how much we would like to go to church on the same weekly Sabbath that He kept! What peace of heart this would bring to us, to be able to keep the Sabbath of Jesus!

And, my friend, we can. For we know enough from Biblical, historical and other records, that we today can know of a certainty the Sabbath of Jesus.

TRACING THE WEEKLY CYCLE

In order to trace back to the Sabbath of Jesus, *we must know the truth about the weekly cycle itself.* Here are the facts:

The seven-day week, as well as the Bible Sabbath that terminates it, both originated during Creation Week. **But has that weekly cycle changed down through the centuries?**

We are going to discover that **God has guarded both the Sabbath and the weekly cycle of seven days.** It is because the seventh-day Sabbath has been kept by God's people—ever since Eden—that we can know that the weekly cycle has not changed.

THE WEEK IN MOSES' TIME

If the weekly cycle were lost between Adam's time and Moses', when God wrote the Ten Commandments and gave them manna for forty years,— the weekly cycle would have been corrected at that time.

THE WEEK IN JESUS' TIME

For all the centuries from Moses to Christ, there were Jews who faithfully kept it. But if the Sabbath could possibly have been lost between Moses' time and Jesus' time, **we would have the example of the Saviour Himself to guide us as to the correctness of the weekly cycle—and the Sabbath day—when He was on earth.**

Scripture tells us, "He that saith he abideth in Him ought himself also so to walk, even as He walked" *(1 John 2:6).* Throughout His earthly life, Jesus gave "us an example, that ye should follow His steps" *(1 Peter 2:21).* And Jesus' steps were obedient in Sabbath observance.

"As His custom was" (Luke 4:16, 31), Jesus kept the Bible Sabbath according to the commandment.

"If ye keep My commandments, ye shall abide in My love; even as I have kept My Father's commandments, and abide in His love."—*John 15:10.*

If the Sabbath had been lost, Jesus would have found it for His followers. They would have known which day of the week was the correct Sabbath.

Jesus was crucified on the sixth day of the week, which was the day before the Sabbath. We today would call it "Friday." On this same sixth day, which was also called the "preparation day," His followers prepared "spices and ointments" to anoint His body for burial, but then stopped when sundown came, "and rested on the Sabbath according to the commandment."

"And that day was the preparation, and the Sabbath drew on. And the women also, which came with Him from Galilee, followed after, and beheld the sepulchre, and how His body was laid. And they returned, and prepared spices and ointments; **and rested the Sabbath day according to the commandment.**"—*Luke 23:54-56.*

This is an important fact, for **it is obvious that Jesus never told His followers to stop keeping the Bible Sabbath, and that they knew which day to keep holy!** —They wanted so badly to anoint His body with precious ointment; but, because it was almost sunset, they went home, planning to try to do it Sunday morning.

In death, Jesus rested in the tomb on the seventh day, the Sabbath *(Matthew 28:1-7).* Then, "as it began to dawn toward the first day of the week" *(Matthew 28:1),* **Christ arose on the first working day in the week—for He had a lot of things to tend to.** It was the first day of a new, working week, the day after the Bible Sabbath.

"He will magnify the law and make it honorable."—*Isaiah 42:21.*

Truly, throughout His life, Jesus magnified the importance of keeping God's Ten Commandment law!

TO BE KEPT NEARLY 40 YEARS LATER

In fact, when He gave His prophecy of the coming destruction of Jerusalem and the Temple, **Christ warned His disciples that—even in the midst of that terrible crisis—nearly forty years later—they should continue sacredly observing the Bible Sabbath.**

"But pray ye that your flight be not in the winter, neither on the Sabbath day."—*Mat-*

thew 24:20.

—Yet that destruction did not occur until A.D. 70—nearly a half-century after Christ's death on the cross! Jonathan Edwards, a leading Protestant revivalist in the eighteenth-century American Colonies, wrote this:

"Christ is here speaking of the flight of the apostles and other Christians out of Jerusalem and Judea, just before their final destruction . . But the final destruction of Jerusalem was after the dissolution of the Jewish constitution, and after the Christian dispensation was fully set up. Yet it is plainly implied in these words of the Lord, that even then—40 years later—Christians would still be bound to a strict observation of the Sabbath."—*Jonathan Edwards, Works, Vol. 4, pp. 621-622.*

It is an astounding fact that the week only exists because God made our world and gave us the Bible Sabbath!

"In connection only with the week is religion obviously the explanation of its origin, and the week only is uniformly attributed to command of God. **The week exists because of the Sabbath.** It is historically and scientifically true that the Sabbath was made by God."—*W.O. Carver, Sabbath Observance, pp. 34-35; published 1940 by the Sunday School Board of the Southern Baptist Convention.*

THE WEEKLY CYCLE
FROM CHRIST'S TIME TO OURS

But could the weekly cycle have been changed after the death and resurrection of Christ? Here are the facts about this:

The *Julian calendar* was in use when Jesus Christ was upon the earth. Its originator, Julius Caesar, died March 14, 44 B.C., several decades before Christ was born. **This calendar which continued in use for fifteen centuries was not accurate in the length of its year**, being nearly one quarter of an hour too long. What it needed was our method of "leap years." By 1582, the vernal equinox of March 21 had receded to March 11, or was 10 days off schedule.

Yet all this time, the length of the week had not changed. Through God's providential care, the weekly cycle has remained unchanged since the Creation of our world.

A change was made to correct the length of the year at the time that Gregory XIII was the pope, and so it was called the *Gregorian calendar.* **This new calendar began to function on Friday, October 5, 1582. Friday the 5th was changed to the 15th. October 1582 only had 21 days. But in all of this, the week remained untouched, and the days of the week were undisturbed.** On a nearby page is what the calendar looked like that particular month:

Folk in Portugal who retired to sleep on Thursday, October 4, awoke the next morning on Friday the 15th. Some nations began the use of the new calendar at once. This included Spain, Portugal and Italy. France waited until December to adopt it. Part of Germany made the changeover in 1583 and the rest of the nation waited until 1700. About that time the Netherlands, Sweden and Denmark also accepted it. Then in 1752, England and the American Colonies made the changeover. By that time eleven days had to be changed, instead of ten. Wednesday, September 2 was followed by Thursday, September 14. Russia and Greece continued to use the old style calendar—the Julian Calendar—for over a hundred and fifty more years. Finally in 1919, Romania, Serbia, and Turkey changed to the new calendar, and Soviet Russia made the change soon after. By then there was a 14-day difference.

For 337 years, the calendars of Europe were mixed up—with dates which were totally confused. *But all this time the days of the week were alike everywhere! They had never changed.*

That which the *Encyclopedia Britannica* called the "unalterable uniformity" of the week has never been affected by calendar changes. And because of this, the seven-day week, given by God at the Creation has never been touched by the calendar changes of mankind.

EVEN MORE POWERFUL EVIDENCE

But there is yet even more powerful evidence that the weekly cycle has never changed, and the seventh day today is the same that it was in the time of Christ, and back to the time of Moses when manna was sent only on six days, and the finger of God etched the commandments on stone.

Our heavenly Father has given us more than written proof;—He has given us living proof—the Jewish race.

Nearly every other Near Eastern ethnic group has disappeared: the Hittites, Sumarians, Babylonians, Assyrians, Moabites, and Philistines—all are gone.

But the Jews remain—and with them the Bible Sabbath. It has been 3,400 years since they arrived at Mount Sinai—but all during those long centuries, down to the time of Christ and beyond to our own time, they have been keeping the Sabbath. Week after week, month after month, year after year, century after century.

Ask any Jewish acquaintance what day is the Sabbath. He will tell you that it is Saturday—the seventh day.

Orthodox Jews, scattered throughout the world, have kept strict record of time. They have carefully obeyed the Sabbath commandment down through the ages. The existence and testimony of the Jewish race is alone enough to settle the matter.

HISTORIANS AND ASTRONOMERS

AGREE

But there are others who have kept records also:

Historians have amassed an accurate record of time. Astronomers have also kept careful records, and theirs is one of the most accurate that you will find anywhere.

And then we have the calendars themselves. **All calendars agree. There is no evidence whatsoever to support the false claim that "time has been lost."** The standard reference works all tell us the same thing: No time has been lost in the weekly cycle. An example of this is to be found in all the major encyclopedias, and the reports of astronomers.

"The week is a period of seven days . . It has been employed from time immemorial."—*The Encyclopedia Britannica, 11th Edition, Vol. 4, p. 988, art. "Calendar."*

"**In the various changes of the calendar, there has been no change in the seven day rota of the week**, which has come down from very early times."—*(signed) F.W. Dyson, Astronomer Royal, Royal Observatory, Greenwich, London. Letter dated March 4, 1932.*

"There has been no change in our calendar in past centuries that has affected in any way the cycle of the week."—*(Signed) James Robertson, Director American Ephemeris, Navy Department, U.S. Naval Observatory, Washington, D.C. Letter dated March 12, 1932.*

In the official *League of Nations Report on the Calendar,* published at Geneva, August 17, 1926, are the following statements from leading astronomers:

"**The week has been followed for thousands of years and therefore has been hallowed by immemorial use.**"—*Anders Dooner (formerly Professor of Astronomy), University of Helsingfors, p. 51.*

"I have always hesitated to suggest breaking the continuity of the week, which without a doubt is the most ancient scientific institute bequeathed to us by antiquity."—*Edouard Baillaud (Director of the Paris Observatory), p. 52.*

"In spite of all of our dickerings with the calendar, it is patent that the human race never lost the septenary [seven day] sequence of week days and that **the Sabbath of these latter times comes down to us from Adam, through the ages, without a single lapse.**"—*Dr. Toten, Professor of Astronomy, Yale University.*

"The continuity of the week has crossed the centuries and all known calendars,—still intact."—*Professor D. Eginitis, Director of the Greek Observatory in Athens, Greece.*

"Having been time calculator at Greenwich for many years, I can testify . . that **this daily period of rotation does not vary one-thousandth part of a second in thousands of years . . Consequently, it can be said with assurance that not a day has been lost since Creation**, and all the calendar changes notwithstanding, **there has been no break in the weekly cycle.**"—*Frank Jeffries, Fellow of the Royal Astronomical Society, and Research Director of the Royal Observatory, Greenwich, England.*

SUMMARY

In summary, we have learned four important facts: First, **Jesus Christ faithfully kept the Bible Sabbath and commanded His followers to keep it** after His death and resurrection. Second, **the Sabbath He kept was the same day that Moses kept and God commanded** on Mount Sinai. Third, **there has been no change in the weekly cycle all through the centuries.** Fourth,—**you and I can keep the same Sabbath that Jesus kept!**

"O day of sweet reflection, thou art a day of love; A day to raise affection from earth to things above. New graces ever gaining from this our day of rest, We seek the rest remaining, in mansions of the blest."

The Sabbath is God's flag, the symbol of His sovereignty, woven in the loom of heaven, and raised over His newly completed creation of our world. And today, after the passing of long years, it still remains the symbol of His right to rule as Creator and Redeemer.

IN THE LAST DAYS AND THROUGHOUT ETERNITY

And there are two more wonderful truths: First, it is predicted that, in spite of all the earlier attempts to destroy knowledge of it, **God will have a people on earth in the last days who will keep the Bible Sabbath.**

"And they that shall be of thee shall build the old waste places: **thou shalt raise up the foundations of many generations; and thou shalt be called, the repairer of the breach**, the restorer of paths to dwell in.

"If thou turn away thy foot from the Sabbath, from doing thy pleasure on My holy day; and call the Sabbath a delight, the holy of the Lord, honourable; and shalt honour him, not doing thine own ways, nor finding thine own pleasure, nor speaking thine own words:

"Then shalt thou delight thyself in the Lord; and I will cause thee to ride upon the high places of the earth, and feed thee with the heritage of Jacob thy father: for the mouth of the Lord hath spoken it."—*Isaiah 58:12-14.*

Second, **God's faithful ones will keep this same seventh-day Sabbath in the New Earth!**

"**Blessed are they that do His command-**

ments, that they may have right to the tree of life, and may enter in through the gates into the city."—*Revelation 22:14.*

"For as the new heavens and the new earth, which I will make, shall remain before Me, saith the Lord, so shall your seed and your name remain. And it shall come to pass, that from one new moon to another, and from one Sabbath to another, shall all flesh come to worship before Me, saith the Lord."—*Isaiah 66:22-23.*

What a glorious future opens up before us, to be accounted as God's faithful children who love and obey Him and trust in Jesus for enabling strength to keep His commandments. One day soon God's faithful ones will enter through the gates into the City and live eternally with Christ!

"Safely through another week, God has brought us on our way; Let us now a blessing seek, Waiting in His courts today; Day of all the week the best, Emblem of eternal rest."

COMING NEXT—Since God the Father and God the Son considered the Bible Sabbath to be an essential part of the unchangeable Ten Commandment law, no disciple or Apostle would dare try to change it to some other day. We will now learn exactly what Christ's disciples, as well as the Apostles, thought of it. Did they cherish and obey it after Christ's death on the cross?

Chapter Twenty

The Sabbath of the Apostles

Is Sunday Sacredness in the Bible?

THE SABBATH OF CHRIST'S DISCIPLES

Among the disciples of Christ, none were more faithful than those that were present at His burial, and two days later when He arose from the dead.

Four were women who with the Apostle John stood at the cross in sad vigil as Jesus suffered and died.

"Now there stood by the cross of Jesus His mother and His mother's sister, Mary the wife of Cleophas, and Mary Magdalene . . and the disciple standing by, whom He loved."—*John 19:25-26.*

As the body of Jesus was laid in the grave, these women were there, along with the close friends who buried Him.

"And that day was the preparation, and the Sabbath drew on. And the women also, which came with Him from Galilee, followed after, and beheld the sepulchre, and how His body was laid. And they returned, and prepared spices and ointments; and rested the Sabbath day according to the commandment."—*Luke 23:54-56.*

(Notice that these verses teach that the Sabbath is the day between Friday and Sunday, and that Christ rested in the tomb on the Bible Sabbath, and then arose on Sunday to begin His activities again on behalf of the human race. While He rested in the tomb, they rested at home.)

Here were the closest friends of Jesus—yet they were very careful to keep the Bible Sabbath.

By the time that Nicodemus and Joseph of Arimathea had, on the sixth day, arranged the burial of Jesus, the sun had almost set on that fateful day of the week. "The Sabbath drew on." They knew that, according to Bible reckoning, the Sabbath begins at evening; that is, sunset.

This pattern was first given us during Creation Week: Genesis 1:5, 8, 13, 19, 23, 31. "And the evening and the morning were the first day," etc. It is also mentioned elsewhere.

"From even unto even, shall ye celebrate your Sabbath."—*Leviticus 23:32.*

"And at even, when the sun did set."—*Mark 1:32.*

Those women were deeply concerned to anoint Christ's body for the burial,—but the Sabbath was about to begin, so they stopped their planned work, went home "and rested the Sabbath day according to the commandment," with the intention of returning to complete their task as soon as they could on the first day of the week, which would be Sunday morning. For it would be the beginning of another work week.

But their hearts were heavy, for not only was Jesus dead, but as they were leaving on Friday afternoon, they saw an immense stone rolled in front of the entrance to the tomb. How could they get the stone rolled away after the Sabbath ended?

"And when the Sabbath was past, Mary Magdalene, and Mary the mother of James, and Salome, had bought sweet spices, that they might come and anoint Him. And very early in the morning the first day of the week, they came unto the sepulchre at the rising of the sun. And they said among themselves, Who shall roll us away the stone from the door of the sepulchre?"—*Mark 16:1-3.*

To their utter astonishment, when they arrived, they found the stone rolled away—and the tomb empty.

Let no one tell you that Christ had taught His followers to keep the first day of the week—Sunday—holy! For it simply is not true. Christ did not change any of the Ten Commandments.

Indeed, instead He commanded His disciples to

make sure they kept the Bible Sabbath nearly forty years after His death and resurrection, even amid the terrible crisis of the siege and destruction of Jerusalem in A.D. 70! "But pray ye that your flight be not . . on the Sabbath day" (*Matthew 24:20*).

It should be noted that **Christ's other disciples, including John and Peter, also carefully kept the Bible Sabbath. They also did not return to the tomb until Sunday morning** (*Luke 24:12; Mark 16:1-2*).

THE SABBATH OF PAUL

But now, let us turn our attention to the Apostle Paul. **Surely, as the apostle to the Gentiles, if any of the apostles observed Sunday, it would be Paul.**

Paul was God's special chosen messenger to the Gentiles. As such **he would be careful to set before them correct principles of Sabbath observance. Was Paul faithful in keeping the Bible Sabbath?**

Arriving at Antioch (where the followers of Christ were first called "Christians"; *Acts 11:26*), Paul "went into the synagogue on the Sabbath day" (*Acts 13:14*). There he delivered a powerful appeal for everyone to accept Christ as the Saviour of the world.

Then came the Gentiles, and "besought that these words might be preached to them the next Sabbath" (*verse 42*).

There is no word or hint that Paul stopped keeping the seventh-day Sabbath in order to reach the Gentiles.

Later called to Philippi in Macedonia, Paul and his company "on the Sabbath . . went out of the city by a riverside, where prayer was wont to be made" (*Acts 16:13*). **This was a Sabbath service that Christ's followers regularly attended. There is no word of controversy about the Sabbath, or any effort to get people to keep another day.**

Thessalonica was the next stop.

"And Paul, as his manner was, went in unto them, and three Sabbath days reasoned with them out of the Scriptures, opening and alleging, that Christ must needs have suffered, and risen again from the dead; and that this Jesus, whom I preach unto you, is Christ."—*Acts 17:2-3*.

Paul preached Christ crucified and risen. **No argument about the Sabbath. No new day was proposed. "As his manner was," he went to church on the Sabbath.**

Persecution drove him to Berea, and from there to Athens. Finally, he arrived in Corinth, where he remained for eighteen months. The Scriptures tell us that **throughout that entire time—a full year and a half,—as he always did, Paul carefully kept the Bible Sabbath.**

"After these things Paul departed from Athens, and came to Corinth . . And he reasoned in the synagogue every Sabbath, and persuaded the Jews and the Greeks . . **And he continued there a year and six months**, teaching the Word of God among them."—*Acts 18:1, 4, 11*.

Just in these few Scriptures alone, we find that Paul kept the Sabbath 84 times; all the while preaching the gospel of Jesus Christ. It was his custom to keep the Bible Sabbath, as it was the custom of Jesus, who at Damascus called him to preach to the Gentiles.

In fact, Paul knew no other Sabbath. He regularly kept the Sabbath and preached for a year and a half at this city, and encouraged others to keep it,—yet **Paul was at Corinth a full 23 years after the cross.**

In Hebrews 4:4, the Sabbath is once again mentioned by Paul: "For he spake in a certain place of the seventh day on this wise, **And God did rest the seventh day from all His works.**" And in verse 9, he declares: "**There remaineth therefore a rest to the people of God.**" Verse 10 tells us that to enter into "His rest," we must cease from our work as God did from His. This is obviously referring to how God rested on the seventh day of Creation Week and blessed it for our use.

God rested on the seventh day of Creation Week, not on the first day. The first day is not God's rest day. Therefore it can never be the Sabbath of rest for the people of God.

Throughout his ministry, **Paul preached Christ as the Saviour who alone could enable men to keep God's moral law. Repeatedly, Paul taught that, apart from Christ's strengthening grace, men were not able to resist temptation and sin, and obey God's law.**

"Be it known unto you therefore, men and brethren, that through this man is preached unto you the forgiveness of sins, And by Him all that believe are justified from all things, from which ye could not be justified by the law of Moses."—*Acts 13:38-39*.

"But this I confess unto thee, that after the way which they call heresy, so worship I the God of my fathers, believing all things which are written in the law and in the prophets."—*Acts 24:14*.

"**Do we then make void the law through faith? God forbid: yea, we establish the law.**"—*Romans 3:31*.

"What shall we say then? **Shall we continue in sin, that grace may abound? God forbid.** How shall we, that are dead to sin, live any longer therein?"—*Romans 6:1-2*.

"**What then? shall we sin, because we are not under the law, but under grace? God forbid.** Know ye not, that to whom ye yield yourselves servants to obey, his servants ye are to whom ye obey; whether of sin unto death, or of obedience unto righteousness?"—*Romans 6:15-16*.

As the above verse explains, **when, through the**

enabling grace of Christ, we obey the Ten Commandments, *we are not under the condemnation of the law*, but instead, we are in a state of humble, enabled obedience. We are under grace—living a life in daily resistance of temptation and sin.

"But God be thanked, that ye were the servants of sin, but ye have obeyed from the heart . . **Being then made free from sin**, ye became the servants of righteousness."—*Romans 6:17-18*.

Paul clarified that the moral law leads men to Christ, who then enables them to obey it; at the same time he spoke not one word against the keeping of the Bible Sabbath—which is in the heart of that Ten Commandment law.

THE SABBATH OF JAMES

The Apostle James was very strong in his defense of the moral law of God. In all that he said, there was no hint that any part of the Ten Commandments had been changed.

"**For whosoever shall keep the whole law, and yet offend in one point, he is guilty of all**. For he that said, Do not commit adultery, said also, Do not kill. Now if thou commit no adultery, yet if thou kill, thou art become a transgressor of the law. **So speak ye, and so do, as they that shall be judged by the law of liberty**."—*James 2:10-12*.

What does James mean in calling the Ten Commandments the "law of liberty"? There are those who declare that freedom from law provides them with the greatest "liberty." When enough people who believed that error got together in 1793, the result was misery to millions and death to thousands in the French Revolution—a revolt against God and His laws.

In reality, disobedience to God's moral law results in slavery to sin and Satan.

In stark contrast, only God's "law of liberty" *(James 2:12)*, **the Ten Commandments, can free a man to live a happy, worthwhile life in this world, and inherit a home in the next.**

In his day, Paderewski was one of the greatest concert pianists in the world. Yet most of us could sit down at his piano and bang on it all we wanted, and only make noise. Although we might imagine ourselves "liberated" from being guided by the rules of piano playing, Paderewski was obedient to them. **His obedience to those rules enabled him to enter upon a level of genuine liberty at the piano which you and I cannot experience.**

Obedience to God's moral law enables us to truly control ourselves and become all that He wants us to be.

THE SABBATH OF JOHN

In the first chapter of Revelation, **the Apostle John was careful to mention that it was on the** "Lord's day" that Christ appeared to him in vision on the Isle of Patmos. **The only day in Scripture that the Lord ever said was His is the Bible Sabbath.** And, in various ways, He said this repeatedly.

"I was in the Spirit on the Lord's day."—*Revelation 1:10*.

The Fourth Commandment clearly explains what day this is:

"But **the seventh day is the Sabbath of the Lord** thy God."—*Exodus 20:10*.

The seventh day is the Sabbath of the Lord **is mentioned six times in the Bible**: Exodus 16:26; 23:12; 31:15; 35:2; Leviticus 23:3; and Deuteronomy 5:14.

The only day which the Bible has ever mentioned as being the Lord's day is the seventh day of the week. The expression found in Isaiah 58:13 is a good example of this:

"If thou turn away thy foot from the Sabbath, from doing thy pleasure on *My holy day* . . then shalt thou delight thyself in the Lord."—*Isaiah 58:13-14*.

What day is the "Lord's day" in the Scriptures? The Bible tells us that the Sabbath is *the day unto the Lord (Exodus 16:23, 25; 31:15; 35:2)*. It is *the day of the Lord (Exodus 20:10; Leviticus 23:3; Deuteronomy 5:14), and His own day—His holy day (Isaiah 58:13)*.

Jesus called Himself the Lord of the Sabbath.

"The Son of man is Lord also of the Sabbath."—*Mark 2:28*.

The Apostle John speaks of it as "the Lord's day" (Revelation 1:10).

"I was in the Spirit on the Lord's day."—*Revelation 1:10*.

John well knew which day was the Lord's day. This day is the memorial day of the Creator (Genesis 2:1-3; Exodus 31:17), and the memorial day of the Redeemer (Ezekiel 20:12, 20).

It is the Lord's Day! God's own day. The day which He wants to share with us.

Repeatedly in his writings, the Apostle John declared that men must obey the moral law of God, which has the Bible Sabbath in its heart. Here are a few of those passages:

"He that saith he abideth in Him ought himself also so to walk, even as He walked." *1 John 2:6*.

"And hereby we do know that we know Him, if we keep His commandments. **He that saith, I know Him, and keepeth not His commandments, is a liar, and the truth is not in him.** But whoso keepeth His Word, in him verily is the love of God perfected: hereby know we that we are in Him. He that saith he abideth in Him ought himself also so to walk, even as He walked."—*1 John 2:3-6*.

"And every man that hath this hope in him purifieth himself, even as He is pure. **Whosoever committeth sin transgresseth also the law: for sin is the transgression of the law.**

"And ye know that He was manifested to take away our sins; and in Him is no sin. **Whosoever abideth in Him sinneth not**: whosoever sinneth hath not seen Him, neither known Him. Little children, let no man deceive you: he that doeth righteousness is righteous, even as He is righteous."—*1 John 3:3-7.*

"By this we know that we love the children of God, when we love God, and keep His commandments. **For this is the love of God, that we keep His commandments**: and His commandments are not grievous. For whatsoever is born of God overcometh the world."—*1 John 5:2-4.*

And we do not want to forget these other words of truth in the book of Revelation, penned by the Apostle John:

The remnant of believers, in the last days, will be distinguished by the fact that they keep all ten of God's commandments! —And they do it by the enabling grace of Christ!

"And the dragon was wroth with the woman, and went to make war with **the remnant of her seed, which keep the commandments of God**, and have the testimony of Jesus Christ."—*Revelation 12:17.*

"Here is the patience of the saints: **here are they that keep the commandments of God**, and the faith of Jesus."—*Revelation 14:12.*

The promise is rich and abundant. Those who faithfully obey God—will inherit eternal life!

"**Blessed are they that do His commandments, that they may have right to the tree of life, and may enter in through the gates into the city**."—*Revelation 22:14.*

SUNDAY IN THE NEW TESTAMENT

We have learned that the seventh-day Sabbath was faithfully kept by Christ's followers after the cross. The Sabbath of the New Testament is the Sabbath of Creation. **Nowhere in Scripture had Sunday, the first day of the week been substituted for the seventh day. From Matthew to Revelation no record of any such change can be found.**

The example and writings of Christ and the Apostles testify that no such change was ever made or even contemplated by them. **Those who observe another day as a day of rest and worship do so without any Scriptural warrant whatsoever, and fail to honor the memorial of Christ's creative and redeeming power.**

It is a solid fact that the character of God and His moral law never change. His moral standard is always the same. Changing ages, and the fallible

customs of men, have had no effect on the law that is the foundation of God's kingdom.

In 1884, a Roman Catholic priest, Thomas Enright, CSSR, of Des Moines, Iowa (formerly president of Redemptorist College, Kansas City, Missouri) offered a thousand dollars to anyone who could give him one verse from the Bible which said that the sanctity of the Bible Sabbath had been transferred to Sunday. He also offered to give it to anyone who could prove from the Bible that Sunday, the first day of the week, should be observed as a holy day. He later declared:

"The Bible says 'Remember the Sabbath day to keep it holy,' but the Catholic Church says, 'No, keep the first day of the week,' and all the world bows down in silent obedience to the mandates of the Catholic Church!"— *Priest Thomas Enright, CSSR president of Redemptorist College, Kansas City, Mo., in a lecture at Hartford, Kansas, February 18, 1884, and published in The American Sentinel R.C. journal, June 1893, p. 173.*

As you might expect, this challenge provoked widespread comment. But no one ever claimed the reward.

It is very clear that all of Christ's disciples, as well as His Apostles, remained true to the Bible Sabbath, and never taught that men should keep any other day. Indeed, they would have no right to do so, for only the Creator, the Lawgiver, would have a right to change His law!

But then, where did Sunday sacredness come from? If any Christians were keeping it before the last book of the Bible ended, we should surely be able to find it in the Word of God.

The question before us here is this: *What does the Bible say about the first day of the week?* There are **nine passages** which mention the first day of the week:

The first one is in Genesis.

"And God said, Let there be light: and there was light. And God saw the light, that it was good: and God divided the light from the darkness. And God called the light Day, and the darkness He called Night. **And the evening and the morning were the first day**."—*Genesis 1:3-5.*

Nothing here about the first day being sacred.

The second one is in Matthew.

"In the end of the Sabbath, **as it began to dawn toward the first day of the week**, came Mary Magdalene and the other Mary to see the sepulchre."—*Matthew 28:1.*

The two women had come to Christ's tomb on Sunday morning with the specific purpose of anointing His body. They had not been able to do it Friday afternoon, because the Bible Sabbath was about to begin, and, as were all of Christ's followers, they were careful to faithfully keep the Sabbath.

Notice in the above verse that **the Bible Sabbath ended before the first day of the week began. This clearly shows that the two are distinct from one another, and not the same! There is no slightest hint of any sacredness attached to the first day of the week in this verse.** Matthew wrote his book several years after the resurrection of Christ.

The third and fourth are in Mark.

"**And when the Sabbath was past**, Mary Magdalene, and Mary the mother of James, and Salome, had bought sweet spices, that they might come and anoint Him. And **very early in the morning the first day of the week**, they came unto the sepulchre at the rising of the sun."—*Mark 16:1-2.*

"Now when Jesus was risen **early the first day of the week**, He appeared first to Mary Magdalene, out of whom He had cast seven devils."—*Mark 16:9.*

Here again there is no word from Christ, but only Mark's record of the resurrection. **The Sabbath was past before the first day came. They are two different days! One is holy; the other is one of the six working days.** After the Sabbath was past, the women arrived, carrying a jar of ointment so they could tend to some work. But Jesus, risen from the dead, also had work to do this first working day of the week.

Thus we see that many years after the resurrection of Christ, when Mark wrote his book, he knew of no Sunday sacredness.

The fifth one is in Luke.

"Now **upon the first day of the week, very early in the morning**, they came unto the sepulchre, bringing the spices which they had prepared, and certain others with them."—*Luke 24:1.*

As with the other Gospel writers, **Luke gives no mention in his book that Jesus ever said anything about Sunday sacredness.**

But he points out, in the two preceding verses, that **Jesus' followers rested on the Bible Sabbath "according to the commandment."**

"And the women also, which came with Him from Galilee, followed after, and beheld the sepulchre, and how His body was laid. And they returned, and prepared spices and ointments; and rested the Sabbath day according to the commandment."—*Luke 23:55-56.*

Naturally, **that was according to the Fourth of the Ten Commandments.**

The sixth one is in John.

"**The first day of the week** cometh Mary Magdalene early, when it was yet dark, unto the sepulchre."—*John 20:1.*

John gives the same story, a simple record of that early morning experience.

Notice that **it was still "dark," although it was the first day of the week. This is because, according to the Bible pattern, each day ends at sunset and the next day begins.**

Christ's disciples knew that, according to Bible reckoning, the Sabbath begins at evening; that is, sunset.

This pattern was first given during Creation Week (*Genesis 1:5, 8, 13, 19, 23, 31*). "And the evening and the morning were the first day," etc. It is also mentioned elsewhere.

"From even unto even, shall ye celebrate your Sabbath."—*Leviticus 23:32.*

"And at even, when the sun did set."—*Mark 1:32.*

So when the sun set the night before, the first day of the week began. **Very early the next morning, while it was still dark, Christ arose and the two women arrived at the tomb.**

The seventh one is also in John.

"Then **the same day at evening, being the first day of the week**, when the doors were shut where the disciples were assembled for fear of the Jews, came Jesus and stood in the midst, and saith unto them, Peace be unto you."—*John 20:19.*

Here again **there is no indication that Jesus ever mentioned the first day of the week as being anything important.**

There are some who say that this was a Sunday church service! But read again what it says: **The disciples were huddled in that upper room, "for fear of the Jews."** They were trying to hide out, lest they be the next to be slain by the murderous Pharisees.

But Jesus knew where they were hiding, and He suddenly appeared there before them.

It has been said that they were celebrating Christ's resurrection; but, **up to the time that He appeared before them, they still did not believe that Jesus had risen.**

Mark makes this unmistakably clear. Mary Magdalene, having seen the resurrected Christ, told the disciples, but they "believed not" (*Mark 16:11*).

Then we are told this:

"**After that He appeared in another form unto two of them, as they walked, and went into the country.** And they went and told it unto the residue: neither believed they them."—*Mark 16:12-13.*

Luke writes that these same two men saw Christ, and explains that, after discovering that their new friend was indeed Jesus,—they hurried back down the road to Jerusalem and went to the upper room where the disciples were hiding. But, as soon as they

W
A
Y

had told them the news that Christ was alive—Jesus suddenly stood in their midst. The entire thrilling story is in Luke 24:13-49. Here is a little of it:

"And it came to pass, as He sat at meat with them, He took bread, and blessed it, and brake, and gave to them. **And their eyes were opened, and they knew Him; and He vanished out of their sight** . . And they rose up the same hour, and returned to Jerusalem, and found the eleven gathered together, and them that were with them . . **And as they thus spake, Jesus Himself stood in the midst of them, and saith unto them, Peace be unto you.** But they were terrified and affrighted, and supposed that they had seen a spirit."—*Luke 24:30-31, 33, 36-37.*

So it is clear that the disciples had not gathered in the upper room because they believed Christ had risen from the dead. As soon as they saw Him, they were terrified.

To the honest seeker after truth, it is clear that Matthew, Mark, Luke, and John, who wrote the four biographies of Christ's life and teachings, knew nothing of Sunday sacredness. They were totally silent on the holiness of any day other than the Sabbath.

The eighth one is in Acts.

"And **upon the first day of the week**, when the disciples came together to break bread, Paul preached unto them, ready to depart on the morrow; and continued his speech until midnight. **And there were many lights in the upper chamber**, where they were gathered together."—*Acts 20:7-8.*

Luke wrote the book of Acts, and in it gave an inspired account of the early Christian church. **Luke recorded eighty-four Sabbath services (after Christ's ascension), and only one first-day meeting**, the one referred to in the above passage. Notice that **no holy title is used for this day. It is simple called "the first day of the week."** There is nothing here about Sunday sacredness.

Here is the entire story of what happened here:

Paul and his missionary companions had spent seven days at Troas (*verse 6*). **Their farewell gathering was held at night. We know this because there were lights in this upper chamber** where the meeting was held. We are told that Paul preached till midnight. According to the Bible pattern (*Genesis 1:5, 8, 13, 19, 23, 31; Leviticus 23:32*), **the first day of the week begins at sundown** and ends Sunday night at sundown. **Since this meeting was held on the first day of the week—and it was night,—it must therefore have been held on what we call "Saturday night."** Had it been held on what we call Sunday night (after sunset on Sunday), it would have been on the second day of the week.

This was Paul's last opportunity to visit with

them, so he continued speaking till midnight. *What happened after this was significant:*

"When he therefore was come up again, and had broken bread, and eaten, and talked a long while, **even till break of day, so he departed.** And they brought the young man alive, and were not a little comforted. And we went before to ship, and sailed unto Assos, there intending to take in Paul: **for so had he appointed, minding himself to go afoot.** And when he met with us at Assos, we took him in, and came to Mitylene."—*Acts 20:11-14.*

On this busy Sunday, Paul's companions took ship and sailed around a point of land to Assos with all the luggage. But Paul remained with his friends at Troas until dawn on Sunday, **and then he walked straight overland, 19 miles to Assos**. He apparently needed the exercise.

Notice that both Paul and his companions were working on Sunday! They sailed to Assos that day, while he walked overland and met them there. Arriving there, he boarded their ship and they headed off to Mitylene. **They considered the first day of the week a common working day**, in accordance with the commandment.

"Remember the Sabbath day, to keep it holy. **Six days shalt thou labour, and do all thy work.**"—*Exodus 20:8-9.*

The reason for this, also given in the Fourth Commandment, is because God spent day one through six creating the world, and then rested the seventh day. He worked on the first day also.

"For in six days the Lord made heaven and earth, the sea, and all that in them is, and rested the seventh day."—*Exodus 20:11.*

The Bible is always consistent with itself! God's plan is a beautiful one—and, if we will cooperate, we can be part of it!

Nothing is said about this Troas meeting being a church service. Nor are we told that it was a communion service, as some suggest. Acts 20:7 says that they did "break bread" together, and then Paul preached. This was just a common evening meal, for **"to break bread" was the Bible expression for partaking of food.** They broke bread daily from house to house (*Acts 2:46*), and they "did eat their meat [meal, in the Greek] with gladness" (*verse 46*).

It is to be noted that even had they held the actual communion service that night, this would in no way make it a holy day. **The Lord's Supper may be celebrated on any day** (*1 Corinthians 11:26*). And, in any case, **that special service commemorates Christ's death, not His resurrection.** "Ye do show the Lord's death till He come" (*verse 26*).

The ninth one is the only instance in all the writings of Paul!

"Now concerning the collection for the saints,

as I have given order to the churches of Galatia, even so do ye. **Upon the first day of the week let every one of you lay by him in store**, as God hath prospered him, **that there be no gatherings** when I come."—*1 Corinthians 16:1-2.*

Is not this remarkable? The only place in all of the Apostle Paul's books, where he even mentioned the first day of the week! **But what does it mean?**

Paul had earlier sent an urgent request to all the Christian churches in the region of Galatia (consisting primarily of Gentiles), to donate money for the poor and persecuted Christian Jews living in Jerusalem.

It is evident that **Paul was a preacher who did not like to give appeals for money from the pulpit. So he said, "that there be no gatherings when I come."** Gatherings of money, of course. **He wanted each family to set aside a certain amount ahead of time. Each family was to do this at home. "Let every one of you lay by him in store."** Another version (RSV) says, "Put something aside and save." Thus **this plan had no connection with a weekly collection at a church service. Quite to the contrary, this money was to be laid aside at home.**

In addition, it was to be on a basis of "as God hath prospered." How simple and clear is the picture.

A church member runs a small shop all week, let us say. **Friday afternoon he closes early enough to prepare for the Sabbath. There is no time to tally up his money and figure accounts.**

But when the Sabbath is past, and the first day of the week comes, he is to check his net earnings and lay aside a proper sum, not at church, but at home.

This text also teaches us to total up our money and figure our budgets on the first day of each week, since there is not time on Friday afternoon to do it, before the Sabbath begins at sunset.

This last of the nine first-day texts in the Bible, like the other eight, gives no shred of evidence for a new holy day, or a regular first-day church gathering.

Here is a summary of what we have learned here: **In the Bible, Sunday is never called the Christian Sabbath; never called the Sabbath day at all; never called the Lord's day; never even called a rest day. No sacred title whatever is applied to it. It is simply called "the first day of the week." And, by the way, the word, "Sunday," does not occur in the Bible.**

Above and beyond all the arguments of man, stands the command of God:

"Remember the Sabbath day, to keep it holy. Six days shalt thou labour, and do all thy work. But the seventh day is the Sabbath of the Lord thy God: in it thou shalt not do any work."—*Exodus 20:8-10.*

I can place a small, upright post on a table. Then I can place a second, and a third. Now I can sight along these posts and they point me in a certain direction.

We have placed post after post, as we have examined Bible verse after Bible verse,—and they all point us in the same direction. They all point to the seventh-day of the week as the only hallowed Sabbath which God ever gave to mankind.

The Sabbath and marriage are the only two institutions which God gave to man in the garden of Eden before his fall. And the enemy of God is determined to distort and destroy both.

George Vandeman shares this story:

"I shall never forget the Lutheran man and his daughter who came up to me after a meeting in which this truth about the Bible Sabbath was shared. They had waited until others had gone. He was a big man, twice my size, and he took me by the lapel of my coat. He simply shook, and the tears rolled down his face as he said, *'Pastor Vandeman, tell me it isn't so! Tell me it isn't so!'*

"I knew what a shock it was to him. *But I could not tell him it isn't so. I dared not hold back truth.* The minister of the gospel whose eyes have seen the truth of this Sabbath question, who feels his responsibility before God as he leads men and women forward to judgment and eternity, cannot tell any man it isn't so. He can only say, 'God has spoken in His Word, Will you follow?' "—*George Vandeman, Truth Makes a Difference.*

"Don't forget the Sabbath, The Lord our God hath blest, Of all the week the brightest, Of all the week the best.

"It brings repose from labor, It tells of joy divine, Its beams of light descending, With heav'nly beauty shine."

COMING NEXT—The only Sabbath in the Bible was the seventh day. Yet nearly every Christian today keeps the first day of the week. Just what did happen in earlier centuries, after the Bible ended? This is the question that will be answered next.

Chapter Twenty-One

How the Sabbath Was Changed

Historians Explain What Happened

One of the czars of Russia while walking in his park came upon a sentry standing guard over a little patch of weeds. "What are you doing here?" he asked.

The sentry replied, "I don't know. All I know is

that the captain of the guard ordered me to stand over this spot."

The czar sent for the captain.

"Captain! —What is this man guarding?"

The captain answered, "All I know is that the regulations call for a sentry to be posted here."

The czar then ordered an investigation, but no one in the government of Russia could discover why that spot needed guarding. **Then they opened the royal archives, which contained historical records going back centuries.**

The archives showed that a hundred years before, in the late eighteenth century, Catherine the Great had planted a rosebush on that plot of ground and ordered a sentry posted there to keep people from trampling on it. Eventually, the rosebush died, but nobody thought to cancel the order.

And for a hundred years men stood guard, carefully protecting something that did not need guarding. And they didn't know why.

Year after year. At first, no one knew how long. Guarding something that wasn't there.

We must open the archives of God's Word that we may understand God's will today. *There are some mysteries that need to be solved.*

MEN WOULD WANT TO MAKE CHANGES

Millions of people are reverently keeping Sunday, the first day of the week,—yet we have discovered that there is not one slightest hint in Scripture that either God nor any Bible writer ever considered it to have the slightest sacredness. *How did Sunday gain this remarkable honor?*

Searching back through the history books, we will discover that **the changeover began with the urging of half-converted Christians who wanted to "modernize" the church, and ended with church councils exalting the first day of the week**—accompanied by intense persecution of those who determined to keep the true Sabbath.

It is clear from the Bible that **if God had wanted to make such a change, He would have definitely stated it** in Scripture.

"Surely the Lord God will do nothing, but He revealeth His secret unto His servants the prophets."—*Amos 3:7.*

The change of the Sabbath from the seventh to the first day of the week was not made upon any divine or Scriptural authority. *God does not alter His moral precepts.*

"I know that, whatsoever God doeth, it shall be forever: nothing can be put to it, nor any thing taken from it: and God doeth it, that men should fear before Him."—*Ecclesiastes 3:14.*

"My covenant will I not break, nor alter the thing that is gone out of My lips."—*Psalm 89:34.*

"It is easier," said Jesus, "for heaven and earth to pass, than for one tittle of the law to fail" *(Luke 16:17).*

But while the Bible gives no record of God's changing the day, historians tell how it happened after the last book in the Bible ended.

Tragically, without any Bible authority for their actions, men have dared to tamper with the law of God, by substituting Sunday, the first day of the week, for the Bible Sabbath, the seventh day.

In the early centuries after the Bible ended, professed Christians arose who wanted to blend Bible principles with heathen traditions. Gradually, this increased, especially from about A.D. 175 to 300.

Many of these half-converted pagans were living in or near Alexandria, Egypt. Some of them started a Christian seminary, where they trained pastors. But this only spread the errors the more widely to Christian churches in other major cities.

THIS APOSTASY HAD BEEN FORETOLD

This great apostasy which, gradually increased after the Bible ended, had been foretold in several Bible passages:

"For I know this, that after my departing shall grievous wolves enter in among you, not sparing the flock. Also of your own selves shall men arise, speaking perverse things, to draw away disciples after them. Therefore watch."—*Acts 20:29-31.*

"For the time will come when they will not endure sound doctrine; but after their own lusts shall they heap to themselves teachers, having itching ears; and they shall turn away their ears from the truth, and shall be turned unto fables."—*2 Timothy 4:3-4.*

"Let no man deceive you by any means: for **that day shall not come, except there come a falling away first, and that man of sin be revealed, the son of perdition; who opposeth and exalteth himself above all that is called God**, or that is worshiped; **so that he as God sitteth in the temple of God, showing himself that he is God."**—*2 Thessalonians 2:3-4.*

In the prophecy of Daniel 7, God had predicted that this apostasy would occur. Under the symbol of "a little horn," a power would later arise in the world that would exalt itself against the God of heaven and would seek to destroy both God's truth and His people.

"I considered the horns, and, behold, there came up among them another little horn . . In this horn were eyes like the eyes of man, and **a mouth speaking great things.**"—*Daniel 7:8,*

Daniel was especially concerned about this

strange little horn power.

"Then I would know the truth of the fourth beast, which was diverse from all the others, . . and of the ten horns that were in his head, and of the other which came up, and before whom three fell; even of that horn that had eyes, and **a mouth that spake very great things**, whose look was more stout than his fellows.

"**I beheld, and the same horn made war with the saints, and prevailed against them**; until the Ancient of days came, and judgment was given to the saints of the Most High; and the time came that the saints possessed the kingdom."—*Daniel 7:19-22.*

"**And he shall speak great words against the Most High**, and shall wear out the saints of the Most High, **and think to change times and laws**: and they shall be given into his hand until a time and times and the dividing of time.

"But the judgment shall sit, and they shall take away his dominion."—*Daniel 7:25-26.*

"**He shall think to change times and laws." This would, of course, be God's moral law and God's special time—the Bible Sabbath.** The little horn's words are spoken against the "Most High," and **his efforts are to destroy the power and authority of the great Lawgiver. It was recognized that this could be best done by altering God's law and changing the Sabbath, which is the sign of the Creator's power.**

Because the Sabbath is the seal of the living God, by it the great moral code of Ten Commandments is stamped as belonging to God. It shows Him to be its Author, as well as the Creator of heaven and earth. **Satan knew that the best way to get rid of men's recognition of the Creator's authority was to do away with the Sabbath.**

NEW-MODELING THE CHURCH

Christ had been crucified in A.D. 31. Most of His disciples and apostles were dead by A.D. 65. John the last of the Apostles, died just before A.D. 100, after completing Revelation, the last book of the Bible.

In the early centuries after that, **the decline of spirituality led to the adoption of many pagan rites and ceremonies by Christians "who wanted to appear modern."** The *"mystery of iniquity"* had began its work in the church.

"Toward the latter end of the second century, many of the churches assumed a new form; the first simplicity disappeared; and insensibly, **as the old disciples retired to their graves, their children came forward and new-modeled the cause**."—*Ecclesiastical Researches, p. 51.*

Tragically, we will discover that modernists in the church decided to substitute the memorial day in honor of Mithra, the Sun god, for the memorial day in honor of the true God, our Creator.

In order to provide you with an accurate understanding of how this great apostasy began, *a number of statements by respected historians will be quoted.*

We want to learn how the predicted little horn power of Daniel 7 would "think to change" the law of God and the Bible Sabbath.

"It must be confessed that there is no law in the New Testament concerning the first day."—*McClintock and Strong, Cyclopedia of Biblical, Theological and Ecclesiastical Literature, Vol. 9, p. 196.*

"**Until well into the second century [a hundred years after Christ] we do not find the slightest indication in our sources that Christians marked Sunday by any kind of abstention from work**."—*W. Rordorf, Sunday, p. 157.*

"**Rites and ceremonies, of which neither Paul nor Peter ever heard, crept silently into use**, and then claimed the rank of divine institutions. [Church] officers for whom the primitive disciples could have found no place, and titles which to them would have been altogether unintelligible, began to challenge attention, and to be named apostolic."—*William D. Killen, The Ancient Church, p. xvi.*

THE ALLUREMENT OF SUN WORSHIP

In the early centuries after Christ there was a struggle between the infant church and paganism. Mithraism, which was the worship of the Sun god, was a special problem. Satan had used it to counterfeit many Bible practices.

The first day of the week had been honored by sun worshipers for centuries. They called this day "Sun day", the *"venerable day of the Sun god."* It was on this day that they conducted their wildest and most immoral ceremonies in honor of their god.

But all the while, the worshipers of the Creator God clung to the Bible and kept the Bible Sabbath.

There had been attempts to introduce sun worship into the church in the Old Testament.

"Sun worship was the earliest idolatry."—*Fausset Bible Dictionary, p. 666.*

Satan had even tried to introduce sun worship into ancient Israel (*Leviticus 26:30; Isaiah 17:8*). King Manasseh practiced direct Sun worship (*2 Kings 21:3, 5*). Josiah destroyed the chariots and horses dedicated to the Sun and its worship (*2 Kings 23:5, 11-12*). Sun altars and incense were burned on the housetops for the Sun (*Zephaniah 1:5*), and **Ezekiel beheld the "greatest abomination": direct Sun worship at the entryway to the Temple of the true God. This was done by facing eastward and praying to the rising sun** (*Ezekiel 8:16-17*).

W
A
Y

THE BEGINNINGS OF SUNDAY SACREDNESS IN THE CHRISTIAN CHURCH

By the year 200, pagan compromises and practices were beginning to come into some of the Christian churches in a decided way.

Sun worship among Christians first started in Alexandria, Egypt, which was a leading Christian center of worldly "higher education." The largest pagan university was located there, and compromising Christians founded a Christian seminary nearby to train pastors. **The bishop of the church at Rome was the first to adopt the pagan practices adopted by the liberal Christians at Alexandria.** He was quick to see the worldly advantage of compromise with paganism. By bringing in pagan customs, he could get more people attending church so it could become wealthier.

About A.D. 196, Victor, bishop of the Roman church, sent out a letter to all the Christian churches in the empire—demanding that they celebrate the resurrection of Christ on a certain Sunday every spring.

This was the first attempt by the bishop of the church at Rome to require Christians to keep Sunday for some special purpose. **It also marked the first time that the bishop of Rome tried to assume authority over the other churches.** Dr. Bower, in his *History of the Popes (Vol. 1, p. 18)*, said this was "the first essay of papal usurpation."

Eventually, the name *"Easter"* became the name of this celebration; which was copied from the pagan spring celebration of the birth of Ishtar, a pagan goddess. (The word *"Easter"* in Acts 12:4 in the KJV is a mistranslation. The Greek word there is "Passover," not "Easter." No Christians observed "Easter" until after the Bible ended.)

"CHURCH GROWTH" BY COMPROMISE

The church leaders at Alexandria and Rome recognized that, by adopting pagan customs, pagans would feel at home in the church. They decided that, by switching over from holding church services on the Bible Sabbath to the pagan day of worship, the day of Mithra the Sun god, the pagans would more likely start coming to church. They succeeded all too well, for those compromising city churches became more wealthy, as large numbers of non-Christians began attending church.

"The [Catholic] Church made a sacred day of Sunday . . largely because it was the weekly festival of the sun;—for **it was a definite policy to take over the pagan festivals endeared to the people by tradition, and give them a Christian significance.**"—*Authur Weigall, The Paganism in Our Christianity, 1928, p. 145.*

But this changeover was gradual, for **the great majority of local churches throughout the Empire** refused to modernize, and worship on Sunday. Recognizing that compromise with paganism was a dangerous threat, those Christians who were faithful to God believed that they should only obey what the Bible said.

"The festival of Sunday, like all other festivals was always only a human ordinance, and it was far from the intentions of the apostles to establish a Divine command in this respect, far from them, and from the early apostolic church, to transfer the laws of the Sabbath to Sunday."—*Augustus Neander, The History of the Christian Religion and Church, 1843, p. 186.*

Unfortunately, by A.D. 250, paganizing customs were becoming somewhat more common in several Christian churches.

DIRECT COMPETITION WITH MITHRA

Ancient Rome had, what was called emperor worship. But emperors were so dissolute that the heathens turned to the worship of gods and goddesses of Egypt, Babylonia, and Asia Minor. **The pagan religion which grew the fastest in popularity was Mithraism**, a religion from Persia which was the worship of the Sun god on Sunday, the first day of the week. Mithraism had absorbed rites and ceremonies from the other pagan religions, and kept increasing in the number of its adherents. It was a very attractive religion to worldlings.

Because Mithra, the Sun god, was said to be a great warrior, most of the Roman soldiers worshiped him, and prayed that he would help them in battle. Mithra, their unconquerable, warrior god, was named *"Sol Invictus"* (Latin for "Invincible Sun"). They also called him *"Lord Mithra."*

Mithraites would worship a statue of Mithra stabbing a huge bull to death. **New converts were required to be "baptized"** by standing under an iron grating—while a bull, slain above them, dripped blood down upon them.

Because their god appeared to "die" every December as the sun dipped lower in the skies, they said Mithra was a "dying, rising Saviour." The first time, in its yearly cycle, that the sun would appear to be getting higher in the sky was **December 25**. So they had a great celebration on that day in honor of the birth of their Saviour. **They also had sunrise worship services on Sunday**, when they would face toward the rising sun and pray to Mithra. **These and many other counterfeits made Mithraism very similar to Christianity.**

The special attraction of Mithraism was their Sunday worship service. This set them apart from all other religions—until compromising Christians began worshiping on that day in order to attract Mithraites to attend their services.

Because "Lord Mithra" was worshiped on Sunday, **by the third century, his worshipers were calling Sunday "the Lord's Day."** This is a known historical fact.

Christians, to excuse their own adoption of Sunday worship services, gave the flimsy excuse that John in Revelation 1:10 was referring to Sunday, even though it was obvious that this verse said nothing about that day.

By the third century, Mithraism had become the primary religion of the heathen in the Roman empire. Emperor Aurelian (A.D. 270-275), whose mother was a priestess of the Sun, made this solar cult the official religion of the empire. His biographer, Flavius Vopiscus, said that **the priests of the Temple of the Sun at Rome were called** *pontiffs.* **They were priests of their dying-rising saviour**, Mithra, **and were called** *vicegerents* in religious matters. In order to learn the will of Mithra, the people had to consult his priests.

"Sun worship was one of the oldest components of the Roman religion."—*Gaston H. Halsberge, The Cult of Sol Invictus, 1972, p. 26.*

ENTER CONSTANTINE

An extremely important series of events occurred when Constantine I became emperor.

The previous emperor, Diocletian, had appointed four generals to become co-rulers in different parts of the empire. When he retired in A.D. 305, while some co-rulers abdicated, others fought battles to see who would gain control of the empire.

Fighting continued on and off for years, but Constantine became the victor. The crucial battle occurred just north of Rome in October 312, at the Battle of Mulvian Bridge.

While some of the emperors before him had persecuted the Christians, Constantine shrewdly recognized that desperate measures were needed in order to strengthen the empire against the increasing invasions of heathen tribes from the north. —He decided that combining the leading religions of the empire into one would greatly strengthen the nation.

By this time, there were only two powerful religions remaining: Mithraism and Christianity. **It is known that Constantine worked closely with Sylvester I, the bishop of the Christian church at Rome, who strongly encouraged him in his objective to combine the two religions into one.**

The year after his victory in 312, by a special edict, **Constantine gave Christianity full legal equality with every other religion in the empire**—something it had never had before. More favors to the church soon followed. **The church had entered the courts of kings, and full apostasy was to follow.**

Yet Constantine remained a heathen, retaining the pagan title of *Pontifex Maximus,* **which meant that he was the supreme priest of the pagan religion of Mithraism.** The title meant that he was the greatest pontiff (Mithraic chieftain) among all the pontiffs of the Sun god. Although his mother, Helena, was a Christian, **Constantine continued to favor his father's god, Mithra.** In his court, he consulted pagan philosophers, as well as Christian ones.

"He continued to use vague monotheistic language that any pagan could accept . . he restored pagan temples, and ordered the taking of the *auspices* by examining livers of freshly killed animals. He used pagan as well as Christian rites in dedicating Constantinople. He used pagan magic formulas to protect crops and heal disease."—*Will Durant, Caesar and Christ, p. 656.*

After showing such favor to the Christians, **Constantine issued an order for his soldiers to stand, facing the rising sun, and pray with their eyes closed to Mithra** for several minutes every morning. Worshiping the the sun as it arose in the east every morning was a regular practice of the Mithrites.

In an unreasonable rage, later in life Constantine had his son killed, because he feared the young man might become a rival. Constantine was definitely not a Christian.

Yet, in spite of this mixing of Christianity and paganism in the mind of Constantine,—*he became the most influential determinant of Christianity for more than a thousand years!*

THE SUNDAY LAW

Constantine's most powerful "contribution" to Christianity was his Sunday Law, which placed the Roman bishop in a position of leadership over the other Christian churches.

"**Unquestionably the first law, either ecclesiastical or civil, by which the Sabbatical observance of that day is known to have been ordained, is the edict of Constantine, A.D. 321.**"—*Chamber's Encyclopedia, article, "Sabbath."*

Bishop Sylvester (314-337) of Rome, and his counselor Eusebius, recognized that the key to control by the Roman pastor, over all the other Christian churches of the Empire, depended on requiring Sunday worship. This would solidify the pagan innovations which the Roman church had been trying to establish everywhere for decades.

It was by their direct request that Constantine enacted his Sunday laws. He was very willing to do this; for **Constantine saw in it a way to unify the Empire under a single religion**, believing that religious unity would help the Empire resist the increasing attacks from the barbarian hordes in the north. The wording of the law was carefully selected, so that both Mithraists and Christians could accept it and come together.

Sylvester heartily cooperated with him in bringing the Mithraists into the Christian churches.

"**Sylvester . . decreed that the rest of the Sabbath should be transferred rather to the**

Lord's day, in order that on that day we should rest from worldly works."—*Rabanus Maurus, De Clericorum Institutione (Concerning the Instruction of the Clergymen), Book 2, Chapter 46.*

Here is the first Sunday law in history, a legal enactment by Constantine I (reigned 306-337):

"**On the Venerable Day of the Sun** ["*Venerable die Solis*"—the sacred day of the Sun] let the magistrates and people residing in cities rest, and let all workshops be closed. In the country, however, persons engaged in agriculture may freely and lawfully continue their pursuits; because it often happens that another day is not so suitable for grain-sowing or for vine-planting; lest by neglecting the proper moment for such operations the bounty of heaven should by lost— given the 7th day of March [A.D. 321], Crispus and Constantine being consuls each of them for the second time."—*The First Sunday Law of Constantine I, in "Codex Justianianus," lib. 3, tit. 12,3; trans. in Phillip Schaff, History of the Christian Church, Vol. 3, p. 380.*

In this decree, Constantine was careful to use wording which would be acceptable to both Christians and Mithraists. (In one of his later five Sunday laws, Constantine required that farmers keep Sunday sacred also.)

"**The retention of the old pagan name 'Dies Solis'** [Day of the Sun], **or 'Sunday,' for the weekly Christian festival, is, in great measure, owing to the union of pagan and Christian sentiment with which the first day of the week was recommended by Constantine to his subjects**, pagan and Christian alike, as the 'venerable day of the sun' . . **It was his mode of harmonizing the discordant religions of the empire under one common institution.**"—*Arthur P. Stanley, Lectures on the History of the Eastern Church, p. 184.*

"**Constantine labored at this time untiringly to unite the worshipers of the old and the new into one religion.** All his laws and contrivances are aimed at promoting this amalgamation to melt together a purified heathenism and a moderated Christianity . . **Of all his blending and melting together of Christianity and heathenism, none is more easy to see through than this making of his Sunday law**: The Christians worshiped their Christ, the heathen their sun-god [so they should now be combined]."—*H.G. Heggtveit, Illustreret Kirkehistorie (Illustrated History of the Church), 1895, p. 202.*

This first of Constantine's six Sunday laws was extremely important in church history!

"**This [Constantine's Sunday decree of March 321] is the 'parent' Sunday law** making it a day of rest and release from labor. For from that time to the present there have been decrees about the observance of Sunday which have profoundly influenced European and American society. **When the Church became a part of State under the Christian emperors, Sunday observance was enforced by civil statutes, and later when the Empire was past, the Church in the hands of the papacy enforced it by ecclesiastical and also by civil enactments.**"—*Walter W. Hyde, Paganism to Christianity in the Roman Empire, 1946, p. 261.*

"Constantine's decree marked the beginning of a long, though intermittent, series of imperial decrees in support of Sunday rest."—*Vincent J. Kelly, Forbidden Sunday and Feast-Day Occupations, 1943, p. 29.*

COMING NEXT—It is an astounding fact that leading Catholic and Protestant churchmen and writers openly admit that there is no Biblical authority for the attempted change of the Sabbath to Sunday. A number of their statements reveal that they clearly understand this historical fact, and freely admit it, but they seem uninterested to returning to God's holy day.

Chapter Twenty-Two

Church Authorities Speak Up
Important Catholics and Protestants

It was in the early part of the 20th century. Workmen were digging in the basement of an ancient building in Jerusalem. This building, which runs alongside the *Via Dolorosa*, said to be the street on which Jesus walked on His way to Calvary, had been built above and around the arch that once rang with the words of Pilate: *"Behold the Man!"*

Over the centuries, since the time of Christ, the surface level had gradually risen higher as new buildings were erected on top of the ruins of older ones.

The workmen were working in a subbasement,—when all at once they came upon the original pavement of the Lithostrotos. When the building was strengthened so nothing would collapse, and the floor was cleared,—there were the stones, *the very stones* upon which our Saviour stood as He was condemned by Pilate!

Jesus endured the agonizing torture of this entire experience, from Gethsemane, through the court trials, and the agonizing torture of the cross;

all this so He could vindicate His Father's moral law and make it possible for you and me to be forgiven and, by His enabling grace, obey that law—so we can become like Him.

How very thankful we can be for the love of God, as revealed in Jesus Christ His Son!

Yet in later centuries, professed Christians dared to change God's moral code, and require men and women to keep their man-made rites and ceremonies, adopted from paganism, on pain of death.

In this chapter, we will discover that, *without hesitation, both Catholic and Protestant authorities clearly state* that the attempted change of the Bible Sabbath to Sunday was actually made.

Frankly admitting that the Bible recognizes only one Sabbath, they claim that the church had the right and the power to change God's true Sabbath to another day of the week. —**The church organization which did the changing has repeatedly said that this act is the mark of its power and authority** in religious matters.

ROMAN CATHOLIC STATEMENTS

Cardinal Gibbons (1834-1921), who was (until his death) considered the highest Catholic authority in America, said this:

"The Catholic Church by its own infallible authority created Sunday a holy day to take the place of the Sabbath of the old law."—*Kansas City Catholic, February 9, 1893.*

"Now the [Catholic] Church . . instituted, by God's authority, Sunday as the day of worship. The same Church, by the same divine authority, taught the doctrine of Purgatory . . **We have, therefore, the same authority for Purgatory as we have for Sunday.**"—*Martin J. Scott, Things Catholics Are Asked About, 1927, p. 236.*

"**Sunday is a Catholic institution, and its claim to observance can be defended only on Catholic principles** . . From beginning to end of Scripture there is not a single passage that warrants the transfer of weekly public worship from the last day of the week to the first."—*Catholic Press, Sydney, Australia, August 1900.*

"**Protestantism, in discarding the authority of the [Roman Catholic] Church, has no good reason for its Sunday theory**, and ought logically to keep Saturday as the Sabbath."—*John Gilmary Shea, in the American Catholic Quarterly Review, January 1883.*

"**They [Protestants] deem it their duty to keep the Sunday holy. Why?—Because the Catholic Church tells them to do so.** They have no other reason."—*The Ecclesiastical Review [RC], February 1914, Vol. 50, No. 2, p. 236.*

"It is well to remind the Presbyterians, Baptists, Methodists, and all other Christians that the Bible does not support them anywhere in their observance of Sunday. **Sunday is an institution of the Roman Catholic Church, and those who observe the day observe a commandment of the Catholic Church.**"—*Priest Brady, in an address, reported in the Elizabeth, N.J. News of March 18, 1903.*

"*Ques.*—**Have you any other way of proving that the [Catholic] Church has power** to institute festivals of precept [to command holy days]?

"*Ans.*—**Had she not such power, she could not have done that in which all modern religionists agree with her**: She could not have substituted the observance of Sunday, the first day of the week, for the observance of Saturday, the seventh day, a change for which there is no Scriptural authority."—*Stephen Keenan, Doctrinal Catechism, p. 176.*

"Reason and common sense demand the acceptance of one or the other of these two alternatives: **either Protestantism and the keeping holy of Saturday or Catholicity and the keeping holy of Sunday**. Compromise is impossible."—*The Catholic Mirror, December 23, 1893.*

"God simply gave His [Catholic] Church the power to set aside whatever day or days she would deem suitable as Holy Days. **The Church chose Sunday, the first day of the week**, and in the course of time added other days, as holy days."—*Vincent J. Kelly, Forbidden Sunday and Feast-Day Occupations, p. 2.*

"Protestants . . accept Sunday rather than Saturday as the day for public worship after the Catholic Church made the change . . But the Protestant mind does not seem to realize that **in accepting the Bible, in observing the Sunday, they are accepting the authority of the spokesman for the church, the Pope.**"—*Our Sunday Visitor, February 5, 1950.*

"**Not the Creator of Universe, in Genesis 2:1-3,—but the Catholic Church** can claim the honor of having granted man a pause to his work every seven days."—*S.C. Mosna, Storia della Domenica, 1969, pp. 366-367.*

"If Protestants would follow the Bible, they should worship God on the Sabbath Day. **In keeping the Sunday they are following a law of the Catholic Church.**"—*Albert Smith, Chancellor of the Archdiocese of Baltimore, replying for the Cardinal, in a letter dated February 10, 1920.*

"We define that the Holy Apostolic See (the Vatican) and **the Roman Pontiff hold the primacy over the whole world.**"—*A Decree of the Council of Trent, quoted in Philippe Labbe and*

Gabriel Cossart, "The Most Holy Councils," Col. 1167.

"It was the Catholic Church which, by the authority of Jesus Christ, has transferred this rest [from the Bible Sabbath] to the Sunday . . Thus **the observance of Sunday by the Protestants is an homage they pay, in spite of themselves, to the authority of the [Catholic] Church.**"—*Monsignor Louis Segur, Plain Talk about the Protestantism of Today, p. 213.*

"We observe Sunday instead of Saturday because **the Catholic Church transferred the solemnity from Saturday to Sunday.**"—*Peter Geiermann, CSSR, A Doctrinal Catechism, 1957 edition, p. 50.*

"We Catholics, then, have precisely the same authority for keeping Sunday holy instead of Saturday as we have for every other article of our creed, namely, the authority of the Church . . **whereas you who are Protestants have really no authority for it whatever; for there is no authority for it [Sunday sacredness] in the Bible**, and you will not allow that there can be authority for it anywhere else."—*The Brotherhood of St. Paul, "The Clifton tracts," Volume 4, tract 4, p. 15.*

"**The Church changed the observance of the Sabbath to Sunday** by right of the divine, infallible authority given to her by her founder, Jesus Christ. The Protestant, claiming the Bible to be the only guide of faith, has no warrant for observing Sunday. In this matter the Seventh-day Adventist is the only consistent Protestant."—*The Catholic Universe Bulletin, August 14, 1942, p. 4.*

"**Of course, the Catholic Church claims that the change was her act**; it could not have been otherwise, as none in those days would have dreamed of doing anything in matters spiritual and ecclesiastical and religious without her. ***And the act is a MARK of her ecclesiastical power and authority in religious matters***."—*Cardinal Gibbons, letter dated July 7, 1895.*

PROTESTANT STATEMENTS

The Bible is your only safe guide. Jesus can help you obey it. Trust God's Word more than man's traditions. **Here are a few of many statements by Protestant leaders agreeing that Sunday is not in the Bible:**

BAPTIST: "There was and is a command to keep holy the Sabbath day, but that Sabbath day was not Sunday. It will however be readily said, and with some show of triumph, that the Sabbath was transferred from the seventh to the first day of the week, with all its duties, privileges and sanctions. Earnestly desiring information

on this subject, which I have studied for many years, I ask, **where can the record of such a transaction be found? Not in the New Testament—absolutely not.** There is no Scriptural evidence of the change of the Sabbath institution from the seventh to the first day of the week."—*Dr. E.T. Hiscox, author of the Baptist Manual.*

Congregationalist: "It is quite clear that however rigidly or devotedly we may spend Sunday, **we are not keeping the Sabbath . . The Sabbath was founded on a specific divine command. We can plead no such command for the observance of Sunday** . . There is not a single line in the New Testament to suggest that we incur any penalty by violating the supposed sanctity of Sunday."—*Dr. R.W. Dale, The Ten Commandments, pp. 106-107.*

Protestant Episcopal: "The day is now changed from the seventh to the first day . . but as **we meet with no Scriptural direction for the change**, we may conclude it was done by the authority of the church."—*The Protestant Episcopal Explanation of the Catechism.*

Baptist: "The Scriptures nowhere call the first day of the week the Sabbath . . There is no Scriptural authority for so doing, nor of course, any Scriptural obligation."—*The Watchman.*

Presbyterian: "There is no word, no hint in the New Testament about abstaining from work on Sunday. The observance of Ash Wednesday, or Lent, stands exactly on the same footing as the observance of Sunday. **Into the rest of Sunday no Divine Law enters.**"—*Canon Eyton, Ten Commandments.*

Anglican: "And where are we told in the Scriptures that we are to keep the first day at all? **We are commanded to keep the seventh; but we are nowhere commanded to keep the first day.**"—*Isaac Williams, Plain Sermons on the Catechism, pp. 334, 336.*

Methodist: "It is true that there is no positive command for infant baptism. **Nor is there any for keeping holy the first day of the week.** Many believe that Christ changed the Sabbath. But, from His own words, we see that He came for no such purpose. **Those who believe that Jesus changed the Sabbath base it only on a supposition.**"—*Amos Binney, Theological Compendium, pp. 180-181.*

Episcopalian: "We have made the change from the seventh to the first day, from Saturday to Sunday, on the authority of the one holy, catholic, apostolic church of Christ."—*Bishop Seymour, Why We Keep Sunday.*

Southern Baptist: "The sacred name of the

seventh day is Sabbath. This fact is too clear to require argument [Exodus 20:10, quoted] . . On this point the plain teaching of the Word has been admitted in all ages . . **Not once did the disciples apply the Sabbath law to the first day of the week,**—that folly was left for a later age, nor did they pretend that the first day supplanted the seventh."—*Joseph Judson Taylor, The Sabbatic Question, pp. 14-17, 41.*

American Congregationalist: "**The current notion, that Christ and His apostles authoritatively substituted the first day for the seventh, is absolutely without any authority in the New Testament.**"—*Dr. Lyman Abbot, Christian Union, June 26, 1890.*

Christian Church: "**Now there is no testimony in all the oracles of heaven that the Sabbath is changed**, or that the Lord's Day came in the room of it."—*Alexander Campbell, Reporter, October 8, 1921.*

Disciples of Christ: "**There is no direct Scriptural authority for designating the first day 'the Lord's Day.'** "—*Dr. D.H. Lucas, Christian Oracle, January 23, 1890.*

Baptist: "To me it seems unaccountable that **Jesus,** during three years' discussion with His disciples, often conversing upon the Sabbath question, discussing it in some of its various aspects, freeing it from its false [Jewish traditional] glosses, **never alluded to any transference of the day**; also, no such thing was intimated. Nor, so far as we know, did the Spirit, which was given to bring to their remembrance all things whatsoever that He had said unto them, deal with this question. **Nor yet did the inspired apostles**, in preaching the gospel, founding churches, counseling and instructing those founded, discuss or approach the subject.

"**Of course I quite well know that Sunday did come into use in early Christian history** as a religious day, as we learn from the Christian Fathers and other sources. **But what a pity that it comes branded with the mark of paganism, and christened with the name of the sun god, then adopted and sanctified by the Papal apostasy, and bequeathed as a sacred legacy to Protestantism!**"—*Dr. E.T. Hiscox, report of his sermon at the Baptist Ministers' Convention, in the New York Examiner, November 16, 1893.*

From the cornerstone of the Lutheran faith, the *Augsburg Confession*, are these words written in 1530. They are no less true today:

"They [the Catholics] allege **the change of the Sabbath into the Lord's Day, contrary, as it seemeth to the Decalogue**; and they have no example more in their mouths than the change of the Sabbath. **They will needs have the Church's power to be very great, because it hath dispensed with a precept of the Decalogue.**"—*Augsburg Confession, quoted in Philip Schaff, The Creeds of Christendom, Vol. 3, p. 64.*

IN CONCLUSION

The great question is, What does the Bible say? If the Bible is not a safe guide, then we are all lost. There is no other anchor for the soul. Upon this old Book, which has weathered the storms of the ages, we must take our stand.

The promise is given that the voice of Jesus will call to the keepers of the gates of Paradise, **"Open ye the gates, that the righteous nation which keepeth the truth may enter in"** (Isaiah 26:2).

God will admit everyone through those gates who is repentant and humble enough to accept Him as their God and their Lord; it matters not whether he be Jew or Gentile, atheist or professed Christian. Whoever is willing to fall at the feet of Jesus and confess his sins, and in Christ's enabling strength resist temptation and obey God's moral code of Ten Commandments will receive fulfillment of the promises.

"**The sons of the stranger, that join themselves to the Lord**, to serve Him, and to love the name of the Lord, to be His servants, **every one that keepeth the Sabbath from polluting it**, and taketh hold of My covenant; even them will I bring to My holy mountain."—*Isaiah 56:6-7.*

"**Blessed are they that do His commandments, that they may have right to the tree of life, and may enter in through the gates into the city.**"—*Revelation 22:14.*

Turning from the statements of men, let us take our stand on the Word of God:

"**Know ye not, that to whom ye yield yourselves servants to obey, his servants ye are to whom ye obey**; whether of sin unto death, or of obedience unto righteousness?"—*Romans 6:16.*

"**Thou shalt worship the Lord thy God, and Him only shalt thou serve**."—*Matthew 4:10.*

"And Elijah came unto all the people, and said, **How long halt ye between two opinions? if the Lord be God, follow Him**: but if Baal, then follow him. And the people answered him not a word."—*1 Kings 18:21.*

God is calling us back to obedience to His holy, moral law. Through the enabling grace of Christ, the Ten Commandments can be obeyed by each of us. It must govern our lives.

"**Long should pause the erring hand of man before it dares to chip away with the chisel of human reasonings one single word graven on the enduring tables of the Ten Commandments by the hand of the infinite God.** What is proposed? To make an erasure in a heaven-born code; to expunge one article from the recorded will of the Eternal! Is the eternal tablet of His law to be defaced by a creature's hand? He who proposes such an act should fortify himself by reasons as holy as God and as mighty as His power."—*George Elliot, The Abiding Sabbath (prize essay), part 2, p. 128, American Tract Society, 1884.*

COMING NEXT—Several questions still remain, and they will be answered next. A specially important one is how we should keep the Bible Sabbath today. This is a very practical question, which you will want to have answered.

Chapter Twenty-Three

Questions Answered

The Bible Has the Answers

After sailing the ship, *Bounty* to Tahiti, Captain Bligh spent a number of months there collecting breadfruit plants, to be transplanted to the British colonies in the Caribbean islands.

But shortly after the ship weighed anchor and set sail for England, the most famous mutiny in British naval history occurred.

Captain Bligh, with eighteen of his men, were set adrift,—and the ship sailed back to Tahiti.

Eventually, a few of the mutineers, and some Tahitian women, sailed with Fletcher Christian east to a destination known only by Fletcher—an island that had been discovered and marked on the charts about ten years earlier—and then forgotten.

Landing at Pitcairn Island, the mutineers hauled everything onto the land and then burned the ship. They were not discovered for years.

But, although quickly forgotten, something special was also taken from the ship—a Bible.

The early days of Pitcairn were a story of drunken revelry and murder. **At last, only one of the mutineers—John Adams—was left.** Surrounded by the children of the fugitives, himself the only link between those young people and a frightful future, Adams felt a solemn responsibility.

Turning to that Bible, which he found in the bottom of a sea chest, he began reading it,—and then, heartbroken at his former life, dedicated his life to Christ. As the undisputed leader of the small colony, he now began teaching the children and women from the Bible. Then they built a church and a school.

Every person on the island became a Christian. Decades later, the Sabbath truth was discovered and everyone became a Sabbathkeeper.

Such is the transforming power of the Book of books. You and I may also experience that power in our lives, as we study it and obey it.

We earlier learned that **the Bible Sabbath originated at the end of Creation Week, when our world was made.** At that time, God established the weekly cycle and set aside the seventh day as a sacred rest day which His obedient people on earth should always keep. He placed this command in the heart of the Ten Commandment law; and, throughout the history of this world, **men and women have repeatedly been tested to see if they will obey His moral law. This includes this special requirement, the Seventh-day Sabbath, as a test of their loyalty.**

We learned that **this Sabbath was never revoked or changed**, that **it is the "Lord's day,"** that **it was faithfully kept by Jesus and His disciples**, and that **it will be kept holy in the last days—and even in the New Earth.**

We learned that **the weekly cycle has never changed** and **the seventh day of each week today is the same Sabbath as in the time of Moses and Christ.**

We learned that the papacy tried to change the Sabbath to Sunday; but we also discovered the startling fact that **the only basis for the Catholic Church's authority and the primacy of its rites and ceremonies ("Tradition") as more sacred and requiring more obedience than the Bible is the fact that the command of God which they dared to change—is obeyed by Protestants!** *This means that if all Protestants would keep the Bible Sabbath, the papacy would lose the basis of its church authority!* Its authority to do what it does is based, not on a command of God, but on the permission of men!

Just now, we want to consider a few other questions which could be asked about the Bible Sabbath.

THE TWO COVENANTS

Question: "If we are living under the new covenant, do we need to keep the Bible Sabbath?"

A covenant is a contract. When we accept Christ as our Saviour, we enter into a contract, or covenant, with Him. The Bible mentions two covenants; one is called "old," and the other "new."

"In that He saith, A new covenant, He hath made the first old. Now that which decayeth and waxeth old is ready to vanish away." "For if that first covenant had been faultless, then should no place have been sought for the second."—*Hebrews 8:13, 7.*

The "old covenant" is the name for a covenant based on the terms and promises stated by the people. It was flawed because they attempted to obey God in their own strength, and utterly failed.

The "new covenant," which was also the original covenant, and is also called the "everlasting covenant," is based on God's requirements and promises. Obedience on our part to the Ten Commandments is the basis of this covenant. God promises eternal life to those who will obey the covenant. They will receive the covenant promises. But, as part of this covenant, Christ provides them with all the grace needed to fulfill their part of the contract.

A special example of the "old covenant" experience occurred when, after hearing the Ten Commandments at Mount Sinai and promising to obey God, the people did not do so—but instead made a golden calf shortly afterward.

"Now therefore, if ye will obey My voice indeed, and keep My covenant, then ye shall be a peculiar treasure unto Me above all people."—*Exodus 19:5.*

"And all the people answered together, and said, All that the Lord hath spoken we will do."—*Exodus 19:8.*

The ten commandments, which was the basis of this contract, is therefore called "the covenant."

"And He declared unto you His covenant, which He commanded you to perform, even ten commandments; and He wrote them upon two tables of stone."—*Deuteronomy 4:13.*

Less than 40 days after making this covenant, the people demanded that an idol be made which they could worship. They had abandoned their covenant with God.

"When the people saw that Moses delayed to come down out of the mount, the people gathered themselves together unto Aaron, and said unto him, **Up, make us gods**, which shall go before us."—*Exodus 32:1.*

The new covenant is different: It is based on God's abundant promises and man's continued, willing submission and obedience.

"He [Christ] is the mediator of a better covenant, which was established upon better promises."—*Hebrews 8:6.*

Under the new covenant, God writes His law on our hearts. That means that we voluntarily submit our lives to obeying His law, through the enabling grace of Christ.

"But this shall be the covenant that I will make with the house of Israel: After those days, saith the Lord, I will put My law in their inward parts, and write it in their hearts; and will be their God, and they shall be My people."—*Jeremiah 31:33.*

The fault of the old covenant was with the people, not with God. **Here is a nice summary of both covenants:**

"For if that first covenant had been faultless, then should no place have been sought for the second. **For finding fault with them**, He saith, Behold, the days come, saith the Lord, when I will make a new covenant with the house of Israel and with the house of Judah: Not according to the covenant that I made with their fathers in the day when I took them by the hand to lead them out of the land of Egypt; **because they continued not in My covenant**, and I regarded them not, saith the Lord.

"**For this is the covenant that I will make** with the house of Israel after those days, saith the Lord; **I will put My laws into their mind, and write them in their hearts**: and I will be to them a God, and they shall be to Me a people."—*Hebrews 8:7-10.*

THE END OF THE LAW

Question: "Paul says that the law has ended, so why should we keep it now?"

The moral law identifies sin. This is the purpose of the law.

"Nay, **I had not known sin, but by the law . . for by the law is the knowledge of sin**."—*Romans 7:7; 3:20.*

"What shall we say then? Is the law sin? God forbid. Nay, **I had not known sin, but by the law**: for I had not known lust, except the law had said, Thou shalt not covet."—*Romans 7:7.*

That truth helps us understand a puzzling verse. In one passage, **Paul says that Christ is the "end of the law."**

"For Christ is the end of the law for righteousness to every one that believeth."—*Romans 10:4.*

Well, that surely does not agree with dozens, even hundreds of other passages of Scripture! Looking closer, we ask, What does Paul mean when he uses the word, "end"? Checking on this, we discover that **Paul said it correctly, but that the KJV translated it by an old English expression which, in 1611, could mean something quite different** than the way it is commonly used today. The Greek word for "end" is *telos*. **Paul actually said, "For Christ is the goal or aim of the law."**

Because the law points out sin, it leads the sinner to Christ who alone can enable him to obey it. By beholding and accepting Christ, the sinner may become a converted, humble, obedient child of God.

Here are three other Bible passages where aim or goal is translated "end" in the KJV:

"Whom having not seen, ye love; in whom, though now ye see Him not, yet believing, ye rejoice with joy unspeakable and full of glory: **Receiving the end of your faith, even the salvation of your souls**."—*1 Peter 1:8-9.*

"Now **the end of the commandment is charity** out of a pure heart, and of a good conscience, and of faith unfeigned."—*1 Timothy 1:5.*

W
A
Y

"Behold, we count them happy which endure. Ye have heard of the patience of Job, **and have seen the end of the Lord**; that the Lord is very pitiful, and of tender mercy."—*James 5:11.*

When a minister visited a prison quarry, one of the prisoners told him this: "Parson, do you see these stones? They're just like the ten commandments; you can keep on breaking 'em, but you can't get rid of them."

The moral law of God is the simplest of all tests in separating the true from the false: "To the law and to the testimony: if they speak not according to this Word, it is because there is no light in them" *(Isaiah 8:20).* That is why they will be the standard in the Judgment. **Who is that man who dares to judge the law that is the judge of truth, and by which law he himself must be judged?**

CHURCH FATHERS AND SUNDAY

Question: "The early church fathers gave us Sunday. They lived closer to the time of the Apostles than we do, so should we keep Sunday also?"

It is true that, by the third century after the Bible ended, in Alexandria and Rome the Christians were keeping Sunday, and prior to that, **by A.D. 200, three or four compromising Christian writers (called "early church fathers") wrote letters, containing a mixture of pagan and Christian sentiments, and recommended Sundaykeeping.**

But we must obey the commands of God, as given in the Bible, not the commands of professed Christians, whenever they might live.

After the time of the Apostles, there arose such men as Clement of Alexandria, Justin Martyr, Irenaeus, and Tertullian who urged the keeping of Sunday by Christians. Shall we build our faith on the writings of such men? **Shall tradition take the place of Holy Scripture?**

(Tertullian was the first authentic "church father" who advocated Sundaykeeping for Christians. Here are several other heathen practices which he recommended to the church: offerings for the dead as birthday honors; prohibiting fasting on Sunday, "the Lord's Day"; the keeping of Easter and Whitsunday; and making the sign of the cross continually throughout the day.)

Here is what knowledgeable historians, who have studied those writings, tell us about these so-called "church fathers"—both early and later:

"**There are but few of them whose pages are not rife with errors**—errors of method, errors of fact, errors of history, of grammar, and even of doctrine. This is the simple truth about them."—*Archdeacon Farrar, History of Interpretation, pp. 162-163.*

"When God's Word is by the Fathers ex-pounded, construed, and glossed, then, in my judgment, **it is even as when one strains milk through a coal-sack, which must needs spoil and make the milk black.** God's Word of itself is pure, clean, bright and clear; but, through the doctrines, books, and writings of the Fathers, it is darkened, falsified, and spoiled."—*Martin Luther, quoted in The Table-Talk of Martin Luther, Hazlitt translation, p. 281.*

Tertullian, who lived west of Alexandria, was one of the few professed Christian writers before A.D. 300 who advocated the keeping of Sunday. Primarily writing in A.D. 196-220, he **wrote careful instructions for how Christians should keep holy the pagan worship day, Sunday**, instead of the Bible Sabbath. Here is part of his instruction:

"At every forward step and movement, at every going in and out, when we put on our clothes and shoes, when we bathe, when we sit at table, when we light the lamps, on couch, on seat, in all the ordinary actions of daily life, we trace upon the forehead the sign of the cross."—*Collected Writings of Tertullian.*

Such theories are not Biblical!

Alexandria, Egypt was the center of apostate Christianity in the early centuries, which supplied the bishop of Rome with many of the pagan rites and ceremonies which he tried to command the other churches to do.

The other earliest, bold advocate of Sunday-keeping was Clement of Alexandria, who (from A.D. 190 to 215) was head of the most apostate Christian seminary in existence at that time.

Clement tried to unite the allegorical errors of Plato's *Republic* with the pagan worship rites of Mithra and Isis—and teach the resulting heresies to Christians. His writings were a cesspool of error. Here are two of Clement's most important statements about Sundaykeeping. As you read them, keep in mind that *he was the first, influential, modernizing Christian to urge the keeping of Sunday.* Here is his "proof" that the sacredness of the seventh day has passed to the eighth day, or Sunday.

"And the Lord's day Plato prophetically speaks of in the tenth book of the *Republic*, in these words, 'And when seven days have passed to each of them in the meadow, on the eighth day they are to set out and arrive in four.' "—*Clement, Miscellanies, Book 5, Chapter 14.*

"And the fourth word [in the Ten Commandments] is that which intimates that the world was created by God, and that He gave us the seventh day as a rest . . The seventh day, therefore, is proclaimed a rest—abstraction from ills—preparing for the primal day, our true rest; which, in truth, is the first creation of light, in which all things are viewed and possessed . . The eighth may possibly turn out to be properly the seventh, and the seventh a day of work. For the creation of the world was concluded in six days . . The Pythagoreans, as I think, reckon six the perfect number. As marriage generates from male to female, so six is generated from the odd number three, which is called the masculine number, and the even number two, which is considered feminine. For twice three is six."—*Clement, Miscellanies, Book, Chapter 16.*

Because first day sanctity is totally missing from the Bible, in order to adopt the sacred day of the Sun god into Christianity, **the church fathers invented every possible theory, declaring that the "eighth day" was superior to the seventh, because it comes after it,—while at the same time they said that the first day is superior to the seventh, because it comes before it**—and first in the week. Those men were pagan-loving philosophers, who used words and logic in irrational ways in order to confuse people who thought they were very wise.

Take God's divinely inspired book, the Bible, as your guide for life, and, clinging to Christ for help and strength, you will safely travel to your heavenly home.

"The grass withereth, the flower fadeth: because the spirit of the Lord bloweth upon it: surely the people is grass. The grass withereth, the flower fadeth: but **the Word of our God shall stand forever**."—*Isaiah 40:7-8.*

"**Forever, O Lord, Thy Word is settled in heaven**."—*Psalm 119:89.*

Countless laws have been enacted by men, but there is only one perfect law—God's law. The justice of that perfect law was met with God's own perfect sacrifice—"a Lamb without blemish and without spot."

"Not silver nor gold hath obtained my redemption, No riches of earth could have saved my poor soul; The blood of the cross is my only foundation, The death of my Saviour now maketh me whole."—*James McGray.*

THE RESURRECTON OF CHRIST

Question: "Should we not keep Sunday holy instead of the Bible Sabbath because Christ rose from the dead on the first day?"

Neither the first advent of Christ, His death, nor His resurrection in any way affected the great Sabbath rest that Christ as Creator had set up four thousand years earlier at the close of Creation Week.

We well agree that the resurrection of Christ was considered worthy of a memorial that would serve to remind men of that marvelous event. —But the Bible says that the ordinance of baptism was chosen for that purpose! It symbolizes *both* Christ's death *and* resurrection.

Genuine baptism (by immersion) is, as Paul explains in Romans 6:1-13, *a real burial and resurrection*, and very fittingly represents the burial and resurrection of Christ. But nowhere has Christ or any apostle said that the first day of the week should be kept in commemoration of the resurrection.

Not only is baptism a memorial of both the death and resurrection of Christ; **it is also a symbol of our victory over sin as we accept Christ.** Paul mentions all three here:

"Know ye not, that so many of us as were baptized into Jesus Christ were baptized into His death? **Therefore we are buried with Him by baptism into death: that like as Christ was raised up from the dead by the glory of the Father, even so we also should walk in newness of life.** For if we have been planted together in the likeness of His death, we shall be also in the likeness of His resurrection: Knowing this, that our old man is crucified with Him, that the body of sin might be destroyed, **that henceforth we should not serve sin**."—*Romans 6:3-6.*

In the above passage, five times baptism is a symbol of death; two times it is a symbol of the resurrection; and two times it symbolizes the clean, obedient life we should live thereafter.

God does not overthrow one sacred memorial of creation and proceed to set up another on its ruins. He makes no mistakes, nor does He have to alter His plans. "For I am the Lord, I change not." *Malachi 3:6.* With Him "is no variableness, neither shadow of turning" *(James 1:17).* Jesus Christ is "the same yesterday, and today, and forever" *(Hebrews 13:8).*

The only important event in the Bible which occurred on the first day—the resurrection of Christ—was seized by the early church fathers, and later by the papacy, as a reason why the Mithraic holy day should be kept by Christians. **Although Christ's resurrection was a certainty; yet it was His crucifixion which was pivotal in the plan of salvation.**

Significantly, the apostate Christians did not try to change the Sabbath to Friday, in honor of the crucifixion, for that would not have brought huge numbers of Mithraists into the church. They also adopted Easter from the worship of Ishtar, and the Queen of Heaven error from Egypt, in order to bring large numbers of other pagans into the church.

HOW JESUS KEPT THE SABBATH

Question: "Did Jesus always carefully keep the Bible Sabbath?"

Jesus was a careful Sabbathkeeper.

"As His custom was, He went into the synagogue on the Sabbath day, and stood up for to read."—*Luke 4:16.*

We also have examples of Jesus providing for basic needs on the Sabbath. In Matthew 12:1-12 is recorded the criticism by the Pharisees of Christ and His disciples. They criticized the disciples for snapping off a few heads of wheat as they walked through a field on the Sabbath.

"Behold, Thy disciples do that which is not lawful to do upon the Sabbath day."—*Matthew 12:2.*

Actually, Jewish law permitted anyone to obtain food from fields not their own; but, since they were doing this on the Sabbath, the caviling Pharisees complained. **Over the years, they had invented a multitude of senseless rules to hedge in the Sabbath, which made it difficult to keep.**

Here are a couple examples of their foolish regulations: A person could not carry a handkerchief on the Sabbath; but, if he pinned it to his clothing, he could. A person could not travel over a mile and a half on the Sabbath. But, if he took food and ate some at the end of that distance, it became his "home;" so he could then journey another mile and a half.

Such senseless theories were ignored by Christ, who kept the Sabbath in accordance with Bible principles.

You will recall that Jesus also cautioned His followers to carefully keep the Sabbath after His death, and avoid doing any worldly business or major activities on that holy day. Just prior to the predicted destruction of Jerusalem, nearly forty years later, the disciples were to try to avoid having to pack up and flee from the city on the Sabbath day.

"Pray ye that your flight be not in the winter, neither on the Sabbath day."—*Matthew 24:20.*

The Pharisees also criticized Jesus for healing a man on the Sabbath.

"And the scribes and Pharisees watched Him, whether He would heal on the Sabbath day; that they might find an accusation against Him."—*Luke 6:7.*

Jesus met their false ideas of Sabbathkeeping with these words:

"Is it lawful on the Sabbath days to do good, or to do evil? to save life, or to destroy it?"—*Luke 6:9.*

Jesus then healed the man *(verse 10)*. **Jesus insisted that it was all right to minister to basic and urgent needs of others on the Sabbath.** He also said that He was "Lord even of the Sabbath day" *(Matthew 12:8; Mark 2:28)*. As the Creator of the Sabbath *(John 1:3)*, the Sabbath was His day. **The Sabbath was made to be a blessing to man.**

"The Sabbath was made for man, and not man for the Sabbath."—*Mark 2:27.*

Throughout His life, Jesus told His disciples that they should obey the Ten Commandments, and He gave them a perfect example of obeying them Himself.

"If ye keep My commandments, ye shall abide in My love; even as I have kept My Father's commandments, and abide in His love."—*John 15:10.*

WHAT DO I DO NOW?

Question: "I did not know about the Bible Sabbath until now, what am I to do?"

God can forgive our past ignorance; but, when we learn the truth about His Sabbath commandment, He requires that we keep it holy. We will let God speak in His Word:

"**The times of this ignorance God winked at; but now commandeth all men everywhere to repent**."—*Acts 17:30.*

"**Whom therefore ye ignorantly worship, Him declare I unto you.** God that made the world and all things therein, seeing that He is Lord of heaven and earth."—*Acts 17:23-24.*

"Turn from these vanities unto the living God, which made heaven, and earth, and the sea, and all things that are therein."—*Acts 14:15.*

"**Beware that thou forget not the Lord thy God, in not keeping His commandments**, and His judgments, and His statutes, which I command thee this day."—*Deuteronomy 8:11.*

"**Hallow My Sabbaths; and they shall be a sign between Me and you**, that ye may know that I am the Lord your God."—*Ezekiel 20:20.*

You and I were once lost in sin, and God leads us out—not merely to be His adopted children, but also to keep His Bible Sabbath.

"And remember that thou wast a servant in the land of Egypt, and that the Lord thy God brought thee out thence through a mighty hand and by a stretched out arm: therefore the Lord thy God commanded thee to keep the Sabbath day."—*Deuteronomy 5:15.*

HOW TO KEEP THE BIBLE SABBATH

Question: "I want to begin keeping the true Sabbath, which God gave us. How do I do it?"

Did you know that **not only has the weekly cycle never been changed,—but it is even part of the functioning of our physical bodies!** It was H.L. Hastings, in his book *(Will the Old Book Stand?)*, who drew attention to the fact that some fevers (for instance, typhoid) run seven, fourteen, twenty-one, and twenty-eight days, changing every seventh day, as do some other diseases that, to one degree or another, result from physical exhaustion.

Many believe that man is built on this seven-day plan and therefore needs a weekly rest day, just as an eight-day clock needed to be wound up every week. **It seems there is a law of sevens inwrought in our nature**, as well as revealed in the Fourth Commandment. **God designed our bodies so they would**

need the Sabbath rest which He commanded us to take.

But, back to the question: "How should we keep the Sabbath?" Let us consider several of the principles involved in genuine Sabbathkeeping:

"Remember the Sabbath day, to keep it holy. **Six days shalt thou labour, and do all thy work.**

"But the seventh day is the Sabbath of the Lord thy God: in it thou shalt not do any work, thou, nor thy son, nor thy daughter, thy manservant, nor thy maidservant, nor thy cattle, nor thy stranger that is within thy gates.

"For in six days the Lord made heaven and earth, the sea, and all that in them is, and rested the seventh day: wherefore the Lord blessed the Sabbath day, and hallowed it."—*Exodus 20:8-11.*

The Fourth Commandment calls our attention to God's creatorship of the world. On this day, we should try to be out in nature with our families during part of the Sabbath hours.

"**The Sabbath calls our thoughts to nature, and brings us into communion with the Creator.** In the song of the bird, the sighing of the trees, and the music of the sea, we still may hear His voice who talked with Adam in Eden in the cool of the day. And **as we behold His power in nature we find comfort, for the word that created all things is that which speaks life to the soul**."—*Desire of Ages, 281-282.*

"**The value of the Sabbath as a means of education is beyond estimate.** Whatever of ours God claims from us, He returns again, enriched, transfigured, with His own glory . . The Sabbath and the family were alike instituted in Eden, and in God's purpose they are indissolubly linked together. **On this day more than on any other, it is possible for us to live the life of Eden** . .

"**God's love has set a limit to the demands of toil. Over the Sabbath He places His merciful hand.** In His own day He preserves for the family opportunity for communion with Him, with nature, and with one another. Since the Sabbath is the memorial of creative power, it is the day above all others when we should acquaint ourselves with God through His works. In the minds of the children the very thought of the Sabbath should be bound up with the beauty of natural things."—*Education, 250-251.*

We are to keep this special day holy, and in order to do this properly we need to live close to God.

"**In order to keep the Sabbath holy, men must themselves be holy.** Through faith they must become partakers of the righteousness of Christ. When the command was given to Israel, 'Remember the Sabbath day, to keep it holy,' the Lord said also to them, 'Ye shall be holy men unto Me.' Ex. 20:8; 22:31."—*Desire of Ages, 283.*

The commandment also tells us that we should spend the other six days working at various tasks, for they are not rest days.

"Six days shalt thou labour, and do all thy work."—*Exodus 20:9.*

Friday is the special day when we are to prepare for the coming Sabbath hours.

"It was the preparation, that is, the day before the Sabbath."—*Mark 15:42.*

"That day was the preparation, and the Sabbath drew on."—*Luke 23:54.*

All through the week, we are to have the Sabbath in mind, but on Friday we are to specially prepare for its holy hours. (Some do part of this preparation on Thursday, to lighten the Friday load.) **Preparations should be entirely completed before the Sabbath begins**; so we can enter it in a peaceful atmosphere, not hurriedly trying to get last things done.

All secular work should be laid aside, and our Sabbath clothes should be laid out. Unnecessary cooking should be avoided on the Sabbath. However, living in colder climates than where the Israelites lived in the desert, warming some food on the Sabbath may be needed.

We should guard the edges of the Sabbath; for, due to trees and buildings between our home and the horizon, it may be easy to not know with certainty the exact moment of sunset.

It is best not to overeat on the Sabbath, so our minds will be clear to better appreciate the spiritual blessings we can receive during these holy hours. The meals should be simple but attractive.

Before the setting of the sun, let the members of the family assemble to read God's Word, to sing and pray. At family worships, let the children take a part. Let them bring their Bibles, and each read a verse or two. Then sing a familiar song or two, followed by prayer.

Let not the precious hours of the Sabbath be wasted in bed. On Sabbath, it is well for the family to arise early, so there is no confusion and rushing about in preparation to leave for Sabbath School and church.

The morning church service only occupies a part of the day. The portion remaining to the family may be made the most sacred and precious season of all the Sabbath hours. Much of this time should be spent by parents with their children. It is not best for parents to attend Sabbath afternoon meetings, while their children run around outside loose.

If your children come to love the precious hours of the Sabbath, they will want to remain faithful when they are grown.

W
A
Y

In pleasant weather, let the parents walk with their children in the fields and groves. Repeat Bible stories, point out the things of nature which call to mind our Creator. Look for nature nuggets to share with one another, such as beautiful leaves. Tell them again about Jesus and how He lived and died for them; and how He is ministering in the Sanctuary above, so they can be empowered to live humble, obedient lives in service to Him and to others. Question them as to what they learned in Sabbath School and church.

Thus parents can make the Sabbath, as it should be, the most joyful, peaceful day of the week. They can lead their children to regard it as a delight, the holy of the Lord.

Those who do not have children, may use these hours to write missionary letters, visit the sick, give Bible studies, or hand out missionary literature from door to door.

There are times when an emergency arises, and someone urgently needs our help on the Sabbath. Helping them and drawing them closer to Jesus is worthwhile during the Sabbath hours. **If a family member is infirm, his basic needs must be cared for** during the Sabbath, as they would on other days. Basic needs must be met.

When it is necessary to be in the company of unbelievers on the Sabbath, we should keep our minds stayed upon God and commune with Him. Whenever there is opportunity, we should speak to others in regard to the truths of the Bible.

We should always be ready to relieve suffering and help those in need. But we should not talk about matters of business or engage in common, worldly conversation. At all times and in all places God requires us to prove our loyalty to Him by honoring the Sabbath.

A Sabbathkeeper cannot allow men in his employ, paid by his money, to work on the Sabbath. If he is in partnership with an unbeliever who is doing this, he must cancel the business relationship.

God will bless our efforts as we seek to be obedient to His plan, and an example and blessing to others.

"And they that shall be of thee shall build the old waste places: thou shalt raise up the foundations of many generations; **and thou shalt be called, The repairer of the breach, the restorer of paths to dwell in.**

"**If thou turn away thy foot from the Sabbath, from doing thy pleasure on My holy day; and call the Sabbath a delight**, the holy of the Lord, honourable; and shalt honour Him, not doing thine own ways, nor finding thine own pleasure, nor speaking thine own words;

"**Then shalt thou delight thyself in the Lord**; and I will cause thee to ride upon the high places of the earth, and feed thee with the heritage of Jacob thy father: for the mouth of the Lord hath spoken it."—*Isaiah 58:12-14.*

In conclusion, it should be mentioned that we live in a very difficult and evil world. It is easier to keep the Bible Sabbath when one lives in the country and everyone in the home is a Sabbathkeeper. But, unfortunately, many have to live in a city and in a home with unbelievers. **Satan will try to do whatever he can to make the life of every Sabbathkeeper difficult, in order to discourage him. But God will provide encouragement and help as you try to do the best you can.**

Please understand that **there is a vast difference between the person who has no respect for the Bible Sabbath, and the one who is trying to keep it holy.** Yes, you may encounter difficulties and discouragements. **But God knows your heart, that you love Him and are determined to be loyal to Him to the end.**

The day is coming when you will inherit a home in the better world, and all of earth's problems will be past.

As Columbus skirted the shores of the New World, he approached the mouth of the River Orinoco. It was suggested that they faced an island. But the famed explorer said, "No such river flows from an island. That mighty torrent must drain the waters of a continent."

In a similar manner, **in these studies, we have discovered the glorious truth about the Bible Sabbath. In doing so, we have encountered a massive amount of evidence showing it to be the only Sabbath we are commanded to keep today.**

Awed by our discovery, we exclaim, "Thank God for revealing this great truth to us! We accept it and make it our own. We will be loyal, obedient children of God to the end!"

"A wooden cross bore a changeless Christ, On the face of Golgotha's hill, Where He died for my sins against a changeless law, And fulfilled His Father's will."—*Author unknown.*

"I will follow Thee, my Saviour, Wheresoever my lot may be. Where Thou goest I will follow; Yes, my Lord, I'll follow Thee.

"I will follow Thee, my Saviour, Thou didst shed Thy blood for me; And though all men should forsake Thee, By Thy grace I'll follow Thee."—*J. Lawson.*

Just now, while this is fresh in your mind, is the time to make this decision. You have wanted to improve your life for a long time, and determining to prove true to Christ will bring you peace of heart.

"Were you there when they crucified my Lord? Were you there when they nailed Him to the tree? Oh, how this causes me to tremble, tremble, tremble. Were you there when they crucified my Lord?"

The explorer, Nansen, tried with a long measuring line to measure the depth of the ocean in the far North. When he could not, he wrote, "Deeper than that." He did this repeatedly, each time, making the same note in his journal, "Deeper than that."

The love of Christ for mankind is deeper far than any measuring line which we can use. It is as measureless as Calvary.

"Through all the depth of sin and loss, Drops the plummet of the cross! Never yet abyss was found, Deeper than that cross could sound."—*Whittier.*

"Could we with ink the ocean fill, And were the skies of parchment made; Were every stalk on earth a quill, And every man a scribe by trade: To write the love of God above Would drain the ocean dry, Nor could the scroll contain the whole, Though stretched from sky to sky."—*M.E. Lehman.*

COMING NEXT—The Bible presents us with important information about the work of the Holy Spirit,—and also about the sin against the Holy Spirit. What is the truth about this? We want to know this.

Chapter Twenty-Four

The Presence of the Holy Spirit
And the Unpardonable Sin

On one occasion, Charles Spurgeon, the leading British preacher of the nineteenth century, preached a dismally poor sermon. He stammered and floundered all the way through it. **That evening, he pled with God to send the Holy Spirit to help it reach hearts and bring conversions. He continued praying that prayer throughout the week.** On the next weekend, he once again delivered a powerful sermon, but he did not afterward pray that the Holy Spirit would use it to convict souls. "I'll watch the results of those two sermons," he said. **Spurgeon was later able to trace forty-one conversions from the first one, and none from the second. He was convinced anew of the power of the Holy Spirit to use us to the degree that we let Him.**

How thankful we can be for the Holy Spirit! Shortly before His crucifixion, Christ promised the gift of the Holy Spirit to guide His followeres as they studied the Scriptures, tried to minister to the needs of others, and shared the truths of how to become followers of Jesus.

"If ye love Me, keep My commandments. And

I will pray the Father, and He shall give you another Comforter, that He may abide with you forever; even the Spirit of truth; whom the world cannot receive, because it seeth Him not, neither knoweth Him: but ye know Him; for He dwelleth with you, and shall be in you."—*John 14:15-17.*

THE GIFT OF THE HOLY SPIRIT

How kind it is of Jesus who, when He was about to go back to heaven,—left the Holy Spirit to help us! "If I depart," Christ said, "I will send Him unto you" *(John 16:7).* This divine "Comforter" would bring encouragement to the faithful.

"But the Comforter, which is the Holy Ghost, whom the Father will send in My name, He shall teach you all things, and bring all things to your remembrance, whatsoever I have said unto you.

"Peace I leave with you, My peace I give unto you: not as the world giveth, give I unto you. Let not your heart be troubled, neither let it be afraid."—*John 14:26-27.*

Also called "the Spirit of truth" *(John 15:26),* **the Holy Spirit also convicts sinners that they are doing wrong.** He moves on their hearts to want to live a better life, and warns men of the coming Judgment.

"And when He is come, He will reprove the world of sin, and of righteousness, and of judgment."—*John 16:8.*

The Holy Spirit speaks *(1 Timothy 4:1);* teaches *(1 Corinthians 2:3-4);* bears witness *(Romans 8:16);* makes intercession *(Romans 8:26);* distributes gifts *(1 Corinthians 12:11);* and invites the sinner to return to God *(Revelation 22:17).*

It was the Holy Spirit who moved on the prophets to give their messages.

"For the prophecy came not in old time by the will of man: but holy men of God spake as they were moved by the Holy Ghost."—*2 Peter 1:21.*

By helping us better understand the Word of God and how to live better lives, the Holy Spirit glorifies Christ.

"Eye hath not seen, nor ear heard, neither have entered into the heart of man, the things which God hath prepared for them that love Him. But God hath revealed them unto us by His Spirit: for the Spirit searcheth all things, yea, the deep things of God."—*1 Corinthians 2:9-10.*

The Holy Spirit will strengthen those who cry to God for help in winning souls. Oh, that this may be your experience and mine!

Back in the old days, there were trolley cars on the streets of many of our cities. They were powered by electricity generated from the powerhouse, which was sent through overhead lines. The trolley car moved forward when the conductor raised the diagonal connector up to touch the overhead wire, called the trolley. *Years ago, L.G. Broughton wrote this:*

"When we would come to a cross street, I noticed that by a touch of the handle the car would almost stop, and yet would not quite stop, but just go creeping along like a snail. Then all at once the motorman would touch the handle again, the car would go very fast. Unable to understand how, if he touched the overhead wire at all, he did not get full power, I asked him.

" 'Why,' he said, 'when I squeeze this handle I open the mouth that grips the trolley. When I want to go slow, I open the mouth that contacts the trolley so it just touches it. We call this "skinning the wire." But when I touch it solidly,—I get all the power in the powerhouse.'

There are thousands of Christians who are just "skinning the wire." **They only want just enough help from God to get through the day. Yet there are those who plead earnestly for the Holy Spirit to use them to help others, that souls may be saved—and they receive power from the powerhouse.** Christ said, "All power is given unto Me in heaven and in earth. Go ye therefore, and teach all nations" *(Matthew 28:18-19).* We can have so much more help from the Holy Spirit if we will *really dedicate* our lives to God's service.

"He [the Holy Spirit] shall glorify Me: for He shall receive of Mine, and shall show it unto you. All things that the Father hath are Mine: therefore said I, that He shall take of Mine, and shall show it unto you."—*John 16:14-15.*

We dare not be like many in the world who live in such a way that the Holy Spirit cannot effectively reach their hearts.

"The Spirit of truth; whom the world cannot receive, because it seeth Him not, neither knoweth Him: but ye know Him; for He dwelleth with you, and shall be in you."—*John 14:17.*

THE SIN AGAINST THE HOLY SPIRIT

Did you ever try out a new alarm clock which, on the first morning startled you out of bed? But if you should turn it off and go back to sleep, and repeat the process day after day, you would soon sleep through its warning. The bell does not ring any less loudly. It is your relationship to the bell that has changed. So it is when we continually ignore the promptings of the Holy Spirit.

We have been given warning not to grieve the Holy Spirit, who pleads with us to come to Christ and obey His Written Word. We are told, "Quench not the Spirit" *(1 Thessalonians 5:19).* "There is a sin unto death" *(1 John 5:16).* We are told:

"And grieve not the holy Spirit of God, whereby ye are sealed unto the day of redemption."—*Ephesians 4:30.*

Alexander MacLaren describes the process by which the conscience becomes seared and hardened in words which one cannot forget:

"An old historian says about the Roman armies that marched through a country, burning and destroying every living thing: *'They make it a solitude, and they call it peace.'*

"And so do men with their consciences. They stifle them, sear them, forcibly silence them, somehow or other; *and then, when there is a dread stillness* in their hearts, broken by no voice of either approbation or blame, but doleful, like the unnatural quiet of a deserted city,—then they say it is peace!"

It is urgent, each day, that we wholeheartedly determine that we shall serve God fully. If we do not, unconsciously we will keep sliding back and erelong Satan will have us in his clutches again.

When we learn important new Bible truths, which are plainly presented,—we must obey them. Let our prayer be that of David:

"Create in me a clean heart, O God; and renew a right spirit within me. Cast me not away from Thy presence; and take not Thy Holy Spirit from me."—*Psalm 51:10-11.*

We are told, "My Spirit shall not always strive with man" *(Genesis 6:3).* We do not want to do "despite unto the Spirit of grace" *(Hebrews 10:29).* **Our probation in this world is short. None of us can know when we might die. Today, while it is today, we must make decisions that will help us press ever upward**, ever close to God in Christ.

"Wherefore as the Holy Ghost saith, Today if ye will hear His voice, Harden not your hearts."—*Hebrews 3:7-8.*

"Take heed, brethren, lest there be in any of you an evil heart of unbelief, in departing from the living God. But exhort one another daily, while it is called today; lest any of you be hardened through the deceitfulness of sin.

"For we are made partakers of Christ, if we hold the beginning of our confidence steadfast unto the end; while it is said, today if ye will hear His voice, harden not your hearts."—*Hebrews 3:12-15.*

"There is a time, we know not when, A place we know not where, That marks the destiny of men, To glory or despair.

"There is a line by us unseen, That crosses every path; The hidden boundary between, God's patience and His wrath.

"How far may we go on in sin? How long will God forbear? **Where does hope end, and where do the confines of despair begin?**

"An answer from the skies is sent; 'Ye that from God depart, **While it is called today, repent, And harden not your heart**.' "—*J. Addison Alexander.*

A continual refusal to submit to the prompt-

ings of the Holy Spirit to repent—leads to the sin against the Holy Spirit. *Here is a powerful description of the priceless treasure in Christ which we can have—and also lose:*

"**When the soul surrenders itself to Christ, a new power takes possession of the new heart.** A change is wrought which man can never accomplish for himself. It is a supernatural work, bringing a supernatural element into human nature. **The soul that is yielded to Christ becomes His own fortress, which He holds in a revolted world**, and He intends that no authority shall be known in it but His own. **A soul thus kept in possession by the heavenly agencies is impregnable to the assaults of Satan.**

"**But unless we do yield ourselves to the control of Christ, we shall be dominated by the wicked one.** We must inevitably be under the control of the one or the other of the two great powers that are contending for the supremacy of the world. It is not necessary for us deliberately to choose the service of the kingdom of darkness in order to come under its dominion. **We have only to neglect to ally ourselves with the kingdom of light.** If we do not co-operate with the heavenly agencies, Satan will take possession of the heart, and will make it his abiding place.

"The only defense against evil is the indwelling of Christ in the heart through faith in His righteousness. Unless we become vitally connected with God, we can never resist the unhallowed effects of self-love, self-indulgence, and temptation to sin. We may leave off many bad habits, for the time we may part company with Satan; but **without a vital connection with God, through the surrender of ourselves** to Him moment by moment, we shall be overcome. Without a personal acquaintance with Christ, and a continual communion, we are at the mercy of the enemy, and shall do his bidding in the end.

" 'The last state of that man is worse than the first. Even so,' said Jesus, 'shall it be also unto this wicked generation.' There are none so hardened as those who have slighted the invitation of mercy, and done despite to the Spirit of grace. **The most common manifestation of the sin against the Holy Spirit is in persistently slighting Heaven's invitation to repent.** Every step in the rejection of Christ is a step toward the rejection of salvation, and toward the sin against the Holy Spirit."—*Desire of Ages, 324.*

COMING NEXT—In the next chapter, we will view the end of the world - and a brief glimpse of the heaven for God's faithful ones that lies beyond it.

Chapter Twenty-Five

Preparing for What is Ahead

As It Was in the Days of Noah

Dionysius II (397–343 B.C.) ruled Syracuse, Sicily, from 367 B.C. to 357 B.C. and again from 346 B.C. to 344 B.C. **During his reign, Dionysius met with repeated attacks on his life and his throne.**

According to an ancient legend, one of the king's servants, Damocles, expressed a desire to sit on his throne for a day. To this, Dionysius agreed.

But the next day, while sitting there enjoying a big meal, **Damocles happened to look up and see a sharpened sword suspended above his head by a single hair.**

Jumping up, Damocles begged Dionysius, sitting nearby, that he no longer wanted to be so fortunate as to sit on the throne!

As for Dionysius, the historical reality, due to his own corrupt activities and repeated attempts by others to slay him, resulted in his being driven from his throne. At the age of only 54, he died an impoverished man in a shack in Corinth, Greece, in 343 B.C.

Several years later Greek and Roman writers, including Cicero, referred to this legend about Damocles.

The story of the sword over Damocles has come down through the ages as a striking illustration of the nearness of a deadly peril.

In the opinion of many thinking people today, the entire human race is now sitting in that chair, with total destruction suspended above by a hair, ready to fall. **A delicate trigger of chance seems to be keeping us going on, day by day**, in our ordinary round of activities, waiting, wondering, worrying.

No ordinary peril threatens mankind today. *For we are living on the edge of the end!*

Down through history, nations—and even entire civilizations—have fallen due to their refusal to acknowledge the God of heaven and to obey His Moral Law.

The first terrible example of this was the Flood which covered the earth in Noah's time. Based on the Hebrew text, it began 1,656 years after Creation Week, which, by our dating, would be about 2348 B.C.

"**And God saw that the wickedness of man was great in the earth**, and that every imagination of the thoughts of his heart was only evil continually."—*Genesis 6:5.*

"**The earth also was corrupt before God, and the earth was filled with violence.** And God looked upon the earth, and, behold, it was corrupt; for all flesh had corrupted his way upon the earth. And God said unto Noah, **The end of all flesh is come before Me; for the earth is filled with violence** through them; and, behold, I will destroy them with the earth."—*Genesis 6:11-13.*

But Noah was different. He loved God and obeyed His every command. That is what God wants us to do now.

"But Noah found grace in the eyes of the Lord." **"Thus did Noah; according to all that God commanded him**, so did he." "And the Lord said unto Noah, . . for thee have I seen righteous before Me in this generation."—*Genesis 6:8, 22; 7:1.*

For the next 120 years, Noah warned the antediluvians to return to God before it was too late. But nearly all of them ignored or ridiculed the warning. They saw him gradually building the Ark, a gigantic boat, and laughed at what he was doing. They mocked his messages, pleading with them to repent, because God was going to send a flood of waters to cover the earth. As in our own day, every form of evil was in the ascendancy. Wickedness of every type was practiced.

"But Noah stood like a rock amid the tempest. Surrounded by popular contempt and ridicule, he distinguished himself by his holy integrity and unwavering faithfulness. A power attended his words, for it was the voice of God to man through His servant. **Connection with God made him strong in the strength of infinite power**, while for one hundred and twenty years his solemn voice fell upon the ears of that generation in regard to events, which, so far as human wisdom could judge, were impossible."—*Patriarchs and Prophets, p. 96.*

Had the people repented, God would have turned away His wrath, as He afterward did when the city of Nineveh repented. But their reply to Noah's final call to repent was to plunge the more deeply into immorality.

Then one afternoon, some of the wildlife, along with Noah and his family entered the Ark—and the giant door on the front of the ship was silently closed by unseen hands.

Everyone was startled; but, as the days passed and nothing happened, the wicked grew yet more bold in their rebellion and their evil words against Noah. Their period of probation was about to expire.

And then it began.

"And it came to pass after seven days, that the waters of the flood were upon the earth . . The same day were all the fountains of the great deep broken up, and the windows of heaven were opened."—*Genesis 7:10, 11.*

On the eighth day, clouds formed in the skies. This was remarkable, for clouds had never been seen before. The earth had always been watered each evening from beneath *(Genesis 2:6).*

Then came the muttering of thunder, flashes of lightning, and soon large drops of water began falling.

"The world had never witnessed anything like this, and the hearts of men were struck with fear. **All were secretly inquiring, 'Can it be that Noah was in the right**, and that the world is doomed to destruction?'

"**Darker and darker grew the heavens, and faster came the falling rain.** The beasts were roaming about in the wildest terror, and their discordant cries seemed to moan out their own destiny and the fate of man.

"Then 'the fountains of the great deep' were 'broken up, and the windows of heaven were opened.' **Water appeared to come from the clouds in mighty cataracts.** Rivers broke away from their boundaries, and overflowed the valleys. Jets of water burst from the earth with indescribable force, throwing massive rocks hundreds of feet into the air, and these, in falling, buried themselves deep in the ground."—*Patriarchs and Prophets, p. 99.*

As the violence increased, rocks, trees, and buildings were hurled in every direction. The terror of the wicked was beyond expression. —*Noah, who had faithfully warned them all those years, was right after all!* **They should have heeded that call to repent of their sins and worship only the Creator. They should have obeyed God's Moral Law after all!**

From the highest peaks, the few who had reached them looked abroad upon a shoreless sea. And then they too were covered by the angry waters.

"The world that then was, being overflowed with water, perished. But the heavens and the earth, which are now, by the same word are kept in store, reserved unto fire against the day of judgment and perdition of ungodly men."—*2 Peter 3:6-7.*

Down through the centuries, God's method of dealing with overwhelming evil has not changed.

While the godly Shemites remained in the higher hill country, the others left the Ararat Mountains where the Ark had settled after the Flood, and settled in the Mesopotamian Valley by the Tigris and Euphrates Rivers. **On this great Plain of Babylonia, they rapidly descended into great wickedness and, in their rebellion against God, began constructing the gigantic Tower of Babel.** They wanted to form a gigantic confederacy of evil which should control the world from a single location. **But Genesis 11:1-9 tells how God destroyed their temple and gave them multiple languages, so they would scatter throughout the world.** (Many scholars believe that Genesis 10:25, which speaks of a division of the world in the days of Peleg, refers to when the Babel builders were scattered in little groups to far lands.)

We will briefly mention two other mighty kingdoms which followed—and also fell due to their immorality.

Having conquered ancient Babylonia, the shattered kingdom which remained in Mesopotamia after God's judgments destroyed the Tower of Babel (*Genesis 11:1-9*), **Assyria was one of the most feared empires in ancient history.** Nineveh, its capital, was immense. Its rulers had inherited the land of Nimrod (*Micah 5:6*), the first great empire builder, who had founded Babel (*Genesis 10:8-10*).

Nineveh today is but a vast, irregular rectangle of mounds lying near Mosul on the left bank of the Tigris River. Standing there on the central mound and looking out over the outlines of Nineveh, we can see why God called it a "great city" (*Jonah 1:2*). **The ancient walls in the distance, seven-and-a-half miles in length, encompassed 1,640 acres of buildings and streets.**

But not much is left now. Archaeologists were able to find Sennacherib's palace—containing no less than seventy-one halls, chambers, and passages whose walls, almost without exception, were originally paneled with sculptured slabs of alabaster.

You will recall how **Jonah was told to go to this politically strong and powerful seat of a vast empire, and warn it that, unless its inhabitants repented—God would permit it to be destroyed.**

"Arise, go to Nineveh, that great city, and cry against it; for their wickedness is come up before Me."—*Jonah 1:2.*

His message was a simple, clear call for repentance of sin. For a brief time the people of Nineveh accepted the message. **But later, scorning their former fears, the Ninevites plunged all the more deeply into sin.** It eventually dared to plan an attack on God's people—and a single angel from God destroyed 185,000 Assyrian soldiers in one night (*2 Kings 19; Isaiah 37; 2 Chronicles 32*).

"Against whom hast thou exalted thy voice, and lifted up thine eyes on high? even against the Holy One of Israel."—*2 Kings 19:22.*

And so it was that Assyria and its proud capital, Nineveh, was finally destroyed—blotted from the earth—in 609 B.C.

After this, arose the empire of Babylon. Would it learn the lesson that morality and obedience to God was their only safety?

Shortly after conquering Assyria, Nabopolassar, and his son Nebuchadnezzar, massively rebuilt the capital city of Babylon. Excavations a hundred years ago showed that the old, inner city lay on the east bank of the Euphrates and was about a square mile in size. In its northwest corner was the royal palace, and south of that a massive temple with its 300-foot temple tower. The splendid hanging gardens were nearby. Then Nebuchadnezzar added an immense addition to the city on the western side of the river, along with a second new palace a mile-and-a-half north of the city.

What did this king later say? And what happened?

"**Is not this great Babylon, that I have built** for the house of the kingdom by the might of my power, and **for the honour of my majesty**?"—*Daniel 4:30.*

—Nebuchadnezzar was stripped of his reasoning powers for several years, "by the decree of the watchers, and . . the holy ones" (*verse 17*).

Although he repented, his descendants did not learn the lesson; and, **in Daniel 5, we are told the story of how God's judgments fell on proud Babylon, as the forces of Cyrus poured in through the mysteriously open gates** in 538 B.C. God named Cyrus and said he would conquer Babylon—173 years before it happened (*Isaiah 44:24; 45:1-3*).

"**Thus saith the Lord to His anointed, to Cyrus**, whose right hand I have holden, to subdue nations before him; and I will loose the loins of kings, to open before him the two leaved gates; and the gates shall not be shut."—*Isaiah 45:1.*

Over the centuries, great cities and empires arose and collapsed. Immorality destroyed them all. They refused to obey God's Ten Commandment law.

But now we come down to our own time in history. God has said, "My spirit shall not always strive with man" (*Genesis 6:3*). When will God's mercy end today? How much longer will He plead with the human heart? Where is that line, beyond which even divine love cannot go?

The warnings of the faithful to return to obedience to God's Ten Commandment Law, the pleadings of God's Spirit are being rejected. Hearts are becoming harder and men and women are daily plunging deeper into sin.

A massive increase of evil has poured in upon us on a scale before unknown. The older ones among us are well-aware that the wickedness exploded into vast amounts since the mid-1960s.

Pornography, abortion, crime, violence, vile lusts, rebellion, and warfare. Gambling casinos or lotteries in nearly every state. Narcotics which stupefy and ruin minds and bodies. Bribery of government officials. Political, business and governmental corruption—all on a scale never before seen.

On and on the list goes. It keeps getting bigger and worse. Every form of evil is condoned or encouraged. The heart is sickened by the sight. We are now in the 21st century, and the sheer magnitude of wickedness threatens to overwhelm civilization.

"Now the Spirit speaketh expressly, that in the latter times some shall depart from the faith, giving heed to seducing spirits, and doctrines of

W
A
Y

devils; speaking lies in hypocrisy; having their conscience seared with a hot iron."—*1 Timothy 4:1-2.*

It is of deepest significance, that accompanying this dramatic increase of evil,—has come an ever-increasing number of natural disasters, especially since the early 1990s. The God of heaven has a line drawn, and mankind is crossing that line.

We are now in the midst of increasing judgments from heaven, in the form of volcanoes, tornadoes, hurricanes, tsunamis, fires, violent wind storms, and floods. **God is trying to wake up the world to its terrible moral crisis. He is calling on men and women to repent, but they are not listening.**

God is withdrawing His Spirit from the wicked, and **Satan is bringing these natural disasters upon the world.**

Friends, I tell you: We are rapidly nearing the end of God's merciful pleading. Our world is about to cross over the line between God's patience and His wrath.

"**There is a time, we know not when, A place we know not where, That marks the destiny of men**, To glory or despair.

"**There is a line by us unseen, That crosses every path; The hidden boundary between, God's patience and His wrath.**

"How far may we go on in sin? How long will God forbear? Where does hope end, and where begin The confines of despair?

"**An answer from the skies is sent; 'Ye that from God depart, While it is called today, repent, And harden not your heart.' "**—*J. Addison Alexander.*

The modern world, sinful, sorrowful, diseased, crime-ridden. Proud, reckless, abandoned, filled with sports and pleasure seeking, fleeing from criminals, enjoying the miseries of sin. Great cities, splattered with neon lights, filled with bars and nightclubs, discos and brothels. Course laughter mingled with shrieks of terror. **But, in the midst of it all, God says, "Repent!"**

"**And as it was in the days of Noe, so shall it be also in the days of the Son of man.** They did eat, they drank, they married wives. They were given in marriage, until the day that Noe entered into the ark, and the flood came, and destroyed them all.

"**Likewise also as it was in the days of Lot;** they did eat, they drank, they bought, they sold, they planted, they builded. But the same day that Lot went out of Sodom it rained fire and brimstone from heaven, and destroyed them all.

"Even thus shall it be in the day when the Son of man is revealed."—*Luke 17:26-30.*

Like a great bell tolling, the voice of God is heard above the intense excitement, groanings, and carnage, calling men to return to obedience to the moral principles He gave on Mount Sinai. **And the bell tolls loudest just before it is forever silenced!**

We are nearing the end of time, soon human probation will close—and then will follow the Seven Last Plagues and other judgments, predicted in Revelation 15:6 to 18:24.

"**The cities of the nations fell: and great Babylon came in remembrance before God, to give unto her the cup of the wine of the fierceness of His wrath.** And every island fled away, and the mountains were not found. And there fell upon men a great hail out of heaven, every stone about the weight of a talent: and men blasphemed God because of the plague of the hail; for the plague thereof was exceeding great."—*Revelation 16:19-21.*

Where will you and I stand when the voice of mercy is no more heard? The time is coming when never another heart shall be touched by the pleadings of the Spirit of God, and God says, "He that is unjust, let him be unjust still" *(Revelation 22:11).*

"**For when they shall say, Peace and safety; then sudden destruction cometh upon them**, as travail upon a woman with child; and they shall not escape."—*1 Thessalonians 5:3.*

As long as there is hope, we may be chastened by God for our profit *(Hebrews 12:9-11).* But it is possible for us to reach a point of hopelessness. **"He, that being often reproved hardeneth his neck, shall suddenly be destroyed, and that without remedy"** *(Proverbs 29:1).*

"**In the last days perilous times shall come.** For men shall be lovers of their own selves, covetous, boasters, proud, blasphemers, disobedient to parents, unthankful, unholy, without natural affection, trucebreakers, false accusers, incontinent, fierce, despisers of those that are good, traitors, heady, highminded, lovers of pleasures more than lovers of God; **having a form of godliness, but denying the power thereof: from such turn away.**"—*2 Timothy 3:1-5*

If, just now, you are outside the safety of Christ's care, do not blame God; blame yourself. *The door is still open, but it will not always be so.* —It may be closed early for you, if you die suddenly.

The world has had six thousand years to prove itself; that is, *it has been on probation.* The love of God and the law of God have been pitted against Satan's hate and his rebellion against God and His law. But time is now running out.

"**Behold, now is the accepted time**; behold, now is the day of salvation."—*2 Corinthians 6:2.*

When that final opportunity ends, probation

will forever close, and not only will Satan intensify the number of natural disasters,—but, in addition, God will send the **Seven Last Plagues.**

These plagues are mentioned in Revelation 16. At that time, those who choose to cling to the cross of Christ and the commandments of God will not worship the beast or his image or receive his mark. They will have the victory. Those who yield will receive the plagues.

Please note that throughout the entire description in Scripture of what happens to the wicked after probation closes—*they never repent.* Their choice has been made and at that time they share Satan's hatred of God.

After the plagues begin to fall, it will be too late for any to get right with God. The Son of God, our Mediator, will leave the Sanctuary in heaven. At that time, His priestly robes of intercession are laid aside and He prepares to return to earth in the clouds of heaven—as "King of kings and Lord of lords" *(Revelation 19:16)*—for His own.

Will God's faithful ones be protected during the falling of the plagues? God will take care of His children. His promise of protection during the falling of the plagues is found in that wonderful chapter, Psalm 91, which we should all know by heart.

"He that dwelleth in the secret place of the Most High shall abide under the shadow of the Almighty. **I will say of the Lord, He is my refuge and my fortress**: my God; in Him will I trust. Surely He shall deliver thee from the snare of the fowler, and from the noisome pestilence."—*Psalm 91:1-3.*

The above verses promise protection against the first plague *(Revelation 16:2)*. But, in addition, protection against the "burning sun" or "destruction . . at noonday" of the fourth plague *(Revelation 16:8-9)* is promised in Psalm 91:5-6. Protection against the "darkness" or "terror by night" of the fifth plague *(Revelation 16:10)* is promised in Psalm 91:5. **Even though thousands fall nearby, God promises to protect you through it all** *(Psalm 91:4-11).*

"**For in the time of trouble He shall hide me in His pavilion**: in the secret of His tabernacle shall He hide me."—*Psalm 27:5.*

As soon as Christ declares that probation has ended, His promise is that He will return soon after for the redeemed.

"**He that is unjust, let him be unjust still**: and he which is filthy, let him be filthy still: and he that is righteous, let him be righteous still: and he that is holy, let him be holy still.

"**And, behold, I come quickly**; and My reward is with Me, to give every man according as his work shall be."—*Revelation 22:11-12.*

Each one of us individually must "prepare to

meet thy God"** *(Amos 4:12).* **How do we prepare?**

By faith: "Without faith it is impossible to please Him: for **he that cometh to God must believe that He is, and that He is a rewarder of them that diligently seek Him**."—*Hebrews 11:6.*

By repentance: "Except ye repent, ye shall all likewise perish."—*Luke 13:3.*

"Repent, and be baptized every one of you."—*Acts 2:38.*

By obedience: "Not every one that saith unto Me, Lord, Lord, shall enter into the kingdom of heaven; **but he that doeth the will of My Father** which is in heaven."—*Matthew 7:21.*

"**Blessed are they that do His commandments, that they may have right to the tree of life**, and may enter in through the gates into the city."—*Revelation 22:14.*

By working with Christ: "Go ye therefore, and teach all nations . . **and, lo, I am with you alway**, even unto the end of the world."—*Matthew 28:19-20.*

To say it in another way, every morning earnestly dedicate yourself anew to God and, in a spirit of prayer, open and study His Inspired Writings. **As you go through the day**, walk closely by the side of Christ, praying as you go, and obeying His Moral Code. **Frequently** send up prayers of thankfulness and requests for guidance. **When in doubt** as to what you should do next, do the next duty. **Share the messages** of truth you have learned. **Fellowship** with God's people. **On Friday, prepare** for the Sabbath **and keep the Bible Sabbath holy.**

Surely right now is the day of salvation; **this is the time, while probation lingers, to accept Christ**—for He is still ministering in the heavenly Sanctuary in our behalf.

"Five bleeding wounds He bears, Received on Calvary; They pour effectual prayers, They strongly speak for me. 'Forgive him, O, forgive!' they cry, Nor let the contrite sinner die.' "—*Charles Wesley.*

Up there in the judgment court in heaven, Christ will plead your case if you will let Him. But that court is nearing the end of the great ledger of names. "Today if ye will hear His voice, harden not your hearts" *(Hebrews 3:15).*

Today Christ ministers for us in the Most Holy Place of the Sanctuary in heaven.

"**Which hope we have as an anchor of the soul**, both sure and steadfast, and which entereth into that within the veil."—*Hebrews 6:19.*

Let us anchor our faith up there in that heavenly Sanctuary, before our High Priest ends His mediation and comes out, and before the seven angels come down with the Seven Last Plagues.

The next great event after the falling of the plagues is the Second Coming of Christ in the clouds of heaven to call forth His sleeping saints from their graves and translate the living righteous, so they can meet Him in the air *(1 Corinthians 15:51-57; 1 Thessalonians 4:16-17)*. He will then take them to heaven for a thousand years where they will decide the cases of the wicked *(Revelation 20:4; 1 Corinthians 6:2-3)*.

After that, Christ, His faithful ones, and the Holy City will return to earth *(Revelation 21:2)*. The dead will be resurrected and marshaled into forces in an attempt to destroy the faithful in the Holy City *(Revelation 20:7-9)*.

When that has happened, everyone in the universe will fully understand that God is good, and the devil, his angels, and his followers are incorrigibly wicked. So all the wicked will be slain in the lake of fire which covers the earth's surface *(Revelation 20:10, 14-15)*. When it has ended the wicked will be totally blotted out—destroyed—for eternity *(Malachi 4:1-3; Psalm 37:20, 37-38; 145:20; 73:17-19)*. Then God will make a new world *(Revelation 21:1; Psalm 37:37-38)*, which will be entirely like the Garden of Eden for His people to enjoy forever.

Notice that it is on the surface of the earth that the wicked are burned up and destroyed. Then, after that fire, brief for many, goes out, the righteous will inherit the surface of the earth, which God will make new, as their eternal home. *So if the wicked will burn forever, the righteous could not inherit the earth!*

Here are several Bible passages which tell us that **the wicked will be blotted out before the redeemed inherit the earth:**

"For evildoers shall be cut off: but **those that wait upon the Lord, they shall inherit the earth**. For yet a little while, and **the wicked shall not be**: yea, thou shalt diligently consider his place, and it shall not be. **But the meek shall inherit the earth**; and shall delight themselves in the abundance of peace."—*Psalm 37:9-11*.

"For, behold, **the day cometh, that shall burn as an oven**; and all the proud, yea, and all that do wickedly, shall be stubble: **and the day that cometh shall burn them up**, saith the Lord of hosts, **that it shall leave them neither root nor branch.**

"But unto you that fear My name shall the Sun of righteousness arise with healing in His wings; **and ye shall go forth**, and grow up as calves of the stall. And **ye shall tread down the wicked; for they shall be ashes** under the soles of your feet in the day that I shall do this, saith the Lord of hosts."—*Malachi 4:1-3*.

Eternal life forever in the earth made new! You and I can inherit if we will remain true to our Creator! To live with Christ and holy beings forever; how glorious it will be!

One evening a little girl, walking hand in hand with her father, looked up at the brilliant shining stars in the night sky. With an enraptured sigh, she said, "Heaven must be beautiful!" When her father asked her why she thought so, she replied, " 'Cause the lights coming through the cracks in the floor are so pretty."

God's faithful children are soon to inherit "an everlasting kingdom" *(Psalm 145:13)* and, with immortal bodies *(1 Corinthians 15:53)*, have "everlasting life" *(Romans 6:22; Galatians 6:8)*.

"**And this is the promise that He hath promised us, even eternal life**."—*1 John 2:25*.

"For God so loved the world, that He gave His only begotten Son, **that whosoever believeth in Him should not perish, but have everlasting life**."—*John 3:16*.

"**And this is the record, that God hath given to us eternal life, and this life is in His Son**."—*1 John 5:11*.

"And I give unto them eternal life; **and they shall never perish**."—*John 10:28*.

"**O the beautiful hills where the saints will rest, When the Lord has made all things new**; Where we shall forget, in the smiles of God, The toils we have journeyed through."

We can hardly imagine how wonderful will be this new land.

"But as it is written, **Eye hath not seen, nor ear heard**, neither have entered into the heart of man, **the things which God hath prepared for them** that love Him."—*1 Corinthians 2:9*.

Those who remain faithful to God, in spite of the difficulties of earth, will receive every possible good thing in heaven.

"For the Lord God is a sun and shield: **the Lord will give grace and glory: no good thing will He withhold from them that walk uprightly**."—*Psalm 84:11*.

It will be a place of total happiness for all.

"But the meek shall inherit the earth; and shall delight themselves in the abundance of peace."—*Psalm 37:11*.

"**Thou wilt show me the path of life: in Thy presence is fullness of joy**; at Thy right hand there are pleasures for evermore."—*Psalm 16:11*.

Even the animals will be peaceful and contented.

"The wolf and the lamb shall feed together, and the lion shall eat straw like the bullock: and dust shall be the serpent's meat. They shall not hurt nor destroy in all My holy mountain, saith the Lord."—*Isaiah 65:25.*

Peaceful country living will be our inheritance. It will include gardening, which will be a source of great happiness to the redeemed.

"And they shall build houses, and inhabit them; and they shall plant vineyards, and eat the fruit of them. They shall not build, and another inhabit; they shall not plant, and another eat: for as the days of a tree are the days of My people, and **Mine elect shall long enjoy the work of their hands**. They shall not labour in vain, nor bring forth for trouble; for they are the seed of the blessed of the Lord, and their offspring with them. And it shall come to pass, that **before they call, I will answer**; and while they are yet speaking, I will hear."—*Isaiah 65:21-24.*

Every Sabbath day, the redeemed will gather to worship their Creator.

"For as the new heavens and the new earth, which I will make, shall remain before Me, saith the Lord, so shall your seed and your name remain. And it shall come to pass, that from one new moon to another, and **from one Sabbath to another, shall all flesh come to worship before Me, saith the Lord**."—*Isaiah 66:22-23.*

"And the ransomed of the Lord shall return, and come to Zion with songs and everlasting joy upon their heads: **they shall obtain joy and gladness, and sorrow and sighing shall flee away**."—*Isaiah 35:10.*

"All hail the power of Jesus' name! Let angels prostrate fall; Bring forth the royal diadem, And crown Him Lord of all!"—*Edward Perronet.*

—*Eden was heaven in miniature*. This is what we will find in the earth made new! We dare not miss having this! It is our decisions and our actions now that determine what our future will be.

Oh, my friend, we must be there! God wants us there! Jesus wants us there! All the angels of heaven want us there! It is an individual choice. If you have not done so already, make that decision now—and, in the strength of Christ, remain firm to the end.

"Just think of stepping on shore and finding it Heaven. Of taking hold of a hand, and finding it God's hand. Of breathing new air and finding it celestial. Of feeling invigorated and finding it immortality. Of passing from storm and tempest to an unbroken calm. Of looking up—and finding it home!"

—Myrtle Erickson

MY COMMITMENT

Oh, Father! I must be there! I must permit nothing to come between my soul and my Saviour! I give Thee all, just now! Take me, hold me, guide me in the days ahead. Help me to remain obedient to Thy Word, and to cling to Christ's hand all along the path that leads all the way to the earth made new! In Jesus' name, I send this earnest petition. I give Thee all; I give Thee all, just now. Amen.

From the author's book, The Bible Guide. Available in single or boxful quantities from the publisher.
Harvestime Books
Boxx 300 Altamont, TN 37301
931-692-2777

"For whatsoever is born of God overcometh the world."
—1 John 5:4

"To him that overcometh will I give to eat of the tree of life, which is in the midst of the paradise of God." —Revelation 2:7

"Blessed are the meek: for they shall inherit the earth."
—Matthew 5:5

"Blessed is the man that endureth temptation: for when he is tried, he shall receive the crown of life, which the Lord hath promised to them that love him." — James 1:12

"If ye be willing and obedient, ye shall eat the good of the land:."
— Isaiah 1:19

"He that overcometh shall inherit all things; and I will be his God." —Revelation 21:7

W
A
Y

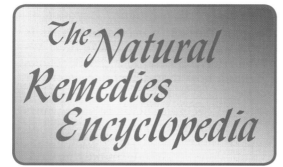

FOR CONVENIENCE IN FINDING WHAT YOU ARE LOOKING FOR,
THIS IS A TABLE OF CONTENTS TO THE PRECEDING SECTION (1080-1209)

W
A
Y

THIS ENTIRE CHAPTER WAS TAKEN FROM THE AUTHOR'S BOOK, THE BIBLE GUIDE
COPIES OF THE ENTIRE BOOK MAY BE OBTAINED FROM THE PUBLISHER OF THIS ENCYCLOPEDIA

The Natural Remedies Encyclopedia

Disease Index

There are over 1,500 entries in this Disease Index, to help you quickly locate the disease or disorder you are looking for.

An outstanding quality of this book is not only its broad coverage of over 730 disorders but the fact that the diseases and problems are grouped together, so you can easily compare them. Few books do this. However, this makes this *Disease Index* very important, when you are looking for a disease by its name.

A

ABDOMINAL CAVITY — 650
Abdominal Hernia   641
Abnormal Pap Smear   675
Abnormally Small Breasts
    675
Achlorhydria   439
Acidosis   434
Acne   328
Acne Rosacea   339
Acne Vulgaris   328

Acquired Immune Deficiency
    Syndrome   806
Actinic Keratoses   355
Acute Bronchitis   500
    —Chronic Bronchitis   501
Acute Gastritis   440
Acute Muscular Rheumatism 626
ADD (Attention Deficit Disorder)
    590
ADDICTIONS (Narcotics) — 824-
    826, 880-883
Addison's Disease   654
Adenitis   740
Adenoid Hypertrophy   742
Adenoids   742
ADHD (Attention Deficit
    Hyperactivity Disorder)   591
Adhesions   318
Adrenal Overactivity   655
Adrenal Underactivity   654
ADRENALS — 653-655
Aerophagia   432
Age Spots   331
Aging   312
Agoraphobia   593
AIDS   806
Alcohol Withdrawal   821, 881

Allergic Rhinitis   850
Allergies   848
ALLERGIES — 846-860
Alopecia   383
Altitude Sickness   287
Aluminum Poisoning   871
Alzheimer's Disease   587
Amblyopia   393
Amebiasis   864
Amenorrhea   681
Amenorrhea, Dysmenorrhea
    678
Ammoniacal Dermatitis   727
Amyotrophic Lateral Sclerosis
    577
Anal Eczema   472
Anal Fistula   733
Anaphylactic Shock   846
Anaphylaxis   846
Anemia   537-541, 713
Angina Pectoris   521
Angular Stomatitis, Geographic
    Tongue   429
Ankylosing Spondylitis   630
Anorexia Nervosa   472
Anosmia   404
Ant bite   833
Anthrax   812
ANUS — 469-472
Anus Itch   471
Anxiety Disorder   595
Aphthous Ulcers   321
Aphonia   416
Apoplexy   529
Appendicitis, Acute   455
Appendicitis, Chronic   456
Appendix / Intestines 453-456
Arsenic Poisoning   871
Arteriosclerosis   523
Arthritis   618
Articular Rheumatism, Acute
    624
Ascaris   862
Asthma   852, 714
Atherosclerosis   523
Athlete's Foot   377
Atrophic Vaginitis   695
Attention Deficit Disorder (ADD)
    590
Attention Deficit Hyperactivity
    Disorder (ADHD) 591
Autism   604

WHERE TO FIND IMPORTANT THINGS IN THE ENCYCLOPEDIA

DISEASES - List: 9-26 / Indexes: 1211- / HERBS - Contents: 129- / Preparing: 132 / Using: 141-189 (dose: often 1 tsp. mixed herbs in 1 cup boiled water) / VITAMINS-MINERALS - Index: 100- / Dosages: 124 / HYDRO-THERAPY - Therapy index: 206- / Disease index: 263- / CARE OF SICK - 28-39 / EMERGENCIES - 973-, 990-

WHERE TO FIND IMPORTANT THINGS IN THIS FRONT TABLE OF CONTENTS

WHERE TO FIND IMPORTANT THINGS IN THE ENCYCLOPEDIA
DISEASES - List: 9-26 / Indexes: 1211- / HERBS - Contents: 129- / Preparing: 132 / Using: 141-189 (dose: often 1 tsp. mixed herbs in 1 cup boiled water) / VITAMINS-MINERALS - Index: 100- / Dosages: 124 / HYDRO-THERAPY - Therapy index: 206- / Disease index: 263- / CARE OF SICK - 28-39 / EMERGENCIES - 973-, 990-

WHERE TO FIND IMPORTANT THINGS IN THE ENCYCLOPEDIA
DISEASES - List: 9-26 / Indexes: 1211- / HERBS - Contents: 129- / Preparing: 132 / Using: 141-189 (dose:
often 1 tsp. mixed herbs in 1 cup boiled water) / VITAMINS-MINERALS - Index: 100- / Dosages: 124 / HYDRO-
THERAPY - Therapy index: 206- / Disease index: 263- / CARE OF SICK - 28-39 / EMERGENCIES - 973-, 990-

Post-Febrile Insanities   602
Post-Menopausal Bleeding   687
Post-Menstrual Syndrome   685
Postnasal Drip   498
Post-Operative Insanities   602
Post-partum Depression   721
Post-partum Psychosis   721
Post-Polio Syndrome   585
Post-Traumatic Stress Disorder   595
Pox   742
Pre-eclampsia   716
PREGNANCY AND CHILDBIRTH — 705-716
Pregnancy Nausea   708
Pregnancy Related Problems   706
Pregnancy Toxemia   716
Pregnancy, Special Problems during:
Premature Labor   715
Premenstrual Syndrome (PMS)   676
Pressure Problems   414
Pressure Sores   324
Prickly Heat   339
Profuse Menstruation   682
Prolapse of the Uterus   693
Prostate Cancer   789
Prostate, Enlarged   668
Prostatitis   670
Protein starvation   480
Pruritis Ani   471
Psilosis   461
Psoriasis   351
Ptomaine Poisoning   878
Puerperal Confusional   602
Puffy Eyes   390
Pyorrhea   426

Q ——————

Q Fever   509
Quinsy   740

R ——————

Rabbit Fever   846
Rabies   844
Radiation Exposure   875
Radiation Poisoning   812, 875
Raynaud's Disease   368
Read, disturbance of ability to read   592
Receding Gums   425
Recent Memory Loss   587
Rectal Abscesses   470
Rectal Fissures   470
Rectal Itching   471
Rectal Prolapse   737
Red Eyes   390
Red, Cracking Lips   431
Regional Enteritis   464
Regurgitation   730
Renal Colic   491-492
Repetitive Strain Injury (RSI)   636

Restless Leg Syndrome   634
Retinal Detachment   397
Retinitus Pigmentosa   401
Reye's Syndrome   750
Rheumatic Fever   750
Rheumatism   623
Rheumatoid Arthritis   623
Rheumatoid Spondylitis   629
Rhinitis; Runny, Stuffy Nose   404
Rickets   614
Rickets in adults   614
Ringing in the Ears   411
Ringworm   335
Rocky Mountain Spotted Fever   840
Rosacea   339
Roseola (Roseola Infantum)   730
RSI   636
Rubella   745
Rubeola   744
Rupture Hernia   641

S ——————

SAD   571
Saliva Problems   428
Salpingitis and Ovaritis   693
SARS   814
Scabies   334
Scalding Urine   489
Scalds   325
Scanty Menstruation   681
Scarlatina   745
Scarlet Fever   745
Scarring   318
Schistosomiasis   864
Schizophrenia   602
Sciatica   566, 626, 645, 713
Scleroderma   355
Scoliosis   649
Scotoma   397
Scrofula (Lymph TB)   665
Scurvy   479
Sea Sickness   287
Seasonal Affective Disorder (SAD)   571
Sebaceous Cysts   338
Seborrhea   346
Seborrheic Dermatitis   346
Seizures   573
Senile Dementia   589
Senile Lentigines   331
Senility   589
Septicemia (Blood Poisoning)   544
Severe Acute Respiratory Syndrome (SARS)
   814
SEXUALLY TRANSMITTED DISEASES — 802-806
Shaking Palsy   582
Shark Attack   814
Sharkskin   353
Shingles   350
Shinsplints   633

WHERE TO FIND IMPORTANT THINGS IN THE ENCYCLOPEDIA
DISEASES - List: 9-26 / Indexes: 1211- / HERBS - Contents: 129- / Preparing: 132 / Using: 141-189 (dose: often 1 tsp. mixed herbs in 1 cup boiled water) / VITAMINS-MINERALS - Index: 100- / Dosages: 124 / HYDRO-THERAPY - Therapy index: 206- / Disease index: 263- / CARE OF SICK - 28-39 / EMERGENCIES - 973-, 990-

Tonsillitis   740
Tooth Decay   423
Tooth Sensitivity   422
Toothache   422
Toxemia   880
Toxic Amblyopia   397
Toxic Shock Syndrome   699
Toxoplasmosis   846, 864
Transient Ischemic Attacks   554
TRANSMITTED DISEASES — 839-846
Traveler's Diarrhea   460
Strep Throat   740
Trichomoniasis   695, 805
Trigeminal Neuralgia   565
Tuberculosis   505
Tularemia   846
TUMORS — 781-782
Tumors (including Fibroids)   782
Tunnel Vision   401
Turista   460
Typhoid Fever   307
Typhus   839

U

Ulcerated Eye and Lid   395
Ulcerative Colitis   463-465
Umbilical Hernia   642
Underactive Thyroid   659
Underweight   482
Uric-acid Diathesis   489
Urinary Stress Incontinence   487
URINE — 486-489
Urine Problems   486
Urine Retention   487
Urticaria   346, 830
Uterine   792
Uterine Bleeding   691
Uterine Fibroids   692
Uterine Fibroma   692
Uterine Polyps   692
Uterine Prolapse   693
Uterus, Prolapse   693
Uterus, Inflammation of   690

V

Vaccination Poisoning   876
Vaccination Problems   752
Vaginal Candidiasis   695
Vaginal Discharge   698
Vaginal Douche   688
Vaginitis   695
Varicella Zoster   742
Varicose Veins   535
Varicose Veins   710
Varicosities   535
Variola   305, 812
Venereal Diseases   802
Venereal Herpes   805
Venereal Warts   805

Vertigo   550
Viral Infections   296
Vitamin C deficiency   479
Vitiligo   353
Vomiting   431-438
Vomiting in Children   735

W

Warts   336, 373
Water Retention   494
Wax Blockage   409
Weak, Debilitated Conditions   278
Weakened Autoimmune System   309
WEIGHT — 480-484
Weil's Disease   449
Wens   338
Wernicke-Korsakoff Syndrome   554
West Nile Encephalitis   813
West Nile Virus   813
Whitlow   367
Whooping Cough   748
Wilson's Disease   476
Womb, Displaced   693
Women's sections   639-736
Worms   861
WOUNDS, BRUISING— 315-319
Wounds, Cuts, and Scrapes   316
Wrinkles   340

X

Xerophthalmia   393, 395
Xerostomia   430

Y

Yeast Infection   281
Yeast Vaginitis   695
Yellow Eyes   390
Yellow Fever   308
Yellow Nail Syndrome   371

WHERE TO FIND IMPORTANT THINGS IN THE ENCYCLOPEDIA
DISEASES - List: 9-26 / Indexes: 1211- / HERBS - Contents: 129- / Preparing: 132 / Using: 141-189 (dose: often 1 tsp. mixed herbs in 1 cup boiled water) / VITAMINS-MINERALS - Index: 100- / Dosages: 124 / HYDRO-THERAPY - Therapy index: 206- / Disease index: 263- / CARE OF SICK - 28-39 / EMERGENCIES - 973-, 990-

The *Natural*
Remedies
Encyclopedia

General
Index

WHERE TO FIND IMPORTANT THINGS IN THE FRONT TABLE OF CONTENTS
REMEDIES CHAPTERS - 10-15 / DISEASE CHAPTERS - 16-23 / WOMEN'S CHAPTERS - 24-26 / TOXIC
PROBLEMS CHAPTERS - 26-29 / EMERGENCIES CHAPTERS - 30-31 / ADDITIONAL HELPS - 31-32 /

G
I
N
D
E
X

WHERE TO FIND IMPORTANT THINGS IN THE ENCYCLOPEDIA

DISEASES - List: 15-26 / Indexes: 1211- / HERBS - Contents: 129- / Preparing: 132 / Using: 141-189 (dose: often 1 tsp. mixed herbs in 1 cup boiled water) / VITAMINS-MINERALS - Index: 100- / Dosages: 124 / HYDRO-THERAPY - Therapy index: 206- / Disease index: 263- / CARE OF SICK - 28-39 / EMERGENCIES - 973-, 990-

Amazing grace! how sweet the sound
That saved a wretch like me!
I once was lost, but now am found;
Was blind, but now I see.

'Twas grace that taught my heart to fear,
And grace my fears relieved;
How precious did that grace appear,
The hour I first believed!

Through many dangers, toils, and snares,
I have already come;
'Tis grace hath brought me safe thus far,
And grace will lead me home.

The Lord has promised good to me,
His Word my hope secures;
He will my shield and portion be,
As long as life endures.

The earth shall soon dissolve like snow,
The sun forbear to shine;
But God, who called me here below,
Will be for ever mine.

When we've been there ten thousand years,
Bright shining as the sun,
We've no less days to sing God's praise
Than when we first begun!

— John Newton

For additional information on this and other fine books, please contact the seller you purchased this book from, or the publisher.
Harvestime Books - Box 300 - Altamont, TN 37301

FIND IT FAST – 126 MOST IMPORTANT HERBS

RED = THE 25 MOST USED HERBS / RED = THE NEXT 25 FREQUENTLY USED HERBS / BLUE = THE OTHER 76 MOST IMPORTANT HERBS

FIND IT FAST – HYDROTHERAPY TREATMENTS

TOC
PRIN
LAWS
DIET
NUTR
HERBS
HYDRO
GEN
SKIN
EXTR
HEAD
G-I
URIN
RESP
CARD
N-M
S-M
ENDO
LYMP
REP-M
REP-W
PREG
CHILD
W HRE
DELIV
CANCER
STD
NEW
DELIV
POIS
HARMF
EMER
PHYS
CHARTS
WAY
SOURCE
D INDEX
G INDEX